a LANGE medical book

# CURRENT
## Pediatric Diagnosis
## & Treatment

17th Edition

**Edited by**

**William W. Hay, Jr., MD**
*Professor, Department of Pediatrics*
*Section of Neonatology and the Division of Perinatal*
*Medicine and Research*
*University of Colorado School of Medicine and*
*The Children's Hospital, Denver*

**Myron J. Levin, MD**
*Professor, Departments of Pediatrics and Medicine*
*University of Colorado School of Medicine and*
*The Children's Hospital, Denver*

**Judith M. Sondheimer, MD**
*Professor, Department of Pediatrics, and Head, Section*
*of Pediatric Gastroenterology, Hepatology, and Nutrition*
*University of Colorado School of Medicine and*
*The Children's Hospital, Denver*

**Robin R. Deterding, MD**
*Associate Professor, Department of Pediatrics, Section of*
*Pediatric Pulmonary Medicine*
*University of Colorado School of Medicine and*
*The Children's Hospital, Denver*

**and Associate Authors**
*The Department of Pediatrics at the University of*
*Colorado School of Medicine is affiliated with*
*The Children's Hospital of Denver, Colorado.*

**Lange Medical Books/McGraw-Hill**
Medical Publishing Division

New York   Chicago   San Francisco   Lisbon   London   Madrid   Mexico City   Milan   New Delhi
San Juan   Seoul   Singapore   Sydney   Toronto

**Current Pediatric Diagnosis & Treatment, Seventeenth Edition**

Copyright © 2005, 2001, by The McGraw-Hill Companies, Inc. All rights reserved. Printed in the United States of America. Except as permitted under the United States Copyright Act of 1976, no part of this publication may be reproduced or distributed in any form or by any means, or stored in a data base or retrieval system, without the prior written permission of the publisher.

Previous editions copyright © 2003, 2001 by The McGraw-Hill Companies, Inc.; copyright © 1999, 1997, 1995, 1991, 1987 by Appleton & Lange

1 2 3 4 5 6 7 8 9 0 DOC/DOC 0 9 8 7 6 5 4

ISBN: 0-07-142960-3
ISSN: 0093-8556

This book was set in Adobe Garamond by Pine Tree Composition, Inc.
The editors were Shelley Reinhardt, Harriet Lebowitz, and Barbara Holton.
The production supervisor was Catherine H. Saggese.
The illustration manager was Charissa Baker.
The cover designer was Mary McKeon.
The text designer was Eve Siegel.
The indexer was Katherin Unger.
RR Donnelley was printer and binder.

INTERNATIONAL EDITION ISBN 0-07-111688-5

Copyright © 2005. Exclusive rights by The **McGraw-Hill Companies**, Inc., for manufacture and export. This book cannot be reexported from the country to which it is consigned by McGraw-Hill. The International Edition is not available in North America.

This book is printed on acid-free paper.

# Contents

# Authors

**Frank J. Accurso, MD**
Professor, Department of Pediatrics, and Head, Section of Pediatric Pulmonary Medicine, University of Colorado School of Medicine; The Mike McMorris Cystic Fibrosis Center and The Children's Hospital, Denver
accurso.frank@tchden.org
*Respiratory Tract & Mediastinum*

**Edythe A. Albano, MD**
Associate Professor, Department of Pediatrics, Section of Pediatric Hematology, Oncology and Bone Marrow Transplantation, University of Colorado School of Medicine and The Children's Hospital, Denver
albano.edythe@tchden.org
*Neoplastic Disease*

**Daniel R. Ambruso, MD**
Professor, Department of Pediatrics, Section of Pediatric Hematology, Oncology and Bone Marrow Transplantation, University of Colorado School of Medicine and The Children's Hospital; Associate Medical Director, Bonfils Blood Center, Denver
daniel.ambruso@uchsc.edu
*Hematologic Disorders*

**Marsha S. Anderson, MD**
Assistant Professor, Department of Pediatrics, Section of Pediatric Infectious Diseases, University of Colorado School of Medicine and The Children's Hospital, Denver
anderson.marsha@tchden.org
*Emergencies & Injuries: Bioterrorism Section; Infections: Bacterial & Spirochetal*

**Vivek Balasubramaniam, MD**
Assistant Professor, Department of Pediatrics, Section of Pediatric Pulmonary Medicine, Pediatric Heart Lung Center, University of Colorado School of Medicine and The Children's Hospital, Denver
vivek.balasubramaniam@uchsc.edu
*Respiratory Tract & Mediastinum*

**Jennifer Barker, MD**
Fellow in Pediatric Endocrinology, Department of Pediatrics, Section of Pediatric Endocrinology, Barbara Davis Center for Childhood Diabetes, University of Colorado Health Sciences Center, Denver
jennifer.barker@uchsc.edu
*Endocrine Disorders*

**Mylène Bassal, MDCM**
Fellow in Pediatric Hematology, Oncology and Bone Marrow Transplantation, Department of Pediatrics, Section of Pediatric Hematology, Oncology and Bone Marrow Transplantation, University of Colorado School of Medicine and The Children's Hospital, Denver
mylene.bassal@uchsc.edu
*Neoplastic Disease*

**F. Keith Battan, MD**
Associate Professor, Department of Pediatrics, Section of Emergency Medicine, University of Colorado School of Medicine; Associate Director, Emergency and Trauma Services, The Children's Hospital, Denver
*Emergencies & Injuries*

**Donald W. Bechtold, MD**
Medical Director, Jefferson Center for Mental Health, Arvada, Colorado; Associate Clinical Professor, University of Colorado School of Medicine, Denver
donaldb@jcmh.org
*Child & Adolescent Psychiatric Disorders & Psychosocial Aspects of Pediatrics*

**Tim A. Benke, MD, PhD**
Assistant Professor, Departments of Pediatrics, Neurology & Pharmacology, University of Colorado School of Medicine and The Children's Hospital, Denver
tim.benke@uchsc.edu
*Neurologic & Muscular Disorders*

**Mark Boguniewicz, MD**
Professor, Department of Pediatrics, University of
Colorado School of Medicine and National Jewish
Medical and Research Center, and The Children's
Hospital, Denver
boguniewiczm@njc.org
*Allergic Disorders*

**Robert M. Brayden, MD**
Associate Professor, Department of Pediatrics, Section
of General Academic Pediatrics, University of
Colorado School of Medicine and The Children's
Hospital, Denver
brayden.robert@tchden.org
*Ambulatory & Community Pediatrics*

**Jeffrey M. Brown, MD, MPH**
Professor, Department of Pediatrics, University of
Colorado School of Medicine; Director, General
Pediatrics Division, Denver Health Medical Center,
Denver
jeff.brown@dhha.org
*Ambulatory & Community Pediatrics*

**Todd C. Carpenter, MD**
Assistant Professor, Department of Pediatrics,
Section of Pediatric Critical Care Medicine,
University of Colorado School of Medicine
and The Children's Hospital, Denver
todd.carpenter@uchsc.edu
*Critical Care*

**H. Peter Chase, MD**
Professor of Pediatrics, University of Colorado Health
Sciences Center, Barbara Davis Center for Child-
hood Diabetes, Denver
peter.chase@uchsc.edu
*Diabetes Mellitus*

**Matthew F. Daley, MD**
Assistant Professor, Department of Pediatrics, Section
of General Academic Pediatrics, University of Colorado School of Medicine and The Children's Hospital, Denver
daley.matthew@tchden.org
*Ambulatory & Community Pediatrics; Immunization*

**Richard C. Dart, MD, PhD**
Professor of Surgery, Medicine, and Pharmacy,
University of Colorado School of Medicine; Director,
Rocky Mountain Poison and Drug Center, Denver
Health Authority, Denver
rdart@rmpdc.org
*Poisoning*

**Robin R. Deterding, MD**
Associate Professor, Department of Pediatrics, Section
of Pediatric Pulmonary Medicine, University of Colorado School of Medicine and The Children's Hospital, Denver
deterding.robin@tchden.org
*Respiratory Tract & Mediastinum*

**Emily L. Dobyns, MD**
Associate Professor, Department of Pediatrics, Section
of Pediatric Critical Care Medicine, University of
Colorado School of Medicine and The Children's
Hospital, Denver
dobyns.emily@tchden.org
*Critical Care*

**Arlene Drack, MD**
Associate Professor, Department of Ophthalmology;
Chief, Section of Pediatric Ophthalmology, Univer-
sity of Colorado School of Medicine and The
Children's Hospital, Denver
*Eye*

**Robert E. Eilert, MD**
Professor, Department of Pediatrics, University of
Colorado Health Sciences Center; Rose Brown
Professor, Department of Orthopedic Surgery, Uni-
versity of Colorado School of Medicine; Chairman,
Department of Orthopedic Surgery, The Children's
Hospital, Denver
eilert.robert@tchden.org
*Orthopedics*

**George S. Eisenbarth, MD, PhD**
Professor, Departments of Pediatrics, Medicine, and
Immunology, University of Colorado School of
Medicine; Executive Director, Barbara Davis Center
for Childhood Diabetes, Denver
george.eisenbarth@uchsc.edu
*Diabetes Mellitus*

**Allan M. Eisenbaum, MD**
Pediatric Ophthalmologist, Wichita Clinic, Wichita,
Kansas; Clinical Assistant Professor, Departments of
Internal Medicine and Pediatrics, University of
Kansas School of Medicine, Wichita
eisenbauma@wichitaclinic.com
*Eye*

**Ellen Roy Elias, MD**
Associate Professor, Departments of Pediatrics and
Genetics, Section of Clinical Genetics and Metabo-
lism, University of Colorado School of Medicine;
Director, Special Care Clinic, The Children's Hos-
pital, Denver
elias.ellen@tchden.org
*Genetics & Dysmorphology*

**Margaret A. Ferguson, MD**
Assistant Professor, Department of Pediatrics, Section of Pediatric Critical Care Medicine, University of Colorado School of Medicine and The Children's Hospital, Denver
ferguson.margaret@tchden.org
*Critical Care*

**Douglas N. Fish, PharmD**
Associate Professor, Department of Pharmacy Practice and Division of Pulmonary Sciences & Critical Care Medicine, University of Colorado Schools of Pharmacy and Medicine; Clinical Pharmacy Specialist in Critical Care/Infectious Diseases, University of Colorado Hospital, Denver
doug.fish@uchsc.edu
*Drug Therapy*

**Douglas M. Ford, MD**
Professor, Department of Pediatrics, Section of Pediatric Nephrology, University of Colorado School of Medicine and The Children's Hospital, Denver
ford.douglas@tchden.org
*Fluid, Electrolyte, & Acid-Base Disorders & Therapy*

**Nicholas K. Foreman, MD**
Associate Professor, Department of Pediatrics, Section of Pediatric Hematology, Oncology and Bone Marrow Transplantation, University of Colorado School of Medicine; Seebaum-Tschetter Chair of Pediatric Neuro-Oncology and Director of Neuro-Oncology, The Children's Hospital, Denver, Colorado
foreman.nicholas@tchden.org
*Neoplastic Disease*

**Norman R. Friedman, MD**
Assistant Professor, Departments of Otolaryngology and Pediatrics, University of Colorado School of Medicine and The Children's Hospital, Denver
friedman.norman@tchden.org
*Ear, Nose, & Throat*

**Roger H. Giller, MD**
Professor, Department of Pediatrics, Section of Pediatric Hematology, Oncology and Bone Marrow Transplantation, University of Colorado School of Medicine; Director, Pediatric Bone Marrow Transplant Program, The Children's Hospital, Denver
giller.roger@tchden.org
*Neoplastic Disease: Hematopoietic Stem Cell Transplantation*

**Edward Goldson, MD**
Professor, Department of Pediatrics, Section of Developmental and Behavioral Pediatrics, University of Colorado School of Medicine and The Children's Hospital, Denver
goldson.edward@tchden.org
*Child Development & Behavior*

**Stephen I. Goodman, MD**
Professor, Department of Pediatrics, Head, Section of Clinical Genetics and Metabolism, University of Colorado School of Medicine and The Children's Hospital, Denver
stephen.goodman@uchsc.edu
*Inborn Errors of Metabolism*

**Douglas K. Graham, MD, PhD**
Assistant Professor, Department of Pediatrics, Section of Hematology, Oncology and Bone Marrow Transplant, University of Colorado Health Sciences Center and The Children's Hospital, Denver
doug.graham@uchsc.edu
*Neoplastic Disease: Hematopoietic Stem Cell Transplantation*

**Carol L. Greene, MD**
Clinical Professor, Department of Pediatrics, George Washington University School of Medicine, Washington, D.C.
cgreene@cnmc.org
*Inborn Errors of Metabolism*

**Brian S. Greffe, MD**
Associate Professor, Department of Pediatrics, Section of Pediatric Hematology, Oncology and Bone Marrow Transplantation, University of Colorado School of Medicine and The Children's Hospital, Denver
greffe.brian@tchden.org
*Neoplastic Disease*

**Jennifer Hagman, MD**
Associate Professor, Department of Psychiatry, University Of Colorado School of Medicine; Co-Director, Eating Disorders Treatment Program; Medical Director, Clinical Services, Department of Psychiatry and Behavioral Sciences, The Children's Hospital, Denver
hagman.jennifer@tchden.org
*Child & Adolescent Psychiatric Disorders & Psychosocial Aspects of Pediatrics*

**K. Michael Hambidge, MD, BChir, ScD**
Professor Emeritus, Department of Pediatrics, Section of Nutrition, University of Colorado Health Sciences Center, Denver
michael.hambidge@uchsc.edu
*Normal Childhood Nutrition & Its Disorders*

**Taru Hays, MD**
Professor of Pediatrics, Department of Pediatrics, Section of Hematology, Oncology and Bone Marrow Transplant, University of Colorado Health Sciences Center and The Children's Hospital, Denver
hays.taru@tchden.org
*Hematologic Disorders*

**Anthony R. Hayward, MD, PhD**
Previously Professor of Pediatrics, University of Colorado Health Sciences Center, Denver
a.hayward@verizon.net
*Immunodeficiency*

**J. Roger Hollister, MD**
Professor, Department of Pediatrics, University of Colorado School of Medicine; Head, Section of Pediatric Rheumatology, University of Colorado School of Medicine and The Children's Hospital, Denver
*Rheumatic Diseases*

**Candice E. Johnson, MD, PhD**
Professor, Department of Pediatrics, Division of General Academic Pediatrics, University of Colorado School of Medicine and The Children's Hospital, Denver
*Ear, Nose, & Throat*

**Carol S. Kamin, MS, EdD**
Associate Professor, Department of Pediatrics, Section of Medical Education and Director, Project L.I.V.E., University of Colorado School of Medicine, Denver
kamin.carol@tchden.org
*Information Technology in Pediatrics*

**David W. Kaplan, MD, MPH**
Professor, Department of Pediatrics, and Head, Section of Adolescent Medicine, University of Colorado School of Medicine and The Children's Hospital, Denver
kaplan.david@tchden.org
*Adolescence; Information Technology in Pediatrics*

**Michael S. Kappy, MD, PhD**
Professor, Department of Pediatrics, and Head, Section of Pediatric Endocrinology, University of Colorado Health Sciences Center and The Children's Hospital, Denver
*Endocrine Disorders*

**Paritosh Kaul, MD**
Assistant Professor, Department of Pediatrics, Section of Adolescent Medicine, University of Colorado Health Sciences Center; Westside Teen Clinic, Denver Health and Hospitals
paritosh.kaul@dhha.org
*Substance Abuse*

**Peggy Kelley, MD**
Assistant Professor, Department of Otolaryngology, University of Colorado School of Medicine and The Children's Hospital, Denver
kelley.peggy@tchden.org
*Ear, Nose, & Throat*

**Gwendolyn S. Kerby, MD**
Assistant Professor, Department of Pediatrics, Section of Pediatric Pulmonary Medicine, University of Colorado School of Medicine and The Children's Hospital, Denver
kerby.gwendolyn@tchden.org
*Respiratory Tract & Mediastinum*

**Nancy F. Krebs, MD, MS**
Professor, Department of Pediatrics, and Head, Section of Nutrition, University of Colorado School of Medicine and The Children's Hospital, Denver
nancy.krebs@uchsc.edu
*Normal Childhood Nutrition & Its Disorders*

**Richard D. Krugman, MD**
Professor, Department of Pediatrics, and Dean, University of Colorado School of Medicine, Denver
richard.krugman@uchsc.edu
*Child Abuse & Neglect*

**Peter A. Lane, MD**
Professor, Department of Pediatrics, Emory University School of Medicine; Director of Hematology, AFLAC Cancer Center and Blood Disorders Service, Children's Healthcare of Atlanta, Atlanta, Georgia
plane@emory.edu
*Hematologic Disorders*

**Gary L. Larsen, MD**
Professor, Department of Pediatrics, Section of Pediatric Pulmonary Medicine, University of Colorado School of Medicine; Senior Faculty Member and Head, Division of Pediatric Pulmonary Medicine, National Jewish Medical and Research Center, Denver
*Respiratory Tract & Mediastinum*

**Myron J. Levin, MD**
Professor, Departments of Pediatrics and Medicine, University of Colorado School of Medicine and The Children's Hospital, Denver
myron.levin@uchsc.edu
*Infections: Viral & Rickettsial; Infections: Parasitic & Mycotic; Sexually Transmitted Infections*

**Kathryn Love-Osborne, MD**
Assistant Professor, Department of Pediatrics, Section of Adolescent Medicine, University of Colorado Health Sciences Center; Medical Director, Eastside Teen Clinic, Denver Health and Hospitals, Denver
kathryn.love-osbo@dhha.org
*Adolescence*

**Gary M. Lum, MD**
Professor, Departments of Pediatrics and Medicine, and Head, Section of Pediatric Nephrology, University of Colorado School of Medicine and The Children's Hospital, Denver
lum.gary@tchden.org
*Kidney & Urinary Tract*

**David K. Manchester, MD**
Professor, Department of Pediatrics and Director, Clinical Services, Section of Clinical Genetics and Metabolism, The Children's Hospital, Denver, Colorado
manchester.david@tchden.org
*Genetics & Dysmorphology*

**Stephanie N. Mateev, MD**
Instructor, Department of Pediatrics, Section of Pediatric Critical Care Medicine, University of Colorado School of Medicine and The Children's Hospital, Denver
stephanie.mateev@uchsc.edu
*Critical Care*

**Dennis J. Matthews, MD**
Associate Professor and Chairman, Department of Rehabilitation Medicine, University of Colorado School of Medicine; Chairman and Medical Director, The Children's Hospital Rehabilitation Center, Denver
matthews.dennis@tchden.org
*Rehabilitation & Sports Medicine*

**Elizabeth J. McFarland, MD**
Associate Professor, Department of Pediatrics, Section of Pediatric Infectious Diseases, University of Colorado School of Medicine; Director, Children's Hospital HIV Program, The Children's Hospital, Denver
betsy.mcfarland@uchsc.edu
*Human Immunodeficiency Virus Infection*

**Jerrod Milton, RPh, BSc**
Adjunct Assistant Clinical Professor, Department of Pharmacy Services, The Children's Hospital, Denver, Colorado
milton.jerrod@tchden.org
*Drug Therapy*

**Shelley D. Miyamoto, MD**
Fellow in Pediatric Cardiology, Department of Pediatrics, Section of Pediatric Cardiology, University of Colorado School of Medicine and The Children's Hospital, Denver
miyamoto.shelley@tchden.org
*Cardiovascular Diseases*

**Paul G. Moe, MD**
Professor, Departments of Pediatrics and Neurology, University of Colorado School of Medicine and The Children's Hospital, Denver
moe.paul@tchden.org
*Neurologic & Muscular Disorders*

**Joseph G. Morelli, MD**
Professor, Departments of Dermatology and Pediatrics, University of Colorado School of Medicine, Denver
joseph.morelli@uchsc.edu
*Skin*

**Peter M. Mourani, MD**
Instructor, Department of Pediatrics, Section of Pediatric Critical Care Medicine, University of Colorado School of Medicine and The Children's Hospital, Denver
peter.mourani@uchsc.edu
*Critical Care*

**William A. Mueller, DMD**
Clinical Associate Professor of Applied Dentistry, University of Colorado School of Dentistry, Denver
williammueller@earthlink.net
*Oral Medicine & Dentistry*

**Kristen Nadeau, MD**
Fellow in Pediatric Endocrinology, Department of Pediatrics, Section of Pediatric Endocrinology, University of Colorado School of Medicine and The Children's Hospital, Denver
kristen.nadeau@uchsc.edu
*Endocrine Disorders*

**Michael R. Narkewicz, MD**
Professor of Pediatrics, Section of Pediatric Gastroenterology, Hepatology and Nutrition, University of Colorado School of Medicine; Hewit-Andrews Chair in Pediatric Liver Disease; Medical Director, The Pediatric Liver Center, The Children's Hospital, Denver
narkewicz.michael@tchden.org
*Liver & Pancreas*

**Rachelle Nuss, MD**
Professor, Department of Pediatrics, Section of
Pediatric Hematology, Oncology and Bone Marrow
Transplantation, University of Colorado School of
Medicine and The Children's Hospital, Denver
rachelle.nuss@uchsc.edu
*Hematologic Disorders*

**Ann-Christine Nyquist, MD, MSPH**
Assistant Professor, Departments of Pediatrics and
Preventive Medicine/Biometrics, Section of
Pediatric Infectious Diseases, University of Colorado
School of Medicine; Medical Director, Infection
Control and Epidemiology, The Children's
Hospital, Denver
nyquist.ann-christine@tchden.org
*Immunization; Sexually Transmitted Infections*

**John W. Ogle, MD**
Professor and Vice Chairman, Department of
Pediatrics, University of Colorado School of
Medicine; Director, Department of Pediatrics,
Denver Health Medical Center, Denver
jogle@dhha.org
*Antimicrobial Therapy; Infections: Bacterial
& Spirochetal*

**Patricia Orma, PharmD**
Adjoint Professor, School of Pharmacy, University
of Colorado Health Sciences Center, Denver;
Pediatric Clinical Pharmacist, The Children's
Hospital, University of California Davis Medical
Center, Sacramento
patricia.orma@ucdmc.ucdavis.edu
*Drug Therapy*

**Iris M. Osberg, MT**
Technical Director, Pediatrics General Clinical
Research Center Core Laboratory, and Director,
Cystic Fibrosis Foundation/Therapeutics
Development Network Labs, University of
Colorado School of Medicine and The Children's
Hospital, Denver
iris.osberg@uchsc.edu
*Chemistry & Hematology Reference Ranges*

**Christopher C. Porter, MD**
Fellow in Pediatric Hematology, Oncology and Bone
Marrow Transplantation, Department of Pediatrics,
Section of Pediatric Hematology, Oncology and
Bone Marrow Transplantation, University of
Colorado School of Medicine and The Children's
Hospital, Denver
*Neoplastic Disease*

**Laura E. Primak, RD, CNSD, CSP**
Professional Research Assistant, Department of
Pediatrics; University of Colorado School of
Medicine and The Children's Hospital, Denver
Nutritionist, Nutrition Academic Award Program,
University of Colorado Health Sciences Center,
Denver
laura.primak@uchsc.edu
*Normal Childhood Nutrition & Its Disorders*

**Ralph R. Quinones, MD**
Associate Professor, Department of Pediatrics;
Director, Scientific Development, Blood and
Marrow Processing Laboratory, Bone Marrow
Transplant Program, Section of Pediatric Hematol-
ogy, Oncology and Bone Marrow Transplantation,
University of Colorado School of Medicine and The
Children's Hospital, Denver
quinones.ralph@tchden.org
*Neoplastic Disease: Hematopoietic Stem Cell Transplan-
tation*

**Ann Reynolds, MD**
Assistant Professor, Department of Pediatrics, Child
Development Unit, University of Colorado School
of Medicine and The Children's Hospital, Denver
reynolds.ann@tchden.org
*Child Development & Behavior*

**Adam A. Rosenberg, MD**
Professor, Department of Pediatrics, Section of
Neonatology; Medical Director, Newborn Service,
University of Colorado Hospital; Director,
Training Program in Pediatrics; University of
Colorado School of Medicine and The Children's
Hospital, Denver
adam.rosenberg@uchsc.edu
*The Newborn Infant*

**Barry H. Rumack, MD**
Clinical Professor of Pediatrics, University of Colorado
School of Medicine, Denver; Director Emeritus,
Rocky Mountain Poison and Drug Center, Denver
barry@rumack.com
*Poisoning*

**Scott D. Sagel, MD**
Assistant Professor, Department of Pediatrics, Section
of Pediatric Pulmonary Medicine, University of
Colorado School of Medicine and The Children's
Hospital, Denver
sagel.scott@tchden.org
*Respiratory Tract & Mediastinum*

**Rebecca Sands, MD**
Assistant Professor, Department of Ophthalmology, University of Colorado Health Sciences Center, Denver; Pediatric Ophthalmologist, Rocky Mountain Lions Eye Institute and The Children's Hospital, Aurora, Colorado
rebecca.sands@uchsc.edu
*Eye*

**Eric J. Sigel, MD**
Associate Professor, Department of Pediatrics, Section of Adolescent Medicine; Co-Director, Eating Disorders Program at The Children's Hospital, Denver, and Clinical Director, Adolescent Clinic, University of Colorado School of Medicine and The Children's Hospital, Denver
sigel.eric@tchden.org
*Eating Disorders; Sexually Transmitted Infections*

**Eric A. F. Simoes, MD, DCH**
Professor, Department of Pediatrics, Section of Pediatric Infectious Diseases, University of Colorado School of Medicine and The Children's Hospital, Denver; Professor of Paediatric Infectious Diseases and Tropical Child Health, Departments of Paediatrics and Obstetrics and Gynaecology, Imperial College, London, England
eric.simoes@uchsc.edu
*Immunization*

**Andrew P. Sirotnak, MD**
Associate Professor, Department of Pediatrics, University of Colorado School of Medicine; Director, Kempe Child Protection Team, The Children's Hospital and Kempe Children's Center, Denver
sirotnak.andrew@tchden.org
*Child Abuse & Neglect*

**Ronald J. Sokol, MD**
Professor, Department of Pediatrics, Section of Pediatric Gastroenterology, Hepatology, and Nutrition and the Pediatric Liver Center and Liver Transplantation Programs; Program Director, Pediatric General Clinical Research Center, University of Colorado School of Medicine and The Children's Hospital, Denver
sokol.ronald@tchden.org
*Liver & Pancreas*

**Henry M. Sondheimer, MD**
Professor, Department of Pediatrics, Section of Pediatric Cardiology, University of Colorado School of Medicine; Clinical Director, Pediatric Cardiology, The Children's Hospital, Denver
sondheimer.henry@tchden.org
*Cardiovascular Diseases*

**Judith M. Sondheimer, MD**
Professor, Department of Pediatrics, and Head, Section of Pediatric Gastroenterology, Hepatology, and Nutrition, University of Colorado School of Medicine and The Children's Hospital, Denver
sondheimer.judith@tchden.org
*Gastrointestinal Tract*

**Kurt R. Stenmark, MD**
Professor, Department of Pediatrics, and Head, Section of Pediatric Critical Care Medicine, University of Colorado School of Medicine and The Children's Hospital, Denver
kurt.stenmark@uchsc.edu
*Critical Care*

**Catherine Stevens-Simon, MD**
Associate Professor, Department of Pediatrics, Section of Adolescent Medicine, University of Colorado School of Medicine and The Children's Hospital, Denver
stevens-simon.catherine@tchden.org
*Substance Abuse*

**Linda C. Stork, MD**
Associate Professor, Department of Pediatrics, Oregon Health and Science University, Portland
storkl@ohsu.edu
*Neoplastic Disease*

**Elizabeth H. Thilo, MD**
Associate Professor, Department of Pediatrics, Section of Neonatology, University of Colorado School of Medicine and The Children's Hospital, Denver
thilo.elizabeth@tchden.org
*The Newborn Infant*

**Janet A. Thomas, MD**
Assistant Professor, Department of Pediatrics, Section of Genetics and Metabolism, University of Colorado School of Medicine and The Children's Hospital, Denver
thomas.janet@tchden.org
*Inborn Errors of Metabolism*

**Sharon H. Travers, MD**
Associate Professor, Department of Pediatrics, Section of Pediatric Endocrinology, University of Colorado School of Medicine and The Children's Hospital, Denver
travers.sharon@tchden.org
*Endocrine Disorders*

**Anne Chun-Hui Tsai, MD, MSc**
Assistant Professor, Department of Pediatrics, Section
   of Clinical Genetics and Metabolism, University of
   Colorado School of Medicine and The Children's
   Hospital, Denver
tsai.chun-hui@tchden.org
*Genetics & Dysmorphology*

**Adriana Weinberg, MD**
Professor, Departments of Pediatrics and Medicine,
   University of Colorado School of Medicine;
   Director, Clinical Virology Laboratory, University
   of Colorado Hospital, Denver
adriana.weinberg@uchsc.edu
*Infections: Viral & Rickettsial; Infections: Parasitic
& Mycotic*

**William L. Weston, MD**
Professor, Departments of Dermatology and Pediatrics,
   University of Colorado School of Medicine, Denver
william.weston@uchsc.edu
*Skin*

**Pamela E. Wilson, MD**
Assistant Professor, Department of Rehabilitation
   Medicine, University of Colorado School of
   Medicine and The Children's Hospital, Denver
wilson.pamela@tchden.org
*Rehabilitation & Sports Medicine*

**Anji T. Yetman, MD**
Associate Professor, Department of Pediatrics, Section
   of Pediatric Cardiology; Director, Adult Congenital
   Cardiac Program, University of Colorado School of
   Medicine and The Children's Hospital, Denver
yetman.angela@tchden.org
*Cardiovascular Diseases*

**Philip S. Zeitler, MD, PhD**
Associate Professor, Department of Pediatrics, Section
   of Pediatric Endocrinology, University of Colorado
   School of Medicine and The Children's Hospital,
   Denver
phil.zeitler@uchsc.edu
*Endocrine Disorders*

# Preface

The seventeenth edition of *Current Pediatric Diagnosis & Treatment* features practical, up-to-date, well-referenced information on the care of children from birth through infancy and adolescence. *CPDT* emphasizes the clinical aspects of pediatric care while also covering the important underlying principles. Its goal is to provide a guide to diagnosis, understanding, and treatment of the medical problems of all pediatric patients in an easy-to-use and readable format.

## INTENDED AUDIENCE

Like all Lange medical books, *CPDT* provides a concise yet comprehensive source of current information. Students will find *CPDT* an authoritative introduction to pediatrics and an excellent source for reference and review. *CPDT* provides excellent coverage of The Council on Medical Student Education in Pediatrics (COMSEP) Curriculum used around the country in Pediatric clerkships. Residents in pediatrics (and other specialties) will appreciate the detailed descriptions of diseases and diagnostic and therapeutic procedures. Pediatricians, family practitioners, nurses and nurse practitioners, and other health-care providers who work with infants and children also will find *CPDT* a useful reference on management aspects of pediatric medicine.

## COVERAGE

Forty-four chapters cover a wide range of topics, including neonatal medicine, child development and behavior, emergency and critical care medicine, and diagnosis and treatment of specific disorders according to major problems and organ systems. A wealth of tables and figures summarizes important information, such as acute and critical care procedures in the delivery room, the office, the emergency room, and the critical care unit; anti-infective agents; drug dosages; immunization schedules; differential diagnosis; and developmental screening tests. The final chapter is a handy guide to normal laboratory values.

## NEW TO THIS EDITION

The seventeenth edition of *CPDT* has been revised comprehensively by the editors and contributing authors. New references as well as up-to-date and useful Web sites have been added, permitting the reader to consult original material and to go beyond the confines of the textbook. As editors and practicing pediatricians, we have tried to ensure that each chapter reflects the needs and realities of day-to-day practice.

**New Editor:** We are delighted to welcome Dr. Robin Deterding as a *CPDT* Editor. Robin brings a wealth of experience in pediatric education methods and in-depth experience in pulmonary medicine and patient diagnosis and management protocols.

**Chapter Revisions:** Eight chapters have been extensively revised, with new authors added in several cases, reflecting substantial new information in each of their areas of pediatric medicine. Especially important is new material added to the chapters on infectious diseases, including information on methicillin-resistant staphylococcus, SARS, human metapneumovirus, and West Nile virus infections. Chapters with major revisions include:

15. Eye
28. Neoplastic Disease
35. Antimicrobial Therapy
36. Infections: Viral & Rickettsial
37. Human Immunodeficiency Virus (HIV) Infections
38. Infections: Bacterial & Spirochetal
39. Infections: Parasitic & Mycotic
40. Sexually Transmitted Infections
43. Information Technology in Pediatric Practice

All other chapters are substantially revised and references have been updated. Seventeen new authors have contributed to these revisions.

**Acknowledgment:** The Editors would like to thank Dr. Anthony Hayward—-who has assumed a position with the General Clinical Research Centers program at the National Institutes of Health—-for his work as Editor of *CPDT*. Anthony served *CPDT* with outstanding scholarship and editorship for five editions (twelfth-sixteenth). We miss his attention to detail in the editorial work, but especially his friendship.

William W. Hay, Jr., MD
Myron J. Levin, MD
Judith M. Sondheimer, MD
Robin R. Deterding, MD

Denver, Colorado
October, 2004

# The Newborn Infant

1

*Elizabeth H. Thilo, MD, & Adam A. Rosenberg, MD*

The first 28 days of life are usually considered the newborn period. In practice, however, neonatal care may extend to many months for sick or very immature infants. Levels of newborn care are classified from level 1 (well newborns) to level 3 (critically ill newborns). Level 3 nurseries are often part of a perinatal center offering critical care to the mother and fetus as well as the newborn infant.

## ■ EVALUATION OF THE NEWBORN INFANT HISTORY

Taking the history in newborn medicine involves three key areas: (1) the medical history of the mother and father, including a relevant genetic history; (2) the history of the mother's previous pregnancies; and (3) the history of the current pregnancy, including antepartum and intrapartum events.

The mother's medical history should include any chronic medical conditions, medications taken during pregnancy, unusual dietary habits, smoking history, occupational exposures to chemicals or infections of potential risk to the fetus, and pertinent aspects of the social history that may suggest increased risks for parenting problems and child abuse. Family illnesses with genetic implications should be sought. The past pregnancy history should include maternal age, gravidity and parity, blood type, and pregnancy outcomes. The current obstetric history should include documentation and results of procedures such as ultrasound, amniocentesis, screening tests (eg, hepatitis B surface antigen [HBsAg], antibody screen, serum alpha fetoprotein [AFP], human immunodeficiency virus [HIV]), and antepartum tests of fetal well-being (eg, biophysical profiles nonstress tests, or Doppler assessment of fetal blood flow patterns). Information should be sought regarding pregnancy-related illnesses in the mother such as urinary tract infection, pregnancy-induced hypertension or preeclampsia, eclampsia, vaginal bleeding, and preterm labor. Peripartum events of importance include duration of ruptured membranes, maternal fever, fetal distress or meconium-stained amniotic fluid, type of delivery (vaginal or cesarean section), anesthesia and analgesia used, reason for operative or forceps delivery, and condition of the infant at birth, including any resuscitation needed and Apgar scores.

## ASSESSMENT OF GROWTH & GESTATIONAL AGE

It is important to know an infant's gestational age because its behavior and anticipated problems can be predicted on this basis. Accurate recall of the date of the last menstrual period is the best indicator of gestational age. Other obstetric observations, such as fundal height and early ultrasound examination, provide supporting information. A postnatal examination can also be used because fetal physical characteristics and neurologic development progress in predictable fashion. Table 1–1 lists the physical and neurologic criteria to be examined. The upper panel is the neuromuscular examination, assessing primarily muscle tone and strength. The lower panel catalogs a variety of physical characteristics. Adding the scores assigned to each characteristic yields a total score that corresponds to the gestational age.

Disappearance of the anterior vascular capsule of the lens is also helpful in determining gestational age. Until 27–28 weeks' gestation, the lens capsule is covered by vessels; by 34 weeks, this vascular plexus is completely atrophied. Foot length, measured carefully from the heel to the tip of the longest toe, also correlates with gestational age in appropriately grown infants. The foot measures 4.5 cm at 25 weeks' gestation and increases by 0.25 cm/week until term.

By convention, unless the physical examination indicates a gestational age more than 2 weeks different (in either direction) from the obstetric dates, the gestational age is as assigned by the dates. The birth weight and gestational age must be plotted on an appropriate standard to determine if the infant's weight is appropriate for gestational age (AGA), small for gestational age (SGA) or intrauterine growth restricted (IUGR), or large for gestational age (LGA) (Figure 1–1). Birth weight and gestational age distributions vary from one population to the next, depending on factors such as those listed in Table 1–2. Whenever possible, standards should be prepared from data derived from the local population, but when such information is not available,

**Table 1–1.** New Ballard Score for assessment of fetal maturation of newly born infants.[a]

### Neuromuscular Maturity

| Neuromuscular Maturity Sign | Score | | | | | | | Record Score Here |
|---|---|---|---|---|---|---|---|---|
| | −1 | 0 | 1 | 2 | 3 | 4 | 5 | |
| Posture | | | | | | | | |
| Square window (wrist) | >90° | 90° | 60° | 45° | 30° | 0° | | |
| Arm recoil | | 180° | 140° to 180° | 110° to 140° | 90° to 110° | <90° | | |
| Popliteal angle | 180° | 160° | 140° | 120° | 100° | 90° | <90° | |
| Scarf sign | | | | | | | | |
| Heel to ear | | | | | | | | |

Total Neuromuscular Maturity Score

### Physical Maturity

| Physical Maturity Sign | Score | | | | | | | Record Score Here |
|---|---|---|---|---|---|---|---|---|
| | −1 | 0 | 1 | 2 | 3 | 4 | 5 | |
| Skin | Sticky, friable, transparent | Gelatinous, red, translucent | Smooth, pink, visible veins | Superficial peeling &/or rash; few veins | Cracking, pale areas; rare veins | Parchment, deep cracking; no vessels | Leathery, cracked, wrinkled | |
| Lanugo | None | Sparse | Abundant | Thinning | Bald areas | Mostly bald | | |
| Plantar surface | Heel toe 40–50 mm: −1 < 40 mm: −2 | > 50 mm: no crease | Faint red marks | Anterior transverse crease only | Creases anterior $^2/_3$ | Creases over entire sole | | |
| Breast | Imperceptible | Barely perceptible | Flat areola; no bud | Stippled areola; 1- to 2-mm bud | Raised areola; 3- to 4-mm bud | Full areola; 5- to 10-mm bud | | |
| Eye/Ear | Lids fused loosely: −1 tightly: −2 | Lids open; pinna flat; stays folded | Slightly curved pinna; soft; slow recoil | Well-curved pinna; soft but ready recoil | Formed & firm instant recoil | Thick cartilage; ear stiff | | |
| Genitals (male) | Scrotum flat, smooth | Scrotum empty; faint rugae | Testes in upper canal; rare rugae | Testes descending; few rugae | Testes down; good rugae | Testes pendulous; deep rugae | | |
| Genitals (female) | Clitoris prominent & labia flat | Prominent clitoris & small labia minora | Prominent clitoris & enlarging minora | Majora & minora equally prominent | Majora large; minora small | Majora cover clitoris & minora | | |

Total Physical Maturity Score

| Maturity | Score | −10 | −5 | 0 | 5 | 10 | 15 | 20 | 25 | 30 | 35 | 40 | 45 | 50 |
|---|---|---|---|---|---|---|---|---|---|---|---|---|---|---|
| Rating | Weeks | 20 | 22 | 24 | 26 | 28 | 30 | 32 | 34 | 36 | 38 | 40 | 42 | 44 |

[a]See text for a description of the clinical gestational age examination.
Reproduced, with permission, from Ballard JL et al: New Ballard Score, expanded to include extremely premature infants. J Pediatr 1991;119:417.

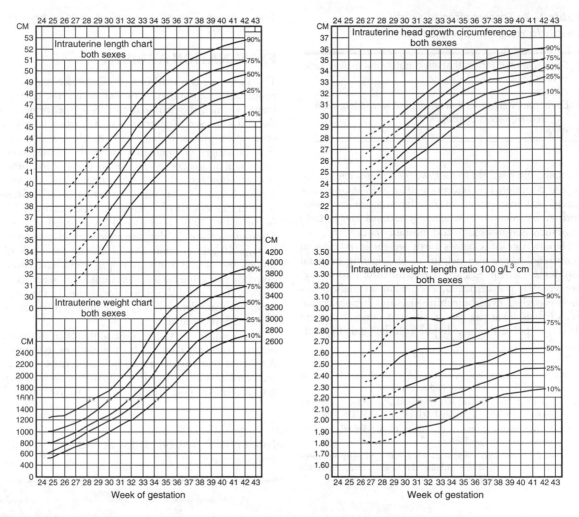

**Figure 1–1.** Intrauterine growth curves for weight, length, and head circumference for singleton births in Colorado. (Reproduced, with permission, from Lubchenco LO et al: Intrauterine growth in length and head circumference as estimated from live births at gestational ages from 26 to 42 weeks. Pediatrics 1966;37:403.)

any regional standard may be used. The birth weight-gestational age distribution of an infant is a screening tool that should be supplemented by clinical data confirming a tentative diagnosis of intrauterine growth restriction or excessive fetal growth. These data include not only the clinical features of the infant determined during the physical examination but also factors such as the size of the parents and the birth weight-gestational age distribution of infants previously born to the parents.

Table 1–3 lists causes of variations in neonatal size in relation to gestational age. An important distinction, particularly in SGA infants, is whether the growth dis-

order is symmetrical (weight, length, and occipitofrontal circumference [OFC] all ≤ 10%) or asymmetrical (only weight ≤ 10%). Asymmetrical growth retardation implies a problem late in the pregnancy, such as pregnancy-induced hypertension or placental insufficiency. Symmetrical growth restriction implies an event of early pregnancy: chromosomal abnormality, drug or alcohol use, congenital viral infections. In general, the outlook for normal growth and development is better in the asymmetrically growth-restricted infant whose intrauterine brain growth has been spared.

The fact that SGA infants have fewer problems (such as respiratory distress syndrome) than AGA infants of

**Table 1–2.** Factors affecting birth weight/gestational age distributions.

---

1. Socioeconomic factors that affect nutritional level and access to health care
2. Altitude
3. Environmental factors that affect birth weight (eg, smoking, alcohol, illicit drug use)
4. Race

---

the same birth weight but a lower gestational age has led to the common misconception that SGA infants have accelerated maturation. SGA infants, when compared with AGA infants of the same gestational age, actually have increased morbidity and mortality rates.

Knowledge of a baby's birth weight in relation to gestational age is also helpful in anticipating neonatal problems. LGA babies are at risk for birth trauma, hypoglycemia, polycythemia, congenital anomalies, cardiomyopathy, hyperbilirubinemia, and hypocalcemia. SGA babies are at risk for fetal distress during labor and delivery, polycythemia, hypoglycemia, and hypocalcemia.

American Academy of Pediatrics: *Guidelines for Perinatal Care,* 5th ed. American Academy of Pediatrics, 2002.

Ballard JL et al: New Ballard score, expanded to include extremely premature infants. J Pediatr 1991;119:417 [PMID:1880657].

Cowett RM: Neonatal care of the infant of the diabetic mother. Neoreviews 2002;3:e190.

McIntire DD et al: Birth weight in relation to morbidity and mortality among newborn infants. N Engl J Med 1999;340:1234 [PMID: 10210706].

**Table 1–3.** Causes of variations in neonatal size in relation to gestational age.

---

**Infants large for gestational age**
  Infant of a diabetic mother
**Infants small for gestational age**
  Asymmetrical
    Placental insufficiency secondary to pregnancy-induced hypertension or other maternal vascular disease
    Maternal age > 35 years
    Poor weight gain during pregnancy
    Multiple gestation
  Symmetrical
    Maternal drug use
      Narcotics
      Cocaine
      Alcohol
    Chromosomal abnormalities
    Intrauterine viral infection (eg, cytomegalovirus)

---

Thureen PJ et al: The small-for-gestational age infant. Neoreviews 2001;2:e139.

## EXAMINATION AT BIRTH

The extent of the newborn physical examination depends on the condition of the infant and the environment in which the examination is being performed. In the delivery room, the examination consists largely of observation plus auscultation of the chest and inspection for congenital anomalies and birth trauma. Major congenital anomalies are present in 1.5% of live births and account for 20–25% of perinatal and neonatal deaths. Because the infant is recovering from the stress of birth, the examination should not be extensive. The Apgar score (Table 1–4) should be recorded at 1 and 5 minutes of age. In the case of severely depressed infants, a 10-minute score should also be recorded. Although the 1- and 5-minute Apgar scores have almost no predictive value for long-term outcome, serial scores do provide a useful shorthand description of the severity of perinatal depression and the quality of the resuscitative efforts needed.

The color of the skin is a useful indicator of cardiac output. Normally there is a high blood flow to the skin. Any stress that triggers a catecholamine response redirects cardiac output away from the skin to preserve oxygen delivery to more critical organs. Cyanosis and pal-

**Table 1–4.** Infant evaluation at birth—Apgar score.[a]

|  | Score | | |
|---|---|---|---|
|  | **0** | **1** | **2** |
| Heart rate | Absent | Slow (< 100) | > 100 |
| Respiratory effort | Absent | Slow, irregular | Good, crying |
| Muscle tone | Limp | Some flexion | Active motion |
| Response to catheter in nostril[b] | No response | Grimace | Cough or sneeze |
| Color | Blue or pale | Body pink; extremities blue | Completely pink |

© 1958 American Medical Association.
[a]One minute and 5 minutes after complete birth of the infant (disregarding the cord and the placenta), the following objective signs should be observed and recorded.
[b]Tested after oropharynx is clear.
Reproduced, with permission, from Apgar V et al: Evaluation of the newborn infant—Second report. JAMA 1958;168:1985.

lor are thus two signs reflecting inadequate skin oxygenation and cardiac output.

The skeletal examination immediately after delivery serves two purposes: (1) to detect any obvious congenital anomalies and (2) to detect signs of birth trauma, particularly in LGA infants or those born after a protracted second stage of labor—in whom a fractured clavicle or humerus might be found.

The umbilical cord should be examined for the number of vessels. Normally, there are two arteries and one vein. In 1% of deliveries (5–6% of twin deliveries), the cord has only two vessels: an artery and a vein. The latter configuration may be considered a minor anomaly and, as with other minor anomalies, carries a slightly increased risk of associated defects. The placenta is usually examined by the physician delivering it. Small placentas are always associated with small infants. The placental examination emphasizes the identification of membranes and vessels—particularly in multiple gestations—as well as the presence and severity of placental infarcts or evidence of clot (placental abruption) on the maternal side.

## GENERAL EXAMINATION IN THE NURSERY

It is important that the examiner have warm hands and a gentle approach. Start with observation, then auscultation of the chest, and then palpation of the abdomen. Examination of the eyes, ears, throat, and hips should be done last, since these maneuvers are most disturbing to the infant. The heart rate should range from 120 to 160 beats/min, and the respiratory rate from 30 to 60 breaths/min; blood pressure is affected by perinatal asphyxia and the need for mechanical ventilation more than by gestational age or birth weight. Systolic blood pressure on day 1 ranges from 50 to 70 mm Hg and increases steadily during the first week of life. *Note:* An irregularly irregular heart rate, usually caused by premature atrial contractions, is common. This irregularity should resolve in the first days of life and is not of pathologic significance.

The presence of minor anomalies (those occurring in < 4% of the population) should be noted. Approximately 15–20% of healthy newborns have one minor anomaly, with a 3% risk of having an associated major anomaly. Approximately 0.8% of newborns have two minor anomalies, and 0.5% have three or more, with a risk of 10% and 20%, respectively, of a major malformation. Common minor anomalies that require no further diagnostic evaluation if isolated in an otherwise normal infant include preauricular pits (although hearing should be assessed), a sacral dimple without other cutaneous abnormality that occurs within 2.5 cm of the anus, a single transverse palmar crease, and three or fewer café-au-lait spots in a white infant or five or fewer in an African American infant.

## Skin

Observe for bruising, petechiae (common over the presenting part), meconium staining, and jaundice. Peripheral cyanosis is commonly present when the extremities are cool or the infant is polycythemic. Generalized cyanosis merits immediate evaluation. Pallor may be caused by acute or chronic blood loss or by acidosis. In dark-skinned infants, pallor and cyanosis should be assessed in the oral region and nail beds. Plethora suggests polycythemia. Note vernix caseosa (a whitish, greasy material covering the body that decreases as term approaches) and lanugo (the fine hair covering the preterm infant's skin). Dry skin with cracking and peeling of the superficial layers is common in postterm infants. Edema may be generalized (hydrops) or localized (eg, on the dorsum of the feet in Turner syndrome). Check for birthmarks such as capillary hemangiomas (lower occiput, eyelids, forehead) and mongolian spot (bluish black pigmentation over the back and buttocks). Milia—small white keratogenous cysts—can be found scattered over the cheeks, forehead, nose, and nasolabial folds. Miliaria (blocked ducts of sweat glands) occurs in intertriginous areas and on the face or scalp. It can appear as small vesicles (crystallina), small erythematous papules (rubra), or pustules. Erythema toxicum is a benign rash characterized by fleeting erythematous papules and pustules filled with eosinophils. Pustular melanosis leaves pigmented macules when the pustules rupture. The pustules are noninfectious but contain neutrophils. Jaundice presenting in the first 24 hours is considered abnormal and should be evaluated (see section on Neonatal Jaundice).

## Head

Check for cephalohematoma (a swelling over one or both parietal bones contained within suture lines) and caput succedaneum (edema over the presenting part that crosses suture lines). Subgaleal hemorrhages (beneath the scalp) are uncommon but can lead to extensive blood loss into this large potential space with resultant hypovolemic shock. Skull fractures may be linear or depressed and may be associated with cephalohematoma. Check the size and presence of the fontanelles. The anterior fontanelle varies from 1 to 4 cm in any direction, whereas the posterior fontanelle should be less than 1 cm. A third fontanelle is a bony defect along the sagittal suture in the parietal bones and may be a feature of certain syndromes, such as trisomy 21. Sutures should be freely mobile. Craniosynostosis is a prematurely fused suture.

## Face

Odd facies may be associated with a specific syndrome. Bruising from birth trauma (especially with face presentation) and forceps marks should be identified. Face presentation may be associated with considerable soft tissue swelling around the nose and mouth, causing considerable distortion. Facial nerve palsy is observed when the infant cries; the unaffected side of the mouth moves normally, giving a distorted grimace.

## Eyes

Subconjunctival hemorrhages are seen frequently as a result of the birth process. Less commonly, a corneal tear may occur, presenting as a clouded cornea. Ophthalmologic consultation is indicated in such cases. Extraocular movements should be assessed. Occasional uncoordinated eye movements are common, but persistent irregular movements are abnormal. The iris should be inspected for abnormalities such as Brushfield spots (trisomy 21) and colobomas. Examine for the red reflex of the retina. The red reflexes should be symmetrical. Dark spots, a blunted reflex on one side, lack of a reflex, and a white reflex are all indications for referral to an ophthalmologist. Leukokoria can be caused by glaucoma (cloudy cornea), cataract, or tumor (retinoblastoma). Infants at risk for chorioretinitis (congenital viral infection) should undergo a formal retinal examination with pupils dilated prior to nursery discharge or as an outpatient.

## Nose

Examine the nose for size and shape. In utero compression can cause deformities. Because babies under age 1 month are obligate nose breathers, any nasal obstruction (eg, bilateral choanal atresia or stenosis) can cause respiratory distress. Unilateral choanal atresia can be diagnosed by occluding each naris. Patency is best checked by holding a cold metal surface (eg, a chilled laryngoscope blade) under the nose, and observing the fog from both nares on the metal. Purulent nasal discharge at birth suggests congenital syphilis.

## Ears

Malformed or malpositioned (low-set or posteriorly rotated) ears are often associated with other congenital anomalies. The tympanic membranes should be visualized. Preauricular pits and tags are also common minor variants that can be associated with hearing loss.

## Mouth

Epithelial (Epstein) pearls are retention cysts along the gum margins and at the junction of the hard and soft palates. Natal teeth may be present and sometimes need to be removed to avoid the risk of aspiration. Check the integrity and shape of the palate; rule out cleft lip and cleft palate. A small mandible and tongue with cleft soft palate is seen with Pierre-Robin syndrome and can result in respiratory difficulty as the tongue occludes the airway. Prone positioning can be very beneficial. A prominent tongue can be seen in trisomy 21 and Beckwith–Wiedemann syndrome. Excessive drooling suggests esophageal atresia.

## Neck

Redundant skin or webbing is seen in Turner syndrome. Sinus tracts may be seen as remnants of branchial clefts. Check for masses: midline (thyroid), anterior to the sternocleidomastoid (branchial cleft cysts), within the sternocleidomastoid (hematoma, torticollis), and posterior to the sternocleidomastoid (cystic hygroma).

## Chest & Lungs

Check for fractured clavicles (crepitus, bruising, and tenderness). Increased anteroposterior diameter (barrel chest) can be seen with aspiration syndromes. Check air entry bilaterally and the position of the mediastinum and heart tones. Decreased breath sounds with respiratory distress and a shift in the mediastinum suggests pneumothorax (tension) or a space-occupying lesion (eg, diaphragmatic hernia). With pneumomediastinum, the heart sounds are muffled. Expiratory grunting and decreased air entry are observed in hyaline membrane disease. Rales are not of clinical significance at this age.

## Heart

Examination of the heart is described in detail in Chapter 19. **Note:** Murmurs are commonly present in the first hours and are most often benign. Severe congenital heart disease in the newborn infant may be present with no murmur at all. The two most common presentations of heart disease in the newborn infant are cyanosis and congestive heart failure with abnormalities of pulses. In hypoplastic left heart and critical aortic stenosis, pulses are diminished at all sites. In aortic coarctation and interrupted aortic arch, pulses are diminished in the lower extremities.

## Abdomen

Check for softness, distention, and bowel sounds. If polyhydramnios was present or excessive oral secretions are noted, pass a soft catheter into the stomach to rule out esophageal atresia. Palpate for kidneys—most abdominal masses in the newborn infant are associated with kidney disorders (eg, multicystic or dysplastic, hydronephrosis). When the abdomen is relaxed, normal-sized kidneys may be felt but are not prominent. A markedly scaphoid abdomen plus respiratory distress suggests diaphragmatic hernia. Absence of abdominal musculature (prune belly syndrome) may occur in association with renal abnormalities. Check the size of the liver and the spleen. These organs are superficial and discernible by light palpation in the newborn infant. The outline of a distended bladder may be seen and palpated above the pubic symphysis.

## Genitalia & Anus

Male and female genitals show characteristics according to gestational age (see Table 1–1). In the female during the first few days, a whitish vaginal discharge with or without blood is normal. Check the patency and location of the anus.

## Skeleton

Check for obvious anomalies, for example, the absence of a bone, clubfoot, fusion or webbing of digits, and extra digits. Examine for hip dislocation by attempting to dislocate the femur posteriorly and then abducting the legs to relocate the femur. Look for extremity fractures and for palsies (especially brachial plexus injuries). Rule out myelomeningoceles and other spinal deformities (eg, scoliosis). Arthrogryposis (multiple joint contractures) results from chronic limitation of movement in utero, which may result from lack of amniotic fluid or from a congenital neuromuscular disease.

## Neurologic Examination

Normal newborns are endowed with a set of reflexes that facilitate survival (eg, rooting and sucking reflexes), as well as sensory abilities (eg, hearing and smell) that allow them to recognize their mother within a few weeks of birth. Although the retina is well developed at birth, visual acuity is poor (20/400) because of a relatively immobile lens. Acuity improves rapidly over the first 6 months, with fixation and tracking becoming well developed by 2 months.

In examining the newborn, observe resting tone (normal-term newborns should exhibit flexion of the upper and lower extremities) and spontaneous movements. Look for symmetry of movements. Extension of extremities should result in spontaneous recoil to the flexed position. Assess the character of the cry; a high-pitched cry may be indicative of disease of the central nervous system (CNS) (eg, hemorrhage). Hypotonia and a weak cry are indicative of systemic disease or a congenital neuromuscular disorder. Check for newborn reflexes:

1. Sucking reflex in response to a nipple or the examiner's finger in the mouth. This reflex is observed by 14 weeks' gestation.
2. Rooting reflex: Head turns to the side of a facial stimulus. This reflex develops by 28 weeks' gestation.
3. Traction response: The infant is pulled by the arms to a sitting position. Initially, the head lags, then with active flexion comes to the midline briefly before falling forward.
4. Palmar grasp with placement of the examiner's finger in the palm. This reflex develops by 28 weeks' gestation and disappears by age 4 months.
5. Deep tendon reflexes: Several beats of ankle clonus and an upgoing Babinski reflex may be normal.
6. Placing: Rub the dorsum of one foot on the underside of a surface. The infant will flex the knee and bring the foot up.
7. Moro (startle) reflex: Hold the infant and support the head. Allow the head to drop 1–2 cm suddenly. The arms will abduct at the shoulder and extend at the elbow. Adduction with flexion will follow. The hands show a prominent spreading or extension of the fingers. This reflex develops by 28 weeks' gestation (incomplete) and disappears by age 3 months.
8. Tonic neck reflex: Forcibly turn the infant's head to one side, and the arm and leg on that side extend while the opposite arm and leg flex ("fencing position"). This reflex disappears by age 8 months.

Adam M, Hudgins L: The importance of minor anomalies in the evaluation of the newborn. Neoreviews 2003;4:e99.

Ackerman LL, Menezes AH: Spinal congenital dermal sinuses: A 30-year experience. Pediatrics 2003;112:641 [PMID: 12949296].

American Academy of Pediatrics Committee on Quality Improvement, Subcommittee on Developmental Dysplasia of the Hip: Early detection of developmental dysplasia of the hip. Pediatrics 2000;105:896 [PMID: 10742345].

American Academy of Pediatrics Section on Ophthalmology: Red reflex examination in infants. Pediatrics 2002;109:980 [PMID: 11986467].

Eichenfield LF et al (editors): Textbook of Neonatal Dermatology. WB Saunders, 2001.

Hernandez JA, Morelli JG: Birthmarks of medical significance. Neoreviews 2003;4:e270.

# ■ CARE OF THE WELL NEWBORN INFANT

The primary responsibility of the level 1 nursery is care of the well infant. This includes promoting mother–infant bonding, establishing feeding, and teaching the techniques of newborn care. Surveillance of the infant is a key function of the staff; they must be alert for the signs and symptoms of illness, including temperature instability, change in activity, refusal to feed, pallor, cyanosis, early or excessive jaundice, tachypnea and respiratory distress, delayed (beyond 24 hours) passage of first stool or voiding of urine, and bilious vomiting. Several preventive measures are undertaken routinely in the normal newborn nursery.

Eye prophylaxis to prevent gonococcal ophthalmia is routinely administered within 1 hour after birth with either erythromycin ointment or silver nitrate 1% drops. Because of the severe chemical conjunctivitis caused by silver nitrate, erythromycin is preferred.

Vitamin K, 1 mg, is given intramuscularly or subcutaneously within 4 hours after birth to prevent hemorrhagic disease of the newborn. The area to be injected must be cleansed thoroughly before injection to prevent infection.

All infants should be vaccinated against hepatitis B, but the first dose can wait until 1–2 months of age if the mother is HBsAG-negative. Hepatitis B vaccine and hepatitis B immune globulin (HBIG) are administered if the mother is known to be HBsAg-positive. If maternal HBsAg status is unknown at birth, the vaccine should be given. The mother's blood should be tested and HBIG given at less than 7 days of age if the test is positive.

Cord blood is collected on all infants at birth and used for blood typing and Coombs' testing if the mother is type O or Rh-negative. Cord blood is useful also for other tests, such as toxicology screens.

Rapid glucose testing should be performed in infants at risk for hypoglycemia (eg, infants of diabetic mothers [IDMs], preterm, SGA, LGA, or stressed infants). Values less than 45 mg/dL should be confirmed by laboratory blood glucose testing and treated. Hematocrit should be measured at age 3–6 hours in infants at risk for or those who have symptoms of polycythemia or anemia.

The state-sponsored newborn genetic screen (for inborn errors of metabolism such as phenylketonuria [PKU], galactosemia, sickle cell disease, hypothyroidism, and cystic fibrosis) is performed just prior to discharge, after 24–48 hours in hospital if possible. In many states, a repeat test is required at 8–14 days of age because the PKU test is often falsely negative when obtained before 48 hours of age. Not all state-mandated screens include the same panel of diseases; the most recent addition in some states is a screen for congenital adrenal hyperplasia. In infants with prolonged hospital stays, the test should be performed by 1 week of age. In addition to the state-mandated screen, some centers offer expanded newborn screening by tandem mass spectrometry that looks for a variety of other inborn errors such as fatty acid oxidation defects.

Infants should routinely be positioned supine or lying on the right side with the dependent arm forward to minimize the risk of sudden infant death syndrome (SIDS). Prone positioning is contraindicated unless specific problems, such as gastroesophageal reflux or respiratory distress, are present. Bed sharing with adults and prone positioning are both associated with increased risk of SIDS.

## FEEDING THE WELL NEWBORN INFANT

Indications that the baby is ready for feeding include (1) alertness and vigor, (2) absence of abdominal distention, (3) good bowel sounds, and (4) normal hunger cry. All of these usually occur within 6 hours after birth, but fetal distress or traumatic delivery may prolong this period.

The healthy full-term infant should be allowed to feed every 2–5 hours on demand. The first feeding usually occurs by 3 hours of life, often as early as in the delivery room. Breast milk or formula (20 kcal/oz) can be given. For formula-fed babies, the volume generally increases from 0.5–1 oz per feeding initially to 1.5–2 oz per feeding on day 3. By day 3, the average full-term newborn takes in about 100 mL/kg/d of milk.

Although a wide range of infant formulas can satisfy the nutritional needs of most neonates, breast milk is the standard on which formulas are based (see also Chapter 10). The distribution of calories in human milk is 55% fat, 38% carbohydrate, and 7% protein, with a whey-to-casein ratio of 60:40, allowing for easy protein digestion. Despite the low concentrations of several vitamins and minerals, their bioavailability is high. All of the necessary nutrients, vitamins, minerals, and water are provided by human milk for the first 6 months of life except vitamin K (thus, 1 mg IM is administered at birth), vitamin D (200–300 IU/d if minimal sunlight exposure), fluoride (0.25 mg/d after 6 months if water supply not fluoridated), and vitamin $B_{12}$ (0.3–0.5 mg/d if the mother is a strict vegetarian and takes no $B_{12}$ supplement). Other advantages of breast milk include (1) the presence of immunologic, antimicrobial, and antiinflammatory factors, including IgA, cellular, and protein or enzymatic components that decrease the incidence of upper respiratory and gastrointestinal (GI) infections in infancy; (2) the possibility that breast feeding may decrease the frequency and severity of childhood eczema and asthma; (3) promotion of mother–infant bonding; and (4) evidence that breast milk as a nutritional source improves neurodevelopmental outcomes.

Although approximately 65% of mothers in the United States initiate breast feeding, only 25% continue to breastfeed at 6 months. Hospital practices that facilitate the successful initiation of breast feeding include rooming-in, nursing on demand, and avoiding the use of pacifiers and supplemental formula (unless medically indicated). The nursery staff must be cognizant of problems associated with breast feeding and be able to provide help and support for mothers in the hospital. It is essential that an experienced professional observe and assist with at least one feeding to document good latch-on, important in preventing the common breast-feeding problems of sore nipples, unsatisfied babies, engorgement, poor milk supply, and excessive hyperbilirubinemia ("lack-of-breast-milk jaundice").

Table 1–5 presents recommendations the nursing mother and health care provider can use to achieve successful breast feeding.

American Academy of Pediatrics Committee on Fetus and Newborn: Controversies concerning vitamin K and the newborn. Pediatrics 2003;112:191 [PMID: 12837888].

American Academy of Pediatrics Committee on Nutrition: Iron fortification of infant formulas. Pediatrics 1999; 104:119 [PMID: 10390274].

American Academy of Pediatrics Task Force on Infant Sleep Position and Sudden Infant Death Syndrome: Concepts of sudden infant death syndrome: Implications for infant sleeping environment and sleep position. Pediatrics 2000; 105:650 [PMID: 10699127].

Anderson JW et al: Breast-feeding and cognitive development: A meta-analysis. Am J Clin Nutr 1999;70:525 [PMID: 10500022].

Dewey KG et al: Risk factors for suboptimal infant breastfeeding behavior, delayed onset of lactation, and excess neonatal weight loss, Pediatrics 2003;112:607 [PMID: 12949292].

Hoffman DR et al: Visual function in breast-fed term infants weaned to formula with or without long-chain polyunsaturates at 4 to 6 months: A randomized clinical trial. J Pediatr 2003;142:669 [PMID: 12838196].

Kunz C et al: Nutritional and biochemical properties of human milk. Part 1: General aspects, proteins, and carbohydrates. Clin Perinatol 1999;26:307 [PMID: 10394490].

Neifert MR: Clinical aspects of lactation: Promoting breast feeding success. Clin Perinatol 1999;26:281 [PMID: 10394489].

Rodriquez-Palmero M et al: Nutritional and biochemical properties of human milk. II: Lipids, micronutrients, and bioactive factors. Clin Perinatol 1999;26:335 [PMID: 10394491].

# EARLY DISCHARGE OF THE NEWBORN INFANT

Discharge at 24–36 hours of age appears safe and appropriate for most infants if there are no contraindications (Table 1–6) and a follow-up visit at 48–72 hours after discharge is ensured. Most infants with severe cardiorespiratory disorders and infections are identified in the first 6 hours of life. The exception may be the infant treated with intrapartum antibiotic prophylaxis for maternal group B streptococcal (GBS) colonization or infection. The Centers for Disease Control and Prevention (CDC) and the American Academy of Pediatrics (AAP) have recommended that these infants be observed in hospital for 48 hours because of the possibility of "partial treatment" with delayed onset of symptoms of infection. However, recent data show that exposure to antibiotics in labor does not appear to change the type or timing of symptoms related to GBS infection in full-term infants, and that hospital observation beyond 24 hours is unnecessary for the asymptomatic full-term infant who received intrapartum chemoprophylaxis. Other problems, such as jaundice and difficulties in breast feeding, typically occur after 48 hours and can usually be dealt with on an outpatient basis provided good follow-up has been arranged.

The AAP recommends a follow-up visit within 48–72 hours for any newborn discharged before 48 hours of age. Infants who are small or slightly premature—especially if breast feeding—are at particular risk for inadequate intake. Suggested guidelines for the follow-up interview and physical examination are presented in Table 1–7. The optimal timing of discharge must be determined in each case based on medical, social, and financial factors.

# CIRCUMCISION

Circumcision is an elective procedure to be performed only in healthy, stable infants. The procedure probably has medical benefits, including prevention of phimosis, paraphimosis, balanoposthitis, and urinary tract infection. Later benefits include decreased incidence of cancer of the penis, cervical cancer (in partners of circumcised men), and sexually transmitted diseases (including HIV). Most parents decide on circumcision for nonmedical reasons. The risks of the procedure include local infection, bleeding, removal of too much skin, and urethral injury. The combined incidence of these complications is less than 1%. Local anesthesia (dorsal penile nerve block or circumferential ring block with 1% lidocaine without epinephrine) or topical application of an anesthetic cream are safe and effective and should always be used. Techniques that allow visualization of the glans throughout the procedure (eg, Plas-

*Table 1–5.* Guidelines for successful breast feeding.

| | First 8 Hours | 8–24 Hours | Day 2 | Day 3 | Day 4 | Day 5 | Day 6 Onward |
|---|---|---|---|---|---|---|---|
| Milk supply | You may be able to express a few drops of milk. | | Milk should come in between the second and fourth days. | | | Milk should be in. Breasts may be firm or leak milk. | Breasts should feel softer after feedings. |
| Baby's activity | Baby is usually wide-awake in the first hour of life. Put baby to breast within 30 min after birth. | Wake up your baby. Babies may not wake up on their own to feed. | Baby should be more cooperative and less sleepy. | Look for early feeding cues such as rooting, lip smacking, and hands to face. | | | Baby should appear satisfied after feedings. |
| Feeding routine | Baby may go into a deep sleep 2–4 h after birth. | Feed your baby every 1–4 h or as often as wanted—at least 8–12 times a day. | | Use chart to write down time of each feeding. | | May go one longer interval (up to 5 h between feeds) in a 24-h period. | |
| Breast feeding | Baby will wake up and be alert and responsive for several more hours after initial deep sleep. | As long as the mother s comfortable, nurse at both breasts as long as baby is actively sucking. | Try to nurse both sides each feeding, aiming at 10 min per side. Expect some nipple tenderness. | Consider hand expressing or pumping a few drops of milk to soften the nipple if the breast is too firm for the baby to latch on. | Nurse a minimum of 10–30 min per side every feeding for the first few weeks of life. Once milk supply is well established, allow baby to finish the first breast before offering the second. | | Mother's nipple tenderness is improving or is gone. |
| Baby's urine output | | Baby must have a minimum of one wet diaper in first 24 h. | Baby must have at least one wet diaper every 8–11 h. | You should see an increase in wet diapers (up to four to six) in 24 h. | Baby's urine should be light yellow. | Baby should have six to eight wet diapers per day of colorless or light yellow urine. | |
| Baby's stool | | Baby should have a black-green (meconium) stool. | Baby may have a second very dark (meconium) stool. | Baby's stools should be in transition from black-green to yellow. | | Baby should have three or four yellow, seedy stools a day. | The number of stools may decrease gradually after 4–6 wk of life. |

Modified, with permission, from Gabrielski L: Lactation support services. The Children's Hospital, Denver, 1999.

**Table 1–6.** Criteria for early newborn discharge.

**Contraindications to early newborn discharge**
1. Jaundice at ≤ 24 h
2. High risk for infection (eg, maternal chorioamnionitis); discharge allowed at 24 h with a normal transition
3. Known or suspected narcotic addiction or withdrawal
4. Physical defects requiring evaluation
5. Oral defects (clefts, micrognathia)

**Relative contraindications to early newborn discharge (infants at high risk for feeding failure, excessive jaundice)**
1. Prematurity or borderline prematurity (< 38 weeks' gestation)
2. Birth weight < 2700 g (6 lb)
3. Baby difficult to arouse for feeding; not demanding regularly in nursery
4. Medical or neurologic problems that interfere with feeding (Down syndrome, hypotonia, cardiac problems)
5. Twins or higher multiples
6. ABO blood group incompatibility or severe jaundice in previous child
7. Mother whose previous breast-fed infant gained weight poorly
8. Mother with breast surgery involving periareolar areas (if attempting to nurse)

**Table 1–7.** Guidelines for early outpatient follow-up evaluation.

**History**
  Rhythmic sucking and audible swallowing for at least 10 minutes total per feeding?
  Baby wakes and demands to feed every 2–3 h (at least eight to ten feedings per 24 h)?
  Do breasts feel full before feedings, and softer after?
  Are there at least six noticeably wet diapers per 24 h?
  Are there yellow bowel movements (no longer meconium)—at least four per 24 h?
  Is baby still acting hungry after nursing (frequently sucks hands, rooting)?

**Physical assessment**
  Weight, unclothed: should not be more than 8–10% below birth weight
  Extent and severity of jaundice
  Assessment of hydration, alertness, general well-being
  Cardiovascular examination: murmurs, brachial and femoral pulses, respirations

tibell and Gomco clamp) are preferred to a blind technique (eg, Mogen clamp) because occasional amputation of the glans can occur with the latter technique. Circumcision is contraindicated in infants with genital abnormalities (eg, hypospadias). Coagulation screen should be performed prior to the procedure in infants with a confirmed family history of serious bleeding disorders.

## HEARING SCREENING

Normal hearing is critical to normal language development. Significant bilateral hearing loss is present in 1–3 infants per 1000 in the well nursery and in 2–4 infants per 100 in the neonatal intensive care unit population. All infants should be screened for hearing loss by auditory brainstem evoked responses or evoked otoacoustic emissions as early as possible. Primary care providers and parents need to be advised of the possibility of hearing loss and offered ready referral in suspect cases.

American Academy of Pediatrics Joint Committee on Infant Hearing: Year 2000 position statement: Principles and guidelines for early hearing detection and intervention programs. Pediatrics 2000;106:798 [PMID: 11015525].

American Academy of Pediatrics Section on Endocrinology and Committee on Genetics: Technical report: Congenital adrenal hyperplasia. Pediatrics 2000;106:1511 [PMID: 11099616].

American Academy of Pediatrics Task Force on Circumcision: Circumcision policy statement. Pediatrics 1999;103:686 [PMID: 10049981].

Bromberger P et al: The influence of intrapartum antibiotics on the clinical spectrum of early-onset group B streptococcal infection in term infants. Pediatrics 2000;106:244 [PMID: 10920146].

Farrell PA et al: SIDS, ALTE, apnea and the use of home monitors. Pediatr Rev 2002;23:3 [PMID: 11773587].

Schulze A et al: Expanded newborn screening for inborn errors of metabolism by electrospray ionization–tandem mass spectrometry: Results, outcome, and implications. Pediatrics 2003;111:1399 [PMID: 12777559].

Sokol J, Hyde M: Hearing screening. Pediatr Rev 2002;23:155 [PMID: 11986491].

Thompson DC et al: Universal newborn hearing screening. Summary of evidence. JAMA 2001;286:2000 [PMID: 11667937].

## ■ COMMON PROBLEMS IN THE TERM NEWBORN INFANT

## NEONATAL JAUNDICE

### General Considerations

Jaundice is a common neonatal problem. Sixty-five percent of newborns develop clinical jaundice with a bilirubin level above 5 mg/dL during the first week of life. From an evolutionary standpoint, hyperbilirubinemia ought to confer some biologic advantage if it occurs so often. Bilirubin is a potent antioxidant and peroxyl scavenger that may help the newborn, who is deficient in most antioxidant substances such as vitamin E, catalase, and superoxide dismutase, to avoid oxygen toxicity in the days after birth. Hyperbilirubinemia can also be toxic, with high levels resulting in an encephalopathy known as kernicterus.

## Metabolism of Bilirubin

Heme (iron protoporphyrin) is broken down by heme oxygenase to iron, which is conserved; carbon monoxide, which is exhaled; and biliverdin, which is then further metabolized to bilirubin by the enzyme bilirubin reductase. Each 1 g of hemoglobin breakdown results in the production of 34 mg of bilirubin (1 mg/dL = 17.2 mmol/L of bilirubin). Bilirubin is carried bound to albumin to the liver, where, in the presence of the enzyme uridyldiphosphoglucuronyl transferase (UDPGT; glucuronyl transferase), it is taken up by the hepatocyte and conjugated with two glucuronide molecules. The conjugated bilirubin is then excreted through the bile to the intestine. In the presence of normal gut flora, the conjugated bilirubin is metabolized further to stercobilins and excreted in the stool. In the absence of gut flora—and with slow intestinal motility, as in the first few days of life—the conjugated bilirubin remains in the intestinal lumen, where a mucosal enzyme (β-glucuronidase) can cleave off the glucuronide molecules, leaving unconjugated bilirubin to be reabsorbed (the enterohepatic circulation of bilirubin).

## Bilirubin Toxicity

The exact mechanism by which bilirubin is toxic to cells is unknown. It is assumed that if the amount of lipid-soluble unconjugated bilirubin exceeds the available binding sites on albumin, "free" bilirubin will be available to enter neurons and damage them. The blood–brain barrier probably plays an important role in protecting an individual from brain damage, but its integrity is impossible to measure clinically. It is unknown whether a level of bilirubin exists above which brain damage always occurs even in a healthy individual.

The syndrome of bilirubin encephalopathy was well described in the era before exchange transfusion as treatment for Rh isoimmunization (see later discussion). The pathologic correlate is known as kernicterus, named for the yellow staining of the subthalamic nuclei (kerns) seen at autopsy. The early symptoms of bilirubin encephalopathy consist of lethargy, hypotonia, and poor sucking, progressing to hypertonia, opisthotonos,

and a high-pitched cry. Long-term sequelae include athetoid cerebral palsy, sensorineural deafness, limitation of upward gaze, and dental dysplasia—a syndrome that has been described as an intelligent mind trapped within an uncontrollable body wracked by painful spasms. Whether or not bilirubin causes more subtle neurologic abnormalities remains debatable.

Bilirubin encephalopathy is rare with current neonatal management, although upwards of 120 cases have been reported to an informal registry since 1990. A specific bilirubin level of 20 mg/dL [344 mmol/L] and above has been associated with an increased risk of kernicterus in the Rh-isoimmunized infant. For decades, the strategy of keeping bilirubin under 20 mg/dL with phototherapy and exchange transfusion if needed eliminated kernicterus in the United States. The reappearance of kernicterus over the past decade has been ascribed to early discharge of breast-feeding infants without appropriate follow-up or appreciation of the early signs of bilirubin encephalopathy. The risk of bilirubin encephalopathy is probably very small for full-term infants without hemolysis even at bilirubin levels of 25 mg/dL (430 mmol/L). Premature infants are probably at some increased risk because of associated illnesses that may affect the integrity of the blood–brain barrier as well as because of reduced albumin levels. For this reason, a lower level of bilirubin is generally assumed to represent the "exchange level" in these infants and is usually determined arbitrarily based on the infant's birth weight and gestational age. One common approach is to use 1% of the birth weight in grams as the exchange level in milligrams per deciliter (mg/dL) (eg, 12 mg/dL for a 1200-g infant) down to a low of 10 mg/dL. Many other arbitrary approaches exist as well.

## Causes of Unconjugated Hyperbilirubinemia

The causes of unconjugated hyperbilirubinemia can be grouped into two main categories: overproduction of bilirubin and decreased conjugation of bilirubin (Table 1–8).

### A. INCREASED BILIRUBIN PRODUCTION

Increased production of bilirubin results from an increased rate of red blood cell destruction (hemolysis) due to the presence of maternal antibodies against fetal cells (Coombs' test-positive), abnormal red cell membrane shape (ie, spherocytosis), or abnormal red cell enzymes (ie, glucose-6-phosphate dehydrogenase [G6PD] deficiency). Antibodies can be directed against the major blood group antigens (the type A or type B infant of a type O mother) or the minor antigens (the Rh system: D, E, C, d, e, c, Kell, Duffy, and so on).

*Table 1–8.* Causes of jaundice secondary to unconjugated hyperbilirubemia.

---

**Overproduction of bilirubin**
1. Increased rate of hemolysis (reticulocyte count elevated)
   a. Patients with a positive Coombs test
      Rh incompatibility
      ABO blood group incompatibility
      Other blood group sensitizations
   b. Patients with a negative Coombs test
      Abnormal red cell shapes
         Spherocytosis
         Elliptocytosis
         Pyknocytosis
         Stomatocytosis
      Red cell enzyme abnormalities
         Glucose-6-phosphate dehydrogenase deficiency
         Pyruvate kinase deficiency
         Hexokinase deficiency
         Other metabolic defects
   c. Patients with bacterial or viral sepsis
2. Nonhemolytic causes of increased bilirubin load (Unconjugated bilirubin elevated, reticulocyte count normal.)
   a. Extravascular hemorrhage
      Cephalohematoma
      Extensive bruising
      Central nervous system hemorrhage
   b. Polycythemia
   c. Exaggerated enterohepatic circulation of bilirubin
      Gastrointestinal tract obstruction
      Functional ileus

**Decreased rate of conjugation**
(Unconjugated bilirubin elevated, reticulocyte count normal.)
   Physiologic jaundice
   Crigler-Najjar syndrome
      Type I glucuronyl transferase deficiency, autosomal-recessive
      Type II glucuronyl transferase deficiency, autosomal-dominant
   Gilbert syndrome
   ?Hypothyroidism

---

**1. Antibody-mediated hemolysis (Coombs' test-positive)**—ABO blood group incompatibility is common, usually not severe, and can accompany any pregnancy in a type O mother. The severity is unpredictable because of variability in the amount of naturally occurring anti-A or anti-B IgG antibodies in the mother. Although 20% of pregnancies are the appropriate "setups" for ABO incompatibility (mother O, baby A or B), only about 33% of such infants are Coombs' test-positive and only about 20% of these develop excessive jaundice. In addition to hyperbilirubinemia in the first days of life, these infants may develop a significant ane-

mia over the first several weeks and on occasion may need to be transfused at a few weeks of age.

Rh isoimmunization is much less common and increases in severity with each immunized pregnancy because of an increased maternal IgG antibody production each time. Most Rh disease can be prevented by administering high-titer $Rh_o$ (D) immune globulin to an Rh-negative woman after any invasive procedure during pregnancy as well as after any miscarriage, abortion, or delivery of an Rh-positive infant. In severe cases, erythroblastosis fetalis (hydrops or generalized edema with heart failure related to severe anemia in the fetus) occurs, often resulting in fetal or neonatal death without appropriate antenatal intervention. In less severe cases, hemolysis is the main problem, with resultant hyperbilirubinemia and anemia. The cornerstone of antenatal management once isoimmunization has been diagnosed is transfusion of the fetus with Rh-negative cells, either directly into the umbilical vein via percutaneous cordocentesis or into the fetal abdominal cavity. Following delivery, phototherapy is usually started immediately, with exchange transfusion (see later discussion) as needed. A 500–750 mg/kg dose of intravenous immune globulin (IVIG) given to the infant as soon after delivery as the diagnosis is made has been shown to decrease the need for exchange transfusion. Ongoing hemolysis will still occur until all maternal antibody is gone; therefore, these infants need to be followed carefully over the first 2 months of life for development of anemia severe enough to require transfusion. The role of erythropoietin therapy in treating late anemia is under investigation.

**2. Nonimmune hemolysis (Coombs' test-negative)**—Hereditary spherocytosis is the most common red cell membrane defect, resulting in hemolysis because of decreased red cell deformability. These infants may have hyperbilirubinemia severe enough to require exchange transfusion. Mild to moderate splenomegaly may be present. Diagnosis is suspected by peripheral blood smear and confirmed by red cell osmotic fragility study. A family history of anemia, jaundice, and gallstones may be elicited.

G6PD deficiency is the most common red cell enzyme defect resulting in hemolysis and should be suspected in a male (it is X-linked) of African, Mediterranean, or Asian descent, particularly when the onset of jaundice is later than usual. The importance of this enzyme deficiency in cases of severe neonatal jaundice has likely been underestimated. In most cases, no triggering agent is found, although those infants who develop severe jaundice with G6PD deficiency also are found to have Gilbert syndrome.

**3. Nonhemolytic increased bilirubin production**—Enclosed hemorrhage, such as cephalohematoma, intracranial hemorrhage, or extensive bruising in the skin, can lead to jaundice as the red blood cells are broken down and removed. Polycythemia leads to jaundice by increased red cell mass, with increased numbers of cells reaching senescence daily. Ileus, either paralytic or mechanical, related to a bowel obstruction, leads to hyperbilirubinemia secondary to increased enterohepatic circulation.

## B. DECREASED RATE OF CONJUGATION

**1. UDPGT deficiency [Crigler–Najjar syndrome type I (complete deficiency, autosomal recessive) and type II (partial deficiency, autosomal dominant)]**—These syndromes result from a mutation in the exon or encoding region of the gene that codes for the enzyme UDPGT, resulting in complete absence or nearly complete absence of the enzyme. Both are rare and result in severe unconjugated hyperbilirubinemia, bilirubin encephalopathy, and death without therapy. In type II, the enzyme can be induced with phenobarbital, lowering bilirubin levels 30–80%. There is no cure, although phototherapy and hepatic transplantation prolong survival in type I.

**2. Gilbert syndrome**—This syndrome is a mild autosomal dominant disorder affecting 6% of the population and is characterized by decreased hepatic UDPGT levels, resulting from a genetic variant of polymorphism in the promoter region (a noncoding area that regulates the amount of structurally normal enzyme produced) of the UDPGT gene. Affected individuals have a greater propensity in the presence of other icterogenic factors such as G6PD deficiency, hereditary spherocytosis, or other factors that increase bilirubin production to develop significant hyperbilirubinemia. They may also be more likely to manifest prolonged jaundice.

## C. HYPERBILIRUBINEMIA CAUSED BY UNKNOWN OR MULTIPLE FACTORS

**1. Physiologic jaundice**—The contributing factors to physiologic jaundice include UDPGT inactivity at birth, a relatively high red cell mass even in the nonpolycythemic neonate, and an absence of intestinal flora, with initially slow intestinal motility leading to an active enterohepatic circulation of bilirubin. For jaundice to be physiologic rather than pathologic, the following criteria should be satisfied: (1) clinical jaundice appears after 24 hours of age; (2) total bilirubin rises by less than 5 mg/dL (86 mmol/L) per day; (3) peak bilirubin occurs at 3–5 days of age, with a total bilirubin of no more than 15 mg/dL (258 mmol/L); and (4) clinical jaundice is resolved by 1 week in the full-term infant and by 2 weeks in the preterm infant. Hyperbilirubinemia outside of these parameters—or jaundice that requires treatment—is not physiologic and must be evaluated further (see later discussion).

**2. High altitude**—Infants at 3100 m (10,000 ft) have twice the frequency of bilirubin > 12 mg/dL (206 mmol/L) as infants at 1600 m (5200 ft) and four times that of infants at sea level: 39% versus 16% versus 8%, respectively. Possible mechanisms include increased bilirubin production secondary to increased hematocrit and decreased clearance caused by hypoxemia.

**3. Racial differences**—Asians are more likely than whites or blacks to have a bilirubin level > 12 mg/dL (206 mmol/L): 23% versus 10–13% versus 4%, respectively.

**4. Prematurity**—Premature infants frequently have poor enteral intake, delayed stooling, and increased enterohepatic circulation. Even at 37 weeks' gestation, they are four times more likely than at 40 weeks to have a bilirubin > 13 mg/dL (224 mmol/L).

**5. Breast feeding and jaundice**—Two syndromes of jaundice are associated with breast feeding: breast milk jaundice and breast feeding-associated jaundice ("lack-of-breast-milk jaundice").

**a. Breast milk jaundice**—This uncommon syndrome of prolonged unconjugated hyperbilirubinemia is believed to be caused by a prolonged increased enterohepatic circulation of bilirubin in some breast-fed infants, perhaps related to increased free fatty acids in the milk. Homozygosity for the Gilbert syndrome 7/7 promoter genotype may also be involved. The presence of moderate unconjugated hyperbilirubinemia for 6–8 weeks in a thriving infant without evidence for hemolysis, hypothyroidism, or other disease strongly suggests this diagnosis.

**b. Breast feeding-associated jaundice**—This common entity is also known as "lack-of-breast-milk jaundice." Breast-fed infants have a higher incidence (9%) of unconjugated serum bilirubin levels > 13 mg/dL (224 mmol/L) than formula-fed infants (2%) and are more likely to have bilirubin > 15 mg/dL (258 mmol/L) than formula-fed infants: 2% versus 0.3%. The pathogenesis appears to be decreased enteral intake and increased enterohepatic circulation. No increase in bilirubin production is seen, as measured by carbon monoxide exhalation. Although rarely severe enough to result in bilirubin encephalopathy, nearly 100% of the infants with kernicterus reported to the registry were breast-fed, and in 50% of them breast feeding was the only known risk factor. Jaundice should be considered a possible sign of failure to establish an adequate milk supply and should prompt specific inquiries into this possibility (Table 1–9). If intake is inadequate, the infant should receive supplementa-

***Table 1–9.*** Signs of inadequate breast milk intake.

---

Weight loss of > 8–10% from birth
Fewer than six noticeably wet diapers per day
Fewer than four stools per day
Nursing fewer than eight times per 24 h for at least 10 min
  each feed

---

tion with formula if needed, and the mother should be instructed to nurse more frequently and to pump her breasts with an electric breast pump every 2 hours to enhance milk production. A consultation with a certified lactation specialist should be considered, because many physicians feel inadequately prepared to handle these situations. Because hospital discharge of normal newborns occurs before the milk supply is established, a follow-up visit 2–3 days after discharge is of obvious importance.

These two entities may sometimes overlap in the same infant, because prolonged jaundice is common in breast-fed infants (20–30%), and high bilirubin levels in many of these infants with high initial levels also persist longest.

### D. PROLONGED HYPERBILIRUBINEMIA

Causes of prolonged unconjugated hyperbilirubinemia include hemolytic disease, breast milk jaundice, Crigler–Najjar or Gilbert syndrome, bowel obstruction, and congenital hypothyroidism. Galactosemia generally presents with hepatomegaly in an ill-appearing, often septic infant, and the hyperbilirubinemia is usually mixed.

## Evaluation of Hyperbilirubinemia

Because most newborns are discharged at 24–36 hours of age prior to establishing a good milk supply or showing the extent of their jaundice, a predischarge bilirubin measurement, either transcutaneous or drawn with the newborn genetic screen, may help predict which infants are at risk for severe hyperbilirubinemia. Clinical jaundice appears at a bilirubin level of 5 mg/dL (86 mmol/L) and appears first on the head, progressing down the chest and abdomen as the level increases. By the time jaundice is noted on the distal extremities, the level is likely to be at least 15 mg/dL (258 mmol/L). When checking serum bilirubin levels, the level should be assessed based on the age in hours at which the sample was obtained. Infants with a total serum bilirubin level greater than the 95th percentile for age in hours have a 40% risk of developing subsequent significant hyperbilirubinemia (Figure 1–2). Infants who develop

clinical jaundice on the first day of life or who develop excessive jaundice require evaluation. The minimal evaluation consists of a feeding and elimination history, weight (and comparison with birth weight), examination for any source of excessive heme breakdown, and laboratory evaluation for blood type, Coombs' testing, complete blood count (CBC) with smear, and total bilirubin level. A G6PD test should be considered if the infant is a male of African, Asian, or Mediterranean racial background, particularly if the jaundice presents later than usual. A fractionated bilirubin level should be obtained if the infant appears acutely ill, if jaundice is prolonged, or if the infant has dark urine with light stools.

Because of large interlaboratory variability, serial bilirubin levels should be obtained from a single laboratory whenever possible to make interpretation of serial measurements more accurate.

## Treatment of Hyperbilirubinemia

### A. PROTOPORPHYRINS

Tin and zinc protoporphyrin or mesoporphyrin (Sn-PP, Zn-PP; Sn-MP, Zn-MP) are inhibitors of heme oxygenase, the enzyme that begins the catabolism of heme (iron protoporphyrin). Studies are underway involving a single injection of these substances shortly after birth to prevent the formation of bilirubin. Although early results are promising, these drugs are still experimental in the United States.

### B. PHOTOTHERAPY

Phototherapy is used most commonly, because it is relatively noninvasive and safe. Light at a wavelength absorbed by bilirubin (blue or white spectrum) is used. The unconjugated bilirubin in the skin is converted by such light to a stereoisomer compound that is water-soluble and able to be excreted in the bile without conjugation. A minimum of 10–14 mW/cm$^2$ irradiance is required, and efficacy is dose-dependent. The dose can be raised by increasing the body surface area exposed to the light and by moving the lights closer to the baby. Fiberoptic blankets are effective, but are inadequate alone for full-term infants. The infant's eyes should be shielded from the light to prevent damage to retinal cells. A frequent side effect of phototherapy is diarrhea, which is managed by feeding a non-lactose-containing formula for the duration of the treatment.

Phototherapy is started when the bilirubin level is approximately 3–5 mg/dL (52–86 mmol/L) lower than the exchange level for that infant (eg, at levels of 15–18 mg/dL [258–310 mmol/L] for a full-term infant), depending also on the infant's age. Guidelines for the use of phototherapy in the full-term infant with and without ABO incompatibility are shown in Tables

***Figure 1–2.*** Risk designation of full-term and near-term newborns based on their hour-specific bilirubin values. (Reproduced, with permission, from Bhutani VK et al: Predictive ability of a predischarge hour-specific serum bilirubin test for subsequent significant hyperbilirubinemia in healthy term and near-term newborns. Pediatrics 1999;103:6.)

1–10 and 1–11. Although phototherapy has been shown to decrease the likelihood of exchange transfusion, the long-term benefits of its use in infants with less severe jaundice are unknown.

### C. Exchange Transfusion

Double-volume exchange transfusion (approximately 160–200 mL/kg body weight) remains necessary in some cases of hemolysis resulting from Rh isoimmunization, ABO incompatibility, or hereditary spherocytosis. In addition to decreasing the bilirubin level by approximately 50% acutely, the exchange also removes nearly 80% of the sensitized or abnormal red blood cells and offending antibody so that ongoing hemolysis will be decreased. The procedure is invasive and not without risk. The risk of mortality is 1–5% and is greatest in the smallest, most immature, and otherwise unstable infants, but sudden death during the proce-

***Table 1–10.*** Guidelines for treatment of the full-term infant with ABO blood group incompatibility.

| |
|---|
| Phototherapy if– |
|   Bilirubin ≥ 10 mg/dL at < 12 h |
|   Bilirubin ≥ 14 mg/dL at 12–24 h |
|   Bilirubin ≥ 15 mg/dL at > 24 h |
| Consider IVIG if hemoglobin is ≤ 13 g/dL and despite ≥ 4 h of phototherapy: |
|   Bilirubin ≥ 12 mg/dL at < 12 h |
|   Bilirubin ≥ 16 mg/dL at 12–24 h |
|   Bilirubin ≥ 18 mg/dL at 24–72 h |
| IVIG = intravenous immune globulin. |

**Table 1–11.** Guidelines for use of phototherapy in the full-term infant without hemolysis.

---

Bilirubin ≥ 15 mg/dL, age < 2 d: Evaluation, phototherapy
Bilirubin ≥ 18 mg/dL, age > 2–3 d: Evaluation, phototherapy
Bilirubin ≥ 20 mg/dL: Evaluation, phototherapy; consider interruption of nursing and formula supplementation; have mother use electric breast pump during interruption of breast feeding
Bilirubin ≥ 25 mg/dL: As above, plus consider exchange transfusion

---

dure can occur in any infant. Risk of serious complications such as necrotizing enterocolitis (NEC), infection, electrolyte disturbances, or thrombocytopenia is 12%. Because of the rarity of the procedure and its inherent risk, it should be performed very cautiously, preferably at a referral center.

For the typical exchange transfusion, the umbilical vein is catheterized, and reconstituted whole blood with a hematocrit of approximately 50% is used in aliquots of 8–10 mL per pass. Albumin 1 g/kg can be given first to aid in binding and removal of bilirubin. Hypocalcemia occurs during the procedure because of binding to the citrate-phosphate-dextrose anticoagulant and needs to be corrected periodically. Hypoglycemia is common following the procedure and requires close monitoring. Thrombocytopenia occurs because of the removal of platelets. The entire procedure should take 1–2 hours and should be performed using aseptic technique.

American Academy of Pediatrics Subcommittee on Neonatal Hyperbilirubinemia: Neonatal jaundice and kernicterus. Pediatrics 2001;108:763 [PMID: 11533348].

Davidson L, Thilo E: How to make kernicterus a never event. Neoreviews 2003;4:e308.

Dennery PA et al: Neonatal hyperbilirubinemia. N Engl J Med 2001;344:581 [PMID: 11207355].

Gottstein R, Cooke RWI: Systematic review of intravenous immunoglobulin in hemolytic disease of the newborn. Arch Dis Child Fetal Neonatal Ed 2003;88:F6 [PMID: 12496219].

Gourley GR: Breast feeding, diet, and neonatal hyperbilirubinemia. Neoreviews 2000;1:e25.

Hammerman C, Kaplan M: Recent developments in the management of neonatal hyperbilirubinemia. Neoreviews 2000; 1:e19.

Johnson LH, Bhutani VK: System-based approach to management of neonatal jaundice and prevention of kernicterus. J Pediatr 2002;140:396 [PMID: 12006952].

Kaplan M et al: Bilirubin genetics for the nongeneticist: Hereditary defects of neonatal bilirubin conjugation. Pediatrics 2003;111:886 [PMID: 12671128].

Newman TB et al: Infants with bilirubin levels of 30 mg/dL or more in a large managed care organization. Pediatrics 2003;111:1303 [PMID: 12777545].

Stevenson DK et al: Prediction of hyperbilirubinemia in near-term and term infants. Pediatrics 2001;108:31 [PMID: 11433051].

# HYPOGLYCEMIA

### ESSENTIALS OF DIAGNOSIS & TYPICAL FEATURES

- *Defined as blood glucose < 40–45 mg/dL.*
- *LGA, SGA, preterm, and stressed infants at risk.*
- *May be asymptomatic.*
- *Infants can present with lethargy, poor feeding, irritability, or seizures.*

## General Considerations

Blood glucose concentration in the fetus is approximately 15 mg/dL less than the maternal glucose concentration. Glucose concentration normally decreases in the immediate postnatal period, with concentrations below 40–45 mg/dL being considered indicative of hypoglycemia. By 3 hours, the glucose concentration in normal full-term babies stabilizes between 50 and 80 mg/dL. After the first few hours of life, concentrations below 40–45 mg/dL should be considered abnormal. The two most commonly encountered groups of full-term newborn infants at high risk for neonatal hypoglycemia are IDMs and IUGR infants.

## Infants of Diabetic Mothers

The IDM has abundant glucose stores in the form of glycogen and fat but develops hypoglycemia because of hyperinsulinemia induced by maternal and fetal hyperglycemia. Other tissues also grow abnormally in utero, probably as a consequence of increased flow of nutrients from the maternal circulation. The result is a macrosomic infant who is at increased risk for trauma during delivery. Other problems related to the in utero metabolic environment include a cardiomyopathy (asymmetrical septal hypertrophy), which can present as a murmur with or without cardiac failure and respiratory distress, and, more rarely, microcolon, which presents as low intestinal obstruction. Infants whose mothers have diabetes at conception are also at increased risk for congenital anomalies probably related to first-trimester glucose control. Other neonatal problems include a hypercoagulable state and polycythemia, a combination that predisposes the infant to large venous thromboses (eg, renal vein thrombosis). Finally, these infants are somewhat immature for their gestational age and are at increased risk for hyaline membrane disease, hypocalcemia, and hyperbilirubinemia.

## Intrauterine Growth Restricted Infants

The IUGR infant has reduced glucose stores in the form of glycogen and body fat and therefore is prone to hypoglycemia despite relatively appropriate endocrine adjustments at birth. In addition to hypoglycemia, marked hyperglycemia and a transient diabetes mellitus-like syndrome may occasionally develop, particularly in the very premature SGA infant. These problems can usually be handled by adjusting glucose intake, though insulin is sometimes needed transiently.

## Other Causes of Hypoglycemia

Hypoglycemia occurs with disorders associated with islet cell hyperplasia (Beckwith–Wiedemann syndrome [macroglossia, omphalocele, macrosomia], erythroblastosis fetalis, nesidioblastosis], inborn errors of metabolism [glycogen storage disease, galactosemia], and endocrine disorders [panhypopituitarism, other deficiencies of counterregulatory hormones]). It may also occur as a complication of birth asphyxia, hypoxia, or other stresses, including bacterial and viral sepsis. Premature infants are also at risk for hypoglycemia because of decreased glycogen stores.

## Clinical Findings

The signs of hypoglycemia in the newborn infant are relatively nonspecific and may be subtle: lethargy, poor feeding, irritability, tremulousness, jitteriness, apnea, and seizures. The disorder is most severe and resistant to treatment if due to hyperinsulinemia. Cardiac failure may occur in severe cases, particularly in IDMs with cardiomyopathy. Infants with hyperinsulinemic states can experience the onset of hypoglycemia very early (within the first 30–60 minutes of life).

Blood glucose can be measured by heelstick using a bedside glucometer. All infants at risk should be screened, including IDMs, IUGR infants, premature infants, and any infant with symptoms that could be due to hypoglycemia. All low or borderline values should be confirmed by direct measurement of blood glucose concentration determined in the laboratory. It is important to continue surveillance of glucose concentration until the baby has been on full enteral feedings without intravenous (IV) supplementation for a 24-hour period. Relapse of hypoglycemia thereafter is unlikely.

Infants with hypoglycemia requiring IV glucose infusions for more than 5 days should be evaluated for the less common causes of hypoglycemia. This work-up should include evaluation for inborn errors of metabolism, hyperinsulinemic states, and deficiencies of counterregulatory hormones.

## Treatment

Therapy is based on provision of glucose either enterally or intravenously. Table 1–12 presents suggested treatment guidelines. In hyperinsulinemic states, boluses of glucose should be avoided and a higher glucose infusion rate used. After initial correction with a bolus of $D_{10}W$, 2 mL/kg, glucose infusion should be increased gradually as needed from a starting rate of 6 mg/kg/min. Finally, in both IDMs and IUGR infants, those with high hematocrits and hypoglycemia are most likely to show clinical signs of hypoglycemia. In such infants, both the hypoglycemia and the polycythemia should be treated—with IV glucose infusion and partial exchange transfusion, respectively.

***Table 1–12.*** Hypoglycemia: suggested therapeutic regimens.

| Screening Test[a] | Presence of Symptoms | Action |
|---|---|---|
| 20–45 mg/dL | No symptoms of hypoglycemia | Draw blood glucose;[b] if the infant is alert and vigorous, feed; follow with frequent glucose monitoring. If the baby continues to have blood glucose < 40 mg/dL or is unable to feed, provide intravenous glucose at 6 mg/kg/min ($D_{10}W$ at 3.6 mL/kg/h). |
| < 45 mg/dL | Symptoms of hypoglycemia present | Draw blood glucose;[b] provide bolus of $D_{10}W$ (2 mL/kg) followed by an infusion of 6 mg/kg/min (3.6 mL/kg/h). |
| < 20 mg/dL | With or without symptoms of hypoglycemia | Draw blood glucose;[b] provide bolus of $D_{10}W$ followed by an infusion of 6 mg/kg/min. If intravenous access cannot be obtained immediately, an umbilical vein line should be used. |

[a]Rapid bedside determination.
[b]Laboratory confirmation.

## Prognosis

The prognosis of hypoglycemia is good if therapy is prompt. CNS sequelae are seen in infants with neonatal seizures resulting from hypoglycemia and are more likely in neonates with persistent hyperinsulinemic hypoglycemia.

Cornblath M: A personal view of a bittersweet journey, Neoreviews 2003;4:e2.

Cornblath M et al: Controversies regarding definition of neonatal hypoglycemia: Suggested operational thresholds. Pediatrics 2000;105:1141 [PMID: 10790476].

Cornblath M, Ichord R: Hypoglycemia in the neonate. Semin Perinatol 2000;24:136 [PMID: 10805169].

Cowett RM: Neonatal care of the infant of the diabetic mother. Neoreviews 2002;3:e190.

Menni F et al: Neurologic outcomes of 90 neonates and infants with persistent hyperinsulinemic hypoglycemia. Pediatrics 2001;107:476 [PMID: 11230585].

Sunehag AL, Haymond MW: Glucose extremes in newborn infants. Clin Perinatol 2002;29:245 [PMID: 12168240].

# RESPIRATORY DISTRESS IN THE TERM NEWBORN INFANT

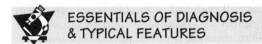

### ESSENTIALS OF DIAGNOSIS & TYPICAL FEATURES

- *Tachypnea, respiratory rate > 60 breaths/min.*
- *Retractions (intercostal, sternal).*
- *Expiratory grunting.*
- *Cyanosis on room air.*

## General Considerations

Respiratory distress is among the most common symptom complexes seen in the newborn infant. It may result from both noncardiopulmonary and cardiopulmonary causes (Table 1–13). Chest radiography, arterial blood gases, and pulse oximetry are useful in assessing both the cause and the severity of the problem. It is important to consider the noncardiopulmonary causes listed in Table 1–13 because the natural tendency is to focus on the heart and lungs. Most of the noncardiopulmonary causes can be ruled out by the history, physical examination, and a few simple laboratory tests. The evaluation of cardiovascular disorders is discussed in a subsequent section.

The most common pulmonary causes of respiratory distress in the full-term infant are transient tachypnea,

***Table 1–13.*** Causes of respiratory distress in the newborn.

| |
| --- |
| Noncardiopulmonary |
|   Hypothermia or hyperthermia |
|   Hypoglycemia |
|   Polycythemia |
|   Metabolic acidosis |
|   Drug intoxications or withdrawal |
|   Insult to the central nervous system |
|     Asphyxia |
|     Hemorrhage |
|   Neuromuscular disease |
|   Phrenic nerve injury |
|   Asphyxiating thoracic dystrophy |
| Cardiovascular |
|   Left-sided outflow tract obstruction |
|     Hypoplastic left heart |
|     Aortic stenosis |
|     Coarctation of the aorta |
|   Cyanotic lesions |
|     Transposition of the great vessels |
|     Total anomalous pulmonary venous return |
|     Tricuspid atresia |
|     Right-sided outflow obstruction |
| Pulmonary |
|   Upper airway obstruction |
|     Choanal atresia |
|     Vocal cord paralysis |
|     Lingual thyroid |
|   Meconium aspiration |
|   Clear fluid aspiration |
|   Transient tachypnea |
|   Pneumonia |
|   Pulmonary hypoplasia |
|   Hyaline membrane disease |
|   Pneumothorax |
|   Pleural effusions |
|   Mass lesions |
|     Lobar emphysema |
|     Cystic adenomatoid malformation |

aspiration syndromes, congenital pneumonia, and air leaks.

### A. TRANSIENT TACHYPNEA (RETAINED FETAL LUNG FLUID)

Respiratory distress is typically present from birth, usually associated with a mild to moderate oxygen requirement (25–50% $O_2$). The infant may be full-term or near-term, nonasphyxiated, and born following a short labor or cesarean section without labor. Chest radiograph shows perihilar streaking and fluid in interlobar fissures. Resolution usually occurs within 12–24 hours.

## B. ASPIRATION SYNDROMES

The infant is typically full-term or near-term, frequently with some fetal distress prior to delivery or depression at delivery. Blood or meconium is usually present in the amniotic fluid, but occasionally the fluid is clear. Respiratory distress is present from birth, in many cases manifested by a barrel chest appearance and coarse breath sounds. An increasing $O_2$ need from pneumonitis may require intubation and ventilation. Chest radiograph shows coarse irregular infiltrates, hyperexpansion, and, in the worst cases, lobar consolidation. In some cases, secondary surfactant deficiency can ensue, with progression to a diffuse homogeneous infiltrate pattern.

When the amniotic fluid contains meconium or blood, suctioning of the infant's mouth and nose as the head is delivered and before delivery of the chest is recommended to prevent aspiration of these secretions with the onset of breathing. If the infant is not vigorous at birth, suctioning of the trachea under direct vision is recommended, especially before commencing resuscitation with positive-pressure ventilation. Although these procedures are recommended, they will not prevent all cases of meconium or blood aspiration. Aspiration often occurs in utero as the stressed infant gasps. Babies with aspirations are at risk of air leak (pneumothorax) because of uneven aeration with segmental overdistention and are at risk for persistent pulmonary hypertension (see section on Cardiac Problems). Standard treatment includes ventilatory support, antibiotics, and pressor support of systemic blood pressure.

## C. CONGENITAL PNEUMONIA

Infants may be of any gestational age, with or without a maternal history of prolonged rupture of the membranes, chorioamnionitis, or maternal antibiotic administration. Onset of respiratory distress may be at birth or may be delayed for several hours. Chest radiograph may resemble that of retained lung fluid or hyaline membrane disease; rarely, there may be a lobar infiltrate.

The lungs are the most common site of infection in the neonate. Most commonly, infections ascend from the genital tract before or during labor, with the vaginal or rectal flora the most likely infectious agents (group B streptococci, *Escherichia coli, Klebsiella*). Shock, poor perfusion, absolute neutropenia (< 2000/mL), and an elevated C reactive protein provide corroborating evidence for pneumonia. Gram stain of tracheal aspirate may be helpful. Because no signs or laboratory findings can confirm the presence or absence of pneumonia with certainty, all infants with respiratory distress should receive a blood culture and broad-spectrum antibiotic therapy (ampicillin 100 mg/kg in two divided doses and gentamicin 4 mg/kg q24h or 2.5 mg/kg q12h) until the diagnosis of a bacterial infection can be ruled out.

## D. SPONTANEOUS PNEUMOTHORAX

Respiratory distress (primarily tachypnea) is present from birth, typically not severe, and requires mild to moderate supplemental $O_2$. Breath sounds may be decreased on the affected side; heart tones may be shifted toward the opposite side and may be distant. Chest radiograph will show pneumothorax or pneumomediastinum.

This entity occurs in 1% of all deliveries. The risk is increased by manipulations such as positive-pressure ventilation in the delivery room. Treatment usually consists of supplemental $O_2$ and watchful waiting. Breathing 100% $O_2$ for a few hours may accelerate reabsorption of the extrapulmonary gas by creating a diffusion gradient for nitrogen across the surface of the lung (nitrogen washout technique). This is effective only if the infant was breathing room air or $O_2$ at low concentration at the time of the pneumothorax. Drainage by needle thoracentesis or tube thoracostomy is occasionally required. A small increased risk of renal abnormalities is associated with spontaneous pneumothorax; therefore, a careful physical examination of the kidneys and observation of urine output are indicated. If pulmonary hypoplasia with pneumothorax is suspected, renal ultrasound would also be indicated.

## E. OTHER PULMONARY CAUSES

The other pulmonary causes of respiratory distress are fairly rare. Bilateral choanal atresia should be suspected if there is no air movement when the infant breathes through the nose. These infants present in the delivery room with good color and heart rate while crying but become cyanotic and bradycardiac when they quiet down and resume normal nasal breathing. Other causes of upper airway obstruction are usually characterized by some degree of stridor or poor air movement despite good respiratory effort. Pleural effusions can be suspected in hydropic infants (eg, those with erythroblastosis fetalis or nonimmune hydrops). Space-occupying lesions cause a shift of the mediastinum and asymmetrical breath sounds and would be apparent on chest radiograph.

## Treatment

Whatever the cause, the cornerstone of treatment of neonatal respiratory distress is provision of adequate supplemental oxygen to maintain a PaO₂ of 60–70 mm

Hg and a saturation by pulse oximetry ($SpO_2$) of 92–96%. $PaO_2$ levels less than 50 mm Hg are associated with pulmonary vasoconstriction, which can exacerbate hypoxemia, whereas those greater than 100 mm Hg may increase the risk of oxygen toxicity without additional benefit. Oxygen should be warmed, humidified, and delivered through an air blender. Concentration should be measured with a calibrated oxygen analyzer. An umbilical or peripheral arterial line should be considered in any infant requiring more than 45% $FiO_2$ by 4–6 hours of life to allow frequent blood gas determinations. Noninvasive monitoring with a pulse oximeter should be used.

Other supportive treatment includes IV provision of glucose and water. Unless infection can be unequivocally ruled out, blood cultures should be obtained and broad-spectrum antibiotics started. Volume expansion (normal saline) can be given in infusions of 10 mL/kg over 30 minutes for low blood pressure, poor perfusion, and metabolic acidosis. Sodium bicarbonate (1–2 mEq/kg) is indicated for treatment of documented metabolic acidosis that has not responded to oxygen, ventilation, and volume. Specific work-up should be pursued as indicated by the history and physical findings. In most cases, a chest radiographic study, blood gas measurements, CBC, and blood glucose allow a diagnosis.

Intubation and ventilation should be undertaken for signs of respiratory failure ($PaO_2$ < 60 mm Hg in 60–80% $FiO_2$, $PaCO_2$ > 60 mm Hg, or repeated apnea). Peak pressures should be adequate to produce chest wall expansion and audible breath sounds (usually 18–24 cm $H_2O$). Positive end-expiratory pressure (4–6 cm $H_2O$) should also be used. Ventilation rates of 20–50 breaths/min are usually required. The goal is to maintain a $PaO_2$ of 60–70 mm Hg and a $PaCO_2$ of 45–55 mm Hg.

## Prognosis

Most of the respiratory conditions affecting the full-term infant are acute and resolve in the first several days. Meconium aspiration syndrome and congenital pneumonia are associated with significant long-term pulmonary morbidity (chronic lung disease) and mortality (approximately 10–20%). Mortality rates in these disorders have been reduced by use of high-frequency ventilation, inhaled nitric oxide to treat pulmonary hypertension, and extracorporeal membrane oxygenation (ECMO).

Ghidini A, Spong CY: Severe meconium aspiration syndrome is not caused by aspiration of meconium. Am J Obstet Gynecol 2001;185:931 [PMID: 11641681].

# HEART MURMURS (SEE ALSO SECTION ON CARDIAC PROBLEMS)

Heart murmurs are common in the first days of life and do not usually signify structural heart problems. If a murmur is present at birth, however, it should be considered a valvular problem until proved otherwise because the common benign transitional murmurs (eg, patent ductus arteriosus) are not audible until minutes to hours after birth.

If an infant is pink, well-perfused, and in no respiratory distress and has palpable and symmetrical pulses (right brachial pulse no stronger than the femoral pulse), the murmur is most likely transitional. Transitional murmurs are soft (grade 1–3/6), heard at the left upper to midsternal border, and generally loudest during the first 24 hours. If the murmur persists beyond 24 hours, blood pressure in the right arm and a leg should be determined. If there is a difference of more than 15 mm Hg (arm > leg) or if the pulses in the lower extremities are difficult to appreciate, cardiology consultation should be arranged to evaluate for coarctation of the aorta. If there is no difference, the infant can be discharged home with follow-up in 2–3 days for auscultation and evaluation for signs of congestive failure. If signs of failure or cyanosis are present, the infant should be referred for evaluation without delay. If the murmur persists without these signs, the infant can be referred for elective evaluation at age 2–4 weeks. Some centers now recommend routine pulse oximetry screening in the nursery to identify infants with congenital heart disease, with a saturation < 95% at sea level triggering an echocardiogram. Further studies will need to be performed to document the accuracy, specificity, and cost-effectiveness of this technique.

Koppel RI et al: Effectiveness of pulse oximetry screening for congenital heart disease in asymptomatic newborns. Pediatrics 2003;111:451 [PMID: 12612220].

Reich JD et al: The use of pulse oximetry to detect congenital heart disease. J Pediatr 2003;142:268 [PMID: 12640374].

# BIRTH TRAUMA

Most birth trauma is associated with difficult delivery, particularly with a large infant, abnormal position, or fetal distress requiring rapid extraction. The most common injuries are soft tissue bruising, fractures (clavicle, humerus, or femur), and cervical plexus palsies, although skull fractures, intracranial hemorrhage (primarily subdural and subarachnoid), and cervical spinal cord injuries can also occur.

Fractures are often diagnosed by the obstetrician, who may feel and hear a snap during delivery. Clavicular fractures may cause decreased spontaneous movement of the arm, with tenderness and crepitus over the area. Humeral or femoral fractures may cause tenderness and swelling over the shaft with a diaphyseal fracture, with limited spontaneous extremity motion in all cases. Epiphyseal fractures are harder to diagnose radiographically owing to the cartilaginous nature of the epiphysis. After 8–10 days, callus appears and is visible on radiographs. Treatment in all cases is gentle handling, with immobilization for 8–10 days: the humerus against the chest with elbow flexed; the femur with a posterior splint from below the knee to the buttock.

Brachial plexus injuries may result from traction as the head is pulled away from the shoulder during delivery. Injury to the C5-6 roots is most common and results in Erb–Duchenne paralysis. The arm is limp, adducted and internally rotated, extended and pronated at the elbow, and flexed at the wrist (so-called waiter's tip posture). Grasp is present. If the lower nerve roots (C8-T1) are involved, the hand is flaccid (Klumpke palsy). Isolated involvement of these roots is rare. If the entire plexus is injured, the arm and hand are flaccid, with an associated sensory deficit.

Early treatment for brachial plexus injury is conservative, because function usually returns over several weeks. Referral should be made to a physical therapist so that the parents can be instructed on range-of-motion exercises and splinting and for further evaluation if needed. Return of function begins in the deltoid and biceps, with recovery by 3 months in most cases.

Spinal cord injury can occur at birth, especially in difficult breech extractions with hyperextension of the neck, or in midforceps rotations when the body fails to turn with the head. Infants are flaccid, quadriplegic, and without respiratory efforts at birth, although facial movements are preserved. The long-term outlook for such infants is grim.

Facial nerve palsy is sometimes associated with forceps use but more often results from chronic in utero pressure of the baby's head against the mother's sacrum. The infant has asymmetrical mouth movements and eye closure with poor movement on the affected side. Most cases resolve spontaneously within a few days to 3 weeks.

Subgaleal hemorrhage into the large potential space under the scalp (Figure 1–3) is associated with difficult vaginal deliveries and repeated attempts at vacuum extraction. It can lead to hypovolemic shock and death from ongoing blood loss and severe coagulopathy triggered by both consumption of clotting factors and release of thromboplastin from accompanying brain injury. This is an emergency requiring rapid replacement of blood and clotting factors.

Gardella C et al: The effect of sequential use of vacuum and forceps for assisted vaginal delivery on neonatal and maternal outcomes. Am J Obstet Gynecol 2001;185:896 [PMID: 11641674].

Rosenberg AA: Traumatic birth injuries. Neoreviews 2003;4:e270.

Towner D et al: Effect of mode of delivery in nulliparous women on neonatal intracranial injury. N Engl J Med 1999;341: 1709 [PMID: 10580069].

# INFANTS OF MOTHERS WHO ABUSE DRUGS

The problem of newborn infants born to mothers who abuse drugs is increasing in all communities. The drugs most commonly abused are tobacco, alcohol, marijuana, and cocaine. Because these mothers may abuse many drugs and give an unreliable history of drug usage, it may be difficult to pinpoint which drug is causing the morbidity seen in a newborn infant. Early hospital discharge makes discovery of these infants based on physical findings and abnormal behavior much more difficult.

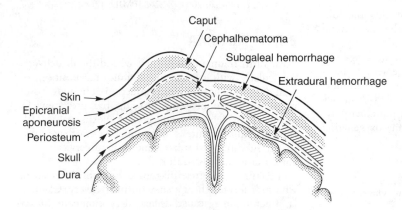

*Figure 1–3.* Sites of extracranial bleeding in the newborn. (Adapted and reproduced, with permission, from Pape KE, Wigglesworth JS: Haemorrhage Ischemia and the Perinatal Brain. JB Lippincott, 1979.)

## 1. Cocaine

Cocaine is currently the most commonly abused hard drug, identified in up to 20–40% of infants on urban delivery services by anonymous screening of urine or meconium; moreover, cocaine is often used in association with other drugs. The obstetric effects include maternal hypertension, decreased uterine blood flow, fetal hypoxemia, and uterine contractions. The rates of stillbirth, placental abruption, and preterm delivery are increased two- to fourfold over rates for nonusers, and IUGR is increased two- to fourfold over that for nonusers. In high-risk populations (no prenatal care, placental abruptions, and preterm labor), urine toxicology screens should be performed in mothers and infants. Analysis of meconium enhances diagnosis by indicating cumulative drug use prior to delivery.

As with other illegal drugs, cocaine may have long-term neurobehavioral effects, but multiple drug use and environmental factors preclude assigning specific effects to cocaine with certainty. The risk of SIDS is increased three to seven times over the risk in nonusers (0.5–1% of exposed infants), but may be lessened by supine infant positioning.

## 2. Opioids

### ESSENTIALS OF DIAGNOSIS & TYPICAL FEATURES

- Irritability, hyperactivity, incessant hunger and salivation.
- Vomiting, diarrhea, excessive weight loss.
- Tremors, seizures.
- Nasal stuffiness, sneezing.
- Often IUGR.

### Clinical Findings

The withdrawal signs in infants born to mothers who are addicted to heroin or who have been in maintenance methadone programs are similar. The clinical findings in infants born to methadone-maintained mothers may actually be more severe and prolonged than those seen with heroin. Clinical manifestations begin usually within 1–2 days. The clinical picture is typical enough to suggest a diagnosis even if a maternal history of drug abuse has not been obtained, although onset may not occur prior to discharge at 24 hours. Confirmation should be attempted with urine toxicol-ogy, but results will be negative unless the last drug dose was within a few days before delivery. Meconium can also be tested for illicit drugs and is more likely to be positive because the substances accumulate throughout pregnancy.

### Treatment

Careful observation of the infant is a requirement. If opioid abuse or withdrawal is suspected, the baby is not a candidate for early discharge. Supportive treatment includes swaddling the infant and providing a quiet, dimly lighted environment. In general, specific treatment should be avoided unless the infant has severe symptoms or excessive weight loss. No single drug has been uniformly effective, and the first choice varies among nurseries. The drugs that have been used include phenobarbital at an initial loading dose of 15–20 mg/kg IM, followed by a maintenance dose of 5 mg/kg/d in two divided doses, usually given orally. Opioids, diazepam, and clonidine have also been used, although the present authors prefer phenobarbital for irritability alone because of its safety and predictability. If diarrhea and weight loss are prominent findings, or if adequate control of symptoms has not been achieved, tincture of opium (25-fold dilution to 0.4 mg/mL morphine equivalent; 0.1 mL/kg qh4 to start) titrated to improve symptoms or methadone 0.05–0.1 mg/kg q6h will be more beneficial than phenobarbital alone. Treatment can be tapered over several days to a week. Both handling and procedures in the nursery should be kept to a minimum. It is also important to review maternal tests for syphilis, HIV, hepatitis B, and gonorrhea as all are common in women who use cocaine or opiates.

### Prognosis

These infants demonstrate long-term neurobehavioral handicaps. However, it is difficult to distinguish the effects of in utero drug exposure from those of environmental influences during upbringing. Infants of opioid abusers have a four- to fivefold increased risk of SIDS.

## 3. Alcohol

The legal substances alcohol and tobacco have much greater effects on perinatal outcome than any illicit substances. Alcohol is the only recreational drug of abuse that is clearly teratogenic and is the most common preventable cause of mental retardation. The effects of alcohol on the fetus and the newborn are roughly proportionate to the degree of ethanol abuse, but there is no established safe dose. Fetal growth and development are adversely affected, and infants can experience with-

***Table 1–14.*** Features observed in fetal alcohol syndrome in the newborn.

| |
|---|
| Craniofacial |
|    Short palpebral fissures |
|    Short, upturned nose |
|    Flat midface |
|    Thin vermillion of upper lip |
|    Flattened philtrum |
| Growth |
|    Prenatal and postnatal growth deficiency (SGA, failure to thrive) |
| Central nervous system |
|    Microcephaly |
|    Partial or complete agnesis of the corpus callosum |
|    Optic nerve hypoplasia |
|    Hypotonia, poor feeding |

drawal similar to that associated with maternal opioid abuse. Features observed are listed in Table 1–14. Clinical features of fetal alcohol syndrome (FAS) are often not obvious in the newborn period.

Children with full-blown FAS demonstrate postnatal growth deficiency and mild to moderate mental retardation. Those with lesser effects are at increased risk for attention-deficit/hyperactivity disorder and subtle developmental delays.

## 4. Tobacco Smoking

Smoking has been shown to have a negative effect on the growth rate of the fetus. The more the mother smokes, the greater the degree of IUGR. There is a twofold increase in low birth weight even in light smokers (< 10 cigarettes/day). More recently, smoking during pregnancy has been associated with mild neurodevelopmental handicaps. The possible effects of multiple drug abuse apply to this category as well, and the potential interaction of multiple factors on fetal growth and development must be considered.

## 5. Toluene Embryopathy

Solvent abuse (paint, lacquer, or glue sniffing) is relatively common. The active organic solvent in these agents is toluene. Features attributable to in utero toluene exposure include prematurity, IUGR, microcephaly, craniofacial abnormalities similar to those associated with in utero alcohol exposure (see Table 1–14), nail hypoplasia, and renal anomalies. Long-term effects include postnatal growth deficiency and developmental delay.

## 6. Marijuana

Marijuana is the most frequently used illegal drug. It does not appear to be teratogenic, and although a mild abstinence-type syndrome has been described, infants exposed to marijuana in utero rarely require treatment. Some long-term neurodevelopmental problems, particularly disordered sleep patterns, have been noted.

## 7. Other Drugs

Drugs and their effects on the newborn should be considered in two categories. In the first are drugs to which the fetus is exposed because of the mother's exposure. In many cases these are drugs prescribed for therapy of maternal conditions. The human placenta is relatively permeable, particularly to lipophilic solutes. Whenever possible, maternal drug therapy should be postponed until after the first trimester. Drugs with potential fetal toxicity include antineoplastics, antithyroid agents, benzodiazepines, warfarin, lithium, angiotensin-converting enzyme inhibitors (eg, captopril, enalapril), and immunosuppressants.

In the second category are drugs the infant acquires from the mother during breast feeding. Most drugs taken by the mother at this time achieve some concentrations in breast milk, although they usually do not present a problem to the infant. If the drug is one that could have adverse effects on the baby, timing breast feeding to coincide with trough concentrations in the mother may be useful. The AAP (see second reference in the following list) has reviewed drugs contraindicated in the breast-feeding mother.

American Academy of Pediatrics Committee on Drugs. Neonatal drug withdrawal. Pediatrics 1998;101:1079 [PMID: 9614425].

American Academy of Pediatrics Committee on Drugs: The transfer of drugs and other chemicals into human milk. Pediatrics 2001;108:776 [PMID: 11533352].

American Academy of Pediatrics Committee on Drugs: Use of psychoactive medication during pregnancy and possible effects on the fetus and newborn. Pediatrics 2000;105:880 [PMID: 10742343].

American Academy of Pediatrics Committee on Substance Abuse and Committee on Children with Disabilities: Fetal alcohol syndrome and alcohol-related neurodevelopmental disorders. Pediatrics 2000;106:358 [PMID: 10920168].

Boyle RJ: Effects of certain prenatal drugs on the fetus and newborn. Pediatr Rev 2002;23:17 [PMID: 11773589].

Coyle MG et al: Diluted tincture of opium (DTO) and phenobarbital versus DTO alone for neonatal opiate withdrawal in term infants. J Pediatr 2002;140:561 [PMID: 12032522].

Frank DA et al: Growth, development, and behavior in early childhood following prenatal cocaine exposure. A systematic review. JAMA 2001;285:1613 [PMID: 11268270].

Gleason CA: Fetal alcohol exposure: Effects on the developing brain. Neoreviews 2001;2:e231.

Holmes LB et al: The teratogenicity of anticonvulsant drugs. N Engl J Med 2001;344:1132 [PMID: 11297704].

Ito S: Drug therapy for breast-feeding women. N Engl J Med 2000; 343:118 [PMID: 10891521].

Johnson K et al: Treatment of neonatal abstinence syndrome. Arch Dis Child Fetal Neonatal Ed 2003;88:F2 [PMID: 12496218].

Singer LT et al: Cognitive and motor outcomes of cocaine-exposed infants. JAMA 2002;287:1852 [PMID: 11960537].

Sokol RH et al: Fetal alcohol spectrum disorder. JAMA 2003;290:2996 [PMID: 14665662].

Thackray HM, Tifft C: Fetal alcohol syndrome. Pediatr Rev 2001; 22:47 [PMID: 11157101].

Ventura SJ et al: Trends and variations in smoking in pregnancy and low birth weight: Evidence from the birth certificate, 1999–2000. Pediatrics 2003;111:1176 [PMID: 12728134].

## MULTIPLE BIRTHS

Twinning has historically occurred as a demographic variation in one of 80 pregnancies (1.25%). The incidence of twinning and higher-order multiple births in the United States has been increasing as a consequence of the increased use of in vitro fertilization and other assisted reproductive technologies. In 1999, twins occurred in 1/43 live births in the United States, with the multiple births accounting for 3% of all births.

A clear distinction should be made between dizygotic (fraternal) and monozygotic (identical) twins. Race, maternal parity, and maternal age affect the incidence only of dizygotic twinning. Drugs that induce ovulation, such as clomiphene citrate and gonadotropins, increase the incidence of dizygotic or polyzygotic twinning quite strikingly. Monozygotic twinning can be viewed as a birth defect; the incidence of malformations is also increased in identical twins and may affect only one of the twins. If a defect is found in one, the other should be examined carefully for lesser degrees of the same defect.

Examination of the placenta can help establish the type of twinning: Two amnionic membranes and two chorionic membranes are found in all cases of dizygotic twins and in one third of monozygotic twins; a single chorionic membrane always indicates monozygotic twins.

### Complications of Multiple Births

#### A. INTRAUTERINE GROWTH RESTRICTION

There is some degree of IUGR in most multiple pregnancies after 34 weeks. If prenatal care is good, however, the growth restriction is rarely significant. There are two exceptions: The first is the monochorial twin pregnancy in which an arteriovenous shunt occurs from one twin's circulation to that of the other (twin–twin transfusion syndrome). The infant on the venous side becomes plethoric and considerably larger than the smaller anemic twin. Morbidity and mortality rates are considerable in twin–twin transfusion syndrome. Discordance in size—birth weights that are significantly different—can also occur when separate placentas are present. One placenta develops poorly, presumably because of a poor implantation site. In this instance, no fetal exchange of blood takes place but the growth rates of the two infants are significantly different.

#### B. PRETERM DELIVERY

Gestation length tends to be inversely related to the number of fetuses. The prematurity rate is 5–10 times that of singletons, with 50% of twins and 90% of triplets born before 37 weeks. The prematurity rate tends to increase the mortality or morbidity rates occurring in twin pregnancies.

#### C. OBSTETRIC COMPLICATIONS

Polyhydramnios, pregnancy-induced hypertension, premature rupture of membranes, abnormal fetal presentations, and prolapsed umbilical cord occur more frequently in women with multiple fetuses. In general, most of the complications can be avoided or minimized by good obstetric management. Multiple pregnancy should always be identified prenatally with ultrasound examinations; doing so allows the obstetrician and pediatrician or neonatologist to plan management jointly. The neonatal complications are usually related to prematurity. Prolongation of pregnancy, therefore, leads to a significant reduction in neonatal morbidity.

Follow-up studies of twin pregnancies have yielded conflicting results. In general, the studies do not suggest that twinning has a significant effect on later development, especially if prematurity is excluded as a separate risk factor.

Banek CS et al: Long-term neurodevelopmental outcome after intrauterine treatment for severe twin–twin transfusion syndrome. Am J Obstet Gynecol 2003;188:876 [PMID: 1272079].

Blondel B, Kaminski M: Trends in the occurrence, determinants and consequences of multiple births. Semin Perinatol 2002;26:239 [PMID: 12211614].

Mari G et al: Perinatal morbidity and mortality rates in severe twin–twin transfusion syndrome: Results of the International Amnioreduction Registry. Am J Obstet Gynecol 2001;185:708 [PMID: 11568802].

Reynolds MA et al: Trends in multiple births conceived using assisted reproductive technology, United States, 1997–2000. Pediatrics 2003;111:1159 [PMID: 12728130].

# ■ NEONATAL INTENSIVE CARE

## PERINATAL RESUSCITATION

Perinatal resuscitation consists of the steps taken by the obstetrician to support the infant during labor and delivery as well as the traditional resuscitative steps taken by the pediatrician after delivery. Intrapartum support includes maintaining maternal blood pressure with volume expanders if needed, maternal oxygen therapy, positioning the mother to improve placental perfusion, readjusting oxytocin infusions or administering a tocolytic if appropriate, minimizing trauma to the infant (particularly important in infants of very low birth weight), suctioning the nasopharynx upon delivery of the head if meconium is present in the amniotic fluid, obtaining all necessary cord blood samples, and completing an examination of the placenta.

Steps taken by the pediatrician or neonatologist focus on temperature support, initiation and maintenance of effective ventilation, maintenance of perfusion and hydration, and glucose regulation.

A number of conditions associated with pregnancy, labor, and delivery place the infant at risk for birth asphyxia: (1) maternal diseases such as diabetes, pregnancy-induced hypertension, heart and renal disease, and collagen–vascular disease; (2) fetal conditions such as prematurity, multiple births, growth retardation, and fetal anomalies; and (3) labor and delivery conditions, including fetal distress with or without meconium in the amniotic fluid, and administration of anesthetics and opioid analgesics.

## Physiology of Birth Asphyxia

Birth asphyxia can be the result of several mechanisms: (1) acute interruption of umbilical blood flow (eg, prolapsed cord with cord compression), (2) premature placental separation, (3) maternal hypotension or hypoxia, (4) chronic placental insufficiency, and (5) failure to execute newborn resuscitation properly.

The neonatal response to asphyxia follows a predictable pattern that has been demonstrated in a variety of species (Figure 1–4). The initial response to hypoxia is an increase in frequency of respiration and a rise in heart rate and blood pressure. Respirations then cease (primary apnea) as heart rate and blood pressure begin to fall. This initial period of apnea lasts 30–60 seconds. Gasping respirations (3–6/min) then begin, while heart rate and blood pressure gradually decline. Secondary or terminal apnea then ensues, with further decline in heart rate and blood pressure. The longer the duration of secondary apnea, the greater the risk for hypoxic

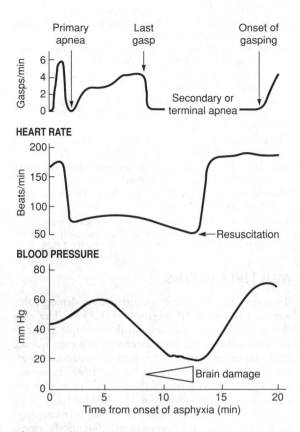

**Figure 1–4.** Schematic depiction of changes in rhesus monkeys during asphyxia and on resuscitation by positive-pressure ventilation. (Adapted and reproduced, with permission, from Dawes GS: *Fetal and Neonatal Physiology.* Year Book, 1968.)

organ injury. A cardinal feature of the defense against hypoxia is the underperfusion of certain tissue beds (eg, skin, muscle, kidneys, GI tract), which allows the perfusion of core organs (ie, heart, brain, adrenals) to be maintained.

The response to resuscitation also follows a predictable pattern. During the period of primary apnea, almost any physical stimulus causes the baby to initiate respirations. Infants in secondary apnea require positive-pressure ventilation. The first sign of recovery is an increase in heart rate, followed by an increase in blood pressure with improved perfusion. The time required for rhythmic, spontaneous respirations to occur is related to the duration of the secondary apnea. As a rough rule, for each 1 minute past the last gasp, 2 minutes of positive-pressure breathing is required before gasping begins, and 4 minutes is required to reach rhythmic breathing. These times can vary depending on the degree and duration of intrauterine asphyxia. Not until some time later do spinal and corneal reflexes return. Muscle tone gradually improves over the course of several hours.

## Delivery Room Management

When asphyxia is anticipated, a resuscitation team of at least two persons should be present: one to manage the airway and one to monitor the heartbeat and provide assistance. The necessary equipment and drugs are listed in Table 1–15.

***Table 1–15.*** Equipment for neonatal resuscitation.

| Clinical Needs | Equipment |
|---|---|
| Thermoregulation | Radiant heat source with platform, mattress covered with warm sterile blankets, servocontrol heating, temperature probe |
| Airway management | **Suction:** Bulb suction, mechanical suction with sterile catheters (6F, 8F, 10F), meconium aspirator<br>**Ventilation:** Manual infant resuscitation bag connected to manometer or with a pressure-release valve capable of delivering 100% oxygen, appropriate masks for term and preterm infants, oral airways, stethoscope<br>**Intubation:** Neonatal laryngoscope with No. 0 and No. 1 blades; endotracheal tubes (2.5, 3.0, 3.5 mm outer diameter with stylet): extra bulbs and batteries for laryngoscope; scissors, adhesive tape, gloves, end tidal $CO_2$ detection device |
| Gastric decompression | Nasogastric tube: 8F with 20-mL syringe |
| Administration of drugs and volume replacement | Sterile umbilical catheterization tray, umbilical catheters (3.5F and 5F), volume expanders, normal saline, drug box[a] with appropriate neonatal vials and dilutions, sterile syringes, needles, and alcohol sponges |
| Transport | Warmed transport isolette with oxygen source |

[a]Epinephrine 1:10,000; naloxone hydrochloride 1 mg/mL; sodium bicarbonate 4.2% (5 mEq/10 mL); 10% dextrose.
Modified, with permission, from Rosenberg AA: Neonatal adaptation. In: Gabbe SG et al (eds). *Obstetrics: Normal and Problem Pregnancies.* Churchill Livingstone, 1996.

### A. STEPS IN THE RESUSCITATION (SEE FIGURE 1–5.)

1. Dry the infant well, and place him or her under the radiant heat source. Do not allow the infant to become hyperthermic.

2. Gently suction the mouth, then the nose.

3. Quickly assess the infant's condition. The best criteria are the infant's respiratory effort (apneic, gasping, regular) and heart rate (> 100 or < 100 beats/min). A depressed heart rate—indicative of hypoxic myocardial depression—is the single most reliable indicator of the need for resuscitation.

4. Infants who are breathing and have heart rates over 100 beats/min usually require no further intervention. Infants with heart rates less than 100 beats/min and apnea or irregular respiratory efforts should be stimulated vigorously. The baby's back should be rubbed with a towel while oxygen is provided near the baby's face.

5. If the baby fails to respond to tactile stimulation within a few seconds, begin bag and mask ventilation, using a soft mask that seals well around the mouth and nose. For the initial inflations, pressures of 30–40 cm $H_2O$ may be necessary to overcome surface-active forces in the lungs. Adequacy of ventilation is assessed by observing expansion of the infant's chest accompanied by an improvement in heart rate, perfusion, and color. After the first few breaths, lower the peak pressure to 15–20 cm $H_2O$. The baby's chest movement should resemble that of an easy breath rather than a deep sigh. The rate of bagging should be 40–60 breaths/min.

6. Most neonates can be resuscitated effectively with a bag and mask. If the infant does not respond to bag and mask ventilation, try to reposition the head (slight extension), reapply the mask to achieve a good seal, consider suctioning the mouth and the oropharynx, and try ventilating with the mouth open. If the infant does not respond within 30 seconds, intubation is appropriate.

Failure to respond to intubation and ventilation can result from (1) mechanical difficulties (Table 1–16), (2) profound asphyxia with myocardial depression, and (3) inadequate circulating blood volume.

Quickly rule out the mechanical causes listed in Table 1–16. Check to ensure the endotracheal tube passes through the vocal cords. A $CO_2$ detector placed between the endotracheal tube and the bag can be very helpful as a rapid confirmation of tube position in the airway. Occlusion of the tube

APPROXIMATE
TIME

Birth

30 SECONDS

- Clear of meconium?
- Breathing or crying?
- Good muscle tone?
- Color pink?
- Term gestation?

*No*

- Provide warmth
- Position; clear airway*
  (as necessary)
- Dry, stimulate, reposition
- Give O₂ (as necessary)

- Evaluate respirations,
  heart rate (HR), and color

*Apnea     or HR < 100*

30 SECONDS

- Provide positive-pressure ventilation*

*HR < 60        HR > 60*

30 SECONDS

- Provide positive-pressure ventilation*
- Administer chest compressions

*HR < 60*

- Administer
  epinephrine*   *HR < 60*

*Endotracheal intubation may
be considered at several steps

Recheck effectiveness of
- Ventilation
- Chest compressions
- Endotracheal intubation
- Epinephrine delivery
Consider possibility of
- Hypovolemia
- Severe metabolic acidosis

*HR < 60 or persistent cyanosis
or failure to ventilate*

Consider:
- Depressed respiratory
  neuromuscular drive
- Airway malfunctions
- Lung problems, such as
  – Pneumothorax
  – Diaphragmatic hernia
- Congenital heart disease

**Figure 1–5.** Delivery room management. (Reproduced, with permission, from American Heart Association, *American Academy of Pediatrics: Neonatal Resuscitation Textbook,* 4th ed, 2000.)

**Table 1–16.** Mechanical causes of failed resuscitation.

| Cause | Examples |
|---|---|
| Equipment failure | Malfunctioning bag, oxygen not connected or running |
| Endotracheal tube malposition | Esophagus, right main stem bronchus |
| Occluded endotracheal tube | |
| Insufficient inflation pressure to expand lungs | |
| Space-occupying lesions in the thorax | Pneumothorax, pleural effusions, diaphragmatic hernia |
| Pulmonary hypoplasia | Extreme prematurity, oligohydramnios |

Reproduced, with permission, from Rosenberg AA: Neonatal adaptation. In: Gabbe SG et al (eds): *Obstetrics: Normal and Problem Pregnancies.* Churchill Livingstone, 1996.

should be suspected when there is resistance to bagging and no chest wall movement. Very few neonates (approximately 0.1%) require either cardiac massage or drugs during resuscitation. Almost all newborns respond to ventilation with 100% oxygen if done effectively.

7. If mechanical causes are ruled out and the heart rate remains below 60 beats/min after intubation and positive-pressure ventilation for 30 seconds, cardiac compression should be initiated. Simultaneous delivery of chest compressions and positive-pressure ventilation is likely to decrease the efficiency of ventilation. Therefore, chest compressions should be interspersed with ventilation at a 3:1 ratio (90 compressions and 30 breaths/min).

8. If drugs are needed (rarely), the drug and dose of choice is epinephrine 1:10,000 solution, 0.1–0.3 mL/kg given via the endotracheal tube or through an umbilical venous line. Sodium bicarbonate, 1–2 mEq/kg of the neonatal dilution (0.5 mEq/mL), can be used in prolonged resuscitation efforts in which the response to other measures is poor. If volume loss is suspected, 10 mL/kg of a volume expander (normal saline) should be administered through an umbilical vein line.

**B. CONTINUED RESUSCITATIVE MEASURES**

The appropriateness of continued resuscitative efforts should be reevaluated in an infant who fails to respond to the previously described efforts. In current practice, resuscitative efforts are made even in apparent stillbirths (ie, infants whose Apgar score at 1 minute is 0–1). Modern resuscitative techniques have led to an increasing survival rate for these infants, with 60% of survivors showing normal development. It is clear from a number of studies that initial resuscitation of these infants should proceed; however, subsequent continued support must depend on response to resuscitation. All studies emphasize that if the Apgar score is not improving markedly over the first 10–15 minutes of life, the mortality rate and the incidence of severe developmental handicaps among survivors are high.

### C. SPECIAL CONSIDERATIONS

**1. Preterm infants–**

**a.** Minimizing heat loss improves survival, so prewarmed towels should be available. The environmental temperature of the delivery suite should be raised to > 25°C (especially for infants weighing < 1500 g).

**b.** In the extremely low birth weight infant (< 1000 g), proceed quickly to intubation.

**c.** Volume expanders and sodium bicarbonate (if needed) should be infused more slowly to minimize rapid swings in blood pressure and serum osmolality.

**2. Narcotic depression—**In the case of opioid administration to the mother during labor, perform the resuscitation as described earlier. When the baby is stable with good heart rate, color, and perfusion but still has poor respiratory effort, a trial of naloxone (0.1 mg/kg IM, SQ, IV, or IT) is indicated. Naloxone should not be administered in place of positive-pressure ventilation. Naloxone should not be used in the infant of an opioid-addicted mother because it will precipitate withdrawal.

**3. Meconium-stained amniotic fluid—**

**a.** The obstetrician carefully suctions the oropharynx and the nasopharynx after delivery of the head with a suction apparatus attached to wall suction.

**b.** The delivery is then completed, and the baby is given to the resuscitation team.

**c.** If the baby is active and breathing, requiring no resuscitation, and if obstetric suctioning has been performed, the airway need not be inspected—only further suctioning of the mouth and nasopharynx is required.

**d.** The airway of any depressed infant requiring ventilation must be checked and cleared (by passage of a tube below the vocal cords) before positive-pressure ventilation is instituted. Special adapters are available for use with regulated wall suction to allow suction to be applied directly to the endotracheal tube.

**4. Universal precautions—**In the delivery room, universal precautions should always be observed.

## Treatment of the Asphyxiated Infant

Asphyxia is manifested by multiorgan dysfunction, seizures and hypoxic-ischemic encephalopathy, and metabolic acidemia. The infant who has experienced a significant episode of perinatal hypoxia and ischemia is at risk for dysfunction of multiple end organs (Table 1–17). The organ of greatest concern is the brain.

The clinical features of hypoxic-ischemic encephalopathy progress over time: birth to 12 hours, decreased level of consciousness, poor tone, decreased spontaneous movement, periodic breathing or apnea, and possible seizures; 12–24 hours, more seizures, apneic spells, jitteriness, and weakness; after 24 hours, decreased level of consciousness, further respiratory abnormalities (progressive apnea), onset of brainstem signs (oculomotor and pupillary disturbances), poor feeding, and hypotonia.

The severity of clinical signs and the length of time the signs persist correlate with the severity of the insult. Other evaluations helpful in assessing severity in the full-term infant include electroencephalogram (EEG), computed tomography (CT) scan, and evoked responses. Magnetic resonance imaging (MRI), particularly diffusion-weighted imaging, is becoming useful, especially in the early evaluation of the infant with perinatal asphyxia.

Markedly abnormal EEGs with voltage suppression and slowing evolving into a burst-suppression pattern are associated with severe clinical symptomatology. A CT scan early in the course may demonstrate diffuse hypodensity and loss of gray/white matter tissue differentiation, whereas later scans may demonstrate brain atrophy and focal ischemic lesions. Visual and so-

**Table 1–17.** Signs and symptoms caused by asphyxia.

---

Hypoxic-ischemic encephalopathy, seizures
Respiratory distress due to aspiration or secondary surfactant deficiency, pulmonary hemorrhage
Persistent pulmonary hypertension
Hypotension due to myocardial dysfunction
Transient tricuspid valve insufficiency
Anuria or oliguria due to acute tubular necrosis
Feeding intolerance; necrotizing enterocolitis
Elevated aminotransferases due to liver injury
Adrenal insufficiency due to hemorrhage
Disseminated intravascular coagulation
Hypocalcemia
Hypoglycemia
Persistent metabolic acidemia
Hyperkalemia

---

matosensory evoked potentials provide information about function. In most instances, it is not necessary to use all of these tests, but some are obtained to confirm an ominous prognosis. Management is directed at supportive care and treatment of specific abnormalities. Fluids should be restricted initially to 60–80 mL/kg/d; oxygenation should be maintained (with mechanical ventilation if necessary); blood pressure should be supported with judicious volume expansion (if hypovolemic) and pressors; and glucose should be in the normal range of 40–100 mg/dL. Hypocalcemia, coagulation abnormalities, and metabolic acidemia should be corrected and seizures treated with IV phenobarbital (20 mg/kg as loading dose, with total initial 24-hour dosing up to 40 mg/kg). Phenobarbital in large doses (40 mg/kg IV 1–6 hours after the event) given as a neuroprotective therapy is associated with improvement in neurologic outcome with minimal adverse effects on blood pressure, respirations, or blood gases. Other anticonvulsants should be reserved for refractory seizures. The role of hypothermia (in particular, selective head cooling), free oxygen radical scavengers, excitatory amino acid antagonists, and calcium channel blockers in minimizing cerebral injury after asphyxia is under active investigation.

## Birth Asphyxia: Long-Term Outcome

Fetal heart rate tracings, cord pH, and 1-minute Apgar scores are imprecise predictors of long-term outcome. Apgar scores of 0–3 at 5 minutes in full-term infants result in an 18–35% risk of death in the first year of life and an 8% risk of cerebral palsy among survivors. The risks of mortality and morbidity increase with more prolonged depression of the Apgar score. The single best predictor of outcome is the severity of clinical hypoxic-ischemic encephalopathy (severe symptomatology including coma carries a 75% chance of death and a 100% rate of neurologic sequelae among survivors). The major sequela of hypoxic-ischemic encephalopathy is cerebral palsy with or without associated mental retardation and epilepsy. Other prognostic features include elevated nucleated red blood cell counts, prolonged seizures refractory to therapy, markedly abnormal EEGs, and CT or MRI scans with evidence of major ischemic injury. Other clinical features required to support perinatal hypoxia as the cause of cerebral palsy include the presence of fetal distress prior to birth, a low cord pH of < 7.00, evidence of other end organ dysfunction, and absence of a congenital brain malformation.

Allan WC: The clinical spectrum and prediction of outcome in hypoxic-ischemic encephalopathy. Neoreviews 2002;3:e108.

American Heart Association and American Academy of Pediatrics: Textbook of Neonatal Resuscitation, 4th ed. American Heart Association/American Academy of Pediatrics, 2000.

Battlin MR et al: Treatment of term infants with head cooling and mild hypothermia (35.0 degrees C and 34.5 degrees C) after perinatal asphyxia. Pediatrics 2003;111:244 [PMID: 12563046].

Croen LA et al: Congenital abnormalities among children with cerebral palsy: More evidence for prenatal antecedents. J Pediatr 2001;138:804 [PMID: 11391320].

Grow J, Barks JDE: Pathogenesis of hypoxic-ischemic cerebral injury in the term infant: Current concepts. Clin Perinatol 2002;29:585 [PMID:12516737].

Gunn AJ, Bennet L: Cerebral hypothermia in the management of hypoxic–ischemic encephalopathy. Neoreviews 2002;3:e116.

Hamkins GDV, Spear M: Defining the pathogenesis and pathophysiology of neonatal encephalopathy and cerebral palsy. Obstet Gynecol 2003;102:628 [PMID: 12962954].

Huppi PS: Advances in postnatal neuroimaging: Relevance to pathogenesis and treatment of brain injury. Clin Perinatol 2002;29:827 [PMID: 12516748].

Mosler D et al: The association of Apgar score with subsequent death and cerebral palsy: A population-based study in term infants. J Pediatr 2001;138:798 [PMID: 11391319].

Niermeyer S: Evidence based guidelines for neonatal resuscitation. Neoreviews 2001;2:e38.

Shankaran S: The postnatal management of the asphyxiated term infant. Clin Perinatol 2002;29:675 [PMID: 12516741].

Willoughby RE Jr, Nelson KB: Chorioamnionitis and brain injury. Clin Perinatol 2002;29:603 [PMID: 12516738].

Wiswell TE et al: Delivery room management of the apparently vigorous meconium-stained neonate: Results of the multicenter, international collaborative trial. Pediatrics 2000;105:1 [PMID: 10617696].

## THE PRETERM INFANT

Premature infants account for the majority of high-risk newborns. The preterm infant faces a variety of physiologic handicaps:

1. The ability to suck, swallow, and breathe in a coordinated fashion is not achieved until 34–36 weeks' gestation. Therefore, enteral feedings must be provided by gavage. Furthermore, preterm infants frequently have gastroesophageal reflux and an immature gag reflex, which increases the risk of aspiration of feedings.

2. Decreased ability to maintain body temperature.

3. Pulmonary immaturity-surfactant deficiency, often with structural immaturity in infants of less than 26 weeks' gestation. Their condition is complicated by the combination of noncompliant lungs and an extremely compliant chest wall.

4. Immature control of respiration, leading to apnea and bradycardia.

5. Persistent patency of the ductus arteriosus, leading to further compromise of pulmonary gas exchange because of overperfusion of the lungs.

6. Immature cerebral vasculature, predisposing the infant to subependymal or intraventricular hemorrhage and periventricular leukomalacia.

7. Impaired substrate absorption by the GI tract, compromising nutritional management.

8. Immature renal function (including both filtration and tubular functions), complicating fluid and electrolyte management.

9. Increased susceptibility to infection.

10. Immaturity of metabolic processes, predisposing to hypoglycemia and hypocalcemia.

## Delivery Room Care

See section on Perinatal Resuscitation.

## Care in the Nursery

### A. THERMOREGULATION

Maintaining a stable body temperature is a function of heat production and conservation balanced against heat loss. Heat production in response to cold stress can occur through voluntary muscle activity, involuntary muscle activity (shivering), and thermogenesis not caused by shivering. Newborns produce heat mainly through the last of these three mechanisms. This metabolic heat production depends on the quantity of brown fat present, which is very limited in the preterm infant. Heat loss to the environment can occur through the following mechanisms: (1) radiation—transfer of heat from a warmer to a cooler object not in contact; (2) convection—transfer of heat to the surrounding gaseous environment, influenced by air movement and temperature; (3) conduction—transfer of heat to a cooler object in contact; and (4) evaporation—cooling secondary to water loss through the skin. Heat loss in the preterm newborn is accelerated because of a high ratio of surface area to body mass, reduced insulation of subcutaneous tissue, and water loss through the immature skin.

The thermal environment of the preterm neonate must be regulated carefully. The infant can be kept warm in an isolette, in which the air is heated and convective heat loss is minimized. Alternatively, the infant can be kept warm on an open bed with a radiant heat source. Although evaporative and convective heat losses are greater when the radiant warmer is used, this system allows easy access to a critically ill neonate. Ideally, the infant should be kept in a neutral thermal environment (Figure 1–6). The neutral thermal environment allows

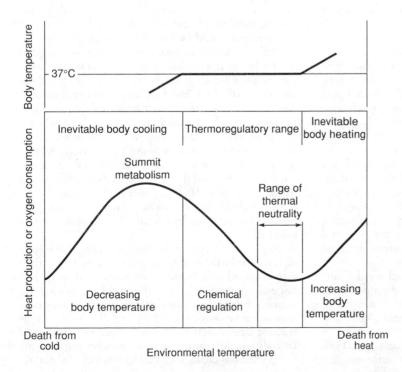

***Figure 1–6.*** Effect of environmental temperature on oxygen consumption and body temperature. (Adapted and reproduced, with permission, from Klaus MH, Fanaroff AA, Martin RJ: The physical environment. In: Klaus MH, Fanaroff AA [editors]: *Care of the High-Risk Neonate,* 5th ed. WB Saunders, 2001.)

the infant to maintain a stable core body temperature with a minimum of metabolic heat production through oxygen consumption. The neutral thermal environment for a given infant depends on size, gestational age, and postnatal age. The neutral thermal environment (for either isolette or radiant warmer care) can be obtained by maintaining an abdominal skin temperature of 36.5°C. Generally, when infants reach 1700–1800 g, they can maintain temperature while bundled in an open crib.

## B. MONITORING THE HIGH-RISK INFANT

Care of the high-risk preterm infant requires sophisticated monitoring techniques. At a minimum, equipment to monitor heart rate, respirations, and blood pressure should be available. Oxygen saturation can be assessed continuously using pulse oximetry. This determination can be correlated with arterial oxygen tension ($PaO_2$) as needed. Transcutaneous $PO_2$ and $PCO_2$ can also be used to assess oxygenation and ventilation. Finally, arterial blood gases, electrolytes, glucose, calcium, bilirubin, and other chemistries must be measured on small volumes of blood. Early in the care of a sick preterm infant, the most efficient way to sample blood for tests as well as to provide fluids and monitor blood pressure is through an umbilical arterial line. Once the infant is stable and the need for frequent blood samples is reduced (usually 4–7 days), the umbilical line should be removed. All indwelling lines are associated with morbidity from thrombosis or embolism, infection, and bleeding.

## C. FLUID AND ELECTROLYTE THERAPY

Fluid requirements in preterm infants are a function of (1) insensible losses (skin and respiratory tract), (2) urine output, (3) stool output (< 5% of total), and (4) others, such as nasogastric losses. In most circumstances, the fluid requirement is determined largely by insensible losses plus urine losses. The major contribution to insensible water loss is evaporative skin loss. The rate of water loss is a function of gestational age (body weight), environment (losses are greater under a radiant warmer than in an isolette), and the use of phototherapy. Respiratory losses are minimal when infants are breathing humidified oxygen. The renal contribution to water requirement is influenced by the decreased ability of the preterm neonate to concentrate the urine and conserve water.

Electrolyte requirements are minimal for the first 24–48 hours until there is excretion in the urine. Basal requirements are as follows: sodium, 3 mEq/kg/d; potassium, 2 mEq/kg/d; chloride, 2–3 mEq/kg/d; and bicarbonate, 2–3 mEq/kg/d.

In the infant born before 30 weeks' gestation, sodium and bicarbonate losses in the urine are frequently elevated, increasing the infant's requirement for these electrolytes.

Initial fluid management after birth is determined by the infant's size. Infants weighing more than 1500 g should start at 80–100 mL/kg/d of 10% dextrose in water ($D_{10}W$), whereas those weighing less should start at 100–120 mL/kg/d of either $D_{10}W$ or 5% dextrose in water ($D_5W$) (infants < 800 g and < 26 weeks' gestation often become hyperglycemic on $D_{10}W$). The most critical issue in fluid management is monitoring. Measurements of body weight, urine output, fluid and electrolyte intake, serum and urine electrolytes, and glucose allow fairly precise determinations of the infant's water, glucose, and electrolyte needs. Parenteral nutrition should be started early and continued until an adequate enteral intake is achieved.

## D. NUTRITIONAL SUPPORT

The average caloric requirement for the growing premature infant is 120 kcal/kg/d. Expected weight gain for the adequately nourished preterm infant is 10–30 g/d. Infants initially require IV glucose infusions to maintain blood glucose concentration in the range of 60–100 mg/dL. Infusions of 5–7 mg/kg/min (approximately 80–100 mL/kg/d of a $D_{10}W$ solution) are usually needed. Nutritional support in the very low birth weight infant should be started as soon as possible after birth, with parenteral alimentation solutions given either peripherally or centrally via an umbilical vein line or percutaneous catheter (Table 1–18). Small-volume trophic feeds with breast milk or 20 kcal/oz of premature formula should be started by gavage at ≤ 10% of the infant's nutritional needs as soon as possible. After several days of trophic feeds the infant can be slowly advanced to full caloric needs over 5–7 days. Even extremely small feed volumes can enhance intestinal readiness to ultimately accept larger feeding volumes. Intermittent bolus feedings are preferred because these appear to stimulate the release of gut-related hormones and may accelerate maturation of the GI tract. A more rapid advancement schedule is used for infants weighing over 1500 g and the slowest schedule in the infant weighing less than 1000 g. *Note:* In the extremely low birth weight infant (< 1000 g) or the postsurgical neonate, continuous-drip feeds are sometimes better tolerated.

In general, long-term nutritional support for infants of very low birth weight consists either of breast milk supplemented to increase protein, caloric density, and mineral content or of infant formulas modified for preterm infants. In all of these formulas, protein concentrations (approximately 2 g/dL) and caloric concentrations (approximately 24 kcal/oz) are relatively high. In addition, premature formulas contain some of the fat as medium-chain triglycerides—which do not re-

***Table 1–18.*** Use of parenteral alimentation solutions.

| | Volume (mL/kg/d) | Carbohydrate (g/dL) | Protein (g/kg) | Lipid (g/kg) | Calories (kcal/kg) |
|---|---|---|---|---|---|
| **Peripheral: Short-term (7–10 days)** | | | | | |
| Starting solution | 100–150 | $D_{10}W$ | 2 | 1 | 46–64 |
| Target solution | 150 | $D_{12.5}W$ | 3–3.5 | 3 | 102 |
| **Central: Long-term (>10 days)** | | | | | |
| Starting solution | 100–150 | $D_{10}W$ | 2 | 1 | 46–64 |
| Target solution | 130 | $D_{20}W$ | 3–3.5 | 3 | 123 |

***Notes:***
1. Protein calories should be no more than 10% of total calories.
2. Advance dextrose in central hyperalimentation as tolerated by 2.5% per day as long as blood glucose remains normal.
3. Advance lipids by 1.0 g/kg/d as long as triglycerides are normal. Use 20% concentration.
4. Total water should be 100–150 mL/kg/d, depending on the child's fluid tolerance.

***Monitoring:***
1. Blood glucose two or three times a day when changing dextrose concentration, then daily.
2. Electrolytes daily, then twice a week when the child is receiving a stable solution.
3. Every other week blood urea nitrogen and serum creatinine; total protein and serum albumin; serum calcium, phosphate, magnesium, direct bilirubin, and CBC with platelet counts.
4. Triglyceride level after 24 h at 2 g/kg/d and 24 h at 3 g/kg/d; then every other week.

quire bile for emulsification—as an energy source. Increased amounts of calcium and phosphorus are provided to enhance bone mineralization. In addition, as with formula for full-term infants, formulas for premature infants are now being enriched with long-chain polyunsaturated fatty acids in the hope of enhancing brain and retinal development. The infant should be advanced gradually to feedings of higher caloric density after a substantial volume (100–120 mL/kg/d) of either breast milk or formula (20 kcal/oz) is tolerated. Success of feedings is assessed by passage of feeds out of the stomach, abdominal examination free of distention, and normal stool pattern.

When the preterm infant approaches term, the nutritional source for the bottle-fed infant can be changed to a transitional formula (22 kcal/oz) until age 6–9 months. Iron supplementation (2–4 mg/kg/d) is recommended for premature infants, beginning at about age 2 months. This can be provided by iron-supplemented formulas. In some infants, iron supplementation may be indicated earlier. In particular, infants treated with erythropoietin (epoetin alfa) for prevention or treatment of anemia of prematurity require a higher dosage of 4–8 mg/kg/d.

Anderson JW et al: Breast-feeding and cognitive development: A meta-analysis. Am J Clin Nutr 1999;70:525 [PMID: 10500022].

Berseth CL et al: Prolonging small feeding volumes early in life decreases the incidence of necrotizing enterocolitis in very low birth weight infants. Pediatrics 2003;111:529 [PMID: 12612232].

Carver JD et al: Growth of preterm infants fed nutrient-enriched or term formula after hospital discharge. Pediatrics 2001;107:683 [PMID: 11335744].

Embleton NE et al: Postnatal malnutrition and growth retardation: An inevitable consequence of current recommendations in preterm infants. Pediatrics 2001;107:270 [PMID: 11158457].

Innis SM et al: Docosahexaenoic acid and arachidonic acid enhance growth with no adverse effects in preterm infants fed formula. J Pediatr 2002;140:547 [PMID: 12032520].

Thureen PJ, Hay WW: Intravenous nutrition and postnatal growth of the micropremie. Clin Perinatol 2000;27:197 [PMID: 10690572].

Williams AF: Early enteral feeding of the preterm infant. Arch Dis Child Fetal and Neonatal Ed 2000;83:F219 [PMID: 11040173].

Yeung MY: Nutritionally regulated hormonal factors in prolonged postnatal growth retardation and its associated adverse neurodevelopmental outcome in extreme prematurity. Biol Neonate 2003;84:1 [PMID: 12890931].

Zeigler EE et al: Aggressive nutrition of the very low birth weight infant. Clin Perinatol 2002;29:225 [PMID: 12168239].

# 1. Apnea in the Preterm Infant

> **ESSENTIALS OF DIAGNOSIS**
> **& TYPICAL FEATURES**
>
> • Respiratory pause of sufficient duration to result in cyanosis or bradycardia.
> • Most common in infants born at < 34 weeks' gestation with onset at < 2 weeks of age.
> • Methylxanthines (eg, caffeine) provide effective treatment for apnea of prematurity.

## General Considerations

In preterm infants, recurrent apneic episodes are a common problem. Apnea is defined as a respiratory pause lasting more than 20 seconds—or any pause accompanied by cyanosis and bradycardia. Shorter respiratory pauses associated with cyanosis or bradycardia also qualify as significant apnea but must be differentiated from periodic breathing, which is common in full-term as well as preterm infants. Periodic breathing is defined as regularly recurring ventilatory cycles interrupted by short pauses not associated with bradycardia or color change. Although apnea in premature infants is often not associated with a predisposing factor, a variety of processes may precipitate apnea (Table 1–19). These

**Table 1–19.** Causes of apnea in the preterm infant.

Temperature instability—both cold and heat stress
Response to passage of a feeding tube
Gastroesophageal reflux
Hypoxemia
    Pulmonary parenchymal disease
    Patent ductus arteriosus
    ?Anemia
Infection
    Sepsis (viral or bacterial)
    Necrotizing enterocolitis
Metabolic causes
    Hypoglycemia
    Hyponatremia
Intracranial hemorrhage
Posthemorrhagic hydrocephalus
Seizures
Drugs (eg, morphine)
Apnea of prematurity

processes should at least be considered before a diagnosis of apnea of prematurity can be established.

Apnea of prematurity is the most frequent cause of apnea. Most apnea of prematurity is mixed apnea characterized by a centrally (brainstem) mediated respiratory pause preceded or followed by airway obstruction. Less common is pure central or pure obstructive apnea. Apnea of prematurity is the result of immaturity of both the central respiratory regulatory centers and protective mechanisms that aid in maintaining airway patency.

## Clinical Findings

Onset, typically during the first 2 weeks of life, is gradual, with the frequency of spells increasing over time. Pathologic apnea can be suspected in an infant with a sudden onset of frequent or very severe apneic spells. Apnea presenting from birth or on the first day of life is unusual but can occur in the preterm infant who does not require mechanical ventilation for respiratory distress syndrome. In the full-term or near-term infant, this presentation can suggest neuromuscular abnormalities of an acute (asphyxia, birth trauma, or infection) or chronic (eg, congenital hypotonia, structural CNS lesion) nature.

The work-up depends on the clinical presentation. All infants—regardless of the severity and frequency of apnea—require a minimum screening evaluation, including a general assessment of well-being (eg, tolerance of feedings, stable temperature, normal physical examination), a check of the association of spells with feeding, measurement of $PaO_2$ or $SaO_2$, blood glucose, hematocrit, and a review of the drug history. Infants with severe apnea of sudden onset may require a more extensive evaluation, including a work-up for infection. Other specific tests are dictated by relevant signs, for example, evaluation for necrotizing enterocolitis in an infant with apnea and abdominal distention or feeding intolerance.

## Treatment

The physician should first address any underlying cause. If the apnea is due simply to prematurity, treatment is dictated by the frequency and severity of apneic spells. Apneic spells frequent enough to interfere with other aspects of care (eg, feeding), or severe enough to necessitate bag and mask ventilation to relieve cyanosis and bradycardia, require treatment. First-line therapy is with methylxanthines. Caffeine citrate (20 mg/kg as loading dose and then 5–10 mg/kg/d) is the drug of choice because of once-daily dosing, wider therapeutic index, and fewer side effects than theophylline. Side effects of methylxanthines include tachycardia, feeding intolerance, and (with overdosing) seizures. The dose used should be the smallest dose necessary to decrease the frequency of apnea and eliminate severe spells. Desired drug levels are usually in the range of 10–20 mg/mL for caffeine. Nasal CPAP (continuous positive airway pressure), by treating the obstructive component of apnea, can be effective treatment for some infants. Intubation and ventilation can eliminate symptomatic apneic spells but carry the risks associated with long-term endotracheal intubation.

## Prognosis

In the majority of premature infants, apneic and bradycardiac spells cease by 34–37 weeks postconception. Spells that require intervention cease prior to self-resolved episodes. In infants born at less than 28 weeks' gestation, episodes may continue past term postconceptual age. Whether to provide home monitoring or outpatient methylxanthine therapy for such infants is controversial. Apneic and bradycardiac episodes in the nursery are not predictors of later SIDS. However, home monitoring in infants still experiencing self-resolving apnea and bradycardia at the time of hospital discharge may be indicated in some cases. The incidence of SIDS is slightly increased in preterm infants. Research in full-term infants has shown an increased incidence of SIDS in infants who sleep in the prone position. Whether this can be extrapolated to the preterm infant (in particular those with gastroesophageal reflux or persistent respiratory symptoms) is unclear. When possible, a supine sleeping position or one that is slightly to the right side seems prudent unless contraindicated by reflux or respiratory symptoms.

## 2. Hyaline Membrane Disease

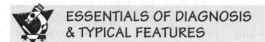

### ESSENTIALS OF DIAGNOSIS & TYPICAL FEATURES

- *Tachypnea, cyanosis, and expiratory grunting.*
- *Poor air movement despite increased work of breathing.*
- *Chest radiograph showing hypoexpansion and air bronchograms.*

## General Considerations

The most common cause of respiratory distress in the preterm infant is hyaline membrane disease. The incidence increases from 5% of infants born at 35–36 weeks' gestation to more than 50% of infants born at 26–28 weeks' gestation. This condition is caused by a deficiency of surfactant. Surfactant decreases surface tension in the alveolus during expiration, allowing the alveolus to remain partly expanded and in that way maintaining a functional residual capacity. The absence of surfactant results in poor lung compliance and atelectasis. The infant must expend a great deal of effort to expand the lungs with each breath, and respiratory failure ensues (Figure 1–7).

## Clinical Findings

Infants with hyaline membrane disease demonstrate all the clinical signs of respiratory distress. On auscultation, air movement is diminished despite vigorous respiratory effort. Chest radiograph demonstrates diffuse bilateral atelectasis, causing a ground-glass appearance. Major airways are highlighted by the atelectatic air sacs, creating air bronchograms. In the unintubated child, doming of the diaphragm and underexpansion occur.

## Treatment

Supplemental oxygen, use of nasal CPAP, early intubation for surfactant administration and ventilation, and placement of umbilical artery and vein lines are the initial interventions required. A ventilator that can deliver breaths synchronized with the infant's respiratory efforts (synchronized intermittent mandatory ventilation) should be used if available. High-frequency ventilators

**Figure 1–7.** Pressure-volume relationships for the inflation and deflation of surfactant-deficient and surfactant-treated preterm rabbit lungs. (Reproduced, with permission, from Jobe AH: The developmental biology of the lung. In: Fanaroff AA, Martin RJ [editors]: *Neonatal-Perinatal Medicine: Diseases of the Fetus and Infant,* 6th ed. Mosby, 1997.)

are also available for rescue of infants doing poorly on conventional ventilation or who have air leak problems.

Four exogenous surfactants (colfosceril palmitate [Exosurf Neonatal], beractant [Survanta], calf lung surfactant extract [Infasurf]), and poractant a (Curosurf) are approved in the United States by the Food and Drug Administration for use in infants with hyaline membrane disease. Surfactant replacement therapy, used both in the delivery room as prophylaxis and with established hyaline membrane disease as rescue, decreases the mortality rate in preterm infants and decreases air leak complications of the disease. During the acute course, ventilator settings and oxygen requirements are significantly less in surfactant-treated infants than in control subjects. The dose of the bovine-derived Survanta is 4 mL/kg, the calf-derived Infasurf is 3 mL/kg, and the porcine-derived Curosurf is 1.25–2.5 mL/kg, given intratracheally. When the first dose is given in the delivery room to prevent hyaline membrane disease the usual dosing schedule is a total of two or three doses given 6–12 hours apart as long as the infant remains ventilated on over 30–40% inspired oxygen concentration. Rescue surfactant is given as two to four doses 6–12 hours apart. The first dose is administered as soon as possible after birth, preferably before 2–4 hours of age. As the disease process evolves, proteins that inhibit surfactant function leak into the air spaces, making surfactant replacement less effective. The second dose should be administered to infants who continue to require ventilation and more than 30–40% inspired oxygen concentration. A prophylactic strategy offers some advantage in those infants born at 26 weeks' gestation or less. For infants over 26 weeks' gestation, early rescue therapy (as soon as a diagnosis of surfactant deficiency can be made) is the strategy of choice. In stable infants, a trial of nasal CPAP at 5–6 cm H$_2$O pressure can be attempted prior to intubation and surfactant administration. For those who do ultimately require intubation, extubation to nasal CPAP should be done as early as possible to minimize lung injury and evolution of chronic lung disease. Antenatal administration of corticosteroids to the mother is an important strategy used by obstetricians to accelerate lung maturation. Infants whose mothers were given corticosteroids more than 24 hours prior to preterm birth have less respiratory distress syndrome and a lower mortality rate. Antenatal corticosteroids and exogenous surfactant administration after birth appear to have a synergistic effect on outcome.

## 3. Chronic Lung Disease in the Premature Infant

### ESSENTIALS OF DIAGNOSIS & TYPICAL FEATURES

- *Oxygen requirement, respiratory symptoms, and abnormal chest radiograph at age 1 month.*
- *Incidence greatest in infants of the lowest gestational ages.*

### General Considerations

Chronic lung disease in the premature infant, defined as respiratory symptoms, oxygen requirement, and chest radiograph abnormalities at age 1 month, occurs in about 20% of infants ventilated for surfactant deficiency. The incidence is higher at lower gestational ages. The development of chronic lung disease is a function of lung immaturity at birth and exposure to high oxygen concentrations and ventilator volutrauma. The use of surfactant replacement therapy or early nasal CPAP has, in general, diminished the severity of the chronic lung disease. The mortality rate from this complication is now very low, but significant morbidity still exists secondary to reactive airway symptoms, hospital readmissions during the first 2 years of life for intercurrent respiratory infection, and systemic hypertension.

### Treatment

The mainstay of therapy for chronic lung disease has been dexamethasone, 0.3–0.5 mg/kg/d, used to decrease lung inflammation. Recently, however, more attention has been focused on the detrimental effects of dexamethasone therapy on long-term neurodevelopment. Attempts are being made to avoid this intervention unless the infant is on very high concentrations of supplemental oxygen and ventilator support with little response to other therapies such as diuretics (furosemide [Lasix] 1–2 mg/kg/d), inhaled $\beta_2$-adrenergic bronchodilators, and inhaled corticosteroids. Inhaled steroids such as beclomethasone, fluticasone, or budesonide are unproven treatments, but may be helpful without the risk of systemic side effects. If it is necessary to use dexamethasone, a dose of 0.2 mg/kg/d for no more than 3 days is recommended. After hospital discharge, some of these infants will continue to require oxygen at home. This can be monitored by pulse oximetry with a target SaO$_2$ of 94–96%.

American Academy of Pediatrics Committee on Fetus and Newborn, Canadian Paediatric Society: Postnatal corticosteroids to treat or prevent chronic lung disease in preterm infants. Pediatrics 2002;109;330 [PMID: 11826218].

American Academy of Pediatrics Committee on Fetus and Newborn: Apnea, sudden infant death syndrome, and home monitoring. Pediatrics 2003;111:914 [PMID: 12671135].

Baird TM et al: Clinical association, treatment, and outcome of apnea of prematurity. Neoreviews 2002;3:e66.

Bancalari E: Epidemiology and risk factors for the "new" bronchopulmonary dysplasia. Neoreviews 2000;1:e2.

Cole CH, Fiascone JM: Strategies for prevention of neonatal chronic lung disease. Semin Perinatol 2000;24:445 [PMID: 11153905].

Durand M et al: A randomized trial of moderately early low-dose dexamethasone therapy in very low birth weight infants: Dynamic pulmonary mechanics, oxygenation, and ventilation. Pediatrics 2002;109:962 [PMID: 11826205].

Eichenwald EC et al: Apnea frequently persists beyond term gestation in infants delivered at 24–28 weeks. Pediatrics 1997; 100:354 [PMID: 9282705].

Herting E et al: Surfactant treatment of neonates with respiratory failure and group B streptococcal infection. Pediatrics 2000; 106:957 [PMID:11061760].

Jobe AH, Bancalari E: Bronchopulmonary dysplasia. Am J Respir Crit Care Med 2001;163:1723 [PMID: 11401896].

Kattwinkel J et al: High- versus low-threshold surfactant replacement for neonatal respiratory distress syndrome. Pediatrics 2000;106:282 [PMID: 10920152].

Kotecha S, Allen J: Oxygen therapy for infants with chronic lung disease. Arch Dis Child Fetal Neonatal Ed 2002;87:F11 [PMID: 12091281].

Martin RJ et al: Pathophysiologic mechanisms underlying apnea of prematurity. Neoreviews 2002;3:e59.

Merrill JD, Ballard RA: Clinical use of antenatal corticosteroids: Benefits and risks. Neoreviews 2000;1:e91.

Murphy BP et al: Impaired cerebral cortical gray matter growth after treatment with dexamethasone for neonatal chronic lung disease. Pediatrics 2001;107:217 [PMID: 11158449].

Narendran V et al: Early bubble CPAP and outcomes in ELBW preterm infants. J Perinatol 2003;23:195 [PMID: 12732855].

Peter CS et al: Gastroesophageal reflux and apnea of prematurity: No temporal relationship. Pediatrics 2002;109:8 [PMID: 11773535].

Ramanathan R et al: Cardiorespiratory events recorded on home monitors: Comparison of healthy infants with those at increased risk for SIDS. JAMA 2001;285:2199 [PMID: 11325321].

Suresh GK, Soll RF: Current surfactant use in premature infants. Clin Perinatol 2001;28:671 [PMID: 11570160].

Tauman R, Sivan Y: Duration of home monitoring for infants discharged with apnea of prematurity. Biol Neonate 2000; 78:168 [PMID: 11044764].

Vaucher Y: Bronchopulmonary dysplasia: An enduring challenge. Pediatr Rev 2002;23:349 [PMID: 12359869].

# 4. Patent Ductus Arteriosus

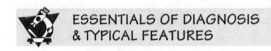

## ESSENTIALS OF DIAGNOSIS & TYPICAL FEATURES

- *Hyperdynamic precordium.*
- *Widened pulse pressure.*
- *Hypotension.*
- *Presence of a systolic heart murmur in many cases.*

## General Considerations

Clinically significant patent ductus arteriosus usually presents on days 3–7 as the respiratory distress from hyaline membrane disease is improving. Presentation can be on days 1 or 2, especially in infants born at less than 28 weeks' gestation and in those who have received surfactant replacement therapy. The signs include a hyperdynamic precordium, increased peripheral pulses, and a widened pulse pressure with or without a systolic heart murmur. Early presentations are sometimes manifested by systemic hypotension without a murmur or hyperdynamic circulation. These signs are often accompanied by an increase in respiratory support. The presence of significant patent ductus arteriosus can be confirmed by echocardiography. Before undertaking medical or surgical ligation, other structural heart disease should be ruled out.

## Treatment

The ductus arteriosus is managed by medical or surgical ligation. A clinically significant ductus causing compromise in the infant can be closed (in about two thirds of cases) with indomethacin, 0.1–0.2 mg/kg IV q12–24h for three doses. If the ductus reopens or fails to close completely, a second course of drug may be used. If indomethacin fails to close the ductus or if a ductus reopens a second time, surgical ligation is called for. In some cases, a more prolonged course of indomethacin is being used to prevent recurrences. In addition, in the extremely low birth weight infant (< 1000 g) who is at very high risk of developing a symptomatic ductus, a prophylactic strategy starting indomethacin (0.1 mg/kg q24h for 3–5 days) on the first day of life can be used. The major side effect of indomethacin is transient oliguria, which can be managed by fluid restriction until urine output improves. There may also be an increased incidence of necrotizing enterocolitis with more prolonged therapy. Transient decreases in intestinal and cerebral blood flow caused by indomethacin can be ameliorated by giving the drug as a slow infusion over 1–2 hours. The drug should not be used if the infant is hyperkalemic, if the creatinine is > 2 mg/dL, or if the platelet count is < 50,000/mL.

Lee J et al: Randomized trial of prolonged low dose versus conventional dose indomethacin for treating patent ductus arteriosus in very low birth weight infants. Pediatrics 2003;112:345 [PMID: 12897285].

Narayan-Sankar M, Clyman RI: Pharmacologic closure of patent ductus arteriosus in the neonate. Neoreviews 2003;4:e215.

Schmidt B et al: Long-term effects of indomethacin prophylaxis in extremely-low-birth-weight infants. N Engl J Med 2001;344: 1966 [PMID: 11430325].

## 5. Necrotizing Enterocolitis

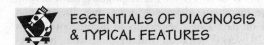

### ESSENTIALS OF DIAGNOSIS & TYPICAL FEATURES

- Feeding intolerance with gastric aspirates or vomiting.
- Bloody stools.
- Abdominal distention and tenderness.
- Pneumatosis intestinalis on abdominal radiograph.

## General Considerations

Necrotizing enterocolitis is the most common acquired GI emergency in the newborn infant; it most often affects preterm infants, with an incidence of 10% in infants of birth weight < 1500 g. In full-term infants, it occurs in association with polycythemia, congenital heart disease, and birth asphyxia. The pathogenesis of the disease is multifactorial. Previous intestinal ischemia, bacterial or viral infection, and immunologic immaturity of the gut are thought to play a role in the genesis of the disorder. In up to 20% of affected infants, the only risk factor is prematurity.

## Clinical Findings

The most common presenting sign is abdominal distention. Other signs include vomiting or increased gastric residuals, heme-positive stools, abdominal tender-

ness, temperature instability, increased apnea and bradycardia, decreased urine output, and poor perfusion. The CBC may show an increased white blood cell count with an increased band count or, as the disease progresses, absolute neutropenia. Thrombocytopenia is often observed along with stress-induced hyperglycemia and metabolic acidosis. Diagnosis is confirmed by the presence of pneumatosis intestinalis (air in the bowel wall) on radiograph. There is a spectrum of disease, and milder cases may exhibit only distention of bowel loops with bowel wall edema (thickened-appearing walls on radiograph).

## Treatment

### A. MEDICAL TREATMENT

Necrotizing enterocolitis is managed by decompression of the gut by nasogastric tube, maintenance of oxygenation, mechanical ventilation if necessary, and IV fluids (normal saline) to replace third-space GI losses. Enough fluid should be given to restore a good urine output. Other measures consist of broad-spectrum antibiotics (usually ampicillin, a third-generation cephalosporin, or an aminoglycoside and possibly additional anaerobic coverage), close monitoring of vital signs, serial physical examinations, and laboratory studies (blood gases, white blood cell count, platelet count, and radiographs).

### B. SURGICAL TREATMENT

Indications for surgery are evidence of perforation (free air present on a left lateral decubitus or crosstable lateral film), a fixed dilated loop of bowel on serial radiographs, abdominal wall cellulitis, or progressive deterioration despite maximal medical support. All of these signs are indicative of necrotic bowel. In the operating room, necrotic bowel is removed and ostomies are created. Reanastomosis is performed after the disease is resolved and the infant is bigger (usually > 2 kg and after 4–6 weeks).

## Course & Prognosis

Infants treated either medically or surgically should not be refed until the disease is resolved (normal abdominal examination, resolution of pneumatosis on radiograph), usually in 10–14 days. Nutritional support during this time should be provided by total parenteral nutrition.

Death occurs in 10% of cases. Surgery is needed in less than 25% of cases. Long-term prognosis is determined by the amount of intestine lost. Infants with short bowel require long-term support with IV nutrition and therefore have very long hospitalizations. Even for those infants, however, the outcome is favorable because of improved parenteral nutrition formulations.

Late strictures—about 3–6 weeks after initial diagnosis—occur in 8% of patients whether treated medically or surgically and generally require operative management.

Berseth CL et al: Prolonged small feeding volumes early in life decreases the incidence of necrotizing enterocolitis in very low birth weight infants. Pediatrics 2003:111:529 [PMID: 12612232].

Caplan MS, Jilling T: The pathophysiology of necrotizing enterocolitis. Neoreviews 2001;2:e103.

Dimmit RA, Moss LR: Clinical management of necrotizing enterocolitis. Neoreviews 2001;2:e110.

## 6. Anemia in the Premature Infant

### General Considerations

In the premature infant, the hemoglobin reaches its nadir at approximately 8–12 weeks and is 2–3 g/dL lower than that in the full-term infant. The lower nadir in premature infants appears to be the result of a decreased erythropoietin response to the low red cell mass. Symptoms of anemia include poor feeding, lethargy, increased heart rate, poor weight gain, and perhaps apnea.

### Treatment

The decision to transfuse is based on the presence of clinical symptoms. Transfusion is not indicated in an asymptomatic infant simply because of an arbitrary hematocrit number. Most infants become symptomatic if the hematocrit drops below 20%. With risks of transfusion, alternative therapies have been explored. Epoetin alfa, 250 units/kg, given subcutaneously three times per week or added daily with iron dextran to parenteral nutrition, has been shown to increase hematocrit and reticulocyte count and to decrease the frequency and volume of transfused blood. This treatment should be reserved for the highest risk infants (those born at less than 28–30 weeks' gestation and below 1000–1200 g). For optimal effect, supplemental iron at a dosage of 4–8 mg/kg/d should be given. Other options include rescue epoetin alfa at 300 IU/kg/d for 7–10 days for hematocrits < 28% or a late transfusion from the same blood unit used for an infant's early transfusions.

Ohls RK: Human recombinant erythropoietin in the preterm and treatment of anemia of prematurity. Paediatr Drugs 2002;4:111 [PMID: 11888358].

## 7. Intraventricular Hemorrhage

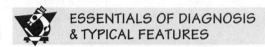

### ESSENTIALS OF DIAGNOSIS & TYPICAL FEATURES

- *Large bleeds are accompanied by hypotension, metabolic acidosis, and altered neurologic status. Smaller bleeds can be asymptomatic.*
- *Routine cranial ultrasound scanning is essential for diagnosis in infants born at less than 32 weeks' gestation.*

### General Considerations

Periventricular-intraventricular hemorrhage occurs almost exclusively in premature infants. The incidence is 20–30% in infants born at less than 31 weeks' gestation and weighing less than 1500 g at birth. The highest incidence is observed in babies of the lowest gestational age (< 26 weeks). Bleeding most commonly occurs in the subependymal germinal matrix (a region of undifferentiated cells adjacent to or lining the lateral ventricles). Bleeding can extend into the ventricular cavity. The proposed pathogenesis of bleeding is presented in Figure 1–8. The critical event is ischemia with reperfusion injury to the capillaries in the germinal matrix that occurs in the immediate perinatal period. The actual amount of bleeding is also influenced by a variety of factors that affect the pressure gradient across the injured capillary wall. This pathogenetic scheme applies also to intraparenchymal bleeding (venous infarction in a region rendered ischemic) and to periventricular leukomalacia (ischemic white matter injury in a watershed region of arterial supply). Central nervous system complications in preterm infants are more frequent in infants exposed antenatally to intrauterine infection.

### Clinical Findings

Up to 50% of hemorrhages occur at less than 24 hours of age, and virtually all occur by the fourth day. The clinical syndrome ranges from rapid deterioration (coma, hypoventilation, decerebrate posturing, fixed pupils, bulging anterior fontanelle, hypotension, acidosis, acute drop in hematocrit) to a more gradual deterioration with more subtle neurologic changes to absence of any specific physiologic or neurologic signs.

The diagnosis can be confirmed by real-time ultrasound scan. This can be performed whenever bleeding is clinically suspected. If symptoms are absent, routine

**Figure 1–8.** Pathogenesis of periventricular and intraventricular hemorrhage.

scanning should be done at 10–14 days in all infants born at < 29 weeks' gestation. Hemorrhages are graded as follows: grade I, germinal matrix hemorrhage only; grade II, intraventricular bleeding without ventricular enlargement; grade III, intraventricular bleeding with ventricular enlargement; and grade IV, any infant with intraparenchymal bleeding. The amount of bleeding is minor (grade I or II) in 75% of infants and major in the remainder.

Follow-up ultrasound examinations are based on the results of the initial scan. Infants with no bleeding or germinal matrix hemorrhage require only a single late scan at age 4–6 weeks to look for periventricular leukomalacia. Any infant with blood in the ventricular system is at risk for posthemorrhagic ventriculomegaly. This is usually the result of impaired absorption of cerebrospinal fluid (CSF), but it can also occur secondary to obstructive phenomena. An initial follow-up scan should be done 1–2 weeks after the initial scan. Infants with intraventricular bleeding and ventricular enlargement should be followed every 7–10 days until ventricular enlargement stabilizes or decreases. Infants without ventriculomegaly should have one additional scan at age 4–6 weeks. In addition, all infants born at 29–32 weeks' gestation should have at least a late scan (4–6 weeks) to look for ventriculomegaly and periventricular leukomalacia.

## Treatment

During acute hemorrhage, supportive treatment (including restoration of volume and hematocrit, oxygenation, and ventilation) should be provided to avoid further cerebral ischemia. Progressive posthemorrhagic hydrocephalus (if it develops) is treated initially with a subgaleal shunt. When the infant is large enough, this can be converted to a ventriculoperitoneal shunt.

Although the incidence and severity of intracranial bleeding have decreased in premature infants, strategies to prevent this complication are still needed. Use of antenatal corticosteroids appears to be important in decreasing this complication, and phenobarbital may have a role in the mother who has not been prepared with steroids and is delivering at less than 28 weeks' gestation. The route of delivery may also play a role, with babies delivered by cesarean section showing a decreased rate of intracranial bleeds, but this issue remains controversial. Postnatal strategies appear less promising. Early indomethacin administration may have some benefit in minimizing bleeding, but does not affect long-term outcome.

## Prognosis

No deaths occur as a result of grade I and grade II hemorrhages, whereas grade III and grade IV hemorrhages carry a mortality rate of 10–20%. Posthemorrhagic ventricular enlargement is rarely seen with grade I hemorrhages but is seen in 54–87% of grade II—IV hemorrhages. Very few of these infants will require a ventriculoperitoneal shunt. Long-term neurologic sequelae are seen no more frequently in infants with grade I and grade II hemorrhages than in preterm infants without bleeding. In infants with grade III and grade IV hemorrhages, severe sequelae occur in 20–25% of cases, mild sequelae in 35% of cases, and no sequelae in 40% of cases. The presence of severe periventricular leukomalacia, large parenchymal bleeds, and progressive ventriculomegaly greatly increases the risk of neurologic sequelae.

Bada HS: Prevention of intracranial hemorrhage. Neoreviews 2000;1:e48.

Ment LR et al: Outcome of children in the indomethacin intraventricular hemorrhage prevention trial. Pediatrics 2000;105: 485 [PMID: 10699097].

Ramsey PS, Rouse DJ: Therapies administered to mothers at risk for preterm birth and neurodevelopmental outcome in their infants. Clin Perinatol 2002;29:725 [PMID: 12616743].

Schmidt B et al: Long-term effects of indomethacin prophylaxis in extremely-low-birth-weight infants. N Engl J Med 2001;344: 1966 [PMID: 11430325].

Shankaran S: Complications of neonatal intracranial hemorrhage. Neoreviews 2000;1:e44.

Thorp JA et al: Perinatal factors associated with severe intracranial hemorrhage. Am J Obstet Gynecol 2001;185:859 [PMID: 11641666].

Volpe JJ: Cerebral white matter injury of the premature infant— More common than you think. Pediatrics 2003;112:176 [PMID: 12737883].

Whitelaw et al: Post haemorrhagic ventricular dilation. Arch Dis Child Fetal Neonatal Ed 2002;86:72 [PMID: 11882544].

## 8. Retinopathy of Prematurity

Retinopathy of prematurity occurs only in the incompletely vascularized retina of the premature infant. The incidence of any acute retinopathy in infants weighing < 1250 g is 66%, whereas only 6% have retinopathy severe enough to warrant intervention. The incidence is highest in babies of the lowest gestational age. The condition appears to be triggered by an initial injury to the developing retinal vessels. Hypoxia, shock, asphyxia, vitamin E deficiency, and light exposure have been associated with this initial injury. After the initial injury, normal vessel development may follow or abnormal vascularization may occur with ridge formation on the retina. The process can still regress at this point or may continue, with growth of fibrovascular tissue into the vitreous associated with inflammation, scarring, and retinal folds or detachment. The disease is graded by stages of abnormal vascular development and retinal detachment (I–V), by the zone of the eye involved (1–3, with zone 1 the posterior region around the macula), and by the amount of the retina involved, in "clock hours" (eg, a detachment in the upper, outer quadrant of the left eye would be defined as affecting the left retina from 12 to 3 o'clock).

Initial eye examination should be performed at 4–6 weeks of age in infants with a birth weight < 1500 g or in those born at < 28 weeks' gestation, as well as in infants weighing > 1500 g with an unstable clinical course. Follow-up is done at 2- to 4-week intervals until the retina is fully vascularized. Infants with zone 1 disease need to be followed at 1- to 2-week intervals. Infants with threshold disease (stage III, zone 1 or 2, in five or more continuous clock hours, with inflammatory changes of "plus" disease) are candidates for laser therapy. Although this treatment does not always prevent retinal detachment, it reduces the incidence of poor outcomes based on visual acuity and anatomic outcomes.

American Academy of Pediatrics Section on Ophthalmology: Screening examination of premature infants for retinopathy of prematurity. Pediatrics 2001;108:809 [PMID: 11533356].

Phelps DL: Retinopathy of prematurity: History, classification, and pathophysiology. Neoreviews 2001;2:e153.

The STOP-ROP Multicenter Study Group: Supplemental therapeutic oxygen for prethreshold retinopathy of prematurity (STOP-ROP), a randomized, controlled trial. I: Primary outcomes. Pediatrics 2000;105:295 [PMID: 10654946].

## 9. Discharge & Follow-Up of the Premature Infant

### Hospital Discharge

Medical criteria for discharge of the premature infant include the ability to maintain temperature in an open crib, nippling all feeds and gaining weight, and the absence of apneic and bradycardiac spells requiring intervention. Infants going home on supplemental oxygen should not desaturate too badly (< 80%) in room air or should demonstrate the ability to arouse in response to hypoxia. Factors such as support for the mother at home and the stability of the family situation play a role in the timing of discharge. Home nursing visits and early physician follow-up can be used to hasten discharge.

### Follow-Up

With advances in obstetric and maternal care, survival for infants born at < 28 weeks' gestation or with birth weights as low as 1000 g is now better than 90%. Seventy to 80% survive at 26–27 weeks' gestation and birth weights of 800–1000 g. Survival at gestational age

**Figure 1–9.** Mortality rates before discharge by 100-g birth weight subgroups in 2001. (Reproduced, with permission, from the Vermont Oxford Network, 2002.)

25 weeks and birth weight 700–800 g is 50–70%, with a considerable drop-off below this level (Figure 1–9).

These high rates of survival do come with a price in terms of morbidity. Major neurologic sequelae, including cerebral palsy, cognitive delay, and hydrocephalus, is reported in 10–25% of survivors with birth weights < 1500 g. The rate of these sequelae tends to be higher in infants with lower birth weights. In addition to a higher incidence of severe neurologic sequelae, infants with birth weights < 1000 g have an increased rate of lesser disabilities, including learning and behavioral problems. Risk factors for neurologic sequelae include seizures, grade III or IV intracranial hemorrhage, periventricular leukomalacia, severe IUGR, poor early head growth, need for mechanical ventilation, and low socioeconomic class. In addition, maternal fever and chorioamnionitis have been associated with an increased risk of cerebral palsy. Other morbidities in these infants include chronic lung disease and reactive airway disease, resulting in an increased risk from respiratory infections and hospital readmissions in the first 2 years, retinopathy of prematurity with associated loss of visual acuity and strabismus, hearing loss, and growth failure. All of these issues require close multidisciplinary outpatient follow-up. Infants with residual lung disease are candidates for monthly palivizumab (Synagis) injections during their first winter after hospital discharge to prevent severe infection with respiratory syncytial virus. Routine immunizations should be done by chronologic age and not age-corrected for prematurity.

American Academy of Pediatrics. Committee on Infectious Diseases and Committee on Fetus and Newborn: Revised indications for the use of palivizumab and respiratory syncytial virus immune globulin intravenous for the prevention of respiratory syncytial virus infection. Pediatrics 2003;112:1442 [PMID: 14654628].

Bhutta AT et al: Cognitive and behavioral outcomes of school-aged children who were born preterm. A meta-analysis. JAMA 2002;288:728 [PMID: 12169077].

D'Angio CT et al: Longitudinal, 15-year follow-up of children born at less than 29 weeks gestation after introduction of surfactant therapy into a region: Neurologic, cognitive, and educational outcomes. Pediatrics 2002;110:1094 [PMID: 12456905].

Doyle LW and the Victorian Infant Collaborative Study Group: Outcome at 5 years of age of children 23–27 weeks gestation: Refining the prognosis. Pediatrics 2001;108:134 [PMID: 11433066].

Gross SJ et al: Impact of family structure and stability on academic outcome in preterm children at 10 years of age. J Pediatr 2001;138:169 [PMID: 11174612].

Hack M et al: Functional limitations and special health care needs of 10- to 14-year old children weighing less than 750 grams at birth. Pediatrics 2000;106:554 [PMID: 10969102].

Hack M et al: Outcomes in young adulthood for very-low-birth-weight infants. N Engl J Med 2002;346:149 [PMID: 11796848].

Horbar JD et al: Trends in mortality and morbidity for very low birth weight infants 1991–1999. Pediatrics 2002;110:143 [PMID: 12093960].

Lorenz JM: Survival of the extremely preterm infant in North America in the 1990s. Clin Perinatol 2000;27:255 [PMID: 10863649].

Ment LR et al: Change in cognitive function over time in very-low-birth-weight infants. JAMA 2003;289:705 [PMID: 12585948].

O'Connor AR et al: Long-term ophthalmic outcome of low birth weight children with and without retinopathy of prematurity. Pediatrics 2002;109:12 [PMID: 11773536].

Saari TN and the Committee on Infectious Diseases: Immunization of preterm and low birth weight infants. Pediatrics 2003;112:193 [PMID: 12837889].

Saigal S et al: School difficulties at adolescence in a regional cohort of children who were extremely low birth weight. Pediatrics 2000;105:325 [PMID: 10654950].

Saigal S et al: Physical growth and current health status of infants who were of extremely low birth weight and controls at adolescence. Pediatrics 2001;108:407 [PMID: 11483807].

Schmidt B et al: Impact of bronchopulmonary dysplasia, brain injury, and severe retinopathy on the outcome of extremely low-birth-weight infants at 18 months: Results from the trial of indomethacin prophylaxis in preterms. JAMA 2003;289:1124 [PMID: 12622582].

Vohr BR et al: Neurodevelopmental and functional outcomes of extremely low birth weight infants in the National Institute of Child Health and Human Development Neonatal Research Network 1993–1994. Pediatrics 2000;105:1216 [PMID: 10835060].

Wood NS et al: Neurologic and developmental disability after extremely preterm birth. N Engl J Med 2000;343:378 [PMID: 10933736].

# CARDIAC PROBLEMS IN THE NEWBORN INFANT

## STRUCTURAL HEART DISEASE

### 1. Cyanotic Presentations

 ESSENTIALS OF DIAGNOSIS & TYPICAL FEATURES

- *Cyanosis, initially without associated respiratory distress.*
- *Failure to increase $Pa_{O_2}$ with supplemental oxygen.*
- *Chest radiograph with decreased lung markings suggests right heart obstruction, while increased lung markings suggest transposition or venous obstruction.*

## General Considerations

The causes of cyanotic heart disease that occur in the newborn period are transposition of the great vessels (TOGV), total anomalous pulmonary venous return (TAPVR), truncus arteriosus (some types), tricuspid atresia, and pulmonary atresia or critical pulmonary stenosis.

## Clinical Findings

Infants with these disorders present with early cyanosis. The hallmark of many of these lesions is cyanosis in an infant without associated respiratory distress. In most of these infants, tachypnea develops over time either because of increased pulmonary blood flow or secondary to metabolic acidemia from progressive hypoxemia. Diagnostic aids include comparing the blood gas or oxygen saturation in room air to that in 100% $Fi_{O_2}$. Failure of $Pa_{O_2}$ or $Sa_{O_2}$ to increase suggests cyanotic heart disease. *Note:* A $Pa_{O_2}$, if feasible, is the preferred measure. Saturation in the newborn may be misleadingly high due to the left-shifted oxyhemoglobin dissociation curve seen with fetal hemoglobin. Other useful aids are chest radiograph, electrocardiography, and echocardiography.

TOGV is the most common form of cyanotic heart disease presenting in the newborn period. Examination generally reveals a systolic murmur and single $S_2$. Chest radiograph shows a generous heart size and a narrow mediastinum with normal or increased lung markings.

There is little change in $PaO_2$ or $SaO_2$ with supplemental oxygen. Total anomalous pulmonary venous return, in which venous return is obstructed, presents early with severe cyanosis and tachypnea because the pulmonary venous return is obstructed, resulting in pulmonary edema. The chest radiograph typically shows a small to normal heart size with marked pulmonary edema. Infants with right heart obstruction (pulmonary and tricuspid atresia, critical pulmonary stenosis, and some forms of truncus arteriosus) have decreased lung markings on chest radiograph and, depending on the severity of hypoxia, may develop metabolic acidemia. Those forms with an underdeveloped right heart will have left-sided predominance on electrocardiography. Although tetralogy of Fallot is the most common form of cyanotic heart disease, the obstruction at the pulmonary valve is often not severe enough to result in cyanosis in the newborn. In all cases, diagnosis can be confirmed by echocardiography.

## 2. Acyanotic Presentations

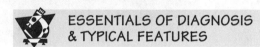

### ESSENTIALS OF DIAGNOSIS & TYPICAL FEATURES

- *Most newborns who present with acyanotic heart disease have left-sided outflow obstruction.*
- *Differentially diminished pulses (coarctation) or decreased pulses throughout (aortic atresia).*
- *Metabolic acidemia.*
- *Chest radiograph showing large heart and pulmonary edema.*

### General Considerations

Newborn infants who present with serious acyanotic heart disease usually have congestive heart failure secondary to left-sided outflow tract obstruction. Infants with left-to-right shunt lesions (eg, ventricular septal defect) may have murmurs in the newborn period, but clinical symptoms do not occur until pulmonary vascular resistance drops enough to cause significant shunting and subsequent congestive heart failure (usually at 3–4 weeks of age).

### Clinical Findings

Infants with left-sided outflow obstruction generally do well the first day or so until the ductus arteriosus—the source of all or some of the systemic flow—narrows.

Tachypnea, tachycardia, congestive heart failure, and metabolic acidosis develop. On examination, all of these infants have abnormalities of the pulses. In aortic atresia (hypoplastic left heart syndrome) and stenosis, pulses are all diminished, whereas in coarctation syndromes, differential pulses (diminished or absent in the lower extremities) are evident. Chest radiographic films in these infants show a large heart and pulmonary edema. Diagnosis is confirmed with echocardiography.

## 3. Treatment of Cyanotic & Acyanotic Lesions

Early stabilization includes supportive therapy as needed (eg, IV glucose, oxygen, ventilation for respiratory failure, pressor support). Specific therapy includes infusions of prostaglandin $E_1$, 0.025–0.1 µg/kg/min, to maintain ductal patency. In some cyanotic lesions (eg, pulmonary atresia, tricuspid atresia, critical pulmonary stenosis) in which lung blood flow is ductus-dependent, this improves pulmonary blood flow and $PaO_2$ by allowing shunting through the ductus to the pulmonary artery. In left-sided outflow tract obstruction, systemic blood flow is ductus-dependent; prostaglandins improve systemic perfusion and resolve the acidosis. Further specific management—including palliative surgical and cardiac catheterization procedures—is discussed in Chapter 19.

## PERSISTENT PULMONARY HYPERTENSION IN THE NEWBORN INFANT

### ESSENTIALS OF DIAGNOSIS & TYPICAL FEATURES

- *Onset of symptoms on day 1 of life.*
- *Hypoxia with poor response to high concentrations of inspired oxygen.*
- *Right-to-left shunts through the foramen ovale, ductus arteriosus, or both.*
- *Most often associated with parenchymal lung disease.*

### General Considerations

Persistent pulmonary hypertension (PPHN) results when the normal decrease in pulmonary vascular resistance after birth does not occur. Most infants so affected are full term or postterm, and many have experienced perinatal asphyxia. Other clinical associations include hypothermia, meconium aspiration syndrome, hyaline membrane disease, polycythemia, neonatal sepsis, chronic intrauterine hypoxia, and pulmonary hypoplasia.

There are three causes of PPHN: (1) acute vasoconstriction resulting from perinatal hypoxia, (2) prenatal increase in pulmonary vascular smooth muscle development, and (3) decreased cross-sectional area of the pulmonary vascular bed because of inadequate vessel number. In the first, an acute perinatal event leads to hypoxia and failure of the pulmonary vascular resistance to drop. In the second, abnormal muscularization of the pulmonary resistance vessels results in persistent hypertension after birth. The third category includes infants with pulmonary hypoplasia (eg, diaphragmatic hernia).

## Clinical Findings

Clinically, the syndrome is characterized by onset on the first day of life, usually from birth. Respiratory distress is prominent, and $PaO_2$ is usually poorly responsive to high concentrations of inspired oxygen. Many of the infants have associated myocardial depression with resulting systemic hypotension. Echocardiography reveals right-to-left shunting at the level of the ductus arteriosus or foramen ovale (or both). Chest radiograph usually shows lung infiltrates related to associated pulmonary pathology (eg, meconium aspiration, hyaline membrane disease). If the majority of right-to-left shunt is at the ductal level, pre- and postductal differences in $PaO_2$ and $SaO_2$ will be observed.

## Treatment

Therapy for PPHN involves supportive therapy for other postasphyxia problems (eg, anticonvulsants for seizures, careful fluid and electrolyte management for renal failure). IV glucose should be provided to maintain normal blood sugar, and antibiotics should be administered for possible infection. Specific therapy is aimed at both increasing systemic arterial pressure and decreasing pulmonary arterial pressure to reverse the right-to-left shunting through fetal pathways. First-line therapy includes oxygen and ventilation (to reduce pulmonary vascular resistance) and crystalloid infusions (10 mL/kg, up to 30 mL/kg) to improve systemic pressure. Ideally, systolic pressure should be greater than 60 mm Hg. With compromised cardiac function, systemic pressors can be used as second-line therapy (eg, dopamine, 5–20 µg/kg/min; dobutamine, 5–20 µg/kg/min; or both). Metabolic acidemia should be corrected with sodium bicarbonate because acidemia exacerbates pulmonary vasoconstriction. In some cases, a mild respiratory alkalosis may improve oxygenation. Pulmonary vasodilation can be enhanced using the inhaled gas nitric oxide, which is identical or very similar to endogenous endothelium-derived relaxing factor, at doses of 5–20 ppm. In addition, use of high-frequency oscillatory ventilation has proved effective in many of these infants, particularly those with severe associated lung disease.

Infants for whom conventional therapy is failing (poor oxygenation despite maximum support) may require extracorporeal membrane oxygenation (ECMO). The infants are placed on bypass, with blood exiting the baby from the right atrium and returning to the aortic arch after passing through a membrane oxygenator. The lungs are essentially at rest during the procedure, and with resolution of the pulmonary hypertension the infants are weaned from ECMO back to ventilator therapy. This therapy can save infants who might otherwise die but has major side effects that must be considered prior to its institution. Neurodevelopmental outcome among survivors of ECMO is similar to that of infants with PPHN managed without the procedure. Approximately 10–15% of survivors have significant neurologic sequelae, with cerebral palsy or cognitive delays. Other sequelae such as chronic lung disease, sensorineural hearing loss, and feeding problems have also been described in this population.

## ARRHYTHMIAS

Irregularly irregular heart rates, commonly associated with premature atrial contractions and less commonly with premature ventricular contractions, are noted often in the first days of life in well newborns. These arrhythmias are benign and of no consequence. Clinically significant bradyarrhythmias are seen in association with congenital heart block. Heart block can be seen in an otherwise structurally normal heart (associated with maternal lupus) or with structural cardiac abnormalities. If fetal hydrops is absent, the bradyarrhythmia has been well tolerated. Indications for cardiac pacing include symptoms of inadequate cardiac output.

On electrocardiography, tachyarrhythmias can be either wide complex (eg, ventricular tachycardia) or narrow complex (eg, supraventricular tachycardia). Supraventricular tachycardia is the most common tachyarrhythmia in the neonate and may be a sign of structural heart disease, myocarditis, left atrial enlargement, and aberrant conduction pathways. Acute treatment is ice to the face and, if unsuccessful, adenosine given IV at a dose of 50–200 µg/kg. If there is no response, the dose can be increased up to 300 µg/kg. Long-term therapy is with digoxin or propranolol. Digoxin should not be used in cases with Wolff–Parkinson–White syndrome. Cardioversion is rarely needed for supraventricular tachycardia but is needed acutely for hemodynamically unstable ventricular tachycardia.

Beck AE, Hudgins L: Congenital cardiac malformations in the neonate: Isolated or syndromic? Neoreviews 2003;4:e105.

Kinsella JP, Abman SH: Inhaled nitric oxide: Current and future uses in neonates. Semin Perinatol 2000;24:387 [PMID: 11153900].

Marino BS et al: Diagnosis and management of the newborn with suspected congenital heart disease. Clin Perinatol 2001;28: 91 [PMID: 11265513].

Schumacher RE, Baumgart S: Extracorporeal membrane oxygenation 2001: The odyssey continues. Clin Perinatol 2001;28: 629 [PMID: 11570158].

Tanel RE, Rhodes LA: Fetal and neonatal arrhythmias. Clin Perinatol 2001;28:187 [PMID: 11265506].

Walsh MC, Stork EK: Persistent pulmonary hypertension of the newborn: Rationale therapy based on pathophysiology. Clin Perinatol 2001;28:609 [PMID: 11570157].

# GASTROINTESTINAL & ABDOMINAL SURGICAL CONDITIONS IN THE NEWBORN INFANT (SEE ALSO CHAPTER 20.)

## ESOPHAGEAL ATRESIA & TRACHEOESOPHAGEAL FISTULA

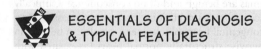

### ESSENTIALS OF DIAGNOSIS & TYPICAL FEATURES

- *Polyhydramnios.*
- *Baby with excessive drooling and secretions, choking with attempted feeding.*
- *Unable to pass an orogastric tube to the stomach.*

## General Considerations

These associated conditions are characterized by a blind esophageal pouch and a fistulous connection between the proximal or distal esophagus (or both) and the airway. In 85% of affected infants, the fistula is between the distal esophagus and the airway. Polyhydramnios is common because of the high level of GI obstruction.

## Clinical Findings

Infants present in the first hours of life with copious secretions, choking, cyanosis, and respiratory distress. Diagnosis can be confirmed with chest radiograph after careful placement of a nasogastric tube to the point at which resistance is met. On chest radiograph, the tube will be seen in the blind pouch. If a tracheoesophageal fistula is present to the distal esophagus, gas will be present in the bowel. In cases of esophageal atresia without tracheoesophageal fistula, there is no gas in the bowel.

## Treatment

The tube in the proximal pouch should be placed on continuous suction to drain secretions and prevent aspiration. The head of the bed should be elevated to prevent reflux of gastric contents through the distal fistula into the lungs. IV glucose and fluids should be provided and oxygen administered as needed. Definitive treatment is by operation and depends on the distance between the segments of esophagus. If the distance is not too great, the fistula can be ligated and the ends of the esophagus anastomosed. In instances in which the ends of the esophagus cannot be brought together, the initial surgery entails fistula ligation and a gastrostomy for feeding. Echocardiography should be performed prior to surgery to rule out a right-sided aortic arch. In those cases, a left-sided thoracotomy would be preferred.

## Prognosis

Prognosis is determined primarily by the presence or absence of associated anomalies. Vertebral, anal, cardiac, renal, and limb anomalies are the most likely anomalies to be observed (VACTERL association). Evaluation for associated anomalies should be done early.

## INTESTINAL OBSTRUCTION

### ESSENTIALS OF DIAGNOSIS & TYPICAL FEATURES

- *Infants with high intestinal obstruction present soon after birth with emesis.*
- *Bilious emesis represents a malrotation with midgut volvulus until proved otherwise.*
- *Low intestinal obstruction is characterized by abdominal distention and late onset of emesis.*

## General Considerations

A history of polyhydramnios is common, and the fluid, if bile-stained, can easily be confused with thin meconium staining. The higher the obstruction in the intestine, the earlier the infant will present with vomiting and the less prominent the distention will be. The opposite is true for lower intestinal obstructions. Most obstructions are bowel atresias, believed to be caused by an ischemic event during development. Approximately 30% of cases of duodenal atresia are associated with Down syndrome. Meconium ileus is a distal small bowel obstruction caused by the exceptionally viscous meconium produced by fetuses with cystic fibrosis. Hirschsprung disease is caused by a failure of neuronal migration to the myenteric plexus of the distal bowel so that the distal bowel lacks ganglion cells, causing a lack of peristalsis in that region with a functional obstruction.

Malrotation with midgut volvulus is a surgical emergency that appears in the first days to weeks as bilious vomiting without distention or tenderness. If malrotation is not treated promptly, torsion of the intestine around the superior mesenteric artery will lead to necrosis of the entire small bowel. For this reason, bilious vomiting in the neonate always demands immediate attention and evaluation.

## Clinical Findings

Diagnosis of intestinal obstructions depends on plain abdominal radiographs with either upper GI series (high obstruction suspected) or contrast enema (lower obstruction apparent) to define the area of obstruction. Table 1–20 summarizes the findings expected.

All infants with meconium ileus are presumed to have cystic fibrosis. Infants with pancolonic Hirschsprung disease, colon pseudo-obstruction syndrome, or colonic dysgenesis or atresia may also present with meconium impacted in the distal ileum. Definitive diagnosis of cystic fibrosis is by the sweat chloride test ($Na^+$ and $Cl^-$ concentration > 60 mEq/L) or by genetic testing. Approximately 10–20% of infants with cystic fibrosis present with meconium ileus. Infants with cystic fibrosis and meconium ileus generally have a normal immunoreactive trypsinogen test result on their newborn screen because of the associated severe exocrine pancreatic insufficiency in utero.

Any in utero perforation results in meconium peritonitis with residual intraabdominal calcifications. Many of these are completely healed at birth. If the infant has no signs of obstruction, no further immediate evaluation is needed. A sweat test to rule out cystic fibrosis should be done at a later date.

Low intestinal obstruction may present with delayed stooling (> 24 hours in term infants is abnormal) with mild distention. Radiograph findings of gaseous distention should prompt contrast enema to diagnose (and treat) meconium plug syndrome. If no plug is found, the diagnosis may be small left colon syndrome (occurring in IDMs) or Hirschsprung disease. Rectal biopsy will be required to make this diagnosis. Imperforate

*Table 1–20.* Intestinal obstruction.

| Site of Obstruction | Clinical Findings | Plain Radiographs | Contrast Study |
|---|---|---|---|
| Duodenal atresia | Down syndrome (30%); early vomiting, sometimes bilious | "Double bubble" (dilated stomach and proximal duodenum, no air distal) | Not needed |
| Malrotation and volvulus | Bilious vomiting with onset anytime in the first few weeks | Dilated stomach and proximal duodenum; paucity of air distally (may be normal gas pattern) | UGI shows displaced duodenojejunal junction with "corkscrew" deformity of twisted bowel |
| Jejunoileal atresia, meconium ileus | Bilious gastric contents > 25 mL at birth; progressive distention and bilious vomiting | Multiple dilated loops of bowel; intraabdominal calcifications if in utero perforation occurred (meconium peritonitis) | Barium or osmotic contrast enema shows microcolon; contrast refluxed into distal ileum may demonstrate and relieve meconium obstruction (successful in about 50%) |
| Meconium plug syndrome; Hirschsprung's disease | Distention, delayed stooling (> 24 h) | Diffuse bowel distention | Barium or osmotic contrast enema outlines and relieves plug; may show transition zone in Hirschsprung's disease; delayed emptying (> 24 h) suggests Hirschsprung's disease |

UGI = upper gastrointesinal tract

anus should be apparent on physical examination, although a rectovaginal fistula with a mildly abnormal-appearing anus can occasionally be confused with normal.

## Treatment

Nasogastric suction to decompress the bowel, IV glucose, fluid and electrolyte replacement, and respiratory support as necessary should be instituted. Antibiotics are usually indicated. The definitive treatment for most of these conditions (with the exception of meconium plug syndrome, small left colon syndrome, and some cases of meconium ileus) is surgery.

## Prognosis

Up to 10% of infants with meconium plug syndrome are subsequently found to have cystic fibrosis or Hirschsprung disease. For this reason, some surgeons advocate performance of a sweat chloride test and rectal biopsy in all of these infants before discharge. The infant with meconium plug syndrome who is still symptomatic after contrast enema should have a rectal biopsy.

In cases of duodenal atresia associated with Down syndrome, the prognosis will depend on associated anomalies (eg, heart defects) and the severity of prestenotic duodenal dilation. Otherwise, these conditions usually carry an excellent prognosis after surgical repair.

## ABDOMINAL WALL DEFECTS

### 1. Omphalocele

Omphalocele is a membrane-covered herniation of abdominal contents into the base of the umbilical cord. There is a high incidence of associated anomalies (cardiac, GI, chromosomal—eg, trisomy 13). The sac may contain liver and spleen as well as intestine.

Acute management of omphalocele involves covering the defect with a sterile dressing soaked with warm saline to prevent fluid loss, nasogastric decompression, IV fluids and glucose, and antibiotics. If the contents of the omphalocele will fit into the abdomen, a primary surgical closure is done. If not, a staged closure is performed, with gradual reduction of the omphalocele contents into the abdominal cavity and a secondary closure. Postoperatively, third-space fluid losses may be extensive; fluid and electrolyte therapy, therefore, must be monitored carefully.

### 2. Gastroschisis

In gastroschisis, the intestine extrudes through an abdominal wall defect lateral to the umbilical cord. There is no membrane or sac and no liver or spleen outside the abdomen. Gastroschisis is associated with no anomalies except intestinal atresias in approximately 10%. The herniation is thought to be related to abnormal involution of the right umbilical vein, although the exact cause is unknown.

Therapy is as described for omphalocele.

## DIAPHRAGMATIC HERNIA

This congenital malformation consists of herniation of abdominal organs into the hemithorax (usually left) through a posterolateral defect in the diaphragm. It presents in the delivery room as severe respiratory distress in an infant with poor breath sounds and scaphoid abdomen. The rapidity and severity of presentation—as well as ultimate survival—depend on the degree of pulmonary hypoplasia, which is a result of compression by the intrathoracic abdominal contents in utero. Affected infants are prone to development of pneumothorax.

Treatment includes intubation and ventilation as well as decompression of the GI tract with a nasogastric tube to intermittent suction. An IV infusion of glucose and fluid should be started. Chest radiograph confirms the diagnosis. Surgery to reduce the abdominal contents from the thorax and to close the diaphragmatic defect is performed after the infant is stabilized. The postoperative course is often complicated by severe pulmonary hypertension, requiring therapy with high-frequency ventilation, inhaled NO, or ECMO. The mortality rate for this condition is 25–40%, with survival dependent on the degree of pulmonary hypoplasia and presence of congenital heart disease.

## GASTROINTESTINAL BLEEDING

### Upper Gastrointestinal Bleeding

Upper GI bleeding is not uncommon in the newborn nursery. Old blood ("coffee-ground" material) may be either swallowed maternal blood or infant blood from a bleeding gastric irritation such as gastritis or stress ulcer. Bright red blood from the stomach is most likely acute bleeding, again due to gastritis. Treatment generally consists of gastric lavage (a sample can be sent for Apt testing to determine if it is mother's or baby's blood) and antacid medication. If the volume of bleeding is large, intensive monitoring, fluid and blood replacement, and endoscopy are indicated (see Chapter 20).

### Lower Gastrointestinal Bleeding

Rectal bleeding is less common than upper GI bleeding in the newborn and is associated with infections (eg, *Salmonella* acquired from the mother perinatally), milk intolerance (blood streaks with diarrhea), or, in stressed infants, necrotizing enterocolitis. An abdominal radiograph should be obtained to rule out pneumatosis intestinalis (air in the wall of the bowel) or other abnormalities in gas pattern (eg, obstruction). If the radiograph is negative and the examination is benign, a protein hydrolysate or predigested formula (eg, Nutramigen or Pregestamil) should be tried or the mother instructed to avoid all dairy products in her diet if nursing. If the amount of rectal bleeding is large or persistent, endoscopy will be needed.

## GASTROESOPHAGEAL REFLUX (See also Chapter 20.)

All people reflux occasionally, and physiologic regurgitant reflux is extremely common in infants. Reflux is pathologic and should be treated when it results in failure to thrive owing to excessive regurgitation, poor intake due to dysphagia and irritability, apnea or cyanotic episodes (acute life-threatening events), or chronic respiratory symptoms of wheezing and recurrent pneumonias. Diagnosis is clinical, with confirmation by barium swallow or pH probe study.

Initial steps in treatment include prone positioning and thickened feeds (rice cereal, 1 tbsp/oz of formula) for those with frequent regurgitation and poor weight gain. Gastric acid suppressants such as ranitidine (2 mg/kg bid) or lansoprazole (1.5 mg/kg/d), along with a prokinetic agent such as metaclopramide (0.1 mg/kg tid–qid), can also be used. Because most infants improve by 12–15 months of age, surgery is reserved for the most severe cases, especially those with chronic neurologic or respiratory conditions that exacerbate reflux and those who have life-threatening events caused by reflux.

Bohn D: Congenital diaphragmatic hernia. Am J Respir Crit Care Med 2002;166:911 [PMID: 12359645].

Cass DL, Wesson DE: Advances in fetal and neonatal surgery for gastrointestinal anomalies and disease. Clin Perinatol 2003;29:1 [PMID: 11917733].

Cohen MS et al: Influence of congenital heart disease on survival in children with congenital diaphragmatic hernia. J Pediatr 2002;141:25 [PMID: 12091847].

Jadcherla SR: Gastroesophageal reflux in the neonate. Clin Perinatol 2002;29:135 [PMID: 11917735].

Rodgers BM: Upper gastrointestinal hemorrhage. Pediatr Rev 1999;20:171 [PMID: 10233176].

Squires RH: Gastrointestinal bleeding. Pediatr Rev 1999; 20:95 [PMID: 10073071].

# ■ INFECTIONS IN THE NEWBORN INFANT

The fetus and the newborn infant are very susceptible to infections. There are three major routes of perinatal infection: (1) blood-borne transplacental infection of the fetus (eg, cytomegalovirus [CMV], rubella, syphilis); (2) ascending infection with disruption of the barrier provided by the amniotic membranes (eg, bacterial infections after 12–18 hours of ruptured membranes); and (3) infection on passage through an infected birth canal or exposure to infected blood at delivery (eg, herpes simplex, hepatitis B, HIV, bacterial infections).

Susceptibility of the newborn infant to infection is related to immaturity of both the cellular and humoral immune systems at birth. This feature is particularly evident in the preterm neonate. Passive protection against some organisms is provided by transfer of IgG across the placenta during the third trimester of pregnancy. Preterm infants, especially those born at less than 30 weeks' gestation, do not have the benefit of the full amount of this passively acquired antibody.

## BACTERIAL INFECTIONS

### 1. Bacterial Sepsis

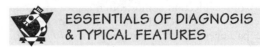

**ESSENTIALS OF DIAGNOSIS & TYPICAL FEATURES**

- *Most infants with early-onset sepsis present at < 24 hours of age.*
- *Respiratory distress is the most common presenting symptom.*
- *Hypotension, acidemia, and neutropenia are associated clinical findings.*
- *The presentation of late-onset sepsis is more subtle.*

### General Considerations

The incidence of early-onset (< 5 days) neonatal bacterial infection is 4–5 per 1000 live births. If rupture of the membranes occurs more than 24 hours prior to delivery, the infection rate increases to 1 per 100 live births. If early rupture of membranes with chorioamnionitis occurs, the infection rate increases further to 1 per 10 live births. Irrespective of membrane rupture, infection rates are five times higher in preterm than in full-term infants.

### Clinical Findings

Early-onset bacterial infections appear most commonly on day 1 of life, and the majority of cases appear at <

12 hours. Respiratory distress due to pneumonia is the most common presenting sign. Other features include unexplained low Apgar scores without fetal distress, poor perfusion, and hypotension. Late-onset bacterial infection (at > 5 days of age) presents in a more subtle manner, with poor feeding, lethargy, hypotonia, temperature instability, altered perfusion, new or increased oxygen requirement, and apnea. Late-onset bacterial sepsis is more often associated with meningitis or other localized infections.

Low total white counts, absolute neutropenia (< 1000/mL), and elevated ratios of immature to mature neutrophils are suggestive of neonatal bacterial infection. Thrombocytopenia is also a common feature. Other laboratory signs are hypoglycemia or hyperglycemia with no change in glucose administration, unexplained metabolic acidosis, and elevated C reactive protein. In early-onset bacterial infection, pneumonia is invariably present; chest radiograph films show infiltrates, but these infiltrates cannot be distinguished from those resulting from other causes of neonatal lung disease. Definitive diagnosis is made by positive cultures from blood, CSF, and the like.

Early-onset infection is most often caused by group B β-hemolytic streptococci (GBS) and gram-negative enteric pathogens (most commonly *Escherichia coli*). Other organisms to consider are *Haemophilus influenzae* and *Listeria monocytogenes*. Late-onset sepsis is caused by coagulase-negative staphylococci (most common in infants with indwelling central venous lines), *Staphylococcus aureus*, GBS, *Enterococcus, Pseudomonas,* and other gram-negative organisms.

## Treatment

A high index of suspicion is important in the diagnosis and treatment of neonatal infection. Table 1–21 presents guidelines for the evaluation and treatment of full-term infants with risk factors or clinical signs of infection. Because the risk of infection is greater in the preterm infant and because respiratory disease is a common sign of infection, any preterm infant with respiratory disease requires blood cultures and broad-spectrum antibiotic therapy for 48–72 hours pending the results of cultures. An examination of CSF should be performed when infection is highly suspected on a clinical basis (eg, associated hypotension, persistent metabolic acidosis, neutropenia) or if the blood culture is positive. Antibiotic coverage should be directed initially toward suspected organisms. Early-onset sepsis is usually caused by GBS or gram-negative enteric organisms; broad-spectrum coverage, therefore, should include ampicillin plus an aminoglycoside or third-generation cephalosporin—for example, ampicillin, 100–150 mg/kg/d divided q12h, and gentamicin,

**Table 1–21.** Guidelines for evaluation of neonatal bacterial infection in the full-term infant.

| Risk Factor | Clinical Signs of Infection | Evaluation and Treatment |
|---|---|---|
| Delivery 12–18 h after rupture of membranes | None | Observation |
| Delivery > 12–18 h after rupture of membranes, chorioamnionitis | None | Complete blood count (CBC), blood culture, broad-spectrum antibiotics for 48–72 h[c] |
| Delivery > 12–18 h after rupture of membranes, chorioamnionitis, maternal antibiotics[a] | None | CBC, blood culture, broad-spectrum antibiotics for 48–72 h[c] |
| With or without risk factors | Present | CBC, blood and CSF cultures, perhaps urine culture (see below); broad-spectrum antibiotics[b] |

[a]Minimum of 24 h of observation is indicated if no treatment is given.
[b]Irrespective of age at presentation, any infant who appears infected by clinical criteria should undergo cerebrospinal fluid (CSF) examination. Urine culture is indicated in the evaluation of infants who were initially well but have developed symptoms after 2–3 d of age.
[c]If clinical signs are absent, close observation without treatment may be sufficient.

2.5 mg/kg/dose q12–24h (depending on gestational age), or cefotaxime, 100 mg/kg/d divided q12h. In infants > 34 weeks' gestation, gentamicin can also be given at a dose of 4 mg/kg q24h. Late-onset infections can also be caused by the same organisms, but coverage may need to be expanded to include staphylococci. In particular, the preterm infant with an indwelling line is at risk for infection with coagulase-negative staphylococci, for which vancomycin is the drug of choice in a dosage of 10–15 mg/kg q8–24h depending on gestational and postnatal ages. Initial broad-spectrum coverage should also include a third-generation cephalosporin (cefotaxime or ceftazidime 100 mg/kg/day divided q12h when *Pseudomonas aeruginosa* is strongly suspected). To prevent the development of vancomycin-resistant organisms, vancomycin should be stopped as soon as cultures and sensitivities indicate it is not needed for ongoing therapy. Other supportive therapy includes the administration of IVIG

(500–750 mg/kg) to infants with known overwhelming infection. The duration of treatment for proved sepsis is 10–14 days of IV antibiotics. In addition, recombinant human granulocyte colony-stimulating factor (rhG-CSF) is under investigation for treatment of neutropenia in the septic infant. In sick infants, the essentials of good supportive therapy should be provided: IV glucose and nutritional support, volume expansion, use of pressors as needed, and oxygen and ventilator support.

Prevention of neonatal GBS infection has been achieved with intrapartum administration of penicillin given > 4 hours prior to delivery. The current clinical guideline (Figure 1–10) is to perform a vaginal and rectal GBS culture at 35–37 weeks' gestation for all pregnant women. Prophylaxis with penicillin is given to GBS-positive women as well as those who have unknown GBS status at delivery with risk factors for infection. Figure 1–11 presents a suggested strategy for the infant born to a mother who received intrapartum prophylaxis for prevention of early-onset GBS or for suspected chorioamnionitis. Some authors also recommend selective neonatal prophylaxis with 50,000 U/kg of penicillin G given IM if adequate intrapartum treatment has not been given.

## 2. Meningitis

Any newborn with bacterial sepsis is also at risk for meningitis. The incidence is low in infants with early-onset sepsis but much higher in infants with late-onset infection. The work-up for any newborn with signs of infection should include a spinal tap. Diagnosis is suggested by a CSF protein > 150 mg/dL, glucose < 30 mg/dL, > 25 leukocytes/mL, and a positive Gram stain. The diagnosis is confirmed by culture. The most common organisms are GBS and gram-negative enteric bacteria. Although sepsis can be treated with antibiotics for 10–14 days, meningitis often requires 21 days. The mortality rate of neonatal meningitis is approximately 10%, with significant neurologic morbidity present in one third of the survivors.

## 3. Pneumonia

The respiratory system can be infected in utero or on passage through the birth canal. Early-onset neonatal infection is usually associated with pneumonia. Pneumonia should also be suspected in older neonates with a recent onset of tachypnea, retractions, and cyanosis. In infants already receiving respiratory support, an in-

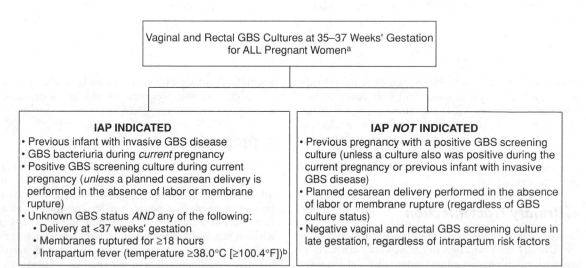

**Vaginal and Rectal GBS Cultures at 35–37 Weeks' Gestation for ALL Pregnant Women[a]**

**IAP INDICATED**
- Previous infant with invasive GBS disease
- GBS bacteriuria during *current* pregnancy
- Positive GBS screening culture during current pregnancy (*unless* a planned cesarean delivery is performed in the absence of labor or membrane rupture)
- Unknown GBS status *AND* any of the following:
  - Delivery at <37 weeks' gestation
  - Membranes ruptured for ≥18 hours
  - Intrapartum fever (temperature ≥38.0°C [≥100.4°F])[b]

**IAP *NOT* INDICATED**
- Previous pregnancy with a positive GBS screening culture (unless a culture also was positive during the current pregnancy or previous infant with invasive GBS disease)
- Planned cesarean delivery performed in the absence of labor or membrane rupture (regardless of GBS culture status)
- Negative vaginal and rectal GBS screening culture in late gestation, regardless of intrapartum risk factors

[a] Exceptions: women with GBS bacteriuria during the current pregnancy or women with a previous infant with invasive GBS disease.

[b] If chorioamnionitis is suspected, broad-spectrum antimicrobial therapy that includes an agent known to be active against GBS should replace GBS IAP.

GBS = group B streptococcus, IAP = intrapartum antimicrobial prophylaxis.

***Figure 1–10.*** Indications for intrapartum antimicrobial prophylaxis to prevent early-onset GBS disease using a universal prenatal culture screening strategy at 35–37 weeks' gestation for all pregnant women. (Reproduced, with permission, from the American Academy of Pediatrics: *Red Book 2003 Report of the Committee on Infectious Disease,* 2003.)

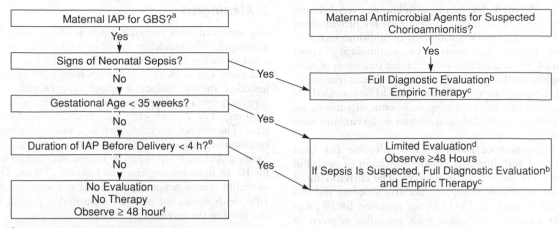

**Figure 1–11.** Empiric management of a neonate born to a mother who received intrapartum antimicrobial prophylaxis (IAP) for prevention of early-onset GBS (group B streptococcal) disease or chorioamnionitis. (Reproduced, with permission, from the American Academy of Pediatrics: *Red Book 2003 Report of the Committee on Infectious Disease,* 2003.)

crease in the requirement for oxygen or ventilator support may indicate pneumonia. Not only common bacteria but also viruses (CMV, respiratory syncytial virus, adenovirus, influenza, herpes simplex, parainfluenza) and *Chlamydia* can cause the disease. In infants with preexisting respiratory disease, intercurrent pulmonary infections may contribute to the ultimate severity of chronic lung disease.

### 4. Urinary Tract Infection

Infection of the urine is uncommon in the first days of life. Urinary tract infection in the newborn can occur in association with genitourinary anomalies and is caused by gram-negative enteric pathogens, *Enterococcus,* or other organisms. Urine should be evaluated as part of the work-up for late-onset infection. Culture should be obtained either by suprapubic aspiration or bladder catheterization. Antibiotic IV therapy is continued for 7–10 days if the blood culture is negative and clinical signs resolve quickly. Evaluation for genitourinary

anomalies, starting with an ultrasound examination and a voiding cystourethrogram, should be done subsequently.

### 5. Otitis Media

Otitis media occurs in a significant number of long-term nursery occupants. It is particularly common in infants who have had prolonged endotracheal intubation or an indwelling nasogastric feeding tube. Evaluation for infection in such an infant is not complete without an ear examination. Gram-negative enteric pathogens are more commonly found infecting agents in nursery occupants than in outpatients.

### 6. Omphalitis

A normal umbilical cord stump will atrophy and separate at the skin level. A small amount of purulent material at the base of the cord is common but can be minimized by keeping the cord open to air and cleaning the base with alcohol several times a day. The cord can become colonized with streptococci, staphylococci, or gram-negative organisms that can cause local infection. Infections are more common in cords manipulated for venous or arterial lines. Omphalitis is diagnosed when redness and edema develop in the soft tissues around the stump. Local and systemic cultures should be obtained. Treatment is with broad-spectrum IV antibiotics (usually nafcillin 50–75 mg/kg/d divided q8–12h and a third-generation cephalosporin). Complications are determined by the degree of infection of the cord vessels and include septic thrombophlebitis, hepatic abscess, necrotizing fasciitis, and portal vein thrombosis. Surgical consultation should be obtained because of the potential for necrotizing fasciitis.

Baltimore RS et al: Early-onset neonatal sepsis in the era of group B streptococcal prevention. Pediatrics 2001;108:1094 [PMID: 11694686].

Philip AGS: Neonatal meningitis in the new millennium. Neoreviews 2003;4:e73.

Schrag S et al: Prevention of perinatal group B streptococcal disease: Revised guidelines from CDC. MMWR Aug 16, 2002;51(RR11):1 [PMID: 12211284].

Schrag SJ et al: Group B streptococcal disease in the era of intrapartum antibiotic prophylaxis. N Engl J Med 2000;342:15 [PMID: 10620644].

Schrag SJ et al: A population based comparison of strategies to prevent early-onset group B streptococcal disease in neonates. N Engl J Med 2002;347:233 [PMID: 12140298].

Sinha A et al: Intrapartum antibiotics and neonatal invasive infections caused by organisms other than group B streptococcus. J Pediatr 2003;142:492 [PMID:12756379].

Stoll BJ et al: Late onset sepsis in very low birth weight neonates: The experience of the NICHD neonatal research network. Pediatrics 2002;110:285 [PMID: 12165580].

Stoll BJ et al: Changes in pathogens causing early onset sepsis in very-low-birth-weight infants. N Engl J Med 2002;347:240 [PMID: 12140299].

Velaphi S et al: Early-onset group B streptococcal infection after a combined maternal and neonatal group B streptococcal chemoprophylaxis strategy. Pediatrics 2003;111:541 [PMID: 12612234].

Young TE: Aminoglycoside therapy in neonates: With particular reference to gentamicin. Neoreviews 2002;3:e243.

## FUNGAL SEPSIS

With the survival of smaller, sicker infants, infection with *Candida* species has become more common. Infants of low birth weight with central lines who have had repeated exposures to broad-spectrum antibiotics are at highest risk. For infants of birth weight < 1500 g, colonization rates of 27–64% have been demonstrated, with many of these infants developing cutaneous lesions although the GI tract appears to be the initial site of colonization. A much smaller percentage (2–5%) develop systemic disease.

Clinical features of fungal sepsis can be indistinguishable from those of late-onset bacterial sepsis but may be more subtle. Thrombocytopenia may be the earliest and only sign. Deep organ involvement (renal, eye, endocarditis) is commonly associated with systemic candidiasis. Treatment is with amphotericin B (0.5–1.5 mg/kg/d). In severe infections, flucytosine (50–150 mg/kg/d) can be added for synergistic coverage. (See Chapter 39.) Prophylaxis with oral mycostatin at 0.5–1 mL PO qid or fluconazole at 3–6 mg/kg/d as a single dose diminishes intestinal colonization with yeast and decreases the frequency of systemic disease.

*Malassezia furfur* is also seen in infants with central lines receiving IV fat emulsion. To eradicate this organism, as well as *Candida* species, it is necessary to remove the indwelling line.

Benjamin DK et al: When to suspect fungal infection in neonates: A clinical comparison of *Candida albicans* and *Candida parasilosis* fungemia with coagulase-negative staphylococcal bacteremia. Pediatrics 2000;106:712 [PMID: 11015513].

Kicklighter SD: Antifungal agents and fungal prophylaxis in the neonate. Neoreviews 2002;3:e249.

## CONGENITAL VIRAL & PARASITIC INFECTIONS (SEE ALSO CHAPTERS 36 & 39.)

### 1. Cytomegalovirus Infection

CMV is the most common virus transmitted in utero. The incidence of congenital infection ranges from 0.2% to 2.2% of live births. Transmission of CMV can occur during either primary or reactivated infection in the mother. An important source of infection is children (especially those in a day care setting), who transmit the virus to parents and workers. The incidence of primary infection in pregnancy is 1–4%, with a 40% transplacental transmission rate to the fetus. Of these infants, 85–90% are asymptomatic at birth, whereas 10–15% have clinically apparent disease—hepatosplenomegaly, petechiae, small size for gestational age, microcephaly, direct hyperbilirubinemia, thrombocytopenia, intracranial calcifications, and chorioretinitis. The risk of neonatal disease is higher when the mother acquires the infection in the first half of pregnancy. The incidence of reactivated infection in pregnancy is less than 1%, with an incidence of clinically apparent disease of 0–1%. Diagnosis in the neonate should be confirmed by culture of the virus from urine. Rapid diagnosis is possible with antigen detection techniques and polymerase chain reaction (PCR) testing. Diagnosis can also be confirmed in utero from an amniocentesis specimen. Although experimental and not routinely recommended, ganciclovir therapy has been used in some severely ill neonates.

The mortality rate in patients with symptomatic congenital CMV may be as high as 20%. Sequelae such as hearing loss, mental retardation, delayed motor development, chorioretinitis and optic atrophy, seizures, language delays, and learning disability occur in 90% of symptomatic survivors. The incidence of complications is 5–15% in asymptomatic infants; the most frequent complication is hearing loss, which can be progressive.

Perinatal infection can also occur with acquisition of virus around the time of delivery. These infections are generally asymptomatic and without sequelae. Postnatal infection is usually asymptomatic but can cause hepatitis, pneumonitis, and neurologic illness in compromised seronegative premature infants. The virus can be acquired postnatally through transfusions or ingestion of CMV-infected breast milk. Transfusion risk can be minimized by using frozen, washed red blood cells or CMV antibody-negative donors.

## 2. Rubella

Congenital rubella infection occurs as a result of rubella infection in the mother during pregnancy. The frequency of infection and damage in the fetus is as high as 80% in mothers infected during the first trimester. Fetal infection rates decline in the second trimester before increasing again in the third trimester. Fetal damage generally does not occur in infections acquired after 18 weeks' gestation. Clinical features of congenital rubella include adenopathy, bone radiolucencies, encephalitis, cardiac defects (pulmonary arterial hypoplasia and patent ductus arteriosus), cataracts, retinopathy, growth retardation, hepatosplenomegaly, thrombocytopenia, and purpura. Affected infants can be asymptomatic at birth but develop clinical sequelae during the first year of life. The diagnosis should be suspected in cases of a characteristic clinical illness in the mother (rash, adenopathy, arthritis) confirmed by serologic testing. Diagnosis can be confirmed by an increase in serum rubella-specific IgM or culture of pharyngeal secretions in the baby. Congenital rubella is now rare because of widespread immunization.

## 3. Varicella

Congenital varicella infection is rare (< 5% after infection acquired during the first or second trimester) but may cause a constellation of findings, including limb hypoplasia, cutaneous scars, microcephaly, cortical atrophy, chorioretinitis, and cataracts. Perinatal exposure (5 days before to 2 days after delivery) can cause severe to fatal disseminated varicella in the infant. If maternal

varicella infection develops within this perinatal risk period, 1.25 mL of varicella immune globulin should be given to the newborn. If this has not been done, the illness can be treated with IV acyclovir (30 mg/kg/d divided q8h).

Hospitalized premature infants of at least 28 weeks' gestation whose mothers have no history of chickenpox—and all infants of less than 28 weeks' gestational age—should receive varicella immune globulin following any postnatal exposure. Susceptible women of childbearing age should be immunized with varicella vaccine.

## 4. Toxoplasmosis

Toxoplasmosis is caused by the protozoan *Toxoplasma gondii*. Maternal infection occurs in 0.1–0.5% of pregnancies and is usually asymptomatic. When primary infection occurs during pregnancy, up to 40% of the fetuses become infected, of whom 15% have severe damage. The sources of transmission include exposure to cat feces and ingestion of raw or undercooked meat. Although the risk of transmission increases to 90% near term, fetal damage is most likely to occur when maternal infection occurs in the second to sixth month of gestation.

Clinical findings include growth retardation, chorioretinitis, seizures, jaundice, hydrocephalus, microcephaly, cerebral calcifications, hepatosplenomegaly, adenopathy, cataracts, maculopapular rash, thrombocytopenia, and pneumonia. The majority of affected infants are asymptomatic at birth but show evidence of damage (chorioretinitis, blindness, low IQ, hearing loss) at a later time. The serologic diagnosis is based on a positive IgA or IgM in the first 6 months of life or a persistent IgG beyond 12 months. Infants with suspected infection should have eye and auditory examinations and a CT scan of the brain. Organism isolation from placenta or cord blood and PCR tests are also available for diagnosis in the neonate and from amniocentesis specimens.

Spiramycin treatment of primary maternal infection is used to try to reduce transmission to the fetus. Neonatal treatment using pyrimethamine and sulfadiazine with folinic acid can improve long-term outcome. (See Chapter 39.)

## PERINATALLY ACQUIRED VIRAL INFECTIONS

### 1. Herpes Simplex (See also Chapter 36.)

Herpes simplex virus (HSV) infection is most commonly acquired at the time of birth during transit through an infected birth canal. The mother may have either primary or reactivated secondary infection. Primary maternal infection, because of the high titer of organism and the absence of maternal antibodies, poses the greatest risk to the infant. The risk of neonatal infection with vaginal delivery in this setting is 33–50%. Seventy percent of mothers with primary herpes at the time of delivery are asymptomatic. The risk to an infant born to a mother with recurrent herpes simplex is much lower (< 0–5%). Time of presentation of localized (skin, eye, mouth) or disseminated disease (pneumonia, shock, hepatitis) in the infant is usually 5–14 days of age. CNS disease usually presents at 14–28 days with lethargy and seizures. In about 10% of cases, presentation can be as early as day 1 of life. Disease appearing this early suggests in utero infection. In about one third of patients, localized skin, eye, and mouth disease is the first indication of infection. In another third, disseminated or CNS disease precedes skin, eye, and mouth findings, whereas the remaining third have disseminated or CNS disease in the absence of skin, eye, and mouth disease. Preliminary diagnosis can be made by scraping the base of a vesicle and finding multinucleated giant cells. Viral culture from vesicles, usually positive in 24–72 hours, makes the definitive diagnosis. PCR technology can assist in diagnosis.

Acyclovir (60 mg/kg/d given q8h) is the drug of choice for neonatal herpes infection. Localized disease is treated for 14 days, and a 21-day course is used for disseminated or CNS disease. Treatment improves survival of neonates with CNS and disseminated disease and prevents the spread of localized disease. Prevention is possible by not allowing delivery through an infected birth canal (eg, by cesarean section within 6 hours after rupture of the membranes). However, antepartum cervical cultures are poor predictors of the presence of virus at the time of delivery. Furthermore, given the low incidence of infection in the newborn from secondary maternal infection, cesarean section is not indicated for asymptomatic mothers with a history of herpes. Cesarean sections are performed in mothers with active lesions (either primary or secondary) at the time of delivery. Infants born to mothers with a history of HSV infection but no active lesions can be observed closely after birth. Cultures should be obtained and acyclovir treatment initiated only for clinical signs consistent with herpes virus infection. Infants born to mothers with active lesions—irrespective of the route of delivery—should be cultured (eye, oropharynx, umbilicus, rectum) 24 hours after delivery. If the infant is colonized (positive cultures) or if symptoms consistent with herpes infection develop, treatment with acyclovir should be started. In cases of maternal primary infection at the time of vaginal delivery, the infant should be cultured and started on acyclovir pending the results of cultures. The major problem facing perinatologists is the high percentage of asymptomatic primary maternal infection. In these cases, infection in the neonate is currently not preventable. Therefore, any infant who presents at the right age with symptoms consistent with neonatal herpes should be cultured and started on acyclovir pending the results of those cultures.

The prognosis is good for localized skin and mucosal disease that does not progress. The mortality rate for both disseminated and CNS herpes is high, with significant rates of morbidity among survivors despite treatment.

## 2. Hepatitis B & C (See also Chapter 21.)

Infants can be infected with hepatitis B at the time of birth. Clinical illness is rare in the neonatal period, but infants exposed in utero are at high risk of becoming chronic HBsAg carriers, developing chronic active hepatitis and, later, hepatocellular carcinoma. The presence of HBsAg should be determined in all pregnant women. If the result is positive, the infant should receive HBIG and hepatitis B vaccine as soon as possible after birth, followed by two subsequent vaccine doses at 1 and 6 months of age. If HBsAg has not been tested prior to birth in a mother at risk, the test should be run after delivery and hepatitis B vaccine given within 12 hours after birth. If the mother is subsequently found to be positive, HBIG should be given as soon as possible (preferably within 48 hours, but not later than 1 week after birth). Subsequent vaccine doses should be given at 1 and 6 months of age. In premature infants born to HBsAg-positive mothers, vaccine and HBIG should be given at birth, but a three-vaccine hepatitis B series should be given after a weight of 2000 g is attained.

Hepatitis C perinatal transmissions occur in about 5% of infants born to mothers who carry the virus. At the present time, no prevention strategies exist. Up to 12 months of age, the only reliable screen for hepatitis C infection is PCR. After that time, the presence of hepatitis C antibodies in the infant strongly suggests that infection has occurred.

## 3. Enteroviral Infection

Enteroviral infections occur with greatest frequency in the late summer and early fall. Infection is usually acquired in the perinatal period. There is often a history of maternal illness (fever, diarrhea, rash) in the week prior to delivery. The illness appears in the infant in the first 2 weeks of life and is most commonly characterized by fever, lethargy, irritability, diarrhea, and rash but is not severe. More severe forms occasionally occur, especially if infection occurs before 1 week of age, including meningoencephalitis and myocarditis, as well as a disseminated illness with hepatitis, pneumonia, shock, and disseminated intravascular coagulation. Diagnosis can be confirmed by culture (rectum, CSF, blood) or by the more rapid PCR techniques.

No therapy has proved efficacy. The prognosis is good for all symptom complexes except severe disseminated disease, which carries a high mortality rate.

## 4. HIV Infection (See also Chapter 37.)

Human immunodeficiency virus (HIV) can be acquired in utero or at the time of delivery, or can be transmitted postpartum via breast milk. The majority of transmission occurs during the 2 weeks prior to delivery and during delivery. Transmission of virus occurs in 13–30% of births. Administration of zidovudine during pregnancy starting at 14–34 weeks' gestation, intrapartum, and for the first 6 weeks of life in the newborn at a dosage of 2 mg/kg PO qid decreases vertical transmission to 7%. Shorter courses of zidovudine are also associated with decreased disease transmission, as is cesarean delivery. The combination of zidovudine treatment and cesarean delivery can lower transmission to 2%. The addition of other anti-HIV therapy may further reduce the risk of ante- and intrapartum viral transmission. Current guidelines for use of antiretroviral drugs in pregnant HIV-infected women are similar to those for nonpregnant patients (eg, highly active retroviral combination therapy). The risk of transmission is increased in mothers with advanced disease, high viral loads, low CD4 counts, and p24 antigenemia. Prematurity, vaginal delivery, ruptured membranes over 4 hours, and chorioamnionitis also increase the transmission rate. Diagnosis is based on clinical, immunologic, and serologic findings. Newborns with congenitally acquired HIV are often free of symptoms. Jaundice, neonatal giant-cell hepatitis, and thrombocytopenia have been reported at birth. Failure to thrive, lymphadenopathy, hepatosplenomegaly, oral thrush, chronic diarrhea, bacterial infections with common organisms, and an increased incidence of upper and lower respiratory diseases, including lymphoid interstitial pneumonitis, may appear early in life or may be delayed for months to years.

Infants born to HIV-infected women should be tested by HIV DNA PCR at < 48 hours, at 1–2 months of age, and at 2–4 months old. In an infant who is age 4 months with no positive PCR, infection can be reasonably excluded. HIV-positive mothers should be counseled not to breast-feed their infants.

Protection of health care workers is an important issue. Testing should be performed in all pregnant women. Because such testing will fail to identify some infected patients, however, universal precautions should be used. Gloves should be worn during all procedures involving blood and blood-contaminated fluids, intubation, and any invasive procedures using needles. When a splash exposure is possible (eg, in the delivery room), a mask and eye covers should be used.

## OTHER INFECTIONS

### 1. Congenital Syphilis

The infant is usually infected in utero by transplacental passage of *Treponema pallidum*. Active primary and secondary maternal syphilis leads to fetal infection in nearly 100% of infants; latent disease in 40%; and late disease in 10%. Fetal infection is rare at under 18 weeks' gestation. Fetal infection can result in stillbirth or prematurity. Findings consistent with early congenital syphilis (presentation at under 2 years) include mucocutaneous lesions, lymphadenopathy, hepatosplenomegaly, bony changes, and hydrops. However, in the newborn period, infants are often asymptomatic, so that diagnosis is based on maternal and infant serologic testing and is only presumptive. Later manifestations (at over age 2 years) include Hutchinson teeth and mulberry molars, keratitis, chorioretinitis, glaucoma, hearing loss, saddle nose, saber shins, and mental retardation. An infant should be evaluated for congenital syphilis if it is born to a mother with positive nontreponemal tests confirmed by a positive treponemal test but without documented adequate treatment (parenteral penicillin G), including the expected fourfold decrease in nontreponemal antibody titer. Infants of mothers treated less than 1 month before delivery also require evaluation. Evaluation should include physical examination, a quantitative nontreponemal serologic test for syphilis, CSF examination for cell count, protein and VDRL, long bone radiographs, and antitreponemal IgM. A definitive diagnosis can be made on rare occasions when the organism is identified by dark-field microscopy or pathologic examination of the placenta. Guidelines for therapy are presented in Table 1–22. Infants should be treated for congenital syphilis if they have proven or probable disease, as evidenced by (1) physical or radiographic evidence, (2) quantitative nontreponemal antibody titers four times higher than the mother, (3) elevated CSF protein or cell count or positive VDRL, or (4) a positive antitreponemal IgM test. Asymptomatic infants should be treated if the mother did not receive adequate treatment for syphilis.

### 2. Tuberculosis (See also Chapter 38.)

Congenital tuberculosis (TB) is rare but may occur in the infant of a mother with hematogenously spread TB

**Table 1–22.** Recommended treatment of neonates ($\leq$ 4 wk of age) with proven or possible congenital syphilis.

| Clinical Status | Antimicrobial Therapy[a] |
|---|---|
| Proven or highly probable disease[b] | Aqueous crystalline penicillin G, 100,000–150,000 U/kg/d, administered as 50,000 U/kg per dose, IV, every 12 h during the first 7 d of life and every 8 h thereafter for a total of 10 d<br>**OR**<br>Penicillin G procaine,[c] 50,000 U/kg/d, IM, in a single dose for 10 d |
| Asymptomatic: normal CSF examination results, CBC and platelet count, and radiographic examination; and follow-up is certain with the following maternal treatment history: | |
| • (a) No penicillin treatment or inadequate or no documentation of penicillin treatment[d]; (b) mother was treated with erythromycin or other nonpenicillin regimen; (c) mother received treatment $\leq$ 4 wk before delivery; (d) sequential serologic tests on the mother do not demonstrate a fourfold or greater decrease in a nontreponemal antibody titer | Aqueous crystalline penicillin G, IV, for 10–14 d[b]<br>**OR**<br>Penicillin G procaine,[c] 50,000 U/kg/d, IM, in a single dose for 10 d<br>**OR**<br>Clinical, serologic follow-up, and penicillin G benzathine,[c] 50,000 U/kg, IM in a single dose |
| • (a) Adequate therapy given >1 mo before delivery; (b) mother's nontreponemal titers decreased fourfold after appropriate therapy for early syphilis and remained stable and low for late syphilis; (c) mother has no evidence of reinfection or relapse | Clinical, serologic follow-up, and penicillin G benzathine, 50,000 U/kg, IM in a single dose[e] |

IV indicates intravenously; IM, intramuscularly; CSF, cerebrospinal fluid; and CBC, complete blood cell.
[a]See text for details.
[b]If more than 1 day of therapy is missed, the entire course should be restarted.
[c]Penicillin G benzathine and penicillin G procaine are approved for IM administration *only*.
[d]See text for definition (includes infants in whom a serum quantitative nontreponemal serologic titer is the same or less than fourfold the maternal titer). If any part of the infant's evaluation is abnormal or not performed or if the CSF analysis is uninterpretable, the 10-day course of penicillin is required.
[e]Some experts would not treat the infant but would provide close serologic follow-up.
Reprinted, with permission, from the American Academy of Pediatrics: Red Book 2003 Report on Infectious Diseases; 2003.

or by aspiration of infected amniotic fluid in cases of tuberculous endometritis. Women with pulmonary TB are not likely to infect the fetus until after delivery. Postnatal acquisition is the most common mechanism of neonatal infection. Management in these cases is based on the mother's evaluation.

1. Mother or other household contact with a positive skin test and negative chest radiograph, or mother with an abnormal chest radiograph but no evidence of tuberculous disease after clinical evaluation: Investigate family contacts. Treat the mother with isoniazid (INH).

2. Mother has an abnormal chest radiograph consistent with tuberculous disease: Mother and infant should be separated until the mother is evaluated for active TB. If active TB is found, maintain sep-

aration until the mother is receiving antituberculosis therapy for 2 weeks. Investigate family contacts.

3. Mother with clinical or radiographic evidence of acute and possibly contagious TB: Evaluate the infant for congenital TB (skin test, chest radiograph, lumbar puncture, cultures) and HIV. Treat the mother and infant. If the infant is receiving INH and the mother has no risk for multidrug-resistant TB, separation is not necessary.

If congenital TB is suspected, multidrug therapy should be initiated.

## 3. Conjunctivitis

*Neisseria gonorrhoeae* may colonize an infant during passage through an infected birth canal. Gonococcal ophthalmitis presents at 3–7 days with copious purulent conjunctivitis. The diagnosis can be suspected when gram-negative intracellular diplococci are seen on a Gram-stained smear and confirmed by culture. Treatment is with IV or IM ceftriaxone, 25–50 mg/kg (not to exceed 125 mg) given once. Prophylaxis at birth is with 1% silver nitrate or 0.5% erythromycin ointment. Infants born to mothers with known gonococcal disease should also receive a single dose of ceftriaxone.

*Chlamydia trachomatis* is another important cause of conjunctivitis, appearing at 5 days to several weeks of age with congestion, edema, and minimal discharge. The organism is acquired at birth after passage through an infected birth canal. Acquisition occurs in 50% of infants born to infected women, with a 25–50% risk of conjunctivitis. Prevalence in pregnancy is over 10% in some populations. Diagnosis is by isolation of the organism or by rapid antigen detection tests. Treatment is with oral erythromycin (30 mg/kg/d in divided doses q8–12h) for 14 days. Topical treatment alone will not eradicate nasopharyngeal carriage, leaving the infant at risk for the development of pneumonitis.

American Academy of Pediatrics Committee on Infectious Diseases: Report of the committee on infectious diseases, 26th ed. Red Book 2003. American Academy of Pediatrics, 2003.

Boppana SB et al: Intrauterine transmission of cytomegalovirus to infants of women with preconceptional immunity. N Engl J Med 2001;344:1366 [PMID: 12359792].

Brown ZA et al: Effect of serologic status and cesarean delivery on transmission rates of herpes simplex virus from mother to infant. JAMA 2003;289:203 [PMID: 12517231].

Centers for Disease Control and Prevention. US Public Health Service Task Force recommendations for use of antiretroviral drugs in pregnant HIV-1 infected women for maternal health and interventions to reduce perinatal HIV-1 transmission in the US. MMWR 2002;51(RR-18):1 [PMID: 12489844].

Darville T: Syphilis. Pediatr Rev 1999;20:160 [PMID: 10233174].

Foulon W et al: Treatment of toxoplasmosis during pregnancy: A multicenter study of impact on fetal transmission and children's sequelae at age 1 year. Am J Obstet Gynecol 1999; 180:410 [PMID:9988811].

Fowler KB et al: Maternal immunity and prevention of congenital cytomegalovirus infection. JAMA 2003;289:1008 [PMID: 12597753].

Hadzic N: Hepatitis C in pregnancy. Arch Dis Childhood Fetal Neonatal Ed 2001;84:F201 [PMID: 11320050].

International Perinatal HIV Group: The mode of delivery and the risk of vertical transmission of human immunodeficiency virus type 1. N Engl J Med 1999;340:977 [PMID: 10099139].

Kimberlin DW et al: Natural history of neonatal herpes simplex virus infections in the acyclovir era. Pediatrics 2001;108:223 [PMID: 11483781].

Kimberlin DW et al: Effect of ganciclovir therapy on hearing in symptomatic cytomegalovirus disease involving the central nervous system: A randomized, controlled trial. J Pediatr 2003;143:16 [PMID: 12915819].

Michelow IC et al: Central nervous system infection in congenital syphilis. N Engl J Med 2002;346:1792 [PMID: 12050339].

Noyola DE et al: Early predictors of neurodevelopmental outcome in symptomatic congenital cytomegalovirus infection. J Pediatr 2001;138:325 [PMID: 11241037].

Pass RF: Cytomegalovirus infection. Pediatr Rev 2002;23:163 [PMID: 11986492].

Peters V et al: Missed opportunities for perinatal HIV prevention among HIV-exposed infants born 1996–2000, pediatric spectrum of HIV disease cohort. Pediatrics 2003;111:1186 [PMID: 12728136].

Tuomala RE et al: Antiretroviral therapy during pregnancy and the risk of an adverse outcome. N Engl J Med 2002;346:1863 [PMID: 12063370].

Watts H: Management of human immunodeficiency virus infection in pregnancy. N Engl J Med 2002;346:1879 [PMID: 12063373].

# ■ HEMATOLOGIC DISORDERS IN THE NEWBORN INFANT

## BLEEDING DISORDERS

Neonatal coagulation is discussed in Chapter 27. Bleeding in the newborn infant may result from inherited clotting deficiencies (eg, factor VIII deficiency) or acquired disorders—hemorrhagic disease of the newborn, disseminated intravascular coagulation (DIC), liver failure, and thrombocytopenia.

### 1. Vitamin K Deficiency Bleeding of the Newborn

Vitamin K deficiency bleeding (VKDB) is caused by the deficiency of the vitamin K-dependent clotting factors (II, VII, IX, and X). Bleeding occurs in 0.25–1.7% of newborns who do not receive vitamin K prophylaxis after birth, generally in the first 5 days to 2 weeks but as late as 12 weeks in an otherwise well infant. Early VKDB (0–2 weeks) can be prevented by either parenteral or oral vitamin K administration, whereas late disease is most effectively prevented by administering parenteral vitamin K. Sites of ecchymoses and surface bleeding include the GI tract, umbilical cord, circumcision site, and nose, although devastating intracranial hemorrhage can occur. Bleeding from vitamin K deficiency is more likely to occur in exclusively breast-fed infants because of very low amounts of vitamin K in breast milk, with slower and more restricted intestinal colonization. Differential diagnosis includes disseminated intravascular coagulation (DIC) and hepatic failure, both occurring in ill infants (Table 1–23).

**Table 1–23.** Features of infants bleeding from vitamin K deficiency (VKDB), disseminated intravascular coagulation (DIC), or liver failure.

|  | VKDB | DIC | Liver Failure |
|---|---|---|---|
| Clinical | Well infant; no prophylactic vitamin K | Sick infant; hypoxia, sepsis, etc | Sick infant; hepatitis, inborn errors of metabolism, shock liver |
| Bleeding | GI tract, umbilical cord, circumcision, nose | Generalized | Generalized |
| Onset | 2–3 d | Any time | Any time |
| Platelet count | Normal | Decreased | Normal or decreased |
| Prothrombin time (PT) | Prolonged | Prolonged | Prolonged |
| Partial thromboplastin time (PTT) | Prolonged | Prolonged | Prolonged |
| Fibrinogen | Normal | Decreased | Decreased |
| Factor V | Normal | Decreased | Decreased |

GI = gastrointestinal.

Treatment consists of 1 mg of vitamin K SQ or IV. IM injections should be avoided in infants who are actively bleeding.

## 2. Thrombocytopenia

Infants with thrombocytopenia have generalized petechiae (not just on the presenting part) and platelet counts < 150,000/mL (usually < 50,000/mL, may be < 10,000/mL). Neonatal thrombocytopenia can be isolated or may occur in association with a deficiency of clotting factors. The differential diagnosis for thrombocytopenia with distinguishing clinical features is presented in Table 1–24. Treatment of neonatal thrombocytopenia is transfusion of platelets (10 mL/kg of platelets increases the platelet count by approximately 70,000/mL). Indications for transfusion in the full-term infant are clinical bleeding or a total platelet count < 10,000–20,000/mL. In the preterm infant at risk for intraventricular hemorrhage, transfusion is indicated for counts < 40,000–50,000/mL.

**Table 1–24.** Differential diagnosis of neonatal thrombocytopenia.

| Disorder | Clinical Tips |
|---|---|
| **Immune**<br>Passively acquired antibody; idiopathic thrombocytopenic purpura, systemic lupus erythematosus, drug-induced | Proper history, maternal thrombocytopenia |
| Isoimmune sensitization to HPA-1a antigen | No rise in platelet count from random donor platelet transfusion. Positive antiplatelet antibodies in baby's serum, sustained rise in platelets by transfusion of mother's platelets |
| **Infections**<br>Bacterial infections<br>Congenital viral infections | Sick infants with other signs consistent with infection |
| **Syndromes**<br>Absent radii<br>Fanconi's anemia | Congenital anomalies, associated pancytopenia |
| Disseminated intravascular coagulation (DIC) | Sick infants, abnormalities of clotting factors |
| Giant hemangioma | |
| Thrombosis | Hyperviscous infants, vascular catheters |
| High-risk with respiratory distress syndrome, pulmonary hypertension, etc | Isolated decrease in platelets is not uncommon in sick infants even in the absence of DIC (? localized trapping) |

HPA = human platelet antigen.

Isoimmune thrombocytopenia (analogous to Rh isoimmunization, with a human platelet antigen (HPA)-1a-negative mother and HPA-1a-positive fetus) requires transfusion of maternal platelets, because 98% of the random population will also be HPA-1a-positive. The mother would be the most readily available known HPA-1a-negative donor. Treatment with steroids has been disappointing. Treatment with IVIG infusion, 1 g/kg/d for 2–3 days or until the platelet count has doubled or is over 50,000/mL, is recommended. Antenatal therapy of the mother with IVIG with or without steroids is also beneficial, since 20–30% of infants with isoimmune thrombocytopenia will experience intracranial hemorrhage, half of them before birth.

Infants born to mothers with idiopathic thrombocytopenic purpura are at low risk for serious hemorrhage despite the thrombocytopenia, and treatment is usually unnecessary. If bleeding does occur, IVIG can be used.

## ANEMIA

The newborn infant with anemia from acute blood loss presents with signs of hypovolemia (tachycardia, poor perfusion, hypotension), with an initially normal hematocrit that falls after volume replacement. Anemia from chronic blood loss is evidenced by pallor without signs of hypovolemia, with an initially low hematocrit and reticulocytosis.

Anemia can be caused by hemorrhage, hemolysis, or failure to produce red blood cells. Anemia occurring in the first 24–48 hours of life is the result of hemorrhage or hemolysis. Hemorrhage can occur in utero (fetoplacental, fetomaternal, or twin-to-twin), perinatally (cord rupture, placenta previa, incision through placenta at cesarean section), or internally (intracranial hemorrhage, cephalohematoma, ruptured liver or spleen). Hemolysis is caused by blood group incompatibilities, enzyme or membrane abnormalities, infection, and DIC and is accompanied by significant hyperbilirubinemia.

Initial evaluation should include a review of the perinatal history, assessment of the infant's volume status, and a complete physical examination. A Kleihaur-Betke test for fetal cells in the mother's circulation should be done. A CBC, blood smear, reticulocyte count, and direct and indirect Coombs' tests should be performed. This simple evaluation should suggest a diagnosis in most infants. It is important to remember that hemolysis related to blood group incompatibility can continue for weeks after birth. Serial hematocrits should be followed.

## POLYCYTHEMIA

Polycythemia in the newborn is manifested by plethora, cyanosis, mild respiratory distress with tachypnea and oxygen need, hypoglycemia, poor feeding, emesis, and lethargy. The capillary hematocrit is > 68%, the venous hematocrit > 65%.

Elevated hematocrits occur in 2–5% of live births. Although 50% of polycythemic infants are AGA, the prevalence of polycythemia is greater in the SGA and LGA populations. Causes of increased hematocrit include (1) twin–twin transfusion, (2) maternal–fetal transfusion, (3) intrapartum transfusion from the placenta, and (4) chronic intrauterine hypoxia (SGA infants, LGA infants of diabetic mothers).

The consequence of polycythemia is hyperviscosity with decreased perfusion of the capillary beds. Clinical symptomatology can affect several organ systems (Table 1–25). Screening can be done by measuring a capillary (heelstick) hematocrit. If the value is greater than 68%,

**Table 1–25.** Organ-related symptoms of hyperviscosity.

| | |
|---|---|
| Central nervous system | Irritability, jitteriness, seizures, lethargy |
| Cardiopulmonary | Respiratory distress, secondary to congestive heart failure, or persistent pulmonary hypertension |
| Gastrointestinal | Vomiting, heme-positive stools, distention, necrotizing enterocolitis |
| Renal | Decreased urinary output, renal vein thrombosis |
| Metabolic | Hypoglycemia |
| Hematologic | Hyperbilirubinemia, thrombocytopenia |

a peripheral venous hematocrit should be measured. Values greater than 65% should be considered consistent with hyperviscosity.

Treatment is recommended for symptomatic infants. Treatment for asymptomatic infants based strictly on hematocrit is controversial. Definitive treatment is accomplished by an isovolemic partial exchange transfusion with normal saline, effectively decreasing the hematocrit. The amount to exchange (in milliliters) is calculated using the following formula:

$$\frac{PVH - DH}{PVH} \times \frac{BV}{kg} \times Wt$$

where PVH = peripheral venous hematocrit, DH = desired hematocrit, BV = blood volume, and Wt = weight.

Blood is withdrawn at a steady rate from an umbilical venous line while the replacement solution is infused at the same rate through a peripheral IV line over 15–30 minutes. The desired hematocrit value is 50–55%; the assumed blood volume is 80 mL/kg.

American Academy of Pediatrics Committee on the Fetus and Newborn: Controversies concerning vitamin K and the newborn. Pediatrics 2003;122:191 [PMID: 12837888].

Manco-Johnson M, Nuss R: Hemostasis in the neonate. Neoreviews 2000;1:e191.

Murray NA: Evaluation and treatment of thrombocytopenia in the neonatal intensive care unit. Acta Paeditr Scand Suppl 2002;438:74 [PMID: 12477267].

Nuss R, Manco-Johnson M: Bleeding disorders in the neonate. Neoreviews 2000;e196.

Sackey K: Hemolytic anemia: Part 1. Pediatr Rev 1999; 20:152 [PMID: 10233172].

Widness JA: Pathophysiology, diagnosis, and prevention of neonatal anemia. Neoreviews 2000;1:e61.

# RENAL DISORDERS IN THE NEWBORN INFANT

Renal function depends on postconceptional age. The glomerular filtration rate (GFR) is 20 mL/min/1.73 m$^2$ in full-term neonates and 10–13 mL/min/1.73 m$^2$ in infants born at 28–30 weeks' gestation. The speed of maturation after birth also depends on postconceptional age. Creatinine can be used as a clinical marker of GFR. Values in the first month of life are shown in Table 1–26. Creatinine at birth reflects the maternal level and should decrease slowly over the first 3–4 weeks. An increasing serum creatinine is never normal. The ability to concentrate urine and retain sodium also depends on gestational age. Infants born at less than 28–30 weeks' gestation are compromised in this respect and if not observed carefully can become dehydrated and hyponatremic. Preterm infants also have an increased bicarbonate excretion and a low tubular maximum for glucose (approximately 120 mg/dL).

## RENAL FAILURE

Renal failure is most commonly seen in the setting of birth asphyxia, hypovolemia, or shock from any cause. The normal rate of urine flow is 1–3 mL/kg/h. After a hypoxic or ischemic insult, acute tubular necrosis may ensue. Typically, 2–3 days of anuria or oliguria is associated with hematuria, proteinuria, and a rise in serum creatinine. The period of anuria or oliguria is followed by a period of polyuria and then gradual recovery. During the polyuric phase, excessive urine sodium and bicarbonate losses may be seen.

The initial step in management is restoration of the infant's volume status as needed. Thereafter, restriction of fluids to insensible water loss (40–60 mL/kg/d) without added electrolytes, plus milliliter-for-milliliter urine replacement, should be instituted. Serum and urine electrolytes and body weights should be followed frequently. These measures should be continued through the polyuric phase. After urine output has been reestablished, urine replacement should be decreased to between 0.5 and 0.75 mL for each milliliter of urine output to see if the infant has regained normal function. If that is the case, the infant can be returned to maintenance fluids.

Finally, many of these infants experience fluid overload and should be allowed to lose enough water through urination to return to birth weight. Hyperkalemia, which may become life-threatening, may occur in this situation despite the lack of added IV potassium. If the serum potassium reaches 7–7.5 mEq/L, therapy should be started with glucose and insulin infusion, giving 1 unit of insulin for every 3 g of glucose administered, in addition to binding resins. Calcium chloride (20 mg/kg bolus) and correction of metabolic acidosis with bicarbonate are also be helpful for arrhythmia resulting from hyperkalemia.

Peritoneal dialysis is occasionally needed for the management of neonatal acute renal failure.

## URINARY TRACT ANOMALIES

Abdominal masses in the newborn are most frequently caused by renal enlargement. Most common is a multicystic or dysplastic kidney; congenital hydronephrosis is second in frequency. Chromosomal abnormalities and syndromes with multiple anomalies frequently include renal abnormalities. An ultrasound examination is the first step in diagnosis. In pregnancies associated with oligohydramnios, renal agenesis or obstruction secondary to posterior urethral valves should be considered. Only bilateral disease or disease in a solitary kidney is associated with oligohydramnios, significant morbidity, and death. Such infants will generally also have pulmonary hypoplasia and die from pulmonary rather than renal insufficiency.

Prenatal ultrasonography identifies infants with renal anomalies (most often hydronephrosis) prior to birth. Postnatal evaluation of these infants should include renal ultrasound and a voiding cystourethrogram at about 1–6 weeks of age, depending on the severity of the antenatal findings. Until genitourinary reflux is ruled out, these infants should receive antibiotic prophylaxis with low-dose penicillin or amoxicillin.

## RENAL VEIN THROMBOSIS

Renal vein thrombosis occurs most often in IDMs and in the context of dehydration and polycythemia. Of particular concern is the IDM who is also poly-

**Table 1–26.** Normal values of serum creatinine (mg/dL).

| Gestational Age at Birth (weeks) | Postnatal Age (days) | |
|---|---|---|
| | 0–2 | 28 |
| < 28 | 1.2 | 0.7 |
| 29–32 | 1.1 | 0.6 |
| 33–36 | 1.1 | 0.45 |
| 36–42 | 0.8 | 0.3 |

cythemic. If fetal distress is superimposed on these problems, prompt reduction in blood viscosity is indicated. Thrombosis usually begins in intrarenal venules and can extend into larger veins. Clinically, the kidney may be enlarged, and blood and protein may be in the urine. With bilateral renal vein thrombosis, anuria ensues. Diagnosis can be confirmed with an ultrasound examination that includes Doppler flow studies of the kidneys. Treatment involves correcting the predisposing condition and systemic heparinization for the thrombosis. Use of thrombolytics for this condition is controversial. Prognosis for a full recovery is uncertain. Some infants will go on to develop significant atrophy of the affected kidney and systemic hypertension.

Kennedy WA: Assessment and management of fetal hydronephrosis. Neoreviews 2002;3:e214.

Saphier CJ et al: Prenatal diagnosis and management of abnormalities in the urologic system. Clin Perinatol 2000;27:921 [PMID: 11816494].

Schmidt B: The etiology, diagnosis, and treatment of thrombotic disorders in newborn infants: A call for international and multi-institutional studies. Semin Perinatol 1997;21:86 [PMID: 9190037].

# ■ NEUROLOGIC PROBLEMS IN THE NEWBORN INFANT

## SEIZURES

### ESSENTIALS OF DIAGNOSIS & TYPICAL FEATURES

- *Usual onset at 12–48 hours*
- *Most common seizure type is characterized by a constellation of findings*
- *Most common causes include hypoxic-ischemic encephalopathy, intracranial bleeds, and infection*

Newborns rarely have well-organized tonic-clonic seizures because of their incomplete cortical organization and a preponderance of inhibitory synapses. The most common type of seizure is characterized by a constellation of findings, including horizontal deviation of the eyes with or without jerking; eyelid blinking or fluttering; sucking, smacking, drooling, and other oral-buccal movements; swimming, rowing, or paddling

movements; and apneic spells. Strictly tonic or multifocal clonic episodes are also seen.

## Clinical Findings

The differential diagnosis of neonatal seizures is presented in Table 1–27. Most neonatal seizures occur between 12 and 48 hours of age. Later onset seizures suggest meningitis, benign familial seizures, or hypocalcemia. Information regarding antenatal drug use, the presence of birth asphyxia or trauma, and family history (regarding inherited disorders) should be obtained. Physical examination focuses on neurologic features, other signs of drug withdrawal, concurrent signs of infection, dysmorphic features, and intrauterine growth. Screening work-up should include blood glu-

**Table 1–27.** Differential diagnosis of neonatal seizures.

| Diagnosis | Comment |
| --- | --- |
| Hypoxic-ischemic encephalopathy | Most common cause (60%), onset in first 24 hours |
| Intracranial hemorrhage | Up to 15% of cases, periventricular-intraventricular hemorrhage, subdural or subarachnoid bleeding, stroke |
| Infection | 12% of cases |
| Hypoglycemia | Small for gestational age, infant of a diabetic mother (IDM) |
| Hypocalcemia, hypomagnesemia | Infant of low birth weight, IDM |
| Hyponatremia | Rare, seen with syndrome of inappropriate secretion of antidiuretic hormone (SIADH) |
| Disorders of amino and organic acid metabolism, hyperammonemia | Associated acidosis, altered level of consciousness |
| Pyridoxine dependency | Seizures refractory to routine therapy; cessation of seizures after administration of pyridoxine |
| Developmental defects | Other anomalies, chromosomal syndromes |
| Drug withdrawal | |
| No cause found | 10% of cases |
| Benign familial neonatal seizures | |

cose, ionized calcium, and electrolytes in all cases. Further work-up depends on diagnoses suggested by the history and physical examination. If there is any suspicion of infection, a spinal tap should be done. Hemorrhages and structural disease of the CNS can be addressed with real-time ultrasound and CT scan. Infarctions are most easily seen on diffusion-weighted MRI scan. Metabolic work-up should be pursued when appropriate. EEG should be done; the presence of spike discharges must be noted and the background wave pattern evaluated. Not infrequently, correlation between EEG changes and clinical seizure activity is absent.

### Treatment

Adequate ventilation and perfusion should be ensured. Hypoglycemia should be treated immediately with a 2 mL/kg infusion of $D_{10}W$ followed by 6 mg/kg/min of $D_{10}W$ (100 mL/kg/d). Other treatments such as calcium or magnesium infusion and antibiotics are indicated to treat hypocalcemia, hypomagnesemia, and suspected infection. Electrolyte abnormalities should be corrected. Phenobarbital, 20 mg/kg IV, should be administered to stop seizures. Supplemental doses of 5 mg/kg can be used if seizures persist, up to a total of 40 mg/kg. In most cases, phenobarbital controls seizures. If seizures continue, therapy with phenytoin, sodium valproate, or lorazepam may be indicated. For refractory seizures, a trial of pyridoxine is indicated.

### Prognosis

Outcome is related to the underlying cause of the seizure. The outcomes for hypoxic-ischemic encephalopathy and intraventricular hemorrhage have been discussed earlier in this chapter. In these settings, seizures that are difficult to control carry a poor prognosis for normal development. Seizures resulting from hypoglycemia, infection of the CNS, some inborn errors of metabolism, and developmental defects also have a high rate of poor outcome. Seizures caused by hypocalcemia or isolated subarachnoid hemorrhage generally resolve without sequelae.

## HYPOTONIA

One should be alert to the diagnosis of congenital hypotonia when a mother has polyhydramnios and a history of poor fetal movement. The newborn may present with poor respiratory effort and birth asphyxia. For a discussion of causes and evaluation, see Chapter 23.

## INTRACRANIAL HEMORRHAGE[1]

### 1. Subdural Hemorrhage

Subdural hemorrhage is related to birth trauma; the bleeding is caused by tears in the veins that bridge the subdural space. Prospective studies relating incidence to specific obstetric complications are not available.

The most common site of subdural bleeding is in ruptured superficial cerebral veins with blood over the cerebral convexities. These hemorrhages can be asymptomatic or may cause seizures, with onset on days 2–3 of life, vomiting, irritability, and lethargy. Associated findings include retinal hemorrhages and a full fontanelle. The diagnosis is confirmed by CT scan.

Specific treatment entailing needle drainage of the subdural space is rarely necessary. Most infants survive; 75% are normal on follow-up.

### 2. Primary Subarachnoid Hemorrhage

Primary subarachnoid hemorrhage is the most common type of neonatal intracranial hemorrhage. In the full-term infant, it can be related to trauma of delivery, whereas subarachnoid hemorrhage in the preterm infant is seen in association with germinal matrix hemorrhage. Clinically, these hemorrhages can be asymptomatic or can present with seizures and irritability on day 2 or, rarely, a massive hemorrhage with a rapid downhill course. The seizures associated with subarachnoid hemorrhage are very characteristic—usually brief, with a normal examination interictally. Diagnosis can be suspected on spinal tap and confirmed with CT scan. Long-term follow-up is uniformly good.

### 3. Neonatal Stroke

Focal cerebral ischemic injury can occur in the context of intraventricular hemorrhage in the premature infant and hypoxic ischemic encephalopathy. Neonatal stroke has also been described in the context of underlying disorders of thrombolysis and maternal drug use (cocaine). In some cases, the origin is unclear. The injury often occurs antenatally. The most common clinical presentation of an isolated cerebral infarct is with seizures, and diagnosis can be confirmed acutely with diffusion-weighted MRI scan. The most frequently described distribution is that of the middle cerebral artery.

Treatment is directed at controlling seizures. Long-term outcome is variable, ranging from normal to hemiplegias and cognitive deficits.

---

[1]Intraventricular hemorrhage is discussed in the section on Care of the Premature Infant.

Brunquell PJ et al: Prediction of outcome based on clinical seizure type in newborn infants. J Pediatr 2002;140:707 [PMID: 12072874].

Hill A: Neonatal seizures. Pediatr Rev 2000;21:117 [PMID: 10756174].

Levene M: The clinical conundrum of neonatal seizures. Am J Dis Child Fetal Neonatal Ed 2002;86:F75 [PMID: 11882546].

Mercuri E et al: Prothrombotic disorders and abnormal neurodevelopmental outcome in infants with neonatal cerebral infarction. Pediatrics 2001;107:1400 [PMID: 11389264].

# METABOLIC DISORDERS IN THE NEWBORN INFANT[2]

## HYPERGLYCEMIA

Hyperglycemia may develop in preterm infants, particularly those of extremely low birth weight who are also SGA. Glucose concentrations may exceed 200–250 mg/dL, particularly in the first few days of life. This transient diabetes-like syndrome usually lasts approximately 1 week.

Management may include simply reducing glucose intake while continuing to supply IV amino acids to prevent protein catabolism with resultant gluconeogenesis. IV insulin infusions will be needed in infants who remain hyperglycemic despite glucose infusion rates of only 5–6 mg/kg/min or less.

## HYPOCALCEMIA

Calcium concentration in the immediate newborn period decreases in all newborn infants. The concentration in fetal plasma is higher than that of the neonate or adult. Hypocalcemia is usually defined as a total serum concentration less than 7 mg/dL (equivalent to a calcium activity of 3.5 mEq/L), although the physiologically active fraction, ionized calcium, should be measured whenever possible. Ionized calcium is usually normal even when total calcium is as low as 6–7 mg/dL. An ionized calcium of greater than 0.9 mmol/L (1.8 mEq/L; 3.6 mg/dL) is not likely to be detrimental.

### Clinical Findings

The clinical signs of hypocalcemia and hypocalcemic tetany include a high-pitched cry, jitteriness, tremulousness, and seizures.

Hypocalcemia tends to occur at two different times in the neonatal period. Early-onset hypocalcemia occurs in the first 2 days of life and has been associated with prematurity, maternal diabetes, asphyxia, and, rarely, maternal hypoparathyroidism. Late-onset hypocalcemia occurs at approximately 7–10 days and is observed in infants receiving modified cow's milk rather than infant formula (high phosphorus intake) or in infants with hypoparathyroidism (DiGeorge syndrome, 22q11 deletion). Mothers in Third-World countries often have vitamin D deficiency, which can also contribute to late-onset hypocalcemia.

## TREATMENT

### A. ORAL CALCIUM THERAPY

The oral administration of calcium salts, often along with vitamin D, is the preferred method of treatment for chronic forms of hypocalcemia resulting from hypoparathyroidism (see Chapter 30).

### B. INTRAVENOUS CALCIUM THERAPY

IV calcium therapy is usually needed for infants with symptomatic hypocalcemia or an ionized calcium less than 0.9 mmol/L. A number of precautions must be observed when calcium gluconate is given intravenously. The infusion must be given slowly so that there is no sudden increase in calcium concentration of blood entering the right atrium, which could cause severe bradycardia and even cardiac arrest. Furthermore, the infusion must be observed carefully, because an IV infiltrate containing calcium can cause full-thickness skin necrosis requiring grafting. For these reasons, IV calcium therapy should be given judiciously and through a central venous line if possible. IV administration of 10% calcium gluconate is usually given as a bolus of 100–200 mg/kg (1–2 mL/kg) over approximately 10–20 minutes, followed by a continuous infusion (0.5–1 g/kg/d) over 1–2 days. Ten percent calcium chloride (20 mg/kg or 0.2 mL/kg per dose) may result in a larger increment in ionized calcium and greater improvement in mean arterial blood pressure in sick hypocalcemic infants and thus may have a role in the newborn. *Note:* Calcium salts cannot be added to IV solutions that contain sodium bicarbonate because they precipitate as calcium carbonate.

## Prognosis

The prognosis is good for neonatal seizures entirely caused by hypocalcemia that is promptly treated.

[2]Hypoglycemia is discussed in the section on Common Problems in the Term Newborn Infant.

# INBORN ERRORS OF METABOLISM

The individual inborn errors of metabolism are rare, but collectively have an incidence of 1/1000 live births. Expanded newborn genetic screening will undoubtedly aid in the diagnosis of these disorders. Nevertheless, many infants will present prior to these results being available. The diseases are considered in detail in Chapter 32. These diagnoses should be entertained when infants who were initially well present with sepsis-like syndromes, recurrent hypoglycemia, neurologic syndromes (seizures, altered levels of consciousness), or unexplained acidosis (suggestive of organic acidemias).

In the immediate neonatal period, urea cycle disorders present as an altered level of consciousness secondary to hyperammonemia. A clinical clue that supports this diagnosis is hyperventilation with primary respiratory alkalosis, along with a lower than expected blood urea nitrogen. The other major diagnostic category to consider consists of infants with severe acidemia secondary to organic acidemias.

Burton BK: Inborn errors of metabolism in infancy: A guide to diagnosis. Pediatrics 1998;102:e69 [PMID: 9832597].

Enns GM, Packman S: Diagnosing inborn errors of metabolism in the newborn: clinical features. Neoreviews 2001;2:e183.

Hemachandra AH, Cowett RM: Neonatal hyperglycemia. Pediatric Rev 1999;20:e16.

# REFERENCES

Christensen RD (ed): *Hematologic Problems of the Neonate.* WB Saunders, 2000.

Eichenfeld LF et al (eds): *Textbook of Neonatal Dermatology.* WB Saunders, 2001.

Fanaroff AA, Martin RJ (eds): *Neonatal-Perinatal Medicine. Diseases of the Fetus and Infant,* 7th ed. Mosby, 2002.

Goldsmith JP, Karotkin EH (eds): *Assisted Ventilation of the Neonate,* 4th ed. WB Saunders, 2003.

Jones KL (ed): *Smith's Recognizable Patterns of Human Malformation,* 5th ed. WB Saunders, 1997.

Klaus MH, Fanaroff AA (eds): *Care of the High-Risk Neonate,* 5th ed. WB Saunders, 2001.

Remington JS, Klein JO (eds): *Infectious Diseases of the Fetus and Newborn Infant,* 5th ed. WB Saunders, 2001.

Thureen PJ et al (eds): *Assessment and Care of the Well Newborn.* WB Saunders, 1999.

Volpe JJ (ed): *Neurology of the Newborn,* 4th ed. WB Saunders, 2000.

Young TE, Mangum OB (ed): *Neofax 2002,* 15th ed. Acorn Publishing, 2000.

### Web Resources

[Cochrane neonatal database]
www.nichd.nih.gov/cochraneneonatal/
[Neoreviews]
http://neoreviews.aapjournals.org/
[Neonatal resuscitation program]
www.aap.org/profed/nrp/nrpmain.html

# Child Development & Behavior

2

*Edward Goldson, MD, & Ann Reynolds, MD*

Child development encompasses all aspects of pediatrics. It applies to somatic, psychological, and cognitive growth and to behavior. The developmental principle, that is, the concept of ongoing change and maturation, is integral to the daily practice of pediatrics. For example, we recognize that a 3-month-old infant is very different from a 3-year-old and from a 13-year-old adolescent, not only with respect to what the child can do but also in terms of the kind of illness he or she might have. This perspective is unique to pediatrics, separating it from other fields of medicine. Although the principles of child development have been the domain of the general pediatrician, the field of developmental and behavioral pediatrics has emerged as a subspecialty that addresses not only typical development but also the diagnosis and evaluation of atypical behavior and development.

This chapter does not attempt to cover the entire field of developmental and behavioral pediatrics. Instead, it focuses on three distinct areas. First, it discusses normal development but does not cover the newborn period or adolescence (see Chapters 1 and 3, respectively). Second, it addresses behavioral variations, emphasizing that these variations reflect the spectrum of normal development and not pathology. Third, it deals with developmental and behavioral disorders and their treatment.

## ■ I. NORMAL DEVELOPMENT

### THE FIRST YEAR

Normal children follow a trajectory of increasing physical size (Figures 2–1 to 2–10) and increasing complexity of function (Figures 2–7, 2–8 and Tables 2–1, 2–2). Growth charts provide an overview of the normal growth trajectory of children, thus alerting the clinician to what is atypical. Table 2–3 provides the theoretical perspectives of human behavior, taking into consideration the work of Freud, Erikson, and Piaget.

The first 5 years of life are a period of extraordinary physical growth and increasing complexity of function. The child triples his or her birth weight within the first year and achieves two thirds of his or her brain size by age 2½ to 3 years. The child progresses from a totally dependent infant at birth to a mobile, verbal person who is able to express his or her needs and desires by age 2–3 years. In the ensuing 2–3 years the child further develops the capacity to interact with peers and adults, achieves considerable verbal and physical prowess, and becomes ready to enter the academic world of learning and socialization.

It is critical for the clinician to identify disturbances in development during these early years because there may be windows of time or sensitive periods when appropriate interventions may be instituted to effectively treat developmental problems. Numerous screening tools are available to identify children with developmental disturbances; however, the clinician can use certain principles to identify problems without resorting to formal screening measures. From a motor perspective, children develop in a cephalocaudal direction. They can lift their heads with good control at 3 months, sit independently at 6 months, crawl at 9 months, walk at 1 year, and run by 18 months. The child learning to walk has a wide-based gait at first. Next, he or she walks with legs closer together, the arms move medially, a heel–toe gait develops, and the arms swing symmetrically by 18 to 24 months.

Clinicians often focus on gross motor development, but an appreciation of fine motor development and dexterity, particularly the grasp, can be instructive not only in monitoring normal development but also in identifying deviations in development. The grasp begins as a raking motion involving the ulnar aspect of the hand at age 3–4 months. The thumb is added to this motion at about age 5 months as the focus of the movement shifts to the radial side of the hand. The thumb opposes the fingers for picking up objects just before age 7 months, and the neat pincer grasp emerges at about age 9 months. Most young children have symmetrical movements. Asymmetries of movement noted in the first 2–3 years of life, be they facial asymmetries or gross motor asymmetries, should be investigated. This is particularly true if other developmental delays are present or if the child has a history of adverse experiences such as prematurity or intracranial hemorrhage. Children should not have a hand preference at 1 year of age and typically develop handedness between 18 and 30 months.

*Figure 2–1.* Percentile standards for length for age and weight for age in girls, birth to age 36 months. (Centers for Disease Control and Prevention.)

**Girls, birth to 36 months**

Name _____

HEAD CIRCUMFERENCE FOR AGE AND WEIGHT FOR LENGTH PERCENTILES

Record # _____

***Figure 2–2.*** Percentile standards for head circumference for age and weight for length in girls, birth to age 36 months. (Centers for Disease Control and Prevention.)

## Boys, birth to 36 months

Name _____

**LENGTH FOR AGE AND WEIGHT FOR AGE PERCENTILES**

Record # _____

***Figure 2–3.*** Percentile standards for length for age and weight for age in boys, birth to age 36 months. (Centers for Disease Control and Prevention.)

## Boys, birth to 36 months

Name _____

**HEAD CIRCUMFERENCE FOR AGE AND WEIGHT FOR LENGTH PERCENTILES**     Record # _____

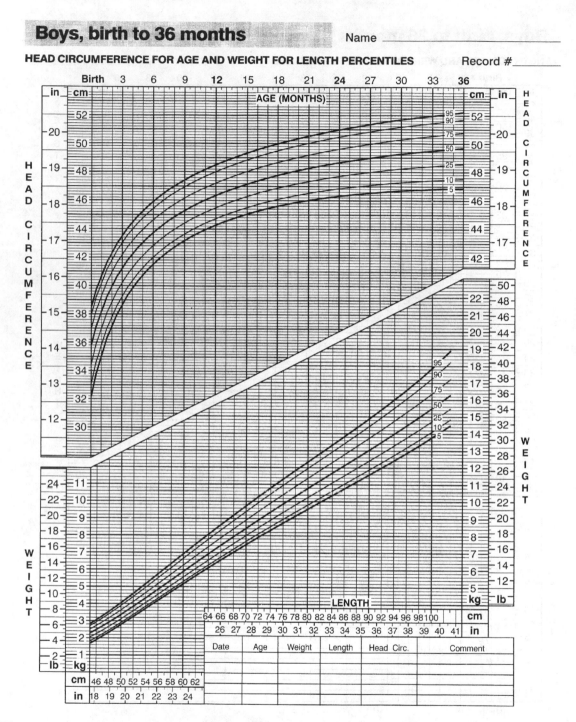

***Figure 2–4.*** Percentile standards for head circumference for age and weight for length in boys, birth to age 36 months. (Centers for Disease Control and Prevention.)

# Girls, 2 to 20 years

Name _____

## STATURE FOR AGE AND WEIGHT FOR AGE PERCENTILES

Record # _____

*Figure 2–5.* Percentile standards for stature for age and weight for age in girls, 2–20 years. (Centers for Disease Control and Prevention.)

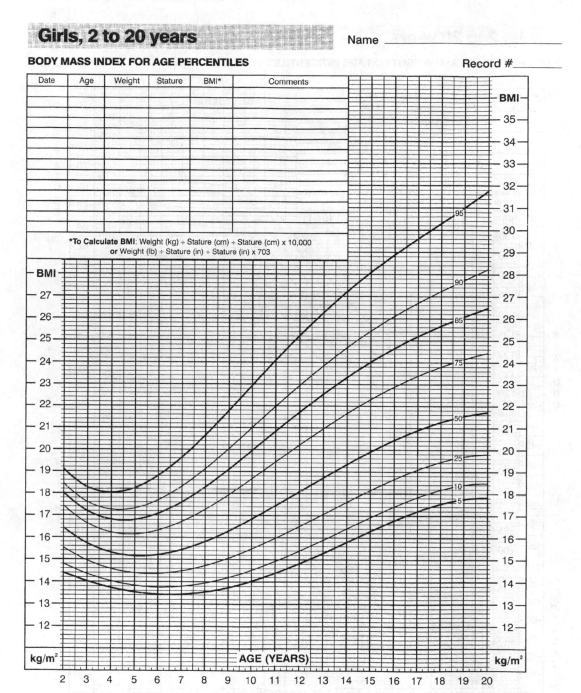

**Girls, 2 to 20 years**                                      Name _____

**BODY MASS INDEX FOR AGE PERCENTILES**                      Record #_____

| Date | Age | Weight | Stature | BMI* | Comments |
|------|-----|--------|---------|------|----------|
|      |     |        |         |      |          |

*To Calculate BMI: Weight (kg) ÷ Stature (cm) ÷ Stature (cm) x 10,000
or Weight (lb) ÷ Stature (in) ÷ Stature (in) x 703

***Figure 2–6.*** Percentile standards for body mass index for age in girls, 2–20 years. (Centers for Disease Control and Prevention.)

# Boys, 2 to 20 years

Name _____

**STATURE FOR AGE AND WEIGHT FOR AGE PERCENTILES**

Record # _____

***Figure 2–7.*** Percentile standards for stature for age and weight for age in boys, 2–20 years. (Centers for Disease Control and Prevention.)

**Figure 2–8.** Percentile standards for body mass index for age in boys, 2–20 years. (Centers for Disease Control and Prevention.)

***Figure 2–9.*** Head circumference of girls. (Modified and reproduced, with permission, from Nelhaus G: Pediatrics 1968;41:106.)

Language is a critical area to consider as well. Children usually have 5–10 comprehensible words by age 1 year; by age 2 years they are putting 2–3 words into phrases, 50% of which their caregivers can understand (see Tables 2–1 and 2–2 and Figure 2–11).

One may easily memorize the developmental milestones that characterize the trajectory of the typical child; however, these milestones become more mean-

ingful and clinically useful if placed in empirical and theoretical contexts. The work of Piaget and others is quite instructive and provides some insight into behavioral and affective development (see Table 2–3). Piaget described the first 2 years of life as the sensorimotor period, during which Infants learn with increasing sophistication how to link sensory input from the environment with a motor response. Infants build on primitive

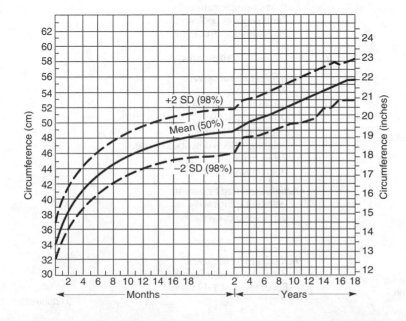

***Figure 2–10.*** Head circumference of boys. (Modified and reproduced, with permission, from Nelhaus G: Pediatrics 1968;41:106.)

***Table 2–1.*** Developmental charts.

___

**1–2 months**

***Activities to be observed:***
Holds head erect and lifts head.
Turns from side to back.
Regards faces and follows objects through visual field.
Drops toys.
Becomes alert in response to voice.

***Activities related by parent:***
Recognizes parents.
Engages in vocalizations.
Smiles spontaneously.

**3–5 months**

***Activities to be observed:***
Grasps cube—first ulnar then later thumb opposition.
Reaches for and brings objects to mouth.
Makes "raspberry" sound.
Sits with support.

***Activities related by parent:***
Laughs.
Anticipates food on sight.
Turns from back to side.

**6–8 months**

***Activities to be observed:***
Sits alone for a short period.
Reaches with one hand.
First scoops up a pellet then grasps it using thumb opposition.
Imitates "bye-bye."
Passes object from hand to hand in midline.
Babbles.

***Activities related by parent:***
Rolls from back to stomach.
Is inhibited by the word *no.*

**9–11 months**

***Activities to be observed:***
Stands alone.
Imitates pat-a-cake and peek-a-boo.
Uses thumb and index finger to pick up pellet.

***Activities related by parent:***
Walks by supporting self on furniture.
Follows one-step verbal commands, eg, "Come here," "Give it to me."

**1 year**

***Activities to be observed:***
Walks independently.
Says "mama" and "dada" with meaning.
Can use a neat pincer grasp to pick up a pellet.
Releases cube into cup after demonstration.

Gives toys on request.
Tries to build a tower of 2 cubes.

***Activities related by parent:***
Points to desired objects.
Says 1 or 2 other words.

**18 months**

***Activities to be observed:***
Builds tower of 3–4 cubes.
Throws ball.
Scribbles spontaneously.
Seats self in chair.
Dumps pellet from bottle.

***Activities related by parent:***
Walks up and down stairs with help.
Says 4–20 words.
Understands a 2-step command.
Carries and hugs doll.
Feeds self.

**24 months**

***Activities to be observed:***
Speaks short phrases, 2 words or more.
Kicks ball on request.
Builds tower of 6–7 cubes.
Points to named objects or pictures.
Jumps off floor with both feet.
Stands on either foot alone.
Uses pronouns.

***Activities related by parent:***
Verbalizes toilet needs.
Pulls on simple garment.
Turns pages of book singly.
Plays with domestic mimicry.

**30 months**

***Activities to be observed:***
Walks backward.
Begins to hop on one foot.
Uses prepositions.
Copies a crude circle.
Points to objects described by use.
Refers to self as I.
Holds crayon in fist.

***Activities related by parent:***
Helps put things away.
Carries on a conversation.

**3 years**

***Activities to be observed:***
Holds crayon with fingers.
Builds tower of 9–10 cubes.

(*continued*)

***Table 2–1.*** Developmental charts. (continued)

Imitates 3-cube bridge.
Copies circle.
Gives first and last name.

**Activities related by parent:**
Rides tricycle using pedals.
Dresses with supervision.

### 3–4 years

**Activities to be observed:**
Climbs stairs with alternating feet.
Begins to button and unbutton.
"What do you like to do that's fun?" (Answers using plurals, personal pronouns, and verbs.)
Responds to command to place toy *in, on,* or *under* table.
Draws a circle when asked to draw a person.
Knows own sex. ("Are you a boy or a girl?")
Gives full name.
Copies a circle already drawn. ("Can you make one like this?")

**Activities related by parent:**
Feeds self at mealtime.
Takes off shoes and jacket.

### 4–5 years

**Activities to be observed:**
Runs and turns without losing balance.
May stand on one leg for at least 10 seconds.
Buttons clothes and laces shoes. (Does not tie.)
Counts to 4 by rote.
"Give me 2 sticks." (Able to do so from pile of 4 tongue depressors.)
Draws a person. (Head, 2 appendages, and possibly 2 eyes. No torso yet.)
Knows the days of the week. ("What day comes after Tuesday?")
Gives appropriate answers to: "What must you do if you are sleepy? Hungry? Cold?"
Copies + in imitation.

**Activities related by parent:**
Self-care at toilet. (May need help with wiping.)
Plays outside for at least 30 minutes.
Dresses self except for tying.

### 5–6 years

**Activities to be observed:**
Can catch ball.
Skips smoothly.
Copies a + already drawn.
Tells age.
Concept of 10 (eg, counts 10 tongue depressors). May recite to higher number by rote.

Knows right and left hand.
Draws recognizable person with at least 8 details.
Can describe favorite television program in some detail.

**Activities related by parent:**
Does simple chores at home (eg, taking out garbage, drying silverware).
Goes to school unattended or meets school bus.
Good motor ability but little awareness of dangers.

### 6–7 years

**Activities to be observed:**
Copies a Δ.
Defines words by use. ("What is an orange?" "To eat.")
Knows if morning or afternoon.
Draws a person with 12 details.
Reads several one-syllable printed words. (My, dog, see, boy.)
Uses pencil for printing name.

### 7–8 years

**Activities to be observed:**
Counts by 2s and 5s.
Ties shoes.
Copies a ◊.
Knows what day of the week it is. (Not date or year.)
Reads paragraph #1 Durrell:

*Reading:*
Muff is a little yellow kitten. She drinks milk. She sleeps on a chair. She does not like to get wet.

*Corresponding arithmetic:*

$$\begin{array}{cccc} 7 & 6 & 6 & 8 \\ +4 & +7 & -4 & -3 \end{array}$$

No evidence of sound substitution in speech (eg, *fr* for *thr*).
Adds and subtracts one-digit numbers.
Draws a man with 16 details.

### 8–9 years

**Activities to be observed:**
Defines words better than by use. ("What is an orange?" "A fruit.")
Can give an appropriate answer to the following:
"What is the thing for you to do if . . .
—you've broken something that belongs to someone else?
—a playmate hits you without meaning to do so?"
Reads paragraph #2 Durrell:

*Reading:*
A little black dog ran away from home. He played with two big dogs. They ran away from him. It began to rain. He

*(continued)*

**Table 2–1.** Developmental charts. (continued)

went under a tree. He wanted to go home, but he did not know the way. He saw a boy he knew. The boy took him home.

*Corresponding arithmetic:*

$$\begin{array}{cccc} 45 & & & \\ 67 & 16 & 14 & 84 \\ +\ 4 & +27 & -\ 8 & -36 \\ \hline \end{array}$$

Is learning borrowing and carrying processes in addition and subtraction.

### 9–10 years

**Activities to be observed:**
Knows the month, day, and year.
Names the months in order. (15 seconds, 1 error.)
Makes a sentence with these 3 words in it: (1 or 2. Can use words orally in proper context.)
   1. work . . . money . . . men
   2. boy . . . river . . . ball
Reads paragraph #3 Durrell:

*Reading:*
Six boys put up a tent by the side of a river. They took things to eat with them. When the sun went down, they went into the tent to sleep. In the night, a cow came and began to eat grass around the tent. The boys were afraid. They thought it was a bear.

*Corresponding arithmetic:*

$$\begin{array}{ccc} 5204 & 23 & 837 \\ -\ 530 & \times\ 3 & \times\ 7 \\ \hline \end{array}$$

Should comprehend and answer the question: "What was the cow doing?"
Learning simple multiplication.

### 10–12 years

**Activities to be observed:**
Should read and comprehend paragraph #5 Durrell:
*Reading:*
In 1807, Robert Fulton took the first long trip in a steamboat. He went one hundred and fifty miles up the Hudson River. The boat went five miles an hour. This was

faster than a steamboat had ever gone before. Crowds gathered on both banks of the river to see this new kind of boat. They were afraid that its noise and splashing would drive away all the fish.

*Corresponding arithmetic:*

$$\begin{array}{ccc} 420 & & \\ \times\ 29 & 9\overline{)72} & 31\overline{)62} \\ \hline \end{array}$$

Answer: "What river was the trip made on?"
Ask to write the sentence: "The fishermen did not like the boat."
Should do multiplication and simple division.

### 12–15 years

Activities to be observed:
Reads paragraph #7 Durrell:

*Reading:*
Golf originated in Holland as a game played on ice. The game in its present form first appeared in Scotland. It became unusually popular and kings found it so enjoyable that it was known as "the royal game." James IV, however, thought that people neglected their work to indulge in this fascinating sport so that it was forbidden in 1457. James relented when he found how attractive the game was, and it immediately regained its former popularity. Golf spread gradually to other countries, being introduced in America in 1890. It has grown in favor until there is hardly a town that does not boast of a private or public course.

*Corresponding arithmetic:*

$$\begin{array}{ccc} 536\overline{)4762} & \dfrac{1}{3} & 7\dfrac{1}{6} \\ & +\dfrac{1}{3} & -\dfrac{3}{4} \end{array}$$

Reduce fractions to lowest forms.

Ask to write a sentence: "Golf originated in Holland as a game played on ice."
Answers questions:
"Why was golf forbidden by James IV?"
"Why did he change his mind?"
Does long division, adds and subtracts fractions.

Modified from Leavitt SR, Goodman H, Harvin D: Pediatrics 1963;31:499.

reflex patterns of behavior (termed schemata; sucking is an example) and constantly incorporate or assimilate new experiences. The schemata evolve over time as infants accommodate new experiences and as new levels of cognitive ability unfold in an orderly sequence. Enhancement of neural networks through dendritic branching occurs in spurts throughout the sensorimotor period. In the first year of life, the infant's percep-

tion of reality revolves around itself and what it can see or touch. The infant follows the trajectory of an object through the field of vision, but before age 6 months the object ceases to exist once it leaves the infant's field of vision. At age 9–12 months, the infant gradually develops the concept of object permanence, or the realization that objects exist even when not seen. The development of object permanence correlates with enhanced

**Table 2–2.** Normal speech and language development.

| Age | Speech | Language | Articulation |
|---|---|---|---|
| 1 month | Throaty sounds | | Vowels: \ah\, \uh\, \ee\ |
| 2 months | Vowel sounds ("eh"), coos | | |
| 2½ months | Squeals | | |
| 3 months | Babbles, initial vowels | | |
| 4 months | Guttural sounds ("ah," "go") | | Consonants, m, p, b |
| 5 months | | | Vowels: \o\, \u\ |
| 7 months | Imitates speech sounds | | |
| 8 months | | | Syllables: da, ba, ka |
| 10 months | | "Dada" or "mama" nonspecifically | Approximates names: baba/bottle |
| 12 months | Jargon begins (own language) | One word other than "mama" or "dada | Understandable: 2–3 words |
| 13 months | | Three words | |
| 16 months | | Six words | Consonants: t, d, w, n, h |
| 18–24 months | | Two-word phrases | Understandable 2-word phrases |
| 24–30 months | | Three-word phrases | Understandable 3-word phrases |
| 2 years | Vowels uttered correctly | Approximately 270 words; uses pronouns | Approximately 270 words; uses phrases |
| 3 years | Some degree of hesitancy and uncertainty common | Approximately 900 words; intelligible 4-word phrases | Approximately 900 words; intelligible 4 word phrases |
| 4 years | | Approximately 1540 words; intelligible 5-word phrases or sentences | Approximately 1540 words; intelligible 5-word phrases |
| 6 years | | Approximately 2560 words; intelligible 6- or 7-word sentences | Approximately 2560 words; intelligible 6- or 7-word sentences |
| 7–8 years | Adult proficiency | | |

Data on articulation from Berry MF: *Language Disorders of Children.* Appleton-Century-Crofts, 1969; and from Bzoch K, League R: *Receptive-Expressive Emergent Language Scale.* University Park Press, 1970.

frontal activity on the electroencephalogram. The concept attaches first to the image of the mother or primary caregiver because of his or her emotional importance and is a critical part of attachment behavior (discussed later). In the second year, children extend their ability to manipulate objects by using instruments, first by imitation and later by trial and error.

Freud described the first year of life as the oral stage because so many of the infant's needs are fulfilled by oral means. Nutrition is obtained through sucking on the breast or bottle, and self-soothing occurs through sucking on fingers or a pacifier. During this stage of symbiosis with the mother, the boundaries between mother and infant are blurred. The baby's needs are totally met by the mother, and the mother has been de-

scribed as manifesting "narcissistic possessiveness" of the infant. This is a very positive interaction in the bidirectional attachment process called bonding. The parents learn to be aware of and to interpret the infant's cues, which reflect its needs. A more sensitive emotional interaction process develops that can be seen in the mirroring of facial expressions by the primary caregiver and infant and in their mutual engagement in cycles of attention and inattention, which further develop into social play. A parent who is depressed or cannot respond to the baby's expressions and cues can have a profoundly adverse effect on the child's future development. Erikson's terms of basic trust versus mistrust are another way of describing the reciprocal interaction that characterizes this stage.

***Table 2–3.*** Perspectives of human behavior.

| Age | Theories of Development | | | Skill Areas | | Psychopathology |
|---|---|---|---|---|---|---|
| | **Freud** | **Erikson** | **Piaget** | **Language** | **Motor** | |
| Birth to 18 months | Oral | Basic trust versus mistrust | Sensorimotor | Body actions; crying; naming; pointing | Reflex sitting, reaching, grasping, walking | Autism; anaclitic depression, colic; disorders of attachment; feeding, sleeping problems |
| 18 months–3 years | Anal | Autonomy versus shame, doubt | Symbolic (preoperational) | Sentences; telegraph jargon | Climbing, running | Separation issues; negativism; fearfulness; constipation; shyness, withdrawal |
| 3–6 years | Oedipal | Initiative versus guilt | Intuition (preoperational) | Connective words; can be readily understood | Increased coordination; tricycle; jumping | Enuresis; encopresis; anxiety; aggressive acting out; phobias; nightmares |
| 6–11 years | Latency | Industry versus inferiority | Concrete operational | Subordinate sentences; reading and writing; language reasoning | Increased skills; sports, recreational cooperative games | School phobias; obsessive reactions; conversion reactions; depressive equivalents |
| 12–17 years | Adolescence (genital) | Identity versus role confusion | Formal operational | Reason abstract; using language; abstract manipulation | Refinement of skills | Delinquency; promiscuity; schizophrenia; anorexia nervosa; suicide |

Adapted and reproduced, with permission, from Dixon S: Setting the stage: Theories and concepts of child development. In Dixon S, Stein M (eds): *Encounters with Children,* 2nd ed. Year Book, 1992.

Turn-taking games, which occur between ages 3 and 6 months, are a pleasure for both the parents and the infant and are an extension of mirroring behavior. They also represent an early form of imitative behavior, which is important in later social and cognitive development. More sophisticated games, such as peek-a-boo, occur at approximately age 9 months. The infant's thrill at the reappearance of the face that vanished momentarily demonstrates the emerging understanding of object permanence.

Age 8–9 months is also a critical time in the attachment process because this is when separation anxiety and stranger anxiety become marked. The infant at this stage is able to appreciate discrepant events that do not match previously known schemata. These new events cause uncertainty and subsequently fear and anxiety. The infant must be able to retrieve previous schemata and incorporate new information over an extended time. These abilities are developed by age 8 months and give rise to the fears that subsequently develop: stranger anxiety and separation anxiety. In stranger anxiety, the infant analyzes the face of a stranger, detects the mismatch with previous schemata, and responds with fear or anxiety, leading to crying. In separation anxiety, the child perceives the difference between the primary caregiver's presence and her absence by remembering the schema of her presence. Perceiving the inconsistency, the child first becomes uncertain and then anxious and fearful. This begins at age 8 months, reaches a peak at 15 months, and disappears by the end of 2 years in a relatively orderly progression as central nervous system (CNS) maturation facilitates the development of new skills. A parent can put the child's understanding of object permanence to good use by placing a picture of the mother near the child or by leaving an object (eg, her sweater) where the child can see it during her absence. A visual substitute for the mother's presence may comfort the child.

## THE SECOND YEAR

Once the child can walk independently, it can move away from the parent and explore the environment. Although the child uses the mother as "home base," returning to her frequently for reassurance, he or she has now taken a major step toward independence. This is the beginning of mastery over the environment and an emerging sense of self. The "terrible twos" and the frequent self-asserting use of "no" are the child's attempt to develop a better idea of what is or might be under its

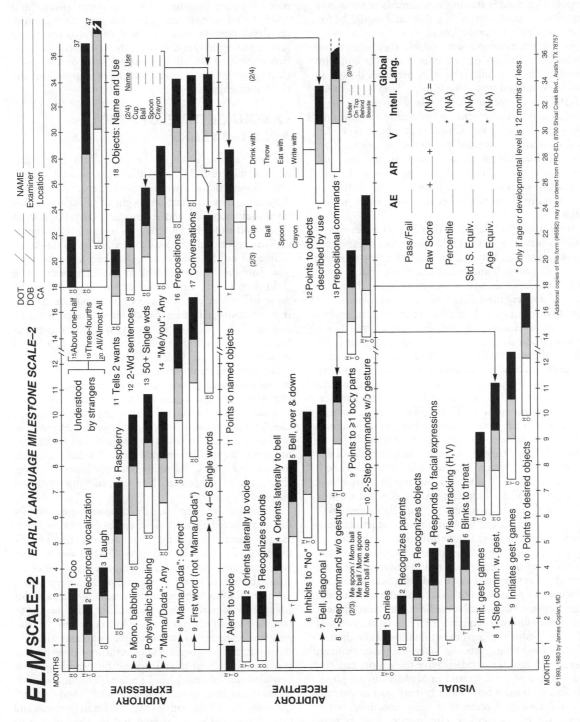

**Figure 2–11.** Early Language Milestone Scale-2. (Reproduced, with permission, from Coplan J: *Early Language Milestone Scale.* Pro Ed, 1993.)

81

control. The child is starting to assert his or her autonomy. Ego development during this time should be fostered but with appropriate limits.

As children develop a sense of self, they begin to understand the feelings of others and develop empathy. They hug another child who is in perceived distress or become concerned when one is hurt. They begin to understand how another child feels when he or she is harmed, and this realization helps them to inhibit their own aggressive behavior. Children also begin to understand right and wrong and parental expectations. They recognize that they have done something "bad" and may signify that awareness by saying "uh-oh" or with other expressions of distress. They also take pleasure in their accomplishments and become more aware of their bodies.

An area of child behavior that has often been overlooked is play. Play is the child's work and a significant means of learning. Play is a very complex process whose purpose can include the practice and rehearsal of roles, skills, and relationships; a means of revisiting the past; a means of actively mastering a range of experiences; and a way to integrate the child's life experiences. It involves emotional development (affect regulation, gender identification and roles), cognitive development (nonverbal and verbal function, executive functioning and creativity), and social/motor development (motor coordination, frustration tolerance, and social interactions such as turn taking). Of interest is the fact that play has a developmental progression. The typical 6- to 12-month-old engages in the game of peek-a-boo, which is a form of social interaction. During the next year or so, although children engage in increasingly complex social interactions and imitation, their play is primarily solitary. However, they do begin to engage in symbolic play such as by drinking from a toy cup and then by giving the doll a drink from a toy cup. By the second to third year children begin to engage in parallel play (engaging in behaviors that are imitative). This form of play gradually evolves into more interactive or collaborative play by the fourth year and is also more thematic in nature. There are of course wide variations in the development of play, reflecting cultural, educational, and socioeconomic variables. Nevertheless, the development of play does follow a sequence that can be assessed and can be very informative in the evaluation of the child.

Brain maturation sets the stage for toilet training. After age 18 months, toddlers have the sensory capacity for awareness of a full rectum or bladder and are physically able to control bowel and urinary tract sphincters. They also take great pleasure in their accomplishments, particularly in appropriate elimination, if it is reinforced positively. Children must be given some control over when elimination occurs. If parents impose severe restrictions, the achievement of this developmental milestone can become a battle between parent and child. Freud termed this period the anal stage because the developmental issue of bowel control is the major task requiring mastery. It encompasses a more generalized theme of socialized behavior and overall body cleanliness, which is usually taught or imposed on the child at this age.

# LANGUAGE DEVELOPMENT: AGES 1–4 YEARS

Communication is important from birth (see Table 2–2 and Figure 2–11), particularly the nonverbal, reciprocal interactions between infant and caregiver. By age 2 months, these interactions begin to include vocalizations such as cooing and reciprocal vocal play between parent and child. Babbling begins by age 6–10 months, and the repetition of sounds such as "da-da-da-da" is facilitated by the child's increasing oral muscular control. Babbling reaches a peak at age 12 months. The child then moves into a stage of having needs met by using individual words to represent objects or actions. It is common at this age for children to express wants and needs by pointing to objects or using other gestures. The acquisition of expressive vocabulary varies greatly between 12 and 24 months of age. As a group, males and children who are bilingual tend to develop expressive language more slowly during that time. It is important to note, however, that for each individual, milestones should still fall within the expected range. Gender and exposure to two languages should never be used as an excuse for failing to refer a child who has significant delay for further evaluation. It is also important to note that most children are not truly bilingual. Most children have one primary language, and any other languages are secondary.

Receptive language usually develops more rapidly than expressive language. Word comprehension increases at age 9 months, and by age 13 months the child's receptive vocabulary may be as large as 20–100 words. After age 18 months, expressive and receptive vocabularies increase dramatically, and by the end of the second year a quantum leap in language development permits a major advance in cognitive development. The child begins to put together words and phrases and begins to use language to represent a new world, the symbolic world. At this time, children begin to put verbs into their phrases and focus much of their language on describing their new abilities, for example, "I go out." They incorporate prepositions into speech and ask "why?" and "what?" questions more frequently. They also begin to appreciate time factors and to understand and use this concept in their speech (see Table 2–1).

The Early Language Milestone (ELM) Scale (see Figure 2–11) is a simple tool for assessing early language development in the pediatric office setting. It is scored in the same way as the Denver II (Figure 2–12) but tests receptive and expressive language areas in greater depth.

Piaget characterized the 2- to 6-year-old stage as preoperational. This stage begins when language has facilitated the creation of mental images in the symbolic sense. The child begins to manipulate the symbolic world; sorts out reality from fantasy imperfectly; and may be terrified of dreams, wishes, and foolish threats. Most of the child's perception of the world is egocentric or interpreted in reference to his or her needs or influence. Cause–effect relationships are confused with temporal ones or interpreted egocentrically. For example, children may focus their understanding of divorce on themselves ("My father left because I was bad" or "My mother left because she didn't love me"). Illness and the need for medical care are also commonly misinterpreted at this age. The child may make a mental connection between a sibling's illness and a recent argument, a negative comment, or a wish for the sibling to be ill. The child may experience significant guilt unless the parents are aware of these misperceptions and take time to deal with them.

At this age, children also endow inanimate objects with human feelings. They also assume that humans cause or create all natural events. For instance, when asked why the sun sets, they may say, "The sun goes to his house" or "It is pushed down by someone else." Magical thinking blossoms between ages 3 and 5 years as symbolic thinking incorporates more elaborate fantasy. Fantasy facilitates development of role playing, sexual identity, and emotional growth. Children test new experiences in fantasy, both in their imagination and in play. In their play, children often create magical stories and novel situations that reflect issues with which they are dealing, such as aggression, relationships, fears, and control. Children often invent imaginary friends at this time, and nightmares or fears of monsters are common. At this stage, other children become important in facilitating play, such as in a preschool group. Play gradually becomes more cooperative; shared fantasy leads to game playing. Freud described the oedipal phase between ages 3 and 6 years, when there is strong attachment to the parent of the opposite sex. The child's fantasies may focus on playacting the adult role with that parent, although by age 6 years oedipal issues are usually resolved and attachment is redirected to the parent of the same sex.

## EARLY SCHOOL YEARS: AGES 5–7 YEARS

Attendance at kindergarten at age 5 years marks an acceleration in the separation–individuation theme initiated in the preschool years. The child is ready to relate to peers in a more interactive manner. The brain has reached 90% of its adult weight. Sensorimotor coordination abilities are maturing and facilitating pencil-and-paper tasks and sports, both part of the school experience. Cognitive abilities are still at the preoperational stage, and children focus on one variable in a problem at a time. However, most children have mastered conservation of length by age 5½ years, conservation of mass and weight by 6½ years, and conservation of volume by 8 years.

By first grade, there is more pressure on the child to master academic tasks—recognizing numbers, letters, and words and learning to write. Piaget described the stage of concrete operations beginning after age 6 years, when the child is able to perform mental operations concerning concrete objects that involve manipulation of more than one variable. The child is able to order, number, and classify because these activities are related to concrete objects in the environment and because these activities are stressed in early schooling. Magical thinking diminishes greatly at this time, and the reality of cause–effect relationships is better understood. Fantasy and imagination are still strong and are reflected in themes of play.

## MIDDLE CHILDHOOD: AGES 7–11 YEARS

Freud characterized ages 7–11 years as the latency years, during which children are not bothered by significant aggressive or sexual drives but instead devote most of their energies to school and peer group interactions. In reality, throughout this period there is a gradual increase in sex drive, manifested by increasingly aggressive play and interactions with the opposite sex. Fantasy still has an active role in dealing with sexuality before adolescence, and fantasies often focus on movie and music stars. Organized sports, clubs, and other activities are other modalities that permit preadolescent children to display socially acceptable forms of aggression and sexual interest.

For the 7-year-old child, the major developmental tasks are achievement in school and acceptance by peers. Academic expectations intensify and require the child to concentrate on, attend to, and process increasingly complex auditory and visual information. Children with significant learning disabilities or problems of attention span may have difficulty in these tasks and subsequently may receive negative reinforcement from teachers and even parents. Such children may develop a poor self-image manifested as behavioral difficulties. The pediatrician must evaluate potential learning disabilities in any child who is not developing adequately at this stage or who presents with emotional or behav-

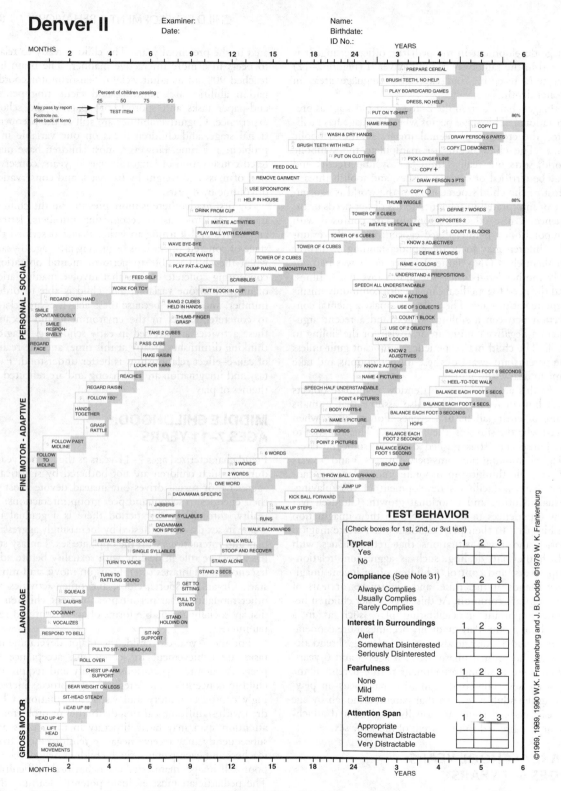

**Figure 2–12.** Denver II. (Copyright © 1969, 1989, 1990 WK Frankenburg and JB Dodds. © 1978 WK Frankenberg.)

ioral problems. The developmental status of school-age children is not documented as easily as that of younger children because of the complexity of the milestones. In the school-age child, the quality of the response, the attentional abilities, and the child's emotional approach to the task can make a dramatic difference in success at school. The clinician must consider all of these aspects in the differential diagnosis of learning disabilities.

Bayley N (ed): *Bayley Scales of Infant Development,* 2nd ed. Psychological Corporation, 1993.

Billeaud FP: *Communication Disorders in Infants and Toddlers,* Andover Medical, 1993.

Bjorklund FP: *Children's Thinking.* Brooks/Cole, 1995.

Dixon SD, Stein MT: *Encounters with Children: Pediatric Behavior and Development,* 3rd ed. Mosby-Year Book, 2000.

Frankenberg WK et al. The Denver II: A major revision and restandardization of the Denver Developmental Screening Test. Pediatrics 1991;89:91.

Glascoe FP, Dworkin PH: The role of parents in the detection of developmental and behavioral problems. Pediatrics 1995;95:829 [PMID: 7539122].

Green M, Palfrey JS (eds): *Bright Futures: Guidelines for Health Supervision of Infants, Children, and Adolescents,* 2nd ed revised. National Center for Education in Maternal and Child Health Georgetown University, 2002.

Levine MD, Carey WB, Crocker AC (eds): *Developmental-Behavioral Pediatrics,* 3rd ed. WB Saunders, 1999.

Parker S, Zuckerman B (eds): *Behavioral and Developmental Pediatrics: A Handbook for Primary Care.* Little, Brown, 1995.

## ■ II. BEHAVIORAL & DEVELOPMENTAL VARIATIONS

Behavioral and developmental variations and disorders encompass a wide range of issues of importance to pediatricians. Practitioners will be familiar with most of the problems discussed in this chapter; however, with increasing knowledge of the factors controlling normal neurologic and behavioral development in childhood, new perspectives on these disorders and novel approaches to their diagnosis and management are emerging.

Variations in children's behavior reflect a blend of intrinsic biologic characteristics and the environments with which the children interact. The next section focuses on some of the more common complaints about behavior encountered by those who care for children. These behavioral complaints are by and large normal variations in behavior, a reflection of each child's individual biologic and temperament traits and the parents' responses. There are no cures for these behaviors, but management strategies are available that can enhance

the parents' understanding of the child and the child's relationship to the environment. These strategies also facilitate the parents' care of the growing infant and child.

The last section of this chapter discusses developmental disorders of cognitive and social competence. Diagnosis and management of these conditions requires a comprehensive and often multidisciplinary approach. The health care provider can play a major role in diagnosis, in coordinating the child's evaluation, in interpreting the results to the family, and in providing reassurance and support.

Capute AJ, Accardo PJ (eds): *Developmental Disabilities in Infancy and Childhood,* 2nd ed. Vol 1, *Neurodevelopmental Diagnosis and Treatment.* Vol. 2, *The Spectrum of Developmental Disabilities.* Brookes/Cole, 1996.

Greydanus DE, Wolraich ML (eds): *Behavioral Pediatrics.* Springer, 1992.

Levine MD, Carey WB, Crocker AC (eds): *Developmental-Behavioral Pediatrics,* 3rd ed. WB Saunders, 1999.

Parker S, Zuckerman B (eds): *Behavioral and Developmental Pediatrics: A Handbook for Primary Care.* Little, Brown, 1995.

Wolraich ML (ed): *Disorders of Development and Learning: A Practical Guide to Assessment and Management,* 2nd ed. Mosby, 1996.

Wolraich ML, Felice ME, Drotar D: *The Classification of Child and Adolescent Mental Diagnoses in Primary Care: Diagnostic and Statistical Manual for Primary Care (DSM-PC) Child and Adolescent Version.* American Academy of Pediatrics, 1996.

## NORMALITY & TEMPERAMENT

The physician confronted by a disturbance in physiologic function rarely has doubts about what is abnormal. Variations in temperament and behavior are not as straightforward. Labeling such variations as disorders implies that a disease entity exists.

The behaviors described in this section are viewed as part of a continuum of responses by the child to a variety of internal and external experiences. Variations in temperament have been of interest to philosophers and writers since ancient times. The Greeks believed there were four temperament types: choleric, sanguine, melancholic, and phlegmatic. In more recent times, folk wisdom has defined temperament as a genetically influenced behavioral disposition that is stable over time. Although a number of models of temperament have been proposed, the one usually used by pediatricians in clinical practice is that of Thomas and Chess, who describe temperament as being the "how" of behavior as distinguished from the "why" (motivation) and the "what" (ability). Temperament is an independent psychological attribute that is expressed as a response to an external stimulus. The influence of temperament is bidirectional: The effect of a particular experience will be influenced by the child's temperament, and the child's temperament will influence the responses of others in the child's environment. Temperament is the style with which the child interacts with the environment.

The perceptions and expectations of parents must be considered when a child's behavior is evaluated. A child that one parent might describe as hyperactive might not be characterized as such by the other parent. This truism can be expanded to include all the dimensions of temperament. Thus, the concept of "goodness of fit" comes into play. For example, if the parents want and expect their child to be predictable but that is not the child's behavioral style, the parents may perceive the child as being bad or having a behavioral disorder rather than as having a developmental variation. An appreciation of this phenomenon is important because the physician may be able to enhance the parents' understanding of the child and influence their responses to the child's behavior. When there is goodness of fit, there will be more harmony and a greater potential for healthy development not only of the child but also of the family. When goodness of fit is not present, tension and stress can result in parental anger, disappointment, frustration, and conflict with the child.

Other models of temperament include those of Rothbart, Buss and Plomin, and Goldsmith and Campos (Table 2–4). All models seek to identify intrinsic behavioral characteristics that lead the child to respond to the world in particular ways. One child may be

**Table 2–4.** Theories of temperament.

| Thomas and Chess | Temperament is an independent psychologic attribute, biologically determined, which is expressed as a response to an external stimulus. It is the child's behavioral style: an interactive model. |
|---|---|
| Rothbart | Temperament is a function of biologically based individual differences in reactivity and self-regulation. It is subsumed under the concept of "personality" and goes beyond mere "behavioral style." |
| Buss and Plomin | Temperament is a set of genetically determined personality traits that appear early in life and are different from other inherited and acquired personality traits. |
| Goldsmith and Campos | Temperament is the individual's differences in the probability of experiencing emotions and arousal. |

highly emotional and another less so (ie, calmer) in response to a variety of experiences, stressful or pleasant. The clinician must recognize that each child brings some intrinsic, biologically based traits to its environment and that such characteristics are neither good nor bad, right nor wrong, normal nor abnormal; they are simply part of the child. Thus, as one looks at variations in development, one should abandon the illness model and consider this construct as an aid to understanding the nature of the child's behavior and its influence on the parent–child relationship.

Barr RG: Normality: A clinically useless concept: The case of infant crying and colic. J Dev Behav Pediatr 1993;14:264 [PMID: 8408670].

Goldsmith HH et al: Roundtable: What is temperament? Four approaches. Child Dev 1987;58:505 [PMID: 3829791].

Prior M: Childhood temperament. J Child Psychol Psychiatr 1992;33:249 [PMID: 1737829].

Thomas A, Chess S: *Temperament and Development.* Brunner/Mazel, 1977.

# COMMON DEVELOPMENTAL CONCERNS

## COLIC

Infant colic is characterized by severe and paroxysmal crying that occurs mainly in the late afternoon. The infant's knees are drawn up and its fists are clenched, flatus is expelled, the facies is "pained," and there is minimal response to attempts at soothing. Studies in the United States have shown that among middle-class infants, crying occupies about 2 hours per day at 2 weeks of age, about 3 hours per day by 6 weeks, and gradually decreases to about 1 hour per day by 3 months. The word "colic" is derived from Greek *kolikos* ("pertaining to the colon"). Although colic has traditionally been attributed to gastrointestinal disturbances, this has never been proved. Colic is a behavioral sign or symptom that begins in the first few weeks of life and peaks at age 2–3 months. In about 30–40% of cases, colic continues into the fourth and fifth months.

A colicky infant, as defined by Wessel, is one who is healthy and well fed but cries for more than 3 hours a day, for more than 3 days a week, and for more than 3 weeks—commonly referred to as the rule of threes. The important word in this definition is "healthy." Thus, before the diagnosis of colic can be made, the pediatrician must rule out diseases that might cause crying. With the exception of the few infants who respond to elimination of cow's milk from its own or the mother's diet, there has been little firm evidence of an association of colic with allergic disorders. Gastroesophageal reflux is often suspected as a cause of colicky crying in young infants. Undetected corneal abrasion, urinary tract infection, and unrecognized traumatic injuries including child abuse must be among the physical causes of crying considered in evaluating these infants. Some attempts have been made to eliminate gas with simethicone and to slow gut motility with dicyclomine. Simethicone has not been shown to ameliorate colic. Dicyclomine has been associated with apnea in infants and is contraindicated.

This then leaves characteristics intrinsic to the child (ie, temperament) and parental caretaking patterns as contributing to colic. Behavioral states have three features: (1) they are self-organizing—that is, they are maintained until it is necessary to shift to another one; (2) they are stable over several minutes; and (3) the same stimulus elicits a state-specific response that is different from other states. The behavioral states are (among others) a crying state, a quiet alert state, an active alert state, a transitional state, and a state of deep sleep. The states of importance with respect to colic are the crying state and the transitional state. During transition from one state to another, infant behavior may be more easily influenced. Once an infant is in a stable state (eg, crying), it becomes more difficult to bring about a change (eg, to soothe). How these transitions are accomplished is probably influenced by the infant's temperament and neurologic maturity. Some infants move from one state to another easily and can be diverted easily; other infants sustain a particular state and are resistant to change.

The other component to be considered in evaluating the colicky infant is the feeding and handling behavior of the caregiver. Colic is a behavioral phenomenon that involves interaction between the infant and the caregiver. Different caregivers perceive and respond to crying behavior differently. If the caregiver perceives the crying infant as being spoiled and demanding and is not sensitive to or knowledgeable about the infant's cues and rhythms—or is hurried and "rough" with the baby—the infant's ability to organize and soothe itself or respond to the caregiver's attempts at soothing may be compromised. Alternatively, if the temperament of an infant with colic is understood and the rhythms and cues deciphered, crying can be anticipated and the caregiver can intervene before the behavior becomes "organized" in the crying state and more difficult to extinguish.

## Management of Colic

A number of approaches can be taken to the management of colic.

1. Parents may need to be educated about the developmental characteristics of crying behavior and made aware that crying increases normally into the second month and abates by the third to fourth month.

2. Parents may need reassurance, based on a complete history and physical examination, that the infant is not sick. Although these behaviors are stressful, they are a normal variant and are usually self-limited. This discussion can be facilitated by having the parent keep a diary of crying and weight gain. If there is a diurnal pattern and adequate weight gain, an underlying disease process is less likely to be present. Parental anxiety must be relieved, because it may be contributing to the problem.

3. For parents to effectively soothe and comfort the infant, they need to understand the baby's cues. The pediatrician can help by observing the infant's behavior and devising interventions aimed at calming both the infant and the parents. One can encourage a quiet environment without excessive handling. Rhythmic stimulation such as gentle swinging or rocking, soft music, drives in the car, or walks in the stroller may be helpful, especially if the parents are able to anticipate the onset of crying. Another approach is to change the feeding habits so that the infant is not rushed, has ample opportunity to burp, and, if necessary, can be fed more frequently so as to decrease gastric distention if that seems to be contributing to the problem.

4. Medications such as phenobarbital elixir and dicyclomine have been found to be somewhat helpful, but their use is to be discouraged because of the risk of adverse reactions and overdosage. A trial of ranitidine hydrochloride might be of help if gastroesophageal reflux is contributing to the child's discomfort.

5. For colic that is refractory to behavioral management, a trial of changing the feedings, eliminating cow's milk from the formula, or from the mother's diet if she is nursing, may be indicated.

Barr RG et al (eds): *Crying as a Sign, a Symptom, and a Signal: Clinical, Emotional, and Developmental Aspects of Infant and Toddler Crying.* MacKeith Press, 2000.

Barr RG, Geertsma MA: Colic: The pain perplex. In: Schechter NL et al (eds): *Pain in Infants, Children and Adolescents.* Williams & Wilkins, 1993.

Barr RG: Colic and crying syndromes in infants. Pediatrics 1998;102:1282 [PMID: 9794970].

Dhigo SK: New strategies for the treatment of colic: Modifying the parent–infant interaction. J Pediatr Health Care 1998;12:256.

Lucassen PL et al: Effectiveness of treatments for infantile colic: A systematic review. Br Med J 1998;316:1563 [PMID: 1945549].

Miller AR, Barr RG: Infantile colic: Is it a gut issue? Pediatr Clin North Am 1991;38:1407.

Treem WR: Infant colic: A pediatric gastroenterologist's perspective. Pediatr Clin North Am 1994;41:1121 [PMID: 7936776].

# FEEDING DISORDERS IN INFANTS & YOUNG CHILDREN

Children have feeding problems for various reasons. The common denominator, however, is usually food refusal. Infants and young children may refuse to eat if they find eating painful or frightening. They may have had unpleasant experiences (emotional or physiologic) associated with eating, they may be depressed, or they may be engaged in a developmental conflict with the caregiver that is being played out in the arena of feeding. The infant may refuse to eat if the rhythm of the feeding experience with the caregiver is not harmonious. The child who has had an esophageal atresia repair and has a stricture may find eating uncomfortable. The very young infant with severe oral candidiasis may refuse to eat because of pain. The child who has had a choking experience associated with feeding may be terrified to eat (oral motor dysfunction or aspiration). The child who is forced to eat by a maltreating parent or an overzealous caregiver may refuse feeds. Children who have required nasogastric feedings or who have required periods of fasting and intravenous nutrition in the first 1–2 months of life are more likely to display food refusal behavior upon introduction of oral feedings.

Depression in children may be expressed through food refusal. Food refusal may develop when the infant's cues around feeding are not interpreted correctly by the parent. The baby who needs to burp more frequently or who needs time between bites but instead is rushed will often passively refuse to eat. Some will be more active refusers, turning their heads away to avoid the feeder, spitting out food, or pushing away food.

Chatoor and coworkers have proposed a developmental and interactive construct of the feeding experience. The stages through which the child normally progresses are establishment of homeostasis (0–2 months), attachment (2–6 months), and separation and individuation (6 months to 3 years). During the first stage, feeding can be accomplished most easily when the parent allows the infant to determine the timing, amount, pacing, and preference of food intake. During the attachment phase, allowing the infant to control the feeding permits the parent to engage the infant in a positive manner. This paves the way for the separation and individuation phase. When a disturbance occurs in the parent–child relationship at any of these developmental levels, difficulty in feeding may ensue, with both the parent and the child contributing to the dysfunctional interaction. One of the most striking manifestations of food refusal occurs during the stage of separation and individuation. Conflict may arise if the parent seeks to dominate the child by intrusive and controlling feeding behavior at the same time the child is striving to achieve autonomy. The scenario then observed is of the parent forcing food on the child while the child refuses to eat. This often leads to extreme parental frustration and anger, and the child may be inadequately nourished and developmentally and emotionally thwarted.

When the pediatrician is attempting to sort out the factors contributing to food refusal, it is essential first to obtain a complete history, including a social history. This should include information concerning the parents' perception of the child's behavior and their expectations of the child. Second, a complete physical examination should be performed, with emphasis on oral–motor behavior and other clues suggesting neurologic, anatomic, or physiologic abnormalities that could make feeding difficult. The child's emotional state and developmental level must be determined. This is particularly important if there is concern about depression or a history of developmental delays. If evidence of oral–motor difficulty is suspected, evaluation by an occupational therapist is warranted. Third, the feeding interaction needs to be observed live, if possible. Finally, the physician needs to help the parents understand that infants and children may have different styles of eating and different food preferences and may refuse foods they do not like. This is not necessarily abnormal but reflects temperamental differences and variations in the child's way of processing olfactory, gustatory, and tactile stimuli.

## Management of Feeding Disorders

The goal of intervention is to identify factors contributing to the disturbance and to work to overcome them. The parents may be encouraged to view the child's behavior differently and try not to impose their expectations and desires. Alternatively, the child's behavior may need to be modified so that the parents can provide adequate nurturing.

When the chief complaint is failure to gain weight, a different approach is required. The differential diagnosis should include not only food refusal but also medical disorders and maltreatment. The most common reason for failure to gain weight is inadequate caloric intake. Excessive weight loss may be due to vomiting or diarrhea, to malabsorption, or to a combination of these factors. In this situation more extensive diagnostic evaluation may be needed. Laboratory studies may include a complete blood count; erythrocyte sedimentation rate; urinalysis and urine culture; blood urea nitrogen; serum electrolytes and creatinine; and stool examination for fat, occult blood, and ova and parasites. Some practitioners also include liver and thyroid profiles. Occasionally an assessment of swallowing function or evaluation for the presence of gastroesophageal reflux may be indicated. Because of the complexity of the problem, a team approach to the diagnosis and treatment of failure to thrive, or poor weight gain, may be most appropriate. The team should include a physician, nurse, social worker, and dietitian. Occupational and physical therapists, developmentalists, and psychologists may be required.

The goals of treatment of the child with poor weight gain are to establish a normal pattern of weight gain and to establish better family functioning. Guidelines to accomplishing these goals include the following: (1) establish a comprehensive diagnosis that considers all factors contributing to poor weight gain; (2) monitor the feeding interaction and ensure appropriate weight gain; (3) monitor the developmental progress of the child and the changes in the family dynamics that facilitate optimal weight gain and psychosocial development; and (4) provide support to the family as they seek to help the child.

Benoit D: Phenomenology and treatment of failure to thrive. Child Adolesc Psychiatr Clin North Am 1993;2:61.

Macht J: *Poor Eaters*. Plenum, 1990.

Reilly SM et al: Oral–motor dysfunction in children who fail to thrive: Organic or non-organic. Dev Med Child Neurol 1999;41:115.

Skuse D: Epidemiologic and definitional issues in failure to thrive. Child Adolesc Psychiatr Clin North Am 1993;2:37.

Stevenson RD: Failure to thrive. In Greydanus DE, Wolraich ML (eds): *Behavioral Pediatrics*. Springer, 1992.

Wolraich ML (ed): *Disorders of Development and Learning*, 3rd ed. Hamilton: BC Decker, 2003

# SLEEP DISORDERS

Sleep is a complex physiologic process influenced by intrinsic biologic properties, temperament, cultural norms and expectations, and environmental conditions. Between 20% and 30% of children experience sleep disturbances at some point in the first 4 years of life. The percentage decreases to 10–12% in school-age children. Sleep disorders fall into two categories. Dyssomnias refer to problems with initiating and maintaining sleep or to excessive sleepiness. Parasomnias refer to abnormalities of arousal, partial arousal, and transitions between stages of sleep.

Sleep is controlled by two different biologic clocks. The first is a circadian rhythm—sleep occurs daily. The second is an ultradian rhythm that occurs several times per night—the stages of sleep. Sleep stages cycle every 50 to 60 minutes in infants to every 90 minutes in adolescents. The circadian clock has a 25-hour cycle. Environmental cues entrain the sleep–wake cycle into a 24-hour cycle. The cues are light–dark, ambient temperature, core body temperature, noise, social interaction, hunger, pain, and hormone production. Without the ability to perceive these cues (ie, blindness, autism) a child might have difficulty entraining a 24-hour sleep–wake cycle. Two major sleep stages have been identified clinically and with the use of polysomnography (electroencephalography, electro-oculography, and electromyelography): rapid eye movement (REM) and nonrapid eye movement (NREM) sleep. In REM sleep, muscle tone is relaxed, the sleeper may twitch and grimace, and the eyes move erratically beneath closed lids. In adults and children, REM sleep occurs throughout the night but is increased during the latter half of the night. NREM sleep is divided into four stages. In the process of falling asleep, the individual enters stage 1, light sleep, characterized by reduced bodily movements, slow eye rolling, and sometimes opening and closing of the eyelids. Stage 2 sleep is characterized by slowing of eye movements, slowing of respirations and heart rate, and relaxation of the muscles but with repositioning of the body. Some dreaming may occur in this stage. Most mature individuals spend about half of their sleep time in this stage. Stages 3 and 4 (also called delta or slow-wave sleep) are the deepest NREM sleep stages, during which the body is relaxed, breathing is slow and shallow, and the heart rate is slow.

The deepest NREM sleep occurs during the first 1–3 hours after going to sleep. Parasomnias occur during deep NREM sleep. Dreams and nightmares occur during REM sleep.

Sleep is clearly a developmental phenomenon. Infants are not born with a sleep–wake cycle. REM sleep is more common than NREM sleep in newborns and decreases by 3 to 6 months of age. Sleep spindles and vertex waves are usually not seen until 9 weeks of age. By 3 to 6 months, stage 1 through 4 NREM sleep can be seen. By 6 to 12 months an infant's electroencephalogram (EEG) can be read using adult criteria. Infants also do not make melatonin until 9 to 12 weeks of age. Melatonin is a hormone that decreases core body temperature and that appears to play a role in sleep onset and sleep maintenance. This hormone is sensitive to light, does cross the placenta, and is present in breast milk.

## 1. Parasomnias

Parasomnias, consisting of arousal from deep NREM sleep, are probably the most frightening for parents. They include night terrors, sleeptalking, and sleepwalking (somnambulism) (see Chapter 22).

## Night Terrors & Sleepwalking

Night terrors commonly occur within 2 hours after falling asleep, during the deepest stage of NREM sleep, and are often associated with sleepwalking. They occur in about 3% of children. During a night terror, the child may sit up in bed screaming, thrashing about, and exhibiting rapid breathing, tachycardia, and sweating. The child is often incoherent and unresponsive to comforting. The episode may last up to half an hour, after which the child goes back to sleep and has no memory of the event the next day. The parents must be reassured that the child is not in pain and that they should let the episode run its course.

Management of night terrors is by reassurance of the parents plus measures to avoid emotional and psychosocial stressors that might be contributing to the problem. Because sleepwalking can result in injury, the parents should determine, if possible, when the attacks usually occur and awaken the child to full arousal about 15 minutes before that time. After 4–5 minutes, the child may be allowed to return to sleep. The waking is discontinued once the terrors stop, which is usually within a week. In severe cases, pharmacologic interventions may be needed temporarily. Imipramine (25–50 mg at bedtime) may be useful. However, behavioral approaches to increase the total amount of sleep and to address the sources of anxiety and stress are of more long-term benefit.

## Nightmares

Nightmares are frightening dreams during REM sleep, typically followed by awakening, which usually occur in the latter part of the night. The peak occurrence is between ages 3 and 5 years, with an incidence between 25% and 50%. A child who awakens during these episodes is usually alert. He or she can often describe the frightening images, recall the dream, and talk about it during the day. The child seeks and will respond positively to parental reassurance. The child will often have difficulty going back to sleep and will want to stay with the parents. Nightmares are usually self-limited and need little treatment. If the child has recurrent nightmares, the pediatrician may have to make a more extensive investigation. Nightmares are often associated with stressful or frightening daytime events or anxieties such as frightening television programs, traumatic life events, and chronic stresses in the family. In severe cases, a psychologist or psychiatrist should be consulted.

## 2. Dyssomnias

The dyssomnias include problems going to sleep and nighttime awakenings. Although parasomnias are frightening, dyssomnias tend to be only annoying and frustrating. They can result in daytime fatigue for both the parents and the child, parental discord about management, and family disruption. A number of factors contribute to these disturbances. The quantity and timing of feeds in the first years of life will influence nighttime awakening. Most infants beyond age 6 months can go through the night without being fed. Thus, under normal circumstances, night waking for feeds is probably a learned behavior and is a function of the child's arousal and the parents' response to that arousal. Cosleeping (ie, sleeping with the parents) can play a role in night waking. In many cultures, cosleeping is accepted behavior. It is inappropriate behavior when it intrudes on the parents' rest and their sexual relationship. Bedtime habits can influence settling in for the night as well as nighttime awakening. If the child learns that going to sleep is associated with pleasant parental behavior such as rocking, singing, reading, or nursing, going back to sleep after nighttime arousal without these pleasant parental attentions may be difficult. The child's temperament is another factor contributing to sleep. It has been reported that children with low sensory thresholds and less rhythmicity are more prone to night waking. Children who have had perinatal difficulties such as intracranial hemorrhage and hyaline membrane disease have a greater incidence of night waking and difficulties returning to sleep. Finally, psychosocial stressors can play a role in night waking.

## Management of Sleep Disorders

A complete medical and psychosocial history should be obtained and a physical examination performed. A detailed sleep history and diary should be maintained to which both parents contribute. Some clinicians use polysomnography to complete the evaluation. Problems often arise when parents try to put the child to bed before he or she is biologically ready. The child might then lie awake and cry. In managing sleep difficulties, the child's individual sleep behavior characteristics must be taken into account and the parents' expectations and fears identified and addressed. Counseling is then provided on the following basis:

1. Sleep is a highly active and organized process that matures during the first years of life. One-week-old infants sleep about 16 hours a day, 6 of those hours during the daylight hours. A 2-year-old child sleeps a total of 13 hours a day, only 1 hour during the day.

2. Individual circadian rhythms do not change immediately; they require consistency and regularity over a period of time before change will occur.

**3.** The duration of sleep for a given individual does not vary significantly from day to day, but there is a wide range of normal.

**4.** The duration of nighttime sleep is correlated inversely with daytime sleep, and bedtimes and awakening times are correlated positively with each other.

**5.** Night waking occurs in 40–60% of infants and young children. If the child does not cry or wake up the parents, such behavior should not be considered a sleep disturbance.

Parents need to set limits for the child while acknowledging the child's individual biologic rhythms. They should resist the child's attempts to put off bedtime or to engage them during nighttime awakenings. Putting a child to bed after prolonged rocking, feeding, or when the child has already fallen asleep frequently results in disturbances of settling down at night or going back to sleep after a nighttime awakening. The goal is to establish clear bedtime rituals, to put the child to bed while still awake, and to create a quiet, secure bedtime environment.

For the child who has a delayed sleep phase—that is, difficulty in falling asleep and waking at desired times but no difficulty at a later hour—a regular schedule and consistent, nonstimulating bedtime rituals must be provided. Approaches used to alter the child's behavior include having the parents withdraw the attention elicited by the wakeful child and having them offer positive reinforcement of the desired behavior. Another strategy to alter this sleep pattern is to gradually move the bedtime to an earlier hour and awaken the child earlier in the morning. However, there is nothing intrinsically normal or abnormal in the delayed sleep phase. It becomes a problem only when it differs from parental expectations.

Some children are afraid to go to sleep. The parents need to help the child identify what is frightening about going to sleep and may need to stay near the child, reassuring the child that he or she is safe. Over a period of time, the child can be reassured and the parents may not need to be so involved. This also applies to nighttime awakenings.

The key to treatment of children who have difficulty going to sleep or who awaken during the night and disturb others is to recognize that both the child and the parents play significant roles in initiating and sustaining what may be an undesirable behavior. Thus, it becomes important for the physician and parents to understand normal sleep patterns, the parents' responses that inadvertently reinforce undesirable sleep behavior, and the child's individual temperament traits.

Chervin RD et al: Inattention, hyperactivity, and symptoms of sleep-disordered breathing. Pediatrics 2002;109(3):449 [PMID: 11875140].

Ferber R: Clinical assessment of child and adolescent sleep disorder. Child Adolesc Psychiatr Clin North Am 1996;5:569.

France KG et al: Fact, act, and tact: A three-stage approach to treating the sleep problems of infants and young children. Child Adolesc Psychiatr Clin North Am 1996;5:581 .

Mindel JA, Owens JA: *A Clinical Guide to Pediatric Sleep: Diagnosis and Management of Sleep Problems.* Lippincott Williams & Wilkins, 2003.

Mindell JA: Treatment of child and adolescent sleep disorders. Child Adolesc Psychiatr Clin North Am 1996;5:741.

Rosen GM et al: Evaluation of parasomnias in children. Child Adolesc Psychiatr Clin North Am 1996;5:601.

Wolfson AR: Sleeping patterns of children and adolescents: Development trends, disruptions and adaptations. Child Adolesc Psychiatr Clin North Am 1996;5:549.

www.kidzzzsleep.org

# TEMPER TANTRUMS & BREATH-HOLDING SPELLS

## 1. Temper Tantrums

Temper tantrums are common between ages 12 months and 4 years, occurring about once a week in 50–80% of children in this age group. The child may throw himself or herself down, kick and scream, strike out at people or objects in the room, and hold his or her breath. These behaviors may be considered normal as the young child seeks to achieve autonomy and mastery over the environment. They are often a reflection of immaturity as the child strives to accomplish age-appropriate developmental tasks and meets with difficulty because of inadequate motor and language skills, impulsiveness, or parental restrictions. In the home, these behaviors may be annoying. In public, they are embarrassing.

Some children tolerate frustration well, are able to persevere at tasks, and cope easily with difficulties; others have a much greater problem dealing with experiences beyond their developmental level. Parents can minimize tantrums by understanding the child's temperament and what he or she is trying to communicate. Parents must also be committed to supporting the child's drive to master his or her feelings.

## Management of Temper Tantrums

Appropriate intervention can provide an opportunity for enhancing the child's growth. The tantrum is a loss of control on the child's part that may be a frightening event and a blow to the child's self-image. The parents and the physician need to view these behaviors within the child's developmental context rather than from a negative, adversarial, angry perspective.

Several suggestions can be offered for parents and physicians in managing tantrums:

1. Minimize the need to say "no" by "child-proofing" the environment so that fewer restrictions need be enforced.

2. Use distraction when frustration increases; direct the child to other, less frustrating activities; and reward the positive response.

3. Present options within the child's capabilities so that he or she can achieve mastery and autonomy.

4. Fight only those battles that need to be won, and avoid those that arouse unnecessary conflict.

5. Do not abandon the preschool child when a tantrum occurs. Stay nearby during the episode without intruding. A small child may need to be restrained. An older child can be asked to go to his or her room. Threats serve no purpose and should not be used.

6. Do not use negative terms when the tantrum is occurring. Instead, point out that the child is out of control and give praise when he or she regains control.

7. Never let a child hurt himself or herself, or others.

8. Do not "hold a grudge" after the tantrum is over, but do not grant the child's demands that led to the tantrum.

9. Seek to maintain an environment that provides positive reinforcement for desired behavior. Do not overreact to undesired behavior, but set reasonable limits and provide responsible direction for the child.

10. Approximately 5–20% of young children have severe temper tantrums that are frequent and disruptive. Such tantrums may result from a disturbance in the parent–child interaction, poor parenting skills, lack of limit-setting, and permissiveness. They may be part of a larger behavioral or developmental disorder or may emerge under adverse socioeconomic conditions, in circumstances of maternal depression and family dysfunction, or when the child is in poor health. Referral to a psychologist or psychiatrist is appropriate while the pediatrician continues to support and work with the family.

## 2. Breath-Holding Spells

Whereas temper tantrums can be frustrating to parents, breath-holding spells can be terrifying. The name for this behavior may be a misnomer in that it connotes prolonged inspiration. In fact, breath-holding occurs during expiration and is reflexive—not volitional—in nature. It is a paroxysmal event occurring in 0.1–5% of healthy children from age 6 months to 6 years. The spells usually start during the first year of life, often in response to anger or a mild injury. The child is provoked or surprised, starts to cry—briefly or for a considerable time—and then falls silent in the expiratory phase of respiration. This is followed by a color change. Spells have been described as either pallid (acyanotic) or cyanotic, with the latter usually associated with anger and the former with an injury such as a fall. The spell may resolve spontaneously, or the child may lose consciousness. In severe cases, the child may become limp and progress to opisthotonos, body jerks, and urinary incontinence. Only rarely does a spell proceed to asystole or a seizure.

## Management of Breath-Holding Spells

For the child with frequent spells, underlying disorders such as seizures, orthostatic hypotension, obstructive sleep apnea, abnormalities of the CNS, tumors, familial dysautonomia, and Rett syndrome need to be considered. An association exists among breath-holding spells, pica, and iron deficiency anemia. These conditions can be ruled out on the basis of the history, physical examination, and laboratory studies. Once it has been determined that the child is healthy, the focus of treatment is behavioral. Parents should be taught to handle the spells in a matter-of-fact manner and monitor the child for any untoward events. The reality is that parents cannot completely protect the child from upsetting and frustrating experiences and probably should not try to do so. Just as in temper tantrums, parents need to help the child control his or her responses to frustration. Parents need to be careful not to be too permissive and submit to the child's every whim for fear the child might have a spell. If loss of consciousness occurs, the child should be placed on his or her side to protect against head injury and aspiration. Maintaining a patent oral airway is essential, but cardiopulmonary resuscitation should be avoided. There are no prophylactic medications. Atropine, 0.01 mg/kg given subcutaneously, has been used with some benefit in spells accompanied by bradycardia or asystole.

Breningstall GN: Breath holding spells. Pediatr Neurol 1996;14:91 [PMID: 8703234].

DiMario FJ Jr: Breath-holding spells in childhood. Am J Dis Child 1992;146:125 [PMID: 1736640].

Greene RW: *The Explosive Child.* Quill, 2001.

Needleman R et al: Temper tantrums: When to worry. Contemporary Pediatrics 1989;6:12.

Needleman R et al: Psychosocial correlates of severe temper tantrums. J Dev Behav Pediatr 1991;12:77.

# ■ III. DEVELOPMENTAL DISORDERS

Developmental disorders include problems with one or more aspects of development, such as verbal, motor, visual–spatial, attentional, and social abilities. These problems are diagnosed by comparing the child's performance level with norms accumulated from observation and testing of children of the same age. Problems with development are often noted by parents when a child does not meet normal motor and language milestones. Developmental disorders may also include difficulties with behavior or attention. Attention-deficit/hyperactivity disorder (ADHD) is the most common neurodevelopmental problem known. ADHD occurs in 2–10% of school-age children and may occur in combination with a variety of other learning or developmental problems. Mild developmental disorders are often not noted until the child is of school age.

Many biologic and psychosocial factors may influence a child's performance on developmental tests. In the assessment of the child, it is important to document adverse psychosocial factors, such as neglect or poverty, which can negatively influence developmental progress. Many of the biologic factors that influence development are genetic and are discussed throughout this section.

## Evaluation

The neurodevelopmental evaluation must focus on (1) defining the child's level of developmental abilities in a variety of domains, including language, motor, visual–spatial, attentional, and social abilities; (2) characterizing the reason for the child's developmental delays; and (3) planning a treatment program for the developmental problems. These objectives are best achieved by a multidisciplinary team that includes the physician, a psychologist, a speech or language therapist, an occupational therapist, and an educational specialist. The psychologist will usually carry out standardized testing of intellectual ability appropriate to the child's age. The motor and language specialists will also carry out clinical testing to document the deficits in their areas and to organize a treatment program. The educational specialist will usually carry out academic testing for the school-age child and plan a course of special education support through the school. The physician is usually the integrator of the information from the team and

must also obtain a detailed medical and developmental history and conduct the physical and neurologic exam.

## Medical and Neurodevelopmental Examination

The medical history should begin with pregnancy, labor, and delivery to identify conditions that might compromise the child's CNS. The physician must ask the child's parents about exposures to toxins, alcohol, drugs, smoking, and infections; maternal chronic illness; prematurity; subsequent newborn course; and complications (eg, intraventricular hemorrhage or hypoxic insult). Problems such as failure to thrive, chronic illnesses, hospitalizations, and abuse can interfere significantly with normal development. If the newborn course has been complicated, then information should be obtained from the hospital where treatment was provided. The occurrence of problems such as apnea, bradycardic episodes, and hyperbilirubinemia should be documented.

The physician should review and document the child's temperament, difficulties with feeding, and subsequent developmental milestones. The child's development in expressive and receptive language skills, motor coordination, and emotions should be discussed in detail. The child's difficulties with tantrums, attentional problems, impulsivity, hyperactivity, or aggression should be documented.

Major illnesses or hospitalizations should be discussed. Any CNS problems, such as trauma, infection, or encephalitis should be documented. The presence of metabolic diseases, such as diabetes or phenylketonuria, and exposure to environmental toxins such as lead should be determined. Chronic diseases such as chronic otitis media infections, hyper- or hypothyroidism, and chronic renal failure can interfere with normal development. The presence of motor or vocal tics, seizures, or sleep disturbances should be documented. In addition, parents should be questioned about any motor, cognitive, or behavioral regression.

A detailed history of school-related events should be recorded, including previous special education support, evaluations through the school, history of repeating grades, difficulties with specific academic areas, problems with peers, and the teacher's impressions of the child's difficulties, particularly related to attentional problems, impulsivity, or hyperactivity.

Perhaps the most important aspect of the medical history is a detailed family history of learning strengths and weaknesses, emotional or behavioral problems, learning disabilities, or mental retardation. The presence of more severe psychopathology, such as schizophrenia, bipolar disorder, depression, anxiety, or ADHD, should be noted for all family members.

Parental learning strengths and weaknesses, temperament difficulties, or attentional problems may be passed on to the child. For instance, dyslexia (deficits in decoding skills resulting in reading difficulties) may be genetic. Autosomal dominant genes on chromosomes 6 and 15 have been associated with dyslexia.

The neurodevelopmental examination should include a careful assessment of dysmorphic features such as epicanthal folds, palpebral fissure size, shape of the philtrum, low set or posteriorly rotated ears, prominent ear pinnae, unusual dermatoglyphics (eg, a single palmar crease), hyperextensibility of the joints, syndactyly, clinodactyly, or other unusual features. A detailed physical and neurologic examination needs to be carried out with an emphasis on both soft and hard neurologic findings. Soft signs can include motor incoordination, which can relate to handwriting problems and academic delays in written language or drawing. Visual motor coordination abilities can be assessed by having the child write, copy designs, or draw a person.

The child's growth parameters, including height, weight, and head circumference, need to be assessed, along with hearing and visual acuity. Cranial nerve abnormalities and oral motor coordination problems need to be noted. The examiner should watch closely for motor or vocal tics, which are quite common in individuals with Tourette syndrome. Both fine and gross motor abilities should be assessed. Dyspraxic movements in fine motor coordination are fairly common. Tandem walking, one-foot balancing, and coordinating a skip may often show surprising abnormalities.

The developmental aspects of the examination can include an assessment of auditory processing and perceptual ability with simple tasks, such as twofold to fivefold directions, assessing right and left directionality, memory for a series of spoken words or digit span, and comprehension of a graded paragraph. In assessing expressive language abilities, the examiner should look for difficulties with word retrieval, formulation and articulation, and adequacy of vocabulary. Visual–perceptual abilities can be assessed by simple visual memory tasks, puzzles, or object assembly, evaluating the child's ability to decode words or organize math problems. Visual motor integration and coordination can be assessed again with handwriting, design copying, and drawing a person. Throughout the assessment the clinician should pay special attention to the child's ability to focus attention and concentrate, and to other aspects of behavior such as evidence of depression or anxiety.

Additional questionnaires and checklists—such as the Child Behavior Checklist by Achenbach; ADHD scales such as the Conners' (or Parent/Teacher) Rating Scale; and the SNAP-IV, which includes the *Diagnostic and Statistical Manual* (DSM-IV) criteria for ADHD—can be used to help with this assessment.

Levine MD et al (eds): *Developmental-Behavioral Pediatrics,* 3rd ed. WB Saunders, 1999.

Reynolds CR, Mayfield JW: Neuropsychological assessment in genetically linked neurodevelopmental disorders. In Goldstein S, Reynolds CR (eds): *Handbook of Developmental and Genetic Disorders in Children.* Guilford, 1999.

Wolraich ML (ed): Disorders of Development and Learning, 3rd ed. Hamilton: BC Decker, 2003

http://www.nichcy.org

# ATTENTION-DEFICIT/HYPERACTIVITY DISORDER

ADHD is a common neurodevelopmental disorder that may affect 2–10% of school-age children and may persist into adolescence and adulthood. It is associated with a triad of symptoms: impulsivity, inattention, and hyperactivity. DSM-IV has described two ADHD subtypes: impulsive and inattentive. To be classified according to either subtype, the child must exhibit six or more of the symptoms listed in Table 2–5. The majority of children with ADHD have a combined type with symptoms of inattention as well as hyperactivity and impulsivity. Although symptoms begin in early childhood, they can diminish between ages 10 and 25 years. Hyperactivity declines more quickly, and impulsivity and inattentiveness often persist in adolescence and adulthood. ADHD may be combined with other psychiatric condi-

***Table 2–5.*** Attention deficit/hyperactivity disorder subtypes.

| Subtype | Symptoms[a] |
|---------|-------------|
| Impulsivity-hyperactivity | Fidgetiness<br>Difficulty remaining seated in the class<br>Excessive running or climbing<br>Difficulty in engaging quiet activities<br>Excessive talking and blurting out answers before questions have been completed<br>Difficulty awaiting turns<br>Interrupting and intruding on others |
| Inattentive | Failure to give close attention to detail<br>Difficulty sustaining intention in task<br>Failure to listen when spoken to directly<br>Failure to follow instructions<br>Difficulty organizing tasks and activities<br>Reluctance to engage in tasks<br>Losing utensils necessary for tasks or activities<br>Easy distractibility<br>Forgetfulness in daily activities |

[a]The child must exhibit six or more of these symptoms.
Adapted, with permission, from American Psychiatric Association, 1994.

tions, such as mood disorder in approximately 20% of patients, conduct disorders in 20%, and oppositionally defiant disorder in up to 40%. Approximately 25% of children with ADHD seen in a referral clinic have tics or Tourette syndrome. Conversely, well over 50% of individuals with Tourette syndrome also have ADHD.

ADHD has a substantial genetic component, with a heritability of 0.75 to 0.91. Several candidate genes have been identified, although there is strong evidence that ADHD is a disorder involving multiple genes. ADHD is also associated with a variety of genetic disorders related to developmental disorders, including fragile X syndrome, Williams syndrome, Angelman syndrome, XXY syndrome (Klinefelter syndrome), and Turner syndrome. Fetal alcohol syndrome (FAS) is also strongly associated with ADHD. CNS trauma, CNS infections, prematurity, and a difficult neonatal course with brain injury can also be associated with later ADHD. Metabolic problems such as hyperthyroidism can sometimes cause ADHD. These organic causes of ADHD should be considered in the evaluation of any child presenting with attentional problems, hyperactivity, or impulsivity. However, in the majority of children who have ADHD the cause remains unknown.

## Treatment

The treatment of ADHD varies depending on the complexity of the individual case. It is important to educate the family regarding the symptoms of ADHD and to clarify that this is a neurologic disorder that at times is difficult for the child to control. Behavior modification techniques usually help these children and should include structure with consistency in daily routine, positive reinforcement whenever possible, and time out for negative behaviors. It is important to try to boost the child's self-esteem because psychological complications are common in this disorder.

A variety of educational interventions can be helpful, including preferential seating in the classroom, a system of consistent positive behavior reinforcement, consistent structure, the repetition of information when needed, and the use of instruction that incorporates both visual and auditory modalities. Many children with ADHD have significant social difficulties, and social skills training can be helpful. Individual counseling is beneficial in alleviating poor self-esteem, oppositional behavior, and conduct problems.

The use of medication, specifically stimulant medication such as methylphenidate (Ritalin) and dextroamphetamine, can be helpful. A new medication, atomoxatine a noncontrolled substance, has been found to be effective in some children with ADHD. Pemoline is no longer recommended because of its association with liver injury.

It is most important that, no matter what medication is used, the diagnosis is correct and the correct dosage is prescribed. A recent study has demonstrated that one of the major factors contributing to treatment failure is inadequate dosing or the failure to recognize the presence of comorbid conditions such as learning disability, anxiety disorders, and depression.

In children with normal intellectual abilities, 70–90% respond well to stimulant medications. Stimulants enhance both dopamine and norepinephrine neurotransmission, which seems to improve impulse control, attention, and hyperactivity. Metabolic studies of the CNS (eg, using positron emission tomography scanning) have demonstrated enhanced metabolism in several areas of the brain, including the caudate and the frontal regions.

The side effects of methylphenidate and dextroamphetamine include appetite suppression and resulting weight loss as well as sleep disturbances. Some individuals experience increased anxiety, particularly with higher doses of stimulant medications. Stimulants may exacerbate psychotic symptoms. They may also exacerbate motor tics in 30% of patients, but in 10% motor tics may be improved. Long-acting and short-acting forms of stimulant medication are available. The initial dose of methylphenidate is 0.3 mg/kg/dose given two or three times daily. Adderall is a relatively new stimulant that combines four dextro and levo amphetamine salts. This is a long-acting medication, and often a single morning dose suffices for the day.

Alternative medications for the treatment of ADHD include clonidine or guanfacine, which are $\alpha_2$-adrenergic presynaptic agonists that decrease norepinephrine levels. They are particularly helpful for individuals who are hyperreactive to stimuli and may be helpful in decreasing motor tics in patients who have Tourette syndrome. Tricyclic antidepressant medications such as imipramine may also be an effective treatment for ADHD, but the cardiovascular side effects at high dosage can include severe arrhythmias. Bupropion is an antidepressant medication that can also be effective for treatment of ADHD symptoms. Its use is contraindicated in patients with a history of seizures, because it will lower the seizure threshold. It has also been known to cause seizures in individuals who have anorexia or bulimia. It is used more commonly in adolescents and adults with ADHD than in children with the disorder.

American Academy of Pediatrics: Clinical practice guideline: Diagnosis and evaluation of the child with attention-deficit/hyperactivity disorder. Pediatrics 2000;105:1117 [PMID: 10836893].

American Psychiatric Association: *Diagnostic and Statistical Manual of Mental Disorders,* 4th ed. American Psychiatric Association, 1994.

Barkley RA: *Attention Deficit Hyperactivity Disorder: A Clinical Workbook,* 2nd ed. Guilford, 1998.

Barkley RA: *Your Defiant Child: Eight Steps to Better Behavior.* Guilford, 1998.

Elia J et al: Treatment of attention deficit hyperactivity disorder. N Engl J Med 1999;340:780 [PMID: 1007214].

Goldman LS et al: Diagnosis and treatment of attention deficit hyperactivity disorder in children and adults. JAMA 1998;79:1100 [PMID: 9546570].

Goldstein S, Mather N: *Overcoming Underachieving: An Action Guide to Helping Your Child Succeed in School.* Wiley, 1998.

Jensen PS et al. Findings from the NIMS Multimotal Treatment Study of ADHD (MTA): Implications and applications for primary care providers. J Develop Behav Pediatr 2001;22:60 [PMID: 11265923].

http://www.chadd.org

http://www.add.org

## MENTAL RETARDATION

Severe deficits in the development of language, motor skills, attention, abstract reasoning, visual–spatial skills, and academic or vocational achievement are associated with mental retardation. Deficits on standardized testing in cognitive and adaptive functioning greater than 2 standard deviations below the mean for the population are considered to fall in the range of mental retardation (Table 2–6). The most common way of reporting the results of these tests is by using an intelligence quotient (IQ). The IQ is a statistically derived number reflecting the ratio of age-appropriate cognitive function and the child's level of cognitive function. A number of accepted standardized measurement tools, such as the Wechsler Intelligence Scale for Children, 3rd edition (WISC-III), can be used to assess these capacities. To receive a diagnosis of mental retardation a child must not only have an IQ of less than 70, but also must demonstrate adaptive skills more than 2 standard deviations below the mean. Adaptive function refers to the child's ability to function in his or her environment and can be measured by a parent or teacher interview-recorded using an instrument such as the Vineland Adaptive Behavior Scales.

The prevalence of mental retardation is approximately 3% in the general population, although some states have reported a prevalence of less than 2%. Mild levels of mental retardation are more common and more likely to have a sociocultural cause than are more severe levels. Poverty, deprivation, or a lack of exposure to a stimulating environment can contribute to developmental delays and poor performance on standardized tests. In addition, physical problems such as hearing loss, blindness, and brain trauma can lead to developmental delays and low IQ test scores. Great strides in our identification of genetic causes of mental retardation have been made since the 1990s because of the Human Genome Project. Over 750 genetic disorders have been associated with mental retardation, and over 200 of those disorders are carried on the X chromosome alone. In approximately 60% of cases, the cause of the mental retardation can be identified. Table 2–7 summarizes the findings of several studies on the causes of mental retardation.

## Evaluation

Children who present with developmental delays should be evaluated by a team of professionals as described at the beginning of this section. For children 0–3½ years of age, the Bayley Scales of Infant Development, second edition, is a well-standardized developmental test. For children older than 3 years of age standardized cognitive testing, such as the Wechsler Preschool and Primary Scale of Intelligence–Revised (WPPSI-R), the WISC-III, the Stanford–Binet IV, or the Kaufman Assessment Battery for Children (K-ABC) should be administered to assess cognitive function over a broad range of abilities, including verbal and

**Table 2–6.** Categories of mental retardation.

| Mental Retardation Range | Intelligence Quotient (IQ) |
| --- | --- |
| Mild mental retardation | 50–69 |
| Moderate mental retardation | 35–49 |
| Severe mental retardation | 20–34 |
| Profound mental retardation | < 20 |

**Table 2–7.** Causes of mental retardation.

| Cause | Percentage of Cases |
| --- | --- |
| Chromosomal abnormalities | 4–28 |
| Fragile X syndrome | 2–5 |
| Monogenetic conditions | 4–14 |
| Structural CNS abnormalities | 7–17 |
| Complications of prematurity | 2–10 |
| Environmental or teratogenic causes | 5–13 |
| "Cultural-familial" mental retardation | 3–12 |
| Metabolic or endocrine causes | 1–5 |
| Unknown | 30–50 |

Adapted from Curry CJ et al: Evaluation of mental retardation: Recommendations for a consensus conference. Am J Med Genet 1997;72:468.

nonverbal scales. For the nonverbal patient, a scale such as the Leiter-R will assess skills that do not involve language.

A full psychological evaluation in school-age children should include an emotional assessment if psychiatric or emotional problems are suspected. Such problems are common in children with developmental delays or mental retardation. A hearing test and a vision screening or ophthalmologic evaluation are important to determine whether hearing and vision are normal.

Diagnostic testing should be carried out in an effort to find the cause of mental retardation. Because chromosomal abnormalities occur in 4–28% of patients with mental retardation, cytogenetic testing is important in cases without a known cause. A consensus panel has recommended a high-resolution karyotype so that small deletions or duplications can be visualized. In addition, fluorescent in situ hybridization (FISH) studies are available. These studies use a fluorescent DNA probe that hybridizes to a region of DNA where a deletion or duplication is suspected. Microdeletion syndromes—such as Prader–Willi syndrome or Angelman syndrome, caused by a deletion at 15q; velocardiofacial syndrome, caused by a deletion at 22q; Smith–Magenis syndrome, caused by a deletion at 17p; and Williams syndrome, caused by a 7p deletion—can be assessed with FISH studies. Sometimes the deletion is so small that it may not be visualized through the microscope even with high-resolution cytogenetic studies. If clinical features consistent with any of the microdeletion syndromes are present, then FISH studies should be ordered to look for a small deletion in a specific region. In addition, duplications may be present. For example, a duplication at 15q has been associated with pervasive developmental disorder or autistic spectrum disorders and with general mental retardation. This duplication can be identified by FISH testing.

Structural abnormalities of the brain can occur in many individuals with mental retardation. Magnetic resonance imaging (MRI) is superior to computed tomography (CT) in identifying structural and myelination abnormalities. CT is the study of choice in evaluation of intracranial calcifications, such as those seen in congenital infections or tuberous sclerosis. The value of CT and MRI studies in a child with a normal-sized head and no focal neurologic signs is unclear, and they are not routinely carried out. Neuroimaging is important in patients with microcephaly, macrocephaly, seizures, loss of psychomotor skills, or specific neurologic signs such as spasticity, dystonia, ataxia, or abnormal reflexes. Neuroimaging is not routinely carried out in known genetic disorders such as Down syndrome, fragile X syndrome, or microdeletion syndromes because the CNS abnormalities have been well described and documentation of the abnormalities usually does not add to management.

Metabolic screening has a relatively low yield (0–5%) in children who present with developmental delay or mental retardation. Many patients with metabolic disorders such as hypothyroidism, phenylketonuria, and galactosemia are identified through newborn screening. Most patients with metabolic problems will present with specific indications for more focused testing, such as failure to thrive, recurrent unexplained illnesses, plateauing or loss of developmental skills, coarse facial features, cataracts, recurrent coma, abnormal sexual differentiation, arachnodactyly, hepatosplenomegaly, deafness, structural hair abnormalities, muscle tone changes, and skin abnormalities. Thyroid function studies should be carried out in any patient who has a palpably abnormal thyroid or exhibits clinical features associated with hypothyroidism. Serum amino acids, urine organic acid, and mucopolysaccharide screens should be considered in children with developmental delays and a suggestive history. Preliminary laboratory findings such as lactic acidosis, hyperuricemia, hyperammonemia, or a low or high cholesterol level require additional metabolic work-up.

Serial follow-up of patients is important because the physical and behavioral phenotype changes over time and diagnostic testing improves with time. Although cytogenetic testing may have been negative 10 years earlier, advances in high resolution techniques, FISH testing, and fragile X DNA testing may now reveal an abnormality that was not identified previously. A stepwise approach to diagnostic testing may also be more cost-effective, so that the test most likely to be positive is done first.

## Treatment

Once a diagnosis of mental retardation is made, treatment should include a combination of individual therapies, such as speech and language therapy, occupational therapy or physical therapy, special education support, behavioral therapy or counseling, and medical intervention, which may include psychopharmacology. To illustrate how these interventions work together, three disorders are described in detail in the next section.

Burack JA et al (eds): *Handbook of Mental Retardation and Development.* Cambridge University Press, 1999.

Curry CJ et al: Evaluation of mental retardation: Recommendations of a consensus conference. Am J Med Genet 1997;72:468 [PMID: 9375733].

Hagerman RJ: *Neurodevelopmental Disorders: Diagnosis and Treatment.* Oxford University Press, 1999.

http:www//TheArc.org

# SPECIFIC FORMS OF MENTAL RETARDATION & ASSOCIATED TREATMENT ISSUES

## 1. Fragile X Syndrome

The most common inherited cause of mental retardation is fragile X syndrome, which is caused by a trinucleotide expansion (CGG repeated sequence) within the fragile X mental retardation I (*FMR1*) gene. Individuals with mental retardation of unknown origin should receive *FMR1* DNA testing to see if they have an expansion of the CGG repeat causing dysfunction of this gene. The CGG sequence at *FMR1* in the normal population includes 5–50 repeats. Carriers of the premutation have 54–200 repeats, and have been considered unaffected. However, there is mounting evidence for a specific phenotype in these individuals. Women with the premutation have a higher incidence of premature ovarian failure, anxiety, and mild facial dysmorphisms. Individuals with the premutation have normal levels of FMR1 protein but increased levels of mRNA. It should be noted that seemingly unaffected females can pass an expansion of the CGG repeat to the next generation. Approximately 1 in 250 women and 1 in 700 men in the general population are premutation carriers. When a premutation of more than 90 repeats is passed on by a female to her offspring, it will expand to a full mutation (more than 200 repeats) 100% of the time, which usually causes mental retardation or learning disabilities. The full mutation is associated with methylation of the gene, which turns off transcription, resulting in a deficiency in the FMR1 protein product. These deficiencies result in mental retardation or significant learning and emotional problems.

Fragile X syndrome includes a broad range of symptoms. Patients can present with shyness, social anxiety, and learning problems, or they can present with mental retardation. Girls are usually less affected by the syndrome because they have a second X chromosome that is producing FMR1 protein. Approximately 70% of girls with the full mutation have cognitive deficits in addition to emotional problems, such as mood lability, ADHD, anxiety, and shyness. Approximately 85% of males with the syndrome have mental retardation and autistic-like features, such as poor eye contact, hand flapping, hand biting, and tactile defensiveness. About 20% of fragile X males meet the criteria for autism.

Children with fragile X syndrome usually present with language delays, hyperactivity, and tantrum behavior in early childhood. Although prominent ears and hyperextensible finger joints are common, approximately 30% of children with the syndrome may not have these features, and the diagnosis must be suspected because of behavioral problems and developmental delays alone. As the boys move into puberty, macro-orchidism develops with an average adult volume of 50 mL, or twice the normal volume. The child's face may become longer during puberty, and the majority of these children continue to have prominent ears.

## Treatment

All young children with fragile X syndrome benefit from language and motor therapy because delays in these areas are universal. Because approximately 10% of boys with the syndrome will be nonverbal at age 5 years, the use of augmentative communication techniques—such as signing; the use of pictures to represent food, toys, or activities; or the use of computers that can be programmed for communication—are helpful. Tantrums and hyperarousal to stimuli, along with hyperactivity, are common. Sensory integrative occupational therapy can be helpful in calming hyperarousal to stimuli and in improving the child's fine and gross motor coordination and motor planning. Speech and language therapy can decrease oral hypersensitivity, improve articulation, enhance verbal output and comprehension, and stimulate abstract reasoning skills.

If the behavioral problems are severe, it can be helpful to involve a behavioral psychologist who emphasizes positive reinforcement, time outs, consistency in routine, and the use of both auditory and visual modalities, such as a picture sequence, to help with difficult transition times and new situations.

Psychopharmacology can also be useful to treat ADHD, aggression, anxiety, or severe mood instability. Clonidine or guanfacine may be helpful in low doses, beginning in the preschool period to treat hyperarousal, tantrums, or severe hyperactivity. Stimulant medications such as methylphenidate, dextroamphetamine, and Adderall are usually beneficial by age 5 years and occasionally earlier. Relatively low doses are used (eg, 0.2–0.3 mg/kg/dose of methylphenidate) because irritability is often a problem with higher doses.

Shyness and social anxiety combined with mild ADHD are commonly seen in girls who have fragile X syndrome. The social anxiety is sometimes so severe that selective mutism (refusal to speak in some environments, especially school) is seen in girls who have the full mutation. The treatment for selective mutism includes fluoxetine, language therapy, and counseling.

Anxiety may also be a significant problem for boys with fragile X syndrome, and the use of a selective serotonin reuptake inhibitor (SSRI) such as fluoxetine, sertraline, fluvoxamine, or paroxetine is often helpful. SSRIs may also decrease aggression or moodiness, although in approximately 25% of cases, an increase in agitation or even hypomania may occur. The use of a more limited serotonin agent, buspirone, may also be helpful for anxiety, particularly if the patient cannot tolerate SSRIs.

Anticonvulsants such as carbamazepine, valproic acid, and gabapentin can be used to treat seizures, which occur in 20% of children with fragile X syndrome. They can also be helpful in treating more severe mood instability that does not improve with an SSRI, clonidine, or a stimulant medication. The use of carbamazepine and valproic acid requires careful monitoring of blood levels, liver function studies, electrolytes, blood count, and platelet level.

Aggression may become a significant problem in childhood or adolescence for boys with fragile X syndrome. Counseling can often be helpful, although medication may be needed. Stimulants, clonidine, and an SSRI may decrease aggression, although sometimes an atypical antipsychotic may be needed. If psychotic features are present, such as paranoia, delusions, or hallucinations, or if thinking is severely disorganized, then an atypical antipsychotic is usually helpful. Risperidone has been used most frequently in pediatrics and has a low risk for extrapyramidal symptoms. Side effects include sedation, excessive appetite and subsequent weight gain, and an increase in prolactin, which can cause breast tenderness and gynecomastia in boys. Usually a low dose of risperidone is well tolerated, and 0.5–2 mg at bedtime usually improves aggression, decreases hyperactivity, and stabilizes mood.

An important component of treatment is genetic counseling. Parents should meet with a genetic counselor after the diagnosis of fragile X syndrome is made because there is a high risk that other family members are carriers or may be affected by the syndrome. A detailed family history is essential, and all siblings of the proband should have *FMR1* DNA testing. If the mother received the gene from her father, then all of her sisters are obligate carriers, and their children are at 50% risk of having the fragile X mutation.

It is also helpful to link up a newly diagnosed family to a parent support group. Educational materials and parent support information may be obtained by calling The National Fragile X Foundation at 1-800-688-8765.

Hagerman RJ: *Fragile X Syndrome in Neurodevelopmental Disorders: Diagnosis and Treatment.* Oxford University Press, 1999.

Hagerman RJ, Cronister AC (eds): *Fragile X Syndrome: Diagnosis, Treatment, and Research,* 3rd ed. Johns Hopkins University Press, 2001.

http://www.FragileX.org

http://www.fraxa.org

## 2. Fetal Alcohol Syndrome

Significant alcohol exposure in utero is associated with a broad spectrum of developmental problems, ranging from learning disabilities to severe mental retardation. The Institute of Medicine has carefully defined diagnostic categories in patients with documented prenatal maternal alcohol consumption as follows:

### A. FETAL ALCOHOL SYNDROME

The diagnosis of FAS requires growth retardation; evidence of CNS neurodevelopmental abnormalities; and a characteristic pattern of facial anomalies, including short palpebral fissures, thin upper lip, indistinct or smooth philtrum, and midface hypoplasia.

### B. PARTIAL FETAL ALCOHOL SYNDROME

The diagnosis of partial fetal alcohol syndrome (PFAS) requires the presence of some but not all components of the facial anomalies as well as growth retardation, CNS neurodevelopmental abnormalities, or behavioral or cognitive abnormalities that are inconsistent with the child's developmental level and cannot be explained by familial background or environment.

### C. ALCOHOL-RELATED NEURODEVELOPMENTAL DISORDER

Alcohol-related neurodevelopmental disorder (ARND) does not require the presence of facial dysmorphic features, but it does require the presence of CNS neurodevelopmental abnormalities (eg, microcephaly, CNS structural defects, neurologic hard and soft signs) or evidence of a complex pattern of behavioral or cognitive abnormalities as outlined earlier. These abnormalities may include learning disabilities; poor impulse control; and problems in memory, attention, or judgment.

### D. ALCOHOL-RELATED BIRTH DEFECTS

The diagnosis of alcohol-related birth defects (ARBD) requires the presence of congenital anomalies including malformations and dysplasias in cardiac, skeletal, renal, ocular, or auditory areas (ie, sensorineural hearing loss). Strong animal and human evidence supports all of these diagnostic categories, including the controversial ARND diagnosis, which does not involve dysmorphic features. The prevalence of FAS, PFAS, and ARND combined is approximately 1 per 100 in the general population. These are common problems, and the physician must always ask about alcohol intake during pregnancy in a nonjudgmental way to obtain an accurate answer. The exact amount of alcohol consumption that leads to teratogenesis remains unclear. There is strong evidence that binge drinking during early critical periods of embryogenesis leads to alcohol-related syndromes.

## Evaluation & Treatment

The majority of children with alcohol-related syndromes present with ADHD symptoms, with or without significant developmental delays. To adequately assess involvement in other organs the following tests are recommended: an ophthalmologic examination, a hearing test, and a careful cardiac examination, with ultrasonography if abnormalities are detected. A careful examination for dysmorphic features and bony abnormalities is necessary. Renal function studies (ie, creatinine) should be conducted and a renal ultrasound obtained. Mental health problems are observed in over 90% of children and adolescents affected by alcohol in utero. Depression, panic attacks, anxiety, and mood instability are common. Because psychotic ideation is present in 20–40% of individuals with alcohol-related syndromes, a thorough emotional or psychiatric evaluation is essential. Long-term therapy and special education services are usually needed, and psychopharmacologic intervention may be helpful.

For treatment of ADHD symptoms, a dextroamphetamine preparation should be tried initially, although methylphenidate may also be helpful. SSRI agents can help relieve anxiety, panic attacks, and depression, although mania or hypomanias, a side effect, may occur in 25–50% of patients. Mood instability may be severe, although it usually responds to a mood stabilizer, such as valproate, or carbamazepine. One should be cautious with lithium because kidney dysfunction, secondary to malformations or hypoplasia, occasionally occurs. Psychotic features should be treated with an atypical antipsychotic such as risperidone. Consultation with a psychiatrist is helpful because the mental health problems associated with these syndromes are complex.

A speech and language evaluation and an occupational therapy evaluation in childhood usually lead to documentation of problems, and ongoing therapy is usually helpful. The most significant problem in alcohol-related syndromes is the high rate of legal problems, incarceration, and alcohol or drug abuse in adolescence and adulthood. An intensive treatment program must be mobilized to improve the outcome of this disorder. Long-term counseling and advocacy, along with intensive job training, usually keeps these adolescents out of trouble, but the failure rate is high.

Hagerman RJ: *Fetal Alcohol Syndrome in Neurodevelopmental Disorders: Diagnosis and Treatment.* Oxford University Press, 1999.

Hagerman RJ, Cronister AC (eds): *Fragile X Syndrome: Diagnosis, Treatment, and Research,* 2nd ed. Johns Hopkins University Press, 1996.

Stratton KR et al: *Fetal Alcohol Syndrome: Diagnosis, Epidemiology, Prevention, and Treatment.* National Academy Press, 1996.

Streissguth AP: *Fetal Alcohol Syndrome: A Guide for Families and Communities.* Brookes/Cole, 1997.

http://www.nofas.org

## 3. Autistic Spectrum Disorders

Autism is a neurologic disorder characterized by (1) qualitative impairments in social interaction; (2) qualitative impairments in communication; and (3) restricted repetitive and stereotyped patterns of behavior, interests, and activities. It is a relatively common disorder, occurring in approximately 1 in 500 children. There is a higher incidence of autistic spectrum disorders in disorders such as fragile X syndrome, tuberous sclerosis, Cornelia de Lange syndrome, Down syndrome, and 15q duplication. Despite this, in as many as 90% of cases of autism, no cause can be identified. There is a strong familial component. Parents of one child with autism have a 2–9% chance of having a second child with autism. The concordance rate among monozygotic twins is high, and there is an increased incidence of speech, language, reading, attention, and affective disorders in family members of children with autism.

## Evaluation & Treatment

Children with autism are often not diagnosed until age 3 to 4 years, when their disturbances in reciprocal social interaction and communication become more apparent. However, impairments in communication and behavior can sometimes be recognized in the first 12 to 18 months of life. Behaviors noted during this period include a lack of motor imitation, a lack of joint attention and social referencing, a lack of affect sharing, poor eye contact, and a lack of symbolic play. The three most striking characteristics during the first year are a consistent failure to orient to one's name, failure to regard people directly, and failure to develop speech. Because of evidence that early intervention is particularly important for children with autism, great interest has arisen in developing a screening instrument that can be used in very young children. The Checklist for Autism in Toddlers (CHAT) is administered at 18 months and includes a short parent questionnaire and direct observation. It evaluates pretend play and joint attention (which includes pointing for interest and following gaze). This instrument is quick and easy to administer and has good specificity and positive predictive value (83%). Unfortunately, its sensitivity is poor (18%). Work is being done to modify this test or develop others with greater sensitivity. When behaviors consistent with autism are noted, the child should be referred to a team of specialists experienced in the assessment of autistic spectrum disorders as soon as possible.

All children with autism should have a formal audiology evaluation because of their language disorder. For children with autism and mental retardation, tests for high-resolution chromosomes, DNA for fragile X syndrome, FISH for 15q duplication, as well as metabolic screening, lead level, and thyroid studies should be considered. A Woods lamp test for tuberous sclerosis may also be done. Other tests should be considered as indicated by findings in the history and physical examination. Neuroimaging is not routinely indicated even in the presence of macrocephaly since children with autism often have relatively large heads. Approximately 15–30% of children with autism demonstrate plateauing or loss of skills (usually language and social skills only) between 12 and 24 months of age. This usually occurs before attaining 10 words. Children who have a history of regression should have a sleep-deprived EEG, or an overnight EEG, with adequate sampling of slow-wave sleep to rule out epileptiform discharges during slow-wave sleep. It should be noted that the recommendations for treatment of that type of EEG abnormality are still being debated.

Much controversy surrounds the appropriate treatment and educational approaches for children with autistic spectrum disorders. As with any child, treatment should be based on the individual needs of the child. It is clear, however, that intervention must begin early and must be comprehensive and intensive. Some advocate 25 hours or more per week of treatment that targets development of social attention, peer interactions, functional language, and appropriate play. It should be noted that psychotropic medications have been helpful in some children with autism. However, these medications should not take the place of behavioral interventions.

Baird G et al: A screening instrument for autism at 18 months of age: A 6-year follow-up study. J Am Acad Child Adolesc Psychiatr 2000;39:694 [PMID: 108946303].

Baird G et al: Current topic: Screening and surveillance for autism and pervasive developmental disorders. Arch Dis Child 2001;84:468 [PMID: 11369559].

Cohen DJ, Volkman FR (eds): *Handbook of Autism and Pervasive Developmental Disorders,* 2nd ed. John Wiley & Sons, Inc. 1997.

Dawson G, Osterling J: Early intervention in autism: Effectiveness and common elements of current approaches. In Guralnick MJ (ed): *The Effectiveness of Early Intervention: Second Generation Research.* Brookes/Cole, 1997.

Filipek PA et al: Practice parameter: Screening and diagnosis of autism: Report of the Quality Standards Subcommittee of the American Academy of Neurology and Child Neurology Society. Neurology 2000;55:468 [PMID: 10953176].

Gabriels RL, Hill DE (eds): *Autism: From Research to Individualized Practice.* Jessica Kingsley Publishers, 2002.

Gilberg C, Coleman M (eds): *The Biology of the Autistic Syndromes.* MacKeith Press, 2000.

Lord C, McGee JP (eds): *Educating Children with Autism.* National Academy of Sciences Press, 2001.

Ozonoff S et al (eds): *Autism Spectrum Disorders: A Research Review for Practioners.* American Psychiatric Publishing, 2003.

Rapin I: Autism. N Engl J Med 1997;337:97 [PMID: 9211680].

Rogers SJ: Empirically supported comprehensive treatments for young children with autism. J Clin Child Psychol 1998;27:168 [PMID: 9648034].

http://www.autism-society.org

http://teacch.com

http://firstsigns.org

### Web Resources

[Title V Program Information: Institute for Child Health Policy]

www.ichp.edu

[Parent Training and Information Centers: Alliance Coordinating Office]

www.taalliance.org

[Advocacy: The Arc of the United States]

www.TheArc.org

[American with Disabilities Act Information: National Access for Public Schools Project]

www.adaptenv.org

[General: NADDC-National Association of Developmental Disabilities Councils]

www.naddc.org

# Adolescence

*David W. Kaplan, MD, MPH, & Kathryn Love-Osborne, MD*

Adolescence is a period of rapid physical, emotional, cognitive, and social growth and development. Generally, adolescence begins at age 11–12 years and ends between ages 18 and 21. Most teenagers complete puberty by age 16–18 years; in western society, however, for educational and cultural reasons, the adolescent period is prolonged to allow for further psychosocial development before the individual assumes adult responsibilities.

The developmental passage from childhood to adulthood encompasses the following steps: (1) completing puberty and somatic growth; (2) developing socially, emotionally, and cognitively, moving from concrete to abstract thinking; (3) establishing an independent identity and separating from the family; and (4) preparing for a career or vocation.

## DEMOGRAPHY

In the United States in 2003, there were 20.3 million adolescents between ages 15 and 19 years and 19.8 million between ages 20 and 24 years. Adolescents and young adults (ages 15–24 years) constitute 14% of the US population. Over the next several decades, the proportion of racial and ethnic minority adolescents is expected to increase. It is projected that by 2040 the percentage of non-Hispanic whites will drop below 50%. Hispanics are becoming the second most populous racial/ethnic group.

## MORTALITY DATA

For the adolescent population, cultural and environmental rather than organic factors pose the greatest threats to life. The three leading causes of death in the adolescent population (ages 15–19 years) in 2000 were unintentional injury (49.8%), homicides (14.1%), and suicides (12.0%). These three causes of violent death accounted for 76.0% of all adolescent deaths. Deaths resulting from homicide among black 15- to 19-year-olds increased 328% between 1983 and 1993. Although the homicide rate has decreased significantly since the high in 1993, homicide is still the leading cause of death for black adolescents age 15–19 years, accounting for 38.0% of all deaths. Although deaths from automobile crashes have decreased over the last

decade, alcohol use remains the underlying cause of most teenage motor vehicle deaths. Almost two thirds of motor vehicle deaths involving young drinking drivers occur on Friday, Saturday, or Sunday, and 70% occur between 8:00 PM and 4:00 AM.

There is continued concern in the United States with the problem of youth violence. This concern is rooted in the high rate of homicides involving handguns among young males, the number of firearm-related suicides, and school shootings. Youths ages 12 to 17 are twice as likely as adults to be victims of serious violent crimes, which include aggravated assault, rape, robbery, and homicide. Violent crimes committed by juveniles constitute about 1 in 4 of all violent crimes. Nationally, 17.4% of high-school students reported carrying a weapon at least once in the preceding 30 days. However, since the peak rate of serious violent crime involving juvenile offenders in 1993, the rate has decreased. The rate of serious violent crimes among youth victims decreased from 37.6 in 1980 to 16.0 in 2000.

## MORBIDITY DATA

Demographic and economic changes in the American family since the mid-1970s have had a profound effect on children and adolescents. Between 1955 and 1990, the divorce rate rose from about 400,000 to nearly 1.2 million a year. Between 1960 and 1990, the number of children involved in divorce each year increased from 460,000 to 1.1 million. The percentage of children and adolescents living in two-parent households has decreased significantly, from 79% in 1980 to 69% in 2001. Sixty-five percent of Hispanic and 38% of black children and adolescents younger than age 18 lived in a two-parent household in 2001. In 2002, 16.7% of children and adolescents younger than age 18 years in the United States were living below the poverty level, compared with 12% in 1970. Forty percent of children in mother-only families were living in poverty.

The major causes of morbidity during adolescence are psychosocial: unintended pregnancy, sexually transmitted infections (STIs), substance abuse, smoking, dropping out of school, depression, running away from home, physical violence, and juvenile delinquency.

High-risk behavior in one area is often associated with problems in another (Figure 3–1). For example, teenagers who live in a dysfunctional family (eg, problems related to drinking or physical or sexual abuse) are much more likely than other teenagers to be depressed. A depressed teenager is at greater risk for drug and alcohol abuse, academic failure, inappropriate sexual activity, STIs, pregnancy, and suicide.

Early identification of the teenager at risk for these problems is important in preventing immediate complications and future associated problems. Early indicators for problems related to depression include the following:

1. Decline in school performance.
2. Excessive school absences or cutting class.
3. Frequent or persistent psychosomatic complaints.
4. Changes in sleeping or eating habits.
5. Difficulty in concentrating or persistent boredom.
6. Signs or symptoms of depression, extreme stress, or anxiety.
7. Withdrawal from friends or family, or change to a new group of friends.
8. Unusually severe violent or rebellious behavior, or radical personality change.
9. Conflict with parents.
10. Sexual acting-out.
11. Conflicts with the law.
12. Suicidal thoughts or preoccupation with themes of death.
13. Drug and alcohol abuse.
14. Running away from home.

American Academy of Pediatrics Committee on Injury and Poison Prevention: Firearm-related injuries affecting the pediatric population. Pediatrics 2000;105:888 [PMID: 10742344].

Anderson RN: Deaths: Leading causes for 2000. Natl Vital Stat Rep 2002;50(16):1 [PMID: 12355905].

Emery RE, Laumann-Billings L: Practical and emotional consequences of parental divorce. Adolesc Med: State of the Art Reviews 1998;9:271 [PMID: 10961235].

Grunbaum JA et al: Youth risk behavior surveillance—United States, 2001. MMWR Surveill Summ 2002;51(4):1 [PMID: 12102329].

O'Malley PM, Johnston LD: Drinking and driving among US high school seniors, 1984–1997. Am J Public Health 1999;89:678 [PMID: 10224978].

Resnick MD et al: Protecting adolescents from harm: Findings from the national longitudinal study on adolescent health. JAMA 1997;278:823 [PMID: 9293990].

*Figure 3–1.* Interrelation of high-risk adolescent behavior.

Steinberg L: Gallagher lecture. The family at adolescence: Transition and transformation. J Adolesc Health 2000;27(3):170 [PMID: 10960215].

Suicide and suicide attempts in adolescents. Committee on Adolescents. American Academy of Pediatrics. Pediatrics 2000;105 (4 Pt 1):871 [PMID: 10742340].

## DELIVERY OF HEALTH SERVICES

How, where, why, and when adolescents seek health care depends on ability to pay, distance to health care facilities, availability of transportation, accessibility of services, time away from school, and privacy. Many common teenage health problems, such as unintended pregnancy and the need for contraception; STIs; and substance abuse, depression, and other emotional problems, have moral, ethical, and legal implications. Teenagers are often reluctant to confide in their parents for fear of punishment or disapproval. Recognizing this reality, health care providers have established many specialized programs such as teenage family planning clinics, drop-in centers, STI clinics, hotlines, and adolescent clinics. For the physician, establishing a trusting and confidential relationship is basic to meeting an adolescent patient's health care needs. A patient who senses that the physician will inform the parents about a confidential problem may lie or fail to disclose information essential for proper diagnosis and treatment.

## ■ GUIDELINES FOR ADOLESCENT PREVENTIVE SERVICES

The American Medical Association guidelines for adolescent preventive services (GAPS) and the National Center for Education in Maternal and Child Health *Bright Futures* cover health screening and guidance, immunization, and health care delivery. The goals of these guidelines are (1) to deter adolescents from participating in behaviors that jeopardize health; (2) to detect physical, emotional, and behavioral problems early and intervene promptly; (3) to reinforce and encourage behaviors that promote healthful living; and (4) to provide immunization against infectious diseases. The guidelines recommend that adolescents between ages 11 and 21 years have annual routine health visits. Health services should be developmentally appropriate and culturally sensitive, and confidentiality between patient and physician should be ensured. A complete schedule of the recommended guidelines is shown in Figure 3–2A.

## RELATING TO THE ADOLESCENT PATIENT

Adolescence is one of the physically healthiest periods in life. The challenge of caring for adolescents lies not in managing complex organic disease but in accommodating to the cognitive, emotional, and psychosocial growth that influences health behavior.

How the physician initially approaches the adolescent may determine the success or failure of the visit. The physician should behave simply and honestly, without an authoritarian or excessively professional manner. Because the self-esteem of many young adolescents is fragile, the physician must be careful not to overpower and intimidate the patient. To establish a comfortable and trusting relationship, the physician should strive to present the image of an ordinary person who has special training and skills.

Because individuals vary greatly in the onset and termination of puberty, chronologic age may be a poor indicator of physical, physiologic, and emotional development. In communicating with an adolescent, the physician must be sensitive to the patient's developmental level, recognizing that outward appearance and chronologic age may not give an accurate assessment of cognitive development.

Working with teenagers can be emotionally draining. Adolescents have a unique ability to identify hidden emotional vulnerabilities. The physician who has a personal need to control patients or foster dependency may be disappointed in caring for teenagers. Because teenagers are consumed with their own emotional needs, they rarely provide the physician with the ego rewards that younger or older patients do.

The physician should be sensitive to the issue of countertransference, the emotional reaction elicited in the physician by the adolescent. How the physician relates to the adolescent patient often depends on the physician's personal characteristics. This is especially true of physicians who treat families that are experiencing parent–adolescent conflicts. It is common for young physicians to overidentify with the teenage patient and for older physicians to see the conflict from the parents' perspective.

Overidentification with the parents is readily sensed by the teenager, who is likely to view the physician as just another authority figure who cannot understand the problems of being a teenager. Assuming a parental-authoritarian role may jeopardize the establishment of a working relationship with the patient. In the case of the young physician, overidentification with the teenager may cause the parents to become defensive about their parenting role and discount the physician's experience and ability.

## Preventive Health Services by Age and Procedure

Adolescents and young adults have a unique set of health care needs. The recommendations for Guidelines for Adolescent Preventive Services (GAPS) emphasize annual clinical preventive services visits that address both the developmental and psychosocial aspects of health, in addition to traditional biomedical conditions. These recommendations were developed by the American Medical Association with contributions from a Scientific Advisory Panel, comprised of national experts, as well as representatives of primary care medical organizations and the health insurance industry. The body of scientific evidence indicates that the periodicity and content of preventive services can be important in promoting the health and well-being of adolescents.

| Procedure | Age of Adolescent | | | | | | | | | | |
| --- | --- | --- | --- | --- | --- | --- | --- | --- | --- | --- | --- |
| | Early | | | | Middle | | | Late | | | |
| | 11 | 12 | 13 | 14 | 15 | 16 | 17 | 18 | 19 | 20 | 21 |
| **Health Guidance** | | | | | | | | | | | |
| Parenting* | | | ● | | | ● | | | | | |
| Development | ● | ● | ● | ● | ● | ● | ● | ● | ● | ● | ● |
| Diet and Physical Activity | ● | ● | ● | ● | ● | ● | ● | ● | ● | ● | ● |
| Healthy Lifestyle** | ● | ● | ● | ● | ● | ● | ● | ● | ● | ● | ● |
| Injury Prevention | ● | ● | ● | ● | ● | ● | ● | ● | ● | ● | ● |
| **Screening** | | | | | | | | | | | |
| **History** | | | | | | | | | | | |
| Eating Disorders | ● | ● | ● | ● | ● | ● | ● | ● | ● | ● | ● |
| Sexual Activity*** | ● | ● | ● | ● | ● | ● | ● | ● | ● | ● | ● |
| Alcohol and Other Drug Use | ● | ● | ● | ● | ● | ● | ● | ● | ● | ● | ● |
| Tobacco Use | ● | ● | ● | ● | ● | ● | ● | ● | ● | ● | ● |
| Abuse | ● | ● | ● | ● | ● | ● | ● | ● | ● | ● | ● |
| School Performance | ● | ● | ● | ● | ● | ● | ● | ● | ● | ● | ● |
| Depression | ● | ● | ● | ● | ● | ● | ● | ● | ● | ● | ● |
| Risk for Suicide | ● | ● | ● | ● | ● | ● | ● | ● | ● | ● | ● |
| **Physical Assessment** | | | | | | | | | | | |
| Blood Pressure | ● | ● | ● | ● | ● | ● | ● | ● | ● | ● | ● |
| BMI | ● | ● | ● | ● | ● | ● | ● | ● | ● | ● | ● |
| Comprehensive Exam | | | ● | | | ● | | | ● | | |
| **Tests** | | | | | | | | | | | |
| Cholesterol | | | 1 | | | 1 | | | | 1 | |
| TB | | | 2 | | | 2 | | | | 2 | |
| GC, Chlamydia, Syphilis, & HPV | | | 3 | | | 3 | | | | 3 | |
| HIV | | | 4 | | | 4 | | | | 4 | |
| Pap Smear | | | 5 | | | 5 | | | | 5 | |
| **Immunizations** | | | | | | | | | | | |
| MMR | | ● | | | | | | | | | |
| Td | | ● | | | | O | | | | | |
| HepB | | ● | | | | 6 | | | | 6 | |
| Hep A | | | 7 | | | 7 | | | | 7 | |
| Varicella | | | 8 | | | 8 | | | | 8 | |

1. Screening test performed once if family history is positive for early cardiovascular disease or hyperlipidemia.
2. Screen if positive for exposure to active TB or lives/works in high-risk situation, eg homeless shelter, jail, health care facility.
3. Screen at least annually if sexually active.
4. Screen if high risk for infection.
5. Screen annually if sexually active or if 18 years or older.
6. Vaccinate any adolescent not previously vaccinated.

7. Vaccinate if at risk for hepatitis A infection.
8. Offer vaccine if no reliable history of chickenpox or previous immunization.
\* A parent health guidance visit is recommended during early and middle adolescence.
\** Includes counseling regarding sexual behavior and avoidance of tobacco, alcohol, and other drug use.
\*** Includes history of unintended pregnancy and STD.
O Do not give if administered in last five years.

**A**

***Figure 3–2.*** **A:** Guidelines for preventive health services. (Reproduced, with permission, from *AMA Guidelines for Adolescent Preventive Services: Recommendations and Rationale.* American Medical Association, 1995.)

# TEEN HEALTH HISTORY

This information is *strictly confidential.* Its purpose is to help your caregiver give you better care. We request that you fill out the form completely, but you may skip any question that you do not wish to answer.

NAME _____ DATE _____
       FIRST          MIDDLE INITIAL     LAST

BIRTHDATE _____ AGE _____ GRADE _____ Name that you like to be called _____

1. Why did you come to the clinic today? _____
_____
_____

**Medical History**                                   **STRICTLY CONFIDENTIAL**
2. Are you allergic to any medicines? . . . . . . . . . . . . . . . . . . . . . . . . YES  NO
   Name of medicines _____
3. Are you taking any medicines now? . . . . . . . . . . . . . . . . . . . . . . YES  NO
   Name of medicines _____
4. Do you have any long-term health conditions? . . . . . . . . . . . . . . . . YES  NO
   Conditions _____
5. Date or age at your last tetanus (or dT) shot_____

**School Information**
6. What grade do you usually make in English? _____
   (Example: A, B, C, D, E, F)
7. What grade do you usually make in Math? _____
8. How many days were you absent from school last semester?_____
9. How many days were you absent last semester because of illness? _____
10. How do you get along at school? _____
_____

| 1 | 2 | 3 | 4 | 5 | 6 | 7 |
|---|---|---|---|---|---|---|
| TERRIBLE | | | | | | GREAT |

11. Have you ever been suspended? . . . . . . . . . . . . . . . . . . . . . . . . . YES  NO
12. Have you ever dropped out of school? . . . . . . . . . . . . . . . . . . . . . YES  NO
13. Do you plan to graduate from high school? . . . . . . . . . . . . . . . . . . YES  NO

**Job/Career Information**
14. Are you working? . . . . . . . . . . . . . . . . . . . . . . . . . . . . . . . . . . . YES  NO
    If YES, What is your job?_____
    How many hours do you work per week?_____
15. What are your future plans or career goals?_____

**Family Information**
16. Who do you live with? (Check all that apply.)
   _____ Both natural parents   _____ Stepmother   _____ Brother(s)-ages:_____
   _____ Mother                 _____ Stepfather   _____ Sister(s)-ages:_____
   _____ Father                 _____ Guardian     _____ Other:Explain _____
   _____ Adoptive parents       _____ Alone
17. Have there been any changes in your family? Check all that apply.
   _____ a. Marriage        _____ d. Serious illness      _____ g. Births
   _____ b. Separation      _____ e. Loss of job          _____ h. Deaths
   _____ c. Divorce         _____ f. Move to new home     _____ i. Other
18. Father's/stepfather's occupation or job: _____
    Mother's/stepmother's occupation or job: _____

B

*Figure 3–2.* **B:** Adolescent medical history questionnaire.

106

19. How do you get along at home?

| 1 | 2 | 3 | 4 | 5 | 6 | 7 |
|---|---|---|---|---|---|---|
| TERRIBLE | | | | | | GREAT |

20. Have you ever run away from home? . . . . . . . . . . . . . . . . . . . . . . . . . . .    YES  NO
21. Have you ever lived in foster care or an institution? . . . . . . . . . . . . . . . .    YES  NO

**Self Information**

22. On the whole, how do you like yourself?

| 1 | 2 | 3 | 4 | 5 | 6 | 7 |
|---|---|---|---|---|---|---|
| NOT VERY MUCH | | | | | | A LOT |

23. What do you do best?_____

24. If you could, what would you like to change about yourself? _____

_____

25. List any habits you would like to break. _____

_____

26. Do you feel people expect too much from you? . . . . . . . . . . . . . . . . . . . . .    YES  NO
27. How do you get along with your friends/peers?

| 1 | 2 | 3 | 4 | 5 | 6 | 7 |
|---|---|---|---|---|---|---|
| TERRIBLE | | | | | | GREAT |

28. Do you feel you have friends you can count on? . . . . . . . . . . . . . . . . . . . .    YES  NO
29. Have you ever felt really sad or depressed for more than 3 days in a row? . .    YES  NO
30. Have you ever thought of suicide as a solution to your problems? . . . . . . . . .    YES  NO
31. Have you gotten into any trouble because of your anger/temper? . . . . . . . . .    YES  NO

**Health Concern**

32. On a scale of 1–7, how would you rate your general health?

| 1 | 2 | 3 | 4 | 5 | 6 | 7 |
|---|---|---|---|---|---|---|
| TERRIBLE | | | | | | GREAT |

33. Do you have any questions or concerns about any of the following? (Check those that apply.)

| | | |
|---|---|---|
| ____ Height/weight | ____ Skin rash | ____ Family violence/physical abuse |
| ____ Blood pressure | ____ Arms, legs/muscle or joint pain | ____ Feeling down or depressed |
| ____ Head/headaches | | ____ Dating |
| ____ Dizziness/passing out | ____ Frequent or painful urination | ____ Sex |
| ____ Eyes/vision | | ____ Worried about VD/STD |
| ____ Ears/hearing/earaches | ____ Wetting the bed | ____ Masturbation |
| ____ Nose/frequent colds | ____ Sexual organs/genitals | ____ Sexual abuse/rape |
| ____ Mouth/teeth | ____ Trouble sleeping | ____ Having children/parenting/adoption |
| ____ Neck/back | ____ Tiredness | |
| ____ Chest/breathing/coughing | ____ Diet food/appetite | ____ Cancer/or dying |
| ____ Breasts | ____ Eating disorder | ____ Other (explain) _____ |
| ____ Heart | ____ Smoking/drugs/alcohol | _____ |
| ____ Stomach/pain/vomiting | ____ Future plans/jobs | |
| ____ Diarrhea/constipation | ____ Worried about parents | |

**Health Behavior Information**

34. Have you lost or gained any weight in the last year? . . . . . . . . . . . . . . . . . .    YES  NO
    Gained (  ) How much? _____
    Lost (  ) How much? _____
35. In the past year, have you tried to lose weight or control your weight by vomiting,
    taking diet pills or laxatives, or starving yourself? . . . . . . . . . . . . . . . . . . . . .    YES  NO
36. Do you ever drive after drinking or when high? . . . . . . . . . . . . . . . . . . . . . .    YES  NO
37. Do you ever smoke cigarettes or use snuff or chewing tobacco? . . . . . . . . . .    YES  NO
38. Do you ever smoke marijuana? . . . . . . . . . . . . . . . . . . . . . . . . . . . . . . . . .    YES  NO
39. Do you ever drink alcoholic beverages? . . . . . . . . . . . . . . . . . . . . . . . . . . .    YES  NO
40. Do you ever use street drugs (speed, cocaine, acid, crack, etc.)? . . . . . . . . .    YES  NO
41. Does anyone in your household smoke? . . . . . . . . . . . . . . . . . . . . . . . . . . .    YES  NO
42. Does anyone in your family have a problem with drugs or alcohol? . . . . . . . .    YES  NO

*Figure 3–2.* Continued

43. Have you ever been in trouble with the police or the law? . . . . . . . . . . . . . .   YES NO
44. Have you begun dating? . . . . . . . . . . . . . . . . . . . . . . . . . . . . . . . . . . . . .   YES NO
45. Do you currently have a boyfriend or girlfriend? . . . . . . . . . . . . . . . . . . . . .   YES NO
    If YES, how old is he/she? _____
46. Do you think you might be gay/lesbian/homosexual? . . . . . . . . . . . . . . . . . .   YES NO
47. Have you ever had sex (sexual intercourse)? . . . . . . . . . . . . . . . . . . . . . . .   YES NO
48. Are you interested in receiving information on preventing pregnancy? . . . . . .   YES NO
49. If you have had sex, are you (or your partner) using any kind of birth control?   YES NO
50. If you have had sex, have you ever been treated for gonorrhea or chlamydia
    or any other sexually transmitted disease? . . . . . . . . . . . . . . . . . . . . . . . .   YES NO

**For males only**
51. Have you been taught how to use a condom correctly? . . . . . . . . . . . . . . . .   YES NO
52. If you have had sex, do you use a condom every time or almost every time?   YES NO
53. Have you ever fathered a child? . . . . . . . . . . . . . . . . . . . . . . . . . . . . . . . .   YES NO

**For females only**
54. How old were you when your periods began? . . . . . . . . . . . . . . . . . . . . . . .   _____
55. What date did your last period start? . . . . . . . . . . . . . . . . . . . . . . . . . . . . .   _____
56. Are your periods regular (once a month)?. . . . . . . . . . . . . . . . . . . . . . . . . .   YES NO
57. Do you have painful or excessively heavy periods? . . . . . . . . . . . . . . . . . . .   YES NO
58. Have you ever had a vaginal infection or been treated for a female disorder?   YES NO
59. Do you think you might be pregnant? . . . . . . . . . . . . . . . . . . . . . . . . . . . . .   YES NO
60. Have you ever been pregnant? . . . . . . . . . . . . . . . . . . . . . . . . . . . . . . . . .   YES NO

**Everyone**
61. Do you have any other problems you would like to discuss with the caregiver?   YES NO

**Past Medical History**
62. Were you born prematurely or did you have any serious problems as an infant?   YES NO
63. Are you allergic to any medicines? . . . . . . . . . . . . . . . . . . . . . . . . . . . . . .   YES NO
    If YES, what? _____
    _____

64. List any medications that you are taking and the problems for which the
    medication was given:

| MEDICATION | REASON | HOW LONG |
|---|---|---|
| _____ | _____ | _____ |
| _____ | _____ | _____ |
| _____ | _____ | _____ |

65. Have you ever been hospitalized? . . . . . . . . . . . . . . . . . . . . . . . . . . . . . . .   YES NO
    If YES, describe your problem and your age at the time.
    AGE          PROBLEM
    _____      _____
    _____      _____
    _____      _____

66. Have you had any injuries? . . . . . . . . . . . . . . . . . . . . . . . . . . . . . . . . . . . .   YES NO
    If YES, describe the injury and your age when it occurred.
    AGE          KIND OF INJURY
    _____      _____
    _____      _____

67. Have you had any serious illnesses? . . . . . . . . . . . . . . . . . . . . . . . . . . . . .   YES NO
    If YES, state the kind of illness and your age when it started.
    AGE          ILLNESS
    _____      _____
    _____      _____

*Figure 3–2.* Continued

## Family History

Have any members of your family, alive or dead (parents, grandparents, uncles, aunts, brothers or sisters), had any of the following problems? If YES, please state the age of the person when the condition occurred and the person's relationship to you.

| PROBLEM | YES | NO | DON'T KNOW | AGE | RELATIONSHIP |
|---|---|---|---|---|---|
| A. Seizure disorder Epilepsy | | | | | |
| B. Mental retardation Birth defects | | | | | |
| C. Migraine headaches | | | | | |
| D. High blood pressure High cholesterol | | | | | |
| E. Heart attack or stroke at less than age 60 | | | | | |
| F. Lung disease Tuberculosis | | | | | |
| G. Liver or intestinal disease | | | | | |
| H. Kidney disease | | | | | |
| I. Allergies Asthma Eczema | | | | | |
| J. Arthritis | | | | | |
| K. Diabetes | | | | | |
| L. Endocrine problems Other glandular problems | | | | | |
| M. Obesity Eating disorder | | | | | |
| N. Cancer | | | | | |
| O. Blood disorders Sickle cell anemia | | | | | |
| P. Emotional problems Suicide | | | | | |
| Q. Alcoholism Drug problems | | | | | |

*Figure 3-2.* Continued

# THE SETTING

Adolescents respond positively to a setting and to services that communicate a sensitivity to their age. A pediatrician's waiting room with toddlers' toys and examination tables too short for a young adult make adolescent patients feel they have outgrown the practice. Similarly, a waiting room filled with geriatric or pregnant patients can make a teenager feel out of place.

It is not uncommon to see a teenage patient who has been brought to the office against his or her wishes, especially for evaluations of drug and alcohol use, parent–child conflict, school failure, depression, or a suspected eating disorder. Even in cases of acute physical illness, the adolescent may feel anxiety about having a physical examination. If future visits are to be successful, the physician must spend time on the first visit to foster a sense of trust and an opportunity to feel comfortable.

# CONFIDENTIALITY

It is helpful at the beginning of the visit to talk with the adolescent and the parents about what to expect. The physician should address the issue of confidentiality, telling the parents that two meetings, one with the teenager alone and one with only the parents, will take place. Adequate time must be spent with both the patient and the parents, or important information may be missed. At the beginning of the interview with the patient, it is useful to say, "I am likely to ask you some personal questions. This is not because I am trying to pry into your personal affairs but because these questions may be important to your health. I want to assure you that what we talk about is confidential, just between the two of us. If there is something I feel we should discuss with your parents, I will ask your permission first unless I feel it is life-threatening."

# THE STRUCTURE OF THE VISIT

Caring for adolescents is a time-intensive process. In many adolescent practices, a 40–50% no-show rate is not unusual. The stated chief complaint may conceal the patient's real concern. For example, a 15-year-old girl may say she has a sore throat but actually may be worried about being pregnant.

By age 11 or 12 years, patients should be seen alone. This gives them an opportunity to ask questions they may be embarrassed to ask in front of a parent. Because of the physical changes that take place in early puberty, some adolescents are too self-conscious to undress in front of a parent. If an adolescent comes in willingly, either for an acute illness or for a routine physical examination, it may be helpful to meet with the adolescent and parent together to obtain the history. In the case of angry adolescents, brought in against their will, it is useful to meet with the parents and patient just long enough to have the parents describe the conflict and voice their concerns. This meeting should last no longer than 3–5 minutes, and the adolescent should then be seen alone. This approach conveys that the physician is primarily interested in the adolescent patient, yet gives the physician an opportunity to acknowledge the parents' concerns.

# The Interview

The first few minutes may dictate the success of the visit, whether or not a trusting relationship can be established. A few minutes just getting to know the patient is time well spent. For example, immediately asking, "Do you smoke marijuana?" when a teenager is brought in for suspected marijuana use confirms the adolescent's negative preconceptions about the physician and the purpose of the visit.

It is preferable to spend a few minutes asking nonthreatening questions. "Tell me a little bit about yourself so I can get to know you." "What do you like to do most?" "Least?" "What are your friends like?" Neutral questions help defuse some of the patient's anger and anxiety. Toward the end of the interview, the physician can ask more directed questions about psychosocial concerns.

Medical history questionnaires for the patient and the parents are useful in collecting historical data (Figure 3–2B).

The history should include an assessment of progress with psychodevelopmental tasks and of behaviors potentially detrimental to health. The review of systems should include questions about the following:

1. Nutrition: Number and balance of meals; calcium, iron, cholesterol intake, body image.

2. Sleep: Number of hours, problems with insomnia or frequent waking.

3. Seat belt or helmet: Regularity of use.

4. Self-care: Knowledge of testicular or breast self-examination, dental hygiene, and exercise.

5. Family relationships: Parents, siblings, relatives.

6. Peers: Best friend, involvement in group activities, gangs, boyfriends, girlfriends.

7. School: Attendance, grades, activities.

8. Educational and vocational interests: College, career, short-term and long-term vocational plans.

9. Tobacco: Use of cigarettes, snuff, chewing tobacco.

10. Substance abuse: Frequency, extent, and history of alcohol and drug use.

11. Sexuality: Sexual activity, contraceptive use, pregnancies, history of sexually transmitted disease, number of sexual partners, risk for HIV infection.

12. Emotional health: Signs of depression and excessive stress.

The physician's personal attention and interest is likely to be a new experience for the teenager, who has probably received medical care only through a parent. The teenager should leave the visit with a sense of having a personal physician.

## Physical Examination

During early adolescence, many teenagers may be shy and modest, especially with a physician of the opposite sex. The examiner should address this concern directly, because it can be allayed by acknowledging the uneasiness verbally and by explaining the purpose of the examination, for example, "Many boys that I see who are your age are embarrassed to have their penis and testes examined. This is an important part of the examination

for a couple of reasons. First, I want to make sure that there aren't any physical problems, and second, it helps me determine if your development is proceeding normally." This also introduces the subject of sexual development for discussion.

A pictorial chart of sexual development is useful in showing the patient how development is proceeding and what changes to expect. Figure 3–3 shows the relationship between height, penis and testes development, and pubic hair growth in the male, and Figure 3–4 shows the relationship between height, breast development, menstruation, and pubic hair growth in the female. Many teenagers do not openly admit that they are interested in this subject, but they are usually attentive when it is raised. This discussion is particularly useful in counseling teenagers who lag behind their peers in physical development.

Because teenagers are sensitive about their changing bodies, it is useful to comment during the examination: "Your heart sounds fine. I feel a small lump under your right breast. This is very common during puberty in boys. It is called gynecomastia and should disappear in

**Figure 3–3.** Adolescent male sexual maturation and growth. (Adapted and reproduced, with permission, from Tanner JM: *Growth at Adolescence.* Blackwell Scientific, 1962.)

**GIRLS**

HEIGHT SPURT

PEAK
Height 3 in/y
Weight 17.5 lb/y

GROWTH RATE
Height 2 in/y
Weight 6 lb/y

AGE RANGE
11.5–16.5 y

MENARCHE

Age Range 10–16.5 y
Average Height 62.5 in (158.5 cm)
Average Weight 106 lb (48 kg)

BREAST

| Breast buds begin. AGE RANGE 8–13 years | Breast and areola grow. | Nipple and areola form separate mound, protruding from breast. | Areola rejoins breast contour and development is complete. AGE RANGE 12.5–18.5 years |

SEXUAL MATURITY RATING

PUBIC HAIR

| 2 | 3 | 4 | 5 |
| Initial hair is straight and fine. AGE RANGE 8–14 years | Pubic hair coarsens, darkens and spreads. | Hair looks like adults but limited in area. | Inverted triangular pattern is established AGE RANGE 12.5–16.5 years |

AGE   11 years   12 years   13 years   14 years   15 years

*Figure 3–4.* Adolescent female sexual maturation and growth. (Adapted and reproduced, with permission, from Tanner JM: *Growth at Adolescence.* Blackwell Scientific, 1962.)

6 months to a year. Don't worry, you are not turning into a girl."

If a teenage girl has not been sexually active and has no gynecologic complaints or abnormalities, a pelvic examination is usually not necessary until about age 18 years. The following are indications for a pelvic examination in a younger teenage girl:

1. A history of sexual intercourse. (The pelvic examination should be done for purposes of contraceptive counseling and to rule out sexually transmitted disease.)

2. Abnormal vaginal discharge.

3. Menstrual irregularities.

4. Suspicion of anatomic abnormalities, such as imperforate hymen.

5. Pelvic pain.

6. Patient request for an examination.

Green M (ed): *Bright Futures: Guidelines for Health Supervision of Infants, Children, and Adolescents.* National Center for Education in Maternal and Child Health, 1994.

Metzl JD: Preparticipation examination of the adolescent athlete: Part 1. Pediatr Rev 2001;22:199 [PMID: 11389307].

Metzl JD: Preparticipation examination of the adolescent athlete: Part 2. Pediatr Rev 2001;22:227 [PMID: 11435624].

Sigman G et al: Confidential health care for adolescents: Position paper of the Society for Adolescent Medicine. J Adolesc Health 1997;21:408 [PMID: 9401860].

# ■ GROWTH & DEVELOPMENT

## PUBERTY

Pubertal growth and physical development are a result of activation of the hypothalamic–pituitary–gonadal axis in late childhood. Before the onset of puberty, pituitary and gonadal hormone levels are low. With the onset of puberty, the inhibition of gonadotropin-releasing hormone (GnRH) in the hypothalamus is removed, allowing pulsatile production and release of the gonadotropins: luteinizing hormone (LH) and follicle-stimulating hormone (FSH). In early to middle adolescence, pulse frequency and amplitude of LH and FSH secretion increase, which stimulates the gonads to produce sex steroids (estrogen or testosterone). In the female, FSH stimulates ovarian maturation, granulosa cell function, and estradiol secretion. LH is important in ovulation and is involved also in corpus luteum formation and progesterone secretion. Initially, estradiol has an inhibitory effect on the release of LH and FSH. Eventually, estradiol becomes stimulatory, and the secretions of LH and FSH become cyclic. Estradiol levels progressively increase, resulting in maturation of the female genital tract and breast development.

In the male, LH stimulates the interstitial cells of the testes, which produce testosterone. FSH stimulates the production of spermatocytes in the presence of testosterone. The testes also produce inhibin, a Sertoli cell protein that also inhibits the secretion of FSH. During puberty, circulating testosterone levels increase more than 20-fold. Levels of testosterone correlate with the physical stages of puberty and the degree of skeletal maturation.

## PHYSICAL GROWTH

During adolescence, a teenager's weight almost doubles, and height increases by 15–20%. During puberty, major organs double in size, with the exception of lymphoid tissue, which decreases in mass. Before puberty, there is little difference in the muscular strength of boys and girls. The body's musculature increases both in size and in strength during puberty, with maximal strength lagging behind the increase in size by many months. Boys attain greater strength and mass, and strength continues to increase into late puberty. Although motor coordination lags behind growth in stature and musculature, it continues to improve as strength increases.

The pubertal growth spurt begins nearly 2 years earlier in girls than in boys. Girls reach their peak height velocity (PHV) between ages 11½ and 12 years; boys, between ages 13½ and 14 years. Linear growth at peak velocity is 9.5 cm/y ± 1.5 cm for boys and 8.3 cm/y ±

1.2 cm for girls. Pubertal growth usually takes 2–4 years and continues longer in boys than in girls. By age 11 years in girls and age 12 years in boys, 83–89% of ultimate height has been attained. An additional 18–23 cm in females and 25–30 cm in males will be achieved during further pubertal growth. Following menarche, growth is rarely more than 5–7.5 cm.

In boys, the quantity of body fat increases before onset of the height spurt. They then lose fat until the growth spurt has finished and gradually again increase in fat. Muscle mass doubles between ages 10 and 17 years. Girls, by contrast, gradually store fat from about age 6 years and do not decrease the quantity of fat, although its location changes, with an increase of subcutaneous fat in the region of the pelvis, breasts, and upper back.

## SEXUAL MATURATION

Sexual maturity rating (SMR) is useful clinically for categorizing genital development. SMR staging includes age ranges of normal development and specific descriptions for each stage of pubic hair growth, penis and testis development in boys, and breast maturation in girls. Figures 3–3 and 3–4 graphically represent this chronologic development with reference to each sexual maturity stage. SMR 1 is prepuberty; SMR 5, adult maturity. In SMR 2 is the pubic hair is sparse, fine, non-pigmented, and downy; in SMR 3, the hair becomes pigmented and curly and increases in amount; and in SMR 4, the hair is adult in texture but limited in area. The appearance of pubic hair precedes that of axillary hair by more than 1 year. Male genital development begins with SMR 2, in which the testes become larger and the scrotal skin reddens and coarsens. In SMR 3, the penis lengthens; and in SMR 4, the penis enlarges in overall size and the scrotal skin becomes pigmented.

Female breast development follows a predictable sequence. Small, raised breast buds appear in SMR 2. In SMR 3, the breast and areolar tissue generally enlarge and become elevated. The areola and papilla (nipple) form a separate mound from the breast in SMR 4, and in SMR 5 the areola assumes the same contour as the breast.

Great variability exists in the timing and onset of puberty and growth, and psychosocial development does not necessarily parallel physical changes. Because of this variability, chronologic age may be a poor indication of physiologic and psychosocial development. Skeletal maturation correlates well with growth and pubertal development.

Teenagers have been entering puberty at increasingly earlier ages during the last century because of better nutrition and improved socioeconomic conditions. In the United States, the average age at menarche is 12.16 years in African American girls and 12.88 in white girls. Among girls reaching menarche, the average weight is 48 kg, and the average height is 158.5 cm. However, menarche may be delayed until age 16 years or may begin as early as age 10. Although the first measurable sign of puberty in girls is the beginning of the height spurt, the first conspicuous sign usually is development of breast buds between ages 8 and 11 years. Although breast development usually precedes the growth of pubic hair, in some girls the sequence may be reversed. A common concern for girls at this time is whether the breasts will be of the right size and shape, especially because it is not unusual for one breast to grow faster than the other. Among girls, the growth spurt starts at about age 9 years and reaches a peak at age 11½, usually at SMR 3–4 breast development and stage 3 pubic hair development. The spurt usually ends by age 14 years. Girls who mature early will reach their PHV sooner and attain their final height earlier. Girls who mature late will attain a greater ultimate height because of the longer period of growth before the growth spurt. Final height is related to skeletal age at onset of puberty as well as genetic factors. The height spurt correlates more closely with breast developmental stages than with pubic hair stages.

The first sign of puberty in the male, usually between ages 10 and 12 years, is scrotal and testicular growth. Pubic hair usually appears early in puberty but may do so any time between ages 10 and 15 years. The penis begins to grow significantly a year or so after the onset of testicular and pubic hair development, usually between ages 10 and 13½. The first ejaculation usually occurs about 1 year after initiation of testicular growth, but its timing is highly variable. About 90% of boys have this experience between ages 11 and 15 years. Gynecomastia, a hard nodule under the nipple, occurs in a majority of boys, with a peak incidence between ages 14 and 15 years. Gynecomastia usually disappears within 6 months to 2 years. The height spurt begins at age 11 years but increases rapidly between ages 12 and 13, with the PHV reached at age 13½ years. The period of pubertal development lasts much longer in boys and may not be completed until age 18 years. The height velocity is higher in males (8–11 cm/y) than in females (6.5–9.5 cm/y). The development of axillary hair, deepening of the voice, and the development of chest hair in boys usually occur in mid-puberty, about 2 years after onset of growth of pubic hair. Facial and body hair begin to increase at age 16–17 years.

Herman-Giddens ME et al: Secondary sexual characteristics and menses in young girls seen in office practice: A study from the Pediatric Research in Office Settings Network. Pediatrics 1997;99:505 [PMID: 9093289].

Kaplowitz PB et al: Earlier onset of puberty in girls: Relation to increased body mass index and race. Pediatrics 2001;108:347 [PMID: 11483799].

Molgaard C et al: Influence of weight, age and puberty on bone size and bone mineral content in healthy children and adolescents. Acta Paediatr 1998;87:494 [PMID: 9641728].

Tanner JM, Davies PW: Clinical longitudinal standards for height and height velocity for North American children. J Pediatr 1985;107:317 [PMID: 3875704].

## PSYCHOSOCIAL DEVELOPMENT

Adolescents are struggling to find out who they are, what they want to do in the future, and, in relation to that goal, what their personal strengths and weaknesses are. These questions arise primarily because teenagers are in the process of establishing their own identity. Adolescence is a period of progressive individuation and separation from the family. Because of the rapid physical, emotional, cognitive, and social growth occurring during adolescence, it is useful to divide the period into three sequential phases of development. Early adolescence occurs roughly between ages 10 and 13 years; middle adolescence, between ages 14 and 16 years; and late adolescence, at age 17 years and later.

### Early Adolescence

Early adolescence (ages 10–13 years) is characterized by rapid growth and development of secondary sex characteristics. Because of the rapid physical changes during this period, body image, self-concept, and self-esteem fluctuate dramatically. Concerns about how personal growth and development deviate from that of peers may be a great worry, especially short stature in boys and delayed breast development or delayed menarche in girls. Although there is a certain curiosity about sexuality, young adolescents tend to feel more comfortable with members of the same sex. Peer relationships become increasingly important. Young teenagers still think concretely and cannot easily conceptualize about the future. They may have vague and unrealistic professional goals, such as becoming a movie star or a lead singer in a rock group.

### Middle Adolescence

During middle adolescence (ages 14–16 years), as the rapid pubertal growth rate subsides, teenagers become more comfortable with their new bodies. Intense emotions and wide swings in mood are typical. Although some teenagers go through this experience relatively peacefully, others struggle desperately. Cognitively, teenagers move from concrete thinking to formal operations and develop the ability to think abstractly. With this new mental power comes a sense of omnipotence and a belief that the world can be changed by merely thinking about it. Sexually active teenagers may believe they do not need to worry about using contraception because they can't get pregnant, "it won't happen to me." Sixteen-year-old drivers believe they are the best drivers in the world and think the insurance industry is conspiring against them by charging such high rates for automobile insurance. With the onset of the ability to think abstractly, teenagers begin to see themselves as others see them and may become extremely self-centered. Because they are establishing their own identities, relationships with other people, including peers, are primarily narcissistic, and experimenting with different images is quite common. Peers determine the standards for identification, behavior, activities, and fashion and provide emotional support, intimacy, empathy, and the sharing of guilt and anxiety during the struggle for autonomy. The struggle for independence and autonomy is often a difficult and stressful period for both the teenager and the parents.

As sexuality increases in importance during this time, adolescents may begin dating and experimenting with sex. Relationships usually tend to be one-sided and narcissistic.

## Late Adolescence

During late adolescence (age 17 years and older), the young person generally becomes less self-centered and begins caring more about others. Social relationships shift from the peer group to the individual. Dating becomes much more intimate. By age 18 years, nearly half of American girls and two-thirds of boys have had sexual intercourse. The older adolescent becomes more independent from the family. The ability to think abstractly allows older adolescents to think more realistically in terms of future plans, actions, and careers. Older adolescents have rigid concepts of what is right or wrong. This is a period of idealism.

## Sexual Orientation

Sexual orientation develops during early childhood. One's gender identity is established by age 2 years, and a sense of masculinity or femininity usually solidifies by age 5 or 6 years. Homosexual adults describe homosexual feelings during late childhood and early adolescence, years before engaging in overt homosexual acts.

Although only 5–10% of American young people acknowledge having had homosexual experiences and only 5% feel that they are or could be gay, homosexual experimentation is common, especially during early and middle adolescence. Experimentation may include mutual masturbation and fondling the genitals and does not by itself cause or lead to adult homosexuality. Theories about the causes of homosexuality include genetic, hormonal, environmental, and psychological models.

The development of homosexual identity in adolescence commonly progresses through two stages. The adolescent feels different, develops a crush on a person of the same sex without clear self-awareness of a gay identity, and then goes through a coming-out phase in which the homosexual identity is defined for the individual and revealed to others. The coming-out phase may be a very difficult period for the young person and the family. The young adolescent is afraid of society's bias and seeks to reject homosexual feelings. This struggle with identity may include episodes of both homosexual and heterosexual promiscuity, STIs, depression, substance abuse, attempted suicide, school avoidance and failure, running away from home, and other crises.

In a clinical setting, the issue of homosexual identity most often surfaces as a result of a teenager being seen for an STI, family conflict, school problem, attempted suicide, or substance abuse rather than as a result of a consultation about sexual orientation. Pediatricians should be aware of the psychosocial and medical implications of homosexual identity and be sensitive to the possibility of these problems in gay adolescents. Successful management depends on the physician's ability to gain the trust of the gay adolescent and on the physician's knowledge of the wide range of medical and psychological problems for which gay adolescents may be at risk. Pediatricians must be nonjudgmental in posing sexual questions if they are to be effective in encouraging the teenager to share concerns. Physicians who for religious or other personal reasons cannot be objective must refer the homosexual patient to another professional for treatment and counseling.

American Academy of Pediatrics Committee on Adolescence: Homosexuality and adolescence. Pediatrics 1993;92:631 [PMID: 8414844].

Friedman RC, Downey JI: Homosexuality. N Engl J Med 1994;331:923 [PMID: 8078554].

Garofalo R et al: Sexual orientation and risk of suicide attempts among a representative sample of youth. Arch Pediatr Adolesc Med 1999;153:487 [PMID: 10323629].

Ghai K, Rosenfeld RL: Disorders of pubertal development: Too early, too much, too late, or too little. Adolesc Med 1994;5:19 [PMID: 10358258].

Russell ST, Joyner K: Adolescent sexual orientation and suicide risk: Evidence from a national study. Am J Public Health 2001;91:1276 [PMID: 11499118].

# ■ BEHAVIOR & PSYCHOLOGICAL HEALTH

It is not unusual for adolescents to seek medical attention for seemingly minor complaints. During early adolescence, teenagers may worry about normal developmental changes such as gynecomastia. They may present with vague symptoms, whereas the hidden agenda may be concerns about pregnancy or an STI. Adolescents with emotional disorders often present with somatic symptoms, for example, abdominal pain, headaches, dizziness or syncope, fatigue, sleep problems, and chest pain, that appear to have no biologic cause. The emotional basis of such complaints may be varied: somatoform disorder, depression, or stress and anxiety.

## PSYCHOPHYSIOLOGIC SYMPTOMS & CONVERSION REACTIONS

The most common somatoform disorders during adolescence are conversion disorders or conversion reactions. (A conversion reaction is a psychophysiologic process in which unpleasant feelings, especially anxiety, depression, and guilt, are communicated through a physical symptom.) Psychophysiologic symptoms result when anxiety activates the autonomic nervous system, resulting in tachycardia, hyperventilation, and vasoconstriction. The emotional feeling may be threatening or unacceptable to the individual, who expresses it as a physical symptom rather than verbally. This process is unconscious, and the anxiety or unpleasant feeling is dissipated by the somatic symptom. The degree to which the conversion symptom lessens anxiety, depression, or the unpleasant feeling is referred to as primary gain. Conversion symptoms not only diminish unpleasant feelings but also release the adolescent from conflict or an uncomfortable situation. This is referred to as secondary gain. Secondary gain may intensify the symptoms, especially with increased attention from concerned parents and friends. Adolescents with conversion symptoms tend to have overprotective parents and become increasingly dependent on their parents as the symptom becomes the major focus concern in the family.

### Clinical Findings

The symptom may appear at times of stress. Nervous, gastrointestinal, and cardiovascular symptoms are common and include paresthesias, anesthesia, paralysis, dizziness, syncope, hyperventilation, abdominal pain, nausea, and vomiting. Specific symptoms may reflect existing or previous illness (eg, pseudoseizures in adolescents with epilepsy) or modeling of a close relative's symptom (eg, chest pain in a boy whose grandfather died of a heart attack).

Conversion symptoms are more common in girls than boys. They occur in patients from all socioeconomic levels; however, the complexity of the symptom may vary with the sophistication and cognitive level of the patient.

### Differential Diagnosis

The history and physical findings are usually inconsistent with anatomic and physiologic concepts. Conversion symptoms are exhibited most frequently at times of stress and in the presence of individuals meaningful to the patient. The patient often exhibits a characteristic personality pattern, including egocentricity, emotional lability, and dramatic and attention-seeking behaviors.

Conversion reactions must be differentiated from hypochondriasis, which is a preoccupation with developing or having a serious illness despite medical reassurance that there is no evidence of disease. Over time, the fear of one disease may give way to concern about another. In contrast to patients with conversion symptoms, who seem relieved if an organic cause is considered, patients with hypochondriasis become more anxious when such a cause is considered.

Malingering is uncommon during adolescence. The malingering patient consciously and intentionally produces false or exaggerated physical or psychological symptoms. Such patients are motivated by external incentives such as avoiding work, evading criminal prosecution, obtaining drugs, or obtaining financial compensation. These patients may be hostile and aloof. Parents of patients with conversion disorders and malingering have a similar reaction to illness. They have an unconscious psychological need to have sick children and reinforce their child's behavior.

Somatic delusions are physical symptoms, often bizarre, that accompany other signs of mental illness. Examples are visual or auditory hallucinations, delusions, incoherence or loosening of associations, rapid shifts of affect, and confusion.

### Treatment

The physician must emphasize from the onset that both physical and emotional causes of the symptom need to be considered. The relationship between physical causes of emotional pain and emotional causes of physical pain should be described to the family, using examples such as stress causing an ulcer or making a severe headache worse. The patient should be encouraged to understand that the symptom may persist and that at least a short-term goal is to continue normal daily activities. Medication is rarely helpful. If the family will accept it, psychological referral is often the best initial step toward psychotherapy. If the family resists psychiatric or psychological referral, the pediatrician may need to begin to deal with some of the emotional factors responsible for the symptom while building rapport with the patient and family. Regular appointments should be scheduled. During the sessions, the teenager should be seen first and encouraged to talk about school, friends, the relationship with the parents, and the stresses of life. Discussion of the symptom itself should be minimized; however, the physician should be supportive and must never suggest that the pain is not real. As the parents gain further insight into the cause of the symptom, they will become less indulgent of the complaints, facilitating the resumption of normal activities. If management is successful, the adolescent will increase coping skills and become more independent, while decreasing secondary gain.

If the symptom continues to interfere with daily activities and if the patient and parents feel that no progress is being made, psychological referral is indicated. A psychotherapist experienced in treating adolescents with conversion reactions is in the best position to establish a strong therapeutic relationship with the patient and family. After referral is made, the pediatrician should continue to follow the patient to ensure compliance with psychotherapy.

American Psychiatric Association: *Diagnostic and Statistical Manual of Mental Disorders,* 4th ed. American Psychiatric Press, 1994.

Gold MA, Friedman SB: Conversion reactions in adolescents. Pediatr Ann 1995;24:296 [PMID: 7659461].

Silber TJ, Pao M: Somatization disorders in children and adolescents. Pediatr Rev 2003;24(8):255 [PMID: 12897265].

Wood BL: Physically manifested illness in children and adolescents: A biobehavioral family approach. Child Adolesc Psychiatr Clin North Am 2001;10:543 [PMID: 11449811].

# DEPRESSION (See also Chapter 6.)

Symptoms of clinical depression (lethargy, loss of interest, sleep disturbances, decreased energy, feelings of worthlessness, and difficulty concentrating) are common during adolescence. The intensity of feelings, often in response to seemingly trivial events such as a poor grade on an examination or not being invited to a party, makes it difficult to differentiate severe depression from normal sadness or dejection. In less severe depression, sadness or unhappiness associated with problems of everyday life is generally short-lived. The symptoms usually result in only minor impairment in school performance, social activities, and relationships with others. Symptoms respond to support and reassurance.

## Clinical Findings

The presentation of serious depression in adolescence may be similar to that in adults, with vegetative signs such as depressed mood, crying spells or inability to cry,

discouragement, irritability, a sense of emptiness and meaninglessness, negative expectations of oneself and the environment, low self-esteem, isolation, a feeling of helplessness, diminished interest or pleasure in activities, weight loss or weight gain, insomnia or hypersomnia, fatigue or loss of energy, feelings of worthlessness, and diminished ability to think or concentrate. However, it is not unusual for a serious depression to be masked because the teenager cannot tolerate the severe feelings of sadness. Such a teenager may present with recurrent or persistent psychosomatic complaints, such as abdominal pain, chest pain, headache, lethargy, weight loss, dizziness and syncope, or other nonspecific symptoms. Other behavioral manifestations of masked depression include truancy, running away from home, defiance of authorities, self-destructive behavior, vandalism, drug and alcohol abuse, sexual acting out, and delinquency.

## Differential Diagnosis

A complete history and physical examination, including a careful review of the patient's medical and psychosocial history, should be performed. The family history should be explored for psychiatric problems.

The teenager should be questioned about the previously listed symptoms of depression, and specifically about suicidal ideation or preoccupation with thoughts of death. The history should include an assessment of school performance, looking for signs of academic deterioration, excessive absence or cutting class, changes in work or other outside activities, and changes in the family (eg, separation, divorce, serious illness, loss of employment by a parent, a recent move to a new school, increasing quarrels or fights with parents, the death of a close relative). The teenager may have withdrawn from friends or family or switched allegiance to a new group of friends. The physician should seek to develop a history of drug and alcohol abuse, conflicts with the police, sexual acting out, running away from home, unusually violent or rebellious behavior, or radical personality changes. Patients with vague somatic complaints or concerns about having a fatal illness may have an underlying affective disorder.

Adolescents presenting with symptoms of depression require a thorough medical evaluation to rule out any contributing or underlying medical illness. Among the medical conditions associated with affective disorders are eating disorders, organic central nervous system (CNS) disorders (tumors, vascular lesions, closed head trauma, and subdural hematomas), metabolic and endocrinologic disorders (systemic lupus erythematosus, hypothyroidism, hyperthyroidism, Wilson disease, hyperparathyroidism, Cushing syndrome, Addison disease, premenstrual syndrome), infections (infectious mononucleosis, syphilis), and mitral valve prolapse. Marijuana use, phencyclidine abuse, amphetamine withdrawal, and excessive caffeine intake can cause symptoms of depression. Common prescription and over-the-counter medications, including birth control pills, anticonvulsants, and β-blockers, may cause depressive symptoms.

Some routine laboratory studies are indicated in the depressed patient to rule out organic disease: a complete blood count (CBC) and erythrocyte sedimentation rate (ESR), urinalysis, serum electrolytes, blood urea nitrogen (BUN), serum calcium, thyroxine and thyroid-stimulating hormone (TSH), Venereal Disease Research Laboratory (VDRL) or rapid plasma reagin (RPR), and liver enzymes. Although metabolic markers such as abnormal secretion of cortisol, growth hormone, and thyrotropin-releasing hormone have been useful in confirming major depression in adults, these neurobiologic markers are less reliable in adolescents.

The risk of depression appears to be greatest in families with a history of early onset and chronic depression. Depression of early onset and bipolar illness are more likely to occur in families with a strong multigenerational history of depression. The lifetime risk of depressive illness in first-degree relatives of adult depressed patients has been estimated to be between 18% and 30%.

## Treatment

The primary care physician may be able to counsel adolescents and parents if depression is mild or is the result of an acute personal loss or frustration and if the patient is not contemplating suicide or other life-threatening behaviors. If, however, there is evidence of a long-standing depressive disorder, suicidal thoughts, or psychotic thinking, or if the physician does not feel competent or has no interest in counseling the patient, psychological referral should be made.

Counseling involves establishing and maintaining a positive supportive relationship; following the patient at least weekly; remaining accessible to the patient at all times; encouraging the patient to express emotions openly, defining the problem and clarifying negative feelings, thoughts, and expectations; setting realistic goals; helping to negotiate interpersonal crises; teaching assertiveness and social skills; reassessing the depression as it is expressed; and staying alert to the possibility of suicide.

Patients with a clinical course consistent with bipolar disease or those who have a significant depression that is unresponsive to supportive counseling should be referred to a psychiatrist for evaluation of antidepressant medication.

Brent DA, Birmaher B: Clinical practice. Adolescent depression. N Engl J Med 2002;347(9):667 [PMID: 12200555].

Jellinek MS, Snyder JB: Depression and suicide in children and adolescents. Pediatr Rev 1998;19:255 [PMID: 9707715].

Labellarte MJ et al: The new antidepressants: Selective serotonin reuptake inhibitors. Pediatr Clin North Am 1998;45:1137 [PMID: 9884679].

Whooley MA, Simon GE: Managing depression in medical outpatients. N Engl J Med 2000;343:1942 [PMID: 11136266].

## ADOLESCENT SUICIDE (See also Chapter 6.)

In 2000, 3994 people age 15–24 years committed suicide, 1621 suicides among those age 15–19 years and 2378 among those age 20–24 years. In the younger group, males had a suicide rate 5 times higher than females, and white males had the highest rate, 15.5 per 100,000. The incidence of unsuccessful suicide attempts is three times higher in females than in males. The estimated ratio of attempted suicides to actual suicides is estimated to be 100:1–50:1. Firearms account for 67% of suicide deaths in both males and females.

With the normal mood swings of adolescence, short periods of depression are common, and a teenager may have thoughts of suicide. Normal mood swings during this period rarely interfere with sleeping, eating, or participating in normal activities. Acute depressive reactions (transient grief responses) to the loss of a family member or friend may result in depression lasting for weeks or even months. An adolescent who is unable to work through this grief can become increasingly depressed. A teenager who is unable to keep up with schoolwork, does not participate in normal social activities, withdraws socially, has sleep and appetite disturbances, and has feelings of hopelessness and helplessness should be considered to be at increased risk for suicide.

Another group of suicidal adolescents is composed of angry teenagers attempting to influence others by their actions. They may be only mildly depressed and may not have a long-standing wish to die. Teenagers in this group, usually females, may attempt suicide or make a suicidal gesture as a way of getting back at someone or gaining attention by frightening another person.

The last group at risk for suicide are adolescents with a serious psychiatric problem such as acute schizophrenia or a true psychotic depressive disorder.

### Risk Assessment

The physician must determine the extent of the teenager's depression and assess the risk of inflicting self-harm. The evaluation should include interviews with both the teenager and the family. The history should include the medical, social, emotional, and academic background (see Table 6–16). The physician should inquire about

1. Common signs of depression
2. Recent events that could be the cause of an underlying depression
3. Evidence of long-standing problems in the home, at school, or with peers
4. Drug or substance use and abuse
5. Signs of psychotic thinking, such as delusions or hallucinations
6. Evidence of masked depression, such as rebellious behavior, running away from home, reckless driving, or other acting-out behavior.

When seeing depressed patients, the physician should always inquire about thoughts of suicide, for example, by asking, "Are things ever so bad that life doesn't seem worth living?" If the response is affirmative, a more specific question should be asked, for example, "Have you thought of taking your life?" If the patient has thoughts of suicide, the immediacy of risk can be assessed by determining if the patient has a concrete, feasible plan. Although patients who are at greatest risk have a concrete plan that can be carried out in the near future, especially if they have rehearsed the plan, the physician should not dismiss the potential risk of suicide in the adolescent who does not describe a specific plan. The physician should pay attention to his or her gut feelings. Subtle nonverbal signs may indicate that the patient is at greater risk than may be apparent.

## Treatment

The primary care physician is often in a unique position to identify an adolescent at risk for suicide, because many teenagers who attempt suicide seek medical attention in the weeks preceding the attempt. These visits are often for vague somatic complaints. If is the patient shows evidence of depression, the physician must assess the severity of the depression and suicidal risk. The pediatrician should always seek emergency psychological consultation for any teenager who is severely depressed, psychotic, or acutely suicidal. It is the psychologist's or psychiatrist's responsibility to assess the seriousness of suicidal ideation and decide whether hospitalization or out-patient treatment is most appropriate. Adolescents with mild depression and at low risk for suicide should be followed closely, and the extent of the depression should be assessed on an ongoing basis. If at any point it appears that the patient is worsening or the teenager is not responding to supportive counseling, referral should be made.

American Academy of Child and Adolescent Psychiatry: Summary of the practice parameters for the assessment and treatment of children and adolescents with suicidal behavior. J Am Acad Child Adolesc Psychiatry 2001;40:495 [PMID: 11314578].

American Academy of Pediatrics Committee on Adolescence: Suicide and suicide attempts in adolescents. Pediatrics 2000;105:871 [PMID: 10742349].

Blumenthal SJ: Youth suicide: The physician's role in suicide prevention. JAMA 1990;264:3194 [PMID: 2255029].

Grossman DC et al: Self-inflicted and unintentional firearm injuries among children and adolescents: The source of the firearm. Arch Pediatr Adolesc Med 1999;153:875 [PMID: 10437764].

The Committee on Adolescence: *Adolescent Suicide.* American Psychiatric Press, 1996.

Zametkin AJ et al: Suicide in teenagers: Assessment, management, and prevention. JAMA 2001;286(24):3120 [PMID: 11754678].

## SUBSTANCE ABUSE

Substance abuse is a complex problem for adolescents and the broader society. See Chapter 4 for an in-depth look at this issue.

## EATING DISORDERS (See Chapter 5.)

## EXOGENOUS OBESITY (See Chapter 10: Normal Childhood Nutrition & Its Disorders)

Overweight, or at risk for obesity, is defined as body mass index (BMI) greater than the 85th percentile for age (Figures 3–5 and 3–6). It is important to note that mean BMI changes dramatically with age. For a 13-year-old, a BMI greater than 25 constitutes obesity, whereas in adolescents older than 18, the adult standard of BMI greater than 30 accurately defines obesity (Figure 3–7).

## Background

Recent data from the National Health and Nutrition Examination Survey (NHANES)-IV showed an increase in obesity in adolescents ages 12–19 from 5% in 1966–1970 to 14% in 1999. The changes in BMI during and after adolescence have been shown to be important predictors of adult adiposity. In general, the longer a child remains obese, the more likely obesity will persist into adulthood. The medical risks associated with obesity are discussed in Chapter 10. The psychosocial hazards of obesity tend to be the greatest consequence for adolescents, who may experience alienation, distorted peer relations, poor self-esteem, guilt, depression, or altered body image.

**2 to 20 years: Girls**
**Body mass index-for-age percentiles**

NAME _____

RECORD # _____

*To Calculate BMI: Weight (kg) ÷ Stature (cm) ÷ Stature (cm) x 10,000
or Weight (lb) ÷ Stature (in) ÷ Stature (in) x 703

***Figure 3–5.*** Percentile values for BMI (kg/m²) in girls. (Centers for Disease Control and Prevention.)

**2 to 20 years: Boys**
**Body mass index-for-age percentiles**

NAME _____

RECORD # _____

*To Calculate BMI: Weight (kg) ÷ Stature (cm) ÷ Stature (cm) x 10,000
or Weight (lb) ÷ Stature (in) ÷ Stature (in) x 703

*Figure 3–6.* Percentile values for BMI (kg/m²) in boys. (Centers for Disease Control and Prevention.)

**Figure 3–7.** Nomogram for determining body mass index (BMI) from height and weight. A straight-edge connecting weight and height allows one to read BMI (weight in kg ÷ [height in m²]). The three dots on the left side of the BMI line represent 50th percentile values for females age 20 years (top), 15 years (middle), and 10 years (bottom). The dots on the right side are for similar-aged males. (Reproduced, with permission, from Forbes GR: Nutrition and growth. In: McAnarney ER et al [eds]: *Textbook of Adolescent Medicine.* WB Saunders, 1992.)

## Diagnosis

An adolescent with a BMI above the 85th percentile is considered at risk for obesity; BMI above the 95th percentile is considered obese. Patients can be identified as at risk for obesity based on current weight relative to height, growth and weight trend, and weight of family members. In addition, the provider needs to assess a patient's readiness to make lifestyle changes. When obesity is diagnosed, the following database can be collected: height; weight; BMI; blood pressure; condition of the skin, thyroid, heart, and abdomen; hematocrit; and urinalysis. Acanthosis nigricans is a cutaneous finding characterized by velvety hyperpigmentation, most prominent behind the neck, in the axilla, and in the groin. Acanthosis is more commonly seen in dark-skinned persons and is a marker for insulin resistance. Endocrine causes of obesity, such as hypothyroidism and Cushing disease, can generally be excluded on the basis of the history and physical examination. If an adolescent is healthy and has no delay of growth or sexual maturation, an underlying endocrinologic, neurologic, or genetic cause is unlikely.

## Treatment

Poorly motivated adolescents may be alienated by an aggressive discussion of weight loss. Instead, providers may give basic information about healthy diet and regular exercise and be available for future visits if patients become interested in weight loss. For the highly motivated patient, treatment should be appropriate to age and developmental level. The adolescent should be taught appropriate eating and exercise habits to maintain weight reduction yet meet nutritional needs for growth and development. You may be more likely to engage the average adolescent by helping him or her to choose concrete, obtainable goals (eg, decreasing soda from three to two per day, or walking with a friend 3 days a week instead of watching television). Appetite-suppressing drugs, fasting, and bypass surgery have no role in the management of obese adolescents unless severe comorbidities of obesity are present. An age-appropriate behavior modification program incorporating good dietary counseling and exercise is optimal. Studies indicate that increased activity may be more important than dietary changes in long-term weight management. Lifestyle activity recommendations, such as walking and taking the stairs, may be more effective in the long run than regimented exercise programs. Avoiding labeling any food as "forbidden" may improve long-term success with healthy eating behaviors. Behavioral treatment involving parents has been shown to improve long-term maintenance of weight loss in children; parental involvement in adolescent weight loss programs has shown mixed results. In general, the most important factor in successful weight loss and weight maintenance is motivation of the adolescent. Monthly follow-up visits may help to maintain motivation, especially initially. Unfortunately, no program has been proven effective for long-term weight reduction.

Styne D: Childhood and adolescent obesity. Pediatr Clin North Am 2001;48:823 [PMID 11494639].

Yanovski JA: Intensive therapies for pediatric obesity. Pediatr Clin North Am 2001;48:1041 [PMID 11494637].

## SCHOOL AVOIDANCE

Any teenager who has missed more than 1 week of school for a physical illness or symptom, and whose clinical picture is inconsistent with a serious illness, should be suspected of harboring primary or secondary emotional factors that contribute to the absence. Investigation of absences may show a pattern, such as missing morning classes or missing the same days at the beginning or end of the week. Emotional factors for school absenteeism are usually attributed to physical symptoms in this age group.

School avoidance should be suspected in children who are consistently absent in spite of parents' and professionals' attempts to encourage school attendance. Adolescents with school avoidance problems often have a history of excessive absences or separation difficulties as a younger child. They may also have a record of recurrent somatic complaints. Parents of a school avoider often feel helpless to compel their adolescent to attend school, may lack the sophistication to distinguish malingering from illness, or may have an underlying need to keep the teenager at home.

A complete history and physical examination should be performed, reviewing the patient's medical, educational, and psychiatric history. Signs of emotional problems should be explored. After obtaining permission from the patient and parents, the physician may find it helpful to speak directly with school officials and some key teachers. The adolescent may be having problems with particular teachers or subjects or experiencing adversity at school (eg, schoolyard bullying, an intimidating instructor). Some students get so far behind academically that they see no way of catching up and feel overwhelmed. Separation anxiety, sometimes of long duration, may be manifested in subconscious worries that something may happen to the mother while the teenager is at school.

The school nurse may give useful information, including the number of visits to the nurse during the last school year. An important part of the history is how the parents respond to the absences and somatic complaints. The parent(s) may be making a subconscious attempt to keep the adolescent at home, which may be coupled with secondary gains for the patient, such as increased parental attention.

### Treatment

The importance of returning to school quickly after a period of school avoidance needs to be emphasized. The pediatrician should facilitate this process by offering to speak with school officials to excuse missed examina-

tions, homework, and papers. The pediatrician should speak directly with teachers who are punitive. The objective is to make the transition back to school as easy as possible. The longer adolescents stay out of school, the more anxious they may become about returning and the more difficult the return becomes. If an illness or symptom becomes so severe that an adolescent cannot go to school, the patient and the parents must be informed that a visit to a medical office is necessary. The physician focuses visits on the parents as much as on the adolescent to alleviate any parental guilt about sending the child to school. If the adolescent cannot stay in school, hospitalization should be recommended for an in-depth medical and psychiatric evaluation. Parents should be cautioned about the possibility of relapse after school holidays, summer vacation, or an acute illness.

Klerman LV: School absence: A health perspective. Pediatr Clin North Am 1988;35:1253 [PMID: 3059298].

## SCHOOL FAILURE

When children graduate from grade school to middle school or junior high school, the amount and complexity of course work increase significantly. This occurs at about the same time as the rapid physical, social, and emotional changes of puberty. To perform well academically, young adolescents must have the necessary cognitive capacity, study habits, concentration, motivation, interest, and emotional focus. Academic failure presenting at adolescence has a broad differential:

1. Limited intellectual abilities
2. Specific learning disabilities
3. Depression or emotional problems
4. Physical causes such as visual or hearing problems
5. Excessive school absenteeism secondary to chronic disease such as asthma or neurologic dysfunction
6. Lack of ability to concentrate
7. Attention-deficit/hyperactivity disorder
8. Lack of motivation
9. Drug and alcohol problems.

Each of these possible causes must be explored in depth (Table 3–1). Evaluation of this differential requires a careful history, physical examination, and appropriate laboratory tests as well as standardized educational and psychological testing.

### Treatment

Treatment depends on the cause. Management must be individualized to address specific needs, foster strengths, and implement a feasible program. For children with specific learning disabilities, an individual prescription

***Table 3–1.*** A classification of common developmental dysfunctions in adolescence.

| Dysfunction | Subtypes | Frequent Manifestations[a] |
|---|---|---|
| 1. Attention deficits | a. Primary<br>b. Secondary (to anxiety or poor information processing)<br>c. Situational (only evident in certain settings) | Weak attention to detail; distractibility; impulsivity, restlessness; task impersistence; performance inconsistency; organizational problems; reduced working capacity |
| 2. Memory impairments | a. Generalized retrieval problems<br>b. Modality-specific retrieval problems<br>c. Attention-retention deficiencies | Deficient, undependable, or slow recall of data from long- or short-term memory<br>Problems with revisualization or auditory, motor, or sequential recall<br>Poor recall associated with superficial initial registration |
| 3. Language disorders | a. Receptive<br>b. Expressive | Poor verbal and reading comprehension; poor listening; trouble following directions and explanations<br>Problems with word finding, sentence formulation<br>Difficulty with written expression |
| 4. Higher-order cognitive disabilities | a. Inferential weakness<br>b. Poor verbal reasoning<br>c. Poor nonverbal reasoning<br>d. Difficulty with abstraction, symbolization<br>e. Weak generalization and rule application | Problems understanding and assimilating new concepts; tendency to think "concretely," delays in mathematics, reading comprehension, science, social studies |
| 5. Fine motor incoordination | a. Eye:hand coordination problems<br>b. Impaired propriokinesthetic feedback<br>c. Dyspraxia<br>d. Motor memory impairment | Slow, labored, sometimes illegible writing; awkward pencil grip; dyssynchrony between cognitive tempo and writing speed; output failure—reduced productivity |
| 6. Organizational deficiencies | a. Temporal-sequential disorientation<br>b. Material disarray<br>c. Integrative dysfunction<br>d. Resynthesis problems<br>e. Attentional disorganization | Problems with time allocation, schedules, planning, arranging ideas in writing<br>Tendency to lose, misplace, forget books, papers; trouble organizing notebook<br>Varying inability to integrate data from multiple sources or sensory modalities<br>Trouble extracting most salient details, retelling and adapting data to current demands<br>Impulsivity, erratic tempo, poor self-monitoring, careless errors |
| 7. Socialization disabilities | a. Wide range of subtypes, including conduct disorder, social impulsivity, impaired social cognition or feedback, egocentricity | Antisocial behaviors; delinquency; withdrawal; excessive dependency on peer support |

[a]Manifestations are likely to vary somewhat depending on compensatory strengths, quality of educational experience, and motivation.
Modified and reproduced, with permission, from Levine MD, Zallen BG: Learning disorders of adolescence. Pediatr Clin North Am 1984;31:2.

for regular and special education courses, teachers, and extracurricular activities is important. Counseling helps these adolescents gain coping skills, raise self-esteem, and develop socialization skills. If the patient has a history of hyperactivity or attention deficit disorder along with poor ability to concentrate, a trial of stimulant medication (eg, methylphenidate, dextroamphetamine) may be useful. If the teenager appears to be depressed or if other serious emotional problems are uncovered, further psychological evaluation should be recommended.

Brown FR et al: AD/HD: A neurodevelopmental perspective. Contemp Pediatr 1996;13:25.

Goldman LS et al: Diagnosis and treatment of attention-deficit/hyperactivity disorder in children and adolescents. JAMA 1998;279:1100 [PMID: 9546570].

Kube DA, Shapiro BK: Persistent school dysfunction: Unrecognized comorbidity and suboptimal therapy. Clin Pediatr (Phila) 1996;45:571 [PMID: 8953132].

Reiff MI: Adolescent school failure. Failure to thrive in adolescence. Pediatr Rev 1998;19:199 [PMID: 9613171].

Shaywitz BA et al: Attention-deficit/hyperactivity disorder. Adv Pediatr 1997;44:331 [PMID: 9265975].

Shaywitz SE: Dyslexia. N Engl J Med 1998;338:307 [PMID: 9445412].

## ■ BREAST DISORDERS

The breast examination should become part of the routine physical examination in girls as soon as breast budding occurs. The preadolescent thus comes to accept breast examination as a routine part of health care, and the procedure serves as an opportunity to offer reassurance about any concerns she may have. The breast examination begins with inspection of the breasts for symmetry and Tanner or sexual maturity rating (SMR) stage. Asymmetrical breast development is common, especially in young adolescents, and is generally transient, although 25% of women may continue to have some degree of asymmetry into adulthood. Unusual causes of breast asymmetry include unilateral breast hypoplasia, amastia, absence of the pectoralis major muscle, and unilateral virginal hypertrophy (massive enlargement of the breast during puberty).

Palpation of the breasts can be performed with the patient in the supine position and the patient's ipsilateral arm placed behind her head. The examiner palpates the breast tissue with the flat of the fingers in concentric circles from the sternum, clavicle, and axilla in to the areola. The areola should be compressed gently to check for discharge.

Instructions for breast self-examination and its purpose can be given to older adolescents approaching age 18 years during this portion of the physical examination, and the patient should be encouraged to begin monthly self-examination after each menstrual flow after age 18 years. Because the vast majority of breast lesions in teens are benign, teaching young adolescents breast self-examination may lead to unnecessary anxiety and overconcern with normal variants.

### BREAST MASSES

Most breast masses in adolescents are benign (Table 3–2); however, cancer does occasionally occur in adolescents. A large study in Greece of 684 females ages 14–20 with breast masses showed only 2.5% to be malignant. The malignant cases included hemangiosarcoma, rhabdomyosarcoma, ductal carcinoma, cystosarcoma phyllodes, and metastatic tumor.

#### Fibroadenoma

Fibroadenoma (which accounts for approximately two-thirds of all breast masses in adolescents) presents as a rubbery, well-demarcated, slowly growing, nontender

**Table 3–2.** Breast masses in adolescent females.

| |
|---|
| **Common** |
|     Fibroadenoma |
|     Fibrocystic changes |
|     Breast cysts |
|     Breast abscess/mastitis |
| **Less common or rare (benign)** |
|     Lymphangioma |
|     Hemangioma |
|     Giant fibroadenoma |
|     Neurofibromatosis |
|     Nipple adenoma/keratoma |
|     Mammary duct actasia |
|     Lipoma |
|     Hematoma |
| **Rare (malignant potential)** |
|     Adenocarcinoma |
|     Cystosarcoma phyllodes |
|     Intraductal papilloma |
|     Rhabdomyosarcoma |
|     Lymphosarcoma |
|     Hemangiosarcoma |
|     Metastatic cancer |

mass that may occur in any quadrant, but is most commonly found in the upper outer quadrant. The average size is 2–3 cm in diameter. In 10–25% of cases, multiple or recurrent lesions occur. Quiescence can be expected after the teenage years.

#### Cysts

Breast cysts are generally tender and spongy, with exacerbation of symptoms premenstrually and improvement after menses. Often they are multiple. Spontaneous regression occurs over two or three menstrual cycles in about 50% of cases.

It is reasonable to follow breast masses that are consistent with fibroadenoma or cyst in adolescents for two or three menstrual cycles. Approximately 25% of fibroadenomas become smaller, and approximately 50% of cysts resolve. If a presumed fibroadenoma does not change after this time, ultrasound will differentiate a solid tumor from a cyst. Patients with solid tumors larger than 2.5 cm in diameter should be referred for fine-needle aspiration or excisional biopsy. Those with tumors less than 2.5 cm in diameter may be followed every 3–6 months, because many of these tumors will shrink or remain the same. Persistent cystic lesions may be drained by needle aspiration. Patients with suspicious lesions should be referred immediately to a breast surgeon (Table 3–3).

***Table 3–3.*** Breast lesions.

| | |
|---|---|
| Fibroadenoma | Rubbery, well demarcated, nontender, slowly growing; most commonly found in the upper outer quadrant of the breast. Usually < 5 cm. |
| Adenocarcinoma | Hard, nonmobile, well-circumscribed, painless mass; generally indolent clinical course; occurs also in males but less frequently. |
| Cystosarcoma phyllodes | Firm, rubbery mass that may suddenly enlarge; associated with skin necrosis; most often benign. |
| Giant juvenile fibroadenoma | Remarkable large fibroadenoma with overlying dilated superficial veins; accounts for 5–10% of fibroadenomas in adolescents; benign but requires excision to prevent breast atrophy and for cosmetic reasons. |
| Intraductal papilloma | A cylindric tumor arising from the ductal epithelium; often subareolar but may be in the periphery of the breast in adolescents, with associated nipple discharge. Most are benign but require excision for cytologic diagnosis. |
| Fat necrosis | Localized inflammatory process in one breast; follows trauma in about half of cases. Subsequent scarring may be confused with cancer. |
| Virginal or juvenile hypertrophy | Massive enlargement of both breasts or, less often, one breast; attributed to end-organ hypersensitivity to normal hormonal levels just before or within a few years after menarche. |
| Miscellaneous | Fibroma, galactocele, hemangioma, intraductal granuloma, interstitial fibrosis, keratoma, lipoma, granular cell myoblastoma, papilloma, sclerosing adenosis. |

## Fibrocystic Breasts

Fibrocystic breast disease sometimes occurs in older adolescents and becomes more common with age. It is characterized by cyclic tenderness and nodularity bilaterally and is believed to be influenced by the estrogen–progesterone balance.

Reassuring the young woman about the benign nature of the process and emphasizing the importance of breast self-examination as she becomes an adult may be all that is needed. Support bras may provide sympto-matic relief. Oral contraceptives (OCPs) often improve symptoms. Studies have shown no association between methylxanthines and fibrocystic breasts; however, some women report reduced symptoms when they discontinue caffeine intake. The efficacy of vitamins E, $B_1$, and A is unknown. Evening primrose oil has been beneficial in 44% of patients. A trial of 1000 mg three times a day for 3 months may be helpful.

## Breast Abscess

The female with a breast abscess usually complains of unilateral breast pain, and examination reveals overlying inflammatory changes. Often the examination is misleading in that the infection may extend much deeper than suspected. A palpable mass is found only late in the course. Although breast feeding is the most common cause of mastitis, trauma and eczema involving the areola are frequent factors in teenagers. *Staphylococcus aureus* is the most common pathogen, but other aerobic and anaerobic organisms have also been implicated.

Cyclic mastodynia, fibrocystic disease, or chest wall pain may also be causes of breast pain, but no associated inflammatory signs should be present.

Fluctuant abscesses should be surgically incised and drained. Oral antibiotics with appropriate coverage (dicloxacillin or a cephalosporin) should be given for 2–4 weeks. Ice packs for the first 24 hours and heat thereafter may relieve symptoms.

## GALACTORRHEA

In teenagers, galactorrhea is most often benign; however, a careful history and work-up are necessary. Prolactinomas are the most common pathologic cause of galactorrhea in adolescents of both sexes and generally present as amenorrhea or failure of sexual maturation. Hypothyroidism is the second most common cause in the adolescent years but has been reported only in girls, usually prepubertally.

Galactorrhea may be present after spontaneous or induced abortions as well as postpartum. Numerous prescribed and illicit drugs are associated with galactorrhea (Table 3–4). In addition, stimulation of the intercostal nerves (following surgery or due to herpes zoster infection), stimulation of the nipples, CNS disorders (hypothalamic injury), or significant emotional distress may produce galactorrhea.

## Clinical Findings

If the teenager has no history of pregnancy or drug use, TSH and serum prolactin levels should be determined. An elevated TSH confirms the diagnosis of hypothy-

**Table 3–4.** Medications and herbs associated with galactorrhea.

| Antidepressants and anxiolytics | Other drugs |
|---|---|
| Alprazolam (Xanax) | Amphetamines |
| Buspirone (BuSpar) | Anesthetics |
| Monoamine oxidase inhibitors | Arginine |
|   Moclobemide (Manerix; available in Canada) | Cannabis |
| | Cisapride (Propulsid) |
| Selective serotonin reuptake inhibitors | Cyclobenzaprine (Flexeril) |
|   Citalopram (Celexa) | Danazol (Danocrine) |
|   Fluoxetine (Prozac) | Dihydroergotamine (DHE 45) |
|   Paroxetine (Paxil) | |
|   Sertraline (Zoloft) | Domperidone (Motilium; available in Canada and Mexico) |
| Tricyclic antidepressants | |
| Antihypertensives | Isoniazid (INH) |
|   Atenolol (Tenormin) | Metoclopramide (Reglan) |
|   Methyldopa (Aldomet) | |
|   Reserpine (Serpasil) | Octreotide (Sandostatin) |
|   Verapamil (Calan) | Opiates |
| Antipsychotics | Rimantadine (Flumadine) |
| Histamine H$_2$-receptor blockers | Sumatriptan (Imitrex) |
|   Cimetidine (Tagamet) | Valproic acid (Depakene) |
|   Famotidine (Pepcid) | |
|   Ranitidine (Zantac) | Herbs |
| Hormones | Anise |
|   Conjugated estrogen and medroxyprogesterone (Premphase, Prempro) | Blessed thistle |
| | Fennel |
| | Fenugreek seed |
| Medroxyprogesterone contraceptive injections (Depo-Provera) | Marshmallow |
| | Nettle |
| Oral contraceptive formulations | Red clover |
| | Red raspberry |
| Phenothiazines | |
|   Chlorpromazine (Thorazine) | |
|   Prochlorperazine (Compazine) | |
|   Others | |

Reprinted, with permission, from American Family Physician.

roidism. An elevated prolactin and normal TSH, often accompanied by amenorrhea, suggest a hypothalamic or pituitary tumor, and magnetic resonance imaging (MRI) scan is indicated. When the prolactin level is normal, uncommon causes such as adrenal, renal, or ovarian tumors should be considered. Males with a negative work-up and normal puberty need to be followed intensively. Males with elevated prolactin levels require an MRI scan every 12–18 months even if the galactorrhea resolves, because of the significant risk of a small pituitary adenoma that may become apparent with serial examinations.

## Treatment

Treatment depends on the underlying cause. Prolactinomas may be removed surgically or suppressed with bromocriptine. Bromocriptine may also be beneficial to some amenorrheic females with normal serum prolactin levels. The female with a negative work-up and persistent galactorrhea may be followed with menstrual history and serum prolactin level every 6–12 months. In many cases, symptoms resolve spontaneously and no diagnosis is made. The female with an elevated serum prolactin concentration but negative prolactinoma work-up may be treated with bromocriptine if her symptoms are bothersome or may be observed with MRI scan every 1–2 years for several years.

## GYNECOMASTIA

Gynecomastia is a common concern of male adolescents, most of whom (60–70%) develop transient subareolar breast tissue during SMR stages 2 and 3. Proposed causes include testosterone–estrogen imbalance, increased serum prolactin level, and abnormal serum protein binding levels.

### Clinical Findings

In type I idiopathic gynecomastia, the adolescent presents with a unilateral (20% bilateral) tender, firm mass beneath the areola. More generalized breast enlargement is classified as type II. Pseudogynecomastia is the term for excessive fat tissue or prominent pectoralis muscles.

### Differential Diagnosis

Gynecomastia may be drug-induced (Table 3–5). Testicular, adrenal, or pituitary tumors, Klinefelter syndrome, primary hypogonadism, thyroid or hepatic dysfunction, or malnutrition may also be associated with gynecomastia (Table 3–6). Onset of gynecomastia in late (rather than early or middle) adolescence is more likely indicative of pathology.

### Treatment

If gynecomastia is idiopathic, reassurance about the common and benign nature of the process can be given. Resolution may take up to 2 years. Medical reduction has been achieved with pharmacotherapeutic agents, such as dihydrotestosterone, danazol, clomiphene, and tamoxifen, but these agents should be reserved for patients in whom no decrease in breast size occurs after 2 years. Surgery is reserved for those with significant psychological trauma or severe breast enlargement.

Lazala C, Saenger P: Pubertal gynecomastia. J Pediatr Endocrinol Metab 2002;15(5):553 [PMID: 12014513].

***Table 3–5.*** Drugs associated with gynecomastia.

| Antibiotics | Drugs and substances of abuse |
|---|---|
| Isoniazid | Alcohol |
| Ketoconazole | Amphetamines |
| Metronidazole | Marijuana |
| **Anti-ulcer drugs** | Opiates |
| Cimetidine | **Hormones or related agents** |
| Omeprazole | Anabolic steroids |
| Ranitidine | Estrogens |
| **Cardiovascular drugs** | Chorionic gonadotropin |
| Captopril | **Psychoactive medications** |
| Digoxin | Tricyclic antidepressants, eg, |
| Enalapril | amitriptyline |
| Methyldopa | Antipsychotics, eg, |
| Reserpine | chlorpromazine, fluphena- |
| Verapamil | zine, haloperidol |
| **Chemotherapeutic drugs** | Anxiolytics, eg, chlordiaze- |
| Busulfan | poxide, diazepam |
| Vincristine | |

***Table 3–6.*** Disorders associated with gynecomastia.

Klinefelter syndrome
Traumatic paraplegia
Male pseudohermaphroditism
Testicular feminization syndrome
Reifenstein syndrome
17-Ketosteroid reductase deficiency
Endocrine tumors (seminoma, Leydig cell tumor, teratoma, feminizing adrenal tumor, hepatoma, leukemia, hemophilia, bronchogenic carcinoma, leprosy, etc)
Hypothyroidism
Hyperthyroidism
Cirrhosis
Herpes zoster
Friedreich ataxia

Pena K, Rosenfeld J: Evaluation and treatment of galactorrhea. Am Fam Physician 2001;63:1763 [PMID: 11352287].

Templeman C, Hertweck S: Breast disorders in the pediatric and adolescent patient. Obstet Gynecol Clin North Am 2000;27:19 [PMID: 10693180].

# ◼ GYNECOLOGIC DISORDERS IN ADOLESCENCE

## PHYSIOLOGY OF MENSTRUATION

The ovulatory menstrual cycle is divided into three consecutive phases: follicular (the first 14 days), ovulatory (midcycle), and luteal (days 16–28). During the follicular phase, pulsatile GnRH from the hypothalamus stimulates anterior pituitary secretion of FSH and LH. Under the influence of FSH and LH, a dominant ovarian follicle emerges by days 5–7 of the menstrual cycle, and the other follicles become atretic. Rising estradiol levels produced by the maturing follicle cause proliferation of the endometrium. By the midfollicular phase, FSH is beginning to decline secondary to estradiol-mediated negative feedback, whereas LH continues to rise as a result of estradiol-mediated positive feedback.

The rising LH initiates progesterone secretion and luteinization of the granulosa cells of the follicle. Progesterone in turn further stimulates LH and FSH. This leads to the LH surge, which causes the follicle to rupture and expel the oocyte.

During the luteal phase, LH and FSH gradually decline. The corpus luteum secretes progesterones. The endometrium enters the secretory phase in response to rising levels of estrogen and progesterone, with maturation 8–9 days after ovulation. If no pregnancy occurs or placental human chorionic gonadotropin (HCG) is released, luteolysis begins; estrogen and progesterone levels decline; and the endometrial lining is shed as menstrual flow approximately 14 days after ovulation (Figure 3–8).

During the first 2 years after menarche, the majority of cycles are anovulatory (50–80%). Between 10% and 20% of cycles remain anovulatory for up to 5 years after menarche.

## PELVIC EXAMINATION

A pelvic examination may be indicated to evaluate abdominal pain or menstrual disorders or to detect a suspected STI in the adolescent. It has previously been recommended that a routine pelvic examination be done at age 18 years to obtain the first Papanicolaou (Pap) smear and to evaluate reproductive anatomy. Recently recommendations have changed to delay the first Pap smear until age 21 years in the absence of menstrual problems in patients who have never had intercourse. The first Pap smear should be performed within 3 years of the initiation of sexual activity. Pap smears should be performed earlier in adolescents with a history of sexual abuse with penile penetration. The adolescent may be apprehensive about the first examination. It should not be rushed, and an explanation of the procedure and its purpose should precede it. The patient can be encour-

**Figure 3–8.** Physiology of the normal ovulatory menstrual cycle; gonadotropin secretion, ovarian hormone production, follicular maturation, and endometrial changes during one cycle. FSH = follicle-stimulating hormone, LH = luteinizing hormone. (Reproduced, with permission, from Emans SJH et al: *Pediatric and Adolescent Gynecology*, 4th ed. Little, Brown, 1998.)

aged to relax by slow, deep breathing and by relaxation of her lower abdominal and inner thigh muscles. A young adolescent may wish to have her mother present during the examination, but the history should be taken privately. A female chaperone should be present with male examiners.

The pelvic examination begins by placing the patient in the dorsal lithotomy position after equipment and supplies are ready (Table 3–7). The examiner inspects the external genitalia, noting the pubic hair maturity rating, the size of the clitoris (2–5 mm is normal), Skene glands just inside the urethral meatus, and Bartholin glands at 4 o'clock and 8 o'clock outside the hymenal ring. In cases of alleged sexual abuse or assault, the horizontal measurement of the relaxed prepubertal hymenal opening should be recorded and the presence of any lacerations, bruises, scarring, or synechiae about the hymen, vulva, or anus should be noted.

A vaginal speculum is then inserted at a 45-degree twist and angled 45 degrees downward. (A medium Pedersen speculum is most often used in sexually experienced patients; a narrow Huffman is used for virginal patients.) The vaginal walls are inspected for estrogen effects, inflammation, or lesions. The cervix should be dull pink. Cervical ectropion is commonly observed in adolescents; the columnar epithelium extends outside the cervical os onto the face of the cervix until later adolescence, when it recedes.

Specimens are obtained, including a wet preparation for leukocytes, trichomonads, and clue cells (vaginal epithelial cells stippled with adherent bacteria); potassium hydroxide (KOH) preparation for yeast and whiff test; cervical swab for gonorrhea and *Chlamydia*; and endocervical and cervical samples for Pap smear. A cervical brush provides a higher yield of cells for the endocervi-

**Table 3–7.** Items for pelvic exam tray.

Medium and virginal speculums (warm)
Gloves
Applicator sticks, sterile
Large swabs to remove excess discharge
Cervical spatulas, cervical brushes
Microscope slides and cover slips (frosted and labeled)
Centrifuge tube or test tube (if swab is to be placed in drop of saline and slide prepared later)
NaCl dropper bottle
KOH dropper bottle
Slide container to send to lab
Gonorrhea test media
*Chlamydia* test media
Lubricant
Kleenex

cal Pap slide. Pap smears should be interpreted by a cytopathologist at a laboratory using the Bethesda system of classification.

The speculum is then removed, and bimanual examination is performed to assess uterine size and position, adnexal enlargement or tenderness, or cervical motion tenderness. Bimanual examination may reveal beading in the adnexa secondary to endometriosis.

## MENSTRUAL DISORDERS

### 1. Amenorrhea

Amenorrhea is the lack of onset of menses when normally anticipated. Primary amenorrhea is no menstrual periods or secondary sex characteristics by age 14 years or no menses in the presence of secondary sex characteristics by age 15 years. Constitutional delay is normal pubertal progression at a delayed onset or rate. Secondary amenorrhea is defined as the absence of menses for at least three cycles after regular cycles have been present. In some instances, evaluation should begin immediately, without waiting for the specified age or duration of lapsed periods, such as in patients with suspected pregnancy, short stature with the stigmata of Turner syndrome, or an anatomic defect.

### Evaluation for Primary Amenorrhea

Primary amenorrhea may be the result of anatomic abnormalities, chromosomal deviations, or physiologic delay (Table 3–8).

The history should include whether puberty has commenced, level of exercise, nutritional intake, presence of stressors, and the age at menarche for female relatives. Adrenal androgens are largely responsible for axillary and pubic hair; estrogen is responsible for breast development, maturation of the external genitalia, vagina, and uterus, and menstruation.

A careful physical examination should be done, noting the percentage of ideal body weight for height and age, SMR stage, vaginal patency, presence of the uterus (assessed through rectoabdominal examination or ultrasonography if pelvic examination is not appropriate), signs of virilization (acne, clitoromegaly of > 5 mm, hirsutism), or stigmata of Turner syndrome (< 152 cm tall, shield-like chest, widely spaced nipples, increased carrying angle of the arms, webbed neck). If pelvic examination reveals normal female external genitalia and pelvic organs, the patient should be given a challenge of medroxyprogesterone, 10 mg orally bid for 5 days (or 10 mg/d for 7–10 days) (Figure 3–9). If withdrawal bleeding occurs within 7 days after administration of medroxyprogesterone, normal anatomy and adequate estrogen effect are implied. If physical examination reveals an absent uterus

**Table 3–8.** Causes of amenorrhea.

**Hypothalamic–pituitary axis**
Hypothalamic repression
  Emotional stress
  Depression
  Chronic disease
  Weight loss
  Obesity
  Severe dieting
  Strenuous athletics
  Drugs (post–birth control pills, phenothiazines)
CNS lesion
  Pituitary lesion: adenoma, prolactinoma
  Craniopharyngioma, brainstem, or parasellar tumors
  Head injury with hypothalamic contusion
  Infiltrative process (sarcoidosis)
  Vascular disease (hypothalamic vasculitis)
Congenital conditions[a]
  Kallmann syndrome
**Ovaries**
Gonadal dysgenesis[a]
  Turner syndrome (XO)
  Mosaic (XX/XO)
Injury to ovary
  Autoimmune disease
  Infection (mumps, oophoritis)
  Toxins (alkylating chemotherapeutic agents)
  Irradiation
  Trauma, torsion (rare)
Polycystic ovary syndrome
Ovarian failure
  Premature menopause
  Resistant ovary
**Uterovaginal outflow tract**
Müllerian dysgenesis[a]
  Congenital deformity or absence of uterus, uterine tubes, or vagina
  Imperforate hymen, transverse vaginal septum, vaginal agenesis, agenesis of the cervix[a]
Testicular feminization (absent uterus)[a]
Uterine lining defect
  Asherman syndrome (intrauterine synechiae postcurettage or endometritis)
  Tuberculosis, brucellosis
**Defect in hormone synthesis or action (virilization may be present)**
Adrenal hyperplasia[a]
Cushing disease
Adrenal tumor
Ovarian tumor (rare)
Drugs (steroids, ACTH)

[a]Indicates condition that usually presents as primary amenorrhea.
ACTH = adrenocorticotropic hormone.

***Figure 3–9.*** Evaluation of primary amenorrhea in a normal female. FSH = follicle-stimulating hormone, IBW = ideal body weight, LH = luteinizing hormone.

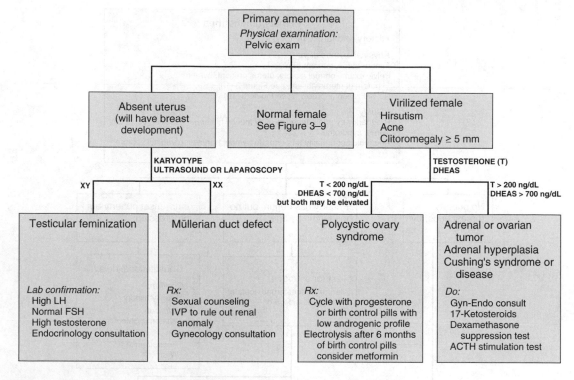

**Figure 3–10.** Evaluation of primary amenorrhea in a female without a uterus or with virilization. ACTH = adrenocorticotropic hormone, DHEAS = dehydroepiandrosterone sulfate, FSH = follicle-stimulating hormone, IVP = intravenous pyelogram, LH = luteinizing hormone.

(Figure 3–10), karyotyping should be performed to differentiate testicular feminization from müllerian duct defect, because these two entities are managed differently.

Laboratory studies should include CBC, ESR, and TSH. If systemic illness is suspected, a urinalysis and a chemistry panel including renal and liver function tests should be obtained. If short stature is present, a bone age should be done. If the diagnosis remains unclear after preliminary evaluation, or if no withdrawal bleed occurs after a medroxyprogesterone challenge, FSH, LH, and prolactin levels should be obtained. Low levels of gonadotropins indicate a more severe hypothalamic suppression, caused by anorexia nervosa, chronic disease, or a CNS tumor. Involvement of a gynecologist or endocrinologist is helpful at this point. If gonadotropin levels are high, ovarian failure or gonadal dysgenesis is implied, and karyotype should be obtained.

## Evaluation & Treatment of Secondary Amenorrhea

Secondary amenorrhea results when estrogen stimulation is unopposed, maintaining the endometrium in the proliferative phase. The most common causes are pregnancy, stress, and polycystic ovary syndrome (PCOS). Ovarian failure can also present as secondary amenorrhea, caused by mosaic Turner syndrome or autoimmune oophoritis.

The history should focus on issues of stress, chronic illness, drugs, weight change, strenuous exercise, sexual activity, and contraceptive use. A review of systems should include questions about headaches, visual changes, hirsutism, constipation, cold intolerance, and galactorrhea.

Physical examination should include ophthalmoscopic and visual field examination, palpation of the thyroid, determination of blood pressure and heart rate, compression of the areola to check for galactorrhea, and a search for signs of androgen excess (eg, hirsutism, clitoromegaly, severe acne, ovarian enlargement).

The first laboratory study obtained is a pregnancy test, even if the patient denies sexual activity. If the teenager is not pregnant, a progesterone challenge (medroxyprogesterone, 10 mg orally bid for 5 days or 10 mg/d for 7–10 days) should be done to determine whether the uterus is primed with estrogen (Figure 3–11).

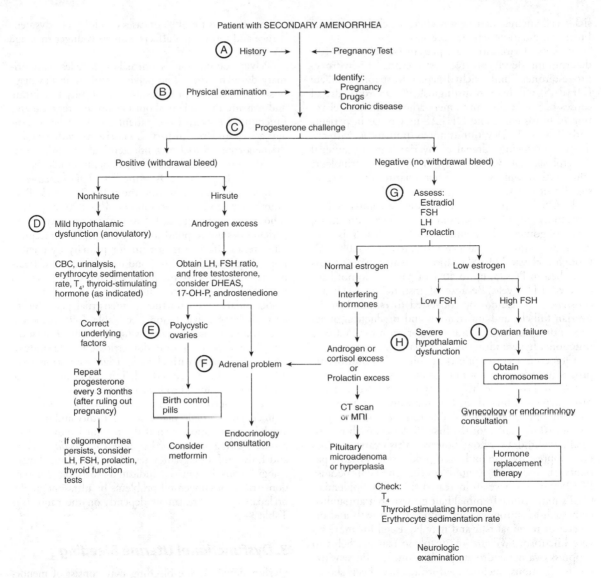

**Figure 3–11.** Evaluation of secondary amenorrhea. CBC = complete blood count, DHEAS = dehydroepiandro-sterone sulfate, FSH = follicle-stimulating hormone, LH = luteinizing hormone, T₄ = thyroxine.

Most patients who have withdrawal flow after progesterone challenge have mild hypothalamic suppression due to weight change, athletics, stress, or illness; however, disorders such as PCOS, adrenal disorders, ovarian tumors, thyroid disease, and diabetes mellitus should be excluded by history and physical examination and appropriate laboratory studies. (See section on Primary Amenorrhea and Figure 3–11.)

If withdrawal flow occurs after the progesterone challenge (see Figure 3–11), serum levels of estradiol,

FSH, LH, and prolactin should be checked. An elevated FSH level accompanied by a low estrogen level implies ovarian failure, in which case blood for karyotype and antiovarian antibodies (if the karyotype is normal) should be obtained and laparoscopy considered. If gonadotropin levels are low or normal and the estradiol level is low, hypothalamic amenorrhea is likely; however, one must consider the possibilities of a CNS tumor (prolactinoma or craniopharyngioma), pituitary infarction from postpartum hemorrhage or sickle cell anemia, uterine synechiae, or chronic disease. Further evaluation may be necessary.

If signs of virilization are present (see Figure 3–10), determining levels of free testosterone, 17-hydroxy-progesterone, and dehydroepiandrosterone sulfate (DHEAS) will help to distinguish PCOS from adrenal causes of virilization and amenorrhea. Although elevation of testosterone and DHEAS may occur in patients with PCOS, the elevation is not as dramatic as with androgen-producing adrenal or ovarian tumors, adrenal hyperplasia, or Cushing syndrome. Endocrinologic consultation will assist in differentiating the cause of significantly elevated androgens.

PCOS is a spectrum of disorders accompanied by symptoms of obesity, insulin resistance, hirsutism, acne, oligomenorrhea, and infertility. PCOS is very common, with a prevalence estimated at 5–10%. Although a classic LH:FSH ratio of greater than 2.5:1 is described in PCOS, up to 40% of patients do not have elevated LH levels. Because of insufficient FSH, androstenedione cannot be converted to estradiol in the ovarian follicle, and anovulation and production of excess androgens result. Thus another term for PCOS is functional hyperandrogenic anovulation.

Oral contraceptive pills containing a low androgenic progestin (desogestrel or norgestimate) such as Desogen or Ortho Tri-Cyclen help to regulate menses and improve acne and hirsutism. Patients who do not wish to take an oral contraceptive pill can be given progesterone, 10 mg daily, for the first 10 days of each month to allow withdrawal flow; however, this treatment does not suppress ovarian androgen production. Hirsute patients should have a lipid profile checked, because PCOS patients have an increased risk of dyslipidemias. OCPs may reduce terminal hair growth, but antiandrogens such as spironolactone reduce the growth and diameter of terminal hair and may be useful for more severe hirsutism. Weight loss in obese patients helps to suppress ovarian androgen production. Insulin sensitizing medications, such as metformin, have been shown in recent studies to improve menstrual regularities in adolescents with PCOS.

## 2. Dysmenorrhea

Dysmenorrhea is the most common gynecologic complaint of adolescent girls, with an incidence of about 80% by age 18 years. Yet many teenage girls do not seek help from a physician, relying instead on female relatives, friends, and the media for advice. Therefore, the physician should ask about menstrual cramps when taking a review of systems.

Dysmenorrhea can be divided into primary and secondary dysmenorrhea on the basis of whether underlying pelvic disease exists (Table 3–9). Primary dysmenorrhea accounts for 80% of cases of adolescent dysmenorrhea and most often affects women younger than age 25 years.

Pelvic examination is normal in females with primary dysmenorrhea. The pelvic examination has diagnostic benefits and provides an opportunity to educate and reassure the patient about her normal reproductive function. However, if the patient has never been sexually active and the history is consistent with primary dysmenorrhea, a trial of a nonsteroidal anti-inflammatory drug (NSAID) is justified. Patients should be instructed to begin NSAIDs at the first sign of menses or dysmenorrhea and continue them for 2–3 days. Recommended doses are ibuprofen 400–800 mg every 6 hours or naproxen (220–550 mg) twice a day. If the patient does not respond to NSAIDs, oral contraceptive pills are an effective treatment for primary dysmenorrhea. If patients do not respond to either of these treatments, secondary dysmenorrhea is more likely and a pelvic examination is indicated.

Secondary dysmenorrhea is menstrual pain due to an underlying pelvic lesion (see Table 3–9). Although uncommon in adolescents, when present it is most often due to infection or endometriosis. In one study of adolescent females with chronic pelvic pain, more than 40% who had not received a definitive diagnosis by the third visit were found to have endometriosis.

The clinician evaluating a patient with secondary dysmenorrhea should take a sexual history and conduct a pelvic examination even if the patient is not sexually active. Testing for gonorrhea and *Chlamydia,* a CBC and ESR, and a pregnancy test should be done. Gynecologic consultation is indicated to look for endometriosis or congenital problems by ultrasonography or laparoscopy. Treatment depends on the cause (see Table 3–9).

## 3. Dysfunctional Uterine Bleeding

Dysfunctional uterine bleeding may consist of menorrhagia (normal intervals with excessive flow) or metrorrhagia (irregular intervals with excessive flow). It results when an endometrium that has proliferated under unopposed estrogen stimulation finally begins to slough, but does so incompletely, causing irregular, painless bleeding. The unopposed estrogen stimulation occurs during anovulatory cycles, common in younger adolescents who have not been menstruating for long. Anovulation may also occur in older adolescents during times of stress or illness (Figure 3–12).

### Clinical Findings

Typically, the adolescent has had several years of regular cycles and then begins to have menses every 2 weeks, or

**Table 3–9.** Dysmenorrhea in the adolescent.

| Primary Dysmenorrhea—no pelvic pathology | | | | |
| Etiology | Onset and Duration | Symptoms | Pelvic Exam | Treatment |
|---|---|---|---|---|
| **Primary** — Excessive amount of prostaglandin F2α, which attaches to myometrium, causing uterine contractions, hypoxia, and ischemia. Also, directly sensitizes pain receptors. | Begins with onset of flow or just prior and lasts 1–2 d. Does not start until 6–18 mos after menarche, when cycles become ovulatory. | Lower abdominal cramps radiating to lower back and thighs. Associated nausea, vomiting, diarrhea, and urinary frequency also due to excess prostaglandins. | Normal. May wait to examine if never sexually active and history is consistent with primary dysmenorrhea. | Mild—heating pad, warm baths, nonprescription analgesics. Moderate to severe—prostaglandin inhibitors at onset of flow or pain. Consider oral contraceptives. |

**Secondary Dysmenorrhea**—underlying pathology present. (Always perform pelvic exam if secondary dysmenorrhea suspected or patient is sexually active. Tests for *Chlamydia* and gonorrhea, CBC, and ESR should be obtained.)

| | Etiology | Onset and Duration | Symptoms | Pelvic Exam | Treatment |
|---|---|---|---|---|---|
| **Infection** | Most often due to a sexually transmitted disease such as chlamydia or gonorrhea. | Recent onset of pelvic cramps. | Pelvic cramps, excessive bleeding, intermenstrual spotting or vaginal discharge. | Mucopurulent or purulent discharge from cervical os, cervical friability, cervical motion tenderness, adnexal tenderness, positive test for STI. | Appropriate antibiotics. |
| **Endometriosis** | Aberrant implants of endometrial tissue in pelvis or abdomen; may result from reflux. | Generally starts more than 2 y after menarche. | Pelvic pain, may occur intermenstrually. | Two thirds are tender on exam, especially during late luteal phase. | Hormonal suppression by oral contraceptives or danazol. Surgery may be necessary for extensive disease. |
| **Complication of pregnancy** | Spontaneous abortion, ectopic pregnancy. | Acute onset. | Pelvic cramps associated with a delay in menses. | Positive HCG, enlarged uterus or adnexal mass. | Immediate gynecologic consult. |
| **Congenital anomalies** | Transverse vaginal septum, septate uterus, or cervical stenosis. | Onset at menarche. | Pelvic cramps. | Underlying congenital anomaly may be apparent. May require exam under anesthesia. | Gynecologic consult for ultrasound, hysteroscopy, or laparoscopy. |
| **IUD** | Increased uterine contractions, or increased risk for pelvic infection. | Onset after placement of IUD or acutely if due to infection. | Pelvic cramps, heavy menstrual bleeding, may have vaginal discharge. | Normal, or see infection earlier. | Prostaglandin inhibitors of mefenamic acid may be drug of choice because they also reduce flow. Appropriate antibiotics and consider removal of IUD if infection is present. |
| **Pelvic adhesions** | Previous abdominal surgery or pelvic inflammatory disease. | Delayed onset after surgery or PID. | Abdominal pain, may or may not be associated with menstrual cycles; possible alteration in bowel pattern. | Variable. | Surgery. Consider a trial of tricyclic antidepressants. |

CBC = complete blood count; ESR = erythrocyte sedimentation rate; HCG = human chorionic gonadotropin; STI = sexually transmitted infection; IUD = intrauterine device; PID = pelvic inflammatory disease.

**Figure 3–12.** Evaluation of dysfunctional uterine bleeding. CBC = complete blood count, Hgb = hemoglobin, OCP = oral contraceptive pills.

complains of bleeding for 2–3 weeks after 2–3 months of amenorrhea. A history of painless, irregular periods at intervals of less than 3 weeks may also be elicited. Bleeding for more than 10 days should be considered abnormal. Dysfunctional uterine bleeding must be considered a diagnosis of exclusion (Table 3–10).

## Management

A pregnancy test and pelvic examination with appropriate tests for sexually transmitted infections should be performed in sexually active patients. A CBC, including a platelet count, should be obtained. The history and physical findings may suggest the need for additional coagulation or hormonal studies. Coagulation studies should be done if the patient presents with severe anemia, especially within 1 year after menarche. Management depends on the severity of the problem (Table 3–11). It is important to treat for a minimum of 3–4 months to progressively reduce the endometrium to baseline thickness.

**Table 3–10.** Differential diagnosis of dysfunctional uterine bleeding in adolescents.

| |
| --- |
| Anovulation |
| Sexually transmitted infections |
|   Cervicitis |
|   Pelvic inflammatory disease |
| Pregnancy complications |
|   Ectopic pregnancy |
|   Spontaneous abortion |
| Bleeding disorders |
|   von Willebrand disease |
|   Thrombocytopenia |
|   Coagulopathy |
| Endocrine disorders |
|   Hypothyroidism |
|   Hyperprolactinemia |
|   Adrenal hyperplasia |
|   Polycystic ovary syndrome |
| Anatomical abnormalities |
| Uterine fibroids |
| Trauma |
| Foreign body |
| Chronic illness |
| Malignancy |
|   Leukemia |
|   Carcinoma |
| Drugs |
|   Birth control pills |
|   Depo-Provera |

## 4. Mittelschmerz

Mittelschmerz is midcycle pain caused by irritation of the peritoneum due to spillage of fluid from the ruptured follicular cyst at the time of ovulation. The patient presents with a history of midcycle, unilateral dull or aching abdominal pain lasting a few minutes to as long as 8 hours. This pain rarely mimics the abdominal findings of acute appendicitis, torsion or rupture of an ovarian cyst, or ectopic pregnancy. The patient should be reassured and treated symptomatically. If the findings are severe enough to warrant consideration of the previously mentioned diagnoses, laparoscopy may be done.

## 5. Premenstrual Syndrome

Premenstrual syndrome (PMS) refers to a cluster of physical and psychological symptoms that are temporally related to the luteal phase of the menstrual cycle and are alleviated by the onset of menses. PMS should be distinguished from major depression, idiopathic cyclic edema, fibromyalgia, chronic fatigue syndrome, and psychosomatic disorders. This may be difficult because of the diversity of symptoms ascribed to PMS and the variability from month to month in the same patient. Premenstrual behavioral symptoms most commonly cited include emotional lability, anxiety, depression, irritability, impulsivity, hostility, and impaired social function. Physical symptoms include bloating, breast tenderness, fatigue, and appetite changes. Previously thought to be a disorder limited to adult women, studies indicate that adolescents also experience premenstrual symptoms. Although a number of causes have been proposed (progesterone deficiency, hyperprolactinemia, estrogen excess or imbalance of the estrogen–progesterone ratio, vitamin $B_{12}$ deficiency, fluid retention, low levels of endorphins and prostaglandins, hypoglycemia, psychosomatic factors), none has been proven. Hormones may play a role; women who have undergone hysterectomy but not oophorectomy may have cyclic symptoms resembling PMS, whereas postmenopausal women have no such symptoms.

Several treatments have been advocated but are without consistent benefits. OCPs or NSAIDs may be beneficial for some women. Sertraline (50–100 mg) has been shown to be significantly better than placebo for treatment of premenstrual dysphoria.

## 6. Ovarian Cysts

Functional cysts account for 20–50% of ovarian tumors in adolescents and are a result of the normal physiologic process of ovulation. They may be asymptomatic or may cause menstrual irregularity, constipation,

***Table 3–11.*** Management of dysfunctional uterine bleeding.[a]

|  | **Mild** | **Moderate** | **Severe** |
|---|---|---|---|
|  | Hgb > 12 g/dL | Hgb 9–12 g/dL | Hgb < 9 g/dL (or dropping); orthostatic symptoms and signs |
| Acute treatment | Menstrual calendar<br>Iron supplementation<br>NSAID with menses may help reduce flow<br>Consider oral contraceptive pills if patient is sexually active and desires contraception | Monophasic oral contraceptive pills up to four pills per day and taper over 2–3 wk; may need antiemetic. Bleeding should stop in a few days. Begin tapering dose 2–3 d after bleeding stops. Expect withdrawal flow a few days after last dose. | Fluids, blood transfusion as needed, admit to hospital if Hgb < 7 or patient is hemodynamically unstable<br>For hemostasis, consider: conjugated estrogens (Premarin), 25 mg IV every 4–6 h for 24 h or until bleeding stops. Provide antiemetic medication.<br>Then: oral contraceptive pills (1/50) cycle:<br>    4 pills/d for 4 d<br>    3 pills/d for 4 d<br>    2 pills/d for 17 d<br>    withdrawal bleeding for 7 d[b] |
| Long-term management | Monitor menstrual calendar and Hgb<br>Follow-up in 2–3 mos | Cycle with either:<br>(1) Medroxyprogesterone acetate, 10 mg PO daily for 10 d starting on day 14 of each cycle for 3–6 mos, or<br>(2) Oral contraceptive pills for 3–6 mos beginning the Sunday after withdrawal bleeding starts.<br>Provide iron supplementation.<br>Monitor Hgb<br>Follow-up within 2–3 wk and every 3 mos | Next: Oral contraceptive pills cycle (using 28-d packs) for 3 mos<br>Begin the Sunday after withdrawal bleeding begins. Length of use dependent on resolution of anemia.<br>Monitor hemoglobin<br>Follow-up within 2–3 wks and every 3 mos |

[a]Diagnosis: Prolonged (> 8 d) painless menses; heavy flow (> 6 tampons/pads per day); short cycles (< 21 d); no cause found.
[b]This schedule will use three 21-d packages.
Hgb = hemoglobin; PO = by mouth; NSAID = nonsteroidal anti-inflammatory drug.
Modified from Blythe M: Common menstrual problems. Part 3. Abnormal uterine bleeding. Adolescent Health Update 1992;4:1.

or urinary frequency. Functional cysts, unless large, rarely cause abdominal pain; however, torsion or hemorrhage of an ovarian cyst may present as an acute abdomen. Follicular cysts account for the majority of ovarian cysts. They are produced every cycle but occasionally are not resorbed. Follicular cysts are unilateral, usually not larger than 4 cm in diameter, and resolve spontaneously. If the patient is asymptomatic, she can be reexamined monthly. The patient should be referred to a gynecologist for laparoscopy if she is premenarcheal, if the cyst has a solid component or is larger than 5 cm by ultrasonography, if she has symptoms or signs suggestive of hemorrhage or torsion, or if the cyst fails to regress within 2 months. Luteal cysts occur less

commonly and may be 5–10 cm in diameter. The patient may have associated amenorrhea or, as the cyst becomes atretic, heavy vaginal bleeding. The patient may be monitored for 3 months but should have a laparoscopy if the cyst is larger than 5 cm, does not resolve within 2 months, or if there is pain or bleeding from the cyst.

Dickerson LM et al: Premenstrual syndrome. Am Fam Physician 2003;67(8):1743 [PMID: 12725453].

Slap GB: Menstrual disorders in adolescence. Best Pract Res Clin Obstet Gynaecol 2003;17(1):75 [PMID: 12758227].

## CONTRACEPTION

According to the Youth Risk Behavior Survey, by 12th grade 60.5% of adolescents in 2001 had had sexual intercourse. This percentage had decreased from 66.7 in 1991. For female adolescents, reported use of a condom at last intercourse increased from 38% in 1991 to 51.3% in 2001. For male adolescents, this percentage increased from 54.5% to 65.1%. However, the percentage of adolescents reporting use of alcohol or drugs before last intercourse increased 18% between 1991 and 2001.

### Abstinence & Decision Making

Many adolescents have given little thought to how they feel about their developing sexuality or how they will handle sexual situations. By talking with teenagers about sexual intercourse and its implications, and alternatives to intercourse, providers can help teens make informed decisions before they find themselves with an unplanned pregnancy or a sexually transmitted infection.

If an adolescent chooses to remain abstinent, the clinician should reinforce that decision. Encouraging adolescents to use contraception when they do engage in sexual intercourse does not lead to higher rates of sexual activity. Another approach to decreasing teen pregnancy is to educate adolescent males on the importance of hormonal contraception and emergency contraception for their partners, in addition to condom use. The teen pregnancy, birth, and abortion rates are higher in the United States than in any other developed country, despite similar rates of sexual experience.

### Emergency Contraception

A discussion of emergency contraception (EC), which could potentially prevent 50–90% of unintended pregnancies and elective abortions, should be part of anticipatory guidance given to both female and male teenagers. Indications for EC include unprotected intercourse within the past 120 hours (5 days), condom breakage, more than two missed oral contraceptive pills, and greater than 14 weeks since the last Depo-Provera injection. The pregnancy rate after EC is 1.8%, compared with 6.8% without such intervention. (See Table 3–12 for dosages.) EC works best within 24 hours of intercourse but can be taken up to 120 hours afterward. It should be verified that other instances of unprotected intercourse beyond 120 hours have not occurred. The only contraindication to the use of EC is pregnancy. Plan B is a progestin-only method that causes significantly less nausea and vomiting than combined estrogen/progesterone methods. Preven is a

**Table 3–12.** Emergency postcoital contraception regimens.

| Pill | Dosage | Each Dose Achieves: |
|---|---|---|
| Plan B[a] | Two tablets orally | Levonorgestrel 1.5 mg |
| Preven[b] | Two tablets orally, repeat in 12 h | Levonorgestrel 0.5 mg |
| Nordette[b] | Four tablets orally and repeat in 12 h | Levonorgestrel 0.6 mg |
| Lo-Ovral[b] | Four tablets orally and repeat in 12 h | Norgestrel 1.2 mg |
| Alesse[b] | Five pink pills orally and repeat in 12 h | Levonorgestrel 0.5 mg |
| Triphasil[b] | Four yellow pills orally and repeat in 12 h | Levonorgestrel 0.5 mg |

[a]Both doses can be given at the same time.
[b]An antiemetic drug taken 30 minutes before the dose may help reduce nausea.

combined estrogen/progesterone product marketed specifically for EC. If these methods are not available, certain combined OCPs can be used for EC. It is important to note that the newer progestin-containing contraceptives are **not** approved for EC. A follow-up appointment should be held in 2–3 weeks, to test for pregnancy if menses have not occurred, to screen for STI if indicated, and to counsel regarding contraceptive use.

### Condoms & Spermicides

The use of condoms has gained popularity as a result of the educational and marketing efforts driven by the acquired immunodeficiency syndrome (AIDS) epidemic. Condom use has increased over the past several decades. Regardless of whether another method is used, all sexually active adolescents should be counseled to use condoms. Condoms offer protection against STIs by decreasing the transmission of gonorrhea, *Chlamydia,* syphilis, herpes simplex, hepatitis, and human immunodeficiency virus (HIV). Spermicides containing nonoxynol-9 are no longer recommended, as recent evidence has suggested that repeated use of spermicide may increase transmission of HIV. Aside from the diaphragm and cervical cap, barrier methods do not require a medical visit or prescription and are widely available. The polyurethane vaginal pouch, or female condom, is also available. Although it has pregnancy and STI prevention properties similar to those of the male condom, its higher cost and greater difficulty of insertion make it less appealing to adolescents.

## Oral Contraceptives

OCPs have a three-pronged mechanism of action: (1) suppression of ovulation; (2) thickening of the cervical mucus, thereby making sperm penetration more difficult; and (3) atrophy of the endometrium, which diminishes the chance of implantation. The latter two actions are progestin effects.

### A. Combination Oral and Cutaneous Contraceptives

Combination OCPs contain both estrogen and progestin. Ethinyl estradiol is the estrogen currently used in nearly all OCPs in the United States. A number of progestins are used in OCPs and differ in their estrogenic, antiestrogenic, and androgenic effects. As estrogen doses decreased in OCPs, the androgenic side effects of progestins became more apparent, leading to the development of two progestins (desogestrel and norgestimate) with lower androgenic potential. Ortho Tri-Cyclen is being advertised as a treatment for acne. All of the lower androgenic pills improve acne and may especially benefit patients with polycystic ovary syndrome. Reports of increased risk of thromboembolism associated with the newer progestins are likely related to an excess of first-time users among desogestrel patients. Factor V Leiden has been identified as a risk factor for venous thrombosis; 5% of patients of European ancestry are carriers of factor V Leiden. Carriers have a 30- to 50-fold increased risk for thrombosis. Testing family members with a history of venous thrombosis for factor V Leiden and other conditions such as the prothrombin gene mutation, protein C and S, and antithrombin III before prescribing estrogen-containing OCPs to the adolescent may prevent these complications. OCPs have many noncontraceptive benefits, including improvement of dysmenorrhea, acne, and PMS; suppression of ovarian and breast cysts; and lower risk of anemia, pelvic inflammatory disease, and ectopic pregnancy. A pill containing 30–35 mg of ethinyl estradiol with norgestimate, desogestrel, or 0.5 mg norethindrone is recommended for adolescents beginning OCPs.

Ortho Evra is a newly released combined estrogen/progesterone patch, which is worn 3 weeks out of every 4. It releases 150 μg of norelgestromin and 20 μg of ethinyl estradiol per day. Side effects are similar to those of combined OCPs. Five percent of patients report having a patch come off. Two percent report skin irritation. Efficacy may be reduced in patients weighing more than 200 pounds. The patch is an attractive alternative to OCPs for adolescents who have difficulty remembering to take a pill every day, as compliance is increased. The failure rate for the patch is reported to be 1%.

### B. Progestin-Only Pills

Progestin-only pills contain no estrogen. Their chief use is in women who experience unacceptable estrogen-related side effects with combination OCPs or who have a contraindication to estrogen-containing pills. Their lack of estrogen, however, is also responsible for the main side effect, less predictable menstrual patterns. For this reason, progestin-only pills are not often appropriate for adolescents. Their mechanism of action relies on the progestin-mediated actions, and ovulation is suppressed in only 15–40% of cycles.

### C. Indications and Contraindications

Combined OCPs may be the method of choice for sexually active adolescents who frequently have unplanned intercourse; however, the patient must be able to comply with a daily dosing regimen. Most states allow OCPs to be prescribed to minors confidentially. Ideally, it is best to wait until 6–12 regular menstrual cycles have occurred before beginning hormonal contraception; however, if the teenager is already sexually active, the medical and social risks of pregnancy outweigh the risks of hormonal contraception.

OCPs or the contraceptive patch may also be used to treat dysmenorrhea, menorrhagia, dysfunctional uterine bleeding, and acne (see previous discussion).

Contraindications to combined OCPs or the contraceptive patch can be categorized as absolute and relative (Table 3–13). When use of estrogenic agents is contraindicated, progestin-only pills and Depo-Provera are alternatives.

### D. Beginning Birth Control Pills or the Contraceptive Patch and Follow-Up

Before a patient begins taking OCPs or the patch, a careful menstrual history, medical history, and family medical history should be taken. In addition, baseline weight and blood pressure should be established; breast and pelvic examination should be performed; and specimens for urinalysis, Pap smear, and gonorrhea and *Chlamydia* testing should be obtained. If patients have not yet initiated intercourse, pelvic examination can be deferred until after intercourse is initiated. If time constraints are present and a patient has no symptoms suggesting an STI, OCPs or the patch may be started and a pelvic exam scheduled as soon as possible.

If the teen has no contraindications (see Table 3–13), she may begin her first pack of pills or the patch with her next menstrual period (either the first Sunday after flow begins or the first day of flow, depending on the brand). A low-dose monophasic combined oral

**Table 3–13.** Contraindications to combined birth control pills.

---

**Absolute contraindications**

Pregnancy

Lactation (wait 6 wk postpartum)

History of thrombophlebitis, thromboembolic disorder, cerebrovascular disease, or ischemic heart disease

Structural heart disease complicated by endocarditis, atrial fibrillation, or pulmonary hypertension

Breast cancer

Severe migraine headaches with neurologic changes (numbness, weakness)

History of benign or malignant liver tumor, active hepatitis or severe cirrhosis

Severe hypertension SBP > 160 mmHg or DBP > 100 mmHg

Major surgery with prolonged immobilization or surgery on legs or pelvis

**Relative contraindications**

Recent pregnancy (wait 3 wk postpartum)

Lactation (6 wk–6 mos) OCPs may decrease milk supply

Undiagnosed vaginal bleeding

Active gallbladder disease

Use of drugs that affect liver enzymes (rifampin, griseofulvin, phenytoin, carbamazepine, barbiturates)

---

SBP = systolic blood pressure; DBP = diastolic blood pressure; OCPs = oral contraceptives.

Reprinted with permission from Hatcher RA et al: *Contraceptive Technology*, 17th ed. Ardent Media, 1998.

**Table 3–14.** Noncontraceptive health benefits of oral contraceptive pills.

---

**Protection against life-threatening conditions**

Ovarian cancer

Endometrial cancer

Pelvic inflammatory disease

Ectopic pregnancy

Morbidity and mortality due to unintended pregnancies

**Alleviate conditions affecting quality of life**

Iron deficiency anemia

Benign breast disease

Dysmenorrhea

Irregular cycles

Functional ovarian cysts

Premenstrual syndrome

Improved acne

**Mounting evidence**

Improved bone density

---

contraceptive or a triphasic pill of low androgenic profile is used for those without contraindications to use of estrogen. With adolescents, it is wise to use 28-day packs rather than 21-day packs to reduce the chance of missing pills. The patient should be instructed on the use of her pills and on the possible risks and side effects and their warning signs. To ensure protection, she should use a back-up method, such as condoms, for the first 2 weeks. In addition, the patient should be advised to use condoms at every intercourse to prevent STIs. A follow-up visit every 3 months for the first year may improve compliance, because teenagers often discontinue birth control pills because of nonmedical reasons or minor side effects. Teenagers may need reassurance about the safety of birth control pills and their added benefits (Table 3–14).

**E. MANAGEMENT OF SIDE EFFECTS**

A different type of combined oral contraceptive should be tried if a patient has a persistent minor side effect for more than the first 2–3 months. Adjustments should be made on the basis of hormonal effects desired (Table 3–15). Changes are most often made for persistent breakthrough bleeding not related to missed pills.

## Injectable and Implantable Hormonal Contraceptives

The depot form of medroxyprogesterone acetate (DMPA), or Depo-Provera, is a long-acting injectable progestational contraceptive. It is given as a deep intramuscular injection of 150 mg into the gluteal or deltoid muscle every 12 weeks. The first injection should be given within the first 5 days of the menstrual cycle to ensure immediate contraceptive protection. Patients more than 1 week late for their injection should have two pregnancy tests 2 weeks apart before restarting DMPA, unless they have not been sexually active since missing the DMPA injection. DMPA works chiefly by blocking the LH surge, thereby suppressing ovulation, but it also thickens cervical mucus and alters the endometrium to inhibit implantation. With a failure rate of less than 0.3%, minimal compliance issues, long-acting nature, reversibility, lack of interference with intercourse, and lack of estrogen-related side effects, it may be an attractive contraceptive for many adolescents. Patients should be warned about unpredictable menstrual patterns, the possibility of weight gain or mood changes, and the potential for decreased bone density, which remains under investigation. DMPA may reduce intravascular sickling and increase hemoglobin and red cell survival in patients with sickle cell disease. Moreover, DMPA may be the preferred method for patients

**Table 3–15.** Estrogenic, progestogenic, and androgenic effects of oral contraceptive pills.

| Estrogenic Effects | Progestogenic Effects | Androgenic Effects |
|---|---|---|
| Nausea | Both the estrogenic and the progestational components of oral contraceptives may contribute to the development of the following adverse effects: | All low-dose combined pills suppress a woman's production of testosterone, which has a beneficial effect on acne, oily skin, and hirsutism. The progestin component may have androgenic as well as progestational effects: |
| Increased breast size (ductal and fatty tissue) |  |  |
| Cyclic weight gain due to fluid retention |  |  |
| Leukorrhea | Breast tenderness | Increased appetite and weight gain |
| Cervical eversion or ectopy | Headaches | Depression, fatigue |
| Hypertension | Hypertension | Decreased libido and/or enjoyment of intercourse |
| Rise in cholesterol concentration in gallbladder bile | Myocardial infarction (rare) | Acne, oily skin |
| Growth of leiomyoma |  | Increased breast tenderness or breast size |
| Telangiectasia |  | Increased LDL cholesterol levels |
| Hepatocellular adenomas or hepatocellular carcinoma (rare) |  | Decreased HDL cholesterol levels |
| Cerebrovascular accidents (rare) |  | Decreased carbohydrate tolerance; increased insulin resistance |
| Thromboembolic complications including pulmonary emboli (rare) |  | Pruritus |
| Stimulation of breast neoplasia (exceedingly rare) |  |  |
| (Most pills with less than 50 µg of ethinyl estradiol do not produce troublesome estrogen-mediated side effects or complications.) |  |  |

LDL = low-density lipoprotein; HDL = high density lipoprotein.
Reproduced with permission from Hatcher RA et al: *Contraceptive Technology*, 17th ed. Ardent Media, 1998.

with seizure disorders, because it has been found to reduce the number of seizures in some patients. DMPA may also be helpful for adolescents with von Willebrand disease, since amenorrhea (which decreases blood loss) is a common effect of DMPA. Studies have shown no increased risk of liver cancer, breast cancer, or invasive squamous cell cervical cancer among users of DMPA, and the risk of endometrial and ovarian cancers is reduced.

Lunelle is a monthly combined estrogen/progesterone injectable contraceptive that was approved in the United States in 2000; however, the manufacturer recently discontinued production of Lunelle. There is potential for another company to produce this contraceptive in the future. Lunelle contains 5 mg of estradiol cypionate and 25 mg of medroxyprogesterone acetate. Its advantages over progestin-only injectable contraceptives include faster return to fertility and less amenorrhea, which theoretically should lower the risk of osteoporosis. Side effects include weight gain, irregular

bleeding, breast pain, menorrhagia, and dysmenorrhea. Efficacy is excellent, with a reported failure rate of 0.2%. Monthly injections may make this method less attractive for adolescents.

The levonorgestrel-containing nonbiodegradable subdermal implant (Norplant System), which is inserted under the skin of the upper arm using a trocar, is effective for 5 years, with pregnancy rates ranging from 0.04 per 100 woman-years in the first year of use to 1.1 per 100 woman-years in the fifth year. It acts through ovulation inhibition and thickening of the cervical mucus. Menstrual irregularities (including prolonged bleeding, intermenstrual spotting, and amenorrhea) are the most common side effects, although headache, acne, weight gain or loss, and depression may occur. Its ease of use, lack of compliance issues, high efficacy, and long-term protection make the subdermal implant an ideal contraceptive for adolescents who can tolerate the menstrual irregularities. In 2000, Norplant was removed from the market because of concern over decreased efficacy in the fifth year in some lots. No implantable contraceptive methods are currently marketed in the United States.

## Implantable Contraceptive Methods Available Outside of the United States

Implanon is a single implant, effective for 3 years. It contains etonogestrel. It has been used in Europe and has a failure rate approaching 0%. Side effects include irregular bleeding, headache, nausea, breast pain, and depression. Return to fertility is rapid following removal. Insertion and removal are reportedly significantly easier than Norplant. Other implantable progesterones used in other countries include Norplant II and Jadelle (levonorgestrel) and Uniplant and Surplant (nomegestrol acetate).

## Contraceptive Vaginal Ring

The Nuva Ring is a vaginal ring that releases 15 µg of ethinyl estradiol and 120 µg of etonogestrel per day. The ring is placed inside the vagina for 3 weeks, followed by 1 week without the ring to allow for withdrawal bleeding. A new ring is inserted each month. Failure rate is 1%. Side effects include vaginitis in 5%, headache in 6%, and foreign body sensation in 2.5%. The vaginal ring is easier to insert correctly than the diaphragm. However, like the diaphragm, adolescents are often reluctant to use contraception requiring insertion into the vagina.

## Contraceptive Methods Not Usually Recommended for Teenagers

Adolescents should understand the menstrual cycle and be taught that ovulation typically occurs 2 weeks before the next menstrual period and may be difficult to predict. Because teenagers frequently have irregular cycles, the rhythm, or calendar, method is not effective. Adolescents also need to be taught that withdrawal is not a reliable method of contraception. Diaphragms and cervical caps require professional fitting and skill with insertion and are not popular among teenagers. Adolescents who have never been pregnant or who engage in behaviors that carry a risk of STIs should not use an intrauterine device. Sterilization is rarely appropriate for adolescents.

Gallo MF et al: Skin patch and vaginal ring versus combined oral contraceptives for contraception. Cochrane Database Syst Rev 2003;(1):CD003552 [PMID: 12535478].

Greydanus DE et al: Contraception in the adolescent: An update. Pediatrics. 2001;107(3):562 [PMID: 11230601].

Petitti DB: Clinical practice: Combination estrogen–progestin oral contraceptives. N Engl J Med 2003;349(15):1443 [PMID: 14534338].

MMWR: Trends in sexual risk behaviors among high school students—United States, 1991–2001. MMWR 2002;51(38): 856 [PMID: 12363337].

Meirik O et al: Implantable contraceptives for women. Hum Reprod Update 2003;9(1):49 [PMID: 12638781].

# PREGNANCY

The teen birth rate in the United States has been steadily decreasing since the early 1990s, with a historic low in 2001. From 1991 to 2001, the birth rate for adolescents age 15–19 years decreased from 61.8 to 45.3/1000. Abortions have also decreased over the past decade. In 1997, 16.3% of pregnancies in 15- to 17-year-olds ended in abortion, as did 37.5% of pregnancies in 18- to 19-year-olds. Despite decreasing rates, the United States still has the highest adolescent pregnancy rate of any developed country. Over 800,000 adolescents younger than age 19 become pregnant every year. Young maternal age and associated maternal risk factors have been linked to adverse neonatal outcome, including higher rates of low-birth-weight babies (< 2500 g) and neonatal mortality. The psychosocial consequences for the teenage mother and her infant are listed in Table 3–16. Teenagers who are pregnant require additional support from their caregivers. Clinics for young mothers may be the best providers.

## Presentation

Adolescents may present with delayed or missed menses or may even request a pregnancy test, but often they present with an unrelated concern or have a hidden agenda. Because of the high level of denial, they may come in with complaints of abdominal pain, urinary frequency, dizziness, or other nonspecific symptoms and have no concern about pregnancy. A history of symptoms such as weight gain, engorged breasts, an unusually light or mistimed period, and urinary frequency may be present. Denial contributes to the delay in seeking prenatal care. Clinicians need to have a low threshold for suspicion of pregnancy. If any suspicion exists, a urine pregnancy test should be obtained.

## Diagnosis

The history and physical examination may assist in making the diagnosis. Bluish coloring and softening of the cervix may be noted on speculum examination. The uterine fundus may be palpable on abdominal examination if sufficient time has elapsed. If uterine size on bimanual examination does not correspond to dates, one

*Table 3–16.* Psychosocial consequences of pregnancy for the adolescent mother and her infant.

| Mother | Infant |
|---|---|
| **Increased morbidity related to pregnancy** | **Greater health risks** |
| Greater risk of toxemia, anemia, prolonged labor, premature labor | Increased chance of low birth weight or prematurity |
| Increased chance of miscarriages, stillbirths | Increased risk of infant death |
| Increased change of maternal mortality | Increased risk of injury and hospitalization by age 5 |
| **Decreased educational attainment** | **Decreased academic achievement** |
| Less likely to get high school diploma, go to college, or graduate | Lower cognitive scores |
| **Lower occupational attainment and prestige** | Decreased development |
| | Greater chance of being behind grade or needing remedial help |
| Less chance of stable employment (some resolution over time) | Lower chance of advanced academics |
| Lower job satisfaction | Lower academic aptitude as a teenager and perhaps a higher probability of dropping out of school |
| Lower income/wages | |
| Greater dependence on public assistance | |
| **Less stable marital relationships** | **Psychosocial consequences** |
| Higher rates of single parenthood | Greater risk of behavior problems |
| Earlier marriage (though less common than in the past) | Poverty |
| | Higher probability of living in a nonintact home while in high school |
| Accelerated pace of marriage, separation, divorce, and remarriage | Greater risk of adolescent pregnancy |
| **Faster pace of subsequent childbearing** | |
| High rate of repeat unintended pregnancy | |
| More births out of marriage | |
| Closer spacing of births | |
| Larger families | |

must consider ectopic pregnancy, incomplete or missed abortion, twin gestation, or inaccurate dates.

Enzyme-linked immunoassay test kits specific for the β-HCG subunit and sensitive to less than 50 mIU/mL of HCG can be performed on urine (preferably the first morning-voided specimen, because it is more concentrated) in less than 5 minutes and are accurate by the expected date of the missed period in almost 100% of patients. Serum radioimmunoassay is also specific for the β subunit, is accurate within 7 days after conception, and is helpful in ruling out ectopic pregnancy or threatened abortion.

The timing of pregnancy tests is important, because HCG levels rise initially after conception, peak at about 60–70 days, then drop to levels not detected by routine office slide tests after 16–20 weeks.

## Special Issues in Management

When an adolescent presents for pregnancy testing, it is helpful, before performing the test, to find out what she hopes the result will be and what she thinks she will do if the test is positive. If she wants to be pregnant and the test is negative, further counseling about the implications of teen pregnancy should be offered. Prenatal vitamins should be prescribed. For those who do not wish to be pregnant, contraception should be discussed, because teens with a negative pregnancy test have a high risk of pregnancy within the next 2 years.

If the adolescent is pregnant, the physician must discuss her support systems and her options with her (abortion, adoption, raising the baby). Many teenagers need help in telling and involving their parents. It is important to remain available for further assistance with decision making. Patients should be informed of the gestational age and time frames required for the different options. If the patient knows what she wants to do, she should be referred to the appropriate resources. Because teenagers are often ambivalent about their plans and may have a high level of denial, it is prudent to follow up in 1 week to be certain that a decision has been made. Avoiding a decision reduces the adolescent's options and may result in poor pregnancy outcomes. Providers can help ensure that the patient obtains prenatal care if she has chosen to continue the pregnancy. In addition, brief counseling about healthy diet; folic acid supplementation (400 μg/d); and avoiding alcohol, tobacco, and other drugs is helpful.

Young maternal age, low maternal prepregnancy weight, poor weight gain, delay in prenatal care, and low socioeconomic status contribute to low birth weight and poor fetal outcome. The poor nutritional status of some teenagers; their erratic diets, smoking, drinking, or substance abuse; and their high incidence of STIs also play a role. Teenagers are also at greater risk than adult women for pre-eclampsia, eclampsia, iron deficiency anemia, cephalopelvic disproportion, prolonged labor, premature labor, and maternal death. Early prenatal care and good nutrition can make a difference with a number of these problems.

Because of the high risk of a second unintended pregnancy within the next 2 years, postpartum contraceptive counseling and follow-up are imperative. Combined OCPs or the contraceptive patch can be started 3 weeks after delivery in adolescents who are not breast feeding; progestin-only methods can be started immediately postpartum, even in breastfeeding adolescents. Pregnancy prevention is the most cost-effective means of reducing the consequences of teenage pregnancy. Sexual decision making, contraceptive counseling, and close follow-up of sexually active adolescents of both sexes can make a difference. Adolescents who receive sexuality and contraceptive education are not more likely to have intercourse but are less likely to become pregnant than their counterparts who do not receive such instruction.

## Ectopic Pregnancy

In the United States, 100,000 ectopic pregnancies occur each year, accounting for 2% of pregnancies. Adolescents have the highest mortality rate from ectopic pregnancy, most likely related to delayed entry into health care. Risk factors include history of pelvic inflammatory disease or chlamydial infection. Conception while on progestin-only methods of contraceptives also increases risk of ectopic pregnancy, because of the progestin-mediated decrease in tubal motility. Providers should keep a high level of suspicion with any adolescent presenting with vaginal bleeding and abdominal pain.

Abma JC, Sonenstein FL: Sexual activity and contraceptive practices among teenagers in the United States, 1988 and 1995. Vital Health Stat 2001;21:1 [PMID: 11478202].

Elfenbein DS et al: Adolescent pregnancy. Pediatr Clin North Am 2003;50(4):781-800, viii [PMID: 12964694].

Hamilton BE et al: Revised birth and fertility rates for the 1990s and new rates for Hispanic populations, 2000 and 2001: United States. Natl Vital Stat Rep 2003;51(12):1 [PMID: 12918931].

# VULVOVAGINITIS

Vaginitis may be due to pathogens or to indigenous flora after a change in milieu of the vagina. Candidal vulvovaginitis and bacterial vaginosis (formerly called *Gardnerella, Haemophilus,* or nonspecific vaginitis) may occur in patients who are not sexually active. These are examples of indigenous flora that may cause symptoms. Bacterial vaginosis, however, is more prevalent in those who are sexually active. In sexually active patients, *Trichomonas* infection or cervicitis due to sexually transmitted pathogens must be considered (see Chapter 40). For this reason, appropriate specimens should be taken from sexually active patients or suspected victims of sexual abuse in order to detect STIs, even if yeast forms are present or bacterial vaginosis is identified.

## 1. Physiologic Leukorrhea

Leukorrhea is the normal vaginal discharge that begins around the time of menarche. The discharge is typically clear or whitish, and its consistency may vary according to cyclic hormonal influences. There should be no odor. Girls in early adolescence may have concerns about such a discharge and need reassurance that it is normal. This may be a good time to tell girls that there is no need for douching. If a vaginal wet preparation is examined, a few squamous epithelial cells may be revealed, but there should be fewer than five polymorphonuclear cells per high-power field.

## 2. Candidal Vulvovaginitis

Candidal vulvovaginitis is caused by yeast (*Candida albicans*). It typically occurs after a course of antibiotics, after which the normal perineal flora are altered and yeast is allowed to proliferate. Diabetic patients, those with compromised immune systems, and those who are pregnant or receiving OCPs are more prone to develop candidal infections.

### Clinical Findings

The patient usually complains of vulvar pruritus or dyspareunia and a thick vaginal discharge, frequently beginning the week before menses. Examination of the vulva reveals erythematous mucosa, sometimes with excoriation, and a thick, white, cheesy discharge. The discharge may be adherent to the walls of the vagina. Leukocytes may be seen on a wet preparation, and a KOH preparation may reveal budding yeast or mycelia. The vaginal preparations are often not helpful, and the patient should be treated on the basis of the clinical examination. Vaginal culture for yeast is usually unnecessary.

### Treatment

Butoconazole, clotrimazole, miconazole, terconazole, or tioconazole vaginal creams or suppositories designed for seven nightly doses are effective in most patients. Fluconazole (150 mg once orally) is also effective and may be beneficial on a monthly prophylactic basis for women with recurring infections. Patients with recurrent episodes should be given prophylactic treatment whenever they take antibiotics. It may be helpful to simultaneously treat the partners of sexually active patients with recurrent candidal infections.

## 3. Bacterial Vaginosis

Bacterial vaginosis may be caused by any of the indigenous vaginal flora, such as *Gardnerella, Bacteroides, Pep-*

*tococcus, Mycoplasma hominis,* lactobacilli, or other anaerobes.

## Clinical Findings

The patient generally complains of a malodorous discharge. On examination, a thin, homogeneous, grayish white discharge is found adhering to the vaginal wall. A whiff test, in which a drop of KOH is added to a smear of the discharge on a slide, results in the release of amines, causing a fishy odor. Wet preparation reveals an abundance of clue cells and small pleomorphic rods.

## Treatment

Treatment for bacterial vaginosis is with metronidazole (500 mg orally bid for 7 days) or clindamycin (300 mg orally bid for 7 days). Topical metronidazole or clindamycin may also be effective. Ampicillin (500 mg orally four times a day for 7 days) is the alternative for pregnant patients.

## 4. Other Causes Of Vulvovaginitis

### Sexually Transmitted Infections

STIs are a common cause of vaginal discharge in adolescents (see Chapter 40). *Chlamydia* and gonorrhea

testing should be done whenever a sexually active adolescent complains of vaginal discharge even when the cervix appears normal.

## Foreign Body Vaginitis

Foreign bodies (most commonly retained tampons or condoms) cause extremely malodorous vaginal discharges. Treatment consists of removal, for which ring forceps may be useful. Further treatment is generally not necessary.

## Allergic or Contact Vaginitis

Bubble baths, feminine hygiene sprays, or vaginal contraceptive foams or suppositories may cause chemical irritation of the vaginal mucosa. Discontinuing use of the offending agent is indicated.

## REFERENCES

Brook I: Microbiology and management of polymicrobial female genital tract infections in adolescents. J Pediatr Adolesc Gynecol 2002;15(4):217 [PMID: 12459228].

# Substance Abuse

*Paritosh Kaul, MD, & Catherine Stevens-Simon, MD*

The use and abuse of mood-altering substances—alcohol, marijuana, opioids, cocaine, amphetamines, sedative-hypnotics, hallucinogens, inhalants, nicotine, anabolic steroids, γ-hydroxybutyrate (GHB), and 3,4-methylenedioxymethamphetamine (ecstasy)—continues to be a serious public health problem. The short- and long-term health, social, emotional, legal, and behavioral consequences of substance abuse are particularly damaging during childhood and adolescence. Not only does early substance use portend chronic, severe polysubstance abuse later in life, but substance use may also compromise physical, cognitive, and psychosocial aspects of adolescent development if this maladaptive behavior becomes the preferred response to environmental stressors.

Substance abuse tends to be a chronic, progressive disease. The first or initiation stage—from nonuser to user—is such a common feature of becoming an American adult that many authorities call it normative behavior. At this stage, substance use is typically limited to experimentation with tobacco or alcohol (so-called gateway substances). During adolescence, young people are expected to establish an independent, autonomous identity. They try out a variety of behaviors within the safety of their family circles and peer groups. This process often involves experimentation with psychoactive substances, usually in culturally acceptable circumstances. Progression to the second or continuation stage of substance abuse is a nonnormative risk behavior with the potential to compromise adolescent development. The American Psychiatric Association criteria listed in Table 4–1 can be used to judge the severity of substance use that progresses beyond the experimentation stage to substance abuse or substance dependency. Maintenance and progression within a class of substances (eg, from beer to liquor) and progression across classes of substances (eg, from alcohol to marijuana) represent the third and fourth stages of substance abuse. Individuals at these stages are polysubstance abusers, and most manifest one or more of the symptoms of dependency listed in Table 4–1. The transition from one stage to the next is typically a cyclic process of regression, cessation, and relapse. Common symptoms and physiologic effects of intoxication (which can occur at any stage) and withdrawal (a symptom of dependency)

for the major classes of substances are presented in Tables 4–2 and 4–3.

American Psychiatric Association: *Diagnostic and Statistical Manual of Mental Disorders,* 4th ed. Text Revised. American Psychiatric Association, 2000.

Comerci GD, Schwebel R: Substance abuse: An overview. Adolescent Medicine: State of the Art Reviews 2000;11(1): 79 [PMID: 10640340].

DuRant RH et al: The relationship between early age of onset of initial substance use and engaging in multiple health risk behaviors among young adolescents. Arch Pediatr Adolesc Med 1999;153:286 [PMID: 10086407].

US Department of Health and Human Services. *Healthy People 2010,* 2nd ed. With Understanding and Improving Health and Objectives for Improving Health (2 vols). Washington, DC: U.S. Government Printing Office, 2000.

## SCOPE OF THE PROBLEM

The best source of information about the prevalence of substance abuse among American children and adolescents is the annual Monitoring the Future Study, which tracks health-related behaviors in a sample of 44,000 8th, 10th, and 12th graders in about 400 public and private schools across the United States. This study probably understates the magnitude of the problem of substance abuse because it excludes two of the most abuse-prone groups of young people—school dropouts and runaways. Although the exclusion of these youngsters may minimize prevalence estimates only moderately for the entire population, errors in estimating drug use among subgroups with high rates of school dropout (eg, urban minority youths) are thought to be substantial. Data from this survey and others show that alcohol is the most frequently abused substance in our society. Experimentation with alcohol typically begins in or before middle school; is more common among boys than girls; and is most common among whites, less common among Hispanics and Native Americans, and least common among blacks and Asians. Over 50% of children consume alcohol before high school, and over 90% do so before graduation. Over 25% of eighth graders and over 50% of high-school students seen in an average American pediatric practice have used alcohol within the last 30 days, and half have consumed five or more drinks on at least

***Table 4–1.*** Substance abuse and substance dependency.

**Diagnostic criteria for substance abuse**

A. A maladaptive pattern of substance use leading to clinically significant impairment or distress, as manifested by one or more of the following occurring within a 12-month period:

1. Recurrent substance use resulting in a failure to fulfill major role obligations at work, school, or home (eg, repeated absences or poor work performance related to substance use; substance-related absences, suspensions, or expulsions from school; neglect of children or household).

2. Recurrent substance use in situations in which it is physically hazardous (eg, driving an automobile or operating a machine when impaired by substance use).

3. Recurrent substance-related legal problems (arrests for substance-related disorderly conduct).

4. Continued substance use despite having persistent or recurrent social or interpersonal problems caused or exacerbated by the effects of the substance (eg, arguments with spouse about consequences of intoxication, physical fights).

B. The symptoms have never met criteria for substance dependence for this class of substance.

**Diagnostic criteria for substance dependency**

A maladaptive pattern of substance use, leading to clinically significant impairment or distress, as manifested by three or more of the following, occurring at any time in the same 12-month period:

1. Tolerance, as defined by either of the following:
   a. Need for markedly increased amounts of the substance to achieve intoxication or desired effect.
   b. Markedly diminished effect with continued use of the same amount of the substance.

2. Withdrawal, as manifested by either of the following:
   a. The characteristic withdrawal syndrome for the substance (criteria A and B of the criteria for withdrawal from the specific substance).
   b. The same (or closely related) substance taken to relieve or avoid withdrawal symptoms.

3. The substance often taken in larger amounts or over a longer period than was intended.

4. There is a persistent desire or unsuccessful efforts to cut down or control substance use.

5. A great deal of time spent in activities necessary to obtain the substance (eg, visiting multiple doctors, driving long distances), use the substance (chain-smoking), or recover from its effects.

6. Important social, occupational, or recreational activities given up or reduced because of substance use.

7. The substance use is continued despite knowledge of having a persistent or recurrent physical or psychological problem that is likely to have been caused or exacerbated by the substance (eg, current cocaine use despite recognition of cocaine-induced depression, or continued drinking despite recognition that an ulcer was made worse by alcohol consumption).

Reprinted, with permission, from the *Diagnostic and Statistical Manual of Mental Disorders,* 4th ed. Text Revision. Copyright 2000. American Psychiatric Association.

one occasion. Use of tobacco, marijuana, and other mood-altering substances is less common (Table 4–4). Marijuana is the most commonly used illicit drug in the United States. First experiences with marijuana and the substances listed in Table 4–4 typically occur during middle school and early high school. Initiation of substance abuse is rare after age 20 years.

The level of substance abuse among American youth rose in the 1960s and 1970s, declined in the 1980s, reached a nadir in 1990, and rose again in the early and mid-1990s, peaking among eighth graders in 1996 (see Table 4–4). Use declined slightly in the late 1990s and was stable in 2000. Marijuana accounted for most of the increased drug use during the 1990s. Table 4–4 shows that marijuana use is still widespread among American youth. Use of most other drugs, including crack cocaine, declined during the 1990s. The major exception to this encouraging trend has been the increased use of ecstasy and anabolic steroids in 1999 and

2000. However, use of both drugs showed a decline in 2002. Overall drug and alcohol use also decreased in 2002. Studies indicate that the rise and fall in use of a substance is heralded by changes in the perceived risks and benefits of using the substance. Increased availability has been a major factor in the rising use of anabolic steroids and ecstasy. The age at initiation of alcohol and other substance abuse dropped significantly in the early 1990s. Currently, most first-time users are between 12 and 14 years of age. Inhalants such as glue and gasoline are predominantly a choice of younger adolescents. This statistic is particularly worrisome because early-onset substance use is one of the best predictors of persistent abuse later in life.

Bachman JG et al: Explaining recent increases in students' marijuana use: Impacts of perceived risks and disapproval, 1976–1996. Am J Public Health 1998;88:887 [PMID: 9618614].

***Table 4–2.*** Physiologic effects of commonly abused mood-altering substances.[1]

| | |
|---|---|
| **EYES/PUPILS** | |
| Mydriasis | Amphetamines, MDMA, or other stimulants, cocaine, glutethimide, jimsonweed, LSD Withdrawal from alcohol and opioids |
| Miosis | Alcohol, barbiturates, benzodiazepines, opioids, PCP |
| Nystagmus | Alcohol, barbiturates, benzodiazepines, inhalants, PCP |
| Conjunctival injection | LSD, marijuana |
| Lacrimation | Inhalants, LSD. Withdrawal from opioids. |
| **CARDIOVASCULAR** | |
| Tachycardia | Amphetamines, MDMA, or other stimulants, cocaine, LSD, marijuana, PCP. Withdrawal from alcohol, barbiturates, benzodiazepines. |
| Hypertension | Amphetamines, MDMA, or other stimulants, cocaine, LSD, marijuana, PCP. Withdrawal from alcohol, barbiturates, benzodiazepines. |
| Hypotension | Barbiturates, opioids. Orthostatic: marijuana. Withdrawal from depressants. |
| Arrhythmia | Amphetamines, MDMA, or other stimulants, cocaine, inhalants, opioids, PCP |
| **RESPIRATORY** | |
| Depression | Opioids, depressants, GHB |
| Pulmonary edema | Opioids, stimulants |
| **CORE BODY TEMPERATURE** | |
| Elevated | Amphetamines, MDMA, or other stimulants, cocaine, PCP. Withdrawal from alcohol, barbiturates, benzodiazepines, opioids. |
| Decreased | Alcohol, barbiturates, benzodiazepines, opioids, GHB |
| **PERIPHERAL NERVOUS SYSTEM RESPONSE** | |
| Hyperreflexia | Amphetamines, MDMA, or other stimulants, cocaine, LSD, marijuana, methaqualone, PCP Withdrawal from alcohol, barbiturates, benzodiazepines |
| Hyporeflexia | Alcohol, barbiturates, benzodiazepines, inhalants, opioids |
| Tremor | Amphetamines or other stimulants, cocaine, LSD Withdrawal from alcohol, barbiturates, benzodiazepines, cocaine |
| Ataxia | Alcohol, amphetamines, MDMA, or other stimulants, barbiturates, benzodiazepines, inhalants, LSD, PCP, GHB |
| **CENTRAL NERVOUS SYSTEM RESPONSE** | |
| Hyperalertness | Amphetamines, MDMA, or other stimulants, cocaine |
| Sedation, somnolence | Alcohol, barbiturates, benzodiazepines, inhalants, marijuana, opioids, GHB |
| Seizures | Alcohol, amphetamines, MDMA, or other stimulants, cocaine, inhalants, methaqualone, opioids (particularly meperidine, propoxyphene) Withdrawal from alcohol, barbiturates, benzodiazepines |
| Hallucinations | Amphetamines, MDMA, or other stimulants, cocaine, inhalants, LSD, marijuana, PCP Withdrawal from alcohol, barbiturates, benzodiazepines |
| **GASTROINTESTINAL** | |
| Nausea, vomiting | Alcohol, amphetamines or other stimulants, cocaine, inhalants, LSD, opioids, peyote, GHB Withdrawal from alcohol, barbiturates, benzodiazepines, cocaine, opioids |

[1]GHB = gamma hydroxybutyrate, LSD = lysergic acid diethylamide, MDMA = methylenedioxymethamphetamine (ecstasy), PCP = phencyclidine hydrochloride.
Adapted with permission from: Schwartz B, Alderman EM: Substance abuse. Pediatr Rev 1997;18:215.

Dyer JE, Roth B, Hyman BA: Gamma-hydroxybutyrate withdrawal syndrome. Ann Emerg Med 2001;37(2):147 [PMID: 11174231].

Gilpin EA, Choi WS, Berry C, et al: How many adolescents start smoking each day in the United States? J Adolesc Health 1999;25:248 [PMID: 10505842].

Johnston LD, O'Malley PM, Bachman JG: (2003). *The Monitoring the Future National Survey Results on Adolescent Drug Use:* *Overview of Key Findings, 2002* (NIH Publication No. 03-5375). Bethesda, MD: National Institute on Drug Abuse. www.monitoringthefuture.org

Kurtzman TL, Otsuka KN, Wahl RA: Inhalant abuse by adolescents. J Adolesc Health 2001;28:1616 [PMID: 11226839].

O'Malley PM, Johnston LD: Drinking and driving among US high school seniors, 1984–1997. Am J Public Health 1999;89:678 [PMID: 10224978].

*Table 4–3.* Effects of commonly abused mood-altering substances.

| Substance | Pharmacology | Intoxication | Withdrawal | Chronic Use |
|---|---|---|---|---|
| Alcohol (ethanol) | Depressant; 10 g/drink Drink: 12 oz beer, 4 oz wine, 1½ oz liquor; one drink increases blood level by approximately 0.025 g/dL (varies by weight) | Legal: 0.05–0.1 g/dL (varies by state) Mild: < 0.1 g/dL; disinhibition, euphoria, mild sedation and impaired coordination Moderate: 0.1–0.2 g/dL; impaired mentation and judgment, slurred speech ataxia Severe: > 0.3 g/dL; confusion, stupor; > 0.4 g/dL; coma, depressed respiration | Mild: headache, tremors, nausea and vomiting ("hangover") Severe: fever, sweaty, seizure, agitation, hallucination, hypertension, tachycardia Delirium tremens (chronic use) | Hepatitis, cirrhosis, cardiac disease, Wernicke encephalopathy, Korsakoff syndrome |
| Marijuana (cannabis) | Delta-9-tetrahydro-cannabinol (THC); 4–6% in marijuana; 20–30% in hashish | Low: euphoria, relaxation, impaired thinking High: mood changes, depersonalization, hallucinations Toxic: panic, delusions, paranoia, psychosis | Irritability, disturbed sleep, tremor, nystagmus, anorexia, diarrhea, vomiting | Cough, gynecomastia, low sperm count, infertility, amotivational syndrome, apathy |
| Cocaine | Stimulant; releases biogenic amines; concentration varies with preparation and route of administration | Hyperalert, increased energy, confident, insomnia, anxiety, paranoia, dilated pupils, tremors, seizures, hypertension, arrhythmia, tachycardia, fever, dry mouth Toxic: coma, psychosis, seizure, myocardial infarction, stroke, hyperthermia, rhabdomyolysis | Drug craving, depression, dysphoria, irritability, lethargy, tremors, nausea, hunger | Nasal septum ulceration, epistaxis, lung damage, intravenous drug use |
| Opioids (heroin, morphine, codeine, methadone, opium, fentanyl, meperidine, propoxyphene) | Depressant; binds central opioid receptor; variable concentrations with substance | Euphoria, sedation, impaired thinking, low blood pressure, pinpoint pupil, urinary retention Toxic: hypotension, arrhythmia, depressed respiration, stupor, coma, seizure, death | Only after > 3 weeks of regular use: drug craving, rhinorrhea, lacrimation, muscle aches, diarrhea, anxiety, tremors, hypertension, tachycardia. | Intravenous drug use: cellulitis, endocarditis, embolisms, HIV |
| Amphetamines | Stimulant; sympatho-mimetic | Euphoria, hyperalert state, hyperactive, hypertension, arrhythmia, fever, flushing, dilated pupils, tremor, ataxia, dry mouth | Lethargy, fatigue, depression, anxiety, nightmares, muscle cramps, abdominal pain, hunger | Paranoia, psychosis |

(continued)

*Table 4–3.* Effects of commonly abused mood-altering substances. (continued)

| Substance | Pharmacology | Intoxication | Withdrawal | Chronic Use |
|---|---|---|---|---|
| | | Toxic: coma, circulatory collapse, hypertensive crisis, cerebral hemorrhage | | |
| MDMA (ecstasy) | Stimulant, psychedelic; releases serotonin, dopamine, and nor-epinephrine; inhibits reuptake of neuro-transmitters; increases dopamine synthesis; inhibits MAO | Enhanced empathy, euphoria, increased energy and self-esteem, tachycardia, hyperten-tion, increased pyscho-motor drive, sensory enhancement, illusions, difficulty concentrating and retaining informa-tion, headaches, palpi-tations, flushing, hyper-thermia<br>Toxic: frank psychosis, coma, seizures, intra-cranial hemorrhage, cerebral infarction, asystole, pulmonary edema, multisystem organ failure, acute re-nal or heptic failure, ARDS, DIC, SIADH, death | None | Paranoid pyschosis |
| GHB (liquid ecstasy) | Depressant, endogen-ous CNS transmitter; influences dopamin-ergic activity, higher levels of GABA-B ac-tivity | 10 mg/kg: sleep<br>30 mg/kg: memory loss<br>50 mg/kg: general anes-thesia<br>Toxic: CNS and respiratory depression, aggressive-ness, seizures, brady-cardia, apnea | Only after chronic use with dosing every 3 hrs<br>Early: mild tremor, tachy-cardia, hypertension, diaphoresis, moderate anxiety, insomnia, nau-sea, vomiting<br>Progressive: confusion, delirium, hallucinations autonomic instability, death | Wernicke–Korsakoff |
| Sedative-hypnotics (barbiturates, ben-zodiazepines, methaqualone) | Depressant | Sedation, lethargy, slurred speech, pin-point pupils, hypoten-sion, psychosis, sei-zures<br>Toxic: stupor, coma, cardiac arrest, seizure, pulmonary edema, death | Only after weeks of use: agitation, delirium, psychosis, hallucina-tions, fever, flushing, hyper- or hypotension, death | Paranoia |

*(continued)*

***Table 4–3.*** Effects of commonly abused mood-altering substances. (continued)

| Substance | Pharmacology | Intoxication | Withdrawal | Chronic Use |
|---|---|---|---|---|
| Hallucinogens (LSD, peyote, mescaline, mushrooms, nutmeg, jimsonweed) | Inhibition of serotonin release | Illusions, depersonalization, hallucination, anxiety, paranoia, ataxia, dilated pupils, hypertension, dry mouth<br>Toxic: coma, terror, panic, "crazy feeling" | None | Flashbacks |
| Phencyclidine | Dissociative anesthetic | Low dose (< 5 mg): illusions, hallucinations, ataxia, hypertension, flushing<br>Moderate dose (5–10 mg): hyperthermia, salivation, myoclonus<br>High dose: (> 10 mg): rigidity, seizure, arrhythmia, coma, death | None | Flashbacks |
| Inhalants (toluene, benzene, hydrocarbons and fluorocarbons) | Stimulation progressing to depression | Euphoria, giddiness, impaired judgment, ataxia, rhinorrhea, salivation, hallucination<br>Toxic: respiratory depression, arrhythmia, coma, stupor, delirium, sudden death | None | Permanent damage to nerves, liver, heart, kidney, brain |
| Nicotine | Releases dopamine, 1 mg nicotine per cigarette | Relaxation, tachycardia, vertigo, anorexia | Drug craving, irritability, anxiety, hunger, impaired concentration | Permanent damage to lung, heart, cardiovascular system |
| Anabolic steroids[a] | Bind steroid receptor<br>Stacking: use many types simultaneously; pyramiding: increase dosage | Increased muscle bulk, strength, endurance, increased drive, hypogonadism, low sperm count, gynecomastia, decreased libido, virilization, irregular menses, hepatitis, early epiphysial closure, aggressiveness | Drug craving, dysphoria, irritability, depression | Tendon rupture, cardiomyopathy, atherosclerosis, peliosis hepatis (orally active C17 derivatives of testosterone are especially hepatotoxic) |

[a]Despite conventional assumptions, scientific studies show that anabolic steroids do not improve aerobic athletic performance and improve strength only in athletes trained in weight lifting before they begin using steroids who continue to train and take a high-protein diet.

Swaim R et al: The effect of school dropout rates on estimates of adolescent substance use among three racial/ethnic groups. Am J Public Health 1997;87:51 [PMID: 9065226].

Tomar SL, Giovino GA: Incidence and predictors of smokeless tobacco use among US youth. Am J Public Health 1998;88:20 [PMID: 9584028].

## MORBIDITY ASSOCIATED WITH SUBSTANCE ABUSE

Use and abuse of alcohol or other mood-altering substances is associated with the leading causes of adolescent and young adult deaths and injuries in the United States (ie, motor vehicle accidents, other unintentional injuries, homicide, and suicide), which are typically

*Table 4–4.* Prevalence of pediatric substance use and abusers by year.

| | Lifetime | | | | | Annual | | | | | 30-day | | | | |
|---|---|---|---|---|---|---|---|---|---|---|---|---|---|---|---|
| | 1991 | 1996 | 2000 | 2001 | 2002 | 1991 | 1996 | 2000 | 2001 | 2002 | 1991 | 1996 | 2000 | 2001 | 2002 |
| **Any Illicit Drug** | | | | | | | | | | | | | | | |
| 8th grade | 18.7 | 31.2 | 26.8 | 26.8 | 24.5 | 11.3 | 23.6 | 19.5 | 19.5 | 17.7 | 5.7 | 14.6 | 11.9 | 11.7 | 10.4 |
| 10th grade | 30.6 | 45.4 | 45.6 | 45.6 | 44.6 | 21.4 | 37.5 | 36.4 | 37.2 | 34.8 | 11.6 | 23.2 | 22.5 | 22.7 | 20.8 |
| 12th grade | 44.1 | 50.8 | 54.0 | 53.9 | 53.0 | 29.4 | 40.2 | 40.9 | 41.4 | 41.0 | 16.4 | 24.6 | 24.9 | 25.7 | 25.4 |
| **Marijuana/Hashish** | | | | | | | | | | | | | | | |
| 8th grade | 10.2 | 23.1 | 20.3 | 20.4 | 19.2 | 6.2 | 18.3 | 15.6 | 15.4 | 14.6 | 3.2 | 11.3 | 9.1 | 9.2 | 8.3 |
| 10th grade | 23.4 | 39.8 | 40.3 | 40.1 | 38.7 | 16.5 | 33.6 | 32.2 | 32.7 | 30.3 | 8.7 | 20.4 | 19.7 | 19.8 | 17.8 |
| 12th grade | 36.7 | 44.9 | 48.8 | 49.0 | 47.8 | 23.9 | 35.8 | 36.5 | 37.0 | 36.2 | 13.8 | 21.9 | 21.6 | 22.4 | 21.5 |
| **Inhalants** | | | | | | | | | | | | | | | |
| 8th grade | 17.6 | 21.2 | 17.9 | 17.1 | 15.2 | 9.0 | 12.2 | 9.4 | 9.1 | 7.7 | 4.4 | 5.8 | 4.5 | 4.0 | 3.8 |
| 10th grade | 15.7 | 19.3 | 16.6 | 15.2 | 13.5 | 7.1 | 9.5 | 7.3 | 6.6 | 5.8 | 2.7 | 3.3 | 2.6 | 2.4 | 2.4 |
| 12th grade | 17.6 | 16.6 | 14.2 | 13.0 | 11.7 | 6.6 | 7.6 | 5.9 | 4.5 | 4.5 | 2.4 | 2.5 | 2.2 | 1.7 | 1.5 |
| **MDMA (Ecstasy)** | | | | | | | | | | | | | | | |
| 8th Grade | — | 3.4 | 4.3 | 5.2 | 4.3 | — | 2.3 | 3.1 | 3.5 | 2.9 | — | 1.0 | 1.4 | 1.8 | 1.4 |
| 10th Grade | — | 5.6 | 7.3 | 8.0 | 6.6 | — | 4.6 | 5.4 | 6.2 | 4.9 | — | 1.8 | 2.6 | 2.6 | 1.8 |
| 12th Grade | — | 6.1 | 11.0 | 11.7 | 10.5 | — | 4.6 | 8.2 | 9.2 | 7.4 | — | 2.0 | 3.6 | 2.8 | 2.4 |

Reprinted, with permission, from *Monitoring the Future Study*, 2003 (www.monitoringthefuture.org).

outcomes of high-risk or violent behaviors combined with impaired judgment. Substance abuse is also associated with physical and sexual abuse. Up to two thirds of sexual assaults and acquaintance or date rapes are linked to alcohol or other drug use. Drug use and abuse also contribute to other high-risk behaviors, such as unsafe and increased sexual activity, leading to unintended pregnancy and sexually transmitted diseases. The use of drugs during periods of low self-esteem and depression increases the risk of suicide.

The well-known long- and short-term risks associated with tobacco, alcohol, and cocaine are listed in Table 4–3. Less well known are the long- and short-term morbidities connected with the currently most popular illicit drugs among adolescents (eg, marijuana and ecstasy). The active ingredient in marijuana, δ-9-tetrahydrocannabinol (THC), transiently causes tachycardia, mild hypertension, and bronchodilation. Regular use can cause lung changes similar to those seen in tobacco smokers. Heavy use decreases fertility in both sexes, leads to immunosuppression, and can cause the destruction of hippocampal and basal ganglia nuclei, resulting in disruption in cognition, learning, coordination, and memory. This may explain the development of so-called amotivational syndrome in heavy users, characterized by decreased attention to environmental stimuli and impaired goal-directed thinking and behavior. Also of concern is the increasing potency of available marijuana. Recent analysis of confiscated marijuana has shown a three- to five-fold increase in the concentration of THC since the 1970s and 1980s.

Ecstasy, which is gaining in popularity with teens and becoming more accessible, can cause permanent brain damage. Chronic use destroys the serotonin system of the brain and has been associated with progressive decline of immediate and delayed memory and with alterations in mood, sleep, and appetite. Even first-time users may develop frank psychosis indistinguishable from schizophrenia. Irreversible cardiomyopathy, noncardiogenic pulmonary edema, and pulmonary hypertension may occur with long-term use. Overdose can cause hyperthermia and multiorgan system failure.

Environmental and prenatal exposure to abused substances carry significant health risks. Parental tobacco smoking has been associated with low birth weight in newborns, sudden infant death syndrome, bronchiolitis, asthma, otitis media, and fire-related injuries. Paternal use of marijuana during pregnancy is associated with an increase the risk of sudden infant death syndrome. In utero exposure to cocaine and alcohol can result in fetal malformations, intrauterine growth retardation, and brain injury.

American Academy of Pediatrics Committee on Substance Abuse: Tobacco's Toll: Implications for the pediatrician. Pediatrics 2001:794 [PMID: 11335763].

Gouzoulis-Mayfrank et al: Impaired cognitive performance in drug free use of recreational Ecstasy. J Neurol Neurosurg Psychiatr 2000;68:719 [PMID: 10811694].

Graeme K: New drugs of abuse. Emerg Med Clin North Am 2000;18:625 [PMID: 11130930].

Heyman RB et al, American Academy of Pediatrics Committee on Substance Abuse: Marijuana: A continuing concern for pediatricians. Pediatrics 1999;104:982 [PMID: 10506247].

Klonoff-Cohen H, Lam-Kruglick P: Maternal and paternal recreational drug use and sudden infant death syndrome. Arch Pediatr Adolesc Med 2001;155:765 [PMID:11434841].

Ownby DR, Johnson CC, Peterson EL: Passive cigarette smoke exposure in infants. Arch Pediatr Adolesc Med 2000;154:1237 [PMID: 11115309].

Tapert SF et al: Adolescent substance use and sexual risk-taking behavior. J Adolesc Health 2001;28:181 [PMID: 11226840].

## SUPPLEMENT USE AND ABUSE

Use of supplements or special diets to enhance athletic performance dates back to antiquity, when warriors and athletes ate certain animals to acquire their characteristics. Today, many elite and casual athletes use ergogenic supplements in an attempt to improve performance. The most popular products among the pediatric population are protein supplements, creatine, and the prohormones. Strength athletes (ie, weight lifters) use protein powders and shakes to enhance muscle repair and mass. The typical amount of protein consumed by athletes far exceeds the recommended daily allowance for resistance-training athletes (1.6–1.7 g/kg/d). Excess consumption of protein provides no added strength or muscle mass and can provoke renal failure in teens with underlying renal dysfunction.

Creatine is the most popular nutritional supplement, with annual sales of $400 million. It is a combination of glycine, arginine, and methionine. Creatine is produced naturally in the liver, kidneys, and pancreas. It facilitates the production of adenosine triphosphate and increases free energy for muscle contraction. It maximizes power during short-duration, intense exercise, and improves baseline strength in adults. In contrast, creatine does not improve performance in longer duration, aerobic exercise; nor has its effectiveness been analyzed in children. Although the American College of Sports Medicine discourages use of the synthetic product by people under 18 years of age, recent studies show that creatine is extensively used by athletes in grades 6–12. Use by high-school juniors and seniors mirrors that of collegiate athletes. Side effects include weight gain, headache, abdominal pain, diarrhea, and increased muscle strain. There are conflicting reports about the risk of renal damage.

Most disturbing for health care providers is the growing availability and use of prohormones, specifically dehydroepiandrosterone (DHEA) and androstene-

dione. Sold as dietary supplements, these precursors to testosterone and other sex hormones are sold without federal regulation. Endogenous DHEA is produced in the adrenal cortex as a precursor of gonadal hormones. Putative benefits of DHEA include increased fat catabolism; increased muscle mass; increased libido; "improved" immune function; and decreased memory loss, heart disease, cancer, type II diabetes mellitus, Alzheimer, and Parkinson disease. Although its effects on strength and performance in athletes remain unstudied and unproven, the advertised benefits are attractive to many athletes. Its effect on young, healthy individuals (ie, those with higher baseline DHEA levels) has not been studied. In adults, two studies have shown that usage at 50 mg/d and 100 mg/d increases androgenic steroid plasma levels and improves subjective perception of physical and psychological well-being. Users of DHEA report few adverse effects.

Androstenedione, which is banned by the International Olympic Committee, National Collegiate Athletic Association, and National Football League, is converted to testosterone by the liver. A recent study of young athletes concluded that oral androstenedione does not increase plasma testosterone concentrations and, in young eugonadal men, has no anabolic effect on muscle protein metabolism. Other studies have shown increased biologically active estrogen levels. No long-term studies of androstenedione have been conducted. Its side effects are believed to be similar to those of other anabolic and androgenic agents. Most side effects are secondary to androgen excess—hyperlipidemia, hypertension, insulin resistance, hyperinsulinism, depression, aggression, paranoia, acne, male pattern baldness, alopecia, priapism, and others. Most effects are reversible with cessation of the product's use. Irreversible side effects include virilization in females (hair loss, clitoromegaly, hirsutism, voice-deepening) and gynecomastia in males.

As the use of supplements and herbs increases, it will be increasingly important for pediatric care providers to be familiar with their common side effects. The Internet has become a source of information and sales of these products, which could lead to their increased use. The easy accessibility, perceived low risk, and low cost of these products significantly increase the likelihood that they will become significant substances of abuse by the pediatric population.

Ahrendt DM: Ergogenic aids: Counseling the athlete. Am Fam Physician 2001;63:913 [PMID: 11261867].

Metzl JD et al: Creatine use among young athletes. Pediatr 2001;108:421 [PMID: 11483809].

Morris CA, Avorn J: Internet marketing of herbal products. JAMA 2003;290:1505 [PMID: 13129992].

Rasmussen BB: Androstenedione does not stimulate muscle protein anabolism in young healthy men. J Clin Endocrinol Metab 2000;85:55 [PMID: 10634363].

Sturmi JE: Anabolic agents. Clin Sports Med 1998;17:261 [PMID: 9580841].

Volek JS, Kraemer WJ: Creatine supplementation: Its role in human performance. Clin Sports Med 1999;18:651 [PMID: 10410847].

## RESPONSE TO THE PROBLEM

Federal, state, and local governments attempt to control the damage caused by substance abuse by prohibiting use and by legislating against associated high-risk behaviors (eg, enacting drunk-driving laws and nighttime curfews). However, neither these legal actions nor the large sums of money spent on school- and community-based drug abuse prevention and treatment programs have curbed the problem. Hence, the American Academy of Pediatrics (AAP) recommends that pediatricians become knowledgeable about the extent and nature of drugs used in their community, provide anticipatory guidance to parents starting with the first prenatal visit, and be aware of community referral and treatment resources for adolescents. The Internet makes this task more difficult. For example, poor methods for age verification make it easy for minors to purchase tobacco products online.

American Academy of Pediatrics Committee on Substance Abuse: Tobacco, alcohol, and other drugs: The role of the pediatrician in prevention and management of substance abuse. Pediatrics 1998;101:125 [PMID: 11345974].

Hogan MJ: Diagnosis and treatment of teen drug use. Med Clin North Am 2000;84:927 [PMID: 10928196].

Ribisl KM et al: Internet sales of cigarettes to minors. JAMA 2003;290:1356 [PMID: 12966128].

Siegel M: The effect of local tobacco sales laws on adolescent smoking initiation. Prev Med 1999;29:334 [PMID: 10564624].

## PREDICTING THE PROGRESSION FROM USE TO ABUSE

Most adolescents who use mood-altering substances do so only intermittently or experimentally. The challenge to pediatric health care providers is to recognize the warning signs, identify potential abusers early, and intervene in an effective and timely fashion before acute or chronic use results in morbidity. The best predictors of ethanol and drug abuse are male sex, young age at first use, and associating with drug-using peers. It is still unclear why only a minority of the young people exhibiting the high-risk characteristics listed in Table 4–5 go on to abuse substances. Substance abuse is a symptom of personal and social maladjustment as often as it is a cause. Because a direct relationship exists between the number of risk factors listed in Table 4–5 and the frequency of substance abuse, a combination of risk factors is the best indicator of risk. Even so, most teenagers who exhibit multiple risk characteristics never develop a substance abuse problem, presumably because the protective factors listed in Table 4–5 give them enough resiliency to cope with stress in more socially adaptive ways.

Being aware of the risk domains listed in Table 4–5 will help physicians identify youngsters most apt to need counseling about substance abuse. Theories concerning the mechanisms responsible for the association between the risk factors listed in Table 4–5 and substance abuse are listed in Table 4–6. These theories provide a framework for understanding why individual patients may be at risk for progressing from occasional to established or compulsive substance abuse. Most theories emphasize social influences as the most reliable predictors of both the onset and the progression of substance abuse. For example, most teenage smokers report smoking at home and cite smoking parents or relatives as a reason to continue smoking.

Problem behavior theory is one of the most frequently cited concepts in the substance abuse literature. Its main argument is that socially disapproved behaviors tend to cluster and to resist intervention because they have both negative and positive consequences for the individual. Expectancy theory, which takes up where problem behavior theory leaves off, proposes a potentially modifiable mechanism by which learning experiences influence substance abuse. Measuring alcohol- and drug-related expectations has been found to provide a more accurate assessment of risk than any of the factors listed in Table 4–5. Expectations about the effects of substances are important determinants of social and psychological reactions to them. Furthermore, these expectations are longitudinally related to different patterns of substance abuse. For example, within homogeneous groups of nondrinkers, low-risk drinkers, and high-risk drinkers, expectations about outcomes differ significantly both at entry into college and 3 years later. At each level alcohol abusers who progress to the next level of drinking expect more positive outcomes from the drinking. Conversely, evidence that negative experiences with alcohol transform some high-risk freshmen drinkers into nondrinking seniors suggests that it may be possible to influence indulgence patterns by altering expectancies. Here intervention is critical. Without guidance, most youngsters do not draw sobering conclusions from their negative experiences with drugs and alcohol. Despite serious accidents and socially unrewarding experiences, positive expectancies about the effects of alcohol tend to increase rather than decrease during the first 3 years of college. Similarly the expectation of weight loss and improved mood leads to initiation of smoking or reluctance to quit.

**Table 4–5.** Factors that influence the progression from substance use to substance abuse.

| Enabling Risk Factors | Potentially Protective Factors |
|---|---|
| **SOCIETAL AND COMMUNITY** | |
| Experimentation encouraged by media | Regular involvement in church activities |
| Illicit substances available | Support for norms and values of society |
| Extreme economic deprivation | Strict enforcement of laws prohibiting substance |
| Neighborhood disorganization, crowding | use among minors and abuse among adults |
| Tolerance of licit and illicit substance use | Neighborhood resources, supportive adults |
| **SCHOOL** | |
| Lack of commitment to school or education | Strong commitment to school or education |
| Truancy | Future-oriented goals |
| Academic failure | Achievement oriented |
| Early, persistent behavior problems | |
| **FAMILY** | |
| Models of substance abuse and other unconventional behavior | Models of conventional behavior |
| Dysfunctional parenting styles; excessive authority or permissiveness | Attachment to parents |
| High family conflict; low bonding | Cohesive family |
| | Nurturing parenting styles |
| **PEERS** | |
| Peer rejection in elementary grades | Popular with peers |
| Substance use prevalent among peers | Abstinent friends |
| Peer attitudes favorable to substance abuse and unconventional behavior | Peer attitudes favor conventional behavior |
| **INDIVIDUAL** | |
| Genetic predisposition | Positive self-concept, good self-esteem |
| Psychological diagnoses (attention-deficit/hyperactivity disorder; antisocial personality) | Intolerance of deviance |
| Depression and low self-esteem | Internally motivated, takes charge of problems |
| Alienation and rebelliousness | |
| Sexual or physical abuse | |
| Early onset of deviant behavior or delinquency | |
| Early onset of sexual behavior | |
| Aggressive | |

Belcher H, Shinitzky H: Substance abuse in children: Prediction, protection, and prevention. Arch Pediatr Adolesc Med 1998;152:952 [PMID: 9790604].

Comerci GD, Schwebel R: Substance abuse: An overview. Adolesc Med 2000;11:79 [PMID: 10640340].

Patton GC et al: Depression, anxiety and smoking initiation: A prospective study over 3 years. Am J Public Health 1998;88:1518 [PMID: 9772855].

## MANAGEMENT OF SUBSTANCE ABUSE

It is critical that pediatric care providers have the knowledge and skill to diagnose, treat, and advocate for their substance-using and abusing patients. The AAP Committee on Substance Abuse recommends that pediatricians include discussions of substance abuse as part of their anticipatory care, starting with parents at the prenatal visit.

## Office Screening

Given the high incidence of substance abuse and the subtlety of its early signs and symptoms, a general psychosocial assessment is the best way to screen for substance abuse. Interviewing and counseling techniques and methods for taking a psychosocial history are discussed in Chapter 3. In an atmosphere of trust and confidentiality, physicians must ask routine screening questions of all patients and be alert for addictive diseases, especially in light of the high level of denial often present in addicted patients. The universal screening approach outlined in the American Medical Association guidelines for adolescent preventive services (GAPS) is a good guide for routine screening and diagnosis. Clues to possible substance abuse include truancy, failing grades, problems with interpersonal relationships, delinquency, depressive affect, chronic fatigue, recurrent abdominal pains, chest pains or palpitations, headache, chronic

**Table 4–6.** Theories accounting for the progression from substance use to substance abuse.[a]

| Theory | Key Constructs and Assumptions | Major Protagonist |
|---|---|---|
| Problem Behavior | Socially problematic behaviors[b] occur together and reflect a common underlying cause. The common antecedent is the reflection of the interaction among individual personality traits (eg, unconventionality), the perceived environment (eg, models of deviance), and a nondominant pattern of socialization (eg, low value on education). | Jessor R, Jessor R: *Problem Behavior and Psychosocial Development.* Academic Press, 1977. |
| Social Learning | Problem behavior theory plus a scheme to explain reinforcement of these behaviors. The risk of problem behavior increases when youngsters have the opportunity to become skillful in unconventional settings and are rewarded for doing so. | Bandura A: *Social Learning Theory.* Prentice-Hall, 1977. |
| Reasoned Action | Behavior is determined by the interaction between perceived consequences and attitudes toward those consequences. The risk of problem behavior increases when the perceived costs are low or the perceived benefits high. | Ajzen I, Fishbein M: *Understanding Attitudes and Predicting Behavior.* Prentice-Hall, 1980. |
| Health Belief | Health behaviors reflect assessments of perceived risk or harm, potential to avoid that harm through alternative behaviors, and ability to access requisite resources. The risk of unhealthy behavior increases when the perceived health risk is low or the ability to avoid that risk is perceived to be low or unrelated to the behavior. | Becker MH: The health belief model and personal health behavior. Health Education Monograph 1974;2:324. |
| Social Control | Behavior is determined by the bonds an individual establishes with society. The risk of problem behavior increases when attachment to those who express conventional values is weak, commitment to participation in conventional activities is low, little time is spent in these activities, and the central value system of society is not fully accepted. | Hirschi T: *Causes of Delinquency.* Univ California Press; 1969. |
| Peer Cluster | The socialization process that accompanies adolescent development results in the formation of peer clusters. Family sanctions, religious identifications, and school adjustment affect behavior indirectly through their effects on peer clusters. | Oetting ER, Beauvais F: Peer cluster theory. Counseling Psychol 1987; 34:205. |
| Expectancy | Problem behavior and reasoned action theories plus a mechanism by which learning experiences exert an influence on future behavior. The risk of problem behavior increases when experiences reinforce preexisting positive expectancies about the effects of deviant behavior. | Werner MJ: Relation of alcohol expectancies to change in problem drinking among college students. Arch Pediatr Adolesc Med 1995;149: 733. |
| Self-Medication | Individuals are predisposed to addiction when they experience painful affective states or psychiatric disorders; symptom relief perpetuates the use of specific substances. | Khantzian EJ: The self-medication hypothesis. Am J Psychiatry 1985;142:1259. |

[a]Ordered by frequency of citation in the literature.
[b]A problem behavior is defined as any behavior compromising the accomplishment of normal developmental tasks of adolescence; most are hard to change because they also serve functions central to the psychosocial development of adolescents who lack conventional alternatives.

cough, persistent nasal discharge, and recurrent complaints of sore throat. Substance abuse should be included in the differential diagnosis of all behavioral, family, psychosocial, and medical problems. Pediatricians seeing patients in emergency departments, trauma units, or prison must have an especially high index of suspicion. A family history of drug addiction or abuse should raise the level of concern about drug abuse in the pediatric patient. Possession of promotional products such as T-shirts and caps with cigarette or alcohol logos should also be a red flag as teenagers who own these items are more likely to use the products they advertise.

Albers AB, Biener L: Adolescent participation in tobacco promotions: Role of psychosocial factors. Pediatrics 2003;111: 402 [PMID: 12563070].

Altman DG et al: Tobacco promotion and susceptibility to tobacco use among adolescents aged 12 through 17 years in a nationally representative sample. Am J Public Health 1996;86: 1590 [PMID: 8916525].

## Diagnosis

Although few children and adolescents will have been abusing substances long enough to have developed overt signs and symptoms, it is important to look for them on physical examination. Positive physical findings can be a tool to penetrate a patient's denial and convince him or her of the significant extent of the alcohol or drug use.

When the psychosocial history suggests the possibility of substance use, the primary tasks of the diagnostic interview are the same as the evaluation of other medical problems (Table 4–7).

First, specific information about the extent of the problem must be gathered. Eliciting multiple-choice answers is a useful technique. For example, "Has anything really good ever happened to you when you are high?" or "Some of my patients like to get high because they feel good; others find it helps them relax and be sociable with friends; and some find it helps them forget their problems. Are any of these things true for you?"

Second, the provider needs to determine why the patient has progressed from initiation to the continuation or maintenance phase of substance abuse. The cause may be different at different periods of development. Although peer group characteristics are one of the best predictors of substance use among early and middle adolescents, this is not so among older adolescents and young adults.

Brief questionnaires can be used if time does not allow for more detailed investigation. Two instruments evaluated rigorously in primary care settings are the CAGE questionnaire and the Perceived Benefits of Drinking Scale. CAGE is a mnemonic derived from the first four questions listed in Table 4–8. A score of 2 or more is highly suggestive of substance abuse. The Perceived-Benefits-of-Drinking Scale consists of the next five statements listed in Table 4–8. Patients who endorse more than three statements deserve further evaluation. Because CAGE is more predictive of substance use problems among males and the Perceived-Benefits-of-Drinking Scale is more predictive among females, many clinicians combine the two scales. Including an additional question about use of tobacco and a question about the patient's best friend's use of mood-altering

**Table 4–7.** Diagnostic interview for substance abuse.

---

**I. Define the extent of the problem by determining:**

Age at onset of substance use

Which substances are being used

Circumstances of use

  Where?

  When?

  With whom?

To what extent substances are being used

  How frequently?

  How much (quantity)?

  With what associated symptoms (eg, tolerance, withdrawal)?

With what result?

  What does the patient gain from becoming high?

  Does the patient get into risky situations while high?

  Does the patient engage in behaviors while high that are later regretted?

**II. Define the cause of the problem by developing a differential diagnosis**

**Table 4–8.** Substance abuse screening questionnaires.

| CAGE Questionnaire |
| --- |
| **CUT DOWN:** Have you ever felt you ought to cut down on your drinking (drug use)? |
| **ANNOYED:** Have people annoyed you by criticizing your drinking (drug use)? |
| **GUILTY:** Have you ever felt bad about your drinking (drug use)? |
| **EYE OPENER:** Have you ever had a drink (used drugs) to steady your nerves in the morning? |
| **(Score 1 point for each positive answer; refer if total points ≥ 2)** |

Used, with permission, from Ewing JE: Detecting alcoholism: The CAGE questionnaire. JAMA 1984;252:1905.

| Perceived Benefits Scales |
| --- |
| 1. Drinking (drug use) helps me forget my problems. |
| 2. Drinking (drug use) helps me be friendly. |
| 3. Drinking (drug use) helps me feel good about myself. |
| 4. Drinking (drug use) helps me relax. |
| 5. Drinking (drug use) helps me be friends with others who drink (use drugs). |
| **(Score 1 point for each positive answer; refer if total points ≥ 3)** |

Used, with permission, from Petchers MK, Singer MI: Perceived-Benefit-of-Drinking Scale. J Pediatr 1987;110:977.

substances further enhances the diagnostic accuracy of these screening tools.

Although constructed as screening tools for alcohol abuse in adults, the questions in Table 4–8 can be adapted to elicit similar information about use of other mood-altering substances by pediatric patients and by their close contacts (eg, parents and older siblings). Finally, clinicians may find it helpful to use these questionnaires to stimulate discussion of the patient's self-perception of his or her substance use. For example, if an adolescent admits to a previous attempt to cut down on drinking, this provides an opportunity to inquire about events that may have led to the attempt.

Additional screening instruments include the following:

1. The Simple Screening Instrument for Alcohol and Other Drug Abuse (SSI-AOD), from the Center for Treatment of Substance Abuse, is a quick, 16-item screen that has proven reliable among adolescent medical patients.
2. The Personal Experience Inventory is a comprehensive, standardized 260-item self-report measure of chemical involvement and the psychosocial aspect of substance use.
3. The Personal Experience Screening Questionnaire is a quick, 38-item screen that evaluates the severity of the problem and associated psychosocial risks.
4. The Adolescent Diagnostic Interview is a structured interview based on the American Psychiatric Association's diagnostic criteria for substance abuse (see Table 4–1).

Although these instruments may be too time-consuming for routine office use, they may prove helpful in the evaluation of patients who pose diagnostic or therapeutic dilemmas.

Fuller PG Jr, Cavanaugh RM Jr: Basic assessment and screening for substance abuse in the pediatrician's office. Pediatr Clin North Am 1995;42(2):295 [PMID: 7724260].

Knight JR et al: Reliabilities of short substance abuse screening tests among adolescent medical patients. Pediatrics 2000;105(4 Pt 2):948 [PMID: 10742352].

Miller NS: The role of the physician in addiction prevention and treatment. Psychiatr Clin North Am 1999;22:489 [PMID: 10385946].

Werner MJ: Screening, early identification, and office-based intervention with children and youth living in substance-abusing families. Pediatrics 1999;103:1099 [PMID: 10224197].

## Comorbidity

It is important for pediatric care providers to recognize the possibility of multiple diagnoses in patients who are abusing substances. Alcohol and substance abusers are more likely than are their nonabusing counterparts to have another psychiatric disorder. Affective disorders, anxiety disorders, and mania rank among the disorders most strongly associated with alcohol and drug dependence. Adolescents with depression are likely to use drugs in an attempt to feel pleasure, but this type of self-medication may exacerbate their condition. In addition to identifying psychiatric comorbidities, it is imperative that providers look for medical conditions that can mimic symptoms of drug withdrawal or intoxication. Patients with significant primary medical conditions may use illicit substances to relieve symptoms (severe pain, chemotherapeutic side effects). Although it is often difficult to determine which diagnosis is primary, it is important for pediatric health care providers to recognize the possibility of a comorbid condition and provide appropriate treatment.

Bucholz KK: Nosology and epidemiology of addictive disorders and their comorbidity. Psychiatr Clin North Am 1999;22: 221 [PMID: 10385930].

Comerci GD, Schwebel R: Substance abuse: An overview. Adolesc Med 2000;11(1):79 [PMID: 10640340].

Jellinek MS: Depression and suicide in children and adolescents. Pediatr Rev 1998;19:255 [PMID: 9797715].

## Pharmacologic Screening

The use of urine and blood testing for detecting substance abuse is controversial. The consensus is that pharmacologic screening should be reserved for situations where behavioral dysfunction is of sufficient concern to outweigh the practical and ethical drawbacks of testing. The AAP recommends screening under certain circumstances (eg, an inexplicably obtunded patient in the emergency department) but discourages routine screening for the following reasons: (1) Voluntary screening programs are rarely truly voluntary owing to the negative consequences for those who decline to participate. (2) Infrequent users or individuals who have not used substances recently may be missed. (3) Confronting substance-abusing individuals with objective evidence of their use has little or no effect on their behavior. (4) The AAP reminds providers that their role is counseling and treatment, not law enforcement, so that drug testing should not be done for the purpose of detecting illegal use. If testing is to be performed, the provider should discuss the plan for screening with the patient, explain the reasons for it, and obtain informed consent. The AAP does not consider parental request and permission sufficient justification for involuntary screening of mentally competent minors.

Beyond the ethical concerns, there are also practical concerns. If testing is to be performed, it is imperative that it be done accurately and that the limitations of testing be understood by all parties. Tests range from simple, inexpensive, chromatographic spot tests, which can be performed in the office, to gas chromatography and mass spectrometry, which require specialized laboratory equipment and are usually reserved for forensic investigations. Most commercial medical laboratories use the enzyme multiplication immunoassay technique, in which a sample of the fluid to be tested is added to a test reagent consisting of a known quantity of the radiolabeled index drug (ie, the drug being tested for). If the index drug is also present in the patient's urine or serum, it competes with the radiolabeled drug for binding sites on the test kit antibody. The unbound or excess drug can then be quantified with a spectrophotometer. Most of the commonly abused mood-altering substances, with the exception of solvents and inhalants, can be detected by this method.

Caution is necessary in interpreting results because false-positives may be obtained as a result of antibody cross-reactions with the medications and substances listed in Table 4–9 or from passive exposure to illicit substances. The most common cause of false-negative tests is infrequent use. Table 4–10 shows the duration of detectability in the urine after last use by class of substance and duration of use. Detectability ranges from a few hours for alcohol to several weeks for regular marijuana use. False-negative results can occur if the patient alters or adulterates the specimen, either by drinking a large volume of fluid or adding such substances as bleach, vinegar, or golden seal powder to the specimen. (Teenagers should be advised that despite street lore,

**Table 4–9.** Causes of false-positive drug screens.

**Opioids**
  Poppy seeds
  Dextromethorphan
  Chlorpromazine
  Diphenoxylate
**Amphetamines**
  Ephedrine
  Phenylephrine
  Pseudophedrine
  N-Acetylprocainamide
  Chloroquine
  Procainamide
**Phencyclidines**
  Dextromethorphan
  Diphenhydramine
  Chlorpromazine
  Doxylamine
  Thioridazine

**Table 4–10.** Duration of urine positivity for selected drugs.

| Drug Class | Detection Time |
| --- | --- |
| Amphetamines | < 48 hours |
| Barbiturates | Short-acting: 1 d Long-acting: 2–3 wk |
| Benzodiazepines | Single dose: 3 d Habitual use: 4–6 wk |
| Cocaine metabolites | Acute use: 2–4 d Habitual use: 2 wk |
| Ethanol | 2–14 h |
| Methadone | Up to 3 d |
| Opioids | Up to 2 d |
| Propoxyphene | 6–48 h |
| Cannabinoids | Moderate use: 5 d Habitual use: 10–20 d |
| Methaqualone | 2 wk |
| Phencyclidine | Acute use: 1 wk Habitual use: 3 wk |
| Anabolic steroids | Days to weeks |

Reprinted, with permission, from Woolf A, Shannon M: Clinical toxicology for the pediatrician. Pediatr Clin North Am 1995;42:317.

ingesting these compounds is an ineffective and potentially dangerous way to prevent drug detection in the urine.) Close observation during collection and pretesting the temperature, specific gravity, and pH of urine samples may detect attempts at deception.

American Academy of Pediatrics Committee on Substance Abuse: Testing for drugs of abuse in children and adolescents. Pediatrics 1996;98:305 [PMID: 8692638].

Perrone J: Drug screening versus history in detection of substance use in ED psychiatric patients. Am J Emerg Med 2001;19: 49 [PMID: 11146019].

Woolf A, Shannon M: Clinical toxicology for the pediatrician. Pediatr Clin North Am 1995;42:317 [PMID: 7724261].

## TREATMENT & REFERRAL

### Office-Based Treatment

The AMA and the AAP recommend that all children and adolescents receive counseling about the dangers of substance use and abuse from their primary health care providers. By offering confidential health care services and routinely counseling about the risks associated with drug abuse, pediatricians can help most of their patients avoid the adverse consequences of experimentation with mood-altering substances. However, more intervention is required for youngsters in environments where substance abuse is regarded as acceptable recreational behavior. Because substance use is often deeply embedded in the fabric of these young peoples' lives, most have little interest in prevention or treatment. Counseling strategies appropriate for patients who wish to change their behavior may be ineffective for a patient who does not consider use of mood-altering substances to be a problem. It may therefore be preferable to begin discussions about treatment by helping youngsters consider alternative ways of meeting the needs that substance use is currently providing. The clinician may in this way help the patient devise alternatives that are more attractive than substance use. Realistically, few substance-abusing teenagers will choose to quit because of a single conversation with even a highly respected health care provider. The message is most effective when offered repeatedly from a variety of sources—family, peers, guidance counselors, and teachers.

Because an assessment of the patient's readiness to change is the critical first step in office-based intervention, clinicians should consider the construct presented in Table 4–11. In theory, individuals pass through this series of stages in the course of changing problem behaviors. Thus, to be maximally effective, providers should tailor their counseling messages to the patient's stage of readiness to change.

Once it has been established that a patient is prepared to act on information about treatment, the next step is to select the program that best fits his or her individual needs. Most drug treatment programs are not designed to recognize and act on the individual vulnerabilities that have predisposed the patient to substance abuse. When programs are individualized, even brief (5- to 10-minute) counseling sessions may promote reductions in cigarette smoking and drinking. This strategy appears to be most effective when the health care provider's message is part of an office-wide program so that the entire staff reinforces the cessation message with every patient. Specific steps to help youngsters quit smoking are discussed in the next section and summarized in Table 4–12. These same strategies and principles can be applied to the treatment of drug and alcohol use.

## Smoking Cessation in Pediatrics

Although more than half of adolescents who smoke regularly say they want to quit and have tried to quit, only a minority report that they have been advised or helped to do so by a health care provider. Practitioners unfa-

**Table 4–11.** Stages of change and intervention tasks.

| Patient Stage | Motivation Tasks |
| --- | --- |
| Precontemplation | Create doubt, increase the patient's awareness of risks and problems with current patterns of substance use |
| Contemplation | Help the patient weigh the relative risks and benefits of changing substance use; evoke reasons to change and risks of not changing; strengthen the patient's self-efficacy for changing current use |
| Determination | Help the patient determine the best course of action to change substance use from among available alternatives |
| Action | Help the patient establish a clear plan of action toward changing substance use |
| Maintenance | Help the patient identify and use strategies to prevent relapse |
| Relapse | Help the patient renew the process of change starting at contemplation |

Reprinted from Werner MJ: Principles of brief intervention for adolescent alcohol, tobacco, and other drug use. Pediatr Clin North Am 1995;42:341. With permission of the publisher.

miliar with approaches to smoking cessation may feel that smoking cessation interventions are time-consuming, nonreimbursable, and impractical in a busy office. In reality, studies conducted by the National Cancer Institute indicate that health care providers can help their patients stop smoking with short office interventions. Some of the most effective smoking cessation interventions are self-help programs consisting of a series of short (typically under 5 minutes) physician interventions reinforced by the entire office staff using the simple protocol outlined in Table 4–12.

The first step is motivational. Provide patients with a list of reasons for quitting. Suggest that they call 1-800-4CANCER to obtain the National Cancer Institute's "Quit for Good" or "Why Do You Smoke?" pamphlets and materials.

However, motivation alone is not enough. Learning to use coping skills to prevent relapse and to avoid discouragement at the time of relapse appear to be important to ultimate success. Smoking cessation is a process that takes time. Relapse must be regarded as a normal part of quitting rather than evidence of personal failure or a reason to forgo further attempts. Patients can actually benefit from relapses if they are helped to identify the circumstances that led to the relapse and to devise

***Table 4–12.*** How to help your patients stop smoking.

---

**Ask** about smoking at every opportunity.
1. Do you smoke? How old were you when you started?
2. How much?
3. How soon after waking do you have your first cigarette?
4. Do you have friends who smoke? family members? relatives? role models?
5. Are you interested in stopping smoking?
6. Have you ever tried to stop before? If so, what happened?

**Advise** all smokers to stop.
1. State your advice clearly, for example: "As your physician, I must advise you to stop smoking now."
2. Personalize the message to quit. Refer to the patient's clinical condition, smoking history, family history, personal interests, or social roles (see Table 4–13).

**Assist** the patient in stopping.
1. Set a quit date. Help the patient pick a date within the next 4 weeks, acknowledging that no time is ideal.
2. Provide self-help materials. The smoking cessation coordinator or support staff member can review the materials with the patient.
3. Discuss the importance of a smoke-free environment.
4. Rehearse through role-playing how to respond to social situations where others are smoking.
5. Elicit support of parents and relatives; encourage them to stop smoking with their teen.
6. Encourage participation in activities that are incompatible with smoking.
7. Consider prescribing replacement therapy (patch or gum) for highly addicted patients (those who smoke a pack or more daily or who smoke their first cigarette within 30 minutes after waking).
8. Consider signing a stop-smoking contract with the patient.
9. If the patient is not willing to quit now, provide motivating literature and flag the chart and do remember to ask again at the next visit.

**Arrange** follow-up visits.
1. Set a follow-up visit within 1–2 weeks after the quit date.
2. Have a member of the office staff call or write the patient within 7 days after the initial visit, reinforcing the decision to stop and reminding the patient of the quit date.
3. At the first follow-up visit, ask about the patient's smoking status to provide support and help prevent relapse.
4. Set a second follow-up visit in 1 month.
5. Remind the teen that relapse is common—indeed the norm. When it happens, discuss the circumstances and encourage the patient to think of alternative responses and to try again.

---

Adapted, with permission, from Glynn T, Manley M: *How to Help Your Patients Stop Smoking: A National Cancer Institute Manual for Physicians.* National Institutes of Health, 1989.

strategies to prevent subsequent relapses or respond to them in a different manner. Because nicotine is a physically and psychologically addictive substance, replacement therapy may relieve withdrawal symptoms. Three types of nicotine replacement therapies (NRT) are available. Nicotine gum and transdermal nicotine patches are recommended for teens. NRT improves smoking cessation rates and provides relief from withdrawal symptoms. Providers should be aware that adolescents may not exhibit the same symptoms of nicotine dependence as adults, that symptoms may occur rapidly, with autonomy lost within as little as 4 weeks. Those who are not comfortable prescribing and monitoring NRT should limit their involvement with patients who smoke to those who do not exhibit signs of nicotine dependency (eg, patients who smoke less than a pack of cigarettes a day or do not feel a craving to smoke their first cigarette within 30 minutes after waking). In addition to NRT, sustained-release forms of the antidepressants bupropion, clonidine, and nortriptyline have been shown in randomized trials to help smokers quit and to decrease relapse rates fivefold.

Two tobacco-use prevention curricula have been selected by The Division of Adolescent and School Health (DASH) of the CDC for adoption by schools—Botvin's Life Skills Training Program and Project Toward No Tobacco (TNT). The first is the more comprehensive of the two curricula. It is designed to target the primary causes of substance use, including tobacco, alcohol, and other drugs, by teaching a combination of health information, general life skills, and skills in resisting tobacco and other drugs. Program effectiveness has been demonstrated among white, African-American, and Hispanic youth.

Project TNT, the second curriculum and the more effective of the two, was designed to target the primary causes of cigarette smoking, smokeless tobacco use, and cigar and pipe smoking among teens. Compared with the subjects who received the standard school health education, subjects in Project TNT were less likely to start using smokeless tobacco or cigarettes, and less likely to use them regularly. The program was equally effective in boys and girls, and was effective during the transitional period from junior to senior high school.

American Academy of Pediatrics Committee on Substance Abuse: Tobacco's toll: Implications for the pediatrician. Pediatrics 2001;107:794 [PMID: 11335763].

DiFranza JR et al: Initial symptoms of nicotine dependence in adolescents. Tobacco Control 2000;9:313 [PMID: 10982576].

DiFranza JR et al: Measuring the loss of autonomy over nicotine use in adolescents: The DANDY (development and assessment of nicotine dependence in youth) Study. Arch Pediatr Adolesc Med. 2002;156:397 [PMID: 11929376].

DuRant RH: Adolescent tobacco use and cessation. Prim Care 1999;26:553 [PMID: 10436287].

Moolchan ET: A review of tobacco smoking in adolescents: Treatment implications. J Am Acad Child Adolesc Psychiatry 2000 Jun;39:682 [PMID: 10846302].

## Referral

There is no consensus about which substance-abusing patients can be adequately treated in the office, which require referral, and which require hospitalization. Factors to be considered are summarized in Table 4–13. When doubt exists about the seriousness of the problem or the advisability of office management, consultation with a specialist should be sought.

Although most primary pediatric providers will not assume responsibility for the treatment of substance-abusing youngsters, clinicians can be instrumental in motivating their patients to seek treatment and in guiding them to appropriate treatment resources. Substance-abusing teenagers must be treated in teen-oriented treatment facilities. Despite the similarities between adult and adolescent substance abuse, adult programs are usually developmentally inappropriate and ineffective for adolescents. As discussed in Chapter 3, many adolescents are concrete thinkers. Their inability to reason deductively, especially about emotionally charged issues, makes it difficult for them to understand the abstract concepts (such as denial) that are an integral component of most adult-oriented programs. This invariably frustrates counselors who misinterpret lack of comprehension as resistance to therapy, and concrete responses as evidence of deceit.

Treatment programs range from low-intensity, outpatient, school-based student assistance programs, which rely heavily on peers and nonprofessionals, to residential, hospital-based programs staffed by psychiatrists and other professionals. Outpatient counseling programs are most appropriate for motivated patients who do not have significant mental health or behavioral problems and are not at risk for withdrawal. Some investigators have raised the concern that in pediatric settings, low-problem users may actually experience a strengthening of the drug subculture by associating with high-problem users in group therapy. More intensive day treatment programs are available for those who require a structured environment. Inpatient treatment should be considered for patients who need medical care and detoxification in addition to counseling, education, and family therapy.

Finally, special dual-diagnosis facilities are available for substance-abusing patients who also have other psychological conditions. These patients are difficult to diagnose and treat because it is often unclear whether their symptoms are a consequence of substance use or a symptom of a comorbid psychological disorder. Recognition of such disorders is critical because they must be treated in programs that include psychiatric expertise.

Approaches to the treatment of substance abuse in children and adolescents are typically modeled after adult treatment programs. Most notable are the 12-step programs modeled after Alcoholics Anonymous. These programs are attractive because they demand total abstinence and acknowledge that substance abuse is a chronic disease requiring a lifelong commitment to abstinence and long-term support from family, peers, and community. Although treatment is usually effective, relapse is common. Because efficacy research has lagged behind practice and implementation (especially among low-intensity programs), there is little empirical evidence on which to base recommendations for one program or another. Various forms of treatment appear to have the potential to be effective. Thus, in practice, referral recommendations should be based on the significance of the problem for the individual and the availability of affordable programs in the community.

**Table 4–13.** Factors to consider prior to referral for substance abuse.

---

Duration and frequency of substance use
The type of substances being used
Presence of other psychological disorders
    Attention-deficit/hyperactivity disorder
    Depression
    Antisocial personality disorder
Presence of other social morbidities
    School failure
    Delinquency
    Homelessness
    Ongoing or past physical or sexual abuse
Program Evaluation
    View on substance abuse as primary disorder vs symptom
    Offers comprehensive evaluation of patient and can manage associated problems identified in initial assessment (eg, comorbid conditions)
    Adherence to abstinence philosophy
    Patient-to-staff ratios
    Separate adolescent and adult treatment programs
    Follow-up and continuing care

---

Fleming M et al: Brief physician advice for problem alcohol drinkers. JAMA 1997;277:1039 [PMID: 9091691].

Garbutt JC et al: Pharmacological treatment of alcohol dependence: A review of the evidence. JAMA 1999;281:1318 [PMID: 10208148].

Heyman RB: Turning the tide: Tobacco and the 21st. Adolesc Med 2000;11:69 [PMID: 10640339].

Hughes JR et al: Recent advances in the pharmacotherapy of smoking. JAMA 1999;281:72 [PMID: 9892454].

Hurt RD et al: A comparison of sustained-release bupropion and placebo for smoking cessation. N Engl J Med 1997; 337:1195 [PMID: 9337378].

Swift RM: Drug therapy for alcohol dependence. N Engl J Med 1999;340:1482 [PMID: 10320388].

## PREVENTION OF SUBSTANCE ABUSE

Prevention of substance abuse has been a public health priority since the 1980s. Pediatric health care providers are important as advocates and educators of the community and government on developmentally appropriate programs. *Primary level* programs focus on preventing the initiation of substance use. The Drug Awareness and Resistance Education (DARE) program is a familiar example of a primary prevention program that attempts to educate elementary and middle school students about the adverse consequences of substance abuse and enable them to resist peer pressures.

*Secondary level* programs target populations at increased risk for substance use. The aim is to prevent progression from initiation to continuance and maintenance, relying on individualized intervention to reduce the risk and enhance the protective factors listed in Table 4–5. This approach enables the provider to focus scarce resources on those who are most likely to benefit from them. Alateen, which supports the children of alcoholic parents typifies secondary level prevention.

*Tertiary level* prevention programs target young people who have been identified as substance abusers. The aim is to prevent the morbid consequences of substance use. One example is identifying adolescents who misuse alcohol and drugs at parties and providing them with a safe ride home. Because prevention is more effective when targeted at reducing the initiation of substance use than at decreasing use, tertiary prevention is the least effective approach.

Very few population-based programs undergo rigorous scientific evaluation. It is the consensus among drug educators that primary prevention programs, such as DARE, have minimal effect in decreasing the use of illicit substances. During the 1990s, when these programs were most popular, a smaller proportion of middle- and high-school students perceived illicit drug and alcohol use as dangerous, and substance use actually increased. Even when knowledge- and resistance-based programs do increase student understanding of adverse consequences, there is no evidence that they change attitudes or abuse rates.

The failure of resistance education programs has fostered interest in a potentially more effective type of program, exemplified by the Adolescents Training and Learning to Avoid Steroids (ATLAS) program. This program, a same-sex, peer-educator program designed to simultaneously reduce the use of steroids and improve dietary and exercise habits of teen athletes has proven effective in randomized controlled trials. Pediatric health care providers should promote developmentally appropriate prevention programs like this one that address the social and psychological problems predisposing youngsters to substance abuse and which provide realistic alternative solutions.

Parents and others should understand that most adolescents who abuse alcohol and drugs do not do so just for the high. Rather, these behaviors are often purposeful, developmentally appropriate coping strategies. To the extent that these behaviors meet young peoples' developmental needs, they are not apt to be abandoned unless equally attractive alternatives are available. For example, even though many teenagers cite stress and anxiety as reasons for smoking, teen-oriented smoking cessation programs rarely address the young smoker's need for alternative coping strategies by offering stress management training. Similarly, for the youngster growing up in an impoverished urban environment, the real costs of substance abuse may be too low and the rewards too high to be influenced by talk and knowledge alone. It is unreasonable to expect a talk-based intervention to change attitudes and behaviors in a direction that is opposite to that of the child's own social milieu. The efficacy of the most promising prevention models and interventions is apt to decay over time unless changes in the social environment provide substance-abusing children and adolescents with realistic alternative ways to meet their developmental needs.

Ennett S et al: How effective is drug abuse resistance education? A meta-analysis of project DARE outcome evaluations. Am J Public Health 1994;84:1394 [PMID: 8092361].

Goldberg L et al: The adolescents' training and learning to avoid steroids program: Preventing drug use and promoting health behaviors. Arch Adolesc Med 2000:154(4):332 [PMID: 10768668].

Goldman LK, Glantz SA: Evaluation of antismoking advertising campaigns. JAMA 1998;279:722 [PMID: 9508154].

### Web Resources

[Monitoring the future Study detailed information and longitudinal data] www.monitoringthefuture.org

[Information on trends from National Institute on Drug Abuse] www.nida.nih.gov

[National Clearinghouse Drug and Alcohol Abuse Gives information and resources including free publications for providers, parents, and adolescents] www.health.org

[Substance use and mental health services administration resources for both substance use and mental health services] www.samhsa.org

# Eating Disorders

*Eric J. Sigel, MD*

Teenagers and younger children continue to develop eating disorders at an alarming rate. The spectrum of eating disorders includes anorexia nervosa, bulimia nervosa, eating disorders not otherwise specified, and binge-eating disorder. The relationship between biology and environment in the development of eating disorders is complex, so these disorders are best defined in a biopsychosocial context.

## ETIOLOGY

Some evidence supports a genetic predisposition for eating disorders. There is a 7% incidence of anorexia nervosa in first-degree relatives of anorexic patients compared with a 1–2% incidence in the general population. Twin studies have shown a 55% concordance rate in monozygotic twins, compared with 7% in dizygotic twins. A study of males with anorexia nervosa showed a relative risk of 20 for first degree female relatives. Most studies have found a higher incidence of eating disorders among first-degree relatives of bulimic patients as well. Several genetic markers have been associated with an increased susceptibility to anorexia nervosa, though no clinically relevant genetic test is available to date. Genetics and eating disorders continue to be an active area of investigation, with a national study underway that will define the genetic aspect more specifically.

Leptin, a hormone produced in adipocytes and involved with satiety signaling, may play a role in the evolution of eating disorders. Anorexic patients have a decreased amount of leptin initially, which increases to excessive levels as they regain weight. One hypothesis is that there may be an abnormality in leptin receptors, with satiety indicators not responding normally. Other neurotransmitters, such as serotonin and neuropeptide Y, which are involved in satiety, are abnormal in some anorexic patients. An alteration in dopamine has also been recognized, though its significance has not been elucidated. Grehlin, a gut peptide, has been shown to be elevated in patients with anorexia nervosa and is also hypothesized to play a role in the pathophysiology of anorexia. Patients with bulimia nervosa or binge-eating disorder appear to have a blunted serotonin response to eating and satiety. With a decreased satiety response, patients continue to eat, leading to a binge. Treatment with selective serotonin reuptake inhibitors (SSRIs)

tends to equilibrate satiety regulation. More research is needed to determine which factors are causative and which are results of the eating disorder.

Traditional psychological theory has suggested many factors that might lead to the development of eating disorders. Enmeshment of mother with daughter to the point that the teenager cannot develop her own identity (a key developmental marker of adolescence) may be a predisposing factor. The teenager may cope by asserting control over food, as she senses her lack of control in the developmental realm. A second theory involves father–daughter distancing. As puberty progresses and a girl's sexuality blossoms, a father may experience difficulty in dealing with his daughter as a sexual being and may respond by withdrawing both emotionally and physically. The teenage girl may intuitively recognize this and subconsciously decrease her food intake in order to become prepubertal again. A third theory is related to puberty itself. Some teenagers may fear or dislike their changing bodies. By restricting food intake they lose weight, stop menstruating, and effectively reverse pubertal development.

In addition, society has provided the message that being thin or muscular is necessary for attractiveness and success. The ease of access to diet products—foods and diet pills—as well as Internet instructions (proanorexia sites) makes it simple for adolescents to embark on a quest for thinness or muscularity.

Genetic predisposition, psychological factors, and environmental factors combine to create a milieu that promotes adolescent eating disorders.

Bailer UF, Kaye WH: A review of neuropeptide and neuroendocrine dysregulation in anorexia and bulimia nervosa. Curr Drug Target CNS Neurol Disord 2003;2(1):53 [PMID: 12769812].

Brambilla F et al: Central dopaminergic function in anorexia and bulimia nervosa: A psychoneuroendocrine approach. Psychoneuroendocrinology 2001;26(4):393 [PMID:11259859].

Strober M et al: Males with anorexia nervosa: A controlled study of eating disorders in first-degree relatives. Int J Eat Disord 2001;29(3)263 [PMID 11262504].

Tolle V et al: Balance in ghrelin and leptin plasma levels in anorexia nervosa patients and constitutionally thin women. J Clin Endocrinol Metab 2003;88(1):109 [PMID: 12519838].

Urwin RE et al: Anorexia nervosa (restrictive subtype) is associated with a polymorphism in the novel norepinephrine transporter gene promoter polymorphic region Mol Psychiatry 2002; 7(6):652 [PMID: 12140790].

Woodside DB: Specificity of eating disorders diagnoses in families of probands with anorexia nervosa and bulimia nervosa. Compr Psychiatry 1998;39;261 [PMID: 9777277].

## INCIDENCE

Among teenage girls in the United States, anorexia nervosa is the third most common chronic illness. The incidence in the United States has been increasing steadily since the 1930s. Ascertaining exact incidence is difficult. It is thought that 1–2% of teenagers have anorexia nervosa and 2–4% have bulimia nervosa. Adolescents outnumber adults 5 to 1, although the number of adults with eating disorders is rising. The incidence is also increasing among younger children. Often prepubertal patients have significant associated psychiatric diagnoses. Females outnumber males 8 to 1. The number of males diagnosed with eating disorders has also increased, which correlates with the increased media emphasis on muscular, chiseled appearance as the male ideal. In the recent Youth Risk Behavior Survey (2001) of US teenagers, 62% of females and 29% of males were attempting to lose weight, a 3% increase compared with 1999. Fourteen percent of youth did not eat for more than 24 hours to lose weight. Overall, 9.2% of youth had used diet pills as a weight loss method in the previous 30 days—12.6% of girls and 5.5% of boys. Self-induced vomiting or laxative use (or both) was also common; 7.8% of females and 2.9% of males were using one or the other to lose weight. Concern about weight, and harmful attempts to lose weight all increased from 1999 to 2001. Binge-eating disorder has a 1.1% incidence in the teenage population. Forty-six percent of females and 30% of males report at least one bingeing episode during their lifetime.

Centers for Disease Control and Prevention. Youth Risk Behavior Surveillance System 2001.

http://www.cdc.gov/mmwr/pdf/ss/ss5104.pdf.

Pawluck D: Secular trends in the incidence of anorexia nervosa: Integrative review of population-based studies. Int J Eat Disord 1998;23:347 [PMID: 9561424].

## PREDISPOSING FACTORS

In the past, the typical anorexic patient was described as a high-achieving, athletic, straight-A student from a middle class socioeconomic background. Demographics have changed somewhat, and anorexia nervosa now occurs in all races and socioeconomic classes. Children involved in gymnastics, figure skating, and ballet—activities that emphasize (and in which coaches often require) thin bodies—are at higher risk for anorexia than are children in sports that do not emphasize body image. Sudden changes in dietary habits, such as becoming vegetarian, may be a first sign of anorexia, especially if the change is abrupt and without good reason.

The typical bulimic patient is more impulsive, tending to engage in risk-taking behavior such as alcohol use, drug use, and sexual experimentation. Bulimic patients are often an appropriate weight for height or slightly overweight, and they get average grades. Some studies have found that 50% of bulimic patients have been sexually abused. In males, wrestling and homosexual orientation predispose to bulimia nervosa.

## DIAGNOSIS

### 1. Anorexia Nervosa

Table 5–1 lists the diagnostic criteria for anorexia nervosa, according to the *Diagnostic and Statistical Manual of Mental Disorders,* 4th edition (DSM-IV). There are two forms of anorexia nervosa. In the restricting type, patients do not regularly engage in binge eating or purging. In the purging type, classic anorexia nervosa is combined with binge eating or purging behavior (or both). Differentiating the two is important because of differing implications for prognosis and treatment.

### Clinical Findings

#### A. SYMPTOMS AND SIGNS

Clinicians should recognize the early symptoms and signs of anorexia nervosa because intervention may pre-

**Table 5–1.** Diagnostic criteria for anorexia nervosa.

---

A. Refusal to maintain body weight at or above a minimally normal weight for age and height (eg, weight loss leading to maintenance of body weight less than 85% of that expected; or failure to make expected weight gain during period of growth, leading to body weight less than 85% of that expected).

B. Intense fear of gaining weight or becoming fat, even though underweight.

C. Disturbance in the way in which one's body weight or shape is experienced, undue influence of body weight or shape on self-evaluation, or denial of the seriousness of the current low body weight.

D. In postmenarchal females, amenorrhea, ie, the absence of at least three menstrual cycles. (A woman is considered to have amenorrhea if her periods occur only following hormone, eg, estrogen, administration.)

---

Reprinted, with permission, from the *Diagnostic and Statistical Manual of Mental Disorders,* 4th ed. Text Revision. Copyright 2000. American Psychiatric Association.

vent the full-blown syndrome from developing. Patients may show some of the behaviors and psychology of anorexia nervosa, such as reduction in dietary fat and intense concern with body image, even before weight loss or amenorrhea occurs.

Making the diagnosis of anorexia nervosa can be challenging because adolescents may try to conceal their illness. Assessing the patient's body image is essential to determining the diagnosis. Table 5–2 lists screening questions that help to tease out a teenager's perceptions of body image. Additional diagnostic screening tools include the Eating Attitudes Test (EAT) or other questionnaires that assess a range of eating and dieting behaviors. Parental observations are critical in determining whether a patient has expressed dissatisfaction over body habitus as well as revealing what weight loss techniques the child has attempted. In the teenager who is not ready to share his or her concerns about body image, the clinician may find clues to the diagnosis by carefully considering other presenting symptoms. Weight loss from a baseline of normal body weight is an obvious red flag and should raise the clinical suspicion of an eating disorder. Additionally, anorexia nervosa should be considered in any girl with secondary amenorrhea who has lost weight.

Physical symptoms are usually secondary to weight loss and proportional to the degree of malnutrition. The body effectively goes into hibernation, becoming functionally hypothyroid (euthyroid sick) to save as much energy as possible. Body temperature decreases, and patients report being colder than normal. Patients become bradycardic, especially in the supine position. Dizziness, lightheadedness, and occasional syncope may

ensue, as orthostasis and hypotension secondary to impaired cardiac function occur. Left ventricular mass is decreased, (as all striated muscle throughout the body loses mass), stroke volume is compromised, and peripheral resistance is increased. Patients can develop prolonged QT syndrome, putting them at risk for cardiac arrhythmias. Peripheral circulation is reduced. Hands and feet may be blue and cool. Hair thins, nails become brittle, and the skin is dry. Lanugo develops as a primitive response to starvation. The gastrointestinal tract may be affected. Inability to take in normal quantities of food, early satiety, and gastroesophageal reflux can develop as the body adapts to reduced intake. The normal gastrocolic reflex may be temporarily lost due to lack of stimuli, leading to delayed gastric emptying and constipation.

Neurologically, patients may experience decreased cognition, inability to concentrate, increased irritability, and depression, which may be related to structural brain changes and decreased cerebral blood flow.

A combination of malnutrition and stress causes hypothalamic hypogonadism. The hypothalamic–pituitary–gonadal axis shuts down as the body struggles to survive, directing finite energy resources to support more vital functions. Both males and females experience decreased libido and interruption of pubertal development, depending on the timing of the illness. Skeletal growth may be interrupted as well.

Nutritional assessment is vital. Often patients eliminate fat from their diets and may eat as little as 100–200 kcal/d. A gown-only weight after urination is the most accurate way to assess weight. Patients tend to wear bulky clothes and may hide weights in their pockets or drink excessive amounts of fluid (water-loading) to trick the practitioner. Calculating body mass index (BMI)—weight in kilograms divided by height in meters squared—is an efficient way to interpret degree of malnutrition. A BMI less than the fifth percentile (using the new BMI growth curves) indicates significant malnutrition. Additionally, ideal body weight (IBW) for height should be calculated. A weight less than 85% IBW is one of the diagnostic criteria for anorexia nervosa. Ideal body weight should be calculated using the 50th percentile of BMI for age.

A hallmark physical feature of anorexia nervosa in girls is amenorrhea, which occurs for two reasons. The hypothalamic–pituitary–ovarian axis shuts down under stress, causing hypothalamic amenorrhea. Additionally, adipose tissue is needed to convert estrogen to its activated form. When weight loss is significant, adipose tissue is lost and there is not enough substrate to activate estrogen. Resuming normal menses depends on increasing both body weight and body fat. Approximately 73% of postmenarcheal girls will resume menstruating if they reach 90% of their IBW. An adolescent female

**Table 5–2.** Screening questions to help diagnose anorexia and bulimia nervosa.

---

How do you feel about your body?

Are there parts of your body you might change?

When you look at yourself in the mirror, do you see yourself as overweight, underweight, or satisfactory?

If overweight, how much do you want to weigh?

If your weight is satisfactory, has there been a time that you were worried about being overweight?

If overweight/underweight, what would you change?

Have you ever been on a diet?

What have you done to help yourself lose weight?

Do you count calories or fat grams?

Do you keep your intake to a certain number of calories?

Have you ever used nutritional supplements, diet pills, or laxatives to help yourself lose weight?

Have you ever made yourself vomit to get rid of food or lose weight?

needs, on average, 17% body fat to restart menses and 22% body fat if she has primary amenorrhea.

## B. LABORATORY FINDINGS

Most organ systems can potentially suffer some degree of damage in the anorexic patient, related both to severity and duration of illness (Table 5–3). Initial screening should include complete blood count with differential, and serum levels of electrolytes, blood urea nitrogen/creatinine, phosphorus, calcium, magnesium, and thyroid-stimulating hormone, as well as liver function tests and urinalysis. An electrocardiogram should be performed, because significant electrocardiographic abnormalities may be present, most importantly prolonged QT syndrome. Bone densitometry should be done if amenorrhea has persisted for 6 months, as patients begin to accumulate risk for osteoporosis.

## Differential Diagnosis

If the diagnosis is unclear (ie, the patient has lost a significant amount of weight but does not have typical body image distortion or fat phobia), then the clinician must consider the differential diagnosis for weight loss in adolescents. This includes inflammatory bowel disease, diabetes, hyperthyroidism, malignancy, and depression. Less common diagnoses include adrenal insufficiency and malabsorption syndromes such as celiac

**Table 5–3.** Laboratory findings: anorexia nervosa.

Increased blood urea nitrogen/creatinine secondary to renal insufficiency

Decreased white blood cells, platelets, and less commonly red blood cells/hematocrit secondary to bone marrow suppression or fat atrophy of the bone marrow

Increased AST and ALT secondary to malnutrition.

Increased cholesterol, thought to be related to fatty acid metabolism

Decreased alkaline phosphatase secondary to zinc deficiency

Low to low-normal thyroid-stimulating hormone and thyroxine

Decreased follicle-stimulating hormone, luteinizing hormone, estradiol, and testosterone secondary to shutdown of hypothalamic–pituitary–gonadal axis

Abnormal electrolytes related to hydrational status

Decreased phosphorus

Decreased insulin-like growth factor

Increased cortisol

Decreased urine specific gravity in cases of intentional water intoxication

ALT = alanine aminotransferase; AST = aspartate aminotransferase.

disease. The history and physical examination should direct laboratory and radiologic evaluation.

## 2. Bulimia Nervosa

Table 5–4 lists the diagnostic criteria for bulimia nervosa. Binge eating is either eating excessive amounts of food during a normal mealtime or having a meal (or other eating episode) last longer than usual, consuming food throughout. Bulimic individuals feel out of control while eating, unable or unwilling to recognize satiety signals. Any type of food may be included in a binge, though typically it is either carbohydrates or junk food. Extreme guilt is often associated with the episode. At some point, either prior to or during a binge, bulimic individuals often decide to purge. The amount of food consumed feels overwhelming, and they do not want to gain weight. The most common ways to purge are self-induced vomiting, exercise, and laxative use. Some individuals will vomit multiple times during a purge episode, after using large amounts of water to cleanse their system. This can induce significant electrolyte abnormalities such as hyponatremia and hypokalemia, which may put the patient at acute risk for arrhythmia or seizure. Other methods of purging include diuretics, diet pills, cathartics, and nutritional supplements, including Metabolife.

**Table 5–4.** Diagnostic criteria for bulimia nervosa.

A. Recurrent episodes of binge eating. An episode of binge eating is characterized by both of the following:
 (1) eating, in a discrete period of time (eg, within any 2-hour period), an amount of food that is definitely larger than most people would eat during a similar period of time and under similar circumstances.
 (2) a sense of lack of control over eating during the episodes (eg, a feeling that one cannot stop eating or control what or how much one is eating)
B. Recurrent inappropriate compensatory behavior in order to prevent weight gain, such as self-induced vomiting; misuse of laxatives, diuretics, enemas, or other medications; fasting; or excessive exercise.
C. The binge eating and inappropriate compensatory behaviors both occur, on average, at least twice a week for 3 months.
D. Self-evaluation is unduly influenced by body shape and weight.
E. The disturbance does not occur exclusively during episodes of anorexia nervosa.

Reprinted, with permission, from the *Diagnostic and Statistical Manual of Mental Disorders,* 4th ed. Text Revision. Copyright 2000. American Psychiatric Association.

Diagnosing bulimia nervosa can be difficult unless the teenager is forthcoming or parents or caregivers can supply direct observations. Often bulimic patients are average or slightly above average in body weight, without any physical abnormalities. Screening all teenagers for body image concerns is crucial. If the teenager expresses concern about being overweight, then the clinician needs to screen the patient about dieting methods. Asking whether patients have binged, feel out of control while eating, or whether they cannot stop eating can clarify the diagnosis. Parents may report that significant amounts of food are missing or disappearing more quickly than normal. If the physician is suspicious, direct questioning about all the ways to purge should follow. Indicating first that the behavior in question is not unusual can make the questioning less threatening and more likely to elicit a truthful response. For example, the clinician might say, "Some teenagers who try to lose weight make themselves vomit after eating. Have you ever considered or done that yourself?"

## Clinical Findings

### A. SYMPTOMS AND SIGNS

Symptoms are related to the mechanism of purging. Gastrointestinal problems are most prominent. Abdominal pain is a frequent complaint. This can be due to gastroesophageal reflux, because frequent vomiting may result in esophagitis. Early satiety, involuntary vomiting, and complaints of food "coming up" on its own are frequent. Less common but more serious is hematemesis or esophageal rupture. Patients may report bowel problems—diarrhea or constipation—if laxatives have been used. Sialadenosis—parotid pain and enlargement—may occur secondary to frequent vomiting. Erosion of dental enamel may result from increased exposure to acidity during vomiting. Because comorbid depression is common in bulimia nervosa, patients may report difficulty sleeping, decreased energy, decreased motivation, and headaches. Lightheadedness or syncope may develop secondary to dehydration.

It is important to note that most purging methods are ineffective. When patients binge, they may consume thousands of calories. Digestion begins rapidly. Although the patient may be able to vomit some of the food, much is actually digested and absorbed. Laxatives work on the large intestine, leading to fluid and electrolyte loss. Consumed calories are still absorbed from the small intestine. Use of diuretics may result in decreased fluid weight and electrolyte imbalance.

On physical examination, bulimic patients may be dehydrated and have orthostatic hypotension. Sialadenosis, tooth enamel loss, dental caries, and abdominal tenderness are the most common findings.

Abrasion of the proximal interphalangeal joints may occur secondary to scraping the fingers against teeth while inducing vomiting. Rarely a heart murmur is heard. An irreversible cardiomyopathy can develop secondary to ipecac use. Tachycardia and hypertension may occur secondary to caffeine and diet pill use.

### B. LABORATORY FINDINGS

Electrolyte disturbances are characteristic of bulimic patients. The method of purging results in specific abnormalities. Vomiting causes metabolic alkalosis, hypokalemia, and hypochloremia. If laxatives are used, then a metabolic acidosis develops with hypokalemia and hypochloremia. Amylase may be increased secondary to chronic parotid stimulation.

American Psychiatric Association: *Diagnostic and Statistical Manual of Mental Disorders,* 4th ed. Text Revision. American Psychiatric Association, 2000.

Kreipe RE, Birndorf SA: Eating disorders in adolescents and young adults. Med Clin North Am Jul 2000;84(4):1027 [PMID: 10928200].

Panagiotopoulos C et al: Electrocardiographic findings in adolescents with eating disorders. Pediatrics 2000;105(5):1100 [PMID: 10790469].

## 3. Binge-Eating Disorder

The diagnostic category of binge-eating disorder was created in DSM-IV. Officially, it is still considered a research diagnosis. Studies show that most adults who have binge-eating disorder (a prevalence of 2–4%) develop symptoms during adolescence Table 5–5 lists the diagnostic criteria.

## Clinical Findings

### A. SYMPTOMS AND SIGNS

Binge-eating disorder is a new eating disorder category. It occurs most often in patients who are overweight or obese. Eighteen percent of such patients report bingeing at least once in the past year. Patients with binge-eating disorder have an increased incidence of depression and substance abuse. Using the DSM-IV diagnostic criteria as a guide for evaluation, the suspicion of binge-eating disorder should be raised for any significantly overweight patient. Specific questionnaires are available for evaluating patients suspected of having binge-eating disorder.

### B. LABORATORY FINDINGS

The clinician should assess causes and complications of obesity, and laboratory evaluation should include thyroid function tests and measurement of cholesterol and triglyceride levels.

**Table 5–5.** Diagnostic criteria for binge-eating disorder.

A. Recurrent episodes of binge eating. An episode of binge eating is characterized by both of the following:
   (1) eating, in a discrete period of time (eg, within any 2-hour period), an amount of food that is definitely larger than most people would eat in a similar period of time under similar circumstances.
   (2) a sense of lack of control over eating during the episode (eg, a feeling that one cannot stop eating or control what or how much one is eating)
B. The binge-eating episodes are associated with three (or more) of the following:
   (1) eating much more rapidly than normal
   (2) eating until feeling uncomfortably full
   (3) eating large amounts of food when not feeling physically hungry
   (4) eating alone because of being embarrassed by how much one is eating
   (5) feeling disgusted with oneself, depressed, or very guilty after overeating
C. Marked distress regarding binge eating at present.
D. The binge eating occurs, on average, at least 2 days a week for 6 months.
E. The binge eating is not associated with regular use of inappropriate compensatory behaviors (eg, purging, fasting, excessive exercise) and does not occur exclusively during the course of anorexia nervosa or bulimia nervosa.

Reprinted, with permission, from the *Diagnostic and Statistical Manual of Mental Disorders*, 4th ed. Text revised. Copyright 2000. American Psychiatric Association.

Fairburn CG et al: The natural course of bulimia nervosa and binge eating disorder in young women. Arch Gen Psych 2000;57: 659. [PMID: 10891036].

Johnson WG et al: Measuring binge eating in adolescents: Adolescent and parent versions of the questionnaire of eating and weight patterns. Int J Eat Disord 1999;26:301 [PMID 10441246].

Schneider M: Bulimia nervosa and binge eating disorder in adolescents. Adolesc Med State of the Art Reviews 2003;14(1): 119 [PMID: 12529196].

## 4. Eating Disorder Not Otherwise Specified

An additional diagnostic category found in DSM-IV is eating disorder not otherwise specified. Patients do not meet all the criteria for either anorexia nervosa or bulimia nervosa, but have features of either or both. Table 5–6 lists the diagnostic criteria. Individuals require similar treatment intervention depending on the clinical features.

**Table 5–6.** Diagnostic criteria for eating disorder not otherwise specified.

The eating disorder not otherwise specified category is for disorders of eating that do not meet the criteria for any specific eating disorder. Examples include
  1. For females, all of the criteria for anorexia nervosa are met except that the individual has regular menses.
  2. All of the criteria for anorexia nervosa are met except that, despite significant weight loss, the individual's current weight is in the normal range.
  3. All of the criteria for bulimia nervosa are met except that the binge eating and inappropriate compensatory mechanisms occur at a frequency of less than twice a week or for a duration of less than 3 months.
  4. The regular use of inappropriate compensatory behavior by an individual of normal body weight after eating small amounts of food (eg, self-induced vomiting after the consumption of two cookies).
  5. Repeatedly chewing and spitting out, but not swallowing, large amounts of food.

Reprinted with permission from the *Diagnostic and Statistical Manual of Mental Disorders*, 4th ed. Text Revision. Copyright 2000. American Psychiatric Association.

## COMPLICATIONS (Table 5–7)

### 1. Anorexia Nervosa

### Short-Term Complications

#### A. EARLY SATIETY

Patients may have significant difficulty digesting modest quantities as their bodies adapt to increased caloric intake. Patients may benefit from a gastric-emptying agent such as metoclopramide. This complication usually resolves after a patient has become used to larger meals.

#### B. SUPERIOR MESENTERIC ARTERY SYNDROME

As patients become malnourished, the fat pad between the superior mesenteric artery and the duodenum may shrink, compressing the transverse duodenum and causing vomiting and intolerance of oral intake, especially solids. Diagnosis is made by an upper GI series, which shows to and fro movement of barium in the descending and transverse duodenum proximal to the obstruction. Treatment involves a liquid diet or nasoduodenal feedings until restoration of the fat pad has occurred, coincident with weight gain.

#### C. CONSTIPATION

Patients may have prolonged constipation, often not having a bowel movement for a week or longer. Two

**Table 5–7.** Complications of anorexia and bulimia nervosa.

| | |
|---|---|
| **Cardiovascular** | **Hematologic** |
| Bradycardia | Leukopenia |
| Postural hypotension | Anemia |
| Arrhythmia, sudden death | Thrombocytopenia |
| Congestive heart failure | ↓ESR |
|   (during refeeding) | Impaired cell-mediated |
| Pericardial effusion |   immunity |
| Mitral valve prolapse | **Metabolic** |
| ECG abnormalities | Dehydration |
|   (prolonged QT, low volt- | Acidosis |
|   age, T-wave abnormali- | Hypokalemia |
|   ties, conduction defects) | Hyponatremia |
| **Endocrine** | Hypochloremia |
| ↓LH, FSH | Hypochloremic alkalosis |
| ↓$T_3$, ↑$rT_3$; ↓ $T_4$, TSH | Hypocalcemia |
| Irregular menses | Hypophosphatemia |
| Amenorrhea | Hypomagnesemia |
| Hypercortisolism | Hypercarotenemia |
| Growth retardation | **Neurologic** |
| Delayed puberty | Cortical atrophy |
| **Gastrointestinal** | Peripheral neuropathy |
| Dental erosion | Seizures |
| Parotid swelling | Thermoregulatory |
| Esophagitis, esophageal |   abnormalities |
|   tears | ↓REM and slow-wave |
| Delayed gastric emptying |   sleep |
| Gastric dilatation (rarely | **Renal** |
|   rupture) | Hematuria |
| Pancreatitis | Proteinuria |
| Constipation | ↓Renal concentrating |
| Diarrhea (laxative abuse) |   ability |
| Superior mesenteric artery | **Skeletal** |
|   syndrome | Osteopenia |
| Hypercholesterolemia | Fractures |
| ↑Liver function tests (fatty | |
|   infiltration of the liver) | |

LH = luteinizing hormone; ECG = electrocardiogram; FSH = follicle-stimulating hormone; $T_3$ = triiodothyronine; $rT_3$ = resin triiodothyronine uptake; $T_4$ = tetraiodothyronine; TSH = thyroid-stimulating hormone; ESR = erythrocyte sedimentation rate; REM = rapid eye movement.

mechanisms contribute to this symptom: loss of gastrocolic reflex and loss of colonic muscle tone. Typically stool softeners do not help because the colon has decreased peristaltic amplitude. Agents that induce peristalsis, such as bisacodyl and polyethylene glycol-electrolyte solution (Miralax), are helpful. Constipation can persist for up to 6–8 weeks after refeeding. Occasionally patients need enemas.

### D. REFEEDING SYNDROME

Described in the Treatment section.

## Long-Term Complications

### A. OSTEOPOROSIS

Approximately 90% of females with anorexia nervosa have reduced bone mass at one or more sites. The development of osteopenia and osteoporosis is multifactorial. Estrogen and testosterone are essential to potentiate bone development. Teenagers are particularly at risk as they accrue 40% of their bone mineral during adolescence. Low body weight is most predictive of bone loss. Amenorrhea, an indicator of estrogen deficiency, is also highly correlated with osteoporosis. Bone minerals begin to resorb without estrogen. Elevated cortisol levels and decreased insulin-like growth factor-1 (IGF-1) also contribute to bone resorption. Studies show that as little as 6 months of amenorrhea can lead to osteopenia or osteoporosis. In one study, 44% of adolescents with anorexia had osteopenia of the lumbar spine. Males also can develop osteoporosis due to decreased testosterone.

The only proven treatment for osteoporosis in anorexia nervosa in girls is regaining sufficient weight and body fat to restart the menstrual cycle. Controversy exists regarding the use of hormone replacement therapy (HRT). Most studies do not support use of HRT to improve bone recovery; however, some evidence indicates that use of HRT may stop further bone loss and may be of particular benefit for patients with extremely low body weight (less than 70% IBW). Some practitioners use HRT if amenorrhea is prolonged (> 1 year) and the patient is not able to achieve normal body weight. The bisphosphonates used to treat postmenopausal osteoporosis are currently being studied in adolescents. Newer treatments in research trials have shown some promise, including recombinant IGF-1 injection and use of dehydroepiandrosterone, though they are both still under investigation.

### B. BRAIN CHANGES

As malnutrition becomes more pronounced, brain tissue—both white and gray matter—is lost and a concomitant increase in cerebrospinal fluid occurs in the sulci and ventricles. Follow-up studies of weight-recovered anorexic patients show a persistent loss of gray matter, although white matter returns to normal. Functionally there does not seem to be a specific relationship between cognition and brain tissue loss, though studies have shown a decrease in cognitive ability, as well as decreased cerebral blood flow in more severe malnourished states. Communicating to the patient and the family that brain tissue can be lost can have a significant effect on the perception of the seriousness of this disorder.

Castro J et al: Bone mineral density in male adolescents with anorexia nervosa. J Am Acad Child Adolesc Psychiatry 2002; 41(5) 613 [PMID: 12014794].

Golden NH: Osteopenia and osteoporosis in anorexia nervosa. Adolesc Med State of the Art Reviews. 2003;14(1):97 [PMID::12529194].

Karlsson MK: Bone size and volumetric density in women with anorexia nervosa receiving estrogen replacement therapy and in women recovered from anorexia nervosa. J Clin Endocrinol Metab 2000;85:3177 [PMID: 10999805].

Kerem NC, Katzman DK: Brain structure and function in adolescents with anorexia nervosa. Adolesc Med State of the Art Reviews. 2003;14(1):109 [PMID: 12529195].

## Mortality

Patients with eating disorders are at a higher risk of dying than the general population. Meta-analysis has shown the risk of dying to be 5.9% in such patients. Mortality estimates vary between 0% and 18%, depending on the patient population studied and the length of the study. One study showed the risk of dying to be 0.56% per year. Death in anorexic patients is due to suicide, abnormal electrolytes, and resultant cardiac arrhythmias.

Herzog DB et al: Mortality in eating disorders: A descriptive study. Int J Eat Dis 2000;28(1):20 [PMID: 10800010].

## 2. Bulimia Nervosa

### Short-Term & Long-Term Complications

Complications for normal-weight bulimic patients are related to their mechanisms of purging, and many of these complications were listed earlier in the Symptoms and Signs section. If the bulimic patient is significantly malnourished, the complications may be the same as those encountered in the anorexic patient. Other complications of bulimia include esophageal rupture, acute or chronic esophagitis, and, rarely, Barrett syndrome. Chronic vomiting can lead to metabolic alkalosis, and laxative abuse may cause metabolic acidosis. Patients may develop aspiration pneumonia from vomiting. Diet pill use can cause insomnia, hypertension, tachycardia, palpitations, seizures, and sudden death.

Patients who stop taking laxatives can have trouble with bowel function, most often constipation. Treating constipation can be difficult psychologically, because the practitioner may need to prescribe agents similar to the drugs of abuse used during the eating disorder.

## Mortality

The mortality rate in bulimic patients is similar to that in anorexic patients. Death usually results from suicide or electrolyte derangements.

## TREATMENT

Many treatment modalities are available. Factors that determine treatment interventions are severity of illness, length of illness, specific manifestations of disease, previous treatment approaches and outcomes, program availability, financial resources, and insurance coverage. Treatment options include outpatient management, day treatment hospitalization, and inpatient hospitalization of either a medical or psychiatric nature. Residential treatment is most often used when outpatient management or short-term hospitalization fails and the eating disorder becomes chronic. Residential treatment usually lasts 2–6 months. Day treatment programs are a good intervention for patients who do not yet need inpatient care but who are not improving with outpatient management. Treatment is costly. Many patients do not have insurance benefits that adequately cover the cost of treatment, leaving parents and practitioners with profound dilemmas as to how to best provide treatment in the face of financial constraints.

Regardless of type of treatment program, a multidisciplinary approach is most effective. Treatment should include medical monitoring, nutrition therapy, and individual and family psychotherapy by practitioners experienced with eating disorder patients. Family therapy is especially helpful with younger teenagers, whereas older teenagers tend to benefit more from individual therapy, although both should be encouraged. Family therapy is an important means by which to help families understand the development of the disease and address the issues that may be barriers to recovery. Both types of therapy are encouraged in most treatment programs, and recovery without psychotherapy is unusual. The average length of therapy is roughly 6–9 months, although some individuals continue therapy for extended periods. Adjunctive modalities include art and horticulture therapy, therapeutic recreation, and massage therapy.

Careful instruction in nutrition is important in helping the teenager dispel misconceptions about nutrition, identify realistic nutritional goals, and normalize eating. Initially, nutrition education may be the most important intervention as the teenager slowly works through his or her fears of fat-containing foods and weight gain. The teenager begins to trust the nutrition therapist and begins to restore body weight, by eventually eating in a well-balanced, healthy manner.

## 1. Anorexia Nervosa

The key to determining level of intervention depends on the degree of malnutrition, the rapidity of weight loss, the degree of medical compromise, and presence of life-threatening electrolyte abnormalities. No absolute criteria determine level of intervention. The practitioner must examine the degree of medical compromise, consider immediate risks, and the potential for an individual to reverse the situation on his or her own.

### A. INPATIENT TREATMENT

Table 5–8 lists the criteria for hospital admission generally used in the medical community. It is usually quite difficult for a patient who is losing weight rapidly (> 2 lb/wk) to reverse the weight loss because the body is in a catabolic state.

If a patient is hospitalized the initial goal is to stop weight loss. The clinician can begin a meal plan containing approximately 250 kcal more than the patient has been routinely eating. Depending on the sophistication of the program and support staff, this can usually be accomplished orally. Ideally, with the help of a nutritionist, patients should start with a well-balanced meal plan, with appropriately divided carbohydrates, proteins, and fats. Usually patients tolerate oral meals. If the patient resists, a nasogastric tube or intravenous alimentation can be used for a short time. Aside from caloric needs, the clinician needs to pay attention to the patient's hydration status, including the appropriate amount of fluid with the meal plan. Dehydration should be corrected slowly. The oral route is usually adequate. Aggressive intravenous fluid administration should be avoided because left ventricular mass is compromised and rapid increase in volume may not be tolerated. Regulating fluid intake is important, because water intoxication can contribute to abnormal electrolytes and falsified weights.

During the initial introduction of food, the clinician needs to monitor the patient for refeeding syndrome, a phenomenon that occurs if caloric intake is increased too rapidly. Signs of refeeding syndrome are decreased

**Table 5–8.** Criteria for inpatient treatment of anorexia nervosa.

Body weight < 75% of ideal body weight
Supine heart rate < 45/min
Symptomatic hypotension or syncope
Hypokalemia: K⁺ < 2.5 mEq/L
Rapid weight loss that cannot be interrupted as outpatient
Failure of outpatient management
Acute food refusal

serum phosphate (as the body finally starts making adenosine triphosphate), decreased serum potassium (as increased insulin causes shifting of K⁺ from extracellular fluid into K⁺-depleted cells), and edema related to fluid shifts as well as from congestive heart failure.

Caloric intake can be increased 250 kcal/d as long as refeeding syndrome does not occur. Weight goals vary depending on programmatic approach. Typically intake is adjusted to reach a goal of 0.1–0.25 kg/d weight gain.

Overnight monitoring for bradycardia is helpful in assessing degree of metabolic compromise. Usually the more rapid and severe the weight loss, the worse the bradycardia. Improving bradycardia correlates with weight recovery. Orthostatic hypotension is most severe around hospital day 4, improving steadily and correcting by the third week of nutritional rehabilitation. An electrocardiogram should be obtained because the patient is at risk for prolonged QT syndrome and junctional arrhythmias related to the severity of bradycardia.

It usually takes 2–3 weeks to reach the initial goals of hospitalization—steady weight gain, toleration of oral diet without signs of refeeding syndrome, corrected bradycardia (heart rate > 45/min for three consecutive nights), and orthostasis. Specific weight criteria are used by many programs when considering discharge. This depends partly on admission weight. Ideally a patient gains at least 5% of his or her ideal weight. Some programs set discharge at 80%, 85%, or 90% IBW. Patient outcomes are improved with discharge at a higher body weight. One study has shown that patients do better if discharged at 95% IBW. Frequently, insurance companies do not cooperate and will not pay beyond strict medical stabilization (normal vital signs and normal electrolytes). In many practitioners' experience, relapse rate is high if patients are discharged at less than 75% IBW.

Extremely malnourished patients may not benefit from individual psychotherapy or nutritional instruction initially because they may be cognitively impaired. Beginning family psychotherapy at first, with the addition of individual psychotherapy after the first week of refeeding, may prove more effective.

Medications (specifically SSRIs) are not helpful in treating anorexia nervosa independently. Once the patient has achieved approximately 85% IBW, then SSRIs (fluoxetine, citalopram, or sertraline) help prevent relapse.

Several open label trials support the use of atypical antipsychotics (risperidone, olanzapine), which target specifically the body image distortion that these patients experience.

To help address the malnourished state, a multivitamin with iron and zinc supplementation may be beneficial. Zinc has been found to be depleted in anorexia nervosa. Supplementation helps restore appetite as well as improve depressive moods. Symptomatic treatment for disturbances in the gastrointestinal system should be used appropriately until symptoms resolve.

## B. OUTPATIENT TREATMENT

Not all patients diagnosed with anorexia nervosa need inpatient treatment, especially if parents and clinicians recognize the warning signs early. These patients can receive treatment in the outpatient setting, employing the same multidisciplinary team approach. Appropriate nutrition counseling is vital in guiding a patient and family through the initial stages of recovery. As the nutrition therapist is working at increasing the patient's caloric intake, a practitioner needs to monitor the patient's weight and vital signs. Often activity level needs to be decreased to help reverse the catabolic state. A reasonable weight gain goal may be 0.2–0.5 kg/wk. If weight loss persists, careful monitoring of vital signs, including supine heart rate, is important in determining whether an increased level of care is needed. Concomitantly, the patient should be referred to a psychotherapist, and, if indicated, assessed by a psychiatrist.

## 2. Bulimia Nervosa

Treatment of bulimia nervosa depends on the frequency of bingeing and purging and the severity of biochemical and psychiatric derangement. If $K^+$ is less than 3.0 mEq/L, then inpatient medical admission is warranted. Typically extracellular $K^+$ is spared at the expense of intracellular $K^+$, so that a patient may become hypokalemic several days after the serum $K^+$ concentration appears to be corrected. Usually cessation of purging is sufficient to correct $K^+$ concentration and is the recommended intervention for $K^+$ greater than 3.0 mEq/L; if $K^+$ is 2.5–2.9 mEq/L, oral supplementation is suggested; if $K^+$ is less than 2.5 mEq/L, then intravenous therapy is recommended. Supplements can be stopped once $K^+$ levels are greater than 3.5 mEq/L. Once serum $K^+$ corrects and remains normal 2 days after supplements are stopped, the clinician can be confident that total body $K^+$ has returned to normal. Continued hospitalization depends on the patient's psychological status.

Many of these patients abuse laxatives and may be chronically dehydrated. The renin–angiotensin–aldosterone axis, as well as the antidiuretic hormone level, may be elevated to compensate. These systems do not shut down automatically when laxatives are stopped, and fluid retention of up to 10 kg/wk may result. This puts patients at risk for congestive heart failure and can scare them as their weight increases dramatically. A diuresis often occurs after approximately 7–10 days. Parents and patients should be advised of this possible

complication of initial therapy to help maintain their confidence in the care plan.

Another reason to hospitalize bulimic patients is failure of outpatient management. The binge–purge cycle is addictive and can be difficult for patients to interrupt on their own. Hospitalization can offer a forced break from the cycle, allowing patients to normalize their eating, interrupt the addictive behavior, and regain ability to recognize satiety signals.

Outpatient management can be pursued if patients are medically stable. Cognitive-behavioral therapy is crucial to help bulimic patients understand their disease and to offer suggestions for decreasing bingeing and purging. Nutrition therapy offers patients ways to regulate eating patterns so that they can avoid the need to binge. Medical monitoring should be done to check electrolytes periodically, depending on the purging method used.

SSRIs are generally quite helpful in treating the binge–purge cycle. Fluoxetine has been studied most extensively; a dose of 60 mg/day is most efficacious in teenagers. Other SSRIs are thought to work similarly and are worth trying if the patient experiences side effects while taking fluoxetine. Treatment for gastro-esophageal reflux and gastritis should be used when appropriate. The pain and swelling of enlarged parotid glands can be helped by sucking on tart candy and by the application of heat.

Bacaltchuk J et al: Antidepressant versus placebo for the treatment of bulimia nervosa: A systematic review. Aust NZ J Psychiatry 2000;34:310 [PMID: 10789536].

Kaye W et al: Double blind placebo-controlled administration of fluoxetine in restricting- and restricting–purging-type anorexia nervosa. Biol Psychiatry 2001;49(7):644 [PMID: 11297722].

Mehler P: Bulimia nervosa. N Engl J Med 2003;349:875 [PMID: 12944574].

Newman-Toker J: Risperidone in anorexia nervosa. J Am Acad Child Adolesc Psychiatry 2000;39(8):941 [PMID: 10939220].

## 3. Binge-Eating Disorder

A combination of cognitive-behavioral therapy and antidepressant medication has been helpful in treating binge-eating disorder in adults. Use of SSRIs for binge-eating disorder in adolescents has not been studied, but in adults, fluoxetine and citalopram help decrease binge episodes, improve depression, and the decreased appetite that contributes to weight loss. This evidence suggests that SSRIs in adolescents with binge eating disorder may be helpful as well.

McElroy SL et al: Citalopram in the treatment of binge-eating disorder: A placebo-controlled trial J Clin Psychiatry 2003; 64(7):807 [PMID: 12934982].

# PROGNOSIS

Outcome in eating disorders, especially anorexia nervosa, has been studied extensively. Unfortunately, most studies have focused on specific inpatient treatment programs, and few have evaluated the less ill patients who do not need hospitalization. About 40–50% of patients receiving treatment recover; 20–30% have intermittent relapses; and 20% have chronic, unremitting illness. As time from initial onset lengthens, the recovery rate decreases and mortality associated with anorexia nervosa and bulimia nervosa increase.

The course of anorexia nervosa often includes significant weight fluctuations over time, and it may be a matter of years until recovery is certain. The course of bulimia nervosa often includes relapse episodes of bingeing and purging, although bulimic patients initially recover faster than do anorexic patients. Up to 50% of anorexic patients may develop bulimia, as well as major psychological sequelae, including depression, anxiety, and substance abuse disorders. Bulimic patients also develop similar psychological illness but rarely develop anorexia. Long-term medical sequelae, aside from low body weight and amenorrhea, have not been studied in an outcome format, although anorexia nervosa is known to have multiple medical consequences including osteoporosis and structural brain changes.

It is unclear whether age at onset affects disease course. Shorter length of time between symptom onset and therapy tends to improve outcome. Various treatment modalities can be equally effective. Favorable outcomes have been found with brief medical hospitalization and long psychiatric or residential hospitalization. Higher discharge weight seems to improve the initial outcome. It is difficult to compare treatment regimens, because the numbers are small and the type of patient and illness varies between studies. No existing studies compare outpatient to inpatient treatment or the effects of day treatment on recovery.

Binge-eating disorder has been recognized only recently, and outcomes have not been studied. Intervention with an SSRI appears to help the bingeing, but little is known regarding long-term prognosis.

Fisher M: The course and outcome of eating disorders in adults and in adolescents: A review. Adolesc Med State of the Art Reviews 2003;14(1):149 [PMID: 12529198].

Herzog D et al: Recovery and relapse in anorexia and bulimia nervosa: A 7.5 year follow-up study. J Am Acad Child Adolesc Psychiatry 1999;38:829 [PMID: 10405500].

# REFERENCES

Kreipe RE, Birndorf SA: Eating disorders in adolescents and young adults. [Review] [32 refs] Med Clin North Am 2000; 84(4)1027 [PMID 10928200].

Rome E et al: Children and adolescents with eating disorders: State of the art. Pediatrics 2003;111;e98 [PMID: 12509603].

Strober M, Freeman R, Morrell W: The long-term course of severe anorexia nervosa in adolescents: Survival analysis of recovery, relapse, and outcome predictors of 10–15 years in a prospective study. Int J Eat Disord 1997;22:339 [PMID: 9356884].

# Child & Adolescent Psychiatric Disorders & Psychosocial Aspects of Pediatrics

**6**

*Jennifer Hagman, MD, & Donald W. Bechtold, MD*

The task of the primary care provider is often to discern when symptoms are indicative of a problem versus a normal variant of development. When the symptoms include changes in behavior, thoughts, and emotions, the task becomes one of determining if a psychiatric disorder is present and what the contributing role of genetic and biologic factors, family and peer relationships, and environment may be.

## ■ PSYCHOSOCIAL ASPECTS OF CHILD DEVELOPMENT AND FAMILY LIFE

### FAMILY LIFE

The structure of families has changed significantly over the past two decades, with an increase in the number of single-parent homes, mothers who work outside the home, blended families, alternative lifestyles including gay and lesbian parents, and a decline in extended families living in close proximity. The family serves the following functions: (1) rearing children to become autonomous adults and eventually competent parents and (2) meeting the needs of family members for nurturing, protection, feedback, recognition (mirroring), promoting adaptive behaviors, and emotional closeness and support. Evidence suggests that the lifestyle preferences of the parent figures are less important to healthy development than is the parents' ability to serve parental functions consistently.

### THE PARENTAL UNIT

The cornerstone of family functioning is the parental unit, which optimally serves as the primary source of stability, consistency, and authority during childhood and adolescence. Effective parents (or adults in the parental role) should be aware of and responsive to the emotional and physical needs of other, more dependent family members while defining the norms of behavior that will lead to independent adaptive functioning in the future. The ways in which parents function in their roles within the family determines in large part the health or impairment of the family and its individual members.

Support systems, which include relatives, friends, and caregivers, serve an important function to help parents through life transitions from birth to the young adult years and beyond. In the case of a two-parent unit, the partners in a healthy relationship can provide the necessary emotional support, respite, and adult companionship for each other. The women's movement has helped men expand their parental roles and personal identities to include more nurturing activities. Because single parents often have no in-house source of adult support, relatives, friends, and other external support systems such as church, school, and childcare providers are critical. In single-parent families or families in which the parents are not able to meet each other's needs, the child is at risk of becoming a pseudoadult companion, thus completing the parental unit.

The lack of a solid parental partnership or effective support system for the family can be an important factor in virtually any child-centered problem. To function successfully as a couple, both partners must find the relationship satisfying through mutual nurturing and affirmation, trust and respect, conflict recognition and resolution, and intimacy and sexual satisfaction.

When the parental unit is weakened by dissatisfaction or by persistent conflict, children are at risk of becoming the focus of heightened parental attention and concern, thus displacing the conflict from within the relationship onto the child. Concern about the child distracts the parents from their own problems, and the child may function as a buffer between the adults. Questions designed to screen the quality of the marital and parental relationship are outlined in Table 6–6.

Beeber LS, Miles MS: Maternal mental health and parenting in poverty. Annu Rev Nurs Res 2003;21:303 [PMID: 12858701].

Hunfeld JA, Fauser BC, deBeaufort ID, Passchier JP: Child development and quality of parenting in lesbian families: No psychosocial indications for a-priori withholding of infertility treatment: A systematic review. Hum Reprod Update 2002;8(6):579 [PMID: 12498426].

Leinonen JA, Solantaus TS, Punamaki RL: Parental mental health and children's adjustment: The quality of marital interaction and parenting as mediating factors. J Child Psychology Psychiatry 2003;44(2)227 [PMID: 12587859].

Schor EL: American Academy of Pediatrics Task Force on the Family: Family Pediatrics, report of the Task Force on the Family. Pediatrics 2003;111(6 Pt 2):1541 [PMID: 12777595].

Wamboldt MZ, Wamboldt FS: Role of the family in the onset and outcome of childhood disorders: Selected research findings. J Am Acad Child Adolesc Psychiatry 2000;39(10):1212 [PMID: 11026173].

# EFFECTS OF MARITAL SEPARATION AND DIVORCE

Currently, about 40% of marriages will end in divorce. Seventy-five percent of divorced parents remarry, and another 50% divorce a second time. Approximately 90% of single parents are mothers, and in about half of such cases the children have little or no contact with the father.

## Clinical Effects of Separation and Divorce

The adverse emotional effects of divorce can be far-reaching for both adults and children. Many women who have been through a divorce report that it takes a minimum of 3 years for a sense of order and stability to return.

Effects on the parent–child relationship include a decrease in parenting capacity manifested by irregularity of schedules, flares of temper, lessening of emotional sensitivity and support of the child, inconsistent discipline, and decreased pleasure in the parent–child relationship. A tendency exists for the divorced parent to look to the child as a source of emotional support or even as a surrogate spouse. In the course of separation and divorce one parent may not be able to contain their angry thoughts about the other, and the child is subjected to a litany of complaints and negative statements, which can be confusing and painful for the child and significantly affect his or her ability to cope with the divorce. Some children may become inappropriately close to their parents by acting as little helpers and parental advisors. Adolescents, in contrast, may rebel in order to distance themselves from the emotional needs of their distressed parents.

The effects of divorce on children are seen most dramatically in the 2 years following dissolution of the marriage and depend largely on the parents' ability to maintain a working relationship with respect to parenting and financial issues related to the children. Few children experience the dissolution of even turbulent marriages as a relief, because the breakup of the nuclear family is perceived as a loss of the structure that provides for their safety and support. Children would rarely choose divorce as a solution for their parents' problems.

The effects of divorce on a child vary with the child's age and developmental level. Preschoolers may display symptoms of behavioral regression, expressing fears of separation at night and when they are with babysitters, sleep disturbances, and irritability. Children age 5–8 years may express their grief with sadness and weeping. Children often wish for reconciliation of the parents and may develop symptoms or behaviors that serve a secondary purpose of causing the parents to communicate or be together.

Approximately 50% experience a decrease in school performance, and some may become aggressive. Children age 9–12 years often respond with anger and blame and are at greatest risk of becoming a surrogate companion. In adolescence, anger often is accompanied by depression. Teenagers rely heavily on their peers during this time and can become pessimistic about their own future involvement in intimate relationships.

## Outcome

The most favorable outcome is for the parents to avoid discussion of their personal conflicts in the presence of the child and resume caregiving relationships with their children in a collaborative manner. Children do not cope well in a setting of unremitting marital strife, and overall development can be significantly affected. It is important that parents develop predictable routines for the children despite the challenges of separation and divorce. Younger children fare best, particularly when they have a support network (eg, siblings, grandparents) while the parents are preoccupied with their own problems. A brief course of psychotherapy should be considered for all parents and children who are going through separation and divorce. Therapy will assist with coping and communication during this difficult time and give the parents and children a place to discuss their fears and emotions with someone who is not directly involved in the situation.

Children of divorced parents experience increased rates of depression and anxiety, especially if the parents are not able to maintain a nonhostile working relationship regarding visitation and decisions related to the children's needs. At 10-year follow-up, 40% of such children report worry, underachievement, self-deprecation, and lingering anger. The effect of divorce on children may be far-reaching in scope and long-term in duration.

On reaching adulthood, children often fear repeating their parents' unhappy marriages and may struggle with issues of commitment and trust in intimate relationships.

Braver SL, Ellman IM, Fabricius WV: Relocation of children after divorce and children's best interests: New evidence and legal considerations. J Fam Psychol 2003;17(2):206 [PMID: 12828017].

Cohen GJ: American Academy of Pediatrics. Committee on Psychosocial Aspects of Child and Family Health: Helping children and families deal with divorce and separation. Pediatrics 2002;110(5):1019 [PMID: 12415046].

Kelly JB: Children's adjustment in conflicted marriage and divorce: A decade review of research. J Am Acad Child Adolesc Psychiatry 2000;39(8):963 [PMID: 10939225].

Pruett MK, Williams TY, Insabella G, Little TD: Family and legal indicators of child adjustment to divorce among families with young children. J Fam Psychol 2003;17(2):169 [PMID: 12828014].

Wallerstein JS: The long-term effects of divorce on children: A review. J Am Acad Child Adolesc Psychiatry 1991;30:349.

Wolchik SA et al: Six-year follow-up of preventive interventions for children of divorce: A randomized controlled trial. JAMA 2002;288(15):1874 [PMID: 12377086].

# CAREGIVER DYSFUNCTION

## Primary Caregiver Dysfunction

Primary caregiver dysfunction can be defined as a failure to provide parenting functions (usually, but not necessarily, by the mother) because of parental vulnerability or disability. Caregiver dysfunction can result from domestic violence, mental illness, and substance abuse. Caregivers can experience significant impairment because of anxiety, depression, exhaustion, anger, or indifference in relation to the demands of child care. Caregiver dysfunction can lead to a number of symptoms in the child (Table 6–1) and includes the risk of

another generation of children who may themselves display caregiver dysfunction as parents.

These individuals frequently have difficult psychosocial histories, find themselves without emotional or physical support, and have unmet personal needs (Table 6–2). Characteristics of the child may also contribute to the parent's failure to nurture and meet the child's needs. Risk factors from the child include prematurity, perinatal complications, birth defects, multiple births, chronic medical or mental illness, and a difficult temperament. These characteristics frequently define the child as different, defective, or disappointing in the parent's eyes.

Caregiver dysfunction is identified by interviewing the parents and observing the interaction between parent and child. The child should be evaluated for organic disorders that could explain the presenting symptoms. A history aimed at identifying specific parental risk factors should be obtained directly from the parent (see Table 6–2), with emphasis on feelings of stress or of being overwhelmed by the needs of the child or the demands of daily life. Attention should be paid to the parent's description of the child and to parental symptoms of anxiety or depression manifested by tension, irritability, fatigability, tearfulness, sleep disturbance, and a wish to avoid or withdraw from daily activities.

In observing the parent–child interaction, the physician should look for reciprocity, mutual enthusiasm, and enjoyment in the relationship, as opposed to pathologic signs of tension, irritability, or apathy on either side of the relationship. Physical disorders that may explain the presenting symptoms must be ruled out, but it should also be noted that caregiver dysfunction and organic disease often coexist.

Interventions are focused primarily on supporting and educating the parents and arranging referrals for as-

**Table 6–1.** Signs and symptoms suggesting primary caregiver dysfunction.

| |
|---|
| Failure to thrive |
| Feeding problems |
| Delays in development |
| Signs of abuse |
| Frequent physician visits, especially for nonspecific concerns |
| Excessive parental worry about illness in the child |
| Inadequate physical care |
| Child perceived as "difficult to deal with" |
| Sleep problems |

**Table 6–2.** Parental risk factors contributing to primary caregiver dysfunction.

| |
|---|
| History of inadequate relations with own mother |
| Isolation from an adult support system (eg, single parent) |
| Psychiatric disorders (particularly acute or chronic depression) |
| Chronic psychosocial or cognitive dysfunctions (eg, unstable relationships, school problems, legal problems, employment problems) |
| Unresolved grief over past losses |
| Marital discord |
| Poverty or financial problems |
| Personal or family illnesses |
| Unwanted or difficult pregnancy |
| Current life stresses (eg, loss of a relationship, recent illness, job loss) |

sessment and treatment of physical or mental illness when appropriate. The physician should empathize, explaining that being a parent is difficult and tiring work and that it requires health, energy, and emotional support. The task is to help the parent feel well physically and emotionally and then to facilitate the development of appropriate childcare skills. A social support system should be sought through friends, family, and community resources. Parenting skills can be taught and positively reinforced over time. Referrals can be made to parenting classes in the community or through mental health centers. Reports are necessary to the department of social services in cases where neglect or abuse is suspected.

The prognosis depends on the parent's receptiveness to professional interventions, support, and education. Follow-up by the physician's office regarding recommendations will increase the chance that interventions to support optimal family functioning will be successful.

American Academy of Child and Adolescent Psychiatry: Practice parameters for the psychiatric assessment of infants and toddlers (0–36 months). J Am Acad Child Adolesc Psychiatry 1997;36 supplement:21S.

Benjet C, Azar ST, Kuersten-Hogan R: Evaluating the parental fitness of psychiatrically diagnosed individuals: Advocating a functional-contextual analysis of parenting. J Fam Psychol 2003;17(2):238 [PMID: 12828020].

Keren M et al: Assessment of caregiver-child interaction in the context of a preschool psychiatric evaluation. Child Adolesc Psychiatr Clin N Am 1999;8:281.

Langrock AM et al: Coping with the stress of parental depression: Parents' reports of children's coping, emotional and behavioral problems. J Clin Child Adolesc Psychol 2002;31(3): 312 [PMID: 12149969].

Mayes LC: Addressing mental health needs of infants and young children. Child Adolesc Psychiatr Clin N Am 1999;8:209.

Zeanah CH, Boris NW, Larrieu JA: Infant development and developmental risk: A review of the past 10 years. J Am Acad Child Adolesc Psychiatry 1997;36:165.

# CHALLENGES IN PARENTING RELATED TO CHILD AND ADOLESCENT DEVELOPMENT

Parenting is challenging, rewarding, and frustrating. Physical and emotional exhaustion as well as unfulfilled expectations about parenting and family life can be avoided or mitigated if both partners share the parenting responsibilities, or if there is a strong support system available to the parents. Primary caregivers are also partly replenished emotionally by the child's positive responses and by memories of their own positive experiences as children. Children who are developmentally disabled or temperamentally difficult may be more unpredictable and challenging for the parent to respond to, and difficulty in the parent–child relationship may result. A mild consequence may be a state of tension in the family. In extreme situations, child abuse and neglect may result. Some parents have unrealistic fantasies about the children that may reflect their own unmet needs. Children with illnesses, disabilities, or temperamental difficulties call for modified expectations so that the parents can meet the special needs of the child.

Developmental disturbances are variations in normal child development that cause distress or concern. Parents frequently contact their physicians with questions about the terrible twos, childhood fears and anxieties, and adolescent rebellion. The health care provider is faced with making the correct diagnosis, educating the parents about normal developmental variations, and developing strategies to facilitate optimal parent–child interactions.

Each new phase of child development presents unique challenges. The infancy years are a time of irregular sleep–wake cycles and a need for almost constant care and attendance. During the toddler years, the child's strivings for autonomy and independence should be supported and encouraged within appropriate limits and without letting the child become the family tyrant. In the subsequent years, parents are faced with competitive challenges, requiring a balanced respect for the child's evolving wishes to be independent while still setting limits that maintain safety and respect for others.

## THE PUSHY PRESCHOOLER

The push for independence and autonomy that begins in the second year of life can pose problems for parents who are insecure in the parental role. Preschool children typically want to have their way even when it poses a danger or is not in their best interest. Children may try to decide when and what the family eats, what time is bedtime, and who sleeps in which bed, all as part of their rudimentary push to become independent. The parents' task is to respect the child's wish for self-determination while setting limits and providing guidance so that the child does not become tyrannical or out of control.

Parents who are having difficulty placing limits on behavior will come in with one of the following types of complaints:

1. Discipline won't work with this child.
2. I can't get her to do what I ask without getting mad.

3. He says, "I don't have to do it if I don't want to."
4. She won't sleep in her own bed.
5. Other children his age don't like him. He always wants his own way.

Parents who have difficulty saying no may be emotionally drained or may believe that confrontation must be avoided. In the former case, parental depression or emotional exhaustion from working and single parenthood is common. In the latter case, the parent typically overidentifies with the frustrated child's distress and is then reminded of painful conflicts or unhappiness in his or her own life. Keeping the child happy (ie, avoiding conflict) keeps the parent from feeling distressed and unhappy, but inevitably leads to more power struggles and defiant behavior.

In planning interventions, the physician must educate the parents about the sometimes pushy nature of preschool children within a healthy developmental context. With that explanation comes the need for external limits, because a child's judgment and self-control are as yet underdeveloped. Parents need to know that a child's disappointment and frustration with limits are a necessary component of growth and development.

Parents who are emotionally depleted or depressed need to be cared for themselves, either through rest, emotional support, and assistance with parenting or through referrals for therapy. In the case of a parent who avoids conflict, the physician should suggest addressing one or two discipline problems. For example, if toys are not picked up after a reminder, they are put away out of the child's reach for some specific period of time. As the parent begins to feel more comfortable with providing limits and appropriate consequences, the child's behavior typically becomes less oppositional; at this point, the parent should use positive reinforcement, such as, "I like the way you picked up your toys; let's read a story together."

## CHILDHOOD FEARS & ANXIETIES

During the elementary school years, parents must begin to let their children experience the challenges that await them outside the home. Parental support of development of these social and emotional skills must be balanced with realistic definitions of success. Persistent separation anxiety on the part of parents and unrealistic standards of performance can contribute to problems for the child in regulating anxiety and developing self-esteem during these years.

The vast majority of childhood fears are not associated with psychological disorders; in fact, the fearful stimuli tend to evolve and change with age in a devel-

**Table 6–3.** Sequence of developmental anxieties.

| Age at First Appearance | Source of Anxieties |
|---|---|
| Early infancy | Sudden loud noises, unpredictable stimuli, loss of postural support, heights. |
| 1 year | Stranger, unfamiliar situations and objects. Beginning of separation distress. |
| 2–6 years | Animals, darkness, imaginary creatures (ghosts and monsters). |
| School age | Bodily injury, physical danger. Fear of loss of loved one. |
| Teens and adulthood | Fear of failure (eg, test anxiety), concerns about social acceptance, loss of a loved one, physical danger, natural disasters. |

opmental sequence (Table 6–3) and, overall, tend to decrease in frequency and intensity with age.

Although the manifestations of many developmental anxieties, such as separation distress and fear of the dark, may wax and wane over months or years, most specific childhood fears are transient (days to weeks in duration) and not associated with substantial interference with daily life. In most cases, all that is needed is to reassure the parents about the developmental nature of fears; the parents can then reassure their children that they will be fine even though they feel frightened at times. Fears become a source of greater concern to health care providers when they appear outside the normal developmental sequence of fears, when they are persistent, when they cause severe distress, or when they interfere with adaptive functioning such as poor attendance at school or avoidance of peer relationships. Approximately 2–3% of preschool age children have fears troublesome enough to require specific mental health interventions such as referral to a child and adolescent psychiatrist.

Fraiberg SH: *The Magic Years: Understanding and Handling the Problems of Early Childhood.* Scribner, 1959.

Gilliam WS: Developmental assessment: Its role in comprehensive psychiatric assessment of young children. Child Adolesc Psychiatr Clin North Am 1999;8:225 [PMID: 10202587].

Hack S, Jellinek MS: Historical clues to the diagnosis of the dysfunctional child and other psychiatric disorders in children. Pediatr Clin North Am 1998;45(1):25 [PMID: 9491085].

Shapiro T, Hertig ME: Normal child and adolescent development. In Hales RE, Yudofsky SC (eds): *Essentials of Clinical Psychiatry.* American Psychiatric Press, 1999.

# ADOLESCENT REBELLION & TURMOIL

Adolescence is a time of considerable physical and emotional change. General theoretic impressions and sampling bias at one time tended to exaggerate the turmoil of normal adolescence. A longitudinal study of normal suburban middle-class boys through their high-school years identified only 21% as experiencing tumultuous unrest. On closer examination, this segment was distinguished from the remainder of the sample by lower socioeconomic status, more overt marital conflicts in the family, and a higher than normal incidence of mental illness in the family. Overall, approximately 20% of adolescents have a stormy course; another 20% progress continuously and smoothly through adolescence; and the remainder show normal overall adjustment but have transient difficulties during times of stress.

The early adolescent has unpredictable changes of mood, intense attachment to peers, and a self-centered point of view, all of which can diminish positive aspects of the parent–child relationship and lead to increased tension between the parent and the adolescent. Not since infancy and the toddler years have parents received so little gratitude for their efforts. Like parents of toddlers, the parents of young adolescents need to support autonomy while providing the structure and limits necessary to maintain safety and promote good decision making on the part of the adolescent.

The sexual interests of the middle adolescent can elicit parental reactions related to the parent's own comfort or concerns about sexuality and can range from pride to fear to envy or even confusion about sexual boundaries with the adolescent. The parents' own past experience may influence their reactions and ability to negotiate this developmental phase in a manner that facilitates communication while helping the teen make responsible decisions.

Finally, as the late adolescent prepares to leave home for college or other independent living, parents face, in addition to anxiety and excitement, the sense of loss and grief associated with their child going out into the world.

Of particular concern to physicians today, as well as to society at large, is the tragic increase in teen violence, including school shootings. Although the prediction of violent behavior remains a difficult and imprecise endeavor, physicians can support and encourage several important prevention efforts.

- The vast majority of the increase in youth violence including suicides and homicides involves the use of firearms. Thus the presence of firearms within the home, the method of storage and safety measures when present, and access to firearms outside the home should be explored regularly with all adolescents as part of their routine medical care.

- Although violence toward others remains difficult to predict, its association with suicidal impulses should not be overlooked. In general, the suicidal youth is somewhat easier to identify than the homicidal youth, and in many cases may be one and the same (see the section on Suicide in Children & Adolescents). Any comment about wishes to be dead or hopelessness should be taken seriously and help sought.

- Parents and guardians should be aware of their child's school attendance and performance and peer groups. They should know their children's friends and be aware of who they are going out with, where they will be, what they will be doing, and when they will be home. Any concerns should be discussed with the teen and interventions sought if necessary.

- Most students involved in school violence could have benefited from earlier interventions to address problems in social and educational functioning in the school environment. Many communities and school districts have increased their efforts to identify and intervene with students whom teachers, peers, or parents recognize as having difficulty.

Anderson M et al: School-associated violent deaths in the United States, 1994–1999. JAMA 2001;286(21):2695 [PMID: 11730445].

Birnbaum AS et al: School functioning and violent behavior among young adolescents: A contextual analysis. Health Educ Res 2003;18(3):389 [PMID: 12828239].

D'Angelo SL, Omar HA: Parenting adolescents. Int J Adolesc Med Health 2003;15(1):11 [PMID: 12723444].

Denninghoff KR et al: Emergency medicine: Competencies for youth violence prevention and control. Acad Emerg Med 2002;9(9):947 [PMID: 12208685].

Grant KE et al: Stressors and child and adolescent psychopathology: Moving from markers to mechanisms of risk. Psychol Bull 2003;129(3)447 [PMID: 12784938].

Group for the Advancement of Psychiatry, Committee on Preventive Psychiatry: Violent behavior in children and youth: Preventive intervention from a psychiatric perspective. J Am Acad Child Adolesc Psychiatry 1999;38:235 [PMID: 10087683].

Kruesi MJP et al: Suicide and violence prevention: Parent education in the emergency department. J Am Acad Child Adolesc Psychiatry 1999;38:250 [PMID: 10087685].

Monasterio EB: Enhancing resilience in the adolescent. Nurs Clin North Am 2002;37(3):373 [PMID: 12448999].

Olsson CA et al: Adolescent resilience: A concept analysis. J Adolesc 2003;26(1):1 [PMID 12550818].

Pontin LE: The Romance of Risk, Why Teenagers Do the Things They Do. Basic Books, 1997.

Twemlow SW, Fonagy P, Sacco FC: An innovative psychodynamically influenced approach to reduce school violence. J Am

Acad Child Adolesc Psychiatry 2001;49(3):377 [PMID: 11288781].

# ■ THE CHRONICALLY ILL CHILD

## Reactions to Chronic Physical or Mental Illness and Disability

Between 5% and 10% of individuals experience a prolonged period of medical illness or disability during childhood, and another 5–10% experience the onset of mental illness in childhood. The psychosocial effects for the child and the family are often profound. Although the specific effect of illness on children and their families depends on the characteristics of the illness, the age of the child, and premorbid functioning, it can be expected that both the child and the parents will go through predictable stages toward eventual acceptance of the disease state. Shock and disbelief at the time of diagnosis give way in time to anger and to mourning the loss of the normal, healthy child. It may take months for a family to accept the disease, to cope with the stresses, and to resume normal life to the extent possible. These stages resemble those that follow the loss of a loved one. If anxiety and guilt remain prominent within the family, a pattern of overprotection can evolve. Likewise, when the illness is not accepted as a reality to be dealt with, a pattern of denial may become prominent. The clinical manifestations of these patterns of behavior are presented in Table 6–4.

Children are very observant and intuitive when it comes to understanding their illness and its general

**Table 6–4.** Patterns of coping with chronic illness.

---

**Overprotection**
  Persistent anxiety or guilt
  Few friends and peer activities
  Poor school attendance
  Overconcern with somatic symptoms
  Secondary gain from the illness
**Effective coping**
  Realistic acceptance of limits imposed by illness
  Normalization of daily activities with peers, play, and school
**Denial**
  Lack of acceptance of the illness
  Poor medical compliance
  Risk-taking behaviors
  Lack of parental follow-through with medical instructions
  General pattern of acting-out behavior

---

prognosis. At the same time, their primary concerns are the effects of the illness on everyday life, feeling sick, and limitations on normal activities. Children are also keenly aware of the family's reactions and may be reluctant to bring up issues they know are upsetting to their parents. Whenever possible, parents should be encouraged to discuss the child's illness and to answer questions openly and honestly, including exploration of the child's fears and fantasies. Such interactions promote closeness and relieve the child's sense of isolation. Even with these active attempts to promote effective sharing between the child and the family, ill children frequently experience fear, anxiety, irritability, and anger over their illness and guilt over causing family distress. Sleep disturbances, tears, and clinging, dependent behavior are not infrequent or abnormal.

# THE TERMINALLY ILL CHILD

The diagnosis of fatal illness in a child is a severe blow even to families who have reason to suspect that outcome. The discussion with parents (and the child) about terminal illness is one of the most difficult tasks for a physician working with children and adolescents. Although parents want and need to know the truth, they are best told in stepwise fashion beginning with temporizing phrases such as, "The news is not good" and "This is a life-threatening illness." The parent's reactions and questions can then be observed for clues to how much they want to be told at any one time. The physician must also attempt to gauge how much of the information the parents are able to comprehend during the initial discussion and consider involvement of appropriate support services. Parent's reactions may proceed in a grief sequence including initial shock and disbelief lasting days to weeks, followed by anger, despair, and guilt over weeks to months, and ending in acceptance of the reality of the situation. These responses vary in intensity, duration, and sequence within the family.

Although children probably do not fully understand the permanency of death until about age 8, most ill children experience a sense of danger and doom that is associated with death before that age. Even so, the question of whether to tell a child about the fatal nature of a disease should in most cases be answered in the affirmative unless the parents object. When the parents object, this should alert the physician to involve the unit social worker, who can work with the family to ensure their decision is in the best interest of the child. Refusal of the adults to tell the child, especially when the adults themselves are very sad, leads to a conspiracy of silence that increases fear of the unknown in the child and leads to feelings of loneliness and isolation at the time of greatest need. In fact, children who are able to discuss their illness with family members are less depressed, have fewer behavior problems, have higher self-esteem, feel closer to their families, and adapt better to the challenges of their disease and its treatment.

The siblings of dying children are also significantly affected. They may feel neglected and deprived because of the time their parents must spend with the sick child. Anger and jealousy may then give rise to feelings of guilt over having such feelings about their sick sibling. Awareness of the emotional responses, coping abilities, and available resources for support of other family members can diminish these feelings and make a significant difference in the family's overall ability to cope with the illness.

After the child dies, the period of bereavement may last for years. Family members may need outside help in dealing with their grief through supportive counseling services or peer-support groups. Bereavement usually does not substantially interfere with overall life functioning for more than 2–3 months. Most parents and siblings are able to return to work and school within a month, although their emotional state and thoughts may continue to be dominated by the loss for some time. When the individual is unable to function in his or her societal and family role beyond this time frame, a diagnosis of complicated bereavement, major depression, posttraumatic stress disorder (PTSD), or adjustment disorder should be considered and appropriate interventions recommended, such as referral for counseling or psychotherapy and possibly antidepressant medication.

## Long-Term Coping

The process of coping with a chronic or terminal illness is complex and varies with the dynamics of each individual child and family. Each change in the course of the illness and each new developmental stage for the child present different challenges. It is important for health care providers to continually assess the family and child's needs and coping abilities over time and to provide appropriate support, information, and access to interventions.

## Assistance from Health Care Providers

### A. EDUCATE THE PATIENT AND FAMILY

Children and their families should be given information about the illness, including its course and treatment, at frequent intervals. Factual, open discussions minimize anxieties. The explanation should be comprehensible to all, and time should be set aside for questions and answers. The setting can be created with an invitation such as, "Let's take some time together to review the situation again."

### B. PREPARE THE CHILD FOR CHANGES AND PROCEDURES

The physician should explain, in an age-appropriate manner, what could be expected with a new turn in the illness or with upcoming medical procedures. This explanation enables the child to anticipate and in turn to master the new development and promotes trust between the patient and the health care providers.

### C. ENCOURAGE NORMAL ACTIVITIES

The child should attend school and play with peers as much as the illness allows. Individual education plans (IEP) should be requested from the school if accommodation beyond the regular classroom is necessary. At the same time, parents should be encouraged to apply the same rules of discipline and behavior to the ill child as are applied to well siblings.

### D. ENCOURAGE COMPENSATORY ACTIVITIES, INTERESTS, AND SKILL DEVELOPMENT

For example, a child whose athletic development has been interrupted by the disability might pursue the acquisition of computer skills.

### E. PROMOTE SELF-RELIANCE

The health care provider should guide and encourage parents in helping ill children assume responsibility for some aspects of their medical care.

### F. PERIODICALLY REVIEW FAMILY COPING

From time to time, the physician should ask, "How is everyone doing with this?" The feelings of the patient, the parents, and other children in the family are explored, as well as concerns about finances and the status of the marriage. Feelings of fear, guilt, anger, and grief should be watched for and accepted as normal reactions to difficult circumstances.

### G. RECOMMEND SUPPORT GROUPS

Appropriate lay support groups for the patient and family should be recommended. Many hospitals have such groups, and hospital social workers can facilitate participation for the patient and family.

Browning D: To show our humanness—Relational and communicative competence in pediatric palliative care. Bioethics Forum 2002;18(3-4):23 [PMID: 12744267].

Christian B: Growing up with chronic illness: Psychosocial adjustment of children and adolescents with cystic fibrosis. Annu Rev Nurs Res 2003;21:151 [PMID: 12858696].

Geist R, Grdisa V, Otley A: Psychosocial issues in the child with chronic conditions. Best Pract Res Clin Gastroenterol 2003;17(2):141 [PMID: 12676111].

Kubler-Ross E: *On Children and Death.* Collier Books, Macmillan Publishing, 1983.

Meyer EC et al: Parental perspective on end-of-life care in the pediatric intensive care unit. Crit Care Med 2002;30(1):226 [PMID: 11902266].

Oliver RC et al: Beneficial effects of a hospital bereavement intervention program after traumatic childhood death. J Trauma 2001;50(3):440 [PMID: 11265051].

Stewart JL: Children living with chronic illness; An examination of their stressors, coping responses and health outcomes. Annu Rev Nurs Res 2003;21:203 [PMID: 12858698].

Suris JC: Chronic conditions and adolescence. J Pediatr Endocrinol Metab 2003;16 (Suppl) 2:247 [PMID: 12729399].

Van Riper M: The sibling experience of living with childhood chronic illness and disability. Annu Rev Nurs Res 2003;21:279 [PMID: 12858700].

Waugh S: Parental views on disclosure of diagnosis to their HIV-positive children. AIDS Care 2003;15(2):169 [PMID 12856338].

# ■ SCREENING FOR PSYCHOSOCIAL PROBLEMS & PSYCHIATRIC DISORDERS WITHIN THE CONTEXT OF HEALTH MAINTENANCE VISITS

Between 5% and 15% of children in the United States have psychiatric disorders, and nearly 50% of pediatric office visits are related to psychosocial or developmental problems. These statistics underscore the importance of screening for mental illness and psychosocial problems in children and their families.

Most families seek help from their primary care providers when they are concerned about a child's health, growth, or development. It is thus critical that primary care providers be able to identify the need for, and initiate the evaluation of, mental health problems in children and adolescents.

The most efficient indicator in screening for psychosocial problems is the history provided by caregivers. Psychosocial information can be obtained from checklists, general questioning, and direct questioning. The most effective method is a combination of these three information-gathering techniques. Questions can be incorporated into the general pediatric office screening forms, or specific questionnaires can be used. The 34-item pediatric symptom checklist (Table 6–5) screens children age 6–12 years for psychosocial dysfunction. The checklist is to be completed in the waiting room by a parent or other caregiver. Each item is rated by the parents as often present (2 points), sometimes present (1 point), or never present (0 points). The information can be used in two ways: first, as a psychosocial review of symptoms and point of depar-

ture for the discussion of problems that often or sometimes occur; and second, as a general screening device, with a total score of 28 or higher indicating a need for in-depth psychosocial evaluation of the child.

Five questions forming the mnemonic PSYCH can be addressed to parents as a means of uncovering areas of concern. The questions can be rephrased slightly and then directed to children as well.

1. **P**arent–child interaction: How are things going with you and your child?
2. **S**chool: How are things going in school? (Academically and behaviorally.)
3. **Y**outh: How are things going with peer relationships?
4. **C**asa: How are things going at home? (Including siblings, the marriage, and parents as individuals.)
5. **H**appiness: How would you describe your child's mood? (Comfortable and happy versus tense and unhappy.)

Direct questions regarding age-appropriate behavior norms can then be reviewed. Concerns about infant attachment, the terrible twos, childhood fears, school problems, and adolescent behavioral problems can in this way be brought into the open for further discussion.

## ASSESSMENT OF BEHAVIORAL AND EMOTIONAL SIGNS AND SYMPTOMS

When an emotional or behavioral sign or symptom is present, a thorough evaluation is indicated. Information must be collected from caregivers, the child, and sometimes school personnel and others acquainted with the child's functioning. At least 30 minutes should be scheduled, and additional appointments may be necessary. Screening questions and guidelines for observation are given in Table 6–6.

It is useful to see both parents and the child first together, then the parents alone, and then the child alone. This sequence enables the physician to observe interactions among family members and gives the parents and the child an opportunity to talk confidentially about their concerns. Parents and children often feel shame and guilt about some personal inadequacy they perceive to be causing the problem. The physician can ease that burden and facilitate the assessment by acknowledging that the family is trying to cope and that the ultimate task of assessment is to seek solutions and not to assign blame. An attitude of nonjudgmental inquiry can be communicated with supportive statements such as, "Let's see if we can figure out what might be happening here and find some ways to make things better."

**Table 6–5.** Pediatric symptom checklist.[a]

| | Never | Sometimes | Often |
|---|---|---|---|
| 1. Complains of aches or pains | | | |
| 2. Spends more time alone | | | |
| 3. Tires easily, little energy | | | |
| 4. Fidgets, is unable to sit still | | | |
| 5. Has trouble with a teacher | | | |
| 6. Is less interested in school | | | |
| 7. Acts as if driven by a motor | | | |
| 8. Daydreams too much | | | |
| 9. Is distracted easily | | | |
| 10. Is afraid of new situations | | | |
| 11. Feels sad, unhappy | | | |
| 12. Is irritable, angry | | | |
| 13. Feels hopeless | | | |
| 14. Has trouble concentrating | | | |
| 15. Has less interest in friends | | | |
| 16. Fights with other children | | | |
| 17. Is absent from school | | | |
| 18. Experiences a drop in school grades | | | |
| 19. Is down on himself or herself | | | |
| 20. Visits doctor, with doctor finding nothing wrong | | | |
| 21. Has trouble with sleeping | | | |
| 22. Worries a lot | | | |
| 23. Wants to be with you more than before | | | |
| 24. Feels he or she is bad | | | |
| 25. Takes unnecessary risks | | | |
| 26. Gets hurt frequently | | | |
| 27. Seems to be having less fun | | | |
| 28. Acts younger than children the same age | | | |
| 29. Does not listen to rules | | | |
| 30. Does not show feelings | | | |
| 31. Does not understand other people's feelings | | | |
| 32. Teases others | | | |
| 33. Blames others for his or her troubles | | | |
| 34. Takes things that belong to others | | | |

[a]Parents are asked to indicate which category—Never, Sometimes, or Often—best fits their child, with 0, 1, or 2 points assigned to each answer, respectively. For interpretation of scores, see text.

Modified and reproduced, with permission, from Murphy JM, Jellinek M: Screening for psychosocial dysfunction in economically disadvantaged and minority children: Further validation of the pediatric symptom checklist. Am J Orthopsychiatry 1988;58:450. Copyright © 1988 by the American Orthopsychiatric Association.

*Table 6–6.* Screening for psychosocial problems.

**Developmental history**
1. Review the landmarks of psychosocial development
2. Summarize the child's temperamental traits
3. Review stressful life events and the child's reactions to them
   a. Separations
   b. Losses
   c. Marital conflict
   d. Illnesses, injuries, and hospitalizations
4. Obtain details of past mental health problems and their treatment

**Family history**
1. Marital history
   a. Overall satisfaction with the marriage
   b. Conflicts or disagreements within the relationship
   c. Quantity and quality of time together away from children
   d. Whether the child comes between or is a source of conflict between the parents
   e. Marital history prior to having children
2. Parenting history
   a. Feelings about parenthood
   b. Whether parents feel united in dealing with the child
   c. "Division of labor" in parenting
   d. Parental energy or stress level
   e. Sleeping arrangements
   f. Privacy
   g. Attitudes about discipline
   h. Interference with discipline from outside the family (eg, ex-spouses, grandparents)
3. Stresses on the family
   a. Problems with employment
   b. Financial problems
   c. Changes of residence
   d. Illness, injuries, and deaths
4. Family history of mental health problems
   a. Depression? Who?
   b. Suicide attempts? Who?
   c. Psychiatric hospitalizations? Who?
   d. "Nervous breakdowns"? Who?
   e. Substance abuse or problems? Who?
   f. Nervousness or anxiety? Who?

**Observation of the parents**
1. Do they agree on the existence of the problem or concern?
2. Are they uncooperative or antagonistic about the evaluation?
3. Do the parents appear depressed or overwhelmed?
4. Can the parents present a coherent picture of the problem and their family life?
5. Do the parents accept some responsibility for the child's problems, or do they blame forces outside the family and beyond their control?
6. Do they appear burdened with guilt about the child's problem?

**Observation of the child**
1. Does the child acknowledge the existence of a problem or concern?
2. Does the child want help?
3. Is the child uncooperative or antagonistic about the assessment?
4. What is the child's predominant mood or attitude?
5. What does the child wish could be different (eg, "three wishes")?
6. Does the child display unusual behavior (activity level, mannerisms, fearfulness)?
7. What is the child's apparent cognitive level?

**Observation of parent–child interaction**
1. Do the parents show concern about the child's feelings?
2. Does the child control or disrupt the joint interview?
3. Does the child respond to parental limits and control?
4. Do the parents inappropriately answer questions addressed to the child?
5. Is there obvious tension between family members?

**Data from other sources**
1. Waiting room observations by office staff
2. School (teacher, nurse, social worker, counselor)
3. Department of social services

## History of the Presenting Problem

First, obtain a detailed description of the problem.

- When did it start?
- Were there unusual stresses at that time?
- How are the child's life and the family's functioning affected?
- What does the child say about the problem?

- What attempts have been made to alleviate the problem?
- Do the parents have any opinions about the cause of the problem?

Questions to screen for other psychosocial problems, listed in Table 6–6, can be asked when additional information is sought.

## Interviewing the Preschool Child

Preschool children should be interviewed with their parents. As the parents discuss their concerns, the physician can look for the following behaviors:

1. Does the child use the parents as a source of security and support?
2. Does the 2- to 5-year-old child warm up to the strange environment and begin to explore the room and even interact with the physician from a distance?
3. How does the child relate to toys that are offered?
4. What is the child's activity level?
5. Does the child display unusual mannerisms (eg, intense clinging, stereotypical motor behaviors)?
6. Does the child disrupt or attempt to control the interview?
7. Do the parents attempt to place appropriate limits on behavior? How does the child respond?

It is helpful to have toy human figures, animals, or puppets, and crayons and paper available that the child can use to portray emotional states and interpersonal interactions. After hearing the history from the parents and after observing the child, the physician may question the 3- to 5-year-old child about toy figures who appear to be feeling sad, worried, angry, or bossy. Children age 3–5 years are frequently able to confirm important interpersonal relationships and attitudes in such symbolic play activities.

## Interviewing the School-Age Child

Most school-age children have mastered separation anxiety sufficiently to tolerate at least a brief interview alone with the physician. In addition, they may have important information to share about their own worries. The child should be told beforehand by the parents or physician (or both) that the doctor will want to talk to the child about his or her feelings. School-age children understand and even appreciate parental concern about unhappiness, worries, and difficulty in getting along with people. At the outset, it is useful to confirm that the purpose of the interview is to explore the child's own opinions about certain issues raised by the parents. Rapport can be enhanced by asking if the child has ever talked with anyone else about how he or she feels. If the answer is affirmative, the child may explain more about what he or she liked or did not like about that discussion. If the child has never before talked about personal feelings with a professional, the physician can acknowledge that it is often not easy to talk with a stranger about some kinds of problems. The physician should then ascertain whether the child

agrees that a problem exists (eg, unhappiness, anxiety, sleep disturbance).

- The physician should ask the child to describe the problem in his or her own words, or ask what he or she thinks is causing the problem.
- It is important to ask the child how the problem affects the child and the family.
- Asking directly about how mom and dad get along can yield information about parental conflicts.
- Questions about school can yield information about life outside the home and with peers.
- Questions about worries, unhappy feelings, and what makes the child angry can elicit clues to the child's emotional life.
- Asking a child to make three wishes can uncover important concerns that may not have been apparent from the history: Let's pretend you could have anything or change anything. What would you wish for and why?

At the end of the interview with the child, it is important to share or reiterate the central points derived from the interview and to state that the next step is to talk with the parents about ways to make things better for the child. At that time, it is good to discuss any concerns or misgivings the child might have about sharing information with parents so that the child's right to privacy is not arbitrarily violated. Most children want to make things better and thus will allow the physician to share appropriate concerns with the parents.

## Interviewing the Adolescent

Because the central developmental task of adolescence is to create an identity separate from that of the parents, the physician must show respect for the teen's point of view. That process usually begins with the physician meeting briefly with the parents and adolescent together to define the concerns. The physician should then meet alone with the adolescent. After the physician has interviewed the adolescent and talked further with the parents, he or she should formulate thoughts and recommendations. Whenever possible, it is helpful to discuss these with the adolescent before presenting them to the parents and teen together. The issue of confidentiality must be approached during the first interview. A good policy is to say, "What we talk about today is between you and me unless we decide someone should know or unless it appears to me that you might be in a potentially dangerous situation."

The interview with the adolescent alone might then start with a restatement of the parents' concern. The patient is then encouraged to describe the situation in his or her own words. The physician should then ask questions about:

1. Predominant mood state
2. Nature of relationships with family members
3. Level of satisfaction with school and peer relationships
4. Plans for the future
5. Drug and alcohol use
6. Sexual activity
7. Worries or concerns
8. What the adolescent would like to be different

In concluding the interview, the physician should summarize his or her thoughts and develop a plan with the teenager to present to the parents. If teenagers participate in the solution, they are more likely to work with the family in improving the situation. This should include a plan either for further investigation or for ways of dealing with the problem and arranging subsequent appointments with the physician or an appropriate referral to a mental health provider.

## DIAGNOSTIC FORMULATION AND INTERPRETATION OF FINDINGS

Diagnosis starts with a description of the presenting problem, which is then evaluated within the context of the child's age, developmental needs and tasks, and temperament; the stresses and strains on the child and the family; and the functioning of the family system and family history of mental illness. The physician then develops an etiologic hypothesis based on the information gathered:

1. The behavior falls within the range of normal given the child's developmental level.
2. The behavior is a temperamental variation.
3. The behavior is related to central nervous system impairment (eg, prematurity, exposure to toxins in utero, seizure disorder, genetic disorders).
4. The behavior is a normal reaction to stressful circumstances (eg, medical illness, change in family structure, loss of a loved one).
5. The problem is primarily a reflection of family dysfunction (eg, the child is the symptom bearer, or scapegoat, or the identified patient for the family).
6. The problem indicates a possible psychiatric disorder.
7. The problem is complicated by an underlying medical condition.
8. Some combination of the preceding.

The physician's first task is to decide whether a problem exists. For example, how hyperactive must a 5-year-old child be before he or she is too hyperactive? Functional impairment may be the single best marker of the difference between symptomatology and normal variation. When a child's function is impaired in major domains of life, such as learning, peer relationships, family relationships, authority relationships, and recreation, or when a substantial deviation from the trajectory of normal developmental tasks occurs, a differential diagnosis should be sought based on the symptom profile. The physician's interpretation is then presented to the family. The interpretive process includes the following components:

1. An explanation of how the presenting problem or symptom is a reflection of a suspected cause
2. A suggested plan of intervention based on the presumed cause
3. A discussion of any further evaluation necessary to confirm or refine a diagnosis

A joint plan involving the physician, parents, and child is then negotiated to address the child's symptoms and developmental needs in light of the family structure and stresses. If an appropriate plan cannot be developed, or if the physician feels that further diagnostic assessment is required, referral to a mental health practitioner should be recommended.

Cassidy SJ, Jellinek M: Approaches to recognition and management of childhood psychiatric disorders in pediatric primary care. Pediatr Clin North Am 1998;45(5):1037 [PMID: 9884674].

Fritz G: Promoting effective collaboration between pediatricians and child and adolescent psychiatrists. Pediatr Ann 2003; 32(6):387 [PMID: 12846016].

Gardner W et al: Primary care clinicians' use of standardized tools to asses child psychosocial problems. Ambul Pediatr 2003; 3(4):191 [PMID: 12882596].

Hack S, Jellinek M: Early identification of emotional and behavioral problems in a primary care setting. Adolesc Med: State of the Art Reviews 1998,9(2):335 [PMID: 10961240].

Murphy JM et al: Screening for psychosocial dysfunction in pediatric practice. Clin Pediatr 1992;31:660 [PMID: 10961240].

Weist MD, Ginsburg, Shafer M: Progress in adolescent mental health. Adolesc Med: State of the Art Reviews 1999;10(1): 165 [PMID: 10086173].

# ■ PSYCHIATRIC DISORDERS OF CHILDHOOD & ADOLESCENCE

A psychiatric disorder is defined as a characteristic cluster of signs and symptoms (eg, emotions, behaviors, thought patterns, and mood states) that are associated with subjective distress or maladaptive behavior. This definition presumes that the individual's symptoms are of such intensity, persistence, and duration that the ability to adapt to life's challenges is compromised.

Psychiatric disorders have their origins in neurobiology, genetics, psychological (life experience), or environmental sources. The neurobiology of childhood disorders is today one of the most active areas of investigation in child and adolescent psychiatry. Although much remains to be clarified, data from genetic studies point to heritable transmission of attention-deficit/hyperactivity disorder (ADHD), schizophrenia, mood and anxiety disorders, pervasive developmental disorders, learning disorders, and tic disorders, among others. About 3–5% of children and 10–15% of adolescents are personally affected by psychiatric disorders and will benefit from psychiatric treatment.

The Diagnostic and Statistical Manual IV—text revision (DSM-IV-TR) is the formal reference text for psychiatric disorders and includes the criteria for each of the mental illnesses, including those that begin in childhood and adolescence. Psychiatric diagnoses are given on five axes to allow the physician to address the developmental, medical, psychosocial, and overall adaptive issues that contribute to the primary diagnosis on axis I or II.

**Axis I:** Clinical disorders and other conditions that may be a focus of clinical attention

**Axis II:** Personality disorders, mental retardation, learning disabilities

**Axis III:** General medical conditions

**Axis IV:** Psychosocial and environmental problems

**Axis V:** Global assessment of functioning (on a scale of 0–100, with 100% being the highest level of functioning)

Primary care physicians often are the first to identify and recommend treatment for mental illness in children and adolescents. Criteria for referral to a child and adolescent psychiatrist are listed in Table 6–7.

American Psychiatric Association: *Diagnostic and Statistical Manual of Mental Disorders—Text Revision.* American Academy of Pediatrics, 2000.

# PERVASIVE DEVELOPMENTAL DISORDERS & AUTISM

Pervasive developmental disorders (PDD) and childhood autism are early-onset, severe neuropsychiatric disorders that were once referred to as childhood psychoses. PDD (including autistic disorder) are now distinguished from childhood schizophrenia on the basis

**Table 6–7.** When to consider consultation or referral to a child and adolescent psychiatrist.

---

Diagnosis is not clear
Pediatrician feels further assessment is needed
Pediatrician believes medication may be needed, but will not be prescribing
Pediatrician has started medications and needs further psychopharmacologic consultation
Individual, family, and/or group psychotherapy is needed.
Psychotic symptoms (hallucinations, paranoia) are present
Bipolar affective disorder is suspected.

---

of clinical differences and family histories. The term PDD denotes a group of disorders with the common findings of impairment of socialization skills and characteristic behavioral abnormalities. Speech and language deficits are common as well.

## 1. Autistic Disorder

### ESSENTIALS OF DIAGNOSIS & TYPICAL FEATURES

- Severe deficits in social responsiveness and interpersonal relationships.
- Abnormal speech and language development.
- Behavioral peculiarities such as ritualized, repetitive, or stereotyped behaviors; rigidity; and poverty of age-typical interests and activities.
- Onset in infancy or early childhood (before age 3 years).

### General Considerations

Autistic disorder is uncommon, with an incidence of approximately 4 cases per 10,000 school-age children. More boys than girls are affected (3:1). Although the cause of autistic disorder is unknown, central nervous system dysfunction is suggested by its higher incidence in populations affected by perinatal disorders: rubella, phenylketonuria, tuberous sclerosis, infantile spasms, encephalitis, and fragile X syndrome. Studies of twins reveal over 90% concordance for autistic disorder in monozygotic twins compared with 24% in dizygotic twins. Twenty-five percent of families with an autistic child have other family members with language-related disorders. (See also Chapter 2.)

## Clinical Findings

Severe deficits in reciprocal social interaction (eg, delayed or absent social smile, failure to anticipate interaction with caregivers, and a lack of attention to a primary caregiver's face) are often evident even in the first year of life. In toddlers, findings include deficiencies in imitative play and a relative lack of interest in interactions with others. Language development is often quite delayed. In fact, children are often first referred for audiologic evaluation because of failure to respond as expected to sounds. When speech does begin to develop, it may be echolalic or nonsensical. Autistic children often display peculiar interests; bizarre responses to sensory stimuli; repetitive, stereotypical motor behaviors (eg, twirling, hand-flapping); odd posturing; self-injurious behavior; abnormal patterns of eating and sleeping; and unpredictable mood changes. Thematic pretend play is often impaired. An intense preoccupation with an age-unusual interest (eg, power poles) may replace the usual broad range of interests of the child's agemates. About 70% of autistic children have intelligence quotients under 70.

## Differential Diagnosis

Although most autistic children function at the mentally retarded level, the vast majority of mentally retarded children do not show the essential characteristics of autistic disorder. A hearing or visual impairment must be ruled out with appropriate screening. Children with developmental speech and language disorders typically show better interpersonal interactions than autistic children. Evaluation should include investigations for metabolic disorders and fragile X syndrome.

## Complications

Approximately 25% of autistic individuals eventually develop a seizure disorder. Comorbid psychiatric disorders such as mood disorders should be screened for if significant changes in behavior occur. Some autistic adolescents who have higher cognitive skills become depressed as they become partially aware of their deficits.

## Treatment

Parents and families need strong support as well as education in caring for a child with autism. Early interventions to facilitate the development of reciprocal interactions, language, and social skills are critical. Occupational therapy for sensory integration is also an integral component of the comprehensive assessment. Sensory integration interventions help the autistic child and help the family better support the child and adapt the environment to their specific needs.

Behaviorally oriented special education classes or day treatment programs are vital in helping the autistic child acquire more appropriate social, linguistic, self-care, and cognitive skills.

No specific medications are available to treat autistic disorder. Pharmacotherapy is aimed at reducing specific target symptoms and must be continually assessed and reevaluated for efficacy and side effects. Coexisting diagnoses must be carefully considered. Neuroleptic medications (eg, risperidone, olanzapine, and haloperidol) may modify a variety of disruptive symptoms, including hyperactivity, aggressiveness, and negativism. Fenfluramine may help the subset of autistic children with low serotonin levels (although serotonin levels are very difficult to measure). Psychostimulants may benefit concurrent ADHD symptoms but can sometimes worsen behavior or mood. Antidepressants—especially the selective serotonin reuptake inhibitors (SSRIs)—may benefit both mood symptoms and symptoms of excessive rigidity or obsessive behavior. Mood stabilizers may diminish irritability, lability, or episodic dyscontrol. Naltrexone may help control severe self-injurious behavior or stereotypes. Controlled studies do not support the use of secretin for autism.

Parents and families need strong support as well as education in caring for a child with autism. Early interventions to facilitate the development of reciprocal interactions, language, and social skills are critical. Occupational therapy for sensory integration is also an integral component of the comprehensive assessment. Sensory integration interventions help the autistic child and help the family better support the child and adapt the environment to their specific needs.

## Prognosis

Autism is a lifelong disorder. The best prognosis is for children who have normal intelligence and have developed symbolic language skills by age 5 years. Most individuals with autism will not be able to live independently and will require significant support and supervision throughout their lives. Approximately one sixth of autistic children become gainfully employed as adults, and another one sixth are able to function in sheltered workshops or special work and school environments. The remainder need ongoing supervision and support, often in a milieu-based therapeutic environment to provide a structured day. Placement in specialized residential homes or programs may be necessary for some individuals whose guardians are unable to meet their special needs or provide a secure and safe home environment.

Chakrabarti S, Fombonne E: Pervasive developmental disorders in preschool children. JAMA 2002;285(24):3093 [PMID: 11427137].

Dunn-Geier J, Ho H, Auersperg E, et al: Effect of secretin on children with autism: A randomized controlled trial. Dev Med Child Neurol 2000;42:796 [PMID: 11132252].

McDougle CJ et al: Research Units on pediatric psychopharmacology (RUPP) Autism Network: Background and rationale for an initial controlled study of risperidone. Child Adolesc Psychiatr Clin North Am 2000;9(1):201 [PMID: 10674197].

Practice parameters for the assessment and treatment of children, adolescents and adults with autism and other pervasive developmental disorders. J Am Acad Child Adolesc Psychiatry 1999;38(12, Suppl):32S [PMID: 10624084].

Prater CD, Zylstra RG: Autism: A medical primer. Am Fam Physician 2002;66(9):1667 [PMID: 12449265].

Santosh PJ, Baird G: Pharmacotherapy of target symptoms in autistic spectrum disorders. Indian J Pediatr 2002;68(5):427 [PMID: 11407159].

## 2. Nonautistic Pervasive Developmental Disorders

Asperger syndrome, childhood disintegrative disorder, pervasive developmental disorder not otherwise specified (PDD-NOS), and Rett syndrome (Table 6–8).

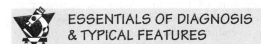

### ESSENTIALS OF DIAGNOSIS & TYPICAL FEATURES

- Substantial social impairment, either primary or representing a loss of previously acquired social skills.
- Abnormalities in speech and language development or behavior resembling autistic disorder.
- Onset by early childhood (may be as late as age 9 years in childhood disintegrative disorder).

### General Considerations

Children with nonautistic PDDs display a wide range of deficits in social, language, and behavioral skills that are similar to those in children with autistic disorder. However, these children deviate from the clinical profile for autistic disorder by failing to meet all the necessary diagnostic criteria, by failing to fulfill severity threshold (ie, milder functional impairment), by manifesting atypical symptomatology (eg, the characteristic hand-wringing or gender distribution in Rett syndrome), or by experiencing onset at a later age. In the past, many of these children would have been classified in the group manifesting so-called atypical development. Children with nonautistic PDDs probably outnumber autistic children by as much as 2–3:1.

### Differential Diagnosis

Specific developmental speech and language disorders should be distinguished. Hearing impairment should be ruled out with appropriate screening.

### Treatment

The backbone of treatment for Asperger syndrome and PDD-NOS is an adaptive behavioral approach aimed at teaching and reinforcing more appropriate social and language skills and behaviors. Rett syndrome and childhood disintegrative disorder have much worse prognoses and call for multidisciplinary, often milieu-based interventions (as for autistic disorder). Occupational therapy for sensory integration interventions may be helpful. In all cases, family education and support are important.

Children should be screened for the presence of other psychiatric conditions, including mood disorders, obsessive–compulsive disorder (OCD), ADHD, and

**Table 6–8.** Characteristics of nonautistic pervasive developmental disorders.

| Disorder | Age at Onset | Clinical Features |
|---|---|---|
| Asperger's syndrome | Early childhood | "Odd" individuals (probably more common in males) with normal intelligence, motor clumsiness, eccentric interests, and a limited ability to appreciate social nuances |
| Childhood disintegrative disorder | 3–4 years | Profound deterioration to severe autistic disorder |
| Pervasive developmental disorder | Early childhood | Two to three times more common than autistic disorder, with similar but less severe symptoms |
| Rett syndrome | 5 months to 4 years old | Females with reduced head circumference and loss of social relatedness who develop stereotyped hand movements and have impaired language and mental functioning |

anxiety disorders, and appropriate interventions should be initiated. Psychoactive medications may be helpful for treating specific target symptoms as described for autistic disorder.

## Prognosis

These are lifelong disorders. The prognosis is variable depending on the severity of social and language deficits and response to treatment interventions.

Starr E et al: Stability and change among high-functioning children with pervasive developmental disorders: A 2-year outcome study. J Autism Dev Disord 2003;33(1):15 [PMID: 12708576].

Tanguay P: Pervasive developmental disorders: A 10 year review. J Am Acad Child Adolesc Psychiatry 2000;39(9):1079 [PMID: 10986804].

Volkmar FR et al: Nonautistic pervasive developmental disorders. In Coffey CE, Brombach RA (eds): *Textbook of Pediatric Neuropsychiatry.* American Psychiatric Press, 1998.

# MOOD DISORDERS

## 1. Depression in Children & Adolescents

### ESSENTIALS OF DIAGNOSIS & TYPICAL FEATURES

- Dysphoric mood, mood lability, irritability or depressed appearance, persisting for days to months at a time.
- Characteristic neurovegetative signs and symptoms (changes in sleep, appetite, concentration, and activity levels).
- Suicidal ideation, feeling of hopelessness

## General Considerations

The incidence of depression in children increases with age, from 1–3% before puberty to around 8% for adolescents. The rate of depression in females approaches adult levels by age 15. The lifetime risk of depression ranges from 10–25% for women and 5–12% for men. The incidence of depression in children is higher when other family members have been affected by depressive disorders. The sex incidence is equal in childhood, but with the onset of puberty the rates of depression for females begin to exceed those for males by 5:1.

## Clinical Findings

Clinical depression can be defined as a persistent state of unhappiness or misery that interferes with pleasure or productivity. The signs and symptoms of depression are surprisingly constant from early childhood to adolescence and adulthood (Table 6–9). The dysphoria of depression in children and adolescents is as likely to be an irritable mood state accompanied by tantrums or verbal outbursts, as it is to be a sad mood. Typically, a child or adolescent with depression begins to look unhappy and may make comments such as "I have no friends," "Life is boring," "There is nothing I can do to make things better," or "I wish I were dead." A change in behavior patterns usually takes place that includes social isolation, deterioration in schoolwork, loss of interest in usual activities, and flashes of anger and irritability. Sleep and appetite patterns commonly change, and the child may complain of tiredness and nonspecific pain such as headaches or stomachaches.

## Differential Diagnosis

Clinical depression can be identified by asking about the symptoms. Children are often more accurate than their caregivers in assessing their own mood state. When several depressive symptoms cluster together over time and are persistent (2 weeks or more) and severe, a diagnosis of major depressive disorder is appropriate. When symptoms are fewer and of lesser severity

**Table 6–9.** Clinical manifestations of depression in children and adolescents.

| Depressive Symptom | Clinical Manifestations |
|---|---|
| Anhedonia | Loss of interest and enthusiasm in play, socializing, school, and usual activities; boredom; loss of pleasure |
| Dysphoric mood | Tearfulness; sad, downturned expression; unhappiness; slumped posture; quick temper; irritability; anger |
| Fatigability | Lethargy and tiredness; no play after school |
| Morbid ideation | Self-deprecating thoughts, statements; thoughts of disaster, abandonment, death, suicide, or hopelessness |
| Somatic symptoms | Changes in sleep or appetite patterns; difficulty in concentrating; bodily complaints, particularly headache and stomachache |

but have persisted for months or years, a diagnosis of dysthymic disorder is justified. Milder symptoms of short duration in response to some stressful life event warrant a diagnosis of adjustment disorder with depressed mood (See Table 6–9).

Rating scales of mood can be helpful in assessing child and adolescent patients. The Child Depression Inventory (CDI), the BECK Depression Rating Scale, and the Reynolds Adolescent Depression Scale are easily used in primary care.

Substantial rates of comorbidity of depression are associated with ADHD, conduct disorders, anxiety disorders, eating disorders, and substance abuse disorders. Medically ill patients also have an increased incidence of depression. Every child and adolescent with a depressed mood state should be asked directly about suicidal ideation and physical and sexual abuse. Depressed adolescents should also be screened for hypothyroidism and substance abuse.

## Complications

Because the emotional pain associated with depression can be intensely distressing, the child or adolescent may consider suicide (see section on Suicide in Children & Adolescents). In addition, adolescents have a propensity to avoid the pain of depression through substance abuse or excitement-seeking behaviors (eg, partying, negativism and defiance, reckless behavior). School performance usually suffers during a depressive episode as children are unable to concentrate or motivate themselves to complete homework or projects. The irritability, isolation, and withdrawal that often result from the depressive episode can lead to loss of peer relationships and tense dynamics within the family.

## Treatment

Treatment includes identifying the symptoms of depression and developing a comprehensive plan to treat the depressive episode and help the caregivers to respond more effectively to the patient's emotional needs. Referrals should be made for individual and family therapy. In therapy, efforts are made to resolve conflicts between family members, improve communication skills within the family, and increase the opportunity for enjoyable time spent together. Attitudes, expectations, and disciplinary methods are evaluated. The child is encouraged to become involved in activities and to pursue opportunities for maximizing skills and talents. Individual psychotherapy aimed at identifying pervasively negative thoughts and correcting negativistic cognitive distortions can increase the patient's awareness of care and concern on the part of adults. It

also helps the young person to identify, label, and verbalize feelings and misperceptions.

Antidepressant medications should be considered for all patients with a depressive diagnosis (Table 6–10). When the symptoms of depression are moderate to severe and persistent and have begun to interfere with relationships and school performance, antidepressant medications may be indicated. Mild depressive symptoms often do not require antidepressant medications and may improve with psychotherapy alone. A positive family history of depression increases the risk of early-onset depression in children and adolescents and chances of a positive response to antidepressant medication.

## Prognosis

A comprehensive treatment intervention, including psychotherapy, medication assessment, and evaluation of school and home environments, often leads to complete remission of depressive symptoms over a 1- to 2-month period. If medications are started and prove effective, they must be continued for 6–9 months after remission of symptoms to prevent relapse. Early-onset depression (before age 15) is associated with increased risk of recurrent episodes and the potential need for longer term treatment with antidepressants. Education of the family and child (or adolescent) will help them identify depressive symptoms sooner and limit the severity of future episodes with earlier interventions. Some studies suggest that up to 30% of preadolescents with major depression manifest bipolar disorder at 2-year follow-up. It is important to reassess the child or adolescent with depressive symptoms regularly for at least 6 months and to maintain awareness of the depressive episode in the course of well-child care.

American Academy of Child and Adolescent Psychiatry: Practice parameters for the assessment and treatment of children and

**Table 6–10.** Interventions for the treatment of depression.

| Adjustment disorder | Refer for psychotherapy | Medications usually not needed |
|---|---|---|
| Mild depression | Refer for psychotherapy | Medications may not be needed |
| Moderate depression | Refer for psychotherapy | Consider antidepressant medication |
| Severe depression | Refer for psychotherapy | Strongly encourage antidepressant medication |

adolescents with depressive disorders. J Am Acad Child Adolesc Psychiatry 1998;37(10, Suppl:63S [PMID: 9785729].

Asarnow JR, Jaycox LH, Tompson MC: Depression in youth: Psychosocial interventions. J Clin Child Psychol 2001;30(1): 33 [PMID: 11294076].

Birmaher B, Arbalaez C, Brent D: Course and outcome of child and adolescent major depressive disorder. Child Adolesc Psychiatr Clin North Am 2002;11(3):619 [PMID: 12222086].

Emslie GJ et al: Fluoxetine for acute treatment of depression in children and adolescents: A placebo-controlled randomized clinical trial. J Am Acad Child Adolesc Psychiatry 2002;41(10):1205 [PMID: 12364842].

Olsen AL et al: Primary care pediatrician's roles and perceived responsibility in the identification and management of depression in children and adolescents. Ambulatory Pediatr 2001; 1(2):91 [PMID: 11888379].

Practice parameters for the assessment and treatment of children and adolescents with depressive disorders. J Am Acad Child Adolesc Psychiatry 1998;31(10, supp):63S.

Ryan ND: Diagnosing pediatric depression. Biol Psychiatry 2001;49(12):1050 [PMID: 11430846].

Ryan ND: Medication treatment for depression in children and adolescents. CNS Spectr 2003;8(4):283 [PMID: 1267943].

Stingard RJ: The neuroscience of depression in adolescence. J Affect Disord 2000;61 (Suppl 1):15 [PMID: 11155964].

Strober M et al: The course of major depressive disorder in adolescents: I. Recovery and risk of manic switching in a follow-up of psychotic and non-psychotic subtypes. J Am Acad Child Adolesc Psychiatry 1993;32:34.

## 2. Bipolar Affective Disorder

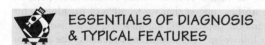

ESSENTIALS OF DIAGNOSIS & TYPICAL FEATURES

- *Periods of abnormally and persistently elevated, expansive, or irritable mood, and heightened levels of energy and activity.*
- *Not caused by prescribed or illicit drugs.*
- *Associated symptoms: grandiosity, diminished need for sleep, pressured speech, racing thoughts, impaired judgment.*

## General Considerations

Bipolar affective disorder (previously referred to as manic–depressive disorder) is an episodic mood disorder manifested by alternating periods of mania or hypomania and depressive episodes or, less commonly, manic episodes alone. Children and adolescents often exhibit a variable course of mood instability combined with misconduct and impulsivity. At least 20% of bipolar adults experience onset of symptoms before age 20 years. Onset of bipolar disorder before puberty is thought to be uncommon, whereas the lifetime prevalence of bipolar disorder in middle to late adolescence approaches 1%.

## Clinical Findings

In about 70% of patients, the first symptoms are primarily those of depression; in the remainder, manic, hypomanic, or mixed states dominate the presentation. Manic patients display a variable pattern of elevated, expansive, or irritable mood along with more rapid speech, higher energy levels, some difficulty in sustaining concentration, and a decreased need for sleep. Patients often do not acknowledge any problem with their mood or behavior. The clinical picture can be quite dramatic, with florid psychotic symptoms of delusions and hallucinations (a full-blown manic psychosis), more subtle changes and lability in mood or behavior (cyclothymia), or milder symptoms of psychomotor activation (hypomania).

## Differential Diagnosis

ADHD is thought to be highly comorbid with bipolar disorder in prepubertal children. Physical or sexual abuse and exposure to domestic violence can often cause children to appear mood labile, hyperactive, and aggressive, and PTSD should be considered by reviewing the history for traumatic life events in children with these symptoms. Diagnostic considerations should also include an acute organic process, particularly substance abuse disorder. Individuals with manic psychosis may resemble those with schizophrenia. Psychotic symptoms associated with bipolar disorder should clear with resolution of the mood symptoms, which should also be prominent. Hyperthyroidism should be ruled out. In prepubescent children, mania may be difficult to differentiate from ADHD and other disruptive behavior disorders. Preoccupation with violence, decreased need for sleep, intense and prolonged rages or dysphoria, and some periodicity of symptom activity suggest bipolar disorder. Table 6–11 further defines points of differentiation between ADHD, conduct disorder, and bipolar disorder.

## Complications

Children and adolescents with bipolar disorder are more likely to be aggressive or assaultive toward peers and family members. This may also result in significant interference with academic learning and peer relationships. The poor judgment associated with manic episodes predisposes to dangerous, impulsive, and sometimes criminal activity. Legal difficulties can arise

*Table 6–11.* Differentiating behavior disorders.

| | ADHD | Conduct Disorder | Bipolar Disorder |
|---|---|---|---|
| School problems | Yes | Yes | Yes |
| Behavior problems | Yes | Yes | Yes |
| Defiant attitude | Occasional | Constant | Episodic |
| Motor restlessness | Constant | May be present | May wax and wane |
| Impulsivity | Constant | May be present | May wax and wane |
| Distractibility | Constant | May be present | May wax and wane |
| Anger expression | Short-lived (minutes) | Plans revenge | Intense rages (minutes to hours) |
| Thought content | May be immature | Blames others | Morbid or grandiose ideas |
| Sleep disturbance | May be present | No | May wax and wane |
| Self-deprecation | Briefly, with criticism | No | Prolonged, with or without suicidal ideation |
| Obsessed with ideas | No | No | Yes |
| Hallucinations | No | No | Diagnostic, if present |
| Family history | May be a history of school problems | May be a history of antisocial behavior | May be a history of mood disorders |

ADHD = attention-deficit/hyperactivity disorder.

from impulsive acts, such as excessive spending, acts of vandalism, theft, or aggression, associated with grandiose thoughts. Affective disorders are associated with a 30-fold greater incidence of successful suicide. Substance abuse may be a further complication, often representing an attempt at self-medication for the mood problem.

## Treatment & Prognosis

Most patients with bipolar disorder respond to pharmacotherapy with mood stabilizers such as lithium, carbamazepine, or valproate, either alone or in combination. The atypical neuroleptic, olanzapine, has been approved by the Food and Drug Administration (FDA) for the treatment of bipolar affective disorder. Neuroleptic medications may be necessary in addition to a mood stabilizer if psychotic symptoms or significant aggression is present. In cases of severe impairment, hospitalization is required to maintain safety and initiate treatment. Although it is often possible to discontinue the neuroleptic medication after remission of symptoms, it is usually necessary to continue the mood stabilizer for at least a year, and longer if the individual has had recurrent episodes. It is not uncommon for the patient to need lifelong medication. Supportive psychotherapy for the patient and family and education about the recurrent nature of the illness are critical. In its adult form, bipolar

disorder is an illness with a remitting course of alternating depressive and manic episodes. The time span between episodes can be years or months depending on the severity of illness and ability to comply with medication interventions. In childhood, the symptoms may be more pervasive and not fall into the intermittent episodic pattern until after puberty.

American Academy of Child and Adolescent Psychiatry: Practice parameters for the assessment and treatment of children with bipolar disorder. J Am Acad Child Adolesc Psychiatry 1997;36 (Suppl):157S [PMID: 9432516].

Emslie GJ et al: Predictors of response to treatment in children and adolescents with mood disorders. Psychiatr Clin North Am 2003;26(2):435 [PMID: 12778842].

James AD, Javaloyes AM: The treatment of bipolar disorder in children and adolescents. J Child Psychol Psychiatry 2001;42(4): 439 [PMID: 11383960].

Kent L, Craddock N: Is there a relationship between attention deficit hyperactivity disorder and bipolar disorder? J Affect Disord 2003;73(3):211 [PMID: 12547289].

Kowatch RA, Delbello MP: The use of mood stabilizers and atypical antipsychotics in children and adolescents with bipolar disorders. CNS Spectr 2003;8(4):273 [PMID: 12679742].

Leibenluft E et al: Defining clinical phenotypes of juvenile mania. Am J Psychiatry 2003;160(3):430 [PMID: 12611821].

Weller EB, Danielyan AK, Weller RA: Somatic treatment of bipolar disorder in children and adolescents. Child Adolesc Psychiatr Clin North Am 2002;11(3):595 [PMID: 12222085].

# SUICIDE IN CHILDREN & ADOLESCENTS

The suicide rate in young people has remained high for several decades. In 1997, suicide was the third leading cause of death among children and adolescents age 10–24 years in the United States. The suicide rate among adolescents age 15–19 years quadrupled from approximately 2.7 to 11.3 per 100,000 since the 1960s. It is estimated that each year, approximately 2 million US adolescents attempt suicide, yet only 700,000 receive medical attention for their attempt. Suicide and homicide rates for children in the United States are two to five times higher than those for the other 25 industrialized countries combined, primarily due to the prevalence of firearms in the United States. For children younger than 10 years old, the rate of completed suicide is low, but from 1980 to 1992 it increased by 120%, from 0.8 to 1.7 per 100,000.

Adolescent girls make three to four times as many suicide attempts as boys of the same age, but the number of completed suicides is three to four times greater in boys. Firearms are the most commonly used method in successful suicides, accounting for 40–60% of cases; hanging, carbon monoxide poisoning, and drug overdoses each account for approximately 10–15% of cases.

Suicide is almost always associated with a psychiatric disorder and should not be viewed as a philosophic choice about life or death or as a predictable response to overwhelming stress. Most commonly it is associated with a mood disorder and the hopelessness that accompanies a severe depressive episode. Suicide attempts are often an angry, impulsive, and retaliatory act of aggression in an individual who is unable to exercise better insight and judgment because of an impaired state due to either mental illness or substance abuse. Although suicide attempts are more common in individuals with a history of behavior problems and academic difficulties, other suicide victims are high achievers who are temperamentally anxious and perfectionistic and who commit suicide impulsively after a failure or rejection, either real or perceived. Mood disorders (in both sexes, but especially in females), substance abuse disorders (especially in males), and conduct disorders are commonly diagnosed at psychological autopsy in adolescent suicide victims. Some adolescent suicides reflect an underlying psychotic disorder, with the young person usually committing suicide in response to auditory hallucinations or psychotic delusions.

The vast majority of young people who attempt suicide give some clue to their distress or their tentative plans to commit suicide. Most show signs of dysphoric mood (anger, irritability, anxiety, or depression). Over 60% make comments such as "I wish I were dead" or "I just can't deal with this any longer" within the 24 hours prior to death. In one study, nearly 70% of subjects experienced a crisis event such as a loss (eg, rejection by girlfriend or boyfriend), a failure, or an arrest prior to completed suicide.

## Assessment of Suicide Risk

Any clinical assessment for depression must include questions about suicidal ideation. If a child or adolescent expresses suicidal thinking, the physician must ask if he or she has an active plan. Suicidal ideation accompanied by any plan warrants immediate referral for a psychiatric crisis assessment. This can usually be accomplished at the nearest emergency room.

Assessment of suicide risk calls for a high index of suspicion and a direct interview with the patient and significant others such as family members, peers, and teachers. A format for the interview is provided in Table 6–12. The highest risk of suicide is among older white adolescent boys. High-risk factors include previous suicide attempts, a suicide note, and a viable plan for suicide with the availability of lethal means, close personal exposure to suicide, conduct disorder, and substance abuse. Other risk factors are signs and symptoms of major depression or dysthymia, a family history of suicide, a recent death in the family, and a view of death as a relief from the pain in their lives. Persons who have little or no family support, those who are facing a crisis in their lives at work or school, and those who refuse to agree not to commit suicide are also at high risk.

## Principles of Intervention

Any suicide attempt must be considered a serious matter. The patient should not be left alone, and one should show understanding of the young person's pain and convey a desire to help. The physician should meet with the patient and the family, both alone and together, and listen carefully to their problems and perceptions. It should be made clear that with the assistance of mental health professionals, solutions can be found.

These patients should be referred for psychiatric evaluation and possible hospitalization if there appears to be a high potential for suicide, if they are severely depressed or intoxicated, if the family does not appear appropriately concerned, or if there are practical limitations on providing supervision and support to ensure safety. Any decision to send the patient home without hospitalization should be made only after consultation with a mental health expert. The decision should rest on a perceived lessening of the risk of suicide and assurance of the family's ability to follow through with outpatient therapy and provide appropriate support and supervision. Guns, pills, knives, and razor blades must

***Table 6–12.*** Clinical interview to assess suicide risk.

1. An observation or change has been noted.
2. How have you been feeling (inside, emotionally)?
3. Have you had periods of feeling down or discouraged?
   a. How often?
   b. How long?
   c. How severe?
4. Do they interfere with your life?
   a. Daily activities?
   b. School or work?
   c. Sleep or appetite? Both?
   d. Family life?
5. Do you have feelings of—
   a. Self-criticism or worthlessness?
   b. Helplessness?
   c. Hopelessness?
   d. Wanting to give up?
6. Are the feelings ever so strong that life does not seem worth living? Have you had thoughts of suicide?
   a. Are you having thoughts of suicide now?
   b. How persistent are they?
   c. How much effort does it take to resist?
   d. Can you tolerate the pain you are feeling?
7. Have you made any plans to carry out suicide?
   a. What are the plans?
   b. Have you taken any tentative action (eg, obtaining a gun or rope, stockpiling pills)?
   c. As you have thought about suicide, how have you viewed the idea of death?
8. What deters you from trying suicide?
9. If the suicidal feelings are subsiding, could you resist the feelings if they returned?
10. Is there someone you can turn to for help at those times? Who?
11. Has the idea of suicide come up in the past?
    a. How often?
    b. When and under what circumstances?
    c. What has happened at those times?
12. Can you tolerate the pain that you are feeling right now?

be removed from the home entirely, and, as much as possible, access to them outside the home must be denied. The patient should be restricted from driving for at least the first 24 hours to lessen the chance of impulsive motor vehicle accidents. Instructions and phone numbers for crisis services should be given, and the family must be committed to a plan for mental health treatment.

Suicide prevention should be a community- and school-based effort to increase awareness and provide access to services, including hotlines. Restricting young people's access to firearms is also a critical factor, as firearms are responsible for 85% of deaths due to suicide or homicide in youth in the United States.

Finally, the physician should be aware of his or her own emotional reactions to dealing with potentially suicidal adolescents and their families. Because the assessment takes considerable time and energy, the physician should be on guard against becoming tired, irritable, or angry. The physician need not be afraid of precipitating suicide by direct and frank discussions of suicidal risk.

Borowsky IW: The role of the pediatrician in preventing suicidal behavior. Minerva Pediatr 2002;54(1):41 [PMID: 11862165].

Borowsky IW, Ireland M, Resnick MD: Adolescent suicide attempts: Risks and protectors. Pediatrics 2001;107(3): 485 [PMID: 11230587].

Gould MS et al: Youth suicide risk and prevention interventions: A review of the past 10 years. J Am Acad Child Adolesc Psychiatry 2003;42(4):386 [PMID: 12649626].

Practice Parameters for the assessment and treatment of children and adolescents with suicidal behavior. J Am Acad Child Adolesc Psychiatry 2001;40(7 Suppl):24S [PMID: 11314578].

Schmidt P et al: Suicide in children, adolescents, and young adults. Forensic Sci Int 2002;127(3):161 [PMID: 12175945].

Weller EB et al: Overview and assessment of the suicidal child. Depress Anxiety 2001;14(3):157 [PMID: 11747125]

## ADJUSTMENT DISORDERS

The most frequent and most disturbing stresses for children and adolescents are marital discord, separation and divorce, family illness, the loss of a loved one, a change of residence, and, for adolescents, peer relationship problems. When faced with stress, children can experience many different symptoms, including changes in mood, changes in behavior, anxiety symptoms, and physical complaints. Key findings include the following:

- The precipitating event or circumstance is identifiable.
- The symptoms have appeared within 3 months after the occurrence of the stressful event.
- Although the child experiences distress or some functional impairment, the reaction is not severe or disabling.
- The reaction does not persist more than 6 months after the stressor has terminated.

The range of symptoms associated with adjustment disorders is listed in Table 6–13.

### Differential Diagnosis

When symptoms are a reaction to an identifiable stressor but are severe, persistent, or disabling, depressive disorder, anxiety disorder, and conduct disorders must be considered.

**Table 6–13.** Signs and symptoms of adjustment reactions.

---

Irritable, angry mood
Anxious, worried mood
Unhappy, depressed mood
Angry resistance to authority
Fatigue
Aches and pains
Decreased school performance
Social withdrawal
Any combination of the above

---

## Treatment

The mainstay of treatment is the doctor's assurance that the emotional or behavioral change is a predictable consequence of the stressful event. This validates the child's reaction and encourages the child to talk about the stressful occurrence and its aftermath. Parents are asked to understand the child's reaction and encourage appropriate verbal expression of feelings, while defining boundaries for behavior that prevent the child from feeling out of control.

## Prognosis

The duration of symptoms in adjustment reactions depends on the severity of the stress; the child's personal sensitivity to stress and vulnerability to anxiety, depression, and other psychiatric disorders; and the available support system.

## SCHIZOPHRENIA

The incidence of schizophrenia is about 1 per 10,000 per year. The onset of schizophrenia is typically between the mid- to late teens and early 30s, with onset before puberty being relatively rare. Symptoms usually begin after puberty, although a full "psychotic break" may not occur until the young adult years. Childhood onset (before puberty) of psychotic symptoms due to schizophrenia is uncommon and usually indicates a more severe form of the spectrum of schizophrenic disorders. It affects only one or two children in every 10,000 of the population younger than age 15 years, and boys outnumber girls by approximately 2:1. Childhood schizophrenia appears to be genetically related to the adult type of schizophrenia. Schizophrenia is a biologically based disease with a strong genetic component. Other psychotic disorders that may be encountered in childhood or adolescence include schizoaffective disorder and psychosis not otherwise specified (NOS). Psychosis NOS may be used as a differen-

tial diagnosis when psychotic symptoms are present, but the cluster of symptoms is not consistent with a schizophrenia diagnosis.

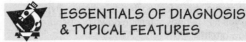

ESSENTIALS OF DIAGNOSIS & TYPICAL FEATURES

- *Delusional thoughts.*
- *Disorganized speech (rambling or illogical speech patterns).*
- *Disorganized or bizarre behavior.*
- *Hallucinations (auditory, visual, tactile, olfactory), negative symptoms (ie, flat affect, avolition, alogia).*

## Clinical Findings

Children and adolescents display many of the symptoms of adult schizophrenia. Hallucinations or delusions, bizarre and morbid thought content, and rambling and illogical speech are typical. Affected individuals tend to withdraw into an internal world of fantasy and may then equate fantasy with external reality. They generally have difficulty with schoolwork and with peer relationships. Adolescents may have a prodromal period of depression prior to the onset of psychotic symptoms. The majority of patients with childhood-onset schizophrenia have had nonspecific psychiatric symptoms or symptoms of delayed development for months or years prior to the onset of their overtly psychotic symptoms.

## Differential Diagnosis

Obtaining the family history of mental illness is critical when assessing children and adolescents with psychotic symptoms. Psychological testing is often helpful in identifying or ruling out psychotic thought processes. Psychotic symptoms in children younger than age 8 years must be differentiated from manifestations of normal vivid fantasy life or abuse-related symptoms. Children with psychotic disorders often have learning disabilities and attention difficulties in addition to disorganized thoughts, delusions, and hallucinations. In psychotic adolescents, mania is differentiated by high levels of energy, excitement, and irritability. Any child or adolescent exhibiting new psychotic symptoms requires a medical evaluation that includes physical and neurologic examinations (including consideration of magnetic resonance imaging and electroencephalogram), drug screening, and metabolic screening for endocrinopathies, Wilson disease, and delirium.

## Treatment

The treatment of childhood and adolescent schizophrenia focuses on four main areas: (1) decreasing active psychotic symptoms, (2) supporting development of social and cognitive skills, (3) reducing the risk of relapse of psychotic symptoms, and (4) providing support and education to parents and family members. Antipsychotic medications (eg, risperidone, olanzapine, haloperidol) are the primary psychopharmacologic intervention. In addition, a supportive, reality-oriented focus in relationships can help to reduce hallucinations, delusions, and frightening thoughts. A special school or day treatment environment may be necessary depending on the child's or adolescent's ability to tolerate the school day and classroom activities. Support for the family emphasizes the importance of clear, focused communication and an emotionally calm climate in preventing recurrences of overtly psychotic symptoms.

## Prognosis

Schizophrenia is a chronic disorder with exacerbations and remissions of psychotic symptoms. It is generally believed that earlier onset (prior to age 13 years) and poor premorbid functioning (oddness or eccentricity) generally predict a poorer outcome.

Calderoni D et al: Differentiating childhood-onset schizophrenia from psychotic mood disorders. J Am Acad Child Adolesc Psychiatry 2001;40(10):1190 [PMID: 11589532].

Jacobsen LK, Rapoport JL: Research update: Childhood-onset schizophrenia: Implications of clinical and neurobiological research. J Child Psychol Psychiatr 1998;39:101 [PMID: 9534088].

Kumra S et al: Childhood-onset schizophrenia: Research update. Can J Psychiatry 2001;46(10):923 [PMID: 11816313].

Practice parameters for the assessment and treatment of children and adolescents with schizophrenia. J Am Acad Child Adolesc Psychiatry 2001;40(7 Suppl):4S [PMID: 11434484].

Shaeffer JL, Ross RG: Childhood onset schizophrenia: Premorbid and prodromal diagnostic and treatment histories. J Am Acad Child Adolesc Psychiatry 2002;41:538 [PMID: 12014786].

# CONDUCT DISORDERS

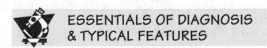

### ESSENTIALS OF DIAGNOSIS & TYPICAL FEATURES

*A persistent pattern of behavior that includes the following:*

- *Defiance of authority.*
- *Violating the rights of others or society's norms.*
- *Aggressive behavior toward persons, animals, or property.*

## General Considerations

Disorders of conduct affect approximately 9% of males and 2% of females younger than 18 years. This is a very heterogeneous population, and overlap occurs with ADHD, learning and other neuropsychiatric disorders, mood disorders, and family dysfunction. Many of these individuals come from homes where domestic violence, child abuse, drug abuse, shifting parental figures, and poverty are environmental risk factors. Although social learning partly explains this correlation, the genetic heritability of aggressive conduct and antisocial behaviors is currently under investigation.

## Clinical Findings

The typical child with conduct disorder is a boy with a turbulent home life and academic difficulties. Defiance of authority, fighting, tantrums, running away, school failure, and destruction of property are common symptoms. With increasing age, fire-setting and theft may occur, followed in adolescence by truancy, vandalism, and substance abuse. Sexual promiscuity, sexual perpetration, and other criminal behaviors may develop. Hyperactive, aggressive, and uncooperative behavior patterns in the preschool and early school years tend to predict conduct disorder in adolescence with a high degree of accuracy, especially when ADHD goes untreated. A history of reactive attachment disorder is an additional childhood risk factor. The risk for conduct disorder increases with inconsistent and severe parental disciplinary techniques, parental alcoholism, and parental antisocial behavior.

## Differential Diagnosis

Young people with conduct disorders, especially those with more violent histories, have an increased incidence of neurologic signs and symptoms, psychomotor seizures, psychotic symptoms, mood disorders, ADHD, and learning disabilities. Efforts should be made to identify these associated disorders (see Table 6–11) because they may suggest specific therapeutic interventions. Conduct disorder is best conceptualized as a final common pathway emerging from a variety of underlying psychosocial, genetic, environmental, and neuropsychiatric conditions. Other diagnoses that may be present or should be differentiated include intermittent explosive disorder and oppositional defiant disorder.

## Treatment

Effective treatment can be complicated by the problematic psychosocial problems often found in the lives of children and adolescents with conduct disorders and difficulty achieving compliance with treatment recommendations. Efforts should be made to stabilize the environment and improve functioning within the home, particularly as it relates to parental functioning and disciplinary techniques. Identification of learning disabilities and placement in an optimal school environment is also critical. Any associated neurologic and psychiatric disorders should be addressed. In severe cases, residential treatment may be needed, often through the juvenile justice system. Medications such as mood stabilizers, neuroleptics, stimulants, and antidepressants have all been studied in youth with conduct disorders, yet none has been found to be consistently effective in this population. Early involvement in programs such as Big Brothers and Sisters, Scouts, and team sports in which consistent adult mentors and role models interact with youth decreases the chances that the youth with conduct disorders will develop antisocial personality disorder. Multisystemic therapy (MST) is being used increasingly as an intervention for youth with conduct disorders and involvement with the legal system. MST is an intensive home-based model of care that seeks to stabilize and improve the home environment and to strengthen the support system and coping skills of the individual and family.

## Prognosis

The prognosis is based on the ability of the child's support system to mount an effective treatment intervention consistently over time. The prognosis is generally worse for children in whom the disorder presents before age 10 years; those who display a diversity of antisocial behaviors across multiple settings; and those who are raised in an environment characterized by parental antisocial behavior, alcoholism or other substance abuse, and conflict. Nearly half of such children become antisocial as adults. Persistent antisocial behavior in childhood or adolescence tends to predict a diagnosable psychiatric disorder in adulthood.

## 1. Oppositional Defiant Disorder

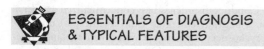

### ESSENTIALS OF DIAGNOSIS & TYPICAL FEATURES

- A pattern of negativistic, hostile, and defiant behavior lasting at least 6 months.

- Loses temper, argues with adults, defies rules.
- Blames others for own mistakes and misbehavior.
- Angry, easily annoyed, vindictive.
- Does not meet criteria for conduct disorder.

Oppositional defiant disorder (ODD) usually is evident before 8 years of age and may be an antecedent to the development of conduct disorder. The symptoms usually first emerge at home, but then extend to school and peer relationships. The disruptive behaviors of ODD are generally less severe than those associated with conduct disorder and do not include hurting other individuals or animals, destruction of property, or theft.

ODD is more common in families where caregiver dysfunction is present, and in children with a history of multiple changes in caregivers; inconsistent, harsh, or neglectful parenting; or serious marital discord.

Interventions include careful assessment of the psychosocial situation and recommendations to support parenting skills and optimal caregiver functioning. Assessment for comorbid psychiatric diagnoses such as learning disabilities, depression, and ADHD should be pursued and appropriate interventions recommended.

American Academy of Child and Adolescent Psychiatry: Practice parameters for the assessment and treatment of children and adolescents with conduct disorder. J Am Acad Child Adolesc Psychiatry 1997;36 (Suppl):122S [PMID: 9334568].

Burke JH, Loeber R, Birmaher B: Oppositional defiant disorder and conduct disorder: Review of the past 10 years, part II. J Am Acad Child Adolesc Psychiatry 2002; 41(11):1275 [PMID: 12410070].

Cunningham CE, Boyle MH: Preschoolers at risk for ADHD and ODD: Family, parenting and behavioral correlates. J Abnorm Child Psychol 2002;30(6):555 [PMID: 12481971].

Farmer EM et al: Review of the evidence base for treatment of childhood psychopathology: Externalizing disorders. J Consult Clin Psychol 2002;70(6):1267 [PMID: 12472301].

Flory K et al: Relation between childhood disruptive behavior disorders and substance use and dependence in young adulthood. Psychol Addictive Behav 2003;17(2):151 [PMID: 12814279].

Greene RW et al: Psychiatric comorbidity, family dysfunction and social impairment in referred youth with oppositional defiant disorder. Am J Psychiatry 2002;159(7):1214 [PMID: 12091202].

Kazdin AE: Treatments for aggressive and antisocial children. Child Adolesc Psychiatr Clin North Am 2000;9(4):841 [PMID: 11005009].

Loeber R et al: Findings on disruptive behavior disorders from the first decade of the developmental trends study. Clin Child Fam Psychol Rev 2000;3(1):37 [PMID: 11228766].

Loeber R et al: Oppositional defiant and conduct disorder: A review of the past 10 years Part 1. J Am Acad Child Adolesc Psychiatry 2000;39(12):1468 [PMID: 11128323].

Waschbusch DA et al: Reactive aggression in boys with disruptive behavior disorders; behavior, physiology and affect. J Abnorm Child Psychol 2002;30(6):641 [PMID: 12481977].

# ANXIETY DISORDERS

## 1. Anxiety-Based School Refusal (School Avoidance)

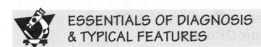

### ESSENTIALS OF DIAGNOSIS & TYPICAL FEATURES

- *A persistent pattern of school avoidance related to symptoms of anxiety.*
- *Somatic symptoms on school mornings, with symptoms resolving if the child is allowed to remain at home.*
- *No organic medical disorder that accounts for the symptoms.*
- *High levels of parental anxiety are commonly observed.*

## General Considerations

Anxiety-based school refusal is a persistent behavioral symptom rather than a diagnostic entity. It refers to a pattern of school nonattendance resulting from anxiety, which may be related to a dread of leaving home (separation anxiety), a fear of some aspect of school, or a fear of feeling exposed or embarrassed at school (social phobia). In all cases, a realistic cause of the fear (eg, an intimidating teacher or a playground bully) should be ruled out. In most cases, anxiety-based school refusal is related to developmentally inappropriate separation anxiety. The incidence between males and females is about equal, and there appear to be peaks of incidence at ages 6–7 years, again at ages 10–11 years, and in early adolescence.

## Clinical Findings

In the preadolescent years, school refusal often begins after some precipitating stress in the family. The child's anxiety is then manifested either as somatic symptoms or in displacement of anxiety onto some aspect of the school environment. The somatic manifestations of anxiety include dizziness, nausea, and stomach distress. Characteristically, the symptoms become more severe as the time to leave for school approaches and then remit if the child is allowed to remain at home for the day. In older children, the onset is more insidious and often associated with social withdrawal and depression. The incidence of anxiety and mood disorders is increased in these families.

## Differential Diagnosis

The differential diagnosis of school nonattendance is presented in Table 6–14. Medical disorders that may be causing the somatic symptoms must be ruled out. Children with learning disorders may wish to stay home to avoid the sense of failure they experience at school. Children may also have transient episodes of wanting to stay at home during times of significant family stress or loss. The onset of school avoidance in middle or late adolescence may herald the onset of schizophrenia or other psychotic disorder. Children who are avoiding school for reasons related to ODD or conduct disorder can be differentiated on the basis of their chronic noncompliance with adult authority and their preference for being with peers rather than at home.

**Table 6–14.** Differential diagnosis of school nonattendance.[a]

---

I. **Emotional or anxiety-based refusal[b]**
  A. Separation anxiety disorder (50–80% of anxious refusers)
  B. Generalized anxiety disorder
  C. Mood/depressive disorder (with or without combined anxiety)
  D. Social phobia
  E. Specific phobia
  F. Panic disorder
  G. Psychosis ("voices" say not to attend)
II. **Truancy[c] behavior disorders**
  A. Oppositional defiant disorder, conduct disorder
  B. Substance abuse disorders
III. **"Realistic" school refusal**
  A. Learning disability, unaddressed or undetected
  B. Marauding students (including gangs)
  C. Psychologically abusive teacher
  D. Family-sanctioned nonattendance
    1. For companionship
    2. For child care
    3. To care for the parent (role-reversal)
    4. To supplement family income
  E. Socioculturally sanctioned nonattendance (school is not valued)
  F. Homosexual attraction, gender concerns
IV. **Undiagnosed medical condition (including pregnancy)**

---

[a]Medically unexplained absence of more than 2 weeks.
[b]Subjectively distressed child who generally stays at home.
[c]Nonsubjectively distressed and not at home.

## Complications

The longer a child remains out of school, the more difficult it is to return and the more strained the relationship between child and parent becomes. Many parents of nonattending children feel tyrannized by their defiant, clinging child. Children often feel accused of making up their symptoms, leading to further antagonism between the child, parents, and medical caregivers.

## Treatment

The goal of treatment is to help the child confront anxiety and overcome it by returning to school. This requires a strong alliance between the parents and the health care provider. The parent must understand that no underlying medical disorder exists, that the child's symptoms are a manifestation of anxiety, and that the basic problem is anxiety that must be faced to be overcome. Parents must be reminded that being good parents in this case means helping a child cope with a distressing experience. Children must be reassured that their symptoms are caused by worry and that they will be overcome on return to school.

A plan for returning the child to school is then developed with parents and school personnel. Firm insistence on full compliance with this plan is essential. The child is brought to school by someone not likely to give in, such as the father or an older sibling. If symptoms develop at school, the child should be checked by the school nurse and then returned to class after a brief rest. The parents must be reassured that school staff will handle the situation at school and that school personnel can reach the primary health care provider if any questions arise.

If these interventions are ineffective, increased involvement of a therapist and consideration of a day treatment program may be necessary. For children with persistent symptoms of separation that do not improve with behavioral interventions, medications such as SSRIs should be considered. Comorbid diagnoses of panic disorder, generalized anxiety, or major depression should be carefully screened for and, if identified, treated appropriately.

## Prognosis

The vast majority of preadolescent children improve significantly with behavioral interventions and return to school. The prognosis is worsened by the length of time the child remains out of school. Long-term outcomes are influenced by comorbid diagnoses and responsiveness to behavioral or medication interventions. A history of school refusal is more common in adults with panic and anxiety disorders and agoraphobia than in the general population.

Egger HL, Coatello EJ, Angold A: School refusal and psychiatric disorders: A community study. J Am Acad Child Adolesc Psychiatry 2003;42(7):797 [PMID: 12819439].

King NJ, Bernstein GA: School refusal in children and adolescents: A review of the past 10 years. J Am Acad Child Adolesc Psychiatry 2001;40(2):197 [PMID: 11211368].

Masi G, Mucci M, Millepiedi S: Separation anxiety disorder in children and adolescents: Epidemiology, diagnosis, and management. CNS Drugs 2001;15(2):93 [PMID: 11460893].

## 2. Generalized Anxiety Disorder & Panic Disorder

Transient developmental fears are common in early childhood. Therefore, the person evaluating the clinical significance of anxiety symptoms in children must consider the age of the child, the developmental fears that can normally be expected at that age, the form of the symptoms and their duration, and the degree to which the symptoms disrupt the child's life.

Anxiety can be manifested either directly or indirectly, as shown in Table 6–15. The characteristics of anxiety in childhood are listed in Table 6–16. Community-based studies of school-age children and adolescents suggest that nearly 10% of children have some type of anxiety disorder. The differential diagnosis of symptoms of anxiety is presented in Table 6–17.

The child's family and school environment should be evaluated for marital discord, family violence, harsh or inappropriate disciplinary methods, sexual abuse, ne-

**Table 6–15.** Signs and symptoms of anxiety in children.

**Psychological**
  Fears and worries
  Increased dependence on home and parents
  Avoidance of anxiety-producing stimuli
  Decreased school performance
  Increased self-doubt and irritability
  Frightening themes in play and fantasy
**Psychomotor**
  Motoric restlessness and hyperactivity
  Sleep disturbances
  Decreased concentration
  Ritualistic behaviors (eg, washing, counting)
**Psychophysiologic**
  Autonomic hyperarousal
  Dizziness and lightheadedness
  Palpitations
  Shortness of breath
  Flushing, sweating, dry mouth
  Nausea and vomiting
  Panic
  Headaches and stomachaches

***Table 6–16.*** Anxiety disorders in children and adolescents.

| Disorder | Major Clinical Manifestations |
|---|---|
| Generalized anxiety disorder | Intense, disproportionate or irrational worry, often about future events |
| Panic disorder | Unprovoked, intense fear with sympathetic hyperarousal, and often palpitations or hyperventilation |
| Posttraumatic stress disorder | Fear of a recurrence of an intense, anxiety-provoking traumatic experience, causing sympathetic hyperarousal, avoidance of reminders, and the re-experiencing of aspects of the traumatic event |
| Separation anxiety disorder | Developmentally inappropriate wish to maintain proximity with caregivers; morbid worry of threats to family integrity or integrity of self upon separation; intense homesickness |
| Social phobia | Painful shyness or self-consciousness; fear of humiliation with public scrutiny |
| Specific phobia | Avoidance of specific feared stimuli |

***Table 6–17.*** Differential diagnosis of symptoms of anxiety.

I. **Normal developmental anxiety**
 A. Stranger anxiety (5 months to 2½ years, with a peak at 6–12 months)
 B. Separation anxiety (7 months to 4 years, with a peak at 18–36 months)
 C. The child is fearful or even phobic of the dark and monsters (3–6 years)
II. **"Appropriate" anxiety**
 A. Anticipating a painful or frightening experience
 B. Avoidance of a reminder of a painful or frightening experience
 C. Child abuse
III. **Anxiety disorder (see Table 6–16), with or without other comorbid psychiatric disorders**
IV. **Substance abuse**
V. **Medications and recreational drugs**
 A. Caffeinism (including colas and chocolate)
 B. Sympathomimetic agents
 C. Idiosyncratic drug reactions
VI. **Hypermetabolic or hyperarousal states**
 A. Hyperthyroidism
 B. Pheochromocytoma
 C. Anemia
 D. Hypoglycemia
 E. Hypoxemia
VII. **Cardiac abnormality**
 A. Dysrhythmia
 B. High-output state
 C. Mitral valve prolapse

glect, and emotional overstimulation. The child's experience of anxiety and its relationship to life events should be explored, and therapy to incorporate specific cognitive and behavioral techniques to diminish the anxiety should be recommended. Finally, when panic attacks or anxiety symptoms do not remit with cognitive, behavioral, and environmental interventions, and they significantly affect life functioning, psychopharmacologic agents may be helpful. SSRIs may be effective across a broad spectrum of anxiety symptoms.

## Prognosis

There appears to be continuity between high levels of childhood anxiety and anxiety disorders in adulthood. Anxiety disorders are thus likely to be lifelong conditions, yet with effective interventions, individuals can minimize their influence on overall life functioning.

American Academy of Child and Adolescent Psychiatry: Practice parameters for the assessment and treatment of children and adolescents with anxiety disorders. J Am Acad Child Adolesc Psychiatry 1997;36 (Suppl):69S [PMID: 9334566].

Blanco C, Antia SX, Lebowitz MR: Pharmacotherapy of social anxiety disorder. Biol Psychiatry 2002;51(1):1098 [PMID: 11801236].

Diler RS: Panic disorder in children and adolescents. Yonsei Med J 2003;44(1):174 [PMID: 12619196].

Gullone E, King NJ, Ollendick TH: Self-reported anxiety in children and adolescents: A three-year follow-up study. J Genet Psychol 2001;162(1):5 [PMID: 11338440].

Rynn MA, Siqueland L, Rickels K: Placebo-controlled trial of sertraline in the treatment of children with generalized anxiety disorder. Am J Psychiatry 2001;158(12):2008 [PMID: 11729017].

Velosa JF, Riddle MA: Pharmacologic treatment of anxiety disorders in children and adolescents. Child Adolesc Psychiatr Clin North Am 2000;9(1):119 [PMID: 10674193].

Wagner KD: Generalized anxiety disorder in children and adolescents. Psychiatr Clin North Am 2001;24(1):139 [PMID: 11225504].

## OBSESSIVE–COMPULSIVE DISORDER

### ESSENTIALS OF DIAGNOSIS & TYPICAL FEATURES

• *Recurrent obsessive thoughts, impulses, or images that cause marked anxiety or distress and are not simply excessive worries about real-life problems.*

- *The individual attempts to ignore or suppress the thoughts or impulses.*
- *Repetitive compulsive behaviors or mental acts that the person feels driven to perform in response to the obsessive thought aimed at preventing or reducing distress.*
- *The obsessions and compulsions cause marked distress, are time-consuming, and interfere with normal routines.*

Obsessive–compulsive disorder (OCD) is an anxiety disorder that often begins in early childhood, but may not be diagnosed until the teen or even young adult years. The essential features of OCD are recurrent obsessions or compulsions that are severe enough to be time-consuming or cause marked distress and functional impairment. Obsessions are persistent ideas, thoughts, or impulses that are intrusive and often inappropriate. Children may have obsessions about contamination or cleanliness; ordering and compulsive behaviors will follow, such as frequent hand-washing, counting, or ordering objects. The goal of the compulsive behavior for the individual with OCD is to reduce anxiety and distress. There may be significant avoidance of situations due to obsessive thoughts or fears of contamination. OCD is often associated with major depressive disorder. The prevalence of OCD is estimated to be around 2%, and the rates are equal between males and females.

## Treatment

OCD is best treated with a combination of cognitive–behavioral therapy (CBT) specific to OCD and medications in more severe cases. SSRIs are effective in diminishing OCD symptoms. Fluvoxamine and sertraline have FDA approval for the treatment of pediatric OCD. The tricyclic antidepressant (TCA) clomipramine has FDA approval for the treatment of OCD in adults.

## Prognosis

Although OCD is usually a lifelong condition, most individuals can achieve significant remission of symptoms with the combination of CBT and medications. A minority of individuals with OCD are completely disabled by their symptoms.

American Academy of Child and Adolescent Psychiatry: Practice parameters for the assessment and treatment of children and adolescents with OCD. J Am Acad Child Adolesc Psychiatry 1998;37(10 Supp):27S [PMID: 9785727].

Cook EH et al: Long-term sertraline treatment of children and adolescents with obsessive–compulsive disorder. J Am Acad Child Adolesc Psychiatry 2001;40(10):1175 [PMID: 11589530].

Geller DA et al: Fluoxetine treatment for OCD in children and adolescents: A placebo controlled trial. J Am Acad Child Adolesc Psychiatry 2001;40(7):773 [PMID: 11437015].

Grados MA, Riddle MA: Pharmacological treatment of childhood obsessive compulsive disorder: From theory to practice. J Clin Child Psychol 2001;30(1):67 [PMID: 11294079].

Kaplan A, Hollander D: A review of pharmacologic treatment for obsessive-compulsive disorder. Psychiatric Serv 2003;54:1111 [PMID: 12883138].

March JS: Cognitive-behavioral psychotherapy for children and adolescents with OCD: A review and recommendations for treatment. J Am Acad Child Adolesc Psychiatry 1995;34(1):7.

March JS et al: Cognitive-behavioral psychotherapy for pediatric obsessive–compulsive disorder. J Clin Child Psychol 2001;30(1):8 [PMID: 11294080].

Riddle MA et al: Fluvoxamine for children and adolescents with OCD: A randomized, controlled, multicenter trial. J Am Acad Child Adolesc Psychiatry 2001;40(2):222 [PMID: 11211371].

Thomsen PH: Obsessions: The impact and treatment of obsessive–compulsive disorder in children and adolescents. J Psychopharmacol 2000;14(2 Suppl 1):S31 [PMID: 10888029].

Waters TL et al: Cognitive-behavioral family treatment of childhood obsessive–compulsive disorder: Preliminary findings. Am J Psychother 2001;55(3):372 [PMID: 11641879].

# POSTTRAUMATIC STRESS DISORDER

### ESSENTIALS OF DIAGNOSIS & TYPICAL FEATURES

- *Signs and symptoms of autonomic hyperarousal such as easy startle, increased heart rate, and hypervigilance.*
- *Avoidant behaviors and numbing of responsiveness.*
- *Flashbacks to a traumatic event, such as nightmares, and intrusive thoughts.*
- *All of the preceding following the experience of traumatic events such as exposure to violence, physical or sexual abuse, natural disasters, car accidents, dog bites, and unexpected personal tragedies.*

## General Considerations

Factors that predispose individuals to the development of posttraumatic stress disorder (PTSD) include proximity to the traumatic event or loss, a history of exposure to trauma, preexisting depression or anxiety disorder, and lack of an adequate support system. PTSD can develop in response to natural disasters, terrorism, motor vehicle accidents, and significant personal injury in addition to physical, sexual, and emotional abuse. Long-overdue attention is now being paid to the substantial effects of family and community violence on the psychological development of children and adolescents. Abused children are most likely to develop PTSD and to suffer wide-ranging symptoms and impaired functioning. Heightened concern about terrorism in the United States has created increased awareness of PTSD and community-based interventions to decrease the risk of PTSD. Studies after the terrorist attacks of September 11, 2001, and Oklahoma City reported up to 40% of children and adolescents experienced PTSD symptoms.

As many as 25% of young people exposed to violence develop symptoms of posttraumatic stress disorder. Factors that predispose to development of PTSD when a person is exposed to a traumatic event include a history of exposure to trauma, preexisting depression or anxiety disorder, and lack of an adequate support system.

## Clinical Findings

Children who have been traumatized show persistent evidence of fear and anxiety and are hypervigilant to the possibility of repetition. They may regress developmentally and experience fears of strangers, of the dark, and of being alone, and avoid reminders of the traumatic event. Children also frequently reexperience elements of the events in dreams and flashbacks. In their symbolic play, one can often notice a monotonous repetition of some aspect of the traumatic event. Children with a history of traumatic experiences or neglect in infancy and early childhood are likely to show signs of reactive attachment disorder and have difficulty forming relationships with caregivers.

## Treatment

The cornerstone of treatment for PTSD is education of the child and family regarding the nature of the disorder so that the child's emotional reactions and regressive behavior are not mistakenly viewed as crazy or manipulative. Support, reassurance, and repeated explanations and understanding are needed. It is critical that the child be living in a safe environment, and if caregivers have been abusive, concerns must be reported to social services. Interventions to maintain safety of the child are imperative. Individual and family psychotherapy are central features of treatment interventions. Specific fears usually wane with time, and behavioral desensitization may help. A supportive relationship with a caregiving adult is essential.

For children with more severe and persistent symptoms, assessment for treatment with medication is indicated. Sertraline has approval for the treatment of PTSD in adults. Target symptoms (eg, anxiety, depression, nightmares, aggression) should be clearly identified and appropriate medications trials initiated with close monitoring. Some of the medications used to treat children with PTSD include clonidine or guanfacine (Tenex), mood stabilizers, and antidepressants and neuroleptics. Children who have lived for an extended time in abusive environments or who have been exposed to multiple traumas are more likely to require treatment with medications. Occupational therapy for sensory integration can also be effective in decreasing reactivity to stimuli and helping the child and caregivers develop and implement self-soothing skills. Individuals who have suffered single-episode traumas usually benefit significantly from psychotherapy and may require limited treatment with medication to address symptoms of anxiety, nightmares, and sleep disturbance. Psychotherapy that includes eye movement desensitization and reprocessing (EMDR) may also be useful.

## Prognosis

At 4- to 5-year follow-up investigations, many children who have been through a traumatic life experience continue to have vivid and frightening memories and dreams and a pessimistic view of the future. The effects of traumatic experiences can be far-reaching. The ability of caregivers to provide a safe, supportive, stable, empathic environment enhances the prognosis for individuals with PTSD. Timely access to therapy and use of therapy over time to work through symptoms also enhance prognosis. Evidence is growing to support a connection between victimization in childhood and unstable personality and mood disorders in later life.

American Academy of Child and Adolescent Psychiatry: Practice parameters for the assessment and treatment of children and adolescents with posttraumatic stress disorder. J Am Acad Child Adolesc Psychiatry 1998;37(Suppl):4S [PMID: 9785726].

Grant KE et al: Stressors and child and adolescent psychopathology: Moving from markers to mechanisms of risk. Psychol Bull 2002;129(3):447 [PMID: 12784938].

Martin SG: Children exposed to domestic violence: Psychological considerations for health care practitioners. Holistic Nurs Pract 2002;16(3):7 [PMID: 11913229].

Meiser-Stedman R: Towards a cognitive-behavioral model of PTSD in children and adolescents. Clin Child Fam Psychol Rev 2002;5(4):217 [PMID: 12495267].

Pine DS: Developmental psychobiology and response to threats: Relevance to trauma in children and adolescents. Biol Psychiatry 2003;53(9):796 [PMID: 12725972].

Pine DS, Cohen JA: Trauma in children and adolescents: Risk and treatment of psychiatric sequelae. Biol Psychiatry 2002;51(7): 519 [PMID: 11950454].

Scheeringa MS et al: New findings on alternative criteria for PTSD in preschool children. J Am Acad Child Adolesc Psychiatry 2003;42(5):561 [PMID: 12707560].

Teicher MH et al: Developmental neurobiology of childhood stress and trauma. Psychiatr Clin North Am 2002;25(2): 397 [PMID: 12136508].

# SOMATOFORM DISORDERS

 ESSENTIALS OF DIAGNOSIS & TYPICAL FEATURES

- *A symptom suggesting physical dysfunction.*
- *No physical disorder accounting for the symptom.*
- *Symptoms causing distress, dysfunction, or both.*
- *Symptoms not voluntarily created or maintained, as in malingering.*

## Clinical Findings

Somatoform disorders are defined by the presence of physical illness or disability for which no organic cause can be identified, although neither the patient nor the caregiver is consciously fabricating the symptoms. The category includes body dysmorphic disorder, conversion disorder, hypochondriasis, somatization disorder, and somatoform pain disorder (Table 6–18).

Conversion symptoms most often occur in school-age children and adolescents. The exact incidence is unclear, but in pediatric practice they are probably seen more often as transient symptoms than as chronic disorders requiring help from mental health practitioners. A conversion symptom is thought to be an expression of underlying psychological conflict. The specific symptom may be symbolically determined by the underlying conflict. Furthermore, the symptom may resolve the dilemma created by the underlying wish or fear (eg, a seemingly paralyzed child need not fear expressing his underlying rage or aggressive retaliatory impulses). Although children can present with a variety of symptoms, the most common include neurologic and gastrointestinal (GI) complaints. Children with conversion disorder may be surprisingly unconcerned about the substantial disability deriving from their symptoms. Symptoms include unusual sensory phenomena, paralysis, vomiting, abdominal pain, intractable headaches, and movement or seizure-like disorders.

**Table 6–18.** Somatoform disorders in children and adolescents.

| Disorder | Major Clinical Manifestations |
|---|---|
| Body dysmorphic disorder | Preoccupation with an imagined defect in personal appearance |
| Conversion disorder | Symptom onset follows psychologically stressful event; symptoms express unconscious feelings and result in secondary gain |
| Hypochondriasis | Preoccupation with worry that physical symptoms manifest unrecognized and threatening condition; medical assurance does not provide relief from worry |
| Somatization disorder | Long-standing preoccupation with multiple somatic symptoms |
| Somatoform pain disorder | Preoccupation with pain that results in distress or impairment beyond what would be expected from physical findings |

In the classic case of conversion disorder, the child's symptoms and examination findings are not consistent with the clinical manifestations of any organic disease process. The physical symptoms often begin within the context of a family experiencing stress, such as serious illness, a death, or family discord. On closer examination, the child's symptoms are often found to resemble symptoms present in other family members. Children with conversion disorder may have some secondary gain associated with their symptoms. A number of reports have pointed to the increased association of conversion disorder with sexual overstimulation or sexual abuse. As with other emotional and behavioral problems, health care providers should always screen for physical and sexual abuse.

## Differential Diagnosis

It is sometimes not possible to rule out medical disease as a source of the symptoms. Medical follow-up is required to monitor for changes in symptoms and response to recommended interventions.

Somatic symptoms are often associated with anxiety and depressive disorders (see Table 6–15). Occasionally, psychotic children have somatic preoccupations and even somatic delusions.

## Treatment & Prognosis

In most cases, conversion symptoms resolve quickly when the child and family are reassured that the symptom is a way of reacting to stress. The child is encouraged to continue with normal daily activities, knowing that the symptom will abate when the stress is resolved.

Treatment of conversion disorders includes acknowledging the symptom rather than telling the child that the symptom is not medically justified and responding with noninvasive interventions such as physical therapy while continuing to encourage normalization of the symptoms. If the symptom does not resolve with reassurance, further investigation by a mental health professional is indicated. Comorbid diagnoses such as depression and anxiety disorders should be addressed, and treatment with psychopharmacologic agents may be helpful.

Campo JV, Fritz G: A management model for pediatric somatization. Psychosomatics 2001;42(6):467 [PMID: 11815681].

Campo JV et al: Somatization in pediatric primary care: Association with psychopathology, functional impairment, and use of services. J Am Acad Child Adolesc Psychiatry 1999;38:1093 [PMID: 10504807].

Dhossche D et al: Somatoform disorders in children and adolescents: A comparison with other internalizing disorders. Ann Clin Psychiatry 2002;14(1):23 [PMID: 12046637].

Fritz GK et al: Somatoform disorders in children and adolescents: A review of the past 10 years. J Am Acad Child Adolesc Psychiatry 1997;36:1329 [PMID: 9334545].

# ELIMINATION DISORDERS

## 1. Enuresis

It is important for the primary care provider to carefully assess the developmental age of the child, the situation in which enuresis is occurring, and to screen for medical concerns before deciding that the enuresis or encopresis is attributable to a behavioral or emotional disorder. It is not uncommon for parents to have unrealistic expectations about toilet training for young children. In many cases of enuresis, the child is simply not developmentally ready or sometimes is unable to remain dry at night. Most children with enuresis are able to remain dry by age 9.

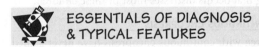

### ESSENTIALS OF DIAGNOSIS & TYPICAL FEATURES

- Urinary incontinence in a child age 5 years (or developmental equivalent) or older.
- No medication or general medical condition causing the urinary incontinence.

## General Considerations

Enuresis is the passage of urine into bedclothes or undergarments, whether involuntary or intentional. At least 90% of enuretic children have primary nocturnal enuresis—that is, they wet only at night during sleep and have never had a sustained period of dryness. Diurnal enuresis (daytime wetting) is much less common, as is secondary enuresis, which develops after a child has had a sustained period of bladder control. The latter two varieties are much more commonly associated with emotional stress, anxiety, and psychiatric disorders. Primary nocturnal enuresis is most often a parasomnia, a deep-sleep (stage 3 or stage 4) event. Etiologically, it is generally viewed as a developmental disorder or maturational lag that children will outgrow. Only infrequently is it associated with a serious psychopathologic disorder.

## Clinical Findings

Primary nocturnal enuresis is common (Table 6–19). The incidence is three times higher in boys than in girls. Most children with enuresis become continent by adolescence or earlier. The family history in such cases frequently reveals other members, especially fathers, who have had prolonged nighttime bed-wetting problems. Although the cause of primary nocturnal enuresis is not established, it appears to be related to maturational delay of sleep and arousal mechanisms or to delay in development of increased bladder capacity.

Daytime wetting most often occurs in timid and shy children or in children with ADHD. It occurs with about equal frequency in boys and girls, and 60–80% of daytime wetters also wet at night. Secondary enuresis typically follows a stressful event, such as the birth of a sibling, a loss, or discord within the family. The symptom can be seen as the result of regression in response

**Table 6–19.** Incidence of enuresis in children.

| Age (years) | Primary Nocturnal Enuresis (%) | Occasional Daytime Enuresis (%)[a] |
|---|---|---|
| 5 | 15 | 8 |
| 7–8 | 7 | — |
| 10 | 3–5 | — |
| 12 | 2–3 | 1 |
| 14 | 1 | — |

[a]Diurnal (daytime) enuresis tends to resolve by developmental age 6 years, with a slight recurrence around age 12 years in early adolescence.

to stress or as a more symbolic expression of the child's feelings.

## Differential Diagnosis

The differential diagnosis includes urinary tract infections, neurologic diseases, seizure disorders, diabetes mellitus, and structural abnormalities of the urinary tract. Urinalysis and urine culture and observing the child's urinary stream can rule out the majority of organic causes of enuresis.

## Complications

The most common complication of enuresis is low self-esteem in response to criticism from caregivers and embarrassment if peers are aware of the problem. Older children with enuresis may be reluctant to attend sleepovers and be self-conscious with peers.

## Treatment

Treatment should emphasize that the symptom of nocturnal enuresis is a developmental lag and often will be outgrown even without treatment. Even with these interventions, many children will have difficulty remaining dry. If the child chooses to pursue treatment, a program of bladder exercises can be prescribed: fluids should be limited after dinner; the child should attempt to hold urine as long as possible during the day and then start and stop the stream at the toilet bowl; the child is instructed to practice getting up from bed and going to the bathroom at bedtime before sleep. These procedures are helpful in perhaps 30–40% of children with nighttime wetting. Another option is a "potty pager." This is a beeper-like object that attaches to the child's underwear and vibrates when the child is wet in an attempt to rouse the child into a wakeful state and increase awareness of the need to urinate.

Desmopressin acetate (DDAVP), administered intranasally at bedtime, can result in complete remission of nocturnal enuresis in 50% of children as long as they continue the treatment. DDAVP is expensive, but can be useful until the child develops the ability to hold urine through the night or awaken to use the bathroom. For others, a trial of the TCA imipramine is worthwhile, at dosages of 25–50 mg at bedtime for children under age 12 years and 50–75 mg for older children. Because many patients relapse once the drug is stopped, its primary use is for camp attendance or overnight visits. Mental health treatment is more often needed for children with daytime wetting or secondary enuresis. The focus is on the verbal expression of feelings that may be associated with perpetuation of the symptom and behavioral interventions to work toward dryness and cope with episodes of wetting.

## 2. Encopresis

### ESSENTIALS OF DIAGNOSIS & TYPICAL FEATURES

- Fecal incontinence in a child age 4 years (or developmental equivalent) or older.
- Not due to medication or medical disorder.

## General Considerations

Functional encopresis is defined as the repeated passage of feces in inappropriate places by a child of at least the developmental equivalent of age 4 years. It may be either involuntary or intentional, although most often it is involuntary. It affects approximately 1–1.5% of school-age children; boys four times more often than girls. Functional fecal incontinence is rare in adolescence.

## Clinical Findings

Functional encopresis can be divided into four types: retentive, continuous, discontinuous, and toilet phobia.

### A. RETENTIVE ENCOPRESIS

In retentive encopresis, also called psychogenic megacolon, the child withholds bowel movements, leading to the development of constipation, fecal impaction, and the seepage of soft or liquid feces around the margins of the impaction into the underclothing. Marked constipation and painful defecation often contribute to a vicious cycle of withholding, thus creating larger impaction and further seepage. These children often have a history of crossing their legs to resist the urge to defecate and of infrequent bowel movements large enough to stop up the toilet, and they are found on examination to have large fecal masses in their rectal vaults. The soiling that occurs distresses most of these children.

### B. CONTINUOUS ENCOPRESIS

Children with continuous encopresis have never gained primary control of bowel function. The bowel movement is usually randomly deposited in underclothing without regard to social norms. Typically, the family structure does not encourage organization and skill training, and for that reason the child has never had adequate bowel training. These children and their parents are more apt to be socially or intellectually disadvantaged.

## C. DISCONTINUOUS ENCOPRESIS

Children with discontinuous encopresis have a history of normal bowel control for an extended period. Loss of control often occurs in response to a stressful event, such as the birth of a sibling, a separation, family illness, or marital disharmony. These children may soil their pants or on occasion defecate on the floor or smear feces as an expression of anger or of a wish to be perceived as younger. They typically display relative indifference to the symptom.

## D. TOILET PHOBIA

In the infrequent case of toilet phobia, a young child views the toilet as a frightening structure to be avoided. These children may view the bowel movement as an extension of themselves, which is then swept away in a frightening manner. They may think that they, too, may be swept away, down the toilet.

## Differential Diagnosis

Differential diagnosis includes the medical causes of constipation and retentive encopresis. Hirschsprung disease can be ruled out with reasonable certainty by the history of passing large-caliber bowel movements in the past and by the presence of palpable stool in the rectal vault. Neurologic disorders, hypothyroidism, hypercalcemia, and diseases of smooth muscle must be considered as well. The child should be examined for anal fissures, which tend to encourage the withholding of bowel movements. In addition, fecal soiling can be a presenting symptom in childhood depression and is sometimes a concomitant finding in children with ADHD. If the child engages in fecal smearing, an underlying psychotic disorder should be considered.

## Treatment

Identifying the type of encopresis is important in treatment planning. Another important variable is the child's own concern about the symptom. Encopresis in children who display denial or indifference is much harder to treat. Children with coexisting depression or ADHD need to receive treatment for those conditions before focusing treatment on soiling.

With the most common type of encopresis, the retentive type, efforts are made to soften stool so that constipation and painful defecation do not perpetuate the behavior. These children are then taught to adopt a regular schedule of sitting on the toilet after meals. A system of positive reinforcement can be added in which the child is rewarded for each day with no soiled under-

clothes. The responsibility for rinsing soiled clothing and depositing it in the appropriate receptacle rests with the child. In the case of continuous encopresis, the family is taught to train the child. For toilet phobia, a progressive series of rewarded desensitization steps is necessary. Children with discontinuous encopresis that persists over a number of weeks often need psychotherapy to help them recognize and verbally express their anger and wish to be dependent, rather than express themselves through fecal soiling.

## Prognosis

Although the ultimate prognosis is excellent, parental distress and parent–child conflict may be substantial prior to the cessation of symptoms. The natural history of soiling is that it resolves by adolescence in all but the most severely disturbed teenagers.

Bonner L, Dobson P: Children who soil: Guidelines for good practice. J Fam Health Care 2003;13(2):32 [PMID: 12793299].

Borowitz SM et al: Treatment of childhood encopresis: A randomized trial comparing three treatment protocols. J Pediatr Gastroenterol Nutr 2002;34(4):378 [PMID: 11930093].

Cedron M: Removing the stigma: Helping reduce the psychosocial impact of bedwetting. Urol Nurs 2002;22(4):286 [PMID: 12242905].

Cox DF et al: Psychological differences between children with and without chronic encopresis. J Pediatr Psychol 2002;27(7):585 [PMID: 12228330].

Fishman L et al: Trends in referral to a single encopresis clinic over 20 years. Pediatrics 2003;111(5 pt 1):e604 [PMID: 12728118].

Fritz G, Rockney R: Summary of the practice parameter for the assessment and treatment of children and adolescents with enuresis. J Am Acad Child Adolesc Psychiatry 2004;43(1):123 [PMID: 14691370].

Gottsegen DN: Curing bedwetting on the spot: A review of one-session cures. Clin Pediatr 2003;42(3):273 [PMID: 12739927].

Loening-Baucke V: Encopresis. Curr Opin Pediatr 2002;14(5):570 [PMID: 12352250].

Mercer R: Dry at night. Treating nocturnal enuresis. Adv Nurs Pract 2003;11(2):26 [PMID: 12640815].

Mikkelson EJ: Enuresis and encopresis: Ten years of progress. Am J Child Adolesc Psychiatr 2001;40(10):1146 [PMID: 11589527].

Thiedke CC: Nocturnal enuresis. Am Fam Physician 2003;67(7):1499 [PMID: 12722850].

Van Ginkel R et al: Childhood constipation: Longitudinal follow-up beyond puberty. Gastroenterology 2003;125(2):357 [PMID: 12891536].

Other psychiatric conditions not covered in this chapter:

Attention-Deficit/Hyperactivity Disorder (ADHD), See Chapter 2

Eating Disorders, See Chapter 5

Mental Retardation, See Chapter 2
Substance Abuse, See Chapter 4
Tourette Syndrome, See Chapter 23

# OVERVIEW OF PEDIATRIC PSYCHOPHARMACOLOGY

Pediatric psychopharmacology has improved significantly over the past decade with increasing study of the effect of psychoactive medications on mental illness in childhood and adolescence. Although relatively few medications are approved for use in children, many of the same psychopharmacologic agents used in adults are now used in children and adolescents.

As with any medication, the risks as well as the benefits of administering psychoactive medications must be discussed with the child's parent or guardian and with the child and adolescent, as is age-appropriate. A recommendation for medication is warranted if the disorder is interfering with psychosocial development, interpersonal relationships, daily functioning, or the patient's sense of personal well-being, and if there is significant potential for benefit with the medication and relatively low risk of harm. Informed consent should be given by the parent or guardian and noted in the record. Adolescents should also provide informed consent for treatment. In some states adolescents age 15 and older must give informed consent. Informed consent includes a discussion of the diagnosis, target symptoms, possible common side effects, any side effects that should be closely monitored, potential benefits associated with the medication, and documentation of informed consent in the medical record. Psychopharmacologic agents are seldom the only treatment for a psychiatric disorder. Most often they are best used adjunctively along with other therapeutic interventions such as individual and family psychotherapy and psychosocial interventions, including assessment of school functioning and special needs.

A good rule when considering the use of psychoactive medications in children and adolescents is, first, to identify target symptoms that can be followed to evaluate the efficacy of treatment. When initiating treatment, start with low doses and increase slowly (in divided doses, if indicated) monitoring for side effects along with therapeutic effects. When drugs are discontinued, dosages should be tapered over 2–4 weeks to minimize withdrawal effects. When multiple choices exist, one should select the medication with the fewest and least ominous risks and side effects. Polypharmacy should be avoided by choosing one drug that might diminish most or all of the target symptoms before considering the simultaneous administration of two or more agents.

Table 6–20 presents an overview of the clinical conditions for which psychopharmacologic agents should be considered and medication categories for which studies have been completed or published case reports have suggested some therapeutic efficacy. Only the stimulants for ADHD and fluvoxamine and sertraline for OCD have FDA approval for specific use in children and adolescents.

In the text that follows, the major classes of psychopharmacologic agents with clinical indications in child and adolescent psychiatry are represented. The more commonly prescribed drugs from each class are reviewed with reference to indications, relative contraindications, initial medical screening procedures (in addition to a general pediatric examination), dosage, adverse effects, drug interactions, and medical follow-up recommendations. This is meant to be a brief reference guide, and the physician should consult a child and adolescent psychopharmacology textbook for additional information on specific medications.

**Table 6–20.** Clinical conditions and appropriate medications

| Diagnosis | Possible Classes of Medications to Target Symptoms |
|---|---|
| ADHD | Stimulants, bupropion, α-agonists |
| Anorexia nervosa | SSRIs, atypical neuroleptics |
| Autism | SSRIs, atypical neuroleptics, clomipramine, naltrexone |
| Bipolar affective disorder | Mood stabilizers, neuroleptics |
| Bulimia nervosa | SSRIs |
| Major depression and dysthymic disorder | Antidepressants |
| Anxiety disorders | Antidepressants, benzodiazepines |
| Posttraumatic stress disorder | Antidepressants, α-agonists, mood stabilizers, atypical neuroleptics |
| Obsessive compulsive disorder | SSRIs, clomipramine |
| Schizophrenia and psychotic disorders | Neuroleptics |
| Conduct disorder and severe aggressive behavior | Mood stabilizers, neuroleptics, α-agonists, stimulants, β blockers |

SSRIs = selective serotonin reuptake inhibitors.

# MEDICATIONS FOR ATTENTION-DEFICIT/HYPERACTIVITY DISORDER (ADHD)

Methylphenidate (Concerta, Metadate, Methylin, Ritalin)

Dextroamphetamine (Dexedrine)

Pemoline (Cylert)

Adderall

Atomoxetine (Strattera)

## A. INDICATIONS

Approximately 75% of children with ADHD experience improved attention span, decreased hyperactivity, and decreased impulsivity when given stimulant medications. Children with ADHD who do not respond favorably to one stimulant may respond well to another. Children and adolescents with ADHD without prominent hyperactivity (ADHD, predominantly inattentive type) are also likely to be responsive to stimulant medications. Atomoxetine (Strattera) and bupropion (Wellbutrin) are nonstimulant medications used to treat ADHD. Strattera has FDA approval for the treatment of ADHD and is a selective noradnergic reuptake inhibitor. Bupropion (Wellbutrin) is primarily used as an antidepressant, and blocks both serotonin and norepinephrine reuptake.

## B. CONTRAINDICATIONS

Use stimulants cautiously in individuals with a personal or family history of motor tics or Tourette syndrome, or if there is a personal or family history of substance abuse, addictive disorders, or psychotic disorders.

## C. INITIAL MEDICAL SCREENING

The initial interview should include screening for personal or family history of motor tics or Tourette syndrome. The child should be observed for involuntary movements. Height, weight, pulse, and blood pressure should be recorded. Liver enzymes should be tested if pemoline is considered.

## D. ADVERSE EFFECTS

Often dose-related and time-limited.

**1. Common adverse effects**—Anorexia, weight loss, abdominal distress, headache, insomnia, dysphoria and tearfulness, irritability, lethargy, mild tachycardia, mild elevation in blood pressure.

**2. Less common effects**—Interdose rebound of ADHD symptoms, emergence of motor tics or Tourette syndrome, behavioral stereotypy, tachycardia or hypertension, depression, mania, and psychotic symptoms. Reduced growth velocity occurs only during active administration. Growth rebound occurs during periods of discontinuation. Ultimate height is not usually noticeably compromised. Treatment with stimulant medications does not predispose to future substance abuse.

## E. DRUG INTERACTIONS

Additive stimulant effects are seen with sympathomimetic amines (ephedrine, pseudoephedrine).

## F. MEDICAL FOLLOW-UP

Pulse, blood pressure, height, and weight should be recorded every 3–4 months and at times of dosage increases. Assess for abnormal movements such as motor tics at each visit.

## G. DOSAGE

**1. Methylphenidate**—The usual starting dose is 5 mg once or twice a day (before school and at noon), gradually increasing to 5–10 mg/wk. Maximum daily dose should not exceed 60 mg, and a single dose should not exceed 0.7 mg/kg. Administration on weekends and during vacations is determined by the need at those times. The duration of action is approximately 3–4 hours. Several extended-release forms can prevent the need for taking medication at school.

**2. Dextroamphetamine sulfate**—The dosage is 2.5–10 mg twice daily, before school and at noon, with or without another dose at 4 PM. A sustained-release preparation may have clinical effects for up to 8 hours. There is also an extended-release form.

**3. Pemoline**—The longer half-life of pemoline allows for the administration of a single dose each morning. The usual starting dose of 37.5 mg is increased weekly by 18.75 mg until the desired clinical effect is achieved or until a maximum daily dose of 112.5 mg is reached. The onset of clinical effect may be delayed for 3–4 weeks. Liver enzymes must be monitored during treatment. Pemoline is contraindicated in individuals with hepatic disease.

Longer acting stimulants (see a psychopharmacology reference source for pharmacologic properties and dosage information): Adderall (dextroamphetamine and amphetamine)

Methylphenidate hydrochloride extended-release tablets (Concerta, Metadate)

**4. Atomoxetine Hydrochloride**—The starting dose for children and adolescents up to 70 kg is 0.5 mg/kg, with titration to a maximum dose of 1.2 mg/kg, in single or divided dosing.

# ANTIDEPRESSANTS

## 1. Selective Serotonin Reuptake Inhibitors

Citalopram, escitalopram (Celexa, Lexapro)
Fluoxetine (Prozac, Sarafem)
Fluvoxamine (Luvox)
Paroxetine (Paxil)
Sertraline (Zoloft)

### A. INDICATIONS

The SSRIs have become the agents of first choice for the treatment of depression and anxiety. Fluvoxamine and sertraline both have approval from the FDA for treatment of pediatric OCD. Although no other SSRIs have FDA approval for pediatric indications, some published studies support the efficacy of SSRIs for the treatment of depression, anxiety, and OCD in pediatric populations. Each SSRI has different FDA indications. However, once an indication is obtained for one SSRI, it is widely believed that other SSRIs are likely to be effective as well for the same indication. The FDA-approved indications are the following:

Major depression (> 18 years of age): fluoxetine, paroxetine, citalopram, sertraline
Panic disorder (> 18 years): paroxetine, sertraline
OCD (> 6 years): sertraline, fluvoxamine
Bulimia (> 18 years): fluoxetine
Posttraumatic stress disorder (> 18 years): sertraline
Premenstrual dysphoric disorder (> 18 years): fluoxetine

### B. CONTRAINDICATIONS

Concern about paroxetine causing a slightly increased incidence of suicidal ideation in children and adolescents in Great Britain led to a 2003 FDA statement regarding caution in prescribing this medication for children and adolescents. Caution should be used in cases of known liver disease, because all SSRIs are metabolized in the liver. Caution should be used when prescribing for an individual with a family history of bipolar disorder, or when the differential diagnosis includes bipolar disorder, because antidepressants can induce manic or hypomanic symptoms.

### C. INITIAL MEDICAL SCREENING

General medical examination only.

### D. ADVERSE EFFECTS

Often dose-related and time-limited: GI distress and nausea (can be minimized by taking medication with food), headache, tremulousness, decreased appetite, weight loss, insomnia, sedation (10%), sexual dysfunction (25%). Irritability, social disinhibition, restlessness, and emotional excitability can occur in approximately 20% of children taking SSRIs.

### E. DRUG INTERACTIONS

All SSRIs inhibit the efficiency of the hepatic microsomal enzyme system. The order of inhibition is: fluoxetine > fluvoxamine > paroxetine > sertraline > citalopram. This can lead to higher than expected blood levels of other drugs, including antidepressants, antiarrhythmics, antipsychotics, β-blockers, opioids, and antihistamines. Taking tryptophan while on an SSRI may result in a serotonergic syndrome of psychomotor agitation and GI distress. A potentially fatal interaction that clinically resembles neuroleptic malignant syndrome may occur when the SSRIs are administered concomitantly with the monoamine oxidase inhibitors (MAOIs). Fluoxetine has the longest half-life of the SSRIs and should not be initiated within 14 days of the discontinuation of an MAOI, or an MAOI initiated within at least 5 weeks of the discontinuation of fluoxetine.

### F. DOSAGE (TABLE 6–21)

The SSRIs are usually given once a day, in the morning with breakfast. One in 10 individuals may experience sedation and prefer to take the medication at bedtime. The alternative antidepressants and fluvoxamine are usually given in twice daily dosing. Bupropion and venlafaxine are now available in a sustained- and extended-release form. Therapeutic response should be expected 4–6 weeks after a therapeutic dose has been reached. The starting dose for a child younger than 12 years old is generally half the starting dose for an adolescent.

## 2. Other Antidepressants

Bupropion (Wellbutrin), bupropion SR (sustained release)
Venlafaxine (Effexor), venlafaxine XR (extended release)
Mirtazapine (Remeron)
Nefazodone (Serzone)

### Bupropion

#### A. INDICATIONS

Bupropion is an antidepressant that inhibits reuptake of primarily serotonin, but also norepinephrine and dopamine. It is approved for treatment of major depression in adults, but is receiving favorable attention for its therapeutic effects with major depressive disorder in adolescents and with ADHD in children and adoles-

*Table 6–21.* Medications used to treat depression in adolescents

| Generic | Trade Name | Adolescent Starting Dose | Target Dose (Average Effective Dose) | Maximum Dose |
|---|---|---|---|---|
| **SSRIs** | | | | |
| Citalopram | Celexa | 20 mg qAM | 20 mg qAM | 40–60 mg qAM |
| Escitalopram | Lexapro | 10 mg | 10 mg | 30 mg |
| Fluoxetine | Prozac | 10 mg qAM | 20 mg qAM | 60 mg qAM |
| Fluvoxamine | Luvox | 50 mg qhs | 100–150 mg qd | 100 mg bid |
| Paroxetine | Paxil | 10 mg qAM | 20 mg qAM | 60 mg qAM |
| Paroxetine CR | Paxil CR | 25 mg | 25 mg | 50 mg |
| Sertraline | Zoloft | 25 mg qAM | 50 mg qAM | 150 mg qAM |
| **Alternative Antidepressants** | | | | |
| Bupropion | Wellbutrin | 75 mg qAM | 150 mg bid | 200 mg bid |
| Bupropion SR | Wellbutrin SR | 100 mg qAM | 100 mg bid | 150 mg bid |
| Mirtazapine | Remeron | 7.5 mg qhs | 15 mg qhs | 30 mg qhs |
| Nefazodone | Serzone | 50 mg qhs | 100 mg bid | 300 mg bid |
| Venlafaxine | Effexor | 37.5 mg qAM | 75 mg bid | 150 mg bid |
| Venlafaxine XR | Effexor XR | 37.5 mg qAM | 150 mg qd | 225 mg qd |

qAM = every morning; qhs = every night at bedtime; qd = every day; bid = twice a day.

cents. Like the SSRIs, bupropion has very few anticholinergic or cardiotoxic effects.

**B. CONTRAINDICATIONS**

History of seizure disorder or bulimia nervosa.

**C. INITIAL MEDICAL SCREENING AND FOLLOW-UP**

General medical examination.

**D. ADVERSE EFFECTS**

Psychomotor activation (agitation or restlessness), headache, GI distress, nausea, anorexia with weight loss, insomnia, tremulousness, precipitation of mania, and induction of seizures with doses above 450 mg/d.

## Venlafaxine

Venlafaxine is an antidepressant that primarily inhibits reuptake of serotonin and norepinephrine.

**A. INDICATIONS**

It is approved for the treatment of major depression in adults.

**B. CONTRAINDICATIONS**

Hypertension.

**C. INITIAL MEDICAL SCREENING AND FOLLOW-UP**

General medical examination.

**D. ADVERSE EFFECTS**

The most common adverse effects are nausea, nervousness, and sweating. Hypertension is likely with doses over 300 mg or over 225 mg of the extended release version. Venlafaxine must be discontinued slowly to minimize withdrawal symptoms: severe headaches, dizziness and significant flu-like symptoms. It is also available in an extended-release form.

## Mirtazapine

Mirtazapine is an $\alpha_2$-antagonist that enhances central noradreneregic and serotonergic activity.

**A. INDICATIONS**

It is approved for the treatment of major depression in adults.

**B. CONTRAINDICATIONS**

Mirtazapine should not be given in combination with MAOIs. Very rare side effects are acute liver failure (1 case per 250–300,000), neutropenia, and agranulocytosis.

**C. INITIAL MEDICAL SCREENING AND FOLLOW-UP**

General medical examination.

**D. ADVERSE EFFECTS**

Dry mouth, increased appetite, constipation, weight gain.

## 3. Tricyclic Antidepressants

Imipramine
Desipramine (Norpramin)
Clomipramine (Anafranil)
Nortriptyline
Amitryptyline (Elavil)

With the introduction of the SSRIs and alternative antidepressants, use of the TCAs has become uncommon for the treatment of depression and anxiety disorders. The TCAs have more significant side-effect profiles, require more substantial medical monitoring, and are quite cardiotoxic in overdose. For these reasons, in general, SSRIs or alternative antidepressants should be considered before recommending a TCA.

### A. INDICATIONS

TCAs have been prescribed for chronic pain syndromes, migraines, headache, depression, anxiety, enuresis, bulimia nervosa, OCD, and PTSD in children and adolescents. Imipramine and desipramine have FDA approval for the treatment of major depression in adults and enuresis for children older than 6 years of age. Some published studies have demonstrated clinical efficacy in the treatment of ADHD, panic disorder, anxiety-based school refusal, separation anxiety disorder, bulimia, night terrors, and sleepwalking. But, as yet, the FDA has not approved their use for these indications. Studies have not supported efficacy in major depression in children and adolescents. Nortriptyline has FDA approval for the treatment of major depression in adults. Clomipramine has FDA approval for the treatment of depression and OCD in adults and may be helpful for obsessive symptoms in autism.

### B. CONTRAINDICATIONS

Known cardiac disease or arrhythmia, undiagnosed syncope, known seizure disorder, family history of sudden cardiac death or cardiomyopathy, known electrolyte abnormality (with bingeing and purging).

### C. INITIAL MEDICAL SCREENING

The family history should be examined for sudden cardiac death; the patient's history for cardiac disease, arrhythmias, syncope, seizure disorder, or congenital hearing loss (associated with prolonged QT interval). Other screening procedures include serum electrolytes and blood urea nitrogen (BUN) in patients who have eating disorders, cardiac examination, and a baseline electrocardiogram (ECG).

### D. MEDICAL FOLLOW-UP

Measure pulse and blood pressure (monitor for tachycardia and orthostatic hypotension) with each dosage increase, and obtain an ECG to monitor for arteriovenous block with each dosage increase; after reaching steady state, record pulse, blood pressure, and ECG every 3–4 months.

### E. ADVERSE EFFECTS

**1. Cardiotoxic effects**—The cardiotoxic effects of TCAs appear to be more common in children and adolescents than in adults. In addition to anticholinergic effects, TCAs have quinidine-like effects that result in slowing of cardiac conduction. Increased plasma levels appear to be weakly associated with an increased risk of cardiac conduction abnormalities. Steady-state plasma levels of desipramine or of desipramine plus imipramine should therefore not exceed 300 ng/mL. In addition, each dosage increase above 3 mg/kg/d must be carefully monitored with pulse, blood pressure, and repeated ECGs to monitor for arteriovenous block. Upper limits for cardiovascular parameters when administering TCAs to children and adolescents are listed in Table 6–22.

**2. Anticholinergic effects**—Tachycardia, dry mouth, stuffy nose, blurred vision, constipation, sweating, vasomotor instability, withdrawal syndrome (GI distress and psychomotor activation).

**3. Other effects**—Orthostatic hypotension and dizziness, lowered seizure threshold, increased appetite and weight gain, sedation, irritability and psychomotor agitation, rash (often associated with yellow dye No. 5), headache, abdominal complaints, sleep disturbance and nightmares, mania.

### F. DRUG INTERACTIONS

TCAs may potentiate the effects of CNS depressants and stimulants; barbiturates and cigarette smoking may decrease plasma levels; phenothiazines, methylphenidate, and oral contraceptives may increase plasma levels; SSRIs given in combination with TCAs will result in higher TCA blood levels due to inhibition of the

**Table 6–22.** Upper limits of cardiovascular parameters with tricyclic antidepressants.

| Heart rate | 130/min |
|---|---|
| Systolic blood pressure | 130 mm Hg |
| Diastolic blood pressure | 85 mm Hg |
| PR interval | 0.2 s |
| QRS interval | 0.12 s, or no more than 30% over baseline |
| QT corrected | 0.45 s |

TCA metabolism by liver enzymes (eg, cytochrome p450 isoenzyme).

## G. DOSAGE

Refer to a pediatric psychopharmacology text for dosages. Daily dosage requirements vary considerably with different clinical disorders.

# MOOD STABILIZERS

Lithium carbonate (Eskalith, Eskalith CR, Lithobid, Lithotabs)

Valproic acid (Depakote, Depakote ER)

Carbamazepine (Tegretol)

Olanzapine (Zyprexa, atypical neuroleptic)

Lithium, valproic acid, and olanzapine (neuroleptic) are FDA approved for the treatment of bipolar disorder. Carbamazepine and oxycarbamazepine, although not FDA approved for treatment of bipolar disorder, may also be effective and carry less risk of weight gain. Lamotrigine (Lamictal) was recently approved for the treatment of bipolar depression in adults. Other antiepileptic medications, such as gabapentin and topiramate, have also been used with varying efficacy. Medications that are effective as mood stabilizers may be helpful also in the treatment of severe aggressive symptoms.

## Lithium

### A. INDICATIONS

Lithium remains a frontline drug in the treatment of bipolar disorder and has been shown to have an augmenting effect when combined with SSRIs for treatment-resistant depression and OCD.

### B. CONTRAINDICATIONS

Lithium is contraindicated in patients with known renal, thyroid, or cardiac disease; those at high risk for dehydration and electrolyte imbalance (eg, vomiting and purging); and those who may become pregnant (teratogenic effects).

### C. INITIAL MEDICAL SCREENING

General medical screening with pulse, blood pressure, height, and weight; complete blood cell count (CBC); serum electrolytes, BUN, and creatinine; and thyroid function tests including thyroid-stimulating hormone levels.

### D. DOSAGE

For children the starting dose is usually 150 mg once or twice a day, with titration in 150–300-mg increments. (Dose may vary with the brand of lithium used, consult a psychopharmacology textbook for medication specific

information.) Oral doses of lithium should be titrated to maintain therapeutic blood levels of 0.8–1.2 mEq/L. The drug is generally given in two doses. Blood samples should be drawn 12 hours after the last dose.

### E. ADVERSE EFFECTS

**1. Lithium toxicity**—Lithium has a narrow therapeutic index. Blood levels required for therapeutic effect are close to those associated with toxic symptoms. Mild toxicity may be indicated by increased tremor, GI distress, neuromuscular irritability, and altered mental status (confusion), and can occur when blood levels exceed 1.5 mEq/L. Moderate to severe symptoms of lithium toxicity are associated with blood levels above 2 mEq/L. Acute renal failure can occur at levels over 2.5–3 mEq/L.

**2. Side effects**—Lithium side effects include intention tremor, GI distress (including nausea and vomiting and sometimes diarrhea), hypothyroidism, polyuria and polydipsia, drowsiness, malaise, weight gain, acne, and granulocytosis.

### F. DRUG INTERACTIONS

Excessive salt intake and salt restriction should be avoided. Thiazide diuretics and nonsteroidal anti-inflammatory agents (except aspirin and acetaminophen) can lead to increased lithium levels. Ibuprofen should be avoided by individuals on lithium due to combined renal toxicity. Precautions against dehydration are required in hot weather and during vigorous exercise.

### G. MEDICAL FOLLOW-UP

Serum lithium levels should be measured 5–7 days following a change in dosage and then quarterly at steady state; serum creatinine and thyroid-stimulating hormone concentrations should be determined every 3–4 months.

## Valproic Acid

### A. INDICATIONS

Valproate has FDA approval for the treatment of bipolar disorder in adults. Its efficacy in acute mania equals that of lithium, but it is generally better tolerated. Valproate is more effective than lithium in patients with rapid-cycling bipolar disorder (more than four cycles per year) and in patients with mixed states (coexisting symptoms of depression and mania). Valproate may be more effective than lithium in adolescents with bipolar disorder because they often have rapid cycling and mixed states.

### B. CONTRAINDICATIONS

Liver dysfunction.

### C. INITIAL MEDICAL SCREENING

CBC and LFTs.

### D. DOSAGE

Usually starts at 15 mg/kg/d and is increased in increments of 5 to 10 mg/kg/d every 1–2 weeks to a range of 500–1500 mg/d in two or three divided doses. Trough levels in the range of 80–120 mg/mL are thought to be therapeutic.

### E. ADVERSE EFFECTS

Between 10% and 20% of patients experience sedation or anorexia, especially early in treatment or if the dose is increased too rapidly. GI upset occurs in 25% of patients and, when severe, can usually be treated with cimetidine. Increased appetite and weight gain can be troublesome for children and adolescents. Blurred vision, headache, hair loss, and tremor occur occasionally. Slight elevations in aminotransferases are frequent. Severe idiosyncratic hepatitis, pancreatitis, thrombocytopenia, and agranulocytosis occur only rarely.

### F. MEDICAL FOLLOW-UP

LFTs should be checked monthly for 3–4 months; subsequently, LFTs, a CBC, and trough valproate levels should be obtained every 3–4 months.

## Carbamazepine

### A. INDICATIONS

Similar to lithium and valproate, carbamazepine may be effective for treating bipolar disorder or for the target symptoms of mood instability, irritability, or behavioral dyscontrol. Some data suggest that it is more effective than valproate for the depressive phases of a bipolar disorder. This may relate to its similarities with the TCAs. A new form of carbamazepine—oxycarbamazepine (Trileptal)—is also being used for pediatric mood disorders; however, without established efficacy. Reportedly, it does not have the worrisome side effects of bone marrow suppression and liver enzyme induction. Blood levels cannot be monitored, and the dose range is similar to that with carbamazepine.

### B. CONTRAINDICATIONS

History of previous bone marrow depression or history of adverse hematologic reaction to another drug; history of sensitivity to a TCA.

### C. INITIAL MEDICAL SCREENING

Obtain a CBC with platelets, reticulocytes, serum iron, and BUN; LFTs; urinalysis.

### D. DOSAGE

Usually start at 10–20 mg/kg/d, in two divided doses, in children younger than age 6 years; 100 mg twice daily in children ages 6–12 years; and 200 mg twice daily in children over age 12 years. Doses may be increased weekly until there is effective symptom control. Total daily doses should not exceed 35 mg/kg/d in children younger than age 6 years; 1000 mg/d in children ages 6–15 years; and 1200 mg/d in adolescents older than age 15 years. Plasma levels in the range of 4–12 mg/mL are thought to be therapeutic.

### E. ADVERSE EFFECTS

Nausea, dizziness, sedation, headache, dry mouth, diplopia, and constipation reflect the drug's mild anticholinergic properties. Rashes are more common with carbamazepine than with other mood stabilizers. Aplastic anemia and agranulocytosis are rare. Leukopenia and thrombocytopenia are more common and, if present, should be monitored closely for evidence of bone marrow depression. These effects usually occur early and transiently and then spontaneously revert toward normal. Liver enzyme induction may significantly change the efficacy of medications given concurrently.

### F. MEDICAL FOLLOW-UP

Conservative management suggests that hematologic, hepatic, and renal parameters should be followed at least every 3 months for the first year. White blood cell counts below 3000/mL and absolute neutrophil counts below 1000/mL call for discontinuation of the drug and referral for hematology consultation.

## Gabapentin

Like valproate and carbamazepine, gabapentin is an anticonvulsant that has been used as a mood stabilizer in some adult populations. It may be used along with either valproate or carbamazepine in individuals with treatment-resistant disorders. The usual adult dose range for seizure disorders is 900–1800 mg/d in three divided doses and may need to be adjusted downward in individuals with renal impairment. Although its use among adolescents and even children is increasing, it is not approved for this indication, and reports of its efficacy remain largely anecdotal. Some reports suggest it may worsen behavioral parameters in children with underlying ADHD.

## NEUROLEPTICS

### 1. Atypical (Newer) Neuroleptics

Aripiprazole (Abilify)
Clozapine (Clozaril)

Olanzapine (Zyprexa)
Risperidone (Risperdal)
Quetiapine (Seroquel)
Ziprasidone (Geodon)

## 2. Conventional Neuroleptics

Chlorpromazine
Thioridazine
Haloperidol
Thiothixene
Molindone
Trifluoperazine
Perphenazine

The neuroleptics, also known as antipsychotics, are indicated for psychotic symptoms in patients with schizophrenia. They are also used for acute mania and as adjuncts to antidepressants in the treatment of psychotic depression (with delusions or hallucinations). The neuroleptics may be used cautiously in refractory PTSD, in refractory OCD, and in individuals with markedly aggressive behavioral problems unresponsive to other interventions. They may also be useful for the body image distortion associated with anorexia nervosa.

The "atypical neuroleptics" differ from conventional neuroleptics in their receptor specificity and effect on serotonin receptors. Conventional neuroleptics are associated with a higher incidence of movement disorders and extrapyramidal symptoms (EPS) due to their wider effect on dopamine receptors. The introduction of the atypical neuroleptics has significantly changed neuroleptic prescribing patterns. The atypical neuroleptics have a better side effect profile for most individuals and comparable efficacy for the treatment of psychotic symptoms and aggression. Atypical neuroleptics have a decreased incidence of EPS and tardive dyskinesias (TD). Significant side effects can include substantial weight gain and sedation. Because of their increased use over conventional neuroleptics, this section will focus primarily on the atypical neuroleptics.

## Aripiprazole (Abilify)

Aripiprazole is the newest atypical neuroleptic and is indicated for the treatment of schizophrenia. It is a partial dopamine blocker and a serotonin agonist. Side effects include nausea and vomiting and fatigue. It is not associated with weight gain. Doses over 30 mg are more likely to be associated with EPS. The dose range is 10 mg–30 mg, and pills can be split.

## Olanzapine (Zyprexa)

The FDA has approved this agent for the treatment of schizophrenia and bipolar disorder in adults. Olanzapine has greater affinity for type-2 serotonin receptors than dopamine-2 receptors and also has an effect on muscarinic, histaminic, and $\alpha$-adrenergic receptors. As with the other atypical neuroleptics, it may be more helpful for treating the negative symptoms of schizophrenia (flat affect, isolation and withdrawal, apathy) than conventional neuroleptics. Anecdotal and case report data support its utility in child and adolescent psychotic disorders. The adult dose range of 5–15 mg/d administered in a single, bedtime dose is probably applicable to adolescents as well. Weight gain can be a significant side effect. The starting dose for children is usually 1.25 mg.

## Quetiapine (Seroquel)

Quetiapine is an antagonist at multiple receptor sites, including serotonin ($5\text{-HT}_{1A}$, $5\text{-HT}_2$), dopamine (D1, D2), histamine, and adrenergic receptors. Quetiapine is given in 25- to 50-mg increments up to 800 mg for the treatment of psychotic symptoms. It is thought to be a "weight-neutral" medication, and the primary side effect is sedation.

## Risperidone (Risperdal)

Risperidone blocks type-2 dopamine receptors (similar to haloperidol) and type-2 serotonin receptors. Adult schizophrenic patients given 2–8 mg/d of risperidone had better symptom relief and fewer side effects than those treated with conventional neuroleptics. Anecdotal reports suggest that similar results may be obtained in adolescents with schizophrenia. Risperidone has also demonstrated good clinical efficacy in the treatment of Tourette syndrome. The initial dose is 1–2 mg/d in two divided doses. Side effects include weight gain and sedation.

## Ziprasidone (Geodon)

Ziprasidone has affinity for multiple serotonin receptors ($5\text{-HT}_2$, $5\text{-HT}_{1a}$, $5\text{-HT}_{1D}$, and $5\text{-HT}_{2C}$) and dopamine-2 receptors, and it moderately inhibits norepinephrine and 5-HT reuptake. It also has moderate affinity for $H_1$ and $\alpha_1$ receptors. Ziprasidone has a greater effect on cardiac QT intervals and requires a baseline ECG and ECG monitoring when a dose of 80 mg is reached and with each dose change above 80 mg to monitor for QT prolongation. Ziprasidone is reported to cause minimal weight gain. The initial dose of ziprasidone is 20 mg, with dose changes 20-mg increments to a total daily dose of 140 mg for the treatment of psychotic symptoms in adults. There are no studies of ziprasidone in children and adolescents at this time.

## Clozapine (Clozaril)

Clozapine is usually reserved for individuals with treatment who have not responded to multiple other neuroleptics due to the side effect of agranulocytosis. Clozapine blocks type-2 dopamine receptors weakly and is virtually free of EPS, apparently including TD. It was very effective in about 40% of adult patients with chronic schizophrenia who did not respond to conventional neuroleptics.

Non–dose-related agranulocytosis occurs in 0.5–2% of subjects. Some case reports note benefit from clozapine in child and adolescent schizophrenic patients who were resistant to other treatment. Contraindications are concurrent treatment with carbamazepine and any history of leukopenia. Initial medical screening should include CBC and LFTs. The daily dose is 200–600 mg in two divided doses. Because of the risk of neutropenia, patients taking clozapine must be registered with the Clozapine Registry and a white blood cell count must be obtained biweekly before a 2-week supply of the drug is dispensed. If the white count falls below 3000/mL, clozapine is usually discontinued. Other side effects include sedation, weight gain, and increased salivation. The incidence of seizures increases with doses above 600 mg/d.

## 3. General Neuroleptic Information

The following adverse effects of neuroleptics apply to both typical and atypical neuroleptics, but are thought to have a significantly lower incidence with the atypical neuroleptics.

### A. Initial Medical Screening

One should observe and examine for abnormal movements and establish baseline values for CBC and LFTs. An ECG should be taken if there is a history of cardiac disease or arrhythmia, and to establish a baseline QT interval (cardiac repolarization) prior to initiation of the neuroleptics that have a greater effect on QT (eg, ziprasidone and thioridazine). Neuroleptics can cause QT prolongation leading to ventricular arrhythmias, such as torsades de pointes. Medications that affect the cytochrome p450 isoenzyme pathway (including SSRIs) may increase the neuroleptic plasma concentration and increase risk of QTc prolongation.

### B. Adverse Effects

The most troublesome adverse effects of the atypical neuroleptics are cognitive slowing, sedation, orthostasis, and weight gain. The conventional neuroleptics have increased incidence of EPS and TD. Sedation, cognitive slowing, and EPS all tend to be dose-related. Because of the risk of side effects, neuroleptic medications should be used with caution and monitored regularly. The risk–benefit ratio of the medication for the identified target symptom should be carefully considered and reviewed with the parent or guardian.

**1. Extrapyramidal side effects**—EPS and acute dystonic reactions are tonic muscle spasms, often of the tongue, jaw, or neck. EPS symptoms can be mildly uncomfortable or may result in such dramatically distressing symptoms as oculogyric crisis, torticollis, and even opisthotonos. The onset usually occurs within days after a dosage change and may occur in up to 25% of children treated with conventional neuroleptics. Acute neuroleptic-induced dystonias are quickly relieved by anticholinergics such as benztropine (Cogentin) and diphenhydramine.

**2. Tardive dyskinesias**—TDs are involuntary movement disorders that are often irreversible and may appear after long-term use of neuroleptic medications. Choreoathetoid movements of the tongue and mouth are most common, but the extremities and trunk may also be involved. The risk of TD is small in patients on atypical neuroleptics, and those on conventional neuroleptics for less than 6 months. There is no universally effective treatment.

**3. Pseudoparkinsonism**—Pseudoparkinsonism is usually manifested 1–4 weeks after the start of treatment. It presents as muscle stiffness, cogwheel rigidity, mask-like facial expression, bradykinesia, drooling, and occasionally pill-rolling tremor. Anticholinergic medications or dosage reductions are helpful.

**4. Akathisia**—Akathisia is usually manifested after 1–6 weeks of treatment. It presents as a unpleasant feeling of driven motor restlessness that ranges from vague muscular discomfort to a markedly dysphoric agitation with frantic pacing. Anticholinergic agents or β-blockers are sometimes helpful.

**5. Neuroleptic malignant syndrome**—Neuroleptic malignant syndrome (NMS) is a very rare medical emergency associated primarily with the conventional neuroleptics, although it has been reported also with atypical neuroleptics. It is manifested by severe muscular rigidity, altered sensorium, hyperpyrexia, autonomic lability, and myoglobinemia. NMS can present without muscle rigidity with atypical neuroleptics and should be considered in the differential diagnosis of any patient on neuroleptics who presents with high fever and altered mental status. Mortality as high as 30% has been reported. Treatment includes immediate medical assessment, withdrawal of the neuroleptic, and may require transfer to an ICU.

**6. Withdrawal dyskinesias**—Withdrawal dyskinesias are reversible movement disorders that appear following withdrawal of neuroleptic medications. Dyskinetic movements develop within 1–4 weeks after withdrawal of the drug and may persist for months.

**7. Other adverse effects**—These include cardiac arrhythmias, irregular menses, gynecomastia and galactorrhea due to increased prolactin, sexual dysfunction, photosensitivity, rashes, lowered seizure threshold, hepatic dysfunction, and blood dyscrasias.

### C. DRUG INTERACTIONS

Potentiation of CNS depressant effects or the anticholinergic effects of other drugs may occur, as well as increased plasma levels of antidepressants.

### D. MEDICAL FOLLOW-UP

One should examine the patient at least every 3 months for signs of the side effects listed. An Abnormal Involuntary Movement Scale (AIMS) can be used to monitor for TD for patients taking neuroleptics.

## ADRENERGIC AGONISTS

### Clonidine and Guanfacine (Tenex)

#### A. INDICATIONS

Clonidine is a nonselective α-adrenergic agonist that is clinically useful in decreasing states of hyperarousal seen in children and adolescents with PTSD and ADHD. Guanfacine is a selective agonist for $\alpha_2$-adrenergic receptors with advantages over the nonselective agonist clonidine. Guanfacine is less sedating and less hypotensive and has a longer half-life, allowing for twice-daily dosing. Case reports find guanfacine effective in ADHD and Tourette syndrome with comorbid ADHD. Bedtime doses of adrenergic agonists can be helpful for the delayed onset of sleep and nightmares that can occur with PTSD, for the difficulty settling for sleep seen in ADHD, or for ameliorating the side effects of stimulant medications. They are also effective in the treatment of tics in Tourette syndrome

#### B. CONTRAINDICATIONS

Adrenergic agonists are contraindicated for patients with known renal or cardiovascular disease and for those with a family or personal history of depression.

#### C. INITIAL MEDICAL SCREENING

The pulse and blood pressure should be recorded prior to starting an adrenergic agonist.

#### D. DOSAGE

Initial dosage of clonidine is usually 0.025–0.05 mg at bedtime. The dosage can be increased after 3–5 days by giving 0.05 mg also in the morning. Further dosage increases are made by adding 0.05 mg first in the morning, then at noon, and then in the evening every 3–5 days to a maximum total daily dose of 0.3 mg in three or four divided doses per day. The half-life of clonidine is in the range of 3–4 hours. Although a clinical response generally becomes apparent by about 4 weeks, treatment effects may increase over 2–3 months. Therapeutic doses of methylphenidate can frequently be decreased by 30–50% when used in conjunction with clonidine. Transdermal administration of clonidine using a skin patch can be quite effective but may result in skin irritation in 40% of patients. Patches are generally changed every 5 days.

The starting dosage of guanfacine is usually 0.5–1 mg once a day, increasing as clinically indicated after 3–5 days to 2–4 mg/d in two or three divided doses per day. Adverse effects include transient headaches and stomachaches in 25% of patients. Sedation and hypertension are mild. For medical follow-up, pulse and blood pressure should be checked every 1–2 weeks for 2 months and then at 3-month intervals.

#### E. ADVERSE EFFECTS

Sedation can be prominent. Side effects include fatigability, dizziness associated with hypotension, increased appetite and weight gain, headache, sleep disturbance, GI distress, skin irritation with transdermal clonidine administration, and rebound hypertension with abrupt withdrawal. Bradycardia can occasionally be marked.

#### F. DRUG INTERACTIONS

Increased sedation with CNS depressants; possible increased anticholinergic toxicity. Several case reports have mentioned cardiac toxicity with clonidine when combined with methylphenidate, although other medications and clinical factors were present in each case.

#### G. MEDICAL FOLLOW-UP

Pulse and blood pressure should be recorded every 2 weeks for 2 months and then every 3 months. The discontinuation of clonidine or guanfacine should occur gradually, with step-wise dosage decreases every 3–5 days to avoid rebound hypertension. Blood pressure should be monitored during withdrawal.

## REFERENCES

Ambrosini PJ et al: Multicenter open-label sertraline study in adolescent outpatients with major depression. J Am Acad Child Adolesc Psychiatry 1999;38:566 [PMID: 10230188].

Baumgartner JL, Emslie GJ, Crismon ML: Citalopram in children and adolescents with depression or anxiety. Ann Pharmacother 2002;36(11):1692 [PMID: 12398561].

Birmaher B et al: Fluoxetine for the treatment of childhood anxiety disorders. J Am Acad Child Adolesc Psychiatry 2003;42(4): 415 [PMID: 12649628].

Campbell M et al: Antipsychotics in children and adolescents. J Am Acad Child Adolesc Psychiatry 1999;38:537 [PMID: 10230185].

Compton SN et al: Sertraline in children and adolescents with social anxiety disorder: An open trial. J Am Acad Child Adolesc Psychiatry 2001;40(5):564 [PMID: 11349701].

Emslie GJ et al: Fluoxetine for acute treatment of depression in children and adolescents; a placebo-controlled randomized clinical trial. J Am Acad Child Adolesc Psychiatry 2002; 41(10):1205 [PMID: 12364842].

Emslie GJ et al: Predictors of response to treatment in children and adolescents with mood disorders. Psychiatr Clin North Am 2003;26(2):435 [PMID: 12778842].

Emslie GJ et al: Nontricyclic antidepressants: Current trends in children and adolescents. J Am Acad Child Adolesc Psychiatry 1999;38:517. [PMID: 10230183].

Emslie GJ, Mayes TL. Mood disorders in children and adolescents; psychopharmacological treatment. Biological Psychiatry 2001; 49(12):1082-90 [PMID: 11430850].

Geller B et al: Critical review of tricyclic antidepressant use in children and adolescents. J Am Acad Child Adolesc Psychiatry 1999;38:513 [PMID: 10230182].

Green WH: *Child and Adolescent Psychopharmacology,* 3rd ed. Lippincott, Williams & Wilkins, 2001.

Galanter CA et al: Response to methylphenidate in children with ADHD and manic symptoms in the multimodal treatment study of children with ADHD titration trial. J Child Adolesc Psychopharmacol 2003;13(2):123 [PMID: 12880507].

Greenhill LL et al: Developing methodologies for monitoring long-term safety of psychotropic medications: Report on the NIMH conference, Sept. 25, 2000. J Am Acad Child Adolesc Psychiatry 2003;42(6):651 [PMID: 12921472].

Hellings JA et al: Weight gain in a controlled study of risperidone in children, adolescents and adults with mental retardation and autism. J Child Adolesc Psychopharmacol 2001;11(3) 229 [PMID: 11642473].

Hughes CW et al: The Texas Children's Medication Algorithm Project: Report of the Texas Consensus Conference Panel on Medication Treatment of Childhood major depressive disorder. J Am Acad Child Adolesc Psychiatry 1999;38(11): 1442 [PMID: 10560232].

Kaftantaris V et al: Lithium treatment of acute mania in adolescents: A large open trial. J Am Acad Child Adolesc Psychiatry 2003;42(9):1038 [PMID: 12960703].

Kastelic EA et al: Selective serotonin reuptake inhibitors for children and adolescents. Curr Psychiatry Rep 2000;2(2): 117 [PMID: 11122943].

Keller MB et al: Efficacy of paroxetine in the treatment of adolescent major depression: A randomized controlled trial. J Am Acad Child Adolesc Psychiatry 2001;40(7):762 [PMID: 11437014].

Kowatch RA et al: Effect size of lithium, divalproex sodium and carbamazepine in children and adolescents with bipolar disorder. J Am Acad Child Adolesc Psychiatry 2000;39(6): 713 [PMID: 10846305].

Kowatch RA et al: Combination pharmacotherapy in children and adolescents with bipolar disorder. Biol Psychiatry 2003; 53(11):978 [PMID: 12788243].

Kowatch RA, Delbello MP: The use of mood stabilizers and atypical antipsychotics in children and adolescents with bipolar disorders. CNS Spectr 2003;8(4):273 [PMID: 12679742].

Kratochvil CJ et al: Pharmacotherapy of childhood anxiety disorders. Curr Psychiatry Rep 2002; (4):264 [PMID: 12126594].

Kutcher S: Practical clinical issues regarding child and adolescent psychopharmacology. Child Adolesc Psychiatr Clin North Am 2000;9(1):245 [PMID: 10674199].

Labellarte MJ et al: The relevance of prolonged QTc measurement to pediatric psychopharmacology. J Am Acad Child Adolesc Psychiatry 2003;42(6):642 [PMID: 12921471].

Leonard HL (ed): *The Brown University Child and Adolescent Pyschopharmacology Update,* (monthly newsletter). Providence RI: Manisses Communications Group, Inc (800-333-7771).

March JS, Vitiello B: Advances in Paediatric neuropsychopharmacology: An overview. Int J Neuropsychopharmacol 2001; 4(2):141 [PMID: 11466164].

Pliszka SR et al: A feasibility study of the children's medication algorithm project (CMAP) for the treatment of ADHD. J Am Acad Child Adolesc Psychiatry 2003;42(3):279 [PMID: 12595780].

Plizka SR. Non-stimulant treatment of attention-deficit/Hyperactivity Disorder. CNS Spectr 2003;8(4):253 [PMID: 12679740].

Remschmidt H et al: Atypical neuroleptics in child and adolescent psychiatry. Eur Child Adolesc Psychiatry 2000;9 (Suppl) 1:9 [PMID: 11140784].

Riddle MA et al: Pediatric psychopharmacology. J Child Psychol Psychiatry 2001;42(1):73 [PMID: 11205625].

Rosenberg DR et al: *Pocket Guide for the Textbook of Child and Adolescent Psychiatric Disorders.* Taylor & Francis, 1998.

Ryan ND: Child and adolescent depression: Short-term treatment effectiveness and long-term opportunities. Int J Methods Psychiatr Res 2003;12(1):44 [PMID: 12830309].

Ryan ND: Medication treatment for depression in children and adolescents. CNS Spectr 2003;8(4):283 [PMID: 12679743].

Ryan ND et al: Mood stabilizers in children and adolescents. J Am Acad Child Adolesc Psychiatry 1999;38:529 [PMID: 10230184].

Scahill L et al: Lithium in children and adolescents. J Child Adolesc Psychiatr Nurs 2001;14(2):89 [PMID: 11883628].

Shoaf TL et al: Childhood depression: Diagnosis and treatment strategies in general pediatrics. Pediatr Ann 2001; 30(3):130 [PMID: 11257942].

Simeon J, Milin R, Walker S: A retrospective chart review of risperidone use in treatment-resistant children and adolescents with psychiatric disorders. Prog Neuropsychopharmacol Biol Psychiatry 2002;26(2):267 [PMID: 11817503].

Steiner H et al: Psychopharmacologic strategies for the treatment of aggression in juveniles. CNS Spectr 2003;8(4):298 [PMID: 12679744].

Vitello B: Current research highlights in child and adolescent psychopharmacology. Curr Psychiatry Rep 2000;2(2):110 [PMID: 11122942].

Walkup J et al: Treatment of pediatric anxiety disorders: An open-label extension of the research units pediatric psychopharmacology anxiety study. J Child Adolesc Psychopharmacol 2002;12(3):175 [PMID: 12427292].

# Child Abuse & Neglect

*Andrew P. Sirotnak, MD, & Richard D. Krugman, MD*

The problem of child abuse and neglect, barely recognized as a significant problem in the early editions of this textbook, has grown to a problem of such serious proportions that in 1990 the US Advisory Board on Child Abuse and Neglect called the present state of the nation's ability to protect children a "national emergency." Over a decade later, the emergency is still with us. What Dr. Henry Kempe and his colleagues first called battered child syndrome was thought to affect 749 children in the United States in 1960. The best data now available suggest that 1–1.5% of American children are abused or neglected annually. In 2002 an estimated 3 million children were reported to child protective service agencies as alleged victims of child abuse and neglect, which translates to an approximate national maltreatment rate of 37 victims per 1000 children. Just under one million of these cases were substantiated by child protective services in 2001, yielding an abuse substantiation rate of 12.3 per 1000 American children. At least 2000 children are victims of fatal child abuse each year. This dramatic increase in cases has resulted from increased recognition of the problem by professionals, partly in response to statutory reporting mandates; a broadening of the definitions of abuse and neglect from the original battered child concept; and changes in the demography and social structure of families and neighborhoods over the past several decades. Substance abuse, poverty and economic strains, parental capacity and skills, and domestic violence are cited as the most common presenting problems in abusive families.

Abuse and neglect of children are best considered in an ecologic perspective, which recognizes the individual, family, social, and psychological influences that come together to contribute to the problem. For most pediatric health care professionals, however, their involvement will be limited to individual cases. This chapter focuses on the knowledge necessary for the recognition, intervention, and follow-up of the more common forms of child maltreatment and highlights the role of pediatric professionals in prevention.

## FORMS OF CHILD MALTREATMENT

Child maltreatment may occur either within or outside the family. The proportion of intrafamilial to extrafamilial cases varies with the type of abuse as well as the gender and age of child. Each of the following conditions may exist as separate or concurrent diagnoses.

## Physical Abuse

Physical abuse of children is most often inflicted by a caregiver or family member but occasionally by a stranger. The most common manifestations include bruises, burns, fractures, head trauma, and abdominal injuries. A small but significant number of unexpected pediatric deaths, particularly in infants and very young children (eg, sudden infant death syndrome), are related to physical abuse.

## Sexual Abuse

Sexual abuse is defined as the engaging of dependent, developmentally immature children in sexual activities that they do not fully comprehend and to which they cannot give consent or activities that violate the laws and taboos of a society. It includes all forms of incest, sexual assault or rape, and pedophilia. This includes fondling, oral–genital–anal contact, all forms of intercourse or penetration, exhibitionism, voyeurism, exploitation or prostitution, and the involvement of children in the production of pornography.

## Emotional Abuse

Emotional or psychological abuse has been defined as the rejection, ignoring, criticizing, isolation, or terrorizing of children, all of which have the effect of eroding their self-esteem. The most common form is verbal abuse or denigration. Children who witness domestic violence should be considered emotionally abused.

## Physical Neglect

Physical neglect is the failure to provide the necessary food, clothing, and shelter and a safe environment in which children can grow and develop. Although often associated with poverty or ignorance, physical neglect involves a more serious problem than just lack of resources. There is often a component of emotional neglect and either a failure or an inability, intentionally or otherwise, to recognize and respond to the needs of the child.

## Emotional Neglect

The most common feature of emotional neglect is the absence of normal parent–child attachment and a subsequent inability to recognize and respond to an infant's or child's needs. A common manifestation of emotional neglect in infancy is nutritional (nonorganic) failure to thrive.

## Medical Care Neglect

Medical care neglect is failure to provide the needed treatment to infants or children with life-threatening illness or other serious or chronic medical conditions.

## Munchausen Syndrome by Proxy

Munchausen syndrome by proxy is a relatively unusual disorder in which a caregiver, usually the mother, either simulates or creates the symptoms or signs of illness in a child. The child can present with a long list of medical problems or often bizarre recurrent complaints. Fatal cases have been reported.

# RECOGNITION OF ABUSE & NEGLECT

The most common features suggesting a diagnosis of child abuse are summarized in Tables 7–1 and 7–2. Obvious signs of injury, sexual abuse, or neglect may be present. Classic radiographic and laboratory findings are discussed later in this chapter. Psychosocial factors may indicate risk for or confirm child maltreatment.

Recognition of any form of abuse and neglect of children can occur only if child abuse is entertained in the differential diagnosis of the child's presenting medical condition. The approach to the family should be supportive, nonaccusatory, and empathetic. The individual who brings the child in for care may not have any involvement in the abuse. Approximately one third

**Table 7–1.** Common historical features in child abuse cases.

Discrepant, evolving, or absent history
Delay in seeking care
Event or behavior by child that triggers a loss of control of caregiver
History of abuse in the caregiver's childhood
Inappropriate affect of the caregiver
Pattern of increasing severity or number of injuries if no intervention
Social or physical isolation of the child or the caregiver
Stress or crisis in the family or the caregiver
Unrealistic expectations of caregiver for the child

**Table 7–2.** Presentations of sexual abuse.

General or direct statements about sexual abuse
Sexualized play or behavior in developmentally immature children
Sexual abuse of other children by the victim
Behavioral changes
   Sleep disturbances (eg, nightmares and night terrors)
   Appetite disturbances (eg, anorexia, bulimia)
   Depression, social withdrawal, anxiety
   Aggression, temper tantrums, impulsiveness
   Neurotic or conduct disorders, phobias or avoidant behaviors
   Guilt, low self-esteem, mistrust, feelings of helplessness
   Hysterical or conversion reactions
   Suicidal, runaway threats or behavior
   Excessive masturbation
Medical conditions
   Recurrent abdominal pain or frequent somatic complaints
   Genital, anal, or urethral trauma
   Recurrent complaints of genital or anal pain, discharge, bleeding
   Enuresis or encopresis
   Sexually transmitted diseases
   Pregnancy
Promiscuity or prostitution, sexual dysfunction, fear of intimacy
School problems or truancy
Substance abuse

of child abuse incidents occur in extrafamilial settings. Nevertheless, the assumption that the caregiver is "nice," combined with the failure to consider the possibility of abuse, can be costly and even fatal. Raising the possibility that a child has been abused is not the same as accusing the caregiver of being the abuser. The health professional who is examining the child can explain to the family that several possibilities might explain the child's injuries or abuse-related symptoms. If the family or presenting caregiver is not involved in the child's maltreatment, they may actually welcome the necessary report and investigation.

## History

### A. PHYSICAL ABUSE

The medical diagnosis of physical abuse is based on the presence of a discrepant history, in which the history offered by the caregiver is not consistent with the clinical findings. The discrepancy may exist because the history is absent, partial, changing over time, or simply illogical or improbable. The presence of a discrepant history should prompt a request for consultation with a multidisciplinary child protection team or a report to the child protective services agency. This agency is mandated by state law to investigate reports of suspected child abuse and neglect. Investigation by social services and possibly law enforcement officers, as well as a home visit, may be required to sort out the circumstances of the child's injuries. Other common historical features in child abuse cases are listed in Table 7–1.

## B. Sexual Abuse

Sexual abuse may come to the clinician's attention in different ways: (1) The child may be brought in for routine care or for an acute problem, and sexual abuse may be suspected by the medical professional as a result of the history or the physical examination. (2) The parent or caregiver, suspecting that the child may have been sexually abused, may bring the child to the health care provider and request an examination to "rule in or rule out" abuse. (3) The child may be referred by child protective services or the police for an evidentiary examination following either disclosure of sexual abuse by the child or an allegation of abuse by a parent or third party. Table 7–2 lists the presentations of child sexual abuse. It should be emphasized that with the exception of acute trauma, certain sexually transmitted infections (STIs), or forensic laboratory evidence, none of these presentations is specific. The presentations listed should arouse suspicion of the possibility of sexual abuse and lead the practitioner to ask the appropriate questions—again, in a compassionate and nonaccusatory manner. The American Academy of Pediatrics has published guidelines for the evaluation of child sexual abuse as well as other guidelines relating to child maltreatment.

## C. Emotional Abuse

Emotional abuse may cause nonspecific symptoms in children. Loss of self-esteem or self-confidence, sleep disturbances, somatic symptoms (eg, headaches, stomachaches), hypervigilance, or avoidant or phobic behaviors (eg, school refusal, running away) may be presenting complaints. These complaints may also be seen in children who experience domestic violence. Emotional abuse can occur in the home or day care, school, sports team, or other settings.

## D. Neglect

Even though in 2002 there were three times as many reports of neglect of children as of physical abuse, neglect is not easily documented on history. Physical neglect—which must be differentiated from the deprivations of poverty—will be present even after adequate social services have been provided to families in need. Emotionally neglectful parents appear to have an inability to recognize the physical or emotional states of their children. For example, an emotionally neglectful parent may ignore an infant's cry if the cry is perceived

incorrectly as an expression of anger. This misinterpretation leads to inadequate nutrition and failure to thrive. The clinician must evaluate the psychosocial history and family dynamics when neglect is a consideration, and a careful social services investigation may be required.

## E. Failure to Thrive

The history offered in cases of failure to thrive is often at odds with the physical findings. Infants who have experienced a significant deceleration in growth are probably not receiving adequate amounts or appropriate types of food despite the dietary history provided. Medical conditions causing poor growth in infancy and early childhood can be ruled out with a detailed history and minimal laboratory tests. A psychosocial history may reveal maternal depression, family chaos or dysfunction, or other previously unknown social risk factors (eg, substance abuse, violence, poverty, psychiatric illness). Placement of the child with another caregiver or hospitalization of the severely malnourished patient is usually followed by a dramatic weight gain.

## Physical Findings

### A. Physical Abuse

The findings on examination of physically abused children may include abrasions, alopecia, bites, bruises, burns, dental trauma, fractures, lacerations, ligature marks, or scars. Injuries may be in multiple stages of healing. Bruises in physically abused children are sometimes patterned (eg, belt marks, looped cord marks, grab or pinch marks) and are typically found over the soft tissue areas of the body. Toddlers or older children typically sustain accidental bruises over bony prominences such as shins and elbows. Any bruise in an infant not developmentally mobile should be viewed with concern. (Other child abuse emergencies are listed in Table 7–3). Lacerations of the frenulum or tongue and bruising of the lips may be associated with force feeding. Pathognomonic burn patterns include stocking or glove distribution; immersion burns of the buttocks, sometimes with a "doughnut hole" area of sparing; and branding burns such as with cigarettes or hot objects (eg, grill, curling iron, or lighter). The absence of splash marks or a pattern consistent with spillage may be helpful in differentiating accidental from nonaccidental scald burns.

Head and abdominal trauma may present with signs and symptoms consistent with those injuries. Inflicted head trauma (eg, shaken baby syndrome) and abdominal injuries may have no visible findings on examination. The finding of retinal hemorrhages in an infant without an appropriate medical condition (eg, leukemia, congenital infection, clotting disorder) should

**Table 7–3.** Potential child abuse medical emergencies.

---

Any infant with bruises (especially head, facial, or abdominal), burns, or fractures

Any infant or child under age 2 years with a history of suspected "shaken baby" head trauma or other inflicted head injury

Any child who has sustained suspicious or known inflicted abdominal trauma

Any child with burns in stocking or glove distribution or in other unusual patterns, burns to the genitalia, and any unexplained burn injury

Any child with disclosure or sign of sexual assault within 48–72 hours after alleged event if the possibility of acute injury is present or if forensic evidence exists

---

arouse concern about possible inflicted head trauma. Retinal hemorrhages are not commonly seen after cardiopulmonary resuscitation in either infants or children.

## B. SEXUAL ABUSE

The genital and anal findings of sexually abused children, as well as the normal developmental changes and variations in prepubertal female hymens, have been described in journal articles and visual diagnosis guides. The majority of victims of sexual abuse exhibit no physical findings. The reasons for this include delay in disclosure by the child, abuse that may cause no physical trauma (eg, fondling, oral–genital contact, exploitation by pornographic photography), or rapid healing of minor injuries such as labial, hymenal, or anal abrasions, contusions, or lacerations. Nonspecific abnormalities of the genital and rectal regions such as erythema, rashes, and irritation may not suggest sexual abuse in the absence of a corroborating history, disclosure, or behavioral changes. Finally, some medical conditions may be misdiagnosed as sexual abuse (eg, lichen sclerosis, dermatitis, labial adhesions, congenital urethral or vulvar disorders, Crohn disease, and accidental straddle injuries to the labia) and can be ruled out by careful history and examination.

Certain STIs should strongly suggest sexual abuse. *Neisseria gonorrhoeae* infection or syphilis beyond the perinatal period are diagnostic of sexual abuse. *Chlamydia trachomatis*, herpes simplex virus, trichomoniasis, and human papillomavirus (HPV) are all sexually transmitted, although the course of these perinatally acquired infections may be protracted. In the case of HPV, an initial appearance of venereal warts beyond the toddler age should raise concerns about sexual abuse. Finally, sexual abuse must be considered with

the diagnosis of human immunodeficiency virus (HIV) infection when other modes of transmission (eg, transfusion, perinatal acquisition) have been ruled out. The Centers for Disease Control and Prevention and sexual abuse atlases list guidelines for the screening of STIs in sexually abused children and adolescents.

## C. NEGLECT AND NONORGANIC FAILURE TO THRIVE

Infants and children with nonorganic failure to thrive have a relative absence of subcutaneous fat in the cheeks, buttocks, and extremities. Other conditions associated with poor nutrient and vitamin intake may be present. If the condition has persisted for some time, these patients may also appear and act depressed. Older children who have been chronically emotionally neglected may also have short stature (ie, deprivation dwarfism). The head circumference is usually normal in cases of nonorganic failure to thrive. Microcephaly may signify a prenatal condition, congenital disease, or chronic nutritional deprivation and increases the likelihood of more serious and possibly permanent developmental delay.

## D. MUNCHAUSEN SYNDROME BY PROXY

Children with Munchausen syndrome by proxy may present with the signs and symptoms of whatever illness is factitiously produced or simulated. They may be actually ill or reported to be ill and have a normal clinical appearance. Among the most common reported presentations are recurrent apnea, dehydration from induced vomiting or diarrhea, sepsis when contaminants are injected into a child, change in mental status, fever, gastrointestinal bleeding, and seizures.

## Radiologic & Laboratory Findings

### A. PHYSICAL ABUSE

Certain radiologic findings are strong indicators of physical abuse. Examples are metaphyseal "corner" or "bucket handle" fractures of the long bones in infants, spiral fracture of the extremities in nonambulatory infants, rib fractures, spinous process fractures, and fractures in multiple stages of healing. Skeletal surveys in children age 3 years or younger should be performed when a suspicious fracture is diagnosed. Computed tomography or magnetic resonance imaging findings of subdural hemorrhage in infants—in the absence of a clear accidental history—are highly correlated with abusive head trauma, especially after the advent of infant seat restraint laws that have reduced the incidence of head trauma in infants. Abdominal CT is the preferred test in suspected abdominal trauma. Any infant or very young child with suspected abuse-related head or abdominal trauma should be evaluated immediately by an emergency physician or trauma surgeon.

Coagulation studies and a complete blood count with platelets are useful in children who present with multiple or severe bruising in different stages of healing. Coagulopathy conditions may confuse the diagnostic picture but can be excluded with a careful history, examination, laboratory screens, and hematologic consultation if necessary.

The differential diagnosis of all forms of physical abuse can be considered in the context of a detailed trauma history, family medical history, radiographic findings, and laboratory testing. The diagnosis of osteogenesis imperfecta or other collagen disorders, for example, may be considered in the child with skin and joint findings or multiple fractures with or without the classic radiographic presentation and is best made in consultation with a geneticist, an orthopedic surgeon, and a radiologist. Trauma—accidental or inflicted—leads the differential diagnosis list for subdural hematomas. Coagulopathy, disorders of copper metabolism, amino acid or organic acid metabolism (eg, Menkes syndrome, glutaric acidemia type 1), chronic or previous central nervous system infection, birth trauma, or congenital central nervous system malformation (eg, arteriovenous malformations, cerebrospinal fluid collections) may need to be ruled out in some cases. It should be recognized, however, that children with these rare disorders can also be abuse victims.

### B. SEXUAL ABUSE

The forensic evaluation of sexually abused children should be performed in a setting that prevents further emotional distress. If the history indicates that the child may have had contact with the ejaculate of a perpetrator within 72 hours, an examination looking for semen or its markers (eg, acid phosphatase) should be performed according to established protocols. More important, if there is a history of possible sexual abuse within the past 48–72 hours, and the child reports a physical complaint or a sign is observed (eg, genital or anal bleeding or discharge), the child should be examined for signs of trauma. The most experienced examiner (pediatrician, nurse examiner, child advocacy center) is preferable. The laboratory and serologic evaluation of STIs should be guided by the type of contact reported and the epidemiology of these infections in the community.

### C. NEGLECT AND GROWTH FAILURE

Children with failure to thrive or malnutrition may not require an extensive work-up. Complete blood count, urinalysis, electrolyte panel, and liver function tests are sufficient screening. Newborn screening should be documented as normal. Other tests should be guided by any clinical history that points to a previously undiagnosed condition (eg, thyroid, metabolic studies). A

skeletal survey may be helpful if concurrent physical abuse is suspected. The best screening method, however, is placement in a setting in which the child can be fed and monitored. Hospital or foster care placement may be required. Weight gain may not occur for several days to a week in severe cases.

Any child with recurrent polymicrobial sepsis (especially in children with indwelling catheters), recurrent apnea, chronic dehydration of unknown cause, or other highly unusual, unexplained laboratory findings should raise the suspicion of Munchausen syndrome by proxy.

## MANAGEMENT & REPORTING OF CHILD ABUSE & NEGLECT

Physical abuse injuries, STIs, and medical sequelae of neglect should be treated immediately. Children with failure to thrive related to emotional and physical neglect need to be placed in a setting in which they can be fed and cared for. Likewise, the child in danger of recurrent abuse or neglect needs to placed in a safe environment.

In the United States, clinicians and many other professionals who come in contact with or care for children are mandated reporters. If abuse or neglect is suspected, a report must be made to the local or state agency designated to investigate such matters. In most cases, this will be the child protective services agency. Law enforcement agencies may also receive such reports. The purpose of the report is to permit professionals to gather the information needed to determine whether the child's environment (eg, home, school, day care setting, foster home) is safe. Many hospitals and communities make child protection teams or consultants available when there are questions about the diagnosis and management in a child abuse case. A listing of pediatric consultants in child abuse is available from the American Academy of Pediatrics.

Except in extreme cases, the reporting of emotional abuse is not likely to generate a response from child protection agencies. This should not deter reporting, especially if the concern is in the context of domestic violence or other forms of abuse or neglect. Practitioners can encourage parents to get involved with parent effectiveness training programs (eg, Parents as First Teachers or Parents Anonymous) or to seek mental health consultation. Support for the child may also include mental health counseling or age-appropriate peer activities in school or the community.

## PREVENTION OF CHILD ABUSE & NEGLECT

Physical abuse is preventable in many cases. Extensive experience and evaluation of high-risk families has shown that the provision of home visitor services to families at risk can prevent abuse and neglect of children. These services can be provided by public health nurses or trained paraprofessionals, although more data are available describing public health nurse intervention. This makes it as easy for the family to pick up the telephone and ask for help before they abuse a child as it is for a neighbor or physician to report an episode of abuse after it has occurred. Parent education and anticipatory guidance may also be helpful, particularly with respect to handling situations that stress parents (eg, colic, crying, behaviors, toilet training), age-appropriate discipline, and general developmental issues. Prevention of abusive injuries perpetrated by nonparent caregivers (eg, babysitters, nannies, unrelated adults in the home) may be addressed by education and counseling of mothers about safe child care arrangements.

The prevention of sexual abuse is more difficult. Most efforts in this area involve teaching children to protect themselves and their "private parts" from harm or interference. These programs are useful but are in general not as efficacious as they are necessary. The age of toilet training is a good anticipatory guidance time to encourage parents to consider this discussion. The most rational approach is to place the burden of responsibility of prevention on the adults who supervise the child and the medical providers rather than on the children themselves.

Efforts to prevent emotional abuse of children have been undertaken through extensive media campaigns. No data are available to assess the effectiveness of this approach.

# REFERENCES

2002 Guidelines for the treatment of sexually transmitted diseases. MMWR 2002 (RR-6);51. Available at: www.cdc.gov/std/treatment/rr5106.pdf

American Academy of Pediatrics: Distinguishing sudden infant death syndrome from child abuse fatalities. Pediatrics 2001;107(2):437 [PMID:11158487].

American Academy of Pediatrics: *Visual Diagnosis of Child Abuse.* [CD ROM], 2nd ed, 2002.

American Academy of Pediatrics: *Visual Diagnosis of Child Sexual Abuse.* [Slide Set Atlas] American Academy of Pediatrics, 2002.

American Academy of Pediatrics: Diagnostic imaging of children abuse. Pediatrics 2000;105(6):1345 [PMID:10835079].

American Academy of Pediatrics: Rotational cranial injury—technical report. Pediatrics 2001;108(1):206 [PMID:11433079].

American Academy of Pediatrics: Guidelines for the evaluation of sexual abuse of children: A subject review. Pediatrics 1999;103:186 [PMID:9917463].

Giardino AP et al (eds): *A Practical Guide to the Evaluation of Child Abuse and Neglect.* Sage, 2001.

Heger A et al (eds): *Evaluation of the Sexually Abused Child: A Medical Textbook and Photographic Atlas,* 2nd ed. Oxford University Press, 2000.

Helfer ME et al (eds): *The Battered Child,* 5th ed. University of Chicago Press, 1997.

Kleinman PK (ed): *Diagnostic Imaging of Child Abuse,* 2nd ed. Williams & Wilkins, 1998.

Olds D et al: Long-term effects of home visitation on maternal life course and child abuse and neglect fifteen year follow-up of a randomized trial. JAMA 1997;278:637.

Olds DL: Prenatal and infancy home visitation by nurses: From randomized trials to community replication. Prev Sci 2002;3(3):153 [PMID: 12387552].

Reece RM, Ludwig S (eds): *Child Abuse: Medical Diagnosis and Management,* 2nd ed. Lippincott, Williams & Wilkins. Philadelphia, 2001.

Reece RM (ed): *Treatment of Child Abuse: Common Ground for Mental Health, Medical, and Legal Practitioners.* Johns Hopkins University Press, 2000.

US Department of Health and Human Services: Administration for Children, Youth, and Families. Child Maltreatment 2001. Available at: http//:www.acf.dhhs.gov/programs/cb

# Ambulatory & Community Pediatrics

8

*Robert M. Brayden, MD, Matthew F. Daley, MD, & Jeffrey M. Brown, MD, MPH*

Pediatric outpatient services provide a child or adolescent with comprehensive longitudinal care and emphasize preventive health care. This chapter discusses common elements of ambulatory visits and offers guidance in the conduct of the health supervision visit, visits for acute and chronic disease management, and consultations. Special attention is paid to the pediatric history and physical examination, normal developmental stages, office telephone management, and community pediatrics.

The development of a physician–patient–parent relationship is of crucial importance if the patient or parent is to effectively confide his or her concerns. The relationship develops over time and with increasing numbers of visits. It is facilitated by the continuity of clinicians and other pediatric staff members. The trust that supports this relationship comes as a result of several experiences in the context of the office visit. Perhaps the greatest factor to facilitate the relationship is for patients or parents to experience advice as valid and effective. Skills such as choosing vocabulary that communicates understanding and competence, commitment of time and attention to the concern, and respect for areas that the patient or parent does not wish to address (assuming the lack of abuse or neglect concerns) are important. Parents and patients often seek evidence that their concerns will be managed confidentially and that the clinician both understands and sympathizes with those concerns. The effective physician–patient–parent relationship is one of the true joys of ambulatory pediatrics.

## PEDIATRIC HISTORY

Pediatrics is unique in that patients seldom provide their own history. Instead, the parent usually describes the child's complaints and behavior to the physician. As with any history, this information may be detailed and accurate or vague and unreliable. A vague exposition of complaints offered by a parent may be a statement of the parent's own concerns. For example, in-

stead of reporting that a child has had a warm, red, tender, swollen knee for 2 days, the parent may say that the child no longer wants to play on the soccer team.

Parents may or may not be able to distinguish whether symptoms are caused by organic illness or a psychological concern. It is often helpful to ask specifically what problems the parents wish to address in order to determine what really prompted the office visit. Some visits are occasioned by problems at school, such as low grades or troublesome peer relationships. Understanding the family and its hopes for and concerns about the child can help in the process of distinguishing organic illness from emotional or behavioral conditions, thus minimizing unnecessary testing and intervention.

Although the parents' concerns need to be understood, it is essential also to obtain as much of the history as possible directly from the patient. Direct histories not only provide firsthand information but also give the child a degree of control over a potentially threatening situation and may reveal important information about the family.

Obtaining a comprehensive pediatric history is time-consuming. Many offices provide questionnaires for parents to complete before the clinician sees the child. Data from questionnaires can make an outpatient visit more productive, allowing the physician to address problems in detail while more quickly reviewing areas that are not of concern. Questionnaires may be more productive than face-to-face interviews in revealing sensitive parts of the history. However, failure to review and assimilate this information prior to the interview may cause a parent or patient to feel that the time and effort have been wasted.

Elements of the history that will be useful over time should be readily accessible in the medical record. Such information can be accumulated on a summary sheet, as illustrated in Figure 8–1. Demographic data; a problem list; information about chronic medications, allergies, and previous hospitalizations; and the names of other physicians providing care for the patient are commonly included. Documentation of immunizations, including all data required by the National

Name _____ Nickname _____ D.O.B. _____
Mother _____ Father _____ Sibs _____
S.S. # _____ Insurance _____

| Problems | | | Chronic Medications | | |
|---|---|---|---|---|---|
| Date of onset | Description | Date resolved | Start date | | Stop date |
| | | | | | |
| | | | | | |
| | | | | | |
| | | | | | |
| | | | | | |
| | | | | | |
| | | | | | |
| | | | **Allergies (Center)** | | |
| | | | Date | | |
| | | | | | |
| **Date** | **Hospitalizations/Injuries/Procedures** | | **Date** | **Consultants** | |
| | | | | | |
| | | | | | |
| | | | | | |
| | | | | | |
| | | | | | |

***Figure 8–1.*** Use of a summary sheet such as this at the front of the record facilitates reorienting the caregiver and his or her partners to the patient. Some practices keep track of health supervision visits on this sheet to tell the physician whether the child is likely to have received the appropriate preventive services. A second page documenting immunizations should record data required by the National Childhood Vaccine Injury Act. When an allergy with potential for anaphylaxis is identified, the patient should wear a medical alert bracelet and obtain an epinephrine kit, if appropriate.

Childhood Vaccine Injury Act, should be kept on a second page.

The components of a comprehensive pediatric history are listed in Table 8–1. The information should, ideally, be obtained at the first office visit. The first seven items are included on the summary pages. Items 8 and 9 are dealt with during each visit. The entire list should be reviewed and augmented with relevant updates at each health supervision visit.

# ◼ PEDIATRIC PHYSICAL EXAMINATION

In approaching the child, time must be taken to allow the patient to become familiar with the examiner. Interactions and instructions help the child understand

**Table 8–1.** Components of the pediatric historical database.[a]

| | |
|---|---|
| 1. Demographic data | Patient's name and nickname, date of birth, social security number, sex, race, parents' names (first and last), siblings' names, and payment mechanism. |
| 2. Problem list | Major or significant problems, including dates of onset and resolution. |
| 3. Allergies | "Triggering allergen," nature of the reaction, treatment needed, and date allergy diagnosed. |
| 4. Chronic medications | Name, concentration, dose, and frequency of chronically used medications. |
| 5. Birth history | Maternal health during pregnancy, medications, street drugs used, complications of pregnancy; duration and ease of labor; form of delivery; analgesics and anesthetics used; need for monitoring; and labor complications. Infant's birth weight, gestational age, Apgar scores, and problems in the neonatal period. |
| 6. Screening procedures | Results of newborn screening, vision and hearing screening, any health screen, or screening laboratory tests. (Developmental screening results are maintained in the development section; see item 14, below.) |
| 7. Immunizations | Date of each immunization administered, vaccine manufacturer and lot number, and name and title of the person administering the vaccine; previous reaction and contraindication to immunization (eg, immunodeficiency or an evolving neurologic problem). |
| 8. Reasons for visit | The patient's or parents' concerns, stated in their own words, serve as the focus for the visit. |
| 9. Present illness | A concise chronologic summary of the problems necessitating a visit, including the duration, progression, exacerbating factors, ameliorating interventions, and associations. |
| 10. Medical history | A statement regarding the child's functionality and general well-being, including a summary record of significant illnesses, injuries, hospitalizations, and procedures. |
| 11. Diet | Eating patterns, likes and dislikes, use of vitamins, and relative amounts of carbohydrates, fat, and protein in the diet. |
| 12. Family history | Information about the illnesses of relatives, preferably in the form of a family tree. |
| 13. Social history | Family constellation, relationships, parents' educational background, religious preference, and the role of the child in the family; socioeconomic profile of the family to identify resources available to the child, access to services that may be needed, and anticipated stressors. |
| 14. Development | (1) Attainment of developmental milestones (including developmental testing results); (2) social habits and milestones (toilet habits, play, major activities, sleep patterns, discipline, peer relationships); (3) school progress and documentation of specific achievements and grades. |
| 15. Sexual history | Family's sexual attitudes, sex education, sexual development and activity, sexually transmitted diseases, and birth control measures. |
| 16. Review of systems (ROS) | This area tends to be overlooked because of the work required to obtain a complete ROS and integrate data into the patient's problems list and care plan. A focused ROS is essential if any problem is to be addressed adequately. |

[a]The components of this table should be included in a child's medical record and structured to allow easy review and modification. The practice name and address should appear on all pages.

what is occurring and what is expected. A gentle, friendly manner and a quiet voice help establish a setting that yields a nonthreatening physical examination. The order in which the child's organ systems are examined should take into consideration the need for a quiet child, the extent of trust established, and the possibility of an emotional response. Painful or unpleasant procedures should be deferred until the end of the examina-

tion. Whether or not the physician can establish rapport with the child, the process should proceed efficiently and systematically.

Because young children may fear the examination and become fussy, simple inspection is very important. For example, during an acute-care visit for fever, the examiner should observe the child's work of breathing prior to beginning the examination. During a health supervision visit, observation will provide the examiner with an opportunity to assess parent–child interactions.

Clothing should be removed slowly and gently to avoid threatening the child. A parent or the child himself or herself is usually the best person to do this. Modesty should always be respected, and gown or drapes should be provided. Examinations of adolescents should be chaperoned whenever a pelvic examination or a stressful or painful procedure is performed.

Examination tables are convenient, but a parent's lap is a safe haven for a young child. For most purposes, an adequate examination can be conducted on a "table" formed by the parent's and examiner's legs as they sit facing each other.

The nature of the physical examination changes as the child develops. Although a thorough physical examination is important at every age, at some ages the examination tends to focus on specific issues and concerns. At any age, an astute clinician can detect signs of important clinical conditions in an asymptomatic child. In infancy, for example, physical examination can reveal the presence of craniosynostosis, congenital heart disease, or congenital hip dysplasia. Similarly, examination of a toddler may reveal pallor (from iron deficiency anemia) or strabismus. The routine examination of an adolescent may reveal scoliosis or acanthosis nigricans (a finding associated with insulin resistance).

# ■ HEALTH SUPERVISION VISITS

One of several timetables for health supervision visits is illustrated in Figure 8–2. (*Note:* A PDF printable format of this figure is available at aap.org.) The federal Maternal and Child Health Bureau has developed comprehensive health supervision guidelines through their Bright Futures program (brightfutures.org). In areas where evidence-based information is lacking, expert opinion has been used as the basis for these plans. For example, immunizations are proven to be effective and necessary (Centers for Disease Control and Prevention, www.cdc.gov/nip), whereas there is disagreement about whether screening for certain metabolic diseases is universally warranted. Practitioners should remember that guidelines are not meant to be rigid; services should be individualized according to the child's needs.

During health supervision visits, the practitioner should review child development and acute and chronic problems, conduct a complete physical examination, order appropriate screening tests, and anticipate future developments. New historical information should be elicited through an interval history. Development should be assessed by parental report and clinician ob-

servation at each visit. Developmental surveillance is facilitated further through the systematic use of parent-directed questionnaires or screening tests. Growth is carefully recorded, and the growth chart is brought up to date (see Chapter 2). Vision and hearing should be assessed subjectively at each visit, with objective assessments at intervals beginning after the child is old enough to cooperate with the screening test. A variety of laboratory screening tests may also be part of the visit.

A major portion of the health supervision visit is anticipatory guidance. This portion of the visit enables the health care provider to address behavioral, developmental, injury prevention, nutritional issues, school problems, and other age-appropriate issues that will arise before the next well child care visit.

American Academy of Pediatrics Committee on Practice and Ambulatory Medicine: Recommendations for Preventive Pediatric Health Care. Pediatrics 2000;105:645.

# DEVELOPMENTAL & BEHAVIORAL ASSESSMENT

At each visit, the parent should be interviewed about aspects of the child's development and behavior. Questionnaires or formal screening tests help to document development objectively. Useful tests include the Denver II, the Parents' Evaluations of Developmental Status (PEDS), the Denver Articulation Screening Examination, and the Early Language Milestone Scale. School-age children's cognitive functions can be assessed through academic achievement and any educational testing that may have been performed. Emotional well-being can be screened by interview and observation. Practices may decide to use screening tools for adolescent depression.

Observation of parent–child interactions (eg, feeding, compliance tasks) may provide the clinician with information to help shape behavioral counseling. Observing the child's temperament and gathering history about the family's disciplinary techniques are other important considerations before providing guidance.

The pediatrician must be familiar with normal development in order to provide effective patient assessment and counsel. The following sections summarize some important motor, language, and emotional milestones of child development.

## Newborns & Infants

Infancy is commonly a period of concern about growth and behavioral and developmental issues, particularly for the first-time parent. Normal motor and language development, feeding, sleep, elimination, and self-stim-

# Recommendations for Preventive Pediatric Health Care (RE9939)

Committee on Practice and Ambulatory Medicine

Each child and family is unique; therefore, these **Recommendations for Preventive Health Care** are designed for the care of children who are receiving competent parenting, have no manifestations of any important health problems, and are growing and developing in satisfactory fashion. **Additional visits may become necessary** if circumstances suggest variations from normal.

These guidelines represent a consensus by the Committee on Practice and Ambulatory Medicine in consultation with national committees and sections of the American Academy of Pediatrics. The Committee emphasizes the great importance of **continuity of care** in comprehensive health supervision and the need to avoid **fragmentation of care.**

| AGE[5] | PRENATAL[1] | NEWBORN[2] | 2-4d[3] | By 1mo | 2mo | 4mo | 6mo | 9mo | 12mo | 15mo | 18mo | 24mo | 3y | 4y | 5y | 6y | 8y | 10y | 11y | 12y | 13y | 14y | 15y | 16y | 17y | 18y | 19y | 20y | 21y |
|---|---|---|---|---|---|---|---|---|---|---|---|---|---|---|---|---|---|---|---|---|---|---|---|---|---|---|---|---|---|
| **HISTORY** Initial/Interval | • | • | • | • | • | • | • | • | • | • | • | • | • | • | • | • | • | • | • | • | • | • | • | • | • | • | • | • | • |
| **MEASUREMENTS** | | | | | | | | | | | | | | | | | | | | | | | | | | | | | |
| Height and Weight | | • | • | • | • | • | • | • | • | • | • | • | • | • | • | • | • | • | • | • | • | • | • | • | • | • | • | • | • |
| Head Circumference | | • | • | • | • | • | • | • | • | • | • | • | | | | | | | | | | | | | | | | | |
| Blood Pressure | | | | | | | | | | | | | • | • | • | • | • | • | • | • | • | • | • | • | • | • | • | • | • |
| **SENSORY SCREENING** | | | | | | | | | | | | | | | | | | | | | | | | | | | | | |
| Vision | | S | S | S | S | S | S | S | S | S | S | S | O | O | O | O | O | O | S | O | S | S | O | S | S | O | S | S | S |
| Hearing | | O | S | S | S | S | S | S | S | S | S | S | S | O | O | O | O | O | S | O | S | S | O | S | S | O | S | S | S |
| **DEVELOPMENTAL/ BEHAVIORAL ASSESSMENT[8]** | | • | • | • | • | • | • | • | • | • | • | • | • | • | • | • | • | • | • | • | • | • | • | • | • | • | • | • | • |
| **PHYSICAL EXAMINATION[9]** | | • | • | • | • | • | • | • | • | • | • | • | • | • | • | • | • | • | • | • | • | • | • | • | • | • | • | • | • |
| **PROCEDURES-GENERAL[10]** | | | | | | | | | | | | | | | | | | | | | | | | | | | | | |
| Hereditary/Metabolic Screening[11] | | ←——•——→ | | | | | | | | | | | | | | | | | | | | | | | | | | | |
| Immunization[12] | | • | | • | • | • | • | • | • | • | • | • | • | • | • | • | • | • | • | • | • | • | • | • | • | • | • | • | • |
| Hematocrit or Hemoglobin[13] | | | | | | | ←——•—————————————————————————————————————————————————————————→ | | | | | | | | | | | | | | | | | | | | | | |
| Urinalysis | | | | | | | | | | | | | | | | • | | | | | | | | | | | | | |
| **PROCEDURES-PATIENTS AT RISK** | | | | | | | | | | | | | | | | | | | | | | | | | | | | | |
| Lead Screening[16] | | | | | | | | | | | | | | | | | | | | | | | | | | | | | |
| Tuberculin Test[17] | | | | | | | | | | | | | | | | | | | | | | | | | | | | | |
| Cholesterol Screening[18] | | | | | | | | | | | | | | | | | | | | | | | | | | | | | |
| STD Screening[19] | | | | | | | | | | | | | | | | | | | | | | | | | | | | | |
| Pelvic Exam[20] | | | | | | | | | | | | | | | | | | | | | ←————————————————————————————————————→ | | | | | | | | |
| **ANTICIPATORY GUIDANCE[21]** | | | | | | | | | | | | | | | | | | | | | | | | | | | | | |
| Injury Prevention[22] | | • | • | • | • | • | • | • | • | • | • | • | • | • | • | • | • | • | • | • | • | • | • | • | • | • | • | • | • |
| Violence Prevention[23] | | • | • | • | • | • | • | • | • | • | • | • | • | • | • | • | • | • | • | • | • | • | • | • | • | • | • | • | • |
| Sleep Positioning Counseling[24] | | ←——•——→ | | | | | | | | | | | | | | | | | | | | | | | | | | | |
| Nutrition Counseling[25] | | • | • | • | • | • | • | • | • | • | • | • | • | • | • | • | • | • | • | • | • | • | • | • | • | • | • | • | • |
| **DENTAL REFERRAL[26]** | | | | | | | | | | | | ←————————————————————————————→ | | | | | | | | | | | | | | | | | |

**Key:**
- • = to be performed
- S = subjective, by history
- O = objective, by a standard testing method
- ←—•—→ = the range during which a service may be provided, with the dot indicating the preferred age.

1. A prenatal visit is recommended for parents who are at high risk, for first-time parents, and for those who request a conference. The prenatal visit should include anticipatory guidance, pertinent medical history, and a discussion of benefits of breastfeeding and planned method of feeding per AAP statement "The Prenatal Visit"(1996).
2. Every infant should have a newborn evaluation after birth. Breastfeeding should be encouraged and instruction and support offered. Every breastfeeding infant should have an evaluation 48-72 hours after discharge from the hospital to include weight, formal breastfeeding evaluation, encouragement, and instruction as recommended in the AAP statement "Breastfeeding and the Use of Human Milk" (1997).
3. For newborns discharged in less than 48 hours after delivery per AAP statement "Hospital Stay for Healthy Term Newborns" (1995).
4. Developmental, psychosocial, and chronic disease issues for children and adolescents may require frequent counseling and treatment visits separate from preventive care visits.
5. If a child comes under care for the first time at any point on the schedule, or if any items are not accomplished at the suggested age, the schedule should be brought up to date at the earliest possible time.
6. If the patient is uncooperative, rescreen within 6 months.
7. All newborns should be screened per the AAP Task Force on Newborn and Infant Hearing Loss: Detection and Intervention" (1999).
8. By history and appropriate physical examination; if suspicious, by specific objective developmental testing. Parenting skills should be fostered at every visit.
9. At each visit, a complete physical examination is essential, with infant totally unclothed, older child undressed and suitably draped.
10. These may be modified, depending upon entry point into schedule and individual need.
11. Metabolic screening (eg, thyroid, hemoglobinopathies, PKU, galactosemia) should be done according to state law.
12. Schedule(s) per the Committee on Infectious Diseases, published annually in the January edition of Pediatrics. Every visit should be an opportunity to update and complete a child's immunizations.
13. See AAP Pediatric Nutrition Handbook (1998) for a discussion of universal and selective screening options. Consider earlier screening for high-risk infants (eg, premature infants and low birth weight infants). See also "Recommendations to Prevent and Control Iron Deficiency in the United States". MMWR. 1998;47 (RR-3):1-29.
14. All menstruating adolescents should be screened annually.
15. Conduct dipstick urinalysis for leukocytes annually for sexually active male and female adolescents.
16. For children at risk of lead exposure consult the AAP statement "Screening for Elevated Blood Levels"(1998). Additionally, screening should be done in accordance with state law where applicable.
17. TB testing per recommendations of the Committee on Infectious Diseases, published in the current edition of Red Book: Report of the Committee on Infectious Diseases. Testing should be done upon recognition of high-risk factors.
18. Cholesterol screening for high-risk patients per AAP statement "Cholesterol in Childhood"(1998). If family history cannot be ascertained and other risk factors are present, screening should be at the discretion of the physician.
19. All sexually active patients should be screened for sexually transmitted diseases (STDs).
20. All sexually active females should have a pelvic examination. A pelvic examination and routine pap smear should be offered as part of preventive health maintenance between the ages of 18 and 21 years.
21. Age-appropriate discussion and counseling should be an integral part of each visit for care per the AAP Guidelines for Health Supervision III (1998).
22. From birth to age 12, refer to the AAP injury prevention program (TIPP®) as described in A Guide to Safety Counseling in Office Practice (1994).
23. Violence prevention and management for all patients per AAP statement "The Role of the Pediatrician in Youth Violence Prevention in Clinical Practice and at the Community Level" (1999).
24. Parents and caregivers should be advised to place healthy infants on their backs when putting them to sleep. Side positioning is a reasonable alternative but carries a slightly higher risk of SIDS. Consult the AAP statement "Changing Concepts of Sudden Infant Death Syndrome: Implications for Infant Sleeping Environment and Sleep Position"(2000).
25. Age-appropriate nutrition counseling should be an integral part of each visit per the AAP

American Academy of Pediatrics

*Figure 8–2.* Recommendations for preventive health care.

ulating behaviors (thumb sucking, rocking, head banging) are frequently of concern. More complete information about developmental milestones and behavioral concerns of infancy is found in Chapter 2.

Attachment is the process by which an infant develops a relationship with a caregiver. Attachment has both biologic and experiential roots and serves as the basis for additional interpersonal interactions. It develops over months to years and shifts in focus as the child develops. Initially the child seeks proximity to the attachment figure but then gradually moves away in distance to meet exploratory needs.

## The Second Year

Using the first year as a template for secure relationships, normal toddlers have an expanding set of relationships with other individuals. The toddler learns a broad set of general and specific behavioral expectations. The child may be dependent on the caregiving figure(s) and at other times may stubbornly wish to be independent. However, children begin to understand parental expectations and what is not permitted.

Children begin to understand feelings of others and develop empathy. They take pleasure in their achievements and express distress when they have misbehaved. Spoken language normally expands rapidly, as do gross motor skills.

## Preschool Years: Ages 2–4 Years

Gross motor development during the preschool years results in children running, jumping, and climbing. Children learn to balance on one foot and hop. Vocabulary continues to expand rapidly with the mastery of hundreds of words. Language development proceeds with multiword sentences, the use of pronouns, and the gradual improvement in articulation skills. Children normally master the concept of numbers 1, 2, and 3 by 3½ years. Four-year-old children should know basic colors and clearly articulate most words.

The social and emotional development of preschool children is characterized by the transition from parallel to group play and the development of magical thinking. Parallel play is the observation of the play of others and initiation of similar activities individually. By age 4 years, most children will begin to prefer the social aspects of group play.

Toileting skills usually are mastered during these years. Toilet training requires a variety of developmental skills. Expressive and receptive language skills are needed to express and respond to questions about the need to use the toilet. Gross motor skills are needed to get to the bathroom and to control urination and defe-

cation. Fine motor skills are needed to dress and undress and to wash the hands.

## Early School Years: Ages 5–7 Years

Separation–individuation is a theme of the early school years. The child is ready to relate to peers in a more interactive manner than he or she did during preschool years. Sensorimotor abilities are maturing and facilitate pencil-and-paper tasks and participation in sports activities.

The first-grader is generally able to recognize numbers, letters, and words; read and write; and understand the concept of conservation of length and mass. Magical thinking tends to decrease during this time.

## Middle Childhood Years: Ages 8–11 Years

Academic skills become more sophisticated. Not only can a child add and subtract multiple-digit numbers, but he or she has a growing ability to perform multiplication and division. The child should also be able to provide effective verbal descriptions. For example, in response to the question "What is an orange?" the child may reply, "A sweet-tasting fruit." Children develop an awareness of month, day, and year. Peers, organized clubs, and sports are important activities for preadolescent children.

## Adolescence

The behavioral and developmental stages of adolescence are outlined in Chapter 3. Familiarity with the child and family over several years makes the pediatrician an excellent professional to screen for the many concerns in this age group.

American Academy of Pediatrics Committee on Children with Disabilities: Developmental Surveillance and Screening of Infants and Young Children. Pediatrics 2001;108:192.

http://paeditrics.aappublications.org

Levine MD et al (eds): *Developmental-Behavioral Pediatrics*, 3rd ed. WB Saunders, 1999.

# GROWTH PARAMETERS

Pediatric growth charts are based on a broad sampling of the US population, with representation of young infants, breastfed infants, and certain ethnic minorities. The 2- to 18-year growth charts include a chart of body mass index (BMI) for age. The BMI is calculated as the weight (in kilograms) divided by the squared height (in meters). The BMI is useful for determining obesity (BMI ≥ 95th percentile for age) and underweight status (BMI ≤ 5th percentile for age). The BMI is highly correlated with secondary complications of obesity.

Height, weight, and head circumference are carefully measured and plotted at each visit during the first 3 years (see growth charts in Chapter 2). For children older than 3 years, height and weight should be measured at each well-child examination. To ensure accurate weight measurements for longitudinal comparisons, infants should be undressed completely, and young children should be wearing underpants only. Recumbent length is plotted on the chart for birth to 3 years (see Figures 2–1 and 2–2). When the child is old enough to be measured upright, height should be plotted on the charts for ages 2–18 years (see Figures 2–3 and 2–4). If circumferential head growth has been steady for the first 2 years, routine measurements may be suspended. However, if a central nervous system problem exists or develops, or if the child has growth deficiency, this measurement continues to be useful. Tracking the growth velocity for each of these parameters allows early recognition of deviations from normal.

Kuczmarski RJ et al: *CDC Growth Charts: United States. Advance Data from Vital and Health Statistics,* no. 314. National Center for Health Statistics, 2000.

www.cdc.gov/growthcharts/default.htm

## BLOOD PRESSURE

Blood pressure screening at well-child visits should start at age 3 years. If the child has a renal or cardiovascular abnormality, a blood pressure reading should be obtained at each visit regardless of age. Accurate determination of blood pressure requires proper equipment (stethoscope, manometer and inflation cuff, or an automated system) and a cooperative, seated subject. Although automated blood pressure instruments are widely available and easy to use, blood pressure readings from these devices are typically 5 mm Hg higher for diastolic and 10 mm Hg higher for systolic blood pressure compared with auscultatory techniques. Therefore, the diagnosis of hypertension should not be made on the basis of automated readings alone. Additionally, blood pressure varies somewhat by the height and weight of the individual. Consequently, hypertension is diagnosed as a systolic or diastolic blood pressure greater than the 95th percentile based on the age and height (or weight) percentile of the patient.

The width of the inflatable portion of the cuff should be 40–50% of the circumference of the limb. Obese children thus need a larger cuff size to avoid a falsely elevated blood pressure reading. Cuffs that are too narrow will overestimate and those that are too wide will underestimate the true blood pressure. Blood pressure norms are provided in Chapter 19.

Norwood VF: Hypertension. Pediatr Rev 2002;23:197 [PMID: 12042594].

Park MK, Menard SW, Yuan C: Comparison of auscultatory and oscillometric blood pressures. Arch Pediatr Adolesc Med 2001;155:50 [PMID: 11177062].

## VISION & HEARING

Examination of the eyes and an assessment of vision should be performed at every health supervision visit. Parents should be queried about any concerns regarding vision, eye alignment, or any other eye problems. For example, parental observation of photophobia or excessive tearing may be suggestive of glaucoma.

For children from birth to 3 years of age, the eyes and eyelids should be inspected, the movement and alignment of the eyes assessed, and the pupils and red reflexes examined. The red reflex, performed on each pupil individually and then on both eyes simultaneously, is used to detect eye opacities (eg, cataracts or corneal clouding) and retinal abnormalities (eg, retinal detachment or retinoblastoma). In children younger than 3 years of age or in nonverbal children of any age, vision can be assessed by testing a child's ability to fixate on and follow an object.

For children 3 years and older, in addition to the eye evaluations, formal testing of visual acuity should be done. This can be performed in the office with a variety of tests, including the tumbling E chart or picture tests such as Allen cards. Each eye is tested separately, with the nontested eye completely covered. Credit is given for any line on which the child gets more than 50% correct. Children 4 years and older who are unable to cooperate should be retested, ideally within 1 month, and those who cannot cooperate with repeated attempts should be referred to an ophthalmologist. Because visual acuity improves with age, results of the test are interpreted using the cutoff values in Table 8–2; however, any two-line discrepancy between the two eyes should be referred to an ophthalmologist. Throughout childhood and adolescence, the clinician should screen for undetected strabismus (ocular misalignment) and decreased visual acuity. The random dot E test is recommended for detecting strabismus. The corneal light re-

***Table 8–2.*** Age-appropriate visual acuity.[a]

| Age (years) | Minimal Acceptable Acuity |
| --- | --- |
| 3–5 | 20/40 |
| 6 and older | 20/30 |

[a]Refer to an ophthalmologist if minimal acuity is not met at a given age or if there is a difference in scores of two or more lines between the eyes.

flex test, the cover test, and visual acuity tests are described further in Chapter 15.

Hearing loss, if undetected, can lead to substantial impairments in speech, language, and cognitive development. Because significant bilateral hearing loss is one of the more common major anomalies found at birth, and early detection and intervention of hearing loss leads to better outcomes for children, universal hearing screening of all infants is required in many parts of the United States. Hearing in infants is assessed using either auditory brainstem responses or evoked otoacoustic emissions. Because universal newborn hearing screening will inevitably be associated with some false-positive test results, confirmatory audiology testing is required for all abnormal tests.

In infants and toddlers, hearing can be assessed by asking the parent to provide examples of sounds to which the baby has responded and by using simple techniques such as shaking rattles or snapping the fingers. Pure tone audiometry in the office is feasible beginning at age 3 years. Any evidence of hearing loss should be substantiated by repeated testing, and if still abnormal, a referral for formal hearing testing should be made. A number of inherited or acquired conditions increase the risk of hearing loss. Children with any risk factors for hearing loss should be closely followed and periodically screened. Additional details are provided in Chapter 17.

American Academy of Pediatrics et al: Eye examination in infants, children, and young adults by pediatricians. Pediatrics 2003;111:902 [PMID: 12671132].

Cunningham M et al: Hearing assessment in infants and children: Recommendations beyond neonatal screening. Pediatrics 2003;111:436 [PMID: 12563074].

Joint Committee on Infant Hearing et al: Year 2000 statement: Principles and guidelines for early hearing detection and intervention programs. Pediatrics 2000;106;798 [PMID: 11015525].

## LABORATORY SCREENING

### Newborn Screening

Newborn screening involves population-wide testing for metabolic and genetic diseases. Blood samples are collected by heelstick from newborns before hospital discharge, and results are usually available within 1 week. States vary in the types of diseases for which they screen, and many states repeat blood testing between 7 and 14 days of life. Repeat testing is necessary to detect such diseases as phenylketonuria (PKU), which may not be discovered if the first newborn blood screen is performed before 24 hours of life.

All state newborn screening programs include tests for PKU and congenital hypothyroidism. If undiagnosed, both diseases result in severe mental retardation. Early treatment maintains cognitive function in the normal range. Also, most states test for galactosemia and sickle cell disease. Additional diseases screened for in some state programs include congenital adrenal hyperplasia, homocystinuria, maple syrup urine disease, biotinidase deficiency, tyrosinemia, other metabolic conditions, cystic fibrosis, and toxoplasmosis. After newborn screening is performed, several additional steps are necessary. Infants with a positive screen result should receive close follow-up, with additional confirmatory studies performed. Screening tests are usually accurate, but the sensitivity and specificity of a particular screening test must be carefully considered. If the screening test result is reported as positive, a confirmatory test must be performed. If symptoms of a disease are present despite a negative screening test, the infant should be tested further. Once a diagnosis is confirmed, the infant will need further evaluation and treatment.

Advances in science and technology, such as the Human Genome Project (http://www.nhgri.nih.gov), have created the potential to test for myriad additional inherited diseases. Any such screening should directly benefit the infant, because not all conditions are worth looking for in current newborn screening programs. To justify testing the entire population for a condition, that condition would have to be a serious and prevalent health problem; early detection and treatment of the disease must improve patient outcomes; and testing would have to be simple, safe, and affordable.

### Lead Screening

The developing infant and child are at risk of lead poisoning because of their propensity to place objects in the mouth and their efficient absorption of the metal. High blood levels (> 70 µg/dL) can cause severe health problems such as seizures and coma. Blood lead levels as low as 10 µg/dL may cause behavioral problems and learning disabilities, and these effects persist into later life. Blood lead levels below 10 µg/dL have been correlated with lower intelligence quotients. The primary source of lead exposure in this country remains lead-based paint, even though most of its uses have been banned since 1977. Typically, children are exposed through chronic ingestion of dust that is contaminated with lead. Environmental controls such as the elimination of leaded gasoline and paints as well as public service educational efforts are thought to be the main reason blood lead levels have declined nationally from a mean of 16 µg/dL in 1976 to 2 µg/dL in 2001. However, considerable variation in lead levels exists in different regions of the United States, and a majority of children at risk of lead toxicity are not currently screened. To eliminate childhood lead poisoning by 2010 (a national health objective—http://www.healthypeople.gov), health care providers need to be vigilant about this environmental health threat.

State public health authorities set policies on childhood lead screening. The Centers for Disease Control and Prevention (www.cdc.gov) recommends universal lead screening for communities with a high percentage of old housing (> 27% of houses built before 1950) or a high percentage of children with elevated blood lead levels (> 12% of children with levels above 10 µg/dL). Communities with inadequate data regarding local blood lead levels should also undergo universal screening. Medicaid requires that all children (ages 1–5 years) be screened twice, once at 1 year of age and a second screen at 2 years of age. In communities with newer housing and a lower percentage of children with elevated lead levels, blood lead screening is recommended only for targeted groups of children. In these areas, caregivers of children between ages 6 months and 6 years may be interviewed by questionnaire about environmental risk factors for lead exposure (Table 8–3), although the data to support the use of this screening are inconclusive. If risk factors are present, a blood lead level should be obtained.

A venous blood sample is preferred over a capillary specimen. An elevated capillary (fingerstick) blood sample should always be confirmed by a venous sample. No action is required for blood lead levels below 10 µg/dL. The cognitive development of children with confirmed blood levels over 14 µg/dL should be evaluated and attempts made to identify the environmental source. Iron deficiency should be treated if present. Chelation of lead should be considered for levels above 25 µg/dL, is always indicated for levels over 44 µg/dL, and is urgently required for levels of 70 µg/dL or more. All families should receive education to decrease the risk of lead exposure. With any elevated lead level (> 10 µg/dL) rescreening should be performed at recommended intervals.

## Iron Deficiency

Iron deficiency is the most common nutritional deficiency in the United States. Severe iron deficiency causes anemia, behavioral problems, and cognitive effects, but recent evidence suggests that even iron deficiency without anemia may cause behavioral and cognitive difficulties. Furthermore, the developmental effects of iron deficiency may be present after 10 years, even if iron deficiency is corrected in infancy. Risk factors for iron deficiency include preterm or low-birth-weight births, multiple pregnancy, iron deficiency in the mother, use of nonfortified formula or cow's milk before age 12 months, and an infant diet that is low in iron-containing foods. Infants and toddlers consuming greater than 24 oz of cow's milk per day are at risk, as are children with chronic illness, restricted diet, or extensive blood loss.

Primary prevention of iron deficiency should be achieved through dietary means, including feeding infants iron-containing cereals by age 6 months, avoiding low-iron formula during infancy, and limiting cow's milk to 24 oz/d in children age 1–5 years. Selective early screening for iron deficiency should be considered with the presence of any of the preceding risk factors. A screening hemoglobin or hematocrit should be obtained for high-risk children between ages 9–12 months and again at 15–18 months, and it should be considered annually through age 5 years. Premature and low-birth-weight infants may need testing before 6 months of age. Universal anemia screening at 9 and 15 months of age is appropriate for children in communities or patient populations in which anemia is found in 5% or more of those tested. Biochemical tests of iron deficiency focusing on ferritin, transferrin saturation, and erythrocyte protoporphyrin may be useful because they are sensitive measures of iron status. Lead poisoning can cause iron deficiency anemia and should be explored as a cause for at-risk infants and children. A screening hematocrit is recommended for pregnant teenagers.

## Hypercholesterolemia & Hyperlipidemia

The benefits of screening and treatment for hypercholesterolemia and hyperlipidemia in children are not

**Table 8–3.** Elements of a lead risk questionnnaire.

**Recommended questions**
1. Does your child live in or regularly visit a house built before 1950? This could include a day care center, preschool, the home of a baby-sitter or relative, and so on.
2. Does your child live in or regularly visit a house built before 1978 with recent, ongoing, or planned renovation or remodeling?
3. Does your child have a sister or brother, housemate, or playmate being followed for lead poisoning?

**Questions that may be considered by region or locality**
1. Does your child live with an adult whose job (eg, at a brass/copper foundry, firing range, automotive or boat repair shop, or furniture refinishing shop) or hobby (eg, electronics, fishing, stained-glass-making, pottery-making) involves exposure to lead?
2. Does your child live near a work or industrial site (eg, smelter, battery recycling plant) that involves the use of lead?
3. Does your child use pottery or ingest medications that are suspected of having a high lead content?
4. Does your child have exposure to burning lead-painted wood?

fully known. However, the American Academy of Pediatrics (www.aap.org) and the American Heart Association (www.americanheart.org) recommend obtaining a total cholesterol measurement in children older than 2 years who have a parent with elevated cholesterol (above 240 mg/dL). If there is a family history of cardiovascular disease before age 55 years, a complete lipoprotein analysis (fasting cholesterol, high-density lipoproteins, low-density lipoproteins, triglycerides) is recommended. For all children, a prudent diet is advised (see Nutrition Counseling section).

## Tuberculosis

In 2002, 15,075 cases of tuberculosis were reported in the United States, with 946 of these cases occurring in children younger than age 15 years. Well-child care should include assessment of the risk of tuberculosis, and tuberculosis screening should be based on high-risk status. High risk is defined as contact with a person with known or suspected tuberculosis; having symptoms or radiographic findings suggesting tuberculosis; birth, residence, or travel to a region with high tuberculosis prevalence (Asia, Middle East, Africa, Latin America); contact with a person with AIDS or HIV; contact with a prisoner, migrant farm worker, illicit drug user, or a person who is or has been recently homeless. The Mantoux test (5 tuberculin units of purified protein derivative) is the only recommended screening test. It can be done as early as 3 months of age and should be repeated annually if the risk persists. The tine test should not be used. Previous vaccination with bacille Calmette Guérin (BCG) is not a contraindication to tuberculosis skin testing.

## Screening of Adolescent Patients

Screening adolescents for blood cholesterol, tuberculosis, and HIV should be offered based on high-risk criteria outlined in this chapter and in Chapter 37. Females with heavy menses, weight loss, poor nutrition, or athletic activity should have a screening hematocrit. During routine visits, adolescents should be questioned sensitively about sexually transmitted infection (STI) risk factors (eg, multiple partners; early onset of sexual activity, including child sexual abuse) and STI symptoms (eg, genital discharge, infectious lesions, pelvic pain). A dipstick urinalysis for leukocytes is generally recommended for sexually active adolescents. Teenage girls who are sexually active and all girls regardless of sexual experience age 18 years and older should have a pelvic examination with Papanicolaou (Pap) smear. A Pap smear should be performed at least every 3 years thereafter and more frequently in patients with STI risk factors. Because females with STIs are often not sympto-

matic, gonococcal and chlamydial cultures and screening tests for syphilis and trichomoniasis are appropriate at the time of each pelvic examination.

American Academy of Pediatrics: Tuberculosis. In Pickering LK (ed): *2000 Red Book: Report of the Committee on Infectious Diseases,* 25th ed. American Academy of Pediatrics 2000, p 593.

American Academy of Pediatrics Committee on Nutrition: Cholesterol in children. Pediatrics 1998;101:141 [PMID: 11345978].

American Academy of Pediatrics Committee on Practice and Ambulatory Medicine: Recommendations for preventive pediatric health care. Pediatrics 2000;105:645.

American Academy of Pediatrics Newborn Screening Task Force: Serving the family from birth to the medical home: Newborn screening: A blueprint for the future—a call for a national agenda on state newborn screening programs. Pediatrics 2000;106:389 [PMID: 10947682].

Recommendations to prevent and control iron deficiency in the United States. MMWR Morb Mortal Wkly Rep 1998; 47(RR-3):1 [PMID: 9563847].

Surveillance for elevated blood lead levels among children—United States, 1997–2001. MMWR Morb Mortal Wkly Rep 2003; 52(SS-10):1 [PMID: 14532866].

## ANTICIPATORY GUIDANCE

A major portion of the health supervision visit is anticipatory guidance. This time enables the clinician to direct the parent's or the older child's attention to issues that may arise in the future. Guidance must be appropriate to age and should focus on, but not be limited to, concerns expressed by the parent or patient. Anticipatory guidance should focus on issues in depth rather than run through a number of issues superficially. A combination of oral and printed presentations may be used. Handouts are an important supplement to anticipatory guidance. A routine schedule for preventive handouts is shown in Table 8–4. Areas of concern include diet, injury prevention, developmental and behavioral issues, and health promotion. Injury prevention is discussed in the next section; other topics are found in other chapters of this book.

### Injury Prevention

Injuries are the leading cause of death in children and adolescents after the first year of life (Figure 8–3). For young people age 15–24 years, injuries are responsible for more than 50% of all deaths. Each year, 16 million visits to emergency departments are occasioned by injuries to children and adolescents, and more than 500,000 of these patients are hospitalized. In the case of physical injury to a young child, the physician must recognize that some injuries may be intentional or the result of parental neglect (see Chapter 7).

**Table 8–4.** Preventive handouts for health supervision visits.

| Age | Suggested Topics |
| --- | --- |
| 2 weeks | Sleep problems: Prevention |
| 2 months | Passive smoking |
| 4 months | Weaning problems: Prevention |
| 6 months | Teething |
| 12 months | Temper tantrums |
| 18 months | Toilet training basics |
| 2 years | Time-out technique |
| 3 years | Spoiled children: Prevention |
| 4 years | Sex education for preschoolers |
| 5 years | Television: Reducing the negative impact |
| 6 years | School work: Preventing problems |
| 8 years | Siblings' arguments and quarrels |
| 10 years | R-rated movies |
| 12 years | Adolescents: Dealing with normal rebellion |

Adapted and reproduced, with permission, from *Contemporary Pediatrics.* These and other topics relevant to preventive health services can be purchased in the *Pediatric Advisor,* a computerized patient handout program. Information about the *Pediatric Advisor* is available by calling Clinical Reference Systems at 1-800-237-8401. The author has a financial interest in this product.

Injury prevention counseling should be part of each health supervision visit and can be reinforced at episodic visits. Counseling should focus on problems that are frequent and age-appropriate. Passive strategies of prevention should be emphasized, because these are more effective than active strategies; for example, encouraging the use of childproof cupboard latches to prevent poisoning will be more effective than instructing parents to watch their children closely.

Informational handouts about home safety, such as The Injury Prevention Program (TIPP; available from the American Academy of Pediatrics), can be provided in the waiting room. Advice can then be tailored to the specific needs of each family, with reinforcement from age-specific TIPP handouts.

The pediatrician's influence can extend beyond the office to advocate for safer communities. For example, a community program in Seattle, Washington, to promote the use of bicycle helmets has increased helmet use from 2% to nearly 40%. The primary care provider is in an ideal position to identify high-risk situations and intervene before injury occurs. If a teenager has emotional problems (eg, depression) and a history of driving violations, for example, the clinician should recommend interventions that could prevent a motor vehicle accident.

## A. MOTOR VEHICLE INJURIES

The primary cause of death of children in the United States is motor vehicle injuries. In 1998, about 57% of children 15 years old or younger killed in motor vehicle accidents were unrestrained. Car safety seats for children are required in this country, and their proper use could reduce vehicle-associated fatalities and hospitalizations by at least 50%. The type of safety seat to be used depends on the child's weight and age: rear-facing infant seat for a child under 20 lb and 1 year of age; forward-facing car seat for a child 20–40 lb and older than 1 year; a belt-positioning booster seat for a child who has outgrown the safety seat. When children have grown enough to properly fit the vehicle seat belts (usually when 4 feet tall), they should use a combination lap/shoulder belt. A rear-facing car seat should never be used in a seat with a passenger air bag. A car seat should never be used if the child has outgrown the seat—for example, ears above the back of the seat or shoulders above the seat strap slots.

Up-to-date information on car seats can be found at www.aap.org/family/carseatguide.htm.

When a child is a passenger in a car crash, the case fatality rate is 1%; for children hit by cars, the risk of fatality increases threefold. Pedestrian safety skills should be taught to children early in childhood; however, parental supervision of children near roadways continues to be required for many years. A final motor vehicle risk for health involves the use of portable electronic devices. Using a cellular telephone while driving is associated with a fourfold increase in motor vehicle accidents. Parents and teenage drivers should avoid this risk.

## B. BICYCLE INJURIES

In 2001, over 400,000 Americans sustained a bicycle injury, and two thirds of these injuries involved children or adolescents. Head trauma accounts for three fourths of all bicycle-related fatalities. More than 85% of brain injuries can be prevented through the use of bicycle helmets, and the rate of fatality to bicyclists is dropping. Therefore, bike riders should wear a helmet every time they ride. Unfortunately, 25% or less of children wear a bike helmet when riding.

## C. FIREARM INJURIES AND VIOLENCE PREVENTION

The United States has a higher rate of firearm-related death than any other industrialized country. Injuries from firearms are more frequent for young people age 15–24 years than for any other age group, and black males are especially vulnerable. Some gun deaths may be accidental, but most are the result of homicide or suicide. A gun in the home doubles the likelihood of a lethal suicide attempt. Although handguns are often kept in homes for protection, a gun is more likely to kill a family member or a friend than an intruder. The most effective way to prevent firearm injuries is to remove guns from the home and community. Families

**Children 1–4 years**

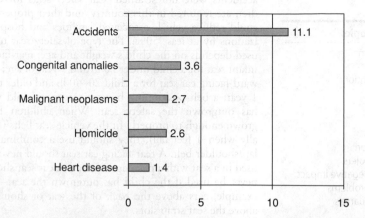

Accidents — 11.1
Congenital anomalies — 3.6
Malignant neoplasms — 2.7
Homicide — 2.6
Heart disease — 1.4

(scale: 0, 5, 10, 15)

**Children 5–14 years**

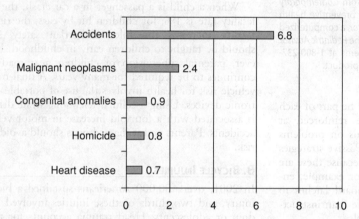

Accidents — 6.8
Malignant neoplasms — 2.4
Congenital anomalies — 0.9
Homicide — 0.8
Heart disease — 0.7

(scale: 0, 2, 4, 6, 8, 10)

**Young adults 15–24 years**

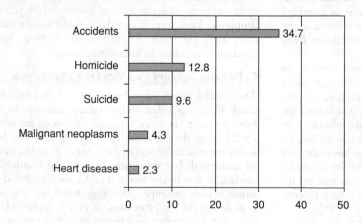

Accidents — 34.7
Homicide — 12.8
Suicide — 9.6
Malignant neoplasms — 4.3
Heart disease — 2.3

(scale: 0, 10, 20, 30, 40, 50)

***Figure 8–3.*** Leading causes of death in children at 1–4 years, at 5–14 years, and at 15–24 years (the 1999 rate per 100,000 population). (National Center for Health Statistics. Used with permission.)

who keep firearms at home should lock them in a cabinet or drawer and store ammunition in a separate locked location.

A nonviolent environment should be provided to all children. Secure parent–infant attachments, social and conflict-resolution skills, and the avoidance of violence (on television or actual) all have a role in promoting nonviolence.

## D. DROWNING AND NEAR DROWNING

Drowning is the second leading cause of injury-related death in children, and those age 1–3 years have the highest rate of drowning. For every death by drowning, six children are hospitalized for near drowning, and up to 10% of survivors experience severe brain damage. Children younger than age 1 year are most likely to drown in the bathtub. Buckets filled with water also present a risk of drowning to the older infant or toddler. For children age 1–4 years, drowning or near drowning occurs most often in home swimming pools; and for school-age children and teens, drowning occurs most often in large bodies of water (eg, swimming pools or open water). After the age of 5 years, the risk of drowning in a swimming pool is much greater for black males than white males. School-age children should be taught to swim, and recreational swimming should always be supervised. Home pools must be fenced securely, and parents should know how to perform cardiopulmonary resuscitation.

## E. FIRE AND BURN INJURIES

Fires and burns are the leading cause of injury-related deaths in the home. Categories of burn injury include smoke inhalation; flame contact; scalding; and electrical, chemical, and ultraviolet burns. Scalding is the most common type of burn in children. Most scalds involve foods and beverages, but nearly one fourth of scalds are with tap water, and for that reason it is recommended that hot water heaters be set to less than 54°C (130°F). The greatest number of fire-related deaths result from smoke inhalation. Smoke detectors can prevent 85% of the injuries and deaths caused by fires in the home. Families should practice emergency evacuation from the home.

Sunburn is a common thermal injury, perhaps because symptoms of excessive sun exposure do not begin until after the skin has been damaged. Sunburn and excessive sun exposure are associated with skin cancers. Prevention of sunburn is best achieved by sun avoidance, particularly during the midday hours of 10 AM, to 3 PM. Sunscreen using a sun protection factor (SPF) of 15 or greater extends the duration of time that a child can spend in the sun without sunburn. Hats, sunglasses, and special precautions for fair-skinned individuals and infants are also important aspects of safe sun

exposure. The safety of sunscreen is not established for infants younger than 6 months; thus sun avoidance, appropriate clothing, and hats are recommended for this age group.

American Academy of Pediatrics, Committee on Injury and Poison Prevention: Bicycle helmets. Pediatrics 2001;108:1030 [PMID: 11581464].

American Academy of Pediatrics, Committee on Injury and Poison Prevention: Firearm-related injuries affecting the pediatric population. Pediatrics 2000;105:888 [PMID: 10742344].

American Academy of Pediatrics, Committee on Injury and Poison Prevention: Reducing the number of deaths and injuries from residential fires. Pediatrics 2000;105:1355 [PMID: 10835082].

Brenner RA et al: Where children drown, United States, 1995. Pediatrics 2001;108:85 [PMID: 11433058].

## NUTRITION COUNSELING

Screening for nutritional problems and guidance for age-appropriate dietary choices should be part of every health supervision visit. Undernutrition, overnutrition, and eating disorders can be detected early by the careful analysis of food choices and eating behaviors, particularly when interpreted in the context of the child's growth pattern. Clinicians should assess the structure of meals (ie, does the family eat three regular meals interspersed with healthy snacks), the type and amounts of food provided, and the degree to which the child grazes or watches television while eating. Iron-fortified formula or breast milk should be used for the first year of life, after which whole cow's milk can be given. Because of continued rapid growth and high energy needs, children should continue to drink whole milk until age 2 years. Baby foods are generally introduced around ages 4–6 months.

For children 2 years old and older, a prudent diet consists of diverse food sources, encourages high-fiber foods (eg, fruits, vegetables, grain products), and limits sodium and fat intake. Foods to be avoided or limited include processed foods, soft drinks, and candy. For additional information on nutritional guidelines, see Chapter 10; for eating disorders, see Chapter 5; for obesity, see Chapter 3.

American Academy of Pediatrics, Committee on Nutrition: Prevention of pediatric overweight and obesity. Pediatrics 2003;112:424 [PMID: 12897303].

Hall RT, Carroll RE: Infant feeding. Pediatr Rev. 2000;21:191 [PMID: 10854314].

## IMMUNIZATIONS

A child's immunization status should be assessed at every clinic visit. Even though parents may keep an immunization record, it is critical that providers also keep an accurate record of a child's immunizations. This information may be written in a prominent location in the chart or kept in a specialized computer database, called an immunization registry.

Despite high overall national immunization coverage levels, areas of underimmunization continue to exist in the United States. Therefore, it is important that clinicians screen records and administer required immunizations at all types of visits, and administer all needed vaccinations simultaneously. Additionally, clinicians should operate reminder/recall systems, in which parents of underimmunized children are prompted by mail or telephone to visit the clinic for immunization. The assessment of clinic-wide immunization levels and feedback of these data to providers has also been shown to increase immunization rates. Finally, clinicians should emphasize to parents the importance of timely immunization.

Immunization schedules and other details of specific vaccines are presented in Chapter 9. A wealth of information for parents and providers about immunizations is also available at the National Immunization Program's website (http://www.cdc.gov/nip).

Santoli JM et al: Immunization pockets of need: Science and practice. Am J Prev Med 2000;19(1S):89 [PMID: 11024333].

Task Force on Community Preventive Services: Recommendations regarding interventions to improve vaccination coverage in children, adolescents, and adults. Am J Prev Med 2000; 18(1S):92 [PMID: 10806981].

# ■ OTHER TYPES OF GENERAL PEDIATRIC SERVICES

## ACUTE-CARE VISITS

Acute-care visits account for 30% or more of the general pediatrician's office visits. These visits must be conducted in an efficient, structured way. Office personnel should determine the reason for the visit, obtain a brief synopsis of the child's symptoms, carefully document vital signs, and list known drug allergies. The physician should document the events related to the presenting problem and note them with the results of the physical examination. The record should include supporting laboratory data and a diagnosis. Treatments and follow-up instructions must be recorded, including when to return to the office if the problem is not ameliorated. Immunization status should be screened and appropriate vaccinations given. As time allows, age-appropriate health maintenance screenings and anticipatory guid-

ance should be provided. Careful documentation of these visits is important for medicolegal reasons.

## PRENATAL VISITS

Ideally, a couple's first trip to a physician's office should take place before the birth of the baby. A prenatal visit goes a long way toward establishing trust and enables the physician to learn about a family's expectations, concerns, and fears regarding the anticipated birth. If the infant develops a problem during the newborn period, the physician who has already met the family is in a better position to maintain rapport and communication with the new parents. If possible, both parents should be present for this visit.

A prenatal visit provides an easy way to acquaint parents with how the practice is conducted, its hours of operation, after-hours coverage, appointment scheduling, and billing. Parents want to know whom they will speak to when they call the office, when they may bring in children for acute-care visits, and how their concerns will be managed.

## SPORTS PHYSICALS

The purpose of the preparticipation health evaluation is to determine whether a child can safely participate in organized sports activity. Attention should be directed toward those parts of the body that are most vulnerable to the stresses of sports. The history and physical examination should focus on the following systems: cardiovascular (stenotic lesions, hypertension, surgery), respiratory (asthma), vision, genitourinary (absence or loss of function of one testicle), gastrointestinal (hepatosplenomegaly, hernia), skin (infection), musculoskeletal (inflammation, dysfunction), and neurologic (concussions, uncontrolled seizures). The sports physical should include counseling about medication usage (eg, diuretic, steroid, and β-blocker abuse, changes in insulin requirements), protective equipment, proper supervision and instruction, injury management, and the emotional aspects of competition and teamwork. The physician should suggest sports that will be compatible with the child's size, strength, endurance, agility, and chronic illness history. The potential for mild menstrual irregularities should be explained to the adolescent female athlete. The athlete with moderate to severe menstrual irregularities should be referred for endocrinologic evaluation. Anticipatory guidance should address nutritional needs to maintain growth, cessation of activity when pain occurs, and fluid and electrolyte availability to avoid dehydration. (See Chapter 24 for a more detailed discussion of sports medicine.)

# CHRONIC DISEASE FOLLOW-UP

Chronic disease is defined as illness that has been present for more than 3 months. When both the history from the parent and the physical examination are used to define chronic disease, 25% of children and 35% of adolescents will meet the definition of chronic illness. The most common chronic illnesses in pediatric practice include asthma, otitis media with effusion, skin disorders, and allergic diseases.

The goal of chronic disease management is to optimize quality of life. The child and family's emotional responses to chronic illness should be addressed, and referrals to counselors should be offered if needed. Specialty referrals need to be monitored and results recorded in the chart in an organized manner. Chronic problems often mean chronic use of medications and the need to monitor their use. Notes should be made in the chart whenever a prescription is refilled. A medication summary page in the chart allows easy access to the drug history and is a convenient place to make notes such as when the anticonvulsant level was last checked and what it was at that time (Figure 8–4). Children with medical appliances such as gastrostomy tubes and indwelling intravenous and bladder catheters need advice on their management. Nutritional intake is often complicated and must be closely and carefully monitored.

Ludder-Jackson P, Vessey JA: *Primary Care of the Child with a Chronic Condition,* 3rd ed. Mosby-Year Book, 2000.

Medication: _____

| Date: Visit (V) or Phone Call (PC) | Tablet Size or Liquid Concentration | Sig. | Disp. | Number of Refills | Approved by | Called by | Pharmacy and Phone No. |
|---|---|---|---|---|---|---|---|
| | | | | | | | |
| | | | | | | | |
| | | | | | | | |
| | | | | | | | |
| | | | | | | | |
| | | | | | | | |

Notes (eg, levels): _____

*Figure 8–4.* Medication summary sheet.

# COUNSELING

Topics amenable to office counseling include behavioral issues such as negativism and noncompliance, temper tantrums, oppositional behavior, and biting; childhood fears and feeding disorders; school problems; family upheavals such as separation, divorce, or remarriage; attention-deficit/hyperactivity disorder; and deaths of family members or close friends. Forty-five minutes is usually enough time for the therapeutic process to evolve, and this time should be protected from interruption. The young child is usually interviewed with the parent; school-age children and adolescents benefit from time alone with the physician. After assessing the situation in one or two sessions, the primary care physician must decide whether the child's and family's needs are within his or her area of expertise or whether referral to another professional such as a psychologist or an education specialist would be appropriate. The pediatrician should know the warning signs for childhood depression and bipolar disorder and have a low threshold for referral of these concerns to the appropriate mental health professional.

# CONSULTATIONS[a]

## Referring Source

Physicians, other professionals, and parents may initiate consultations with a general pediatrician. The general pediatrician may be called on to evaluate many different types of problems both in the hospital and in the ambulatory setting. Parents sometimes desire a second opinion regarding a specific concern while maintaining a relationship with another clinician for their child's primary care. Subspecialists, family physicians, or professionals such as school officials, psychologists, or social workers may also seek second opinions. Finally, an insurance company physician or administrator may want a second opinion before authorizing a set of services.

Consultations usually require one or two 45- to 60-minute appointments. When the patient is referred to a pediatric consultant, the number of visits and the extent of service should be specified. A screening questionnaire, completed in advance by a parent, should delineate the patient's physical, behavioral, and developmental (or school) problems and serve as an initial database.

The types of consultations the general pediatrician may be asked to do include an evaluation only, an evaluation and interpretation, or an evaluation and treatment of an isolated problem. The type of consultation being requested should be clearly determined at the time of referral of the patient. This understanding should be clarified with the patient's insurance company so that appropriate authorization and reimbursement for the visit can occur.

## Communication with the Referring Source

Communication is the key to a satisfactory referral process. The pediatric consultant frequently sends the referral source a brief note acknowledging the referral and requesting additional information. The final consultation report should be sent promptly, with content appropriate for the referring source. School officials usually want to know only whether the patient is physically healthy or, if not, what their responsibility is. A referring physician expects a full report. Recommendations should be specific (eg, drugs, dosages, other forms of therapy, duration of therapy, specific laboratory tests). A copy of or reference to a recent review article on the subject will also be appreciated.

A medical evaluation should contain a factual summary of the history, physical examination, and laboratory and radiologic findings. Families are grateful if a copy is sent to them for their information and records. At the end of the consultation, the parents should be told when the patient should see the primary physician—usually in 1–2 weeks. Positive comments about the referring physician's competence and judgment serve to support the primary physician–patient relationship. The parents must feel confident that the primary physician can provide the necessary follow-up care. If the referring physician had tentatively made the correct diagnosis prior to referral, the consultant's corroboration should be made clear to the parents and included in the consultation report.

# TELEPHONE TRIAGE AND ADVICE[b]

Providing appropriate, efficient, and timely clinical advice over the telephone is a critical element of patient care for all primary care providers. In fact, an estimated 20–30% of all clinical care delivered by general pediatric offices is provided by telephone. Telephone calls to and from patients occur both during regular office hours and after the office has closed (termed afterhours), and the personnel and systems in place to handle office-hours versus before- and after-hours calls may differ. In either circumstance, several principles are important: (1) advice is given only by clinicians or other staff with formal medical education (eg, nurse, medical assistant), (2) staff is given additional training in pro-

[a]Contributed by Barton D. Schmitt, MD.

[b]Contributed by Barton D. Schmitt, MD.

viding telephone care, (3) documentation is made of all pertinent information from calls, (4) standardized protocols covering the most common pediatric symptoms are used, and (5) a physician is always available to handle urgent or difficult calls.

During routine office hours, approximately 20–25% of all telephone calls made to pediatric offices are regarding clinical matters. Many of these calls, however, are routine in nature, and an experienced nurse within the office can screen calls and provide appropriate advice by telephone. Calls from inexperienced or anxious parents about simple concerns should be answered with understanding and respect. Certain types of calls received during office hours should be promptly transferred to a physician: (1) true emergencies, (2) calls regarding hospitalized patients, (3) calls from other medical professionals, and (4) calls from parents who demand to speak with a physician. Nurses should also seek help from a clinician whenever they are uncertain about how to handle a particular call. When in doubt about the diagnosis or necessary treatment, nurses giving telephone advise should err on the side of having the patient seen in the office.

Several different options are available for handling after-hours pediatric telephone care. Clinicians may choose to take all calls from their patients, may rely on "advice" nurses without specific pediatric protocols or training, or may use a system specifically designed for pediatric telephone care, called a pediatric after-hours call center. Pediatric call centers, although not available in all communities and potentially more expensive than other options for after-hours care, have certain benefits. Calls are managed using standardized protocols, the call centers are typically staffed by nurses with abundant pediatric experience, the calls are well-documented, and call centers often perform ongoing quality assurance. Extensive research on pediatric call centers has revealed a high degree of appropriate referrals to emergency departments, and a high level of parent satisfaction with the process.

In general, after-hours pediatric telephone calls tend to be more serious than calls made during regular office hours. Deciding which patients need to be seen, and how urgently, are the most important aspects of these after-hours telephone "encounters." Several factors influence this final patient disposition: (1) the age of the patient, (2) the duration and type of symptom, (3) the presence of any underlying chronic condition, (4) whether the child appears "very sick" to the caller, and (5) the anxiety level of the caller. Once all the pertinent medical information is gathered, a decision is made about whether the child should be seen immediately (by ambulance versus car), seen in the office later (today versus tomorrow), or whether the illness can be safely cared for at home. At the end of the call, it should be confirmed that parents understand and feel comfortable with the plan for their child.

Kempe A et al: Delivery of pediatric after-hours care by call centers: A multicenter study of parental perceptions and compliance. Pediatrics 2001;108:e111 [PMID: 11731638].

Luberti AA: After-hours telephone care: Options for the pediatrician. Pediatr Ann 2001;30:249 [PMID: 11383464].

Poole SR: Creating an after-hours telephone triage system for office practice. Pediatr Ann 2001;30:268 [PMID: 11383466].

## COMMUNITY PEDIATRICS

Community pediatrics is by definition "a concern for all children in the community, especially children who do not get adequate medical care." Pediatricians have historically been very involved in supporting and developing services for vulnerable children in their communities. As a group, pediatricians recognize that communities are integral determinants of a child's health and that the synthesis of public health and personal health principles and practices is important in the practice of community pediatrics. As well, pediatricians have a long commitment to work with other professionals in the community and advocate for the needs of all children.

Pediatricians in practice are frequently instrumental in referring children and families to valuable services and resources. For example, uninsured children can be enrolled in either their state Medicaid program or State Children's Health Insurance Program (SCHIP). Children with special health care needs may be eligible for services typically funded through state health departments and through programs such as those provided based on the Individuals with Disabilities Education Act (IDEA). A variety of community-based immunization programs can provide access to needed immunization for eligible children. Food and nutrition programs such as the federally funded Women, Infant and Children (WIC) program provide sources of free food for eligible families. Finally, subsidized preschool and child care services such as the federally funded Head Start program provide needed preschool programs. Pediatricians are in a unique position to make referrals to these important services from the ambulatory and hospital-based practice settings.

American Academy of Pediatrics, Committee on Child Health Services: The pediatrician's role in community pediatrics. Pediatrics 1999;103:1304 [PMID: 10353949].

Haggerty RJ: Community pediatrics. N Engl J Med 1968;278:15 [PMID: 5634652].

# ■ COMMON GENERAL PEDIATRIC ISSUES

## FEVER

### Definition and Measurement

Fever is one of the most common reasons for pediatric office visits, emergency department encounters, and after-hours telephone calls. Several different definitions of fever exist, but most experts define fever as a rectal temperature of 38°C or above. Temperature in pediatric patients can be measured in a variety of manners: rectal (using a mercury or digital thermometer), oral (mercury, digital), axillary (mercury, digital, or liquid crystal strip), forehead (liquid crystal strip), or tympanic (using a device that measures thermal infrared energy from the tympanic membrane). Tympanic measurement of temperature, because it is quick, not particularly uncomfortable, and requires little patient cooperation, is rapidly becoming the norm in many settings. However, several cautions apply to the use of this technique: tympanic temperatures have been shown to be less accurate in infants younger than 3 months old and are subject to false readings if the instrument is not positioned properly or the external ear canal is occluded by wax.

### Causes of Fever

Fever occurs when there is a rise in the hypothalamic set-point in response to endogenously produced pyrogens. A tremendously broad range of conditions cause fever, including infections, malignancies, autoimmune diseases, metabolic diseases, chronic inflammatory conditions, medications (including immunizations), central nervous system abnormalities, and exposure to excessive environmental heat. In most settings, however, the majority of fevers in pediatric patients are caused by self-limiting viral infections. Teething does not cause fever over 38.4°C.

### Evaluation

#### A. GENERAL CONSIDERATIONS

When evaluating a child with fever, one should elicit from the parents information about the duration of fever, the maximum height of fever documented at home, all associated symptoms, any chronic medical conditions, any medications taken, medication allergies, fluid intake, urine output, exposures and travel, and any additional features of the illness that concern the parents (Table 8–5). In the office, a temperature,

**Table 8–5.** Guidelines for evaluating children with fever.

**A. See immediately if:**
(1) The child is less than 3 months old.
(2) The fever is over 40.6°C.
(3) The child is crying inconsolably or whimpering.
(4) The child is crying when moved or even touched.
(5) The child is difficult to awaken.
(6) The child's neck is stiff.
(7) Purple spots or dots are present on the skin.
(8) The child's breathing is difficult, and not better after the nasal passages are cleared.
(9) The child is drooling saliva and is unable to swallow anything.
(10) A convulsion has occurred.
(11) The child acts or looks "very sick."

**B. See within 24 hours if:**
(1) The child is 3–6 months old (unless fever occurs within 48 hours after a diphtheria-tetanus-pertussis vaccination and the infant has no other serious symptoms).
(2) The fever exceeds 40°C (especially if the child is under age 3 years).
(3) Burning or pain occurs with urination.
(4) The fever has been present for more than 24 hours without an obvious cause or identified site of infection.
(5) The fever has subsided for more than 24 hours and then returned.
(6) The fever has been present for more than 72 hours.

heart rate, respiratory rate, and blood pressure should be documented, as well as an oxygen saturation if the child has any increased work of breathing. A complete physical examination, including a neurologic exam, should then be performed, with particular attention paid to the child's degree of toxicity and hydration status. A well-appearing, well-hydrated child with evidence of a routine viral infection can be safely sent home with symptomatic treatment and careful return precautions. Depending on the age of the patient, presence of underlying conditions, type of infection, and the provider's assessment of toxicity and hydration, many focal bacterial infections can also be treated as outpatients, with appropriate oral antibiotics as discussed in Chapter 38.

#### B. FEVER WITHOUT A FOCUS OF INFECTION

Children who present with fever but without any symptoms or signs of a focal infection are often a diagnostic and management challenge. Literally hundreds of articles have been published in the medical literature about the proper evaluation and treatment of infants and young children with fever. When assessing a child with fever but no apparent source of infection on examination, the provider needs to carefully consider the likelihood of a serious but "hidden" or occult bacterial infection. With the widespread use of effective vaccines against *Haemophilus influenzae* type b and *Streptococcus pneumoniae,* two of the most common causes of invasive bacterial infections in unimmunized children, the incidence of occult bacterial infections appears to be declining. However, vaccines are not 100% effective, and other organisms cause serious occult infections in children; therefore, febrile children will always demand careful evaluation and observation. Appropriate choices for empiric antibiotic therapy of children with fever without focus are discussed in Chapter 35.

Febrile infants 28 days old or younger, because of their likelihood of serious disease including sepsis, should always be treated conservatively. Hospitalization and parenteral antibiotics should be strongly considered in all circumstances. An initial diagnostic evaluation should include complete blood count; blood culture; urinalysis; urine culture; Gram stain, protein, and glucose tests of cerebrospinal fluid (CSF); and CSF culture. Consideration should also be given to the possibility of a perinatal herpes simplex virus infection (neonatal herpes is described in more detail in Chapter 36). A chest radiograph should be obtained for any infant with increased work of breathing.

Infants age 29–90 days are at risk of a variety of invasive bacterial infections, including perinatally acquired organisms (eg, group B streptococci) or infections acquired in the household (eg, pneumococci or meningococci). Febrile infants without a focus of infection can be divided into those who appear toxic versus nontoxic, and those at low risk versus higher risk of invasive bacterial disease. As with febrile neonates, toxic children in this age group should be admitted to the hospital for parental antibiotics and close observation. In nontoxic infants, low risk has been defined as previously healthy; no focal infection on examination; white blood cell (WBC) count between 5000 and 15000/mm$^3$; band cells < 1500/mm$^3$; normal urinalysis; and, when diarrhea is present, < 5 WBCs/hpf. Nontoxic low-risk infants in this age group are typically treated as outpatients with close follow-up. Longstanding practice guidelines, published by Baraff and colleagues in 1993, recommend that nontoxic but high-risk infants be admitted, undergo lumbar puncture, and receive parental antibiotics. Other experts have more recently suggested that in certain circumstances these infants can be safely treated as outpatients.

In an era of increasing immunization coverage against the most commonly invasive pneumococcal serotypes, it is difficult to estimate the risk of occult bacteremia in febrile 3–36-month-olds with no focus of infection. Nevertheless, for children 3–36 months old with temperatures ≥ 39°C, urine cultures should be considered in all male children younger than 6 months of age and in all females younger than 2 years of age. Chest radiographs should be performed in any child with increased work of breathing and should also be considered in children with high (≥ 20,000/mm$^3$) WBC counts but no respiratory symptoms. Depending on the child's appearance, underlying medical condition, and the height of fever, blood cultures should also be obtained. Empiric antibiotic therapy may be considered, particularly for children with temperature ≥ 39°C and WBC count ≥ 15,000/mm$^3$. However, in previously healthy, well-appearing, fully immunized children with reassuring laboratory studies, observation without antibiotics is safe and appropriate in many circumstances.

## Treatment of Fever

Fever phobia is a term that describes parents' anxious response to the fevers that all children experience. In a recent study, 91% of caregivers thought that a fever could cause harmful effects. Seven percent of parents thought that if they did not treat the fever, it would keep going higher. Parents need to be reassured that fevers < 41.7°C cause no brain damage. Parents need to be counseled that, although fevers can occasionally (≈4%) cause seizures, in which case their child needs to be seen, febrile seizures are generally harmless and also cause no brain damage.

Several safe and effective medications are available for the treatment of fever. Acetaminophen is indicated for children older than 2 months of age for fevers ≥ 39°C or if the child is uncomfortable. Acetaminophen is given in a dosage of 15 mg/kg of body weight per dose and can be given every 4–6 hours. The other widely used antipyretic in the United States is ibuprofen. Ibuprofen is given in a dosage of 10 mg/kg of body weight per dose and can be given every 6–8 hours. Ibuprofen and acetaminophen are similar in safety and their ability to reduce fever; however, ibuprofen is longer lasting. Aspirin should not be used for treating fever in any child or adolescent, because of its association with the development of Reye syndrome (particularly during infections with varicella and influenza).

Crocetti M, Moghbeli N, Serwint J: Fever phobia revisited: Have parental misconceptions about fever changed in 20 years? Pediatrics 2001;107:1241 [PMID: 11389237].

Klein JO: Management of the febrile child without a focus of infection in the era of universal pneumococcal immunization. Pediatr Infect Dis J 2002;21:584 [PMID: 12182394].

McCarthy PL: Fever without apparent source on clinical examination. Curr Opin Pediatr 2002;14:103 [PMID: 11880744].

Rehm KP: Fever in infants and children. Curr Opin Pediatr 2001;13:83 [PMID: 11216593].

## GROWTH DEFICIENCY

Growth deficiency—formerly termed failure to thrive—is deceleration of growth velocity resulting in crossing two major percentile lines on the growth chart. The diagnosis is warranted also if a child younger than age 6 months has not grown for 2 consecutive months or if a child older than age 6 months has not grown for 3 consecutive months. Growth deficiency occurs in about 8% of children.

Patterns of growth deficiency suggest, but are not specific for, different causes. In type I growth deficiency, the head circumference is preserved and the weight is depressed more than the height. This most common type results from inadequate caloric intake, excessive loss of calories, excessive intake of calories, or inability to use calories peripherally. Most such cases result from inadequate delivery of calories. This may be the result of poverty, lack of caregiver understanding, poor caregiver–child interaction, abnormal feeding patterns, or a combination of factors. Type II growth deficiency, which is associated with genetically determined short stature, endocrinopathies, constitutional growth delay, heart or renal disease, or various forms of skeletal dysplasias, is characterized by normal head circumference and proportionate diminution of height and weight. In type III growth deficiency, all three parameters of growth—head circumference, weight, and height—are lower than normal. This pattern is associated with central nervous system abnormalities, chromosomal defects, and in utero or perinatal insults.

## Clinical Findings

### A. INITIAL EVALUATION

The history and physical examination will identify the cause of growth reduction in the vast majority of cases (Table 8–6). The physical examination should focus on signs of organic disease or evidence of abuse or neglect: dysmorphic features, skin lesions, neck masses, adventitial breath sounds, heart murmurs, abdominal masses, and neuromuscular tone and strength. Throughout the evaluation, the physician should observe the caregiver–child interaction and the level of family functioning. Developmental screening and laboratory screening tests (complete blood count, blood urea nitrogen, creatinine, electrolytes, urinalysis, and urine culture) complete the initial office evaluation.

**Table 8–6.** Components of initial evaluation.

Birth history: Newborn screening result. Rule out intrauterine growth retardation, anoxia, congenital infections.
Feeding and nutrition: Difficulty sucking, chewing, swallowing. Feeding patterns. Intake of formula, milk, juice, solids.
Stooling and voiding of urine: Diarrhea, constipation, vomiting, poor urine stream.
Growth pattern: Several points on the growth chart are crucial.
Recurrent infections.
Hospitalizations.
HIV risk factors.
Developmental history.
Social and family factors: Family composition, financial status, supports, stresses. Heritable diseases, heights and weights of relatives.
Review of systems.

### B. FURTHER EVALUATION

A prospective 3-day diet record should be a standard part of the evaluation. This is useful in assessing undernutrition even when organic disease is present. The diet history is evaluated by a pediatric dietitian for calories, protein, and micronutrients as well as for the pattern of eating. Additional laboratory tests should be ordered based on the history and physical examination. For example, stool collection for fat determination is indicated if a history of diarrhea suggests malabsorption. Moderate or high amounts of proteinuria should prompt work-up for nephrotic syndrome. Vomiting should suggest a gastrointestinal, metabolic, neurologic, infectious, or renal cause. The tempo of evaluation should be based on the severity of symptoms and the magnitude of growth failure.

## Treatment

A successful treatment plan addresses the child's diet and eating patterns, the child's development, caregiver skills, and any organic disease. High-calorie diets and frequent monitoring (every 1 or 2 weeks initially) are essential. Acceptable weight gain varies by age (Table 8–7).

The child with growth deficiency may also be developmentally delayed because of living in an environment that fails to promote development or from the effect on the brain of nutrient deprivation. Restoring nutrition does not fully reverse the deficit but does reduce the long-term consequences.

Education in nutrition, child development, and behavioral management as well as psychosocial support of the primary caregiver is essential. If family dysfunction

**Table 8–7.** Acceptable weight gain by age.

| Age (months) | Weight Gain (g/d) |
| --- | --- |
| Birth to 3 | 20–30 |
| 3–6 | 15–20 |
| 6–9 | 10–15 |
| 9–12 | 6–11 |
| 12–18 | 5–8 |
| 18–24 | 3–7 |

is mild, behavior modification and counseling will be useful. Day care may benefit the child by providing a structured environment for all activities, including eating. If family dysfunction is severe, the local department of social services can help provide structure and assistance to the family. Rarely, the child may need to be temporarily or permanently removed from the home. Hospitalization is reserved for management of dehydration, for cases in which home therapy has failed to result in expected growth, for children who show evidence of abuse or willful neglect, for management of an illness that compromises a child's ability to eat, or for care pending foster home placement.

Weston JA: Growth deficiency. In Berman S (ed): *Pediatric Decision Making,* 4th ed. Mosby-Year Book, 2003.

# Immunization

*Matthew F. Daley, MD, Ann-Christine Nyquist, MD, MSPH, & Eric A. F. Simoes, MD, DCH*

Immunization is used either to prevent primary infection or to prevent the secondary consequences of an infection. Any assessment of the benefits of a proposed immunization program must take into account the likelihood of occurrence of infection in a defined population or specific individual, the consequence of infection, and the likelihood that the vaccination will prevent that infection. The anticipated benefit of immunization must be weighed against the risk to the individual of adverse consequences. The physician must present this information to the parents so they can give informed consent to immunization. The immunization recommendations outlined in this chapter are current but will change as technology evolves and our understanding of the epidemiology of vaccine-preventable diseases changes. The most useful sources for current information about immunization are the following:

1. *Morbidity and Mortality Weekly Report.* Published weekly by the Centers for Disease Control and Prevention (CDC), Atlanta, GA 30333. Available at http://www.cdc.gov/mmwr.

2. *The Red Book: Report of the Committee on Infectious Diseases.* Published at 2- to 3-year intervals by the American Academy of Pediatrics (AAP). The 2003 *Red Book* is available from the AAP. Updates are published in the journal *Pediatrics* and can be accessed at http://www.aap.org/.

3. CDC: National Immunization Program Information Hotline. Provides services to consumers and health care professionals regarding new vaccines, new schedules, and safety issues. 1-800-232-2522 (Spanish 1-800-232-0233). Operates from 8:00 AM to 11:00 PM Monday through Friday. Printed information can be obtained at http://cdc.gov/nip/.

4. CDC: Advisory Committee on Immunization practice. Available at http://www.cdc.gov/nip/ACIP.

## STANDARDS FOR PEDIATRIC IMMUNIZATION PRACTICES

An estimated 11,000 children are born each day in the United States, each requiring 15–19 doses of vaccine by age 18 months to be protected against 12 childhood diseases. Although 97–98% of these children are vaccinated by or shortly after school entry, about a quarter of the 2-year-olds in this country are not fully immunized. Low immunization coverage has been attributed to difficulties in reaching the urban poor and racial and ethnic minorities, and an increasingly mobile society. However, deficiencies in the health care delivery system are also a contributor, as is limited use of recall systems. Some parents seeking immunization for their children face significant barriers; not all providers take advantage of opportunities to administer vaccines, and inadequate or absent third-party payment for immunizations further reduces coverage. The AAP recommends the following specific proven practices to improve this coverage: (1) sending caretakers reminder and recall notices, (2) using prompts during all visits, (3) periodic measurement of immunization rates, and (4) having standing orders for vaccines.

The National Childhood Vaccine Injury Act of 1986 requires that for each vaccine covered under the Vaccine Injury Compensation Program (VICP) caretakers should be advised about the risks and benefits of vaccination, in a standard manner, using the Vaccine Information Statements (VIS). In addition the CDC and AAP have the requirements and recommendations summarized later on. Each time a VICP covered vaccine is administered the current version of VIS must be provided to the nonminor patient or legal caretaker. Documentation is required in the medical record, including the vaccine manufacturer, lot number, and its date of administration and expiration. The name and address of the person administering the vaccine, VIS version and date, and site and route of administration should also be recorded.

The use of disposable syringes and needles or some other form of single-dose delivery of vaccine is preferred to minimize the opportunity for contamination. A 70% solution of alcohol is appropriate for disinfection of the stopper of the vaccine container and of the skin at the injection site. A 5% topical emulsion of lidocaine–prilocaine (EMLA) cream applied to the site of vaccination for 30–60 minutes prior to the injection minimizes the pain, especially when multiple vaccines are administered.

The manufacturer's recommendations for route and site of administration of injectable vaccines are critical for safety and efficacy. All vaccines containing an adjuvant must be administered intramuscularly to avoid granuloma formation or necrosis. Such injections should be given at a 90-degree angle into the anterolateral thigh (not intragluteally) in infants (< age 18 months) and may be given in the deltoid or triceps in older children. A 22-gauge needle ⅞–1¼ inches long is recommended for children, but a 25-gauge ⅞–1 inch needle may be sufficient for young infants. Aspiration prior to intramuscular injection is suggested by many experts. Vaccines may be administered intramuscularly, subcutaneously, or intradermally. Subcutaneous injections should be administered at a 45-degree angle on the volar surface of the forearm using a 25-gauge ⅝-inch needle. Intradermal injections should be administered with the bevel facing upward using a ⅜- to ¾-inch 25- to 27-gauge needle. A 25-gauge ¾- to ⅝-inch needle is recommended. A separate syringe and needle should be used for each vaccine.

It is safe to administer many combinations of vaccines simultaneously without increasing the risk of adverse effects or compromising response. Up to seven injections may be necessary at the 12- to 15-month visit. (See the following individual preparations for further discussion.) Inactivated vaccines (with the exception of cholera and yellow fever) can be given simultaneously or at any time after a different vaccine. Parenteral live-virus vaccines, if not administered on the same day, should be given at least 30 days apart (eg, measles, mumps, rubella [MMR] and varicella [VAR]). Lapses in the immunization schedule do not call for reinstitution of the series. Extra doses of hepatitis B (HepB), *Haemophilus influenzae* type B (Hib), MMR, or VAR are not harmful, but repetitive exposure to tetanus vaccine beyond the recommended intervals can result in hypersensitivity reactions and should be avoided. If an immunoglobulin (Ig) or blood product has been administered, live-virus vaccination should be delayed 3–10 months, depending on the product, to avoid interference with the immune response (eg, 3 months for tetanus Ig, hepatitis A Ig, and hepatitis B Ig, 5–6 months for measles Ig or cytomegalovirus Ig (CMVIg), 9 months for respiratory syncytial virus immunoglobulin, and 11 months for IgIV for Kawasaki disease).

With the large number of vaccine preparations available, interchangeability of vaccines is an issue. All brands of Hib conjugate, hepatitis B, and hepatitis A vaccines are interchangeable. For vaccines containing acellular pertussis antigens, it is recommended that the same brand be used, but when the brand is unknown or the same brand is unavailable, any DTaP (diphtheria, tetanus toxoids, and acellular pertussis vaccine) should be used to continue vaccination. Longer than recommended intervals between vaccinations does not reduce

final antibody titers, and thus lapsed schedules do not require restarting the series.

Atkinson WL et al: Centers for Disease Control and Prevention: General recommendations on immunization: Recommendations of the Advisory Committee on Immunization Practices (ACIP) and the American Academy of Family Physicians (AAFP). MMWR Recomm Rep 2002;51(RR-2):1.

Halperin BA et al: Use of lidocaine–prilocaine patch to decrease intramuscular injection pain does not adversely affect the antibody response to diphtheria–tetanus–acellular pertussis–inactivated poliovirus–*Haemophilus influenzae* type b conjugate and hepatitis B vaccines in infants from birth to six months of age. Pediatr Infect Dis J 2002;21:399 [PMID: 12150176].

Saari TN, American Academy of Pediatrics Committee on Infectious Diseases: Immunization of preterm and low birth weight infants. Pediatrics 2003;112:193 [PMID: 12837889].

Wood DL, American Academy of Pediatrics Committee on Community Health Services, American Academy of Pediatrics Committee on Practice and Ambulatory Medicine: Increasing immunization coverage. Pediatrics 2003;112:993 [PMID: 14523201].

# ■ THE COMPOSITION OF IMMUNIZING AGENTS

## ACTIVE IMMUNIZATION

The immune response to immunization varies. A small proportion of children receiving certain antigens simply do not mount a response capable of conferring protection. For this reason, every vaccine has a definable failure rate.

The immunogen is suspended or dissolved in sterile water or saline, or in more complex media such as tissue culture medium, which may contain constituents from the biologic system used to produce the immunogen. Most vaccines contain preservatives and trace amounts of antibiotics such as neomycin to prevent bacterial overgrowth. Some vaccines contain adjuvants such as aluminum hydroxide and aluminum phosphate that also help to retain the immunogen at the site of inoculation for a prolonged time, thus increasing antigenic stimulation. The theoretical cumulative toxicity of mercury in thimerosal-containing vaccines has led to the development of thimerosal-free vaccines. All vaccines routinely administered to children are now free of thimerosal.

Although the prospect is unlikely, vaccine administration could have unforeseen adverse consequences. Thus vaccines should be administered where there is ready access to emergency resuscitative equipment and drugs (eg, epinephrine, antihistamines).

## PASSIVE IMMUNIZATION

Immune globulin (Ig) is derived from pooled donations of large numbers of individuals (more than 1000 per lot). Ig is prepared by alcohol fractionation, is sterile, and will not transmit any infectious agents (including hepatitis B and C viruses and HIV). Ig is a 16.5% solution consisting primarily of IgG with very small amounts of IgA and IgM.

## ROUTINE CHILDHOOD & ADOLESCENT IMMUNIZATIONS

Table 9–1 sets forth a schedule of routine immunizations for normal infants and children. Table 9–2 presents recommended schedules for children who did not start vaccination at the recommended time during the first year of life. Variations from these schedules may be necessitated by epidemiologic or individual clinical circumstances. Recommendations for minimum ages and intervals between doses are shown in Table 9–2.

To complete the 2004 schedule, 19 separate injections may be required from birth to age 6 years. Combination vaccines represent a solution to the problem of large numbers of injections during any single clinic visit. Currently available combination vaccines include MMR and various combinations of Hib, HepB, and diphtheria, tetanus, and pertussis vaccines, and more recently a DTaP–HBV–IPV/Hib combination vaccine.

Combination vaccines incorporating hepatitis A, meningococcal, pneumococcal, and varicella vaccines are being developed, and a pentavalent vaccine combining MMR, HepB, and IPV will soon be available. Separate vaccines should not be combined into one syringe by the provider, unless approved by the FDA, because this could decrease the efficacy of each component vaccine.

### Safe Handling of Vaccines

The numerous vaccines and other immunologic substances, such as antibody preparations and immunoglobulins for routine use by the practitioner, vary in the storage temperatures required. Vaccines that require routine freezing are VAR and oral poliovirus (OPV). Yellow fever vaccine may also be stored frozen. Product package inserts should be consulted for detailed information on vaccine storage conditions and shelf life.

American Academy of Pediatrics: Combination vaccines for childhood immunizations: Recommendations of the Advisory Committee on Immunization Practices (ACIP), the American Academy of Pediatrics (AAP), and the American Academy of Family Physicians (AAFP). Pediatrics 1999;103:1064 [PMID: 10224194].

Avdicova M et al: Immunogenicity and reactogenicity of a novel hexavalent DTPa–HBV–IPV/Hib vaccine compared to separate concomitant injections of DTPa–IPV/Hib and HBV Eur J Pediatr 2002;161:581 [PMID: 12424582].

Centers for Disease Control and Prevention: Recommended childhood and adolescent immunization schedule—United States, June–2004. MMWR 2004;53:1 [PMID: 14733209].

FDA licensure of diphtheria and tetanus toxoids and acellular pertussis adsorbed, hepatitis B (recombinant), and poliovirus vaccine combined, (PEDIARIX) for use in infants. MMWR Morb Mortal Wkly Rep 2003;52:203.

Halperin SA et al: Simultaneous administration of meningococcal C conjugate vaccine and diphtheria–tetanus–acellular pertussis–inactivated poliovirus–*Haemophilus influenzae* type b conjugate vaccine in children: A randomized double-blind study. Clin Invest Med 2002;25:243 [PMID: 12516995].

## ■ SAFETY OF IMMUNIZATION

### VACCINE FACTORS

The safety standards for all vaccines licensed for use in the United States are established by the Food and Drug Administration (FDA) and involve regular examination of manufacturing techniques as well as production lots of vaccine. No incidents of bacterial or viral contamination of vaccines at the factory level have been reported in the United States for decades.

### HOST FACTORS

The contraindications and precautions relating to immunization presented in Table 9–3 reflect the current recommendations of the Advisory Committee on Immunization Practices and the Committee of Infectious Diseases of the AAP.

### Healthy Children

Minor acute illnesses, with or without low-grade fever, are not contraindications (see Table 9–3) to vaccination, because there is no evidence that vaccination under these conditions increases the rate of adverse effects or decreases efficacy. A moderate to severe febrile illness may be a reason to postpone vaccination. Routine physical examination and temperature assessment are not necessary before vaccinating healthy infants and children.

### Children with Chronic Illnesses

Most chronic diseases are not contraindications to vaccination; in fact, children with chronic diseases may be at greater risk of complications from vaccine-preventable diseases such as influenza and pneumococcal infections. Premature infants are a good example. They should be immunized according to their chronologic, not gestational, age. Vaccine doses should not be reduced for preterm or low-birth-weight infants. The one exception to this rule may be children with progressive central nervous system (CNS) disorders. Vaccination may be deferred or avoided entirely for such children, whereas children with static CNS diseases are candidates for vaccination.

## Immunodeficient Children

Congenitally immunodeficient children should not be immunized with live-virus or live-bacteria vaccines. Depending on the nature of the immunodeficiency, other vaccines are safe, but may fail to evoke an immune response. Children with cancer and children receiving high-dose corticosteroids or other immunosuppressive agents should not be vaccinated with live-virus or live-bacteria vaccines. This contraindication does not apply if the malignancy is in remission and chemotherapy has not been administered for at least 90 days. Live-virus vaccines may also be administered to previously healthy children receiving low to moderate doses of corticosteroids (defined as up to 2 mg/kg/d of prednisone or prednisone-equivalent, with a 20 mg/d maximum) for less than 14 days; children receiving low to moderate doses of alternate-day corticosteroids; children being maintained on physiologic corticosteroid therapy without other immunodeficiency; and children using only topical, inhaled, or intraarticular corticosteroids.

Contraindication of live-pathogen vaccine also applies to children with HIV infection, with the proviso that MMR is recommended at 12 months of age (after 6 months during an epidemic). The booster dose may be given as early as 1 month later, but doses given before 1 year of age should not be considered part of a complete series. VAR vaccination is recommended for CDC class N1 or A1 (CD4 ≥ 25%). Severely immunocompromised children with HIV infection should not receive the measles or VAR vaccines. OPV is contraindicated and is no longer recommended in the United States. The ACIP recommends routine vaccination for all children with an all inactivated poliovirus vaccine (IPV) vaccination schedule. Thus immunodeficient children should no longer be exposed to oral poliovaccine through household contacts. MMR and VAR are not contraindicated in household contacts of immunocompromised children.

## Allergic or Hypersensitive Children

Hypersensitivity reactions are rare following vaccination, occurring in 1.53 cases/million doses. They are generally attributable to a trace component of the vaccine rather than to the antigen itself. MMR, IPV, and VAR contain microgram quantities of neomycin, and IPV also contains trace amounts of streptomycin and polymyxin B. Children with known anaphylactic responses to these antibiotics should not be given these vaccines. Trace quantities of egg antigens may be present in influenza, and yellow fever vaccines and MMR. Children who have had anaphylactic reactions to eggs should not be given these vaccines; children with less serious reactions to eggs may generally be safely immunized. If doubt exists about the nature of a child's egg sensitivity, a skin testing procedure is outlined in the *Red Book*. Some vaccines (MMR, VAR, and yellow fever) contain gelatin, a substance to which persons with known food allergy may develop an anaphylactic reaction. Skin testing before vaccination may be an option in such cases.

## Special Circumstances

Detailed recommendations for preterm low-birth-weight babies; pediatric transplant recipients; Alaskan Natives/American Indians; children in residential institutions or military communities; or are refugees, new immigrants, or travelers are available in the AAP *Red Book*.

American Academy of Pediatrics: *2003 Red Book: Report of the Committee on Infectious Diseases,* 26th ed. American Academy of Pediatrics, 2003.

Bohlke K et al: Vaccine Safety Datalink Team: Risk of anaphylaxis after vaccination of children and adolescents. Pediatrics 2003;112:815 [PMID: 14523172].

# DIPHTHERIA

The risk for exposure to toxigenic strains of *Clostridium diphtheriae* in the United States is low (2 cases in 2002); however, diphtheria remains endemic in many countries. Diphtheria toxoid is prepared by the formaldehyde inactivation of diphtheria toxin. The protective efficacy of diphtheria toxoid has never been measured on a mass scale, but is estimated to be greater than 85%.

## Preparations Available

1. Diphtheria toxoid is used only when tetanus toxoid and pertussis vaccine are both contraindicated.
2. Diphtheria–tetanus vaccine (DT) (pediatric) is used when pertussis vaccine is contraindicated. DT contains more diphtheria toxoid per dose than preparations used for adults and should not

**Table 9–1.** Recommended childhood and adolescent immunization schedule[a,j]: United States, January–June 2004.

| Vaccine | Birth | 1 mo | 2 mos | 4 mos | 6 mos | 12 mos | 15 mos | 18 mos | 24 mos | 4–6 yrs | 11–12 yrs | 13–18 yrs |
|---|---|---|---|---|---|---|---|---|---|---|---|---|
| | | | | Range of recommended ages | | | catch-up vaccination | | | | Preadolescent assessment | |
| Hepatitis B[b] | HepB #1 | only if mother HBsAg (-) | | | | | | | | | HepB series | |
| | | | HepB #2 | | | HepB #3 | | | | | | |
| Diphtheria, Tetanus, Pertussis[c] | | | DTaP | DTaP | DTaP | | DTaP | | | DTaP | Td | Td |
| Haemophilus influenzae type b[d] | | | Hib | Hib | Hib[d] | Hib | | | | | | |
| Inactivated Polio | | | IPV | IPV | | IPV | | | | IPV | | |
| Measles, Mumps, Rubella[e] | | | | | | MMR #1 | | | | MMR #2 | MMR #2 | |
| Varicella[f] | | | | | | Varicella | | | | | Varicella | |
| Pneumococcal[g] | | | PCV | PCV | PCV | PCV | | | | PCV | PPV | |

-------------- Vaccines below this line are for selected populations --------------

| | | | | | | | | | | | | |
|---|---|---|---|---|---|---|---|---|---|---|---|---|
| Hepatitis A[h] | | | | | | | | | | | Hepatitis A | |
| Influenza[i] | | | | | | Influenza (yearly) | | | | | | |

[a]Indicates the recommended ages for routine administration of currently licensed childhood vaccines, as of December 1, 2003, for children through age 18 years. Any dose not given at the recommended age should be given at any subsequent visit when indicated and feasible. ▨ Indicates age groups that warrant special effort to admister those vaccines not given previously. Additional vaccines may be licensed and recommended during the year. Licensed combination vaccines may be used whenever any components of the combination are indicated and the vaccine's other components are not contraindicated. Providers should consult the manufacturers' package inserts for detailed recommendations. Clinically significant adverse events that follow vaccination should be reported to the Vaccine Adverse Event Reporting System (VAERS). Guidance on how to obtain and complete a VAERS form is available at http://www.vaers.org or by telephone, 800-822-7967.

[b]**Hepatitis B vaccine (HepB).** All infants should receive the first dose of HepB vaccine soon after birth and before hospital discharge; the first dose also may be given by age 2 months if the infant's mother is HBsAg-negative. Only monovalent HepB vaccine can be used for the birth dose. Monovalent or combination vaccine containing HepB may be used to complete the series; 4 doses of vaccine may be administered when a birth dose is given. The second dose should be given at least 4 weeks after the first dose except for combination vaccines, which cannot be administered before age 6 weeks. The third dose should be given at

least 16 weeks after the first dose and at least 8 weeks after the second dose. The last dose in the vaccination series (third or fourth dose) should not be administered before age 24 weeks. *Infants born to HBsAg-positive mothers* should receive HepB vaccine and 0.5 mL hepatitis B immune globulin (HBIG) within 12 hours of birth at separate sites. The second dose is recommended at age 1–2 months. The last dose in the vaccination series should not be administered before age 24 weeks. These infants should be tested for HBsAg and anti-HBs at age 9–15 months. *Infants born to mothers whose HBsAg status is unknown* should receive the first dose of the HepB vaccine series within 12 hours of birth. Maternal blood should be drawn as soon as possible to determine the mother's HBsAg status; if the HBsAg test is positive, the infant should receive HBIG as soon as possible (no later than age 1 week). The second dose is recommended at age 1–2 months. The last dose in the vaccination series should not be administered before age 24 weeks.

[c]**Diphtheria and tetanus toxoids and acellular pertussis vaccine (DTaP).** The fourth dose of DTaP may be administered at age 12 mo provided 6 mo have elapsed since the third dose and the child is unlikely to return at age 15–18 mo. The final dose in the series should be given at age ≥4 y. **Tetanus and diphtheria toxoids (Td)** is recommended at age 11–12 y if at least 5 y have elapsed since the last dose of tetanus and diphtheria toxoid-containing vaccine. Subsequent routine Td boosters are recommended every 10 y.

[d]**_Haemophilus influenzae_ type b (Hib) conjugate vaccine.** Three Hib conjugate vaccines are licensed for infant use. If PRP-OMP (PedvaxHIB or ComVax [Merck]) is administered at ages 2 and 4 months, a dose at age 6 months is not required. DTaP/Hib combination products should not be used for primary vaccination in infants at ages 2, 4, or 6 mo but can be used as boosters after any Hib vaccine. The final dose in the series should be given at age ≥ 12 mo.

[e]**Measles, mumps, and rubella vaccine (MMR).** The second dose of MMR is recommended routinely at age 4–6 y but may be administered during any visit provided that at least 4 weeks have elapsed since the first dose and that both doses are administered beginning at or after age 12 months. Those who have not received the second dose previously should complete the schedule by the visit at age 11–12 years.

[f]**Varicella vaccine (VAR).** Varicella vaccine is recommended at any visit at or after age 12 months for susceptible children (i.e., those who lack a reliable history of chickenpox). Susceptible persons aged ≥13 years should receive 2 doses given at least 4 weeks apart.

[g]**Pneumococcal vaccine.** The heptavalent **pneumococcal conjugate vaccine (PCV)** is recommended for all children aged 2–23 mo and for certain children aged 24–59 mo. The final dose in the series should be given at age ≥12 mo. **Pneumococcal polysaccharide vaccine (PPV)** is recommended in addition to PCV for certain high-risk groups. See _MMWR_ 2000;49(No. RR-9):1–35.

[h]**Hepatitis A vaccine.** Hepatitis A vaccine is recommended for children and adolescents in selected states and regions, and for certain high-risk groups. Consult local public health authority and _MMWR_ 1999;48(No. RR-12):1–37. Children and adolescents in these states, regions, and high-risk groups who have not been vaccinated against hepatitis A can begin the hepatitis A vaccination series during any visit. The two doses in the series should be administered at least 6 months apart.

[i]**Influenza vaccine.** Influenza vaccine is recommended annually for children aged ≥ 6 months with certain risk factors (including but not limited to asthma, cardiac disease, sickle cell disease, HIV, and diabetes), and household members of persons in groups at high risk (see _MMWR_ 2003;52[No. RR-8]:1–36), and can be administered to all others wishing to obtain immunity. In addition, healthy children aged 6–23 mo are encouraged to receive influenza vaccine if feasible because children in this age group are at substantially increased risk for influenza-related hospitalizations. For healthy persons aged 5–49 y, the intranasally administered live-attenuated influenza vaccine (LAIV) is an acceptable alternative to the intramuscular trivalent inactivated influenza vaccine (TIV). See _MMWR_ 2003;52(No. RR-13):1–8. Children receiving TIV should be administered a dosage appropriate for thier age (0.25 mL if 6–35 mo or 0.5 mL if ≥3 y). Children aged ≤8 y who are receiving influenza vaccine for the first time should receive 2 doses (separated by at least 4 weeks for TIV and at least 6 weeks for LAIV).

[j]Additional information about vaccines, including precautions and contraindications for vaccination and vaccine shortages, is available at http://www.cdc.gov/nip or from the National Immunization information hotline, telephone 800-232-2522 (English) or 800-232-0233 (Spanish). Approved by the **Advisory Committee on Immunization Practices** (http://www.cdc.gov/nip/acip), the **American Academy of Pediatrics** (http://www.aap.org), and the **American Academy of Family Physicians** (http://www.aafp.org). Reproduced, with permission, from recommended adulthood and adolescent immunization schedule—United States, January–June 2004. _MMWR_ 2004:53; Q1–4 [PMID 14733209].

---

be used in adults because of potentially severe local adverse reactions.

3. Tetanus–diphtheria vaccine (Td) (adult) is for use in persons age 7 years or older. It is less likely to produce local reactions while still eliciting a good immunogenic response in this population.

4. Diphtheria–tetanus–pertussis vaccine (DTP) was the standard immunizing agent for healthy children prior to availability of DTaP but may still be used when DTaP is unavailable. DTP is no longer manufactured in the United States.

5. Diphtheria–tetanus–acellular pertussis vaccine (DTaP) contains an amount of diphtheria toxins similar to DTP and is recommended as the standard immunizing agent for healthy children.

6. Diphtheria–tetanus–acellular pertussis and _H influenzae_ type b conjugate vaccine (DTaP–Hib) is licensed only for the fourth dose in the DTP–Hib series (age 15–18 months). Earlier use may result in suboptimal response to the Hib component.

7. Diphtheria–tetanus–acellular pertussis–hepatitis B–inactivated poliovirus (DTaP–HepB–IPV) is licensed for use in infants ages 2, 4, and 6 months.

## Dosage & Schedule of Administration

The preceding preparations are given intramuscularly in a dose of 0.5 mL. The use of jet injection may be associated with more local reactions. See Table 9–1 for the routine schedule and Table 9–2 for immunization of children not appropriately immunized during the first year of life.

## Adverse Effects

No significant adverse reactions have been associated with diphtheria toxoid alone.

## Antibody Preparations

Equine diphtheria antitoxin is available for the treatment of diphtheria. Dosage depends on the size and lo-

***Table 9–2.*** Catch-up immunization schedule for children and adolescents who start late or who are >1 month behind.

| Dose 1 (minimum age) | Minimum interval between doses | | | |
|---|---|---|---|---|
| | Dose 1 to dose 2 | Dose 2 to dose 3 | Dose 3 to dose 4 | Dose 4 to dose 5 |
| DTaP (6 wk) | 4 wk | 4 wk | 6 mo | 6 mo[a] |
| IPV (6 wk) | 4 wk | 4 wk | 4 wk[b] | |
| HepB[c] (birth) | 4 wk | 8 wk (and 16 wk after 1st dose) | | |
| MMR (12 mo) | 4 wk[d] | | | |
| VAR (12 mo) | | | | |
| Hib[e] (6 wk) | 4 wk: if 1st dose given at age <12 mo<br>8 wk (as final dose): if 1st dose given at age 12–14 mo<br>No further doses needed: if 1st dose given at age ≥15 mo | 4 wk[f]: if current ag <12 mo<br>8 wk (as final dose)[f]: if current age ≥12 mo and 2nd dose given at age <15 mo<br>No further doses needed: if previous dose given at age ≥15 mo | 8 wk (as final dose): this dose only necessary for children aged 12 mo–5 y who received 3 doses before age 12 mo | |
| PCV[g] (6 wk) | 4 wk: if 1st dose given at age <12 mo and current age <24 mo<br>8 wk (as final dose): if 1st dose given at age ≥12 mo or current age 24–59 mo<br>No further doses needed: for healthy children if 1st dose given at age ≥24 mo | 4 wk: if current age <12 mo<br>8 wk (as final dose): if current age ≥12 mo<br>No further doses needed: for healthy children if previous dose given at age ≥24 mo | 8 wk (as final dose): this dose only necessary for children aged 12 mo–5 y who received 3 doses before age 12 mo | |

### Catch-up schedule for children aged 7–18 years

| Minimal interval between doses | | |
|---|---|---|
| Dose 1 to dose 2 | Dose 2 to dose 3 | Dose 3 to booster dose |
| Td: 4 wk | Td: 6 mo | Td[h]: 6 mo: if 1st dose given at age <12 mo and current age <11 y<br>5 y: if 1st dose given at age ≥12 mo and 3rd dose given at age <7 y and current age ≥11 y<br>10 y: if 3rd dose given at age ≥7 y |
| IPV[i]: 4 wk | IPV[i]: 4 wk | IPV[b,i] |
| HepB: 4 wk | HepB: 8 wk (and 16 wk after 1st dose) | |
| MMR: 4 wk | | |
| VAR[i]: 4 wk | | |

***Note:*** A vaccine series does not require restarting, regardless of the time that has elapsed between doses.

[a]**Diphtheria and tetanus toxoids and acellular pertussis vaccine (DTaP):** The fifth dose is not necessary if the fourth dose was given after the fourth birthday.

[b]**Inactivated polio vaccine (IPV):** For children who received an all-IPV or all-oral poliovirus (OPV) series, a fourth dose is not necessary if third dose was given at age ≥4 years. If both OPV and IPV were given as part of a series, a total of 4 doses should be given, regardless of the child's current age.

cation of the diphtheritic membrane and an estimate of the patient's level of intoxication. Before using this preparation, the presence or absence of equine serum sensitivity must be determined using a scratch test of a 1:1000 dilution. If the test is positive, desensitization must be undertaken. If negative, the doses shown in Table 9–4 are suggested.

As of January 1997, diphtheria antitoxin is no longer commercially available in the United States but may be obtained from the CDC.

## TETANUS

When anaerobic *Clostridium tetani* colonizes devitalized tissue, the exotoxin tetanospasmin is disseminated to inhibitory motor neurons, resulting in tetanus. Tetanus primarily occurs in unvaccinated or inadequately vaccinated persons. Despite the existence of a safe and effective vaccine, 22 cases of tetanus were reported in the United States in 2002. Tetanus-prone wounds include (1) puncture wounds, including those acquired due to body piercing, tattooing, and intravenous drug abuse; (2) animal bites; (3) lacerations or abrasions; and (4) wounds resulting from nonsterile delivery and umbilical cord care (neonatal tetanus). Intravenous drug abusers are an increasing proportion of tetanus patients in the United States, accounting for up to 20–40% of cases in some states.

Tetanus toxoid is prepared by inactivating the toxin with formaldehyde. The protective efficacy of tetanus toxoid has never been measured in any large study, but it is believed to be high.

### Preparations Available

1. Tetanus toxoid (fluid) is used rarely—only when rapid immunization is desirable.
2. Tetanus toxoid adsorbed on aluminum phosphate is the standard single-antigen booster toxoid.
3. Tetanus–diphtheria vaccines (pediatric DT and adult Td) are the standard dual-antigen booster toxoids and are more often used for prophylaxis in routine wound management over the single-antigen preparation.
4. DTaP with or without Hib (discussed in the section on Hib).
5. DTaP–Hep B–IPV.

### Dosage & Schedule of Administration

The preceding preparations are administered intramuscularly in a dose of 0.5 mL. See Table 9–1 for the routine schedule and Table 9–2 for vaccination of children not appropriately immunized during the first year of life. A booster dose of Td should be scheduled at age 11–12 years or at age 14–16 years and every 10 years thereafter to protect against tetanus and diphtheria.

Table 9–5 summarizes recommendations for the use of tetanus prophylaxis in routine wound management. Patients with non–tetanus-prone wounds should be boosted if more than 10 years have elapsed since their last immunization; those with tetanus-prone wounds should receive a booster if more than 5 years have elapsed.

---

cHepatits B vaccine (HepB): All children and adolescents who have not been vaccinated against hepatis B should begin the hepatitis B vaccination series during any visit. Providers should make special efforts to immunize children who were born in, or whose parents were born in, areas of the world where hepatitis B virus infection is moderately or highly endemic.

dMeasles, mumps, and rubella vaccine (MMR): The second dose of MMR is recommended routinely at age 4–6 years, but may be given earlier if desired.

eHaemophilus influenzae type b (Hib) conjugate vaccine: Vaccine generally is not recommended for children aged ≥5 years.

fHib: If current age is <12 months and the first 2 doses were PRP-OMP (PedvaxHIB® or ComVax® [Merck]), the third (and final) dose should be given at age 12–15 months and at least 8 weeks after the second dose.

gPneumococcal conjugate vaccine (PCV): Vaccine generally is not recommended for children age ≥5 years.

hTetanus and diphtheria toxoids (Td): For children aged 7–10 years, the interval between the third and booster dose is determined by the age when the first dose was given. For adolescents aged 11–18 years, the interval is determined by the age when the third dose was given.

iIPV: Vaccine generally is not recommended for persons aged ≥18 years.

jVaricella vaccine (VAR): Give 2-dose series to all susceptible adolescents aged ≥13 years.

Reporting adverse reactions. Clinically significant adverse events that follow vaccination should be reported to the Vaccine Adverse Event Reporting System (VAERS). Guidance on completing a VAERS form is available at http://www.vaers.org or at telephone, 800-822-7967. Disease reporting. Suspected cases of vaccine-preventable diseases should be reported to state or local health departments. Additional information about vaccines, including precautions and contraindications for vaccination and vaccine shortages, is available at http://www.cdc.gov/nip or at the National Immunization information hotline, telephone 800-232-2552 (English) or 800-232-0233 (Spanish).

Reproduced, with permission, from Recommended childhood and adolescent immunization schedule Unted States, January–June 2004. MMWR 2004:53; Q1–4 [PMID 14733209].

***Table 9–3.*** Guide to contraindications and precautions[a] to commonly used vaccines.

| Vaccine | True contraindications and precautions[a] | Untrue (vaccines can be administered) |
|---|---|---|
| General for all vaccines, including diphtheria and tetanus toxoids and acellular pertussis vaccine (DTaP); pediatric diphtheria-tetanus toxoid (DT); adult tetanus-diphtheria toxoid (Td); inactivated poliovirus vaccine (IPV); measles-mumps-rubella vaccine (MMR); *Haemophilus influenzae* type b vaccine (Hib); hepatitis A vaccine; hepatitis B vaccine; varicella vaccine; pneumococcal conjugate vaccine (PCV); influenza vaccine; and pneumococcal polysaccharide vaccine (PPV) | **Contraindications**<br>Serious allergic reaction (eg, anaphylaxis) after a previous vaccine dose<br>Serious allergic reaction (eg. anaphylaxis) to a vaccine component<br>**Precautions**<br>Moderate or severe acute illness with or without fever | Mild acute illness with or without fever<br>Mild to moderate local reaction (ie, swelling, redness, soreness); low-grade or moderate fever after previous dose<br>Lack of previous physical examination in well-appearing person<br>Current antimicrobial therapy<br>Convalescent phase of illness<br>Premature birth (hepatitis B vaccine is an exception in certain circumstances)[b]<br>Recent exposure to an infectious disease<br>History of penicillin allergy, other nonvaccine allergies, relatives with allergies, receiving allergen extract immunotherapy |
| DTaP | **Contraindications**<br>Severe allergic reaction after a previous dose or to a vaccine component<br>Encephalopathy (eg, coma, decreased level of consciousness; prolonged seizures) within 7 days of administration of previous dose of DTP or DTaP<br>Progressive neurologic disorder, including infantile spasms, uncontrolled epilepsy, progressive encephalopathy: defer DTaP until neurologic status clarified and stabilized.<br>**Precautions**<br>Fever of >40.5°C ≤48 h after vaccination with a previous dose of DTP or DTaP<br>Collapse or shock-like state (ie, hypotonic hyporesponsive episode) ≤48 h after receiving a previous dose of DTP/DTaP<br>Seizure ≤3 d of receiving a previous dose of DTP/DTaP[c]<br>Persistent, inconsolable crying lasting ≥3 h ≤48 hours after receiving a previous dose of DTP/DTaP<br>Moderate or severe acute illness with or without fever | Temperature of <40.5°C, fussiness or mild drowsiness after a previous dose of diphtheria toxoid-tetanus toxoid-pertussis vaccine (DTP)/DTaP<br>Family history of seizures[c]<br>Family history of sudden infant death syndrome<br>Family history of an adverse event after DTP or DTaP administration<br>Stable neurologic conditions (eg, cerebral palsy, well-controlled convulsions, developmental delay) |
| DT, Td | **Contraindications**<br>Severe allergic reaction after a previous dose or to a vaccine component<br>**Precautions**<br>Guillain-Barré syndrome ≤6 wk after previous dose of tetanus toxoid-containing vaccine<br>Moderate or severe acute illness with or without fever | |

(continued)

***Table 9–3.*** Guide to contraindications and precautions[a] to commonly used vaccines.

| Vaccine | True contraindications and precautions[a] | Untrue (vaccines can be administered) |
|---|---|---|
| IPV | **Contraindications**<br>Severe allergic reaction to previous dose or vaccine component<br>**Precautions**<br>Pregnancy<br>Moderate or severe acute illness with or without fever | — |
| MMR[d] | **Contraindications**<br>Severe allergic reaction after a previous dose or to a vaccine component<br>Pregnancy<br>Known severe immunodeficiency (eg, hematologic and solid tumors; congenital immunodeficiency; long-term immunosuppressive therapy,[e] or severely symptomatic human immunodeficiency virus [HIV] infection)<br>**Precautions**<br>Recent (≤11 mo) receipt of antibody-containing blood product (specific interval depends on product)[g]<br>History of thrombocytopenia or thrombocytopenic purpura<br>Moderate or severe acute illness with or without fever | Positive tuberculin skin test<br>Simultaneous TB skin testing[f]<br>Breast-feeding<br>Pregnancy of recipient's mother or other close or household contact<br>Recipient is child-bearing–age female<br>Immunodeficient family member or household contact<br>Asymptomatic or mildly symptomatic HIV infection<br>Allergy to eggs |
| Hib | **Contraindications**<br>Severe allergic reaction after a previous dose or to a vaccine component<br>Age <6 wk<br>**Precaution**<br>Moderate or severe acute illness with or without fever | — |
| Hepatitis B | **Contraindication**<br>Severe allergic reaction after a previous dose or to a vaccine component<br>**Precautions**<br>Infant weighing <2000 g[b]<br>Moderate or severe acute illness with or without fever | Pregnancy<br>Autoimmune disease (eg, systemic lupus erythematosus or rheumatoid arthritis) |
| Hepatitis A | **Contraindications**<br>Severe allergic reaction after a previous dose or to a vaccine component<br>**Precautions**<br>Pregnancy<br>Moderate or severe acute illness with or without fever | — |

*(continued)*

***Table 9–3.*** Guide to contraindications and precautions[a] to commonly used vaccines.

| Vaccine | True contraindications and precautions[a] | Untrue (vaccines can be administered) |
|---|---|---|
| Varicella[d] | **Contraindications**<br>Severe allergic reaction after a previous dose or to a vaccine component<br>Substantial suppression of cellular immunity<br>Pregnancy<br>**Precautions**<br>Recent (≤11 mo) receipt of antibody-containing blood product (specific interval depends on product)[g]<br>Moderate or severe acute illness with or without fever | Pregnancy of recipient's mother or other close or household contact<br>Immunodeficient family member or household contact[h]<br>Asymptomatic or mildly symptomatic HIV infection<br>Humoral immunodeficiency (eg, agammaglobulinemia) |
| PCV | **Contraindication**<br>Severe allergic reaction after a previous dose or to a vaccine component<br>**Precautions**<br>Moderate or severe acute illness with or without fever | — |
| Influenza | **Contraindication**<br>Severe allergic reaction to previous dose or vaccine component, including egg protein<br>**Precautions**<br>Moderate or severe acute illness with or without fever | Nonsevere (eg, contact) allergy to latex or thimerosal<br>Concurrent administration of coumadin or aminophylline |
| PPV | **Contraindication**<br>Severe allergic reaction after a previous dose or to a vaccine component<br>**Precaution**<br>Moderate or severe acute illness with or without fever | — |

[a]Events or conditions listed as precautions should be reviewed carefully. Benefits and risks of administering a specific vaccine to a person under these circumstances should be considered. If the risk from the vaccine is believed to outweigh the benefit, the vaccine should not be administered. If the benefit of vaccination is believed to outweigh the risk, the vaccine should be administered. Whether and when to administer DTaP to children with proven or suspected underlying neurologic disorders shoud be decided on a case-by-case basis.

[b]Hepatitis B vaccination should be deferred for infants weighing <2000 g if the mother is documented to be hepatitis B surface antigen (HbsAg)-negative at the time of the infant's birth. Vaccination can commence at chronological age 1 month. For infants born to HbsAg-positive women, hepatitis B immunoglobulin and hepatitis B vaccine should be administered at or soon after birth regardless of weight. See text for details.

[c]Acetaminophen or other appropriate antipyretic can be administered to children with a personal or family history of seizures at the time of DTaP vaccination and every 4–6 h for 24 h thereafter to reduce the possibility of postvaccination fever (**Source:** American Academy of Pediatrics. Active immunization. In: Pickering LK, ed. 2000 red book: report of the Committee on Infectious Diseases. 25th ed. Elk Grove Village, IL: American Academy of Pediatrics, 2000).

[d]MMR and varicella vaccines can be administered on the same day. If not administered on the same day, these vaccines should be separated by ≥28 d.

[e]Substantially immunosuppressive steroid dose is considered to be ≥2 wk of daily receipt of 20 mg or 2 mg/kg body weight of prednisone or equivalent.

[f]Measles vaccination can suppress tuberculin reactivity temporarily. Measles-containing vaccine can be administered on the same day as tuberculin skin testing. If testing cannot be performed until after the day of MMR vaccination, the test should be postponed for ≥4 weeks after the vaccination. If an urgent need exists to do skin test, do so with the understanding that reactivity might be reduced by the vaccine.

[g]See text for details.

[h]If a vaccinee experiences a presumed vaccine-related rash 7–25 d after vaccination, avoid direct contact with immunocompromised persons for the duration of the rash.

Reproduced, with permission, from MMWR Recomm Rep 2002:51(RR-2)1–35 [PMID 11848294].

***Table 9–4.*** Suggested dosing for equine diphtheria antitoxin.[a]

| Site | Duration of Lesion | Toxic (?) | Dose (units) |
|------|--------------------|-----------|--------------|
| Pharyngeal or laryngeal | ≤ 48 h | NA | 20,000–40,000 |
| Nasopharyngeal | NA | NA | 40,000–60,000 |
| Extensive or brawny swelling of the neck | ≥ 72 h | Yes | 80,000–120,000 |
| Cutaneous | NA | NA | 20,000–40,000 |

[a]NA = Not applicable.

## Adverse Effects

Significant reactions to tetanus toxoid, historically an extremely safe preparation, are very unusual. Anaphylaxis, Guillain–Barré syndrome, and brachial neuritis related to tetanus toxoid are extremely rare.

## Antibody Preparations

Tetanus immune globulin (TIg) (human) is indicated in the management of tetanus-prone wounds in individuals who have had an uncertain number or fewer than three tetanus immunizations with tetanus toxoid, as described earlier. Persons fully immunized with at least three doses do not require TIg, regardless of the nature of their wounds (see Table 9–5). The dose is

300–600 units (one or two vials) intramuscularly. Part of the dose may be infiltrated locally.

Tetanus Surveillance—United States, 1998–2000. MMWR 2003;52 (SS-3):1 [PMID: 12825541].

## PERTUSSIS

Pertussis is increasingly recognized as a disease affecting older children and adults, including fully vaccinated persons with waning immunity. Maintaining vaccination in young infants will protect against severe disease in this age group, but because booster vaccination is not approved for children over age 7 years, a reservoir of disease among those with waning immunity is a continuing problem.

Pertussis vaccines currently used in the United States for initial immunization contain purified components of pertussis antigens. The DTaP preparations have a protective efficacy of about 70–90% after three doses, depending on the source. Further epidemiologic evidence of the efficacy of pertussis vaccine is provided by the observation of a large increase in pertussis cases in Great Britain and Japan after those countries reduced or abandoned use of the vaccine.

### Preparations Available

1. DTaP
2. DTaP–Hib
3. DTaP–HepB–IPV

***Table 9–5.*** Summarized recommendations for the use of tetanus prophylaxis in routine wound management—Advisory Committee on Immunization Practices (ACIP), 1991.

| History of Adsorbed Tetanus Toxoid | Clean, Minor Wounds | | All Other Wounds[a] | |
|---|---|---|---|---|
| | Td[b] or DT | TIG[c] | Td or DT | TIG |
| Unknown or < 3 doses | Yes | No | Yes | Yes |
| ≥ 3 doses[d] | No[e] | No | No[f] | No |

[a]Such as, but not limited to, wounds contaminated with dirt, feces, soil, or saliva; puncture wounds; avulsions; and wounds resulting from missiles, crushing, burns, or frostbite.
[b]For children over age 7 y the diphtheria and tetanus toxoids and acellular pertussis vaccines (DTaP)—or pediatric diphtheria and tetanus toxoids (DT), if pertussis vaccine is contraindicated—is preferred to tetanus toxoid (TT) alone. For persons age 7 y or older, the tetanus and diphtheria toxoids (Td) for adults is preferred to TT alone.
[c]TIG-tetanus immune globulin.
[d]If only three doses of fluid toxoid have been received, a fourth dose of toxoid—preferably an adsorbed toxoid—should be administered.
[e]Yes, if more than 10 years have elapsed since the last dose.
[f]Yes, if more than 5 years have elapsed since the last dose. More frequent boosters are not needed and can accentuate side effects.
From: MMWR Morb Mortal Wkly Rep 1998;47(SS-2):11.

## Dosage & Schedule of Administration

Each of the available preparations is administered in a dose of 0.5 mL intramuscularly. See Table 9–1 for the routine schedule and Table 9–2 for vaccination of those children not appropriately immunized during the first year of life.

## Adverse Effects

A large number of adverse reactions have been attributed to pertussis vaccine. These can be divided into three categories: local reactions, mild to moderate systemic reactions (that occur in up to half of children), and severe systemic reactions. The estimated rates of these reactions within the first 48 hours after vaccination are shown in the following discussion. The only absolute contraindications to the further use of pertussis vaccine are an anaphylactic reaction to the vaccine or a severe acute neurologic illness within 7 days after vaccination (see Table 9–3). Precaution is urged for the following associations: a convulsion within 3 days (1:1750); persistent, severe, inconsolable screaming or crying for over 3 hours (1:100); a hypotonic–hyporesponsive episode within 48 hours (1:1750); and an unexplained temperature rise to 40.5°C within 48 hours (1:330).

Controversy continues regarding the causation of serious neurologic illness by pertussis vaccine. The only large-scale case-controlled study with enough statistical power to examine this issue—the British National Childhood Encephalopathy Study (NCES)—has minimized any potential relationship.

It was calculated that although the attributable risk for serious acute neurologic injury ranges from less than 1:1,000,000 to 1:140,000, the risk for permanent brain damage is even lower, if indeed there is any risk. This reassessment, along with new studies, has led the AAP, the Canadian National Advisory Committee, and the British Pediatric Association to conclude that pertussis vaccine has not been proven to cause brain damage and to reaffirm the safety and effectiveness of routine pertussis vaccine in immunization programs for infants and children.

The 1991 National Academy of Sciences Institute of Medicine report concluded that the vaccine was causally related to only four adverse effects: acute encephalopathy, the range of excess risk being nil to 10.5 per million immunizations; shock (and an unusual shock-like state), 3.5–291 cases per 100,000 immunizations; anaphylaxis, 2 cases per 100,000 injections of DTP; and protracted, inconsolable crying, 0.1–6% of recipients. Thus, although epidemiologic evidence may be consistent with a causal relationship, pertussis toxin has no proven role in severe neurologic reactions to DTP.

# DIPHTHERIA–TETANUS–PERTUSSIS VACCINE

DTP has been used for the vaccination of healthy infants against diphtheria, tetanus, and pertussis for more than 40 years. It has the combined clinical efficacy of the three single-dose preparations, and the efficacy of pertussis vaccine may even be enhanced by the adjuvant effect of the diphtheria and tetanus toxoids. DTP is no longer manufactured in the United States.

As of 1999, DTaP is the recommended vaccination against diphtheria, tetanus, and pertussis for all doses in the routine vaccination series (the DTaP–Hib combination vaccine can only be used as the fourth dose).

Two basic types of acellular (DTaP) vaccines have been studied. The T-type vaccines are produced by extraction and purification of *B pertussis* cultures. In contrast, the B-type vaccines contain combinations of pertussis toxin (PT), filamentous hemagglutinin (FHA), pertactin (Prn), and fimbriae (Fim). It has been hypothesized that immunity against PT alone may be sufficient to protect against pertussis, but this view has been challenged, and it has been claimed that antibodies against FHA, Prn, and Fim may be required for optimal protection.

Efficacy trials of various acellular pertussis vaccines in Sweden, Germany, Italy, and Senegal have established a 2- to 10-fold lower frequency of minor adverse events and reduced rates of more serious events (hypotonic–hyporesponsive episodes, persistent crying, temperatures higher than 40°C, and seizures) compared with the whole-cell vaccine, good immunogenicity, and a protective efficacy ranging from 59% to 89%. Tripedia (Aventis Pasteur, Inc) is licensed for use as the complete five-dose series. Infanrix (GlaxoSmithKline) and DAPTACEL (Aventis Pasteur) are approved for use for the first four doses of the five-dose series. Licensure of other DTaP vaccines as a five-dose series is anticipated. For children with adverse reactions in the precaution category to DTP, DTaP may be substituted. In those with a true contraindication, neither vaccine should be used. Studies are underway to evaluate the efficacy and safety of acellular vaccines containing reduced quantities of pertussis antigens for use as boosters in adolescents.

## Preparations Available

1. DTaP (Tripedia [Aventis Pasteur]) contains diphtheria toxoid, tetanus toxoid, PT, and FHA.
2. DTaP (Infanrix [GlaxoSmithKline]) contains diphtheria toxoid, tetanus toxoid, PT, FHA, and Prn.
3. DTaP (DAPTACEL) contains PT, FHA, pertactin, and fimbriae types 2 and 3.

4. DTaP–Hib (TriHIBit [Aventis Pasteur]) has been licensed for use as the fourth dose (booster) in the DPT immunization series.

5. DTaP–Hep B–IPV (Pediarix) contains PT, FHA, and pertactin and is licensed for the first three doses beginning at 2 months of age.

## Dosage & Schedule of Administration

DTaP is administered in a dose of 0.5 mL intramuscularly. See Table 9–1 for the routine schedule and Table 9–2 for the procedure in children not immunized during the first year. The ACIP/AAP and AAFP recommend a series of five vaccinations before age 7 years (at 2, 4, 6, and 15–18 months and at 4–6 years). Whenever feasible, the same brand of DTaP should be used for all doses.

## Adverse Effects

Local reactions, fever, and other mild systemic effects occur with one fourth to two thirds the frequency noted following whole-cell DTP vaccination. Moderate to severe systemic effects, including fever of 40.5°C, persistent inconsolable crying lasting 3 hours or more, and hypotonic–hyporesponsive episodes, are less frequent than with whole-cell DTP. These are without sequelae. Severe neurologic effects have not been temporally associated with DTaP vaccinations in use in the United States. Data are limited regarding differences in reactogenicity among currently licensed acellular pertussis vaccines. With all currently licensed DTaP vaccines, reports of the frequency and magnitude of substantial local reactions at injection sites have increased with increasing dose number (including swelling of the thigh or entire upper arm after receipt of fourth and fifth doses).

Braun M et al: Infant immunization with acellular pertussis vaccines in the US: Assessment of the first two years' data from the Vaccine Adverse Event Reporting System (VAERS). Pediatrics 2000;106:e51 [PMID: 20473510].

Pichichero M et al: Safety and immunogenicity of six acellular pertussis vaccines and one whole-cell pertussis vaccine given as a fifth dose in four- to six-year-old children. Pediatrics 2000;105:e11 [PMID: 20085384].

Use of Diphtheria Toxoid-Tetanus Toxoid-Acellular Pertussis Vaccine as a Five-Dose Series: Supplemental recommendations of the Advisory Committee on Immunization Practices. MMWR Morb Mortal Wkly Rep 2000;49(RR13):1 [PMID: 11106289].

## POLIOMYELITIS

Vaccines directed against poliovirus infections have eliminated the naturally occurring disease in developed countries. In the United States, the number of reported cases of paralytic poliomyelitis has fallen from more than 18,000 in 1954 to 0–10 per year currently. As of November 2003, 556 polio cases were reported worldwide since the beginning of the year, from the Indian subcontinent (India, Pakistan, and Afghanistan), the Middle East (Lebanon and Egypt), and west Africa (Burkina Faso, Nigeria, Chad, Togo, Niger, and Ghana). The World Health Organization (WHO) has reset the target of 2008 for global eradication of poliomyelitis. The injectable poliovirus vaccine of enhanced potency (IPV-E), which has a higher content of antigens than the old IPV, is the only vaccine against poliomyelitis available in the United States.

IPV is incapable of causing poliomyelitis by virtue of being inactivated, whereas OPV can do so rarely. The rate of this in the United States was 1 case of paralytic disease per 760,000 first doses of OPV distributed. Ninety-three percent of recipient cases and 76% of all vaccine-associated paralytic poliomyelitis (VAPP) occurred after administration of the first or second dose of OPV. The risk of paralysis in the immunodeficient recipient may be as much as 6800 times that in normal subjects. However, IPV cannot protect against intestinal infection with wild virus, as OPV does. IPV cannot produce so-called secondary vaccination of close contacts when vaccine-strain virus is shed into the environment. IPV, however, produces a much higher serologic response than OPV, a higher booster response at lower prevaccination levels, and an equivalent mucosal response. IPV has the practical advantage of not requiring freezing for storage, as OPV does. On the basis of these data, the ACIP recommends that all children in the United States receive an all-IPV schedule (four doses of IPV). However, the mass administration of OPV requires no needles and syringes.

Completely immunized adult visitors to areas of continuing wild-type poliovirus circulation should receive a booster dose of IPV-E. Unimmunized or incompletely immunized adults and children should have received two (preferably three) doses of the vaccine prior to travel to these and other areas with circulation of wild-type or vaccine-type virus.

## Preparations Available

1. Inactivated IPV-E (IPOL) [Aventis Pasteur] contains antigens of types 1, 2, and 3 poliovirus.

2. DTaP-HepB-IPV (PEDIARIX), [GlaxoSmithKline Biologicals] contains diphtheria and tetanus toxoids and acellular pertussis adsorbed (DTaP), hepatitis B (HepB), and inactivated poliovirus vaccine (IPV-E)

## Dosage & Schedule of Administration

IPV-E is administered in a dose of 0.5 mL subcutaneously. The DTaP–HepB–IPV combination vaccine can be used in the primary series at 2, 4, and 6 months and can be used to complete the primary series. It can be administered with Hib and pneumococcal conjugate (PCV) vaccines at separate sites, but is not approved for the fourth dose of IPV or fourth and fifth doses of DTaP.

## Adverse Effects

IPV has essentially no adverse effects associated with it other than possible rare hypersensitivity reactions to trace quantities of antibiotics. The DTaP–HepB–IPV combination has similar rates of local and systemic adverse responses to three doses administered separately except for fever, which is higher in the combination vaccinated children.

Aristegui J et al: Comparison of the reactogenicity and immunogenicity of a combined diphtheria, tetanus, acellular pertussis, hepatitis B, inactivated polio (DTPa–HBV–IPV) vaccine, mixed with the *Haemophilus influenzae* type b (Hib) conjugate vaccine and administered as a single injection, with the DTPa-IPV/Hib and hepatitis B vaccines administered in two simultaneous injections to infants at 2, 4, and 6 months of age. Vaccine 2003;21:3593 [PMID: 12922087].

Centers for Disease Control: FDA licensure of diphtheria and tetanus toxoids and acellular pertussis adsorbed, hepatitis B (recombinant), and poliovirus vaccine combined, (PEDIARIX) for use in infants. MMWR Morb Mortal Wkly Rep 2003;52:203.

Pichichero ME et al: Impact of a birth dose of hepatitis B vaccine on the reactogenicity and immunogenicity of diphtheria–tetanus–acellular pertussis–hepatitis B–inactivated poliovirus–*Haemophilus influenzae* type b combination vaccination. Pediatr Infect Dis J 2002;21:854 [PMID: 12352809].

Schmitt HJ et al: The safety, reactogenicity and immunogenicity of a 7-valent pneumococcal conjugate vaccine (7VPnC) concurrently administered with a combination DTaP-IPV-Hib vaccine. Vaccine 2003;21:3653 [PMID: 12922095].

## MEASLES

In the 20 years after the 1963 introduction of measles vaccination in the United States, the annual number of reported cases decreased from 500,000 to fewer than 1500. However, between 1989 and 1991 there was a resurgence of measles, with 55,622 cases reported. The major reasons for the increase in cases and the resulting deaths were failure to provide vaccine to preschool children aged 15 months or older, the presence in the community of susceptible children younger than age 15 months, and the growing number of appropriately vaccinated but nonimmune individuals (primary vaccine failures: 2–10%) in schools and colleges. These reasons have led to recommendations for a two-dose vaccination schedule at 12–15 months and at 4–6 years of age.

Given the efficacy rate of the current vaccine (> 95%), the elimination of indigenous measles from the Americas is an attainable public health goal. Only 116 measles cases (1 death) were reported in the United States during 2001. It is believed there is no endemic circulation of measles in the Americas. In 2002 only Venezuela and Columbia had indigenous transmission.

Recently reports in the medical and lay press have suggested a possible association between MMR vaccination, autism, and gastrointestinal inflammation. This association, has been refuted because of the limited number of patients studied, methods of case and control selection, and means of determining developmental regression. Several large epidemiologic studies subsequently found no association between MMR vaccination and either autism or bowel inflammation. Also, no evidence has been found to support the separate administration of measles, mumps, and rubella vaccines (as opposed to the MMR combination). However, the influence of the lay press is most profound in the United Kingdom, where low vaccination rates with measles vaccine has lead to a resurgence of measles, with a distinct possibility that it will become an endemic disease in the United Kingdom.

## Preparations Available

The Moraten strain is a live attenuated vaccine derived from the Edmonston B strain after multiple passages in chick embryo tissue culture. The Moraten strain is available as a monovalent vaccine or in combination with rubella vaccine (MR) or in the MMR combination.

## Dosage & Schedule of Administration

### A. ROUTINE VACCINATION

Measles vaccine should be given as MMR at 12–15 months and again at 4–6 years of age. A dose of 0.5 mL, whether alone or in combination, should at least be given subcutaneously. The second dose of MMR is recommended at school entry to help prevent school-based measles outbreaks. Children not reimmunized at school entry should receive their second MMR by 11–12 years of age. If an infant receives the vaccine before 12 months of age, two doses are required to complete the series, the first after at least 12 months of age and the second at least 1 month later. Ig interferes with the immune response to the attenuated vaccine strains of MMR. Therefore, MMR immunization after Ig administration should be deferred by 3 to 11 months, depending on the type of Ig product received. Consult the American Academy of Pediatrics' *2003 Red Book* for specific recommendations.

### B. VACCINATION OF TRAVELERS

People traveling abroad should be immune to measles. In high-risk areas, age at primary vaccination should be as soon as possible after the first birthday (ie, at 12 months). However, younger infants 6–11 months of age traveling to high-risk areas should receive the monovalent vaccine followed by two doses at 12–15 months given at least 4 weeks apart, and should complete the series at 4–6 years.

### C. REVACCINATION UNDER OTHER CIRCUMSTANCES

Persons entering college and other institutions for education beyond high school, medical personnel beginning employment, and persons traveling abroad should have documentation of immunity to measles, defined as receipt of two doses of measles vaccine after their first birthday, birth before 1957, or a documented measles history or immunity.

### D. OUTBREAK CONTROL

A community outbreak is defined as a single documented case of measles. Control depends on immediate protection of all susceptible persons (defined as persons who have no documented immunity to measles in the affected community. In the case of unvaccinated individuals, the following recommendations hold: (1) age 6–11 months, monovalent measles vaccine (or MMR) if cases are occurring in children younger than age 1 year, followed by two doses of MMR at age 12–15 months and again at age 4–6 years; and (2) age 12 months or older, MMR followed by revaccination at 4–6 years. A child with an unclear or unknown vaccination history should be reimmunized with MMR. Anyone with a known exposure who is not certain of receiving two doses of MMR should receive an additional dose. Unimmunized persons who are not immunized within 72 hours of exposure should be excluded from contact with potentially infected persons until at least 2 weeks after the onset of rash of the last case of measles.

Measles vaccination is contraindicated in pregnant women, women intending to become pregnant within the next 28 days, immunocompromised persons (except those with asymptomatic HIV or those with HIV infection who are not severely immunocompromised), and persons with anaphylactic egg or neomycin allergy. It is also contraindicated in children receiving high-dose steroid therapy (greater than or equal to 2 mg/kg/d, or 20 mg/day total, for longer than 14 days) with the exception of those receiving physiologic replacement doses. In these patients, an interval of 1 month between cessation of steroid therapy and vaccination is sufficient. Leukemic patients who have been in remission and off chemotherapy for at least

3 months can receive MMR safely. Children with minor acute illnesses (including febrile illnesses), nonanaphylactic egg allergy, or a history of tuberculosis should be immunized. Monovalent measles or MMR may be safely administered simultaneously with other routine pediatric immunizations.

## Adverse Effects

Between 5% and 15% of vaccinees become febrile to 39.5°C or higher about 6–12 days following vaccination, lasting approximately 1–2 days, and 5% may develop a transient morbilliform rash. Transient thrombocytopenia occurs in 1:25,000 to 1:100,000 persons. Encephalitis and other CNS conditions such as aseptic meningitis and Guillain–Barré syndrome are reported to occur at a frequency of 1 case per 3 million doses in the United States. This rate is lower than the rate of these conditions in the general unvaccinated population, implying that the relationship between them and measles vaccination may not be causal. MMR vaccination is associated with an increased risk of febrile seizures 8 to 14 days after vaccination, but no subsequent long-term complications have been seen. A recent study found an increase in female mortality in Guinea Bissau after receiving the high titered measles vaccine at less than 6 months of age.

## Antibody Preparations

If a child is seen within 72 hours after exposure, vaccination is the preferred method of protection. If vaccine is contraindicated, Ig, given intramuscularly at a dose of 0.25 mL/kg (0.5 mL/kg in immunocompromised patients; maximum dose in either circumstance is 15 mL), is effective in preventing or modifying measles if it is given within 6 days after exposure. Measles vaccine should be given 5 months later to children receiving the 0.25 mg/kg dose and 6 months later for the higher dose. For children receiving regular IgIV, a dose of 100–400 mg/kg should be adequate for measles prophylaxis for exposures occurring within 3 weeks of the last dose.

Aaby P et al: Differences in female–male mortality after high-titer measles vaccine and association with subsequent vaccination with diphtheria–tetanus–pertussis and inactivated poliovirus: Reanalysis of West African studies. Lancet 2003;361: 2183 [PMID: 14643138].

Jansen VA et al: Measles outbreaks in a population with declining vaccine uptake. Science 2003;301:804 [PMID: 12907792].

Melvin AJ, Mohan KM: Response to immunization with measles, tetanus, and *Haemophilus influenzae* type b vaccines in children who have human immunodeficiency virus type 1 infection and are treated with highly active antiretroviral therapy. Pediatrics 2003;111:e641[PMID: 12777579].

Stein CE et al: The global burden of measles in the year 2000—A model that uses country-specific indicators. J Infect Dis 2003;187 (Suppl) 1:S8 [PMID: 12721886].

Stratton K et al (eds): Institute of Medicine, Immunization Safety Review Committee: *Immunization Safety Review: Thimerosal-Containing Vaccines and Neurodevelopmental Disorders.* National Academies Press, 2001.

Wilson K et al: Association of autistic spectrum disorder and the measles, mumps, and rubella vaccine: A systematic review of current epidemiological evidence. Arch Pediatr Adolesc Med 2003;157:628 [PMID: 12860782].

## MUMPS

Mumps vaccine has dramatically reduced this infection and its complications in the United States, from 185,691 cases in 1967 to 226 cases in 2001. Most reported cases of mumps are in children age 5–14 years.

### Preparations Available

The Jeryl Lynn Strain is the only mumps vaccine available in the United States. It is prepared from virus isolated from a child and passaged in embryonated eggs and in chick embryo tissue culture. The vaccine is available as a monovalent vaccine and, in its preferred form, in the MMR combination.

### Dosage & Schedule of Administration

Mumps vaccine is given to children in the combination vaccine MMR at age 12–15 months and again at age 4–6 years. Despite the greater than 95% efficacy of the mumps vaccine, outbreaks have been reported in highly vaccinated populations. Most cases were attributed to primary vaccine failure. It is hoped that the two-dose schedule (with the second dose given before school entry) will prevent school-based outbreaks. As monovalent vaccine, it is safe and effective if given after the first birthday. The dose of either monovalent or MMR vaccine is 0.5 mL subcutaneously. Use of the monovalent vaccine is limited to susceptible individuals with proven immunity to the other constituents of MMR. Revaccination with mumps vaccine or any of the vaccines in MMR is not harmful; therefore, anyone with an unclear vaccination history should be immunized with MMR. The same recommendations and contraindications apply to mumps vaccine as to measles vaccine, except as relates to travel. Because maternal antibody to mumps is present in most infants, and the disease is not severe in infancy, infants younger than 12 months of age traveling to endemic countries need not routinely be given mumps vaccine (see previous discussion).

### Adverse Effects

Reactions after mumps vaccination are rare and include parotitis, low-grade fever, and orchitis. In 1989, a nationwide surveillance of neurologic complications after a mumps vaccine was conducted in Japan. At least 311 cases of mild aseptic meningitis (96 had vaccine-type mumps virus in the cerebrospinal fluid) occurred among 630,157 recipients. There were no sequelae. Aseptic meningitis may be more common than was previously suspected (1–4 cases per 10,000 vaccinations). This rate was also found in Brazil but not in Germany, where different vaccine strains were used.

Nolan T et al: Reactogenicity and immunogenicity of a live attenuated tetravalent measles–mumps–rubella–varicella (MMRV) vaccine. Vaccine 2002;21:281 [PMID: 12450703].

Schlipkoter U et al: Surveillance of measles–mumps–rubella vaccine-associated aseptic meningitis in Germany. Infection 2002;30:351 [PMID: 12478324].

## RUBELLA

The use of rubella vaccine represents an important deviation from the public health philosophy underlying the other vaccines discussed in this chapter. It is not intended to protect individuals from rubella infection but rather to prevent the serious consequences of rubella infection during pregnancy: miscarriage, fetal demise, and congenital rubella syndrome (CRS). CRS is a group of birth defects including deafness, cataracts, heart defects, and mental retardation. In the United States, the approach has been to vaccinate young children. The intent is to reduce transmission to susceptible women of childbearing age via a herd immunity effect. Immunity lasts for at least 15 years. Other countries, notably the United Kingdom, vaccinate pubertal girls (age 11–14 years). The relative efficacy of these two strategies in the prevention of CRS is unclear.

With the use of rubella vaccines since 1970, rubella incidence rates have declined more than 99%. Twenty-three cases were reported during 2001 in the United States. However, approximately 10% of young adults are now susceptible to rubella. Outbreaks of rubella continue to occur in the United States, despite widespread use of MMR, but the epidemiology of rubella transmission has changed in the past decade. Currently most cases of rubella are seen in foreign-born adults, and outbreaks have occurred in poultry and meat processing plants that employ many foreign-born workers. Similarly, 92% of infants with CRS during 1997–1999 were born to foreign-born mothers.

## Preparations Available

The RA 27/3 strain is the only vaccine available in the United States. It is grown in human diploid cells. The RA 27/3 strain is available as a monovalent vaccine, in combined preparations with measles vaccine, or in measles and mumps vaccines. In most circumstances, MMR vaccination is the recommended means of immunizing against rubella.

## Dosage & Schedule of Administration

Either the monovalent or combined form should be administered subcutaneously in a dose of 0.5 mL. Current practice is to administer MMR vaccine at age 12–15 months and again at 4–6 years. A person can be considered immune only with documentation of either serologic immunity to rubella or vaccination with at least one dose of rubella vaccine after age 1 year, or if born before 1957. A clinical diagnosis of rubella is unacceptable. Susceptible pubertal girls and postpubertal women identified by premarital or prenatal screening should also be immunized. Whenever rubella vaccination is offered to a woman of childbearing age, pregnancy should be ruled out and the woman advised to prevent conception for 3 months following vaccination. If a pregnant woman is vaccinated or becomes pregnant within 3 weeks of vaccination, she should be counseled regarding the risk to her fetus. It has been estimated that the risk of serious malformations attributable to giving the RA 27/3 vaccine to pregnant women is from zero to 1.6%. This is much less than the 20–85% risk of CRS after maternal infection in the first trimester of pregnancy. All susceptible adults in institutional settings (including colleges), day care center personnel, military personnel, and hospital and health care personnel should be immunized.

## Adverse Effects

In children, adverse effects from rubella vaccination are very unusual. Between 5% and 15% of children develop rash, fever, or lymphadenopathy 5–12 days after vaccination. Rash also occurs alone or as a mild rubella illness in 2–4% of adults. Arthralgia and arthritis occur in 10–25% of adult vaccinees, as opposed to only 0–2% of 6- to 16-year-old vaccinees. Chronic arthritis may be causally related to RA 27/3 vaccinations and occurs more often in women age 45 or older, starting 10–11 days after the vaccination and lasting for up to a year. Rare complications include peripheral neuritis and neuropathy, transverse myelitis, and diffuse myelitis.

Castillo-Solorzano C et al: New horizons in the control of rubella and prevention of congenital rubella syndrome in the Americas. J Infect Dis 2003;187 (Suppl) 1:S146 [PMID: 12721906].

Centers for Disease Control and Prevention: Control and prevention of rubella: Evaluation and management of suspected outbreaks, rubella in pregnant women, and surveillance for congenital rubella syndrome. MMWR Morb Mortal Wkly Rep 2001;50(RR-12):1 [PMID: 11475320].

Centers for Disease Control and Prevention: Revised ACIP recommendation for avoiding pregnancy after receiving a rubella-containing vaccine. MMWR Morb Mortal Wkly Rep 2001;50:1117.

Danovaro-Holliday MC et al: Identifying risk factors for rubella susceptibility in a population at risk in the United States. Am J Public Health 2003;93:289 [PMID: 12554568].

Geier DA, Geier MR: A one-year follow-up of chronic arthritis following rubella and hepatitis B vaccination based upon analysis of the Vaccine Adverse Events Reporting System (VAERS) database. Clin Exp Rheumatol 2002;20:767 [PMID: 12508767].

# HAEMOPHILUS INFLUENZAE TYPE B INFECTION

The first vaccine licensed against *Haemophilus influenzae* type b in the United States, composed of the capsular polysaccharide of *H influenzae* type b polyribosyl ribitol phosphate (PRP), was moderately effective in preventing *H influenzae* type b disease in children older than 18 months of age. Conjugation of the PRP with protein carriers confers T-cell–dependent characteristics on the vaccine and enhances the immunologic response to PRP in infancy. Since 1993, the incidence of *H influenzae* type b invasive disease in children younger than age 5 years has declined 99% in the United States.

Three conjugate vaccines are currently available in the United States (Table 9–6). Studies in infants ages 2–6 months demonstrated the immunogenicity of each of these vaccines except DTaP-Hib, which is approved only for the fourth (booster) dose. A geometric mean titer (GMT) of 1 mcg/mL of antipolysaccharide antibody 3 weeks postvaccination has correlated with long-term protection from invasive disease. After three doses at ages 2, 4, and 6 months, each of the three vaccines (see Table 9–6) produces protective levels of antibody. Regardless of the vaccine used in the primary series, booster vaccination of children older than age 12 months with any licensed vaccine elicits an adequate response. Furthermore, each vaccine is immunogenic as a single dose given after age 15 months. Limited information on interchangeability of different *H influenzae* type b vaccines suggests that any combination of the *H influenzae* type b conjugate vaccines will provide adequate protection.

If PRP-OMP is administered as only part of a primary series, the recommended number of doses to complete the series is determined by the other Hib conjugate vaccine.

***Table 9–6.*** *Haemophilus influenzae* type b conjugate vaccines for children.

| Vaccine | Trade Name and Manufacturer | Polysaccharide | Linkage | Protein Carrier |
|---|---|---|---|---|
| HbOC | HibTITER (Wyeth-Lederle-Praxis) | Small | None | CRM[197] mutant *Corynebacterium diphtheriae* toxin protein |
| PRP-OMP | PedvaxHIB (Merck & Co.) | Medium | Thioether | *Neisseria meningitidis* outer membrane protein complex |
| PRP-T | ACTHIB (Aventis Pasteur) | Large | Six-carbon | Tetanus toxoid |
| PRP-T DTaP | TriHIBit (Aventis Pasteur) | Large | Six-carbon | See above for PRP-T |
| PRP-OMP-Hepatitis B | Comvax (Merck & Co.) | Medium | Thioether | See above for PRP-OMP |

Because of the differences in the immunogenic response and the different regimens used in these trials, the recommendations for use of HbOC, PRP-T, and PRP-OMP differ and are summarized in Table 9–7. Regardless of the regimen implemented, it is crucial to complete the series, because cases of invasive *H influenzae* type b disease have been described in partially vaccinated children. Given the increased risk of disease in early infancy among Native American and Alaskan Native children, the use of PRP-OMP for the first dose in the series is recommended because high antibody responses occur after the first dose in this vaccine.

The FDA has licensed PRP-OMP-HepB (Comvax) for use in infants as young as 6 weeks of age. Antibody responses are comparable to those for HbOC and DTP or PRP-OMP and HepB administered separately. In addition, PRP-T-DTaP (TriHIBit) has been licensed for use as a booster. Use in the primary series may result in insufficient titers to Hib. If the exact conjugate vaccine previously administered is unknown, it is recommended that at least three doses of conjugate vaccine be administered to children between ages 2 and 6 months. Unvaccinated or partially vaccinated children younger than age 2 years who experience invasive *H influenzae* type b disease should receive a complete series of vaccinations. Children older than age 2 years mount an adequate immune response to invasive *H influenzae* type b disease and do not require further vaccinations. Unim-

***Table 9–7.*** Schedule for *Haemophilus influenzae* type b conjugate vaccine administration.

| Vaccine | Age at First Vaccination | Primary Series (Same Vaccine If Possible) | Booster (Any Conjugate Vaccine) |
|---|---|---|---|
| HbOC or PRP-T[a] | 2–6 mo | Three doses 2 mo apart | 12–15 mo |
| | 7–11 mo | Two doses 2 mo apart | 12–19 mo |
| | 12–14 mo | One dose | 2 mo later |
| | 15–59 mo | One dose | ... |
| PRP-OMP[b] | 2–6 mo | Two doses 2 mo apart | 12–15 mo |
| | 7–11 mo | Two doses 2 mo apart | 12–18 mo |
| | 12–14 mo | One dose | 2 mo later |
| | 15–59 mo | One dose | ... |

[a]A booster dose of DTP or DTaP should be administered at 4–6 y of age, before kindergarten or elementary school. This booster is not necessary if the fourth vaccinating dose was administered after the fourth birthday. DTaP-Hib (TriHIBit) is only approved for the fourth (booster) dose.

[b]Comvax may be administered by the same schedule for primary immunization as PRP-OMP. It should only be used in infants of hepatitis B-negative mothers. If the series is started late, three doses should be given if started in infants ($\leq$ 10 mo), two doses if started at 11–14 mo, and one dose if started at age 15–71 mo. However, three doses of hepatitis B vaccine are required regardless of age of starting immunization.

munized children age 5 years or older with a chronic illness known to be associated with invasive *H influenzae* type b disease, such as sickle cell anemia and asplenia, should be given a single dose of any of the licensed conjugate vaccines.

## Preparations Available

See Table 9–6.

## Dosage & Schedule of Administration

The dose for all preparations is 0.5 mL, given intramuscularly.

## Adverse Effects

Fewer than 5% of those immunized develop systemic reactions (including fever) to the vaccine. About 25% of recipients develop mild transient local reactions. Adverse effects following the second dose of PRP-OMP are more frequent than following the first dose and more frequent following the third dose of HbOC than following the first two doses.

Breukels MA et al: Immunological characterization of conjugated *Haemophilus influenzae* type b vaccine failure in infants. Clin Infect Dis 2001;32:1700 [PMID: 21259605].

Edwards KM, Decker MD: Combination vaccines. Infect Dis Clin North Am 2001;15:209 [PMID: 21197372].

# PNEUMOCOCCAL INFECTIONS

*Streptococcus pneumoniae* is the most common cause of invasive bacterial infection in children, with most invasive disease occurring in children younger than age 2 years. Prior to the year 2000, the available pneumococcal polysaccharide vaccine had an overall efficacy of 57%, was not effective in children younger than 2 years, and therefore was only indicated for certain high-risk children age 2 years or older. However, the seven most common serotypes of pneumococcus that cause invasive disease in children in the United States have now been linked to a nontoxic but immunogenic variant of diphtheria toxin. In the largest efficacy and safety trial, the heptavalent pneumococcal conjugate vaccine (PCV7) was 97.4% effective at preventing invasive disease by vaccine serotypes. Additionally, the reduction in total invasive pneumococcal infections in children who had received one or more vaccine doses, regardless of pneumococcal serotype, was 89.1%. PCV7 was much less effective in preventing acute otitis media. Although the vaccine's effect on invasive disease in American Indian children was difficult to demonstrate, PCV7 has been shown to reduce the incidence of invasive disease and carriage of antibiotic-resistant pneumococci in day care centers. Postlicensure, its routine implementation in infancy has led not only to a remarkable 92% reduction in invasive disease in children younger than 2 years, but also a 46% reduction against vaccine type in adults and 47% effectiveness against disease in the elderly caused by the types in the vaccine.

Subsequently studies with a heptavalent pneumococcal polysaccharide-meningococcal outer membrane protein complex conjugate vaccine (PnOMPC) in Finland demonstrated an overall vaccine efficacy of 56% against acute otitis media (AOM) in children age 6–24 months, with vaccine serotype-specific efficacy ranging from 37–82%, but a trial in 383 Dutch children with recurrent AOM showed no efficacy in this population. A trial in South Africa of a nonavalent pneumococcal polysaccharide vaccine (PnCRM9) reduced invasive disease by 83% in children without HIV and 65% in those with HIV. However, it only reduced radiographic pneumonia by 20%

Universal immunization of all infants with PCV7 is now recommended, with four doses given at 2, 4, 6, and 12–15 months of age. Children age 24 to 59 months at high risk of invasive pneumococcal disease should receive both the conjugate vaccine (PCV7) and the 23-valent polysaccharide vaccine (23PS). Although definitive data about using PCV7 and 23PS in combination are not available for invasive disease, it does reduce AOM in one study. It is also known that immunization with PCV7 induces immunologic memory that is boosted by some of the serotypes in 23PS. Additionally, 23PS provides coverage against a broader range of serotypes than does PCV7. Recommendations for using PCV7 and 23PS in high-risk children age 24–59 months are found in Table 9–8. Children at high risk of invasive pneumococcal disease include those with chronic cardiovascular, pulmonary (cystic fibrosis but not asthma), or liver diseases, and those with anatomic and functional asplenia (including sickle cell disease), nephrotic syndrome, chronic renal failure, diabetes mellitus, cerebrospinal fluid leak, or immunosuppression (including those with HIV infection, complement deficiencies, malignancies, prolonged use of steroids, and organ transplants). Penicillin prophylaxis of patients with sickle cell disease should be continued regardless of vaccination with PCV7 or 23PS. Insufficient data are available to provide definitive recommendations for pneumococcal vaccination for immunocompromised children 5 years and older. Providers can consider giving one dose each of PCV7 and 23PS, separated by 6 to 8 weeks, to older children at risk of invasive pneumococcal disease. An additional 23PS booster should be given 3–5 years later. Additionally, because otherwise healthy Alaskan Natives and American Indians are at moderately increased risk of invasive pneu-

**Table 9–8.** Recommended pneumococcal (PCV7 and 23PS) immunization of children at high risk of invasive pneumococcal disease.

| Age | Previous Doses | PCV7 | 23PS |
|---|---|---|---|
| 2–6 mo | None | 3 doses, 6–8 wk apart<br>1 booster dose at 12–15 mo | 1 dose at 24 mo[a]<br>2nd dose 3–5 y after the first dose of 23PS |
| 7–11 mo | None | 2 doses, 6–8 wk apart<br>1 booster dose at 12–15 mo | 1 dose at 24 mo[a]<br>2nd dose 3–5 y after the first dose of 23PS |
| 12–23 mo | None | 2 doses, 6–8 wk apart | 1 dose at 24 mo[a]<br>2nd dose 3–5 y after the first dose of 23PS |
| 24–59 mo | 4 doses of PCV7 | None | 1 dose, 6–8 wk after last dose of PCV7<br>2nd dose 3–5 y after the first dose of 23PS |
| 24–59 mo | 1–3 doses of PCV7 | 1 dose, 6–8 wk after the last dose of PCV7 | 1 dose, 6–8 wk after last dose of PCV7<br>2nd dose 3–5 y after the first dose of 23PS |
| 24–59 mo | 1 dose of 23PS | 2 doses, 6–8 wk apart, starting 6–8 wk after 23PS dose | 1 dose 3–5 y after the first dose of 23PS |
| 24–59 mo | None | 2 doses, 6–8 wk apart | 1 dose, 6–8 wk after last dose of PCV7<br>2nd dose 3–5 y after the first dose of 23PS |

[a]The dose of 23PS should be given at least 8 weeks after the last dose of PCV7.
Modified, with permission, from American Academy of Pediatrics. Pneumococcal infections. In Pickering LK (ed): *Red Book 2003 Report of the Committee on Infectious Diseases,* 20th ed. American Academy of Pediatrics, 2003, p 498.

mococcal disease, they also may benefit from receiving both PCV7 and 23PS.

## Preparations Available

Pneumococcal conjugate vaccine (Prevnar) is composed of seven purified capsular polysaccharides, each coupled to a nontoxic modified diphtheria toxin. Serotypes included in the vaccine and potentially cross-reacting serotypes accounted for 86% of bacteremia, 83% of meningitis, and 65% of AOM cases caused by pneumococcus during the period 1978–1994. The vaccine is licensed for use in children age 6 weeks to 9 years.

The 23-valent polysaccharide vaccine (Pneumovax) is only for use in persons 2 years and older. It contains 25 μg of each purified capsular polysaccharide antigen of 23 serotypes of *S pneumoniae*. These 23 types cause 88% of cases of pneumococcal bacteremia and meningitis in adults and nearly 100% of those in children in the United States. Cross-reactive antibody responses may protect against an additional 8% of bacteremic serotypes in adults.

## Dosage & Schedule of Administration

PCV7 is given as a 0.5-mL intramuscular dose. The first dose can be given as early as 6 weeks of life, with a recommended vaccination schedule of 2, 4, 6, and

12–15 months. Children who receive their first dose of PCV7 at 7–11 months of age should receive two doses separated by 6–8 weeks, followed by a booster dose at 12–15 months. Children who receive their first dose of PCV7 at 12–23 months require two doses total, separated by 6–8 weeks. PCV7 may be given concurrently with the other routinely recommended childhood immunizations.

Children older than 23 months at high risk of invasive pneumococcal disease should receive both PCV7 and 23PS, as outlined in Table 9–8. PCV7 and 23PS should not be given simultaneously, and when both are indicated, they should be given 6–8 weeks apart. The dose of 23PS is 0.5 mL, given intramuscularly. If splenectomy or immunosuppression can be anticipated, vaccination should be done at least 2 weeks beforehand. Revaccination with 23PS may be considered after 3–5 years in children at high risk of fatal pneumococcal infection.

## Adverse Effects

The most common adverse effects associated with PCV7 administration are fever, induration, and tenderness at the site of the injection. When it is given simultaneously with DTaP, no increase in febrile seizures has been seen when compared with administration of DTaP alone. Vaccination with PCV7 is contraindicated for individuals with a known hypersensitivity to any component of the vaccine.

With 23PS, 50% of all vaccine recipients develop pain and redness at the injection site. Fewer than 1% develop systemic side effects such as fever and myalgia. Anaphylaxis is rare. The vaccine is contraindicated during pregnancy.

American Academy of Pediatrics, Committee on Infectious Diseases: Policy statement: Recommendations for the prevention of pneumococcal infections, including the use of pneumococcal conjugate vaccine (Prevnar), pneumococcal polysaccharide vaccine, and antibiotic prophylaxis. Pediatrics 2000;106:362 [PMID: 10920170].

Black S et al: Efficacy, safety and immunogenicity of heptavalent pneumococcal conjugate vaccine in children. Pediatr Infect Dis J 2000;19:187 [PMID: 10749457].

Centers for Disease Control and Prevention: Preventing pneumococcal disease among infants and young children: Recommendations of the Advisory Committee on Immunization Practices (ACIP). MMWR Morb Mortal Wkly Rep 2000;49(No. RR-9):1.

Dagan R et al: Effect of a nonavalent conjugate vaccine on carriage of antibiotic-resistant *Streptococcus pneumoniae* in day-care centers. Pediatr Infect Dis J 2003;22:532 [PMID: 12799510].

Kilpi T et al: Finnish Otitis Media Study Group: Protective efficacy of a second pneumococcal conjugate vaccine against pneumococcal acute otitis media in infants and children: Randomized, controlled trial of a 7-valent pneumococcal polysaccharide-meningococcal outer membrane protein complex conjugate vaccine in 1666 children. Clin Infect Dis 2003;37:1155 [PMID: 14557958].

Klugman KP et al: A trial of a 9-valent pneumococcal conjugate vaccine in children with and those without HIV infection. N Engl J Med 2003;349:1341 [PMID: 14523142].

O'Brien KL et al: Efficacy and safety of seven-valent conjugate pneumococcal vaccine in American Indian children: Group randomised trial. Lancet 2003;362:355 [PMID: 12907008].

Veenhoven R et al: Effect of conjugate pneumococcal vaccine followed by polysaccharide pneumococcal vaccine on recurrent acute otitis media: A randomised study. Lancet 2003;361:2189 [PMID: 12842372].

Whitney CG et al: Active bacterial core surveillance of the emerging infections program network. Decline in invasive pneumococcal disease after the introduction of protein-polysaccharide conjugate vaccine. N Engl J Med 2003;348:1737 [PMID: 12724479].

## HEPATITIS A

In 2001, approximately 11,000 cases of hepatitis A infection were reported in the United States. This represents a substantial decline from the 32,000 cases reported in 1995, the year hepatitis A vaccine (HepA) was first licensed. However, because the incidence of hepatitis A infection varies from year to year and from region to region in the United States, continued surveillance will be needed to determine if the decline in disease will be sustained, and if the decline is the result of HepA vaccination strategies.

Children are known to be an important source of transmission of hepatitis A through a community. Approximately one third of all reported cases occur in children younger than 15 years of age. Additionally, the likelihood of being symptomatic from infection varies inversely with age, with approximately 70% of children younger than 6 years of age being asymptomatic when infected. The predominance of a fecal–oral route of transmission, the less than vigilant hand-washing among young children, and their preponderance of asymptomatic infections all combine to create a potent mechanism for spread of hepatitis A infection.

National hepatitis A vaccination recommendations were revised in 1999, with increased emphasis on childhood immunization as a means of hepatitis A control. Routine vaccination of children 2 years and older is recommended for areas with greater than twice the national average of hepatitis A infection (primarily the western United States), and vaccination should be considered in areas with disease rates exceeding (but less than twice) the national average. Although the long-term effect of this strategy is unknown, one community with recurrent hepatitis A epidemics documented a 94% reduction in infections after instituting routine childhood vaccination, and disease incidence declined in both children and adults.

In addition to the routine immunization of children in areas of increased disease incidence, HepA is indicated for the following groups: (1) international travelers (except to Canada, Western Europe, Japan, Australia, and New Zealand), (2) children with chronic hepatitis B or hepatitis C infections or other chronic liver disease, (3) children with clotting factor disorders, (4) homosexual or bisexual males, (5) persons with an occupational exposure to hepatitis A, and (6) illegal drug users.

Vaccine efficacy is 94–100% at protecting against clinical hepatitis A. HepA is not approved for use in children younger than 2 years old.

## Preparations Available

Two inactivated hepatitis A vaccines are currently available for children: Havrix (GlaxoSmithKline) and Vaqta (Merck). Havrix contains a preservative (2-phenoxyethanol), but Vaqta does not. A combination vaccine against hepatitis A and hepatitis B (Twinrix, GlaxoSmithKline) is also available, but is only licensed in the United States for persons 18 years and older.

## Dosage & Schedule of Administration

Havrix is available in two formulations. For individuals between the ages of 2 and 18 years, 720 ELU (ELISA units) is administered in two doses of 0.5 mL, separated by 6–12 months. For persons older than 18 years, a higher dose (1440 ELU) is recommended, also in two doses.

Vaqta also has two formulations. For persons 2–17 years of age, two doses of 25 ELU (0.5 mL) are given, separated by 6–18 months. Individuals older than 17 years old are given 50 ELU (1.0 mL) in a two-dose schedule.

Both vaccines should be stored and shipped at 2–8°C and should not be frozen. HepA is given intramuscularly, and may be given simultaneously with other vaccines, including hepatitis B vaccine.

## Adverse Effects

Adverse reactions are mild and consist of pain and induration at the injection site, feeding problems, and headache. The vaccine should not be administered to children with hypersensitivity to 2-phenoxyethanol (in the case of Havrix) or alum (for both preparations).

## Antibody Preparations

For children younger than age 2 years at increased risk of hepatitis A infection (eg, those traveling to endemic areas or those with clotting factor disorders), Ig should be used as preexposure prophylaxis. The recommended dosages are 0.02 mL/kg in a single intramuscular dose if the duration of exposure is likely to be less than 3 months and 0.06 mL/kg if exposure is likely to be more than 3 months. For long-term prophylaxis of persons not eligible for vaccination, prophylactic doses can be repeated every 5 months.

Postexposure prophylaxis with Ig should be given to previously unvaccinated persons exposed within the prior 2 weeks to hepatitis A. Postexposure Ig is recommended for household or sexual contacts of persons with serologically confirmed hepatitis A, and for day care staff and attendees in outbreak situations. Individuals given one dose of HepA at least 1 month before exposure do not need Ig. When indicated, a single intramuscular dose of Ig (0.02 mL/kg) should be given as soon as possible, but not more than 2 weeks after the last exposure. If HepA is also indicated, it may be given simultaneously with Ig, but at a different anatomic injection site.

Armstrong GL, Bell BP: Hepatitis A virus infection in the United States: Model-based estimated and implications for childhood immunization. Pediatrics 2002;109:839 [PMID: 11986444].

Averhoff F et al: Control of hepatitis A through routine vaccination of children. JAMA 2001;286:2968 [PMID: 11743837].

Bell BP: Hepatitis A vaccine. Semin Pediatr Infect Dis 2002:13:165 [PMID: 12199612].

## HEPATITIS B

Hepatitis B vaccine (HepB), when given with hepatitis B immune globulin (HBIg), is 95% effective in preventing vertical (perinatal) transmission of hepatitis B virus. HepB alone is 90–95% effective in preventing horizontal hepatitis B transmission in susceptible children and adults. Between 1982 and 2002 an estimated 40 million children and 30 million adults in the United States received hepatitis B vaccine. The use of HepB is also increasing internationally, with 126 (66%) of 191 World Health Organization member countries reporting childhood HepB vaccination programs.

All pregnant women should be routinely screened for hepatitis B surface antigen (HBsAg). Women with positive reactions are highly likely to transmit the infection to their offspring. Infants born to HBsAg-positive mothers should receive both HepB and HBIg immediately after birth. Infants for whom the maternal HBsAg status is unknown should receive HepB (but not HBIg) within 12 hours of birth, and the mother's HBsAg status (and thus the newborn's need for HBIg) should be determined as soon as possible.

Universal HepB immunization of low-risk newborns (those with HBsAg-negative mothers) was temporarily halted in July of 1999 because of concerns about the amount of thimerosal (a mercury-containing preservative) that infants were receiving through vaccination. Once a thimerosal-free vaccine became available, the AAP and ACIP recommended reinstituting HepB vaccination of all infants at birth, using only thimerosal-free vaccine. Despite the updated recommendations, some institutions have been slow to restart their newborn HepB programs, thereby missing an important opportunity to interrupt hepatitis B transmission.

Routine immunization with HepB is recommended for all infants and all previously unvaccinated children 0–18 years of age. A two-dose schedule (as opposed to the standard pediatric three doses) is available for adolescents (see following discussion). Since initiating universal recommendations, the percentage of children age 19–35 months receiving three doses of HepB increased from less than 10% in 1991 to 90% in 2002.

In addition to the universal immunization of children, older persons in several risk categories have been identified as target populations for preexposure vaccination. Those that are relevant to physicians caring for children include residents and staff in institutions for the developmentally delayed, residents and staff of hemodialysis units, recipients of clotting factor concentrates, homosexually active males, users of illicit injectable drugs, household contacts of chronic hepatitis B carriers, incarcerated juveniles, long-term international travelers to endemic areas, and all health care personnel. Screening for markers of past infection before HepB immunization is generally not indicated for children and adolescents, but may be considered for high-risk individuals. Because vaccines consist of a purified inactive subunit of the virus and are not infectious, they are not contraindicated in immunosuppressed individuals or in pregnant women.

HepB is immunogenic in infants, children, and young adults. The protective efficacy of HepB correlates well with antibody levels, and virtually all persons with levels of 10 mIU/mL or more are protected in clinical trials.

## Preparations Available

1. HepB (Recombivax HB, Merck) contains recombinant hepatitis B vaccine only.
2. HepB (Engerix-B, GlaxoSmithKline) contains recombinant hepatitis B vaccine only.
3. HepB-Hib (Comvax, Merck) contains Recombivax HB and *Haemophilus influenzae* type b (PRP-OMP) vaccine.
4. DTaP-IPV-HepB (Pediarix, GlaxoSmithKline) contains diphtheria and tetanus toxoids and acellular pertussis (DTaP), inactivated poliovirus (IPV), and Engerix-B vaccines.
5. HepB-HepA (Twinrix, GlaxoSmithKline) contains Engerix-B and hepatitis A vaccines; only approved for persons 18 years of age or older.

Only the single-antigen vaccines (Recombivax HB, Engerix-B) can be given between birth and 6 weeks of age. Any single or combination vaccine (except Twinrix) may be used to complete the hepatitis B vaccination series. All pediatric formulations contain trace to no thimerosal.

## Dosage & Schedule of Administration

HepB is administered as part of the primary childhood immunization schedule for infants and children, as outlined in Table 9–9. The preferred initial dose is during the postpartum period. For children younger than 11 years of age, three intramuscular doses of HepB are needed. Adolescents age 11–15 years have two options: the standard pediatric three-dose schedule or two doses of adult Recombivax HB (1.0-mL dose), with the second dose administered 4–6 months after the first dose. Simultaneous administration with other vaccines at different sites is safe and effective. HepB should be given intramuscularly in either the anterolateral thigh or deltoid, depending on the age and size of the patient. Administration intradermally or in the buttocks results in poor immune responses in some individuals.

### A. NEONATAL

Infants of HBsAg-positive mothers should be cleansed of blood in the delivery room. Both HepB (see Table 9–9) and HBIg (0.5 mL intramuscularly) should be administered simultaneously at different sites within 12 hours of birth. The vaccine should be repeated at 1 month and 6 months. After completion of the HepB series, at 9 to 15 months of age, immunized infants should be tested for anti-HBs. If the anti-HBs assay is positive, vaccination has been effective. If the result is

**Table 9–9.** Hepatitis B vaccine schedule and dosage.

|  | Recombivax HB | Engerix-B | Dose Schedule and Ages |
|---|---|---|---|
| Infants of HBsAg-negative mothers[a] | 0.5 mL | 0.5 mL | 0–2 d, 1–2 mo, and 6–18 mo |
| Infants of HBsAg-positive mothers[b] (HBIG 0.5 mL should also be given) | 0.5 mL | 0.5 mL | Day 0, 1 mo, and 6 mo |
| Children and adolescents < 20 y old | 0.5 mL[c] | 0.5mL | Day 0, 1 mo, and 4 mo |
| Immunosuppressed persons and dialysis patients | 1.0 mL[d] | 2.0 mL[e] | |

[a]Infants of mothers with unknown HBsAg status should be tested at delivery. The infant should receive hepatitis B vaccine within 12 hours of birth. Preterm and low-birth-weight infants of HBsAg-negative mothers should receive the first vaccine dose at 30 days of chronologic age if medically stable, or at discharge if before 30 days of age.
[b]Preterm and low-birth-weight infants of HBsAg-positive mothers should receive Hepatitis B vaccine and HBIG within 12 hours of birth regardless of birthweight and gestational age; these infants should receive 4 vaccine doses total.
[c]A 2-dose schedule (1.0 mL at 0 months and 4–6 months) is also available for adolescents age 11–15 years.
[d]Special formulation containing 40 micrograms/mL.
[e]Two doses of 1.0 mL at one site in a four-dose schedule at Day 0 and at 1, 2, and 6 months.
HBsAg: hepatitis B surface antigen; HBIG: hepatitis B immune globulin.
Modified from MMWR Vol 40, No RR13;001

negative, HBsAg should be tested for; if that test result is positive, immunization has failed and the infant is a chronic carrier. If both HBsAg and anti-HBs are negative, the series should be repeated at 0, 1, and 6 months, followed by repeat anti-HBs testing 1 month after the third dose.

For infants born to mothers of unknown HBsAg status, the same schedule should be followed, except that HBIg should be withheld until the HBsAg status of the mother is known. If the mother is HBsAg-positive, HBIg should be initiated as soon as possible but no later than 7 days after birth.

For infants born to HBsAg-negative mothers, the first dose should be administered in the newborn period, or, if this is not possible, at least before age 2 months. The doses and the schedule for routine vaccination of these infants are set forth in Table 9–9. For preterm infants with birth weights of less than 2 kg born to HBsAg-negative mothers, initiation of HepB should be delayed until 30 days of chronologic age if the infant is medically stable or prior to hospital discharge if discharged before 30 days of age.

If maternal screening is not possible, the infant should receive the first dose of HepB within 12 hours after birth, the second at age 1–2 months, and the third at 6 months. There should be at least 1 month between first and second doses. The third dose should be administered at least 4 months after the first dose and at least 2 months after the second dose, but not before the child is 6 months old.

### B. Older Children and Adolescents

All children should receive HepB as part of the routine schedule. The universal immunization of all adolescents is recommended, on either a two- or three-dose schedule. (See Table 9–9 for dosages and schedules.)

### C. Immunosuppressed Persons and Dialysis Patients

Hemodialysis patients and other immunocompromised persons should be vaccinated with larger doses or an increased number of doses (or both) (see Table 9–9).

### D. Lapsed Hepatitis B Immunization

The HepB series can be completed regardless of the interval from the last vaccine dose. There is no need to start the series over or to test routinely for anti-HBs in healthy children unless the child's mother is HBsAg-positive.

### E. Postexposure Prophylaxis

Postexposure prophylaxis is indicated for unvaccinated persons with perinatal, sexual, household, percutaneous, or permucosal exposure to hepatitis B. When prophylaxis is indicated, unvaccinated individuals should receive HBIg (0.06 mL/kg) and the first dose of HepB at a separate anatomic site. For sexual contact or household blood exposure with an acute case of hepatitis B, HBIg and HepB should be given. Sexual and household contacts of someone with chronic infection should receive immunization (but not HBIg). For individuals with percutaneous or permucosal exposure to blood, HepB should be given, and HBIg considered depending on the HBsAg status of the person who was the source of the blood and on the vaccination response status of the exposed person. All previously vaccinated persons exposed to hepatitis B should be retested for anti-HBs. If levels are adequate (≥ 10 mIU/mL), no treatment is necessary. If levels are inadequate and the exposure was to HBsAg-positive blood, HBIg and vaccination are required.

## Adverse Effects

The overall rate of adverse effects is low and minor, and effects include fever (1–6%) and pain at the injection site (3–29%). There is no evidence of an association between vaccination and sudden infant death syndrome, multiple sclerosis, autoimmune disease, or chronic fatigue syndrome.

## Antibody Preparations

HBIg is prepared from HIV-negative and hepatitis C virus-negative donors with high titers of hepatitis B surface antibody. The process used to prepare this product inactivates or eliminates HIV and hepatitis C virus. The use of HBIg is described earlier in this section.

Biroscak BJ et al: Impact of the thimerosal controversy on hepatitis B vaccine coverage of infants born to women of unknown hepatitis B surface antigen status in Michigan. Pediatrics 2003;111:e645 [PMID: 12777580].

Centers for Disease Control and Prevention (CDC): Hepatitis B vaccination—United States, 1982–2002. MMWR Morb Mortal Wkly Rep 2002;51:549 [PMID: 12118536].

Centers for Disease Control and Prevention (CDC): Global progress toward universal childhood hepatitis B vaccination, 2003. MMWR Morb Mortal Wkly Rep 2003;52:868 [PMID: 12970620].

## VARICELLA

Prior to the availability of vaccine, about 4 million cases of varicella-zoster virus (VZV) infection occurred annually in the United States, mostly in children younger than 10 years. This resulted in 11,000 hospitalizations and 100 deaths per year due to severe complications such as secondary bacterial infections, pneumonia, encephalitis, hepatitis, and Reye syndrome. A live attenuated (VAR) vaccine was developed in Japan in the

1970s and licensed in the United States by the FDA in 1995 for children older than 12 months. As of 2002, approximately 81% of children age 19–35 months in the United States have received one dose of VAR. In three communities participating in an active disease surveillance program, reported VZV cases declined from 71% to 84% from 1995 to 2000. VZV disease declined by a similar amount in all age groups, including infants and susceptible adults, suggesting that disease transmission has been reduced even among the unvaccinated.

In seven postlicensure studies, vaccine effectiveness ranged from 95% to 100% in preventing moderate and severe disease, and 71% to 100% in preventing any disease among vaccinees. However, a more recent investigation of a VZV outbreak at a day care center revealed vaccine effectiveness of 86% against serious disease and 44% against any disease. Preliminary data suggest that vaccine effectiveness may be somewhat diminished when (1) vaccine is given nonsimultaneously but within 28 days of MMR vaccination or (2) oral steroids have been used in the preceding 3 months. The administration of vaccine at younger than 15 months of age has been suggested as a potential risk factor for diminished protection, but this has not been confirmed. Some concern has also arisen that vaccine-induced immunity may wane over time, although no evidence supports this contention to date. The necessity for and cost-effectiveness of changing to a two-dose schedule for children has not been determined.

In February 1999, the ACIP expanded its recommendations for VZV vaccine to promote wider usage. It is predicted that with 97% coverage rates, transmission of VZV could be ended in 30 years. Updated recommendations include (1) establishing child care and school entry requirements, (2) use of the vaccine following exposure and for outbreak control, (3) use for some children with HIV infection, and (4) use in adults and adolescents at risk for exposure.

Proof of immunity to VZV is recommended as a requirement for day care and school entry, and is now required in 38 states; vaccination, physician diagnosis of VZV infection, and serologic documentation of protective antibody meet this requirement.

Data from US and Japanese studies suggest that vaccine is effective in preventing or modifying VZV severity in susceptible individuals if used within 3–5 days of exposure, and this is now recommended by the ACIP and the AAP. A study in the United States suggests that the efficacy of postexposure vaccination is 95% for prevention of any disease and 100% for prevention of moderate or severe disease. There is no evidence that postexposure prophylaxis will increase the risk for vaccine-related adverse events or interfere with development of immunity. In addition to routine childhood

immunization, susceptible groups targeted for immunization include: (1) adults or adolescents older than 13 years residing in households with susceptible children; (2) those who work as teachers of young children or as day care workers; (3) persons living or working in environments that facilitate transmission (eg, colleges, correctional facilities); (4) international travelers; and (5) nonpregnant women of childbearing age.

## Preparations Available

A cell-free preparation of OKA strain VZV is produced and marketed in the United States (Merck). Each dose of VAR contains not less than 1350 plaque-forming units of VZV and trace amounts of neomycin and gelatin. Storage in a freezer at a temperature of $-15°C$ or colder provides a shelf life of 15 months. VAR may be stored for 72 hours at refrigerator temperature in its lyophilized state, VAR must be administered within 30 minutes after thawing and reconstitution.

## Dosage & Schedule of Administration

One dose (0.5 mL) of VAR is recommended for immunization for all healthy children age 12 months to 12 years who lack a history of VZV infection. Children 13 years or older require two doses of VAR 1 month apart. Asymptomatic or mildly symptomatic HIV-infected children (CDC class N1 or A1) should receive two doses of vaccine (with a 3-month interval between doses). VAR may be given simultaneously with MMR at separate sites. If not given simultaneously, the interval between administration of VAR and MMR must be greater than 28 days. Simultaneous VAR administration does not appear to affect the immune response to other childhood vaccines. VAR should be delayed 5 months after intravenous immunoglobulin infusion.

## Adverse Events

Since the approval of VAR in 1995, more than 30,000,000 doses have been distributed in the United States. The most commonly recognized adverse reactions, occurring in approximately 20% of vaccinees, are minor injection site reactions. Additionally, 3–5% of patients will develop a localized rash, and an additional 3–5% will develop a sparse generalized varicelliform rash. These rashes typically consist of two to five lesions and may appear 5–26 days after immunization. In most cases in which rash occurred within the first 2 weeks after immunization, polymerase chain reaction (PCR) analysis of these lesions has demonstrated the presence of wild-type rather than vaccine-strain virus, suggesting natural infection sometime immediately prior to vaccination. Transmission of vaccine virus from healthy patients to healthy recipients is very rare; has never occurred in the absence of a rash in the index case; and has only resulted in mild disease. One case involved transmission from a vaccinee to a susceptible pregnant female. The pregnancy was terminated, but PCR analysis of the fetus showed no evidence of VZV infection. Based on data from the Vaccine Adverse Event Reporting System (VAERS), rates of serious adverse events following VAR are not increased compared with rates expected after natural infection or the background rates of similar events in the community. Herpes zoster infection has occurred following VAR administration in immunocompetent and immunocompromised persons within 25–722 days after immunization. Many of these cases were due to presumably unappreciated latent wild-type virus. Furthermore, based on preliminary data, the age-specific risk of herpes zoster infection seems to be lower in immunocompetent children following VAR immunization than after natural infection.

## Contraindications

Table 9–3 lists contraindications to VZV immunization, such as known hypersensitivity or allergy to any VAR component, including neomycin. VAR is also contraindicated in children who have cellular immunodeficiencies, including those with leukemia, lymphoma, other malignancies affecting the bone marrow or lymphatic systems, and congenital T-cell abnormalities (although vaccine administration to children with acute lymphocytic leukemia is under investigation). The exception to this rule is the recommendation that VAR be administered to HIV-infected children in CDC immunologic class I (CD4+ T-lymphocyte count of 25% or more) because the vaccine is safe and immunogenic in this group. Children receiving immunosuppressive therapy, including high-dose steroids, should not receive VAR. Household contacts of immunodeficient patients should be immunized. VAR should not be given to pregnant women; however, the presence of a pregnant mother in the household is not a contraindication to immunization of a child within that household.

## Antibody Preparations

Varicella-zoster immune globulin (VZIg) is prepared from plasma harvested from persons known to have high titers of anti-VZV antibody. It is indicated for high-risk susceptible persons who are exposed to VZV, for example, immunocompromised individuals without a history of chickenpox, susceptible pregnant women, newborns whose mothers develop varicella 5 days prior to delivery or within 48 hours after delivery, hospitalized premature infants 28 weeks or more gestation

(whose mother lacks history of chickenpox or is seronegative), and hospitalized premature infants less than 28 weeks gestation (regardless of maternal history or serostatus). Exposure is defined as a household contact or playmate contact (over 1 h/d), hospital contact (in the same or contiguous room or ward), intimate contact with a person with zoster deemed contagious, or a newborn contact. Susceptibility is defined as the absence of anti-VZV antibody by an appropriate test. VZIg should be given as soon as possible after exposure, but should be administered within 96 hours. Newborns should be given one vial (125 U) intramuscularly. The dose for all others is 125 U/10 kg body weight intramuscularly (maximum dose, 625 U). VZIg should be readministered following reexposure of susceptible persons if more than 3 weeks has elapsed since a prior dose of VZIg.

American Academy of Pediatrics. Committee on Infectious Diseases: Varicella vaccine update. Pediatrics 2000;105:136 [PMID: 10617719].

Galil K et al: Outbreak of varicella at a day-care center despite vaccination. N Engl J Med 2002;347:1909 [PMID: 12477940].

Seward JF et al: Varicella disease after introduction of varicella vaccine in the United States, 1995–2000. JAMA 2002;287:606 [PMID: 11829699].

Verstraeten T et al: A retrospective cohort study of the association of varicella vaccine failure with asthma, steroid use, age at vaccination, and measles–mumps–rubella vaccination. Pediatrics 2003;112:e98 [PMID: 12897314].

## INFLUENZA

Influenza occurs each winter and early spring, often associated with significant morbidity and mortality rates in certain high-risk persons. Up to 36,000 deaths per year in the United States are attributable to influenza, and global epidemics (pandemics) can occur. Children at high risk of influenza-related complications include those with hemoglobinopathies and those with chronic cardiac, pulmonary (including asthma), metabolic, renal, and immunosuppressive diseases. Children and adolescents receiving long-term aspirin therapy are also at risk of substantial morbidity from influenza-related Reye syndrome. Additionally, healthy children younger than 2 years of age are at increased risk of hospitalization during influenza season.

Annual influenza vaccination is indicated for all children older than 6 months of age who have a chronic health condition that places them at higher risk of complications from influenza infection. Members (including other children) of households with persons in high-risk groups should also be immunized. The vaccine may be administered to healthy children older than age 6 months, and the inactivated vaccine is now routinely recommended for all children ages 6–23 months.

Physicians should identify high-risk children in their practices and encourage parents to seek influenza vaccination for them each fall. In pandemic years, it may be important to advocate vaccination in all children regardless of their usual state of health. Influenza vaccination has a 65–80% efficacy in protecting against disease. In high-risk groups, it may be even more effective in preventing lower respiratory disease or other secondary complications, thereby decreasing hospitalizations and deaths. Each year, recommendations are formulated in the spring and summer regarding the constituents of influenza vaccine for the coming season. These recommendations are based on the results of surveillance in Asia and the southern hemisphere during the spring and summer. The vaccine each year is a trivalent inactivated vaccine containing antigens from two strains of influenza A and one strain of influenza B, chosen as those likely to circulate in the United States during the upcoming winter.

To eliminate the need for injections, and potentially to enhance mucosal and systemic immune response to vaccination, a live attenuated intranasal vaccine has been developed. This vaccine is trivalent (containing two type A strains and one type B strain), cold-adapted, and temperature-sensitive. These viruses replicate poorly in the lower respiratory tract but well in the nasal mucosa (thereby producing immunity). The vaccine is effective in preventing influenza in healthy children. However, because of questions regarding its possible association with pneumonia and asthma in vaccines aged 12–60 months, it is currently licensed only for otherwise healthy children and adults age 5–49 years of age.

## Preparations Available

The inactivated influenza vaccine virus is grown in eggs, formalin-inactivated, and contains trace quantities of thimerosal as a preservative. These whole-virus preparations may be further treated with detergents to produce split (subvirion) or purified surface antigen vaccines. Only split-virus or purified surface antigen preparations should be used for children age 12 years and younger. Several manufacturers produce similar vaccines each year. Fluzone split-virus (Aventis Pasteur) is approved for children 6 months and older; Fluvirin (Evans Vaccines) is approved only for children 4 years and older.

The intranasal trivalent live attenuated influenza virus vaccine (Flumist, Medimmune) is also produced in a trivalent formulation using identical virus strains to the killed vaccine. It is also made in eggs and comes in a single-use prefilled sprayer. It should be stored at –15°C in a frost-free freezer. It may be thawed and stored in a 4–8°C refrigerator for less than 24 hours prior to use. It should not be refrozen after thawing.

## Dosage & Schedule of Administration

### A. INACTIVATED INFLUENZA VIRUS VACCINE

Because influenza can circulate yearly from November through early March in the United States, the key time to initiate vaccination is between October and early November of each year. However, providers should continue vaccinating individuals as long as vaccine is available and there is still influenza activity in the community. Children younger than age 6 months should not be immunized. Two doses are recommended for children younger than age 9 years who are receiving influenza vaccine for the first time; subsequent seasons require single doses. Older children receiving vaccine for the first time require only a single dose. The dose for children ages 6–35 months is 0.25 mL, given intramuscularly; for older children, 0.5 mL, given intramuscularly. The recommended site of vaccination is the anterolateral aspect of the thigh for younger children and the deltoid for older children. Because this vaccine is inactivated, pregnancy is not a contraindication to its use. The vaccine is recommended for women in the second or third trimester of pregnancy (or those who will enter the second or third trimester) during the influenza season. Influenza vaccine has been shown in some but not all studies to transiently increase HIV replication. Nevertheless, the CDC currently recommends influenza vaccination for all HIV-infected persons. Simultaneous administration with other routine vaccinations is acceptable.

### B. LIVE ATTENUATED INFLUENZA VIRUS VACCINE

This vaccine is supplied in a prefilled single-use sprayer containing 0.5 mL of the vaccine, approximately half of which is sprayed into each nostril. A dose divider clip is provided to assist in dividing the dose. If the patient sneezes during administration, the dose should not be repeated. It can be administered to children with minor illnesses, but should not be given if significant nasal congestion is present. Because it is a live vaccine it should be administered 48 hours after cessation of therapy in children receiving antiinfluenza antivirals, and antivirals should not be given for 2 weeks after vaccination.

## Adverse Effects

### A. INACTIVATED VACCINE

The killed vaccine is safe. A small proportion of children will experience some systemic toxicity, consisting of fever, malaise, and myalgias. These symptoms generally begin 6–12 hours after vaccination and may last 24–48 hours. Cases of Guillain–Barré syndrome followed the swine influenza vaccination program in 1976–1977, but careful study by the Institute of Medicine showed no association with that vaccine in children and young adults—nor in any age with vaccines given in subsequent years. For patients with anaphylactic egg allergies in whom influenza vaccination is indicated, a protocol for influenza vaccination is referenced in later discussion.

## B. LIVE VACCINE

In 20 studies of the vaccine where 28,000 doses were administered to more than 20,000 children, signs and symptoms reported more in vaccinees than placebo recipients were runny nose and nasal congestion (20–75%), headache (2–46%), fevers (0–26%), myalgias (0–21.5%), vomiting (3–13%), and abdominal pain (2%). These were reported more frequently with the first dose and were all self-limited. However, in a study of the vaccine in children age 1–17 years of age, significant increases in asthma or reactive airway disease occurred in the subset age 11–59 months. Hence, it is not recommended in high-risk patients or in children younger than 5 years of age.

## Chemoprophylaxis and Treatment

In the United States four influenza antiviral agents are available: amantadine, rimantidine, zanamivir, and oseltamivir. The prophylactic and therapeutic uses of these drugs are discussed in Chapter 36. Chemoprophylaxis is not a substitute for vaccination, and chemoprophylaxis does not interfere with vaccine immunogenicity.

Bernstein DI et al: Cold-Adapted, Trivalent, Influenza Vaccine Study Group: Effect of yearly vaccinations with live, attenuated, cold-adapted, trivalent, intranasal influenza vaccines on antibody responses in children. Pediatr Infect Dis J 2003;22:28 [PMID: 12544405].

Bridges CB et al: Prevention and control of influenza: Recommendations of the Advisory Committee on Immunization Practices (ACIP). MMWR Recomm Rep 2003;52(RR-8):1 [PMID: 12755288].

Committee on Infectious Diseases, American Academy of Pediatrics: Reduction of the influenza burden in children. Pediatrics 2002;110:1246 [PMID: 12456947].

DeStefano F et al: Vaccine Safety Datalink Research Group, National Immunization Program, Centers for Disease Control and Prevention: Vaccinations and risk of central nervous system demyelinating diseases in adults. Arch Neurol 2003;60:504 [PMID: 12707063].

Harper SA et al: Using live, attenuated influenza vaccine for prevention and control of influenza: Supplemental recommendations of the Advisory Committee on Immunization Practices (ACIP). MMWR Recomm Rep 2003;52(RR-13):1. [PMID: 14557799].

Stratton K et al (eds): *Immunization Safety Review: Influenza Vaccines and Neurological Complications 2003*. Immunization Safety Review Committee, National Research Council. National Academies Press, 2003.

Szilagyi PG et al: Potential burden of universal influenza vaccination of young children on visits to primary care practices. Pediatrics 2003;112:821 [PMID: 14523173].

# ■ VACCINATIONS FOR SPECIAL SITUATIONS

## RABIES

Human rabies infection is almost universally fatal, even with aggressive treatment. Fortunately, the incidence of human rabies in the United States is very low, with fewer than three cases per year in the 1990s. Of the 36 human cases with rabies reported in the United States from 1980 to 1996, bat exposure was suspected in 21 cases. However, there was a definite history of bite in only one or two of these cases. Although dogs represent the most important vector for human rabies worldwide, in the United States, because of widespread vaccination of dogs and cats, bats are the most important cause of human rabies. Rabies is also common in skunks, raccoons, and foxes; it is uncommon in rodents.

Human rabies is preventable with appropriate and timely postexposure prophylaxis. Postexposure care consists of local wound care, passive immunization, and active immunization. Immediately after an animal bite, all wounds should be flushed and aggressively cleaned with soap and water. If possible, the wound should not be sutured. Passive immunization after high-risk exposure consists of the injection of rabies immune globulin near the wound, as described later. Active immunization is accomplished by completing a schedule of immunization with one of the three rabies vaccines available in the United States. It is important to keep in mind that bites from bats are often unrecognized; prophylaxis should be given if a bat is found indoors even if there is no history of contact, especially if found in the same room with a sleeping or unattended child or with an intoxicated or otherwise incapacitated individual.

Local public health officials should be consulted before postexposure rabies prophylaxis is started to avoid unnecessary vaccination and to assist in the proper handling of the animal (if confinement or testing of the animal is appropriate). To facilitate consultation, the physician should know the species of animal, its availability for testing or confinement, the nature of the attack (provoked or unprovoked), and the nature of the exposure (bite, scratch, lick, aerosol of saliva). Preexposure prophylaxis is indicated for veterinarians, animal handlers, and any persons whose work or home environment potentially places them in close contact with animal species in which rabies is endemic—bats, skunks, raccoons, and foxes. Rabies immunization should also be considered for children traveling to countries where rabies is endemic; this is particularly important for travelers who will not have prompt access to medical care should an exposure occur.

## Preparations Available

Rabies vaccines stimulate immunity after 7–10 days, and the immunity persists for 2 years or more postvaccination. Three preparations are available:

1. Human diploid cell vaccine (HDCV) is grown in human cell culture (Imovax, Aventis Pasteur).
2. Rabies vaccine adsorbed (RVA) is prepared in fetal rhesus lung cell culture (BioPort Corporation).
3. Purified chick embryo cell vaccine (PCEC) is grown in chick embryo cells (RabAvert, Chiron).

## Dosage & Schedule of Administration

The three rabies vaccines available in the United States are equally safe and efficacious for both preexposure and postexposure prophylaxis. For all three vaccines, 1.0 mL is given intramuscularly in the deltoid (for adults and older children) or anterolateral thigh (for infants and young children). The volume of the dose is not reduced for children. Vaccine should not be given in the gluteal region. In some parts of the world, because of limited resources, a smaller dose of vaccine is given intradermally; this is not recommended in the United States.

### A. Primary Preexposure Vaccination

Preexposure rabies immunization should be considered for individuals at high risk for exposure to rabies, for example, veterinarians, animal handlers, spelunkers, and people moving to or extensively traveling in areas with endemic rabies. Three intramuscular injections in the deltoid area of 1 mL of any vaccine are given on days 0, 7, and 21 or 28.

### B. Postexposure Prophylaxis

Postexposure prophylaxis is a medical urgency, but there is time for consultation with local or state public health officials. The incubation period for rabies virus is usually several weeks but up to one year.

**1. In unvaccinated individuals**—As soon as possible after exposure (and up to 7 days after the first dose of vaccine), human rabies immune globulin (RIg) should be administered (recommended dose 20 IU/kg). The full dose of RIg should be infiltrated near the wound, if anatomically possible, with the remainder infiltrated intramuscularly at a site distant from vaccine administration. The first dose of rabies vaccine should be administered as soon as possible. Vaccine and RIg should never be mixed in the same syringe or given at the same anatomic site. Postexposure failures occurred only when some deviation from the approved protocol occurred (eg, less than usual amount of RIg, no RIg at wound site, no cleansing of wound, vaccination in the gluteal area). Four subsequent doses of rabies vaccine should be given on days 3, 7, 14, and 28. The WHO recommends an additional dose on day 90, but the ACIP does not concur.

**2. In previously vaccinated individuals**—RIg is not necessary, and only two doses of vaccine on days 0 and 3, are needed.

### C. Booster Vaccination

Previously vaccinated individuals with potential continued exposure to rabies should have a serum sample tested for rabies antibody every 2 years. If the titer is less than 1:5 for complete neutralization by the rapid fluorescent focus inhibition test, a booster dose of rabies vaccine should be administered.

## Adverse Effects

The rabies vaccines are relatively free of side effects. Approximately 15–25% of adults experience pain, swelling, or erythema at the injection site; 10–20% may have mild systemic reactions such as headache, nausea, muscle aches, and dizziness. Three cases of Guillain–Barré syndrome have been described; all three patients recovered fully. Children complain of side effects less frequently. An immune complex-like reaction occurs in about 6% of persons 2–21 days after receiving booster doses of HDCV. Travelers to countries where rabies is endemic may need immediate postexposure prophylaxis and may have to use locally available vaccines and antisera. In many developing countries, the only vaccines readily available may be nerve tissue vaccines (NTV) derived from the brains of adult animals or suckling mice, and the antirabies sera may be of equine origin. Although adverse reactions to antisera are uncommon and typically mild, the NTV may induce neuroparalytic reactions in 1:2000 to 1:8000 vaccinees; this is a significant risk and may justify preexposure vaccination prior to travel.

## Antibody Preparations

RIg is prepared from the plasma of human volunteers hyperimmunized with rabies vaccine. The recommended dose is 20 IU/kg body weight. The rabies-neutralizing antibody content is 150 IU/mL, supplied in 2-mL or 10-mL vials. It is very safe.

Centers for Disease Control and Prevention: Human rabies prevention–United States, 1999. Recommendations of the Advisory Committee on Immunization Practices (ACIP): MMWR Morbid Mortal Wkly Rep 1999;48(RR-1):1 [PMID: 10077411].

Chang HG et al: Public health impact of reemergence of rabies, New York. Emerg Infect Dis 2002;8:909 [PMID: 12194765].

Hanlon CA et al: The incurable wound revisited: Progress in human rabies prevention? Vaccine 2001;19:2273 [PMID: 11257347].

Plotkin SA: Rabies. Clin Infect Dis 2000;30:4 [PMID: 10619725].

# TYPHOID FEVER

Typhoid vaccines have shown variable efficacy in field trials, typically producing protection in the 50–80% range. Two vaccines are currently available in the United States: a parenteral vaccine derived from a virulence (Vi) antigen capsular polysaccharide (ViCPS); and a live attenuated oral vaccine (Ty21a). Moderate protection against invasive *Salmonella typhi*, the causative bacterium of typhoid fever, has been demonstrated for 2–5 years following vaccination.

Routine typhoid vaccination is recommended only for children who reside in households with a documented typhoid carrier or who are going to live or travel extensively in an endemic area. The oral vaccine is most commonly used because of its ease of administration. However, noncompliance with oral vaccine dosing instructions occurs frequently, and correct usage should be stressed or the parenteral ViCPS vaccine used. Travelers should be advised, however, that because none of the vaccines offer total protection, careful selection of food and drink is imperative.

## Preparations Available

1. Parenteral ViCPS (Typhim Vi, Aventis Pasteur) is for intramuscular use.
2. Oral live attenuated Ty21a vaccine (Vivotif Berna Vaccine, Swiss Serum and Vaccine Institute) is supplied as enteric-coated capsules.

## Dosage & Schedule of Administration

ViCPS is administered as a single intramuscular dose (0.5 mL), with boosters needed every 2 years if exposure continues. It is approved for children 2 years and older.

The dose of the oral preparation is one capsule every 2 days for a total of four capsules, taken 1 hour before meals. The capsules should be taken with cool liquids, and should be kept refrigerated. A full course of four capsules is recommended every 5 years if exposure continues. This vaccine is not approved for children younger than age 6 years, and capsules should not be dispensed from a package that has been opened beforehand. The antimalarial drugs mefloquine and chloroquine can be given simultaneously with oral typhoid vaccine; however, the antimalarial proguanil, as well as antimicrobials, should not be given simultaneously with Ty21a.

## Adverse Reactions

The oral and parenteral typhoid vaccines may produce mild adverse reactions such as abdominal complaints (for oral) and injection site swelling or redness (for parenteral). As with all live attenuated vaccines, Ty21a should not be given to immunocompromised patients.

Garmory HS et al: Salmonella vaccines for use in humans: Present and future perspectives. FEMS Microbiol Rev 2002;26:339 [PMID: 12413664].

Lin FY et al: The efficacy of a *Salmonella typhi* Vi conjugate vaccine in 2-to-5-year-old children. N Engl J Med 2001;344: 1263 [PMID: 11320385].

Parry CM et al: Typhoid fever. N Engl J Med 2002;347:1770 [PMID: 12456854].

# MENINGOCOCCAL DISEASE

Infection with *Neisseria meningitidis* causes significant morbidity and mortality, with 120,000 cases worldwide per year, including 2400–3000 cases in the United States. Meningococcal disease has a 10% case-fatality rate in the United States, and up to 19% of survivors are left with serious disabilities, such as neurologic impairment, loss of limb function, or hearing loss. Infants younger than 1 year of age have the highest rate of disease, but college freshmen, particularly those living in dormitories, have a higher incidence than the general US population. Five serogroups of meningococcus (A, B, C, W-135, and Y) cause the vast majority of disease.

In prior years, meningococcal disease in the United States was caused primarily by serogroup B and C strains (45% each), with the remainder of cases due to W-135 and Y serogroups (10%). Now disease due to serogroup B is decreasing, and disease due to Y is increasing (up to 43% in some areas). The majority of disease in developing countries is caused by serogroups A and C.

A polysaccharide-based vaccine against serogroups A, C, Y, and W-135 is available in the United States. The vaccine has 85–100% efficacy in older children and adults against groups A and C disease. The vaccine is not recommended for routine immunization because it is relatively ineffective in children younger than 2 years; it is unable to protect against serogroup B disease; and the immunity it confers appears to be short-lived, and its repeated use may actually decrease antibody response. However, functionally or anatomically asplenic children should be vaccinated, as well as those with terminal complement or properdin deficiencies. Meningococcal vaccine provides some protection for travelers to countries with epidemic or endemic disease (primarily sub-Saharan Africa). The vaccine is also recommended in outbreaks caused by vaccine-preventable serogroups. Because of a moderately increased risk (three- to fourfold) of meningococcal disease in college freshmen, the ACIP and AAP recommend that care providers discuss meningococcal vaccination with incoming and current freshmen, and administer vaccine to those who request it.

Because of the severe disease caused by the meningococcus and the limitations of the currently licensed vaccine, intensive effort is going into the development of new meningococcal vaccines. However, a number of barriers still exist. Because of the global variation in the incidence of different meningococcal serogroups, a vaccine designed for use in the United States and western Europe may provide little benefit to the developing world. The bacterial capsule proteins of serogroup B, which causes a substantial proportion of disease in the United States, particularly in infants younger than 1 year old, are poorly immunogenic in humans. Antibodies to serogroup B capsular proteins cross-react with human embryonal neural tissue, and therefore serogroup B vaccines carry a theoretical risk of producing autoimmunity. Finally, the relatively low incidence of meningococcal disease makes studying vaccine efficacy difficult and costly.

Despite these challenges, there are a number of promising meningococcal vaccine developments. Serogroup A and C polysaccharide have been linked to protein carriers and found to be immunogenic in infants. In 1999, the United Kingdom began routine childhood immunization with a conjugate meningococcal serogroup C vaccine. Early results have shown an 80% reduction in serogroup C disease in targeted age groups.

The only vaccine currently available in the United States is the quadrivalent A, C, W-135, and Y vaccine (Menomune, Aventis Pasteur). Each dose contains 50 μg of the four purified capsular polysaccharides. It is approved for children 2 years of age and older.

## Dosage & Schedule of Administration

Quadrivalent meningococcal vaccine is given as a single 0.5-mL subcutaneous injection. It can be given simultaneously with other vaccines. It should be given to high-risk individuals and to those affected by vaccine-preventable outbreaks. Because reimmunization of young children produces serogroup A but not serogroup C antibodies, reimmunization is only recommended when there is continued risk of serogroup A infection.

## Adverse Effects

With more than 6 million doses of vaccine distributed, few serious adverse events have been reported. A recent national review of meningococcal vaccine safety found that fever, injection site hypersensitivity, and allergic reactions were the most common associated events.

Until better vaccines are available, chemoprophylaxis with rifampin, ceftriaxone, or ciprofloxacin (adults) should be used to prevent meningococcal disease in exposed individuals (see Chapter 38).

Ball R et al: Vaccine Adverse Event Reporting System Working Group: Safety data on meningococcal polysaccharide vaccine from the Vaccine Adverse Event Reporting System. Clin Infect Dis 2001;32:1273 [PMID: 11303261].

Centers for Disease Control and Prevention: Prevention and control of meningococcal disease in college students: Recommendations of the Advisory Committee on Immunization Practices (ACIP). MMWR Morb Mortal Wkly Rep 2000;49(No. RR-7):13 [PMID: 10902835].

Centers for Disease Control and Prevention: Prevention and control of meningococcal disease. Recommendations of the Advisory Committee on Immunization Practices (ACIP). MMWR Morb Mortal Wkly Rep 2000;49(RR-7):1 [PMID: 10902834].

Lingappa JR et al: Active Bacterial Core surveillance (ABCs) team: Surveillance for meningococcal disease and strategies for use of conjugate meningococcal vaccines in the United States. Vaccine 2001;19:4566 [PMID: 11483285].

Soriano-Gabarro M et al: Vaccines for the prevention of meningococcal disease in children. Semin Pediatr Infect Dis 2002; 13:182 [PMID: 12199614].

## CHOLERA

Cholera causes significant morbidity and mortality worldwide. It may present only as travelers diarrhea. For travelers, the risk of developing cholera per month of stay in a developing country is low, ranging from 0.001% to approximately 0.01%. No cholera vaccines are available in the United States. Because the causative bacterium *Vibrio cholerae* is not invasive, and because secretory IgA (sIgA) is crucial, newer vaccines available in other countries are administered orally. Two oral vaccines (one consisting solely of live attenuated bacteria and the other in combination with the B subunit of cholera toxin) are safe and immunogenic. Cholera vaccination is no longer required for international travel or for entry into any countries.

Ryan ET, Calderwood SB: Cholera vaccines. Clin Infect Dis 2000;31:561 [PMID: 20472098].

## TUBERCULOSIS

In 2000, 22 states in the United States had tuberculosis incidence rates of less than 3.5 cases/100,000 population, setting the stage for possible elimination of the disease in these areas. However, of the 11,795 cases reported to the CDC in 2002, nearly 40% of new cases of TB occur in persons born in other countries. Bacille Calmette-Guérin vaccine (BCG) consists of live attenuated *Mycobacterium bovis.* BCG is not currently indicated for mass use in the United States, chiefly because of doubts about its efficacy. BCG is the most widely used vaccine in the world and has been administered to over 2.5 billion people (71% of infants worldwide are vaccinated) with a low incidence of serious complications. It is inexpensive, can be given any time after birth, sensitizes the vaccinated individual for 5–50 years, and stimulates both B-cell and T-cell immune responses. BCG is useful in two circumstances in the United States: (1) in tuberculin-negative infants or older children residing in households with untreated or poorly treated individuals with active infection with isoniazid- and rifampin-resistant *Mycobacterium tuberculosis* and (2) in infants or children found to live under constant exposure without the possibility of removal from continuous exposure or access to prophylaxis and treatment. BCG reduces the risk of tuberculous meningitis and disseminated TB in pediatric populations by 50–100%. BCG appears to have had little epidemiologic effect on TB, despite a reported efficacy of 50% in a meta-analysis of 26 vaccine trials, with the greatest protection against pulmonary disease. The two currently licensed BCG vaccines in the United States are produced by Connaught Laboratories and Organon Teknika Corporation. They are given intradermally in a dose of 0.05 mL for newborns and 0.1 mL for all other children. Mantoux testing is advised 2–3 months later, and revaccination is advised if the Mantoux test is negative. Adverse effects occur in 1–10% of healthy individuals, including local ulceration, regional lymph node enlargement, and lupus vulgaris. The vaccine is contraindicated in pregnant women and in immunocompromised individuals, including those with HIV infection, because it has caused disseminated or fatal infection.

Factors associated with increased probability that a positive TB skin test (TST) is due to *M tuberculosis* infection include (1) larger reactions, (2) contact with an individual known to be infected, (3) family history of TB, (4) longer interval between BCG administration and skin testing, and (5) country of origin with increased incidence of endemic TB. The details and cutoff observations for TB skin testing are described in Chapter 38. To ensure that those infected with TB are evaluated, a 5-mm or greater cutoff for a positive Mantoux test is used in immunocompromised children. In immunocompetent persons, the cutoff is 10 mm or above, whereas it is 15 mm or above when no risk factors are present in the absence of clinical disease (eg,

screening). Recently, a case-control study from New York identified that contact with an adult with active TB, foreign birth, foreign travel, or a relative with a positive TST predicted latent TB (with use of the TST). This may justify routinely testing children with these risk factors as well. In 2001 a new test (Quanti FERON-TB) that measures the release of interferon-γ in whole blood in response to stimulation with purified protein derivative (PPD) was approved by the FDA. This test is not recommended for persons with symptoms of active TB who are at increased risk for progression to active TB, but may be used instead of TST in those at increased or low risk for latent TB infection, including as a screening of recent immigrants. BCG almost invariably causes its recipients to be tuberculin-positive (5–7 mm), but the reaction often becomes negative after 3–5 years. However, a positive Mantoux test in a child with a history of BCG vaccination who is being investigated for TB as a case contact should be interpreted as indicating infection with *M tuberculosis.*

Almeida LMD et al: Use of purified protein derivative to assess the risk of infection in children in close contact with adults with tuberculosis in a population with high Calmette-Guérin bacillus coverage. Pediatr Infect Dis J 2001;20:1061 [PMID: 11734712].

Brewer TF: Preventing tuberculosis with bacillus Calmette-Guérin vaccine: A meta-analysis of the literature. Clin Infect Dis 2000;31 (Suppl) 3:S64 [PMID: 11010824].

Mazurek GH, Villarino ME: CDC. Guidelines for using the QuantiFERON-TB test for diagnosing latent *Mycobacterium tuberculosis* infection. Centers for Disease Control and Prevention. MMWR Recomm Rep 2003;52(RR-2):15 [PMID: 12583541].

Saiman L et al: Risk factors for latent tuberculosis infection among children in New York City. Pediatrics 2001;107:999 [PMID: 11331677].

## YELLOW FEVER

Immunization against yellow fever is indicated for children as young as age 4 months traveling to endemic areas or to countries that require it for entry, but otherwise immunization should be delayed until age 9 months or older. Public health authorities maintain updated information on these requirements and must be consulted. Yellow fever vaccine is a live vaccine made from the 17D yellow fever attenuated virus strain grown in chick embryos. It is contraindicated in infants younger than age 4 months due to an increased susceptibility to vaccine-associated encephalitis, in pregnant women, in persons with anaphylactic egg allergy, and in immunocompromised individuals. It can only be administered at licensed yellow fever vaccination locations (usually public health departments). A single subcutaneous injection of 0.5 mL of reconstituted vaccine is administered. The International Health Regulations require revaccination at 10-year intervals, but immunity may be lifelong. Adverse reactions are generally mild—consisting of fever, mild headache, and myalgia 5–10 days after vaccination occurring in less than 25% of vaccinees. The risk for vaccine-associated encephalitis within 30 days following vaccination has been estimated to be less than 1/8,000,000 persons. Recently, a new serious adverse reaction syndrome was described. This yellow fever vaccine-associated viscerotropic disease consists of severe multiple organ system failure and death within 1–2 two weeks postvaccination, especially in older adults. These reports have caused a reevaluation of the vaccine's use. Health care providers should be careful to administer yellow fever vaccine only to persons truly at risk for exposure to yellow fever. There is no contraindication to giving other live-virus vaccines simultaneously with yellow fever vaccine or at intervals of a day to a month.

Centers for Disease Control and Prevention: Yellow fever vaccine: Recommendations of the Immunization Practices Advisory Committee (ACIP), 2002. MMWR 2002;51(RR-17):1 [PMID: 22324159].

Monath TP: Yellow fever: An update. Lancet Infect Dis 2001;1: 11 [PMID: 21860137].

Thompson MJ: Immunizations for international travel. Prim Care: Clin Office Pract 2002;29:787 [PMID:22574700]

# ANTHRAX

Anthrax is an acute infectious disease caused by the spore-forming bacteria *Bacillus anthracis*. Although it occurs most frequently as a disease of cattle, goats, and sheep, humans may become infected through contact with, ingestion of, or inhalation of spores from infected animals or their products. The spore is durable and can be delivered as an aerosol, with an incubation of 2–30 days. Inhalation causes the most serious form of human anthrax, making it an attractive agent for potential use by bioterrorists (see Chapter 11). In December 2001, the US Department of Health and Human Services obtained a limited supply of anthrax vaccine for potential preexposure civilian vaccination. The only available anthrax vaccine in the United States is an inactivated, noninfectious, cell-free anthrax vaccine (BioPort Corporation). It is prepared from a toxigenic, nonenecapsulated strain and is aluminum hydroxide-adsorbed. Routine preexposure vaccination with anthrax vaccine adsorbed (AVA) is indicated for persons at risk for repeated exposure to *B anthracis* spores, such as laboratory personnel handling environmental specimens for bioterrorism level B and C laboratories, workers making repeated entries into known *B anthracis* spore-contaminated areas after a terrorist attack, and workers in other settings in which repeated exposure to aerosolized *B anthracis* spores might occur. For military personnel, and for other selected populations for which a calculable risk can be assessed, preexposure vaccination has been used.

The recommended vaccination schedule is subcutaneous injections at 0, 2, and 4 weeks; then at 6 months, 12 months, and 18 months. Postexposure vaccination consists of three injections: as soon as possible after exposure and again at 2 and 4 weeks after exposure in combination with antimicrobial chemoprophylaxis for 60 days. The duration of protection in humans is unknown; however, annual booster injections are recommended to maintain immunity. The vaccine has not been evaluated for safety and efficacy in children younger than age 18 years or in adults older than age 60 years.

## Adverse Events

No studies have definitively documented occurrence of chronic diseases (eg, cancer or infertility) following anthrax vaccination. Although controversial, analysis of VAERS data documents no pattern of serious adverse events clearly associated with the vaccine, except mild injection site reactions.

Centers for Disease Control and Prevention: Use of anthrax vaccine in the United States: Recommendations of the Advisory Committee on Immunization Practices (ACIP). MMWR 2000,49(RR15):1 [PMID: 21017696].

Centers for Disease Control and Prevention: Use of anthrax vaccine in response to terrorism: Supplemental recommendations of the Advisory Committee on Immunization Practices. MMWR 2002;51:1024 [PMID: 22346733].

# SMALLPOX (VARIOLA)

Smallpox is a highly contagious infection caused by the variola virus. In 1972, routine smallpox immunization was discontinued in the United States, and in 1980 the World Health Organization declared smallpox to be eradicated worldwide. In recent years, concern that smallpox virus stocks may be in the hands of bioterrorists and potentially released within a nonimmune population has incited a debate about whether a large-scale smallpox immunization should be resumed. A smallpox immunization plan has been implemented in the United States to develop smallpox response teams throughout the nation. The only smallpox vaccine licensed in the United States is a lyophilized, live vaccinia virus preparation. Vaccinia is related to variola and is highly effective in preventing smallpox. Vaccine is administered using a bifurcated needle to deliver vaccine into the epidermis. Vaccine "take" is determined by the development of a papule progressing to vesicle to pustule to scab that heals after 14–21 days. Fever is common after primary immunization and less common after reimmunization. Severe complications of immunization include death, postvaccinal encephalitis, progressive vaccinia, myocarditis, eczema vaccinatum, and accidental inoculation to other body sites. Transmission of vaccine virus from a recently immunized individual to a susceptible contact can occur. Smallpox vaccine is not recommended for people younger than 18 years of age. The US government has contracted for development of 200 million doses of tissue culture-derived vaccinia vaccine and has encouraged development of safer effective smallpox vaccines. Vaccinia immune globulin (VIg) is recommended only for the treatment of complications of vaccination and not for prophylaxis or treatment.

Abramson JS et al: The US smallpox vaccination plan. Pediatrics 2002;110:841 [PMID: 22662823].

Centers for Disease Control and Prevention: Recommendations for using smallpox vaccine in a preevent vaccination program. Supplemental recommendations of the Advisory Committee on Immunization (ACIP) and the Healthcare Infection Control Practices Advisory Committee (HICPAC). MMWR 2003;52:1 [PMID: 22596449].

Centers for Disease Control and Prevention: Smallpox vaccination and adverse reactions: Guidance for clinicians. MMWR 2003;52:1 [PMID: 22504376].

# ■ PASSIVE PROPHYLAXIS

## Intramuscular Immune Globulin

Ig may prevent or modify infection with hepatitis A virus if administered in a dose of 0.02 mL/kg within 14 days after exposure. Measles infection may be prevented or modified in a susceptible person if Ig is given in a dose of 0.25 mL/kg within 6 days after exposure. Special forms of Ig include TIg, HBIg, RIg, VIg, and VZIg. These are obtained from donors known to have high titers of antibody against the organism in question. Their use has been described earlier in this chapter. Palivizumab is a humanized monoclonal antibody against respiratory syncytial virus (RSV) and is used to prevent RSV in high-risk populations with monthly doses during RSV season.

Ig must be given intramuscularly. The dose varies depending on the clinical indication. Adverse reactions include pain at the injection site, headache, chills, dyspnea, nausea, and anaphylaxis, although all but the first are rare.

## Intravenous Immune Globulin

The primary indications for IVIg are for replacement therapy in antibody-deficient individuals, for the treatment of Kawasaki disease, idiopathic thrombocytopenic purpura, Guillain–Barré syndrome, and other autoimmune diseases, and chronic B-cell lymphocytic leukemia. IVIg may be beneficial in some children with HIV infection, toxic shock syndrome, and for anemia caused by parvovirus B19. Specific antibody-enriched IVIg preparations have also been developed for the prevention and treatment of the following viral infections: cytomegalovirus immune globulin (CMVIg) for prevention and treatment of CMV disease and respiratory syncytial virus immune globulin (RSVIg) for prevention of RSV illness in high-risk children. Prophylaxis to prevent RSV in infants and children at increased risk for severe disease is available in either an intravenous (RSV-IVIg) or intramuscular (Palivizumab) preparation. Both products should be considered for (1) infants and children younger than age 2 years with chronic lung disease who have required medical therapy (supplemental oxygen, bronchodilator, diuretic, or corticosteroid therapy) for their disease within 6 months before the anticipated RSV season, (2) infants born between 33 and 35 weeks (32 weeks 1 day and 35 weeks 0 days) gestation or earlier without chronic lung disease with two or more risk factors (child care attendance, school-age siblings, exposure to environmental air pollution, congenital airway abnormalities, or severe neuromuscular disease) up to age 6 months, (3) infants born at 29–32 weeks up to 6 months of age, and (4) up to age 12 months for infants born at 28 weeks or earlier.

Palivizumab is approved for use in children who are 24 months old or younger with hemodynamically significant cyanotic or acyanotic congenital heart disease. Those most likely to benefit from prophylaxis are infants (< 1 year of age) who are receiving medication to control congestive heart disease, with moderate to severe pulmonary hypertension and cyanotic heart disease. An increased number of cyanotic events occurred following RSV-IVIg administration in these infants. RSV prophylaxis should be initiated at the onset of the RSV season and continued until the end of the season, regardless of breakthrough RSV illness during that RSV season.

RSV-IVIg (RespiGam [MedImmune]) is derived from human donors screened for high levels of RSV-neutralizing activity. It is administered intravenously in a dose of 750 mg/kg once a month during the RSV season. RSV intramuscular monoclonal antibody, palivizumab (Synagis [MedImmune]), is a humanized monoclonal antibody directed against the F glycoprotein of RSV, a surface protein that is highly conserved among RSV isolates. It is administered in a dose of 15 mg/kg once a month and is packaged in 50- and 100-mg vials.

Although palivizumab has greater ease of administration and fewer adverse effects, some considerations may favor the use of RSV-IVIg. Specifically, RSV-IVIg provides protection from other non-RSV respiratory infections, including influenza and acute and recurrent otitis media. In contrast, palivizumab avoids the risk of transmission of human pathogens, because it is a pure preparation of RSV antibody. Palivizumab does not interfere with response to routine childhood vaccinations; infants receiving RSV-IVIg should have MMR and VAR deferred for 9 months after their last dose.

IVIg must only be administered intravenously. Adverse reactions include headache, flushing, diaphoresis, hypotension, fever, nausea, vomiting, and anaphylaxis. Since November 1997, a shortage of IVIg has existed in the United States. Distribution and production factors have contributed to the shortage, but increased off-label use of the product is also a factor. Despite FDA, National Institutes of Health, and CDC guidelines, over 50% of IVIg is issued for unapproved purposes.

Feltes TF et al: Palivizumab prophylaxis reduces hospitalization due to respiratory syncytial virus in young children with hemodynamically significant congenital heart disease. J Pediatr 2003;143:532 [PMID: 14571236].

Impact-RSV Study Group: Palivizumab, a human respiratory syncytial virus monoclonal antibody, reduces hospitalization from RSV infection in high-risk infants. Pediatrics 1998;102:531.

Meissner HC, Long SS, American Academy of Pediatrics Committee on Infectious Diseases and Committee on Fetus and Newborn: Revised indications for the use of palivizumab and respiratory syncytial virus immune globulin intravenous for the prevention of respiratory syncytial virus infections. Pediatrics 2003;112(6 Pt 1):1447 [PMID: 14654628].

Simoes EA: Immunoprophylaxis of respiratory syncytial virus: Global experience. Respir Res 2002;3 (Suppl 1):S26 [PMID: 12119055].

## Antitoxins & Antivenins

Igs of animal origin are available for use in certain situations. These include botulinum antitoxin, tetanus antitoxin, diphtheria antitoxin, and snake and spider antivenins. A variety of adverse reactions, including acute febrile responses, anaphylaxis, and serum sickness, may develop after use of these products. A schedule for hypersensitivity testing and desensitization for antisera of equine origin can be found in the *Red Book*.

# ■ LEGAL ISSUES IN IMMUNIZATION

The National Childhood Vaccine Injury Act of 1986 established two programs: the National Vaccine Program (NVP) and the National Vaccine Injury Compensation Program (NVICP). The purpose was to provide no-fault compensation for persons found to have been injured by certain vaccines. Under the terms of the act, liability claims against those who administer or manufacture vaccines must go before a federal compensation board before a civil suit may be filed. Compensation may be sought for certain events following certain immunizations within specified time intervals. The compensation system is funded by a continuing surcharge levied against the manufacturers for each dose sold of the specified vaccines.

Physicians administering the specified vaccines are also obliged by the act to report any of the specified reactions to the VAERS (call 1-800-822-7967 for forms). Compensation forms from the NVICP may be obtained by calling 1-800-338-2382. The act provides no penalty for failure to report.

Recognizing the need to improve its capability to study vaccine safety, the CDC participated in pilot studies using large linked databases of computerized vaccination and medical records. The Vaccine Safety Datalink Project (which is a network of several health maintenance organizations' computerized information on immunization, medical outcomes, and potential confounders) was initiated in 1989 and has served as a useful tool to accumulate and analyze data as new vaccines are introduced.

Vaccine information materials are available from the CDC to meet the requirements of the act. Separate short (1500- to 2000-word) forms are used for DTaP, MMR, and poliovirus vaccines. Patients or parents are legally required to sign these forms if the vaccine is purchased on a federal contract. Informed consent is also needed for physicians who wish to be covered fully by the vaccine compensation program. Current recommendations of the AAP and CDC for VCIP were discussed at the start of this chapter and should be followed.

Atkinson WL et al: Centers for Disease Control and Prevention: General recommendations on immunization: Recommendations of the Advisory Committee on Immunization Practices (ACIP) and the American Academy of Family Physicians (AAFP). MMWR Recomm Rep 2002;51(RR-2):1 [PMID: 11848294].

Chen RT et al: The Vaccine Safety Datalink: Immunization research in health maintenance organizations in the USA. Bull World Health Organ 2000;78:186 [PMID: 10743283].

Chen RT et al: Vaccine Safety Datalink project: A new tool for improving vaccine safety monitoring in the United States: The Vaccine Safety Datalink Team. Pediatrics 1997;99:765 [PMID: 9164767].

# Normal Childhood Nutrition & Its Disorders

*Nancy F. Krebs, MD, MS, Laura E. Primak, RD, CNSD, CSP &
K. Michael Hambridge, MD, BChir, ScD*

## ■ NUTRITIONAL REQUIREMENTS

### NUTRITION & GROWTH

The nutrient requirements of children are influenced by their growth rate and body composition and the composition of new growth. These factors vary with age and are especially important during early postnatal life. Growth rates are higher in early infancy than at any other time, including the adolescent growth spurt (Table 10–1). Growth rates decline rapidly starting in the second month of postnatal life (proportionately later in the premature infant). Because of their more rapid growth rate in early infancy, nutrient requirements are slightly higher in males than in females.

Nutrient requirements also depend on body composition. In the adult, the brain, which accounts for only 2% of body weight, contributes 19% to the total basal energy expenditure. In contrast, in a full-term neonate, the brain accounts for 10% of body weight and for 44% of total energy needs under basal conditions. Thus, in the young infant, total basal energy expenditure and the energy requirement of the brain are relatively high.

Composition of new tissue is a third factor influencing nutrient requirements. For example, fat accounts for about 40% of weight gain between birth and 4 months but for only 3% between 24 and 36 months. The corresponding figures for protein are 11% and 21%; for water, 45% and 68%. The high rate of fat deposition in early infancy has implications not only for energy requirements but also for the optimal composition of infant feedings.

Because of the high nutrient requirements for growth and the body composition, the young infant is especially vulnerable to undernutrition. Slowed physical growth rate is an early and prominent sign of undernutrition in the young infant. The limited fat stores of the very young infant mean that energy reserves are unusually restricted. The relatively large size and continued growth of the brain render the central nervous system (CNS) especially vulnerable to the effects of malnutrition in early postnatal life.

### ENERGY

The major determinants of energy expenditure are basal metabolism, metabolic response to food, physical activity, and growth. The efficiency of energy use may be a significant factor, and thermoregulation may contribute in extremes of ambient temperature if the body is inadequately clothed. Because adequate data on requirements for physical activity in infants and children are unavailable and because individual growth requirements vary, recommendations have been based on calculations of actual intakes by healthy subjects. The recent trend toward lower figures for infants reflects a move away from hypercaloric and possibly inappropriate feeding practices that were in vogue in past decades. Suggested guidelines for energy intake of infants and young children are given in Table 10–2. Also included in this table are calculated energy intakes of infants who are exclusively breast-fed, which have been verified recently in a number of centers. Growth velocity of breast-fed infants during the first 3 months typically equals or exceeds the 50th percentile for the National Center for Health Statistics (NCHS) grids. The recommended dietary allowances (RDAs) of the Food and Nutrition Board, National Academy of Sciences, and National Research Council (10th edition) are not synonymous with requirements. The RDAs do not take into account the rapid changes in requirements that occur during infancy, especially the first 6 months, RDAs should therefore be used cautiously for calculating energy requirements of infants.

After the first 4 years, energy requirements expressed on a body weight basis decline progressively. The estimated daily energy requirement is about 40 kcal/kg/d at the end of adolescence. Approximate daily energy requirements can be calculated by adding 100 kcal per year to the base of 1000 kcal per day at age 1 year. Appetite and growth are reliable indices of caloric needs in most healthy children, but intake also depends to some

**Table 10–1.** Changes in growth rate, energy required for growth, and body composition in infants and young children.

| Age (months) | Growth Rate (g/d) Male | Growth Rate (g/d) Both | Growth Rate (g/d) Female | Energy Requirements for Growth (kcal/kg/d) | Body Composition Water | Body Composition Protein | Body Composition Fat |
|---|---|---|---|---|---|---|---|
| 0–0.25 | | 0[a] | | | 75 | 11.5 | 11 |
| 0.25–1 | 40 | | 35 | 50 | | | |
| 1–2 | 35 | | 30 | 25 | | | |
| 2–3 | 28 | | 25 | 16 | | | |
| 3–6 | | 20 | | 10 | 60 | 11.5 | 26 |
| 6–9 | | 15 | | | | | |
| 9–12 | | 12 | | | | | |
| 12–18 | | 8 | | | | | |
| 18–36 | | 6 | | 2 | 61 | 16 | 21 |

[a]Birth weight is regained by 10 d. Weight loss of more than 10% of birth weight indicates dehydration or malnutrition; this applies to both formula-fed and breast-fed infants.
Data from Fomon SJ (ed): *Infant Nutrition,* 2nd ed. WB Saunders, 1974. Used with permission.

extent on the energy density of the food offered. Individual energy requirements of normal infants and children vary considerably, and malnutrition and disease increase the variability. Premature infant energy requirements can exceed 120 kcal/kg/d, especially during illness or when catch-up growth is desired.

One method of calculating requirements for malnourished patients is to base the calculations on the ideal body weight (ie, 50th percentile weight for the patient's length age or 50th percentile weight-for-height)

rather than actual weight. Alternatively the extra daily energy requirement for catch-up growth can be calculated as:

$$\frac{5 \times \text{Weight (g) deficit below IBW}}{\text{Interval (days) for correction of deficit}}$$

where 5 kcal is the energy cost of each gram of new tissue deposited. These calculations should be adjusted according to the growth response.

**Table 10–2.** Recommendations for energy and protein intake.

| Age | Energy (kcal/kg/d) Based on Measurements of Energy Expenditure | Energy (kcal/kg/d) Intake from Human Milk | Energy (kcal/kg/d) Guidelines for Average Requirements | Protein (g/kg/d) Intake from Human Milk | Protein (g/kg/d) Guidelines for Average Requirements |
|---|---|---|---|---|---|
| 10 days to 1 month | — | 105 | 120 | 2.05 | 2.5 |
| 1–2 months | 110 | 110 | 115 | 1.75 | 2.25 |
| 2–3 months | 95 | 105 | 105 | 1.36 | 2.25 |
| 3–4 months | 95 | 75–85 | 95 | 1.20 | 2.0 |
| 4–6 months | 95 | 75–85 | 95 | 1.05 | 1.7 |
| 6–12 months | 85 | 70 | 90 | — | 1.5 |
| 1–2 years | 85 | — | 90 | — | 1.2 |
| 2–3 years | 85 | — | 90 | — | 1.1 |
| 3–5 years | — | — | 90 | — | 1.1 |

Compiled from Krebs NF et al: Growth and intakes of energy and zinc in infants fed human milk. J Pediatr 1994;124:32–9; Garza C, Butte NF: Energy intakes of human milk-fed infants during the first year. J Pediatr 1990;117:(S)124. Data used with permission.

World Health Organization: Report of a Joint FAO/WHO/UNO Expert Consultation: Energy and Protein Requirements. WHO Tech Rep Ser No. 724, 1985;724.

## PROTEIN

Only amino acids and ammonium compounds are usable as sources of nitrogen in humans. Amino acids are provided through the digestion of dietary protein. Nitrogen is absorbed from the intestine as amino acids and short peptides. Absorption of nitrogen is more efficient from synthetic diets that contain peptides in addition to amino acids. Some intact proteins are absorbed in early postnatal life, a process that may be important in the development of protein tolerance or allergy.

The liver plays a central role in amino acid metabolism, including regulation of the absorbed amino acids. Excess amino acids, including essential amino acids, are degraded in the liver, except for the branched-chain amino acids, which pass into the systemic circulation and are taken up primarily by muscle. Insulin stimulates this uptake and suppresses muscle protein catabolism. Protein turnover rates far exceed intake, indicating a reuse of amino acids. However, some of these amino acids released from protein turnover are degraded. After removal of the amino group, the keto acids are either used directly for energy or converted to carbohydrate and fat. Nitrogen is excreted primarily via the kidney as urea.

Because there are no major stores of body protein, a regular dietary supply of protein is essential. In infants and children, optimal growth depends on an adequate dietary protein supply. Relatively subtle effects of protein deficiency are now recognized, especially those affecting tissues with rapid protein turnover rates, such as the immune system and the GI mucosa.

Relative to body weight, rates of protein synthesis and turnover and accretion of body protein are exceptionally high in the infant, especially the premature infant. Eighty percent of the dietary protein requirement of a premature infant is used for growth, compared with only 20% in a 1-year-old child. Protein requirements per unit of body weight decline rapidly during infancy as growth velocity decreases. The recommendations in Table 10–2 are derived chiefly from the Joint FAO/WHO/UNO Expert Committee and are similar to the RDAs. They deliver a protein intake above the quantity provided in breast milk. The protein intake required to achieve protein deposition equivalent to the in utero rate in very low birth weight infants is 3.7–4.0 g/kg/day simultaneous with adequate energy intake. Protein requirements increase in the presence of skin or gut losses, burns, trauma, and infection. Requirements also increase during times of catch-up growth accompanying recovery from malnutrition (ap-

proximately 0.2 g of protein per gram of new tissue deposited). Young infants experiencing rapid recovery may need as much as 1–2 g/kg/d of extra protein. By age 1 year, the extra protein requirement is unlikely to be more than 0.5 g/kg/d. Inadequate protein intake may occur in breast-fed infants fed low-protein supplements (eg, fruit juices), in infants with protein malabsorption (cystic fibrosis), or in infants fed low-protein weaning food (eg, cassava) as the dietary staple.

The quality of protein depends on its amino acid composition. Infants require 43% of protein as essential amino acids, and children require 36%. Adults cannot synthesize eight essential amino acids: isoleucine, leucine, lysine, methionine, phenylalanine, threonine, tryptophan, and valine. Histidine may be added to this list. Cysteine and tyrosine are considered partially essential because their rates of synthesis are limited and may be inadequate in certain circumstances. In young infants, synthetic rates for cysteine, tyrosine, and perhaps taurine are insufficient for needs. Taurine, an amino acid used to conjugate bile acids, may also be conditionally essential in infancy. Taurine supplementation may improve fat absorption in preterm infants and in infants with cystic fibrosis. Taurine supplements may also improve auditory brainstem evoked potentials in preterm infants. Lack of an essential amino acid leads to weight loss within 1–2 weeks. Wheat and rice are deficient in lysine, and legumes are deficient in methionine. Appropriate mixtures of vegetable protein are therefore necessary to achieve high protein quality.

Because the mechanisms for removal of excess nitrogen are efficient, moderate excesses of protein are not harmful and may help to ensure an adequate supply of certain micronutrients. Adverse effects of excessive protein intake may include increased calcium losses in urine and, over a life span, increased loss of renal mass. Excessive protein intake may also cause elevated blood urea nitrogen, acidosis, hyperammonemia, and, in the premature infant, failure to thrive, lethargy, and fever.

Denne SC: Protein and energy requirements of preterm infants. Semin Neonatal 2001;6:377 [PMID: 11988027].

Heird WC: Determination of nutritional requirements in preterm infants, with special reference to "catch-up" growth. Semin Neonatol 2001;6:365 [PMID: 11988026].

## LIPIDS

Fats are the main dietary energy source for infants and account for up to 50% of the energy in human milk. Over 98% of breast milk fat is triglyceride, which has an energy density of 9 kcal/g. Fats can be stored efficiently in adipose tissue with a minimal energy cost of storage. This is especially important in the young infant. Fats are required for the absorption of fat-soluble vitamins and for myelination of the CNS. Fat also provides essential fatty acids (EFAs) necessary for brain development, for phospholipids in cell membranes, and for the synthesis of prostaglandins and leukotrienes. The EFAs are polyunsaturated fatty acids, linoleic acid (18:2$\omega$6) and linolenic acid (18:3$\omega$3). Arachidonic acid (20:4$\omega$6) is derived from dietary linoleic acid and is present primarily in membrane phospholipids. Oxygenation of arachidonic acid through the lipoxygenase pathway yields leukotrienes, and oxygenation through the cyclooxygenase pathway yields prostaglandins. Important derivatives of linolenic acid are eicosapentaenoic acid (20:6$\omega$3) and docosahexaenoic acid (22:6$\omega$3) found in human milk and brain lipids. Visual attention and possibly psychomotor development of formula-fed premature infants is improved in formulae supplemented with 20:6$\omega$3, which is not derived readily from 18:3$\omega$3.

Clinical features of EFA $\omega$6 deficiency include growth failure, erythematous and scaly dermatitis, capillary fragility, increased fragility of erythrocytes, thrombocytopenia, poor wound healing, and susceptibility to infection. The clinical features of deficiency of $\omega$3 fatty acids are less well defined, but dermatitis and neurologic abnormalities including blurred vision, peripheral neuropathy, and weakness have been reported. Marine oil-supplemented formula improves visual acuity of preterm infants through age 4 months by improving docosahexaenoic acid status. Fatty fish are the best dietary source of $\omega$3 fatty acids. A high intake of fatty fish is associated with decreased platelet adhesiveness and decreased inflammatory response.

Up to 5–10% of fatty acids in human milk are polyunsaturated. Most of these are $\omega$6 series with smaller amounts of long-chain $\omega$3 fatty acids. About 40% of breast milk fatty acids are monounsaturates, primarily oleic acid (18:1), and up to 10% of total fatty acids are medium-chain triglycerides (MCTs) ($C_8$ and $C_{10}$) with a calorie density of 7.6 kcal/g. In general, the percentage of calories derived from fat is a little lower in infant formulas than in human milk. Infant formulas usually contain a relatively high percentage of linoleic acid but very little long-chain $\omega$3 fatty acid. The American Academy of Pediatrics recommends that infants receive at least 30% of calories from fat, with at least 1.7% of total calories from $\omega$6 fatty acids and 0.5% from $\omega$3 fatty acids. It is appropriate that 40–50% of energy requirements be provided as fat during the first 2 years of life. Children older than 2 years should be switched gradually to a diet containing approximately 30% of total calories from fat, with no more than 10% of calories either from saturated fats or polyunsaturated fats.

During digestion, triglycerides are hydrolyzed to monoglycerides, free fatty acids, and glycerol in the lumen of the gut. Substantial hydrolysis of triglycerides in milk formulas occurs in the stomach by the action of lingual and gastric lipases. Pancreatic lipases and bile salt levels are relatively low in early postnatal life, but breast milk contains a bile salt-stimulated lipase that is effective in the lumen of the duodenum. Bile salts promote the formation of the colipase–lipase complex, which adheres to the triglycerides prior to hydrolysis. Bile salts also have a major role in the emulsification of fatty acids, allowing their passage through the unstirred water layer to the surface of the mucosal cell. After passage into the enterocyte, long-chain ($\geq C_{12}$) fatty acids and monoglycerides are reesterified to triglycerides and are packaged with phospholipids, cholesterol, and protein into chylomicrons, which are transported in the lymphatics to the liver and thence the circulation. At the capillary endothelial surface of adipose and muscle tissue, lipoprotein lipase (LPL) hydrolyzes triglycerides from chylomicrons, releasing free fatty acids and glycerol, which are taken up by the adjacent cells. LPL also hydrolyzes triglycerides synthesized in the liver and transported to peripheral tissues as very low density lipoproteins.

Beta-oxidation of fatty acids occurs in the mitochondria of muscle and liver. Carnitine is necessary for oxidation of the fatty acids, which must cross the mitochondrial membranes as acylcarnitine. Carnitine is synthesized in the human liver and kidney from lysine and methionine. Carnitine needs of infants are met by breast milk or formulas, and carnitine is now added routinely to soy-based formulas. In the liver, substantial quantities of fatty acids are converted to ketone bodies, which are then released into the circulation as an important fuel for the brain of the young infant.

MCTs are sufficiently soluble that micelle formation is not required for transport across the intestinal mucosa. They are transported directly to the liver via the portal circulation. MCTs are rapidly metabolized in the liver, undergoing beta-oxidation or ketogenesis. They do not require carnitine to enter the mitochondria. Ketones are formed from MCTs even when provided orally. MCTs are useful for patients with luminal phase defects, absorptive defects, and chronic inflammatory bowel disease. The potential side effects of MCT administration include diarrhea when given in large quantities; high octanoic acid levels in patients with cirrhosis; and, if they are the only source of lipids, deficiency of EFA.

Auestad N et al: Growth and development in term infants fed long-chain polyunsaturated fatty acids: A double-masked, randomized, paralleled, prospective, multivariate study. Pediatrics 2001;108:372 [PMID: 11483802].

Jensen CL, Heird WC: Lipids with an emphasis on long-chain polyunsaturated fatty acids. Clin Perinatol 2002;29:261 [PMID: 12168241].

Willatts P, Forsyth JS: The role of long chain polyunsaturated fatty acids in infant cognitive development. Prostaglandins Leukot Essent Fatty Acids 2000;63:95 [PMID: 10970720].

# CARBOHYDRATES

The energy density of carbohydrate is 4 kcal/g. Approximately 40% of caloric intake in human milk is in the form of lactose, or milk sugar. Lactose supplies 20% of the total energy in cow's milk. The percent of total energy in infant formulas from carbohydrate is similar to that of human milk.

After the first 2 years of life, 55–60% of energy requirements should be derived from carbohydrates, with no more than 10% from simple sugars. These dietary guidelines are, unfortunately, not reflected in the diets of North American children, who typically derive 25% of their energy intake from sucrose and less than 20% from complex carbohydrates.

The rate at which lactase hydrolyzes lactose to glucose and galactose in the intestinal brush border determines how quickly milk carbohydrates, are absorbed. Lactase levels are highest in young infants, declining by more than 50% later in the first year. Lactase levels decline further with age depending on genetic factors. Lactose-intolerant children experience varying degrees of symptoms depending on the specific activity of their own intestinal lactase and the amount of lactose consumed. Lactase is located predominantly at the tip of the intestinal villi, where it is especially vulnerable to the effects of gastroenteritis or malnutrition. Thus, it may be helpful to avoid giving lactose-containing foods to children recovering from gastroenteritis or malnutrition, although this is not universally necessary. Galactose is preferentially converted to glycogen in the liver prior to conversion to glucose for subsequent oxidation. Infants with galactosemia, an inborn metabolic disease caused by deficient galactose-1-phosphate uridyltransferase, require a lactose-free diet starting in the neonatal period.

Starch is broken down in the lumen of the gut into disaccharides and oligosaccharides, which are hydrolyzed into glucose by maltase, isomaltase, and glucoamylase in the brush border. Glucoamylase, which hydrolyzes oligosaccharides of 4–9 glucose units, is located predominantly at the base of the villi, where it may be protected from partial villus atrophy. Glucose polymers of this length are used extensively in infant formulas and as caloric supplements. Advantages include a relatively low osmolality and better hydrolysis by the damaged mucosa. Glucose and galactose are absorbed actively with sodium. This provides the theoretic basis for the composition of oral rehydration solutions in the management of diarrhea. The glucose enhances the absorption of sodium (and thus of water) and also supplies some energy.

During and immediately following a meal, plasma glucose levels are maintained by glucose absorption. If less than 10% of dietary energy is regularly provided by carbohydrate, ketosis results. Between 2–4 hours after a meal, plasma glucose depends increasingly on use of hepatic glycogen stores. These provide only 100–150 g glucose in the adult and only 6 g in the neonate. After liver glycogen is depleted, the body progressively depends on gluconeogenesis. Glucose is the principal fuel for the brain and is the main energy source for other tissues, including red and white blood cells.

Children and adolescents in North America consume large quantities of sucrose in soft drinks, candy, syrups, and sweetened breakfast cereals. A high sucrose intake may predispose a child to obesity and is a major risk factor for dental caries. Sucrase hydrolyzes sucrose to glucose and fructose in the brush border of the small intestine. Fructose is absorbed more slowly than and independently of glucose by facilitated diffusion. This characteristic can be an advantage. Neither fructose nor galactose stimulates insulin secretion. Fructose, however, is easily converted to hepatic triglycerides, which may be undesirable in malnourished patients.

Dietary fiber can be classified in two major types: nondigested carbohydrate ($\beta$1–4 linkages) and noncarbohydrate (lignin). Insoluble fibers (cellulose, hemicellulose, and lignin) increase stool bulk and water content and decrease gut transit time. They may impair mineral absorption. Soluble fibers (pectins, mucilages, oat bran) bind bile acids and reduce lipid and cholesterol absorption. Pectins also slow gastric emptying and the rate of nutrient absorption. Fiber intakes are low in North America. Few data regarding the fiber needs of children are available. Federally recognized standards for dietary fiber intake do not yet exist. However, the American Academy of Pediatrics suggests 0.5 g dietary fiber for every kilogram of the child's weight, up to 35 g/d. The American Health Foundation recommends that children older than 2 years consume in grams per day an amount of fiber equal to 5 plus the age in years.

# MAJOR MINERALS

(See Table 10–3 for recommended intakes.)

## Calcium

The major dietary sources of calcium are milk and other dairy products. Although some calcium is available from legumes, broccoli, some green leafy vegetables, and fortified cereals, it is difficult to achieve an adequate calcium

***Table 10–3.*** Summary of dietary reference intakes for selected minerals and trace elements

| | 0–6 mo | 7–12 mo | 1–3 yr | 4–8 yr | 9–13 yr | 14–18 yr male | 14–18 yr female |
|---|---|---|---|---|---|---|---|
| **Calcium** (mg/d) | 210[a] | 270[a] | 500[a] | 800[a] | 1300[a] | 1300[a] | 1300[a] |
| **Phosphorus** (mg/d) | 100[a] | 275[a] | 460[a] | 500 | 1250 | 1250 | 1250 |
| **Magnesium** (mg/d) | 30[a] | 75[a] | 80 | 130 | 240 | 410 | 360 |
| **Iron** (mg/d) | 0.27[a] | 11 | 7 | 10 | 8 | 11 | 15 |
| **Zinc** (mg/d) | 2[a] | 3 | 3 | 5 | 8 | 11 | 9 |
| **Copper** (µg/d) | 200[a] | 220[a] | 340 | 440 | 700 | 890 | 890 |
| **Selenium** (µg/d) | 15[a] | 20[a] | 20 | 30 | 40 | 55 | 55 |

[a]Adequate Intakes (AI). All other values represent the Recommended Dietary Allowances (RDA). Both the RDA and AI may be used as goals for individual intakes.
National Academy of Sciences, Food and Nutritional Board, Institute of Medicine: *Dietary Reference Intakes, Applications in Dietary Assessment.* National Academy Press, Washington, DC 2000: 287–289. http://www.nap.edu.

intake without dietary dairy products or calcium supplementation. Average calcium absorption, is 20–30%, but calcium absorption from human milk is 60%. Absorption is enhanced by lactose, glucose, and protein and is impaired by phytate, fiber, oxalate, and unabsorbed fat. Control of calcium absorption is exerted primarily by variations in serum 1,25-dihydroxycholecalciferol (calcitriol), which increases in response to increases in circulating parathyroid hormone (PTH). PTH is secreted in response to a fall in plasma ionized calcium. It also promotes the release of calcium from bone. Calcium is excreted primarily via the kidney. It is the most abundant mineral in the body, and more than 99% is in the skeleton. Many vital cellular processes depend on calcium, especially changes in cytosolic free calcium levels. Changes in these levels also occur in various pathologic states and can grossly disturb intracellular metabolism. A deficiency in dietary calcium can occur in premature infants and lactating adolescents as a result of restricted milk intake and also in patients with steatorrhea. Deficient calcium intake results in decreased bone density. Bone density increases with increasing calcium intake up to a daily intake of more than 1000 mg in adolescents. Maximizing bone density in adolescence has im-

portant implications for achieving peak bone density and minimizing postmenopausal osteoporosis.

## Phosphorus

Phosphorus is abundant in meats, eggs, dairy products, grains, legumes, and nuts. Phosphorus levels are high in processed foods and very high in colas and other soft drinks. Approximately 80% of dietary phosphorus is absorbed; the kidney is responsible for homeostatic control. PTH decreases tubular reabsorption of phosphorus. More than 85% of body phosphorus is in bone. Phosphorus is also a component of many organic compounds with vital metabolic roles, including adenosine triphosphate (ATP) and 2,3-diphosphoglycerate. Many of the clinical effects of phosphorus depletion are attributable to cellular energy depletion from lack of ATP or to cellular anoxia secondary to impaired release of oxygen from hemoglobin. Other key compounds containing phosphorus include cell membrane phospholipids and nucleotides.

Nutritional phosphorus deficiency is rare but has occurred in very premature infants fed human milk, in whom it can produce osteoporosis and rickets, and in patients with severe protein-energy malnutrition. Non-nutritional phosphorus depletion may result from chronic diarrhea, Fanconi tubulopathy, and the ingestion of phosphorus-binding antacids. Severe hypophosphatemia results from a deficiency together with an acute extracellular-to-intracellular shift in phosphorus. This shift can be triggered by glucose, by insulin, or during nutritional rehabilitation of the malnourished patient. Phosphorus deficiency affects most organ systems, including muscle (weakness progressing to rhabdomyolysis), cellular components of blood (both physiologic and functional changes), the GI system, the CNS, and bone (bone pain, osteomalacia). Respiratory insufficiency may result from weakness of the diaphragm. Phosphate depletion in the premature infant can cause hypercalcemia. Phosphorus depletion can be treated with phosphorus salts or skim milk. Phosphorus excess may cause neonatal tetany due to decreased serum calcium. Phosphorus retention in chronic renal disease leads to metabolic bone disease.

## Magnesium

Two thirds of dietary magnesium is derived from vegetables, cereals, and nuts. The kidney controls magnesium homeostasis by minimizing excretion when intake is low. Magnesium is the second most abundant intracellular cation; 50% is in bone. Levels in the cytosol are 10 times that in the extracellular fluids and are especially high in mitochondria. Magnesium activates many enzymes, especially phosphorus-hydrolyzing and -transferring enzymes involved in energy metabolism. Magnesium also plays major roles in nucleic acid metabolism.

Dietary magnesium deficiency is not recognized except as a component of protein-energy malnutrition, but magnesium depletion may occur secondary to renal disease, intestinal malabsorption, or medications inducing magnesium loss from the gut or kidney. Hypomagnesemia produces neuromuscular excitability, muscle fasciculation and tremors, personality changes, neurologic abnormalities, and electrocardiographic changes (depression of ST segment and T waves). Disturbances of PTH metabolism can cause secondary hypocalcemia. Acute magnesium depletion can be treated with a 50% solution of $MgSO_4$, providing 0.3–1.0 mEq of magnesium per kilogram given intravenously over a 24-hour period. Magnesium excess can cause respiratory depression, lethargy, and coma.

## Sodium

In the United States and western Europe, only 10% of sodium intake is derived from unprocessed foods; 15% is derived from salt added while cooking and 75% from salt added to processed foods during manufacturing. The 10% derived from unprocessed foods is sufficient to meet normal requirements. Current dietary recommendations suggest that North Americans should reduce sodium intake so as to restore a normal ratio of dietary sodium to potassium. The present ratio is approximately 2:1, but in other cultures and in other mammalian species the ratio is 0.25:1. A high sodium-to-potassium ratio has been implicated in the pathogenesis of hypertension, especially if the intake of dietary calcium is low.

Excessive sweating or high sweat sodium (as in cystic fibrosis) may increase the requirement for dietary sodium. Sodium deficiency occurs most commonly as a result of diarrhea and vomiting. Anorexia, vomiting, and mental apathy may result from chronic depletion of sodium chloride. Hyponatremic and hypernatremic dehydration are discussed in Chapter 42.

Severe malnutrition and severe stress or hypermetabolism can disturb the ionic gradient across cell membranes and lead to excess intracellular sodium, which can adversely affect cellular metabolism. Sodium should be administered with great caution in these circumstances. Suggested dietary intake of sodium for infants is 50 mg/kg/d; for children older than 1 year, it is 250–500 mg/d.

## Chloride

The intake and homeostasis of dietary chloride are closely linked with those of sodium. However, chloride is itself important in the physiologic mechanisms of the kidney and the gut. Active chloride transport in the ascending loop of Henle is necessary for the passive reabsorption of sodium. Deficiency of chloride leads to a decrease in the absorption of sodium in the ascending loop of Henle and an increase in the amount of sodium presented to the distal tubule. This sodium is exchanged for $H^+$ and $K^+$, which can result in hypokalemic alkalosis.

Infants fed formulas low in chloride have experienced a nutritional deficiency of chloride. Other causes of chloride deficiency include cystic fibrosis, pyloric stenosis and other causes of vomiting, familial chloride diarrhea, chronic diuretic (furosemide) therapy, and Bartter syndrome. Chloride deficiency has been associated with failure to thrive and may especially affect head growth. Other features include anorexia, lethargy, muscle weakness, vomiting, dehydration, and hypovolemia. Laboratory features include hypochloremia, hypokalemia, metabolic alkalosis, and hyperreninemia. Suggested dietary intake of chloride for infants is 70 mg/kg/d; for children older than 1 year, it is 700 mg/d.

## Potassium

Potassium is readily available in unprocessed foods, including nuts, whole grains, meats and fish, beans, bananas, and orange juice. Relatively high potassium intakes are encouraged except in the presence of renal failure. The kidneys control potassium homeostasis via the aldosterone–renin–angiotensin endocrine system. Potassium is the principal intracellular cation. The amount of total body potassium, therefore, depends on lean body mass. Potassium deficiency occurs in protein-energy malnutrition and can be a cause of sudden death from cardiac failure if not treated aggressively during the initial phase of rehabilitation. Because of loss of lean body mass, excessive potassium is excreted in the urine in any catabolic state. This too requires aggressive replenishment during recovery. During acidosis, intracellular potassium is exchanged for $H^+$. Potassium is shifted into the extracellular fluid, and large amounts may be lost in the urine (eg, in diabetic ketoacidosis) despite normal or elevated plasma potassium. Other causes of potassium deficiency are diarrhea and diuretics. Potassium deficiency may produce muscle weakness, mental confusion, and sudden death from arrhythmias. Electrocardiographic findings include depression of the ST segment and low T waves. Hyperkalemia may result from renal insufficiency. Suggested dietary intake of potassium for infants is 80 mg/kg/d; for children older than 1 year, it is 800 mg/d.

## TRACE ELEMENTS

Trace elements with a recognized role in human nutrition are iron, iodine, zinc, copper, selenium, manganese, molybdenum, chromium, cobalt (as a component of vitamin $B_{12}$), and fluoride. Dietary requirements of trace elements are summarized in Table 10–3. Iron deficiency is discussed in Chapter 27. In general, good dietary sources of trace elements include human milk, meats, shellfish, legumes, nuts, and whole grain cereals. Fish are a good source of selenium. Absorption of iron, zinc, copper, and probably other trace elements from human milk is especially efficient; healthy full-term breast-fed infants generally do not require exogenous trace elements, including iron, until approximately 6 months. Factors affecting trace element absorption include the quantity in the diet, the simultaneous ingestion of foods promoting the formation of insoluble complexes (phytate, fiber, phosphate, oxalate), the oxidation state of the element (ascorbic acid increases iron absorption and decreases copper absorption), its chemical form in the diet (heme versus nonheme iron), competitive inhibition of mucosal absorption (interactions of iron, zinc, and copper), and host factors such as nutritional status, diarrhea, and in-

testinal function. The GI tract is the major site of homeostatic control for iron and zinc; the liver for copper; the intestinal tract and liver for manganese; and the kidneys for selenium, chromium, and iodine.

Deficiencies of iron, zinc, and possibly copper, occur in the free-living population. In certain geographic regions iodine and selenium deficiency is common because of deficiencies in soil and water. Infants exclusively fed cow's milk are at risk for iron and copper deficiency. Excessive loss and impaired absorption can cause iron, zinc, or copper deficiency. Trace element deficiencies have been associated with the use of synthetic diets and especially intravenous (IV) nutrition. Protein-energy malnutrition may be complicated by deficiencies in iron, zinc, copper, selenium, or chromium. Deficiencies in zinc, copper, iron, and molybdenum occur as a result of specific genetic diseases affecting the absorption or metabolism of these elements (see Chapter 33).

## Zinc

Zinc is a component of many enzymes and plays important roles in nucleic acid metabolism, protein synthesis, and membrane structure and function. Zinc deficiency is the result of diets low in available zinc (high phytate) and synthetic diets (oral or IV) lacking adequate zinc supplements. Diseases associated with impaired absorption (regional enteritis, celiac disease, cystic fibrosis) or excessive loss (chronic diarrhea), and inborn diseases of zinc metabolism may produce a state of zinc deficiency. Although the zinc in human milk is very efficiently absorbed, the zinc concentration in breast milk steadily declines over time. After 6 months, the exclusively breast-fed infant is likely to need additional zinc from complementary foods.

Several recent large trials have shown that zinc supplementation in infants and young children is associated with a significant reduction in the incidence of pneumonia and of acute and chronic diarrhea. Improved zinc status has also been associated with improved immunocompetence. Low-birth-weight infants appear to be particularly vulnerable to zinc deficiency, and randomized trials of zinc supplementation in developing countries have shown significant improvements in growth as well as reduction in the mortality and morbidity associated with infection. Mild deficiency is associated with impaired growth and poor appetite. Severe deficiency is characterized by mood changes, irritability, and lethargy. Impairment of the immune system, especially T-cell function, has been linked to increased susceptibility to infection. The most severe deficiency state is characterized by an acroorificial skin rash, usually accompanied by diarrhea and alopecia. These features occur in patients with acrodermatitis enteropathica, an inborn error of zinc metabolism, in subjects receiving IV feeding without adequate zinc supplements, and in some breast-fed infants whose mothers have a defect in the secretion of zinc by the mammary gland. Plasma zinc collected before breakfast is below 6 μmol/L (40 μg/dL) in patients with severe zinc deficiency and 6–9 μmol/L (40–60 μg/dL) in patients with moderate zinc deficiency. In patients with mild zinc deficiency, plasma zinc concentration may be within the normal range (60–100 μg/dL).

Dietary zinc deficiency can be treated with 1 mg/kg/d of zinc for 3 months (eg, 4.5 mg of $ZnSO_4$ + 7 $H_2O$/kg/d), preferably administered separately from meals and iron supplements. Sustained clinical remission in acrodermatitis enteropathica is usually achieved with 30–50 mg $Zn^{2+}$ per day, but larger quantities may be required.

Black RE: Zinc deficiency, infectious disease and mortality in the developing world. J Nutr 2003;133:1485S [PMID: 12730449].

Gibson RS: Zinc supplementation for infants. Lancet 2000;355: 2008 [PMID: 10885346].

Krebs NF et al: Abnormalities in zinc homeostasis in young infants with cystic fibrosis. Pediatr Res 2000;48:256 [PMID: 10926304].

Sazawal S et al: Zinc supplementation in infants born small for gestational age reduces mortality: A prospective, randomized, controlled trial. Pediatrics 2001;108:1280 [PMID: 11731649].

## Copper

Copper is a vital component of several oxidative enzymes: cytochrome c oxidase, the terminal oxidase in the electron transport chain; cytosolic and mitochondrial superoxide dismutase, which have key roles in the body defense against free radicals; lysyl oxidase, which is necessary for the cross-linking of elastin and collagen; and ferroxidases (including ceruloplasmin) necessary for the oxidation of ferrous storage iron to ferric iron prior to attachment to transferrin for transport to the red cell precursors in the bone marrow. $Cu^{2+}$ is highly reactive and must be transported in the circulation bound to ceruloplasmin so that its oxidative potential can be contained.

Copper deficiency occurs in the following circumstances: in premature infants fed milk preparations low in copper; in association with prolonged feeding with unmodified cow's milk; in association with generalized malnutrition; in patients maintained on prolonged total parenteral nutrition (TPN) without copper supplementation; and in patients with intestinal malabsorption or prolonged diarrhea.

Osteoporosis is an early finding of copper deficiency. Later, enlargement of costochondral cartilages, cupping and flaring of long-bone metaphyses, and spontaneous rib fractures may occur. The radiologic findings must be distinguished from child abuse (asymmetrical fractures), rickets, and scurvy. Neutropenia and hypochromic anemia are other early manifestations. The anemia is unresponsive to iron therapy. Very severe CNS disease is present in Menkes steely (kinky) hair syndrome, in which a profound copper deficiency state results from an X-linked defect in cellular metabolism of copper.

A low plasma copper or ceruloplasmin level helps confirm the diagnosis of copper deficiency. However, these levels are normally very low in the young infant, especially the premature infant, and are higher than adult values in later infancy and early childhood. Hence, age-matched normal data are necessary for comparison. Interleukin-1 grossly elevates both ceruloplasmin and copper levels; the levels are also high in pregnancy.

Copper deficiency can be treated with a 1% copper sulfate solution (2 mg of the salt or 500 mg of elemental copper per day for infants).

Olivares M et al: Copper homeostasis in infant nutrition: Deficit and excess. J Pediatr Gastroenterol Nutr 2000;31(2):102 [PMID: 10941959].

## Selenium

Selenium is an essential component of glutathione peroxidase, which catalyzes the reduction of hydrogen peroxide to water in the cell cytosol by the addition of reducing equivalents derived from glutathione. Hence, selenium plays an important role in protection against free-radical injury.

Selenium deficiency is the major causal factor in Keshan disease, an often fatal cardiomyopathy primarily affecting infants, children, and young women in a large area of China where there is a severe geochemical selenium deficiency. Similar cases have been identified in the United States in patients maintained on long-term TPN without adequate selenium supplement, in whom symptoms also include skeletal muscle pain and tenderness. Macrocytosis and loss of hair pigment occur in milder selenium deficiency. Premature infants have exceptionally low serum selenium levels, which decline further without supplementation. Blood levels are especially low in premature infants with bronchopulmonary dysplasia. The minimum recommended selenium content for full-term infant formulas is 1.5 μg/100 kcal, and that for preterm infant formulas is 1.8 μg/100 kcal.

A plasma selenium level less than 0.5 μmol/L (< 40 μg/L) suggests mild selenium deficiency. A level less than 0.12 μmol/L (< 10 μg/L) indicates a possible severe selenium deficiency.

## Iodine

Endemic goiter resulting from environmental iodine deficiency has been eradicated in North America by prophylactic measures but continues to be a health problem in many developing countries. Goiter occurs when iodine intake is less than 20 mg/d. Most persons with endemic goiter are clinically euthyroid. Maternal iodine deficiency causes endemic neonatal hypothyroidism in about 5–15% of neonates who may have goiter at birth.

Neurologic endemic cretinism, seen in most parts of the world, is characterized by severe mental retardation, deaf–mutism, spastic diplegia, and strabismus. Evidence of hypothyroidism is usually absent, and it is thought that the neurologic damage is due to a direct effect of fetal iodine deficiency or to an imbalance between thyroxine (low) and triiodothyronine (normal or elevated). Myxedematous endemic cretinism occurs in some central African countries. Signs of congenital hypothyroidism are present. Milder neurologic damage occurs in some cases of endemic neonatal goiter.

The use of iodized salt has been highly effective in preventing goiter. In areas where endemic goiter occurs, intramuscular depot injections of iodized oil have also been used for prevention.

## Fluoride

When fluoride is incorporated into the hydroxyapatite matrix of dentin, it effectively reduces the incidence of dental caries. Fluoride is most effectively administered as an additive to drinking water, but in infancy and childhood, fluoride vitamin preparations serve the same purpose. Ready-made formulas contain less than 0.3 ppm of fluoride. The recognized benefits of topical fluoride supplementation in preventing caries must be weighed against the increasing incidence of fluorosis in children in the United States. Fluorosis is characterized by an increased porosity (undermineralization) of the enamel and is evident clinically as discoloration of the teeth. Recommendations for fluoride supplementation in infants have been revised (Table 10–4). The American Academy of Pediatrics Committee on Nutrition, recommends withholding fluoride supplementation until age 6 months.

Centers for Disease Control and Prevention: Recommendations for using fluoride to prevent and control dental caries in the United States. MMWR Morb Mortal Wkly Rep 2001;50(no. RR-14):1.

Klein CJ: Nutrient requirements for preterm infant formulas. J Nutr 2002;132:1472S [PMID: 12042465].

***Table 10–4.*** Supplemental fluoride recommendations (mg/d).

| Age | Concentration of Fluoride in Drinking Water | | |
|---|---|---|---|
| | < 0.3 ppm | 0.3–0.6 ppm | > 0.6 ppm |
| 6 months to 3 years | 0.25 | 0 | 0 |
| 3–6 years | 0.5 | 0.25 | 0 |
| 6–16 years | 1 | 0.5 | 0 |

Reprinted, with permission, from Centers for Disease Control and Prevention: Recommendations for using fluoride to prevent and control dental caries in the United States. MMWR Morb Mortal Wkly Rep 2001;50(RR-14):8.

## VITAMINS

## 1. Fat-Soluble Vitamins

Because they are insoluble in water, the fat-soluble vitamins require digestion and absorption of dietary fat and a carrier system for transport in the blood. Deficiencies in these vitamins develop more slowly than deficiencies in water-soluble vitamins because the body accumulates stores of fat-soluble vitamins. Excessive intakes carry a considerable potential for toxicity (Table 10–5).

### Vitamin A

Dietary sources of vitamin A include dairy products, fortified margarine, eggs, liver, meats, fish oils, and corn. The vitamin A precursor β-carotene is abundant in yellow and green vegetables. Dietary retinyl palmitate requires hydrolysis by pancreatic and intestinal hydrolases. β-Carotene is cleaved in the intestinal mucosal cells by dioxygenase to yield two molecules of retinal (retinaldehyde), which is then reduced to retinol (vitamin A alcohol). Carotene appears to have an important role in its own right as an antioxidant.

Retinol is reesterified in the intestinal mucosa and transported in chylomicrons to the liver for storage. From the liver, vitamin A is exported to the body attached to retinol-binding protein and prealbumin. Retinol-binding protein may be decreased in liver disease or in protein-energy malnutrition. Circulating retinol-binding protein may be increased in chronic renal failure.

Vitamin A has a critical role in the photochemical basis of vision. The photosensitive pigment rhodopsin is formed from retinal and a protein called opsin. Vitamin A also modifies differentiation and proliferation of epithelial cells, especially in the respiratory tract. Vitamin A is necessary for glycoprotein synthesis. Retinol

***Table 10–5.*** Effects of vitamin toxicity.

**Thiamin**
(Very rare.) Anaphylaxis; respiratory depression
**Riboflavin**
None
**Pyridoxine**
Sensory neuropathy at doses > 500 mg/d
**Niacin**
Histamine release → cutaneous vasodilation; cardiac arrhythmias; cholestatic jaundice; gastrointestinal disturbance; hyperuricemia; glucose intolerance
**Pantothenic acid**
Diarrhea
**Biotin**
None
**Folic acid**
May mask $B_{12}$ deficiency, hypersensitivity
**Cobalamin**
None
**Vitamin C**
Interference with copper absorption; decreased tolerance to hypoxia, increased oxalic acid excretion
**Carnitine**
None recognized
**Vitamin A**
(> 20,000 IU/d): Vomiting, increased intracranial pressure (pseudotumor cerebri); irritability; headaches; insomnia; emotional lability; dry, desquamating skin; myalgia and arthralgia; abdominal pain; hepatosplenomegaly; cortical thickening of bones of hands and feet
**Vitamin D**
(> 40,000 IU/d): Hypercalcemia; vomiting; constipation; nephrocalcinosis
**Vitamin E**
(? 25–100 mg/kg/d intravenously): Necrotizing enterocolitis and liver toxicity (but probably due to polysorbate 80 used as a solubilizer)
**Vitamin K**
*Lipid-soluble vitamin K:* Very low order of toxicity.
Water-soluble, synthetic vitamin K: Vomiting, porphyrinuria; albuminuria; hemolytic anemia; hemoglobinuria; hyperbilirubinemia (do not give to neonates)

can be irreversibly oxidized to retinoic acid, which is effective in glycoprotein synthesis but is ineffective for vision.

Vitamin A deficiency occurs in premature infants, in association with IV nutrition with inadequate vitamin A supplement, and in association with protein-energy malnutrition, when the manifestations are frequently made more severe by measles. Other causes of vitamin A deficiency are dietary insufficiency and fat malabsorption.

The features of vitamin A deficiency are primarily related to the eye and vision. Night blindness progresses to xerosis (dryness of cornea and conjunctiva), xerophthalmia (extreme dryness of the conjunctiva), Bitot spots, keratomalacia (clouding and softening of the cornea), ulceration and perforation of the cornea, prolapse of the lens and iris, and eventually blindness. Vitamin A deficiency is the leading cause of blindness in children worldwide. Other features of vitamin A deficiency include follicular hyperkeratosis (dry, thickened, rough skin), pruritus, growth retardation, increased susceptibility to infection, anemia, and hepatosplenomegaly. Vitamin A treatment of children with rubeola in developing countries has been associated with reduction in morbidity and mortality from this viral infection.

Serum retinol levels below 20 μg/dL are low, and levels less than 10 μg/dL indicate deficiency. A ratio of retinol to retinol-binding protein below 0.7 is also indicative of vitamin A deficiency.

Suggested intakes of vitamin A are summarized in Table 10–6. Therapy of xerophthalmia requires 5000–10,000 international units (IU)/kg/d for 5 days orally or intramuscularly. The standard maintenance dose in fat malabsorption syndromes is 2500–5000 IU (800–1600 μg). Doses as high as 25,000–50,000 IU/d may be needed, but monitoring to avoid toxicity is essential. The effects of vitamin A toxicity are summarized in Table 10–5.

Villamor E, Fawzi WW: Vitamin A supplementation: Implications for morbidity and mortality in children. J Infect Dis 2000;182 (Suppl):S122 [PMID: 10944494].

## Vitamin D

Vitamin D requirements are normally met primarily from cholecalciferol (vitamin $D_3$) produced by ultraviolet radiation of dehydrocholesterol in the skin. Similarly, ergocalciferol (vitamin $D_2$) is derived from UV irradiation of ergosterol in the skin. Vitamin D is transported from the skin to the liver attached to a specific carrier protein. The primary dietary source of vitamin D is fortified milk and formulas. Egg yolk and fatty fish contain some vitamin D. Vitamin D absorption depends on normal fat absorption. Absorbed vitamin D is transported to the liver in chylomicrons. Vitamins $D_2$ and $D_3$ undergo 25-hydroxylation in the liver and then 1α-hydroxylation in kidney proximal tubules to yield 1,25-dihydroxycholecalciferol (calcitriol) and calcitriol, respectively. PTH activates the 1α-hydroxylase enzyme in the kidney. 25-Hydroxycholecalciferol (calcidiol) is the major circulating form of vitamin D. Calcitriol is the biologically active form of vitamin D. Calcitriol stimulates the intestinal absorption of cal-

***Table 10–6.*** Summary of dietary reference intakes for select vitamins.

| | 0–6 mo | 7–12 mo | 1–3 yr | 4–8 yr | 9–13 ys | 14–18 yr male | 14–18 yr female |
|---|---|---|---|---|---|---|---|
| Thiamin (mg/d) | 0.2[a] | 0.3[a] | 0.5 | 0.6 | 0.9 | 1.2 | 1.0 |
| Riboflavin (mg/d) | 0.3[a] | 0.4[a] | 0.5[a] | 0.6[a] | 0.9[a] | 1.3[a] | 1.0[a] |
| Pyridoxine (mg/d) | 0.1[a] | 0.3[a] | 0.5 | 0.6 | 1.0 | 1.3 | 1.2 |
| Niacin (mg/d) | 2[a] | 4[a] | 6 | 8 | 12 | 16 | 14 |
| Pantothenic Acid (mg/d) | 1.7[a] | 1.8[a] | 2[a] | 3[a] | 4[a] | 5[a] | 5[a] |
| Biotin (µg/d) | 5[a] | 6[a] | 8[a] | 12[a] | 20[a] | 25[a] | 25[a] |
| Folic Acid (µg/d) | 65[a] | 80[a] | 150 | 200 | 300 | 400 | 400 |
| Cobalamin (µg/d) | 0.4[a] | 0.5[a] | 0.9 | 1.2 | 1.8 | 2.4 | 2.4 |
| Vitamin C (mg/d) | 40[a] | 50[a] | 15 | 25 | 45 | 75 | 65 |
| Vitamin A (µg/d) | 400[a] | 500[a] | 300 | 400 | 600 | 900 | 700 |
| Vitamin D (IU/d) | 200[a] | 200[a] | 200[a] | 200[a] | 200[a] | 200[a] | 200[a] |
| Vitamin E (mg/d) | 4[a] | 5[a] | 6 | 7 | 11 | 15 | 15 |
| Vitamin K (µg/d) | 2[a] | 2.5[a] | 30[a] | 55[a] | 60[a] | 75[a] | 75[a] |

[a]Adequate Intakes (AI). All other values represent the Recommended Dietary Allowances (RDA). Both the RDA and AI may be used as goals for individual intakes.

Reprinted, with permission, from National Academy of Sciences, Food and Nutritional Board, Institute of Medicine: *Dietary Reference Intakes, Applications in Dietary Assessment.* National Academy Press, Washington, DC 2000: 287–89. http://www.nap.edu.

cium and phosphate, the renal reabsorption of filtered calcium, and the mobilization of calcium and phosphorus from bone.

Vitamin D deficiency usually results from a combination of inadequate sunlight exposure and low dietary intake. An infant with light skin pigmentation requires only about 30 minutes per week of total body sun exposure or 2 hours per week of head exposure to maintain adequate vitamin D status. Adequate amounts of sun exposure for infants with more darkly pigmented skin are difficult to quantify. Furthermore, dermatolo-

gists advise caution in exposure to sun, even for young infants. Vitamin D content of human milk is low. In the United States, cow's milk and infant formulas are routinely supplemented with vitamin D. The American Academy of Pediatrics now recommends vitamin D supplementation for all breast-fed infants until they are receiving at least 500 mL/d of vitamin D in fortified formula or milk. Supplementation should be initiated during the first 2 months of life.

Vitamin D deficiency also occurs in fat malabsorption syndromes. Use of P-450–stimulating drugs may decrease hydroxylated vitamin D, which can also be decreased by hepatic and renal disease and by inborn errors of metabolism. End-organ unresponsiveness to calcitriol may also occur.

The clinical effects of vitamin D deficiency are osteomalacia (adults) or rickets (children), in which osteoid (matrix) with reduced calcification accumulates in bone. Cartilage fails to mature and calcify. Clinical findings include craniotabes, rachitic rosary, pigeon breast, bowed legs, delayed eruption of teeth and enamel defects, Harrison groove, scoliosis, kyphosis, dwarfism, painful bones, fractures, anorexia, and weakness. Radiographic findings include cupping, fraying, and flaring of metaphyses. The loss of sharp definition of bone trabeculae accounts for the general decrease in skeletal radiodensity. The diagnosis is supported by characteristic radiologic abnormalities of the skeleton, low serum phosphorus, high serum alkaline phosphatase, and high serum PTH. The diagnosis can be confirmed by a low level of serum 25-hydroxycholecalciferol.

Rickets is treated with 1600–5000 IU/d of vitamin $D_3$ (1 IU = 0.025 μg). If this is poorly absorbed, calcidiol, 25 μg/d (1000 IU), or calcitriol, 0.05–0.2 μg/kg/d, is given. Renal osteodystrophy is treated with calcitriol.

Suggested dietary intakes for vitamin D are summarized in Table 10–6 and toxic effects in Table 10–5.

Gartner LM, Greer FR, Section on Breastfeeding and Committee on Nutrition, American Academy of Pediatrics: Prevention of rickets and Vitamin D deficiency: New Guidelines for Vitamin D intake. Pediatrics 2003;111(4):908 [PMID: 12671133].

Kreiter SR et al: Nutritional rickets in African American breastfed infants. J Pediatr 2000;137:153 [PMID: 10931404].

## Vitamin E

Vegetable oils are the main dietary source of vitamin E. Coconut and olive oils, however, are low in vitamin E. Some vitamin E is present in cereals, dairy products, and eggs. Vitamin activity may decrease with processing, storage, or heating. Vitamin E is a family of compounds, the tocopherols, with four major forms: alpha, gamma, beta, and delta. α-Tocopherol has the highest biologic activity. Vitamin E can donate an electron to a free-radical molecule to stop oxidation reactions. Oxidized vitamin E is then reduced by ascorbic acid or glutathione. The reduced tocopherol is able to scavenge another free radical. The nutrients that participate in antioxidant defenses include β-carotene, vitamin C, selenium, copper, manganese, and zinc. Vitamin E is located at specific sites in the cell to protect polyunsaturated fatty acids in the membrane lipids from lipid peroxidation and to protect thiol groups and nucleic acids. Vitamin E also functions as a cell membrane stabilizer, may function in the electron transport chain, and may modulate chromosomal expression.

Vitamin E deficiency may occur in the following circumstances: prematurity; cholestatic liver disease, pancreatic insufficiency, abetalipoproteinemia, and short bowel syndrome; as an isolated inborn error of vitamin E metabolism; and perhaps as a result of increased use due to oxidant stress.

Vitamin E deficiency shortens red cell half-life and may cause hemolytic anemia. Chronic vitamin E deficiency results in a progressive neurologic disorder with loss of deep tendon reflexes, loss of coordination, vibratory and position sensation, nystagmus, weakness, scoliosis, and retinal degeneration. In premature infants, vitamin E deficiency may contribute to oxidant injury of the lung, retina, and brain (brain hemorrhage). These putative adverse effects in the premature infant require confirmation.

Vitamin E nutritional status can be partially assessed by measuring serum vitamin E (normal range for children is 3–15 mg/mL). The ratio of serum vitamin E to total serum lipid is normally more than 0.8 mg/g. Sensitivity of erythrocytes to hydrogen peroxide-induced hemolysis is also used as a test of vitamin E status.

Suggested dietary intakes of vitamin E are summarized in Table 10–6. Requirements increase if dietary polyunsaturated fatty acids increase. Between 0.4 mg and 0.5 mg of vitamin E is needed per gram of polyunsaturated fatty acids in the diet (1 IU = 1 mg of DL-α-tocopherol acetate).

Large oral doses (up to 100 IU/kg/d) of vitamin E correct the deficiency resulting from most malabsorption syndromes. For abetalipoproteinemia, 100–200 IU/kg/d of vitamin E are needed. Vitamin E therapy in ischemia-reperfusion injury and in the prevention of intracranial hemorrhage in the preterm infant remains controversial. Toxic effects of intravenously administered vitamin E are summarized in Table 10–5.

## Vitamin K

Vitamin $K_1$ (phylloquinone) is obtained from leafy vegetables, soybean oil, fruits, seeds, and cow's milk. Vitamin $K_2$ (menaquinone), which has 60% of the activity of $K_1$, is synthesized by intestinal bacteria. $K_2$ may be a major source of vitamin K in infants and young children, but less is produced in the intestine of breast-fed infants.

Vitamin K is necessary for the posttranslational carboxylation of glutamic acid residues of the vitamin K-dependent coagulation proteins. Carboxylation allows these proteins to bind calcium, leading to activation of the clotting factors. Thus vitamin K is necessary for the maintenance of normal plasma levels of coagulation factors II (prothrombin), VII, IX, and X and is also necessary for maintenance of normal levels of the anticoagulation protein C. Vitamin K deficiency occurs in newborns, especially those who are breast-fed and who do not receive vitamin K prophylaxis at delivery. The deficiency may result in hemorrhagic disease of the newborn. Later, vitamin K deficiency may result from fat malabsorption syndromes and the use of nonabsorbed antibiotics and anticoagulant drugs (eg, warfarin). Clinical features are bruising or bleeding in the GI tract, genital urinary tract, gingiva, lungs, joints, and brain. Vitamin K status can be assessed with plasma levels of protein-induced vitamin K absence or by prothrombin time.

Vitamin K requirements are summarized in Table 10–6. Newborns require prophylactic intramuscular vitamin K (0.5–1 mg). For older children with acute bleeding, 3–10 mg of vitamin K is given intramuscularly or intravenously. For chronic malabsorption syndromes, 2.5 mg twice weekly to 5 mg/d is given orally. To reverse warfarin effect, 25–50 mg of IV vitamin K is given. Toxic effects of vitamin K are summarized in Table 10–5.

Greer FR: Do breastfed infants need supplemental vitamins? Pediatr Clin North Am 2001;48(2):415 [PMID: 11339161].

Miller CA, Committee on Fetus and Newborn, American Academy of Pediatrics: Controversies concerning vitamin K and the newborn. Pediatrics 2003;112(1):191 [PMID: 12837888].

## 2. Water-Soluble Vitamins

Deficiencies of water-soluble vitamins are uncommon in the United States because of the abundant food supply and fortification of prepared foods. Most bread and wheat products are routinely fortified with B vitamins, including the mandatory addition of folic acid to enriched grain products since January 1998. There is conclusive evidence that folic acid supplements (400 μg/d) during the periconceptional period protect against neural tube defects. Dietary intakes of folic acid from natural foods and enriched products also result in protection. Recommended intakes of folic acid during the periconceptional period may also afford protection later against neuroectodermal brain tumors in young children.

The risk of toxicity from water-soluble vitamins is not as great as that associated with fat-soluble vitamins because excesses of the former can be excreted in the urine. However, deficiencies in these vitamins develop more quickly than deficiencies in fat-soluble vitamins because of the limited stores.

Additional salient details are summarized in Tables 10–6 to 10–11. Although dietary intake of the water-soluble vitamins on a daily basis is not necessary, these

**Table 10–7.** Summary of biologic roles of water-soluble vitamins.

**B vitamins involved in production of energy**
Thiamin ($B_1$)
  Thiamin pyrophosphate is coenzyme in oxidative decarboxylation (pyruvate dehydrogenase, α-ketoglutarate dehydrogenase, and transketolase).
Riboflavin ($B_2$)
  Coenzyme of several flavoproteins (eg, flavin mononucleotide [FMN] and flavin adenine dinucleotide [FAD]) involved in oxidative/electron transfer enzyme systems.
Niacin
  Hydrogen-carrying coenzymes: nicotinamide-adenine dinucleotide (NAD), nicotinamide-adenine dinucleotide phosphate (NADP); decisive role in intermediary metabolism.
Pantothenic acid
  Major component of coenzyme A.
Biotin
  Component of several carboxylase enzymes involved in fat and carbohydrate metabolism.
**Hematopoietic B vitamins**
Folic acid
  Tetrahydrofolate has essential role in one-carbon transfers. Essential role in purine and pyramidine synthesis; deficiency → arrest of cell division (especially bone marrow and intestine).
Cobalamin ($B_{12}$)
  Methyl cobalamin (cytoplasm): synthesis of methionine with simultaneous synthesis of tetrahydrofolate (reason for megaloblastic anemia in $B_{12}$ deficiency). Adenosyl cobalamin (mitochondria) is coenzyme for mutases and dehydratases.
**Other B vitamins**
Pyridoxine ($B_6$)
  Prosthetic group of transaminases, etc, involved in amino acid interconversions; prostaglandin and heme synthesis; central nervous system function; carbohydrate metabolism; immune development.
**Other water-soluble vitamins**
L-Ascorbic acid (C)
  Strong reducing agent—probably involved in all hydroxylations. Roles include collagen synthesis; phenylalanine → tyrosine; tryptophan → 5-hydroxytryptophan; dopamine → norepinephrine; $Fe^{3+}$; folic acid → folinic acid; cholesterol → bile acids; leukocyte function; interferon production; carnitine synthesis. Copper metabolism; reduces oxidized vitamin E.
Carnitine
  Transfer of long-chain fatty acids from cytosol to mitochondria (necessary for beta-oxidation).

***Table 10–8.*** Major dietary sources of water-soluble vitamins.

**Thiamin**
   Whole grains, cereals (including fortification), lean pork, legumes
**Riboflavin**
   Dairy products, meat, poultry, wheat germ, leafy vegetables
**Pyridoxine**
   All foods
**Niacin**
   Meats, poultry, fish, legumes, wheat, all foods except fats, synthesized in body from tryptophan
**Pantothenic acid**
   Ubiquitous
**Biotin**
   Yeast, liver, kidneys, legumes, nuts, egg yolks (synthesized by intestinal bacteria)
**Folic acid**
   Leafy vegetables (lost in cooking), fruits, whole grains, wheat germ, orange juice, beans, nuts
**Cobalamin**
   Eggs, dairy products, liver, meats; none in plants
**Vitamin C**
   Fresh fruits and vegetables
**Carnitine**
   Meats, dairy products; none in plants

***Table 10–9.*** Circumstances in which the possibility of vitamin deficiencies merit consideration.

| Circumstance | Possible Deficiency |
| --- | --- |
| Prematurity | All vitamins |
| Protein-energy malnutrition | $B_1$, $B_2$, folate, A |
| Synthetic diets (including total parenteral nutrition) | All vitamins |
| Inherited disorders | Folate, $B_{12}$, D, carnitine |
| Vitamin–drug interactions | $B_6$, biotin, folate, $B_{12}$, carnitine, fat-soluble vitamins |
| Fat malabsorption syndrome | Fat-soluble vitamins |
| Breast-feeding | $B_1$,[a] folate,[b] $B_{12}$,[c] D,[d] K[e] |
| Periconceptional | Folate |

[a]Alcoholic or malnourished mother.
[b]Folate-deficient mother.
[c]Vegan mother or maternal pernicious anemia.
[d]Infant not exposed to sunlight and mother's vitamin D status suboptimal.
[e]Maternal status poor; neonatal prophylaxis omitted.

***Table 10–10.*** Causes of deficiencies in water-soluble vitamins.

**Thiamin**
   Infantile beriberi; seen in infants breast-fed by mothers with history of alcoholism or poor diet; has been described as complication of total parenteral nutrition (TPN); protein-energy malnutrition; prematurity
**Riboflavin**
   General undernutrition; prematurity; inactivation in total parenteral nutrition solutions exposed to light
**Pyridoxine**
   Prematurity (these infants may not convert pyridoxine to pyridoxal-5-P); $B_6$ dependency syndromes; drugs (isoniazid); heat-treated formulas (historical)
**Niacin**
   Maize or millet diets (high leucine and low tryptophan intakes); prematurity
**Pantothenic acid**
   None
**Biotin**
   Suppressed intestinal flora and impaired intestinal absorption
**Folic acid**
   Prematurity; seen in term breast-fed infants whose mothers are folate-deficient and in term infants fed unsupplemented processed cow's milk or goat's milk; kwashiorkor; chronic overcooking; malabsorption of folate because of a congenital defect; sprue; celiac disease; drugs (phenytoin)
   Increased requirements: chronic hemolytic anemias, diarrhea, malignancies, hypermetabolic states, infections, extensive skin disease, cirrhosis, pregnancy
**Cobalamin**
   Rare; seen in breast-fed infants of mothers with latent pernicious anemia or who are on an unsupplemented strict vegetarian diet; absence of luminal proteases; congenital malabsorption of $B_{12}$
**Vitamin C**
   Prematurity; maternal megadoses during pregnancy → deficiency in infants; lack of fresh fruits or vegetables; seen in infants fed formula and pasteurized cow's milk (historical)
**Carnitine**
   Seen in premature infants fed unsupplemented formula or fed intravenously; dialysis; inherited deficits in carnitine synthesis; organic acidemias; valproic acid

**Table 10–11.** Clinical features of deficiencies in water-soluble vitamins.

**Thiamin**
   Infantile beriberi (cardiac; aphonic; pseudomeningitic)
**Riboflavin**
   Cheilosis; angular stomatitis; glossitis; soreness and burning of lips and mouth; dermatitis of nasolabial fold and genitals; ± ocular signs (photophobia → indistinct vision)
**Pyridoxine**
   Listlessness; irritability; seizures; gastrointestinal disturbance; anemia; cheilosis; glossitis
**Niacin**
   Pellagra (weakness; lassitude; dermatitis of exposed areas; diarrhea; dementia)
**Pantothenic acid**
   Weakness; gastrointestinal disturbance; burning feet.
**Biotin**
   Scaly dermatitis; alopecia; irritability; lethargy
**Folic acid**
   Megaloblastic anemia; neutropenia; thrombocytopenia; growth retardation; delayed maturation of central nervous system in infants; diarrhea (mucosal ulcerations); glossitis; jaundice; mild splenomegaly; neural tube defects
**Cobalamin**
   Megaloblastic anemia; neurologic degeneration
**Vitamin C**
   Anorexia, irritability, apathy, pallor; fever; tachycardia; diarrhea; failure to thrive; increased susceptibility to infections; hemorrhages under skin, mucous membranes, into joints and under periosteum; long-bone tenderness; costochondral beading
**Carnitine**
   Increased serum triglycerides and free fatty acids; decreased ketones; fatty liver; hypoglycemia; progressive muscle weakness, cardiomyopathy, hypoglycemia

vitamins, with the exception of vitamin $B_{12}$, are not stored in the body.

Carnitine is synthesized in the liver and kidneys from lysine and methionine. In certain circumstances (see Table 10–10) synthesis is inadequate, and carnitine can then be considered a vitamin. A dietary supply of other organic compounds, such as inositol, may also be required in certain circumstances.

Honein MA et al: Impact of folic acid fortification of the US food supply on the occurrence of neural tube defects. JAMA 2001;285:2981 [PMID: 11410096].

McNulty H et al: Response of red blood cell folate to intervention: Implications for folate recommendations for the prevention of neural tube defects. Am J Clin Nutr 2000;71(5):1308S [PMID: 10799407].

# ■ INFANT FEEDING

## BREAST FEEDING

Breast feeding, one of the most important influences on children's health worldwide, provides optimal nutrition for the normal infant during the early months of life. Numerous immunologic factors in breast milk (including secretory IgA, lysozyme, lactoferrin, bifidus factor, and macrophages) provide protection against GI and upper respiratory infections. In developing countries, lack of refrigeration and contaminated water supplies make formula feeding hazardous. Allergic diseases are less common among breast-fed infants. Although formulas have improved progressively and are made to resemble breast milk as closely as possible, it is impossible to mimic the nutritional or immune composition of human milk. Additional differences of physiologic importance continue to be identified. Furthermore, the relationship developed through breast feeding can be an important part of early maternal interactions with the infant and provides a source of security and comfort to the infant.

Breast feeding has been reestablished as the predominant mode of feeding the young infant in the United States. Unfortunately, breast-feeding rates remain low among several subpopulations, including low-income, minority, and young mothers; many mothers face obstacles in maintaining lactation once they return to work. Skilled use of a breast pump, particularly an electric one, may help to maintain lactation in these circumstances.

Absolute contraindications to breast feeding are rare. They include tuberculosis (in the mother) and galactosemia (in the infant). Breast feeding is associated with maternal-to-child transmission of HIV, but the risk is influenced by duration and pattern of breast feeding and maternal factors, including immunologic status and presence of mastitis. Complete avoidance of breast feeding by HIV-infected women is presently the only mechanism to ensure prevention of maternal–infant transmission. Current recommendations are that HIV-infected mothers in developed countries refrain from breast feeding if safe alternatives are available. In developing countries, the benefits of breast feeding, especially the protection of the child against diarrheal illness and malnutrition outweigh the risk of HIV infection via breast milk.

The newborn weighing less than 1500 g and receiving human milk benefits from the addition of a human milk fortifier designed to increase the protein, calcium, phosphorus, and micronutrient content as well as the caloric density. Breast-fed infants with cystic fibrosis can be breast-fed successfully if exogenous pancreatic enzymes are provided. If normal growth rates are not achieved in the breast-fed child with CF, energy or specific macronutrient supplements may be necessary. All infants should receive supplemental vitamins A, D, E, K, and sodium chloride based on standardized nutrition protocols for cystic fibrosis.

Borowitz D et al: Consensus report on nutrition for pediatric patients with cystic fibrosis. J Pediatr Gastroenterol Nutr 2002;35:246-59 [PMID: 12352509].

Coutsoudis A, Rollins N: Breast-feeding and HIV transmission: The jury is still out. J Pediatr Gastroenterol Nutr 2003;26(4):434 [PMID: 12658031].

Ryan AS et al: Breastfeeding continues to increase into the new millennium. Pediatrics 2002;110(6):1103 [PMID: 12456906].

## Management of Breast Feeding

In developed countries, we cannot assume that the art of breast feeding is being automatically passed from mother to daughter. Health professionals are now playing roles of greater importance in supporting and promoting breast feeding. Organizations such as the La Leche League have been effective in promoting breast feeding and providing education and support for mothers and health professionals.

Perinatal hospital routines and follow-up pediatric care have a great influence on the successful initiation of breast feeding. Breast feeding is promoted by prenatal and postpartum education, frequent mother–baby contact after delivery, one-on-one advice about breast-feeding technique, demand feeding, rooming-in, avoidance of bottle supplements, early follow-up after delivery, maternal confidence, family support, adequate maternity leave, and good advice about common problems such as sore nipples. Breast feeding is undermined by mother and baby separations, bottle-feeding babies in the nursery at night, routinely offering supplemental bottles, conflicting advice from staff, incorrect infant positioning and latch-on, scheduled feedings, lack of maternal confidence or support, delayed follow-up, early return to employment, and inaccurate advice for common breast-feeding difficulties.

It is important for mothers to know that very few women are unable to nurse their babies. The newborn is generally fed ad libitum every 2–3 hours, with longer intervals (4–5 hours) at night. Thus a newborn infant nurses at least eight to ten times a day, so that a generous milk supply is stimulated. This frequency is not an indication of inadequate lactation. Mothers also need reassurance about the stooling patterns of breast-fed babies. In neonates, a loose stool is often passed with each feeding; later (at age 3–4 months), there may be an interval of several days between stools. Failure to pass several stools a day in the early weeks of breast feeding suggests inadequate milk intake and supply.

Expressing milk may be indicated if the mother returns to work or if the infant is premature, cannot suck adequately, or is hospitalized. Modern electric breast pumps are very effective and can be borrowed or rented.

## Technique of Breast Feeding

Breast feeding can be started after delivery as soon as both mother and baby are stable. Correct positioning and breast-feeding technique are necessary to ensure effective nipple stimulation and optimal breast emptying with minimal nipple discomfort.

If the mother wishes to nurse while sitting, the infant should be elevated to the height of the breast and turned completely to face the mother, so that their abdomens touch. The mother's arms supporting the infant should be held tightly at her side, bringing the baby's head in line with her breast. The breast should be supported by the lower fingers of her free hand, with the nipple compressed between the thumb and index fingers to make it more protractile. The infant's initial licking and mouthing of the nipple helps make it more erect. When the infant opens its mouth, the mother should rapidly insert as much nipple and areola as possible.

Some breast-fed infants fail to thrive. The most common cause of early failure to thrive is poorly managed mammary engorgement, which rapidly decreases milk supply. Unrelieved engorgement can result from inappropriately long intervals between feeding, improper infant suckling, a nondemanding infant, sore nipples, maternal or infant illness, nursing from only one breast, and latching difficulties. The mother's ignorance of technique, inappropriate feeding routines, and inadequate amounts of fluid and rest all can be factors. Some infants are too sleepy to do well on an ad libitum regimen and may need waking to feed at night. Primary lactation failure is rare, occurring in less than 5% of women.

A sensible guideline for duration of feeding is 5 minutes per breast at each feeding the first day, 10 minutes on each side at each feeding the second day, and approximately 15 minutes per side thereafter. A vigorous infant can obtain most of the available milk in 5–7 minutes, but additional sucking time ensures breast emptying, promotes milk production, and satisfies the infant's sucking urge. The side on which feeding is commenced should be alternated. The mother may break suction gently after nursing by inserting her finger between the baby's gums.

## Follow-Up

Individualized assessment before discharge should identify the mothers and infants needing additional support. All mother–infant pairs require early follow-up. The onset of copious milk secretion between the second and fourth postpartum days is a critical time in the establishment of lactation. Failure to empty the breasts during this time can cause engorgement, which quickly leads to diminished milk production.

## Common Problems

Nipple tenderness requires attention to proper positioning of the infant and correct latch-on. Ancillary measures include nursing for shorter periods, beginning feedings on the less sore side, air drying the nipples well after nursing, and use of lanolin cream. Severe nipple pain and cracking usually indicate improper infant attachment. Temporary pumping, which is well tolerated, may be needed.

Breast-feeding jaundice is exaggerated physiologic jaundice associated with inadequate intake of breast milk, infrequent stooling, and unsatisfactory weight gain (see Chapter 1). If possible, the jaundice should be managed by increasing the frequency of nursing and, if necessary, augmenting the infant's sucking with regular breast pumping. Supplemental feedings may be necessary, but care should be taken not to decrease breast milk production further.

In a small percentage of breast-fed infants, breast milk jaundice is caused by an unidentified property of the milk that inhibits conjugation of bilirubin. In severe cases, interruption of breast feeding for 24–36 hours may be necessary. The mother's breast should be emptied with an electric breast pump during this period.

The symptoms of mastitis include flu-like symptoms with breast tenderness, firmness, and erythema. Antibiotic therapy covering β-lactamase-producing organisms should be given for 10 days. Analgesics may be necessary, but breast feeding should be continued. Breast pumping may be helpful adjunctive therapy.

Neifert MR: Prevention of breastfeeding tragedies. Pediatr Clin North Am 2001;48(2):273 [PMID: 11339153].

## Maternal Drug Use

Many factors play a role in determining the transmission of drugs in breast milk, including the route of administration, dosage, molecular weight, pH, and protein binding. In general, any drug prescribed to newborns can be consumed via breast milk without ill effect. Very few drugs are absolutely contraindicated in breast-feeding mothers; these include radioactive compounds, antimetabolites, lithium, diazepam, chloramphenicol, antithyroid drugs, and tetracycline. For up-to-date information, a regional drug center should be consulted.

Maternal use of illicit or recreational drugs is a contraindication to breast feeding. Expression of milk for a feeding or two after use of a drug is not an acceptable compromise. The breast-fed infants of mothers taking methadone (but no alcohol or other drugs) as part of a treatment program have generally not experienced ill effects when the daily maternal methadone dose is under 40 mg.

American Academy of Pediatrics, Committee on Drugs: The transfer of drugs and other chemicals to human milk. Pediatrics 2001;108(3):776 [PMID: 11533352].

Case Western Reserve University: (http://www.breastfeedingbasics.org).

Dr. Hales Breastfeeding Pharmacology Page: (http://neonatal.ttuhsc.edu/lact/).

Lactation Education Resources: (http://www.leron-line.com/medications.htm).

Spencer JP et al: Medications in the breast-feeding mother. Am Fam Physician 2001;64(1):119 [PMID: 11456429].

## Nutrient Composition

The nutrient composition of human milk is summarized and compared with that of cow's milk and formulas in Table 10–12. Outstanding characteristics include (1) relatively low but highly bioavailable protein content, which is adequate for the normal infant; (2) generous but not excessive quantity of essential fatty acids; (3) long-chain unsaturated ω3 fatty acids, of which docosahexaenoic acid is thought to be especially important; (4) relatively low sodium and solute load; and (5) lower concentration of highly bioavailable calcium, iron, and zinc, which are adequate for the needs of normal breast-fed infants for approximately 6 months. A source of iron, from iron-fortified cereal, meat, or a supplement, should be introduced by age 6 months.

## Weaning and Complementary Foods

The American Academy of Pediatrics and the World Health Organization recommend the introduction of solid foods in normal infants at about 6 months of age. Gradual introduction of a variety of foods including enriched cereals, fruits, vegetables, and meats should complement the breast milk diet. Although the order of introduction is not critical, single-ingredient complementary foods are introduced one at a time at weekly intervals before a new food is given. Fruit juice is not an essential part of an infant diet. When introduced (ideally at > 6 months and with a cup), the amount should be limited to 4 oz/d. Breast feeding should ideally con-

***Table 10–12.*** The composition of milk (per 100 kcal).

| Nutrient (unit) | Minimal Level Recommended[a] | Mature Human Milk | Typical Commercial Formula | Cow's Milk (mean) |
|---|---|---|---|---|
| Protein (g) | 1.8[b] | 1.3–1.6 | 2.3 | 5.1 |
| Fat (g) | 3.3[c] | 5 | 5.3 | 5.7 |
| Carbohydrate (g) | — | 10.3 | 10.8 | 7.3 |
| Linoleic acid (mg) | 300 | 560 | 2300 | 125 |
| Vitamin A (IU) | 250 | 250 | 300 | 216 |
| Vitamin D (IU) | 40 | 3 | 63 | 3 |
| Vitamin E (IU) | 0.7/g linoleic acid | 0.3 | 2 | 0.1 |
| Vitamin K (µg) | 4 | 2 | 9 | 5 |
| Vitamin C (mg) | 8 | 7.8 | 8.1 | 2.3 |
| Thiamin (µg) | 40 | 25 | 80 | 59 |
| Riboflavin (µg) | 60 | 60 | 100 | 252 |
| Niacin (µg) | 250 | 250 | 1200 | 131 |
| Vitamin $B_6$ (µg) | 15 µg of protein | 15 | 63 | 66 |
| Folic acid (µg) | 4 | 4 | 10 | 8 |
| Pantothenic acid (µg) | 300 | 300 | 450 | 489 |
| Vitamin $B_{12}$ (µg) | 0.15 | 0.15 | 0.25 | 0.56 |
| Biotin (µg) | 1.5 | 1 | 2.5 | 3.1 |
| Inositol (mg) | 4 | 20 | 5.5 | 20 |
| Choline (mg) | 7 | 13 | 10 | 23 |
| Calcium (mg) | 5 | 50 | 75 | 186 |
| Phosphorus (mg) | 25 | 25 | 65 | 145 |
| Magnesium (mg) | 6 | 6 | 8 | 20 |
| Iron (mg) | 1 | 0.1 | 1.5 in fortified | 0.08 |
| Iodine (µg) | 5 | 4–9 | 10 | 7 |
| Copper (µg) | 60 | 25–60 | 80 | 20 |
| Zinc (mg) | 0.5 | 0.1–0.5 | 0.65 | 0.6 |
| Manganese (µg) | 5 | 1.5 | 5–160 | 3 |
| Sodium (mEq) | 0.9 | 1 | 1.7 | 3.3 |
| Potassium (mEq) | 2.1 | 2.1 | 2.7 | 6 |
| Chloride (mEq) | 1.6 | 1.6 | 2.3 | 4.6 |
| Osmolarity (mOsm) | — | 11.3 | 16–18.4 | 40 |

[a]Committee on Nutrition, American Academy of Pediatrics.
[b]Protein of nutritional quality equal to casein.
[c]Includes 300 mg of essential fatty acids.

tinue for at least 12 months, and thereafter for as long as mutually desired. Infants who are not breast-fed should receive standard iron-fortified infant formula. Whole cow's milk can be introduced after the first year of life.

American Academy of Pediatrics, Committee on Nutrition: The use and misuse of fruit juice in pediatrics. Pediatrics 2001;107(5):1210 [PMID: 11331711].

Dewey KG: Nutrition, growth, and complementary feeding of the breastfed infant. Pediatr Clin North Am 2001;48(1): 87 [PMID: 11236735].

Gibson RS, Hotz C: The adequacy of micronutrients in complementary foods. Pediatrics 2000;106(5):1298 [PMID: 11061842].

Kleinman RE: American Academy of Pediatrics recommendations for complementary feeding. Pediatrics 2000;106(5): 1274 [PMID: 11061819].

Kramer MS et al: Infant growth and health outcomes associated with 3 compared with 6 mo of exclusive breastfeeding. Am J Clin Nutr 2003;78:291 [PMID: 12885711].

## SPECIAL DIETARY PRODUCTS FOR INFANTS

### Soy Protein Formulas

A common rationale for the use of soy protein formulas is transient lactose intolerance after acute gastroenteritis. In such cases it is reasonable to recommend a soy protein formula for a period of 2–4 weeks. These formulas are also useful for infants with galactosemia and hereditary lactase deficiency. Lactose-free cow's milk protein-based formulas are also available. Soy protein formulas are often used in cases of suspected intolerance to cow's milk protein. Although infants with true cow's milk protein intolerance may also be intolerant of soy protein, those with documented IgE-mediated allergy to cow's milk protein usually do well on soy formula.

## Semielemental & Elemental Formulas

Semielemental formulas include protein hydrolysate formulas. The major nitrogen source of most of these products is casein hydrolysate, supplemented with selected amino acids. These formulas contains an abundance of EFA from vegetable oil; certain brands also provide substantial amounts of MCTs. Elemental formulas are available with free amino acids and varying levels and types of fat components.

Semielemental and elemental formulas are invaluable for infants with a wide variety of malabsorption syndromes. They are also effective in infants who cannot tolerate cow's milk and soy protein. For specific product information, consult standard pediatric reference texts, formula manufacturers, or a pediatric dietitian.

Hernell O, Lonnerdal B: Nutritional evaluation of protein hydrolysate formulas in healthy term infants: Plasma amino acids, hematology, and trace elements. Am J Clin Nutr 2003;78:296 [PMID: 12885712].

## Formula Additives

Occasionally it may be necessary to increase the caloric density of an infant feeding to provide greater calories or restrict fluid intake. Concentrating formula to 24–26 kcal/oz is usually well tolerated, delivers an acceptable renal solute load, and increases the density of all the nutrients. Beyond this, individual nutrient additives (Table 10–13) are usually employed to achieve the desired caloric density (up to 30 kcal/oz). Adding carbohydrates (eg, glucose polymers, maltodextrin) has the following benefits: they are generally well tolerated, mix readily with the formula, and are reasonably priced. Microlipid (Mead Johnson), a safflower lipid emulsion, also mixes well but is more expensive. MCT oil doesn't mix well and is expensive, but can be very beneficial for patients with cholestasis or malabsorptive disorders. The caloric density of breast milk can be increased by adding infant formula powder or any of the additives used with infant formula. Human milk fortifiers are generally used only for premature infants because of their specialized nutrient composition.

## Special Formulas

Special formulas are those in which one component, often an amino acid, is reduced in concentration or removed for the dietary management of a specific inborn metabolic disease. Also included under this heading are formulas designed for the management of specific disease states, such as hepatic failure, pulmonary failure with chronic carbon dioxide retention, and renal failure. These condition-specific formulas were made primarily with the critically ill adult in mind and are even

***Table 10–13.*** Common infant formula additives.

| Additive | Kcal/g | Kcal/Tbsp | Kcal/mL | Comments |
|---|---|---|---|---|
| Dry rice cereal | 3.75 | 15 | — | Thickens formula but not breast milk |
| Polycose (Ross) | 3.8 | 23 | 2 | Glucose polymers |
| Moducal (Mead Johnson) | 3.75 | 30 | — | Maltodextrin |
| MCT oil (Mead Johnson) | 8.3 | 116 | 7.7 | Not a source of essential fatty acids |
| Microlipid (Mead Johnson) | 9 | 68.5 | 4.5 | Safflower oil emulsion with 0.4 g linoleic acid/mL |
| Vegetable oil | 9 | 124 | 8.3 | Does not mix well |
| Promod (Ross) | 4.3 | 16.8 (3 g protein) | — | Whey protein concentrate |
| Casec (Mead Johnson) | 3.8 | 16.7 (4 g protein) | — | Calcium caseinate |
| Duocal (SHS) | 4.9 | 42 | — | Protein-free mix of hydrolyzed corn starch (60% kcal), and fat (35% MCT) |

MCT = medium-chain triglyceride.

used sparingly in those populations, thus their use in pediatrics should only be undertaken with clear indication and caution.

Complete information regarding the composition of these special formulas, the standard infant formulas, specific metabolic disease formulas, and premature infant formulas can be found in standard reference texts and in the manufacturers' literature.

## PRUDENT DIET

Because of the association of diet with the development of such chronic diseases as diabetes, obesity, and cardiovascular disease, learning a healthy eating behavior at a young age is an important preventative measure.

Salient features of a prudent diet for children older than 2 years include the following:

1. Consumption of three regular meals per day, and 2 or 3 healthful snacks according to appetite, activity, and growth needs.

2. Inclusion of a variety of foods. Diet should be nutritionally complete and promote optimal growth and activity.

3. Fat less than 30% of total calories (though severe fat restriction may result in an energy deficit and growth failure). Saturated fats and polyunsaturated fats each should provide less than 10% of total calories. Monounsaturated fats should provide 10% or more of caloric intake.

4. Cholesterol intake less than 100 mg/1000 kcal/d, to a maximum of 300 mg/d.

5. Carbohydrates should provide 55–60% or more of daily caloric intake, with no more than 10% in the form of simple sugars. A high-fiber, complex carbohydrate diet is recommended.

6. Limitation of grazing behavior, eating while watching television, and the consumption of soft drinks and other high-sugar beverages.

7. Limitation of sodium intake by choosing fresh over highly processed foods.

The consumption of lean cuts of meats, poultry, and fish should be encouraged. Skim milk, soft margarine, and vegetable oils (especially olive oil) should be used. Whole-grain bread and cereals and plentiful amounts of fruits and vegetables are recommended. The consumption of processed foods, soft drinks, desserts, and candy should be limited.

A prudent diet should be only one component of counseling on lifestyles for children. Other aspects are the maintenance of a desirable body weight and body mass index (BMI), regular physical activity, avoidance of smoking, and screening for hypertension. Universal screening for total cholesterol is controversial. Current recommendations are to routinely screen those children who have a positive family history of premature cardiovascular disease, although this approach will identify only about 50% of those with significantly elevated cholesterol levels. If the result is high ($\geq 200$ mg/dL), a fasting lipoprotein analysis should be obtained.

Coon KA et al: Relationships between use of television during meals and children's food consumption patterns. Pediatrics 2001;107:E7 [PMID: 11134471].

Kavey RE et al: American Heart Association guidelines for primary prevention of atherosclerotic cardiovascular disease beginning in childhood. J Pediatr 2003;142(4):368 [PMID: 12712052].

Lauer RM et al: Efficacy and safety of lowering dietary intake of total fat, saturated fat, and cholesterol in children with elevated LDL cholesterol: The Dietary Intervention Study in Children. Am J Clin Nutr 2000;72(Suppl):1332S [PMID: 11063475].

Obarzanek E et al: Long-term safety and efficacy of a cholesterol-lowering diet with elevated low-density lipoprotein cholesterol: Seven-year results of the Dietary Intervention Study in Children (DISC). Pediatrics 2001;107(2):256 [PMID: 11158455].

## ■ PEDIATRIC UNDERNUTRITION

**Failure to thrive** is a term used to describe infants and young children whose weight curve has fallen by two major percentile channels from a previously established rate of growth (see Chapter 8). The acute loss of weight, or failure to gain weight at the expected rate, produces a condition of reduced weight for height known as **wasting.** The reduction in height for age, as is seen with more chronic malnutrition, is termed **stunting.**

The typical pattern for mild pediatric undernutrition is decreased weight, with normal height and head circumference. In more chronic malnutrition, height and eventually head circumference growth will slow relative to the standard for age. Significant calorie deprivation produces severe wasting, called **marasmus.** Significant protein deprivation in the face of adequate energy intake, possibly with additional insults such as infection, may produce edematous malnutrition called **kwashiorkor.**

Pediatric undernutrition is usually multifactorial in origin, and successful treatment depends on accurate identification and management of those factors. The terms "organic" and "nonorganic" failure to thrive, though still used by many medical professionals, are not helpful because any systemic illness or chronic condition can cause growth impairment and yet may also be compounded by psychosocial problems.

A discussion of the multiple medical conditions that can cause pediatric undernutrition are beyond the scope of this chapter. However, the most common cause is inadequate dietary intake. Inappropriate formula mixing or a family's food beliefs may lead to hypocaloric or unbalanced dietary intakes. Highly restricted diets secondary to perceived food allergies or intolerances may result in inadequate intake of calories, protein, or specific micronutrients. Iron and zinc are micronutrients that are often marginal in many patients with undernutrition. Zinc deficiency can depress appetite and affect growth, and can easily be corrected with oral zinc supplements given over 1–2 months. Cases of severe malnutrition and kwashiorkor have occurred in infants of well-intentioned parents who substitute "health food" milk alternatives (eg, rice milk and unfortified soy milk) for infant formula.

Poor eating is often a learned behavior. Families should be counseled regarding choices of foods that are appropriate for the age and developmental level of the child. Children should have structured meal times (eg, three meals and two to three snacks during the day), ideally at the same time other family members eat. Consultation with a pediatric dietitian can be helpful for educating the families. Estimates of calorie needs should be based on the need for catch-up growth rather than on the usual RDA for age. Poor feeding may be related to family dysfunction. Children whose households are chaotic and children who are abused, neglected, or exposed to poorly controlled mental illness may be described as poor eaters, and may fail to gain. Careful assessment of the social environment of such children is critical, and disposition options may include support services, close medical follow-up visits, family counseling, and even foster placement while a parent receives therapy.

Carvalho NF et al: Severe nutritional deficiencies in toddlers resulting from health food milk alternatives. Pediatrics 2001;107(4):1 [PMID: 11335767].

Schwartz ID: Failure to thrive: An old nemesis in the new millennium. Pediatr Rev 2000;21(8):257 [PMID: 10922022].

# PEDIATRIC OVERWEIGHT/OBESITY (See also Chapter 3 for specifics on adolescent obesity.)

## Background

The prevalence of childhood and adolescent obesity has increased rapidly in the United States and many other parts of the world. Currently in the United States, approximately 15% of 6- to 19-year-olds are overweight, with even higher rates among subpopulations of minority and economically disadvantaged children. The increasing incidence of childhood obesity is related to a complex combination of genetic, environmental, psychosocial, biologic, and socioeconomic factors.

Overweight status in the pediatric population is associated with significant comorbidities, which if untreated are likely to persist into adulthood. The probability of obesity persisting into adulthood increases from 20% at 4 years to 80% by adolescence. Obesity is associated with cardiovascular and endocrine abnormalities (eg, dyslipidemia, insulin resistance and type II diabetes), orthopedic problems, pulmonary complications (eg, obstructive sleep apnea), and mental health problems.

## Definitions

BMI is the standard measure of obesity in adults. Its use in children provides a consistent measure across age groups. BMI is correlated with more accurate measures of body fatness and is calculated with readily available information: weight and height (kg ÷ m$^2$). Routine plotting of the BMI on age- and gender-appropriate charts (http://www.cdc.gov/growthcharts) can identify those with excess weight gain relative to linear growth. BMI between the 85th and 95th percentile for age and sex identifies those at risk of being overweight. Overweight or obese is defined as BMI at or above 95% and is associated with increased risk of secondary complications. An upward change in BMI percentiles in any range should prompt an evaluation and possible treatment. Although the degree of change that indicates risk has not been defined, an annual increase of 3–4 BMI units is almost always an indicator of a rapid increase in body fat. For children younger than 2 years old, weight for length greater than 95th percentile indicates overweight and warrants further assessment, especially of energy intake.

## Risk Factors

There are multiple risk factors for developing obesity, reflecting the complex relationships between genetic and environmental factors. Family history is a strong risk factor. If one parent is obese, the odds ratio is approximately 3 for obesity in adulthood, but if both parents are obese, the odds ratio increases to greater than 10.

Environmental risk factors offer potential areas to target for intervention. The absence of family meals, excessive consumption of sweetened beverages, large portion sizes, frequent consumption of foods prepared outside the home, excessive television viewing, and sedentary lifestyle are all associated with a greater prevalence of obesity.

## Assessment

Early recognition of high-risk patterns of weight gain or high-risk behaviors is essential, as it is likely that anticipatory guidance or intervention before weight gain becomes severe will be more successful. Routine evaluation at well-child visits should include:

1. Measurement of weight and height, calculation of BMI, and plotting all three parameters on age- and sex-appropriate growth charts (http://www.cdc.gov/growthcharts). Evaluate for upward crossing of BMI percentile channels.

2. History regarding diet and activity patterns (Table 10–14) Physical exam: Blood pressure, assess distribution of adiposity (central vs generalized); markers of comorbidities, such as acanthosis nigricans, hirsutism, hepatomegaly, orthopedic abnormalities; physical stigmata of genetic syndrome (eg, Prader–Willi syndrome).

3. Laboratory studies are generally reserved for children with BMI in overweight category (> 95th percentile) or those who have evidence of comorbidities; may include fasting lipid profile, insulin and glucose, liver function tests, thyroid function (if evidence of plateau in linear growth). Other studies should be guided by findings in history and physical.

*Table 10–14.* Suggested areas for assessment of diet and activity patterns.

---

**Diet**
  Meal and snack pattern: structured vs grazing, skipping meals
  Portion sizes: adult portions for young children?
  Frequency of meals away from home (restaurants or take out)
  Frequency/amounts of caloric beverages (soda, juice, milk)
  Frequency of eating fruits and vegetables
  Frequency of family meals?
**Activity**
  Time spent in sedentary activity: television, video games
  Time spent in vigorous activity: organized sports, physical education, free play
  Activities of daily living: walking to school, chores, yard work

---

## Treatment

Therapy should be based on risk factors, including age, severity of obesity, and comorbidities, as well as family history and support. For all children with uncomplicated obesity, the primary goal is to achieve healthy eating and activity patterns, not necessarily to achieve ideal body weight. For children with a secondary complication, improvement of the complication is an important goal. For children 2–7 years old with BMI at 95% or above and without complications, the goal should generally be maintenance of baseline weight, allowing the child to "grow into" his or her height, with a gradual normalization of BMI. For children 2–7 years old with BMI at 95% or above and secondary complications, weight loss is indicated. For children older than 7 years with BMI between 85th and 95th percentile, without complications, weight maintenance is an appropriate goal. If secondary complications are present, weight loss is recommended; an appropriate goal is 1 pound weight loss/month until a BMI less than 85% is achieved. Excessive acute weight loss should be avoided, as this may contribute to nutrient deficiencies and linear growth stunting.

There are few studies of the long-term effects of weight control programs for children. Treatment focused on behavior changes in the context of the family has been associated with sustained weight loss and decreases in BMI. Clinicians should assess the family's readiness to take action (stages-of-change model). Concurrent changes in dietary patterns and increasing physical activity are most likely to provide success. The whole family should be encouraged to adopt healthy eating patterns, with parents modeling healthy food choices, controlling foods brought into the home, and guiding appropriate portion sizes. Limiting sedentary activity has been found to be more effective than specifically promoting increased physical activity. The American Academy of Pediatrics recommends no television for children younger than 2 years old, and a maximum of 2 h/d of television and video games for older children.

Treatment may be considered at three different levels depending on the severity of the problem, the age of the child, the ability of the family to implement changes, the preferences of the parents and child, and the skills of the health care provider. (1) General: Counseling regarding problem areas identified by screening questions (see Table 10–14); emphasis on guidelines around healthy eating and physical activity patterns. This is especially appropriate for preventing further weight gain or for mildly overweight children. (2) Structured: Provide more specific and structured dietary pattern, such as meal planning, exercise prescription, behavior change goals. This may be done in the primary care setting or, if resources are available, referred to more specialized treatment program. (3) Group treatment: Generally best for the older child or adolescent, with varying level of parental involvement depending on age of child. Several published programs are available. The Weight Information Network (WIN) is a service available through the National Institutes of Health, which disseminates information on weight control programs and is available online: (http://www.niddk.nih.gosv//NutritionDocs.html). No single prescription is effective for all patients. The physician will do best to assess the severity of the problem, treatment needs in context of the family's preferences and abilities, and local resources, including availability of registered dietitians with expertise in pediatric weight management and behaviorists or family therapists.

Pharmacotherapy can be an adjunct to dietary, activity, and behavioral treatment, but by itself it is unlikely to result in significant or sustained weight loss. For severe obesity in adolescents, particularly with comorbidities, bariatric surgery is being performed in some centers. This is still considered experimental, and there is an urgent need for long-term outcome, safety, and efficacy data. However, there is limited evidence that in carefully selected and closely monitored patients, medications or surgery (or both) can result in significant weight loss with a reduction in comorbidities for those who are severely afflicted.

Barlow SE, Dietz WH: Obesity evaluation and treatment: Expert Committee Recommendations. Pediatrics 1998;102(3):e29 [PMID: 9724677].

Berkowitz RI et al: Behavior Therapy and sibutramine for the treatment of adolescent obesity. JAMA 2003;289(14): 1805. [PMID: 12684359].

Krebs NF, Jacobson MS, Committee on Nutrition, American Academy of Pediatrics: Prevention of Pediatric Overweight and Obesity Policy Statement. Pediatrics 2003;112(2):1 [PMID: 12897303].

Ogden CL et al: Prevalence and trends in overweight among US children and adolescents, 1999–2000. JAMA. 2002;288: 1728 [PMID: 12365956].

# NUTRITION SUPPORT

## 1. Enteral

### Indications

Enteral nutrition support is indicated when a patient cannot adequately meet nutritional needs by oral intake alone and has a functioning GI tract. This method of support can be used for both short- and long-term delivery of nutrition. Even when the gut cannot be used to deliver 100% of nutritional needs, some enteral feed-

ings should be attempted. Enteral nutrition, full or partial, provides multiple physiologic benefits:

1. Maintaining gut mucosal integrity
2. Preserving gut-associated lymphoid tissue
3. Stimulation of gut hormones and bile flow

Most pediatric patients requiring enteral nutrition can have their needs met with standard enteral formulations. Specialized formulas are available for patients of all ages who have conditions such as severe milk protein allergy, single- or multiple-nutrient malabsorption, renal failure, and hepatic failure. The decision to use such specialized formulas must be made in the context of the patient's condition and nutritional needs.

### Access Devices

Nasogastric feeding tubes can be used for supplemental nocturnal drip or daytime bolus feedings, but generally are not used for more than 6 months. Complications such as otitis media and sinusitis may limit the duration of nasogastric tube feedings. Initiation of nasogastric feeding usually requires a brief hospital stay to ensure tolerance to feedings and to allow for parental instruction in tube placement and feeding administration.

If long-term feeding support is anticipated, a more permanent feeding device, such as a gastrostomy tube, may be considered. With either a nasogastric or a gastrostomy tube, insurance coverage is important, as many carriers do not cover the cost of formula for tube feedings. Referral to a homecare company is necessary for equipment and other services such as nursing visits and dietitian follow-up.

Table 10–15 suggests appropriate timing for initiation and advancement of drip and bolus feedings, according to a child's age. Clinical status and tolerance to feedings should ultimately guide their advancement.

### Monitoring

Monitoring the adequacy of enteral feeding depends on nutritional goals. Growth should be frequently assessed, especially for young infants and malnourished children. Hydration status should be monitored carefully at the initiation of enteral feeding. Constipation and diarrhea can be problems, and attention to stool frequency, volume, and consistency can help guide management. When diarrhea occurs, factors such as infection, hypertonic enteral medications, antibiotic use, and alteration in normal gut flora should be addressed before formula changes are tried.

It is important to determine whether the feeding schedule is developmentally appropriate. This will not be possible for all patients, especially those who are crit-

**Table 10–15.** Guidelines for the initiation and advancement of tube feedings.

| Age | Drip Feeds | | Bolus Feeds | |
| --- | --- | --- | --- | --- |
| | Initiation | Advancement | Initiation | Advancement |
| Preterm | 1–2 mL/kg | 1 mL as tolerated | 5–20 mL | 5–10 mL as tolerated |
| Birth–12 mos. | 5–10 mL/h | 5–10 mL q 2–8 h | 10–60 mL | 20–40 mL q 3–4 h |
| 1–6 years | 10–15 mL/h | 10–15 mL q 2–8 h | 30–90 mL | 30–60 mL q feed |
| 6–14 years | 15–20 mL/h | 10–20 mL q 2–8 h | 60–120 mL | 60–90 mL q feed |
| > 14 years | 20–30 mL/h | 20–30 mL q 2–8 h | 60–120 mL | 60–120 mL q feed |

ically ill. However, for children who are more stable, it is recommended that tube feeding schedules mimic as closely as possible an age-appropriate feeding schedule, such as six small feedings per day for a toddler. When night drip feedings are used in conjunction with daytime feeds, it is suggested that less than 50% of goal calories be delivered at night so as to maintain a daytime sense of hunger and satiety. This will be especially important once a transition to oral intake begins. Children who are satiated by tube feedings will be less likely to take significant amounts of food by mouth, thus possibly delaying the transition from tube to oral nutrition.

## 2. Parenteral Nutrition

### Indications

#### A. PERIPHERAL PARENTERAL NUTRITION

Peripheral parenteral nutrition is indicated when complete enteral feeding is not possible or desirable (eg, in the premature infant of very low birth weight during the first few days of postnatal life or in the malnourished surgical patient during the early postoperative period). Short-term partial IV feeding via a peripheral vein is a preferred alternative to dextrose and electrolyte solutions alone. Because of the osmolality of the solutions required, it is usually impossible to achieve total calorie and protein needs with parenteral nutrition via a peripheral vein.

#### B. TOTAL PARENTERAL NUTRITION

TPN should be provided only when clearly indicated. Apart from the expense, numerous risks are associated with this method of feeding (see Complications section). Even when TPN is indicated, every effort should be made to provide at least a minimum of nutrients enterally to help preserve the integrity of the GI mucosa and of GI function.

The primary indication for TPN is the loss of function of the GI tract that prohibits the provision of more than a small proportion of required nutrients by the enteral route. Important examples include short bowel syndrome, some congenital defects of the GI tract, and prematurity.

### Cather Selection & Position

An indwelling central venous catheter is preferred for long-term IV nutrition. For periods of up to 3–4 weeks, a percutaneous central venous catheter threaded into the superior vena cava from a peripheral vein can be used. For the infusion of dextrose concentrations higher than 12.5%, the tip of the catheter should be located in the superior vena cava. Catheter positioning in the right atrium has been associated with complications, including right atrial thrombi formation. After placement, a chest radiograph must be obtained to check this position. If the catheter is to be used for nutrition and medications, a double-lumen catheter should be used if possible.

### Complications

#### A. MECHANICAL COMPLICATIONS

**1. Related to catheter insertion or to erosion of catheter through a major blood vessel**—Complications include trauma to adjacent tissues and organs, damage to the brachial plexus, hydrothorax, pneumothorax, hemothorax, and cerebrospinal fluid penetration. The catheter may slip during dressing or tubing changes, or the patient may manipulate the line.

Chaturvedi A et al: Catheter malplacement during central venous cannulation through arm veins in pediatric patients. J Neurosurg Anesthes 2003;15(3):170 [PMID: 12826963].

**2. Clotting of the catheter**—Addition of heparin (1000 U/L) to the solution is an effective means of preventing this complication. If an occluded catheter does not respond to heparin flushing, filling the catheter with recombinant tissue plasminogen activator or sterile 95% ethanol may be effective.

**3. Related to composition of infusate**—Calcium phosphate precipitation may occur if excess amounts of calcium or phosphorus are administered. Factors that increase the risk of calcium phosphate precipitation include increased pH and decreased concentrations of amino acids. Precipitation of medications incompatible with TPN or lipids can also cause clotting.

Freytes CO: Thromboembolic complications related to indwelling central venous catheters in children. Curr Opin Oncol 2003;15:289 [PMID: 12874506].

Hooke C: Recombinant tissue plasminogen activator for central venous access device occlusion. J Pediatr Oncol Nurs 2000;17(3):174 [PMID: 10944865].

### B. Septic Complications

Septic complications are the most common cause of nonelective catheter removal, but strict use of aseptic technique and limiting entry into the catheter can reduce the rates of line sepsis.

Fever over 38–38.5°C in a patient with a central catheter should be considered a line infection until proved otherwise. Cultures should be obtained and IV antibiotics empirically initiated. Removing the catheter may become necessary with certain infections (eg, fungal), with catheter replacement deferred until the infection is adequately treated.

Benjamin DK et al: Bacteremia, central catheters, and neonates: When to pull the line. Pediatrics 2001;107(6):1272 [PMID: 11389242].

### C. Metabolic Complications

A variety of metabolic complications associated with TPN may occur. Many of the complications are related to deficiencies or excesses of specific nutrients in administered fluids. These complications are less common as a result of experience and improvements in nutrient solutions. However, specific deficiencies still occur, especially in the premature infant. Avoidance of deficiencies and excesses and of metabolic disorders requires attention to the nutrient balance, electrolyte composition, and delivery rate of the infusate and careful monitoring, especially when the composition or delivery rate is changed.

Currently the most challenging metabolic complication is cholestasis, particularly common in premature infants of very low birth weight. The cause of cholestasis associated with TPN is unknown. Patient and med-

ical risk factors include prematurity, sepsis, hypoxia, major surgery (especially GI surgery), absence of enteral feedings, and small bowel bacterial overgrowth. Risk factors related to TPN include amino acid excess or imbalance and prolonged duration of TPN. Amino acid solutions with added cysteine decrease cholestasis. Practices that may minimize cholestasis include initiating even minimal enteral feedings as soon as feasible, avoiding sepsis by meticulous line care, avoiding overfeeding, using cysteine- and taurine-containing amino acid formulations designed for infants, preventing or treating small bowel bacterial overgrowth, protecting TPN solutions from light, and avoiding hepatotoxic medications.

Waitzberg DL et al: Access routes for nutritional therapy. World J Surg 2000;24(12):1468 [PMID: 11193710].

## NUTRIENT REQUIREMENTS & DELIVERY

### Energy

When patients are fed intravenously, no fat and carbohydrate intakes are unabsorbed, and no energy is used in nutrient absorption. These factors account for at least 7% of energy in the diet of the enterally fed patient. The intravenously fed patient also expends less energy in physical activity because of the impediment to mobility. Average energy requirements are therefore at least 7% lower in children fed intravenously, and the decrease in activity probably increases this figure to a total reduction of 10–15%. Caloric guidelines for the IV feeding of infants and young children are as follows:

| Age (months) | Requirements (kcal/kg/d) |
|---|---|
| 0–1 | 100–110 |
| 2–4 | 90–100 |
| 5–60 | 70–90 |
| >5 years | 1500 kcal for 1st 20 kg + 25 kcal for each additional kg/d |

These guidelines are averages; individuals vary considerably. A multitude of factors can significantly increase the energy requirement, including exposure to a cold environment, fever, sepsis, burns, trauma, cardiac or pulmonary disease, and catch-up growth after malnutrition.

With few exceptions, such as some cases of respiratory insufficiency, at least 50–60% of energy requirements are provided as glucose. Up to 40% of calories may be provided by IV fat emulsions.

## Dextrose

The energy density of IV dextrose (monohydrate) is 3.4 kcal/g. Dextrose is the main exogenous energy source provided by total IV feeding. IV dextrose suppresses gluconeogenesis and provides a substrate that can be oxidized directly, especially by the brain, red and white blood cells, and wounds. Because of the high osmolality of dextrose solutions ($D_{10}W$ yields 505 mOsm/kg $H_2O$), concentrations greater than 10–12.5% cannot be delivered via a peripheral vein or improperly positioned central line.

*Dosing guidelines:* The standard initial quantity of dextrose administered will vary by age (Table 10–16). Tolerance to IV dextrose normally increases rapidly, due primarily to suppression of hepatic production of endogenous glucose. Dextrose can be increased by 2.5 g/kg/d; by 2.5%–5%/day; or by 2–3 mg/kg/min/d if there is no glucosuria or hyperglycemia. Standard final infusates for infants via a properly positioned central venous line usually range from 15% to 25% dextrose, though concentrations of up to 30% dextrose may be used especially at low flow rates. Tolerance to IV dextrose loads is markedly diminished in the premature neonate and in hypermetabolic states.

Problems associated with IV dextrose administration include hyperglycemia, hyperosmolality, and glucosuria (with osmotic diuresis and dehydration). Possible causes of unexpected hyperglycemia include the following: (1) inadvertent infusion of higher glucose concentrations than ordered, (2) uneven flow rate, (3) sepsis, (4) a stress situation, and (5) pancreatitis. IV insulin reduces hyperglycemia but does not increase glucose oxidation rates; it may also decrease the oxidation of fatty acids, resulting in less energy for metabolism. Hence, insulin should be used very cautiously. A standard IV dose is 1 U/4 g of carbohydrate, but much smaller quantities may be adequate and, usually, one starts with 0.2–0.3 U/4 g of carbohydrate.

Hypoglycemia may occur after an abrupt decrease in or cessation of IV glucose. When cyclic IV nutrition is provided, the IV glucose load should be decreased steadily for 1–2 hours prior to discontinuing the infusate. If the central line must be removed, the IV dextrose should be tapered gradually over several hours.

Maximum oxidation rates for infused dextrose decrease with age. It is important to note that the ranges for dextrose administration provided in Table 10–16 are guidelines and that individual patient tolerance and clinical circumstances may warrant administration of either less or more dextrose. Quantities of exogenous dextrose in excess of maximal glucose oxidation rates are used initially to replace depleted glycogen stores; hepatic lipogenesis occurs thereafter.

**Table 10–16.** Pediatric macronutrient guidelines for total parenteral nutrition.

| Age | Dextrose | | Amino acids | Lipid |
|---|---|---|---|---|
| | mg/kg/min | g/kg/d | g/kg/d | g/kg/d |
| | 50–60% kcal | | 10–20% kcal | 30–40% kcal |
| Preterm | Initial 5–8 | Initial 7–11 | Initial 1.5–2 | Initial 0.5–1 |
| | Max 11–12.5 | Max 16–18 | Max 3–4 | Max 2.5–3.5 |
| Birth–12 mo. | Initial 6–8 | Initial 9–11 | Initial 1.5–2 | Initial 1 |
| | Max 11–15 | Max 16–21.5 | Max 3 | Max 2.5–3.5 |
| 1–6 yr | Initial 6–7 | Initial 8–10 | Initial 1–1.5 | Initial 1 |
| | Max 10–12 | Max 14–17 | Max 2–2.5 | Max 2.5–3.5 |
| > 6 yr | Initial 5–7 | Initial 8–10 | Initial 1 | Initial 1 |
| | Max 9 | Max 13 | Max 1.5–2 | Max 3 |
| > 10 yr | Initial 4–5 | Initial 5–7 | Initial 1 | Initial 1 |
| | Max 6–7 | Max 8–10 | Max 1.5–2 | Max 2–3 |
| Adolescents | Initial 2–3 | Initial 3–4 | Initial 1 | Initial 0.5–1 |
| | Max 5–6 | Max 7–8 | Max 1.5–2 | Max 2 |

Excess hepatic lipogenesis may lead to a fatty liver. Lipogenesis results in release of carbon dioxide, which when added to the amount of carbon dioxide produced by glucose oxidation (which is 40% greater than that produced by lipid oxidation) may elevate the $PaCO_2$ and aggravate respiratory insufficiency or impede weaning from a respirator.

## Lipids

The energy density of lipid emulsions (20%) is 10 kcal/g of lipid or 2 kcal/mL of infusate. The lipids are derived from either soybean or safflower oil. All consist of more than 50% linoleic acid and 4–9% linolenic acid. It is recognized that this high level of linoleic acid is not ideal, except when small quantities of lipid are being given to prevent an EFA deficiency. Ultimately, improved emulsions are anticipated. Because 10% and 20% lipid emulsions contain the same concentrations of phospholipids, a 10% solution delivers more phospholipid per gram of lipid than a 20% solution. Twenty percent lipid emulsions are preferred.

The level of LPL activity is the rate-limiting factor in the metabolism and clearance of fat emulsions from the circulation. LPL activity is inhibited or decreased by malnutrition, leukotrienes, immaturity, growth hormone, hypercholesterolemia, hyperphospholipidemia, and theophylline. LPL activity is enhanced by glucose, insulin, lipid, catecholamines, and exercise. Heparin releases LPL from the endothelium into the circulation and enhances the rate of hydrolysis and clearance of triglycerides. In small premature infants, low-dose heparin infusions may increase tolerance to IV lipid emulsion.

The advantages of using fat emulsions to provide up to 40% of caloric intake include the following:

1. The high energy density allows more energy to be provided when fluid volume is restricted.
2. The low osmolality (280 mOsm/kg $H_2O$) is of special value when using a peripheral line.
3. EFA deficiencies can be prevented.

4. The production of $CO_2$ is 40% lower per unit of energy, an important consideration in cases of pulmonary insufficiency.
5. The energy cost of fat storage is negligible.
6. The risk of fatty liver is decreased because of decreased hepatic lipogenesis from dextrose.

Potential disadvantages of fat emulsions include the following:

1. Impairment of function of neutrophils, macrophages, and the reticuloendothelial system.
2. Coagulation defects, including thrombocytopenia, elevated prothrombin time, and partial thromboplastin time.
3. Decrease in pulmonary oxygen diffusion.
4. Competition by free fatty acids with bilirubin and drugs for albumin-binding sites.
5. Increase in low-density lipoprotein cholesterol.

In general, these adverse effects can be avoided by starting with modest quantities and advancing cautiously in light of results of triglyceride monitoring and clinical circumstances. In cases of severe sepsis, special caution is required to ensure that the lipid is metabolized effectively. Monitoring with long-term use is also essential.

IV lipid dosing guidelines: Check serum triglycerides before starting and after increasing the dose. Commence with 1 g/kg/d, given over 12–20 hours or 24 hours in small preterm infants. Advance by 0.6–1.0 g/kg/d, every 1–2 days, up to goal (Table 10–16).

As a general rule, do not increase the dose if the serum triglyceride level is above 250 mg/dL during infusion (150 mg/dL in neonates) or if the level is greater than 150 mg/dL 6–12 hours after cessation of the lipid infusion.

Serum triglyceride levels above 400–600 mg/dL may precipitate pancreatitis. In patients for whom normal amounts of IV lipid are contraindicated, 4–8% of calories as IV lipid should be provided (300 mg linoleic acid/100 kcal) to prevent essential fatty acid deficiency.

***Table 10–17.*** Electrolyte requirements for parenteral nutrition.

| Electrolyte | Preterm Infant | Full-Term Infant | Child | Adolescent |
|---|---|---|---|---|
| Sodium | 2–5 mEq/kg | 2–3 mEq/kg | 2–3 mEq/kg | 60–150 mEq/d |
| Chloride | 2–5 mEq/kg | 2–3 mEq/kg | 2–3 mEq/kg | 60–150 mEq/d |
| Potassium | 2–3 mEq/kg | 2–3 mEq/kg | 2–3 mEq/kg | 70–180 mEq/d |

Neonates and malnourished pediatric patients receiving lipid-free parenteral nutrition are at high risk for EFA deficiency because of limited adipose stores.

Crook MA: Lipid clearance and total parenteral nutrition: The importance of monitoring plasma lipids. Nutrition 2000;16:774 [PMID: 10978859].

## Nitrogen

One gram of nitrogen is yielded by 6.25 g of protein (1 g of protein contains 16% nitrogen). Caloric density of protein is equal to 4 kcal/g.

### A. PROTEIN REQUIREMENTS

Protein requirements for IV feeding are the same as those for normal oral feeding (see Table 10–2).

### B. PROTEIN-ENERGY INTERACTIONS

There are important interactions between protein and energy requirements. A positive nitrogen balance cannot be achieved on a hypocaloric diet, because protein will be catabolized for energy. When energy intakes are low, the administration of some amino acid does, however, lessen the severity of the negative nitrogen balance. Conversely, when nitrogen intake is low, the provision of calories improves nitrogen balance to some extent. In infants, the energy necessary to minimize nitrogen loss associated with an amino acid-free diet is approximately 70 kcal/kg/d. At this level of energy intake, positive nitrogen balance depends on the level of nitrogen intake and is independent of further increase in energy intake.

In infants receiving about 50 kcal/kg/d, increasing protein intake up to 3 g/kg/d improves the nitrogen balance. In these circumstances, therefore, a ratio of grams of nitrogen per kilocalorie as low as 1:100 can be advantageous. However, at higher levels of energy intake, ratios of 1:250 to 1:150 or more are optimal. Although these ratios provide a useful crude check, they are not usually the best means of determining protein requirements.

### C. INTRAVENOUS AMINO ACID SOLUTIONS

Nitrogen requirements can be met by one of the commercially available amino acid solutions. For older children and adults, none of the standard preparations has a clear advantage over the others as a source of amino acids. For infants, however, including premature infants, accumulating evidence suggests that the use of TrophAmine (McGaw) is associated with a normal plasma amino acid profile, superior nitrogen retention, and a lower incidence of cholestasis. TrophAmine contains 60% essential amino acids, is relatively high in branched-chain amino acids, contains taurine, and is compatible with the addition of cysteine within

24–48 hours after administration. The dose of added cysteine is 40 mg/g of TrophAmine. The relatively low pH of TrophAmine is also advantageous for solubility of calcium and phosphorus.

### D. DOSING GUIDELINES

Amino acids can be started at 1.0–2.0 g/kg/d in most patients (see Table 10–16). In severely malnourished infants, the initial amount should be 1.0 g/kg/d. Even in very low birth weight infants, there is evidence that higher initial amounts of amino acids are tolerated with little indication of protein "toxicity." Larger quantities of amino acids in relation to calories can minimize the degree of negative nitrogen balance when the infusate is hypocaloric. Amino acid intake can be advanced by 0.5–1.0 g/kg/d toward the goal. Normally the final infusate will contain 2–3% amino acids, depending on the rate of infusion. Concentration should not be advanced beyond 2% in peripheral vein infusates due to osmolality.

### E. MONITORING

Monitoring for tolerance of the IV amino acid solutions should include routine blood urea nitrogen. Serum alkaline phosphatase, γ-glutamyltransferase, and bilirubin should be monitored to detect the onset of cholestatic liver disease.

### F. SPECIAL AMINO ACID PREPARATIONS

Some solutions are designed to provide high concentrations of branched-chain amino acids. These solutions are expensive and should not be ordered without a specific reason, which does not include their routine use in liver disease. They may be indicated in hepatic failure, especially in the presence of encephalopathy, and are also undergoing experimental use in multisystem organ failure. In this circumstance, the branched-chain amino acids are given as a source of metabolizable energy, providing up to 25% of energy intake. Solutions containing only essential amino acids may have some application in the management of acute renal failure.

### G. ALBUMIN

Albumin can be added to the infusate when clinically indicated to restore blood volume or oncotic pressure. If the origin of hypoalbuminemia is considered to be primarily nutritional, however, the hypoalbuminemia should be managed by careful nutritional rehabilitation rather than by IV administration of albumin. Albumin is deficient in isoleucine and tryptophan and has too long a half-life (15–20 days) to be considered a useful nutritional source of amino acids. Potential adverse effects of IV albumin administration include loss of albumin from the circulation into interstitial fluid of the lungs and elsewhere due to increased capillary permeability, coagulation defects secondary to volume expansion and dilution of clotting factors, inhibition of platelet aggregation, increases in prothrombin time and partial thromboplastin time, increased sodium intake in the albumin infusate, and increased binding to serum calcium resulting in decreased ionized calcium.

Albumin is a poor nutritional marker because of the number of nonnutritional factors that contribute to hypoalbuminemia.

Dosing Guidelines: When clinical circumstances warrant, albumin can be added to parenteral nutrition in the amount of 0.5–1.0 g/kg/d. The half-life of IV albumin in critical illness can be as short as under 12 hours. National shortages of albumin are not unusual. Thus its use must be reserved for patients with true therapeutic need who show a clinical response to the intervention.

## Minerals & Electrolytes

### A. CALCIUM, PHOSPHORUS, AND MAGNESIUM

Intravenously fed premature and full-term infants should be given relatively high amounts of calcium and phosphorus. Current recommendations are as follows: calcium, 500–600 mg/L; phosphorus, 400–450 mg/L; and magnesium, 50–70 mg/L. After age 1 year, the recommendations are as follows: calcium, 200–400 mg/L; phosphorus, 150–300 mg/L; and magnesium, 20–40 mg/L. The ratio of calcium to phosphorous should be 1.3:1 by weight or 1:1 by molar ratio. These recommendations are deliberately presented as milligrams per liter of infusate to avoid inadvertent administration of concentrations of calcium and phosphorus that are high enough to precipitate in the tubing. During periods of fluid restriction, care must be taken not to inadvertently increase the concentration of calcium and phosphorus in the infusate. These recommendations assume an average fluid intake of 120–150 mL/kg/d and an infusate of 25 g of amino acid per liter. With lower amino acid concentrations, the concentrations of calcium and phosphorus should be decreased.

### B. ELECTROLYTES

Standard recommendations are given in Table 10–17. After chloride requirements are met, the remainder of the anion required to balance the cation should be given as acetate to avoid the possibility of acidosis resulting from excessive chloride. The required concentrations of electrolytes depend to some extent on the flow rate of the infusate and must be modified if flow rates are unusually low or high and if there are specific indications in individual patients. IV sodium should be administered sparingly in the severely malnourished patient be-

cause of impaired membrane function and high intracellular sodium levels. Conversely, generous quantities of potassium are indicated. Replacement electrolytes and fluids should be delivered via a separate infusate.

### C. TRACE ELEMENTS

Recommended IV intakes of trace elements are as follows: zinc 100 µg/kg, copper 20 µg/kg, manganese 1 µg/kg, chromium 0.2 µg/kg, selenium 2 µg/kg, and iodide 1 µg/kg. Of note, IV zinc requirements may be as high as 400 µg/kg for premature infants and can be up to 250 µg/kg for infants with short bowel syndrome and significant GI losses of zinc. When IV nutrition is supplemental or limited to fewer than 2 weeks, and preexisting nutritional deficiencies are absent, only zinc need routinely be added.

IV copper requirements are relatively low in the young infant because of the presence of hepatic copper stores. These are significant even in the 28-week fetus. Circulating levels of copper and manganese should be monitored in the presence of cholestatic liver disease. If monitoring is not feasible, temporary withdrawal of added copper and manganese is advisable. Copper and manganese are excreted primarily in the bile, but selenium, chromium, and molybdenum are excreted primarily in the urine. These trace elements, therefore, should be administered with caution in the presence of renal failure.

Although low doses of iron are routinely added in some centers to the IV infusate for infants and children, no official recommendation has been made because of the lack of adequate published data regarding compatibility. Iron added to the infusate should be in a diluted form of iron dextran in a concentration of 1 mg/L. After age 2 months, maintenance IV iron requirements for the full-term infant are approximately 100 µg/kg/d. After the first month, the premature infant requires up to 200 µg/kg/d intravenously. Although overload is unlikely to occur during short-term parenteral nutrition, a surreptitious accumulation of extra iron could occur if parenteral nutrition is prolonged. This risk is enhanced if the patient has received blood transfusions. A second concern is that the potential for free iron is increased in malnourished infants with low transferrin levels. Excess iron is thought to enhance the risk of gram-negative septicemia. Iron has powerful oxidant properties and can enhance the demand for antioxidants, especially vitamin E. None of these concerns appear to preclude the routine use of iron supplements during IV nutrition, but they do emphasize the need for a conservative attitude in determining dosage schedules.

## Vitamins

Two vitamin formulations are available for use in pediatric parenteral nutrition: MVI Pediatric and MVI-

12 (AstraZeneca). MVI Pediatric contains the following: vitamin A, 0.7 mg; vitamin D, 400 IU; vitamin E, 7 mg; vitamin K, 200 μg; ascorbic acid, 80 mg; thiamin, 1.2 mg; riboflavin, 1.4 mg; niacinamide, 17 mg; pyridoxine, 1 mg; vitamin $B_{12}$, 1 μg; folic acid, 140 μg; pantothenate, 5 mg; and biotin, 20 μg. This formulation is suboptimal, with too little vitamin A and excessive amounts of water-soluble vitamins, but it is the best one available. Recommended dosing is as follows: 5 mL for children weighing more than 3 kg, 3.25 mL for infants 1–3 kg, and 1.5 mL for infants weighing less than 1 kg. Children older than 11 years old can receive 10 mL of the adult formulation, MVI-12, which contains the following: vitamin A, 1 mg; vitamin D, 200 IU; vitamin E, 10 mg; ascorbic acid, 100 mg; thiamin, 3 mg; riboflavin, 3.6 mg; niacinamide, 40 mg; pyridoxine, 4 mg; vitamin $B_{12}$, 5 μg; folic acid, 400 μg; pantothenate, 15 mg; and biotin, 60 μg. MVI-12 contains no vitamin K.

IV lipid preparations contain enough tocopherol to affect total blood tocopherol levels. The majority of tocopherol in soybean oil emulsion is α-tocopherol, which has substantially less biologic activity than the α-tocopherol present in safflower oil emulsions.

A dose of 40 IU/kg/d of vitamin D (maximum 400 IU/d) is adequate for both full-term and preterm infants.

## Fluid Requirements

The initial fluid volume and subsequent increments in flow rate are determined by basic fluid requirements, the patient's clinical status, and the extent to which additional fluid administration can be tolerated and may be required to achieve adequate nutrient intake. Calculation of initial fluid volumes to be administered should be based on standard pediatric practice. Tolerance of higher flow rates must be determined on an individual basis. If replacement fluids are required for ongoing abnormal losses, these should be administered via a separate line.

## Monitoring

Vital signs should be checked on each shift. With a central catheter in situ, a fever of more than 38.5°C requires that peripheral and central-line blood cultures, urine culture, complete physical examination, and examination of the IV entry point be made. Instability of vital signs, elevated white blood cell count with left shift, and glycosuria suggest sepsis. Removal of the central venous catheter should be considered if the patient is toxic or unresponsive to antibiotics.

### A. Physical Examination

Monitor especially for hepatomegaly (differential diagnoses include fluid overload, congestive heart failure, steatosis, and hepatitis) and edema (differential diagnoses include fluid overload, congestive heart failure, hypoalbuminemia, and thrombosis of superior vena cava).

### B. Intake and Output Record

Calories and volume delivered should be calculated from previous day's intake and output records (that which was delivered rather than that which was ordered). The following entries should be noted on flow sheets: IV, enteral, and total fluid (mL/kg/d); dextrose (g/kg/d or mg/kg/min); protein (g/kg/d); lipids (g/kg/d); energy (kcal/kg/d); percent of energy from enteral nutrition.

### C. Growth, Urine, and Blood

Routine monitoring guidelines are given in Table 10–18. These are minimum requirements, except in the very long-term stable patient. Individual variables should be monitored more frequently as indicated, as should additional variables or clinical indications. For example, a blood ammonia analysis should be ordered for an infant with lethargy, pallor, poor growth, acidosis, azotemia, or abnormal liver test results.

Greene HL et al: Guidelines for the use of vitamins, trace elements, calcium, magnesium, and phosphorus in infants and children receiving total parenteral nutrition: Report of the Subcommittee on Pediatric Parenteral Nutrient Requirements from the Committee on Clinical Practice Issues of the American Society for Clinical Nutrition. Am J Clin Nutr 1988;48: 1324 [PMID: 3142247].

Shulman RJ, Phillips S: Parenteral nutrition in infants and children. J Pediatr Gastroenterol Nutr 2003;36(5):587 [PMID: 12717082].

## INTENSIVE CARE NUTRITION

Severe stress of any kind (eg, large surface area and deep burns, major trauma, major surgery, sepsis) results in common metabolic changes that require special nutritional management. First, several hormones are increased, including thyroid hormone, catecholamines, cortisol, and glucagon. These hormones, acting directly on peripheral tissues or indirectly through an increase in peripheral insulin resistance, produce a hypermetabolic state accompanied by rapid protein catabolism and hyperglycemia. These hormonal changes develop in seconds for the catecholamines, within minutes for insulin and glucagon, and within hours for thyroid and cortisol. Rapid measurements of these hormones and their metabolic effects are not available for routine clinical management, so clinicians anticipate and deal with

***Table 10–18.*** Routine total parenteral nutrition monitoring summary.

| Variables | Acute Stage | Long-Term[b] |
|---|---|---|
| Growth | | |
|   Weight | Daily | Weekly |
|   Length | Weekly | |
|   Head circumference | Weekly | |
| Urine | | |
|   Glucose (dipstick) | With each void | With changes in intake or status |
|   Specific gravity | Void | |
|   Volume | Daily | |
| Blood | | |
|   Glucose | 4 hours after changes,[a] then daily × 2 days | Weekly |
|   $Na^+$, $K^+$, $Cl^-$, $CO_2$, blood urea nitrogen | Daily for 2 days after changes,[a] then twice weekly | Weekly |
|   $Ca^{2+}$, $Mg^{2+}$, P | Initially, then twice weekly | Weekly |
|   Total protein, albumin, bilirubin, aspartate transaminase, and alkaline phosphatase | Initially, then weekly | Every other week |
|   Zinc and copper | Initially according to clinical indications | Monthly |
|   Triglycerides | Initially, 1 day after changes,[a] then weekly | Weekly |
|   Compete blood count | Initially, then twice weekly; according to clinical indications (see text) | Twice weekly |

[a]Changes include alterations in concentration or flow rate.
[b]Long-term monitoring can be tapered to monthly or less often, depending on age, diagnosis, and clinical status of patient.

them. Early and aggressive IV and enteral nutrition are essential, with the goal of providing adequate nonprotein calories (favoring lipids over glucose) and amino acids to preserve essential protein structures. The utility of insulin infusion, including coinfusion of growth hormone and insulin-like growth factor-1 remains controversial.

Agnus MSD, Jaksic T: Nutritional support of the critically ill child. Curr Opin Pediatr 2002;14:470 [PMID: 12130914].

Briassoulis G et al: Energy expenditure in critically ill children. Crit Care Med 2000;28(4):1166 [PMID: 10809300].

## Provision of Nutrients in Hypermetabolic States

Enteral feeding should be continued whenever possible, so that the integrity of the enterocytes can be maintained. The increase in energy requirements varies according to the severity of hypermetabolism and its cause. Requirements are highest in burn patients, but major trauma and sepsis may increase energy requirements by 20–50% over resting energy needs. Mounting evidence suggests that increases in energy needs associated with acute stress are short-lived, and that in most cases energy needs equivalent to resting energy expendi-

ture will be adequate for the stressed patient. Ideally, energy expenditure should be measured in critically ill patients. When this is impossible, the patient should be monitored for weight gain (fluid vs tissue) and signs of overfeeding.

The muscle proteolysis and negative nitrogen balance characteristic of the hypermetabolic state cannot be counteracted totally by aggressive nutrition support, but the adverse effects can be attenuated. Negative nitrogen balance can be improved by providing 1.5–2 times the basal protein requirement for the patient's age. Larger quantities are unlikely to improve nitrogen balance, require substantial energy expenditure for oxidation, and increase $CO_2$ production.

Another metabolic aberration in the stress-induced, hypermetabolic state is uncontrolled hepatic gluconeogenesis, often producing markedly elevated blood glucose concentrations. Gluconeogenesis is not switched off, as would normally be expected, by the administration of IV dextrose. In fact, dextrose administration may aggravate hyperglycemia and increase hepatic lipogenesis. In some patients (especially those who develop multisystem organ failure), only very modest quantities of dextrose (< 45% of energy requirements) are tolerated. If severe hyperglycemia and glycosuria occur, insulin therapy may be necessary. However, the effects of insulin in hypermetabolic states are complex and not well clarified. Hypermetabolism is characterized by insulin resistance. Furthermore, insulin requires the simultaneous administration of greater than normal amounts ($\leq$ 25% of energy needs) of amino acids to limit or partially reverse muscle catabolism and gluconeogenesis. Theoretically, insulin administration could decrease lipolysis and thus deprive the hypermetabolic patient of some of the major sources of usable endogenous fuel.

Although lipolysis is increased in hypermetabolic states, beta-oxidation of fatty acids also is increased, at least initially. IV lipids usually can be metabolized well in early stages, and up to 50% of energy may be provided as lipid. Metabolically, lipid is the preferred fuel in patients with severe sepsis. Lipid tolerance deteriorates in advanced multisystem organ failure.

The metabolic and nutritional advantages of lipid as a fuel must be balanced against potential adverse effects in the septic child (see preceding discussion of IV lipids). It is important not to administer fat emulsion in excess of quantities that can be cleared effectively from the circulation.

Much interest has focused on the potential benefits of dietary factors in conferring an advantage to the immune system, called "immunonutrition." Of the factors studied, glutamine during acute stress has garnered much attention, though clinical trials have failed to show consistent results. Glutamine is a nonessential amino acid that is an important source of nitrogen for nucleic acid synthesis. It may become conditionally essential during acute illness and serve as a preferred energy source for certain tissues. Most glutamine supplementation studies have involved adults and have yielded conflicting results; thus its therapeutic relevance to pediatric populations is unknown. Other factors potentially useful as immune modulators include arginine, which has a central role in nitric oxide metabolism; nucleotides, which may be essential nutrients in formula-fed infants; probiotics, which may shorten the course of bacterial and viral gastroenteritis; and prebiotics, whose fermentation products (short-chain fatty acids) may be a source of nutrition for the colon. The use of these compounds in pediatric nutrition support is still experimental, and further research is needed to show clear safety and efficacy.

Ball PA, Hardy G: Glutamine in pediatrics: Where next? Nutrition 2002;18:451 [PMID: 12044814].

Buchman AL: Glutamine: Commercially essential or conditionally essential? A critical appraisal of the human data. Am J Clin Nutr 2001;74:25 [PMID: 11451714].

Jackson NC et al: Effects of glutamine supplementation, GH, and IGF-I on glutamine metabolism in critically ill patients. Am J Physiol Endocrinol Metab 2000;278:E226 [PMID: 10662706].

# Emergencies & Injuries

*F. Keith Battan, MD, & Marsha S. Anderson, MD*

## ■ I. EMERGENCIES & INJURIES

*F. Keith Battan, MD*

## ADVANCED LIFE SUPPORT FOR INFANTS & CHILDREN

A systematic approach to a seriously ill or injured child will allow rapid determination of the child's physiologic status and concurrent initiation of resuscitative measures. The goal of rapid assessment and intervention is not initially to make a specific clinical diagnosis but to correct any physiologic derangement—Is there airway obstruction or respiratory failure? Is there shock?—and then to intervene rapidly to ensure adequate oxygenation, ventilation, circulation, and thereby cerebral perfusion. Once initial resuscitative measures are begun, consideration of the cause of the arrest begins, with an emphasis on treatable, reversible causes. It is essential to determine whether any directed therapy (eg, glucose administration for hypoglycemia) is needed.

When progressive deterioration leads to bradycardia and ultimately to asystole, sufficient hypoxic and ischemic insult to the brain and other vital organs has occurred to make neurologic recovery extremely unlikely, even in the doubtful event that the child survives the arrest. Children who respond to ventilation and oxygenation alone or to less than 5 minutes of advanced life support are much more likely to survive neurologically intact. Therefore, it is essential to recognize the child who is at risk for progressing to cardiopulmonary arrest and to provide aggressive intervention before asystole occurs.

*Note:* Standard precautions must be maintained during resuscitation efforts.

## THE ABCS OF RESUSCITATION

Severely ill children should be rapidly evaluated in a deliberate sequence of *a*irway patency, *b*reathing adequacy, and *c*irculation integrity. Derangement at each point must be corrected before proceeding to the next function. Thus, if a child's airway is obstructed, the air- way must be opened (eg, by head positioning and the chin lift maneuver) before breathing and then circulation are assessed.

### Airway

Look, listen, and feel for upper airway patency: (1) *Look* for signs of obstruction such as inspiratory work or suprasternal retractions. A patient with significant airway obstruction will have an altered level of consciousness, such as agitation or lethargy. (2) *Listen* for adventitious breath sounds such as stridor, snoring, or gurgling. (3) *Feel* for air movement with your face near the child's mouth and nose.

The airway is managed initially by noninvasive means such as oxygen administration, chin lift, jaw thrust, suctioning, or bag–valve–mask ventilation, then by invasive maneuvers such as endotracheal intubation, laryngeal mask insertion, or, rarely, cricothyroidotomy. If neck injury is suspected, the cervical spine must be immobilized and kept from extension or flexion. (See Approach to the Pediatric Trauma Patient section.) The following discussion assumes that basic life support has been instituted.

Knowledge of pediatric anatomy is important for airway management. Infants are obligate nasal breathers; therefore, secretions or blood in the nasopharynx can cause significant distress. Children's tongues are large relative to their oral cavities, and the larynx is high and anteriorly located.

**A.** Place the head in the sniffing position (Figure 11–1). The neck should be slightly flexed and the head gently extended so as to bring the face forward. This position aligns the oral, pharyngeal, and tracheal planes (Figure 11–2). The head should be repositioned if airway obstruction persists after head tilt and jaw thrust. In an infant, the relatively large occiput puts the head in a sniffing position when supine; in an older child, more head extension is necessary. Avoid hyperextension of the neck, especially in infants.

**B.** Perform the chin lift or jaw thrust maneuver (Figure 11–3). Lift the chin upward while avoiding pressure on the submental triangle, or lift the jaw by traction upward on the angle of the jaw. Jaw thrust without head tilt should be done if cervical spine injury is possible.

**Figure 11-1.** Opening the airway with the head tilt/chin lift. Gently lift the chin with one hand and push down on the forehead with the other hand. (Reproduced, with permission, from *Textbook of Pediatric Life Support.* American Heart Association, 1997.)

**C.** Suction the mouth of secretions, blood, and foreign material.

**D.** Remove visible foreign bodies, using fingers or a Magill forceps—visualizing by means of a laryngoscope if necessary. Blind finger sweeps should not be done.

**E.** Insert an oropharyngeal or, in the conscious patient, a nasopharyngeal airway to relieve upper airway obstruction due to prolapse of the tongue into the posterior pharynx (Figures 11–4 and 11–5). This is the most common cause of airway obstruction in unconscious children. The correct size for an oropharyngeal airway is obtained by measuring from the upper central gumline to the angle of the jaw. Nasopharyngeal airways should fit snugly but not tightly within the nares and should be equal in length to the distance from the nares to the tragus.

## Breathing

Assessment of respiratory status is largely accomplished by inspection. (1) *Look* for adequate and symmetrical chest rise and fall, respiratory rate, increased work of breathing (including retractions, flaring, and grunting), accessory muscle use (eg, abdominal muscles), skin color, and tracheal deviation. Cyanosis is a late finding in children owing to their relative anemia, making pulse oximetry determination highly desirable. Again note mental status. (2) *Listen* for adventitious breath sounds such as wheezing. Auscultate for air entry, symmetry of breath sounds, and rales. (3) *Feel* for subcutaneous crepitus.

If spontaneous breathing is inadequate, initiate positive-pressure ventilation with bag–mask ventilation and 100% oxygen. If some respiratory effort is present but inadequate, coordinate bagging with the patient's efforts. Adequacy of ventilation is reflected in adequate rise and fall of the chest and auscultation of good air entry bilaterally. If the chest does not rise and fall easily with bagging, reposition the airway and repeat the maneuvers described previously in the Airway section. Perform airway foreign body extraction maneuvers if the airway remains obstructed, including visualizing the airway with a laryngoscope and using Magill forceps. The presence of asymmetrical breath sounds in a child in cardiac arrest or in severe distress suggests pneumothorax and is an indication for needle thoracostomy.

**Figure 11–2.** Correct positioning of the child older than 2 years of age for ventilation and tracheal intubation. **A:** With the patient on a flat surface (eg, bed or table), the oral (O), pharyngeal (P), and tracheal (T) axes pass through three divergent planes. **B:** A folded sheet or towel placed under the occiput of the head aligns the pharyngeal and tracheal axes. **C:** Extension of the atlanto-occipital joint results in alignment of the oral, pharyngeal, and tracheal axes. (Reproduced, with permission, from *Textbook of Pediatric Life Support.* American Heart Association, 1997.)

In small children, the transmission of breath sounds throughout the chest may impair the ability to auscultate the presence of a pneumothorax. Bag–mask ventilation is effective in the *vast* majority of cases. *Note:* Effective oxygenation and ventilation are the keys to successful resuscitation.

Using cricoid pressure (Sellick maneuver) during all positive-pressure ventilation, intubate the trachea in patients unresponsive to bag–mask ventilation, those in coma, those who require airway protection, or those who will require prolonged ventilation. Advanced airway management techniques are described in the references accompanying this section. Cricothyroidotomy is rarely necessary. (See Approach to the Pediatric Trauma Patient section.)

## Circulation

The diagnosis of shock must be rapid. Diagnosis can and should be made by clinical examination. Clinical assessments A–E are often referred to as an assessment of perfusion:

### A. Pulses

Check adequacy of peripheral pulses. Pulses become weak and thready only with severe hypovolemia. Compare peripheral pulses to central pulses.

### B. Heart Rate

Compare with age-specific norms. Tachycardia can be a nonspecific sign of distress, whereas bradycardia for age is a prearrest sign and necessitates aggressive resuscitation.

### C. Extremities

As shock progresses, extremities become cooler, from distal to proximal. For example, a child whose extremities are cool distal to the elbows and knees is in severe shock.

### D. Capillary Refill Time

This is an important indicator of perfusion. A refill time longer than 2.0 seconds is abnormal unless the child is cold.

### E. Mental Status

Hypoxia, hypercapnia, or ischemia will result in altered mental status. Remember that other important treatable conditions may also result in altered mental status, such as intracranial hemorrhage, meningitis, and hypoglycemia.

### F. Skin Color

Compromised cardiopulmonary status can cause pallor or gray, mottled, or ashen skin colors.

**Figure 11–3.** Opening the airway with the jaw thrust. Lift the angles of the mandible. This moves the jaw and tongue forward and opens the airway without bending the neck. (Reproduced, with permission, from *Textbook of Pediatric Life Support*. American Heart Association, 1997.)

**Figure 11–4.** **A-D:** Selection of an oral airway. An airway of the proper size will relieve obstruction caused by the tongue without damaging laryngeal structures. The appropriate size can be estimated by holding the airway next to the child's face (**A**). The tip of the airway should end just cephalad to the angle of the mandible (*dashed line*), resulting in proper alignment with the glottic opening (**B**). If the oral airway inserted is too large, the tip will align posterior to the angle of the mandible (**C**) and obstruct the glottic opening by pushing the epiglottis down (*arrow*). If the oral airway is too small, the tip will align well above the angle of the mandible (**D**) and exacerbate airway obstruction by pushing the tongue into the hypopharynx (*arrows*). (Adapted, with permission, from Cote and Todres in *Textbook of Pediatric Life Support*. American Heart Association, 1997.)

*Figure 11–5.* **A:** Nasopharyngeal airways. A shortened tracheal tube may be substituted (to reduce resistance). **B:** Placement of a nasopharyngeal airway. **C:** Shortened (cut) tracheal tube used as a nasopharyngeal airway. Note that the standard 15-mm adapter must be firmly reinserted into the tracheal tube. (Reproduced, with permission, from *Textbook of Pediatric Life Support.* American Heart Association, 1997.)

In the figure labels:
Nasopharyngeal airways (2), shortened endotracheal tube

Nasopharyngeal airway in place

### G. Blood Pressure

Blood pressure determination is not necessary to make the diagnosis of shock. It is important to remember that shock or inadequate perfusion of vital organs may be present before the blood pressure falls below the normal limits for age. As intravascular volume falls, peripheral vascular resistance increases so that blood pressure is maintained until there is 35–40% depletion of blood volume, followed by precipitous and often irreversible deterioration of perfusion (Figure 11–6). Shock that occurs with signs of decreased perfusion (eg, tachycardia and delayed capillary refill time) but normal blood pressure is compensated shock. When blood pressure also falls, decompensated shock is present. The appropriate-size cuff must be used to obtain an accurate blood pressure. Blood pressure determination should be done manually, because automated machines can give erroneous readings in children.

## MANAGEMENT OF SHOCK

Intravenous (IV) access is essential but can be difficult to establish in children with shock. Peripheral access, especially the antecubital veins, should be attempted first, but central cannulation—depending on individual expertise—should follow quickly if peripheral access is unsuccessful. Alternatives are percutaneous cannulation

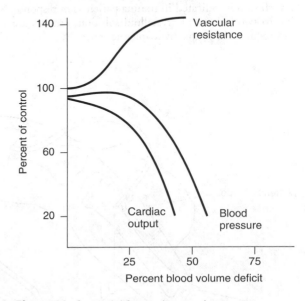

*Figure 11–6.* Model for cardiovascular response to hypovolemia from hemorrhage (based on normative data). (Reproduced, with permission, from *Textbook of Pediatric Life Support.* American Heart Association, 1997.)

of femoral, subclavian, or internal or external jugular veins; cutdown at antecubital, femoral, or saphenous sites; or intraosseous (IO) lines (Figure 11–7). Consider IO needle placement in any severely ill child when venous access cannot be established rapidly. Use short, wide-bore catheters to allow maximal flow rates. Two IV lines should be started in severely ill children. In newborns, the umbilical veins may be cannulated. Consider arterial access if beat-to-beat monitoring or frequent laboratory tests will be needed.

## Differentiation of Shock States & Initial Therapy

Therapy for inadequate circulation is determined by the cause of circulatory failure.

### A. HYPOVOLEMIC SHOCK

The most common type of shock in the pediatric population is hypovolemic. Frequent causes include dehydration, diabetes, or heat illness; hemorrhage; and burns. Initial therapy is with isotonic crystalloid solution, that is, normal saline or lactated Ringer solution. Give 20 mL/kg body weight, repeated as necessary, with frequent reassessments, until perfusion normalizes. Children tolerate large volumes of fluid replacement—the full circulating blood volume of 80 mL/kg could potentially be given safely with appropriate monitoring and reassessment. Typically, in hypovolemic shock, no more than 50 mL/kg is needed. Packed red blood cell transfusion is indicated in trauma patients not responding to two boluses of crystalloid solution. Pressors are not required in simple hypovolemic states.

### B. DISTRIBUTIVE SHOCK

Distributive shock represents relative hypovolemia from increased vascular capacitance of circulating volume. Examples are sepsis, anaphylaxis, and spinal cord injury. Initial therapy is again by limited isotonic volume replacement with crystalloid, but pressors may be necessary if perfusion does not normalize after delivery of two 20 mL/kg boluses of crystalloid. Children in distributive shock must be admitted to a pediatric intensive care unit.

### C. CARDIOGENIC SHOCK

Cardiogenic shock can occur as a complication of congenital heart disease, myocarditis, dysrhythmias, ingestions (eg, clonidine, cyclic antidepressants), or as a sequela of prolonged shock due to any cause. The diagnosis is suggested by any of the following signs: abnormal cardiac rhythm, distended neck veins, rales, abnormal heart sounds such as an $S_3$ or $S_4$, friction rub, narrow pulse pressure, or hepatomegaly. Chest radiographs will show cardiomegaly and pulmonary edema—not seen in shock due to other causes. An initial bolus of crystalloid may be given, but dopamine or other pressors, and possibly agents to reduce afterload, are necessary to improve perfusion. Comprehensive cardiopulmonary monitoring is essential. Children in cardiogenic shock must be admitted to a pediatric intensive care unit.

## Observation & Further Management

Reassess perfusion after each fluid bolus to determine additional fluid needs. Serial central venous pressure

Tibial tuberosity

Anterior border

90° to medial surface

***Figure 11–7.*** IO cannulation technique. (Reproduced, with permission, from *Textbook of Pediatric Life Support.* American Heart Association, 1997.)

determinations or a chest radiograph may aid clinical assessments to help determine volume status. Place an indwelling urinary catheter to monitor urine output.

Caution must be exercised with volume replacement if intracranial pressure is potentially elevated, as in severe head injury, diabetic ketoacidosis, or meningitis. Even in such situations, however, normal intravascular volume must be restored, as reflected by adequate peripheral perfusion and mean arterial pressure, to achieve adequate cerebral perfusion pressure.

## Summary of Cardiopulmonary Resuscitation

Assess the ABCs in sequential fashion and begin interventions as soon as a derangement is detected—before assessing the next system. After each intervention, it is essential that each system be reassessed to ensure improvement and to avoid failing to recognize clinical deterioration.

Chameides L et al (eds): *Textbook of Pediatric Advanced Life Support.* American Heart Association/American Academy of Pediatrics, 2002.

*Textbook of Advanced Pediatric Life Support,* 4th ed. APLS Joint Task Force: American College of Emergency Physicians/ American Academy of Pediatrics, 2003.

http://www.aap.org/apls/aplsmain.htm

# EMERGENCY PEDIATRIC DRUGS

Though careful attention to airway and breathing remains the mainstay of pediatric resuscitation, medications are often needed. Rapid delivery to the central circulation, which can be via peripheral IV catheter, is essential. Infuse medications close to the catheter's hub and flush in with saline to achieve the most rapid systemic effects. If no IV or IO access is achievable, some drugs may be given by endotracheal tube (Table 11–1). The use of length-based emergency measuring tapes that contain preprinted drug dosages, equipment sizes, and IV fluid amounts (Broselow tapes) or preprinted resuscitation drug charts is much more accurate than

**Table 11–1.** Emergency drugs that can be given by endotracheal tube.

| |
|---|
| Lidocaine |
| Epinephrine |
| Atropine |
| Naloxone |

estimation formulas and helps minimize dosing errors. Selected emergency drugs used in pediatrics are summarized in Table 11–2.

# APPROACH TO THE SERIOUSLY ILL CHILD

An unstable patient may present with a known diagnosis, such as a child known to have asthma in status asthmaticus and respiratory failure, or a child with known congenital heart disease. Often a child presents in cardiorespiratory failure of unknown cause. The initial approach is designed to rapidly identify and reverse life-threatening conditions. Children with chronic disease may present with an exacerbation in that system or secondary to a new, unrelated problem.

## Preparation for Emergency Management

Resuscitation occurs simultaneously at two levels: rapid cardiopulmonary assessment, with indicated stabilizing measures, while venous access ("lifelines") are gained and cardiopulmonary monitoring initiated. The technique of accomplishing these concurrent goals is outlined as follows:

**A.** If advance notice of the patient's arrival has been received, prepare a resuscitation room and summon appropriate personnel as needed, such as a neurosurgeon for an unresponsive child after severe head injury or a radiology technician for imaging studies.

**B.** Assign team responsibilities, including a team leader plus others designated to manage the airway, perform chest compressions, achieve access, draw blood for laboratory studies, place monitors, gather additional historical data, and provide family support.

**C.** Age-appropriate equipment should be made ready, including a cardiorespiratory monitor, pulse oximeter, and appropriate blood pressure cuff. Age- and weight-appropriate laryngoscope blades, endotracheal tubes, a naso- or orogastric tube, and an indwelling urinary catheter should be assembled for rapid access. Use a length-based emergency tape if available. See Table 11–3 for sizes.

## Reception & Assessment

When the patient arrives, the team leader begins a rapid assessment as team members perform their preassigned tasks. If the patient is received from prehospital care providers, careful attention must be paid to their report, because they have information that they alone have observed. Interventions and medications should be ordered only by the team leader to avoid confusion, and the leader should refrain from personally perform-

*Table 11-2.* Emergency pediatric drugs.

| Drug | Indications | Dosage and Route | Comment |
|---|---|---|---|
| Atropine | 1. Bradycardia, especially cardiac in origin<br>2. Vagally mediated bradycardia, eg, during laryngoscopy and intubation<br>3. Anticholinesterase poisoning | 0.01–0.02 mg/kg (minimum, 0.1 mg; maximum, 2 mg) IV, IO, ET. May repeat every 5 min. | Atropine may be useful in hemodynamically significant primary cardiac-based bradycardias. Because of paradoxic bradycardia sometimes seen in infants, a minimum dose of 0.1 mg is recommended by the American Heart Association. Epinephrine is the first-line drug in pediatrics for bradycardia caused by hypoxia or ischemia. |
| Bicarbonate | 1. Documented metabolic acidosis<br>2. Hyperkalemia | 1 meq/kg IV or IO; by arterial blood gas: $0.3 \times$ kg $\times$ base deficit. May repeat every 5 min. | Infuse slowly. Sodium bicarbonate will be effective only if the patient is adequately oxygenated, ventilated, and perfused. Some adverse side effects. |
| Calcium chloride 10% | 1. Documented hypocalcemia<br>2. Calcium channel blocker overdose<br>3. Hyperkalemia, hypermagnesemia | 10–30 mg/kg slowly IV, preferably centrally, or IO with caution. | Calcium is no longer indicated for asystole. Potent tissue necrosis results if infiltration occurs. Use with caution. |
| Epinephrine | 1. Bradycardia, especially hypoxic–ischemic<br>2. Hypotension (by infusion)<br>3. Asystole<br>4. Fine ventricular fibrillation refractory to initial defibrillation<br>5. Pulseless electrical activity<br>6. Anaphylaxis | Bradycardia and first dose in arrests: 0.01 mg/kg of 1:10,000 solution IV or IO. Second and subsequent doses in arrests: 0.1–0.2 mg/kg of 1:1000 solution IV or IO. Repeat every 3–5 min.<br>ET: 10x intended IV dose<br>SC: 0.01 mg/kg of 1:1000 solution (= 0.01 mL/kg) (anaphylactic shock). Maximum dose: 0.3–0.5 mL.<br>Constant infusion by IV drip: 0.1–1 µg/kg/min. | Epinephrine is the single most important drug in pediatric resuscitation. Evidence from animal studies and small series of human subjects indicates that the present recommended dose may be insufficient, and some clinicians use doses of 0.1–0.3 mg/kg IV. A randomized controlled trial has not been done. |
| Glucose | 1. Hypoglycemia<br>2. Altered mental status (empirical)<br>3. With insulin, for hyperkalemia | 0.5–1 g/kg IV or, IO. May repeat as necessary. | Neonates: 1 cc/kg $D_{10}W$. Older children: 2–4 cc/kg $D_{25}W$, 6–10 cc/kg $D_{10}W$. |
| Naloxone | 1. Opioid overdose<br>2. Altered mental status (empirical) | 0.1 mg/kg IV, IO, or ET; maximum dose, 2 mg. May repeat as necessary. | Side effects are few. A dose of 2 mg may be given in young children. Repeat as necessary, or give as constant infusion in opioid overdoses. |

ET = endotracheally, IO = intraosseously, IV = intravenously, SC = subcutaneously.

***Table 11–3.*** Equipment sizes and estimated weight by age.

| Age (years) | Weight (kg) | Endotracheal Tube Size (mm)[a] | Laryngoscope Blade (Size) | Chest Tube (Fr) | Foley (Fr) |
|---|---|---|---|---|---|
| Premature | 1–2.5 | 2.5 uncuffed | 0 | 8 | 5 |
| Term newborn | 3 | 3.0 | 0–1 | 10 | 8 |
| 1 | 10 | 3.5–4.0 | 1 | 18 | 8 |
| 2 | 12 | 4.5 | 1 | 18 | 10 |
| 3 | 14 | 4.5 | 1 | 20 | 10 |
| 4 | 16 | 5.0 | 2 | 22 | 10 |
| 5 | 18 | 5.0–5.5 | 2 | 24 | 10 |
| 6 | 20 | 5.5 | 2 | 26 | 12 |
| 7 | 22 | 5.5–6.0 | 2 | 26 | 12 |
| 8 | 24 | 6.0 cuffed | 2 | 28 | 14 |
| 10 | 32 | 6.0–6.5 cuffed | 2–3 | 30 | 14 |
| Adolescent | 50 | 7.0 cuffed | 3 | 36 | 14 |
| Adult | 70 | 8.0 cuffed | 3 | 40 | 14 |

[a]Internal diameter.

ing procedures, which may distract him or her from optimal direction of the resuscitation. A complete timed record should be kept of events, including medications, interventions, and response to intervention.

### A. All Cases

In addition to cardiac compressions and ventilation, ensure that the following are instituted:

1. 100% high-flow oxygen.
2. Monitoring, including cardiorespiratory, pulse oximetry, and end-tidal $CO_2$ if the patient is intubated.
3. IV (peripheral, IO, or central) access. Two lines preferred.
4. Blood drawn and sent. Bedside blood glucose determination is essential.
5. Full vital signs obtained.
6. Clothes removed.
7. Foley catheter and naso- or orogastric tube inserted.
8. Complete history.
9. Notify needed consultants.
10. Family support.
11. Consider law enforcement or security activation and emergency unit lockdown for cases possibly involving terrorism, gang violence, or threats to staff or family.

### B. As Appropriate

1. Immobilize neck.
2. Have chest radiograph taken for line and tube placement.
3. Insert central venous pressure and arterial line.

Patterson M: Resuscitation update for the pediatrician. Pediatr Clin North Am 1999;46:1285 [PMID: 10629685].

## APPROACH TO THE PEDIATRIC TRAUMA PATIENT

Injuries, including motor vehicle crashes, falls, burns, and immersions, account for the greatest number of deaths among children older than age 1 year. All providers of pediatric care must be cognizant of this sobering statistic, become involved, and work with injury prevention specialists, prehospital providers, and emergency, critical care, and rehabilitation physicians and nurses to reduce this terrible loss.

A team approach to the severely injured child, using assigned roles as outlined in the preceding section, will optimize outcomes. A calm atmosphere in the receiving area will contribute to thoughtful care. Conscious children are terribly frightened by serious injury; constant reassurance can help alleviate anxiety. Analgesia and sedation can and should be given to stable patients. It is unconscionable in the modern era to let children suffer pain needlessly. Treat pain expeditiously with oral or parenteral narcotics with appropriate monitoring. Parents are often anxious, angry, or guilty and require ongoing support from the services of staff, social workers or child life workers (therapists knowledgeable about child development). To provide optimal multidisciplinary care, regional pediatric trauma centers provide dedicated teams of pediatric specialists in emergency pediatrics, trauma surgery, orthopedics, neurosurgery, and critical care. Because most children with severe injuries are not seen in these centers, however, primary care providers must be able to provide initial assessment and stabilization of the child with life-threatening injuries before transport to a verified pediatric trauma center.

## Mechanism of Injury

Document the time of occurrence, the type of energy transfer to the child (eg, hit by a car, rapid deceleration), secondary impacts if the child was thrown by the initial impact, appearance of the child at the scene, interventions performed, and clinical condition during transport. The report of emergency service personnel is invaluable. All information of this type must be forwarded with the patient to the referral facility if secondary transport occurs.

Trauma in children is predominantly blunt, although penetrating trauma occurs in 10% of cases. Head and abdominal injuries are particularly common and important in the pediatric age group.

## Initial Assessment & Management

The vast majority of children who reach a hospital alive survive to discharge. Most deaths from trauma in children are due to head injuries. Therefore, cerebral resuscitation must be the foremost consideration when treating children with serious injuries. The ultimate measure of outcome is the child's eventual level of functioning. Strict attention to the ABCs ensures optimal oxygenation, ventilation, and perfusion, and ultimately, cerebral perfusion.

The primary and secondary survey is a method for evaluating and treating injured patients in a systematic way that provides a rapid assessment and stabilization phase, followed by a head-to-toe examination and definitive care phase.

## PRIMARY SURVEY

The primary survey is designed to identify rapidly and treat immediately all physiologic derangements resulting from trauma. It is the resuscitation phase. Priorities are still airway, breathing, and circulation, but with important further considerations in the trauma setting:

*A*irway, with cervical spine control
*B*reathing
*C*irculation, with hemorrhage control
*D*isability (neurologic deficit)
*E*xposure (maintain a warm *E*nvironment, undress the patient completely, and *E*xamine)

Evaluation and treatment of the ABCs are as discussed earlier in this chapter. Modifications in the trauma setting are added in the sections that follow.

### Airway

Failure to manage the airway appropriately is the most common cause of preventable morbidity and death. Administer 100% high-flow oxygen to all patients. During assessment and management of the airway, provide cervical spine protection, initially by manual in-line immobilization, not traction. A hard cervical spine collar is then applied, and the head and body are secured to a backboard, surrounded by a lightweight means of cushioning (eg, rolled blankets) to further immobilize the head and body and allow log-rolling of the child in case of vomiting. Assess the airway for patency as before. Head positioning must avoid flexion or extension of the neck. Use jaw thrust rather than chin lift during intubation. Suction the mouth and pharynx free of blood, foreign material, or secretions, and remove loose teeth. Insert an oropharyngeal airway if upper airway noises are heard or obstruction from posterior prolapse of the tongue occurs. A child with a depressed level of consciousness or a need for prolonged ventilation, hyperventilation, or operative intervention requires endotracheal intubation after bag–mask preoxygenation. Orotracheal intubation is the route of choice and is possible without cervical spine manipulation. Nasotracheal intubation may be possible in children age 12 years or older who have spontaneous respirations—if not contraindicated by midfacial injury with the possibility of cribriform plate disruption. Rarely, if tracheal intubation cannot be accomplished—particularly in the setting of massive midfacial trauma—cricothyroidotomy may be necessary. Needle cricothyroidotomy using a large-bore catheter through the cricothyroid membrane is the procedure of choice in patients younger than age 12 years. Operative revision will be needed for formal controlled tracheostomy.

## Breathing

Most ventilatory problems are resolved adequately by the airway maneuvers described earlier in this chapter and by positive-pressure ventilation. Breathing assessment is as described previously: Assess for an adequate rate and for symmetrical chest rise, increased work of breathing, color, tracheal deviation, crepitus, flail segments, deformity, or penetrating wounds. Sources of traumatic pulmonary compromise include pneumothorax, hemothorax, pulmonary contusion, flail chest, and central nervous system (CNS) depression. Asymmetrical breath sounds, particularly if tracheal deviation, cyanosis, or bradycardia is present, suggest pneumothorax, probably under tension. To evacuate the pneumothorax, insert a large-bore catheter-over-needle assembly attached to a syringe over the fourth rib in the anterior axillary line into the pleural cavity and withdraw air. If a pneumothorax or hemothorax is present, place a chest tube to water seal. Insertion should be over the rib to avoid the neurovascular bundle that runs below the rib margin. Open pneumothoraces can be treated temporarily by taping petrolatum-impregnated gauze on three sides over the wound, creating a flap valve. After airway and breathing interventions have begun, hemodynamic status may be addressed.

## Circulation

Ongoing hemorrhage, external or internal, gives pediatric trauma some of its anxiety-provoking character. During the assessment of circulation, IV access should be achieved, preferably at two sites. If peripheral access is not readily available, a central line, cutdown, or IO line is established. A cardiorespiratory monitor and oximeter should be applied early in the resuscitation. Peripheral perfusion and blood pressure should be recorded at frequent intervals. Determine hematocrit, blood type and cross-match, and serum amylase. Consider blood and urine toxicologic screening.

External hemorrhage can be controlled by direct pressure. To avoid damage to adjoining nerves and vessels, avoid placing hemostats on vessels, except in the scalp.

Determination of the site of internal hemorrhage can be challenging. Sites include the chest, abdomen, retroperitoneum, pelvis, and thighs. Bleeding into the intracranial vault rarely causes shock in children except in infants. An experienced pediatric trauma surgeon and radiologic studies—principally computed tomography (CT) and ultrasound—will localize the site of internal bleeding.

Suspect cardiac tamponade after penetrating or blunt injuries to the chest if shock, pulseless electrical activity, narrowed pulse pressure, distended neck veins, hepatomegaly, or muffled heart sounds are present. Ultrasound may be diagnostic if readily available. Diagnose and treat with pericardiocentesis and rapid volume infusion.

Treat signs of poor perfusion vigorously: A tachycardic child with a capillary refill time of 3 seconds, or other abnormalities in the perfusion examination, is in *shock* and is sustaining vital organ insults. Remember that hypotension is a late finding. Volume replacement is initially accomplished by rapid infusion of normal saline or lactated Ringer solution at 20 mL/kg of body weight, followed by 10 mL/kg of packed red blood cells if perfusion does not normalize after two crystalloid bolus infusions.

Reassessment should be done rapidly following each bolus. If clinical signs of perfusion have not normalized, repeat the bolus. Lack of response or later signs of hypovolemia suggest the need for blood transfusion and possible surgical exploration. For every milliliter of external blood loss 3 mL of crystalloid solution should be administered.

A common problem is the brain-injured child who is at risk for intracranial hypertension and who is also hypovolemic. In such cases, circulating volume must be restored to ensure adequate cerebral perfusion; therefore, fluid replacement is required until perfusion normalizes. Thereafter provide maintenance fluids with careful serial reassessments. Do not restrict fluids for children with head injuries.

## Disability–Neurologic Deficit

Assess pupillary size and reaction to light and the level of consciousness. The level of consciousness can be reproducibly characterized by the AVPU system (Table 11–4). Pediatric Glasgow Coma Scale assessments should be done as part of the secondary survey (Table 11–5; see Secondary Survey section).

## Exposure and Environment

Significant injuries can be missed unless the child is completely undressed and examined fully, front and back. Cutting away clothing as necessary can minimize movement. Because of their high ratio of surface area to

**Table 11–4.** AVPU system for evaluation of level of consciousness.

| | |
|---|---|
| A | Alert |
| V | Responsive to Voice |
| P | Responsive to Pain |
| U | Unresponsive |

*Table 11–5.* Glasgow Coma Scale.[a]

| | |
|---|---|
| **Eye opening response** | |
| Spontaneous | 4 |
| To speech | 3 |
| To pain | 2 |
| None | 1 |
| **Verbal response** | |
| Oriented | 5 |
| Confused conversation | 4 |
| Inappropriate words | 3 |
| Incomprehensible sounds | 2 |
| None | 1 |
| **Best upper limb motor response** | |
| Obeys | 6 |
| Localizes | 5 |
| Withdraws | 4 |
| Flexion in response to pain | 3 |
| Extension in response to pain | 2 |
| None | 1 |

[a]The appropriate number from each section is added to total between 3 and 15. A score less than 8 usually indicates central nervous system depression requiring positive pressure ventilation.

body mass, infants and children cool rapidly. Because hypothermia compromises outcome except with isolated head injuries, it is necessary to continuously monitor the body temperature and to use warming techniques vigorously as necessary. Hyperthermia, conversely, adversely affects outcomes in children with acute brain injuries, so maintain normal body temperatures.

## Monitoring

Cardiopulmonary monitors with pulse oximetry and end-tidal $CO_2$ monitors should be put in place immediately. At the completion of the primary phase, additional "tubes" should be placed.

### A. Nasogastric or Orogastric Tube

Children's stomachs should be assumed to be full, and gastric distention from positive-pressure ventilation increases the chance of vomiting and aspiration.

### B. Urinary Catheter

An indwelling urinary bladder catheter should be placed to monitor urine output. Contraindications are based on the risk of urethral transection; signs include blood at the meatus or in the scrotum or a displaced prostate detected on rectal examination. Urine should be tested for blood. Urine output should exceed 1 mL/kg/h.

## SECONDARY SURVEY

After the resuscitation phase, a head-to-toe examination should be performed to reveal all injuries and determine priorities for definitive care.

### Skin

Search for lacerations, hematomas, swelling, and abrasions. Remove foreign material, and cleanse as necessary. Cutaneous signs may indicate underlying pathology (eg, a flank hematoma overlying a renal contusion) although surface signs may be absent even with significant internal injury. Make certain the child's tetanus immunization status is current. Consider tetanus immune globulin for unimmunized children.

### Head

Check for hemotympanum and for clear or bloody cerebrospinal fluid (CSF) leak from the nares. Battle sign (hematoma over the mastoid) and raccoon eyes are late signs of basilar skull fracture. Explore wounds, excluding foreign bodies and defects in galea or skull. CT scan of the head is an integral part of evaluation for altered level of consciousness, seizure after trauma, or focal neurologic findings (see Head Injury section). Pneumococcal vaccine is indicated for basilar skull fractures.

### Spine

Cervical spine injury must be excluded in all children. This can be done without radiographs in children with normal neurologic findings on examination who are able to deny midline neck pain or midline tenderness on palpation of the neck and who have no other painful injuries that might obscure the pain of a cervical spine injury. Voluntary movement of the extremities must be observed. If radiographs are indicated, a cross-table lateral neck view is obtained initially, followed by anteroposterior and odontoid views. "Normal" studies do not exclude significant injury, which can be bony or ligamentous, or involve the spinal cord itself. Therefore, an obtunded child should be maintained in cervical spine immobilization until the child has awakened and an appropriate neurologic examination can be performed. The entire thoracolumbar spine must be palpated and areas of pain or tenderness examined by radiography.

### Chest

Pneumothoraces are detected and decompressed during the primary survey. Hemothoraces can occur with rib fractures or with injury to intercostal vessels, large pulmonary vessels, or lung parenchyma. Tracheobronchial disruption is suggested by large continued air leak despite chest tube decompression. Pulmonary contusions may require ventilatory support. Myocardial contusions and aortic injuries are unusual in children.

## Abdomen

Blunt abdominal injury is common in multisystem injuries. Significant injury can exist without cutaneous signs or instability of vital signs. Tenderness, guarding, distention, lack of bowel sounds, or poor perfusion mandates immediate evaluation by a pediatric trauma surgeon. Injury to solid viscera frequently can be managed nonoperatively in stable patients; however, in the presence of intestinal perforation or hypotension, operative treatment is indicated. Serial examinations, ultrasound, and CT scan—or, in unstable patients, diagnostic peritoneal lavage—provide diagnostic help. Elevated liver function tests have good specificity but only fair sensitivity for hepatic injury. Serum amylase will rise progressively with pancreatic injury, which may not be easily visualized by initial CT.

## Pelvis

Pelvic fractures are classically manifested by pain, crepitus, and abnormal motion. Pelvic fracture is a relative contraindication to urethral catheter insertion. Perform a rectal examination, noting tone, tenderness, and prostate position in boys. Stool should be tested for blood.

## Genitourinary System

If urethral transection is suspected (see earlier discussion), perform a urethrogram before catheter placement. Diagnostic imaging of the child with hematuria includes CT scan, or occasionally IV urograms. Management of kidney injury is largely nonoperative except for renal pedicle injuries.

## Extremities

Long bone fractures are common but rarely life-threatening. Test for pulses, perfusion, and sensation. Neurovascular compromise requires immediate orthopedic consultation. Delayed diagnosis of fracture sometimes occurs when children are comatose; reexamination is necessary to avoid overlooking previously missed fractures.

## Central Nervous System

Most deaths in children with multisystem trauma are from head injuries, so optimal neurointensive care is important. Significant injuries include diffuse axonal injury; cerebral edema; subdural, subarachnoid, and epidural hematomas; parenchymal hemorrhages; and spinal cord injury. A full sensorimotor examination should be performed. Deficits require immediate neurosurgical consultation. Extensor or flexor posturing represents intracranial hypertension, not seizure activity, until proved otherwise, and should be treated with mild hyperventilation ($PaCO_2$ in the mid-30s mm Hg), and adequate but not excessive volume resuscitation. If accompanied by a fixed and unreactive pupil a herniation syndrome is present, and hyperventilation should be to a $PaCO_2$ in the mid-20s. Diuretics, usually mannitol, should be given if perfusion is normal and signs of herniation are present. Normal peripheral perfusion must be ensured to optimize cerebral perfusion. Level of consciousness by the AVPU system (see Table 11–4) or Glasgow Coma Scale (see Table 11–5) should be assessed serially. Seizure activity warrants exclusion of significant intracranial injury. In the trauma setting, seizures are frequently treated with fosphenytoin. Acute spinal cord injury may benefit from high-dose methylprednisolone therapy. Corticosteroids are not indicated for head trauma.

American College of Surgeons, Committee on Trauma: *Textbook of Advanced Trauma Life Support.* American College of Surgeons, 1997.

http://www.facs.org/trauma/atls/information.html

Junkins E et al: A prospective evaluation of the clinical presentation of pediatric pelvic fractures. J Trauma 2001;51(1):64 [PMID: 11468469].

Schutzman SA, Greenes DS: Pediatric minor head trauma. Ann Emerg Med 2001;37:65 [PMID: 11145776].

Viccellio P et al: A prospective multicenter study of cervical spine injury in children. Pediatrics 2001;108(2):E20 [PMID: 11483830].

# HEAD INJURY

Closed head injuries range in severity from minor asymptomatic trauma without sequelae to intracranial hemorrhage leading to death. Head injury, including the shaken-baby syndrome, is common in cases of child abuse. Even following minor closed head injury, neuropsychiatric sequelae can occur.

## Assessment

The considerations discussed earlier in the Approach to the Pediatric Trauma Patient section apply here as well. The history should include the time and mechanism of injury. How far did the child fall and onto what surface? Was there loss of consciousness? Does the child remember events preceding, during, and following the injury? What have been the child's levels of consciousness and activity since the injury? Has there been vomiting, headache, ataxia, seizures, or visual disturbance?

The physical examination should be complete, keeping in mind the mechanism of injury, and should include a detailed neurologic examination. Look for associated injuries such as mandibular fracture, scalp or skull injury, or cervical spine injury. CSF leak from the ears or nose or the two later-appearing signs of periorbital hematomas (raccoon eyes) and Battle sign, imply basilar skull fracture. Children with suspected basilar skull fractures should receive the pneumococcal vaccine. Obtain vital signs and assess the child's level of consciousness by the AVPU system (see Table 11–4) or Glasgow Coma Scale (see Table 11–5), noting irritability or lethargy; pupillary equality, size, and reaction to light; funduscopic examination; reflexes; body posture; and rectal tone. Always consider child abuse—the injuries observed should be consistent with the history and the child's developmental level.

Radiographic studies may be indicated. Plain films are useful only in cases of penetrating head trauma or for assessing depressed skull fractures and ruling out foreign bodies. Major morbidity does not follow from skull fracture per se but rather from the associated intracranial injury. The presence of a skull fracture on plain films is associated with an increased likelihood of finding a serious intracranial injury demonstrated by CT scanning. CT scan should be performed in the child with persistent vomiting or an abnormal or lateralizing neurologic examination, including an abnormal mental status that does not quickly return to normal. In infants, a normal neurologic exam does not exclude significant intracranial hemorrhage. In the setting of an appropriate mechanism, and if scalp findings such as large hematomas are found, consider performing CT.

## CONCUSSION

A concussion injury is defined as a brief loss or alteration of consciousness followed by a return to normal. Brain tissue is not damaged, and there are no focal findings on detailed neurologic examination. There may be pallor, amnesia, or several episodes of vomiting. Disposition is based on the clinical course and suitability of follow-up. The patient may be discharged when neurologically normal after a period of observation. Parents should closely observe the child at home and return if the child exhibits altered level of consciousness, persistent vomiting, gait disturbances, unequal pupils, seizures, or increasing headache, or if the parents have any concerns.

## CONTUSION

A bruise of the brain matter is a contusion. The child's level of consciousness decreases, and focal findings if any correspond to the area of the brain that is injured.

These patients require CT scan, a period of observation, and consideration of neurorehabilitation follow-up for posttraumatic brain injury sequelae.

## DIFFUSE AXONAL INJURY

Diffuse axonal injury is a potentially severe form of traumatic brain injury characterized by coma without focal signs on neurologic examination. There may be no external signs of trauma. The initial CT scan is normal or may demonstrate only scattered small areas of cerebral contusion and areas of low density. Prolonged disability may follow diffuse axonal injury.

## ACUTE INTRACRANIAL HYPERTENSION

Close observation will detect early signs and symptoms of intracranial pressure elevation. Early recognition is essential to avoid disastrous outcomes. In addition to traumatic causes, intracranial pressure elevation with or without herniation syndromes may be seen in spontaneous intracranial hemorrhage, CNS infection, hydrocephalus, ruptured arteriovenous malformation, metabolic derangement (eg, diabetic ketoacidosis), ventriculoperitoneal shunt obstruction, or tumor. Symptoms include headache, vision changes, vomiting, gait difficulties, and a progressively decreasing level of consciousness. Other signs may include stiff neck, cranial nerve palsies, and progressive hemiparesis. Cushing triad (bradycardia, hypertension, and irregular respirations) is a late and prearrest finding. Papilledema is also a late finding. Consider CT scan before lumbar puncture if there is concern about intracranial pressure elevation because of the risk of precipitating herniation. Lumbar puncture should be deferred if coma or shock is present.

Therapy for intracranial pressure elevation must be swift and aggressive. Strict attention to normal oxygenation, moderate ventilation, and adequate perfusion is paramount. Controlled rapid sequence intubation with appropriate sedation, muscle relaxation, and agents to reduce the intracranial pressure elevation that accompanies intubation is followed by mild hyperventilation ($PaCO_2$ lowered to 35–38 mm Hg) and avoidance of hypoperfusion and hypoxemia. Mannitol (0.5 g/kg intravenously), an osmotic diuretic, will reduce brain water, as will furosemide (0.1–0.2 mg/kg intravenously). These measures may acutely lower intracranial pressure. Fluid infusion and, ultimately, pressors should be used to maintain normal arterial blood pressure and peripheral perfusion, if necessary. Adjunctive measures include elevating the head of the bed 30 degrees, treating hyperpyrexia and pain, and maintaining the head in a midline position. Obtain immediate neurosurgical evaluation. Further details about management of intracranial hypertension (cerebral edema) are presented in Chapter 13.

## DISPOSITION FOR CHILDREN WITH CLOSED HEAD INJURY

Patients with mild head injury may be discharged with detailed written instructions—after a period of brief observation—if the examination remains normal and parental supervision and follow-up are appropriate. Children with persistent deficits require admission or prolonged observation. If the patient responds to voice commands and mental status is improving gradually over a period of several hours, observation may be done without further radiographic studies. If the mental status deteriorates, however, CT scan and neurosurgical consultations are indicated. If the CT scan is normal and the physical findings normalize, these children may also be discharged after a period of observation. Patients with severe head injury require cerebral resuscitation, evaluation by a neurosurgeon, and admission to hospital.

Baker C et al: Evaluation of pediatric cervical spine injuries. Am J Emerg Med 1999;17(3):230 [PMID: 10337876].

Hendey GW et al: Spinal cord injury without radiologic abnormality: Results of the National Emergency X-radiography Utilization Study in blunt cervical study. J Trauma 2002;53.1 [PMID: 12131380].

Holmes JF et al: Identification of children with intra-abdominal injuries after blunt trauma. Ann Emerg Med 2002;39:500 [PMID: 11973557].

Ponsford J et al: Impact of early intervention on outcome after mild traumatic brain injury in children. Pediatrics 2001;108:1297 [PMID: 11731651].

Simon B et al: Pediatric minor head trauma: Indications for computed tomographic scanning revisited. J Trauma 2001;51: 231 [PMID: 11493779].

# BURNS

Thermal injury is a major cause of accidental death and disfigurement in children. Pain, morbidity, the association with child abuse, and the preventable nature of burns constitute an area of major concern in pediatrics. Common causes include hot water or food, appliances, flames, grills, vehicle-related burns, and curling irons. Burns occur commonly in toddlers—in boys more frequently than in girls.

## ELECTRICAL BURNS

Even brief contact with a high-voltage source will result in a contact burn. When an infant or toddler bites an electric cord, burns to the commissure of the lips occur that appear gray and necrotic, with surrounding erythema. If an arc is created with passage of current through the body, the pattern of the thermal injury will depend on the path of the current; therefore, search for an exit wound and internal injuries. Extensive damage to deep tissues may occur. Current traversing the heart may cause nonperfusing arrhythmias. Neurologic effects of electrical burns can be immediate (eg, confusion, disorientation, peripheral nerve injury), delayed (eg, nerve damage in the thrombosed limb after compartment syndrome), or late (eg, impaired concentration or memory).

# EVALUATION OF THE BURNED PATIENT

## Classification

Burns are classified clinically according to the nature of the burn and the extent and thickness; associated injuries are ascertained in the initial evaluation.

Superficial (first-degree) burns are easily recognized and treated. They are painful, dry, red, and hypersensitive. Sunburn is a common example. Healing occurs with minimal damage to epidermis. At the other end of the spectrum are full-thickness (third-degree) burns affecting all epidermal and dermal elements, leaving avascular skin. The wound is dry, depressed, leathery in appearance, and without sensation. Unless skin grafting is provided, the scar will be hard, uneven, and fibrotic. Partial-thickness (second-degree) burns are further classified as superficial or deep, depending on appearance and healing time, with each subgroup treated differently. Superficial partial-thickness burns are red and may blister. Deep partial-thickness burns are white and dry, blanch with pressure, and the involved skin has decreased sensitivity to pain.

## Management

Burn management depends on the depth and extent of thermal injury. Burn extent can be classified as major or minor. Minor burns are less than 10% of the body surface area for superficial and partial-thickness burns, or less than 2% for full-thickness burns. Partial- or full-thickness burns of the hands, feet, face, eyes, ears, and perineum are considered major.

### A. SUPERFICIAL AND PARTIAL-THICKNESS BURNS

These injuries can generally be treated in the outpatient setting. It is *mandatory* that rapid and effective analgesia be provided, and redosed as indicated by the child. Oral codeine may occasionally suffice, but often parenteral narcotics are indicated. Superficial burns are treated with cool compresses and analgesia. Treatment of partial-thickness burns with blisters consists of antiseptic cleansing, topical antimicrobial coverage, and observation for infection. Blisters appear early in deeper partial-thickness burns and, if open, may be debrided. Alternatively, the blister may be used as a protective flap after cleaning and dressing. After debridement, the wound should be cleansed with dilute (1–5%) povidone–iodine solution, thoroughly washed with normal saline, and covered with topical antibiotic, which does not need to be silver sulfadiazine. The wound should be protected with a bulky dressing and reexamined within 24 hours and serially thereafter. Wounds with a potential for causing loss of function or scarring—especially wounds of the hand or digits—should be referred promptly to a burn surgeon. Outpatient analgesia should be provided on discharge.

### B. Full-Thickness and Deep or Extensive Partial-Thickness Burns

Major burns place particular importance on the ABCs of trauma management. Early establishment of an artificial airway is critical with oral or nasal burns because of their association with inhalation injuries and critical airway narrowing.

The trauma resuscitation protocol outlined previously, in the Primary Survey section, should be followed. There may be inhalation injury from carbon monoxide, cyanide, or other toxic products if flames were present. A nasogastric tube and bladder catheter should be placed. The secondary survey should ascertain whether any other injuries are present, including those suggestive of abuse.

Fluid administration is based on several principles. Capillary permeability is markedly increased. Fluid needs are based on examination findings, percentage of body surface area burned, depth, and age. Maintaining normal intravascular pressure and replacing fluid losses are essential. Figure 11–8 shows percentages of body surface area by body part in infants and children. The Parkland formula for fluid therapy is 4 mL/kg/% body surface area burned for the first 24 hours, with half in the first 8 hours, in addition to maintenance rates. Acutely, however, fluid resuscitation should be based on clinical assessment of volume status as described earlier.

Indications for admission include major burns as previously defined; uncertainty of follow-up; suspicion of abuse; presence of upper airway injury; explosion, inhalation, electrical, or chemical burns; burns associated with fractures; or the need for parenteral pain control. Children with chronic metabolic or connective tissue diseases and infants deserve hospitalization.

## Sedation and Analgesia

What more important mission can providers have than relieving pain and anxiety in children in acute care set-

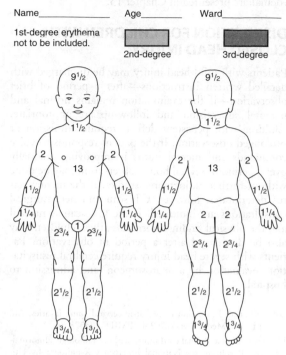

**Infant Less Than One Year of Age**

Name_____ Age_____ Ward_____

1st-degree erythema not to be included.

2nd-degree    3rd-degree

Variations From Adults Distribution in Infants and Children (in Percent).

|  | New-born | 1 Year | 5 Years | 10 Years |
|---|---|---|---|---|
| Head | 19 | 17 | 13 | 11 |
| Both thighs | 11 | 13 | 16 | 17 |
| Both lower legs | 10 | 10 | 11 | 12 |
| Neck | 2 |  |  |  |
| Anterior trunk | 13 |  |  |  |
| Posterior trunk | 13 |  |  |  |
| Both upper arms | 8 | These percentages remain constant at all ages |  |  |
| Both lower arms | 6 |  |  |  |
| Both hands | 5 |  |  |  |
| Both buttocks | 6 |  |  |  |
| Both feet | 7 |  |  |  |
| Genitalia | 1 |  |  |  |
|  | 100 |  |  |  |

**Figure 11–8.** Lund and Browder modification of Berkow scale for estimating extent of burns. (The table under the illustration is after Berkow.)

tings? Consider whether the child needs relief from anxiety (sedation) or relief from pain (analgesia). Many agents also have amnestic properties. Parenteral agents can be effective and safe and produce few side effects if used judiciously.

Conditions such as fracture reduction, laceration repair, burn care, sexual assault examinations, lumbar puncture, and diagnostic procedures such as CT and magnetic resonance imaging may all be performed more effectively and with less trauma to the child if effective sedation or analgesia is used. The clinician should decide whether procedures will require either sedation or analgesia alone, or both, and then choose agents accordingly.

Safe and effective sedation requires thorough knowledge of the selected agent and its side effects; suitable monitoring devices; resuscitative medications, equipment, and personnel; and appropriate informed consent from the parents. This process is now called procedural sedation and analgesia (PSA) and should proceed as follows:

1. Choose the right medication or combination of medications for the procedure.

2. Discuss risks and benefits of the proposed PSA and obtain verbal informed consent from the parents.

3. Ensure appropriate NPO (nothing-by-mouth) status for 4–6 hours. For certain emergency procedures, suboptimal NPO status may be allowed, with attendant risks identified.

4. Establish vascular access as required.

5. Ensure that resuscitative equipment and personnel are readily available.

6. Attach the cardiorespiratory monitor and pulse oximeter, as indicated.

7. Give the agent selected, with continuous monitoring for side effects. A dedicated observer, usually a nurse, should monitor the patient at all times. Respiratory effort, perfusion, and mental status should be assessed and documented serially.

8. Titrate the medication to achieve the desired sedation level. The ideal level is that of "conscious" or "light" sedation—that is, the patient's sensorium is slightly dulled, but eyes are generally open and airway reflexes are preserved.

9. Continue monitoring the patient after finishing the procedure. If a painful stimulus has been eliminated (eg, fracture reduction) mental status can decrease.

10. Criteria for discharge include the child's ability to sit unassisted, to take oral fluids, and to answer verbal commands. A PSA discharge handout should be given, with precautions for close observation and avoidance of potentially dangerous activities.

The following are some commonly used sedatives and analgesics:

**1. Midazolam (Versed)**—This agent has particular usefulness in pediatrics due to its safety, rapid onset, and short half-life. Administration may be oral, rectal, intranasal, intramuscular, or IV. When given slowly intranasally, the drug's kinetics are nearly the same as when given intravenously. Many children report a burning sensation with intranasal administration. Oral or rectal administration results in relatively delayed onset, and titration is difficult. Intramuscular injections can be combined with opioid analgesics if systemic analgesia is desired. IV administration allows optimal ability to titrate dosing to the desired sedation level. Complicated or prolonged procedures are best facilitated by IV placement to facilitate redosing, which also provides IV access if resuscitation becomes necessary. Potential side effects of midazolam include cardiorespiratory depression.

**2. Barbiturates**—This class of agents (eg, pentobarbital [Nembutal]) has the advantage of minimizing movement during procedures, which makes them advantageous for diagnostic studies such as CT or magnetic resonance imaging. Rectal administration of thiopental is safe and effective. Onset of action with IV administration is rapid. Potential side effects, although uncommon, include respiratory and cardiac depression and laryngospasm.

**3. Narcotics**—These agents (eg, morphine, meperidine, and fentanyl) have powerful analgesic and sedative effects. They can be combined with anxiolytics such as benzodiazepines. Desired and adverse effects, such as respiratory depression, are potentiated when benzodiazepines and narcotics or barbiturates are given together. Therefore, sedative doses should be reduced when sedatives and analgesics are given together.

**4. Ketamine**—Increasingly and now commonly used in emergency departments, this agent has the advantage of being a sympathomimetic, that is, increasing heart rate and blood pressure. It is a potent analgesic and anxiolytic and has amnestic properties. Side effects include salivation (therefore, it is usually given with glycopyrrolate as an antisalivation agent), laryngospasm (occasionally), nystagmus, emergence reactions, and vomiting. With comprehensive knowledge of this medication, its use can be a significant advantage to children.

American Academy of Pediatrics, Committee on Drugs: Guidelines for monitoring and management of pediatric patients during and after sedation for diagnostic and therapeutic procedures: An addendum. Pediatrics 2002;110:836 [PMID: 12359805].

Berde CB, Sethna NF: Analgesics for the treatment of pain in children. N Engl J Med 2002;347:1094 [PMID: 12362012].

Singer AJ et al: Parents and practitioners are poor judges of young children's pain severity. Acad Emerg Med 2002;9:609 [PMID: 12045074].

# DISORDERS DUE TO HIGH ENVIRONMENTAL TEMPERATURE

Disorders due to heat range from mild cramps to life-threatening heat stroke. Heat cramps are characterized by brief, severe cramping (not rigidity) of skeletal or abdominal muscles following exertion. Core body temperature is normal or only slightly elevated. Heat cramps may be associated with a relative sodium deficiency. Mild cases can be treated with oral salt-containing solutions; more severe cases require IV infusion of normal saline solution. Heat exhaustion is manifested by constitutional symptoms after exposure to heat and humidity. Patients continue to sweat, and core temperature is normal or only slightly increased. Patients with heat exhaustion have varying proportions of salt and water depletion. Presenting symptoms and signs include weakness, fatigue, headache, disorientation, pallor, thirst, nausea and vomiting, and occasionally muscle cramps. Shock may be present. No major CNS dysfunction should be present. Treat with IV fluids, modified by measured electrolyte levels. Both heat cramps and heat exhaustion can be avoided with acclimatization and liberal water and salt intake during exercise.

Heat stroke represents failure of thermoregulation and is life-threatening. The diagnosis is based on a rectal temperature of over 40°C with associated neurologic signs in a patient with an exposure history. Lack of sweating is not a necessary criterion. Symptoms are similar to those of heat exhaustion, but CNS dysfunction is more prominent. Patients with heat stroke are often incoherent and combative. In more severe cases, vomiting, shivering, coma, seizures, nuchal rigidity, and posturing may be present. Patients can have high, low, or normal cardiac output. Cellular hypoxia, enzyme dysfunction, and disrupted cell membranes lead to global end-organ derangements: rhabdomyolysis, myocardial necrosis, electrolyte abnormalities, acute tubular necrosis and renal failure, hepatic degeneration, adult respiratory distress syndrome, and disseminated intravascular coagulation. Consider sepsis, malignant hyperthermia, and neuroleptic malignant syndrome in the differential diagnosis.

## Heat Stroke Management

1. Immediately cool the patient's body with cool water mist, ice, fans, or other cooling device.
2. If the patient is unresponsive, manage the airway, giving 100% oxygen.
3. Administer IV fluids: isotonic crystalloid for hypotension, 5% dextrose normal saline for maintenance. Consider central venous pressure determination.
4. Place monitors, check rectal temperatures continuously, and place a Foley catheter and nasogastric tube.
5. Obtain laboratory tests: complete blood count; electrolytes; glucose; creatinine; prothrombin time and partial thromboplastin time; creatine kinase; liver function tests; arterial blood gases; urinalysis; and serum calcium, magnesium, and phosphate.
6. Admit to pediatric intensive care unit.

## Malignant Hyperthermia

Malignant hyperthermia is a rare but life-threatening syndrome characterized by a hypermetabolic state including high fever, diaphoresis, malaise, rhabdomyolysis, disseminated intravascular coagulation, hyperreflexia, and psychosis. It is most often associated with anesthetic agents, but can be seen in the outpatient setting in the neuroleptic-malignant syndrome. Drugs such as atropine, lidocaine, meperidine, nonsteroidal anti-inflammatory agents, tricyclic antidepressants, cocaine, and antipsychotics can induce a central hyperthermic syndrome. Treatment includes cooling, rectal acetaminophen, seizure treatment with a benzodiazepine, and, in the case of malignant hyperthermia caused by neuromuscular blockers, dantrolene sodium.

# HYPOTHERMIA

Seriously ill children should have core temperature quickly determined. Hypothermia in children, defined as core body temperature less than 35°C, is frequently associated with cold water submersion accidents. Many other disorders cause incidental hypothermia, including sepsis, metabolic derangements, ingestions, CNS disorders, and endocrinopathies. Neonates, trauma victims, intoxicated patients, and the chronically disabled are particularly at risk. Mortality rates are high and are related to the underlying disorder. Conversely, mild therapeutic hypothermia following hypoxic–ischemic CNS insult and isolated traumatic brain injury may be a recommendation in the near future.

As core temperature falls, a variety of mechanisms begin to conserve and produce heat. Peripheral vasoconstriction allows optimal maintenance of core temperature. Heat production can be increased by a hypothalamic-mediated increase in muscle tone and metabolism. When shivering begins, heat production increases to two to four times basal levels.

## Clinical Findings

Clinical manifestations of hypothermia depend on the severity of body temperature depression. Severe cases (≤

28°C) mimic death: Patients are pale or cyanotic, pupils may be fixed and dilated, muscles are rigid, and there may be no palpable pulses. Heart rates as low as 4–6/min may provide adequate perfusion, because of the lowered metabolic needs in severe hypothermia. If these findings are a result of primary hypothermia and not postmortem changes, the fact of death cannot be ascertained until the patient has been rewarmed and remains unresponsive to resuscitative efforts. Children with a core temperature as low as 19°C have survived neurologically intact.

## Treatment

### A. GENERAL SUPPORTIVE MEASURES

Management of hypothermia is complex but largely supportive. Core body temperature must be documented by continuously monitoring with a low-reading indwelling rectal thermometer. Patients must be handled gently, because the hypothermic myocardium is exquisitely sensitive and prone to arrhythmias. Ventricular fibrillation may occur spontaneously or as a result of minor handling or invasive procedures. If asystole or ventricular fibrillation is present on the cardiac monitor, perform chest compressions and use standard pediatric advanced life support techniques and medications. Spontaneous reversion to sinus rhythm at 28–30°C may occur as rewarming proceeds.

### B. REWARMING

1. Passive rewarming, such as covering with blankets, is appropriate only for mild cases (> 33°C).

2. Active rewarming is achieved by external or core rewarming techniques. External rewarming methods include warming lights, thermal mattresses or electric warming blankets, immersion in warm baths, and hot water bottles or warmed bags of IV solutions. One must be aware of the potential for core temperature depression after rewarming is begun, as warmed peripheral acidemic blood is distributed to the core circulation. Core rewarming techniques are optimal and include the delivery of warmed, humidified oxygen and the use of warmed (to 40°C) fluids for IV replacement, peritoneal dialysis, bladder irrigation, and mediastinal lavage. Extracorporeal blood rewarming achieves controlled core rewarming, can stabilize volume and electrolyte disturbances, and is maximally effective (Table 11–6).

## SUBMERSION INJURIES

Drowning is the second most common cause of death by unintentional injury among children. Water hazards

**Table 11–6.** Management of hypothermia.

**General measures**
Administer warmed and humidified 100% oxygen.
Monitor core temperature, heart and respiratory rates, and blood pressure continuously.
Consider central venous pressure determination for severe hypothermia.
**Laboratory studies**
Complete blood count and platelets
Serum electrolytes, glucose, creatinine, amylase
Prothrombin time, partial thromboplastin time
Arterial blood gases
Consider toxicology screen
**Treatment**
Correct hypoxemia, hypercapnia, pH < 7.2, clotting abnormalities, and glucose and electrolyte disturbances.
Start rewarming techniques: passive, active (core and external), depending on degree of hypothermia.
Replace intravascular volume with warmed intravenous crystalloid infusion at 42°C.
Treat asystole and ventricular fibrillation per PALS protocols. Cardiac massage should be continued at least until core temperature reaches 30°C, when defibrillation is more likely to be effective.

are ubiquitous and include lakes and streams; swimming pools; bathtubs; and even toilets, buckets, and washing machines. Risk factors include epilepsy, alcohol, intentional trauma, and lack of supervision. Males predominate in submersion deaths, as in most other nonintentional deaths. All pediatric care providers must make efforts to prevent these needless tragedies.

Major morbidity stems from CNS and pulmonary insult. Laryngospasm or breath-holding may lead to loss of consciousness and cardiovascular collapse before aspiration can occur (so-called dry drowning).

Anoxia from laryngospasm or aspiration leads to irreversible CNS damage after only 4–6 minutes. A child must fall through ice or directly into icy water for cerebral metabolism to be slowed sufficiently by hypothermia to provide some protection from anoxic damage.

Cardiovascular changes include myocardial depression and arrhythmias. Electrolyte alterations are generally slight. Unless hemolysis occurs, hemoglobin concentrations also change only slightly.

## Assessment & Management

Depending on the duration of submersion and any protective hypothermia effects, children may appear clinically dead or completely normal. Observation over time assists with prognosis. The child who has been rewarmed to at least 33°C and is still apneic and pulseless in the emergency department will probably not survive to discharge or will be left with severe neurologic deficits. Until a determination of brain death can be made, however, aggressive resuscitation should be continued.

One should keep in mind possible associated injuries, such as neck injury from diving into shallow water. For children who appear well initially, observation for 8–12 hours will detect late pulmonary compromise or changes in neurologic status. Respiratory distress, an abnormal chest radiograph, abnormal arterial blood gases, or hypoxemia by pulse oximetry indicates the need for treatment with supplemental oxygen, cardiopulmonary monitoring, and frequent reassessment. Serially assess the degree of respiratory distress and mental status. Signs of pulmonary infection may appear many hours after the submersion event.

Patients who are in coma and who require mechanical ventilation have a high risk of anoxic encephalopathy. The value of therapy with hyperventilation, corticosteroids, intentional hypothermia, and barbiturates remains unproved.

# BITES: ANIMAL & HUMAN

Bites account for a large number of visits to the emergency department. Most fatalities are due to dog bites. However, the majority of infected bite wounds are from human and cat bites.

## DOG BITES

Boys are bitten more frequently than girls, and the dog is known by the victim in most cases. Younger children have a higher incidence of head and neck wounds, whereas school-age children are bitten most often on the upper extremities.

Dog bites are treated largely the same way as other wounds: high-pressure, high-volume irrigation with normal saline, scrubbing, debridement of any devitalized tissue and removal of foreign matter, and tetanus prophylaxis. The risk of rabies from dogs is low in developed countries, but rabies prophylaxis should be considered when appropriate. Wounds should be sutured only if necessary for cosmetic reasons because closure of the wound increases the risk of infection. Prophylactic antibiotics have not been shown to decrease rates of infection in low-risk dog bite wounds not involving the hands or feet. If a bite involves a joint, periosteum, or neurovascular bundle, prompt orthopedic surgery consultation should be obtained.

Pathogens that infect dog bites include *Pasteurella multocida*, streptococci, staphylococci, and anaerobes.

Infected dog bites can be treated with penicillin for *P multocida,* and broad-spectrum coverage can be provided by amoxicillin and clavulanic acid or cephalexin (see dose for cat bites in next section). Complications of dog bites include scarring, CNS infections, septic arthritis, osteomyelitis, endocarditis, and sepsis.

## CAT BITES

Cat-inflicted wounds occur more frequently in girls, and their principal complication is infection. The infection risk is higher in cat bites than dog bites because of the puncture character of the wound produced by cat teeth. Wound management is similar to that for dog bites. Cat wounds should not be sutured except when absolutely necessary for cosmetic reasons. *P multocida* is the most common pathogen. Cat bites create a puncture-wound inoculum, and prophylactic antibiotics (penicillin plus cephalexin, or amoxicillin and clavulanic acid) are recommended. The dose of amoxicillin trihydrate and clavulanic acid should be on the high side of recommended dosage in order to ensure adequate tissue penetration both in dog and cat bites. The dosage of the amoxicillin component should be 80 mg/kg/24 h in three divided doses. The maximum dosage is 2 g/24 h. Scratches or bites from young cats may result in cat scratch fever.

## HUMAN BITES

Most human bites occur during fights. *P multocida* is not a known pathogen in human bites—cultures most commonly grow streptococci, anaerobes, staphylococci,

---

### PEDIATRIC EMERGENCY MEDICINE

Pediatric emergency medicine is a subspecialty with fellowship training and subboard certification that provides resuscitation and urgent care of ill or injured infants, children, and adolescents. The body of emergency research literature is substantial and growing rapidly. EMS-C (Emergency Medical Services for Children) programs exist to enhance the spectrum of care of the severely ill or injured child through, for example, community injury prevention, prehospital care by emergency medical technicians and paramedics, emergency department-based stabilization and critical care, and rehabilitation. Pediatric emergency medicine physicians are intimately involved in the care of injured patients, because trauma is the leading cause of death among children over age 1 year.

and *Eikenella corrodens.* Hand wounds and deep wounds should be treated with antibiotic coverage against *E corrodens* and gram-positive pathogens by a penicillinase-resistant penicillin. Wound management is the same as for dog bites. Only severe lacerations involving the face should be sutured. Other wounds can be managed by delayed primary closure or healing by second intention.

A major complication of human bite wounds is infection of the metacarpophalangeal joints. A hand surgeon should evaluate clenched-fist injuries from human bites. Operative debridement is followed in many cases by IV antibiotics.

Knapp JF: Updates in wound management for the pediatrician. Pediatr Clin North Am 1999 46(6):1201 [PMID: 10629682].

# ■ II. BIOTERRORISM

*Marsha S. Anderson, MD*

Bioterrorism is the intentional use of biological agents to produce disease or intoxication in a susceptible population. Biologic agents have been used frequently throughout history, the most recent instances being the United States anthrax outbreak in 2001 and the ricin contamination of the Dierksen Senate Office Building in 2004. In the anthrax outbreak inhalational and cutaneous anthrax disease resulted from exposures to anthrax spores in envelopes that traveled through the US Postal system. Over 32,000 people were treated or received antibiotic prophylaxis, 22 people contracted anthrax, and 5 died. Several cases involved postal workers, and were believed to be related to high-speed mail sorting and stamping equipment and the compressed air used to clean these machines—all of which were thought to increase aerosolization of spores in the postal facilities.

## General Considerations

Bioterrorism is a concern because at least 17 nations are thought capable of producing biologic weapons. In addition, some cult groups are interested in obtaining these agents. Biologic weapons are attractive to terrorists and rogue states because they are relatively simple and cheap to manufacture, difficult to detect, and capable of inflicting mass casualties over a wide area. Moreover, most target populations are susceptible to candidate disease agents, and mass casualty and medical response systems are unprepared to deal with the effects of these agents.

**Table 11–7.** Potential bioterrorism agents and the diseases produced.

| Agent | Disease Produced |
| --- | --- |
| *Bacillus anthracis* | Anthrax |
| Variola virus | Smallpox |
| *Yersinia pestis* | Plague |
| Botulinum toxin | Botulism |
| *Francisella tularensis* | Tularemia |
| *Brucella* species | Brucellosis |
| *Coxiella burnetti* | Q-fever |
| Filoviradae | Ebola, Marburg |
| Bunyaviridae | Rift Valley fever |
| *Salmonella typhi* | Typhoid fever |

There are many potential biologic agents (Table 11–7). *Bacillus anthracis* (anthrax), variola virus (smallpox), *Yersinia pestis* (plague), and botulinum toxin (botulism) are the most likely attack agents.

Biologic agents can be delivered via aerosolization, food or water contamination, parenteral injection, or direct contact with skin. Aerosolization is thought to be the most efficient exposure method for many agents. The aim is to create an invisible cloud of infectious particles with diameters of 0.5–10 μg. At this particle size, the aerosolized infectious agents reach the alveolar spaces.

Unlike a bomb explosion or a chemical spill, a bioterrorism event is likely to be covert. A covert attack may not have an immediate effect because of the time between exposure and development of disease. Days to weeks later (depending on the agent and incubation period), patients will present to their primary care physicians or local emergency departments. Consequently, first responders to a covert biologic incident will *not* be the military or law enforcement officials. Rather, physicians, nurses, or emergency medical technicians will identify the initial cases. Only after an outbreak has been recognized will the possibility of a biologic attack be considered. For this reason, it is imperative that medical first-responders remain vigilant and report any unusual clustering of disease to their state health departments.

## ANTHRAX

Anthrax is caused by the bacterium *Bacillus anthracis,* a spore-forming gram-positive rod. Anthrax occurs naturally in domesticated and wild herbivores. *B anthracis* spores, common in the soil, are ingested by grazing animals. Three proteins—protective antigen, lethal factor, and edema factor—combine to form two toxins responsible for the morbidity and mortality associated with the disease. Edema toxin (made by the linkage of protective antigen and edema factor) is an adenylate cyclase analogue that promotes generation of cyclic adenosine monophosphate and alters intercellular flux of water and ions. This is responsible for the edema characteristically seen around cutaneous lesions. Lethal toxin, produced by the interaction of protective antigen and lethal factor, is a mitogen-activated protein kinase inhibitor that influences cell signaling.

## A. Cutaneous Anthrax

Ninety-five percent of naturally acquired anthrax cases are acquired by direct skin contact with infected animals, animal parts, or spores. Presumably the bacteria or spores are inoculated through wounds or small breaks in the skin. After an incubation period of 1–12 days, a small macular or papular and sometimes pruritic lesion appears at the site of inoculation. This develops into a vesicle or group of vesicles that ultimately ulcerates, enlarges, and develops a characteristic black center, or eschar. Marked edema surrounding the lesion is typical. The ulcer is depressed, painless, and may have a heaped border. Systemic symptoms such as fever, headache, and myalgias may be present. The differential diagnosis includes brown recluse spider (*Loxosceles reclusa*) bite (where these are endemic), ecthyma gangrenosum (common in neutropenic hosts), ulceroglandular tularemia, and routine wound infection (*Staphylococcus aureus,* group A *Streptococcus*). Diagnosis is made by culture and Gram stain of the vesicular fluid or a biopsy specimen. Cultures obtained prior to antibiotic treatment usually yield the diagnosis. Polymerase chain reaction (PCR) and immunohistochemical tests are available at most state health departments or through the Centers for Disease Control and Prevention (CDC). PCR can be done on formalin-fixed tissue from a biopsy specimen. All suspected anthrax cases should be immediately reported to the state health department. Although person-to-person transmission of any form of anthrax has not been reported, patients are generally placed in contact isolation because they have a draining wound.

Mortality is 10–20% without treatment. Doxycycline and ciprofloxacin are effective first-line therapy (Table 11–8). Ciprofloxacin might be preferred initially, because some investigators have reported genetically engineered B anthracis strains resistant to penicillin and tetracycline. Once the susceptibilities are known, therapy can be tailored (usually penicillin, ciprofloxacin, or doxycycline). Patients who are not systemically ill can be treated orally. If intravenous (IV) therapy is initiated, oral therapy can be used once the patient improves. Patients who develop cutaneous anthrax as a consequence of a bioterrorist attack may also

**Table 11–8.** Empiric treatment of cutaneous anthrax (without systemic involvement[a]) associated with a bioterrorist attack.[b]

|  | Initial therapy | Course |
|---|---|---|
| Children | Ciprofloxacin 10–15 mg/kg orally (maximum 500 mg/dose) | 60 d[d] |
|  | *or* |  |
|  | Doxycycline |  |
|  | ≤ 45 kg: 2.2 mg/kg/dose orally | 60 d[d] |
|  | > 45 kg: 100 mg orally | 60 d[d] |
| Adults[c] | Ciprofloxacin 500 mg orally | 60 d[d] |
|  | *or* |  |
|  | Doxycycline 100 mg orally q12h | 60 d[d] |

[a]Cutaneous anthrax with systemic involvement, extensive edema, or lesions on the head or neck requires a multidrug regimen as in inhalational anthrax (see Table 11–9).
[b]This table is for initial therapy. Each bioterrorist episode is potentially unique, and the organisms may have unique susceptibilities. Regimens may need to be revised once the susceptibility pattern of the organism is known.
[c]Recommendations for pregnant women are the same as for adults, since this is a serious and sometimes life-threatening illness. Doxycycline's adverse effects on bones and teeth is dose related.
[d]At least 60 days is recommended to treat the infection and for prophylaxis for inhalational exposures. Longer prophylaxis (up to 100 days) might be recommended if the patient is judged to be at high risk for exposure to a large number of spores. Anthrax vaccine might also be considered as part of postexposure prophylaxis (currently available under research protocol, discussion with the state health department is recommended).

be at risk for inhalational disease. For this reason, during the 2001 outbreak, the CDC recommended continuation of antibiotics for 60 days (this was later extended to a total of 100 days).

## B. Gastrointestinal

Gastrointestinal anthrax, which is typically acquired by the ingestion of poorly cooked contaminated meat, has an incubation period of 1–7 days. It might be acquired by swallowing aerosolized spores. The oropharyngeal form consists of fever, marked cervical adenopathy, ulcerations at the base of the tongue, dysphagia, and submental swelling. Fever, vomiting, abdominal pain, and bloody diarrhea are characteristics of the abdominal form. Massive ascites may occur. Blood culture results are often positive. Mortality is high, despite antibiotic therapy. Thus antibiotics should be instituted as soon as the diagnosis is considered. Patients should be treated with the same regimen as for inhalational anthrax (Table 11–9).

**Table 11–9.** Initial therapy of invasive or inhalational anthrax secondary to a bioterrorist attack.[a]

| | Empiric therapy |
|---|---|
| Children | Ciprofloxacin[b,c] 20–30 mg/kg/day, intravenously, divided in two daily doses (maximum 1 gram/day) *Plus* one or two additional antibiotics from this list:[d] Vancomycin Rifampin Doxycycline Penicillin[e] Imipenem Clindamycin |
| Adults | Ciprofloxacin[b] 400 mg intravenously every 12 hours *Plus* one or two additional antibiotics from this list:[d] Vancomycin Rifampin Doxycycline Penicillin[e] Imipenem Clindamycin |
| Pregnant Women | Same as for adults above (high mortality outweighs the risks of the antibiotics to the developing fetus). |
| Immunocompromised Persons | Same as for children and adults (above) |

[a]Consult a specialist in infectious disease as well as the state health department. Therapy may need to be modified once susceptibility results are known or in specific outbreak situations. These recommendations also apply to patient with cutaneous anthrax with signs of systemic disease or head/neck lesions, and to patients with gastrointestinal anthrax.
[b]Ciprofloxacin is preferred in a patient with inhalational anthrax secondary to a bioterrorist attack.
[c]If unable to give ciprofloxacin due to patient allergy or unavailability, doxycycline would be the next preferred agent. Doxycycline dose for adults and children > 45 kg is 100 mg, given intravenously every 12 hours. Doxycycline dose for children ≤ 45 kg is 2.2 mg/kg/dose, given intravenously every 12 hours.
[d]Doxycycline and penicillin have in vivo activity with susceptible organisms. The rest of the list has demonstrated activity in vitro. Consider CNS penetration of antibiotics in patients with possible meningitis. Consult with an infectious disease specialist.
[e]*Bacillus anthracis* may have inducible or constitutive beta lactamase production. Penicillin should not be used alone. Consult an infectious disease specialist.

## C. INHALATIONAL

Inhalational anthrax, the most lethal form, occurs after the inhalation of anthrax spores. It is estimated that 8000–40,000 spores can produce lethal disease in 50% of those exposed. Onset of symptoms is typically 1–7 days after exposure, but may be as long as 60 days, depending on inoculum size, host factors, and concurrent antibiotic use (for prophylaxis or other illnesses). Patients initially develop flu-like symptoms of fever, headache, malaise, and myalgias. Vomiting and abdominal pain were observed in the 2001 inhalational anthrax outbreak. Precordial discomfort or chest pain is also common, sometimes first occurring several days after the onset of symptoms. After 2–3 days transient improvement sometimes occurs, followed by abrupt onset of respiratory deterioration, which often leads to respiratory failure, shock, and death. Aggressive antibiotic therapy as well as modern intensive care management reduced mortality from 80% to 45% in the 2001 outbreak. Inhalational anthrax is not transmitted from one person to another.

## Diagnosis

The diagnosis may be difficult early in the illness (outside of a known outbreak) because the symptoms (except rhinorrhea, which is usually absent) are similar to influenza and other acute viral diseases. Almost all patients have abnormalities on either chest radiograph or CT scans. The most common abnormality is a widened mediastinum caused by mediastinitis (Figure 11–9). Pulmonary effusions are present in many patients, probably due to mechanical obstruction of lymphatic vessels (from enlarged nodes) as well as from the effects of edema toxin. Pulmonary infiltrates are seen in some patients, contradicting the classical teaching that infiltrates are not seen in inhalational anthrax.

Blood cultures obtained prior to antibiotics generally will grow *B anthracis* within 24–36 hours. Coagulation studies, blood urea nitrogen, creatinine, and liver function tests should be obtained for severely ill patients. A chest CT scan could be considered if the chest radiograph is normal. Rapid influenza tests can be performed on nasal wash specimens when influenza is in the differential diagnosis. Patients with signs or symptoms suggestive of meningitis should have a lumbar puncture. Pleural fluid may contain the organism. The state health department can arrange specific tests for anthrax, such as PCR or immunohistochemistry tests.

## Treatment

Patients with possible inhalational anthrax should be started on IV antibiotics when the diagnosis is suspected. Most patients will require intensive care moni-

***Figure 11–9.*** Chest radiograph of a patient with inhalational anthrax demonstrates the characteristic widened mediastinum and the presence of pleural effusions. (CDC, Dr PS Brachman, 1961.)

toring. The optimal antibiotic regimen for patients with inhalational anthrax is unknown. There is even less experience with pediatric patients. Table 11–9 lists recommendations for empiric therapy for invasive or inhalational anthrax prior to susceptibility results. These recommendations are for guidance until consultations with an infectious disease specialist and the state health department or CDC are available. Once the susceptibility results are known, therapy may be altered. The specific circumstances of a given bioterrorist event may prompt the CDC to issue alternative recommendations.

Combination therapy was employed during the 2001 outbreak and reduced mortality (compared with historical cases). If susceptibilities are unknown, ciprofloxacin should be used as a first-line agent with one or two other recommended drugs (see Table 11–9). Clindamycin inhibits bacterial protein synthesis and would theoretically inhibit toxin production. Strains of *B anthracis* may produce β-lactamases, so penicillin should not be used alone. If meningitis is suspected, one or two of the drugs used should be able to cross the blood–brain barrier. (If penicillin is used, be sure to use another drug that crosses the blood–brain barrier.) Once susceptibilities of the strain of *B anthracis* are known, the antibiotic regimen may be altered. Antibiotics can be changed from the IV to the oral route once

the patient is improved enough to be discharged from the hospital. Antibiotics should be continued for at least 60 days.

Steroids might be considered for meningitis, based on experience with steroids in other forms of bacterial meningitis. Steroids have been used for severe edema, particularly of the head and neck.

## Postexposure Prophylaxis

### A. ANTIBIOTIC PROPHYLAXIS

Once a bioterrorist attack with anthrax has been identified, the state health department and CDC will identify individuals at high risk for exposure. Possible prophylaxis regimens include oral ciprofloxacin or doxycycline. Once susceptibilities of the offending strain are known, other antibiotics might be recommended. *B anthracis* spores are hardy, and rhesus monkey studies have shown some exposed animals died even after 30 days of antibiotics. For this reason, long prophylaxis regimens are recommended. In the 2001 anthrax outbreak, high-risk individuals were asked to complete 60 days initially and then given the option to extend the prophylaxis regimen by an additional 40 days (100 days total) with or without receiving three doses of the anthrax vaccine.

### B. ANTHRAX VACCINE

Currently, anthrax vaccine is not licensed for postexposure prophylaxis. Protective antigen is the immunogenic agent in a cell-free filtrate of an attenuated strain. This vaccine has been routinely given to active US military personnel and reservists to induce protective immunity *prior* to exposures. It is given subcutaneously at 0, 2 weeks, 4 weeks, 6 months, 12 months, and 18 months. After this series, annual boosters are required. Animal studies have suggested some protective efficacy of the vaccine in postexposure prophylaxis, but there are no data for humans. However, based on animal studies and human immunogenicity studies, it has been suggested that three doses of anthrax vaccine (at 0, 2, and 4 weeks postexposure) might protect against residual anthrax spores in patients receiving postexposure antibiotics. Antibiotics would be continued until about 6 weeks after the first vaccine. Use of vaccine with this approach is available under an investigational new drug protocol (contact Centers for Disease Control and Prevention, Atlanta, GA).

## SMALLPOX

Smallpox is caused by the variola virus. The disease has two forms: variola major, the more severe form, with mortality rates sometimes exceeding 30% in unvaccinated persons (1% if vaccinated); and variola minor, a milder form with a mortality rate of less than 1%.

Smallpox is spread person to person by aerosol or droplet routes. There are no animal reservoirs or human "carrier states." To eliminate smallpox as a human disease, it was essential to disrupt the human-to-human chain of transmission. The World Health Organization (WHO) began a global vaccination campaign in 1967 that eradicated smallpox by 1980. Routine vaccination in the civilian US population stopped in 1972, and the US military ceased vaccination in the late 1980s. In 1999, WHO recommended that all smallpox virus stocks be destroyed or sent for storage to two reference laboratories: CDC in Atlanta and the Institute of Virus Preparations in Moscow. The destruction of these remaining smallpox stores has been postponed, citing the need to maintain the strains for vaccine research.

There is concern that smallpox virus may exist outside the two reference laboratories. The world's population is relatively unprotected from this virus, since no smallpox vaccine has been given worldwide for almost 20 years. Following a single vaccination, neutralizing antibody declines over a 5- to 10-year period. Few people have received more than one vaccine, except as part of travel or military requirements.

In 2002–2003 the United States began a voluntary smallpox vaccination program. The goal of the initiative was to increase the nation's smallpox preparedness capacity by offering vaccination to public health teams and health care workers, who would be the individuals most likely to come in contact with smallpox patients in the event of an outbreak of disease. The plan called for immunization of 450,000 health care and public health workers in the first phase. By August 2003, 38,000 health care and public health workers had received the vaccine. In large part, the effort was stalled by concerns about side effects of vaccination, as well as reports of 22 cases of myocarditis and pericarditis that occurred in vaccine recipients.

## Clinical Signs and Symptoms

The incubation period is 7–17 days (usually 12–14 days). Initial symptoms are similar to those of influenza: fever, headache, and myalgias. By day 4–5, a maculopapular rash develops on the face, then spreads to the extremities, and finally to the trunk. By day 6–7, the characteristic pustules form, which are quite painful and deeply embedded in the skin (Figure 11–10). The rash is most concentrated on the extremities and face, in contrast to varicella (Table 11–10). The lesions develop "in phase" (all at the same time) on a given area of the body. This also contrasts with chickenpox, in which lesions are seen in multiple phases of evolution. At the height of the illness, the patient is toxic. Death occurs from overwhelming viremia or from secondary

***Figure 11–10.*** Typical smallpox lesions. (CDC, James Hicks, 1973.)

infections at the end of the first week or during the second week of the illness. By day 8 or 9, crusts form, and by day 12, scabs are seen. Mortality rates vary with the virulence of the strain and may approach or exceed 30%. As opposed to varicella, smallpox is a disease that affects the deep epithelial structures, including the sebaceous glands. Therefore, scarring is extensive. Smallpox lesions of the cornea can cause scarring and blindness.

Two forms of smallpox are difficult to recognize clinically: hemorrhagic smallpox and malignant smallpox. **Hemorrhagic smallpox** can occur in persons of all ages, but pregnant women are particularly vulnerable. The initial symptoms are typical of smallpox, although more severe, and are followed by a dusky erythema of the skin and the appearance of petechiae and hemorrhages of the mucosal surfaces and gastrointestinal tract. In addition hemorrhage into the skin lesions occurs. Mortality is very high, and death usually occurs within several days of the rash developing. **Malignant smallpox** also begins with the typical constitutional symptoms. Lesions develop and become confluent, but

***Table 11–10.*** Clinical differences between chickenpox and smallpox.

| | Chickenpox | Smallpox |
|---|---|---|
| Rash progression | Occurs in crops | Does not occur in crops |
| Rash distribution | Concentrated on trunk | Concentrated on face and extremities |
| Rash evolution | Lesions are present in multiple forms at the same time: vesicles, pustules, crusts | Lesions all look the same on a given body part—they evolve in phase. |
| Rash presence on palms and soles | Uncommon | Common. Extensive lesions on the palms and soles frequently seen. |

never progress to the vesicular or pustular stage. Instead, they are flat and soft to the touch. The skin develops a crepe paper-like appearance, and petechiae or purpura are sometimes seen. This form of smallpox is difficult to diagnose primarily because the typical "pox" lesions are not seen. Death is common, and the few survivors often have large epidermal losses.

Smallpox is highly contagious. All patients requiring hospitalization need to be isolated in negative-pressure rooms with airborne precautions. In large outbreaks, when the number of patients exceeds isolation capacity, patients can be grouped into cohorts. In addition, a regional "smallpox" hospital or facility might need to be established.

## Differential Diagnosis

The initial differential diagnosis includes influenza and other viral diseases and early anthrax (also presenting with influenza-like symptoms). Later, when the skin lesions are apparent, smallpox must be distinguished from varicella (see Table 11–10).

## Diagnosis

The state health department and the CDC must be notified immediately for any case of suspected smallpox. Because smallpox is an eradicated disease, a single case constitutes a probable bioterrorist event. The reemergence of smallpox would be an international medical emergency because of its potential for spread and the vulnerability of the world's population.

If possible, specimens from the patient should be collected by a person who has been vaccinated within the prior 3 years. In an initial case, however, this may not be possible. Personal protective equipment should be worn (gown, gloves, eye protection, and mask). To obtain vesicle or pustule fluid for viral culture, examination by electron microscopy, or PCR, the lesion will likely need to be opened with a scalpel. The material obtained should be placed in a dry vacutainer tube, the

rubber stopper replaced, and the junction of the tube and stopper sealed with adhesive tape. The whole vacutainer should then be placed in an additional waterproof, sealed container. Smallpox virus isolation and examination require BL-4 level containment facilities, to which these specimens must often be transported. Contact your state health department for specific recommendations on packaging specimens for transport. In a bioterrorist event, this specimen might be considered evidence, and chain of custody must be observed. For all these reasons, it is imperative to notify the state health department immediately if a case is suspected.

## Treatment

No known therapy is effective against human smallpox. The antiviral agent cidofovir appears to prevent disease in mice and monkeys when given in the first 2 days of exposure. However, no studies have been done of its efficacy in humans with smallpox. The drug must be given intravenously and is potentially myelosuppressive and nephrotoxic.

## Infection Control and Postexposure Prophylaxis

Patients who do not need hospitalization should be isolated and cared for at home to minimize spread. Those who require hospitalization should be isolated in negative-pressure rooms with aerosol precautions. Anyone entering the room should wear a gown, mask, gloves, and eye protection. All bed linens, laundry, and wastes should be bagged and autoclaved prior to being laundered or incinerated.

Smallpox vaccination administered within 2–3 days after exposure will prevent the disease in most individuals. Vaccination as late as 4–5 days after exposure may attenuate the disease and prevent death. Therefore, all close contacts of the patient must be identified, vaccinated (if within 4–5 days of exposure), and monitored for development of symptoms. If the contacts become febrile or experience other symptoms, they should be isolated until a diagnosis is made. The Working Group for Civilian Biodefense (Johns Hopkins University) recommends vaccination of all hospital employees (unless contraindicated) at a hospital where a smallpox case is admitted. Currently, the CDC has stockpiled smallpox vaccine that could be released in the event of a smallpox outbreak. In addition to stocks of smallpox vaccine, the CDC maintains control of supplies of vaccinia immune globulin (VIG) to be used in the setting where immunocompromised persons are judged to need immunization. The following groups of patients should be given VIG if smallpox vaccination is required secondary to an exposure: (1) patients who are receiving immunosuppressive agents or radiation, (2) persons with an immunodeficiency syndrome (acquired or congenital, HIV), (3) persons with eczema or other significant exfoliative skin diseases, and (4) pregnant women. VIG should be given intramuscularly at a dose of 0.3 mL/kg in an extremity other than the one used for the smallpox vaccine at the same visit. This will not significantly affect vaccine efficacy. VIG intended for intramuscular administration *cannot* be given intravenously. In addition, VIG is indicated for some types of vaccine complications such as severe generalized vaccinia, progressive vaccinia, and eczema vaccinatum.

## Potential Vaccine Complications

The strain of vaccinia used in the currently stockpiled vaccine has been associated with the lowest complication rate, but complications may still be significant. The number and severity of potential complications of smallpox vaccine are reasons (among others) why routine smallpox vaccination is not currently recommended.

**1. Encephalopathy**—Encephalopathy is most common among children younger than 2 years of age, and 10–25 cases occur per million vaccinees.

**2. Encephalitis**—This occurs in 2–9 vaccinees per million first-time recipients.

**3. Autoinoculation**—Self-inoculation of the vaccinia virus from the vaccine site lesion to other sites of the body is fairly common.

**4. Eczema vaccinatum**—Persons with active or inactive eczema or other exfoliative skin diseases may develop vaccinia lesions (sometimes extensive) at sites of current or previous eczema. This complication can be serious and even fatal.

**5. Generalized vaccinia**—Generalized vaccinia occurs when lesions develop outside the vaccination site in otherwise healthy persons. It is seen only in first-time vaccine recipients. These lesions develop at the same

time as the primary vaccine lesion, thus distinguishing them from autoinoculation variety. They evolve in the same manner as the primary lesion.

**6. Progressive vaccinia**—This occurs in immunocompromised persons who receive smallpox vaccine. It has been seen in patients with humoral (agammaglobulinemia) defects, cell-mediated immunity problems, and patients receiving immunosuppressive agents. The vaccinial lesion does not heal, and the virus spreads to contiguous tissue and systemically to bones and organs. Local tissue destruction is seen. Death occurs in over one third of patients.

Patients with progressive vaccinia, eczema vaccinatum, severe generalized vaccinia, or corneal autoinoculation of vaccinia may benefit from administration of VIG. The recommended dose is 0.6 mL/kg, administered intramuscularly. Due to the large volume of this dose, it can be divided and administered over 24–36 hours. In addition, a second dose (also divided) can be administered if no improvement is noted within 48–72 hours.

A new intravenous vaccinia immune globulin (IV-VIG) is currently available from the CDC under an investigational new drug protocol for treatment of adverse events related to smallpox vaccination (CDC, 1-877-554-4652).

**7. Myocarditis/pericarditis**—Myocarditis or pericarditis (or both) was reported in 22 primary vaccine recipients under the pre-event voluntary health care and public health worker vaccine program. Five civilian patients had cardiac ischemic events after receiving the smallpox vaccine. Review of the data suggested a causal relationship between myocarditis/pericarditis and the vaccine. However, the rate of cardiac ischemic events in vaccine recipients was not above the expected background rate. As a precaution, the Advisory Committee on Immunization Practices (ACIP) and the CDC recommend screening and excluding persons from preevent vaccination if there is a history of cardiac disease or any of the following risk factors: previous myocardial infarction, angina, congestive heart failure, cardiomyopathy, stroke, or transient ischemic attack. In addition, persons with three or more of the following risk factors should not receive vaccine under this program: hypertension, diabetes, hypercholesterolemia, smoking, or an immediate family member who had onset of a heart condition before age 50.

## PLAGUE

Plague is caused by *Yersinia pestis,* a gram-negative bacterium. The clinical manifestations of plague caused by a bioterrorist attack would differ from bubonic plague, the type clinicians are most familiar with. A bioterrorist attack would likely use aerosolized *Y pestis*. Inhalation of 100–500 bacilli could result in primary pneumonic plague (as opposed to "bubonic plague"). Primary pneumonic plague is rare in the United States and has been associated with cats that have acquired pneumonic plague and passed it to their owners. The incubation period for primary pneumonic plague is short: 1–6 days (usually 2–4). Symptoms include fever, malaise, shortness of breath, cough, and sometimes hemoptysis or bloody sputum. Nausea, vomiting, diarrhea, and abdominal pain are common. No buboes usually appear (as seen in bubonic plague), although occasionally cervical buboes may be seen. Chest radiograph typically shows a bilateral, lobar pneumonia. The white blood count is typically elevated with leukocytosis.

## Diagnosis

No widely accessible, rapid diagnostic tests are available for plague. A presumptive diagnosis may be made from the Gram stain of sputum, lymph node aspirate (if bubo present), CSF, or stained blood smear. Gram-negative bacilli or coccobacilli, sometimes with "safety pin" bipolar staining, are characteristic. Blood culture results are usually positive. CSF and lymph node aspirate specimens, if obtained, should be cultured. The laboratory should be alerted to take appropriate precautions with the samples, and they should be informed plague is suspected. The health department should be notified immediately for suspected plague, as pneumonic plague has the potential for rapid spread. The state health department can also facilitate further testing for plague. A direct fluorescent antibody test, as well as PCR, is available through some state health departments and the CDC.

## Treatment

Primary pneumonic plague progresses rapidly. Therefore, antibiotics need to be administered immediately if the diagnosis is suspected. Mortality is quite high if antibiotic therapy is initiated later than 24 hours after symptoms start. Streptomycin has been used historically for plague and is FDA-approved for this use. However, lack of availability of this medicine, coupled with lack of familiarity with its use, has led many experts to recommend gentamicin. In addition, streptomycin must be administered intramuscularly. For patients with sepsis or shock, the intramuscular route may lead to erratic absorption. All these factors make gentamicin a reasonable choice. Doxycycline has been used in some cases with successful results. In the event that streptomycin or gentamicin cannot be given, doxycycline could be used. Ciprofloxacin has shown efficacy in animal studies, but there are no human studies of its use in plague. Antibiotics are usually continued for 10 days or, in late responders, for several days beyond lysis of fever.

All of the medications useful for plague are potentially problematic for pregnant women. Pregnant women should not be treated with streptomycin, if avoidable, as it is associated with fetal deafness. Gentamicin is also not generally recommended in pregnancy, except for serious illness. Doxycycline has been associated with fetal bone developmental problems and maternal liver toxicity. Gentamicin is recommended as the preferred agent in pregnancy, followed by doxycycline as an alternative.

## Infection Control

Primary pneumonic plague is transmitted by respiratory droplets or aerosols. A 7-day course of doxycycline is recommended for plague prophylaxis for individuals who are asymptomatic household (or close) contacts or hospital contacts. Close contacts are those who were within 6 feet an infected person. Contacts who begin prophylaxis should also wear a surgical mask and limit unnecessary contact with others for the first 48 hours of therapy. Masks can be discontinued for asymptomatic contacts that have been on prophylaxis for more than 48 hours. Contacts who develop fever or other symptoms should be promptly evaluated, isolated, and given IV antibiotics while awaiting diagnostic evaluation. Hospital personnel attending to patients with pneumonic plague should wear gowns, gloves, masks, and eye protection.

In the event of a bioterrorist incident, postexposure prophylaxis might be recommended by the CDC or state health department to individuals known to be at high risk for an exposure. Doxycycline and ciprofloxacin would be the agents most likely recommended, because they are oral drugs and readily obtainable.

## BOTULINUM TOXIN

*Clostridium botulinum* is a spore-forming, anaerobic bacterium that makes botulinum toxin. This is the most potent neurotoxin known. There are actually seven different botulinum toxins made by *C botulinum*, designated by the letters A through G. These act by irreversibly binding to the presynaptic cholinergic membrane and inhibiting release of acetylcholine. Botulism is classically a food-borne disease seen when humans ingest preformed toxin present in improperly canned foods. A bioterrorist release of botulinum toxin would likely be aerosolized. Inhalation of the toxin and absorption into the bloodstream carry the toxin throughout the body. The clinical syndrome seen in these patients is very similar to food-borne botulism. The incubation period for an inhalational exposure is unknown, but is probably 12–96 hours.

## Signs and Symptoms

Patients typically present with diplopia, ptosis, difficulty swallowing, and speech abnormalities (see Chapter 38). Loss of head control, symmetrical weakness, and respiratory difficulties may occur as the descending paralysis progresses. Patients may need mechanical ventilation due to loss of gag reflexes and paralysis of respiratory musculature. The toxin does not cross the blood–brain barrier, so patients have a clear sensorium. This may be difficult to establish, however, as these patients may have extreme difficulties communicating because of bulbar palsies. Patients with botulism are afebrile unless they have a secondary infection such as aspiration pneumonia. Deep tendon reflexes are often diminished or absent.

## Diagnosis and Treatment (These are discussed in Chapter 38.)

## Postexposure Prophylaxis

Theoretically, neutralizing antibody present prior to exposure or delivered shortly after could bind to toxins and prevent clinical botulism. This has been demonstrated in primate studies. However, botulism antitoxins are scarce in the United States, and providing antitoxin for widespread exposures would be impossible.

Arnon SS et al: Botulinum toxin as a biological weapon: Medical and public health management. Smallpox as a biological weapon: Medical and public health management. Working Group on Civilian Biodefense. JAMA 2001;285:1059 [PMID: 11209178].

Fulginiti VA et al: Smallpox vaccination: A review, part I. Background, vaccination technique, normal vaccination and re-vaccination, and expected normal reactions. Clin Infect Dis 2003;37(2):241 [PMID: 12856217].

Inglesby T et al: Plague as a biological weapon. JAMA 2000;283: 2281 [PMID: 10807389].

Inglesby TV et al: Anthrax as a biological weapon, 2002: Updated recommendations for management. JAMA 2002;287(17): 2236 [PMID: 11980524].

Jernigan JA et al: Bioterrorism-related inhalational anthrax: The first 10 cases reported in the United States. Emerg Infect Dis 2001;7:993 [PMID: 11747719].

Wharton M et al: Recommendations for using smallpox vaccine in a pre-event program. MMWR 2003;52(RR07):1 [PMID: 12710832].

# Poisoning

**12**

*Richard C. Dart, MD, PhD, & Barry H. Rumack, MD*

Poisonings result from the complex interaction of the agent, the child, and the family environment. The peak incidence is at age 2 years. Most ingestions occur in children younger than age 5 years as a result of insecure storage of drugs, household chemicals, and the like. Twenty-five percent of children will have a second episode of ingestion within 1 year following the first one. Repeated poisonings may require intervention on the child's behalf. Accidental poisonings are unusual after age 5 years. Poisonings in older children and adolescents usually represent manipulative behavior, chemical or drug abuse, or genuine suicide attempts.

Watson WA et al: 2002 annual report of the American Association of Poison Control Centers Toxic Exposure Surveillance System. Am J Emerg Med 2003;21:353 [PMID: 14523881].

## PREVENTING CHILDHOOD POISONINGS

Each year, children are accidentally poisoned by medicines, polishes, insecticides, drain cleaners, bleaches, household chemicals, and garage products. It is the responsibility of adults to make sure that children are not exposed to potentially toxic substances.

Here are some suggestions for parents:

1. Insist on packages with safety closures and learn how to use them properly.
2. Keep household cleaning supplies, medicines, garage products, and insecticides out of the reach and sight of your child. Lock them up whenever possible.
3. Never store food and cleaning products together. Store medicine and chemicals in original containers and never in food or beverage containers.
4. Avoid taking medicine in your child's presence. Children love to imitate. Never suggest that medicine is candy.
5. Read the label on all products and heed warnings and cautions. Never use medicine from an unlabeled or unreadable container. Never pour medicine in a darkened area where the label cannot be seen clearly.
6. If you are interrupted while using a product, take it with you—it takes only a few seconds for your child to get into it.
7. Know what your child can do physically. For example, if you have a crawling infant, keep household products stored above floor level, not beneath the kitchen sink.
8. Keep the phone numbers of your doctor, poison center, hospital, police department, and emergency medical system near the phone.

## PHARMACOLOGIC PRINCIPLES OF TOXICOLOGY

In the evaluation of the poisoned patient, it is important to compare the anticipated pharmacologic or toxic effects with the patient's clinical presentation. If the history is that the patient ingested a tranquilizer 30 minutes ago, but the clinical examination reveals dilated pupils, tachycardia, dry mouth, absent bowel sounds, and active hallucinations—clearly anticholinergic toxicity—diagnosis and therapy should proceed accordingly.

### LD$_{50}$

Estimates of the LD$_{50}$ (the amount per kilogram of body weight of a drug required to kill 50% of a group of experimental animals) or median lethal dose are of little clinical value in humans. It is usually impossible to determine with accuracy the amount swallowed or absorbed, the metabolic status of the patient, or in which patients the response to the agent will be atypical. Furthermore, these values are often not valid in humans even if the history is accurate.

### Half-Life (t$_{1/2}$)

The $t_{1/2}$ of an agent must be interpreted carefully. Most published $t_{1/2}$ values are for therapeutic dosages. The $t_{1/2}$ may increase as the quantity of the ingested substance increases for many common intoxicants such as salicylates and phenytoin. One cannot rely on the published $t_{1/2}$ for salicylate (2 hours) to assume rapid elimination of the drug. In an acute salicylate overdose (150 mg/kg), the apparent $t_{1/2}$ is prolonged to 24–30 hours.

346

## Volume of Distribution

The volume of distribution (Vd) of a drug is determined by dividing the amount of drug absorbed by the blood level. With theophylline, for example, the Vd is 0.46 L/kg body weight, or 32 L in an adult. In contrast, digoxin distributes well beyond total body water. Because the calculation produces a volume above body weight this figure is frequently referred to as an apparent volume of distribution, a designation shared by many drugs (Table 12–1).

The Vd can be useful in predicting which drugs will be removed by dialysis, extracorporeal perfusion, or exchange transfusion. When a drug is differentially concentrated in body lipids or is heavily tissue- or protein-bound and has a high volume of distribution, only a small proportion of the drug will be in the free form and thus accessible to diuresis, dialysis, or exchange transfusion. A drug that is water-soluble and has a low volume of distribution may cross the dialysis membrane well and also respond to diuresis. In general, methods of extracorporeal elimination are not effective for toxic agents with a Vd greater than 1 L/kg.

## Metabolism & Excretion

The route of excretion or detoxification is important for planning treatment. Methanol, for example, is metabolized to the toxic product, formic acid. This metabolic step may be blocked by the antidote fomepizole or ethanol.

## Blood Levels

Care of the poisoned patient should never be guided solely by laboratory measurements. Treatment should be directed first by the clinical signs and symptoms, followed by more specific therapy based on laboratory determinations. Clinical information may speed the identification of a toxic agent by the laboratory.

# GENERAL TREATMENT OF POISONING

The telephone is often the first contact in pediatric poisoning. Proper telephone management can reduce morbidity and prevent unwarranted or excessive treatment. The decision to refer the patient is based on the identity and dose of the ingested agent, the age of the child, the time of day, the reliability of the parent, and whether child neglect or endangerment is suspected.

## Initial Telephone Contact

Basic information that should be written down at the first telephone contact includes the patient's name, age, weight, address and telephone number, the agent and amount of agent ingested, the patient's present condition, and the time elapsed since ingestion or other exposure.

Use the history to evaluate the urgency of the situation and decide whether immediate emergency transportation to a health facility is indicated. An emergency exists if the ingestant is high risk (caustic solutions, hydrogen fluoride, drugs of abuse, or medications such as a calcium channel blocker, opioid, hypoglycemic agent, antidepressant) or if the self-poisoning was intentional. If immediate danger does not exist, obtain more details about the suspected toxic agent. It may be difficult to obtain an accurate history. Obtain names of drugs or ingredients, manufacturers, prescription numbers, names and phone numbers of prescribing physician and

***Table 12–1.*** Some examples of p$K_a$ and Vd.

| Drug | p$K_a$ | Diuresis | Dialysis | Apparent Vd |
|---|---|---|---|---|
| Amobarbital | 7.9 | No | No | 200–300% body weight |
| Amphetamine | 9.8 | No | Yes | 60% body weight |
| Aspirin | 3.5 | Alkaline | Yes | 15–40% body weight |
| Chlorpromazine | 9.3 | No | No | 40–50 L/kg (2800–3500% body weight) |
| Codeine | 8.2 | No | No | 5–10 L/kg (350–700% body weight) |
| Desipramine | 10.2 | No | No | 30–40 L/kg (2100–2800% body weight) |
| Ethchlorvynol | 8.7 | No | No | 5–10 L/kg (350–700% body weight) |
| Glutethimide | 4.5 | No | No | 10–20 L/kg (700–1400% body weight) |
| Isoniazid | 3.5 | Alkaline | Yes | 61% body weight |
| Methadone | 8.3 | No | No | 5–10 L/kg (350–700% body weight) |
| Methicillin | 2.8 | No | Yes | 60% body weight |
| Phenobarbital | 7.4 | Alkaline | Yes | 75% body weight |
| Phenytoin | 8.3 | No | No | 60–80% body weight |
| Tetracycline | 7.7 | No | No | 200–300% body weight |

pharmacy, and so on. Find out whether the substance was shared among several children, whether it had been recently purchased, who had last used it, how full the bottle was, and how much was spilled. If unsure of the significance of an exposure, consult with a certified Poison Control Center.

## FIRST AID FOR POISONING (Advice for Parents)

Syrup of ipecac is used to induce vomiting; the activated charcoal is used to bind poisons. Use them only as instructed by your Poison Control Center or doctor. Consult your physician to decide if you should keep syrup of ipecac and activated charcoal in your home.

### Inhaled Poisons

If smoke, gas, or fumes have been inhaled, immediately drag or carry the victim to fresh air. Then call 911, the Poison Control Center, or your doctor. Do not enter an area where poisonous fumes are present that have caused loss of consciousness. Too often the rescuer becomes a victim as well.

### Poisons on the Skin

If the poison has been spilled on the skin or clothing, remove the clothing and flood the involved parts with water. Wash with soapy water and rinse thoroughly. Then call the Poison Control Center or your doctor.

### Swallowed Poisons

If the substance swallowed is a medicine, give nothing. Milk or water should be administered immediately to any patient who has ingested a strongly acid or alkaline agent. Do not give more than 15 mL/kg (250 mL maximum in a child weighing 16 kg or more). Do not induce vomiting in patients who are comatose, convulsing, or who have lost the gag reflex. Induce emesis with ipecac or administer charcoal **only** if advised to do so by a health care professional. **Caution:** Antidote labels on products may be incorrect. Do not give salt, vinegar, or lemon juice. Call before doing anything else.

### Poisons in the Eye

Rinse out the eye with plain water before the patient arrives at the emergency room. Use plain tap water—do not try to neutralize acids or bases. Pour water into the eye from a drinking glass or pitcher for 15–20 minutes or fill a basin with water and have the patient put his or her face into the water and open the eyes to dilute. Then transport the patient to the hospital.

### Bring the Poison to the Hospital

Everything in the vicinity of the patient that may be a cause of poisoning should be brought to the health care facility.

## OBTAINING INFORMATION ABOUT POISONS

Current data on ingredients of commercial products and medications can be obtained from a certified regional poison center. It is important to have the actual container at hand when calling. **Caution:** Antidote information on labels of commercial products or in the *Physicians' Desk Reference* may be incorrect or inappropriate.

## FOLLOW-UP

In over 95% of cases of ingestion of potentially toxic substances by children, a trip to the hospital is not required. In these cases, it is important to call the parent at 1 and 4 hours after an ingestion. If the child has ingested an additional unknown agent and develops symptoms, a change in management may be needed, including transportation to the hospital. An additional call should be made 24 hours after the ingestion to begin the process of poison prevention.

## PREVENTION OF POISONING

A major goal of pediatricians is to reduce the number of accidental ingestions in the high-risk age group (ie, < age 5 years). A systematic poison education effort should be part of the routine care of every patient. Parents of very young children should be encouraged to search the house and identify all hazardous substances that should be removed from the home or locked up. Pediatric or medical office staff can help families with poison prevention by telephone by asking a few simple questions about storage of hazardous substances in the home. The following is a partial list of potentially poisonous substances that must be stored safely if small children are in the home: drain-cleaning crystals or liquid, dishwasher soap and cleaning supplies, paints and paint thinners, garden spray and other insecticide materials, automobile products (antifreeze, windshield wiper fluid, gasoline), and all medications.

The section entitled Preventing Childhood Poisonings may be copied from this book and given to parents at the 6-month check-up. Although syrup of ipecac is not recommended for all poisonings, it is useful for some types, such as plant material, pills too large to be lavaged, and decontamination in rural areas where health care may be 30 minutes or more away. Reinforcement should occur at the 1-year check-up to make certain that adequate poison-proofing measures have been instituted and maintained.

# INITIAL EMERGENCY DEPARTMENT CONTACT

## Make Certain the Patient Is Breathing

As in all emergencies, the principles of treatment are attention to airway, breathing, and circulation. These are sometimes overlooked under the stressful conditions of a pediatric poisoning.

## Treat Shock

Initial therapy of the hypotensive patient should consist of laying the patient flat and administering intravenous isotonic solutions. Vasopressors should be reserved for poisoned patients in shock who do not respond to these standard measures.

## Treat Burns

Burns may occur following exposure to strong acid or strong alkaline agents or petroleum distillates. Burned areas should be decontaminated by flooding with sterile saline solution or water. A burn unit should be consulted if more than minimal burn damage has been sustained. Skin decontamination should be performed in a patient with cutaneous exposure. Emergency department personnel in contact with a patient who has been contaminated (with an organophosphate insecticide, for example) should themselves be decontaminated if their skin or clothing becomes contaminated.

## Take a Pertinent History

The history should be taken from the parents and all individuals present at the scene. It may be crucial to determine all of the kinds of poisons in the home. These may include drugs used by family members, chemicals associated with the hobbies or occupations of family members, or the purity of the water supply. Unusual dietary or medication habits or other clues to the possible cause of poisoning should also be investigated.

# DEFINITIVE THERAPY OF POISONING

## Prevention of Absorption

### A. EMESIS

Induced vomiting is contraindicated in patients who have ingested a minimally toxic substance (eg, most antibiotics), who are comatose or convulsing, or who have lost the gag reflex or ingested strong acids, strong bases,

some hydrocarbons, or sharp objects. The use of ipecac has decreased dramatically over the past 10 years and is reserved for those instances when medications have been taken within 30–60 minutes prior to contact.

**1. Ipecac method**—This may be effective if administered within an hour of ingestion. Adult dose, 30 mL; pediatric dose, 15 mL. Give orally (PO) and repeat once in 20 minutes if necessary.

**2. Other emetics**—The only approved oral emetic agent is syrup of ipecac. Use of sodium chloride may lead to lethal hypernatremia. Apomorphine, mustard, soap, and other emetics should not be used.

### B. LAVAGE

If the patient is or is becoming unconscious, is convulsing, or has lost the gag reflex, gastric lavage following endotracheal or nasotracheal intubation should be performed rather than induction of vomiting. Lavage is rarely performed in pediatric patients. Emesis and lavage recover an average of about 30% of the stomach contents if performed soon after ingestion. Although these procedures may be helpful in reducing the amount of material available for absorption, approximately 70% of an ingested dose will remain. Additional measures such as charcoal should be instituted to prevent further absorption.

### C. CHARCOAL

The dose of charcoal is 1–2 g/kg (maximum, 100 g) per dose. Repeating the dose of activated charcoal may be useful for those agents that slow passage through the gastrointestinal (GI) tract. When multiple doses of activated charcoal are given, repeated doses of sorbitol or saline cathartics must not be given. Repeated doses of cathartics may cause electrolyte imbalances and fluid loss. Charcoal dosing is repeated every 2–6 hours until charcoal is passed through the rectum.

### D. CATHARSIS

Despite their widespread use, cathartics have not been shown to improve outcome. The use of cathartics should therefore be avoided.

### E. WHOLE GUT LAVAGE

Whole bowel lavage uses an orally administered, nonabsorbable hypertonic solution such as CoLyte or GoLYTELY. The use of this procedure in poisoned patients remains controversial. Preliminary recommendations for use of whole bowel irrigation include poisoning with sustained-release preparations, mechanical movement of items through the bowel (eg, cocaine packets, iron tablets), and poisoning with substances poorly absorbed by charcoal (eg, lithium, iron). Underlying bowel pathology and intestinal obstruction are relative contraindications to its use. Consultation with a certified regional poison center is recommended.

American Academy of Clinical Toxicology, European Association of Poisons Centers and Clinical Toxicologists: Position statement and practice guidelines on the use of multidose activated charcoal in the treatment of acute poisoning. J Toxicol Clin Toxicol 1999;37:731 [PMID: 10584586].

Gielen AC et al: Effects of improved access to safety counseling, products, and home visits on parents' safety practices: Results of a randomized trial. Arch Pediatr Adolesc Med 2002;156:33 [PMID: 11772403].

Hoffman RJ, Nelson L: Rational use of toxicology testing in children. Curr Opin Pediatr 2001;13:183 [PMID: 11317063].

Vale JA: Position statement: Gastric lavage. American Academy of Clinical Toxicology; European Association of Poisons Centres and Clinical Toxicologists. J Toxicol Clin Toxicol 1997;35:711 [PMID: 9482426].

## Enhancement of Excretion

Excretion of certain substances can be hastened by urinary alkalinization or dialysis. It is important to make certain that the patient is not volume-depleted. Volume-depleted patients should receive a normal saline bolus of 10–20 mL/kg, followed by sufficient intravenous (IV) fluid administration to maintain urine output at 2–3 mL/kg/h.

### A. URINARY ALKALINIZATION

**1. Alkaline diuresis**—Urinary alkalinization should be chosen on the basis of the substance's $pK_a$, so that ionized drug will be trapped in the tubular lumen and not reabsorbed (see Table 12–1). Thus, if the $pK_a$ is less than 7.5, urinary alkalinization is appropriate; if it is over 8.0, this technique is not usually beneficial. The $pK_a$ is sometimes included along with general drug information. Urinary alkalinization is achieved with sodium bicarbonate. It is important to observe for hypokalemia, caused by the shift of potassium intracellularly. Follow serum $K^+$ and observe for ECG evidence of hypokalemia. If complications such as renal failure or pulmonary edema are present, hemodialysis or hemoperfusion may be required.

### B. DIALYSIS

Hemodialysis (or peritoneal dialysis if hemodialysis is unavailable) is useful in the poisonings listed below. Dialysis should be considered part of supportive care if the patient satisfies any of the following criteria:

**1. Clinical criteria—**

**a.** Potentially life-threatening toxicity that is caused by a dialyzable drug and cannot be treated by conservative means.

**b.** Hypotension threatening renal or hepatic function that cannot be corrected by adjusting circulating volum.

**c.** Marked hyperosmolality or severe acid–base or electrolyte disturbances not responding to therapy.

**d.** Marked hypothermia or hyperthermia not responding to therapy.

**2. Immediate dialysis**—Immediate dialysis should be considered in ethylene glycol and methanol poisoning only if acidosis is refractory, the patient does not respond to fomepizole treatment, or blood levels of ethanol of 100 mg/dL are consistently maintained.

**3. Dialysis indicated on basis of condition of patient**—In general, dialyze if the patient is in a coma deeper than level 3. Peritoneal dialysis or exchange transfusion may be more useful than hemodialysis in small children—as much for ease of achieving fluid and electrolyte homeostasis as for poison removal. Other drugs not listed here may be dialyzable. Information should be verified prior to institution of dialysis.

## ■ MANAGEMENT OF SPECIFIC COMMON POISONINGS

### ACETAMINOPHEN (PARACETAMOL)

Overdosage of acetaminophen is the most common pediatric poisoning and can produce severe hepatotoxicity. The incidence of hepatotoxicity in adults and adolescents has been reported to be ten times higher than in children younger than age 5 years. In the latter group, less than 0.1% develop hepatotoxicity after acetaminophen overdose. In children, toxicity most commonly results from repeated overdosage arising from confusion about the age-appropriate dose, use of multiple products that contain acetaminophen, or use of adult suppositories.

Acetaminophen is normally metabolized in the liver. A small percentage of the drug goes through a pathway leading to a toxic metabolite. Normally, this electrophilic reactant is removed harmlessly by conjugation with glutathione. In overdosage, the supply of glutathione becomes exhausted, and the metabolite may bind covalently to components of liver cells to produce necrosis. Some authors have proposed that therapeutic doses of acetaminophen may be toxic to children with depleted glutathione stores. However, there is no evidence that administration of therapeutic doses can cause toxicity, and only a few inadequate case reports have been made in this regard.

## Treatment

Treatment is to administer acetylcysteine. In the United States, it may only be given PO. Consultation on difficult cases may be obtained from the Rocky Mountain Poison Center (1-800-525-6115) or any poison center. Blood levels should be obtained as soon as possible after 4 hours and plotted on Figure 12–1. The nomogram is used only for acute ingestion, not repeated supratherapeutic ingestions. If the patient has ingested acetaminophen in a liquid preparation, blood levels obtained 2 hours after ingestion will give an accurate reflection of the toxicity to be expected relative to the standard nomogram (see Figure 12–1). Acetylcysteine is administered to patients whose acetaminophen levels plot in the toxic range on the nomogram. Acetylcysteine is effective even when given more than 24 hours after ingestion although it is most effective when given within 8 hours postingestion.

The dose of acetylcysteine is 140 mg/kg PO, diluted to a 5% solution in sweet fruit juice or carbonated soft drink. The primary problems associated with administration are nausea and vomiting. After this loading dose, 70 mg/kg should be administered PO every 4 hours for 72 hours. Aspartate aminotransferase (AST), alanine aminotransferase (ALT), serum bilirubin, and plasma prothrombin time should be followed daily. Significant abnormalities of liver function may not develop until up to 72 hours after ingestion. Repeated miscalculated overdoses given by parents to treat

fever are the major source of toxicity in children younger than age 10 years, and parents are often unaware of the significance of symptoms of toxicity, thus delaying its prompt recognition and therapy.

Rumack BH: Acetaminophen hepatotoxicity: The first 35 years. J Toxicol Clin Toxicol 2002;40:3 [PMID: 11990202].

Smilkstein M et al: Efficacy of oral N-acetylcysteine in the treatment of acetaminophen overdose. N Engl J Med 1988;319:1557 [PMID: 0003059186].

Sztajnkrycer MJ, Bond GR: Chronic acetaminophen overdosing in children: Risk assessment and management. Curr Opin Pediatr 2001;13:177 [PMID: 11317062].

## ALCOHOL, ETHYL (ETHANOL)

Alcoholic beverages, tinctures, cosmetics, and rubbing alcohol are common sources of poisoning in children. Concomitant exposure to other depressant drugs increases the seriousness of the intoxication. (Blood levels cited here are for adults; comparable figures for children are not available.) In most states, alcohol levels of 50–80 mg/dL are considered compatible with impaired faculties, and levels of 80–100 mg/dL are considered evidence of intoxication.

Complete absorption of alcohol requires 30 minutes to 6 hours, depending on the volume, the presence of food, and the time spent in consuming the alcohol. The rate of metabolic degradation is constant (about 20 mg/h in an adult). Absolute ethanol, 1 mL/kg, re-

**Figure 12–1.** Semilogarithmic plot of plasma acetaminophen levels versus time. (Modified and reproduced, with permission, from Rumack BH, Matthew H: Acetaminophen poisoning and toxicity. Pediatrics 1975;55:871.)

sults in a peak blood level of about 100 mg/dL in 1 hour after ingestion. Acute intoxication and chronic alcoholism increase the risk of subarachnoid hemorrhage.

## Treatment

Management of hypoglycemia and acidosis is usually the only measure required. Start an IV drip of $D_5W$ or $D_{10}W$ if blood glucose is under 60 mg/dL. Fructose has been suggested as an accelerator of metabolism, but it may cause vomiting, intensify lactic acidosis, and decrease blood volume via osmotic diuresis. Glucagon does not correct the hypoglycemia, because hepatic glycogen stores are reduced. Death is usually caused by respiratory failure. In severe cases, cerebral edema should be treated with IV dexamethasone, 0.1 mg/kg every 4–6 hours. Dialysis is indicated in life-threatening intoxication.

Ernst AA et al: Ethanol ingestion and related hypoglycemia in a pediatric and adolescent emergency department population. Acad Emerg Med 1996;3:46 [PMID: 8749967].

Roy M et al: What are the adverse effects of ethanol used as an antidote in the treatment of suspected methanol poisoning in children? J Toxicol Clin Toxicol 2003;41:155 [PMID: 12733853].

## AMPHETAMINES & RELATED DRUGS (METHAMPHETAMINE)

### Clinical Presentation

#### A. ACUTE POISONING

Amphetamine and methamphetamine poisoning is common because of the widespread availability of "diet pills" and the use of "speed," "crank," "crystal," and "ice" by adolescents. (Care must be taken in the interpretation of slang terms because they have multiple meanings.) A new cause of amphetamine poisoning are drugs for treating attention deficit hyperactivity disorder, such as methylphenidate. Symptoms include CNS stimulation, anxiety, hyperactivity, hyperpyrexia, hypertension, abdominal cramps, nausea and vomiting, and inability to void urine. Severe cases often include rhabdomyolysis. A toxic psychosis indistinguishable from paranoid schizophrenia may occur. Methamphetamine laboratories in homes are a potential cause of childhood exposure to a variety of hazardous and toxic substances.

#### B. CHRONIC POISONING

Chronic amphetamine users develop tolerance; more than 1500 mg of IV methamphetamine can be used daily. Hyperactivity, disorganization, and euphoria are followed by exhaustion, depression, and coma lasting 2–3 days. Heavy users, taking more than 100 mg/d, have restlessness, incoordination of thought, insomnia, nervousness, irritability, and visual hallucinations. Psychosis may be precipitated by the chronic administration of high doses. Depression, weakness, tremors, GI complaints, and suicidal thoughts occur frequently.

## Treatment

Standard decontamination procedures should be used: gastric emptying followed by charcoal in recent ingestions; activated charcoal alone if ingestion occurred hours earlier. The treatment of choice is diazepam, titrated in small increments to effect. Very large total doses may be needed. In case of extreme agitation or hallucinations, droperidol (0.1 mg/kg/dose) or haloperidol (up to 0.1 mg/kg) parenterally has been used. When combinations of amphetamines and barbiturates (diet pills) are used, the action of the amphetamines begins first, followed by a depression caused by the barbiturates. In these cases, treatment with additional barbiturates is contraindicated because of the risk of respiratory failure.

Chronic users may be withdrawn rapidly from amphetamines. If amphetamine–barbiturate combination tablets have been used, the barbiturates must be withdrawn gradually to prevent withdrawal seizures. Psychiatric treatment should be provided.

Kolecki P: Inadvertent methamphetamine poisoning in pediatric patients. Pediatr Emerg Care 1998;14:385 [PMID: 9881979].

Schwartz RH, Miller NS: MDMA (ecstasy) and the rave: A review. Pediatrics 1997;100:705 [PMID: 9310529].

## ANESTHETICS, LOCAL

Intoxication from local anesthetics may be associated with CNS stimulation, acidosis, delirium, ataxia, shock, convulsions, and death. Methemoglobinuria has been reported following local dental analgesia. The maximum recommended dose for subcutaneous (SQ) infiltration is 4.5 mg/kg. The temptation to exceed this dose in procedures lasting a long time is great and may result in inadvertent overdosage. PO application of viscous lidocaine may produce toxicity. Hypercapnia may lower the seizure threshold to locally injected anesthetics.

Local anesthetics used in obstetrics cross the placental barrier and are not efficiently metabolized by the fetal liver. Mepivacaine, lidocaine, and bupivacaine can cause fetal bradycardia, neonatal depression, and death. Prilocaine causes methemoglobinemia, which should be treated if levels in the blood exceed 40% or if the patient is symptomatic.

Accidental injection of mepivacaine into the head of the fetus during paracervical anesthesia has caused neonatal asphyxia, cyanosis, acidosis, bradycardia, convulsions, and death.

## Treatment

If the anesthetic has been ingested, mucous membranes should be cleansed carefully and activated charcoal may be administered. Oxygen administration is indicated, with assisted ventilation if necessary. Methemoglobinemia is treated with methylene blue, 1%, 0.2 mL/kg (1–2 mg/kg/dose, IV) over 5–10 minutes; this should promptly relieve the cyanosis. Acidosis may be treated with sodium bicarbonate, seizures with diazepam, bradycardia with atropine. Therapeutic levels of mepivacaine, lidocaine, and procaine are less than 5 mg/mL.

Bozynski MEA et al: Lidocaine toxicity after maternal pudendal anesthesia in a term infant with fetal distress. Am J Perinatol 1987;4:164 [PMID: 3566884].

Spiller HA et al: Multi-center retrospective evaluation of oral benzocaine exposure in children. Vet Hum Toxicol 2000;42:228 [PMID: 10928690].

## ANTIHISTAMINES

Although antihistamines typically cause CNS depression, children often react paradoxically with excitement, hallucinations, delirium, ataxia, tremors, and convulsions followed by CNS depression, respiratory failure, or cardiovascular collapse. Anticholinergic effects such as dry mouth, fixed dilated pupils, flushed face, fever, and hallucinations may be prominent.

Antihistamines are widely available in allergy, sleep, cold, and antiemetic preparations, and many are supplied in sustained-release forms, which increases the likelihood of dangerous overdoses. They are absorbed rapidly and metabolized by the liver, lungs, and kidneys. A potentially toxic dose is 10–50 mg/kg of the most commonly used antihistamines, but toxic reactions have occurred at much lower doses.

## Treatment

Activated charcoal should be used to reduce drug absorption. Emetics may be ineffective if the antihistamine is structurally related to phenothiazines. Whole bowel irrigation may be useful for sustained-release preparations. Physostigmine, 0.5–2 mg IV slowly administered, dramatically reverses the central and peripheral anticholinergic effects of antihistamines, but it should be used only for diagnostic purposes. Diazepam, 0.1–0.2 mg/kg IV, can be used to control seizures. Forced diuresis is not helpful. Exchange transfusion was reported to be effective in one case.

Cetaruk EW, Aaron CK: Hazards of nonprescription medications. Emerg Med Clin North Am 1994;12:483 [PMID: 8187693].

Skare JA: Antihistamine-containing cough/cold medications present a low hazard in pediatric accidental exposure incidents: Analysis of Poison Control Center data. Vet Hum Toxicol 1997;39:367 [PMID: 9397509].

Ten Eick AP et al: Safety of antihistamines in children. Drug Saf 2001;24:119 [PMID: 11235817].

## ARSENIC

Arsenic is used in some insecticides (fruit tree or tobacco sprays), rodenticides, weed killers, and wood preservatives. It is well absorbed primarily through the GI and respiratory tracts, but skin absorption may occur. Arsenic can be found in the urine, hair, and nails by laboratory testing.

Highly toxic soluble derivatives of this compound, such as sodium arsenite, are frequently found in liquid preparations and can cause death in as many as 65% of victims. The organic arsonates found in persistent or preemergence weed killers are relatively less soluble and less toxic. Poisonings with a liquid arsenical preparation that does not contain alkyl methanearsonate compounds should be considered potentially lethal. Patients exhibiting clinical signs other than gastroenteritis should receive treatment until laboratory tests indicate that treatment is no longer necessary.

## Clinical Presentation

### A. ACUTE POISONING

Abdominal pain, vomiting, watery and bloody diarrhea, cardiovascular collapse, paresthesias, neck pain, and garlic odor on breath occur. Convulsions, coma, anuria, and exfoliative dermatitis are later signs. Inhalation may cause pulmonary edema. Death is the result of cardiovascular collapse.

### B. CHRONIC POISONING

Anorexia, generalized weakness, giddiness, colic, abdominal pain, polyneuritis, dermatitis, nail changes, alopecia, and anemia often develop.

## Treatment

In acute poisoning, empty the stomach and administer activated charcoal. Then immediately give dimercaprol (commonly known as BAL), 3–5 mg/kg intramuscularly (IM), and follow with 2 mg/kg IM every 4 hours. The dimercaprol-arsenic complex is dialyzable. A second choice is succimer. The initial dose is 10 mg/kg every 8 hours for 5 days. A third choice is penicillamine, 100 mg/kg PO to a maximum of 1 g/d in four divided doses.

Chronic arsenic intoxication should be treated with succimer or penicillamine. Collect a 24-hour baseline urine specimen and then begin chelation. If the 24-hour urine arsenic level is greater than 50 mg, continue chelation for 5 days. After 10 days, repeat the 5-day cycle once or twice depending on how soon the urine arsenic level falls below 50 mg/24 h.

Abernathy CO et al: Arsenic: Health effects, mechanisms of actions, and research issues. Environ Health Perspect 1999;107: 593 [PMID: 10379007].

Cullen MN et al: Pediatric arsenic ingestion. Am J Emerg Med 1995;13:432 [PMID: 7605532].

## BARBITURATES

The toxic effects of barbiturates include confusion, poor coordination, coma, miotic or fixed dilated pupils, and respiratory depression. Respiratory acidosis is commonly associated with pulmonary atelectasis, and hypotension occurs frequently in severely poisoned patients. Ingestion of more than 6 mg/kg of long-acting or 3 mg/kg of short-acting barbiturates is usually toxic.

### Treatment

Activated charcoal should be administered. Careful, conservative management with emphasis on maintaining a clear airway, adequate ventilation, and control of hypotension is critical. Urinary alkalinization and the use of multiple-dose charcoal may decrease the elimination half-life of phenobarbital but have not been shown to alter the clinical course. Hemodialysis is not useful in the treatment of poisoning with short-acting barbiturates. Analeptics are contraindicated.

Amitai Y, Degani Y: Treatment of phenobarbital poisoning with multiple dose activated charcoal in an infant. J Emerg Med 1990;8:449 [PMID: 2212564].

Cote CJ et al: Adverse sedation events in pediatrics: Analysis of medications used for sedation. Pediatrics 2000;4:633 [PMID: 11015502].

## BELLADONNA ALKALOIDS (Atropine, Jimsonweed, Potato Leaves, Scopolamine, Stramonium)

The effects of anticholinergic compounds include dry mouth; thirst; decreased sweating with hot, dry, red skin; high fever; and tachycardia that may be preceded by bradycardia. The pupils are dilated, and vision is blurred. Speech and swallowing may be impaired. Hallucinations, delirium, and coma are common. Leukocytosis may occur, confusing the diagnosis.

Atropinism has been caused by normal doses of atropine or homatropine eye drops, especially in children with Down syndrome. Many common plants and over-the-counter medications contain belladonna alkaloids.

### Treatment

Emesis or lavage should be followed by activated charcoal. Gastric emptying is slowed by anticholinergics, so that gastric decontamination may be useful even if delayed. Physostigmine, 0.5–2 mg IV, administered slowly, dramatically reverses the central and peripheral signs of atropinism but should be used only as a diagnostic agent. High fever must be controlled. Catheterization may be needed if the patient cannot void.

Burns MJ et al: A comparison of physostigmine and benzodiazepines for the treatment of anticholinergic poisoning. Ann Emerg Med 2000;35:374 [PMID: 10736125].

Schultz U et al: Central anticholinergic syndrome in a child undergoing circumcision. Acta Anaesthesiol Scand 2002;46:224 [PMID: 11942877].

## CARBON MONOXIDE

The degree of toxicity correlates well with the carboxyhemoglobin level taken soon after acute exposure but not after oxygen has been given or when there has been some time since exposure. Onset of symptoms may be more rapid and more severe if the patient lives at a high altitude, has a high respiratory rate (ie, infants), is pregnant, or has myocardial insufficiency or lung disease. Normal blood may contain up to 5% carboxyhemoglobin (10% in smokers).

The most prominent early symptom is headache. Other effects include confusion, unsteadiness, and coma. Proteinuria, glycosuria, elevated serum aminotransferase levels, or electrocardiogram (ECG) changes may be present in the acute phase. Permanent cardiac, liver, renal, or CNS damage occurs occasionally. The outcome of severe poisoning may be complete recovery, vegetative state, or any degree of mental injury between these extremes. The primary mental deficits are neuropsychiatric.

### Treatment

The biologic half-life of carbon monoxide on room air is approximately 200–300 minutes; on 100% oxygen, it is 60–90 minutes. Hyperbaric oxygen therapy at 2–2.5 atm of oxygen shortens the half-life to 30 minutes. After the level has been reduced to near zero, therapy is aimed at the nonspecific sequelae of anoxia. Dexamethasone, 0.1 mg/kg IV or IM every 4–6 hours, should be added if cerebral edema develops.

Chou KJ: Characteristics and outcome of children with carbon monoxide poisoning with and without smoke exposure referred for hyperbaric oxygen therapy. Ped Emerg Care 2000;3:151 [PMID: 10888449].

Walker AR: Emergency department management of house fire burns and carbon monoxide poisoning in children. Curr Opin Pediatr 1996;8:239 [PMID: 8814401].

# CAUSTICS

## 1. Acids (Hydrochloric, Hydrofluoric, Nitric, & Sulfuric Acids; Sodium Bisulfate)

Strong acids are commonly found in metal and toilet bowl cleaners, batteries, and other products. Hydrofluoric acid is the most toxic and hydrochloric acid the least toxic of these household substances. However, even a few drops can be fatal if aspirated into the trachea.

Painful swallowing, mucous membrane burns, bloody emesis, abdominal pain, respiratory distress due to edema of the epiglottis, thirst, shock, and renal failure can occur. Coma and convulsions sometimes are seen terminally. Residual lesions include esophageal, gastric, and pyloric strictures as well as scars of the cornea, skin, and oropharynx.

Hydrofluoric acid is a particularly dangerous poison. Dermal exposure creates a penetrating burn that can progress for hours or days. Large dermal exposure or ingestion may produce life-threatening hypocalcemia abruptly as well as burn reactions.

### Treatment

Emetics and lavage are contraindicated. Water or milk (< 15 mL/kg) is used to dilute the acid, because a heat-producing chemical reaction does not occur. Take care not to induce emesis by excessive fluid administration. Alkalies should not be used. Burned areas of the skin, mucous membranes, or eyes should be washed with copious amounts of warm water. Opioids for pain may be needed. An endotracheal tube may be required to alleviate laryngeal edema. Esophagoscopy should be performed if the patient has significant burns or difficulty in swallowing. Acids are likely to produce gastric burns or esophageal burns. Evidence is not conclusive, but corticosteroids have not proved to be of use.

Hydrofluoric acid burns on skin are treated with 10% calcium gluconate gel or calcium gluconate infusion. Severe exposure may require large doses of IV calcium. Therapy should be guided by calcium levels, the ECG, and clinical signs.

## 2. Bases (Clinitest Tablets, Clorox, Drano, Liquid-Plumr, Purex, Sani-Clor)

Alkalies produce more severe injuries than acids. Some substances, such as Clinitest tablets or Drano, are quite toxic, whereas the chlorinated bleaches (3–6% solutions of sodium hypochlorite) are usually not toxic. When sodium hypochlorite comes in contact with acid in the stomach, hypochlorous acid, which is very irritating to the mucous membranes and skin, is formed. Rapid inactivation of this substance prevents systemic toxicity. Chlorinated bleaches, when mixed with a strong acid (toilet bowl cleaners) or ammonia, may produce irritating chlorine or chloramine gas, which can cause serious lung injury if inhaled in a closed space (eg, bathroom).

Alkalies can burn the skin, mucous membranes, and eyes. Respiratory distress may be due to edema of the epiglottis, pulmonary edema resulting from inhalation of fumes, or pneumonia. Mediastinitis or other intercurrent infections or shock can occur. Perforation of the esophagus or stomach is rare.

### Treatment

The skin and mucous membranes should be cleansed with copious amounts of water. A local anesthetic can be instilled in the eye if necessary to alleviate blepharospasm. The eye should be irrigated for at least 20–30 minutes. Ophthalmologic consultation should be obtained for all alkaline eye burns.

Ingestions should be treated with water as a diluent. Routine esophagoscopy is no longer indicated to rule out burns of the esophagus due to chlorinated bleaches unless an unusually large amount has been ingested or the patient is symptomatic. The absence of oral lesions does not rule out the possibility of laryngeal or esophageal burns following granular alkali ingestion. The use of corticosteroids is controversial, but has not been shown to improve long-term outcome except possibly in partial-thickness esophageal burns. Antibiotics may be needed if mediastinitis is likely, but they should not be used prophylactically. (See Caustic Burns of the Esophagus section in Chapter 20).

Broto J et al: Conservative treatment of caustic esophageal injuries in children: 20 years of experience. Pediatr Surg Int 1999;15: 323 [PMID: 10415278].

Hamza AF et al: Caustic esophageal strictures in children: 30 years' experience. J Pediatr Surg 2003;338:828 [PMID: 12778375].

Lamireau T et al: Accidental caustic ingestion in children: Is endoscopy always mandatory? J Pediatr Gastroenterol Nutr 2001;33:81 [PMID: 11479413].

Lovejoy FH Jr: Corrosive injury of the esophagus in children: Failure of corticosteroid treatment reemphasizes prevention. N Engl J Med 1990;323:668 [PMID: 2385270].

# COCAINE

Cocaine is absorbed intranasally or via inhalation or ingestion. Effects are noted almost immediately when the drug is taken intravenously or smoked. Peak effects are delayed for about an hour when the drug is taken orally or nasally. Cocaine prevents the reuptake of endogenous catecholamines, thereby causing an initial sympathetic discharge, followed by catechol depletion after chronic abuse.

## Clinical Findings

A local anesthetic and vasoconstrictor, cocaine is also a potent stimulant to both the CNS and the cardiovascular system. The initial tachycardia, hyperpnea, hypertension, and stimulation of the CNS are often followed by coma, seizures, hypotension, and respiratory depression. In severe cases of overdose, various dysrhythmias may be seen, including sinus tachycardia, atrial arrhythmias, premature ventricular contractions, bigeminy, and ventricular fibrillation. If large doses are taken intravenously, cardiac failure, dysrhythmias, rhabdomyolysis, or hyperthermia may result in death.

In addition to those poisoned through recreational use of cocaine, others are at risk of overdose. A "body stuffer" is one who quickly ingests the drug, usually poorly wrapped, to avoid discovery. A "body packer" wraps the drug carefully for prolonged transport. A stuffer typically manifests toxicity within hours of ingestion; a packer is asymptomatic unless the package ruptures, usually days later.

## Treatment

Except in cases of body stuffers or body packers, decontamination is seldom possible. Activated charcoal should be administered, and whole bowel irrigation may be useful in selected cases. Testing for cocaine in blood or plasma is generally not clinically useful, but a qualitative analysis of the urine may aid in confirming the diagnosis. For severe cases, an ECG is indicated. In suspected cases of body packing, radiographs of the GI tract may show multiple packets. X-ray films are usually not helpful for identifying stuffers. Seizures are treated with IV diazepam titrated to response. Hypotension is treated with standard agents. Because cocaine abuse may deplete norepinephrine, an indirect agent such as dopamine may be less effective than a direct agent such as norepinephrine. Agitation is best treated with a benzodiazepine.

Delaney-Black V: Prenatal cocaine exposure as a risk factor for later developmental outcomes. JAMA 2001;286:46 [PMID: 11434823].

King TA et al: Neurologic manifestations of in utero cocaine exposure in near-term and term infants. Pediatrics 1995;96: 259 [PMID: 7630680].

Mott SH et al: Neurologic manifestations of cocaine exposure in childhood. Pediatrics 1994;93:557 [PMID: 8134208].

Qureshi AI et al: Cocaine use and the likelihood of nonfatal myocardial infarction and stroke: Data from the Third National Health and Nutrition Examination Survey. Circulation 2001;103:502 [PMID: 11157713].

## CONTRACEPTIVE PILLS

The only known toxic effects following acute ingestion of oral contraceptive agents are nausea, vomiting, and vaginal bleeding in girls.

## COSMETICS & RELATED PRODUCTS

The relative toxicities of commonly ingested products in this group are listed in Table 12–2. Permanent wave neutralizers may contain bromates, peroxides, or perborates. Bromates have been removed from most products because they can cause nausea, vomiting, abdominal pain, shock, hemolysis, renal failure, and convulsions. Perborates can cause boric acid poisoning. Four grams of bromate salts is potentially lethal.

Poisoning is treated by gastric lavage with 1% sodium thiosulfate followed by demulcents to relieve gastric irritation. Sodium bicarbonate, 2%, in the lavage fluid may reduce hydrobromic acid formation. Sodium thiosulfate, 25%, 1.65 mL/kg, can be given intravenously, but methylene blue should not be used to treat methemoglobinemia in this situation, because it increases the toxicity of bromates. Dialysis is indicated in renal failure but does not enhance excretion of bromate.

Fingernail polish removers used to contain toluene, but now usually have an acetone base, which does not require specific treatment other than monitoring CNS status.

Cobalt, copper, cadmium, iron, lead, nickel, silver, bismuth, and tin are sometimes found in metallic hair dyes. In large amounts, they can cause skin sensitiza-

**Table 12–2.** Relative toxicities of cosmetics and similar products.

| High toxicity | Low toxicity |
|---|---|
| Permanent wave neutralizers | Perfume |
|  | Hair removers |
|  | Deodorants |
| **Moderate toxicity** | Bath salts |
| Fingernail polish |  |
| Fingernail polish remover | **No toxicity** |
| Metallic hair dyes | Liquid makeup |
| Home permanent wave lotion | Vegetable hair dye |
| Bath oil | Cleansing cream |
| Shaving lotion | Hair dressing |
| Hair tonic (alcoholic) | (nonalcoholic) |
| Cologne, toilet water | Hand lotion or cream |
|  | Lipstick |

tion, urticaria, dermatitis, eye damage, vertigo, hypertension, asthma, methemoglobinemia, tremors, convulsions, and coma. Treatment for ingestions is to administer demulcents and, only with large amounts, the appropriate antidote for the heavy metal involved.

Home permanent wave lotions, hair straighteners, and hair removers usually contain thioglycolic acid salts, which cause alkaline irritation and perhaps CNS depression.

Shaving lotion, hair tonic, hair straighteners, cologne, and toilet water contain denatured alcohol, which can cause CNS depression and hypoglycemia.

Deodorants usually consist of an antibacterial agent in a cream base. Antiperspirants are aluminum salts, which frequently cause skin sensitization. Zirconium oxide can cause granulomas in the axilla with chronic use.

## CYCLIC ANTIDEPRESSANTS

Cyclic antidepressants (eg, amitriptyline, imipramine) have a very low ratio of toxic to therapeutic doses, and even a moderate overdose can have serious effects. Cyclic antidepressant overdosage causes dysrhythmias, coma, convulsions, hypertension followed by hypotension, and hallucinations. These effects may be life-threatening and require rapid intervention. One agent, amoxapine, differs in that it causes fewer cardiovascular complications, but it is associated with a higher incidence of seizures.

### Treatment

Decontamination should include gastric lavage and administration of activated charcoal.

An ECG should be taken in all patients. A QRS interval greater than 100 ms specifically identifies patients at risk to develop dysrhythmias. If dysrhythmias are demonstrated, the patient should be admitted and monitored until free of irregularity for 24 hours. Another indication for monitoring is persistent tachycardia of more than 110 beats/min. The onset of dysrhythmias is rare beyond 24 hours after ingestion.

Alkalinization with sodium bicarbonate, 0.5–1.0 mEq/kg IV, or hyperventilation may dramatically reverse ventricular dysrhythmias and narrow the QRS interval. Lidocaine may be added for treatment of arrhythmias. Bolus administration of sodium bicarbonate is recommended for all patients with QRS widening to above 120 ms and for those with significant dysrhythmias, to achieve a pH of 7.5–7.6. Forced diuresis is contraindicated. A benzodiazepine should be given for convulsions.

Hypotension is a major problem. Cyclic antidepressants block the reuptake of catecholamines, thereby producing initial hypertension followed by hypotension. Treatment with physostigmine is contraindicated. Vasopressors are generally effective. Dopamine is the agent of choice because it is readily available. If dopamine is ineffective, norepinephrine (0.1–1 µg/kg/min, titrated to response) should be added. Diuresis and hemodialysis are not effective.

Kerr GW et al: Tricyclic antidepressant overdose: A review. Emerg Med J 2001;18:236 [PMID: 11435353].

McKinney PE et al: Reversal of severe tricyclic antidepressant-induced cardiotoxicity with intravenous hypertonic saline solution. Ann Emerg Med 2003;42:20 [PMID: 12827118].

## DIGITALIS & OTHER CARDIAC GLYCOSIDES

Toxicity is typically the result of incorrect dosing or unrecognized renal insufficiency. Clinical features include nausea, vomiting, diarrhea, headache, delirium, confusion, and, occasionally, coma. Cardiac dysrhythmias typically involve bradydysrhythmias, but every type of dysrhythmia has been reported in digitalis intoxication, including atrial fibrillation, paroxysmal atrial tachycardia, and atrial flutter. Death usually is the result of ventricular fibrillation. Transplacental intoxication by digitalis has been reported.

### Treatment

If vomiting has not occurred, induce emesis or provide lavage followed by charcoal. Potassium is contraindicated in acute overdosage unless there is laboratory evidence of hypokalemia. In acute overdosage, hyperkalemia is more common. Hypokalemia is common in chronic toxicity.

The patient must be monitored carefully for ECG changes. The correction of acidosis better demonstrates the degree of potassium deficiency present. Bradycardias have been treated with atropine. Phenytoin, lidocaine, magnesium salts (not in renal failure), amiodarone, and bretylium have been used to correct arrhythmias.

Definitive treatment is with digoxin immune Fab (ovine) (Digibind). Indications for its use include hypotension or any dysrhythmia, typically ventricular dysrhythmias and progressive bradydysrhythmias that produce clinical concern. Elevated T-waves indicated high potassium and may be an indication for digoxin immune Fab (Digibind, DigiFab) use. Techniques of determining dosage and indications related to levels, when available are described in product literature.

Woolf AD et al: The use of digoxin-specific Fab fragments for severe digitalis intoxication in children. N Engl J Med 1992;326:1739 [PMID: 1997016].

## DIPHENOXYLATE WITH ATROPINE (LOMOTIL)

Lomotil contains diphenoxylate hydrochloride, a synthetic narcotic, and atropine sulfate. Small amounts are potentially lethal in children; it is contraindicated in children younger than age 2 years. Early signs of intoxication with this preparation result from its anticholinergic effect and consist of fever, facial flushing, tachypnea, and lethargy. However, the miotic effect of the narcotic predominates. Later, hypothermia, increasing CNS depression, and loss of the facial flush occur. Seizures are probably secondary to hypoxia.

### Treatment

Prolonged monitoring (24 hours) with pulse oximetry is sufficient in most cases. If respiratory depression occurs, an airway should be established with an endotracheal tube. Gastric lavage and administration of activated charcoal may be useful because of the prolonged delay in gastric emptying time.

Naloxone hydrochloride (0.4–2 mg IV in children and adults) should be given. A transient improvement in respiration may be followed by respiratory depression. Repeated doses may be required because the duration of action of diphenoxylate is considerably longer than that of naloxone. The anticholinergic effects do not usually require treatment.

McCarron MM et al: Diphenoxylate-atropine (Lomotil) overdose in children: An update. Pediatrics 1991;87:694 [PMID: 2020516].

## DISINFECTANTS & DEODORIZERS

### 1. Naphthalene

Naphthalene is commonly found in mothballs, disinfectants, and deodorizers. Naphthalene's toxicity is often not fully appreciated. It is absorbed not only when ingested but also through the skin and lungs. It is potentially hazardous to store baby clothes in naphthalene, because baby oil is an excellent solvent that may increase dermal absorption. *Note:* Most moth balls contain *para*-dichlorbenzene and not naphthalene—see next section. Metabolic products of naphthalene may cause severe hemolytic anemia, similar to that due to primaquine toxicity, 2–7 days after ingestion. Other physical findings include vomiting, diarrhea, jaundice, oliguria, anuria, coma, and convulsions. The urine may contain hemoglobin, protein, and casts.

### Treatment

Induced vomiting should be followed by activated charcoal. Urinary alkalinization may prevent blocking of the renal tubules by acid hematin crystals. Anuria may persist for 1–2 weeks and still be completely reversible.

Ostlere L et al: Haemolytic anaemia associated with ingestion of naphthalene-containing anointing oil. Postgrad Med J 1988;64:444 [PMID: 3211822].

Siegel E, Wason S: Mothball toxicity. Pediatr Clin North Am 1986;33:369 [PMID: 3515301].

### 2. p-Dichlorobenzene, Phenolic Acids, & Others

Disinfectants and deodorizers containing *p*-dichlorobenzene or sodium sulfate are much less toxic than those containing naphthalene. Disinfectants containing phenolic acids are highly toxic, especially if they contain a borate ion. Phenol precipitates tissue proteins and causes respiratory alkalosis followed by metabolic acidosis. Some phenols cause methemoglobinemia.

Local gangrene occurs after prolonged contact with tissue. Phenol is readily absorbed from the GI tract, causing diffuse capillary damage and, in some cases, methemoglobinemia. Pentachlorophenol, which has been used in terminal rinsing of diapers, has caused infant fatalities.

The toxicity of alkalies, quaternary ammonium compounds, pine oil, and halogenated disinfectants varies with the concentration of active ingredients. Wick deodorizers are usually of moderate toxicity. Iodophor disinfectants are the safest. Spray deodorizers are not usually toxic, because a child is not likely to swallow a very large dose.

Signs and symptoms of acute quaternary ammonium compound ingestion include diaphoresis, strong irritation, thirst, vomiting, diarrhea, cyanosis, hyperactivity, coma, convulsions, hypotension, abdominal pain, and pulmonary edema. Acute liver or renal failure may develop later.

### Treatment

Activated charcoal may be used prior to gastric lavage. Castor oil dissolves phenol and may retard its absorption. This property of castor oil, however, has not been proved clinically. Mineral oil and alcohol are contraindicated because they increase the gastric absorption of phenol. The metabolic acidosis must be managed carefully. Anticonvulsants or measures to treat shock may be needed.

Because phenols are absorbed through the skin, exposed areas should be irrigated copiously with water. Undiluted polyethylene glycol may be a useful solvent as well.

Mucklow ES: Accidental feeding of dilute antiseptic solution (chlorhexidine 0.05% with cetrimide 1%) to five babies. Hum Toxicol 1988;7:567 [PMID: 3229768].

Van Berkel M, de Wolff FA: Survival after acute benzalkonium chloride poisoning. Hum Toxicol 1988;7:191 [PMID: 3378808].

## DISK-SHAPED BATTERIES

Small, flat, smooth disk-shaped batteries measure between 10 and 25 mm in diameter. About 69% of them pass through the GI tract in 48 hours and 85% in 72 hours. Some may become entrapped. These batteries contain caustic materials and heavy metals.

Batteries impacted in the esophagus may cause symptoms of refusal to take food, increased salivation, vomiting with or without blood, and pain or discomfort. Aspiration into the trachea may also occur. Fatalities have been reported in association with esophageal perforation.

When a history of disk battery ingestion is obtained, radiographs of the entire respiratory tract and GI tract should be taken so that the battery can be located and the proper therapy determined.

### Treatment

If the disk battery is located in the esophagus, it must be removed immediately. If the battery has been in the esophagus for more than 24 hours, the risk of caustic burn is greater.

Location of the disk battery below the esophagus has been associated with tissue damage, but the course is benign in most cases. Perforated Meckel diverticulum has been the major complication. It may take as long as 7 days for spontaneous passage to occur, and lack of movement in the GI tract may not require removal in an asymptomatic patient. Some researchers have suggested repeated radiographs and surgical intervention if passage of the battery pauses, but this approach may be excessive. Batteries that have opened in the GI tract have been associated with some toxicity due to mercury, but the patients have recovered.

Emesis is ineffective. Asymptomatic patients may simply be observed and stools examined for passage of the battery. If the battery has not passed within 7 days or if the patient becomes symptomatic, radiographs should be repeated. If the battery has come apart or appears not to be moving, a purgative, enema, or nonabsorbable intestinal lavage solution should be administered. If these methods are unsuccessful, surgical intervention may be required. Levels of heavy metals (mainly mercury) should be measured in patients in whom the battery has opened or symptoms have developed.

Dane S: A truly emergent problem: Button battery in the nose. Acad Emerg Med 2000;7:204 [PMID: 10691084].

Litovitz TL, Schmitz BF: Ingestion of cylindrical and button batteries: An analysis of 2382 cases. Pediatrics 1992;89:747 [PMID: 2304794].

## GAMMA-HYDROXYBUTYRATE, GAMMA-BUTYROLACTONE, & BUTANEDIOL

Gamma-hydroxybutyrate (GHB), γ-butyrolactone (GBL), and butanediol have become popular drugs of abuse in adolescents and adults. GHB is a CNS depressant that is structurally similar to the inhibitory neurotransmitter γ-aminobutyric acid. GBL and butanediol are converted in the body to GHB. These drugs cause deep but short-lived coma; the coma often lasts only 1–4 hours. Treatment consists of supportive care with close attention to airway and endotracheal intubation if respiratory depression or decreased gag reflex complicates the poisoning. Atropine has been used successfully for symptomatic bradycardia.

Withdrawal from GHB, GBL, or butanediol can cause several days of extreme agitation, hallucination, or tachycardia. Treatment with high doses of benzodiazepines or with butyrophenones (eg, haloperidol or droperidol) or secobarbital may be needed for several days.

Dyer JE et al: Gamma-hydroxybutyrate withdrawal syndrome. Ann Emerg Med 2001;37:147 [PMID: 11174231].

Sporer KA et al: Gamma-hydroxybutyrate serum levels and clinical syndrome after severe overdose. Ann Emerg Med 2003;42:3 [PMID: 12827115].

## HYDROCARBONS (Benzene, Charcoal Lighter Fluid, Gasoline, Kerosene, Petroleum Distillates, Turpentine)

Ingestion of hydrocarbons may cause irritation of mucous membranes, vomiting, blood-tinged diarrhea, respiratory distress, cyanosis, tachycardia, and fever. Although a small amount (10 mL) of certain hydrocarbons is potentially fatal, patients have survived ingestion of several ounces of other petroleum distillates. The more aromatic a hydrocarbon is and the lower its viscosity rating, the more potentially toxic it is. Benzene, gasoline, kerosene, and red seal oil furniture polish are the most dangerous. A dose exceeding 1 mL/kg is likely to cause CNS depression. A history of coughing or choking, as well as vomiting, suggests aspiration with resulting hydrocarbon pneumonia. This is an acute hemorrhagic necrotizing disease that usually develops within 24 hours of the ingestion and resolves without sequelae in 3–5 days. However, several weeks may be required for full resolution of a hydrocarbon pneumonia. Pneumonia may be caused by the aspiration of a few drops of petroleum distillate into the lung or by absorption from the circulatory system. Pulmonary edema and hemorrhage, cardiac dilatation and dysrhythmias, hepatosplenomegaly, proteinuria, and hematuria can occur following large overdoses. Hypoglycemia is occasionally present. A chest radiograph may reveal pneumonia within hours after the ingestion. An abnormal urinalysis in a child with a previously normal urinary tract suggests a large overdose.

## Treatment

Both emetics and lavage should be avoided when only a small amount has been ingested. Mineral oil should not be given, because it can cause a low-grade lipoid pneumonia.

Epinephrine should not be used with halogenated hydrocarbons because it may affect an already sensitized myocardium. The usefulness of corticosteroids is debated, and antibiotics should be reserved for patients with infections. Oxygen and mist are helpful. Extracorporeal membrane oxygenation has been successful in at least two cases of failure with standard therapy.

Anas N et al: Criteria for hospitalizing children who have ingested products containing hydrocarbons. JAMA 1981;246:840 [PMID: 7253158].

Bysani GK et al: Treatment of hydrocarbon pneumonitis. High frequency jet ventilation as an alternative to extracorporeal membrane oxygenation. Chest 1994;106:300 [PMID: 8020296].

Lifshitz M et al: Hydrocarbon poisoning in children: A 5-year retrospective study. Wilderness Environ Med 2003;14:78 [PMID: 12825880].

Lorenc JD: Inhalant abuse in the pediatric populations: A persistent challenge Cur Opin Ped 2003;15:204 [PMID: 12640280].

Sheridan RL: Burns with inhalation injury and petrol aspiration in adolescents seeking euphoria through hydrocarbon inhalation. Burns 1996;22:566 [PMID: 8909762].

## IBUPROFEN

Most exposures in children do not produce symptoms. In one study, for example, children ingesting up to 2.4 g remained asymptomatic. When symptoms occur, the most common are abdominal pain, vomiting, drowsiness, and lethargy. In rare cases, apnea (especially in young children), seizures, metabolic acidosis, and CNS depression leading to coma have occurred.

## Treatment

If a child has ingested less than 100 mg/kg, dilution with water or milk may be all that is necessary to minimize the GI upset. In children, the volume of liquid used for dilution should be less than 4 oz. When the ingested amount is more than 400 mg/kg, seizures or CNS depression may occur; therefore, gastric lavage may be preferred to emesis. Activated charcoal may also be of value. There is no specific antidote. Neither alkalinization of the urine nor hemodialysis is helpful.

Cuzzolin L et al: NSAID-induced nephrotoxicity from the fetus to the child. Drug Safety 2001;242:9 [PMID: 11219488].

Hall AH et al: Ibuprofen overdose in adults. J Toxicol Clin Toxicol 1992;30:23 [PMID: 1542147].

Lesko SM: The safety of ibuprofen suspension in children. Int J Clin Pract (Supp) 2003;135:50 [PMID: 12723748].

Oker EE et al: Serious toxicity in a young child due to ibuprofen. Acad Emerg Med 2000;7:821 [PMID: 10917334].

## INSECT STINGS (Bee, Wasp, & Hornet)

Insect stings are painful but not usually dangerous; however, death from anaphylaxis may occur. Bee venom has hemolytic, neurotoxic, and histamine-like activities that can on rare occasion cause hemoglobinuria and severe anaphylactoid reactions. Massive envenomation from numerous stings may cause hemolysis, rhabdomyolysis, and shock leading to multiple organ failure.

## Treatment

The physician should remove the stinger, taking care not to squeeze the attached venom sac. For allergic reactions, epinephrine 1:1000 solution, 0.01 mL/kg, should be administered IV or SQ above the site of the sting. Three to four whiffs from an isoproterenol aerosol inhaler may be given at 3- to 4-minute intervals as needed. Corticosteroids (hydrocortisone), 100 mg IV, and diphenhydramine, 1.5 mg/kg IV, are useful ancillary drugs but have no immediate effect. Ephedrine or antihistamines may be used for 2 or 3 days to prevent recurrence of symptoms.

A patient who has had a potentially life-threatening insect sting should be desensitized against the Hymenoptera group, because the honey bee, wasp, hornet, and yellow jacket have common antigens in their venom. For the more usual stings, cold compresses, aspirin, and diphenhydramine 1 mg/kg PO, are sufficient.

Reisman RE, Livingstone A: Late-onset allergic reactions, including serum sickness after insect stings. J Allergy Clin Immunol 1989;84:331 [PMID: 2778239].

Ross RN et al: Effectiveness of specific immunotherapy in the treatment of hymenoptera venom hypersensitivity: A meta-analysis. Clin Ther 2000;22:351 [PMID: 10963289].

Vetter RS et al: Mass envenomations by honey bees and wasps. West J Med 1999;170:223 [PMID: 10344177].

## INSECTICIDES

The petroleum distillates or other organic solvents used in these products are often as toxic as the insecticide itself. Decontamination may be performed by aspirating the stomach with a nasogastric tube.

### 1. Chlorinated Hydrocarbons (eg, Aldrin, Carbinol, Chlordane, DDT, Dieldrin, Endrin, Heptachlor, Lindane, Toxaphene)

Signs of intoxication include salivation, GI irritability, abdominal pain, vomiting, diarrhea, CNS depression, and convulsions. Inhalation exposure causes irritation of the eyes, nose, and throat; blurred vision; cough; and pulmonary edema.

Chlorinated hydrocarbons are absorbed through the skin, respiratory tract, and GI tract. Decontamination of skin with soap and evacuation of the stomach contents are critical. All contaminated clothing should be removed. Castor oil, milk, and other substances containing fats or oils should not be left in the stomach because they increase absorption of the chlorinated hydrocarbons. Convulsions should be treated with diazepam, 0.1–0.3 mg/kg IV. Epinephrine should not be used because it may cause cardiac arrhythmias.

### 2. Organophosphate (Cholinesterase-Inhibiting) Insecticides (eg, Chlorthion, Co-Ral, DFP, Diazinon, Malathion, Paraoxon, Parathion, Phosdrin, TEPP, Thio-TEPP)

Dizziness, headache, blurred vision, miosis, tearing, salivation, nausea, vomiting, diarrhea, hyperglycemia, cyanosis, sense of constriction of the chest, dyspnea, sweating, weakness, muscular twitching, convulsions, loss of reflexes and sphincter control, and coma can occur.

The clinical findings are the result of cholinesterase inhibition, which causes an accumulation of acetylcholine. The onset of symptoms occurs within 12 hours of the exposure. Red cell cholinesterase levels should be measured as soon as possible. (Some normal individuals have a low serum cholinesterase level.) Normal values vary in different laboratories. In general, a decrease of red cell cholinesterase to below 25% of normal indicates significant exposure.

Repeated low-grade exposure may result in sudden, acute toxic reactions. This syndrome usually occurs after repeated household spraying rather than agricultural exposure.

Although all organophosphates act by inhibiting cholinesterase activity, they vary greatly in their toxicity. Parathion, for example, is 100 times more toxic than malathion. The toxicity is influenced by the specific compound, the type of formulation (liquid or solid), the vehicle, and the route of absorption (lungs, skin, or GI tract).

### Treatment

Decontamination of skin, nails, hair, and clothing with soapy water is extremely important. Atropine plus a cholinesterase reactivator, pralidoxime, is an antidote for organophosphate insecticide poisoning. After assessment and management of the ABCs, atropine should be given and repeated every few minutes until airway secretions diminish. An appropriate starting dose of atropine is 2–4 mg IV in an adult and 0.05 mg/kg in a child. The patient should receive enough atropine to stop secretions (mydriasis in not an appropriate stopping point). Severe poisoning may require gram quantities of atropine administered over 24 hours.

Because atropine antagonizes the muscarinic parasympathetic effects of the organophosphates but does not affect the nicotinic receptor, it does not improve muscular weakness. Pralidoxime should also be given immediately in more severe cases and repeated every 6–12 hours as needed (25–50 mg/kg diluted to 5% and infused over 5–30 minutes at a rate of no more than 500 mg/min). Pralidoxime should be used in addition to—not in place of—atropine if red cell cholinesterase is less than 25% of normal. Pralidoxime is most useful within 48 hours after the exposure but has shown some effects 2–6 days later. Morphine, theophylline, aminophylline, succinylcholine, and tranquilizers of the reserpine and phenothiazine types are contraindicated. Hyperglycemia is common in severe poisonings.

Eisenstein EM, Amitai Y: Index of suspicion: Case 1. Organophosphate intoxication. Pediatr Rev 2000;21:205 [PMID: 10854316].

Lifshitz M et al: Carbamate and organophosphate; poisoning in young children. Pediatr Emerg Care 1999;15:102 [PMID: 10220078].

### 3. Carbamates (eg, Carbaryl, Sevin, Zectran)

Carbamate insecticides are reversible inhibitors of cholinesterase. The signs and symptoms of intoxication are similar to those associated with organophosphate poisoning but are generally less severe. Atropine titrated to effect is sufficient treatment. Pralidoxime should not be used with carbaryl poisoning but is of value with other carbamates. In combined exposures to organophosphates, give atropine but reserve pralidoxime for cases in which the red cell cholinesterase is depressed below 25% of normal or marked effects of nicotinic receptor stimulation are present.

## 4. Botanical Insecticides (eg, Black Flag Bug Killer, Black Leaf CPR Insect Killer, Flit Aerosol House & Garden Insect Killer, French's Flea Powder, Raid)

Allergic reactions, asthma-like symptoms, coma, and convulsions have been reported. Pyrethrins, allethrin, and rotenone do not commonly cause signs of toxicity. Antihistamines, short-acting barbiturates, and atropine are helpful as symptomatic treatment.

## IRON

Five stages of intoxication may occur in iron poisoning: (1) Hemorrhagic gastroenteritis, which occurs 30–60 minutes after ingestion and may be associated with shock, acidosis, coagulation defects, and coma. This phase usually lasts 4–6 hours. (2) Phase of improvement, lasting 2–12 hours, during which patient looks better. (3) Delayed shock, which may occur 12–48 hours after ingestion. Metabolic acidosis, fever, leukocytosis, and coma may also be present. (4) Liver damage with hepatic failure. (5) Residual pyloric stenosis, which may develop about 4 weeks after the ingestion.

Once iron is absorbed from the GI tract, it is not normally eliminated in feces but may be partially excreted in the urine, giving it a red color prior to chelation. A reddish discoloration of the urine suggests a serum iron level greater than 350 mg/dL.

## Treatment

GI decontamination is based on clinical assessment. Syrup of ipecac may be administered at home, with appropriate follow-up, provided the history does not warrant an emergency department visit. The patient should be referred to a health care facility if symptomatic or if the history indicates toxic amounts. Gastric lavage and whole bowel irrigation should be considered in these patients.

Shock is treated in the usual manner. Sodium bicarbonate and Fleet Phospho-Soda left in the stomach to form the insoluble phosphate or carbonate have not shown clinical benefit and have caused lethal hypernatremia or hyperphosphatemia. Deferoxamine, a specific chelating agent for iron, is a useful adjunct in the treatment of severe iron poisoning. It forms a soluble complex that is excreted in the urine. It is contraindicated

in patients with renal failure unless dialysis can be used. Institute IV deferoxamine chelation therapy if the patient is symptomatic and a serum iron determination cannot be obtained readily, or if the peak serum iron exceeds 400 µg/dL (62.6 µmol/L) at 4–5 hours after ingestion.

Deferoxamine should not be delayed until serum iron levels are available in serious cases of poisoning. IV administration is indicated if the patient is in shock, in which case it should be given at a dosage of 15 mg/kg/h. Infusion rates up to 35 mg/kg/h have been used in life-threatening poisonings. Rapid IV administration can cause hypotension, facial flushing, urticaria, tachycardia, and shock. Deferoxamine, 90 mg/kg IM every 8 hours (maximum, 1 g), may be given if IV access cannot be established, but the procedure is painful. The indications for discontinuation of deferoxamine have not been clearly delineated. Generally, it can be stopped after 12–24 hours if the acidosis has resolved and the patient is improving.

Hemodialysis, peritoneal dialysis, or exchange transfusion can be used to increase the excretion of the dialyzable complex. Urine output should be monitored and urine sediment examined for evidence of renal tubular damage. Initial laboratory studies should include blood typing and cross-matching; total protein; serum iron, sodium, potassium, and chloride; $P_{CO_2}$; pH; and liver function tests. Serum iron levels fall rapidly even if deferoxamine is not given.

After the acute episode, liver function studies and an upper GI series are indicated to rule out residual damage.

Black J et al: Child abuse by intentional iron poisoning presenting as shock and persistent acidosis. Pediatrics 2003;111:197 [PMID: 12509576].

Juurlink DN et al: Iron poisoning in young children: Association with the birth of a sibling. CMAJ 2003;165:1539 [PMID: 12796332].

Morris CC: Pediatric iron poisonings in the United States. South Med J 2000;93:352 [PMID: 11142463].

## LEAD

Lead poisoning (plumbism) causes vague symptoms, including weakness, irritability, weight loss, vomiting, personality changes, ataxia, constipation, headache, and colicky abdominal pain. Late manifestations consist of retarded development, convulsions, and coma associated with increased intracranial pressure, which is a medical emergency.

Plumbism usually occurs insidiously in children younger than age 5 years. The most likely sources of lead include flaking leaded paint, artist's paints, fruit tree sprays, solder, brass alloys, home-glazed pottery, and fumes from burning batteries. Only paint containing less than 1% lead is safe for interior use (eg, furniture, toys). Repetitive ingestions of small amounts of lead are far more serious than a single massive exposure. Toxic effects are likely to occur if more than 0.5 mg of lead per day is absorbed.

Blood lead levels are used to assess the severity of exposure. A complete blood count and serum ferritin concentration should be obtained; iron deficiency increases absorption of lead. Glycosuria, proteinuria, hematuria, and aminoaciduria occur frequently. Blood lead levels usually exceed 80 μg/dL in symptomatic patients. Abnormal blood lead levels should be repeated in asymptomatic patients to rule out laboratory error. Specimens must be meticulously obtained in acid-washed containers. A normocytic, slightly hypochromic anemia with basophilic stippling of the red cells and reticulocytosis may be present in plumbism. Stippling of red blood cells is absent in cases involving only recent ingestion.

The CSF protein is elevated, and the white cell count is usually less than 100 cells/mL. CSF pressure may be elevated in patients with encephalopathy; lumbar punctures must be performed cautiously to prevent herniation.

## Treatment

Standard GI decontamination is indicated if an acute ingestion has occurred or lead is noted on the abdominal radiograph. Succimer is an orally administered chelator approved for use in children and reported to be as efficacious as calcium edetate. Treatment for blood lead levels of 20–45 μg/dL in children has not been determined. Succimer should be initiated at blood lead levels over 45 μg/dL. The initial dose is 10 mg/kg (350 mg/m²) every 8 hours for 5 days. The same dose is then given every 12 hours for 14 days. At least 2 weeks should elapse between courses. Blood lead levels increase somewhat (ie, rebound) after discontinuation of therapy. Courses of dimercaprol (4 mg/kg/dose) and calcium edetate may still be used but are no longer the preferred method, except in cases of lead encephalopathy.

Anticonvulsants may be needed. Mannitol or corticosteroids and volume restriction are indicated in patients with encephalopathy. A high-calcium, high-phosphorus diet and large doses of vitamin D may remove lead from the blood by depositing it in the bones. A public health team should evaluate the source of the lead. Necessary corrections should be completed before the child is returned home.

American Academy of Pediatrics Committee on Drugs: Treatment guidelines for lead exposure in children. Pediatrics 1995;96: 155 [PMID: 7596706].

Markowitz M: Lead poisoning. Pediatr Rev 2000;21:327 [PMID: 11010979].

Rogan WJ et al: Exposure to lead in children—How low is low enough? N Engl J Med 2003;16:1515 [PMID: 12700370].

Rogan WJ et al: Treatment of Lead-Exposed Children Trial Group: The effect of chelation therapy with succimer on neuropsychological development in children exposed to lead. N Engl J Med 2001;344:1421 [PMID: 11346806].

# MUSHROOMS

Toxic mushrooms are often difficult to distinguish from edible varieties. Contact a poison center to obtain identification assistance. Symptoms vary with the species ingested, time of year, stage of maturity, quantity eaten, method of preparation, and interval since ingestion. A mushroom that is toxic to one individual may not be toxic to another. Drinking alcohol and eating certain mushrooms may cause a reaction similar to that seen with disulfiram and alcohol. Cooking destroys some toxins but not the deadly one produced by *Amanita phalloides,* which is responsible for 90% of deaths due to mushroom poisoning. Mushroom toxins are absorbed relatively slowly. Onset of symptoms within 2 hours of ingestion suggests muscarinic toxin, whereas a delay of symptoms for 6–48 hours after ingestion strongly suggests *Amanita* (amanitin) poisoning. Patients who have ingested *A phalloides* may relapse and die of hepatic or renal failure following initial improvement.

Mushroom poisoning may produce muscarinic symptoms (salivation, vomiting, diarrhea, cramping abdominal pain, tenesmus, miosis, and dyspnea), coma, convulsions, hallucinations, hemolysis, and delayed hepatic and renal failure.

## Treatment

Induce vomiting and follow with activated charcoal. If the patient has muscarinic signs, give atropine, 0.05 mg/kg IM (0.02 mg/kg in toddlers), and repeat as needed (usually every 30 minutes) to keep the patient atropinized. Atropine, however, is used only when cholinergic effects are present and not for all mushrooms. Hypoglycemia is most likely to occur in patients with delayed onset of symptoms. Try to identify the mushroom if the patient is symptomatic. Consultation with a certified poison center is recommended. Local botanical gardens, university departments of botany, and societies of mycologists may be able to help. Supportive care is usually all that is needed; however, in the case of *A phalloides,* penicillin, silibinin, or hemodialysis may be indicated.

Lampe KF, McCann MA: Differential diagnosis of poisoning by North American mushrooms, with particular emphasis on

*Amanita phalloides*-like intoxication. Ann Emerg Med 1987;16:956 [PMID: 3631682].

Michelot D et al: *Amanita muscaria*: Chemistry, biology, toxicology and ethnomycology. Mycol Res 2003;107:131 [PMID: 12747324].

Pawlowska J et al: Liver transplantation in three family members after *Amanita phalloides* mushroom poisoning. Transplant Proc 2002;34:3313 [PMID: 12493457].

## NITRITES, NITRATES, ANILINE, PENTACHLOROPHENOL, & DINITROPHENOL

Nausea, vertigo, vomiting, cyanosis (methemoglobinemia), cramping abdominal pain, tachycardia, cardiovascular collapse, tachypnea, coma, shock, convulsions, and death are possible manifestations of nitrite or nitrate poisoning.

Nitrite and nitrate compounds found in the home include amyl nitrite, butyl nitrates, isobutyl nitrates, nitroglycerin, pentaerythritol tetranitrate, sodium nitrite, nitrobenzene, and phenazopyridine. Pentachlorophenol and dinitrophenol, which are found in wood preservatives, produce methemoglobinemia and high fever because of uncoupling of oxidative phosphorylation. Headache, dizziness, and bradycardia have been reported. High concentrations of nitrites in well water or spinach have been the most common cause of nitrite-induced methemoglobinemia. Symptoms do not usually occur until 15–50% of the hemoglobin has been converted to methemoglobin. A rapid test is to compare a drop of normal blood with the patient's blood on a dry filter paper. Brown discoloration of the patient's blood indicates a methemoglobin level of more than 15%.

### Treatment

Induce vomiting and administer activated charcoal. Decontaminate affected skin with soap and water. Oxygen and artificial respiration may be needed. If the blood methemoglobin level exceeds 30%, or if levels cannot be obtained and the patient is symptomatic, give a 1% solution of methylene blue, 0.2 mL/kg IV over 5–10 minutes. Avoid perivascular infiltration, because it causes necrosis of the skin and subcutaneous tissues. A dramatic change in the degree of cyanosis should occur. Transfusion is occasionally necessary. Epinephrine and other vasoconstrictors are contraindicated. If reflex bradycardia occurs, atropine should be used.

Herman MI et al: Methylene blue by intraosseous infusion for methemoglobinemia. Ann Emerg Med 1999;33:111 [PMID: 9867898].

Kennedy N et al: Faulty sausage production causing methaemoglobinaemia. Arch Dis Child 1997;76:367 [PMID: 9166036].

## OPIOIDS (Codeine, Heroin, Methadone, Morphine, Propoxyphene)

Opioid-related medical problems may include drug addiction, withdrawal in a newborn infant, and accidental overdoses. Unlike other narcotics, methadone is absorbed readily from the GI tract. Most opioids, including heroin, methadone, meperidine, morphine, and codeine, are excreted in the urine within 24 hours and can be detected readily.

Narcotic-addicted adolescents often have other medical problems, including cellulitis, abscesses, thrombophlebitis, tetanus, infective endocarditis, HIV infection, tuberculosis, hepatitis, malaria, foreign body emboli, thrombosis of pulmonary arterioles, diabetes mellitus, obstetric complications, nephropathy, and peptic ulcer.

### Treatment of Overdosage

Opioids can cause respiratory depression, stridor, coma, increased oropharyngeal secretions, sinus bradycardia, and urinary retention. Pulmonary edema rarely occurs in children; deaths usually result from aspiration of gastric contents, respiratory arrest, and cerebral edema. Convulsions may occur with propoxyphene overdosage.

Although suggested doses for naloxone hydrochloride range from 0.01 to 0.1 mg/kg, it is generally unnecessary to calculate the dosage on this basis. This extremely safe antidote should be given in sufficient quantity to reverse opioid binding sites. For children under age 1 year, 1 ampoule (0.4 mg) should be given initially; if there is no response, five more ampoules (2 mg) should be given rapidly. Older children should be given 0.4–0.8 mg, followed by 2–4 mg if there is no response. An improvement in respiratory status may be followed by respiratory depression, because the antagonist's duration of action is less than 1 hour. Neonates poisoned in utero may require 10–30 mg/kg to reverse the effect.

### Withdrawal in the Addict

Diazepam, 10 mg every 6 hours PO, has been recommended for the treatment of mild narcotic withdrawal in ambulatory adolescents. Management of withdrawal in the confirmed addict may be accomplished with the administration of clonidine, by substitution with methadone, or with reintroduction of the original addicting agent, if available through a supervised drug withdrawal program. A tapered course over 3 weeks will accomplish this goal. Death rarely, if ever, occurs. The abrupt discontinuation of narcotics (cold turkey method) is not recommended and may cause severe physical withdrawal signs.

## Withdrawal in the Newborn

A newborn infant in opioid withdrawal is usually small for gestational age and demonstrates yawning, sneezing, decreased Moro reflex, hunger but uncoordinated sucking action, jitteriness, tremor, constant movement, a shrill protracted cry, increased tendon reflexes, convulsions, vomiting, fever, watery diarrhea, cyanosis, dehydration, vasomotor instability, seizure, and collapse. The onset of symptoms commonly begins in the first 48 hours but may be delayed as long as 8 days depending on the timing of the mother's last fix and her predelivery medication. The diagnosis can be confirmed easily by identifying the narcotic in the urine of the mother and the baby.

Several treatment methods have been suggested for narcotic withdrawal in the newborn. Phenobarbital, 8 mg/kg/d IM or PO in four doses for 4 days and then reduced by one third every 2 days as signs decrease, may be continued for as long as 3 weeks. Methadone may be necessary in those infants with congenital methadone addiction who are not controlled in their withdrawal by large doses of phenobarbital. Dosage should be 0.5 mg/kg/d in two divided doses but can be increased gradually as needed. After control of the symptoms is achieved, the dose may be tapered over 4 weeks.

It is unclear whether prophylactic treatment with these drugs decreases the complication rate. The mortality rate of untreated narcotic withdrawal in the newborn may be as high as 45%.

American Academy of Pediatrics Committee on Drugs: Naloxone dosage and route of administration for infants and children: Addendum to emergency drug doses for infants and children. Pediatrics 1990;86:484 [PMID: 2388800].

Traub SJ et al: Pediatric "body packing" Arch Pediatr Adolesc Med 2003;157:174 [PMID: 12580688].

## PHENOTHIAZINES (Chlorpromazine, Prochlorperazine, Trifluoperazine)

### Clinical Presentations

#### A. Extrapyramidal Crisis

Episodes characterized by torticollis, stiffening of the body, spasticity, poor speech, catatonia, and inability to communicate although conscious are typical manifestations. These episodes usually last a few seconds to a few minutes but have rarely caused death. Extrapyramidal crises may represent idiosyncratic reactions and are aggravated by dehydration. The signs and symptoms occur most often in children who have received prochlorperazine. They are commonly mistaken for psychotic episodes.

#### B. Overdose

Lethargy and deep prolonged coma commonly occur. Promazine, chlorpromazine, and prochlorperazine are the drugs most likely to cause respiratory depression and precipitous drops in blood pressure. Occasionally, paradoxic hyperactivity and extrapyramidal signs as well as hyperglycemia and acetonemia are present. Seizures are uncommon.

#### C. Neuroleptic Malignant Syndrome

Neuroleptic malignant syndrome is a rare idiosyncratic complication of phenothiazine use that may be lethal. It is a syndrome involving mental status change (confusion, coma), motor abnormalities (lead pipe rigidity, clonus), and autonomic dysfunction (tachycardia, hyperpyrexia).

### Treatment

Extrapyramidal signs are alleviated within minutes by the slow IV administration of diphenhydramine, 1–2 mg/kg (maximum, 50 mg), or benztropine mesylate, 1–2 mg IV (1 mg/min). No other treatment is usually indicated.

Patients with overdoses should receive conservative supportive care. Activated charcoal should be administered. Hypotension may be treated with standard agents, starting with isotonic saline administration. Agitation is best treated with diazepam. Neuroleptic malignant syndrome is treated by discontinuing the drug, giving aggressive supportive care, and administering dantrolene or bromocriptine.

Baker PB et al: Hyperthermia, hypertension, hypertonia, and coma in massive thioridazine overdose. Am J Emerg Med 1988;6:346 [PMID: 3390252].

Dyer KS et al: Use of phenothiazines as sedatives in children: What are the risks? Drug Saf 1999;21:81 [PMID: 10456377].

O'Malley GF et al: Olanzapine overdose mimicking opioid intoxication. Ann Emerg Med 1999;34:279 [PMID: 10424936].

## PLANTS

Many common ornamental, garden, and wild plants are potentially toxic. Only in a few cases will small amounts of a plant cause severe illness or death. Table 12–3 lists the most toxic plants, symptoms and signs of poisoning, and treatment. Contact your poison center for assistance with identification.

*Table 12–3.* Poisoning due to plants.[a]

| | Symptoms and Signs | Treatment |
|---|---|---|
| Arum family: *Caladium, Dieffenbachia,* calla lily, dumb-cane (oxalic acid) | Burning of mucous membranes and airway obstruction secondary to edema caused by calcium oxalate crystals. | Accessible areas should be thoroughly washed. Corticosteroids relieve airway obstruction. Apply cold packs to affected mucous membranes. |
| Castor bean plant (ricin—a toxalbumin) Jequinty bean (abrin—a toxalbumin) | Mucous membrane irritation, nausea, vomiting, bloody diarrhea, blurred vision, circulatory collapse, acute hemolytic anemia, convulsions, uremia. | Fluid and electrolyte monitoring. Saline cathartic. Forced alkaline diuresis will prevent complications due to hemagglutination and hemolysis. |
| Foxglove, lily of the valley, and oleander[b] | Nausea, diarrhea, visual disturbances, and cardiac irregularities (eg, heart block). | See treatment for digitalis drugs in text. |
| Jimsonweed: See Belladonna Alkaloids section in text | Mydriasis, dry mouth, tachycardia, and hallucinations. | Activated charcoal. |
| Larkspur (ajacine, *Delphinium,* delphinine) | Nausea and vomiting, irritability, muscular paralysis, and central nervous system depression. | Symptomatic. Atropine may be helpful. |
| Monkshood (aconite) | Numbness of mucous membranes, visual disturbances, tingling, dizziness, tinnitus, hypotension, bradycardia, and convulsions. | Activated charcoal, oxygen. Atropine is probably helpful. |
| Poison hemlock (coniine) | Mydriasis, trembling, dizziness, bradycardia. Central nervous system depression, muscular paralysis, and convulsions. Death is due to respiratory paralysis. | Symptomatic. Oxygen and cardiac monitoring equipment are desirable. Assisted respiration is often necessary. Give anticonvulsants if needed. |
| *Rhododendron* (grayanotoxin) | Abdominal cramps, vomiting, severe diarrhea, muscular paralysis. Central nervous system and circulatory depression. Hypertension with very large doses. | Atropine can prevent bradycardia. Epinephrine is contraindicated. Antihypertensives may be needed. |
| Yellow jessamine (active ingredient, geisemine, is related to strychnine) | Restlessness, convulsions, muscular paralysis, and respiratory depression. | Symptomatic. Because of the relation to strychnine, activated charcoal and diazepam for seizures are worth trying. |

[a]Many other plants cause minor irritation but are not likely to cause serious problems unless large amounts are ingested. See Lampe KF, McCann MA: *AMA Handbook of Poisonous and Injurious Plants.* American Medical Association, 1985. See also Rumack BH, Spoerke DG (eds): POISINDEX information System. Micromedex, Inc., Denver, CO. [Published quarterly.]
[b]Done AK: Ornamental and deadly. Emerg Med 1973;5:255.

# PSYCHOTROPIC DRUGS

Psychotropic drugs consist of four general classes: stimulants (amphetamines, cocaine), depressants (eg, narcotics, barbiturates), antidepressants and tranquilizers, and hallucinogens (eg, LSD, PCP).

## Clinical Presentations

The following clinical findings are commonly seen in patients abusing drugs. See also other entries discussed in alphabetic order in this chapter.

### A. STIMULANTS

Agitation, euphoria, grandiose feelings, tachycardia, fever, abdominal cramps, visual and auditory hallucinations, mydriasis, coma, convulsions, and respiratory depression.

### B. DEPRESSANTS

Emotional lability, ataxia, diplopia, nystagmus, vertigo, poor accommodation, respiratory depression, coma, apnea, and convulsions. Dilatation of conjunctival blood vessels suggests marijuana ingestion. Narcotics cause miotic pupils and, occasionally, pulmonary edema.

## C. ANTIDEPRESSANTS AND TRANQUILIZERS

Hypotension, lethargy, respiratory depression, coma, and extrapyramidal reactions.

## D. HALLUCINOGENS AND PSYCHOACTIVE DRUGS

Belladonna alkaloids cause mydriasis, dry mouth, nausea, vomiting, urinary retention, confusion, disorientation, paranoid delusions, hallucinations, fever, hypotension, aggressive behavior, convulsions, and coma. Psychoactive drugs such as LSD cause mydriasis, unexplained bizarre behavior, hallucinations, and generalized undifferentiated psychotic behavior.

## Management of the Patient Who Abuses Drugs

Only a small percentage of the persons using drugs come to the attention of physicians; those who do are usually experiencing adverse reactions such as panic states, drug psychoses, homicidal or suicidal thoughts, or respiratory depression.

Even with cooperative patients, an accurate history is difficult to obtain. A drug history is most easily obtained in a quiet spot by a gentle, nonthreatening, honest examiner, and without the parents present. The user often does not really know what drug has been taken or how much. Street drugs are almost always adulterated with one or more other compounds. Multiple drugs are often taken together. Friends may be a useful source of information.

The patient's general appearance, skin, lymphatics, cardiorespiratory status, GI tract, and CNS should be focused on during the physical examination, because they often provide clues suggesting drug abuse.

Hallucinogens are not life-threatening unless the patient is frankly homicidal or suicidal. A specific diagnosis is usually not necessary for management; instead, the presenting signs and symptoms are treated. Does the patient appear intoxicated? In withdrawal? "Flashing back?" Is some illness or injury (eg, head trauma) being masked by a drug effect? (Remember that a known drug user may still have hallucinations from meningoencephalitis.)

The signs and symptoms in a given patient are a function not only of the drug and the dose but also of the level of acquired tolerance, the "setting," the patient's physical condition and personality traits, the potentiating effects of other drugs, and many other factors.

A common drug problem is the "bad trip," which is usually a panic reaction. This is best managed by "talking the patient down" and minimizing auditory and visual stimuli. Allowing the patient to sit with a friend while the drug effect dissipates may be the best treatment. This may take several hours. The physician's job is not to terminate the drug effect but to help the patient through the bad experience.

Drug therapy is often unnecessary and may complicate the clinical course of a drug-related panic reaction. Although phenothiazines have been commonly used to treat bad trips, they should be avoided if the specific drug is unknown, because they may enhance toxicity or produce unwanted side effects. Diazepam is the drug of choice if a sedative effect is required. Physical restraints are rarely indicated and usually increase the patient's panic reaction.

For treatment of life-threatening drug abuse, consult the section on the specific drug elsewhere in this chapter and the section on general management at the beginning of the chapter.

After the acute episode, the physician must decide whether psychiatric referral is indicated; in general, patients who have made suicidal gestures or attempts and adolescents who are not communicating with their families should be referred.

Dar KJ, McBrien ME: MDMA induced hyperthermia: Report of a fatality and review of current therapy. Intensive Care Med 1996;22:995 [PMID: 8905441].

Weir E: Raves: A review of the culture, the drugs and the prevention of harm. CMAJ 2000;162:1843 [PMID: 10906922].

# SALICYLATES

The use of childproof containers and publicity regarding accidental poisoning have reduced the incidence of acute salicylate poisoning. Nevertheless, serious intoxication still occurs and must be regarded as an emergency. In recent years, the frequency of poisoning has begun to rise again.

Salicylates uncouple oxidative phosphorylation, leading to increased heat production, excessive sweating, and dehydration. They also interfere with glucose metabolism and may cause hypoglycemia or hyperglycemia. Respiratory center stimulation occurs early.

Patients usually have signs of hyperventilation, sweating, dehydration, and fever. Vomiting and diarrhea sometimes occur. In severe cases, disorientation, convulsions, and coma may develop.

The severity of acute intoxication can in some measure be judged by serum salicylate levels. High levels are always dangerous irrespective of clinical signs, and low levels may be misleading in chronic cases. Other laboratory values usually indicate metabolic acidosis despite hyperventilation, low serum $K^+$ values, and often abnormal serum glucose levels.

In mild and moderate poisoning, stimulation of the respiratory center produces respiratory alkalosis. In severe intoxication (occurring in severe acute ingestion with high salicylate levels and in chronic toxicity with lower levels), respiratory response is unable to overcome the metabolic overdose.

Once the urine becomes acidic, progressively smaller amounts of salicylate are excreted. Until this process is reversed, the half-life will remain prolonged, because metabolism contributes little to the removal of salicylate.

Chronic severe poisoning may occur as early as 3 days after a regimen of salicylate is begun. Findings usually include vomiting, diarrhea, and dehydration.

## Treatment

Charcoal binds salicylates well, and, after emesis or lavage, it should be given for acute ingestions. Mild poisoning may require only the administration of oral fluids and confirmation that the salicylate level is falling. Moderate poisoning involves moderate dehydration and depletion of potassium. Fluids must be administered at a rate of 2–3 mL/kg/h to correct dehydration and produce urine with a pH of greater than 7.0. Initial IV solutions should be isotonic, with sodium bicarbonate constituting half the electrolyte content. Once the patient is rehydrated, the solution can contain more free water and approximately 40 mEq of $K^+$ per liter.

Severe toxicity is marked by major dehydration. Symptoms may be confused with those of Reye syndrome, encephalopathy, and metabolic acidosis. Salicylate levels may even be in the therapeutic range. Major fluid correction of dehydration is required. Once this has been accomplished, hypokalemia must be corrected and sodium bicarbonate given. Usual requirements are sodium bicarbonate, 1–2 mEq/kg/h over the first 6–8 hours, and $K^+$, 20–40 mEq/L. A urine flow of 2–3 mL/kg/h should be established. Despite this treatment some patients will develop the paradoxical aciduria of salicylism. This is due to hypokalemia and the saving of $K^+$ and excretion of $H^+$ in the renal tubule. Correction of $K^+$ will allow the urine to become alkaline and ionize the salicylate, resulting in excretion rather than reabsorption of nonionized salicylate in acid urine.

Renal failure or pulmonary edema is an indication for dialysis. Hemodialysis is most effective, and peritoneal dialysis relatively ineffective. Hemodialysis should be used in all patients with altered mental status or deteriorating clinical status. Acetazolamide should not be used.

Yip L et al: Concepts and controversies in salicylate toxicity. Emerg Med Clin North Am 1994;12:351 [PMID: 8187688].

## SCORPION STINGS

Scorpion stings are common in arid areas of the southwestern United States. Scorpion venom is more toxic than most snake venoms, but only minute amounts are injected. Although neurologic manifestations may last a week, most clinical signs subside within 24–48 hours.

The most common scorpions in the United States are *Vejovis, Hadrurus, Androctonus,* and *Centruroides* species. Stings by the first three produce edema and pain. Stings by *Centruroides* (the Bark scorpion) cause tingling or burning paresthesias that begin at the site of the sting; other findings include hypersalivation, restlessness, muscular fasciculation, abdominal cramps, opisthotonos, convulsions, urinary incontinence, and respiratory failure.

## Treatment

Sedation is the primary therapy. Antivenom is reserved for severe poisoning. In severe cases, the airway may become compromised by secretions and weakness of respiratory muscles. Endotracheal intubation may be required. Patients may require treatment for seizures, hypertension, or tachycardia.

The prognosis is good as long as the patient's airway is managed appropriately.

Gibly R et al: Continuous intravenous midazolam infusion for *Centruroides exilicauda* scorpion envenomation. Ann Emerg Med 1999;34:620 [PMID: 10533010].

LoVecchio F et al: Incidence of immediate and delayed hypersensitivity to *Centruroides* antivenom. Ann Emerg Med 1999;34:615 [PMID: 10533009].

## SNAKEBITE

Despite the lethal potential of venomous snakes, human morbidity and mortality rates are surprisingly low. The outcome depends on the size of the child, the site of the bite, the degree of envenomation, the type of snake, and the effectiveness of treatment.

Nearly all poisonous snakebites in the United States are caused by pit vipers (rattlesnakes, water moccasins, and copperheads). A few are caused by elapids (coral snakes), and occasional bites occur from cobras and other nonindigenous exotic snakes kept as pets. Snake venom is a complex mixture of enzymes, peptides, and proteins that may have predominantly cytotoxic, neurotoxic, hemotoxic, or cardiotoxic effects but other effects as well. Up to 25% of bites by pit vipers do not result in venom injection. Pit viper venom causes predominantly local injury with pain, discoloration, edema, and hemorrhage.

Swelling and pain occur soon after rattlesnake bite and are a certain indication that envenomation has occurred. During the first few hours, swelling and ecchymosis extend proximally from the bite. The bite is often obvious as a double puncture mark surrounded by ecchymosis. Hematemesis, melena, hemoptysis, and other manifestations of coagulopathy develop in severe cases. Respiratory difficulty and shock are the ultimate causes of death. Even in fatal rattlesnake bite, a period of 6–8 hours usually elapses between the bite and death; as a result, there is usually enough time to start effective treatment.

Coral snake envenomation causes little local pain, swelling, or necrosis; and systemic reactions are often delayed. The signs of coral snake envenomation include bulbar paralysis, dysphagia, and dysphoria; these signs may appear in 5–10 hours and may be followed by total peripheral paralysis and death in 24 hours.

## Treatment

Children in snake-infested areas should wear boots and long trousers, should not walk barefoot, and should be cautioned not to explore under ledges or in holes.

### A. EMERGENCY (FIRST AID) TREATMENT

The most important first aid measure is transportation to a medical facility. Splint the affected extremity and minimize the patient's motion. Tourniquets and ice packs are contraindicated. Incision and suction are not useful for either crotalid or elapid snake bite.

### B. DEFINITIVE MEDICAL MANAGEMENT

Blood should be drawn for hematocrit, clotting time and platelet function, and serum electrolyte determinations. Establish two secure IV sites for the administration of antivenom and other medications.

Specific antivenom is indicated when signs of progressive envenomation are present. Two antivenoms are available for treating pit viper envenomation: polyvalent pit viper antivenom and polyvalent Crotalidae Fab (CroFab). Both are effective, but their indications differ. For coral snake bites, an eastern coral snake antivenom (Wyeth Laboratories) is available. Patients with pit viper bites should receive antivenom if progressive local injury, coagulopathy, or systemic signs (eg, hypotension, confusion) are present. (Antivenom should not be given IM or SQ.) See package labeling or call your certified poison center for details of use. Hemorrhage, pain, and shock diminish rapidly with adequate amounts of antivenom. For coral snake bites, give three to five vials of antivenom in 250–500 mL of isotonic saline solution. An additional three to five vials may be required.

To control pain, administer a narcotic analgesic, such as meperidine, 0.6–1.5 mg/kg/dose, given PO or IM. Cryotherapy is contraindicated because it commonly causes additional tissue damage. Early physiotherapy minimizes contractures. In rare cases, fasciotomy to relieve pressure within muscular compartments is required. The evaluation of function and of pulses will better predict the need for fasciotomy. Antihistamines and corticosteroids (hydrocortisone, 1 mg/kg, given PO for a week) are useful in the treatment of serum sickness or anaphylactic shock. Antibiotics are not needed unless clinical signs of infection occur. Tetanus status should be evaluated and the patient immunized, if needed.

Bond GR: Snake, spider, and scorpion envenomation in North America. Pediatr Rev 1999;20:147 [PMID: 10233171].

Dart RC, McNally J: Efficacy, safety, and use of snake antivenoms in the United States. Ann Emerg Med 2001;37:181 [PMID: 11174237].

# SOAPS & DETERGENTS

## 1. Soaps

Soap is made from salts of fatty acids. Some toilet soap bars contain both soap and detergent. Ingestion of soap bars may cause vomiting and diarrhea, but they have a low toxicity. Induced emesis is unnecessary.

## 2. Detergents

Detergents are nonsoap synthetic products used for cleaning purposes because of their surfactant properties. Commercial products include granules, powders, and liquids. Dishwasher detergents are very alkaline and can cause caustic burns. Low concentrations of bleaching and antibacterial agents as well as enzymes are found in many preparations. The pure compounds are moderately toxic, but the concentration used is too small to alter the product's toxicity significantly, although occasional primary or allergic irritative phenomena have been noted in persons who frequently use such products and in employees manufacturing these products.

## Cationic Detergents (Ceepryn, Diaperene, Phemerol, Zephiran)

Cationic detergents in dilute solutions (0.5%) cause mucosal irritation, but higher concentrations (10–15%) may cause caustic burns to mucosa. Clinical effects include nausea, vomiting, collapse, coma, and convulsions. As little as 2.25 g of some cationic agents have caused death in an adult. In four cases, 100–400 mg/kg of benzalkonium chloride caused death. Cationic detergents are rapidly inactivated by tissues and ordinary soap.

Because of the caustic potential and rapid onset of seizures, emesis is not recommended. Activated charcoal should be administered. Anticonvulsants may be needed.

## Anionic Detergents

Most common household detergents are anionic. Laundry compounds have water softener (sodium phosphate) added, which is a strong irritant and may reduce ionized calcium. Anionic detergents irritate the skin by removing natural oils. Although ingestion causes diarrhea, intestinal distention, and vomiting, no fatalities have been reported.

The only treatment usually required is to discontinue use if skin irritation occurs and replace fluids and electrolytes. Induced vomiting is not indicated following ingestion of electric dishwasher detergent, because of its alkalinity. Dilute with water or milk.

## Nonionic Detergents (Brij Products; Tritons X-45, X-100, X-102, & X-144)

These compounds include lauryl, stearyl, and oleyl alcohols and octyl phenol. They have a minimal irritating effect on the skin and are almost nontoxic when swallowed.

Klasaer AE et al: Marked hypocalcemia and ventricular fibrillation in two pediatric patients exposed to a fluoride-containing wheel cleaner. Ann Emerg Med 1996;28:713 [PMID: 8953969].

Lovejoy FH Jr, Woolf AD: Corrosive ingestions. Pediatr Rev 1995;16:473 [PMID: 8559706].

Vincent JC, Sheikh A: Phosphate poisoning by ingestion of clothes washing liquid and fabric conditioner. Anesthesiology 1998;53:1004 [PMID: 9893545].

## SPIDER BITES

Most medically important bites in the United States are caused by the black widow spider (*Latrodectus mactans*) and the North American brown recluse (violin) spider (*Loxosceles reclusa*). Positive identification of the spider is helpful, because many spider bites may mimic those of the brown recluse spider.

## Black Widow Spider

The black widow spider is endemic to nearly all areas of the United States. The initial bite causes sharp fleeting pain. Local and systemic muscular cramping, abdominal pain, nausea and vomiting, and shock can occur. Convulsions occur more commonly in small children than in older children. Systemic signs of black widow spider bite may be confused with other causes of acute abdomen. Although paresthesias, nervousness, and transient muscle spasms may persist for weeks in sur-

vivors, recovery from the acute phase is generally complete within 3 days. In contrast to popular opinion, death is extremely rare.

Most authors recommend calcium gluconate as initial therapy (50 mg/kg IV per dose, up to 250 mg/kg/24 h), although it is often not effective and the effects are of short duration. Methocarbamol (15 mg/kg PO) or diazepam titrated to effect is useful. Morphine or barbiturates may occasionally be needed for control of pain or restlessness, but they increase the possibility of respiratory depression. Antivenom is available but should be reserved for severe cases in which the above therapies have failed. Local treatment of the bite is not helpful.

## Brown Recluse Spider (Violin Spider)

The North American brown recluse spider is most commonly seen in the central and Midwestern areas of the United States. Its bite characteristically produces a localized reaction with progressively severe pain within 24 hours. The initial bleb on an erythematous ischemic base is replaced by a black eschar within 1 week. This eschar separates in 2–5 weeks, leaving an ulcer that heals slowly. Systemic signs include cyanosis, morbilliform rash, fever, chills, malaise, weakness, nausea and vomiting, joint pains, hemolytic reactions with hemoglobinuria, jaundice, and delirium. Fatalities are rare. Fatal disseminated intravascular coagulation has been reported.

Although of unproved efficacy, the following therapies have been used: dexamethasone, 4 mg IV four times a day, during the acute phase; polymorphonuclear leukocyte inhibitors, such as dapsone or colchicine, and oxygen applied to the bite site; and total excision of the lesion to the fascial level.

Clark RF et al: Clinical presentation and treatment of black widow spider envenomation: A review of 163 cases. Ann Emerg Med 1992;21:782 [PMID: 1351707].

Sams HH et al: Nineteen documented cases of *Loxosceles reclusa* envenomation. J Am Acad Dermatol 2001;44:603 [PMID: 11260528].

## THYROID PREPARATIONS (Thyroid Desiccated, Sodium Levothyroxine)

Ingestion of the equivalent of 50–150 g of desiccated thyroid can cause signs of hyperthyroidism, including irritability, mydriasis, hyperpyrexia, tachycardia, and diarrhea. Maximal clinical effect occurs about 9 days after ingestion—several days after the protein-bound iodine level has fallen dramatically.

Induce vomiting. If the patient develops clinical signs of toxicity, propranolol, 0.01–0.1 mg/kg (maximum, 1 mg), is useful because of its antiadrenergic activity.

Brown RS et al: Successful treatment of massive acute thyroid hormone poisoning with iopanoic acid. J Pediatr 1998;132: 903 [PMID: 9602214].

Golightly LK et al: Clinical effects of accidental levothyroxine ingestion in children. Am J Dis Child 1987;141:1025[PMID: 2887106].

## TOXIC ALCOHOLS

Ethylene glycol and methanol are the toxic alcohols. The primary source of ethylene glycol is antifreeze, while methanol is present in windshield wiper fluid and also as an ethanol denaturant. Ethylene glycol causes severe metabolic acidosis and renal failure. Methanol causes metabolic acidosis and blindness. Onset of symptoms with both agents occurs within several hours after ingestion, longer if ethanol was ingested simultaneously.

### Treatment

The primary treatment is to block the enzyme alcohol dehydrogenase which converts both agents to their toxic metabolites. This is accomplished with fomepizole (loading dose of 15 mg/kg) or ethanol. Fomepizole is preferred for children, due to its reduced side effects in this age group.

Barceloux DG et al: American Academy of Clinical Toxicology Practice Guidelines on the Treatment of Methanol Poisoning. J Toxicol Clin Toxicol 2002;40:415 [PMID: 12216995].

Brent J et al: Fomepizole for the treatment of ethylene glycol poisoning: Methylpyrazole for toxic alcohols study group. N Engl J Med 1999;40:832 [PMID: 10080845].

## VITAMINS

Accidental ingestion of excessive amounts of vitamins rarely causes significant problems. Occasional cases of hypervitaminosis A and D do occur, however, particularly in patients with poor hepatic or renal function. The fluoride contained in many multivitamin preparations is not a realistic hazard, because a 2- or 3-year-old child could eat 100 tablets, containing 1 mg of sodium fluoride per tablet, without experiencing serious symptoms. Iron poisoning has been reported with multivitamin tablets containing iron. Pyridoxine abuse has caused neuropathies; nicotinic acid, myopathy.

Dean BS, Krenzelok EP: Multiple vitamins and vitamins with iron: Accidental poisoning in children. Vet Hum Toxicol 1988; 30:23 [PMID: 3354178].

Fraser DR: Vitamin D. Lancet 1995;345:104 [PMID: 7815853].

## WARFARIN

Warfarin is used as a rodenticide. It causes hypoprothrombinemia and capillary injury. It is absorbed readily from the GI tract but is absorbed poorly through the skin. A dose of 0.5 mg/kg of warfarin may be toxic in a child. A prothrombin time is helpful in establishing the severity of the poisoning.

If bleeding occurs or the prothrombin time is prolonged, give 1–5 mg of vitamin $K_1$ (phytonadione) IM or SQ. For large ingestions with established toxicity, 0.6 mg/kg may be given.

Another group of long-acting anticoagulant rodenticides (brodifacoum, difenacoum, bromadiolone, diphacinone, pinone, valone, and coumatetralyl) have been a more serious toxicologic problem than warfarin. They also cause hypoprothrombinemia and a bleeding diathesis that responds to phytonadione, although the anticoagulant activity may persist for periods ranging from 6 weeks to several months. Treatment with vitamin K1 may be needed for weeks.

Isbister GK, Whyte IM: Management of anticoagulant poisoning. Vet Hum Toxicol 2001;43:117 [PMID: 11308119].

Mullins ME et al: Unintentional pediatric superwarfarin exposures: Do we really need a prothrombin time? Pediatrics 2000;105: 402 [PMID: 10654963].

# Critical Care

*Todd C. Carpenter, MD, Emily L. Dobyns, MD, Stephanie N. Mateev, MD,*
*Peter M. Mourani, MD, Margaret A. Ferguson, MD, & Kurt R. Stenmark, MD*

Caring for critically ill children remains one of the most demanding and challenging aspects of the field of pediatrics. The care of patients with life-threatening conditions, from serious medical illness to traumatic injuries and recovery from major surgery, requires a detailed understanding of the physiology of the body and the pathophysiology of major illnesses, as well as an understanding of and experience with the rapidly changing technologies available in a modern intensive care unit (ICU). In addition, the science of caring for the critically ill patient has evolved rapidly over the last decade, as the molecular mediators of illness have become better defined and new therapies have been devised based on those advances. As a result, critical care is more than ever a multidisciplinary field that requires a team-oriented approach, including critical care physicians and nursing staff, pharmacists, referring physicians, consulting specialists, and social services specialists.

The intensivist plays an essential role in coordinating and directing the care provided by the ICU team, and in so doing stands at the crossroads of the various participating disciplines. There are two primary models of ICU organization: "open" units, where primary responsibility for the patient remains with the referring physician and secondary responsibility lies with the intensivist as consultant; and "closed" units, where only the on-site intensivist is allowed to write orders directing the patient's care. Although the merits of both of these organizational approaches are debated, a substantial and growing body of evidence from studies conducted in adult medical, surgical, and pediatric ICUs suggests that the closed ICU model may lead to significant reductions in ICU length of stay and resource use, as well as to reductions in mortality of as much as 15%.

An additional factor to consider in the provision of critical care services for children is the cost of those services in relation to the outcomes achieved. Critical care services in the United States are estimated to account for 30% of all acute-care hospital costs; some estimates run as high as 1% of the gross national product. One study has examined the cost-effectiveness of pediatric ICU care compared with adult ICU care. Those investigators found that the short- and long-term mortality among pediatric patients was three times lower than it was among adult ICU patients, despite similar ICU

costs and length of stay. These findings suggest that pediatric critical care services are relatively cost-effective compared with similar services provided to adult patients. Along with the preceding discussion of the intensivist's role in ICU practice, the findings of these studies serve to highlight the complexities of this growing field, as well as the key role of the ICU specialist in caring for the sickest children.

Brilli RJ et al: Critical care delivery in the intensive care unit: Defining clinical roles and the best practice model. Crit Care Med 2001;29(10):2007 [PMID: 11588472].

Pollack MM et al: Impact of quality of care factors on pediatric intensive care unit mortality. JAMA 1994;272(12):941 [PMID: 8084061].

Seferian EG et al: Comparison of resource utilization and outcome between pediatric and adult intensive care unit patients. Pediatr Crit Care Med 2001;2:2 [PMID: 12797880].

Tilford JM et al: Volume-outcome relationships in pediatric intensive care units. Pediatr 2000;106:289 [PMID: 10920153].

Young MP, Birkmeyer JD: Potential reduction in mortality rates using an intensivist model to manage intensive care units. Eff Clin Pract 2000;3(6):284 [PMID: 11151525].

## ACUTE RESPIRATORY FAILURE

Acute respiratory failure, defined as the inability of the respiratory system to adequately deliver oxygen or remove $CO_2$, contributes significantly to the morbidity and mortality of critically ill children. This condition accounts for approximately 50% of deaths in children younger than age 1 year. Anatomic and developmental differences place infants at higher risk than adults for respiratory failure. An infant's thoracic cage is more compliant than that of the adult or older child. The intercostal muscles are poorly developed and unable to achieve the "bucket handle" motion characteristic of adult breathing. Furthermore, the diaphragm is shorter, relatively flat with fewer type I muscle fibers, and therefore less effective and more easily fatigued. The infant's airways are smaller in caliber than those in older children and adults, resulting in greater resistance to inspiratory and expiratory airflow and greater susceptibility to occlusion by mucus plugging and mucosal edema. Compared with adults, the alveoli of children are smaller and have less collateral ventilation, resulting in a greater tendency to collapse and develop atelectasis. Finally, young infants may have an especially reactive pulmonary vascular bed, impaired immune system, or residual effects from prematurity, all of which increase the risk of respiratory failure.

Respiratory failure can be classified into two types, which usually coexist in variable proportion. The $PaO_2$ is low in both, whereas the $PaCO_2$ is high only in patients with type II respiratory failure (Table 13–1). Type I respiratory failure is a failure of oxygenation and occurs in three situations: (1) **ventilation–perfusion mismatch,** or V/Q mismatch, which occurs when blood flows to parts of the lung that are inadequately ventilated, or when ventilated areas of the lung are inadequately perfused; (2) **diffusion defects,** caused by thickened alveolar membranes or excessive interstitial fluid at the alveolar–capillary junction; and (3) **intrapulmonary shunt,** which occurs when structural anomalies in the lung allow blood to flow through the lung without participating in gas exchange. Type II respiratory failure generally results from alveolar hypoventilation and is usually secondary to situations such as central nervous system (CNS) dysfunction, oversedation, or neuromuscular disorders (see Table 13–1).

**Table 13–1.** Types of respiratory failure.

| Findings | Causes | Examples |
|---|---|---|
| **Type I**<br>Hypoxia<br>Decreased $PaO_2$<br>Normal $PaCO_2$ | Ventilation/perfusion defect | Positional (supine in bed), adult respiratory distress syndrome (ARDS), atelectasis, pneumonia, pulmonary embolus, bronchopulmonary dysplasia |
| | Diffusion impairment | Pulmonary edema, ARDS, interstitial pneumonia |
| | Shunt | Pulmonary arteriovenous malformation, congenital adenomatoid malformation |
| **Type II**<br>Hypoxia<br>Hypercapnia<br>Decreased $PaO_2$<br>Increased $PaCO_2$ | Hypoventilation | Neuromuscular disease (polio, Guillain–Barré syndrome), head trauma, sedation, chest wall dysfunction (burns), kyphosis, severe reactive airways |

## Clinical Findings

### A. SYMPTOMS AND SIGNS

The clinical findings in respiratory failure are caused by the low $PaO_2$, high $PaCO_2$, and pH changes affecting the lungs, heart, kidneys, and brain. The clinical features of progressive respiratory failure are summarized in Table 13–2. Hypercapnia depresses the CNS, and also results in acidemia that depresses myocardial function. Patients in respiratory failure can exhibit significant changes in CNS and cardiac function. Features of respiratory failure are not always clinically evident, however, and some signs or symptoms may have nonrespiratory causes. Furthermore, a strictly clinical assessment of arterial hypoxemia or hypercapnia is not reliable. As a result, the precise assessment of the adequacy of oxygenation and ventilation must be based on both clinical and laboratory data.

### B. LABORATORY FINDINGS

Laboratory findings are helpful in assessing the severity and acuity of respiratory failure and in determining specific treatment. Arterial oxygen saturation can be measured continuously and noninvasively by **pulse oximetry,** a technique that should be used in the assessment and treatment of all patients with suspected respiratory failure. **End-tidal $CO_2$ monitoring** provides a continuous noninvasive means of assessing arterial $pCO_2$. Because carbon dioxide diffuses freely across the alveo-

**Table 13–2.** Clinical features of respiratory failure.

| |
|---|
| **Respiratory**<br>Wheezing<br>Expiratory grunting<br>Decreased or absent breath sounds<br>Flaring of alae nasi<br>Retractions of chest wall<br>Tachypnea, bradypnea, or apnea<br>Cyanosis |
| **Neurologic**<br>Restlessness<br>Irritability<br>Headache<br>Confusion<br>Convulsions<br>Coma |
| **Cardiac**<br>Bradycardia or excessive tachycardia<br>Hypotension or hypertension |
| **General**<br>Fatigue<br>Sweating |

lar–capillary barrier, the exhaled end-tidal $CO_2$ (ETCO$_2$) level approximates the alveolar $P_{CO_2}$, which should equal the arterial $P_{CO_2}$. Though useful for following trends in ventilation, this technique is susceptible to significant error, particularly with patients who have rapid, shallow breathing or increased dead space ventilation. **Arterial blood gas (ABG) analysis** remains the gold standard for assessment of acute respiratory failure. ABGs give information on the patient's acid–base status (with a measured pH and calculated bicarbonate level) as well as $P_{aO}$ and $P_{aCO_2}$ levels. The $P_{aO_2}$ is a critical determinant of oxygen delivery to the tissues, and the $P_{aCO_2}$ is a sensitive measure of ventilation related inversely to the minute ventilation (Figure 13–1). Although measurement of capillary or venous blood gases may provide some reassurance regarding ventilatory function if blood gas results are normal, these tests yield virtually no useful information regarding oxygenation and may generate highly misleading information about the ventilatory status of patients who have poor perfusion or who had blood draws that were difficult. As a result, ABG analysis is important for all patients with suspected respiratory failure, particularly those with abnormal venous or capillary gases.

Knowing the ABG values and the inspired oxygen concentration also enables one to calculate the difference between alveolar oxygen concentration and the arterial oxygen value, known as the **alveolar–arterial oxygen difference** (A–aDO$_2$, or A–a gradient). The A–a gradient is less than 15 mm Hg under normal conditions, though it widens with increasing inspired oxygen concentrations, to about 100 mm Hg in normal patients breathing 100% oxygen. This number has prognostic value in severe hypoxemic respiratory failure, with A–a gradients over 400 mm Hg being strongly associated with mortality. Diffusion impairment, shunts, and V/Q mismatch all increase the A–aDO$_2$ (Table 13–3).

In addition to the calculation of the A–aDO$_2$, assessment of intrapulmonary shunting (the percentage of pulmonary blood flow that passes through nonventilated areas of the lung) may be helpful. Normal individuals have less than a 5% physiologic shunt from bronchial, thebesian, and coronary circulations. Shunt fractions greater than 15% usually indicate the need for aggressive respiratory support. When intrapulmonary shunt reaches 50% of pulmonary blood flow, $P_{aO_2}$ does not increase regardless of the amount of supplemental oxygen used.

## Treatment

### A. Oxygen Supplementation

Patients with hypoxemia induced by respiratory failure may respond to **supplemental oxygen** administration alone (Table 13–4). Those with hypoventilation and diffusion defects respond better than do patients with shunts or V/Q mismatch. Severe V/Q mismatch generally responds only to aggressive airway management and mechanical ventilation. Patients with severe hypoxemia, hypoventilation, or apnea require assistance with bag and mask ventilation until the airway is successfully intubated and controlled artificial ventilation can be provided. Ventilation may be maintained for some time with a mask of the proper size, but gastric distention, emesis, and inadequate tidal volumes are possible complications. An artificial airway may be lifesaving for patients who fail to respond to simple oxygen supplements.

### B. Intubation

Intubation of the trachea in infants and children requires experienced personnel and the right equipment. A patient in respiratory failure whose airway must be stabilized should first be positioned properly to facilitate air exchange while supplemental oxygen is given. The sniffing position is used in infants. Head extension with jaw thrust is used in older children without neck injuries. If obstructed by secretions or vomitus, the airway must be cleared by suction. When not obstructed, the airway should open easily with proper positioning and placement of an oral or nasopharyngeal airway of the correct size. Patients with a normal airway may be intubated under intravenous (IV) anesthesia by experi-

***Figure 13–1.*** Relationship between alveolar ventilation, arterial oxygen saturation (Sao$_2$), and partial pressures of oxygen and $CO_2$ in the arterial blood (Pao$_2$ and Paco$_2$, respectively). (Reproduced, with permission, from Pagtakhan RD, Chernick V: Respiratory failure in the pediatric patient. Pediatr Rev 1982;3:244.)

***Table 13–3.*** Key equations describing pulmonary function and oxygen delivery.

| | | |
|---|---|---|
| $Pio_2$ | = | (barometric pressure – 47) × % inspired oxygen concentration |
| $AaDo_2$ | = | $Pio_2 - (Paco_2/R) - Pao_2$ (normal = 5–15 mm Hg) |
| $CO_2$ | = | $(1.34 \times$ hemoglobin $\times Sao_2) + (0.003 \times Pao_2)$ |
| $Do_2$ | = | $Cao_2 \times CI \times 10$ (normal 620 + 50 mL/min/m$^2$) |

Oxygen consumption ($Vo_2$) = $(Cao_2 - Cvo_2) \times CI \times 10$ (normal 120–200 mL/min/m$^2$)

$$\frac{Qs}{Qt} = \frac{Cco_2 - Cao_2}{Cco_2 - Cvo_2} \quad \text{(normal} < 5\%)$$

$$Vd = \frac{(Paco_2 - Peco_2)}{Pcco_2} \quad \text{(normal approximately 2 mL/kg)}$$

$$Compliance = \frac{\text{Volume (tidal volume)}}{\text{Pressure (PIP} - \text{PEEP)}} \quad \text{(normals vary with age)}$$

| | | |
|---|---|---|
| $A–aDo_2$ | = | Alveolar–arterial oxygen difference (mm Hg) |
| $Cao_2$ | = | Oxygen content of arterial blood (mL/dL) |
| $Cco_2$ | = | Oxygen content of pulmonary capillary blood (mL/dL) |
| CI | = | Cardiac index (L/min) |
| $CO_2$ | = | Oxygen content of the blood (mL/dL) |
| $Cvo_2$ | = | Oxygen content of mixed venous blood (mL/dL) |
| $Do_2$ | = | Oxygen delivery (mL/min) |
| $Paco_2$ | = | Partial pressure of carbon dioxide in arterial blood (mm Hg) |
| $Pao_2$ | = | Partial pressure of oxygen in arterial blood (mm Hg) |
| $Pcco_2$ | = | Partial pressure of carbon dioxide in capillary blood (mm Hg) |
| $Peco_2$ | = | Partial pressure of carbon dioxide in expired air (mm Hg) |
| $Pio_2$ | = | Partial pressure of oxygen in inspired air (mm Hg) |
| PIP | = | Peak inspiratory pressure |
| Qs/Qt | = | Intrapulmonary shunt (in patients without cardiac shunt) (%) |
| R | = | Respiratory quotient (usually 0.8) |
| $Sao_2$ | = | Arterial oxygen saturation (fractional) |
| Vd | = | Physiologic dead space (anatomic dead space + alveolar dead space) (mL) |
| Ve | = | Expiratory minute volume (L/min) |
| $Vo_2$ | = | Oxygen consumption per minute |

enced personnel (Table 13–5). Patients with obstructed upper airways (eg, patients with croup, epiglottitis, foreign bodies, or subglottic stenosis) should be awake when intubated unless trained airway specialists decide otherwise.

The size of the endotracheal tube is of critical importance in pediatrics (see Table 11–3 for sizes). An inappropriately large endotracheal tube can cause pressure necrosis of the tissues in the subglottic region, leading in some cases to scarring and permanent stenosis of the subglottic region that can require surgical repair. An inappropriately small endotracheal tube can result in inadequate pulmonary toilet and excessive air leak around the endotracheal tube, making optimal ventilation and oxygenation difficult. Two useful methods for calculat-

ing the correct size of endotracheal tube for a child are (1) measuring the child's height with a Broselow tape and then reading the corresponding endotracheal tube size on the tape, or (2) in children older than age 2 years, choosing a tube size equal to the simple computation (16 + age in years) ÷ 4.

Correct placement of the endotracheal tube should be confirmed by auscultation for the presence of equal bilateral breath sounds and if using a colorimetric filter (pH-sensitive indicator that changes from purple to yellow when exposed to carbon dioxide) by the detection of carbon dioxide. An assessment of air leakage around the endotracheal tube is also important. To do this, connect an anesthesia bag and pressure manometer to the endotracheal tube and allow it to inflate, creating

***Table 13–4.*** Supplemental oxygen therapy.

| Source | Maximum % O$_2$ | Range of Rates | Advantages | Disadvantages |
|---|---|---|---|---|
| Nasal cannula | 35–40% | 0.125–4 L/min | Easily applied, relatively comfortable | Uncomfortable at higher flow rates, requires open nasal airways, easily dislodged, lower % O$_2$, nosebleeds |
| Simple mask | 50–60% | 5–10 L/min | Higher % O$_2$, good for mouth breathers | Uncomfortable, dangerous for patients with poor airway control and at risk for emesis, hard to give airway care, unsure of % O$_2$ |
| Face tent | 40–60% | 8–10 L/min | Higher % O$_2$, good for mouth breathers, less restrictive | Uncomfortable, dangerous for patients with poor airway control and at risk for emesis, hard to give airway care, unsure of % O$_2$ |
| Rebreathing mask | 80–90% | 5–10 L/min | Higher % O$_2$, good for mouth breathers, highest O$_2$ concentration | Uncomfortable, dangerous for patients with poor airway control and at risk for emesis, hard to give airway care, unsure of % O$_2$ |
| Oxyhood | 90–100% | 5–10 L/min (mixed at wall) | Stable and accurate O$_2$ concentration | Difficult to maintain temperature, hard to give airway care |

***Table 13–5.*** Drugs commonly used for controlled intubation.

| Drug | Class of Agent | Dose | Advantages | Disadvantages |
|---|---|---|---|---|
| Atropine | Anticholinergic | 0.02 mg/kg, minimum of 0.1 mg | Prevents bradycardia, dries secretions | Tachycardia, fever; seizures and coma with high doses |
| Fentanyl | Narcotic (sedative) | 1–3 μg/kg IV | Rapid onset, hemodynamic stability | Respiratory depression, chest wall rigidity with rapid administration in neonates |
| Midazolam | Benzodiazepine (sedative) | 0.1–0.2 mg/kg IV | Rapid onset, amnestic | Respiratory depression, hypotension |
| Thiopental | Barbiturate (anesthetic) | 3–5 mg/kg IV | Rapid onset, lowers intracranial pressure | Hypotension, decreased cardiac output, no analgesia provided |
| Ketamine | Dissociative anesthetic | 1–2 mg/kg IV 2–4 mg/kg IM | Rapid onset, bronchodilator, hemodynamic stability | Increases oral and airway secretions, may increase ICP and pulmonary artery pressure |
| Rocuronium | Nondepolarizing muscle relaxant | 1 mg/kg | Rapid onset, suitable for rapid sequence intubation, lasts 30 minutes | Requires refrigeration |
| Pancuronium | Nondepolarizing muscle relaxant | 0.1 mg/kg | Longer duration of action (40–60 min) | Tachycardia, slow onset (2–3 min) |

IV = intravenously, IM = intramuscularly.

positive pressure. Check for the leak by auscultating over the throat, noting the pressure at which air escapes around the endotracheal tube. Leaks at pressures of 15–20 cm $H_2O$ are acceptable. Leaks at lower pressures may lead to ineffective ventilation, and the endotracheal tube should be upsized if continued mechanical ventilation is needed. Leaks at higher pressures are acceptable only with patients who have severe lung disease and poor compliance and who thus require high pressures to ventilate and oxygenate. A chest radiograph is necessary for final assessment of endotracheal tube placement.

Artigas A et al: The American-European Consensus Conference on ARDs, Part 2. Am J Respir Crit Care Med 1998;157:1332 [PMID: 9563759].

Bateman ST, Arnold JH: Acute respiratory failure in children. Curr Opin Pediatr 2000;12(3):233 [PMID: 10836159].

Green KE, Peters JI: Pathophysiology of acute respiratory failure. Clin Chest Med 1994;15:1 [PMID: 8200186].

Hedenstierna G, Lattuada M: Gas exchange in the ventilated patient. Curr Opin Crit Care 2002;8:39 [PMID: 12205405].

Sagarin MJ et al; National Emergency Airway Registry (NEAR) investigators: Pediatr Emerg Care 2002;18:417 [PMID: 12488834].

Shapiro MB et al: Respiratory failure. Conventional and high-tech support. Surg Clin North Am 2000;80(3):871 [PMID: 10097266].

Sigillito RJ, DeBlieux PM: Evaluation and initial management of the patient in respiratory distress. Emerg Med Clin North Am 2003;21:239 [PMID: 12793613].

Weiss IK et al: Clinical use of continuous arterial blood gas monitoring in the pediatric intensive care unit. Pediatrics 1999;103:440 [PMID: 9925838].

# MECHANICAL VENTILATION

The increased compliance of an infant's chest wall, the relative alveolar hypoplasia in early childhood, the small caliber of the airways, and the small tidal volumes of young children make mechanical ventilation of the pediatric patient challenging. The goals of mechanical ventilation are to facilitate the movement of gas into and out of the lungs (ventilation) and to improve oxygen uptake into the bloodstream (oxygenation). Modern mechanical ventilators can accomplish these objectives in a variety of ways. Depending on the mode of ventilation selected, the ventilator can deliver a machine-controlled breath (control ventilation), or can assist the patient's own spontaneous respiratory efforts (support ventilation), or can do both (mixed mode ventilation). Additionally, ventilator breaths can be delivered as a targeted tidal volume (volume ventilation) or as a targeted airway pressure (pressure ventilation). Ongoing advances in microprocessor control and ventilator design give the clinician increasingly complex choices in tailoring a mode of mechanical ventilation to particular clinical scenarios. This section will describe the modes of mechanical ventilation most commonly used in pediatric intensive care units.

## Pressure Ventilation

In pressure-controlled modes of ventilation, air flow is begun at the start of the inspiratory cycle and continues until a preset airway pressure is reached. That airway pressure is then maintained until, at the end of the set inspiratory time, the exhalation valve on the ventilator opens and gas exits into the machine. Because airway pressure is the controlling variable with this mode of ventilation, changes in the compliance of the respiratory system will lead to fluctuations in the actual tidal volume delivered to the patient. The advantage of pressure-controlled ventilation lies primarily in the avoidance of high airway pressures that might cause lung injury or barotrauma, particularly in those patients with fragile lung parenchyma, such as premature infants. The main disadvantage of pressure-controlled ventilation is the possibility of delivering either inadequate or excessive tidal volumes during periods of changing lung compliance, as described earlier.

## Volume Ventilation

Volume-controlled ventilation is the most commonly used mode of mechanical ventilation in most pediatric intensive care units (PICUs). In contrast to pressure-controlled modes, volume ventilation delivers a preset tidal volume to the patient. Changes in lung compliance will lead to fluctuations in the airway pressure generated by the tidal volume. The main advantage of volume ventilation is more reliable delivery of the desired tidal volume and thus better control of ventilation. More reliable tidal volume delivery may also help prevent atelectasis from hypoventilation. Disadvantages of volume ventilation include the risk of barotrauma from excessive airway pressures and difficulties overcoming leaks in the ventilator circuit. Older volume ventilators also suffered from a lack of continuous gas flow through the circuit, thus increasing the patient's work of breathing on spontaneous breaths. Most modern machines have overcome that problem by providing a continuous flow through the circuit and by improved triggering mechanisms to deliver the breaths in synchrony with the patient's demands.

## Modes of Ventilation

Most modern ventilators can deliver either a pressure-controlled or a volume-controlled breath in several manners. **Assist-control** modes deliver breaths at a selected rate and duration (inspiratory time) and can be targeted for either volume or pressure set by the clinician (as opposed to the patient). Spontaneous breaths are not assisted, and the patient's own respiratory efforts are not considered. **Synchronized intermittent mandatory ventilation (SIMV)** is a mode in which the rate, inspiratory time, and volume or pressure settings are set by the clinician. But the ventilator allows a window of time around each breath in which it waits for the patient to make an inspiratory effort. The machine breath is then synchronized with the patient's effort, to improve the comfort of those who are breathing spontaneously. In **pressure support,** the patient's own efforts are assisted by the delivery of gas flow to achieve a certain airway pressure. This mode of ventilation allows the patient to determine the rate and inspiratory time of breaths, thus improving patient comfort and decreasing the work of breathing. Perhaps the most common mode of ventilation in PICUs is **SIMV with pressure support,** a mixed mode allowing pressure-supported breaths between the synchronized machine breaths. Whether such mixed modes of ventilation provide any measurable advantage over single modes remains unclear, despite their popularity.

## Setting the Ventilator

When initiating mechanical ventilation, the clinician will vary the parameters according to the mode of ventilation selected. Volume-controlled modes of ventilation generally require a set tidal volume, inspiratory time, rate, and level of positive end-expiratory pressure (PEEP). A typical initial tidal volume is 8–12 mL/ kg, as long as that volume does not cause excessive airway pressures. The inspiratory time is typically set at 1 second or 33% of the respiratory cycle, whichever is shorter. Rate can be adjusted to patient comfort and blood gas measurements of ventilation, but generally patients starting on mechanical ventilation will require full support at least initially with a rate of 20–30 breaths/min.

Pressure-controlled ventilation is set up in similar fashion, though the sufficiency of the inspiratory pressure to provide an adequate tidal volume is assessed by observing the patient's chest rise and by measuring the returned tidal volume. Typically, patients without lung disease will require pressures of 15–20 cm $H_2O$, and patients with respiratory illnesses will initially require 20–30 cm $H_2O$ pressure to provide adequate ventilation.

## Positive End-Expiratory Pressure

The PEEP level is the final major setting required to initiate mechanical ventilation. All mechanical ventila-

tors open their expiratory limbs at the end of inspiration until a preset pressure is achieved; this is the PEEP value. During ventilation of normal lungs, physiologic PEEP is in the range of 2–4 cm $H_2O$ pressure. This pressure helps to prevent the end-expiratory collapse of open lung units, thus preventing atelectasis and shunting. In disease states such as pulmonary edema, pneumonia, or acute respiratory distress syndrome (ARDS), a higher PEEP may increase the patient's functional residual capacity (FRC), open previously collapsed alveoli, increase mean airway pressure, and improve oxygenation. High levels of PEEP, although often valuable in improving oxygenation, may also cause $CO_2$ retention, barotrauma with resultant air leaks, decreased central venous return and thus decreased cardiac output, and increased intracranial pressure (ICP). In general, PEEP should be set at 3–5 cm $H_2O$ initially and titrated up to maintain adequate oxygenation at an acceptable fractional inspiratory oxygen ($FiO_2$), while watching carefully for the adverse effects listed earlier.

## Monitoring the Ventilated Patient

Ventilated patients must be monitored carefully for respiratory rate and activity, chest wall movement, and quality of breath sounds. Oxygenation should be measured either by ABGs or by continuous pulse oximetry. Ventilation should be assessed by blood gas analysis or by noninvasive means, such as transcutaneous monitoring or end-tidal sampling. Transcutaneous $PO_2$ ($PtO_2$) or $PCO_2$ ($PtCO_2$) measurements are most useful with younger patients who have good skin perfusion, but they become problematic with poorly perfused or obese patients. End-tidal $CO_2$ monitoring is done by placing a gas-sampling port on the endotracheal tube and analyzing expired gas for $CO_2$. This technique appears to be more valuable for patients with large tidal volumes, lower respiratory rates, and without leaks around the endotracheal tube. In practice, end-tidal $CO_2$ values may differ significantly from measured $PaCO_2$ values and thus are most useful for following relative fluctuations in ventilation. Frequent, preferably continuous, blood pressure monitoring is also necessary for patients receiving oxygen at a high PEEP, given the risk of adverse cardiovascular effects.

## Adjusting the Ventilator

Mechanical ventilation can assist with both ventilation ($PCO_2$) and oxygenation ($PO_2$). Ventilation is most closely associated with the delivered minute-volume, or the tidal volume multiplied by the respiratory rate. Abnormal $PCO_2$ values can be most effectively addressed by changes in the respiratory rate or the tidal volume. Increased rate or tidal volume should increase minute-volume and thus decrease $pCO_2$ levels; decreases in rate or tidal volume should act in the opposite fashion. In some circumstances, additional adjustments may also be necessary. For example, for patients with disease characterized by extensive alveolar collapse, increasing PEEP may improve ventilation by rerecruiting collapsed lung units. Also, for patients with disease characterized by significant airway obstruction, decreases in respiratory rate may allow more time for exhalation and improve ventilation despite an apparent decrease in the minute-volume provided.

The variables most closely associated with oxygenation are the inspired oxygen concentration and the mean airway pressure during the respiratory cycle. Increases in inspired oxygen concentration will generally increase arterial oxygenation, unless right-to-left intracardiac or intrapulmonary shunting is a significant component of the patient's illness. Concentrations of inspired oxygen above 60–65%, however, may lead to hyperoxic lung injury. Patients with hypoxemic respiratory failure requiring those levels of oxygen or higher to maintain adequate arterial saturations should have their hypoxemia addressed by increases in mean airway pressure.

Mean airway pressure is affected by PEEP, peak inspiratory pressure, and inspiratory time. Increases in any one of those factors will increase mean airway pressure and should improve arterial oxygenation. It is important to bear in mind, however, that increases in mean airway pressure may also lead to decreases in cardiac output. In this circumstance, raising mean airway pressure may increase arterial oxygenation but actually compromise oxygen delivery to the tissues. For patients with severe hypoxemic respiratory failure, these trade-offs highlight the need for careful monitoring of these variables by experienced personnel.

## Managing the Ventilated Patient

Patients undergoing mechanical ventilation generally require the same meticulous supportive care given to all PICU patients. Since mechanical ventilation is often frightening and uncomfortable for patients, leading to dyssynchrony with the ventilator and impaired ventilation and oxygenation, they deserve careful attention directed toward optimizing comfort and decreasing anxiety. Sedative–anxiolytics are typically provided as intermittent doses of benzodiazepines, with or without opioids. Some patients respond better to the steady state of sedation provided by continuous infusion of these agents, although oversedation of the ventilated patient may lead to longer durations of ventilation and difficulties with weaning from the ventilator.

For a patient with severe respiratory illnesses, even small movements by the patient may compromise ventilation and oxygenation. In such cases, muscle paralysis may facilitate oxygenation and ventilation. Nondepolarizing neuromuscular blocking agents are most commonly used for this purpose, and they may be given as intermittent doses or as continuous infusions. When muscle relaxants are given, extra care must be taken to ensure that levels of sedation are adequate, as many of the usual signs of patient discomfort are masked by the paralytics.

## Alternative Methods of Ventilation

**High-frequency oscillatory ventilation (HFOV)** is a mode of mechanical ventilation in which the ventilator provides very small, very rapid tidal volumes. Respiratory rates used during oscillatory ventilation typically range from 5 to 10 Hz (rates of 300–600 breaths/min) in most PICU patients. This mode of ventilation has been used successfully for neonates, older pediatric patients, and adults, and for diseases as diverse as pneumonia, pulmonary contusion, ARDS, and asthma. HFOV is increasingly being used as initial therapy in severe, diffuse lung diseases, such as ARDS, which require high mean airway pressures to maintain oxygenation. The advantage of HFOV is that these high levels of mean airway pressure can be achieved without high peak inspiratory pressures or large tidal volumes, thus theoretically protecting the lung from ventilator-induced lung injury. Disadvantages of HFOV include generally poor tolerance by patients who are not heavily sedated or even paralyzed, the risk of cardiovascular compromise due to high mean airway pressures, and the risk of barotrauma in patients with heterogeneous lung disease. Although HFOV clearly may be useful for selected patients, it remains unsettled whether HFOV provides a clear benefit in outcome compared with carefully managed conventional modes of ventilation.

**Inverse ratio ventilation** is another strategy sometimes employed with patients who have severe hypoxemic respiratory failure. This approach entails increasing the inspiratory time until it exceeds the expiratory time in the respiratory cycle, thus "inverting" the I:E ratio from the usual 1:2 or 1:3 to 2:1 or even 3:1. This practice, most commonly done while using a pressure-controlled mode of ventilation, leads to significant increases in mean airway pressure and may improve oxygenation in selected patients. Disadvantages of this approach are the increased need for sedation and paralysis due to patient discomfort, hypercarbia due to less effective ventilation, and the risk of cardiovascular compromise from high mean airway pressures. While useful for selected patients as a rescue strategy, inverse-ratio ventilation has not yet been shown to provide any significant advantage over conventional modes of ventilation or HFOV in managing severe hypoxemic respiratory failure.

Arnold JH et al: High-frequency oscillatory ventilation in pediatric respiratory failure: A multicenter experience. Crit Care Med 2000;28:3913 [PMID: 11153635].

Cheifetz IM: Invasive and noninvasive pediatric mechanical ventilation. Respir Care 2003;48:442 [PMID: 12667269].

Flaatten H et al: Outcome after acute respiratory failure is more dependent on dysfunction in other vital organs than on the severity of the respiratory failure. Crit Care 2003;7:R72 [PMID: 12930559].

Frank JA, Matthay MA: Science review: Mechanisms of ventilator-induced injury. Crit Care 2003;7:233 [PMID: 12793874].

Gattinoni L et al: Physiologic rationale for ventilator setting in acute lung injury/acute respiratory distress syndrome patients. Crit Care Med 2003;31:S300 [PMID: 12682456].

Kallas HJ: Non-conventional respiratory support modalities applicable in the older child: High frequency ventilation and liquid ventilation. Crit Care Clin 1998;14:655 [PMID:9891632].

Matthews BD, Noviski N: Management of oxygenation in pediatric acute hypoxemic respiratory failure. Pediatr Pulmonol 2001;32:459 [PMID: 11747250].

Riphagen S, Bohn D: High frequency oscillatory ventilation. Intensive Care Med 1999;25(12):1459 [PMID: 10702031].

Thompson BT et al: Clinicians' approaches to mechanical ventilation in acute lung injury and ARDS. Chest 2001;120:1622 [PMID: 11713144].

# ACUTE RESPIRATORY DISTRESS SYNDROME

ARDS is a syndrome of acute respiratory failure characterized by increased pulmonary capillary permeability and pulmonary edema that results in refractory hypoxemia, decreased lung compliance, and bilateral diffuse alveolar infiltrates on chest radiography. Statistics of ARDS reflect one of the true successes of current ICU management, as mortality has decreased over the past decade from approximately 50–60% to less than 40%.

Our understanding of this illness has been hampered over the years by inconsistencies in the case definitions used by various authors. An international consensus conference was convened in 1997 to establish the current guidelines defining diagnostic criteria for ARDS. The diagnosis of ARDS rests on four features: (1) an underlying illness or injury that predisposes to ARDS; (2) bilateral infiltrates on chest radiograph; (3) an absence of evidence of heart failure and, in particular, left ventricular (LV) failure; and, most importantly, (4) severe hypoxemic respiratory failure. Hypoxemia is assessed using the ratio of the arterial oxygen level ($PaO_2$) to the inspired oxygen concentration ($FiO_2$). When the $PaO_2/FiO_2$ ratio is less than 200, and the other two criteria are met, the case is defined as ARDS. When the $PaO_2/FiO_2$ ratio is between 200 and 300, and the other two criteria are met, the case is defined as acute lung injury. This definition is debated, however, particularly since the current criteria do not include any assessment of the airway pressure needed to

oxygenate the patient. Numerous other diagnostic systems have been proposed.

In addition, because the clinical disorder or disorders that led to the development of acute lung injury clearly influence the patient's prognosis for recovery, precise definition of the underlying problem is important. Although the average mortality in this population is 40%, the rate is quite variable and dependent on the associated clinical disorder. Mortality can be as high as 90% among adult ARDS patients with underlying liver failure, and less than 10% among pediatric ARDS associated with respiratory syncytial virus infection. The development of multisystem organ failure is a frequent complicating factor in the care of the patient with ARDS, and the failure of organs outside the lung has a large role in determining the prognosis. In fact, nonpulmonary organ failures are the leading cause of death in the most recent studies of adult or pediatric ARDS patients.

## Clinical Presentation & Pathophysiology

ARDS may be precipitated by a variety of insults (Table 13–6), of which infection is the most common. Despite the diversity of causes, the clinical presentation is remarkably similar in most cases. ARDS can be divided roughly into four clinical phases (Table 13–7). In the earliest phase, the patient may have dyspnea and tachypnea with a relatively normal $PO_2$ and a hyperventilation-induced respiratory alkalosis. No significant abnormalities are noted on physical or radiologic examination of the chest. Experimental studies suggest that neutrophils accumulate in the lungs at this stage and that their products damage lung endothelium.

Over the next few hours, hypoxemia increases and respiratory distress becomes clinically apparent, with

**Table 13–6.** Acute respiratory distress syndrome risk factors.

| Direct Lung Injury | Indirect Lung Injury |
|---|---|
| Aspiration of gastric contents | Sepsis |
| Hydrocarbon ingestion or aspiration | Shock |
| Inhalation injury (heat or toxin) | Pancreatitis |
| Pulmonary contusion | Burns |
| Pneumonia | Trauma |
| Near-drowning | Fat embolism |
| | Drug overdoses (including aspirin, opioids, barbiturates, tricyclic antidepressants) |
| | Transfusion of blood products |

***Table 13–7.*** Pathophysiologic changes of modern acute respiratory distress syndrome (low-pressure pulmonary edema).

| | Symptoms | Laboratory Findings | Pathophysiology |
|---|---|---|---|
| **Phase 1 (early changes)**<br>Normal radiograph | Dyspnea, tachypnea, normal chest examination | Mild pulmonary hypertension, normoxemic or mild hypoxemia, hypercapnia. | Neutrophil sequestration, no clear tissue damage |
| **Phase 2 (onset of parenchymal changes)[a]**<br>Patchy alveolar infiltrates beginning in dependent lung<br>No perivascular cuffs (unless a component of high-pressure edema is present)<br>Normal heart size | Dyspnea, tachypnea, cyanosis, tachycardia, course rales | Pulmonary hypertension, normal wedge pressure, increased lung permeability, increased lung water, increasing shunt, progressive decrease in compliance, moderate to severe hypoxemia. | Neutrophil infiltration, vascular congestion, fibrin strands, platelet clumps, alveolar septal edema, intraalveolar protein, white cells, type I epithelial damage |
| **Phase 3 (acute respiratory failure with progression, 2–10 days)**<br>Diffuse alveolar infiltrates<br>Air bronchograms<br>Decreased lung volume<br>No bronchovascular cuffs<br>Normal heart | Tachypnea, tachycardia, hyperdynamic state, sepsis syndrome, signs of consolidation, diffuse rhonchi | Phase 2 changes persist. Progression of abnormalities, increasing shunt fraction, further decrease in compliance, increased minute ventilation, impaired oxygen extraction of hemoglobin. | Increased interstitial and alveolar inflammatory exudate with neutrophil and mononuclear cells, type II cell proliferation, beginning fibroblast proliferation, thromboembolic occlusion |
| **Phase 4 (pulmonary fibrosis, pneumonia with progression, > 10 days)[b]**<br>Persistent diffuse infiltrates<br>Superimposed new pneumonic infiltrates<br>Recurrent pneumothorax<br>Normal heart size<br>Enlargement with cor pulmonale | Symptoms as above, recurrent sepsis, evidence of multiple organ system failure | Phase 3 changes persist. Recurrent pneumonia, progressive lung restriction, impaired tissue oxygenation, impaired oxygen extraction. Multiple organ system failure. | Type II cell hyperplasia, interstitial thickening; infiltration of lymphocytes, macrophages, fibroblasts; loculated pneumonia or interstitial fibrosis; medial thickening and remodeling of arterioles |

[a]The process is readily reversible at this stage if the initiating factor is controlled.
[b]Multiple organ system failure is common. The mortality rate is greater than 80% at this stage, since resolution is more difficult.
Modified slightly and reproduced, with permission, from Demling RH: Adult respiratory distress syndrome: Current concepts. New Horizons 1993;1:388.

cyanosis, tachycardia, irritability, and dyspnea. Radiographic evidence of early parenchymal change is noted by "fluffy" alveolar infiltrates initially appearing in dependent lung fields, indicative of pulmonary edema. The edema fluid typically has a high concentration of protein (75–95% of plasma protein concentration), which is characteristic of an increased permeability-type edema and differentiates it from cardiogenic or hydrostatic pulmonary edema. Protein in the airspaces acts to inactivate surfactant, which, combined with damage to type 2 alveolar pneumocytes, leads to a marked deficiency in surfactant content in the lung. As a result, the lung is particularly prone to collapse and to shearing injuries due to the high surface tension required to open collapsed alveoli.

Alveolar epithelial injury in ARDS lowers the threshold for alveolar edema formation and impairs gas exchange. The functional integrity of the alveolar epithelium, as measured by the ability of the alveoli to clear liquid out of the airspaces, has prognostic importance in ARDS. Those patients who still show evidence of functional alveolar liquid clearance mechanisms during the first day of their illness have a much higher survival rate than those with evidence of severe epithelial impairment.

Pulmonary hypertension, decreases in lung compliance, and increases in airway resistance are also commonly noted. Clinical studies suggest that airway resistance may be increased in 50% of patients with ARDS.

Computed tomography (CT) studies of adult patients in the acute phases of ARDS have established that this illness is characterized by heterogeneous collapse of the lung, with typical areas of dependent consolidation, overinflation in the upper zones, and relatively small areas of normally expanded lung. These findings have led to the opinion that the lung in ARDS is best viewed as "small" rather than stiff, prompting a shift toward ventilating these patients with smaller tidal volumes and tolerating the relative hypercarbia that may ensue. In addition, a large body of research in recent years has shown that ventilation with large tidal volumes and low PEEP levels allows a pattern of cyclic alveolar overdistention and collapse, which causes a lung injury histologically similar to ARDS even in normal lungs. This phenomenon is now called ventilator-induced lung injury. Taken together, these findings have given rise to the view that acute ARDS can best be treated by rerecruiting those areas of dependent collapse and minimizing the stretch-induced injury, or volutrauma, in the nondependent areas of the lung. This approach has been termed the open-lung strategy and has been the subject of intense scrutiny in recent years (see below).

The subacute phase of ARDS (5–10 days after lung injury) is characterized by type II cell and fibroblast proliferation in the interstitium of the lung. This results in decreased lung volumes and signs of consolidation that are noted clinically and radiographically. Worsening of the hypoxemia with an increasing shunt fraction, as well as a further decrease in lung compliance, are noted. Some patients develop an accelerated fibrosing alveolitis in which fibroblasts and collagen formation in the interstitium are markedly increased. The mechanisms responsible for these changes are unclear. Current investigation centers on the role of growth and differentiation factors, such as transforming growth factor-β and platelet-derived growth factor released by resident and nonresident lung cells such as alveolar macrophages, mast cells, neutrophils, alveolar type II cells, and fibroblasts.

During the chronic phase of ARDS (10–14 days after lung injury), fibrosis, emphysema, and pulmonary vascular obliteration occur. During this phase of the illness, oxygenation defects generally improve, and the lung becomes more fragile and susceptible to barotrauma. Air leak is common among patients still ventilated with high levels of airway pressure at this late stage in their illness. Also, patients have increased amounts of dead space, and difficulties with ventilation are common. Airway compliance remains low, perhaps because of ongoing pulmonary fibrosis and insufficient surfactant production.

Secondary infections are common in the subacute and chronic phases of ARDS and significantly influence the outcome. The mechanisms responsible for increased host susceptibility to infection during this phase are not well understood.

Mortality in the late phase of ARDS exceeds 80%. Death is usually caused by multiple organ failure and systemic hemodynamic instability rather than by hypoxemia.

## Treatment

### A. MONITORING

Multiorgan system monitoring is mandatory for patients with ARDS. ABG analysis is required for accurate assessment of oxygenation and ventilation and for the rational titration of ventilator strategies that may have profound adverse effects. Hemodynamic monitoring should include, at a minimum, central venous pressure (CVP) measurements to help determine the level of cardiac preload, and an indwelling arterial catheter for continuous blood pressure measurements and ABG sampling. For patients with severe disease or concurrent cardiac dysfunction, consideration can be given to pulmonary artery catheterization to help with fluid management and to allow assessment of mixed venous blood saturation as an index of overall tissue oxygenation. Obtaining chest films daily is important for patients receiving vigorous support because severe ARDS is associated with a 40–60% incidence of air leaks. Secondary infections are common and increase mortality rates strikingly. Thus surveillance for infection is important, requiring appropriate cultures and following the temperature curve and white blood cell count. Renal, liver, and gastrointestinal (GI) function should be watched closely because of the great likelihood of multiple organ dysfunction.

### B. FLUID MANAGEMENT

Given the increases in pulmonary capillary permeability in ARDS, pulmonary edema accumulation is likely with any elevation in pulmonary hydrostatic pressures. In this setting, most clinicians reduce intravascular volume to the lowest level that is still compatible with an adequate cardiac output and adequate oxygen delivery to the tissues.

### C. HEMODYNAMIC SUPPORT

Hemodynamic support is directed toward increasing perfusion and oxygen delivery. In those circumstances when volume expansion is necessary to improve oxygen delivery, this can best be achieved by giving packed red blood cells to maintain the hematocrit between 35% and 40%, and by giving colloid or crystalloid solutions to nonanemic volume-depleted patients. Inotropes should be used as needed to optimize oxygen delivery to the tissues.

### D. VENTILATORY SUPPORT

Basic principles of ventilator management were described earlier (see Adjusting the Ventilator section). In addition to those principles, current ventilatory management of ARDS is directed at the rerecruitment of areas of dependent alveolar collapse and the protection of noncollapsed areas from overdistension. Since an FiO$_2$ greater than 60% over 24 hours can cause additional injury to the lung, mean airway pressure should be increased to provide an adequate PaO$_2$ (> 55 mm Hg) at an FiO$_2$ of 60% or less. In general, this can be accomplished by incremental increases in PEEP every 15–30 minutes until adequate oxygenation is achieved or until a limiting side effect of the PEEP is reached. Ventilation with high levels of PEEP acts by helping to prevent dependent collapse of edematous lung units. PEEP levels of 12–14 cm H$_2$O are not unusual, and levels as high as 20–25 cm H$_2$O have been used successfully in these patients. Before increasing PEEP significantly, the physician should optimize conditions by making sure that the patient's intravascular volume is appropriate, the endotracheal tube does not leak, and the patient is heavily sedated and paralyzed.

The actual mode of ventilation employed (volume or pressure) with an ARDS patient is probably unimportant. However, recent work from a large multicenter trial sponsored by the National Institutes of Health suggests that the tidal volumes used may be important. Using a PEEP strategy similar to that described in the preceding paragraph, the investigators compared the effects of a low (6 mL/kg) tidal volume versus a normal (12 mL/kg) tidal volume in 861 adult ARDS patients. Those patients ventilated with the lower tidal volume demonstrated fewer extrapulmonary organ failures and an overall 25% decrease in mortality. In keeping with these findings and with experimental data demonstrating ventilator-induced lung injury at alveolar pressures greater than 30 cm H$_2$O, we suggest that current practice for pediatric ARDS patients should consist of ventilation with tidal volumes in the 6–8 mL/kg range, or at least with tidal volumes small enough to keep alveolar pressures below 30–35 cm H$_2$O.

### E. OTHER THERAPIES

As previously described, HFOV is an increasingly popular technique that has been used successfully in pediatric patients with ARDS. When used as part of a strategy of aggressive increases in mean airway pressure to rerecruit deflated areas of the lung and to prevent cyclic overdistention and collapse, HFOV is a physiologically rational approach to this illness. It has not yet been determined whether HFOV provides additional benefits compared with open-lung strategy ventilation with conventional ventilator modes.

**Prone positioning** is a technique of changing the patient's position in bed from supine to prone, with the goal of allowing postural drainage and improving ventilation of collapsed dependent lung units. This technique often dramatically improves oxygenation, partic-

ularly for patients early in the course of ARDS. The oxygenation improvements are often not sustained, however, necessitating repeat position changes to maintain the effect. Whether prone positioning contributes to improved outcomes for patients with ARDS remains uncertain.

Based on the ability of inhaled **nitric oxide** (iNO) to reduce pulmonary artery pressure and to improve the matching of ventilation with perfusion without producing systemic vasodilation, iNO has been proposed as a beneficial therapy for ARDS. Several recent multicenter trials of iNO in the treatment of ARDS, both in adults and in children, have shown acute improvements in oxygenation in subsets of patients but no significant improvement in overall survival. As a result, the current role of iNO in the treatment of ARDS remains unclear. Additional studies are now focusing on the anti-inflammatory role (by reducing neutrophil adhesion and activation) iNO may play in ARDS. Studies to evaluate the combined effects of several of these alternative therapies are also being planned.

**Surfactant replacement** therapy has been tried with some success in patients with ARDS. Surfactant replacement, in some instances, improves lung compliance and oxygenation, and hastens weaning from mechanical ventilation. In randomized trials of surfactant replacement, there were no differences in outcome (death, length of ventilation, or hospitalization), but there was some evidence of decreased inflammation. A multicenter trial of surfactant treatment for pediatric ARDS is currently in progress.

Although **corticosteroids** have not been found to be beneficial in early stage ARDS, these agents may reduce the inflammation and fibrosis associated with later stage ARDS. Indeed, the use of methylprednisolone in adults whose lung injury was not improving after 7 days of ARDS was associated with in improvement of lung injury and multiple organ dysfunction. Mortality was also reduced, when compared with control subjects receiving placebo. A large multicenter trial is under way to further evaluate the use of steroids in the late phase of ARDS.

**Extracorporeal membrane oxygenation** (ECMO) has been used in pediatric patients with severe ARDS. In older studies, patients who received ECMO had better survival rates than did control subjects. ECMO has not been studied in comparison with current conventional ventilation strategies. In addition, recent improvements in outcome for pediatric ARDS patients receiving conventional therapies have made the role of ECMO less clear and have made further prospective randomized studies of ECMO difficult to complete. For now, ECMO remains a rescue therapy for patients with severe ARDS unresponsive to other modalities.

### F. FOLLOW-UP

Information regarding the long-term outcome of pediatric patients with ARDS remains limited. One report of 10 children followed 1–4 years after severe ARDS showed 3 still symptomatic and 7 with hypoxemia at rest. Until further information is available, all patients with a history of ARDS need close follow-up of pulmonary function.

Acute Respiratory Distress Syndrome Network: Ventilation with lower tidal volumes as compared with traditional tidal volumes for acute lung injury and the acute respiratory distress syndrome. N Engl J Med 2000;342:1301 [PMID: 10793162].

Anderson MR: Update on pediatric acute respiratory distress syndrome. Respir Care 2003;48:261 [PMID: 1266727].

Curley MA et al: The effects of early and repeated prone positioning in pediatric patients with acute lung injury. Chest 2000;118:156 [PMID: 10893373].

ECMO utilization. Pediatrics 2000;106:1339 [PMID: 11099586].

Hintz SR et al: Decreased use of neonatal extracorporeal membrane oxigenation (ECMO): How new treatment modalities have affected ECMO utilization. Pediatrics 2000 Dec; 106(6): 1339 [PMID: 11099586]

Krishnan JA, Brower RG: High-frequency ventilation for acute lung injury and ARDS. Chest 2000:118:795 [PMID: 10988205].

Lewandowski K: Extracorporeal membrane oxygenation for severe acute respiratory failure. Crit Care 2000;4(3):156 [PMID: 11094500].

McIntyre RC Jr et al: Thirty years of clinical trials in acute respiratory distress syndrome. Crit Care Med 2000;28:3314 [PMID: 11008997].

Meduri GU et al: Effect of prolonged methylprednisolone therapy in unresolving acute respiratory distress syndrome: A randomized controlled trial. JAMA 1998;280:159 [PMID: 9669790]. (Classic)

Redding GJ: Current concepts in adult respiratory distress syndrome in children. Curr Opin Pediatr 2001;13(3):261 [PMID: 11389362].

Sachdeva RC, Guntupalli KK: Acute respiratory distress syndrome. Crit Care Clin 1997;13:503 [PMID: 9246528].

Shorr AF et al: D-Dimer correlates with proinflammatory cytokine levels and outcomes in critically ill patients. Chest 2002;121: 1262 [PMID: 11948062].

Sokol J et al: Inhaled nitric oxide for acute hypoxemic respiratory failure in children and adults. Cochrane Database Syst Rev 2000;4:CD002787 [PMID: 11914763].

Vincent JL: New management strategies in ARDS: Immunomodulation. Crit Care Clin 2002;18:69 [PMID: 11910733].

Ware LB, Matthay MA: The acute respiratory distress syndrome. N Engl J Med 2000;342:1334 [PMID: 10793167].

## ASTHMA (LIFE-THREATENING)

Status asthmaticus may be defined as reversible small airway obstruction that is refractory to sympathomimetic and anti-inflammatory agents and that may progress to respiratory failure without prompt and aggressive intervention. Life-threatening asthma is caused by severe bronchospasm, excessive mucous secretion, inflammation, and edema of the airways (see Chapter 17). Reversal of these mechanisms is the key to successful treatment. Status asthmaticus remains a common diagnosis among children admitted to the PICU, and asthma continues to be associated with surprisingly high mortality rates.

The physical examination helps determine the severity of illness. Accessory muscle (sternocleidomastoid) use correlates well with a forced expiratory volume ($FEV_1$) and peak expiratory flow rates (PEFRs) less than 50% of normal predicted values. A pulsus paradoxus of over 22 mm Hg has been correlated with elevated $PaCO_2$ levels. The absence of wheezing may be misleading because, in order to produce a wheezing sound, the patient must take in a certain amount of air. The ABG analysis remains the single most important laboratory determination in the evaluation of a child in severe status asthmaticus. Patients with severe respiratory distress, signs of exhaustion, alterations in consciousness, elevated $PaCO_2$, or acidosis should be admitted to the PICU.

### Treatment

Much of the morbidity associated with the treatment of severe asthma is related to the complications of mechanical ventilation that occur in patients with severe airflow obstruction. As a result, the goal of initial treatment of the patient with life-threatening status asthmaticus is to improve the patient's ability to ventilate without resorting to intubation and mechanical ventilation. The medical therapies described in the following discussion should be undertaken swiftly and aggressively with the goal of reversing the bronchospasm before respiratory failure necessitates invasive ventilation.

Due to inadequate minute-ventilation and V/Q mismatching, patients with severe asthma are almost always hypoxemic and should receive supplemental **humidified oxygen** immediately.

**Inhaled $\beta_2$-agonist** therapy with agents such as albuterol remains first-line therapy to reverse acute bronchoconstriction. If the patient is in severe distress and has poor inspiratory flow rates, thus preventing adequate delivery of nebulized medication, subcutaneous injection of epinephrine or terbutaline may be considered. The frequency of $\beta_2$-agonist administration varies according to the severity of the patient's symptoms and the occurrence of adverse side effects. Nebulized albuterol may be given intermittently at a dose of 0.1 mg/kg per nebulization up to 2.5 mg, or it can be administered continuously at a dose of 0.5 mg/kg/h to a maximum of 20 mg/h, usually without serious side effects. The heart rate and blood pressure of these patients should be monitored closely, because excessive tachycardia and ventricular ectopy may occur.

Systemic **corticosteroids** act by decreasing inflammation, stabilizing mast cells, and increasing $\beta_2$-receptor expression. These agents speed the resolution of severe asthma exacerbations refractory to bronchodilator therapy and should be given to all patients admitted to the hospital with severe asthma. The optimal dose is unknown, although a frequently used dosage is 1 mg/kg of IV methylprednisolone every 6 hours. The acute complications of corticosteroid usage include GI bleeding, hyperglycemia, and hypertension.

Inhaled **anticholinergic agents** may also be helpful in patients with severe asthma. In some patients, cholinergic-related bronchoconstriction is more marked than in others, so not all patients respond. Nebulized ipratropium bromide is the drug of choice, and is given at a dose of 250–500 μg/dose.

**Intravenous β-agonists** should be considered in patients with severe bronchospasm unresponsive to inhaled bronchodilators. The agent most commonly used in the United States is terbutaline, a relatively specific $\beta_2$-agonist, which can be given as a bolus dose or as a continuous infusion. Owing to its relative specificity for $\beta_2$-receptors, terbutaline has fewer cardiac side effects than previously available IV β-agonists like isoproterenol. Terbutaline is given as a bolus or loading dose of 10 μg/kg followed by a continuous infusion of 0.5–5 μg/kg/min. In general, patients receiving IV $\beta_2$-agonist therapy should have indwelling arterial lines for continuous blood pressure and blood gas monitoring.

**Theophylline** remains a controversial agent in the management of severe asthma. Although some studies suggest this drug may confer some additional benefit when given with steroids and $\beta_2$-agonists, other studies of children hospitalized with moderate to severe asthma have not shown a clear benefit in adding theophylline to other therapy. Besides causing bronchodilation, this agent decreases mucociliary inflammatory mediators and reduces microvascular permeability. When the decision to add theophylline to high-dose $\beta_2$-agonist therapy for severe status asthmaticus is being weighed, the increased risk of serious side effects such as tachycardia and cardiac arrhythmias must be considered. Theophylline is given IV as aminophylline. Each 1 mg/kg of aminophylline given as a loading dose will increase the serum level by approximately 2 mg/dL. For a patient who has not previously received aminophylline or oral (PO) theophylline preparations, load with 7–8 mg/kg of aminophylline in an attempt to achieve a level of 10–15 mg/dL; then start a continuous infusion of aminophylline at a dosage of 0.8–1 mg/kg/h. Watch closely for toxicity (gastric upset, tachycardia, seizures) and follow serum levels closely, trying to maintain steady-state levels of 12–16 mg/dL.

**Magnesium sulfate** has been reported to be an effective bronchodilator in patients with severe status asthmaticus and may be considered for patients in danger of worsening respiratory failure. The mechanism of action of magnesium is unclear, but its smooth muscle relaxation properties are probably caused by interference with calcium flux in the bronchial smooth muscle cell. Magnesium sulfate is given IV at a dose of 25–50 mg/kg/dose. Though it is usually well tolerated, hypotension and flushing are side effects.

If the previously described aggressive management fails to result in significant improvement, **mechanical ventilation** may be necessary. In general, if there is steady deterioration (increased acidosis, rising PaCO$_2$) despite intensive therapy for asthma, the patient should be intubated and ventilated mechanically. Mechanical ventilation for patients with asthma is difficult because the severe airflow obstruction often leads to very high airway pressures, air trapping, and resultant barotrauma. The goal of mechanical ventilation with an intubated asthmatic patient is to maintain adequate oxygenation and ventilation with the least amount of barotrauma until other therapies become effective. Worsening hypercarbia after intubation should be anticipated and aggressive efforts to normalize blood gases should be moderated, as such efforts may only lead to complications. Due to the severe air flow obstruction, these patients will require long inspiratory times to deliver a breath and long expiratory times to avoid air trapping. In general, the ventilator rate should be decreased until the expiratory time is long enough to allow emptying prior to the next machine breath. Ventilator rates of 8–12 breaths/min are typical initially. Either volume- or pressure-targeted modes of ventilation can be used effectively in these patients. PEEP should be kept low (0–2 cm H$_2$O). Isolated reports have noted patients who respond to greater PEEP, but these cases are the exception. These ventilator strategies and the resulting hypercarbia typically are uncomfortable, requiring that patients be heavily sedated. Barbiturates should be avoided if possible. If fentanyl and midazolam (Versed) are inadequate, or if ventilating the patient is difficult, bolus or continuous infusion of ketamine should be considered because it has been shown to be beneficial in certain circumstances. Most patients, at least initially, will also require neuromuscular blockade to optimize ventilation and minimize airway pressures.

## Monitoring

Severely asthmatic patients should be monitored for heart rate, blood pressure, O$_2$ saturation, and arterial pH and PaCO$_2$. Continuous blood pressure monitoring is necessary because air-trapping can lead to increased levels of occult PEEP ("auto-PEEP"), an effect that can impair venous return and decrease cardiac output. Close ventilator monitoring is necessary because increases in inspiratory pressure or decreases in pulmonary compliance may signal worsening bronchoconstriction, mucus plugging, or an extrapleural air leak. Chest films of ventilated asthmatic patients should be obtained daily and immediately with sudden changes in patient condition, due to the risk of pneumothorax and pneumomediastinum. In addition, if the patient is receiving neuromuscular blocking agents, the degree of nerve block should be monitored closely because nondepolarizing agents such as pancuronium, when given with corticosteroids, can cause prolonged paralysis and muscle weakness.

Bohn D: Lung salvage and protection ventilatory techniques. Pediatr Clin North Am 2001;48(3):553 [PMID: 11411293].

DiNicola LK et al: Drug therapy approaches in the treatment of acute severe asthma in hospitalized children. Paediatr Drugs 2001;3:509 [PMID: 11513282].

Kercsmar CM: Acute inpatient care of status asthmaticus. Respir Care Clin North Am 2000;6(1):155 [PMID: 10639561].

Kreutzer ML, Louie S: Pharmacologic treatment of the adult hospitalized asthma patient. Clin Rev Allergy Immunol 2001;20: 357 [PMID: 11413904].

Sabato K, Hanson JH: Mechanical ventilation for children with status asthmaticus. Respir Care Clin North Am 2000;6(1): 171 [PMID: 10639562].

Werner HA: Status asthmaticus in children: A review. Chest 2001;119(6):1913 [PMID11399724 ].

# SHOCK

Shock may be defined as failure of the cardiovascular system to deliver critical substrates and to remove toxic metabolites. This failure leads to anaerobic metabolism in cells and ultimately to irreversible cellular damage. Shock has been categorized into a series of recognizable stages: compensated, uncompensated, and irreversible. Patients in compensated shock have relatively normal cardiac output and normal blood pressures, but they have alterations in the microcirculation that increase flow to some organs and reduce flow to others. In infants, compensatory increases in cardiac output are achieved primarily by tachycardia rather than by increases in stroke volume. Heart rates of 190–210/min are common in infants with compensated shock, but heart rates over 220/min raise the possibility of supraventricular tachycardia. In older patients, cardiac contractility (stroke volume) and heart rate increase to improve cardiac output. Blood pressure remains normal initially because of peripheral vasoconstriction and increased systemic vascular resistance. Thus hypotension occurs late and is more characteristic of the uncompensated stage of shock. In the uncompensated stage, the oxygen and nutrient supply to the cells deteriorates fur-

ther with subsequent cellular breakdown and release of toxic substances, causing further redistribution of flow. At this point, the patient is hypotensive, with poor cardiac output.

Shock can be classified by mechanism into hypovolemic (including distributive), cardiogenic, and septic. Often, two or three of these occur together.

## A. Hypovolemic Shock

Hypovolemic shock is caused by decreased circulating blood volume or preload. This may result from loss of whole blood or plasma or from fluid loss from the kidney or gut. These patients usually have intact compensatory mechanisms that maintain normal blood pressure by increasing cardiac output and shunting blood away from certain organs. These responses protect blood flow to the heart and brain. Untreated, hypovolemic shock can progress to an irreversible stage. Additionally, a relative hypovolemia occurs when arterial and capillary shunting past tissue beds occurs with an increase in venous capacitance, causing blood to pool—so-called distributive shock. This results from anaphylaxis or vasodilating drugs.

## B. Cardiogenic Shock/Failure

Age-dependent differences occur in myocardial physiology that are relevant to therapy. Neonatal myocardium has reduced systolic performance and contractility. The sarcolemma, sarcoplasmic reticulum, and T-tubules are less well developed, resulting in a greater dependency on transsarcolemma $Ca^{2+}$ flux (ie, serum $Ca^{2+}$) for contraction. A high resting state of myocardial contractility occurs that limits the response to inotropic agents. Relatively minor increases in afterload can result in diminished stroke volume. Diastolic compliance is diminished, and small changes in volume result in large changes in ventricular wall tension. Consequently preload reserve is limited, and maximization of the Frank–Starling curve occurs relatively quickly (10–15 mm Hg in animal models). Aggressive volume resuscitation beyond this is often ineffective and not tolerated. Stroke volume is relatively fixed, and greater increases in cardiac output are seen through increased heart rate.

Central to the understanding of cardiogenic failure are the progressive nature of ventricular dysfunction and the compensatory mechanisms that occur in the presence of excessive hemodynamic demands. Inadequate cardiac output activates the renin–angiotensin system. The consequent sodium and water retention augments intravascular volume and increases cardiac output through increased preload. With progression, cardiac compliance is decreased and preload augmentation via the Frank–Starling mechanism is maximized. Subsequently, small changes in ventricular volume can lead to large increases in ventricular pressure and, therefore, pulmonary venous pressure with resultant pulmonary edema. Thus, fluids should be cautiously administered in this setting and should possibly be guided by left atrial or pulmonary artery capillary wedge pressure monitoring. The atrial distention that occurs in the failing heart leads to increased production and release of atrial natriuretic peptide (ANP). Though the function of this molecule is not completely understood, ANP is a vasodilator and augments sodium and water excretion.

Heart failure also induces autonomic nervous system changes, including increased activation of the adrenergic sympathetic system and decreased parasympathetic stimulation. Increased adrenergic tone is associated with elevated circulating norepinephrine levels, increased vasoconstriction, and afterload. These combined factors in turn lead to a cycle of increased afterload, increased energy expenditure, decreased cardiac output, myocyte death, and progressive ventricular dysfunction. The cardiomyocyte effects of prolonged adrenergic stimulation include decreased β-receptors, decreased norepinephrine stores, and, therefore, potentially decreased responses to sympathetic stimulation. Increased cellular concentrations of cyclic adenosine monophosphate and inositol triphosphate lead to increased inward $Ca^{2+}$ flux and at least transient increases in contractility. Subsequently, excessive unremoved calcium impairs luciotropy and augments the propensity for arrhythmias. Blood flow is redistributed away from the splanchnic system, skin, and muscles toward the heart, brain, adrenal glands, and diaphragm. Endothelial dysfunction is common and contributes to the abnormal vascular tone. Endothelin-1 production is elevated in the lung and increases pulmonary vascular resistance (PVR) and systemic vascular resistance (SVR). The release of endothelial-derived nitric oxide is also impaired. Circulating arginine vasopressin and tumor necrosis factor alpha (TNF-α) levels have also been reported to be elevated. In the later stages of heart failure, cardiomyocyte hypertrophy, fibroblast hyperplasia, and increases in altered production and accumulation occur in extracellular matrix, leading to impaired myocardial function.

Signs and symptoms of cardiac failure are produced by the body's attempts to compensate for the decreased pump function. The body compensates by activating the sympathetic nervous and renin–angiotensin–aldosterone systems. The child in acute heart failure will present with hypotension and such evidence of poor perfusion as metabolic acidosis and organ dysfunction. In response to the poor output, tachycardia and vasoconstriction will be evident with cool and mottled extremities. Although the extremities are cool, the child's core temperature will be elevated. To improve cardiac output, the body will retain fluid and sodium, resulting in generalized edema. Pulmonary edema will cause tachypnea, and the rales can be heard on auscultation. The pulmonary edema may be severe enough to compromise respiration and lead to hypoxemia and respiratory failure.

The work-up can be performed at the same time treatment is initiated, and it should include an echocardiogram to evaluate cardiac anatomy and function. Serial echocardiograms may also be helpful to specifically assess the improvement in function with treatment. A chest radiograph can reveal the amount of cardiomegaly, pulmonary edema, and the presence of any effusions. Laboratory tests should include electrolyte measurements and renal and liver function tests.

Management of cardiogenic failure in the pediatric patient is complicated by the varied underlying causes that often require disparate therapies. The factors that influence cardiac output are preload, afterload, contractility, and heart rate and rhythm. An analysis of a low cardiac output state should consider the specific cardiac lesion and should use these factors as a framework for therapy.

Cardiogenic failure results from an imbalance of systemic oxygen delivery and demand. Therapy is aimed at restoring oxygen delivery and reducing demand. Sedation, reduced environmental stress, temperature regulation, supplemental $O_2$, red cell transfusion, and augmentation of cardiac output all have roles. The overall goal of increasing cardiac output should include restoring an appropriate sinus rate and rhythm, optimizing preload, augmenting myocardial contractility with minimal increases in myocardial $O_2$ consumption, and maximizing afterload reduction. If bradycardia is excessive, temporary pacing with transthoracic, transesophageal, or intracardiac methods should be considered. Excessive tachycardia is to be avoided, as it shortens ventricular diastole, leading to a reduction in diastolic filling, shortened diastolic coronary perfusion, and increased myocardial $O_2$ consumption.

Cardiogenic failure is associated with elevated ventricular filling pressures (> 20 mm Hg). Thus, although increasing preload can result in augmented cardiac output (to a degree), volume should be administered cautiously—the Frank–Starling curve may remain flat with little further improvement possible, occurring at the expense of elevating pulmonary venous pressure with resultant pulmonary edema. Diuretics can be administered to reduce pulmonary edema and to improve pulmonary compliance, the work of breathing, and oxygenation. Contractility can be augmented through inotropic stimulation of myocardial $β_1$-receptors (Table 13–8). Dopamine is an α- and β-agonist, which, at lower doses (3–5 μg/kg/min), improves blood flow to the renal, coronary, and splanchnic beds (type D1 receptor). At higher doses the α-receptor effects predominate, with vasoconstriction increasing SVR and PVR.

**Table 13–8.** Pharmacologic support of the shock patient.

| Drug | Dose | Alpha-Adrenergic Effect[a] | Beta-Adrenergic Effect[a] | Vasodilator Effect | Actions and Advantages | Disadvantages |
|---|---|---|---|---|---|---|
| Dopamine | 1–20 µg/kg/min | + to +++ (dose-related) | + to +++ (dose-related) | At low doses, renal vasodilation occurs (dopaminergic receptors) | Moderate inotrope, wide and safe dosage range, short half-life. | May cause worsening of pulmonary vasoconstriction |
| Dobutamine | 1–10 µg/kg/min | 0 | +++ | | Moderate inotrope, less chronotropic, fewer dysrhythmias than with isoproterenol or epinephrine. | Marked variation among patients |
| Epinephrine | 0.05–1 µg/kg/min | ++ to +++ (dose-related) | +++ | | Significant increases in inotropy, chronotropy, and systemic vascular resistance. | Tachycardia, dysrhythmias, renal ischemia, systemic and pulmonary vascular resistance |
| Isoproterenol | 0.05–1 µg/kg/min | 0 | +++ | Peripheral vasodilation | Significant increase in inotropy and chronotropy. Systemic vascular resistance can drop, and pulmonary vascular resistance should not increase and may decrease. | Significant myocardial oxygen consumption increases, tachycardia, dysrhythmias |
| Norepinephrine | 0.05–1 µg/kg/min | +++ | +++ | | Powerful vasoconstrictor (systemic and pulmonary); rarely used except possibly in patients with very low systemic vascular resistance or in conjunction with vasodilator. | Reduced cardiac output if afterload is too high, renal ischemia |
| Nitroprusside | 0.05–8 µg/kg/min | 0 | 0 | Arterial and venous dilation (smooth muscle relaxation) | Decreases systemic and pulmonary vascular resistance, very short-acting. Blood pressure returns to previous levels within 1–10 minutes after infusion is stopped. | Toxicities (thiocyanates and cyanide), increased intracranial pressure and ventilation/perfusion mismatch, methemoglobinemia, increased intracranial pressure |
| Milrinone | 0.25–0.75 µg/kg/min | 0 | 0 | Blank | Phosphodiesterase III inhibition. Decreases SVR and PVR, increases myocardial contractility with only mild increase in myocardial $O_2$ consumption. Usually used with low-dose dopamine or dobutamine. | |

[a]0 = no effect, + = small effect, ++ = moderate effect, +++ = potent effect.
SVR = systemic vascular resistance; PVR = pulmonary vascular resistance.

Dobutamine is predominately a β-agonist that additionally effects a dose-dependant vasodilatation (β$_2$-receptor) and has been shown to shift the ventricular pressure–volume loop toward normal, reducing LV filling pressure and hence pulmonary venous pressure. As first-line pharmacotherapy single agents or in combination, low-dose dopamine and dobutamine are often beneficial by improving contractility without increasing afterload and by limiting chronotropic effect. Isoproterenol is a pure β-agonist that causes significant tachycardia (limiting its utility), increased myocardial O$_2$ consumption, and systemic and pulmonary arterial vasodilatation. It is useful in instances of associated bradycardia, such as occur in heart transplantation and heart block. Epinephrine is an α- and β-agonist that causes the greatest increase in myocardial O$_2$ consumption of all inotropes. At a low dose (< 0.05 μg/kg/min) it increases heart rate and contractility and decreases SVR (β$_2$-receptor). At higher doses the α-effects predominate, increasing afterload. Despite these drawbacks, epinephrine can be useful as a second agent in refractory cases. It should be administered in combination with a vasodilator to offset the α-effects. Milrinone (0.25–0.75 μg/kg/min) is a newer agent in the class of phosphodiesterase inhibitors. It causes a number of beneficial effects, including a limited increase in myocardial O$_2$ consumption, decreased SVR and PVR, increased contractility, and improved luciotropy. Theoretically it is the ideal agent and is frequently used as the first-line drug, often in combination with low-dose dopamine or dobutamine.

Afterload reduction is an important additional therapy that increases stroke volume and decreases myocardial O$_2$ consumption. Agents commonly used are nitroprusside, hydralazine, and the angiotensin-converting enzyme (ACE) inhibitors. Nitroprusside is a rapid-acting IV agent, which is readily titratable and causes venodilation and arteriolar dilation, resulting in decreased SVR and PVR. Venodilation can decrease preload, and volume may therefore need to be coadministered to restore an appropriate preload. Nitroprusside is a useful titratable IV agent to start while planning a transition to a PO agent. Hydralazine is a direct systemic arteriolar dilator of coronary, renal, and splanchnic vessels, which can be given IV or PO. It is less titratable intravenously than nitroprusside, and ACE inhibitors have largely replaced it as a PO agent. ACE inhibitors are now the agents of choice for oral afterload reduction and have been shown to improve survival and functional status in adults. Patients should be switched to ACE inhibitors as soon as indicated. LV afterload is a function of systolic transmural pressure (aortic pressure/intrapleural pressure), and mechanical afterload reduction can be attained by delivering positive airway pressure through mechanical ventilation or through continuous positive airway pressure/bilevel positive airway pressure (CPAP/BIPAP). This must be taken into account when weaning a patient with significant LV dysfunction from mechanical ventilation. If cardiac output cannot be augmented sufficiently despite aggressive medical therapy, consideration should be given to mechanical circulatory support as a bridge to cardiac transplantation. Such support is provided by ECMO, ventricular access device, or intraaortic balloon pump counterpulsation.

Congenital heart defects pose special concerns. **Aortic stenosis,** for instance, obstructs flow across the LV outflow tract, elevates intraventricular pressure, and increases systolic workload and LV hypertrophy. Due to the outflow tract gradient and hypertrophy, diastolic flow in the coronaries is decreased, which can result in subendocardial ischemia. Dopamine is indicated for inotropic support. Afterload reduction is relatively contraindicated, as it may further compromise coronary flow.

**Hypertrophic cardiomyopathy** is associated with a hypertrophied nondilated left ventricle, often with dynamic left or biventricular outflow tract obstruction. Coronary abnormalities with luminal compromise are frequent. Systolic function is elevated, ejection fraction is increased, and diastolic dysfunction is evident. Inotropes are contraindicated due to increased dynamic gradient, coronary compromise, and subendocardial ischemia. Preload should be maximized, and pharmacotherapy with β-blockers and calcium channel antagonists is warranted.

**Aortic insufficiency** is associated with retrograde flow into the left ventricle during diastole. The amount of regurgitation depends in part on the pressure gradient across the aortic valve and on the heart rate. With increasing heart rates, diastole is shortened and regurgitation limited. Therapy should include inotropic support to improve overall cardiac output and aggressive afterload reduction to reduce the regurgitant fraction. Heart rate can be increased with isoproterenol or transesophageal pacing.

In **mitral regurgitation,** blood is forced back into the low-pressure left atrium during systole. The regurgitant fraction depends partly on the relative resistance to flow across the mitral and aortic valves during systole. Therapy should include inotropic support to improve total cardiac output, and aggressive afterload reduction to improve antegrade aortic flow.

**Anomalous left coronary artery** typically arises from the pulmonary artery. Patients with this disorder exhibit myocardial dysfunction secondary to myocardial ischemia. Pathophysiology includes blood flow from the right coronary artery to the left coronary artery and into the pulmonary artery, resulting in a "steal" phenomenon in the left coronary distribution. Medical therapy is futile, and urgent surgical correction is indicated. Prior to surgery, limited medical therapy can include inotropic support, although care must be exercised not to reduce pulmonary arterial pressure (and increase steal) or excessively increase myocardial $O_2$ consumption. Dopamine and milrinone have been used with limited success.

Cardiopulmonary bypass (high/low flow) and deep hypothermic circulatory arrest are frequently required to facilitate surgical correction of congenital defects. These techniques are associated with widespread organ system effects, including increased total body water, transient myocardial dysfunction, gas exchange abnormalities, coagulation abnormalities, and hormonal and stress responses. Impairment in myocardial contractility is predictable 6–12 hours following surgery. The myocardium can be supported with increased preload, inotropes, and afterload reduction. Dopamine and milrinone are often used in combination.

## C. Septic Shock

Septic shock has components of both cardiogenic and hypovolemic shock. Septic shock is only indirectly caused by microorganisms. Rather, septic shock is the direct result of the production and secretion of inflammatory mediators. Proinflammatory mediators [TNF-α, interleukin (IL)-1, IL-6, IL-8, and platelet-activating factor] are produced and released in excess of the anti-inflammatory mediators (IL-10, glucocorticoids, and catecholamines), resulting in a proinflammatory cascade that initiates a number of pathophysiologic responses.

Septic shock caused by gram-negative organisms appears to be mediated by endotoxins (lipopolysaccharides) and the subsequent release of cytokines (TNF, IL-1, IL-10), eicosanoid products, bradykinin, and endorphins. These agents can directly mediate many of the manifestations of septic shock and also act to amplify the injury by attracting granulocytes and macrophages—cells that cause further cellular injury. Vasodilators (prostaglandin $I_2$, endorphins) predominate early, causing a drop in systemic vascular resistance. Cardiac output generally is increased to compensate for the decreased systemic vascular resistance. This phase has been described as warm shock, because the skin remains well perfused and warm. As septic shock progresses, the heart is no longer able to maintain such a high output, and vasoconstrictors (thromboxane, leukotrienes, endothelin) predominate, with resultant decreased peripheral perfusion. Extremities become cool, urine output decreases, and oxygen delivery falls.

Shock caused by gram-positive organisms is becoming more common in the PICU. This may be due to use of broad-spectrum empiric antibiotics, the increasing use of long-term intravascular catheters and other surgically implanted foreign bodies, the changing epidemiology of gram-positive pathogens, and antibiotic resistance among gram-positive organisms. It is important to realize that the pathogenesis of gram-positive septic shock is different from that of gram-negative sepsis. Gram-positive infections most often arise from skin wounds, soft tissues, and catheter sites, rather than the GI and genitourinary sources associated with gram-negative infections. Gram-negative bacteria have an outer membrane composed of endotoxin that plays a key role in the pathogenesis of gram-negative infection, but the cell wall of gram-positive bacteria is embedded with molecules of lipoteichoic acid that are able to mimic some properties of endotoxin. Additionally, gram-positive bacteria make a range of soluble extracellular toxins, including the pyrogenic toxin superantigens of staphylococci and streptococci.

These superantigens are unusual because they do not require previous processing and specific presentation by antigen-presenting cells. These superantigens are able to bind and activate more lymphocytes than conventionally processed antigens. It is hypothesized that in gram-positive septic shock, toxins are released, resulting in a massive lymphocyte activation with a release of T-cell cytokines, which then causes cellular injury and organ failure.

The host response to gram-positive sepsis is also different from that to gram-negative sepsis. Gram-negative endotoxin induces a rapid (1–5 hours) release of proinflammatory cytokines. Gram-positive toxins induce a more delayed response (50–75 hours) dominated by TNF-α and interferon-α.

## Other Organ Involvement

Organ dysfunction during and after an episode of shock is common. Systems most often affected include the kidney, the blood coagulation system, the lungs, the CNS, the liver, and the GI tract. The kidney responds to hypotension by increasing plasma renin and angiotensin concentrations, thereby decreasing glomerular filtration rate and urine output. This can progress to damage of the energy-consuming renal parenchyma, causing acute tubular necrosis. Coagulopathies may exist in any type of shock but are especially common in septic shock. They result from the release of mediators that activate the clotting cascade, leading ultimately to a consumptive coagulopathy (ie, disseminated intravascular coagulation). The CNS dysfunction is related to decreased cerebral perfusion pressure and thus to decreased substrate delivery to the brain. Liver dysfunction commonly occurs after shock and may be manifested by increases in liver enzymes and decreased production of clotting factors leading to a bleeding diathesis. GI problems include ileus, bleeding (eg, gastritis, ulcers), and necrosis with sloughing of intestinal mucosa. Evaluation of multiorgan system dysfunction is mandatory in the work-up of shock. Multiple organ system failure secondary to shock greatly increases the mortality of the disease.

## Monitoring

Both noninvasive and invasive monitoring of the patient in shock provides information on the severity, progression, and response to treatment. Extremely valuable information can be derived from examination of the cardiovascular, mucocutaneous, musculoskeletal, renal, and central nervous systems.

### A. CLINICAL FINDINGS

**1. Cardiovascular system**—Tachycardia is not always present even when hypotension is profound. Hypotension occurs late in pediatric shock (median systolic blood pressure for a child older than age 2 years can be estimated by adding 90 mm Hg to twice the age in years). An important part of the cardiovascular examination is simultaneous palpation of distal and proximal pulses. An increase in the amplitude difference of pulses between proximal arteries (carotid, brachial, femoral) and distal arteries (radial, posterior tibial, dorsalis pedis) can be palpated in early shock and reflects increased systemic vascular resistance. Distal pulses may be thready or absent even in the presence of normal blood pressure because of poor stroke volume compensated by tachycardia and increased systemic vascular resistance. In uncompensated shock, hypotension is present and proximal pulses are also diminished. Early shock causes peripheral cutaneous vasoconstriction, which preserves flow to vital organs.

**2. Skin**—Because of peripheral vasoconstriction, the skin is gray or ashen in newborns and pale and cold in older patients. Capillary refilling after blanching is slow (> 3 seconds). Mottling of the skin may also be observed.

**3. Musculoskeletal system**—Decreased oxygen delivery to the musculoskeletal system produces hypotonia. Decreased spontaneous motor activity, flaccidity, and prostration are observed.

**4. Urinary output**—Urine output is directly proportionate to renal blood flow and the glomerular filtration rate and therefore is a good reflection of cardiac output. Catheterization of the bladder is necessary to give accurate and continuous information. (Normal urine output is > 1 mL/kg/h; outputs < 0.5 mL/kg/h are considered significantly decreased.)

**5. Central nervous system**—The patient's level of consciousness reflects the adequacy of cortical perfusion. When cortical perfusion is severely impaired, the infant or child fails to respond first to verbal stimuli, then to light touch, and finally to pain. Lack of motor response and failure to cry in response to venipuncture or lumbar puncture should alert the clinician to the severity of the situation. In uncompensated shock in the presence of hypotension, brainstem perfusion may be decreased. Poor thalamic perfusion can result in loss of sympathetic tone. Finally, poor medullary flow produces irregular respirations followed by gasping, apnea, and respiratory arrest.

### B. INVASIVE MONITORING

Patients with poor cardiac output who are hypovolemic often need invasive monitoring for diagnostic and therapeutic reasons. Arterial catheters give constant blood pressure readings, and, to an experienced interpreter, the shape of the waveform is helpful in evaluating cardiac output. CVP monitoring gives useful information about relative changes in volume status as therapy is given. CVP monitoring does not provide information about absolute volume status because intravascular volume, which is considered preload, is inferred most accurately from LV end-diastolic pressures. Therefore, intravascular volume is assessed more accurately by monitoring pulmonary capillary wedge pressure or left atrial pressure. Measurements of pulmonary capillary wedge pressure can be obtained with a pulmonary artery catheter. The pulmonary artery catheter provides additional valuable information on volume and cardiac status (Table 13–9) but is associated with a higher complication rate than CVP lines. Placement of a pulmonary artery catheter should be considered for patients with fluid-refractory (= 40–60 mL/kg) and dopamine-resistant shock. Measurements of arterial and mixed venous oxygen saturations, along with cardiac output data, are useful in calculating oxygen delivery, consumption, and extraction. Oxygen consumption is frequently reduced long before hypotension is present. With the use of a pulmonary artery catheter, the effects of manipulating hemoglobin, oxygen saturation, and cardiac output (the determinants of oxygen consumption and delivery) can be followed in attempts to achieve independence of oxygen delivery and consumption. Patients receiving significant inotropic or ventilatory support may also benefit from the placement of a pulmonary artery catheter.

## Treatment

Early stabilization of hemodynamics with fluid and inotropes is similar in either gram-positive or gram-negative sepsis.

### A. FLUID RESUSCITATION

Fluid infusion should start with 20-mL/kg boluses titrated to clinical monitors of cardiac output, heart

***Table 13–9.*** Hemodynamic parameters.[a]

| Parameter | Formula | Normal Values | Units |
|---|---|---|---|
| Cardiac output | $CO = HR \times SV$ | Wide age-dependent range | L/min |
| Cardiac index | $CI = CO/BSA$ | 3.5–5.5 | L/min/m$^2$ |
| Stroke index | $SI = SV/BSA$ | 30–60 | mL/m$^2$ |
| Systemic vascular resistance | $SVR = 79.9 \dfrac{(MAP - CVP)}{CI}$ | 800–1600 | dyne s/cm$^{-5}$/m$^2$ |
| Pulmonary vascular resistance | $PVR = 79.9 \dfrac{(MPAP - PCWP)}{CI}$ | 80–240 | dyne s/cm$^{-5}$/m$^2$ |

[a]Formulas and normals from Katz RW, Pollack M, Weibley R: Pulmonary artery catheterization in pediatric intensive care. Adv Pediatr 1983;30:169.
HR = heart rate, SV = stroke volume, BSA = body surface area, MAP = mean arterial pressure, CVP = central venous pressure, MPAP = mean pulmonary artery pressure, PCWP = pulmonary capillary wedge pressure.

rate, urine output, capillary refill, and level of consciousness. Patients who do not respond rapidly to the initial fluid bolus should be considered for invasive hemodynamic monitoring (placement of a CVP, arterial line, and possibly pulmonary artery catheter).

Initially, most patients tolerate crystalloid (salt solution), which is readily available and inexpensive. However, 4 hours after a crystalloid infusion, only 20% of the solution remains in the intravascular space. Patients with serious capillary leaks and ongoing plasma losses (eg, burn cases) should initially receive crystalloid, because in these cases colloid (protein and salt solution) leaks into the interstitium. The protein draws intravascular fluid into the interstitium, thus increasing ongoing losses. Patients with hypoalbuminemia or those with intact capillaries who need to retain volume in the intravascular space (eg, patients at risk for cerebral edema) probably benefit from colloid infusions. Experience with dextran (a starch compound dissolved in salt solution) is limited. Patients with normal heart function tolerate increased volume better than those with poor function. Additionally, large volumes of fluid for acute stabilization in children with shock have not been shown to increase the incidence of ARDS or cerebral edema. Increased fluid requirements may persist for several days.

### B. PHARMACOTHERAPY

Empiric antibiotics are chosen according to the most likely cause of infection. Inotropic support should be considered for patients who continue to have clinical evidence of decreased cardiac output after receiving 60 mL/kg of fluid resuscitation. Dopamine remains the first-line vasopressor. Dopamine causes vasoconstriction by stimulating the release of norepinephrine from sympathetic nerves. Infants younger than 6 months of age may not have fully developed sympathetic vesicles and may therefore be resistant to dopamine. Dopamine can increase renal, coronary, and cerebral blood flow by its action on β-receptors and dopaminergic receptors. At higher doses (15 mg/kg/min), α-vasoconstrictor actions predominate. Dobutamine may be added to dopamine; however, children younger than 12 months of age may be less responsive. Epinephrine should be used for dopamine-refractory shock and is often considered first for patients in cold septic shock. Norepinephrine, and in some instances phenylephrine, can be used to increase peripheral vasoconstriction in patients whose perfusing pressure cannot be increased by dopamine and epinephrine (see Table 13–8). Hypocalcemia is often a contributor to cardiac dysfunction in shock. Calcium replacement should be given to normalize ionized calcium levels.

The role of inflammatory mediators in the pathogenesis of septic shock continues to be defined. Drugs that block some of these mediators appear to be beneficial when given early to animals. Human studies of these same blockers have failed to demonstrate a clear benefit. The differences in pathogenesis and host response to gram-positive or gram-negative sepsis may explain some of the differential responsiveness to anti-inflammatory agents seen in past clinical trials. Additionally, the discrepancies may result from low-affinity binding by these antibodies. The molecular mechanisms by which lipopolysaccharide activates cells are becoming better understood, which may assist in the development of more effective therapies. Modulation of T cells (with glucocorticoids, cyclosporine, and antibodies directed at cytokines) in models of superantigen-induced injury have proven beneficial, but remain experimental. Ibuprofen, because of its ability to block cyclooxygenase (cyclooxygenase metabolites are potent modulators of cell function), has shown a trend toward stabilizing patients with septic shock, although not enough evidence is yet available to recommend for or against the use of ibuprofen for septic shock. Recently, excess production of nitric oxide (NO) has been demonstrated to contribute to the hypotension and poor perfusion occurring in shock. Analogs of L-arginine (L-NMA) have been used to block the production of NO in animal models of septic shock with some improvement in survival. Anecdotal use in adults with severe septic shock has demonstrated some success.

Protein C is a primary regulator of coagulation, fibrinolysis, and coagulation-induced inflammation. Deficits in protein C activation correlate with morbidity and mortality in septic shock. Deficiencies of protein C have been found in children and adults with sepsis. Recombinant activated protein C reduced mortality rates in an animal model of sepsis. A large randomized, double-blind, placebo-controlled trial of recombinant activated protein C in adults with severe sepsis showed a significant reduction in mortality rates in patients treated with activated protein C. A similarly designed clinical trial of activated protein C in pediatric patients with severe sepsis is ongoing.

Corticosteroids, by virtue of their action on many mediators, are thought to play a role in shock and—based on positive results in animal models of septic shock—have been advocated for treatment of shock in humans. Children with meningococcal meningitis and AIDS patients with pneumocystis pneumonia have shown improvement in oxygenation and a trend toward improved survival when treated with corticosteroids. The use of hydrocortisone in adults with relative adrenal insufficiency and septic shock was shown to improve short-term outcome. Importantly, a low aldosterone state may be more common in children with septic shock than previously thought. Hydrocortisone (50 mg/kg) should be considered for children at risk for adrenal insufficiency—those with purpura fulminans or pituitary or adrenal abnormalities, those receiving steroids for chronic illness, and those with septic shock and multiorgan system dysfunction not responding well to traditional inotropic therapy.

ECMO has been considered in the treatment of shock in patients with recoverable cardiac and pulmonary function who require both pulmonary and cardiac support.

Annane D: Corticosteroids for septic shock. Crit Care Med 2001;29(7):S117 [PMID: 11445745].

Auslender M, Artman M: Overview of the management of pediatric heart failure. Prog in Ped Cardiol 2000;11:231 [PMID: 1097876].

Batra AS, Lewis AB: Acute myocarditis. Curr Opin Pediatr 2001;13:234 [PMID: 11389357].

Butt W: Septic shock. Pediatr Clin North Am 2001;48(3):601 [PMID: 114111296].

Carcillo JA: Pediatric septic shock and multiple organ failure. Crit Care Clin 2003;19:413 [PMID: 1284813]

McCarthy RE III et al: Long term outcome of fulminant myocarditis as compared with acute (nonfulminant) myocarditis. N Engl J Med 2000;342:690 [PMID: 10706898].

Patel GP et al: New treatment strategies for severe sepsis and septic shock. Curr Opin Crit Care 2003;9:390 [PMID: 14508152].

Proft T, Fraser JD: Bacterial superantigens. Clin Exp Immunol 2003;133:299 [PMID: 12930353].

Schwartz SM et al: Cellular and molecular aspects of myocardial dysfunction. Crit Care Med 2001;29(10):S214 [PMID: 11593064].

Sessler CN, Shepherd W: New concepts in sepsis. Curr Opin Crit Care 2002;8:465 [PMID: 12357117].

Shekerdemian L: Nonpharmacologic treatment of acute heart failure. Curr Opin Pediatr 2001;13:240 [PMID: 11389358].

Tabbutt S: Heart failure in pediatric septic shock: Utilizing inotropic support. Crit Care Med 2001;29:S231 [PMID: 11593066].

Takala A et al: Markere of inflammation in sepsis. Ann Med 2002;34:614 [PMID: 12553502].

Trager K et al: Metabolic alterations in sepsis and vasoactive drug-related metabolic effects. Curr Opin Crit Care 2003;9:271 [PMID: 12883281].

van Deuren M et al: Update on meningococcal disease with emphasis on pathogenesis and clinical management. Clin Microbiol Rev 2000;13(1):144 [PMID: 10627495].

Vincent JL et al; Recombinant Human Activated Protein C Worldwide Evaluation In Severe Sepsis (PROWESS) Study Group: Effects of drotrecogin alfa (activated) on organ dysfunction in the PROWESS trial. Crit Care Med 2003;31:834 [PMID: 12626993].

# INDICATIONS FOR CENTRAL VENOUS & ARTERIAL CANNULATION

Placement of catheters into the central venous or arterial circulation may be justified for continuous assessment of intravascular volume or cardiac function; blood drawing for lab work; or administration of volume, drugs, or hyperalimentation. One should always weigh the risks of bleeding, infection, and clotting against the expected benefits before placing any indwelling catheter.

## General Rules for Equipment Selection & Technique

1. Set up and examine all equipment needed before getting started. Use of a limited number of kits and equipment will provide greater consistency and success.

2. Apply EMLA cream (eutectic mixture of lidocaine 2.5% and prilocaine 2.5%) to the area of puncture (45 minutes before the procedure) or infiltrate with local anesthetic before prepping the skin.

3. The remainder of the procedure should occur under aseptic technique (including gown, mask, hair cover for operator and assistant).

4. Sterilize and drape the area around the point of entry.

5. When searching for the vessel, make straight passes while maintaining slight negative pressure. Advance and withdraw the needle at the same speed. Frequently, the blood return will occur during withdrawal.

6. Once there is free flow of venous blood into the syringe, remove the syringe without moving the needle and, if using the Seldinger technique, pass the J wire through the needle. When appropriate, watch the electrocardiogram for arrhythmias, because they frequently occur when the J wire touches the right side of the heart.

7. Withdraw the needle over the J wire and clean the wire of blood.

8. Make a nick with a No. 11 blade at the point where the J wire enters the skin. Pass the introducer or the intravascular catheter (or both) over the J wire.

9. With the catheters in place, remove the wire along with the introducer.

10. Check to make sure that blood can be drawn easily through the new line.

11. Verify the position of the line on radiograph.

## Points of Entry for Venous Line Placement

### A. EXTERNAL JUGULAR VEIN

Place a soft cloth roll beneath the patient's shoulder and turn the head to the contralateral side (Figure 13–2). The Valsalva maneuver, Trendelenburg position, and occlusion of the vessel at the clavicular level are ways of temporarily increasing jugular distention and visibility. To overcome the problems of this vessel's mobility and thick wall, apply cephalic retraction of the skin over the vessel superior to the point of needle entry. Maintain gentle negative pressure in the syringe attached to the needle as it is advanced toward the vessel. Needle entry into the vessel lumen is usually signaled by a change in resistance followed by appearance of venous blood in the hub of the needle. Remove the syringe without moving the needle and pass a soft J wire into the vessel lumen. Remove the needle and pass the central line over the J wire.

### B. INTERNAL JUGULAR VEIN

Once the patient has been prepped, draped, and positioned as shown in Figure 13–3, feel for the trachea halfway between the angle of the jaw and the suprasternal notch and then feel lateral to the trachea for the carotid pulse. Just lateral to the carotid pulse, at a 30-degree angle from horizontal, insert a finder needle (25-gauge), aiming between the ipsilateral nipple and shoulder. Once venous return is established, remove the finder needle and repeat the procedure with the appropriate-size larger needle.

**Figure 13–2.** External jugular vein technique. (Reproduced, with permission, from Chameides L: *Textbook of Pediatric Advanced Life Support.* American Heart Association, 1988.)

### C. SUBCLAVIAN VEIN

After the patient has been prepped, draped, and positioned (Figure 13–4), move the needle flat along the chest, entering along the inferior edge of the clavicle just lateral to the midclavicular line and aiming for the suprasternal notch. Once venous return is established, use the Seldinger technique.

### D. FEMORAL VEIN

With the patient's leg slightly abducted (Figure 13–5), find the femoral artery 3–4 cm below the inguinal ligament. The femoral vein is just medial and parallel to the femoral artery. Insert the needle at a 30- to 45-degree angle. Once venous return is established, use the Seldinger technique.

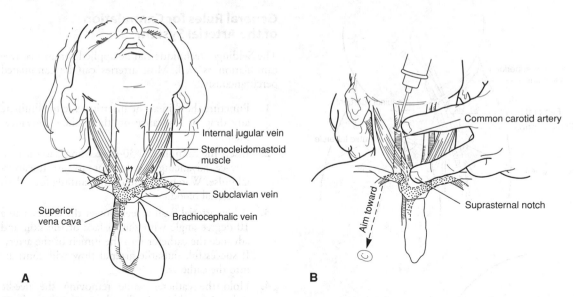

**Figure 13–3.** **A:** The internal jugular vein and its relationship to the surrounding anatomy. **B:** Technique of anterior internal jugular cannulation. (Reproduced, with permission, from Chameides L: *Textbook of Pediatric Advanced Life Support*. American Heart Association, 1988.)

**Figure 13–4.** Subclavian artery. **A:** Anatomy. **B:** Technique. (Reproduced, with permission, from Chameides L: *Textbook of Pediatric Advanced Life Support*. American Heart Association, 1988.)

**A**

**B**

***Figure 13–5.*** Femoral vein. **A:** Anatomy. **B:** Technique. (Reproduced, with permission, from Chameides L: *Textbook of Pediatric Advanced Life Support.* American Heart Association, 1988.)

## E. Antecubital Vein

Peripherally inserted catheter (PIC) lines (2.8–4 Fr) are long, soft, Silastic, styletted catheters most commonly threaded from an antecubital vessel to the right atrium. These lines are not difficult to insert and are easy to dress and keep clean. They are suited for long-term use because they are tolerable for the patient, good for infusion of hyperalimentation and drugs, and less thrombogenic. In general, they are not suitable for obtaining blood for laboratory analysis.

## General Rules for Cannulation of the Arterial System

The Seldinger technique can be applied for arterial tree cannulation as well. Most arteries can be cannulated percutaneously.

1. Puncture the skin at the insertion site to eliminate any drag or resistance on the catheter advancement.
2. Insert the cannula at a 30-degree angle to the skin surface, advancing at a slow rate toward the arterial pulse. Watch the hub of the cannula for a flash of arterial blood.
3. When arterial flash is seen, lower the catheter to a 10-degree angle with the surface of the skin and advance the catheter into the lumen of the artery. If successful, pulsatile arterial flow will continue into the catheter.
4. Hold the catheter while removing the needle stylet. Arterial blood will pulse out of the catheter if the tip is in the arterial lumen.
5. Advance the catheter into the lumen; attach a syringe containing normal saline with 1 unit/mL of heparin; aspirate to make certain that there are no bubbles; and then gently flush the catheter.
6. If arterial flow into the needle stylet stops during catheter advancement, advance this unit an additional centimeter. Remove the needle stylet and place it on a sterile surface. Pull the catheter out slowly. When the tip of the catheter flips into the arterial lumen, the pulsatile arterial blood flow is seen. Rotate the catheter to ensure that the catheter is free within the vessel lumen, then advance the remainder of the catheter length into the vessel.
7. Suture the catheter in place while ensuring that the arterial trace is not damped.
8. Dress the insertion site with sterile gauze, and tape it to the skin.

## Points of Entry for Arterial Line Placement

Always consider whether collateral arterial blood is flowing to the structures distal to the insertion point. The Allen test must be done prior to radial or ulnar artery cannulation.

Arterial sites, listed in order of preference, include:

1. Radial artery (nondominant arm first)
2. Femoral artery (morbidity is the same as for the radial artery beyond the newborn period)
3. Posterior tibial artery
4. Dorsalis pedis artery

5. Ulnar artery (if distal radial filling is present in that hand)
6. Axillary artery
7. Brachial artery (poor collateral flow, used only during cardiac surgery in newborn-sized patients with arterial access limitations)

## Final Considerations

1. Patient benefit should outweigh any risks from central venous or arterial cannulation.
2. Coagulation status of the patient at the time of placement and throughout the time of use must be considered, because deep venous and arterial thrombus formation is partially related to the patient's coagulation status.
3. The incidence of catheter colonization and infection increases if central venous and arterial lines are left in for more than 6 days.

Johnson EM et al: Complications and risks of central venous catheter placement in children. Surgery 1998;124:911 [PMID: 9823406].

Stovroff M, Teague WG: Intravenous access in infants and children. Pediatr Clin North Am 1998;45:1373 [PMID: 9889758].

Vrazas JI: Central venous catheter placement. Hosp Med 1999;60:337 [PMID: 10396408].

## BRAIN INJURY/CEREBRAL EDEMA

Intracranial hypertension is a common feature of many illnesses treated in the PICU (Table 13–10). The early signs and symptoms of intracranial hypertension (Table 13–11) tend to be nonspecific. The classic Cushing triad of bradycardia, hypertension, and apnea occurs late and is often incomplete in children.

Accurate assessment and treatment of elevations in ICP requires an understanding of the basic pathophysiology of intracranial hypertension, as well as the current evidence supporting the various treatment options. Most of our current understanding and approach to treatment is based on studies of patients with traumatic brain injuries. Whether those concepts are directly relevant to the pathophysiologic processes involved in more global CNS injuries, such as hypoxia and metabolic disorders, remains a matter of debate.

Within the constraints of a closed skull, an enlargement of brain tissue, an increased volume of cerebrospinal fluid (CSF), or an increased volume of blood (or the presence of a space-occupying lesion such as a tumor or an abscess) will reduce the size of the other compartments or increase pressure. The factors contributing to intracranial hypertension can be understood by considering each of these three primary compartments.

**Table 13–10.** Pediatric illnesses commonly associated with intracranial hypertension

| **Diffuse processes** |
|---|
| Trauma |
| Hypoxic-ischemic |
|     Near-drowning |
|     Cardiorespiratory arrest |
| Infectious |
|     Encephalitis |
|     Meningitis |
| Metabolic |
|     Reye's syndrome |
|     Liver failure |
|     Inborn error metabolism (IEM) |
| Toxic |
|     Lead |
|     Vitamin A |
| **Focal processes** |
| Trauma |
| Hypoxic-ischemic |
|     Trauma |
|     Stroke |
| Infectious |
|     Abscess |
| Mass lesions |
|     Tumors |
|     Hematomas |

The brain occupies about 80% of the volume of the skull. Apart from solid tumors, increases in the brain compartment are generally a result of cerebral edema. Cerebral edema can be divided into three forms: vasogenic, hydrostatic, and cytotoxic. *Vasogenic* edema occurs in areas of inflamed tissue characterized by increased capillary permeability, and is most typical

**Table 13–11.** Signs and symptoms of intracranial hypertension in children.

| **Early** |
|---|
| Poor feeding, vomiting |
| Irritability, lethargy |
| Seizures |
| Hypertension |
| **Late** |
| Coma |
| Decerebrate responses |
| Cranial nerve palsies |
| Abnormal respirations |
| Bradycardia |
| Hypertension |
| Apnea |

around CNS tumors, abscesses, and infarcts. This form of edema is thought to be at least partially responsive to corticosteroid therapy. *Hydrostatic,* or interstitial, edema is a result of elevated CSF hydrostatic pressures. It occurs primarily in lesions associated with obstruction to CSF flow, and in a typical periventricular distribution. This form of edema is best treated by CSF drainage. The third form of cerebral edema, *cytotoxic* edema, is the most common of the three forms seen in the PICU and is, unfortunately, the least easily treated. Cytotoxic edema occurs as a result of direct injury to brain cells, often leading to irreversible cell swelling and death. This form of cerebral edema is typical of traumatic brain injuries as well as hypoxic-ischemic injuries and metabolic disease.

CSF occupies an estimated 10% of the intracranial space. Intracranial hypertension due primarily to increases in CSF volume (eg, hydrocephalus, primary or secondary) is generally easily diagnosed by CT scan and easily treated with appropriate drainage and shunting.

Cerebral blood volume comprises the final 10% of the intracranial space. Changes in cerebral blood volume generally result from alterations in vascular diameter in response to local metabolic demands or to local vascular pressures—so-called metabolic and pressure autoregulation. These physiologic responses are the means by which the CNS circulation regulates and maintains adequate blood flow to the brain. Given the difficulty in effectively treating cytotoxic brain swelling and the relative rarity of uncomplicated CSF obstructive lesions in the PICU, most of the current therapies aimed at controlling intracranial hypertension rely on altering cerebral blood volume.

Several factors interact to control cerebral blood volume via the autoregulatory responses of the cerebral vasculature. The rate of cerebral metabolism is an important determinant of cerebral blood volume. High metabolic rates lead to vasodilation and increased blood volume, whereas low metabolic rates allow the vessels to constrict and reduce blood flow and blood volume. Partial pressure of carbon dioxide is another important determinant of cerebral blood volume, as elevations in blood $P_{CO_2}$ lead to cerebral vasodilation and decreases in $P_{CO_2}$ lead to vasoconstriction. Finally, cerebral blood volume is linked to cerebral blood flow through the phenomenon of pressure autoregulation. As shown in Figure 13–6, at low systolic blood pressures, the cerebral vessels are maximally dilated and blood flow is only increased by increasing blood pressure. Within the range of autoregulation, the cerebral vessels attempt to maintain a constant flow rate over a range of blood pressures; increased blood pressure results in vasoconstriction, in turn reducing cerebral blood volume. Once the cerebral vessels are maximally constricted, continued increases in pressure may further increase cerebral blood flow and volume.

Treatments for intracranial hypertension are largely derived from experience with traumatic brain injury. An important concept in this regard is that of a "primary" as opposed to a "secondary" brain injury. In this context, primary injury refers to direct damage to brain tissue resulting from the original insult to the CNS, such as physical damage from trauma. This injury is complete before the patient reaches the health care system. As the injured brain swells due to cytotoxic edema, intracranial hypertension develops, potentially limiting cerebral blood flow to portions of the brain and leading to extension of the initial injury (ie, secondary injury). Medical treatment of the patient with intracranial hypertension aims to prevent or reduce secondary injuries.

The primary goal of treatment is to optimize perfusion of areas of the brain that are salvageable. This can

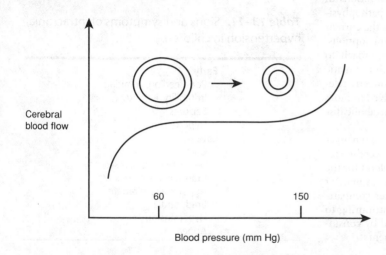

*Figure 13–6.* Pressure autoregulation in the cerebral vasculature.

be accomplished by reducing ICP and by ensuring adequate perfusion. Rational guidance of treatment requires invasive monitoring so that it can be effectively titrated. Although a complete discussion of the indications for ICP monitoring is beyond the scope of this chapter, the topic can be briefly summarized with the suggestion that an ICP monitor be used for patients at significant risk for intracranial hypertension, in whom the treatment of elevated CNS pressures is planned. Monitoring other parameters of CNS oxygen delivery (ie, blood pressure, ABGs, intravascular volume) generally mandates the placement of arterial and central venous catheters. Little evidence exists to support the utility of ICP-directed therapies in conditions associated with global CNS injuries (eg, anoxic brain injuries).

Maintenance of adequate cardiac output and oxygen delivery to the CNS is critical in treating patients with intracranial hypertension. Studies in both adult and pediatric head injury patients show that even a single episode of hypotension or arterial hypoxemia is associated with a marked increase in mortality rates. Although studies have not delineated clear age-appropriate thresholds for blood pressure and arterial $PO_2$ in this setting, a rational starting point for therapy would seem to be maintenance of an adequate circulating blood volume, a blood pressure at least well within the normal range for age, and an arterial $PO_2$ of at least 60 mm Hg. Hypotension and hypoxemia should be treated urgently and aggressively.

In general, the threshold at which treatment for intracranial hypertension should be started is in the range of 15 to 20 cm $H_2O$ pressure. Above this pressure, the compliance of the skull worsens dramatically (Figure 13–7), and very minor increases in intracranial contents lead to large increases in ICP. Initial therapy for intracranial hypertension should always consist of securing the airway and providing adequate sedation. Additional measures would include the removal of any mass lesions (eg, tumors, abscesses, hematomas) and adequate ventricular drainage. Further efforts are then largely directed at reducing cerebral blood volume.

Osmotic diuretics such as mannitol are often used to treat intracranial hypertension. They are thought to act first by decreasing blood viscosity, allowing for increased flow and subsequent autoregulatory vasoconstriction. The osmotic effects on the cells and interstitium of the brain prolong the reduction in ICP. Although mannitol has never been subjected to a placebo-controlled trial, it has been shown to lead to better outcomes than barbiturate therapy in patients with refractory ICP elevations. Current guidelines suggest the use of mannitol in doses of 0.25 to 0.5 g/kg for intracranial hypertension unresponsive to sedation. Renal failure due to acute tubular necrosis can be a treatment-limiting side effect, particularly if serum osmolarity is allowed to rise above 320 and intravascular volume depletion occurs.

Hyperventilation—long a mainstay in the treatment of intracranial hypertension—is controversial. Although acutely effective in causing cerebral vasoconstriction, hyperventilation leads to much larger decreases in blood flow than in blood volume, such that hyperventilation to the point necessary to control ICP may actually compromise CNS perfusion and lead to worsened secondary injury. This concept has been confirmed by studies showing worse outcomes in head-injured patients consistently hyperventilated to a $PCO_2$ of 25 mm Hg or less. Current guidelines suggest that moderate hyperventilation ($PCO_2$ of 30–35 mm Hg) may be used for mild to moderate intracranial hypertension but that extreme hyperventilation ($PCO_2$ < 30 mm Hg) should be reserved for patients with ICP

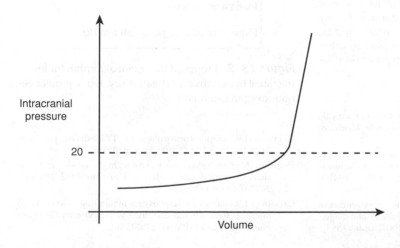

***Figure 13–7.*** Compliance curve of the skull with changing volume of intracranial contents.

elevations unresponsive to other measures, including sedation, paralysis, ventricular drainage, and osmotic diuretics. Due to the risks of worsened CNS ischemia, monitoring cerebral perfusion by blood flow studies or jugular bulb saturation is recommended for patients undergoing extreme hyperventilation.

The use of barbiturates in this setting is based on their suppression of cerebral metabolism and the subsequent metabolic autoregulation effects on cerebral blood volume. Although effective in many instances for ICP elevations, these agents are potent cardiac depressants, and their use often leads to hypotension, necessitating the use of a pressor to maintain perfusion. In addition, plasma barbiturate levels correlate poorly with effect on ICP, suggesting that monitoring of CNS electrical activity by electroencephalography (EEG) is necessary to accurately titrate the use of these agents. Current guidelines suggest the use of barbiturates for treating intracranial hypertension refractory to sedation, paralysis, ventricular drainage, and osmotic diuretics.

Another important concept in the management of intracranial hypertension is that of the cerebral perfusion pressure (CPP). The CPP is the driving pressure across the cerebral circulation and is defined as mean airway pressure – CVP (or ICP, whichever is higher). Some authors have suggested that careful attention to maintenance of a supranormal cerebral perfusion pressure may lead to better outcomes for head-injured patients. Although there are no well-controlled trials to draw from (particularly for pediatric patients), current guidelines suggest that maintenance of a "normal" CPP for age (50–70 mm Hg) is a valid secondary goal of treatment, as long as it is included in a plan to use the other ICP-directed therapies discussed earlier.

A suggested treatment algorithm for patients with documented intracranial hypertension is presented in Figure 13–8. As mentioned earlier, this algorithm represents the current best evidence for the management of intracranial hypertension. The information is largely drawn from experience with traumatic brain injuries, and the direct applicability of these concepts to other illnesses associated with intracranial hypertension remains unclear.

**Figure 13–8.** Proposed treatment algorithm for intracranial hypertension in head injury. $Jvo_2$ = jugular venous oxygen saturation.

Albanese J et al: Decompressive craniectomy for severe traumatic brain injury: Evaluation of the effects at one year. Crit Care Med 2003;31:2535 [PMID: 14530763].

Bayir H et al: Traumatic brain injury in infants and children: Mechanisms of secondary damage and treatment in the intensive care unit. Crit Care Clin 2003;19:529 [PMID: 12848319].

Carney NA et al: Guidelines for the acute medical management of severe traumatic brain injury in infants, children, and adolescents. Pediatr Crit Care Med 2003;4:S1 [PMID: 12847355].

Goldstein LB: Neuropharmacology of TBI-induced plasticity. Brain Inj 2003;17:685 [PMID: 12850953].

Heimann A et al: Effects of hypertonic/hyperoncotic treatment after rat cortical vein occlusion. Crit Care Med 2003;31:2495 [PMID: 14530757].

Littlejohns LR et al: Brain tissue oxygen monitoring in severe brain injury: I. Research and usefulness in critical care. Crit Care Nurse 2003;23:17 [PMID: 12961780].

McIntyre LA et al: Prolonged therapeutic hypothermia after traumatic brain injury in adults: A systematic review. JAMA 2003;289:3007 [PMID: 12799408].

Okonkwo DO, Stone JR: Basic science of closed head injuries and spinal cord injuries. Clin Sports Med 2003;22:467 [PMID: 12852680].

Phillis JW, O'Regan MH: The role of phospholipases, cyclooxygenases, and lipoxygenases in cerebral ischemic/traumatic injuries. Crit Rev Neurobiol 2003;15:61 [PMID: 14513863].

Roberts I et al: Mannitol for acute traumatic brain injury. Cochrane Database Syst Rev 2003;(2):CD001049 [PMID: 12804397].

# ETHICAL DELIBERATION AND END-OF-LIFE CARE IN THE PICU

## Bioethics Consultation in the PICU

Advances in critical care medicine give PICU practitioners the ability to prolong life without being able to ensure a reasonable quality of life. Health care professionals in this setting are often called on to help patients and families wrestle with questions of medical futility. As conflict surrounding care and decision making has arisen, the introduction of ethics consultation in the ICU setting has served to improve the process by helping to identify, analyze, and resolve ethical problems. Ethics consultation can independently clarify views and allow the health care team, patient, and family to make decisions that respect patient autonomy and promote maximum benefit and minimal harm to the patient.

## Managed Withdrawal of Treatment

With increasing frequency, PICU deaths are predictable and result from the withholding or withdrawing of life-sustaining medical therapy (LSMT). Discussions with patients and families regarding the decision to limit resuscitation or to withdraw LSMT should respect the following basic principles:

- Deliberations begin with a clear statement that the patient's good is the goal.
- With the assistance of the health care team, the patient and family can make reasonable decisions about limitation or withdrawal of LSMT based on goals of care for the patient.
- The burden of continued life (pain and suffering) should outweigh any potential benefit from continued therapy.
- Discussions with the patient and family are conducted by experienced personnel with the ability to communicate in a clear and compassionate manner at an appropriate time and place.

- It should be emphasized that decisions are not irrevocable; if at any time the family or health care providers wish to reconsider the decision, full medical therapy should be reinstituted until the situation is clarified.

## Palliative Care

Helping a patient experience a dignified and pain-free death is one of the many unique challenges facing caregivers in the PICU. Pediatric death is characterized by its relative infrequency, by the prognostic uncertainties of many pediatric illnesses, and by the fine line between congenital disorder and incurable disease. When a predictable early death is likely, intensivists are often called on to care for the patient and family during the final days and hours of the patient's life.

In the past several years, palliative medicine has developed as a specialized field of practice to address the needs of dying children. The practice of providing supportive care at end-of-life in pediatrics is fundamentally different from that in adult medicine. In-hospital deaths in pediatrics encompass a more heterogeneous patient population with developmental issues and family dynamics that complicate the process.

Once the inclusive decision is made to limit or withdraw LSMT, a palliative care plan should be agreed on and instituted. The plan should address the following basic principles:

- Adequate pain control and sedation
- Provision of warmth and cleanliness
- Nutrition
- Ongoing patient and family support

The decision to withhold or withdraw LSMT from a pediatric patient does not suggest a plan to hasten the death. The goal of palliative care remains optimization of the patient's and family's experience prior to and following the death.

## Tissue & Organ Donation

Organ transplantation has become standard therapy. Although the demand for tissue and solid organs has increased, donations have remained largely unchanged. The prospect of organ or tissue donation should be considered with all patients dying in the PICU. To be a solid organ donor, the patient must be clinically brain dead and have no conditions contraindicating donation. With patients from whom life-support must be withdrawn, tissue (heart valves, corneas, skin, bone) can be obtained after cardiac death. The Required Request Law mandates that health care professionals approach all donor-eligible families to inquire about organ procurement. The decision to donate must be made free of coercion, with informed consent, and without financial incentive.

## Brain Death (See Chapter 23.)

The development of criteria and expertise in the clinical brain death exam is borne out of the demand for solid organs from patients still receiving LSMT. Currently, the diagnosis of brain death is based on national guidelines that render some clarity and standardization to this critical task.

## Clinical Brain Death Exam

Establish the cause of the disease or injury and exclude potentially reversible syndromes that may produce signs similar to brain death. Also establish the following:

- Coexistence of coma and apnea[a] ("apnea test" ~ 3 minutes with $PCO_2 > 60$ mm Hg)
- Absence of brainstem function
- Normal blood pressure and temperature
- Flaccid muscle tone, no spontaneous movements
- Exam consistent throughout observation period

  Recommended observation periods for children of the following ages:

- Seven days to 2 months old—Two exams over 48 hours; with EEG
- Two months to 1 year—Two exams over 24 hours; with EEG
- Over 1 year—Two exams over 12 to 24 hours

American Academy of Pediatrics Committee on Bioethics and Committee on Hospital Care: Palliative care for children. Pediatrics 2000;106:351 [PMID: 10920167].

Arnold RM et al: Ethical issues in organ procurement: A review for intensivists. Crit Care Clin 1996; 12:29 [PMID: 8821008].

Brody H et al: Withdrawing intensive life-sustaining treatment: Recommendations for compassionate clinical management. N Engl J Med 1997;336:652 [PMID: 9032053].

Canadian Neurocritical Care Group: Guidelines for the diagnosis of brain death. Can J Neurol Sci 1999;26:64 [PMID: 10068812].

Feudtner C et al: Deaths attributed to pediatric complex chronic conditions: National trends and implications for supportive care services. Pediatrics 2001;107:e99 [PMID: 11389297].

Harrison AM, Botkin JR: Can pediatricians define and apply the concept of brain death? Pediatrics 1999;103: e82 [PMID: 10353979].

[a]Cerebral angiography, radionuclide scanning, or transcranial Doppler ultrasonography can be used to assess brain function if apnea testing cannot be performed or if there is need for corroborative studies.

Hynson JL, Sawyer SM: Paediatric palliative care: Distinctive needs and emerging issues. J Paediatr Child Health 2001;37:323 [PMID: 11532048].

Kunin H: Ethical issues in pediatric life-threatening illness: Dilemmas of consent, assent, and communication. Ethics Behavior 1997;7:43 [PMID: 11654857].

McCallum DE et al: How children die in hospital. J Pain Symptom Manage 2000;20:6 [PMID: 11131260].

Schneiderman LJ et al: Impact of ethics consultation in the intensive care setting: A randomized, controlled trial. Crit Care Med 2000;28:12 [PMID: 11153636].

# NUTRITIONAL SUPPORT OF THE CRITICALLY ILL CHILD

## Metabolic and Physiologic Responses

When severely ill pediatric patients are admitted to the intensive care unit, the initial therapy is directed at the primary or underlying problem and at providing cardiorespiratory and hemodynamic support. Although this management is critical to sustaining life in these patients, provision of adequate nutritional support is often overlooked early in the course of therapy. As increasing evidence demonstrates that nutritional status and support affect the morbidity and mortality of critically ill patients, it is vital that this aspect of care be addressed early in the hospital course.

Trauma, surgery, burns, and sepsis impose metabolic and physiologic disturbances that vary in degree, but have many similarities. The insult triggers the afferent limb of the neurophysiologic reflex, which is composed of pain and neurosensory pathways. In response, the efferent limb consisting of neurologic and endocrine pathways, increases autonomic sympathetic activity with norepinephrine and epinephrine secretions and increases pituitary release of a host of hormones including adrenocorticotropic hormone (ACTH), growth hormone (GH), and antidiuretic hormone (ADH). Release of catecholamines inhibits insulin secretion and activity, and stimulates glucagon and ACTH production. ACTH and ADH increase corticosteroid release, inhibit insulin activity, and increase aldosterone. The overall effect is to direct an end-organ increase in metabolic rate and to provide increased substrate availability for energy use (Table 13–12). In addition, the body has a cellular response to tissue injury. Cells migrate to the damaged area to facilitate wound healing and aid in infection control with the release of inflammatory mediators. These cells are mainly dependent on glucose for their energy source, which is an important reason the hypermetabolic state is necessary. These events initiate a hypermetabolic response that influences the mobilization and use of nutrients as substrates. Although all substrates undergo increased use, the fraction of calories derived from glucose is reduced, and the

***Table 13–12.*** Metabolic and physiologic responses to severe illness.

**Physiologic**
   *Cardiovascular*
      Increased cardiac output
      Peripheral vasodilatation and capillary leak
      Expansion of vascular compartment
   *Pulmonary*
      Increased minute ventilation
      Ventilation/perfusion mismatch
      Inefficient gas exchange
      Increased carbon dioxide responsiveness
   *Skeletal muscle*
      Easier fatigability
      Slower relaxation
      Altered force-frequency pattern
   *Renal*
      Salt and water retention
      Impaired concentrating ability

**Metabolic**
   *Hormone and hormone-like levels*
      Increased insulin
      Increased glucocorticoids
      Increased catecholamines
      Increased interleukin-1
      Increased tumor necrosis factor
   *Carbohydrate metabolism*
      Increased blood glucose
      Increased gluconeogenesis
      Increased glucose turnover
      Glucose intolerance
   *Fat metabolism*
      Increased lipid turnover and utilization
      Insuppressible lipolysis
      Decreased ketogenesis
   *Protein metabolism*
      Increased muscle protein catabolism
      Increased muscle branched-chain amino acid oxidation
      Increased serum amino acids
      Increased mitogen losses

fraction derived from protein and lipid breakdown is increased.

Hyperglycemia and glucose intolerance are characteristic traits of the hypermetabolic state. Although glucose use is increased, serum glucose levels are elevated, reflecting neuroendocrine stimulation of glycogenolysis and gluconeogenesis. Gluconeogenesis occurs primarily from lactate, alanine, glutamine, and other amino acids derived from muscle breakdown and from glycerol derived from lipolysis. The hepatic production of glucose is increased, and fails to respond to increased plasma concentrations of glucose or insulin when these sub-

stances are infused intravenously. Hyperglycemia and secondary hyperinsulinemia also inhibit ketosis despite the increased rate of lipolysis. The hyperglycemia does, however, maintain glucose supply to the brain. An elevated glucagon/insulin ratio and increased secretion and plasma concentrations of catecholamines produce relative peripheral insulin resistance. Inefficient glucose and fatty acid uptakes are inadequate to meet increased energy needs, leading to increased oxidation of branched-chain amino acids. Because branched-chain amino acids are essential amino acids, their oxidation depletes a valuable pool of precursors for protein synthesis. Administration of excess glucose can lead to hyperosmolar complications, excess energy expenditure, increased $CO_2$ production, cholestasis, and fatty infiltration of the liver.

Lipids are the major source of energy used during periods of stress starvation. Thus, lipolysis is increased and lipogenesis is decreased despite high levels of glucose and insulin. During stress starvation, peripheral tissues, such as skeletal muscle, myocardium, and respiratory muscles are able to use lipids as their primary energy source. Turnover of medium- and long-chain fatty acids is increased, although the clearance rate of long-chain fatty acid and triglycerides is reduced, primarily through a reduction in peripheral lipoprotein lipase activity that is inhibited by TNF. If excess lipids are administered, complications such as hyperlipidemia, bacteremia, and suppression of in vitro tests of polymorphonuclear and lymphocyte function may occur.

Protein catabolism is the hallmark of the metabolic stress response. Although the rate of protein synthesis is actually increased in the hypermetabolic state, it is significantly reduced compared with the rate of protein breakdown. Protein is broken down mainly to provide carbon skeletons for use in gluconeogenesis, but amino acids are also used to support the cellular inflammatory response, the hepatic synthesis of acute-phase reactant proteins, and wound healing. Thus, the contribution of protein to total caloric expenditure increases from 10% in normal children to 15–20% in critically ill children. The discrepancy between protein catabolism and synthesis leads to a negative nitrogen balance and loss of lean body mass. This condition can be reduced or even reversed with increased nonprotein calorie and protein nutrition. Increased nutrient intake appears to make a difference in the ability of the patient to tolerate stress.

## Nutritional Assessment

The pediatric patient is at a marked disadvantage compared with adults during periods of stress starvation. The child is a growing organism with little metabolic reserve to compensate for the metabolic stresses created by surgery, trauma, and sepsis. Preexisting nutritional status and the degree of stress imposed by the disease process are important factors in estimating nutritional requirements of the critically ill patient. Accurate assessment of nutritional requirements is important as both overfeeding and underfeeding can lead to increased morbidity. One way to estimate nutritional requirements is to apply US recommended dietary allowances (RDA). However, since these recommendations are based on populations of normal healthy subjects, applying RDAs to critically ill patients significantly overestimates their caloric requirements. Therefore, several equations have been formulated in an attempt to predict basal energy needs of the critically ill patient. Some of these formulas estimate the basal metabolic rate (BMR), which is the energy requirement for a fasting (10–12 hours) person who recently awoke from sleep and is at rest with a normal body temperature in the absence of any stress. Other formulas estimate the resting energy expenditure (REE), which is the energy expenditure of a person at rest with a normal body and ambient temperature, but not necessarily fasting. The BMR and REE are similar, usually differing by less than 10%. Harris-Benedict and the World Health Organization have recommended formulas that are among the most commonly used (Table 13–13). Once the basal metabolic demands have been estimated, it is then multiplied by a stress factor correlating to underlying disease process to determine the ultimate energy requirements for the patient (Table 13–14). Compared with RDAs, these formulas better estimate energy requirements in sick patients. However, recent evidence

**Table 13–14.** Activity and stress factors (× REE).

| Condition | Factor | Condition | Factor |
|---|---|---|---|
| ICU on vent | Activity 1.0–1.15 | Peritonitis | Stress 1.2–1.5 |
| Confined to bed | Activity 1.1–1.2 | Cardiac failure | Stress 1.25–1.5 |
| Light activity | Activity 1.2–1.3 | Head injury | Stress 1.3–1.4 |
| Fever, per 1°C | Stress 1.12–1.13 | Liver failure | Stress 1.4–1.5 |
| Major surgery | Stress 1.2–1.3 | Sepsis | Stress 1.4–1.5 |
| Multiple fractures | Stress 1.2–1.35 | Burns | Stress 1.5–2.0 |

REE = resting energy expenditure.

suggests that even they may not be accurate enough to use in critically ill children.

Indirect calorimetry has been used to measure patients' REE and appears to reflect a more accurate method of determining nutritional requirements. Indeed, indirect calorimetry measurements were used to derive the stress factors used with prediction formulas. Though this method was once used strictly for research, technology has enabled the production of portable, accurate devices that can be used anywhere in the hospital. Indirect calorimetry measures the amount of oxygen absorbed across the lung. This value is assumed to be equal to the amount of oxygen consumed in metabolic processes. The metabolic rate determined in milliliters of oxygen consumed per minutes can be converted to calories per hour, thereby providing a measure of REE. Carbon dioxide production is also measured. The ratio of $CO_2$ production to $O_2$ consumption yields the respiratory quotient (RQ), which is a measure of substrate use. Inefficiencies in substrate use can be discovered and corrected by modification of RQ through alteration of energy substrates that are provided to the patient. A recent study with 55 critically ill children was performed comparing two well-known prediction formulas with indirect calorimetry. The data suggest that prediction methods are unreliable for clinical use, and that indirect calorimetry is the only useful way of determining REE in sick children.

## Provision of Nutrition

Once energy requirements are determined, the practitioner must decide to deliver nutritional support through either the enteral or the parenteral route. En-

**Table 13–13.** Estimating needs for critically ill pediatric patients.

| | Age | Resting Energy Expenditure (REE) kcal/kg | Average Range of Energy Needs kcal/kg | Average Range of Protein Needs g/kg |
|---|---|---|---|---|
| Infants | 0–6 mo | 55 | 90–120 | 2–3.5 |
| | 6–12 mo | 55 | 90–120 | 1.5–2.5 |
| Children | 1–3 y | 55 | 75–100 | 1.5–2.5 |
| | 4–6 y | 45 | 65–90 | 1.5–2.0 |
| | 7–10 y | 40 | 55–70 | 1.0–2.0 |
| Males | 11–14 y | 30 | 40–55 | 1.0–2.0 |
| | 15–18 y | 30 | 40–45 | 1.0–1.5 |
| | 19–24 y | 25 | 30–40 | 1.0–1.5 |
| Females | 11–14 y | 30 | 40–55 | 1.0–2.0 |
| | 15–18 y | 25 | 30–40 | 1.0–1.5 |
| | 19–24 y | 25 | 30–40 | 1.0–1.5 |

Based on WHO formulas for protein and energy requirements.

teral feeding is preferred because it is more physiologic, associated with fewer complications, and in some cases, the only way to safely deliver some nutrients. More knowledge exists about enteral feeding in relation to both energy requirements and utilization; and practically, it is less expensive than parental nutrition.

Patients should be screened shortly after admission for nutritional requirements and preferred route of administration. Over the years, many practice patterns have been developed that list specific conditions or therapies in which enteral feeding may not be well tolerated by patients. Recent studies are proving that these may not be based on true physiologic differences and that a majority of patients who are critically ill can tolerate enteral feedings. The list of absolute contraindications for enteral feeding is shrinking and now may include just diseases of the GI tract.

Because it provides for a more physiologic digestive process, direct gastric feeding is preferable to the intestinal route. Patients supported with gastric feeds can usually tolerate higher osmotic loads and larger volumes, and have a lower frequency of diarrhea. Gastric acid also has a bactericidal effect that may decrease a patient's susceptibility to infection. However, for severely ill patients sedated and on mechanical ventilation, the high risk of reflux and aspiration becomes an increasing concern with this manner of feeding. Therefore, transpyloric feeding has been instituted in these patients and in any patient at high risk for aspiration. Although transpyloric feeding may limit reflux and aspiration, it does not entirely eliminate it.

The choice of formulas must be based on age, GI function, history of feeding tolerance, nutrient requirements, and route of feeding. The osmolality, nutrient complexity, caloric density, and cost are all factors that should be taken into consideration. An increasing number of commercially made formulas and additives are now available to meet the nutritional needs of the critically ill patient (Table 13–15).

Parenteral nutrition (PN) is indicated for patients who are unable to meet nutritional needs with enteral feeds. It consists of the IV delivery of nutrients, fluid, carbohydrates, protein, fat, electrolytes, vitamins, minerals, and trace elements. The proportions of these elements are individualized to suit the patient's specific nutritional needs. PN often requires central venous access, and thus this method also carries the risks associated with central venous catheters (infection, clots, and insertion-related complications).

PN can be ordered in many ways, as nutrients can be ordered based on a child's weight or per liter, or a combination of both. Standard ranges and guidelines are usually provided on order forms. Parenteral energy needs can be approximately 10–15% lower than estimated enteral needs due to reduced energy required for digestion, absorption, and fecal losses. The percentage of protein, carbohydrate, and fat that contributes to ideal total energy intake varies with the individual and the disease condition. General guidelines for energy distribution are 8–15% protein, 45–60% carbohydrate, and 25–40% fat. Solutions should be instituted slowly and advanced gradually over several days as tolerated by the patient. Guidelines for the administration of a balanced parenteral diet are provided in Chapter 10. A constant flow rate is important to maintaining steady glucose delivery. If PN must be stopped abruptly, a 10% glucose solution should be started to prevent hypoglycemia. Administration of high glucose and amino

***Table 13–15.*** Pediatric enteral formulas.

| Formula Category | Formula Examples | Typical Uses |
|---|---|---|
| Standard, milk protein-based | Pediasure<br>Pediasure with Fiber<br>Kindercal (with/without fiber)<br>Nutren Junior | Nutritionally complete for ages 1–10 years. Can be used for tube feeds or oral supplements. |
| Food based | Compleat Pediatric | Made with beef protein, fruits, and vegetables—does contain lactose. Fortified with vitamins/minerals. |
| Semielemental | Peptamen Jr. | Indicated for impaired gut function with peptides as protein source, and high MCT content with lower total fat % than standard pediatric formulas. |
| Elemental | Pediatric Vivonex (24 kcal/oz)<br>Elecare<br>Neocate One Plus | Indicated for impaired gut function or protein allergy, and contains free amino acids and lower fat with majority as MCT. |

MCT = medium-chain triglycerides.

acid concentrations in total parenteral nutrition requires central venous access.

Immunonutrition is an area of growing interest and research. The term describes a point of view that dietary factors can confer an advantage to the immune system or other adaptive functions in infants and children. The claims of health benefits ascribed to foods or dietary supplements are not new, but until recently, these claims have not been supported by scientific review. Breast milk, the model for infant formula manufacturers, has long been recognized for its immunonutritive properties, containing such nutrients as secretory immunoglobulins, lysozyme, interferon, and growth factors. However, the contribution of specific components to a positive outcome has yet to be elucidated. Growing evidence supports the immunomodulatory effects of minerals (eg, iron, zinc, selenium, vitamin A), amino acids (arginine and glutamine), and nucleotides. Evidence also points to the emergence of prebiotics, nondigestable food components that favor the colonization and growth of bacteria normally resident in the colon; and probiotics, live microbial feed supplements with beneficial effects to the host. Although some of these concepts hold promise, it is still too early to advocate any specific guidelines, because some of these nutrients used in high doses have been reported to produce possible harmful effects.

Coss-Bu JA et al: Energy metabolism, nitrogen balance and substrate utilization in critically ill children. Am J Clin Nutr 2001;74:664 [PMID: 11684536].

Dominguez-Cherit G et al: Total parenteral nutrition. Curr Opin Crit Care 2002;8:285 [PMID: 12386487].

Fung EB: Estimating energy expenditure in critically ill adults and children. AACN Clin Issues 2000;11:480 [PMID: 11288413].

Griffiths RD: Specialized nutrition support in critically ill patients. Curr Opin Crit Care 2003;9:249 [PMID: 12883278].

Irving SY et al: Nutrition for the critically ill child: Enteral and parenteral support. AACN Clin Issues 2000;11:541 [PMID: 11288418].

Novak F et al: Glutamine supplementation in serious illness: A systematic review of the evidence. Crit Care Med 2002;30:2022 [PMID: 12352035].

Suchner U et al: Immune-modulatory actions of arginine in the critically ill. Br J Nutr 2002;87:S121 [PMID: 11895148].

Wernerman J: Glutamine and acute illness. Curr Opin Crit Care 2003;9:279 [PMID: 12883282].

Wyncoll D, Beale R: Immunologically enhanced enteral nutrition: Current status. Curr Opin Crit Care 2001;7:128 [PMID: 11373522].

# PAIN & ANXIETY CONTROL

Anxiety control and pain relief are important responsibilities of the critical care physician. It is well recognized that infants and children experience pain and require pain relief. Indeed, outcomes are improved in children receiving appropriate pain control. A child's anxiety in the PICU may heighten perception of pain to a level that causes deterioration of his or her condition. It is important to distinguish between anxiety and pain, because pharmacologic therapy may be directed at one or both of these symptoms (Table 13–16). Further, before initiating or increasing sedative drugs, it is important to exclude or address physiologic causes of agitation, such as hypoxemia, hypercapnia, and cerebral hypoperfusion caused by low cardiac output.

## Sedation

Sedative (anxiolytic) drugs are used to induce calmness without producing sleep—although at high doses, all anxiolytics will cause drowsiness and sleep. The five indications for the use of sedative drugs are (1) to allay fear and anxiety; (2) to manage acute confusional states; (3) to facilitate treatment or diagnostic procedures; (4) to facilitate mechanical ventilation; and (5) to obtund physiologic responses to stress—that is, reduce tachycardia, hypertension, or increases in ICP. Parenteral administration (bolus or infusion) allows titration of response in the critically ill child. Sedatives fall into several classes, with the opioid and benzodiazepine classes serving as the mainstay of anxiety treatment in the ICU.

### A. BENZODIAZEPINES

Benzodiazepines possess anxiolytic, hypnotic, anticonvulsant, and skeletal muscle relaxant properties. Although their exact mode of action is unknown, it appears to be located within the limbic system of the CNS and to involve the neuroinhibitory transmitter γ-amino butyric acid. Most benzodiazepines are metabolized in the liver, with their metabolites subsequently excreted in the urine; thus, patients in liver failure are likely to have long elimination times.

Benzodiazepines can cause respiratory depression if given rapidly in high doses, and they potentiate the analgesic and respiratory depressive effects of opioids and barbiturates. Therefore, it is important to monitor cardiorespiratory status and have resuscitation equipment available. Three benzodiazepines with differing half-lives are presently used in the ICU setting:

**1. Midazolam**—Midazolam has the shortest half-life (1½–3½ hours) of the benzodiazepines and is the only benzodiazepine that should be administered as a continuous IV infusion. It produces excellent retrograde amnesia lasting for 20–40 minutes after a single IV dose. Therefore, it can be used either for short-term sedation or for "awake" procedures such as endoscopy or as a continuous infusion in the anxious, restless patient.

***Table 13–16.*** Pain and anxiety control.

| Drug | Dose and Method of Administration[a] | Advantages | Disadvantages | Usual Duration of Effect |
|---|---|---|---|---|
| Morphine | IV, 0.1 mg/kg; continuous infusion, 0.01–0.05 mg/kg/h | Excellent pain relief, reversible | Respiratory depression, hypotension, nausea, suppression of intestinal motility, histamine release | 2–4 h |
| Meperidine | IV, 1 mg/kg | Good pain relief, reversible | Respiratory depression, histamine release, nausea, suppression of intestinal motility | 2–4 h |
| Fentanyl | IV, 1–2 µg/kg; continuous infusion, 0.5–2 µg/kg/h | Excellent pain relief, reversible, short half-life | Respiratory depression, chest wall rigidity, severe nausea and vomiting | 30 min |
| Diazepam | IV, 0.1 mg/kg | Sedation and seizure control | Respiratory depression, jaundice, phlebitis | 1–3 h |
| Lorazepam | IV, 0.1 mg/kg | Longer half-life, sedation and seizure control | Nausea and vomiting, respiratory depression, phlebitis | 2–4 h |
| Midazolam | IV, 0.1 mg/kg | Short half-life, only benzodiazepine given as continuous infusion | Respiratory depression | 30–60 min |

[a]Intravenous (IV) administration is most common in the ICU. The effects of morphine, meperidine, and fentanyl are reversible by administration of naloxone (opioid antagonist).

The single IV dose is 0.1 mg/kg, whereas a continuous infusion should be started at a rate of 0.1 mg/kg/h after an initial loading dose of 0.1 mg/kg. The midazolam infusion dosage must be titrated upward to achieve the desired effect. Midazolam is not an analgesic; therefore, small doses of an analgesic such as morphine or fentanyl may be needed.

**2. Diazepam**—Diazepam has a longer half-life than midazolam and can be given PO as well as by the IV route. Its disadvantage in the ICU is its intermediary metabolite, nordazepam, which has a very long half-life and may accumulate, prolonging sedation. It produces excellent anxiolysis and amnesia. Additionally, it is used to treat acute status epilepticus. The IV dose is 0.1 mg/kg and can be repeated every 15 minutes to achieve the desired effect or until undesirable side effects (somnolence and respiratory depression) occur.

**3. Lorazepam**—Lorazepam possesses the longest half-life of the three benzodiazepines discussed here and can be used to achieve sedation for as long as 6–8 hours. It has less effect on the cardiovascular and respiratory systems than other benzodiazepines and can be given PO, IV, or intramuscularly (IM). The IV route is the most common. The IV dosage is 0.1 mg/kg. Lorazepam can also be used to treat acute status epilepticus.

**B. OTHER DRUGS**

**1. Chloral hydrate**—Chloral hydrate is an enteral sedative and hypnotic agent frequently used in children. After administration, it is rapidly metabolized by the liver to its active form trichloroethanol, which has an 8-hour half-life. A sedative dose is 6–20 mg/kg per dose, usually given every 6–8 hours, whereas the hypnotic dose is up to 50 mg/kg with a maximum dose of 1 g. The hypnotic dose is frequently used to sedate young children for outpatient radiologic procedures such as computed tomography scanning and magnetic resonance imaging. There is little effect on respiration or blood pressure with therapeutic doses of chloral hydrate. The drug is irritating to mucous membranes, however, and may cause gastric upset if administered on an empty stomach.

**2. Ketamine**—Ketamine is a phencyclidine derivative that produces a trance-like state of immobility and amnesia known as dissociative anesthesia. After IM or IV administration, it causes central sympathetic nervous system stimulation with resultant increases in heart rate, blood pressure, and cardiac output. Respiration is not depressed at therapeutic doses. Because salivary and tracheobronchial mucous gland secretions are increased, atropine should be administered 20 minutes prior to the ketamine. A disadvantage of ketamine usage is the occurrence of unpleasant dreams or hallucinations. The incidence is less in children than in adults, and it can be reduced even further by the concurrent administration of a benzodiazepine. Because of its inotropic properties, ketamine is useful for the sedation of certain critically ill patients whose conditions are unstable. Additionally, its bronchodilator effects make it the induction agent of choice for patients with status asthmaticus requiring intubation. It is given as an IV injection of 1–2 mg/kg over 60 seconds, with supplementary doses of 0.5 mg/kg being required every 10–30 minutes to maintain an adequate level of anesthesia. Alternatively, it can be administered as an IM injection of 3–7 mg/kg, which usually produces the desired level of anesthesia within 3–4 minutes. If prolonged anesthesia is required, ketamine can be administered by IV infusion at doses of 3–20 mg/kg/h.

**3. Antihistamines**—The antihistamines diphenhydramine and hydroxyzine can be used as sedatives but are not as effective as the benzodiazepines. Diphenhydramine produces sedation in only 50% of those patients receiving it. It can be given IV, IM, or PO at a dose of 1 mg/kg. Hydroxyzine can be given either IM or PO. It is frequently used concurrently with morphine or meperidine, adding anxiolysis and potentiating the effects of the opioid. The sedative effects of both drugs can last from 4 to 6 hours following a single dose.

**4. Propofol**—Propofol is an anesthetic induction agent whose main advantages are a rapid recovery time and no cumulative effects resulting from its rapid hepatic metabolism. It has no analgesic properties and frequently causes pain on injection. Dose-related hypotension and metabolic acidosis have been reported in pediatric patients, and a recent FDA bulletin has recommended against the use of propofol in pediatric patients outside the controlled environment of the operating room.

**5. Barbiturates**—Barbiturates (phenobarbital, thiopental) can cause direct myocardial and respiratory depression and are, in general, poor choices for sedation of seriously ill patients. Phenobarbital has a very long half-life (up to 4 days), and recovery from thiopental, although it is a short-acting barbiturate, can be prolonged because remobilization of tissue stores occurs.

## Analgesia

### A. OPIOID ANALGESICS

Opioid analgesics (morphine, fentanyl, codeine, meperidine) are the mainstays of therapy for most forms of acute severe pain as well as chronic cancer pain management. They possess both analgesic and dose-related sedative effects, although a range of plasma concentrations produce analgesia without sedation. In addition, opioids can cause respiratory depression, nausea, pruritus, slowed intestinal motility, miosis, urinary retention, cough suppression, biliary spasm, and vasodilation. The dose of opioid required to produce adequate analgesia varies greatly from one individual to the next. Therefore, in the intensive care setting, a continuous infusion of morphine or fentanyl allows dosages to be easily titrated to achieve the desired effect.

In general, infants younger than age 3 months are more susceptible than older children to the respiratory depressant effects of opioids. Starting dosages for these patients should be about one third to one half the usual pediatric dose. Most opioids (except meperidine) have minimal cardiac depressive effects, and critically ill patients generally tolerate them well. Fentanyl does not cause the histamine release that morphine does and thus produces less vasodilation and drop in systemic blood pressure. Opioids are metabolized in the liver, with metabolites excreted in the urine. Thus patients with hepatic or renal impairment may have a prolonged response to their administration. Patients who receive regular doses of opioids for 2 weeks or more frequently develop a physiologic dependence with the development of withdrawal symptoms (agitation, tachypnea, tachycardia, sweating, diarrhea) upon acute termination of the drug. In these patients, gradual tapering of the opioid dosage over a 5- to 10-day period will prevent withdrawal symptoms. As with any potent sedative or analgesic used in the ICU setting, appropriate patient monitoring (pulse oximetry, cardiorespiratory monitoring, blood pressure monitoring) should be used during the period of opioid administration, and equipment should be available to support prompt intervention if undesired side effects occur.

The ICU regimen for sedation and analgesia must be carefully modified when the patient is transferred to the ward or a lower vigilance area. Patients with baseline respiratory, hepatic, or renal insufficiencies are most predisposed to respiratory insufficiency from sedatives or opioid analgesics.

Advantages of continuous infusions of sedatives are that it provides a more constant level of sedation, increases patient comfort, and allows better tolerance of newer approaches to mechanical ventilation. Prolongation of mechanical ventilation, hospitalization, and inability to assess neurologic function and mental status have been recognized as disadvantages of continuous infusions. A recent study of the daily interruption of continuous sedation, allowing the adult patient to "wake up," was associated with a decrease in duration of mechanical ventilation and length of stay in the ICU. Currently, similar data are not available for pediatric patients.

Frequently pediatric patients will require relatively deep levels of sedation while undergoing a procedure (eg, vascular line placement, radiographic studies). Often these patients are not intubated and are not expected to require intubation and ventilatory support—so called conscious sedation. (New American Academy of Pediatric guidelines will recommend a change in terminology to "moderate sedation/analgesia".) A systematic approach should include the following:

1. Pertinent history to elicit underlying illnesses
2. Physical exam focusing on the anatomy and adequacy of the child's airway (ie, large tonsils or facial deformity)
3. Informed consent
4. Appropriate patient fasting from solids (6 hours) and liquids (2 hours)
5. Age- and size-appropriate equipment
6. Drug dosages calculated on a milligram per kilogram basis
7. Monitoring and documentation of vital signs (including continuous pulse oximetry, respiratory rate and pattern, level of arousability)
8. Separate observer to monitor deeply sedated patients
9. Practitioner capable of intubating and treating patients who enter a deeper state of sedation than initially anticipated
10. Discharge criteria ensuring the patient has recovered to his or her baseline level of consciousness.

Short-acting agents are preferred. Agents typically used include an opioid (usually fentanyl or morphine) and a benzodiazepine (most often midazolam). Another option is ketamine and midazolam. It is important to select and become comfortable with a specific combination; learn the indications and potential complications. Using a familiar agent and following the systematic approach outlined earlier have reduced anesthetic complications in this population of patients.

Patient-controlled analgesia (PCA) is a computer-governed infusion pump for constant infusion or patient-regulated bolus infusion of opioid analgesics. The basal infusion mode is intended to provide a constant serum level of analgesic. The bolus mode allows the patient, by pushing a button, to self-administer additional doses for breakthrough pain. The patient is usually permitted six boluses an hour, with 10-minute lockouts. If the patient is using allotted hourly boluses, this usually means that the basal infusion rate is too low. The patient must understand the concept of PCA in order to be a candidate for its use. In some circumstances in pediatrics it is more appropriate for the nurse or parent to administer the bolus dose.

Naloxone reverses the analgesia, sedative, and respiratory depressive effects of opioid agonists. Its administration should be titrated to achieve the desired effect (eg, reversal of respiratory depression) because full reversal using 1–10 µg/kg may cause acute anxiety, dysphoria, nausea, and vomiting. Furthermore, because the duration of effect of naloxone is shorter (30 minutes) than that of most opioids, the patient must be observed carefully for reappearance of the undesired effect.

**B. Nonopioid Analgesics**

Nonopioid analgesics used in the treatment of mild to moderate pain include acetaminophen, aspirin, and other nonsteroidal anti-inflammatory drugs (NSAIDs) such as ibuprofen and naproxen.

**1. Acetaminophen**—Acetaminophen is the most commonly used analgesic in pediatrics in the United States and is the drug of choice for mild to moderate pain because of its low toxicity and lack of effect on bleeding time. It is metabolized by the liver. Suggested doses are 10–15 mg/kg PO to approximately 10–20 mg/kg PR every 4 hours.

**2. Aspirin**—Aspirin is also an effective analgesic for mild to moderate pain at doses of 10–15 mg/kg PO every 4 hours. However, its prolongation of bleeding time, association with Reye syndrome, and propensity to cause gastric irritation limit its usefulness in pediatric practice. Aspirin and other NSAIDs are still useful, especially for pain of inflammatory origin, bone pain, and pain associated with rheumatic conditions.

**3. Other NSAIDs**—Ibuprofen and naproxen are NSAIDs whose use has been limited in pediatrics to date. Naproxen is FDA approved for children aged 2–12 years (5–7 mg/kg PO every 8–12 hours), whereas ibuprofen requires more frequent dosing intervals (4–10 mg/kg PO every 6–8 hours).

All of the NSAIDs have a therapeutic ceiling after which no increase occurs in analgesic potency above the recommended dose. They all can cause gastritis and should be given with antacids or with meals, and they should be used with caution in people at risk for renal compromise. In addition, the analgesic effects of acetaminophen, aspirin, and other NSAIDs are additive to those of opioids. Thus, if additional analgesia is required, their use should be continued and an appropriate PO opioid (codeine, morphine) or parenteral opioid (morphine, fentanyl) begun.

Cote CJ et al: Adverse sedation events in pediatrics: A critical incident analysis of contributing factors. Pediatr 2000;105:805 [PMID: 10742324].

Cote CJ: Conscious sedation: Time for this oxymoron to go away. J Pediatr 2001;139:15 [PMID: 11445787].

Cray SH et al: Lactic acidemia and bradyarrhythmia in a child sedated with propofol. Crit Care Med 1998;26:2087 [PMID: 9875925].

Gehlbach BK, Kress JP: Sedation in the intensive care unit. Curr Opin Crit Care 2002;8:290 [PMID: 12386488].

Kress JP et al: Daily interruption of sedative infusions in critically ill patients undergoing mechanical ventilation. N Engl J Med 2000;342:1471 [PMID: 10816184].

Tobias JD: Sedation and analgesia in paediatric intensive care units. Paediatr Drugs 1999;109 [PMID: 10937446].

# Skin

14

*Joseph G. Morelli, MD, & William L. Weston, MD*

## ■ GENERAL PRINCIPLES OF DIAGNOSIS OF SKIN DISORDERS

Examination of the skin requires that the entire surface of the body be palpated and inspected in good light. The onset and duration of each symptom should be recorded, together with a description of the primary lesion and any secondary changes, using the terminology set forth in Table 14–1. In practice, the characteristics of skin lesions are described in an order opposite that shown in the table. Begin with distribution, then configuration, color, secondary changes, and primary changes. For example, guttate psoriasis could be described as generalized, discrete, red, scaly papules.

## ■ GENERAL PRINCIPLES OF TREATMENT OF SKIN DISORDERS

### TOPICAL THERAPY

Treatment should be simple and aimed at preserving normal skin physiology, keeping in mind that one is treating the child and not the anxious parent or grandparent. Topical therapy is often preferred because medication can be delivered in optimal concentrations to the desired site.

Water is an important therapeutic agent, and optimally hydrated skin is soft and smooth. This occurs at approximately 60% environmental humidity. Because water evaporates readily from the cutaneous surface, skin hydration (stratum corneum of the epidermis) is dependent on the water concentration in the air, and sweating contributes little. However, if sweat is prevented from evaporating (eg, in the axilla, groin), local humidity and hydration of the skin are increased. As humidity falls below 15–20%, the stratum corneum shrinks and cracks; the epidermal barrier is lost and allows irritants to enter the skin and induce an inflammatory response. Replacement of water will correct this condition if evaporation is prevented. Therefore, dry and scaly skin is treated by soaking the skin in water for 5 minutes and then adding a barrier to evaporation (Table 14–2). Oils and ointments prevent evaporation for 8–12 hours, so they must be applied once or twice a day. In areas already occluded (axilla, diaper area), ointments or oils will merely increase retention of water and should not be used.

Overhydration (maceration) can also occur. As environmental humidity increases to 90–100%, the number of water molecules absorbed by the stratum corneum increases and the tight lipid junctions between the cells of the stratum corneum are gradually replaced by weak hydrogen bonds; the cells eventually become widely separated, and the epidermal barrier falls apart. This occurs in immersion foot, diaper areas, axillae, and the like. It is desirable to enhance evaporation of water in these areas by air drying.

### WET DRESSINGS

By placing the skin in an environment where the humidity is 100% and allowing the moisture to evaporate to 60%, pruritus is relieved. Evaporation of water stimulates cold-dependent nerve fibers in the skin, and this may prevent the transmission of the itching sensation via pain fibers to the central nervous system. It also is vasoconstrictive, thereby helping to reduce the erythema and also decreasing the inflammatory cellular response.

The simplest form of wet dressing consists of one set of wet underwear (eg, long johns) worn under a dry pair. The underwear should be soaked in warm (not hot) water and wrung out until no more drops come out. When covered by the dry layer, the wet dressings need to be changed only every 4–6 hours.

### TOPICAL GLUCOCORTICOIDS

Twice-daily application of topical steroids is the mainstay of treatment for all forms of dermatitis (Table 14–3). Topical steroids can also be used under wet dressings. Wet dressings are removed every 4–6 hours, and a topical steroid is applied; the skin is then covered again with wet dressings. If treatment is applied

***Table 14–1.*** Examination of the skin.

| Clinical Appearance | Description and Examples |
|---|---|
| **Primary lesions (first to appear)** | |
| Macule | Any circumscribed color change in the skin that is flat. Examples: white (vitiligo), brown (café au lait spot), purple (petechia). |
| Papule | A solid, elevated area less than 1 cm in diameter whose top may be pointed, rounded, or flat. Examples: acne, warts, small lesions of psoriasis. |
| Plaque | A solid, circumscribed area more than 1 cm in diameter, usually flat-topped. Example: psoriasis. |
| Vesicle | A circumscribed, elevated lesion less than 1 cm in diameter and containing clear serous fluid. Example: blisters of herpes simplex. |
| Bulla | A circumscribed, elevated lesion more than 1 cm in diameter and containing clear serous fluid. Example: bullous erythema multiforme. |
| Pustule | A vesicle containing a purulent exudate. Examples: acne, folliculitis. |
| Nodule | A deep-seated mass with indistinct borders that elevates the overlying epidermis. Examples: tumors, granuloma annulare. If it moves with the skin on palpation, it is intradermal; if the skin moves over the nodule, it is subcutaneous. |
| Wheal | A circumscribed, flat-topped, firm elevation of skin resulting from tense edema of the papillary dermis. Example: urticaria. |
| **Secondary changes** | |
| Scales | Dry, thin plates of keratinized epidermal cells (stratum corneum). Examples: psoriasis, ichthyosis. |
| Lichenification | Induration of skin with exaggerated skin lines and a shiny surface resulting from chronic rubbing of the skin. Example: atopic dermatitis. |
| Erosion and oozing | A moist, circumscribed, slightly depressed area representing a blister base with the roof of the blister removed. Examples: burns, bullous erythema multiforme. Most oral blisters present as erosions. |
| Crusts | Dried exudate of plasma on the surface of the skin following acute dermatitis. Examples: impetigo, contact dermatitis. |
| Fissures | A linear split in the skin extending through the epidermis into the dermis. Example: angular cheilitis. |
| Scars | A flat, raised or depressed area of fibrotic replacement of dermis or subcutaneous tissue. Examples: acne scar, burn scar. |
| Atrophy | Depression of the skin surface caused by thinning of one or more layers of skin. Example: lichen sclerosis. |
| **Color** | The lesion should be described as red, yellow, brown, tan, or blue. Particular attention should be given to the blanching of red lesions. Failure to blanch suggests bleeding into the dermis (petechiae). |
| **Configuration of lesions** | |
| Annular (circular) | Annular nodules represent granuloma annulare; annular scaly papules are more apt to be caused by dermatophyte infections. |
| Linear (straight lines) | Linear papules represent lichen striatus; linear vesicles, incontinentia pigmenti; linear papules with burrows, scabies. |
| Grouped | Grouped vesicles occur in herpes simplex or zoster. |
| Discrete | Discrete lesions are independent of each other. |
| **Distribution** | Note whether the eruption is generalized, acral (hands, feet, buttocks, face), or localized to a specific skin region. |

***Table 14–2.*** Bases used for topical preparations.

| Base | Combined With | Uses |
|------|---------------|------|
| Liquids | | Wet dressings: relieve pruritus, vasoconstrict |
| | Powder | Shake lotions, drying pastes: relieve pruritus, vasoconstrict |
| | Grease and emulsifier; oil in water | Cream: penetrates quickly (10–15 min) and thus allows evaporation |
| | Excess grease and emulsifier; water in oil | Emollient cream: penetrates more slowly and thus retains moisture on skin |
| Grease | | Ointments: occlusive (hold material on skin for prolonged time) and prevent evaporation of water |
| Gel | | Transparent, colorless, semisolid emulsion: nongreasy, more drying and irritating than cream |
| Powder | | Enhances evaporation |

**Characteristics of bases for topical preparations:**
1. Most greases are triglycerides (eg, Aquaphor, petrolatum, Eucerin).
2. Oils are fluid fats (eg, Alpha Keri, olive oil, mineral oil).
3. True fats (eg, lard, animal fats) contain free fatty acids that cause irritation.
4. Ointments (eg, Aquaphor, petrolatum) should not be used in intertriginous areas such as the axillae, between the toes, and in the perineum, because they increase maceration. Lotions or creams are preferred in these areas.
5. Oils and ointments hold medication on the skin for long periods and are therefore ideal for barriers or prophylaxis and for dried areas of skin. Medication gets into the skin more slowly from ointments.
6. Creams carry medication into skin and are preferable for intertriginous dermatitis.
7. Solutions, gels, or lotions should be used for scalp treatments.

throughout the 24-hour period, maximum benefit is obtained after 72 hours; if treatment is applied only at night, maximum benefit is obtained after 7 days. When the condition has improved, the wet dressings are discontinued and a steroid ointment is applied twice daily. Daily application of steroids is not to be continued for more than 1 month. Only low-potency steroids (see Table 14–3) are applied to the face or intertriginous areas.

***Table 14–3.*** Topical glucocorticoids.

| Glucocorticoid | Concentrations |
|----------------|----------------|
| **Low potency[a] = 1–9** | |
| Hydrocortisone | 0.5% and 1% |
| Desonide | 0.05% |
| **Moderate potency = 10–99** | |
| Mometasone furoate | 0.1% |
| Hydrocortisone valerate | 0.2% |
| Fluocinolone acetonide | 0.025% |
| Triamcinolone acetonide | 0.01% |
| Amcinonide | 0.1% |
| **High potency = 100–499** | |
| Desoximetasone | 0.25% |
| Fluocinonide | 0.05% |
| Halcinonide | 0.1% |
| **Super potency = 500–7500** | |
| Betamethasone dipropionate | 0.05% |
| Clobetasol propionate | 0.05% |

[a]1% hydrocortisone is defined as having a potency of 1.

Bikowski J: The use of therapeutic moisturizers in various dermatology disorders. Cutis 2001;68(5 Suppl):3 [PMID: 11845952].

Brazzini B, Pimpinelli N: New and established topical corticosteroids in dermatology: Clinical pharmacology and therapeutic use. Am J Clin Dermatol 2002;3:47 [PMID: 11817968].

Schnopp C et al. Topical steroids under wet-wrap dressings in atopic dermatitis—A vehicle controlled trial. Dermatology 2002 204(1):56 [PMID: 11834851].

# ■ DISORDERS OF THE SKIN IN NEWBORNS

## TRANSIENT DISEASES IN NEWBORNS

### Milia

Multiple white papules 1 mm in diameter scattered over the forehead, nose, and cheeks are present in up to 40% of newborn infants. Histologically, they represent superficial epidermal cysts filled with keratinous material associated with the developing pilosebaceous follicle. Their intraoral counterparts are called Epstein pearls and are even more common than facial milia. All of these cystic structures spontaneously rupture and exfoliate their contents.

## Sebaceous Gland Hyperplasia

Prominent yellow macules at the opening of each pilosebaceous follicle, predominantly over the nose, represent overgrowth of sebaceous glands in response to the same androgenic stimulation that occurs in adolescence.

## Acne Neonatorum

Open and closed comedones, erythematous papules, and pustules identical in appearance to adolescent acne may occur in infants over the forehead, cheeks, and chin. The lesions may be present at birth but usually do not appear until age 4–6 weeks. Spontaneous resolution occurs over a period of 6 months to 1 year. Rarely, severe neonatal acne may be a manifestation of a virilizing syndrome.

## Harlequin Color Change

A cutaneous vascular phenomenon unique to neonates in the first week of life occurs when the infant (particularly one of low birth weight) is placed on one side. The dependent half develops an erythematous flush with a sharp demarcation at the midline, and the upper half of the body becomes pale. The color changes usually subside within a few seconds after the infant is placed supine but may persist for as long as 20 minutes.

## Mottling

A lace-like pattern of dilated cutaneous vessels appears over the extremities and often the trunk of neonates exposed to lowered room temperature. This feature is transient and usually disappears completely on rewarming.

## Erythema Toxicum

Up to 50% of full-term infants develop erythema toxicum. Usually at 24–48 hours of age, blotchy erythematous macules 2–3 cm in diameter appear, most prominently on the chest but also on the back, face, and extremities. These are occasionally present at birth. Onset after 4–5 days of life is rare. The lesions vary in number from a few up to as many as 100. Incidence is much higher in full-term infants than in premature ones. The macular erythema may fade within 24–48 hours or may progress to formation of urticarial wheals in the center of the macules or, in 10% of cases, pustules. Examination of a Wright-stained smear of the lesion will reveal numerous eosinophils. No organisms are seen on Gram stain. This may be accompanied by peripheral blood eosinophilia of up to 20%. All of the lesions fade and disappear within 5–7 days. A similar eruption in newborns of African descent, benign pustular melanosis, shows mostly neutrophils and leaves hyperpigmentation. Herpes simplex virus infection is in the differential diagnosis, but the infants are not ill and multinucleated giant cells are not present.

## Sucking Blisters

Bullae, either intact or as an erosion with a blister base without inflammatory borders, may occur over the forearms, wrists, thumbs, or upper lip. These presumably result from vigorous sucking in utero. They resolve without complications.

## Miliaria

Obstruction of the eccrine sweat ducts occurs often in neonates and produces one of two clinical pictures. Obstruction in the stratum corneum causes miliaria crystallina, characterized by tiny (1- to 2-mm), superficial grouped vesicles without erythema over intertriginous areas and adjacent skin (eg, neck, upper chest). More commonly, obstruction of the eccrine duct deeper in the epidermis results in erythematous grouped papules in the same areas and is called miliaria rubra. Rarely, these may progress to pustules. Heat and high humidity predispose the patient to eccrine duct pore closure. Removal to a cooler environment is the treatment of choice.

## Subcutaneous Fat Necrosis

Reddish or purple, sharply circumscribed, firm nodules occurring over the cheeks, buttocks, arms, and thighs and occurring between 1 and 7 days of life represent subcutaneous fat necrosis. Cold injury is thought to play an important role. These lesions resolve spontaneously over a period of weeks, although as in all instances of fat necrosis they may calcify.

Orchard D: Rashes in infants: Pitfalls and masquerades. Aust Fam Physician 2001;30:1047 [PMID: 11759454].

Verbov J: Common skin conditions in the newborn. Semin Neonatol 2000;5:303 [PMID: 11841650].

## PIGMENT CELL BIRTHMARKS, NEVI, & MELANOMA

Birthmarks may involve an overgrowth of one or more of any of the normal components of skin (eg, pigment cells, blood vessels, lymph vessels). A nevus is a hamartoma of highly differentiated cells that retain their normal function.

## Mongolian Spot

A blue-black macule found over the lumbosacral area in 90% of infants of Native American, African, and Asian descent is called a mongolian spot. These spots are occasionally noted over the shoulders and back and may extend over the buttocks. Histologically, they consist of spindle-shaped pigment cells located deep in the dermis. The lesions fade somewhat with time as a result of darkening of the overlying skin, but some traces may persist into adult life.

## Café au Lait Macule

A café au lait macule is a light brown, oval macule (dark brown on brown or black skin) that may be found anywhere on the body. Café au lait spots over 1.5 cm in greatest diameter are found in 10% of white and 22% of black children. These lesions persist throughout life and may increase in number with age. The presence of six or more such lesions over 1.5 cm in greatest diameter may be a clue to neurofibromatosis 1 (NF-1). Patients with Albright syndrome (see Chapter 30) also have increased numbers of café au lait macules. Most newborns with NF-1 will acquire the macules later.

## Spitz Nevus

A reddish brown solitary nodule appearing on the face or upper arm of a child represents a Spitz nevus. Histologically, it consists of pigment-producing cells of bizarre shape with numerous mitoses.

## Junctional Nevus & Compound Nevus

Dark brown or black macules, usually few in number at birth but becoming more numerous with age, represent junctional nevi. Histologically, these lesions are clones of melanocytes at the junction of the epidermis and dermis. With aging, they may become raised (papules) and contain intradermal melanocytes, creating a compound nevus. The surface may at times become irregular and roughened.

Brown to blue solitary papules with smooth surfaces represent intradermal nevi. When pigmentation is present deeper in the dermis, the lesions appear blue or blue-black and are called blue nevi.

## Melanoma

Pigmented lesions with variegated colors (red, white, blue), notched borders, and nonuniform, irregular surfaces should arouse a suspicion of melanoma. Ulceration and bleeding are advanced signs of melanoma. If melanoma is suspected, excisional biopsy for pathologic examination should be done as the treatment of choice.

## Giant Pigmented Nevus (Bathing Trunk Nevus)

An irregular dark brown to black plaque over at least 5% of the body surface represents a giant pigmented nevus. Often the lesions are of such size as to cover the entire trunk (bathing trunk nevi). Histologically, they are compound nevi. Transformation to malignant melanoma has been reported in as many as 10% of cases in some series, although the true incidence is probably much lower. Malignant change may occur in the neonatal period or at any time thereafter. Two thirds of melanoma in children with giant congenital pigmented nevi develop in areas other than the skin.

Tissue expanders may be useful in excision of large lesions. The risk of melanoma and the potential for cosmetic improvement should be evaluated carefully for each patient.

Fishman C et al: Diagnosis and management of nevi and cutaneous melanoma in infants and children. Clin Dermatol 2002;20: 44 [PMID: 11849894].

Makkar HS, Frieden IJ: Congenital melanocytic nevi: An update for the pediatrician. Curr Opin Pediatr 2002;14:397 [PMID: 12130901].

# VASCULAR BIRTHMARKS
## Capillary Malformations

Flat vascular birthmarks can be divided into two types: those that are orange or light red (salmon patch) and those that are dark red or bluish red (port-wine stain).

The salmon patch is a light red macule found over the nape of the neck, upper eyelids, and glabella. Fifty percent of infants have such lesions over their necks. Eyelid lesions fade completely within 3–6 months; those on the neck fade somewhat but usually persist into adult life.

Port-wine stains are dark red or purple macules appearing anywhere on the body. A bilateral facial port-wine stain or one covering the entire half of the face may be a clue to Sturge–Weber syndrome, which is characterized by seizures, mental retardation, glaucoma, and hemiplegia (Chapter 23). Most infants with smaller, unilateral facial port-wine stains do not have Sturge–Weber syndrome. Similarly, a port-wine stain over an extremity may be associated with hypertrophy of the soft tissue and bone of that extremity (Klippel–Trénaunay syndrome). The pulsed dye laser is the treatment of choice for infants and children with port-wine stains.

Rothfleisch JE et al: Laser treatment of congenital and acquired vascular lesions: A review. Dermatol Clin 2002;20:1 [PMID: 11859585].

## Hemangioma

A red, rubbery nodule with a roughened surface is a hemangioma. The lesion is often not present at birth but is represented by a permanent blanched area on the skin that is supplanted at age 2–4 weeks by red nodules. Histologically, these are benign tumors of capillary endothelial cells. Hemangiomas may be superficial, deep, or mixed. The terms strawberry and cavernous are misleading and should not be used. The biologic behavior of a hemangioma is the same despite its location. Fifty percent resolve spontaneously by age 5 years, 70% by age 7 years, and 90% by age 9 years, leaving redundant skin, hypopigmentation, and telangiectasia. Local complications include superficial ulceration and secondary pyoderma.

Complications that require immediate treatment are (1) airway obstruction (hemangiomas of the head and neck may be associated with subglottic hemangiomas), (2) visual obstruction (with resulting amblyopia), and (3) cardiac decompensation (high-output failure). In these instances, the treatment of choice is with prednisone, 2–4 mg/kg orally daily for 4–6 weeks. Interferon alfa-2a has been used to treat serious hemangiomas unresponsive to prednisone. Ten percent of patients with hemangiomas treated with interferon alfa-2a have developed spastic diplegia. Therefore, interferon alfa-2a therapy should be reserved for truly life-threatening hemangiomas. If the lesion is ulcerated or bleeding, pulsed dye laser treatment may be helpful. The Kasabach–Merritt syndrome, which is platelet trapping with consumption coagulopathy, does not occur with hemangiomas. It is seen only with the very rare vascular tumors called hemangioendotheliomas and tufted angiomas.

Bruckner AL, Frieden IJ: Hemangiomas of infancy. J Am Acad Dermatol 2003;48:477 [PMID: 12664009].

David LR et al: Br J Plast Surg 2003;56:317 [PMID: 12873458].

## Lymphatic Malformations

Lymphatic malformations may be superficial or deep. Superficial lymphatic malformations present as fluid-filled vesicles often described as looking like frog spawn. Deep lymphatic malformations are rubbery, skin-colored nodules occurring in the parotid area (cystic hygromas) or on the tongue. They often result in grotesque enlargement of soft tissues. Surgical excision is the only treatment, although the results are not satisfactory.

Fliegelman LJ et al: Lymphatic malformations: Predictive factors for recurrence. Otolaryngol Head Neck Surg 2000;123:706 [PMID: 11112962].

## EPIDERMAL BIRTHMARKS

### Epidermal Nevus

Linear or groups of linear, warty, papular, unilateral lesions represent overgrowth of epidermis since birth. These areas may range from dirty yellow to brown or may be darkly pigmented. The histologic features of the lesions include thickening of the epidermis and elongation of the rete ridges and hyperkeratosis. Clinically, widespread lesions may be associated with focal motor seizures, mental subnormality, and skeletal anomalies.

Treatment once or twice daily with topical calcipotriene may improve the lesions.

Dosik JS: Epidermal nevus. Dermatol Online J 2001;7:14 [PMID: 11328635].

Happle R, Rogers M: Epidermal nevi. Adv Dermatol 2002;18:175 [PMID: 12528406].

Lee SH, Rogers M: Inflammatory linear verrucous epidermal naevi: A review of 23 cases. Australas J Dermatol 2001;42:252 [PMID: 11903156].

### Nevus Comedonicus

The lesion known as nevus comedonicus consists of linear groups of widely dilated follicular openings plugged with keratin, giving the appearance of localized noninflammatory acne. The treatment of choice is surgical removal. If this is not feasible, topical retinoic acid may be helpful.

Lefkowitz A et al: Nevus comedonicus. Dermatology 1999;199:204 [PMID: 10592398].

### Nevus Sebaceus

The nevus sebaceus of Jadassohn is a hamartoma of sebaceous glands and underlying apocrine glands that is diagnosed by the appearance at birth of a yellowish, hairless, smooth plaque in the scalp or on the face. The lesion may be contiguous with an epidermal nevus on the face and constitute part of the linear epidermal nevus syndrome.

Histologically, nevus sebaceus represents an overabundance of sebaceous glands without hair follicles. At puberty, with androgenic stimulation, the sebaceous cells in the nevus divide, expand their cellular volume, and synthesize sebum, resulting in a warty mass. Because 15% of these lesions become basal cell carcinomas after puberty, excision is recommended before puberty.

Cribier B et al: Tumors arising in nevus sebaceus: A study of 596 cases. J Am Acad Dermatol 2000;42:263 [PMID: 10642683].

## CONNECTIVE TISSUE BIRTHMARKS (Juvenile Elastoma, Collagenoma)

Connective tissue nevi are smooth, skin-colored papules 1–10 mm in diameter that are grouped on the trunk. A solitary, larger (5–10 cm) nodule is called a shagreen patch and is histologically indistinguishable from other connective tissue nevi that show thickened, abundant collagen bundles with or without associated increases of elastic tissue. Although the shagreen patch is a cutaneous clue to tuberous sclerosis (Chapter 23), the other connective tissue nevi occur as isolated events. These nevi remain throughout life and need no treatment.

Batta K: Management of large birthmarks. Semin Neonatol 2000;5:325 [PMID: 11032717].

## HEREDITARY SKIN DISORDERS

### Ichthyosis

Ichthyosis is a term applied to several heritable diseases characterized by the presence of excessive scales on the skin. Major categories are listed in Table 14–4. Treatment consists of controlling scaling with lactic acid with ammonium hydroxide (Lac-Hydrin) 12% applied once daily. Restoring water to the skin is also very helpful.

DiGiovanni JJ, Robinson-Bostom L: Ichthyosis: Etiology, diagnosis and management. Am J Clin Dermatol 2003;4:81 [PMID: 12553849].

### Epidermolysis Bullosa

The diagnostic feature of this group of diseases is the formation of blisters in response to slight trauma. They can be divided into scarring and nonscarring types (Table 14–5).

Treatment usually consists of systemic antibiotics for infection, protection of the skin with petrolatum, zinc oxide, or synthetic dressings, and cooling the skin. If hands and feet are involved, reducing skin friction with 5% glutaraldehyde every 3 days is helpful.

Fine JD et al: Revised classification system for inherited epidermolysis bullosa: Report of the Second International Consensus Meeting on etiology and classification of epidermolysis bullosa. J Am Acad Dermatol 2000;42:1051 [PMID: 10827412].

Moss C: Genetic skin disorders. Semin Neonatol 2000;5:311 [PMID: 11036715].

Pai S, Marinkovich MP: Epidermolysis bullosa: New and emerging trends. Am J Clin Dermatol 2002;3:371 [PMID: 12113646].

## ■ COMMON SKIN DISEASES IN INFANTS, CHILDREN, & ADOLESCENTS

### ACNE

The common forms of acne in pediatric patients occur at two ages: in the newborn period and in adolescence. Neonatal acne is a response to maternal androgen, first appearing at age 4–6 weeks and lasting until age 4–6 months. The lesions are primarily on the face, upper chest, and back, in a distribution similar to that

***Table 14–4.*** Four major types of ichthyosis.

| Name | Age at Onset | Clinical Features | Genetic Defect | Inheritance |
|---|---|---|---|---|
| **Ichthyosis with normal epidermal turnover** | | | | |
| Ichthyosis vulgaris | Childhood | Fine scales, deep palmar and plantar markings | Filaggrin/profilaggrin | Autosomal-dominant |
| X-linked ichthyosis | Birth | Palms and soles spared; thick scales that darken with age; corneal opacities in patients and carrier mothers | Cholesterol sulfatase | X-linked |
| **Ichthyosis with increased epidermal turnover** | | | | |
| Epidermolytic hyper-keratosis | Birth | Verrucous, yellow scales in flexural areas and palms and soles | Keratins 1 and 10 | Autosomal-dominant |
| Lamellar ichthyosis | Birth; collodion baby | Erythroderma, ectropion, large coarse scales; thickened palms and soles | Transglutaminase 1 | Autosomal-recessive |

***Table 14–5.*** Types of epidermolysis bullosa.

| Name | Age at Onset | Clinical Features | Genetic Defect | Inheritance |
|---|---|---|---|---|
| **Nonscarring types** | | | | |
| Epidermolysis bullosa simplex | Birth | Hemorrhagic blisters over the lower legs; cooling prevents blisters | Keratins 5 and 14 | Autosomal-dominant |
| Recurrent bullous eruption of the hands and feet (Weber–Cockayne syndrome) | First few years of life | Blisters brought out by walking | Keratins 5 and 14 | Autosomal-dominant |
| Junctional bullous dermolysis (Herlitz disease) | Birth | Erosions on legs, oral mucosa; severe peri-oral involvement | Laminin V | Autosomal-recessive |
| **Scarring types** | | | | |
| Epidermolysis bullosa dystro-phica, dominant | Infancy | Numerous blisters on hands and feet; milia formation | Type VII collagen | Autosomal-dominant |
| Epidermolysis bullosa dystro-phica, recessive | Birth | Repeated episodes of blistering, secondary infection and scarring—"mitten hands and feet" | Type VII collagen | Autosomal-recessive |

seen in adolescent acne. It has been hypothesized, but not proved, that infants who have severe neonatal acne will develop severe adolescent acne.

The onset of adolescent acne is between ages 8 and 10 years in 40% of children. The early lesions are usually limited to the face and are primarily closed comedones (whiteheads; see following discussion). Eventually, 85% of adolescents develop some form of acne.

## Clinical Findings

Acne occurs in sebaceous follicles, which, unlike hair follicles, have large, abundant sebaceous glands and usually lack hair. They are located primarily on the face, upper chest, back, and penis. Obstruction of the sebaceous follicle opening produces the clinical lesion of acne. If the obstruction occurs at the follicular mouth, the clinical lesion is characterized by a wide, patulous opening filled with a plug of stratum corneum cells. This is the open comedo, or blackhead. Open comedones are the predominant clinical lesion in early adolescent acne. The black color is caused not by dirt but by oxidized melanin within the stratum corneum cellular plug. Open comedones do not often progress to inflammatory lesions. Closed comedones, or white-heads, are caused by obstruction just beneath the follicular opening in the neck of the sebaceous follicle, which produces a cystic swelling of the follicular duct directly beneath the epidermis. The stratum corneum produced

accumulates continuously within the cystic cavity. The resultant lesion is an enlarging sphere just beneath the skin surface. Most authorities believe that closed comedones are precursors of inflammatory acne. If open or closed comedones are the predominant lesions on the skin in adolescent acne, the condition is called comedonal acne.

In typical adolescent acne, several different types of lesions are present simultaneously, for example, open and closed comedones and inflammatory lesions such as papules, pustules, and cysts. Inflammatory lesions may also rarely occur as interconnecting, draining sinus tracts. Adolescents with cystic acne require prompt medical attention, because ruptured cysts and sinus tracts result in severe scar formation. New acne scars are highly vascular and have a reddish or purplish hue. Such scars return to normal skin color after several years. Acne scars may be depressed beneath the skin level, raised, or flat to the skin. In adolescents with a tendency toward keloid formation, keloidal scars can occur following acne lesions, particularly over the sternal area.

## Differential Diagnosis

Consider rosacea, nevus comedonicus, flat warts, miliaria, molluscum contagiosum, and the angiofibromas of tuberous sclerosis.

## Pathogenesis

The primary event in acne formation is obstruction of the sebaceous follicle. Ordinarily the lining of such follicles contains one or two layers of stratum corneum cells, but in acne the stratum corneum is overproduced. This phenomenon is androgen-dependent in adolescent acne. The sebaceous follicles contain an enzyme, testosterone 5α-reductase, which converts plasma testosterone to dihydrotestosterone. This androgen is a potent stimulus for nuclear division of the follicular germinative cells and subsequently of excessive cell production. Thus obstruction requires the presence of both circulating androgens and the converting enzyme. After the production or administration of androgens, a delay results until cellular proliferation occurs, followed by follicular obstruction.

The pathogenesis of inflammatory acne is not well understood. Undoubtedly, physical manipulation of a closed comedo could lead to rupture of the cavity contents into the dermis with a subsequent inflammatory response. Spontaneous inflammation also occurs in obstructed follicles, but the reason for this is unclear. An attractive hypothesis is that overgrowth of gram-positive bacteria in the obstructed follicle (either *Propionibacterium acnes* or *Staphylococcus epidermidis*) might stimulate factors that initiate inflammation. Overproduction of sebum and free fatty acid formation seem unlikely as causes of inflammation in acne as presently understood.

Adolescent acne may be worsened by several external causes. Frictional acne caused by headbands, football helmets, or tight-fitting brassieres or other garments occurs predominantly underneath the area where the garment is worn. Oil-based cosmetics may be responsible for predominantly comedonal acne, and hair sprays may produce acne along the hair margin.

Drug-induced acne should be suspected in teenagers if all lesions are in the same stage at the same time and if involvement extends to the lower abdomen, lower back, arms, and legs. Drugs responsible for acne include corticotropin (ACTH), glucocorticoids, androgens, hydantoins, and isoniazid, each of which increases plasma testosterone.

## Treatment

Different treatment options are listed in Table 14–6.

### A. TOPICAL KERATOLYTIC AGENTS

The mainstay of acne therapy is the use of potent topical keratolytic agents applied to the skin to relieve follicular obstruction. The most effective keratolytic agents are the retinoids; tretinoin (retinoic acid), adapalene, and tazarotene. The agents may be used once

**Table 14–6.** Acne treatment.

| | |
|---|---|
| Comedonal acne | One of the following:<br>Retinoic acid, 0.025, 0.05, or 0.1% cream; 0.01 or 0.025% gel; or 0.1% microgel<br>Adapalene, 0.1% gel or solution |
| Papular inflammatory acne | One from first grouping, plus one of the following:<br>Topical antibiotics<br>Benzoyl peroxide, 2.5, 4, 5, 8, or 10% gel or lotion; 4 or 8% wash<br>Azaleic acid, 20% cream<br>Clindamycin, 1% lotion, solution, or gel |
| Pustular inflammatory acne | One from first grouping, plus one of the following:<br>Oral antibiotics<br>Tetracycline or erythromycin, 250–500 mg, bid<br>Minocycline or doxycycline, 50–100 mg, bid |
| Nodulocystic acne | Accutane, 1 mg/kg/day |

daily, or the combination of a retinoid applied to acne-bearing areas of the skin once daily in the evening and a benzoyl peroxide gel or azaleic acid applied once daily in the morning may be used. This regimen will control 80–85% of cases of adolescent acne.

### B. TOPICAL ANTIBIOTICS

Topical antibiotics are used to avoid the side effects caused by systemic antibiotics. Topical antibiotics are less effective than systemic antibiotics and at best are equivalent in potency to 250 mg of tetracycline orally once a day. One percent clindamycin phosphate solution is the most efficacious topical antibiotic. Most *P acnes* are now resistant to topical erythromycin solutions.

### C. SYSTEMIC ANTIBIOTICS

Antibiotics that are concentrated in sebum, such as tetracycline, minocycline, and doxycycline, are very effective in inflammatory acne. The usual dose of tetracycline is 0.5–1 g; of minocycline and doxycycline, 50–100 mg taken once or twice daily on an empty stomach (nothing to eat 1 hour before or after the medication). Treatment should be continued for 2–3 months until the acne lesions are suppressed.

### D. ORAL RETINOIDS

An oral retinoid, 13-*cis*-retinoic acid (isotretinoin; Accutane), is the most effective treatment for severe cystic acne. The precise mechanism of its action is unknown, but decreased sebum production, decreased follicular obstruction, decreased skin bacteria, and general anti-inflammatory activities have been described. The initial dosage is 40 mg once or twice daily. This drug is not effective in comedonal acne or other mild forms of acne. Side effects include dryness and scaliness of the skin, dry lips, and, occasionally, dry eyes and dry nose. Up to 10% of patients experience mild, reversible hair loss. Elevated liver enzymes and blood lipids have rarely been described. Acute depression may occur. Isotretinoin is teratogenic in young women of childbearing age. Because of this and the other side effects, it is not recommended unless strict adherence to the FDA guidelines is ensured. Accutane prescribers must now be certified.

### E. OTHER ACNE TREATMENTS

No convincing evidence supports the contention that dietary management, mild drying agents, abrasive scrubs, oral vitamin A, ultraviolet light, cryotherapy, and incision and drainage have any beneficial effects in the management of acne.

### F. AVOIDANCE OF COSMETICS AND HAIR SPRAY

Acne can be aggravated by a variety of external factors that result in further obstruction of partially occluded sebaceous follicles. Discontinuing the use of oil-based cosmetics, face creams, and hair sprays may alleviate the comedonal component of acne within 4–6 weeks.

## Patient Education & Follow-Up Visits

The mechanism of acne formation and the treatment plan must be explained to adolescent patients. Time should be set aside at the first visit to answer questions. Explain that there will not be much improvement for 4–8 weeks. Fifty percent improvement at 8–12 weeks is considered average. Establish guidelines for ideal control and explain that the best result the patient can expect is the appearance of only one or two new pimples a month. No drug is available that will prevent an adolescent from ever having another acne lesion. A written education sheet is useful.

Follow-up visits should be made every 6–8 weeks. The criterion for ideal control is a few lesions every 4 weeks. Explain again what medications are being used and what the treatment is intended to achieve, and question the patient to determine whether the medications are being used properly.

Gollnick H, Cunliffe W: Management of acne: A report from a global alliance to improve outcomes in acne. J Am Acad Dermatol 2003;49:S1 [PMID: 12833004].

# BACTERIAL INFECTIONS OF THE SKIN

## Impetigo

Erosions covered by honey-colored crusts are diagnostic of impetigo. Staphylococci and group A streptococci are important pathogens in this disease, which histologically consists of superficial invasion of bacteria into the upper epidermis, forming a subcorneal pustule.

Impetigo should be treated with an antimicrobial agent effective against *Staphylococcus aureus* (β-lactamase-resistant penicillins or cephalosporins, clindamycin, amoxicillin–clavulanate) for 7–10 days. Topical mupirocin (three times daily) is also effective.

## Bullous Impetigo

All impetigo is bullous, with the blister forming just beneath the stratum corneum, but in bullous impetigo there is, in addition to the usual erosion covered by a honey-colored crust, a border filled with clear fluid. Staphylococci may be isolated from these lesions, and systemic signs of circulating exfoliatin are absent. Bullous varicella is a disorder that represents bullous impetigo as a superinfection in varicella lesions. Treatment with oral antistaphylococcal drugs for 7–10 days is effective. Application of cool compresses to debride crusts is a helpful symptomatic measure.

## Ecthyma

Ecthyma is a firm, dry crust, surrounded by erythema that exudes purulent material. It represents deep invasion by group A β-hemolytic streptococci through the epidermis to the superficial dermis. Treatment is with systemic penicillin. This should not be confused with ecthyma gangrenosum. Lesions of ecthyma gangrenosum may be similar in appearance, but they are seen in a severely ill or immunocompromised patient and are due to systemic dissemination of bacteria, usually *Pseudomonas aeruginosa,* through the bloodstream.

## Cellulitis

Cellulitis is characterized by erythematous, hot, tender, ill-defined, edematous plaques accompanied by regional lymphadenopathy. Histologically, this disorder represents invasion of microorganisms into the lower dermis and sometimes beyond, with obstruction of local lymphatics. Group A β-hemolytic streptococci and coagulase-positive staphylococci are the most common causes; pneumococci and *Haemophilus influenzae* are rare causes. Staphylococcal infections are usually more localized and more likely to have a purulent center; streptococcal infections spread more rapidly, but these characteristics cannot be used to specify the infecting agent. An entry site of prior trauma or infection (eg, varicella) is often present. Septicemia is a potential complication. Treatment is with an appropriate systemic antibiotic.

## Folliculitis

A pustule at a follicular opening represents folliculitis. If the pustule occurs at eccrine sweat orifices, it is correctly called poritis. Staphylococci and streptococci are the most frequent pathogens. Treatment consists of measures to remove follicular obstruction—either cool, wet compresses for 24 hours or keratolytics such as those used for acne.

## Abscess

An abscess occurs deep in the skin, at the bottom of a follicle or an apocrine gland, and is diagnosed as an erythematous, firm, acutely tender nodule with ill-defined borders. Staphylococci are the most common organisms. Treatment consists of incision and drainage and systemic antibiotics.

## Scalded Skin Syndrome

This entity consists of the sudden onset of bright red, acutely painful skin, most obvious periorally, periorbitally, and in the flexural areas of the neck, the axillae, the popliteal and antecubital areas, and the groin. The slightest pressure on the skin results in severe pain and separation of the epidermis, leaving a glistening layer (the stratum granulosum of the epidermis) beneath. The disease is caused by a circulating toxin (exfoliatin) elaborated by phage group II staphylococci. The site of action of the exfoliatin is the intracellular area of the granular layer, resulting in a separation of cells. The causative staphylococci may be isolated not from the skin but rather from the nasopharynx, an abscess, sinus, blood culture, and so on. Treatment is with systemic antistaphylococcal drugs.

Chilller K et al: Skin microflora and bacterial infection of the skin. J Investig Dermatol Symp Proc 2001;6:170 [PMID: 11924823].

Oumeish I et al: Acute bacterial skin infections in children. Clin Dermatol 2000;18:667 [PMID: 11173202].

# FUNGAL INFECTIONS OF THE SKIN

## 1. Dermatophyte Infections

Dermatophytes become attached to the superficial layer of the epidermis, nails, and hair, where they proliferate. They grow mainly within the stratum corneum and do not invade the lower epidermis or dermis. Release of toxins from dermatophytes, especially those whose natural host is animals or soil, for example, *Microsporum canis* and *Trichophyton verrucosum*—results in dermatitis. Fungal infection should be suspected with any red and scaly lesion.

## Classification & Diagnosis

### A. TINEA CAPITIS

Thickened, broken-off hairs with erythema and scaling of underlying scalp are the distinguishing features (Table 14–7). In epidemic ringworm, hairs are broken off at the surface of the scalp, leaving a "black dot" appearance. Pustule formation and a boggy, fluctuant mass on the scalp occur in *M canis* and *T tonsurans* infections. This mass, called a kerion, represents an exaggerated host response to the organism. Diffuse scaling of the scalp may also be seen. Fungal culture should be performed in all cases of suspected tinea capitis.

### B. TINEA CORPORIS

Tinea corporis presents either as annular marginated papules with a thin scale and clear center or as an annular confluent dermatitis. The most common organisms are *Trichophyton mentagrophytes* and *M canis*. The diagnosis is made by scraping thin scales from the border of the lesion, dissolving them in 20% KOH, and examining for hyphae.

### C. TINEA CRURIS

Symmetrical, sharply marginated lesions in inguinal areas occur with tinea cruris. The most common organisms are *Trichophyton rubrum*, *T mentagrophytes*, and *Epidermophyton floccosum*.

### D. TINEA PEDIS

The diagnosis of tinea pedis in a prepubertal child must always be regarded with skepticism; atopic feet or con-

**Table 14–7.** Clinical features of tinea capitis.

| Most Common Organisms | Clinical Appearance | Microscopic Appearance in KOH |
|---|---|---|
| *Trichophyton tonsurans* (90%) | Hairs broken off 2–3 mm from follicle; "black dot"; no fluorescence | Hyphae and spores within hair |
| *Microsporum canis* (10%) | Thickened broken-off hairs that fluoresce yellow-green with Wood's lamp | Small spores outside of hair; hyphae within hair |

tact dermatitis is a more likely diagnosis in this age group. Tinea pedis occurs most commonly in postpubertal males with blisters on the instep of the foot. Fissuring between the toes is occasionally seen.

### E. Tinea Unguium (Onychomycosis)

Loosening of the nail plate from the nail bed (onycholysis), giving a yellow discoloration, is the first sign of fungal invasion of the nails. Thickening of the distal nail plate then occurs, followed by scaling and a crumbly appearance of the entire nail plate surface. *T rubrum* and *T mentagrophytes* are the most common causes. The diagnosis is confirmed by KOH examination and fungal culture. Usually only one or two nails are involved. If every nail is involved, psoriasis, lichen planus, or idiopathic trachyonychia is a more likely diagnosis than fungal infection.

## Treatment

The treatment of dermatophytosis is quite simple: If hair is involved, griseofulvin is the treatment of choice. Topical antifungal agents do not enter hair or nails in sufficient concentration to clear the infection. The absorption of griseofulvin from the gastrointestinal tract is enhanced by a fatty meal; thus, whole milk or ice cream taken with the medication increases absorption. The dosage of griseofulvin is 20 mg/kg/d. With hair infections, cultures should be done every 4 weeks, and treatment should be continued for 6–8 weeks following a negative culture. The side effects are few, and the drug has been used successfully in the newborn period. Itraconazole and terbinafine have been used when response to griseofulvin is unsatisfactory. For nails, daily administration of topical ciclopirox 8% (Penlac nail lacquer) can be considered, as can pulsed-dose itraconazole given in three 1-week pulses separated by 3 weeks.

Tinea corporis, tinea pedis, and tinea cruris can be treated effectively with topical medication after careful inspection to make certain that the hair and nails are not involved. Treatment with clotrimazole (Lotrimin), miconazole (Micatin), econazole (Spectazole), terbinafine (Lamisil), or haloprogin (Halotex) applied twice daily for 3–4 weeks is recommended.

Pomeranz AJ, Sabnis SS: Tinea capitis: Epidemiology, diagnosis and management strategies. Paediatr Drugs 2002;4:779 [PMID: 1241130].

## 2. Tinea Versicolor

Tinea versicolor is a superficial infection caused by *Pityrosporum orbiculare* (also called *Malassezia furfur*), a yeast-like fungus. It characteristically causes polycyclic connected hypopigmented macules and very fine scales in areas of sun-induced pigmentation. In winter, the polycyclic macules appear reddish brown.

Treatment consists of application of selenium sulfide (Selsun), 2.5% suspension, or topical antifungals. Selenium sulfide should be applied to the whole body and left on overnight. Treatment can be repeated again in 1 week and then monthly thereafter. It tends to be somewhat irritating, and the patient should be warned about this difficulty.

VanderStraten MR et al: Cutaneous infections dermatophytosis, onychomychosis and tinea versicolor. Infect Dis North Am 2003;17:87 [PMID: 12751262].

## 3. Candida albicans *Infections* (See also Chapter 39.)

In addition to being a frequent invader in diaper dermatitis, *Candida albicans* also infects the oral mucosa, where it appears as thick white patches with an erythematous base (thrush); the angles of the mouth, where it causes fissures and white exudate (perleche); and the cuticular region of the fingers, where thickening of the cuticle, dull red erythema, and distortion of growth of the nail plate suggest the diagnosis of candidal paronychia. *Candida* dermatitis is characterized by sharply defined erythematous patches, sometimes with eroded areas. Pustules, vesicles, or papules may be present as satellite lesions. Similar infections may be found in other moist areas, such as the axillae and neck folds. This infection is more common in children who have recently received antibiotics.

A topical imidazole cream is the drug of first choice for *C albicans* infections. In diaper dermatitis, the cream form can be applied every 3–4 hours. In oral thrush, nystatin suspension should be applied directly to the mucosa with the parent's finger or a cotton-tipped applicator, because it is not absorbed and acts topically. In candidal paronychia, the antifungal agent is applied over the area, covered with occlusive plastic wrapping, and left on overnight after the application is made airtight. Refractory candidiasis will respond to a brief course of oral fluconazole.

Hay RJ: The management of superficial candidiasis. J Am Acad Dermatol 1999;40:S35 [PMID: 10367915].

## VIRAL INFECTIONS OF THE SKIN (See Chapter 36.)

### Herpes Simplex

Grouped vesicles or grouped erosions suggest herpes simplex. The microscopic finding of epidermal giant cells after scraping the vesicle base with a No. 15 blade, smearing on a slide, and staining with Wright stain (Tzanck smear) suggests herpes simplex or varicella-zoster. Rapid immunofluorescent tests for herpes simplex virus and varicella-zoster virus are available. In infants, lesions resulting from herpes simplex type 1 are seen on the gingiva and lips, periorbitally, or on the thumb in children who suck their thumbs. Recurrent erosions in the mouth are usually aphthous stomatitis in children rather than recurrent herpes simplex. Herpes simplex type 2 lesions are seen on the genitalia and in the mouth in adolescents. Cutaneous dissemination of herpes simplex occurs in patients with atopic dermatitis (eczema herpeticum, Kaposi varicelliform eruption). The treatment of herpes simplex virus infections is discussed in Chapter 36.

Whitley RJ: Herpes simplex virus in children. Curr Treat Options Neurol 2002;4:231 [PMID: 11931730].

## Varicella-Zoster

Grouped vesicles in a dermatome, usually on the trunk or face, suggest varicella-zoster infection. Zoster in children may not be painful and usually has a mild course. In patients with compromised host resistance, the appearance of an erythematous border around the vesicles is a good prognostic sign. Conversely, large bullae without a tendency to crusting and systemic illness imply a poor host response to the virus. Varicella-zoster and herpes simplex lesions undergo the same series of changes: papule, vesicle, pustule, crust, slightly depressed scar. Varicella appears in crops, and many different stages of lesions are present at the same time.

Itching is usually the only symptom, and cool baths as frequently as necessary or drying lotions such as calamine lotion are sufficient to relieve symptoms. In immunosuppressed children, intravenous or oral acyclovir should be used.

Chen TM et al: Clinical manifestations of varicella-zoster virus infection. Dermatol Clin 2002;20:267 [PMID: 12120440].

Emmert DH: Treatment of common cutaneous herpes simplex virus infections. Am Fam Physician 2000;15:1697 [PMID: 10750877].

## Human Immunodeficiency Virus Infection (See also Chapter 37.)

The average time of onset of skin lesions after perinatally acquired human immunodeficiency virus (HIV) infection is 4 months; after transfusion-acquired infection, it is 11 months. Persistent oral candidiasis and recalcitrant candidal diaper rash are the most frequent cutaneous features of infantile HIV infection. Severe or recurrent herpetic gingivostomatitis, varicella-zoster infection, and molluscum contagiosum infection occur.

Recurrent staphylococcal pyodermas, tinea of the face, and onychomycosis are also observed. A generalized dermatitis with features of seborrhea is extremely common. In general, persistent, recurrent, or extensive skin infections should make one suspicious of HIV infection.

Garman ME, Tyring SK: The cutaneous manifestations of HIV infection. Dermatol Clin 2002;20:193 [PMID: 12120434].

Laude TA: Manifestations of HIV disease in children. Clin Dermatol 2000;18:457 [PMID: 11024313].

Stefanaki C et al: Skin manifestations of HIV-1 infection in children. Clin Dermatol 2002;20:74 [PMID: 11849897].

Wananukul S et al: Mucocutaneous findings in pediatric AIDS related to degree of immunosuppression. Pediatr Dermatol 2003;20:289 [PMID: 1286945].

## Virus-Induced Tumors

### A. Molluscum Contagiosum

Molluscum contagiosum is a poxvirus that induces the epidermis to proliferate, forming a pale papule. Molluscum contagiosum consists of umbilicated, white or whitish yellow papules in groups on the genitalia or trunk. They are common in sexually active adolescents and in infants and preschool children. Molluscum lesions in general are treated in the same manner as warts. Treatment for molluscum includes benign neglect, topical imiquimod, topical cantharidin, oral cimetidine, and curettage.

Smith KJ, Skelton H: Molluscum contagiosum: Recent advances in pathogenic mechanisms and new therapies. Am J Clin Dermatol 2002;3:535 [PMID: 12358555].

### B. Warts

Warts are skin-colored papules with irregular (verrucous) surfaces. They are intraepidermal tumors caused by infection with human papillomavirus. This DNA virus induces the epidermal cells to proliferate, thus resulting in the warty growth. Flat warts are smoother and smaller than common warts and are often seen on the face.

No therapy for warts is ideal, and some types of therapy should be avoided because the recurrence rate of warts is high. For flat warts, a good response to 0.05% tretinoin cream or topical imiquimod (Aldara) cream, applied once daily for 3–4 weeks, has been reported.

The best treatment for the solitary common (vulgaris) wart is to freeze it with liquid nitrogen. The liquid nitrogen should be allowed to drip from the cotton-tipped applicator onto the wart without pressure. Pressure exaggerates cold injury by causing vasoconstriction and may produce a deep ulcer and scar. Liquid nitrogen is applied by drip until the wart turns completely white and stays white for 20–25 seconds. Large and painful plantar warts are treated most effectively by applying 40% salicylic acid plaster cut with a scissors to fit the lesion. The sticky brown side of the plaster is placed against the lesion, taped on securely with adhesive tape, and left on for 5 days. The plaster is then removed, and the white necrotic warty tissue can be gently rubbed off with a pumice stone and a new salicylic acid plaster applied. This procedure is repeated every 5 days, and the patient is seen every 4 weeks. Most plantar warts resolve in 6–8 weeks when treated in this way. Vascular pulsed dye lasers are a useful adjunct therapy for the treatment of plantar warts.

Sharp scalpel excision, electrosurgery, and nonspecific burning laser surgery should be avoided, because the resulting scar often becomes a more difficult problem than the wart itself and the wart may recur in the area of the scar.

Venereal warts (condylomata acuminata) (see Chapter 40) may be treated with imiquimod, 25% podophyllum resin (podophyllin) in alcohol, or podofilox, a lower concentration of purified podophyllin. Podophyllin should be painted on the lesions and then washed off after 4 hours. Retreatment in 2–3 weeks may be necessary. Podofilox is applied daily, whereas imiquimod is used on Monday, Wednesday, and Friday. A wart not on the vulvar mucous membrane but on the adjacent skin should be treated as a common wart and frozen.

For isolated warts and periungual warts, cantharidin is effective and painless in children. It causes a blister and sometimes is difficult to control. An undesirable complication is the appearance of warts along the margins of the cantharidin blister. Cantharidin is applied to the skin, allowed to dry, and covered with occlusive tape or a bandage for 24 hours.

No wart therapy is immediately and definitively successful, and recurrences are reported in more than 30% of cases even with the best care.

Allen AL, Siegfried EC: What's new in human papillomavirus infection. Curr Opin Pediatr 2000;12:365 [PMID: 10943818].

Savrin C: Human papillomavirus in children. Adv Nurse Pract 2001;9:99 [PMID: 12400281].

# INSECT INFESTATIONS

## Scabies

Scabies is suggested by linear burrows about the wrists, ankles, finger webs, areolas, anterior axillary folds, genitalia, or face (in infants). Often there are excoriations, honey-colored crusts, and pustules from secondary infection. Identification of the female mite or her eggs

and feces is necessary to confirm the diagnosis. Scrape an unscratched papule or burrow with a No. 15 blade and examine microscopically in immersion oil to confirm the diagnosis. In a child who is often scratching, scrape under the fingernails. Examine the parents for unscratched burrows.

Lindane (γ-benzene hexachloride; Kwell) and permethrin are excellent scabicides. However, because lindane is concentrated in the central nervous system, where toxicity from systemic absorption in infants has been reported, the following restricted use of this agent is recommended: (1) For adults and older children, one treatment of lindane lotion or cream applied to the entire body and left on for 4 hours, followed by showering, is sufficient. (2) Infants tend to have more organisms and many more lesions and may have to be retreated in 7–10 days. All family members should be treated simultaneously. Permethrin 5% cream (Elimite) may be substituted for lindane in infants.

## Pediculoses (Louse Infestations)

The presence of excoriated papules and pustules and a history of severe itching at night suggest infestation with the human body louse. This louse may be discovered in the seams of underwear but not on the body. In the scalp hair, the gelatinous nits of the head louse adhere tightly to the hair shaft. The pubic louse may be found crawling among pubic hairs, or blue-black macules may be found dispersed through the pubic region (maculae ceruleae). The pubic louse is often seen on the eyelashes of newborns.

Lindane (γ-benzene hexachloride; Kwell) is recommended: For head lice, a shampoo preparation is left on the scalp for 5 minutes and rinsed out thoroughly. The hair is then combed with a fine-tooth comb to remove nits. This may be repeated in 7 days. Lindane cream or lotion applied to the body for 4 hours may be necessary for body lice, but boiling the clothing for 10 minutes followed by ironing the seams with a hot iron usually eliminates them. Permethrin 1% creme rinse also eliminates lice. Lindane cream or lotion applied to the pubic area for 24 hours is sufficient to treat pediculosis pubis. It may be repeated in 4–5 days. Permethrin 5% cream (Elimite) may be substituted for lindane in infants.

Angel TA et al: Infestations in the pediatric patient. Pediatr Clin North Am 2000;47:921 [PMID: 10943266].

Lafuente CR: Is it scabies? How to tell. Nurse Pract 2003;28: 57 [PMID: 12796625].

Roberts RJ: Clinical practice. Head lice. N Engl J Med 2002; 346:1645 [PMID: 12023998].

Venna S et al: Scabies and lice: Review of the clinical features and management principles. Dermatol Nurs 2001;13:257 [PMID: 11917782].

## Papular Urticaria

Papular urticaria is characterized by grouped erythematous papules surrounded by an urticarial flare and distributed over the shoulders, upper arms, and buttocks in infants. Although not a true infestation, these lesions represent delayed hypersensitivity reactions to stinging or biting insects and can be reproduced by patch testing with the offending insect. Fleas from dogs and cats are the usual offenders. Less commonly, mosquitoes, lice, scabies, and bird and grass mites are involved. The sensitivity is transient, lasting 4–6 months. Usually no other family members are affected. It is often difficult for the parents to understand why no one else is affected. The logical therapy is to remove the offending insect, although in most cases it is very difficult to identify the exact cause. Topical corticosteroids and oral antihistamines will control symptoms.

Demain JG: Papular urticaria and things that bite in the night. Curr Allergy Asthma Rep 2003;3:291 [PMID: 12791206].

Stibich AS, Schwartz RA: Papular urticaria. Cutis 2001;68:89 [PMID: 11534921].

## DERMATITIS (ECZEMA)

The terms *dermatitis* and *eczema* are currently used interchangeably in dermatology, although the term *eczema* truly denotes an acute weeping dermatosis. All forms of dermatitis, regardless of cause, may present with acute edema, erythema, and oozing with crusting, mild erythema alone, or lichenification. Lichenification is diagnosed by thickening of the skin with a shiny surface and exaggerated, deepened skin markings. It is the response of the skin to chronic rubbing or scratching.

Although the lesions of the various dermatoses are histologically indistinguishable, clinicians have nonetheless divided the disease group called dermatitis into several categories based on known causes in some cases and differing natural histories in others.

## 1. Atopic Dermatitis

Atopic dermatitis is a general term for chronic superficial inflammation of the skin that can be applied to a heterogeneous group of patients. Many (not all) patients go through three clinical phases. In the first, infantile eczema, the dermatitis begins on the cheeks and scalp and frequently expresses itself as oval patches on the trunk, later involving the extensor surfaces of the extremities. The usual age at onset is 2–3 months, and this phase ends at age 18 months to 2 years. Only one third of all infants with atopic eczema progress to phase 2 childhood or flexural eczema in which the predominant involvement is in the antecubital and popliteal fossae, the neck, the wrists, and sometimes the hands or feet. This phase lasts from age 2 years to adolescence. Some children will have involvement only of the soles of the feet, with cracking, redness, and pain, so-called atopic feet. Only one third of children with typical flexural eczema will progress to adolescent eczema, which is usually manifested by hand dermatitis only. Atopic dermatitis is quite unusual after age 30 years.

Atopic dermatitis results from an interaction between susceptibility genes, the host environment, skin barrier defects, pharmacologic abnormalities and immunologic response. The case for food and inhalant allergens as specific causes of atopic dermatitis is not strong. However, since the cause of atopic dermatitis remains unknown, there is debate between dermatologists and allergists on the exact role of allergy in atopic dermatitis (see Chapter 34).

A few patients with atopic dermatitis have immunodeficiency with recurrent pyodermas, unusual susceptibility to herpes simplex viruses, hyperimmunoglobulinemia E, defective neutrophil and monocyte chemotaxis, and impaired T-lymphocyte function (see Chapter 29).

A faulty epidermal barrier may predispose the patient with atopic dermatitis to itchy skin. Inability to hold water within the stratum corneum results in rapid evaporation of water, shrinking of the stratum corneum, and cracks in the epidermal barrier. Such skin forms an ineffective barrier to the entry of various irritants—and, indeed, it may be clinically useful to regard atopic dermatitis as a primary-irritant contact dermatitis and simply tell the patient, you have sensitive skin. Chronic atopic dermatitis is frequently infected secondarily with *Staphylococcus aureus* or *Streptococcus pyogenes*.

## Treatment

### A. Acute Stages

Application of wet dressings and topical corticosteroids is the treatment of choice for acute, weeping atopic eczema. A topical steroid preparation is applied two times daily and covered with wet dressings as outlined at the beginning of this chapter. Superinfection or colonization with *S aureus* is common, and appropriate systemic antibiotics may be necessary. If the expected improvement is not seen, bacterial cultures should be obtained to identify the possibility of an organism resistant to standard therapy.

### B. Chronic Stages

Treatment is aimed at avoiding irritants and restoring water to the skin. No soaps or harsh shampoos should be used, and the patient should avoid woolen or any rough clothing. Bathing is minimized to every second or third day. Twice-daily lubrication of the skin is very important.

Nonperfumed lotions or creams are suitable lubricants. Plain petrolatum is an acceptable lubricant, but some people find it too greasy and it may also cause considerable sweat retention. Liberal use of Cetaphil lotion as a soap substitute four or five times a day is also satisfactory as a means of lubrication. A bedroom humidifier is often helpful. Topical corticosteroids should be limited to medium strength (see Table 14–3). There is never any reason to use super- or high-potency corticosteroids in atopic dermatitis. In superinfected atopic dermatitis, systemic antibiotics for 10–14 days are necessary.

Topical tacrolimus and pimecrolimus are new topical immunosuppressive agents that are effective in atopic dermatitis. Tacrolimus should be reserved for children older than 2 years of age with atopic dermatitis unresponsive to medium-potency topical steroids. Pimecrolimus is helpful for chronic eczema of the face.

Treatment failures in chronic atopic dermatitis are most often the result of patient noncompliance. This is a frustrating disease for parent and child.

Cookson WO, Moffatt MF: The genetics of atopic dermatitis. Curr Opin Allergy Clin Immunol 2002;2:383 [PMID: 12582320].

Daniels J, Harper J: The epidemiology of atopic dermatitis. Hosp Med 2002;63:649 [PMID: 12474607].

Eichenfield LF, Beck L: Elidel (pimecrolimus) cream 1%: A nonsteroidal topical agent for the treatment of atopic dermatitis. J Allergy Clin Immunol 2003;111:1153 [PMID: 12743593].

Gianni LM, Sulli MM: Topical tacrolimus in the treatment of atopic dermatitis. Ann Pharmacother 2001;35:943 [PMID: 11485148].

Lee DJ, Eichenfield LF: Atopic, contact, and seborrheic dermatitis in adolescents. Adolesc Med 2001;12:269 [PMID: 11404201].

Leung DY, Bieber T: Atopic dermatitis. Lancet 2003;361: 151 [PMID: 12531593].

Lewis-Jones: Atopic dermatitis in childhood. Hosp Med 2001; 62:136 [PMID: 11291461].

## 2. Nummular Eczema

Nummular eczema is characterized by numerous symmetrically distributed coin-shaped patches of dermatitis, principally on the extremities. These may be acute, oozing, and crusted or dry and scaling. The differential diagnosis should include tinea corporis, impetigo, and atopic dermatitis.

The same topical measures should be used as for atopic dermatitis, although treatment is often more difficult.

## 3. Primary Irritant Contact Dermatitis (Diaper Dermatitis)

Contact dermatitis is of two types: primary irritant and allergic eczematous. Primary irritant dermatitis develops within a few hours, reaches peak severity at 24 hours, and then disappears. Allergic eczematous contact dermatitis (described in the next section) has a delayed onset of 18 hours, peaks at 48–72 hours, and often lasts as long as 2–3 weeks even if exposure to the offending antigen is discontinued.

Diaper dermatitis, the most common form of primary irritant contact dermatitis seen in pediatric practice, is caused by prolonged contact of the skin with urine and feces, which contain irritating chemicals such as urea and intestinal enzymes. The diagnosis of diaper dermatitis is based on the picture of erythema and scaling of the skin in the perineal area and the history of prolonged skin contact with urine or feces. This is frequently seen in the "good baby" who sleeps many hours through the night without waking. In 80% of cases of diaper dermatitis lasting more than 3 days, the affected area is colonized with *C albicans* even before appearance of the classic signs of a beefy red, sharply marginated dermatitis with satellite lesions.

Treatment consists of changing diapers frequently. Because rubber or plastic pants prevent evaporation of the contactant and enhance its penetration into the skin, they should be avoided as much as possible. Air drying is useful. Streptococcal perianal cellulitis and infantile psoriasis should be included in the differential diagnosis. Treatment of long-standing diaper dermatitis should include application of nystatin or an imidazole cream with each diaper change.

Kazaks EL, Lane AT: Diaper dermatitis. Pediatr Clin North Am 2000;47:909 [PMID: 10943265].

Levy M: Diaper rash syndrome or dermatitis. Cutis 2001;67: 37 [PMID: 11398268].

## 4. Allergic Eczematous Contact Dermatitis (Poison Ivy Dermatitis)

Plants such as poison ivy, poison sumac, and poison oak cause most cases of allergic contact dermatitis in children. Allergic contact dermatitis has all the features of delayed-type (T-lymphocyte-mediated) hypersensitivity. Many substances may cause such a reaction; nickel sulfate, potassium dichromate, and neomycin are the most common causes. Nickel is found to some degree in all metals. Nickel allergy is commonly seen on the ears secondary to the wearing of earrings, and near the umbilicus from pants snaps and belt buckles. The true incidence of allergic contact dermatitis in children is unknown. Children often present with acute dermatitis with blister formation, oozing, and crusting. Blisters are often linear and of acute onset.

Treatment of contact dermatitis in localized areas is with topical corticosteroids. In severe generalized involvement, prednisone, 1–2 mg/kg/d orally for 10–14 days, can be used.

Bruckner AL, Weston WL: Allergic contact dermatitis in children: A practical approach to management. Skin Therapy Lett 2002;7:3 [PMID: 12548328].

Weston WL, Bruckner A: Allergic contact dermatitis. Pediatr Clin North Am 2000;47:897 [PMID: 10943264].

## 5. Seborrheic Dermatitis

Seborrheic dermatitis is an erythematous scaly dermatitis accompanied by overproduction of sebum occurring in areas rich in sebaceous glands (ie, the face, scalp, and perineum). This common condition occurs predominantly in the newborn and at puberty, the ages at which hormonal stimulation of sebum production is maximal. Although it is tempting to speculate that overproduction of sebum causes the dermatitis, the exact relationship is unclear.

Seborrheic dermatitis on the scalp in infancy is clinically similar to atopic dermatitis, and the distinction may become clear only after other areas are involved. Psoriasis also occurs in seborrheic areas in older children and should be considered in the differential diagnosis.

Seborrheic dermatitis responds well to low-potency topical corticosteroids.

## 6. Dandruff

Physiologic scaling or mild seborrhea, in the form of greasy scalp scales, may be treated by medicated dandruff shampoos. The cause is unknown.

Warner RR et al: Dandruff has an altered stratum corneum ultrastructure that is improved with zinc pyrithione shampoo. J Am Acad Dermatol 2001;45:897 [PMID: 11712036].

## 7. Dry Skin Dermatitis (Asteatotic Eczema, Xerosis)

Newborns and older children who live in arid climates are susceptible to dry skin, characterized by large cracked scales with erythematous borders. The stratum corneum is dependent on environmental humidity for its water, and below 30% environmental humidity the stratum corneum loses water, shrinks, and cracks. These cracks in the epidermal barrier allow irritating substances to enter the skin, predisposing the patient to dermatitis.

Treatment consists of increasing the water content of the skin in the immediate external environment. House humidifiers are very useful. Minimize bathing to every second or third day.

Frequent soaping of the skin impairs its water-holding capacity and serves as an irritating alkali, and all soaps should therefore be avoided. Frequent use of emollients (eg, Cetaphil, Eucerin, Lubriderm) should be a major part of therapy.

## 8. Keratosis Pilaris

Follicular papules containing a white inspissated scale characterize keratosis pilaris. Individual lesions are discrete and may be red. They are prominent on the extensor surfaces of the upper arms and thighs and on the buttocks and cheeks. In severe cases, the lesions may be generalized. Such lesions are seen frequently in children with dry skin and have also been associated with atopic dermatitis and ichthyosis vulgaris.

Treatment is with keratolytics such as topical retinoic acid, lactic acid, or urea creams followed by skin hydration.

Lateef A, Schwartz RA: Keratosis pilaris. Cutis 1999;63:205 [PMID: 10228747]

## 9. Pityriasis Alba

White, scaly macular areas with indistinct borders are seen over extensor surfaces of extremities and on the cheeks in children with pityriasis alba. Suntanning exaggerates these lesions. Histologic examination reveals a mild dermatitis. These lesions may be confused with tinea versicolor. Low-potency topical steroids may help decrease any inflammatory component and may lead to faster return of normal pigmentation.

Blessman-Weber M et al: Pityriasis alba: A study of pathogenic factors. J Eur Acad Dermatol Venereol 2002;16:463 [PMID: 12428838].

## COMMON SKIN TUMORS

If the skin moves with the nodule on lateral palpation, the tumor is located within the dermis; if the skin moves over the nodule, it is subcutaneous. Seventy-five percent of lumps in childhood will be either epidermal inclusion cysts (60%) or pilomatrichomas (15%).

### Epidermal Inclusion Cysts

Epidermal inclusion cysts are smooth, dome-shaped nodules in the skin that may grow to 2 cm in diameter. In infants, they may be found near the eyes, and in older children and adolescents on the chest, back, or scalp. They are the most common superficial lumps in children. Treatment, if desired, is surgical excision.

**Pilomatrichomas** are benign tumors of the hair matrix. They are most commonly seen on the face and upper trunk. They are firm and may be irregular. Their color varies from flesh-colored to pink or blue. The firmness is secondary to calcification of the tumor. Treatment is by surgical excision.

## Granuloma Annulare

Circles or semicircles of nontender intradermal nodules found over the lower legs and ankles, the dorsum of the hands and wrists, and the trunk, in that order, suggest granuloma annulare. Histologically, the disease appears as a central area of tissue death (necrobiosis) surrounded by macrophages and lymphocytes. No treatment is necessary. Lesions resolve spontaneously within 1–2 years in most children.

## Pyogenic Granuloma

Rapid growth of a dark red papule with an ulcerated and crusted surface over 1–2 weeks following skin trauma suggests pyogenic granuloma. Histologically, this represents excessive new vessel formation with or without inflammation (granulation tissue). It is neither pyogenic nor granulomatous but should be regarded as an abnormal healing response. Pulsed dye laser and curettage followed by electrocautery are the treatments of choice.

## Keloids

Keloids are scars raised above the skin surface with many radial projections of scar tissue. They continue to enlarge over several years. They are often found on the face, earlobes, neck, chest, and back. Keloids show no racial predilection. Treatment includes intralesional injection with triamcinolone acetonide, 20 mg/mL, or excision and injection with corticosteroids.

Wyatt AJ, Hansen RC: Pediatric skin tumors. Pediatr Clin North Am 2000;47:937 [PMID: 10943267].

# PAPULOSQUAMOUS ERUPTIONS

Papulosquamous eruptions (Table 14–8) comprise papules or plaques with varying degrees of scale.

## 1. Pityriasis Rosea

Erythematous papules that coalesce to form oval plaques preceded by a large oval plaque with central clearing and a scaly border (the herald patch) establish the diagnosis of pityriasis rosea. The herald patch has the appearance of ringworm and is often treated as such. It appears 1–30 days before the onset of the generalized papular eruption. The oval plaques are parallel in their long axis and follow lines of skin cleavage. In

**Table 14–8.** Papulosquamous eruptions in children.

| |
|---|
| Psoriasis |
| Pityriasis rosea |
| Tinea corporis |
| Lichen planus |
| Chronic parapsoriasis |
| Dermatomyositis |
| Lupus erythematosus |
| Pityriasis rubra pilaris |
| Secondary syphilis |

whites, the lesions are primarily on the trunk; in blacks, lesions are primarily on the extremities and may be accentuated in the axillary and inguinal areas. This disease is common in school-age children and adolescents and is presumed to be viral in origin. The role of human herpes virus 7 in the pathogenesis of pityriasis rosea is debated. The condition lasts 6 weeks and may be pruritic the first 7–10 days. The major differential diagnosis is secondary syphilis, and a VDRL test should be done if syphilis is suspected. A chronic variant of this disease may last 2–3 years and is called chronic parapsoriasis or pityriasis lichenoides chronica.

Exposing the skin to sunlight until a mild sunburn occurs (slight redness) will hasten the disappearance of lesions. Ordinarily, no treatment is necessary.

Karnath B et al: Pityriasis rosea. Appearance and distribution of macules aid diagnosis. Postgrad Med 2003;113:94 [PMID: 12764899].

Kempf W, Burg G: Pityriasis rosea—A virus-induced skin disease? An update. Arch Virol 2000;145:1509 [PMID: 11003465].

## 2. Psoriasis

Psoriasis is characterized by erythematous papules covered by thick white scales. Guttate (drop-like) psoriasis is a common form in children that often follows an episode of streptococcal pharyngitis by 2–3 weeks. The sudden onset of small papules (3–8 mm), seen predominantly over the trunk and quickly covered with thick white scales, is characteristic of guttate psoriasis. Chronic psoriasis is marked by thick, large scaly plaques (5–10 cm) over the elbows, knees, scalp, and other sites of trauma. Pinpoint pits in the nail plate are seen, as well as yellow discoloration of the nail plate resulting from onycholysis. Thickening of all 20 nails is an uncommon feature. The sacral and seborrheic areas are commonly involved.

Psoriasis has no known cause and demonstrates active proliferation of epidermal cells, with a turnover time of 3–4 days versus 28 days for normal skin. These rapidly proliferating epidermal cells are producing excessive stratum corneum, giving rise to thick, opaque scales. Papulosquamous eruptions that present problems of differential diagnosis are listed in Table 14–8.

## Treatment

All therapy is aimed at diminishing epidermal turnover time. Topical steroids are the initial treatment of choice. Penetration of topical corticosteroids through the enlarged epidermal barrier in psoriasis requires that more potent preparations be used, for example, fluocinonide 0.05% (Lidex) or clobetasol 0.05% (Temovate) ointment twice daily.

The second line of therapy is topical calcipotriene (Dovonex) applied twice daily or the combination of a superpotent topical steroid twice daily on weekends and calcipotriene twice daily on weekdays for 8 weeks.

Anthralin therapy is also useful. Anthralin is applied to the skin for a short contact time (eg, 20 minutes once daily) and then washed off with a neutral soap (eg, Dove). A 6-week course of treatment is recommended.

Crude coal tar therapy is messy and stains bedclothes. The newer tar gels (Estar, psoriGel) cause less staining and are most efficacious. They are applied twice daily for 6–8 weeks. These preparations are sold over the counter and are not usually covered by insurance plans.

Scalp care using a tar shampoo requires leaving the shampoo on for 5 minutes, washing it off, and then shampooing with commercial shampoo to remove scales. It may be necessary to shampoo daily until scaling is reduced. More severe cases of psoriasis are best treated by a dermatologist.

Marcoux D, Prost Y: Pediatric psoriasis revisited. J Cutan Med Surg 2002;6:22 [PMID: 11976986].

Morris A et al: Childhood psoriasis: A clinical review of 1262 cases. Pediatr Dermatol 2001;18:188 [PMID: 11437997].

Rogers M: Childhood psoriasis. Curr Opin Pediatr 2002;14:404 [PMID: 12130902].

## HAIR LOSS (ALOPECIA)

Hair loss in children (Table 14–9) imposes great emotional stress on the patient and the parent. A 60% hair loss in a single area is necessary before hair loss can be detected clinically. Examination should begin with the scalp to determine whether there are color or infiltrative changes. Hairs should be examined microscopically for breaking and structural defects and to see whether growing or resting hairs are being shed. Placing removed hairs in mounting fluid (Permount) on a glass microscope slide makes them easy to examine. Three diseases account for most cases of hair loss in children:

**Table 14–9.** Other causes of hair loss in children.

**Hair loss with scalp changes**
Atrophy:
  Lichen planus
  Lupus erythematosus
Nodules and tumors:
  Epidermal nevus
  Nevus sebaceus
Thickening:
  Burn
**Hair loss with hair shaft defects** (hair fails to grow out enough to require haircuts)
  Monilethrix—alternating bands of thin and thick areas
  Pili annulati—alternating bands of light and dark pigmentation
  Pili torti—hair twisted 180 degrees, brittle
  Trichorrhexis invaginata (bamboo hair)—intussusception of one hair into another
  Trichorrhexis nodosa—nodules with fragmented hair

alopecia areata, tinea capitis (described earlier in this chapter), and trichotillomania.

## Alopecia Areata

Loss of every hair in a localized area is called alopecia areata. This is the most common cause of hair loss in children. An immunologic pathogenic mechanism is suspected because dense infiltration of lymphocytes precedes hair loss. Ninety-five percent of children with alopecia areata completely regrow their hair within 12 months, although as many as 40% may have a relapse in 5–6 years. A rare and unusual form of alopecia areata begins at the occiput and proceeds along the hair margins to the frontal scalp. This variety, called ophiasis, often eventuates in total scalp hair loss (alopecia totalis). The prognosis for regrowth in ophiasis is poor.

Treatment of alopecia areata is difficult. Systemic corticosteroids given to suppress the inflammatory response will result in hair growth, but the hair will fall out again when the drug is discontinued. Superpotent topical steroids, minoxidil (Rogaine), and anthralin are treatment options. In children with alopecia totalis, a wig is most helpful.

Madani S, Shapiro J: Alopecia areata update. J Am Acad Dermatol 2000;42:549 [PMID: 10727199].

Tan E et al: A clinical study of childhood alopecia areata in Singapore. Pediatr Dermatol 2002;19:298 [PMID: 12220271].

## Trichotillomania

Traumatic hair pulling causes the hair shafts to be broken off at different lengths, with an ill-defined area of hair loss, petechiae around follicular openings, and a wrinkled hair shaft on microscopic examination. This behavior may be merely habit, an acute reaction to severe stress, or a sign of a psychiatric disorder. Eyelashes and eyebrows rather than scalp hair may be pulled out. If the behavior has a long history, psychiatric evaluation may be helpful. Oiling the hair to make it slippery is an aid to behavior modification.

O'Sullivan RL et al: Characterization of trichotillomania. A phenomenological model with clinical relevance to obsessive–compulsive spectrum disorders. Psychiatr Clin North Am 2000;23:587 [PMID: 10986729].

Walsh KH, McDougle CJ: Trichotillomania: Presentation, etiology, diagnosis and therapy. Am J Clin Dermatol 2001;2:327 [PMID: 11721651].

## REACTIVE ERYTHEMAS

### Erythema Multiforme

Erythema multiforme begins with papules that later develop a dark center and then evolve into lesions with central blisters and the characteristic target lesions (iris lesions) that have three concentric circles of color change. Primary injury is to endothelial cells, with later destruction of epidermal basal cells and blister formation. Erythema multiforme has sometimes been diagnosed in patients with severe mucous membrane involvement, but Stevens–Johnson syndrome is the usual term when severe involvement of conjunctiva, oral cavity, and genital mucosa also occur.

Many causes are suspected, particularly concomitant herpes simplex virus, drugs, especially sulfonamides, and *Mycoplasma* infections. Recurrent erythema multiforme is usually associated with reactivation of herpes simplex virus. In the mild form, spontaneous healing occurs in 10–14 days, but Stevens–Johnson syndrome may last 6–8 weeks.

Treatment is symptomatic in uncomplicated erythema multiforme. Removal of offending drugs is an obvious measure. Oral antihistamines such as hydroxyzine, 2 mg/kg/d orally, are useful. Cool compresses and wet dressings will relieve pruritus. Steroids have not been demonstrated to be effective. Chronic acyclovir therapy has been successful in decreasing attacks in those patients with herpes-associated recurrent erythema multiforme.

Forman R et al: Erythema multiforme, Stevens–Johnson syndrome and toxic epidermal necrolysis in children: A review of 10 years' experience. Drug Saf 2002;25:965 [PMID: 12381216].

Leaute-Labreze C et al: Diagnosis, classification, and management of erythema multiforme and Stevens–Johnson syndrome. Arch Dis Child 2000;83:347 [PMID: 10999875].

### Drug Eruptions

Drugs may produce urticarial, morbilliform, scarlatiniform, or bullous or fixed skin eruptions. Urticaria may appear within minutes after drug administration, but most reactions begin 7–14 days after the drug is first administered. These eruptions may occur in patients who have received these drugs for long periods, and eruptions continue for days after the drug has been discontinued. Acute drug eruptions usually do not produce fever, elevated sedimentation rate, or serum sickness. If any of these occur, a search for a concomitant infection is warranted. Drugs commonly implicated in skin reactions are listed in Table 14–10.

Millikan LE, Feldman M: Pediatric drug allergy. Clin Dermatol 2002;20:29 [PMID: 11849892].

## MISCELLANEOUS SKIN DISORDERS ENCOUNTERED IN PEDIATRIC PRACTICE

### Aphthous Stomatitis

Recurrent erosions on the gums, lips, tongue, palate, and buccal mucosa are often confused with herpes simplex. A smear of the base of such a lesion stained with Wright stain will aid in ruling out herpes simplex by the absence of epithelial multinucleate giant cells. A culture for herpes simplex is also useful in this difficult differential diagnostic problem. The cause remains un-

**Table 14–10.** Common drug reactions.

**Fixed drug eruption/erythema multiforme/toxic epidermal necrolysis**
   Anticonvulsants
   Nonsteroidal anti-inflammatory drugs
   Sulfonamides
**Urticaria**
   Barbiturates
   Opioids
   Penicillins
   Sulfonamides
**Morbilliform eruption**
   Anticonvulsants
   Cephalosporins
   Penicillins
   Sulfonamides
**Photodermatitis**
   Psoralens
   Sulfonamides
   Tetracyclines
   Thiazides

known, but T-cell-mediated cytotoxicity to various viral antigens has been postulated.

There is no specific therapy for this condition. Rinsing the mouth with liquid antacids will provide relief in most patients. Topical corticosteroids in a gel base (eg, fluocinonide gel) may provide some relief. In severe cases that interfere with eating, prednisone, 1 mg/kg/d orally for 3–5 days, will suffice to abort an episode. Colchicine, 0.2–0.5 mg/d, sometimes reduces the frequency of attacks.

Porter SR et al: Recurrent aphthous stomatitis. Clin Dermatol 2000;18:569 [PMID: 11134852].

## Vitiligo

Vitiligo is characterized clinically by the development of areas of depigmentation. These are often symmetri-cal and occur mainly on extensor surfaces. The depigmentation results from a destruction of melanocytes. The basis for this destruction is unknown, but immunologically mediated damage is likely and vitiligo sometimes occurs in individuals with selective IgA deficiency, graft-versus-host disease, or autoimmune endocrinopathies. Treatment is not very effective. Potent topical steroids for 4 months are the initial treatment. Topical tacrolimus and calcipotriene have also been used. Narrow-band ultraviolet B waves (UVB 311 nm) may be used in severe cases.

Handa S, Dogra S: Epidemiology of childhood vitiligo: A study of 625 patients from north India. Pediatr Dermatol 2003;20: 207 [PMID: 12787267].

Westerhof W: Vitiligo management update. Skin Therapy Lett 2000;5:1 [PMID: 10889569].

# Eye

*Rebecca Sands, MD, Arlene Drack, MD, & Allan M. Eisenbaum, MD*

Normal vision is a skill acquired during infancy and childhood. To become adept requires a normal visual environment. The child must experience equally good visual inputs from well-aligned eyes during this period while the visual nervous system is still exhibiting plasticity. Thus, pediatric ophthalmology emphasizes early diagnosis and treatment of pediatric eye diseases in order to obtain the best possible visual outcome.

But eye disease in children does not always originate in the ocular system. Abnormal eye findings in a child may be a sign of systemic disease. This chapter seeks to increase the reader's awareness of pediatric ophthalmic disease and treatment in order to achieve more favorable visual outcomes and healthier children.

## COMMON NONSPECIFIC SIGNS & SYMPTOMS

Nonspecific signs and symptoms commonly occur as the chief complaint or as an element of the history of a child with eye disease. Five of these findings are presented in the following sections with a sixth—leukocoria—which often has serious implications. Do not hesitate to seek the help of a pediatric ophthalmologist when you believe the diagnosis and treatment of these signs and symptoms require in-depth clinical experience.

### Redness

Redness (injection) of the bulbar conjunctiva or deeper vessels is a common presenting complaint. It may be mild and localized or diffuse and bilateral. Causes include superficial or penetrating foreign bodies, infection, allergy, and conjunctivitis associated with systemic entities such as Stevens–Johnson syndrome or Kawasaki disease. Irritating noxious agents also result in injection. Subconjunctival hemorrhage may be traumatic or spontaneous or may be associated with hematopoietic disease, vascular anomalies, or inflammatory processes. Uncommonly, an injected eye can be due to an intraocular or orbital tumor.

### Tearing

In infants, tearing is usually due to nasolacrimal obstruction, but tearing may also be associated with con-genital glaucoma, in which case photophobia and blepharospasm may also be present. Inflammation, allergic and viral diseases, or conjunctival and corneal irritation can also cause tearing.

### Discharge

Purulent discharge is usually associated with bacterial conjunctivitis. In infants and toddlers with nasolacrimal obstruction, a mucopurulent discharge may be present with low-grade, chronic dacryocystitis. Watery discharge occurs with viral infection, iritis, superficial foreign bodies, and nasolacrimal obstruction. Mucoid discharge may be a sign of allergic conjunctivitis or nasolacrimal obstruction. Histologically, a mucoid discharge due to allergy is expected to show eosinophils; a purulent bacterial discharge will show polymorphonuclear leukocytes.

### Pain & Foreign Body Sensation

Pain in or around the eye may be due to foreign bodies, corneal abrasions, lacerations, acute infections of the globe or ocular adnexa, iritis, and angle closure glaucoma. Large refractive errors, poor accommodative ability, and sinus disease may manifest as headaches. Trichiasis (inturned lashes) and contact lens problems are also causes of ocular discomfort.

### Photophobia

Acute aversion to light may occur with corneal abrasions, foreign bodies, and iritis. Squinting of one eye in bright light is a common sign of intermittent exotropia. Photophobia is present in infants with glaucoma, albinism, aniridia, and retinal dystrophies such as achromatopsia. Photophobia is common after ocular surgery and after dilation of the pupil with mydriatic and cycloplegic agents. Photophobia in individuals with no ocular pathology may be due to migraine headache, meningitis, and retrobulbar optic neuritis.

### Leukocoria

Although not a common sign or complaint, leukocoria (a white pupil) is associated with serious diseases and requires prompt ophthalmologic consultation. Causes

**Figure 15–1.** Leukocoria of left eye caused by retrolental membrane (persistent hyperplastic primary vitreous or persistent fetal vasculature).

of leukocoria include retinoblastoma, retinopathy of prematurity (ROP), pupillary membrane, cataract, vitreous opacities, retinal detachment, *Toxocara* infection, and retinal dysplasia (Figure 15–1).

## REFRACTIVE ERRORS

Refractive error refers to the optical state of the eye (Figure 15 2). It is a physical characteristic like height or weight and can be quantitated. Not all refractive errors require correction, but severe errors can cause amblyopia. Those that do can usually be corrected with glasses. Less often, contact lenses are required, usually for very high or asymmetrical refractive errors, or for adolescents who do not want to wear spectacles. Laser refractive surgery is not currently indicated for most children, although studies are being reported. There are three common refractive errors: myopia, hyperopia, and astigmatism. Inequality of the refractive state between the two eyes (anisometropia) can cause amblyopia (reduced vision with or without an organic lesion; see Amblyopia & Strabismus section). Children at particular risk for refractive errors requiring correction with spectacles include those who were born prematurely, who have Down syndrome, who are offspring of parents with refractive errors, or who have certain systemic conditions such as Stickler, Marfan, or Ehlers–Danlos syndrome.

## Myopia (Nearsightedness)

For the myopic or nearsighted individual, objects nearby are in focus; those at a distance are blurred. This is because the plane of focus is anterior to the retina. The onset is typically at about age 8 years and may progress throughout adolescence and young adulthood. A myopic person may squint to produce a pinhole effect, which improves distance vision. Divergent lenses

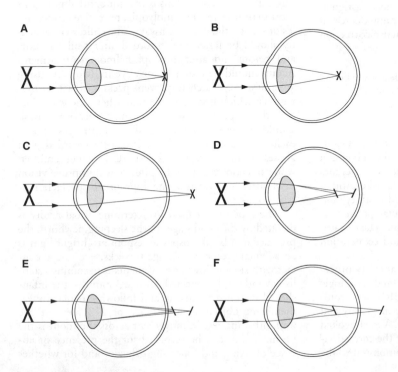

**Figure 15–2.** Different refractive states of the eye . **A:** Emmetropia. Image plane from parallel rays of light falls on retina. **B:** Myopia. Image plane focuses anterior to retina. **C:** Hyperopia. Image plane focuses posterior to retina. **D:** Astigmatism, myopic type. Images in horizontal and vertical planes focus anterior to retina. **E:** Astigmatism, hyperopic type. Images in horizontal and vertical planes focus posterior to retina. **F:** Astigmatism, mixed type. Images in horizontal and vertical planes focus on either side of the retina.

provide clear distance vision. Many studies have been done to determine whether treatment can slow or stop myopic progression. Atropine eyedrops have shown some effect, but produce many side effects. A newer drug, perenzipine, has shown promise in animal studies, and human studies are underway.

Saw SM et al: Myopia: Attempts to arrest progression. Br J Ophthalmol 2002 Nov;86(11):1306 Review [PMID: 12386095].

## Hyperopia (Farsightedness)

Saying that the hyperopic child is sighted for far (not near) is somewhat misleading, because the child can focus on near objects if the hyperopia is not excessive. Large amounts of uncorrected hyperopia can cause esotropia (inward deviation, or crossing, of the eyes) and amblyopia (see Amblyopia & Strabismus section). Most infants have a hyperopic refraction that begins to diminish during the toddler years and does not require correction.

## Astigmatism

When either the cornea or the crystalline lens is not perfectly spherical, an image will not be sharply focused in one plane. Schematically, there will be two planes of focus. Both of the planes can be either in front of or behind the retina, or one of the planes can be in front of the retina and the other behind it. This refractive state is described as astigmatism. Large amounts of astigmatism not corrected at an early age can cause decreased vision from amblyopia, but proper refractive correction can prevent this.

DeRespinis PA: Eyeglasses: Why and when do children need them? Pediatr Ann 2001;30:455 [PMID: 11510343].

## EXAMINATION

Ophthalmic examination of the pediatric patient begins with a calm demeanor and reassuring voice. Having a parent present is invaluable. The examination includes a history, assessment of visual acuity, external examination, observation of ocular alignment and motility, and ophthalmoscopic examination. Intraocular pressure is less frequently measured. Testing of binocular status and near point is desirable when age and cooperation permit.

Circumstances will dictate the use of ancillary procedures such as instilling fluorescein dye and radiologic tests (magnetic resonance imaging [MRI] and computed tomography [CT] scan). Electroretinography and electrooculography test retinal function. Visual evoked response testing assesses the function of the cortical visual pathways. Visual field testing demonstrates the presence or absence of scotomas and visual field defects occurring anywhere along the visual pathway. In the office setting, visual field testing may be done in a gross manner by confrontation, that is, bringing an object from the periphery of the child's field of vision in each of four quadrants or by having an older child count the examiner's fingers as they are presented in two quadrants simultaneously. It must be emphasized that accurate results can be difficult to achieve in young children.

## History

Evaluation begins by ascertaining the chief complaint and taking a history of the present illness. Elements of the history include onset of the complaint, its duration, whether it is monocular or binocular, treatment received thus far, and associated systemic symptoms. If an infectious disease is suspected, ask about possible contact with others having similar findings. The ocular history is obtained, as is the perinatal and developmental history and any history of allergy. The family history should be explored for ocular disorders that may be familial or inherited.

## Visual Acuity

Visual acuity testing is the single most important test of visual function and should be part of every general physical examination. This is the nonophthalmologist's most definitive test for amblyopia, refractive errors, and lesions along the optic pathways. The child's visual acuity should be tested and recorded after ocular trauma and before and after any ophthalmologic treatment. Acuity should be tested in each eye individually, using an adhesive eyepatch to prevent peeking. If latent nystagmus, which becomes apparent when one eye is occluded, is present (see Nystagmus section), vision should be tested simultaneously in both eyes and in each eye individually. Vision is usually recorded with glasses in place (corrected vision). In older children who can cooperate, use of a pinhole will improve vision in children not wearing the appropriate spectacle prescription.

The type of test used to determine visual acuity is dictated by the child's age. In the sleeping newborn, the presence of a blepharospastic response to bright light is an adequate response. At age 6 weeks, eye-to-eye contact with slow following movements is becoming established and can be detected. By age 3 months, the infant should demonstrate fixing and following ocular movements for objects at a distance of 2–3 feet. At age 6 months, interest in movement across the room is the norm. Vision can be recorded for the presence or absence of fixing and following behavior and for whether vision is steady (unsteady when nystagmus is present) and maintained. Vision should be tested and recorded for each eye. Visual acuity can be quantified in infants using other techniques, such as the 15-diopter prism test, preferential looking technique, or the pattern visual evoked response.

In the verbal child, the use of familiar icons will allow for a quantitative test. Allen or Lea symbols with familiar pictures can be used to test children age 2½–3 years. Four-year-olds are often ready to play the tumbling E game (in which the child identifies the orientation of the letter E, which is turned in one of four directions) or the HOTV letters game (in which these four letters are shown individually at a distance and matched on a board that the child is holding). Literate children are tested with letters. Typical acuity levels in developmentally appropriate children are approximately 20/60 or better in 2½-to 3 year-olds, 20/40–20/30 in 3-year-olds, 20/30–20/25 in 4-year-olds, and 20/20 in literate 5- to 6-year-olds. Perhaps more important than the absolute visual acuity is the presence of a difference of acuity between the two eyes, which might be a sign of amblyopia, uncorrected refractive error, or disease. As little as one line difference in acuity should be considered significant.

The practitioner should be aware of two situations complicated by nystagmus. Children who require a face turn or torticollis (in which the head is tilted to the right or left) to quiet the nystagmus will have poor visual acuity results when tested in the absence of the compensatory head posture.

When latent nystagmus is present, acuity testing is particularly challenging (see Nystagmus section). Nystagmus appears or worsens when an eye is occluded, degrading central vision. To minimize the nystagmus, the occluder should be held about 12 inches in front of the eye not being tested. Testing both eyes simultaneously without occlusion often gives a better visual acuity measurement than when either eye is tested individually.

Becker R, et al: Examination of young children with Lea symbols. Br J Ophthalmol 2002;86(5):513 [PMID: 11973243].

Simon JW, Kaw P: Vision screening performed by the pediatrician. Pediatr Ann 2001;30(8):446 [PMID: 11510342].

## External Examination

Inspection of the anterior segment of the globe and its adnexa requires adequate illumination and often magnification. A penlight provides good illumination and should be used in both straight-ahead and oblique illumination. A Wood lamp or a blue filter cap placed over a penlight is needed for evaluation after applying a fluorescent stain. Immobilization of the child may be necessary. A drop of topical anesthetic may facilitate the examination. Assessment of the entire anterior segment except the trabecular meshwork and, to a lesser extent, the lens is possible.

In cases of suspected foreign body, pulling down on the lower lid provides excellent visualization of the inferior cul-de-sac (palpebral conjunctiva). Visualizing the upper cul-de-sac and superior bulbar conjunctiva is possible by having the patient look inferiorly while the upper lid is pulled away from the globe and the examiner peers into the upper recess. Illumination with a penlight is necessary. The upper lid should be everted to evaluate the superior tarsal conjunctiva (Figure 15–3).

When indicated for further evaluation of the cornea, a small amount of fluorescein solution should be instilled into the lower cul-de-sac. Blue light will stain defects yellow-green. Disease-specific staining patterns may be observed. For example, herpes simplex lesions of the corneal epithelium produce a dendrite or branch-like pattern. A foreign body lodged beneath the upper lid shows one or more vertical lines of stain on the cornea due to the constant movement of the foreign body over the cornea. Contact lens overwear produces a central staining pattern. A fine, scattered punctate pattern may be a sign of viral keratitis or medication toxicity. Punctate erosions of the inferior third of the cornea can be seen with staphylococcal blepharitis or exposure keratitis secondary to incomplete lid closure.

***Figure 15–3.*** Eversion of the upper lid. **A:** The patient looks downward. **B:** The fingers pull the lid down, and an index finger or cotton-tip is placed on the upper tarsal border. **C:** The lid is pulled up over the finger. **D:** The lid is everted.

## Pupils

The child's pupils should be evaluated for reaction to light, regularity of shape, and equality of size as well as for the presence of afferent pupillary defect. This defect, occurring in optic nerve disease, is evaluated by the swinging flashlight test (see Diseases of the Optic Nerve section). Irregular pupils are associated with iritis, trauma, pupillary membranes, and structural defects such as iris coloboma (see Iris Coloboma section).

Pupils vary in size due to lighting conditions and also age. In general, infants have miotic (constricted) pupils. Children have larger pupils than either infants or adults, whereas the elderly have miotic pupils.

Anisocoria, a size difference between the two pupils, may be physiologic if the size difference is within 1 mm and is the same in light and dark. Anisocoria occurs with Horner syndrome, third nerve palsy, Adie tonic pupil, iritis, and trauma. Medication could also cause abnormal pupil size or reactivity. For example, contact with atropine-like substances (belladonna alkaloids) will cause pupillary dilation with little or no pupillary reaction. Systemic antihistamines and scopolamine patches, among other medicines, can dilate the pupils and interfere with accommodation (focusing).

## Alignment & Motility Evaluation

Alignment and motility should be tested because amblyopia is associated with strabismus, a misalignment of the visual axes of the eyes. Besides alignment, ocular rotations should be evaluated in the six cardinal positions of gaze (Table 15–1; Figure 15–4). A small toy is an interesting target for testing ocular rotations in infants; a penlight works well in older children.

Alignment can be assessed in several ways. In order of increasing accuracy, these methods are observation, the corneal light reflex test, and cover testing. Observation includes an educated guess about whether the eyes are properly aligned. Corneal light reflex evaluation (Hirschberg test) is performed by shining a beam of a light at the patient's eyes, observing the reflections off each cornea, and estimating whether these "reflexes" appear to be positioned properly. If the reflection of light is noted temporally on the cornea, esotropia is suspected (Figure 15–5). Nasal reflection of the light suggests exotropia (outward deviation). Accuracy of these tests increases with increasing angles of misalignment.

Another way of evaluating alignment is with the cover test, in which the patient fixes on a target while one eye is covered. If an esotropia or an exotropia is present, the deviated eye will make a corrective movement to fixate on the target when the previously fixating eye is occluded. The other eye is tested similarly. When the occluder is removed from the eye just uncov-

**Table 15–1.** Function and innervation of each of the extraocular muscles.

| Muscle | Function | Innervation |
|---|---|---|
| Medial rectus | Adductor | Oculomotor (third) |
| Lateral rectus | Abductor | Abducens (sixth) |
| Inferior rectus | Depressor Adductor Extorter | Oculomotor |
| Superior rectus | Elevator Adductor Intorter | Oculomotor |
| Inferior oblique | Elevator Abductor Extorter | Oculomotor |
| Superior oblique | Depressor Abductor Intorter | Trochlear (fourth) |

ered, a refixation movement of that eye indicates a phoria, or latent deviation if alignment is reestablished. If the uncovered eyes picks up fixation and strabismus is still present, then that eye can be presumed to be dominant and the nonpreferred eye possibly amblyopic. If the eye remains deviated after the occluder is removed, a tropia is noted to be present (Figure 15–6). A deviated eye that is blind or has very poor vision will not fixate on a target. Consequently, spurious results to cover testing may occur, as can happen with disinterest on the part of the patient, small-angle strabismus, and inexperience in administering cover tests.

MR = medial rectus
SR = superior rectus
SO = superior oblique

LR = lateral rectus
IR = inferior rectus
IO = inferior oblique

**Figure 15–4.** Cardinal positions of gaze and muscles primarily tested in those fields of gaze. Arrow indicates position in which each muscle is tested.

**Figure 15–5.** Temporal displacement of light reflection showing esotropia (inward deviation) of the right eye. Nasal displacement of the reflection would show exotropia (outward deviation).

## Ophthalmoscopic Examination

A handheld direct ophthalmoscope allows visualization of the ocular fundus. As the patient's pupil becomes more constricted, viewing the fundus becomes more difficult. Although it is taught that pupillary dilation can precipitate an attack of closed-angle glaucoma in the predisposed adult, children are very rarely predisposed to angle closure. Exceptions include those with a dislocated lens, past surgery, or an eye previously com-

promised by a retrolental membrane, such as in ROP. Therefore, if an adequate view of the fundus is precluded by a miotic pupil, use of a dilating agent (eg, 1 drop each eye of 2.5% phenylephrine or 0.5% or 1% tropicamide) should provide adequate mydriasis (dilation). In infants, 1 drop of a combination of 1% phenylephrine with 0.2% cyclopentolate (Cyclomydril) is safer. Structures to be observed during ophthalmoscopy include the optic disk, blood vessels, the macular reflex, and retinal changes if present, as well as the clarity of the vitreous media. By increasing the amount of plus lens dialed into the instrument, the point of focus moves anteriorly from the retina to the lens and finally to the cornea.

Ophthalmoscopy should include assessment of the clarity of the ocular media, that is, the quality of the red reflex. The practitioner should take the time to become familiar with this reflex. The red reflex test (Brückner test) is useful for identifying disorders such as media opacities (eg, cataracts), large refractive errors, tumors such as retinoblastoma, and strabismus. A difference in quality of the red reflexes between the two eyes constitutes a positive Brückner test and requires referral to an ophthalmologist.

Eyes straight (maintained in position by fusion).

Position of eye under cover in orthophoria (fusion-free position). The right eye under cover has not moved.

Position of eye under cover in esophoria (fusion-free position). Under cover, the right eye has deviated inward. Upon removal of cover, the right eye will immediately resume its straight-ahead position.

Position of eye under cover in exophoria (fusion-free position). Under cover, the right eye had deviated outward. Upon removal of the cover, the right eye will immediately resume its straight-ahead position.

**Figure 15–6.** Cover testing. The patient is instructed to look at a target at eye level 20 feet away. Note that in the presence of constant strabismus (ie, a tropia rather than a phoria), the deviation will remain when the cover is removed. (Reproduced, with permission, from *General Ophthalmology*, 15th ed. Originally published by Appleton & Lange. Copyright © 1999 by The McGraw-Hill Companies, Inc.)

The red reflex of each eye can be compared simultaneously when the observer is approximately 4 feet away from the patient. The largest diameter of light is shown through the ophthalmoscope, and no correction (zero setting) is dialed in the ophthalmoscope unless it is to compensate for the examiner's uncorrected refractive error. A red reflex chart is available through the American Academy of Pediatrics.

## OCULAR TRAUMA

A foreign body of the globe or adnexa may be difficult to visualize due to its small size or location. The clinician should always maintain a high index of suspicion for an occult or intraocular foreign body if the history suggests this. In cases such as these, ophthalmologic referral needs to be considered.

Foreign bodies on the globe and palpebral conjunctiva usually cause discomfort and red eye. Magnification may be needed for inspection. Foreign bodies that lodge on the upper palpebral conjunctiva are best viewed by everting the lid on itself and removing the foreign body with a cotton applicator. The conjunctival surface (palpebral conjunctiva) of the lower lid presents no problem with visualization. After simple removal of a foreign body that is thought not to be contaminated, no other treatment is needed if no corneal abrasion has occurred.

When foreign bodies are noted on the bulbar conjunctiva or cornea (Figure 15–7), removal is facilitated by using a topical anesthetic. If the foreign body is not too adherent, it can be dislodged with a stream of irrigating solution (Dacriose or saline) or with a cotton applicator after instillation of a topical anesthetic. Otherwise, a foreign body spud or needle is used to undermine the foreign body. This must be done with adequate magnification and illumination. An antibiotic ointment is then instilled. Ferrous corneal bodies often have an associated rust ring, which may be removed under slitlamp visualization in cooperative children or under anesthesia if necessary.

Corneal abrasions are evaluated with fluorescein dye and treated with a topical antibiotic, but not necessarily a pressure patch. Patching is not advised for corneal abrasions caused by contact lens wear, and it is being used less frequently for corneal abrasions and after removal of corneal foreign bodies since the moist, hypoxic environment predisposes to bacterial infection. One drop of topical cycloplegic agent such as 5% homatropine, 1% atropine (with appropriate warnings to parents about systemic side effects), or 0.25% scopolamine is useful to relieve the discomfort of ciliary spasm and iritis. Daily follow-up is required until healing is complete.

A

B

*Figure 15–7.* **A:** Corneal foreign body at the nasal edge of the cornea. **B:** Subconjunctival foreign body of graphite.

Suspected intraocular foreign bodies and corneal and scleral lacerations require emergency referral to an ophthalmologist. In cases of suspected perforation of the globe, it may be best to keep the child at rest, gently shield the eye with a metal shield or cut-down paper cup, and keep the extent of examination to a necessary minimum to prevent expulsion of intraocular contents. In this setting, the child should be given nothing by mouth in case eye examination under anesthesia or surgical repair is required. The diagnosis may be difficult if the signs of obvious corneal perforation (shallow anterior chamber with hyphema and irregular pupil) are not present (Figure 15–8). Furthermore, nonradiopaque materials such as glass will not be seen on x-ray film. A CT scan may be useful in evaluating ocular trauma, including bony injury and foreign body wound. MRI will

**Figure 15–8.** Corneal laceration with irregular pupil and vitreous loss.

**Figure 15–9.** Laceration involving right lower lid and canaliculus.

not provide bony detail and must be avoided if a magnetic foreign body is suspected.

Zaidman GW et al: Successful surgical rehabilitation of children with traumatic corneal laceration and cataract. Ophthalmology 2001;108:338 [PMID: 11158810].

## INJURIES TO THE EYELIDS

### Ecchymosis

Orbital and soft tissue trauma may produce so-called black eye or ecchymosis (blue or purplish hemorrhagic areas) of the eyelids. The extent of the injury to the eye and orbit may not correlate fully with its appearance. Blowout fracture, which occurs from blunt trauma fracturing the walls of the orbit, must be suspected. Ocular motility must be assessed, the globe examined, and intraocular pressure measured, usually by an ophthalmologist. Cold compresses or ice packs for brief periods (eg, 10 minutes at a time) are recommended in older children in the first 24 hours after injury to reduce hemorrhage and swelling. Abuse needs to be considered when orbital injury is poorly explained.

### Lacerations

The lids and lacrimal apparatus are susceptible to laceration. Except for superficial lacerations away from the globe, repair in children is best performed in the operating room under general anesthesia. Special consideration must be given to lacerations involving the lid margin, to through-and-through lacerations, to lacerations that may involve the levator muscle in the upper lid, and to those that may involve the canaliculus (Figure 15–9). These injuries are best repaired by an ophthalmologist.

### Burns

Eyelid burns can occur in toddlers from contact with a lighted cigarette. The cornea is often involved as well. Curling irons can cause similar burns. These burns usually heal following application of antibiotic ointment. Severe thermal or chemical burns can cause scars resulting in ectropion or entropion of the lid and scarring of the conjunctiva and cul-de-sac.

Burns of the conjunctiva and cornea may be thermal, radiant, or chemical. Superficial thermal burns cause pain, tearing, and injection. Management is with topical antibiotics and patching. Add a cycloplegic agent if corneal involvement is present, because pain from ciliary spasm and iritis may accompany the injury.

Radiant energy causes ultraviolet keratitis. Typical examples are welder's burn and burns associated with skiing without goggles in bright sunlight. The fluorescein dye pattern will show a uniformly stippled appearance of the corneal epithelium. Antibiotic ointment, pressure patches, and a cycloplegic agent such as 5% homatropine are usually followed by recovery within 24 hours.

Chemical burns with strong acid and alkaline agents can be blinding and constitute a true ocular emergency. Examples are burns caused by exploding batteries, spilled drain cleaner, and bleach. Alkali burns may not cause significant injection because the conjunctival vessels become damaged. Alkalis tend to penetrate deeper than acids into ocular tissue. Immediate treatment consists of copious irrigation and removal of precipitates as soon as possible after the injury. The patient should be referred to an ophthalmologist after immediate first aid has been given.

Forbes BJ: Management of corneal abrasions and ocular trauma in children. Pediatr Ann 2001;30:465 [PMID: 11510344].

## Hyphema

Blunt trauma to the globe may cause hyphema, or bleeding within the anterior chamber from a ruptured vessel located near the root of the iris or in the anterior chamber angle. Bleeding may be microscopic or may fill the entire anterior chamber (Figure 15–10). Blunt trauma severe enough to cause hyphema may be associated with other ocular injury, including iritis, lens subluxation, retinal edema or detachment, and glaucoma. In patients with sickle cell anemia or trait, even moderate elevations of intraocular pressure may quickly lead to optic atrophy and permanent vision loss. Therefore, all African-Americans whose sickle cell status is unknown should be tested if hyphema is observed. These patients require extra vigilance in diagnosing and treating hyphema.

Management of hyphema in an otherwise uninjured patient should include testing of visual acuity and assessment of the integrity of the globe and orbit. A shield should be placed over the eye, the head elevated, and arrangements made for ophthalmologic referral.

Nontraumatic causes of hyphema include juvenile xanthogranuloma and blood dyscrasias. Rarely, hyphema is noted in the newborn after a stressful birth.

***Figure 15–10.*** Hyphema filling approximately 20% of the anterior chamber.

Lai JC et al: Traumatic hyphema in children. Risk factors for complications. Arch Ophthalmol 2001;119:64 [PMID: 11709038].

## Nonaccidental Trauma & Shaken Baby Syndrome

From an ocular standpoint, in both nonaccidental trauma and shaken baby syndrome, the hallmark of diagnosis is retinal hemorrhage, although it need not be present with rotational injury severe enough to cause subdural hematoma. In general, the presence and severity of the retinal hemorrhages correlates with the level of brain injury. Careful evaluation of the posterior and peripheral retina requires pupillary dilation and indirect ophthalmoscopy.

The history of how the injuries or retinal findings occurred is often vague and not well correlated with the extent of injury. Hemorrhages may be unilateral or bilateral and may be located in the posterior pole or periphery. Whereas retinal hemorrhages tend to resolve fairly quickly, those in the vitreous do not. If a blood clot lies over the macula, deprivation amblyopia may occur. Retinal and vitreous hemorrhages associated with intracranial hemorrhage from skull injury are known as Terson syndrome. Retinal hemorrhages are rarely associated with cardiopulmonary resuscitation or seizures. As a rule, retinal hemorrhages do not occur from major accidental trauma such as motor vehicle accidents unless a compressive chest injury is present, but they have been associated with low fibrinogen levels and blood dyscrasias. Other ocular findings associated with nonaccidental trauma include lid ecchymosis, subconjunctival hemorrhage, and hyphema. Additional retinal findings include retinal folds and retinoschisis. Acute-onset esotropia can also occur.

American Academy of Pediatrics. Committee on Child Abuse and Neglect. Shaken baby syndrome: Rotational cranial injuries—Technical report. Pediatrics 2001;108:206 [PMID: 11433079].

Drack AV et al: Unilateral retinal hemorrhages in documented cases of child abuse. Am J Ophthalmol 1999;128(3):340 [PMID: 10511029].

Kivlin JD et al: Shaken baby syndrome. Ophthalmology 2000; 107(7):1246 [PMID: 10889093].

Morris MW et al: Evaluation of infants with subdural hematoma who lack external evidence of abuse. Pediatrics 2001; 105:549 [PMID: 10699108].

## Prevention of Ocular Injuries

Air rifles, paint balls, and fireworks are responsible for many serious eye injuries in children. Golf injuries can also be very severe. Bungee cords have been associated with multiple types of severe ocular trauma, including corneal abrasion, iris tears, hyphema, vitreous hemorrhage, retinal detachment, and blindness. These activities should be avoided or very closely supervised. Safety goggles should be used in laboratories and industrial arts classes and when operating snow blowers, power lawn mowers, and power tools or when using hammers and nails. Sports-related eye injuries can be prevented with protective eyewear. Sports goggles and visors of polycarbonate plastic will prevent injuries in games using fast projectiles such as tennis or racquet balls, or where opponents may swing elbows or poke at the eye.

The one-eyed individual should be specifically advised to wear polycarbonate eyeglasses full time and goggles for all sports. High-risk activities such as boxing and the martial arts should be avoided by one-eyed children.

American Academy of Pediatrics Committee on Sports Medicine and Fitness and American Academy of Ophthalmology Committee on Eye Safety and Sports Ophthalmology: Protective eyewear for young athletes. Pediatrics 1996;98:311 [PMID: 8692640].

American Academy of Pediatrics. Committee on Injury and Poison Prevention: Fireworks-related injuries to children. Pediatrics 2001;108:190 [PMID: 11433076].

Chorich LJ III et al: Bungee cord associated ocular injuries. Am J Ophthalmol 1998;125:270 [PMID: 9467466].

Thompson CG et al: The aetiology of perforating ocular injuries in children. Br J Ophthalmol 2002;86(8):920 [PMID: 12140216].

# DISORDERS OF THE OCULAR STRUCTURES

## Diseases of the Eyelids

Blepharitis is inflammation of the lid margin characterized by crusty debris at the base of the lashes; varying degrees of erythema at the lid margins; and, in severe cases, secondary corneal changes such as punctate erosions, vascularization, and ulcers. When conjunctival injection accompanies blepharitis, the condition is known as blepharoconjunctivitis. *Staphylococcus* is the most common bacterial cause. Treatment includes lid scrubs with a nonburning baby shampoo several times a week and application of a topical antibiotic ointment such as erythromycin or bacitracin at bedtime.

Rosacea can also occur in the pediatric age group and cause chronic blepharoconjunctivitis with corneal changes that decrease vision. Systemic antibiotics and local treatment are required.

Pediculosis of the lids (phthiriasis palpebrarum) is caused by *Phthirus pubis*. Nits and adult lice can be seen on the eyelashes when viewed with appropriate magnification. Mechanical removal and application to the lid margins of phospholine iodide or 1% mercuric oxide

ointment can be effective. Other bodily areas of involvement must also be treated if involved. Family members and contacts may also be infected (see Chapter 14).

Papillomavirus may infect the lid and conjunctiva. Warts may be recurrent, multiple, and difficult to treat. Treatment modalities include cryotherapy, cautery, carbon dioxide laser, and surgery.

Localized staphylococcal infections of the glands of Zeis within the lid cause a sty (hordeolum) (Figure 15–11). When the infection coalesces and points internally or externally, it may discharge itself or require incision. The lesion is tender and red. Warm compresses help to hasten the acute process. Some practitioners prescribe a topical antibiotic ointment. Any coexisting blepharitis should be treated.

A chalazion is an inflammation of the meibomian glands, which may produce a tender nodule over the tarsus of the upper or lower lid. In addition to localized erythema of the corresponding palpebral conjunctiva, there may be a yellow lipogranuloma (Figure 15–12). Treatment includes warm compresses for 10–15 minutes four times a day for up to 6 weeks. If incision and curettage are needed because the lesion is slow to resolve, the child will require a general anesthetic.

## Viral Lid Disease

Herpes simplex virus may involve the lids at the time of primary herpes simplex infection. Vesicular lesions with an erythematous base occur. Primary herpes simplex blepharoconjunctivitis should be treated with systemic acyclovir (liquid formulation available), valacyclovir, or famciclovir. When either the conjunctiva or the cornea is involved, treatment should include topical 1% trifluridine or 3% vidarabine.

***Figure 15–11.*** Hordeolum and blepharitis, left upper lid.

A

B

***Figure 15–12.*** Chalazion. **A:** Right lower lid, external view. **B:** Right lower lid conjunctival surface.

***Figure 15–13.*** Congenital ptosis of severe degree, left upper lid.

Herpes zoster causes vesicular disease in association with a skin eruption in the dermatome of the ophthalmic branch of the trigeminal nerve. In older children, treatment of ophthalmic herpes zoster with oral acyclovir, valacyclovir, or famciclovir within 5 days after onset may reduce the morbidity. When vesicles are present on the tip of the nose with herpes zoster (Hutchinson sign), ocular involvement, including iritis, may develop. Herpes simplex or herpes zoster can be diagnosed by rapid viral culture (24–48 hours) or detection of antigen in skin lesions (3 hours). Impetigo is in the differential diagnosis of vesicular lid disease.

Molluscum contagiosum lesions are typically umbilicated papules. If near the lid margin, the lesions may shed and cause conjunctivitis. Cautery or excision of lesions at the lid margin is useful.

## Lid Ptosis

Ptosis—a droopy upper lid (Figure 15–13)—may be congenital or acquired but is usually congenital in children owing to a defective levator muscle. Other causes of ptosis are myasthenia gravis, lid injuries, third nerve palsy, and Horner syndrome (see next section). Surgical correction is indicated for moderate to severe ptosis. Mild cases require operative management less often than do more severe cases, and comesis may be better if surgery is delayed until most of the facial growth has occurred, usually aorund 5 years old. Ptosis may be associated with astigmatism and amblyopia.

An interesting association sometimes seen with congenital ptosis is the Marcus Gunn jaw-winking phenomenon. An intermittent reduction of the ptosis occurs during mastication or sucking. It is due to a synkinesis or simultaneous firing of either the external or internal pterygoid muscle (innervated by the trigeminal nerve) and the levator muscle (innervated by the oculomotor nerve).

## Horner Syndrome

Horner syndrome, which may be congenital or acquired, is the triad of miosis, ptosis, and anhidrosis. The ptosis is usually mild with a well-defined upper lid crease. This differentiates it from congenital ptosis, which typically has a poorly defined lid crease. Another key finding of congenital Horner syndrome is heterochromia of the two irides, with the lighter colored iris occurring on the same side as the lesion (Figure 15–14). Anhidrosis can occur in congenital and acquired cases. Of note, not all of the three signs must be present to make the diagnosis. The syndrome is caused by an abnormality or lesion to the sympathetic chain. The congenital variety is most commonly the result of birth trauma. Acquired cases may occur in children who have had cardiothoracic surgery, trauma, or brainstem vascular malformation. Most worrisome is a Horner syndrome caused by neuroblastoma of the sympathetic chain in the apical lung region. An excellent screening test for this is the spot urine vanillylmandelic acid/creatinine ratio.

***Figure 15–14.*** Congenital Horner syndrome. Ptosis, miosis, heterochromia. Lighter colored iris is on affected left side.

Pharmacologic assessment of the pupils with topical cocaine and hydroxyamphetamine or epinephrine will help determine whether the Horner syndrome is due to a preganglionic or postganglionic lesion of the sympathetic chain. Physical examination, including palpation of the neck and abdomen for masses, and MRI of structures in the head, neck, chest and abdomen should be considered.

McDonnell JF et al: Pediatric Horner syndrome due to cervical thymic rest. J Pediatr Ophthalmol Strabismus 2002;39(3): 185 [PMID: 12051288].

## Eyelid Tics

Eyelid tics may occur as a transient phenomenon lasting several days to months. Although a tic may be an isolated finding in an otherwise healthy child, it may also occur in children with multiple tics, attention-deficit/hyperactivity disorder, or Tourette syndrome. Caffeine consumption may cause or exacerbate eyelid tics. If the disorder is a short-lived annoyance, no treatment is needed.

# DISORDERS OF THE NASOLACRIMAL SYSTEM

## Nasolacrimal Duct Obstruction

Nasolacrimal obstruction occurs in up to 6% of infants. Most cases clear spontaneously during the first year. Signs and symptoms include a wet eye with mucoid discharge, erythema of one or both lids, and conjunctivitis (Figure 15–15). Obstruction in any part of the drainage system may result from incomplete canalization of the duct or membranous obstructions. Nasolacrimal obstruction may also occur in individuals with craniofacial abnormalities or amniotic band syndrome. Differential diagnosis of tearing includes congenital glaucoma, foreign bodies, nasal disorders, and, in older children, allergies.

Massage over the nasolacrimal sac may empty debris from the nasolacrimal sac and may clear the obstruction, although the efficacy of massage in clearing naso

***Figure 15–15.*** Nasolacrimal obstruction, right eye. Mattering on upper and lower lids.

lacrimal obstruction is debated. Cleansing the lids and medial canthal area decreases the likelihood of infection and irritation. Superinfection may occur, and treatment with topical antibiotics may help decrease the discharge. The mainstay of surgical treatment is probing, which is successful 80% or more of the time, but the success rate may decrease after the infant reaches age 1 year. Other surgical procedures, including infracture of the inferior nasal turbinate, balloon dilation, and silicone tube intubation, may be necessary if probing fails. Much less often, dacryocystorhinostomy is required.

Mandeville JT et al: Obstruction of the lacrimal drainage system. Curr Opin Ophthalmol 2002;13(5):303 [PMID 12218461].
Wagner RS: Management of congenital nasolacrimal obstruction. Pediatr Ann 2001;30:481 [PMID: 11510346].

## Congenital Dacryocystocele

Congenital dacryocystocele is thought to result from obstructions proximal and distal to the nasolacrimal sac. An intranasal duct cyst may be present beneath the inferior turbinate at the valve of Hasner. These cysts may be associated with respiratory distress. At birth, the nasolacrimal sac is distended and has a bluish hue that often leads to an erroneous diagnosis of hemangioma. The tense and swollen sac displaces the medial canthus superiorly (Figure 15–16). Massage and warm compresses are sometimes effective, but probing of the nasolacrimal system often is necessary. Repeated probing and endoscopic marsupialization of the intranasal cyst under general anesthesia may be required. Dacryocystitis and sepsis can result from dacryocystocele.

**Figure 15–16.** Congenital dacryocystocele on left side. Raised, bluish discolored mass of enlarged nasolacrimal sac. Note superiorly displaced medial canthus.

Levin AV et al: Nasal endoscopy in the treatment of congenital lacrimal sac mucoceles. Int J Pediatr Otorhinolaryngol 2003;67(3):255 ?PMID: 12633925?.

## Dacryocystitis

Acute and chronic dacryocystitis are typically bacterial and caused by organisms such as *Staphylococcus aureus, Streptococcus pneumoniae, Streptococcus pyogenes,* viridans streptococci, *Moraxella catarrhalis,* and *Haemophilus* species. Attempts at identifying the offending organism by culture and staining should be made when possible. Acute dacryocystitis presents with inflammation, swelling, tenderness, and pain over the lacrimal sac (located inferior to the medial canthal tendon). Fever may be present. The infection may point externally (Figure 15–17). A purulent discharge and tearing can be expected, because the cause of infection is almost always nasolacrimal obstruction.

Signs of chronic dacryocystitis are mucopurulent debris on the lids and lashes, tearing, injection of the palpebral conjunctiva, and reflux of pus at the puncta when pressure is applied over the sac. Chronic dacryocystitis and recurrent episodes of low-grade dacryocystitis are caused by nasolacrimal obstruction.

Treatment of severe acute dacryocystitis is with intravenous antibiotics. Oral antibiotics can be tried in milder cases. Topical antibiotic administration is ad-

**Figure 15–17.** Acute dacryocystitis in an 11-week-old infant.

junctive and is also used with recurrent chronic infections. Warm compresses are beneficial. After the acute episode subsides—and in chronic cases—the nasolacrimal obstruction must be relieved surgically. If it cannot be drained via the intranasal portion of the nasolacrimal duct, external drainage may be necessary. This should be done as a last resort since a fistula may develop.

## DISEASES OF THE CONJUNCTIVA

Conjunctivitis may be infectious, allergic, or associated with systemic disease. Trauma, irritation of the conjunctiva, and intraocular inflammation also can result in injection of conjunctival vessels that can be confused with conjunctivitis (Table 15–2).

### Ophthalmia Neonatorum

Ophthalmia neonatorum (conjunctivitis in the newborn) occurs during the first month of life. It is characterized by redness and swelling of the lids and conjunctiva and by discharge (Figure 15–18). Ophthalmia neonatorum may be due to inflammation resulting from silver nitrate prophylaxis given at birth, bacterial infection (gonococcal, staphylococcal, pneumococcal, chlamydial), or viral infection. In developed countries, *Chlamydia* is the most common cause. Neonatal conjunctivitis is visually threatening if caused by *Neisseria gonorrhoeae.* Herpes simplex is a rare but serious cause of neonatal conjunctivitis. Gram staining, Giemsa staining for elementary bodies, enzyme immunoassay for chlamydia, and bacterial and viral cultures aid in making an etiologic diagnosis.

Although no single prophylactic medication can eliminate all cases of neonatal conjunctivitis, povidone–iodine may provide broader coverage against the organisms causing this disease than silver nitrate or erythromycin ointment. Silver nitrate is not effective against chlamydia. The choice of prophylactic agent is often dictated by local epidemiology and cost considerations.

Treatment of these infections requires specific systemic antibiotics because they can cause serious infections in other organs. Specifically, *Chlamydia* can cause a delayed-onset pneumonitis. Parents should be examined and receive treatment when a sexually associated pathogen is present.

### Bacterial Conjunctivitis

In general, bacterial conjunctivitis is accompanied by a purulent discharge and viral infection by a watery discharge. One or both eyes may be involved. Regional lymphadenopathy is not a common finding in bacterial

***Table 15–2.*** Clinical and laboratory features of conjunctivitis.

|  | Viral | Bacterial | Chlamydial | Allergic |
|---|---|---|---|---|
| Itching | Minimal | Minimal | Minimal | Severe |
| Hyperemia | Generalized | Generalized | Generalized | Generalized |
| Tearing | Profuse | Moderate | Moderate | Moderate |
| Exudation | Minimal, mucoid | Profuse, purulent | Profuse; mucoid or mucopurulent | Minimal, slight mucus |
| Preauricular adenopathy | Common | Uncommon | Common in inclusion conjunctivitis | None |
| Stained conjunctival smears and scrapings | Lymphocytes, plasma cells, multinucleated giant cells, eosinophilic intranuclear inclusions | Neutrophils, bacteria | Neutrophils, plasma cells, basophilic intracytoplasmic inclusions | Eosinophils |
| Associated sytemic signs and symptoms | Rash, sore throat, fever in some patients | Occasional fever, sore throat | Pneumonia in neonates | Variable—may or may not be present |

Modified from Vaughan D, Asbury T, Riordan-Eva P (eds): *General Ophthalmology*, 15th ed. Appleton & Lange, 1999.

conjunctivitis except in cases of oculoglandular syndrome due to *S aureus,* group A β-hemolytic streptococci, *Mycobacterium tuberculosis* or atypical mycobacteria, *Francisella tularensis* (the agent of tularemia), and *Bartonella henselae* (the agent of cat-scratch fever).

Common bacterial causes of conjunctivitis in older children include nontypable *Haemophilus* species, *S pneumoniae, M catarrhalis,* and *S aureus.* If conjunctivitis is not associated with systemic illness, topical antibiotics such as erythromycin, polymyxin–bacitracin, sulfacetamide, tobramycin, and fluoroquinolones are

usually adequate. Systemic therapy is recommended for conjunctivitis associated with *Chlamydia trachomatis, N gonorrhoeae,* and *N meningitidis.*

## Viral Conjunctivitis

Adenovirus infection is often associated with pharyngitis, a follicular reaction of the palpebral conjunctiva, and preauricular adenopathy (pharyngoconjunctival fever). Epidemics of adenoviral keratoconjunctivitis occur. Treatment is supportive. Children with presumed adenoviral keratoconjunctivitis are considered contagious 10–14 days from the day of onset. They should stay out of school and group activities as long as their eyes are red and tearing. Strict handwashing precautions are recommended.

During the prodromal period of measles infection, conjunctivitis occurs; this is preceded by a transverse marginal line of conjunctival injection across the lower lids.

Herpes simplex virus may cause conjunctivitis or blepharoconjunctivitis. Treatment is with topical trifluridine 1% drops or 3% vidarabine ointment. Oral acyclovir may be used prophylactically in children to reduce recurrence of herpes simplex ocular disease.

Altemeier III WA: The importance of adenoviral infections in pediatrics. Pediatr Ann 2001;30:439 [PMID: 11510341].

## Allergic Conjunctivitis

In hay fever conjunctivitis, the eyes are red and itchy, with mucoid discharge. Symptomatic treatment is with

***Figure 15–18.*** Ophthalmia neonatorum due to *Chlamydia trachomatis* infection in a 2-week-old infant. Note marked lid and conjunctival inflammation.

***Table 15–3.*** Common ocular allergy medications.

| Generic Name | Brand Name | Mechanism of Action | Side Effects | Dosage | Indications |
|---|---|---|---|---|---|
| Lodoxamide tro-methamine 0.1% | Alomide | Mast-cell stabilizer | Transient burning or stinging | 1 drop 4 times daily—taper | Vernal kerato-conjunctivitis |
| Cromolyn Na 4% | Crolom, Opticrom | Mast-cell stabilizer | Transient burning or stinging | 1 drop 4–6 times daily | Vernal kerato-conjunctivitis |
| Olopatidine | Patanol | Mast-cell stabilizer, H1 receptor antagonist | Headache, burning or stinging | twice daily (interval 6–8 hrs) | Itching due to allergic conjunctivitis |
| Ketorolac trometh-amine 0.5% | Acular | NSAID | Transient burning or stinging | 1 drop 4 times daily | Itching due to seasonal allergic conjunctivitis |
| Levocobastine HCl 0.05% | Livostin | H1 receptor antagonist | Transient burning or stinging, headache | 1 drop 4 times daily | Relief of symptoms of seasonal allergic conjunctivitis |
| Naphazoline HCl 0.1% | AK-con, Naphcon, Opcon, Vasocon | Ocular decongestant, vasoconstrictor | Mydriasis, increased redness, irritation, discomfort, punctate keratitis, increased intra-ocular pressure, dizzy, HA, nausea, nervousness, HTN, weakness, cardiac effects, hyperglycemia | Varies by preparation | Temporary relief of redness due to minor eye irritants |
| Pheniramine maleate | Component in AK-Con A, Opcon-A, Naphcon-A | Antihistamine | | 1 drop every 3–4 h, as needed | Relief of symptoms of seasonal allergic conjunctivitis |

a combination topical vasoconstrictor plus an antihistamine (naphazoline–antazoline); a nonsteroidal anti-inflammatory drug such as ketorolac tromethamine 0.5%; a mast cell stabilizer such as lodoxamide tromethamine 0.1%; or prednisolone 0.125% (Table 15–3). Corticosteroids should be used with caution because their extended use causes glaucoma and or cataracts in some patients. Central nervous system (CNS) depression has been reported with accidental ingestion of naphazoline.

Vernal conjunctivitis is a seasonal form of allergic conjunctivitis associated with tearing, itching, and a stringy discharge. It is more common in males. In the palpebral form, dramatic changes of the superior palpebral conjunctiva occur, with cobblestone papillae (Figure 15–19). Corneal ulcers can occur. Topical treatments include a mast cell stabilizer such as 4% cromolyn sodium or 0.1% lodoxamide tromethamine and limited use of a topical corticosteroid. One form of

***Figure 15–19.*** Vernal conjunctivitis. Cobblestone papillae in superior tarsal conjunctiva.

vernal conjunctivitis (limbal vernal) presents with nodules at the limbus (the corneal–conjunctival junction). Contact lens wear may induce a conjunctivitis that appears similar to the palpebral form of vernal conjunctivitis.

## Mucocutaneous Diseases

Conjunctivitis and conjunctival changes are associated with a number of systemic syndromes. Examples are erythema multiforme (Stevens–Johnson syndrome; see Chapter 14), Reiter syndrome (Chapter 40), and Kawasaki disease (Chapter 19), which is also associated with iritis. With Stevens–Johnson syndrome, conjunctival changes include erythema, vesicular lesions that frequently rupture, and symblepharon (adhesions) between the raw edges of the bulbar and palpebral (lid) conjunctiva. Management may include artificial tears and lubricants to provide comfort and a topical corticosteroid to prevent adhesions and dry eye in severe cases of erythema multiforme. Lysis of adhesions or use of a scleral ring by an ophthalmologist may be required. Surgical treatment of severe cases of symblepharon with amniotic membrane grafts are under investigation. Cycloplegic agents and topical corticosteroids are prescribed for iritis in Kawasaki disease.

Honavar SG et al: Amniotic membrane transplantation for ocular surface reconstruction in Stevens–Johnson syndrome. Ophthalmology 2000 May;107(5):975–979 [PMID 10811093].

# DISORDERS OF THE IRIS

## Iris Coloboma

Iris coloboma is a developmental defect due to incomplete closure of the anterior embryonal fissure. The child's pupil will have an elongated shape reminiscent of a keyhole or cat's eye (Figure 15–20). The affected area is located inferonasally but may extend posteriorly, involving the retina and choroid. The effect on visual acuity is variable. Iris coloboma may be an isolated defect or may be associated with a number of chromosomal abnormalities and syndromes. Variable genetic expression of coloboma can include a broad spectrum, from iris coloboma, to microphthalmia-with-cyst, and even clinical anophthalmia.

## Aniridia

Aniridia is a bilateral disorder that includes macular hypoplasia and absence of almost all of the iris (Figure 15–21). Cataract, corneal changes, and glaucoma are often seen. Photophobia and nystagmus occur.

Aniridia may occur as an autosomal dominant inheritance pattern or in a sporadic form that is associated

*Figure 15–20.* Iris coloboma located inferiorly.

with Wilms tumor. Repeated examination and abdominal ultrasonography are thus indicated. The aniridia gene has been isolated to the 11p13 chromosome region. Aniridia, genitourinary abnormalities, and mental retardation have been linked to an 11p deletion.

## Albinism

Albinism is caused by defective melanogenesis. Most cases of albinism are autosomal recessive, but an X-linked form does occur. Tyrosinase is an essential enzyme in the production of melanin. Many cases of complete albinism are caused by mutations of the tyrosinase gene. Albinism with some pigment production, especially in people of African descent, is more commonly caused by mutations of the *p* gene.

Affected individuals are usually legally blind and have nystagmus (see nystagmus section). Iris, skin, and hair color varies according to the type and severity of albinism as well as the individual's race. Iris transillumination may be obvious or may require slitlamp examination with retroillumination to detect focal areas of

*Figure 15–21.* Bilateral aniridia. Iris remnants present temporally in each eye.

transillumination. Other ocular abnormalities include foveal hypoplasia, abnormal optic pathway projections, strabismus, and poor stereoacuity. These children should be evaluated by a pediatric ophthalmologist in order to optimize their visual function.

Albinism may be associated with other systemic manifestations. Bleeding problems occur in individuals with Hermansky–Pudlak syndrome (chromosome 10q23 or 5q13), in which oculocutaneous albinism is associated with a platelet abnormality. Chédiak–Higashi syndrome (chromosome 1q42–44) is characterized by neutrophil defects, recurrent infections, and oculocutaneous albinism. Other conditions associated with albinism are Waardenburg, Prader–Willi, and Angelman syndromes.

The risk of skin cancer is much higher in individuals with albinism. Parents and patients must be advised to use sunscreen and wear protective clothing.

Dorey SE et al: The clinical features of albinism and their correlation with visual evoked potentials. Br J Ophthalmol 2003; 87(6):767–772 [PMID 12770978].

Russell-Eggitt I: Albinism. Ophthalmol Clin North Am 2001;1 4(3):533–546 [PMID 11705153].

## Other Iris Conditions

Heterochromia, or a difference in iris color, can occur in congenital Horner syndrome, after iritis, or with tumors and nevi of the iris and use of topical prostaglandins. Malignant melanoma of the iris may also cause iris heterochromia. Acquired iris nodules (Lisch nodules), which occur in type I neurofibromatosis, usually become apparent by age 8 years. When seen on slitlamp examination, Lisch nodules are 1–2 mm in diameter and often beige in color, although their appearance can vary. Iris xanthogranuloma occurring with juvenile xanthogranuloma can cause hyphema and glaucoma. Patients with juvenile xanthogranuloma should be evaluated by an ophthalmologist for ocular involvement.

DeBella K et al: Use of the National Institutes of Health criteria for diagnosis of neurofibromatosis 1 in children. Pediatrics 2000;105:608 [PMID: 10699117].

## GLAUCOMA

Glaucoma is increased intraocular pressure, which causes damage to ocular structures and loss of vision. Signs of glaucoma presenting within the first year of life include buphthalmos (enlargement of the globe due to low scleral rigidity in the infant eye) as well as tearing, photophobia, blepharospasm, corneal clouding due to edema, and optic nerve cupping. After age 3 years, usually only optic nerve changes occur.

Pediatric glaucoma can be congenital or acquired and unilateral or bilateral. In general, do not expect to see a red, inflamed eye with congenital or infantile glaucoma. Although acute pupillary block glaucoma causes a red, painful eye, pupillary block is quite rare in the pediatric age group.

Glaucoma may be inherited. Glaucoma can be classified on an anatomic basis into two types: open-angle and closed-angle. Precipitating angle-closure glaucoma in a child by dilating the pupil of an otherwise healthy eye is a very rare occurrence.

Glaucoma also occurs with ocular and systemic syndromes. Aniridia and anterior segment dysgenesis are examples. Systemic syndromes associated with glaucoma include Sturge–Weber syndrome, the oculocerebrorenal syndrome of Lowe, and the Pierre Robin syndrome. Glaucoma can also occur with hyphema, iritis, lens dislocation, intraocular tumor, and ROP. Treatment depends on the cause, but surgery is often the choice unless the rise in intraocular pressure is transient, in which case medical treatment is indicated.

Be aware that some individuals are "steroid responders" who develop increased intraocular pressure when challenged with exogenous steroids. The optic nerve of African Americans is probably prone to damage with acute increases in traocular pressure.

## UVEITIS

Inflammation of the uveal tract can be subdivided according to the uveal tissue primarily involved (iris, choroid, retina) or by location, that is, anterior, intermediate, or posterior uveitis. Perhaps the most commonly diagnosed form of uveitis in childhood is traumatic iridocyclitis (iritis).

## Anterior Uveitis

Injection, photophobia, pain, and blurred vision usually accompany iritis (anterior uveitis, iridocyclitis). An exception to this is iritis associated with juvenile rheumatoid arthritis (Chapter 26), when the eye is quiet and asymptomatic, but slitlamp examination will reveal anterior chamber inflammation in which inflammatory cells and protein flare are seen.

Iridocyclitis associated with juvenile rheumatoid arthritis occurs most often in girls with pauciarticular arthritis and a positive antinuclear antibody. All children with juvenile rheumatoid arthritis need to be screened according to a schedule recommended by the American Academy of Pediatrics (www.aap.org). Treatment with a topical corticosteroid and a cycloplegic agent is aimed at quieting the inflammation and preventing or delaying the onset of cataract and glaucoma.

Methotrexate and other immunosuppressive agents can be used in refractory cases.

Inflammatory bowel disease is also associated with iritis—perhaps more commonly with Crohn disease than with ulcerative colitis. Other ocular findings of the anterior segment that can be associated with inflammatory bowel disease include conjunctivitis, episcleritis, and sterile corneal infiltrates. Posterior segment findings may include central serous retinochoroidopathy, panuveitis (inflammation of all uveal tissue), choroiditis, ischemic optic neuropathy, retinal vasculitis, neuroretinitis, and intermediate uveitis (see section on Intermediate Uveitis).

Posterior subcapsular cataracts can develop in patients with or without ocular inflammation. Most, if not all, of these patients have been taking corticosteroids as part of the long-term treatment of inflammatory bowel disease. Children with Crohn disease or ulcerative colitis should have routine periodic ophthalmologic examinations to rule out ocular inflammation, which may be asymptomatic, and cataracts associated with systemic corticosteroids.

Other causes of anterior uveitis in children include syphilis, tuberculosis, sarcoidosis, relapsing fever (borreliosis), and Lyme disease, all but the last also causing posterior uveitis. Juvenile spondyloarthropathies, including ankylosing spondylitis, Reiter syndrome, and psoriatic arthritis, are also associated with anterior uveitis. A substantial percentage of cases are of unknown origin.

Kodsi SR et al: Time of onset of uveitis in children with juvenile rheumatoid arthritis. J AAPOS 2002;6(6):373 [PMID 12506279].

Oren B et al: The prevalence of uveitis in juvenile rheumatoid arthritis. J Am Assoc Pediatr Ophthalmol Strabismus 2001;5:2 [PMID: 11182663].

## Posterior Uveitis

The terms *choroiditis, retinitis,* and *retinochoroiditis* denote the tissue layer primarily involved in posterior uveitis. Characteristic features occur with posterior uveitis as a result of certain organisms. Active toxoplasmosis (see Chapter 39) produces a white lesion appearing as a "headlight in the fog" owing to the overlying vitritis. Inactive lesions have a hyperpigmented border. Contiguous white satellite lesions suggest reactivation of disease. Congenital infections must be treated aggressively with a triple drug regimen (pyramethamine, sulfadiazine, and leukovorin) for 1 year. Studies have shown improved ophthalmic and neurologic outcomes with prolonged treatment. A granular "salt and pepper" retinopathy is characteristic of congenital rubella. In infants, the TORCH complex (toxoplasmosis, rubella, cytomegalovirus [CMV], herpes simplex virus) and syphilis must be suspected in congenital infections that cause chorioretinitis.

Congenital lymphocytic choriomeningitis virus (LCMV) may also present with chorioretinitis. The virus is transmitted to humans by consumption of food contaminated with rodent urine or feces. It most closely resembles congenital toxoplasmosis in presentation. Diagnosis is done by immunofluorescent antibody or enzyme-linked immunosorbent assay (ELISA) laboratory testing. If possible, pregnant women should avoid exposure to rodents.

Ocular candidiasis occurs typically in an immunocompromised host or an infant in the intensive care nursery receiving hyperalimentation. Candidal chorioretinitis appears as multifocal, whitish yellow, fluffy retinal lesions that may spread into the vitreous and produce a so-called cotton/fungus ball vitritis.

Acute retinal necrosis syndrome is caused most often by varicella-zoster virus and occasionally by herpes simplex virus. Patients may present with a red and painful eye. Ophthalmoscopy may show unilateral or bilateral patchy white areas of retina, arterial sheathing, vitreous haze, atrophic retinal scars, retinal detachment, and optic nerve involvement.

CMV is a cause of congenital infection that may be accompanied by retinitis. CMV infection must be considered as a cause of retinitis in immunocompromised and human immunodificiency virus (HIV)-infected children. CMV retinitis appears as a white retinal lesion, typically but not always associated with hemorrhage, or as a granular, indolent-appearing lesion with hemorrhage and a white periphery. Cotton wool spots (nerve fiber layer infarcts) also commonly occur in HIV-positive patients.

In toddlers and older youngsters, *Toxocara canis* or *T cati* infections (ocular larva migrans; see Chapter 39) occur from ingesting soil contaminated with parasite eggs. The disease is usually unilateral. Common signs and symptoms include a red injected eye, leukocoria, and decreased vision. Fundus examination may show endophthalmitis (vitreous abscess) or localized granuloma. Diagnosis is based on the appearance of the lesion and serologic testing using ELISA for *T canis* and *T cati.* Treatment options include periocular corticosteroid injections and vitrectomy.

Bresin AP et al: Ophthalmic outcomes after prenatal and postnatal treatment of congenital toxoplasmosis. Am J Ophthalmol 2003;135(6):779 [PMID 12788116].

Mets MB et al: Lymphocytic choriomeningitis virus: An underdiagnosed cause of congenital chorioretinitis. Am J Ophthalmol 2000;130(2):209 [PMID 11004296].

## Intermediate Uveitis

Pars planitis, often of uncertain cause, can be associated with vitreous floaters. The inflammation is described as snowbanking because a heaped-up white precipitate is located in the far anterior periphery of the retina and vitreous base. Pupillary dilation and indirect ophthalmoscopy are required for observation. Macular edema and decreased vision can result.

*Toxocara* infections with peripheral granuloma can be associated with intermediate uveitis, as can inflammatory bowel disease, multiple sclerosis, and sarcoidosis. Retinoblastoma and other neoplasms can imitate uveitis, causing a so-called masquerade syndrome.

## ACQUIRED IMMUNODEFICIENCY SYNDROME & THE EYE

Ocular infections are important manifestations of acquired immunodeficiency syndrome (AIDS) (see Chapter 37). As CD4 T-lymphocyte counts fall below 200/μL, opportunistic infections increase in these patients. Pathogens commonly causing eye infection include *Toxoplasma gondii* and CMV. Especially when CD4+ counts fall below 50/μL, the patient is at high risk for CMV retinitis, the leading cause of vision loss in AIDS patients (see Posterior Uveitis section) and blindness. Active CMV retinitis must be treated with intravenous foscarnet or ganciclovir. These medications may be required in combination if the retinitis fails to respond to a single drug regimen. Intravitreal ganciclovir or ganciclovir implants in conjunction with oral valganciclovir may be required in severe cases or in individuals intolerant to intravenous therapy. The incidence of CMV retinitis has fallen dramatically with the use of multidrug antiretroviral therapy.

Acute retinal necrosis syndrome (see Posterior Uveitis section) is a severe necrotizing retinitis in AIDS patients that often results in blindness. Most cases are thought to be caused by varicella-zoster virus. Other implicated agents are herpes simplex types 1 and 2 and occasionally CMV. Therapy with antiviral agents is required, but the prognosis is poor. A specific HIV retinopathy not associated with other known infectious agents also occurs. Various retinal abnormalities include cotton wool spots, retinal hemorrhages, microaneurysms, perivasculitis, and decreased visual acuity from ischemic maculopathy.

Frenkel et al: Oral ganciclovir in children: Pharmacokinetics, safety, tolerance, and antiviral effects. The Pediatric AIDS Clinical Trials Group. J Infect Dis 2000;182(6):1616 [PMID 11069232].

Jabs DA et al: Characteristics of patients with cytomegalovirus retinitis in the era of highly active antiretroviral therapy. Am J Ophthalmol 2002;133(1):48 [PMID 11755839].

## DISORDERS OF THE CORNEA
### Conditions Causing Corneal Clouding

The differential diagnosis of corneal clouding in a newborn infant includes forceps trauma, congenital glaucoma, infection, congenital malformation, and tumor. In older children, corneal clouding is associated with mucopolysaccharidoses, Wilson disease, and cystinosis. Infiltrates occur with viral infections, staphylococcal lid disease, corneal dystrophies, and interstitial keratitis due to congenital syphilis.

### Microcornea & Megalocornea

Microcornea—a corneal diameter less than 10 mm in a full-term infant or older child—may be associated with other anterior segment malformations or a microphthalmic globe. Megalocornea—diameter of 12.5 mm or greater—should be regarded as due to congenital glaucoma until proved otherwise.

### Keratitis

Both herpes simplex and herpes zoster can infect the cornea. When the epithelium breaks down, a dendritic or ameboid pattern can be seen with fluorescein staining. Corneal involvement with herpes simplex can be recurrent and lead to blindness. Topical antivirals such as trifluridine and vidarabine are indicated when herpes simplex infection is limited to the corneal epithelium. Topical corticosteroids may be a useful addition when stromal disease is present. The use of corticosteroids in the presence of herpetic disease should be undertaken only by an ophthalmologist because of the danger of worsening the disease. Oral acyclovir started in the early phase (first 5 days) may be helpful in treating herpes zoster eye disease. Acyclovir prophylaxis is helpful in preventing recurrent herpetic epithelial keratitis (see Viral Conjunctivitis section) and stromal keratitis caused by herpes simplex.

Adenovirus conjunctivitis may progress to keratitis 1–2 weeks after onset. Slitlamp examination reveals white infiltrates beneath the corneal epithelium. Vision may be decreased. In most cases no treatment is necessary because adenovirus keratitis is most often self-limiting. However, adenovirus is highly contagious and easily spread (see Conjunctivitis section).

Contact lens wearers are at risk for severe vision-threatening *Acanthamoeba* keratitis from contaminated contact lens solutions. Treatment is difficult and may require corneal transplantation (see Chapter 39).

The Herpetic Eye Disease Study Group: Acyclovir for the prevention of recurrent herpes simplex virus eye disease. N Engl J Med 1998;339:300 [PMID: 9696640].

Schwartz GS et al: Oral acyclovir for the management of herpes simplex virus keratitis in children. Ophthalmology 2000;107:278 [PMID: 10690825].

## Corneal Ulcers

Bacterial corneal ulcers in healthy children who are not contact lens wearers are usually secondary to corneal trauma from corneal abrasion or a penetrating foreign body. Decreased vision, pain, injection, a white corneal infiltrate or ulcer (Figure 15–22), and hypopyon (pus in the anterior chamber) may all be present. Prompt referral to an ophthalmologist is necessary for culture and antibiotic treatment.

# DISORDERS OF THE LENS

Lens disorders involve abnormality of clarity or position. Lens opacification–cataract can affect vision depending on its density, size, and position. Visual potential is also influenced by age at onset and the success of amblyopia treatment.

## Cataracts

Cataracts in children may be unilateral or bilateral, may exist as isolated defects, or may be accompanied by other ocular disorders or systemic disease (Figure 15–23). Congenital and infantile cataracts may also be part of a chromosomal syndrome. Leukocoria, poor fixation, and strabismus or nystagmus (or both) may be the presenting complaints. In the newborn, absence of a red reflex should suggest the possibility of cataract, especially if the infant's pupil has been dilated for the examination.

The appearance of the cataract may sometimes suggest its cause. Anterior capsular cataracts are develop-

***Figure 15–23.*** Cataract causing leukocoria.

mental, that is, not related to infection or metabolic problems. Laboratory investigation for infectious and metabolic causes is often indicated. Such investigation would include cultures or serologic tests for toxoplasmosis, rubella, CMV, herpes simplex virus, and syphilis as well as evaluation for metabolic errors as may occur with galactosemia or Lowe syndrome.

Early diagnosis and treatment are necessary to prevent deprivation amblyopia in children younger than age 9 years, because such children are visually immature. Cataracts that are visually significant require removal. Rehabilitation with an intraocular lens is commonplace, especially with cataracts removed after the age of 2 years. But contact lenses and glasses still play a role, as does occlusion of the better-seeing eye to treat the amblyopia.

Fallaha N et al: Pediatric cataracts. Ophthalmol Clin North Am 2001;14(3):479 [PMID 11705148].

Wilson ME et al: Paediatric cataract blindness in the developing world: Surgical techniques and intraocular lenses in the new millennium. Br J Ophthalmol 2003;87(1):14 [PMID 12488254].

## Dislocated Lenses

Lens dislocation is usually bilateral except when caused by trauma. Subluxation causes refractive errors of large magnitude that are difficult to correct. Another ophthalmologic concern is pupillary block glaucoma. In this disorder, a malpositioned unstable lens interferes with the normal flow of aqueous humor from where it is produced in the ciliary body (posterior to the pupil) into the trabecular meshwork (anterior to the pupillary plane).

Dislocated lenses are associated with other ocular conditions and systemic syndromes, including Marfan syndrome, homocystinuria, Weill–Marchesani syndrome, sulfite oxidase deficiency, hyperlysinemia,

***Figure 15–22.*** Corneal ulcer. Note white infiltrate located on inferior cornea.

syphilis, and Ehlers–Danlos syndrome. Work-up and treatment are multidisciplinary endeavors.

# DISORDERS OF THE RETINA

## Retinal Hemorrhages in the Newborn

Retinal hemorrhages are commonly seen in the otherwise healthy newborn. Although it occurs most often after vaginal delivery, this finding can also be present after suction delivery or cesarean section. The hemorrhages may be unilateral or bilateral and be located anywhere in the retina. They may appear as dot, blot, subretinal, or preretinal hemorrhages. They may also break into the vitreous.

In general, retinal hemorrhages of the newborn disappear quickly, usually within the first month of life, which may help differentiate this condition from retinal hemorrhages that occur in the shaken baby syndrome. Another cause of retinal hemorrhage is coagulopathy.

Emerson AV et al: Incidence and rate of disappearance of retinal hemorrhage in newborns. Ophthalmology 2001;108:36 [PMID: 11150261].

## Retinopathy of Prematurity

Retinopathy of prematurity (ROP) continues to be an important cause of blindness, especially for infants born at less than 28 weeks' gestation and weighing less than 1250 g. Premature infants with incomplete retinal vascularization are at risk for developing abnormal peripheral retinal vascularization, which may lead to retinal detachment. However, most cases of ROP do not progress to retinal detachment and require no treatment.

The CRYO-ROP study outlined a standard nomenclature to describe the progression and severity of ROP (Table 15–4). Since retinal blood vessels emanate from the optic nerve, and do not fully cover the developing retina until term, the optic nerve is used as the central landmark. The most immature zone of retina, zone 1, is the most posterior concentric imaginary circle around the optic nerve. Further out is zone 2, and beyond that is zone 3. Zone 1 disease is, by definition, more high risk than disease in more anterior zones. Similarly, the stages of the abnormal vessels are numbered from zero, or simply incomplete vascularization, through stages I, II, and III. When 5 contiguous, or 8 noncontiguous clock hours of stage 3 disease occur, "threshold" has been reached. At this stage in the CRYO-ROP study, 50% of eyes had a bad outcome without treatment, progressing to stage IV or V. This was therefore chosen as the stage for mandatory treatment. Plus disease (+) refers to dilation and tortuosity of the vessels around the optic nerve, and is an ominous sign of active, worsening ROP. Rush disease refers to cases in which the disease skips intervening stages and goes rapidly to retinal detachment.

The risk of developing visually threatening ROP is inversely proportional to birth weight and gestational age. Infants weighing less than 1500 g at birth or born at less than 33 weeks' gestation may develop visually threatening ROP. The cause of this disorder—including the role of supplemental oxygen in the neonatal period—is still not fully understood. During the first epidemic of ROP in the 1960s, delivery of high levels of oxygen without arterial monitoring appeared to contribute significantly to the development of ROP. Pulse oximetry and better regulation led to a decline in cases, but better survival for the smallest, sickest infants has increased the numbers of affected infants once again, leading to speculation that low birth weight and gestational age may be more important than oxygen in etiology. Anecdotal reports of improvement in near-threshold ROP with high oxygen saturations led to the STOP-ROP study, which investigated whether keeping $PaO_2$ high at this critical stage reduced the need for laser. The results did not show a benefit. A study in which infants were kept at relatively low oxygen saturation from birth did show a reduction in severe ROP cases and showed no increase in cerebral palsy at 18 months follow-up, which had been reported in the past with oxygen curtailment. Further study and follow-up of this method is needed. Other risk factors for severe ROP are bronchopulmonary dysplasia, intraventricular hemorrhage, sepsis, apnea and bradycardia, and mutations of Norrie disease gene. White males, infants with zone 1 disease, and infants with very low birth weight and gestational age have a higher risk of reaching threshold.

Another cofactor that has been investigated is ambient light in the nursery. One early study found a correlation between light exposure and development of ROP, but the multicenter LIGHT-ROP trial found no

**Table 15–4.** Stages of retinopathy of prematurity.

| | |
|---|---|
| Stage I | Demarcation line or border dividing the vascular from the avascular retina. |
| Stage II | Ridge. Line of stage I acquires volume and rises above the surface retina to become a ridge. |
| Stage III | Ridge with extraretinal fibrovascular proliferation. |
| Stage IV | Subtotal retinal detachment. |
| Stage V | Total retinal detachment. |

"Plus disease" signifies arteriolar tortuosity and venular dilation of posterior pole vessels.

correlation. Recent studies suggest that the substance vascular endothelial growth factor (VEGF) may play a key role in ROP development, and methods of modulating VEGF are being investigated.

Screening guidelines and a uniform classification system have been adopted, but alternative screening paradigms have also been suggested. The first retinal examination is recommended at age 4–6 weeks after birth, or 31 weeks postmenstrual age, whichever is earlier. The frequency of follow-up examinations depends on the findings and the risk factors for developing the disease, but for most infants will be every 1–2 weeks. Acute-phase ROP begins to involute at a mean postmenstrual age of 38.6 weeks, but the range for onset of involution is wide. Examinations can be discontinued when the retinas are fully vascularized, or when the baby is 45 weeks' gestational age and has never had prethreshold disease or worse, or is vascularized out to zone 3 and never had zone 1 or 2 disease. The treatment of threshold ROP within 72 hours of diagnosis with cryotherapy reduced the occurrence of bad visual outcomes by 50%. Diode laser treatment has largely replaced cryotherapy because it provides better access for treating zone 1 disease and causes less inflammation. Reported success rates are higher than with cryotherapy. However, some patients still develop blinding retinal detachment. With smaller, sicker infants surviving, treatment guidelines may need to be amended to treat earlier than threshold in some infants. Studies investigating this are underway.

Other findings associated with ROP include strabismus, amblyopia, myopia, glaucoma, and loss of visual field.

American Academy of Pediatrics, the American Association for Pediatric Ophthalmology and Strabismus, and the American Academy of Ophthalmology: A joint statement: Screening examination of premature infants for retinopathy of prematurity. Revised 2001.

http://www.aao.org/aao/education/library/information/rop.cfm

Chow LC et al; CSMC Oxygen Administration Study Group: Can changes in clinical practice decrease the incidence of severe retinopathy of prematurity in very low birth weight infants? Pediatrics 2003;111(2):339 [PMID: 12563061].

Cryotherapy for Retinopathy of Prematurity Cooperative Group: Effect of retinal ablative therapy for threshold retinopathy of prematurity: Results of Goldmann perimetry at the age of 10 years. Arch Ophthalmol 2001;119:1120 [PMID: 11483077].

Cryotherapy for Retinopathy of Prematurity Cooperative Group: Multicenter trial for retinopathy of prematurity: Ophthalmological outcomes at 10 years. Arch Ophthalmol 2001;119:1110 [PMID: 11483076].

Holmstrom G, el Azazi M: Ophthalmologic followup of preterm infants: A population based, prospective study of visual acuity and strabismus. Br J Ophthalmol 1999;83:143 [PMID: 10396188].

Onofrey CB et al: The outcome of retinopathy of prematurity screening for retinopathy using an outcome predictive program. Ophthalmology 2001;108:27 [PMID: 11150259].

Repka MX et al: Involution of retinopathy of prematurity. Arch Ophthalmol 2000;118:645 [PMID: 10815156].

Repka MX et al: The incidence of ophthalmologic intervention in children with birth weights less than 1251 grams: Results through 5½ years: Cryotherapy for retinopathy of prematurity cooperative group. Ophthalmology 1998;105:1621 [PMID: 9754167].

Reynolds JD et al, CRYO-ROP and LIGHT-ROP Cooperative Study Groups: Evidence-based screening criteria for retinopathy of prematurity: Natural history data from the CRYO-ROP and LIGHT-ROP studies. Arch Ophthalmol 2002;120(11):1470 [PMID: 12427059].

STOP-ROP Multicenter Study Group: Supplemental therapeutic oxygen for threshold retinopathy of prematurity (STOP-ROP), a randomized, controlled trial. I: Primary outcomes. Pediatrics 2000;105:420 [PMID: 10654946].

Subhani M et al: Screening guidelines for retinopathy of prematurity: The need for revision in extremely low birth weight infants. Pediatrics 2001;108:27 [PMID: 11335739].

## Retinoblastoma

Retinoblastoma is the most common primary intraocular malignancy of childhood, with an incidence estimated between 1:17,000 and 1:34,000 live births (see Chapter 28). Most patients present before age 3 years; children with hereditary or bilateral retinoblastoma usually present earlier than those with unilateral, sporadic disease.

Inherited forms of retinoblastoma are autosomal dominant with high penetrance. The disease may consist of a solitary mass or multiple tumors in one or both eyes. All bilateral cases and some unilateral cases are caused by germinal mutations; however, most unilateral cases are caused by a somatic retinal mutation. In both situations, the mutation occurs in the retinoblastoma gene (*Rb*) at chromosome 13q14. This is a tumor suppressor gene. One mutated copy may be inherited in an autosomal dominant fashion (germline mutation). If a second mutation spontaneously occurs in any cell, tumorigenesis is likely. Individuals with a germinal mutation are at risk for the development of tumors other than retinoblastoma (pineal tumors, osteosarcoma, and other soft tissue sarcomas). All children with unilateral or bilateral retinoblastoma must be presumed to have the germline form, including being followed expectantly for other tumors in the remaining eye and systemically. Approximately 15% of patients with unilateral disease have germline mutations.

The most common presenting sign in a child with previously undiagnosed retinoblastoma is leukocoria (see Figure 15–1). Evaluation of the pupillary red reflex is important, although a normal red reflex does not rule out retinoblastoma. This examination requires indirect ophthalmoscopy with scleral depression and pupillary dilation, performed by an ophthalmologist. Other children present with strabismus, red eye, glaucoma, or pseudohypopyon (appearance of pus-like material in the anterior chamber).

Treatment of unilateral cases, especially of large tumors, usually has been enucleation, because at the time of presentation the eye is filled with tumor. Vision and eyes can be salvaged in some cases. Chemoreduction of intraocular tumors is a newer treatment technique used to reduce initial tumor volume. In conjunction with local treatment such as laser photocoagulation, cryotherapy, plaque radiotherapy, and thermotherapy, it can preserve vision and spare the patient enucleation and radiation that may lead to disfigurement and the induction of secondary tumors, especially in eyes classified with less extensive disease. Agents used in chemoreduction include carboplatin, etoposide, and vincristine. Eradication of tumor before infiltration into the optic nerve or choroid carries a good prognosis for survival.

Genetic testing is available for patients with retinoblastoma. Once the causative mutation is found in an affected individual, unaffected members of the family may be tested to determine their personal and reproductive risk. This testing may avoid many unnecessary examinations under anesthesia for young relatives of patients of with retinoblastoma.

Ganesh A et al: Retinoblastoma and the 13 q deletion syndrome. J Pediatr Ophthalmol Strabismus 2001;38:247 [PMID: 11495315].

Metz TH Jr et al: Pupillary dilation by pediatricians. Pediatrics 1999;104:958 [PMID: 10506240].

Richter S et al: Sensitive and efficient detection of *RB1* gene mutations enhances care for families with retinoblastoma. Am J Hum Genet 2003;72(2):253 Epub 2002 Dec 18 [PMID:12541220].

Sussman DA et al: Comparison of retinoblastoma reduction for chemotherapy vs external beam radiotherapy. Arch Ophthalmol 2003;121(7):979 [PMID: 12860801].

## Retinal Detachment

Retinal detachment occurs infrequently in children. Common causes are trauma and high myopia. Other causes are ROP, Marfan syndrome, and Stickler syndrome.

Symptoms of detachment are floaters, flashing lights, and loss of visual field; however, children often cannot appreciate or verbalize their symptoms. A detachment may not be discovered until the child is referred after failing a vision screening examination, strabismus supervenes, or leukocoria is noted. Treatment of retinal detachment is surgical. For children with conditions predisposing to retinal detachment, or a strong family history, examinations under anesthesia by an ophthalmologist, with prophylactic laser treatment, are often recommended.

## Diabetes Mellitus

Diabetic retinopathy is a specific vascular complication of diabetes mellitus. Patients with type 1, or insulin-dependent, diabetes are at higher risk of developing severe proliferative retinopathy leading to visual loss than are those with type 2, or non-insulin-dependent, diabetes. The American Diabetes Association recommends annual screening for retinopathy 5 years after onset of diabetes in adults. In children older than age 9 years, referral to an ophthalmologist for screening of retinopathy should be begun 3–5 years after the onset of diabetes. Acute onset of diabetes may be accompanied by sudden myopia and by cataracts. Both conditions may be reversible with systemic glucose control. Young children with type 1 diabetes should be followed for the Wolfram, or DIDMOAD, syndrome, in which diabetes mellitus occurs in conjunction with diabetes insipidus, optic atrophy, and deafness.

American Academy of Pediatrics Section on Endocrinology and Ophthalmology: Screening for retinopathy in the pediatric patient with type 1 diabetes mellitus. Pediatrics 1998;101; 313 [PMID: 9457160].

Raman V et al: Retinopathy screening in children and adolescents with diabetes. Ann N Y Acad Sci 2002;958:387 [PMID: 12021146].

## DISEASES OF THE OPTIC NERVE

Optic nerve function is evaluated by checking visual acuity, color vision, pupillary response, and visual fields. Poor optic nerve function results in decreased central or peripheral vision, decreased color vision, strabismus, and nystagmus.

The swinging flashlight test is used to assess function of each optic nerve. It is performed by shining a light alternately in front of each pupil to check for an afferent pupillary defect or Marcus Gunn pupillary defect. An abnormal response in the affected eye is pupillary dilation when the light is directed into that eye after having been shown in the other eye with its healthy optic nerve. This results from poorer conduction along the optic nerve of the affected eye, which in turn results in less pupillary constriction of both eyes than occurs when the light is shined into the noninvolved eye. Hippus—rhythmic dilating and constricting movements of the pupil—can be confused with an afferent pupillary defect.

The optic nerve is evaluated as to size, shape, color, and vascularity. Occasionally, myelinization past the entrance of the optic nerve head occurs. It appears white, with a feathered edge (Figure 15–24). Myeliniza-

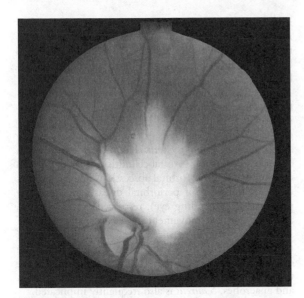

***Figure 15–24.*** Myelinization extending from optic nerve superiorly onto the retina.

tion onto the retina can be associated with myopia and amblyopia. Anatomic defects of the optic nerve include colobomatous defects and pits.

Optic nerve hypoplasia may be associated with absence of the septum pellucidum and hypothalamic–pituitary dysfunction, which is known as septooptic dysplasia, or de Morsier syndrome. Children with septooptic dysplasia and hypocortisolism are at risk for sudden death during febrile illness from thermoregulatory disturbance and dehydration from diabetes insipidus. Optic nerve hypoplasia may occur in infants of diabetic mothers and has also been associated with alcohol use or ingestion of quinine or phenytoin during pregnancy. Anatomically, the size of the involved optic nerve may range from absent (aplasia) to almost full size, with a segmental defect. However, the nerve often appears larger than it is because it is surrounded by a depigmented halo. Visual function with optic nerve hypoplasia ranges from mildly decreased to absent light perception. If only one eye is involved, the child usually presents with strabismus. If both eyes are affected, nystagmus is usually the presenting sign.

Because the optic nerve is an outgrowth of the brain, changes in this structure often reflect CNS disease and defects of central midline structures.

## Papilledema

Papilledema (optic disc edema, choked disc) is associated with increased intracranial pressure due to any cause, such as tumor or intracranial infection. This dysfunction appears as an elevated disc with indistinct margins, increased vessel diameter, and increased capillarity, giving the disc a hyperemic appearance with surrounding hemorrhages and exudates in more severe cases. Observed changes may be subtle to striking. Optic nerve head changes are bilateral and generally symmetrical.

Besides known causes such as hydrocephalus and intracranial tumor, papilledema is associated with so-called benign intracranial hypertension, also known as pseudotumor cerebri or idiopathic intracranial hypertension. Papilledema occurs almost equally in boys and girls and sometimes is associated with obesity or upper respiratory tract infection. Other associated causes are viral infections, corticosteroid use and withdrawal, sinus infection, trauma, tetracycline use, growth hormone, and venous sinus thrombosis. Early in the course of the disorder, the patient may not notice a change in vision, although the blind spot may be enlarged. Transient obscurations of vision (amaurosis fugax) may occur as the process becomes more long-standing. Further effects on vision will occur as the papilledema becomes chronic and ultimately leads to optic atrophy. Work-up and treatment are directed toward finding the underlying systemic or CNS cause. Treatment of idiopathic intracranial hypertension may be pharmacologic—for example, using acetazolamide, a carbonic anhydrase inhibitor, or a corticosteroid. Diagnostic lumbar puncture may also be curative. Optic nerve sheath fenestration and lumboperitoneal shunt are surgical interventions.

Kesler A et al: Idiopathic intracranial hypertension in the pediatric population. J Child Neurol 2002;17(10):745 [PMID 12546428].

Rekate HL et al: Lumboperitoneal shunts in children. Pediatr Neurosurg 2003;38(1):41 [PMID 12476026].

Salman MS et al: Idiopathic "benign" intracranial hypertension: Case series and report. J Child Neurol 2001;16:465 [PMID: 11453440].

## Papillitis

Papillitis is a form of optic neuritis seen on ophthalmoscopic examination as an inflamed optic nerve head. Optic neuritis in the pediatric age group may be idiopathic, associated with multiple sclerosis, acute disseminated encephalomyelitis, Devic disease, or cat-scratch disease.

Papillitis may have the same appearance as papilledema. However, papillitis may be unilateral, whereas papilledema is almost always bilateral. Papillitis can be differentiated from papilledema by an afferent pupillary defect (Marcus Gunn pupil), by its greater effect in decreasing visual acuity and color vision, and by the presence of a central scotoma. Papilledema that is not yet chronic will not have as dramatic an effect on vision. Because increased intracranial pressure can cause both papilledema and a sixth (abducens) nerve palsy, papilledema can be differentiated from papillitis if esotropia and loss of abduction are also present. However, esotropia may also develop secondarily in an eye that has lost vision from papillitis. In pseudopapilledema, a normal variant of the optic disc, the disc appears elevated, with indistinct margins and a normal vascular pattern. Pseudopapilledema sometimes occurs in hyperopic individuals. Retrobulbar neuritis, an inflamed optic nerve but with a normal-appearing nerve head, is associated with pain and the other findings of papillitis.

Work-up of the patient with papillitis includes lumbar puncture and cerebrospinal fluid analysis. *Bartonella henselae* can be detected by serology. MRI is the preferred imaging study. An abnormal MRI is associated with a worse visual outcome. Treatment with corticosteroids is frequently used.

## Optic Atrophy

Optic atrophy, noted as pallor of the nerve head with loss of capillarity, occurs in children most frequently after neurologic compromise during the perinatal period. An example would be a premature infant who develops an intraventricular hemorrhage. Hydrocephalus, glioma of the optic nerve, craniosynostosis, certain neurologic diseases, and toxins such as methyl alcohol can cause optic atrophy, as can certain inborn errors of metabolism, long-standing papilledema, or papillitis.

## DISEASES OF THE ORBIT

### Periorbital & Orbital Cellulitis

The fascia of the eyelids joins with the fibrous orbital septum to isolate the orbit from the lids. This septum serves as a barrier to the posterior spread of infection from preseptal infection. Infections arising anterior to the orbital septum are termed preseptal. Preseptal (periorbital) cellulitis, which indicates infection of the structures of the eyelid, is characterized by lid edema, erythema, swelling, pain, and mild fever. It usually arises from a local exogenous source such as an abrasion of the eyelid, from other infections (hordeolum, dacryocystitis, chalazion), or from infected varicella or insect bite lesions. *Staphylococcus aureus* and *Streptococcus pyogenes* are the most common pathogens cultured from these sources. Preseptal infections in children younger than age 3 years also occur from bacteremia, although this is much less common since *Haemophilus influenzae*

immunization became available. *Streptococcus pneumoniae* bacteremia is still an occasional cause of this infection. Children with periorbital cellulitis from presumed bacteremia must be examined for additional foci of infection.

Infection of the orbit almost always arises from contiguous sinus infection, because the walls of three sinuses make up portions of the orbital walls and infection can breach these walls or extend by way of a richly anastomosing venous system. The orbital contents can develop a phlegmon (orbital cellulitis), or frank pus can develop in the orbit (orbital abscess). When the orbit is infected, the signs of periorbital disease are joined by proptosis (a protruding eye), restricted eye movement, and pain with eye movement. Fever is usually high. CT scanning or MRI is required to establish the extent of the infection within the orbit. Sinus imaging should be obtained at the same time. The pathogenic agents are those of acute or chronic sinusitis—respiratory flora and anaerobes. *S aureus* is also frequently implicated.

Therapy for preseptal and orbital cellulitis infection is with systemic antibiotics. Treatment of orbital infections may require surgical drainage for subperiosteal abscess in conjunction with intravenous antibiotics. Drainage of infected sinuses is often part of the therapy.

Ambati BK et al: Periorbital and orbital cellulites before and after the advent of *Haemophilus influenzae* type B vaccination. Ophthalmology 2000;107(8):1450 [PMID 10919886].

Starkey CR et al: Medical management of orbital cellulites. Pediatr Infect Dis J 2001;20(10):1002 [PMID 11642617].

### Craniofacial Anomalies

Craniofacial anomalies can affect the orbit and visual system. Examples of changes associated with craniofacial disease involving the orbits are proptosis, corneal exposure, hypertelorism (widely spaced orbits), strabismus, amblyopia, lid coloboma, papilledema, and optic atrophy. Craniofacial anomalies occur with craniosynostoses and midface syndromes such as Treacher Collins and Pierre Robin sequence. Fetal alcohol syndrome is associated with similar changes of the ocular adnexa.

### Orbital Tumors

Both benign and malignant orbital lesions occur in children. The most common tumor is capillary hemangioma (Figure 15–25). This type of tumor may be located superficially in the lid or deep in the orbit and can cause ptosis, refractive errors, and amblyopia. Deeper lesions may cause proptosis. Capillary hemangiomas in infants initially increase in size before involuting at about age 2–4 years. Therapy with intralesional

***Figure 15–25.*** Right upper lid hemangioma causing ptosis.

or systemic corticosteroids is indicated if the lesion is large enough to cause amblyopia.

Orbital dermoid cysts vary in size and are usually found temporally at the brow and orbital rim or supranasally. These lesions are firm, well encapsulated, and mobile. Rupture of the cyst causes a severe inflammatory reaction. Treatment is by excision. Lymphangioma occurring in the orbit is typically poorly encapsulated, increases in size with upper respiratory infection, and is susceptible to hemorrhage. Other benign tumors of the orbit are orbital pseudotumor, neurofibroma, teratoma, and tumors arising from bone, connective tissue, and neural tissue.

Of grave concern is orbital rhabdomyosarcoma, the most common primary orbital malignancy in childhood (see Chapter 28). This tumor grows rapidly and displaces the globe. The average age at onset is 6–7 years. The tumor is often initially mistaken for orbital swelling due to insignificant trauma. Radiation and chemotherapy are the mainstays of treatment after biopsy confirms the diagnosis. With expeditious diagnosis and proper treatment, the survival rate of patients with orbital rhabdomyosarcoma confined to the orbit approaches 90%.

Tumors metastatic to the orbit also occur; neuroblastoma is the most common. The patient may exhibit proptosis, orbital ecchymosis (raccoon eyes), Horner syndrome, or opsoclonus (dancing eyes). Ewing sarcoma, leukemia, Burkitt lymphoma, and the histiocytosis X group of diseases may involve the orbit.

Shields JA et al: Pediatric ocular and intraocular tumors. Pediatr Ann 2001;30:491 [PMID: 11510347].

## NYSTAGMUS

Nystagmus is a rhythmic oscillation or jiggling of the eyes. It may be unilateral or bilateral, more pronounced in one eye, or gaze-dependent. Nystagmus may be associated with esotropia or may occur with ocular lesions that cause deprivation amblyopia (eg, cataract, eyelid ptosis) or conditions in which the visual pathways are hypoplastic, sometimes referred to as "sensory nystagmus." Both optic nerve hypoplasia and macular hypoplasia, the latter occurring with aniridia or albinism, are associated with nystagmus. Nystagmus can also occur with normal ocular structures and seemingly normal CNS development, sometimes referred to as "motor nystagmus." In the latter instance, the nystagmus may be blocked in certain positions of gaze, in which case a face turn or torticollis may develop. Latent nystagmus occurs when one eye is occluded. This type of nystagmus occurs in patients with congenital esotropia. An associated amblyopia may be present.

Most nystagmus occurring in childhood is of ocular origin, but CNS disease and, less frequently, inner ear disease are other causes. A CNS cause is likely when the nystagmus is acquired. The clinician should evaluate the fundus for optic nerve abnormalities and the quality of the macular reflex, because both optic nerve hypoplasia and macular hypoplasia can cause nystagmus.

Evaluation of nystagmus begins with the pediatric ophthalmologist. Careful evaluation for iris transillumination defects caused by albinism should be performed. An electroretinogram (ERG) is usually required to rule out retinal pathology as the cause. Some types of nystagmus, usually motor nystagmus, can be treated, generally with surgery; less frequently, prisms are useful. Spasmus nutans, in which a rapid, shimmering, dysconjugate nystagmus occurs with head bobbing and torticollis, is said to improve with time. Glioma of the hypothalamus can mimic spasmus nutans. Neuroimaging may be necessary to determine if the cause of the nystagmus is due to a CNS disease.

## AMBLYOPIA & STRABISMUS

Visual development is a learned function. For it to proceed normally, a child must experience a normal visual environment with well-aligned eyes that are free of visually threatening disease and significant refractive errors. The consequences of not meeting these requirements during the sensitive period of visual development in the first decade of life are strabismus and decreased vision, or amblyopia.

### Amblyopia

Amblyopia is a unilateral or bilateral reduction in central visual acuity due to the sensory deprivation of a well-formed retinal image that occurs with or without a visible organic lesion commensurate with the degree of visual loss. Amblyopia can occur only during the critical period of visual development in the first decade of life when the visual nervous system is plastic. Approximately 3% of the population is amblyopic. Screening for amblyopia should be a component of periodic well-child examinations. The single best screening technique to discover amblyopia is obtaining visual acuity in each eye. In preverbal children unable to respond to visual acuity assessment, amblyogenic factors are sought, including strabismus; media opacities; unequal Brückner reflexes (pupillary red reflexes); and a family history suggestive of strabismus, amblyopia, or ocular disease occurring in childhood (see Examination section).

Amblyopia is classified according to its cause. Strabismic amblyopia can occur in the nondominant eye of a strabismic child. Refractive amblyopia can occur in both eyes if significant refractive errors are untreated (ametropic or refractive amblyopia). Another type of refractive amblyopia can occur in the eye with the worse refractive error when imbalance is present between the eyes (anisometropic amblyopia). Deprivation amblyopia occurs when dense cataracts or complete ptosis prevents formation of a formed retinal image. Of the three types of amblyopia, this form of amblyopia results in the worst vision.

The earlier treatment is begun, the better the chance of improving visual acuity. Treatment is usually discontinued after age 9 years. Amblyogenic factors such as refractive errors are addressed. Because of the extreme sensitivity of the visual nervous system in infants, congenital cataracts and media opacities must be diagnosed and treated within the first few weeks of life. Visual rehabilitation and amblyopia treatment must then be started in order to foster visual development.

After eradicating amblyogenic factors, the mainstay of treatment is patching the sound eye, which causes the visual nervous system to process input from the amblyopic eye and in that way permits the development of useful vision. Other treatment modalities include "fogging" the sound eye with cycloplegic drops (atropine), lenses, and filters.

Pediatric Eye Disease Investigator Group: A randomized trial of atropine vs. patching for treatment of moderate amblyopia in children. Arch Ophthalmol 2002;120(3):268 [PMID 11879129].

Repka MX et al: A randomized trial of patching regimens for treatment of moderate amblyopia in children. Arch Ophthalmol 2003;121(5)603 [PMID 12742836].

## Strabismus

Strabismus is misalignment of the visual axes of the two eyes. Its prevalence in childhood is about 2–3%. Strabismus is categorized by the direction of the deviation and its frequency. Early diagnosis of strabismus and amblyopia, which often coexist, provides the best chance of reaching full visual potential. Strabismus may cause or be due to amblyopia.

Misdiagnosis of strabismus when the eyes are well aligned—pseudostrabismus—can occur when relying on the gross observation of the appearance of the two eyes. If the child has prominent epicanthal folds, pseudoesotropia may be diagnosed erroneously. Observation of the reflection of a penlight on the cornea, corneal light reflex, is a more accurate means of determining if the eyes are straight. If strabismus is present, the corneal light reflex will not be centered in both eyes.

An infant whose eyes are destined to be well aligned may appear intermittently esotropic, but this should occur less frequently over the first few months of life. By age 5 or 6 months, the baby's eyes should be constantly well aligned.

Besides its effect on visual development, strabismus may be a marker of other ocular or systemic disease. Twenty percent of patients with retinoblastoma exhibit strabismus. Patients with CNS disorders such as hydrocephalus, space-occupying lesions, and an amaurotic (blind) eye can also exhibit strabismus. In children younger than age 3 or 4 years, blind eyes tend to assume a position of esodeviation, but after about age 4 years an amaurotic eye tends to show an exotropic shift.

### A. ESOTROPIA

In esotropia, the visual axes of the eyes are excessively convergent. In terms of cause and treatment, esotropia can be categorized by age at onset. Congenital esotropia (infantile esotropia) has its onset in the first year of life in healthy infants. The deviation is large and obvious. Surgery is the mainstay of treatment. Controversy exists as to how young the child should be when surgery is performed so that the child can obtain an optimal binocular result. The age range is from younger than 6 months to 2 years. Esotropia beginning in the first year also occurs in premature infants or in children with a complicated perinatal history associated with CNS problems such as intracranial hemorrhage and periventricular leukomalacia. Esotropia is associated with certain syndromes. In Möbius' syndrome (congenital facial diplegia), a sixth nerve palsy causing esotropia is associated with palsies of the seventh and twelfth cranial nerves and limb deformities. Duane syndrome can affect the medial or lateral rectus muscles (or both). It may be an isolated defect or may be associated with a multitude of systemic defects (eg, Goldenhar syndrome). Duane syndrome is often misdiagnosed as a sixth (abducens) nerve palsy. The left eye is involved more commonly than the right, but both eyes can be involved. Girls are affected more frequently than boys. Children with unilateral paretic or restrictive causes of esotropia may develop face turns toward the affected eye in order to maintain binocularity.

*Figure 15–26.* Accommodative esotropia. Without glasses, esotropic **(A).** With glasses, well-aligned at distance **(B)** and at near with bifocal correction **(C).**

The most frequent type of acquired esotropia is the accommodative type (Figure 15–26). Onset is usually between ages 2 and 5 years. The deviation is variable in magnitude and constancy and is often accompanied by amblyopia. One type of accommodative esotropia is associated with a high hyperopic refraction. In another type, the deviation is worse with near than with distant vision. This type of esodeviation is usually associated with lower refractive errors. Management includes glasses with or without bifocals, amblyopia treatment, and in some cases surgery. After age 5 years, any esotropia of recent onset should arouse suspicion of CNS disease. Infratentorial masses, hydrocephalus, demyelinating diseases, and idiopathic intracranial hypertension are causes of abducens palsy, which appears as an esotropia, lateral rectus paralysis or paresis, and face turn. The face turn is an attempt to maintain binocu-

larity away from the field of action of the paretic muscle. Papilledema is often but not invariably present with increased intracranial pressure. Besides the vulnerability of the abducens nerve to increased intracranial pressure, it is susceptible to infection and inflammation. Otitis media and Gradenigo syndrome (inflammatory disease of the petrous bone) can cause sixth nerve palsy. Less commonly, migraine and diabetes mellitus are considerations in children with sixth nerve palsy. Work-up includes imaging studies and neurologic examination.

### B. Exotropia

Exotropia does not usually offer as many diagnostic pitfalls as esotropia. The visual axes of the two eyes are deviated in a divergent position (Figure 15–27). The deviation most often begins intermittently and occurs after age 2 years. Congenital (infantile) exotropia is extremely rare in an otherwise healthy infant. Early-onset exotropia may occur in infants and children with severe neurologic problems. All children with constant, congenital exotropia require CNS neuroimaging. Treatment of exotropia is with surgery, orthoptic exercises, patching, and occasionally glasses.

Havertape SA et al: Sensory strabismus—eso or exo? J Pediatr Ophthalmol Strabismus 2001;38(6):327 [PMID 11759769].

*Figure 15–27.* Exotropia. **A:** Fixation with left eye. **B:** Fixation with right eye

Ing MR et al: Outcome study of stereopsis in relation to duration of misalignment in congenital esotropia. J AAPOS 2002;6(1):3 [PMID 11907472].

Rubin SE: Management of strabismus in the first year of life. Pediatr Ann 2001;30:474 [PMID: 11510345].

Schworm HD et al: Comitant strabismus. Curr Opin Ophthalmol 2000;11(5):310 [PMID 11148695].

## UNEXPLAINED DECREASED VISION IN INFANTS & CHILDREN

Some infants with delayed visual development during the first few months of life who are otherwise normal neurologically will reach an appropriate level of visual maturation. Occult causes of poor vision and blindness in children are those for which there are no obvious ocular defects: they include Leber congenital amaurosis, a childhood form of retinitis pigmentosa; achromatopsia, the absence of functioning cones in the retina; and optic nerve abnormalities, including optic nerve hypoplasia and atrophy as well as night blindness.

Cerebral visual impairment, also known as cortical blindness, is manifested as decreased visual attentiveness of varying degree. Cerebral visual impairment can be congenital or acquired. Insults to the optic pathways and higher cortical visual centers are responsible. Asphyxia, trauma, intracranial hemorrhage, and periventricular leukomalacia are some of the causes of cortical visual impairment.

Besides an ophthalmologic work-up, ERG and visual evoked response testing may be required in children with decreased vision of unexplained etiology. Imaging studies of the brain and a pediatric neurologic evaluation may be useful. A low-vision assessment may be indicated. Low-vision aids enhance remaining vision. Devices used include magnifiers for both distance and near vision, closed-circuit television, and large-print reading materials.

Hoyt CS: Visual function in the brain-damaged child. Eye 2003;17(3):369 [PMID 12724701].

## THE BLIND CHILD

Vision is the principal route of sensory input. A child's development will therefore be affected profoundly by blindness or very poor vision. There are psychological consequences for the child blind from birth, as well as for the family. It can be devastating to a young family to find out that their newborn is blind. Although acquired blindness may give an individual time to grow as a sighted person and make preparations for life as a nonsighted person if loss of vision is slow and predicted, psychological consequences for the child and family must be addressed. The child blind from birth or from very early childhood has had little or no opportunity to form visual impressions of the physical world. Blind children and their families should receive the benefit of knowledgeable therapists and support groups.

Blind infants reach developmental landmarks on a different schedule from that of sighted children. In addition, some blind children are multiply handicapped. For example, the premature child who is blind from ROP may also have cerebral palsy. Children with Usher syndrome become both deaf and blind.

Leading causes of blindness in the pediatric age group differ among regions of the world and between industrialized nations and developing countries. The most common causes of blindness in the pediatric age group are thought to be cerebral visual impairment, ROP, and optic nerve hypoplasia. Albinism, optic atrophy, cataract, retinitis pigmentosa, microphthalmia or anophthalmia, aniridia, and glaucoma are other diseases causing blindness.

Thompson L et al: The visually impaired child. Pediatr Clin North Am 2003;50(1):225 [PMID 12713115].

## LEARNING DISABILITIES & DYSLEXIA

Visits to the physician because of educational difficulties are common. Evaluation of the child with learning disabilities and dyslexia should include ophthalmologic examination to identify any ocular disorders that could cause or contribute to poor school performance. Most children with learning difficulties have no demonstrable problems on ophthalmic examination.

A multidisciplinary approach as suggested by the American Academy of Pediatrics, the American Association for Pediatric Ophthalmology and Strabismus, and the American Academy of Ophthalmology is recommended in evaluating children with learning disabilities. Although many therapies directed at "training the eyes" exist, scientific support for such approaches is weak.

Mathes PG et al: The prevention and identification of reading disability. Semin Pediatr Neurol 2002;9(3):185 [PMID 12350039].

## VISION SCREENING

Vision screening in the pediatric age group is a challenge, especially in younger and developmentally delayed children. Accuracy of the screening test being administered to a particular population and expense in terms of time, equipment, and personnel are some of the factors that must be considered in screening individuals and groups. Vision screening is consistent with the recommendations of the American Academy of Pediatrics (www.aap.org). Risk factors that should be screened for because they interfere with normal visual development and are amblyogenic include media opacities, strabismus, and refractive errors that are different in the two eyes (anisometropia) or of large magnitude in both eyes.

The practitioner should have an understanding of the limitations of the screening test being administered. For example, one study cites the sensitivity and specificity of visual acuity screening in preschool children as 90% and 44%, respectively. When possible, visual acuity of each eye and alignment of the two eyes should be assessed. (See Visual Acuity section for acceptable acuities at different ages.) Two caveats are to be observed when testing monocular visual acuity. First, in an amblyopic patient who demonstrates the crowding phenomenon, an amblyopic eye may score better when presented with single, isolated targets than with multiple targets on a line. Second, monocular visual acuity is worse in a patient with latent nystagmus. Preschool and young school-age children often test better when looking at a visual acuity chart at a 10-foot distance than at one placed at 20 feet or when looking into the type of machine typically used at a motor vehicle department.

When it is not possible to measure visual acuity or assess alignment in the preschool-age group, random dot stereopsis testing (for depth perception) is effective in screening for manifest strabismus and amblyopia, but this test may miss some cases of anisometropic (unequal refractive error) amblyopia and small-angle strabismus. This test is not designed to detect refractive errors.

An innovative technique that is being used more frequently in the pediatric age group and may prove useful for developmentally delayed children and perhaps infants is photoscreening. Photoscreening relies on the Brückner test of corneal light reflexes. Photoscreening does not screen directly for amblyopia but for amblyogenic factors, which include strabismus, media opacities, and refractive errors. Automated methods of photoscreening are still being validated. Problems exist with sensitivity and specificity of the instruments, and the role of their use in the pediatric population remains a controversy.

Donahue SP et al: Screening for amblyogenic factors using a volunteer lay network and the MTI photoscreener: Initial results from 15,000 preschool children in a statewide effort. Ophthalmology 2000;107(9):1637; discussion 1645. [PMID: 10964820].

Simon JW et al: Vision screening performed by the pediatrician. Pediatr Ann 2001;30:446 [PMID: 11510342].

## REFERENCES

American Academy of Ophthalmology: *Orbit, Eyelids and Lacrimal System: Basic and Clinical Science Course.* Section 7, 1999–2000.

American Academy of Ophthalmology: *Pediatric Ophthalmology and Strabismus: Basic and Clinical Science Course.* Section 6, 2002.

Brodsky MC et al: *Pediatric Neuro-Ophthalmology.* Springer, 1996.

Fraunfelder FT, Roy FH (eds): *Current Ocular Therapy 5.* WB Saunders, 2002.

Isenberg SJ (ed): *The Eye in Infancy,* 2nd ed. Mosby, 1994.

Nussenblatt RB et al (eds): *Uveitis Fundamentals and Clinical Practice,* 2nd ed. Mosby, 1996.

Olitsky SE, Nelson LB: Common ophthalmologic concerns in infants and children. Pediatr Clin North Am 1998;45:993 [PMID: 9728197].

Rhee DJ, Pyfer MF (eds): *The Wills Eye Manual Office and Emergency Room Diagnosis and Treatment of Eye Disease,* 3rd ed. Lippincott Williams & Wilkins, 1999.

Ritch R et al (eds): *The Glaucomas,* 2nd ed, 3 vols. Mosby, 1996.

Simon J, Calhoun J: *A Child's Eye.* Triad, 1998.

Tasman W, Jaeger EA (eds): *Duane's Clinical Ophthalmology,* 6 vols. Lippincott Williams & Wilkins, 1994. (1995 edition on CD-ROM.)

Vaughan DG et al (eds): *General Ophthalmology,* 15th ed. (Originally published by Appleton & Lange.) McGraw-Hill, 1999.

Wright KW, Spiegel PW: *Pediatric Ophthalmology and Strabismus.* Mosby, 1999.

# Oral Medicine & Dentistry

*William A. Mueller, DMD*

The American Academy of Pediatric Dentistry (AAPD) and the American Academy of Pediatrics recommend that a child's first oral examination be performed no later than age 12 months, and optimally within 6 months after eruption of the first tooth. This recommendation is intended to establish the child's dental home and provide an opportunity to implement preventive dental health habits. Because the bacterial infection causing dental caries can be acquired as early as age 14 months, waiting until age 3 years, which was the prior recommendation, allows for significant disease progression before treatment. Pediatric dentists are knowledgeable about nursing caries and other types of caries, and their familiarity with the effectiveness of sealants, fluorides, and cariology makes them the parents' best resource for help in rearing caries-free children. Some experts have even suggested that infant oral health begin with prenatal oral health counseling.

Most oral disease in children is preventable. Oral evaluation of a child should consist of infant risk assessment and anticipatory guidance. This approach advances dental care past tooth monitoring to health promotion. Infant risk assessment determines the danger for each child of developing oral disease. Anticipatory guidance is directed toward individualized cost-effective use of dental services. Because pediatricians and other pediatric health care professionals are far more likely to encounter new mothers and infants than are dentists, it is essential that they be aware of the infectious pathophysiology and associated risk factors of early childhood dental caries to make appropriate decisions regarding effective intervention.

The primary goals for an infant oral health program are (1) to establish with parents the goals of oral health, (2) to inform parents of their role in reaching these goals, (3) to motivate parents to learn and practice good preventive dental care, and (4) to initiate a long-term dental care relationship with parents. Pediatricians should incorporate oral health into anticipatory guidance either by learning to provide this information in their offices or by referring the child to a pediatric dental colleague.

## ORAL EXAMINATION OF THE NEWBORN & INFANT

The mouth of the normal newborn is lined with an intact, smooth, moist, and shiny mucosa (Figure 16–1). The alveolar ridges are continuous and relatively smooth. Within the alveolar bone are numerous tooth buds, which at birth are mostly primary teeth and a few permanent teeth just starting to calcify.

### Teeth

The primary teeth begin to form at approximately 6 weeks' gestation, and their calcification starts in the second trimester. The permanent teeth are just beginning to develop at birth. There is enough development of permanent teeth to permit their damage by perinatal or antenatal insults such as anoxia, severe jaundice, or infection.

The primary teeth usually begin to erupt at approximately age 6–7 months. However, on rare occasions (1:2000), teeth are present at birth (natal teeth) or erupt within the first month (neonatal teeth). These are most common in the anterior mandible and can be "real" primary teeth or supernumerary teeth. These can be differentiated radiographically. On occasion, these teeth must be removed to facilitate nursing, heal persistent ulceration of the tongue, or eliminate the risk of aspiration.

### Frena

Noticeable but small maxillary and mandibular labial frena should be present (Figure 16–2). Several small accessory frena may also be present farther posteriorly. The extreme is multiple thick tightly bound frena, as in oral–facial–digital syndrome. Decisions about if and when a labial frenum should be reduced surgically are best left until adolescence. Many thick frena need not be corrected.

The tongue is connected to the floor of the mouth by the lingual frenum (Figures 16–1 and 16–3). This

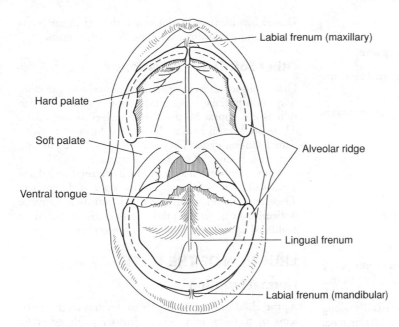

**Figure 16–1.** Normal anatomy of the newborn mouth.

connection should not impede the free movement of the tongue. If the attachment is tight and high up on the alveolar ridge (Figure 16–4), it may restrict movement and cause periodontal damage. This condition is called ankyloglossia (tongue-tie). If it needs to be corrected surgically, earlier (at age 3–4 years) is better than later, but there is usually no urgency for surgery in the neonatal period.

## Palate

The palate of the newborn should be intact and continuous from the alveolar ridge anteriorly to the uvula (see Figure 16–1). Cleft lip and palate are common defects (1:700 live births). The cleft of the palate can be unilateral or bilateral (Figure 16–5). The cleft can involve just the alveolar ridge, as in Figure 16–5, or the ridge

**Figure 16–2.** The frena.

***Figure 16–3.*** Normal position of lingual frenum.

and entire palate. Clefts can also be isolated soft palate defects. This is common in the Pierre Robin syndrome. Cleft palate may also present a submucous cleft, which may be detected by passing a finger posteriorly along the midline of the palate. Normally the posterior nasal spine is detectable, but if a submucous cleft is present, a bony notch will be found. Affected children sometimes have a bifid uvula.

Cleft lip and palate rehabilitation requires an extensive program involving many specialties and can be a lifelong endeavor. Children with cleft palate are best treated by a cleft palate team with coordinated care from relevant specialties. Cleft lip and palate treatment begins immediately after birth with fabrication of a palatal obturator as a feeding aid. This appliance also helps approximate the alveolar segments in order to facilitate the initial lip repair. In the case of bilateral cleft lip and palate, the dentist will often apply extraoral orthopedic traction to guide the protruding premaxilla back into the oral cavity to facilitate surgical lip closure.

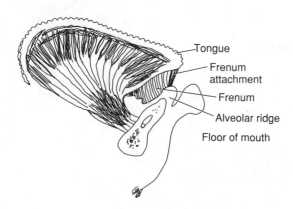

***Figure 16–4.*** Ankyloglossia (tongue-tie).

Dental involvement in children with cleft palate is extensive and is coordinated by the cleft palate team.

## Other Soft Tissue Variations

Other minor soft tissue variations can exist in the newborn mouth. Small (1–2 mm), round, smooth, whitish bumps can appear on the alveolar ridges or the palate. These are keratin cysts and are called Epstein pearls or dental lamina cysts. They are benign and require no treatment because they usually disappear.

Some newborns may have small intraoral lymphangiomas on the alveolar ridge or the floor of the mouth. These and any other soft tissue variations that are more noticeable or larger than those just described should be evaluated by a dentist familiar with neonates.

## ERUPTION OF THE TEETH

### Normal Eruption

As the child grows and begins to develop teeth, problems of teething may occur. Primary teeth generally begin to erupt at about age 6 months. They are usually mandibular incisors, but can be maxillary, and appear as early as age 3–4 months or as late as age 12–16 months. Many side effects are ascribed to teething, such as diarrhea, drooling, fever, and rash. But any real correlation is doubtful.

Common treatment for teething pain has been application of a topical anesthetic or "teething gel." Most of these agents contain benzocaine or, less commonly, lidocaine. They can cause numbness of the entire oral cavity and pharynx, and suppression of the gag reflex can be a serious side effect. Systemic analgesia (acetaminophen or ibuprofen) is safer and more effective. Solid rubber or chilled fluid-filled teething toys are beneficial, if only for distraction purposes. Massaging the gums can be very soothing.

Occasionally, swelling of the gingiva is seen during teething. This condition can appear as red to purple, round, raised, smooth lesions that may be symptomatic but usually are not. They appear in the anterior or posterior alveolar ridge and on the crest. These so-called eruption cysts or eruption hematomas are fluid-filled areas immediately overlying an erupting tooth and generally disappear spontaneously.

### Delayed Eruption

Premature loss of a primary tooth can either accelerate or delay eruption of the underlying secondary tooth. Early eruption occurs when the permanent tooth is beginning its active eruption and the overlying primary tooth is removed. This generally occurs when the primary tooth is within 1 year of its normal exfoliation. If,

**Figure 16–5.** Types of clefts.

however, loss of the primary tooth occurs more than 1 year before expected exfoliation, the permanent tooth will probably be delayed in eruption owing to healing that results in filling in of bone and gingiva over the permanent tooth. The loss of a primary tooth may cause adjacent teeth to tip into the space and lead to impaction of the underlying permanent tooth. A space maintainer should be placed by a dentist to avoid this.

Other local factors delaying or preventing eruption include supernumerary teeth, cysts, tumors, overretained primary teeth, ankylosed primary teeth, and impaction. A generalized delay in eruption may be due to endocrinopathies (hypothyroidism, hypopituitarism) or other systemic conditions (cleidocranial dysplasia, rickets, trisomy 21).

## Ectopic Eruption

Ectopic eruption occurs when the position of an erupting tooth is abnormal. In severe instances, the order in which teeth erupt is affected. If the dental arch provides insufficient room, permanent teeth may erupt abnormally. In the mandible, lower incisors may be lingually placed to such an extent that the primary incisors do not exfoliate. The parents' concern about a "double row of teeth" may be the reason for the child's first dental visit. If the primary teeth are not loose, they may be removed by the dentist; if they are loose, they are generally allowed to exfoliate naturally. In the maxilla, inadequate room for eruption of the permanent first molar may cause abnormal resorption of the distal root structures of the second primary molar. If the problem is severe, the permanent molar may even become caught under the unresorbed enamel crown of the deciduous molar and thus require extraction of the primary tooth and orthodontic repositioning of the permanent first molar after it has erupted. If the first molar is not repositioned, the second premolar is likely to become impacted. If problems are detected early, the dentist may be able to redirect the permanent molar's eruption pathway so that it erupts correctly and the second primary molar is not lost.

## Impaction

Impaction occurs when a tooth is prevented from erupting for any reason. The teeth most often affected are the third molars (wisdom teeth) and the maxillary canines. Patients with impacted third molars are at risk for developing odontogenic tumors or dentigerous cysts. The impacted third molar (along with its opposing third molar) may be removed after it has been determined that eruption cannot occur, but this decision may not be possible until the late teens. Impacted maxillary canines should not be extracted because of their aesthetic importance and key role in facial development and dental occlusion. They can often be brought into correct alignment through surgical exposure and orthodontic treatment.

## Other Variations

Failure of teeth to develop—a condition sometimes called congenitally missing teeth—is rare in the primary dentition. However, it occurs in about 5% of permanent dentitions, with one or more of the third molars missing in about 25% of all individuals. The ones most frequently missing are maxillary lateral incisors and mandibular second premolars. The incidence of congenitally missing teeth varies among different genetic groups.

Occasionally, extra teeth are present, most typically an extra (fourth) molar or extra (third) bicuspid. Mesiodens, which are peg-shaped supernumerary teeth situated at the maxillary midline that occur in about 5% of individuals, may interfere with eruption of permanent incisors. Mesiodens should be considered for removal even if they do not erupt.

## DENTAL CARIES & PERIODONTAL DISEASE

The process of tooth decay (caries) and periodontal disease are among the most common and easily preventable of all infectious diseases. Current research is changing the traditional view of dental caries as the manifestation of caries activity (eg, "holes in the teeth"). Practitioners are now pursuing the more practical objective of diagnosing and treating the caries process in the context of a life continuum, rather than only as cavitated teeth. The traditional "cavity" is irreversible and requires surgical correction. Filling cavities does nothing to address the underlying pathologic process that caused them. Prevention, early diagnosis, and prompt intervention offer greater efficiency and better health outcomes with lower costs.
The basic tenets of cariology are

1. Caries is the most common chronic disease of childhood.

2. Caries is an infectious disease that is transmissible and caused by colonization with *Streptococcus mutans*.

3. *S mutans* is transmitted from a mother to her child and detectable by 26 months on average, with a range of 12–36 months.

4. Caries is a process present in all individuals. The expression of cavities depends on its level of activity and the host's resistance.

5. After establishment of *S mutans* in the oral cavity, caries is a dietary disease.

6. Control of caries before age 3 years is aimed at limiting the establishment of *S mutans* by reducing the number of episodes of direct transmission from highly infected mothers; reducing dietary support for *S mutans* (refined carbohydrates); and ensuring proper levels of fluoride exposure topically and systemically.

7. Control of caries after age 3 years is aimed at limiting the acidogenesis of oral flora by reducing the frequency of carbohydrate ingestion and maintaining a high frequency of fluoride exposures.

8. There is a threshold of caries activity below which clinical disease does not develop.

9. Caries is largely a disease of poverty; the 29 million children and adolescents in low-income families account for 80% of tooth decay.

Teeth can be attacked by acidogenic bacteria, especially *S mutans*. Dental plaque accumulates on the surface of the teeth as an adherent film. As plaque grows, bacteria accumulate within it in close proximity to the tooth. An equally important factor is a substrate for the bacteria. Carbohydrate—especially a refined carbohydrate such as sucrose—is the most effective substrate for caries, since bacteria readily metabolize sucrose to produce acid. The acidic environment causes the enamel of the teeth to dissolve, which is the beginning of caries. After the decay process has penetrated the enamel, there is very little to keep it from affecting the vital tissues (nerve) of the tooth. The tooth subsequently becomes necrotic, and an abscess occurs (Figure 16–6). This process is not always symptomatic, but it can lead to severe pain, fever, and swelling.

In the early stages of decay, the tooth may be sensitive to temperature changes or, especially, to sweets. At this point, the tooth can be repaired by removing the caries and filling the defect. As the decay progresses, more pain may be involved, and root canal therapy may be necessary for both primary or permanent teeth. Once an abscess has formed, with or without swelling, a choice must be made between root canal therapy and removal of the tooth. In the presence of cellulitis or fa-

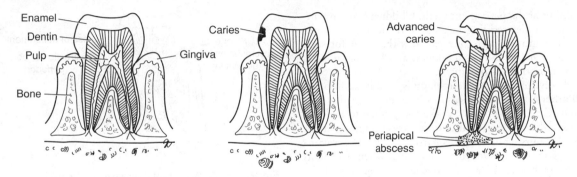

***Figure 16–6.*** Tooth anatomy and progression of caries.

cial space abscess, extraction is usually the treatment of choice.

Many people question the importance of the primary dentition. Baby teeth allow the child to eat properly, speak properly, have a good self-image, and preserve the space for the permanent dentition. Premature loss of primary teeth can cause major orthodontic and dental growth and development problems.

## Preventing Dental Caries

To prevent dental caries, it is necessary to remove the bacteria on a regular basis. Oral hygiene for the infant should start at birth. The gums can be cleaned gently with a moist, soft cloth. Once the teeth begin to erupt, oral hygiene must be practiced in earnest. Again, a moist, soft cloth can be used after feeding to gently rub the teeth. A very small, very soft toothbrush can be used as well. Toothpaste at the start is not necessary but should be added by age 2 years. Prior to age 6 years parents may need to be involved in brushing and flossing. Brushing with a fluoride-containing toothpaste (at least twice daily) and flossing the teeth regularly will minimize the oral flora. A second step is to decrease the amount of substrate

available to the bacteria. Eliminating refined carbohydrates is very effective (low-sugar diets), but limiting exposure to them is also beneficial because each exposure produces an acidic environment for up to 30 minutes. The form of the substrate is important. Caramels, licorice, raisins, gummy bears, and so on are concentrated sugar with a sticky texture that will remain on the teeth much longer than the same sugar in liquid form. The primary care physician can play an invaluable role in disseminating this information and reinforcing these ideas.

## Fluoride

Fluoride prevents dental caries predominantly after eruption of the tooth into the mouth. Its actions are primarily topical for both children and adults. The mechanisms of action include inhibition of demineralization, enhancement of remineralization, and inhibition of bacterial activity in dental plaque. Table 16–1 sets forth the current systemic fluoride dosages to be administered to children as recommended by the American Academy of Pediatrics and the AAPD. It is important not to exceed these recommendations because doing so may lead to fluorosis, which is unsightly

***Table 16–1.*** Fluoride dosages administered to children based on tap water fluoride supply.

| Age (years) | Dose of Fluoride Administered | | |
| --- | --- | --- | --- |
| | If < 0.3 ppm F in Drinking Water | If 0.3–0.6 ppm F in Drinking Water | If > 0.6 ppm F in Drinking Water |
| 6 months to 3 years | 0.25 mg/d | 0 | 0 |
| 3–6 years | 0.5 mg/d | 0.25 mg/d | 0 |
| 6–16 years | 1 mg/d | 0.5 mg/d | 0 |

staining of the permanent teeth. Children from low-income families residing in areas with fluoridated water incur treatment costs one half less than that for such children in nonfluoridated areas, and they require less hospitalization for treatment.

Daily topical fluoride therapy is used in addition to all other oral hygiene measures in certain high-risk children. Children allowed to take their bottle to bed and those who nurse at will and fall asleep nursing are at risk for nursing caries. This particular type of decay involves mostly the maxillary incisors. When a child is lying in bed sucking on a bottle, the contents of the bottle are "trapped" between the backs of the front teeth and the tongue. This allows for more concentrated damage to the teeth as the acid produced by bacteria fails to dissipate. In addition, as the child falls asleep, salivary function decreases dramatically. This further endangers the teeth by eliminating the buffering capacity of saliva and its remineralizing potential. Topical fluoride may slow the decay process and, combined with elimination of high-risk nursing practices and institution of good oral hygiene, can prevent serious dental problems in these infants.

Patients with chronically low oral pH may benefit from daily topical fluoride. This patient group includes those with gastroesophageal reflux, bulimia, or salivary dysfunction from radiation, graft-versus-host disease, or autoimmune disease. Saliva is a very effective oral cavity buffer. It also helps remineralize minor enamel dissolution. Xerostomia can lead to rampant caries. These children need dental care more frequently than healthy children. Multiply handicapped children who cannot maintain proper oral hygiene can also benefit from additional topical fluoride. Any child with a serious medical problem or disability should be referred to a pediatric dentist as early as possible, usually before age 1 year.

## Periodontal Disease

Periodontal disease involves the supporting structures: bone, gums, and ligaments. It begins as inflammation of the gum tissue adjacent to the tooth. Bacterial accumulation in the space between the tooth and gum (gingival sulcus) causes irritation that leads to inflamed tissue. This beginning phase is called gingivitis. As the inflammation spreads through the sulcus, it involves more soft tissue. Eventually soft tissue destruction and loss of bone occur as disease spreads toward the apex of the tooth. This is called periodontitis and requires professional cleaning and often medication or surgery for correction. Figure 16–7 shows the different stages and progression of periodontal disease.

The prevention and initial management of periodontal disease in children involves removal of bacteria from the teeth with proper oral hygiene.

**Figure 16–7.** Periodontal disease.

## OROFACIAL TRAUMA

Orofacial trauma often consists only of abrasions or lacerations of the lips, gingiva, tongue, or mucosa, including the frena, without damage to the teeth. Lacerations should be cleansed and inspected for foreign bodies and sutured if necessary. Occasionally, radiographs of the tongue, lips, or cheeks are used to detect tooth fragments or other foreign bodies.

Tooth-related trauma can result in displacement (luxation), fracture, or loss of teeth (avulsion). Figure 16–8 demonstrates the different luxation injuries, and Figure 16–9 shows the different degrees of tooth fracture.

The least problematic luxation injury is mobility without displacement (subluxation). Unless mobility is extensive, this condition can be followed without active intervention. An intrusive luxation in the primary dentition is usually observed for a period of time to discern whether the tooth or teeth will reerupt (see Figure 16–8). If this has not occurred after several months or if the area becomes infected, the teeth are usually removed. Permanent teeth may be damaged with any intrusive injury of primary teeth. Permanent teeth intrusions are corrected with surgical or orthodontic repositioning of teeth and placement of a splint for 10–14 days. Root canal treatment may be necessary later. Lateral and extrusive luxations of permanent teeth are generally repositioned and splinted. Severe luxations in any direction in primary teeth are treated with extraction.

Avulsed primary dentition is not replanted. The area is investigated for fractured roots or foreign bodies. Avulsed permanent teeth are gently cleansed and replanted with splinting. If replaced into the alveolar bone within 1 hour, the prognosis for these teeth is good. The prognosis worsens rapidly with increased time outside of the mouth. Hank solution is the best storage and transport medium for avulsed teeth that

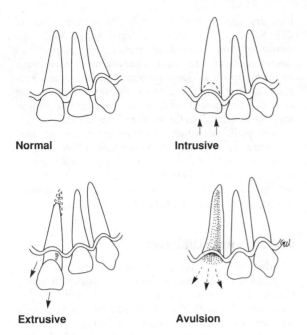

**Figure 16–8.** Patterns of luxation injuries.

will be replanted. Milk or saline can be used if Hank solution is not accessible.

All luxated and replanted teeth need to be followed carefully and regularly by a dentist. These teeth can become abscessed or fused to the bone (ankylosed) at any time during the healing process.

A patient with fractured teeth should be seen promptly by a dentist. Fractured teeth need to be protected quickly to avoid sensitivity, pain, or infection of exposed pulp. Severe fracture may require immediate root canal surgery.

All facial trauma needs to be evaluated for jaw fracture. Blows to the chin are among the most common childhood orofacial traumas. They are also a leading

cause of condylar fracture in the pediatric population. Condylar fracture should be suspected when pain or deviation occurs when the jaw is opened.

## DENTAL EMERGENCIES

Dental emergencies other than trauma are usually associated with pain or swelling due to advanced caries. Odontogenic pain usually responds to acetaminophen, ibuprofen, codeine, or, in severe cases, hydrocodone. As with teething, topical application of medicaments is of limited value.

Swelling confined to the gum tissue above or below the tooth is usually not an urgent situation. This "gumboil" or parulis represents infection that has spread outward from the root of the tooth through the bone and periosteum into the gum. Usually it will begin to drain and leave a fistulous tract. If the infection invades the facial spaces, cellulitis can occur. Swelling of the midface—especially the bridge of the nose and the lower eyelid—should be urgently evaluated as a potential dental infection. Extraction of teeth or root canal therapy combined with antibiotics is the usual treatment. With extensive facial cellulitis, many young children require hospitalization and intravenous antibiotics.

## ANTIBIOTICS IN PEDIATRIC DENTISTRY

The antibiotics of choice for odontogenic infection are amoxicillin and clindamycin. Several patient groups require prophylactic antibiotic coverage prior to any invasive dental manipulation, including tooth cleaning. Children with heart diseases that place them at risk for subacute bacterial endocarditis head this list. Some immunosuppressed patients also receive coverage during dental procedures. Although there is some controversy regarding the need for antibiotics in children with indwelling central venous catheters (eg, Broviac, Quinton, Hickman, and other lines), some experts medicate them prior to invasive dental treatment.

Children with a ventriculoperitoneal shunt should not receive prophylaxis because there is no circulatory connection to such a shunt.

## SPECIAL PATIENT POPULATIONS

### Children with Cancer

Children with cancer should be evaluated by a dentist knowledgeable about pediatric oncology soon after diagnosis. The aim is to eliminate all existing and potential sources of infection before the child receives chemotherapy and becomes neutropenic. Areas of concern include abscessed teeth, teeth with extensive caries, teeth that will soon exfoliate, ragged or broken teeth or

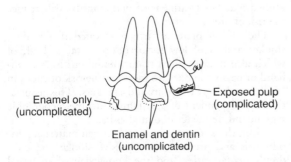

Enamel only
(uncomplicated)

Exposed pulp
(complicated)

Enamel and dentin
(uncomplicated)

**Figure 16–9.** Patterns of crown fractures.

fillings, and orthodontic appliances. Once chemotherapy begins, there is a brief interval before its myelosuppressive effects reach their nadir (7–14 days). Once the child becomes neutropenic, abscessed, infected, or severely carious teeth can no longer be considered innocent, even if asymptomatic. A loose tooth that will soon exfoliate can become a nidus for infection as well as a cause of bleeding for a thrombocytopenic patient. Sharp, ragged teeth can be an irritation that leads to infection. Chemotherapeutic drugs and local irradiation are cytotoxic to the oral mucosa, which becomes atrophic and ulcerates with ease (mucositis). This is painful and often leads to inadequate oral intake and nutrition. Once the mucosal barrier is breached by ulceration, the patient can become septic, especially with α-hemolytic streptococci and other mouth flora. Herpes simplex virus is another pathogen that can enhance drug-induced mucositis. Friction and damage to the mucosa is the main concern with braces. Therefore, all orthodontic hardware is removed prior to chemotherapy.

The pediatric oncology patient should be monitored throughout therapy to screen for infection, manage oral bleeding, and control oral pain. These children can experience spontaneous oral hemorrhaging, especially when the platelet count is below 20,000/mL. Poor oral hygiene or areas of irritation can increase the chances of bleeding.

Children receiving radiation therapy to the head and neck are prone to develop extensive salivary dysfunction (xerostomia) when salivary tissue is in the path of the primary beam of radiation. Xerostomia should be managed aggressively to avoid rapid extensive destruction of dentition. Customized fluoride applicators are used in this situation in combination with close follow-up.

Children undergoing bone marrow transplantation may have acute graft-versus-host reaction as another contributor to severe oral mucositis. Long-term follow-up includes managing salivary dysfunction from total body radiation and treatment of oral graft-versus-host disease.

The pediatric oncology patient also needs to be followed by a dentist who is familiar with young children and their growth and development. Oral and maxillofacial growth disturbances can occur after therapy. Late effects of therapy include morphologic changes in tooth development (microdontia or extensive hypocalcification) and disturbances in eruption (blunted roots or delayed eruption).

## Children with Hematologic Problems

The child with hemophilia needs to have the appropriate clotting factor provided before and after any invasive dental procedures (including the administration of local anesthesia, even for simple fillings) (see Chapter 27). Some patients with very mild factor VIII deficiency or von Willebrand disease may respond to desmopressin acetate. Antifibrinolytic medications such as aminocaproic acid and tranexamic acid are used successfully after dental treatment. Postoperative bleeding can also be treated with a wide variety of topical medicaments, such as Gelfoam and thrombin.

The pediatric patient receiving anticoagulant therapy must undergo dosage adjustment before invasive dental treatment. This is a relatively simple matter when dealing with heparin, with its short half-life of 4–6 hours. It is a much more difficult problem with warfarin, which has a half-life of 40–70 hours.

## Children with Diabetes

Children who are insulin-dependent are prone to dental problems. They have an impaired capacity to heal, a higher incidence of periodontal disease, and a higher caries rate. These children need to be followed carefully on a routine basis. Care must be taken not to disturb the regular cycle of eating and insulin dosage. Anxiety associated with dental appointments can cause a major upset in the diabetic child's routine. Postoperative pain or pain from dental abscess can prevent them from eating. Warnings about eating until the numbness wears off or until the filling gets hard can also alter their normal schedule of food intake and insulin dosage. Insulin levels must be adjusted to conform to treatment needs and vice versa.

## MATERNAL–FETAL RELATIONSHIP

In addition to the discovery that childhood caries is an infectious disease transmitted by bacteria from the mother to the child, a number of other maternal–fetal relationships related to the oral cavity have been identified. A recent large prospective study has shown a significant association between maternal periodontitis at 21–24 weeks' gestation and preterm birth. It is unknown whether treatment of periodontitis will reduce the risk of preterm birth.

The risk of preterm birth is elevated if a mother smokes and is of low socioeconomic status, both of which also increase the risk for periodontitis. Secondhand or passive smoke also increases the risk of caries in children who grow up around smokers. This association is independent of age, family income, geographic region, and frequency of dental visits.

Given the known association between maternal periodontitis and preterm birth, passive smoke and children's dental caries, and the knowledge of maternal transmission of caries-causing bacteria, it is important to advise expectant teenage mothers about these risk factors.

Moreover, low-birth-weight, preterm children have a greater predisposition to many oral developmental anomalies than normal-birth-weight children. These include generalized enamel hypoplasia associated with increased predisposition to early childhood caries, localized enamel hypoplasia, crown dilaceration of the maxillary left incisors, and palatal deformations associated with laryngoscopy and endotracheal intubation. Dental development in preterm infants is retarded in the eruption of the primary dentition and in the development of the permanent teeth.

## DENTAL REFERRAL

Referral to a dentist is appropriate whenever there is a question about a child's oral and maxillofacial health and development. Most pediatric dentists will want to see a child for a first visit by age 12 months. The average child should be seen every 6 months for dental follow-up. Any child with additional risk factors should be seen earlier and more frequently.

## REFERENCES

Hale KJ, American Academy of Pediatrics Section on Pediatric Dentistry: Oral health risk assessment timing and establishment of the dental home. Pediatrics 2003;111:1113 [PMID: 12728101].

Jeffcoat M et al: Periodontal infection and preterm birth: Results of a prospective study. J Am Dent Assoc 2001;132:875 [PMID: 11480640].

Seow W et al: A controlled study of the morphometric changes in the primary dentition of pre-term, very-low-birthweight children. J Dent Res 2000;79:63 [PMID: 10690662].

# Ear, Nose, & Throat

*Candice E. Johnson, MD, PhD, Peggy Kelley, MD, & Norman R. Friedman, MD*

## ■ I. THE EAR

## INFECTIONS OF THE EAR

The spectrum of ear diseases includes the structures of the outer ear (otitis externa), the middle ear (acute otitis media), the mastoid bone (mastoiditis), and the inner ear (labyrinthitis).

### 1. Otitis Externa

Otitis externa is inflammation of the skin lining the ear canal and surrounding soft tissue. The most common cause is loss of the protective function of cerumen, leading to maceration of the underlying skin. Other causes are trauma to the ear canal from using cotton-tipped applicators for cleaning or from using poorly fitted ear plugs while swimming; contact dermatitis due to hair sprays, perfumes, or self-administered ear drops; secondary infection of the canal from otitis media with a patent tympanostomy tube; and chronic drainage from a perforated tympanic membrane (TM). Infections due to *Staphylococcus aureus* or *Pseudomonas aeruginosa* are the most common.

Symptoms include pain and itching in the ear, especially with chewing or pressure on the tragus. Movement of the pinna or tragus causes considerable pain. Drainage may be minimal unless the otitis externa is from a draining PE tube or TM perforation. The ear canal may be grossly swollen, and the patient may resist any attempt to insert an ear speculum. Debris is noticeable in the canal. It is often impossible to visualize the TM. Hearing is normal unless complete occlusion has occurred.

### Treatment

Topical treatment usually suffices. The crucial initial step is removal of desquamated epithelium and moist cerumen. This debris can be irrigated out or suctioned out using warm Burow solution (one packet of Domeboro powder [aluminum acetate and acetic acid] to 250 mL tap water) or normal saline, as long as it is known that the TM is intact. If the TM cannot be seen, then a perforation may be presumed to exist. Children

with otitis externa secondary to draining tubes or perforations should be treated with topical therapy only in the absence of systemic symptoms. The topical therapy chosen must be safe for the inner ear because the perforation or the patent tube allows the drops access to the middle and inner ear. Safe drops, such as fluoroquinolone drops, have no aminoglycoside or toxic preservatives. Once the ear canal is open, instill antibiotic ear drops two or three times daily. A corticosteroid may reduce the inflammatory response, but this is debated. If the canal is too edematous to allow the ear drop to get in, an ear wick for the first few days may be helpful. Oral antibiotics are indicated if any signs of invasive infection, such as fever, cellulitis of the auricles, or tender postauricular lymph nodes, are present. Prescribe an antistaphylococcal antibiotic while awaiting the results of culture of the ear canal discharge. Systemic antibiotics alone without topical treatment will not clear up otitis externa. Analgesics may be required temporarily.

During the acute phase, the patient should avoid swimming. A cotton ear plug is not helpful and may prolong the infection. Schedule a follow-up visit in 1 week to document an intact tympanic membrane (Figure 17–1). Children who have intact TMs and are predisposed to this problem should receive 2 or 3 drops of a 1:1 solution of white vinegar and 70% ethyl alcohol into the ears before and after swimming.

Hannley MT et al: Use of ototopical antibiotics in treating 3 common ear diseases. Otolaryngol Head Neck Surg 2000;6:934 [PMID: 10828818].

Hughes E, Lee JH: Otitis externa. Pediatr Rev 2001;22:191 [PMID:11389206 ].

### 2. Otitis Media

### Classification & Clinical Findings

Otitis media is an infection associated with middle ear effusion (a collection of fluid in the middle ear space) or with otorrhea (a discharge from the ear through a perforation in the TM or a ventilating tube). Otitis media can be further classified by its associated clinical symptoms, otoscopic findings, duration, frequency, and complications. These more specific classifications are

**Right Tympanic Membrane**

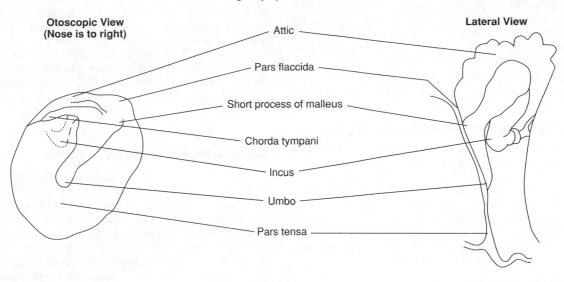

Otoscopic View (Nose is to right)

Lateral View

Attic
Pars flaccida
Short process of malleus
Chorda tympani
Incus
Umbo
Pars tensa

***Figure 17–1.*** Tympanic membrane.

acute otitis media, otitis media with effusion, and chronic suppurative otitis media.

## A. ACUTE OTITIS MEDIA

Acute otitis media (AOM) is commonly defined as inflammation of the middle ear resulting in an effusion and associated with rapid onset of symptoms such as otalgia, fever, irritability, anorexia, or vomiting. An ear effusion is best documented by pneumatic otoscopy or tympanometry. To distinguish AOM from otitis media with effusion (OME), signs of inflammation of the TM or symptoms of acute infection must be present. Otoscopic findings specific for AOM are a bulging TM; impaired visibility of the ossicular landmarks; a yellow, white, or bright red color; opacification of the eardrum; and squamous exudate or bullae on the eardrum. OME is associated with a nonbulging eardrum, which may be retracted or neutral, but always has decreased mobility, may have opacification, and may have white or amber discoloration. Children with OME may develop acute infection, but they will then exhibit inflammation of the eardrum as described for AOM.

## B. OTITIS MEDIA WITH EFFUSION

Otitis media with effusion is defined as an asymptomatic middle ear effusion that often follows AOM, but may have no such antecedent history. Otoscopic findings that suggest OME include visualization of air–fluid levels or bubbles, and a clear or amber middle ear fluid. Effusion is usually associated with either a mild or a moderate conductive hearing impairment of 15 dB or higher. OME can also be associated with negative middle ear pressure, which results in prominence of the malleus and a negative pressure peak on tympanometry.

## C. CHRONIC SUPPURATIVE OTITIS MEDIA

This type of otitis media is defined as persistent otorrhea lasting longer than 6 weeks. Most often it occurs in children with tympanostomy tubes or TM perforations. Occasionally, it is an accompanying sign of cholesteatoma. Organisms commonly isolated are *Pseudomonas aeruginosa* and *Staphylococcus aureus,* but fungi and anaerobic bacteria may also play a role.

## Pathogenesis of Acute Otitis Media

Factors that make otitis media more common in children than in adults include bacterial nasopharyngeal colonization in the absence of antibody, frequent upper respiratory infections (URI), exposure to parental cigarette smoke, unfavorable eustachian tube function, and allergies.

## A. BACTERIAL COLONIZATION

Nasopharyngeal colonization with *Streptococcus pneumoniae, Haemophilus influenzae,* or *Moraxella catarrhalis* increases the risk of otitis media. Colonization with normal flora such as viridans streptococci may prevent otitis episodes by inhibiting the growth of these pathogens, and a nasal spray of viridans streptococci is under study. Colonization usually occurs sequentially with different serotypes of pathogen, and there is a risk of AOM with each new serotype acquired. Infants in daycare acquire these serotypes at a younger age than those in home care. Since younger children are at higher risk of AOM, the increased number of children in daycare over the last 3 decades has played a major role in the increase in AOM.

### B. Viral Upper Respiratory Infections

These infections increase the colonization of the nasopharynx with otitis pathogens, perhaps because of increased adherence to the mucosa. Viral infection also impairs eustachian tube function by adenoidal swelling and edema. Therefore, factors that increase the frequency of viral respiratory infections, such as child care attendance, smoke exposure, later birth order, and absence of breast-feeding, promote colonization with otitis pathogens and predispose to otitis.

### C. Smoke Exposure

Passive smoking increases the risk of persistent middle ear effusion by enhancing attachment of the pathogen, prolonging the inflammatory response, and impeding drainage through the eustachian tube. For infants age 12–18 months, exposure to each additional pack of cigarettes smoked at home is associated with an 11% increase in the duration of a middle ear effusion.

### D. Eustachian Tube Dysfunction

Infants born with craniofacial disorders, such as Down syndrome or a cleft palate, are often affected by AOM and OME. The patency of the tube allows aeration of the middle ear. When the tube is obstructed, a vacuum develops, which can pull nasopharyngeal secretions into the middle ear.

### E. Host Immune Defenses

Immunocompromised children usually experience recurrent AOM and sinusitis, as well as pneumonia. However, children who experience recurrent or persistent otitis may have selective impairments of immune defenses against specific otitis pathogens. For example, a recent study showed some such children have low-to-absent IgG2 or IgA pneumococcal polysaccharide antibody responses (or both) after vaccination, despite normal serum levels of total IgG2 and IgA.

### F. Breast-Feeding

Breast-feeding reduces the incidence of acute respiratory infections, provides IgA antibodies that reduce colonization with otitis pathogens, and decreases the aspiration of contaminated secretions into the middle ear space.

### G. Genetic Susceptibility

Although we know AOM to be multifactorial, and no gene for susceptibility has yet been identified, recent studies of twins and triplets suggest that as much as 70% of the risk is genetically determined. This has implications for the subsequent offspring of parents with a child experiencing recurrent AOM. These families might wish to consider breast-feeding and home care for later children.

## Microbiology of Acute Otitis Media

The role of respiratory viral infection in precipitating otitis media is unquestionable, yet fewer that 12% of ear effusions grow viruses. Recent studies with sensitive viral antigen or nucleic acid tests have detected virus in over 40% of infected ears. The viral infection may precede the bacterial otitis media by 3–14 days and presumably causes adenoid hypertrophy and eustachian tube dysfunction. The two viruses most clearly shown to precipitate otitis media are respiratory syncytial virus and influenza, accounting for the annual surge in otitis media cases in January to April in temperate climates.

About 50% of AOM in the Midwestern and northeastern United States is due to *S pneumoniae*, while the warmer, drier climates of southern Israel and Denver report a preponderance of nontypable *H influenzae*—the same two organisms most frequently associated with sinusitis. Another pathogen, *M catarrhalis*, may cause up to 25% of AOM in colder climates, but is much less common in Denver and southern Israel, possibly because of the drier, hotter climate (Table 17–1). The fourth organism found is *Streptococcus pyogenes;* this organism and *S pneumoniae* are the predominant causes of mastoiditis. The microbiologic causes of AOM in early infancy differ only slightly from those in later life. The risk of gram-negative enteric infection is increased in infants younger than age 4 weeks who are or have been hospitalized in a neonatal intensive care nursery.

Resistant *S pneumoniae* is a common pathogen in acute otitis, representing up to 40% of isolates, as well as in persistent effusions and chronic suppurative otitis. Children with resistant strains tend to be younger and to have had more unresponsive infections. Antibiotic treatment in the preceding 3 months also increases the risk of harboring resistant pathogens. Penicillin resistance develops through stepwise mutations in the structure of the penicillin-binding proteins. Strains for which minimum inhibitory concentrations (MICs) of penicillin range between 0.12 and 1.0 µg/mL are said to exhibit "intermediate" resistance. Strains for which MICs are equal to or higher than 2 µg/mL are said to have a "high-level resistance." The prevalence of resis-

*Table 17-1.* Bacteriology of acute otitis media in two U.S. cities and Israel.

| | Minneapolis, MN (Personal correspondence)[a] | Southern Israel (Lebowitz and Dagan)[b] | Denver, CO (Author)[a] |
|---|---|---|---|
| *Streptococcus pneumoniae* | 49 | 22 | 23 |
| *Haemophilus influenzae* | 14 | 30 | 37 |
| *Moraxella catarrhalis* | 14 | 4 | 5 |
| *Streptococcus pyogenes* | 5 | 3 | 3 |
| *S pneumoniae + H influenzae* | Not reported | 14 | 3 |
| *Staphylococcus aureus* or other | 6 | 0 | 0 |
| No growth | 6 | 30 | 28 |

[a]Unpublished data. Updated 1998–2002.
[b]Dagan R et al: Bacteriologic efficacies of oral azithromycin and oral cefaclor in treatment of acute otitis media in infants and young children. Antimicrob Agents Chemother 2000;44:43.

tant strains no longer varies significantly among geographic areas within the United States. These strains are also resistant to other drug classes. Approximate rates of resistance are 60% for trimethoprim–sulfamethoxazole, 15% for macrolides, and 2% for amoxicillin (dosed at 90 mg/kg/d). Between 90% and 100% of highly penicillin-resistant strains are susceptible to clindamycin and rifampin, and 97% are susceptible to fluroquinolones. Second-generation fluroquinolones such as ciprofloxacin and norfloxacin are much less active against *S pneumoniae* than are the third-generation agents such as gatifloxacin and levofloxacin. Unfortunately, fluroquinolones are not approved for children younger than 16 years; however, studies are under way to assess their safety and efficacy in this age group.

## Diagnosis

### A. PNEUMATIC OTOSCOPY

Acute otitis media is overdiagnosed. Contributing to errors in diagnosis are the temptation to accept the diagnosis without removing enough cerumen to adequately visualize the eardrum, and the mistaken belief that a red eardrum establishes the diagnosis. In fact, redness of the eardrum can be caused by a viral URI, the child's crying, or even efforts to remove cerumen. Failure to achieve an adequate seal with the otoscope, poor visualization due to low light intensity, and mistaking the ear canal wall for the membrane can make it difficult to assess eardrum mobility.

A pneumatic otoscope with a rubber suction bulb and tube is used to assess mobility of the TM. The speculum inserted into the patient's ear canal must be large enough to provide an airtight seal. Placing a piece of rubber tubing 0.25–0.5 cm wide near the end of the ear speculum helps to create an adequate pneumatic seal. The tubing should fit snugly on the speculum at a distance about 0.5 cm from its end. The largest possible speculum (usually 3 or 4 mm) should be used to maximize the field of view, avoiding disposable specula if possible. When the rubber bulb is squeezed, the TM will move freely to and fro if no fluid is present; if fluid is present in the middle ear space, the mobility of the TM will be absent or resemble a fluid wave. The ability to assess mobility is compromised by low light intensity; a halogen source is necessary. These bulbs dim, but rarely ever "burn out."

Disposable ear specula have become popular but are not needed for infection control, because reusable specula can be easily disinfected. The disposable specula are sharp at the tip and often cause pain when pushed to get an airtight seal.

### B. CERUMEN REMOVAL

Cerumen removal is an essential skill for anyone who cares for children. Impacted cerumen can cause itching, pain, hearing loss, or otitis externa. Parents should be advised that earwax protects the ear (cerumen contains lysozymes and immunoglobulins that inhibit infection) and will come out by itself; therefore, parents should never put anything solid into the ear canal to remove the earwax. Eardrops (discussed later) may be used.

The physician may remove cerumen under direct vision through the operating head of an otoscope, provided two adults are present to hold the child. Cerumen that obstructs the view of the TM can often be pushed aside, the pneumatic seal reestablished, and mobility assessed without removing the speculum. Alternatively, a plastic disposable ear curette of about size 0 (often green) may be used.

Irrigation can also be used to remove cerumen. Very hard cerumen may adhere to the wall of the ear canal and cause pain or bleeding if one attempts to remove it with a curette. This type of wax can be softened with carbamyl peroxide solutions, mineral oil, or a few drops of detergent before irrigation is attempted. After 20 minutes, irrigation with a soft bulb syringe can be started with water warmed to 35–38°C to prevent vertigo. A commercial jet tooth cleanser (eg, Water Pik) is also an excellent device for removing cerumen, but it is important to set it at low power (2 or less) to prevent damage to the TM. A perforated TM is a contraindication to any form of irrigation. In difficult cases, it may be necessary to consult an otolaryngologist.

## C. TYMPANOMETRY

Tympanometry can identify an effusion, and it requires little training. It should supplement and not replace pneumatic otoscopy because it does not identify inflammation. Because of the compliance of the cartilaginous canal of the infants, tympanometry should be reserved for children older than age 6 months. Tympanometry uses an electroacoustic impedance bridge to measure TM compliance and display it in graphic form (along the $y$-axis, expressed in mm $H_2O$). Compliance is determined at air pressures from +200 to –400 mm $H_2O$ that are created in the sealed external ear canal. The existing middle ear pressure can be measured by determining the ear canal pressure at which the TM is most compliant. Because total visualization of the TM is not necessary, tympanometry does not require removal of cerumen unless the canal is completely blocked.

Tympanograms can be classified into four major patterns, as shown in Figure 17–2. The pattern shown in Figure 17–2A, characterized by maximum compliance at normal atmospheric pressure, indicates a normal TM, good eustachian tube function, and absence of effusion. The pattern shown in Figure 17–2B identifies a nonmobile TM, which indicates middle ear effusion. The pattern shown in Figure 17–2C indicates an intact mobile TM with poor eustachian tube function and excessive negative pressure (> –300 mm $H_2O$ air pressure) in the middle ear. Figure 17–2D shows a flat tracing, which would have a very large middle ear volume on the printout, due to a patent tube or large perforation.

## D. ACOUSTIC REFLECTOMETRY

Acoustic reflectometry measures the spectral gradient of the TM using a handheld instrument, without requiring an airtight seal. However, recent data suggest that this method cannot reliably distinguish negative middle ear pressure from effusion. Much more study is required before this method can be recommended, and the instrument is presently not being sold.

## Treatment of Acute Otitis Media

An algorithm for the management of AOM is presented in Figure 17–3. Drugs commonly used are listed in Table 17–2.

## A. THE OBSERVATION OPTION

*Nontreatment:* Few issues in clinical medicine are as controversial as antibiotic treatment of otitis media, because of the increasing prevalence of resistant organisms since 1990 and questions about how to measure efficacy. The natural history of AOM is that it improves clinically through host defenses; however, bacteriologic cure rates (determined by a second tympanocentesis while on therapy) were only 32% at 2–7 days on placebo in Dr Howie's classic studies. In children receiving a placebo, the cure rate is 16% for *S pneumoniae,* 84% for *M catarrhalis,* and 50% for nontypable *H influenzae.* Therefore, the absence of overt symptoms does not necessarily mean that the bacterial infection has been cured. In a meta-analysis of 33 trials of antibiotic treatment of AOM, only 4 trials contained a placebo. Eighty-one percent of patients who received a placebo became asymptomatic by 7–14 days, and treatment with antibiotics increased the resolution rate by 14%. This study has led to the assertion that seven children must be treated with antibiotics to benefit one child. However, the age group younger than 2 years, who experience the highest rate of AOM, were barely included in this meta-analysis. Although most clinicians routinely treat acute otitis with antibiotics, it is also reasonable to individualize this decision and involve the family in the process. This calls for a trade-off between the risks of antibiotic treatment (allergic reactions, side effects, and colonization with an antibiotic-resistant pathogen) and the benefit of a more rapid clinical response. More rapid pain relief may be a reasonable justification for treatment. Patients not receiving treatment who fail to improve within 48 to 72 hours should be reassessed and given antibiotics if symptoms of AOM are still present. It is advisable to treat otitis media in all children younger than age 2 years with antibiotics because they respond less well to bacterial polysaccharide and are more likely to develop complications. Of three recent studies of placebo compared with antibiotics in children younger than 2 years, clinical cure rates were 28–42% with placebo and 41–74% with an antibiotic.

One can avoid the antibiotic treatment dilemma by not overdiagnosing AOM. To summarize, to accurately diagnose otitis media, cerumen must first be thor-

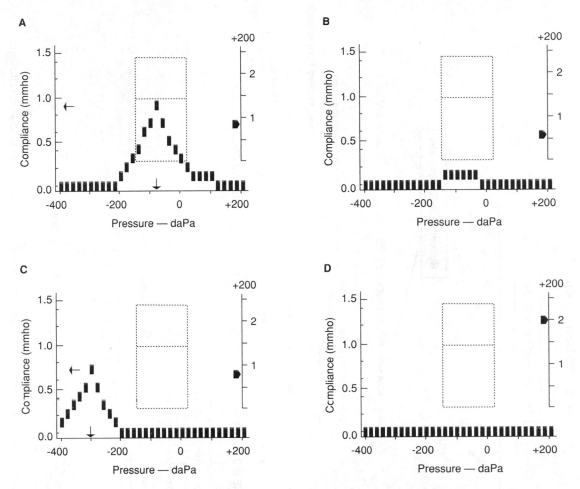

***Figure 17–2.*** Four types of tympanograms obtained with Welch–Allyn MicroTymp 2. **A:** Normal middle ear. **B:** Otitis media with effusion or acute otitis media. **C:** Negative middle ear pressure due to eustachian tube dysfunction. **D:** Patent tympanostomy tube or perforation in the tympanic membrane. Same as B except for a very large middle ear volume.

oughly removed. Pneumatic otoscopy is mandatory to avoid misinterpreting red ears.

## B. ANTIBIOTIC THERAPY

Amoxicillin remains the first-line antibiotic for treating otitis media, even with a high prevalence of drug-resistant *S pneumoniae,* because resistance to β-lactam antibiotics, such as amoxicillin, develops as a stepwise process over many years. A bacterial strain resistant to low levels of amoxicillin will usually be eradicated by a higher dosage. Amoxicillin dosage may be raised considerably without toxicity; for example, a dosage of 200 mg/kg/d has been used to treat meningitis in children, and a maximum daily dose of 4 g has been used

in adults. Studies have shown that increasing the dosage from 40 mg/kg to 90 mg/kg yields a drug concentration in middle ear fluid that surpasses the minimal level needed to inhibit 98% of all pneumococcal otitis media. A second advantage is that dosing amoxicillin at these higher levels may help delay stepwise emergence of resistance. In recognition of this new pharmacodynamic data, the federal government in June 1999 doubled the MIC used to define resistance to amoxicillin to 8 μg/mL or greater. Because otitis media is not a life-threatening disease, it is not necessary for a first-line antibiotic to achieve 100% cure. High-dose amoxicillin will usually eradicate the most invasive pathogen, *S pneumoniae,* and if no improvement occurs, a second-

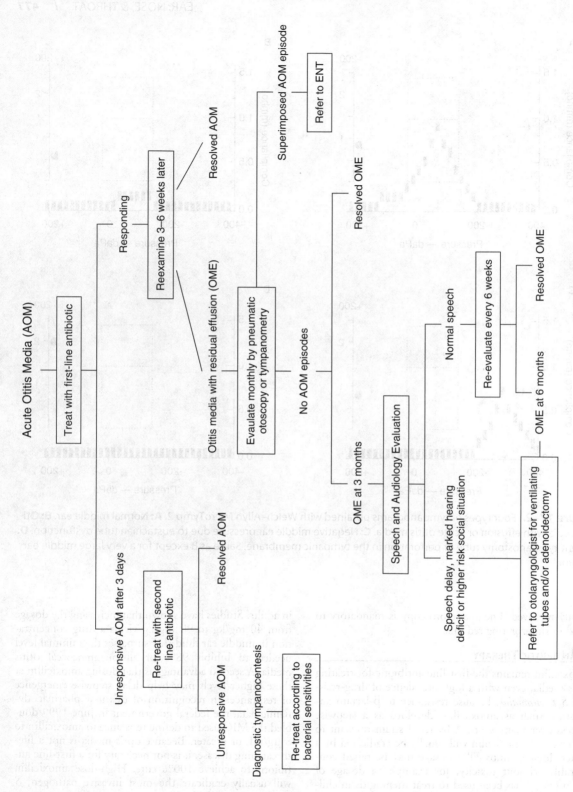

**Figure 17–3.** Algorithm for acute otitis media. AOM = acute otitis media; ENT = ear, nose, and throat consult; OME = otitis media with effusion.

**Table 17–2.** Treatment of acute otitis media in an era of drug resistance.

---

#### First-line therapy

1. Amoxicillin 90 mg/kg/d, up to 4 g d. For children over 2 years of age, give for 5 days; under 2 years of age, for 10 days.
2. If amoxicillin has caused a rash, give cefuroxime (Ceftin), cefdinir (Omnicef), or cefpodoxime (vantin).
3. If urticaria or other IgE-mediated events have occurred, give trimethoprim-sulfa or azithromycin (Zithromax).
4. If the child is unable to take oral medication, give single intramuscular dose of ceftriaxone (Rocephin).

#### Second-line therapy

This is for clinical failure after 48–72 hours of treatment, or for recurrences within 4 weeks.

1. Amoxicillin-clavulanate (Augmentin ES-600), given so that the patient receives amoxicillin at 90 mg/kg/d.
2. If amoxicillin has caused allergic symptoms, see recommendations above.

#### Third-line therapy

1. Tympanocentesis is recommended to determine the cause.
2. Ceftriaxone (Rocephin), two doses given intramuscularly, 48 hours apart, with the option of a third dose.

#### Recurrences > 4 weeks after the first episode

1. A new pathogen is likely, so restart first-line therapy.
2. Be sure the diagnosis is not OM with effusion (OME), which may be observed for 3–6 months without treatment.

---

line antibiotic may be chosen to cover *M catarrhalis* and β-lactamase-producing *H influenzae.*

Amoxicillin–clavulanate enhanced strength (ES), with 90 mg/kg/d of amoxicillin dosing and unchanged amounts of clavulanic acid, is an appropriate choice as a second-line antibiotic when a child is clinically failing after 48 to 72 hours on amoxicillin (see Table 17–2). If generic dosing is preferred to reduce costs, two prescriptions are required: low-dose amoxicillin–clavulanate and 45 mg/kg of amoxicillin. The generic amoxicillin–clavulanate should never be doubled in dosage, since the amount of clavulanate will be too high In this situation, the most likely pathogen is *H influenzae,* and the addition of clavulanate to amoxicillin will broaden the coverage while retaining efficacy against *S pneumoniae.*

Three oral cephalosporins are more β-lactamase-stable (cefuroxime, cefpodoxime, and cefdinir), and these are alternative choices for second-line therapy for children who develop papular rashes with amoxicillin (see Table 17–2). Unfortunately, these do not cover highly penicillin-resistant pneumococci, only the intermediately resistant class. Of these three drugs, only cefdinir is palatable in the liquid form; the other two drugs have a bitter aftertaste which is difficult, but not impossible, to conceal with milk or sweet food given after the drug. A second-line agent is also indicated when a child experiences symptomatic infection within 1 month of stopping amoxicillin; however, repeat use of high-dose amoxicillin is indicated if more than 4 weeks has passed without symptoms, because a new pathogen is usually present. Macrolides and sulfonamides are not recommended as second-line agents due to poor coverage of *H influenzae.* The major use of these drug classes is in children with urticaria or anaphylactic reactions to β-lactams.

If a child remains symptomatic longer than 3 days while taking a second-line agent, a tympanocentesis may be useful to identify the causative pathogen or to prove sterility. The parents may be noncompliant or the child may not have absorbed the antibiotic well, in which case an organism sensitive to many drugs may be found. If a highly resistant pneumococcus is found or if tympanocentesis is not feasible, intramuscular ceftriaxone at 50 mg/kg/day for 3 consecutive days is the best choice. Further studies are needed in children failing second-line therapy. Table 17–2 also lists alternative drugs for penicillin-allergic children. If the child has experienced anaphylaxis to amoxicillin, cephalosporins should not be substituted. However, the maculopapular rash frequently seen with amoxicillin is not IgE-mediated, and cephalosporins may be used.

Figure 17–3 shows the recommended follow-up of AOM that resolves with a residual effusion at 3–4 weeks. Children, particularly those young enough to still be developing language skills, should be seen every 8 weeks for otoscopic exams to determine if the effusion is persistent or occurs only with symptomatic infections. Prophylactic antibiotics and corticosteroids are no longer recommended for OME. A hearing test should be performed after approximately 3 months of continuous bilateral effusion in children younger than 3 years and those at risk of language delay due to poverty or craniofacial anomalies. Children with hearing loss or speech delay should be referred to an otolaryngologist for possible ventilation tubes.

### C. Duration of Therapy

The duration of antibiotic treatment is controversial. Only three recent trials have used stringent entry and outcome criteria. Success rates were higher at 12–14 days following 10 days of therapy in all three studies, particularly for children younger than 2 years of age, and for those in daycare. At this time, short-course (5-day) therapy can only be recommended for children older than 2 years and not in daycare.

A recent study of preschoolers by Schrag and colleagues demonstrated that drug-resistant pneumococcal carriage at day 28 posttherapy was lower in a short-course high-dose amoxicillin group compared with a group given a standard course of therapy. This is an important finding, because we now know that the nasopharyngeal flora determines the pathogen of the next AOM. Efforts to reduce drug-resistant pneumococci include use of Prevnar vaccine and the 23-valent pneumococcal vaccine in children older than 2 years.

### D. PAIN MANAGEMENT

Children with pain related to AOM may obtain relief from acetaminophen, ibuprofen, or a topical anesthetic drop. In a randomized controlled trial, Auralgan (benzocaine and antipyrine) ear drops were superior to olive oil in reducing pain. A recent study of 88 children, all older than 2 years of age, found that Auralgan eardrops provided enough pain relief that the majority did not need antibiotic therapy. When pain persists after antimicrobial treatment, tympanocentesis should be considered for pain relief and to diagnose the causative pathogen.

### E. FOLLOW-UP VISITS

The optimal timing for follow-up visits depends on the response to therapy. Children should be reassessed when symptoms of AOM continue beyond 72 hours or recur during treatment. The follow-up visit for preschool children should be 3–6 weeks after start of therapy. The need for follow-up visits for asymptomatic school-age children without risk factors of recurrent disease should be based on the history of speech delay or the presence of OME in the past.

### F. TYMPANOCENTESIS OR MYRINGOTOMY

Tympanocentesis is performed by placing a needle through the TM and aspirating the middle ear fluid. Myringotomy involves making an incision in the drum with a myringotomy knife to drain the fluid. Indications for tympanocentesis or myringotomy are (1) AOM in a patient with compromised host resistance, (2) painful bulging of the TM, particularly in a toddler younger than 48 months, (3) a complete workup for presumed sepsis or meningitis, such as in a neonate, (4) unresponsive otitis media despite courses of two appropriate antibiotics, and (5) acute mastoiditis or other suppurative complications. The technique of tympanocentesis is as follows:

**1. Premedication**—In the conditions mentioned, the pain associated with tympanocentesis is only slightly greater than the pain of existing acute inflammation of the TM. Therefore, no premedication is generally indi-

cated. The patient who is extremely difficult to hold may be premedicated with meperidine, 1 mg/kg intramuscularly. Tetracaine has been used, but no studies are available on its efficacy in children with acute inflammation, which rapidly removes locally administered drugs. Unquestionably, the best pain minimization method is to perform the procedure rapidly and return the child immediately to the parent's arms.

**2. Restraint**—The patient must be completely immobile while the procedure is being performed. A papoose board or a sheet can be used to immobilize the patient's body, and an extra attendant is required to hold the child's head steady. It is helpful to have the parent remain in sight of the child for reassurance.

**3. Site selection**—With an open-headed operating otoscope (Figure 17–4), the operator carefully selects a target. This is best done in the anteroinferior quadrant, although the posteroinferior quadrant is a safe but shallower alternative. These sites avoid damage to the ossicles during the procedure.

***Figure 17–4.*** Operating head and Alden-Senturia trap for tympanocentesis. 18 gauge spinal needle attached and bent.

**4. Aspiration**—An 8.8-cm spinal needle (No. 18 or No. 20) with a short bevel is attached to a 3-mL syringe. Alternatively, either an Alden-Senturia trap (Storz Instrument Co., St. Louis, Mo.) or the Tymp-Tap aspirator (Xomed Surgical Products, Jackson, Florida) is attached to a suction pump. The operator then aspirates the middle ear effusion from the anterior inferior quadrant. Aspirate should be placed directly onto culture plates for maximum recovery, and chocolate agar suffices to grow all common pathogens.

## G. Nonvaccine Prophylaxis

Chemoprophylaxis has been used successfully since the 1960s, and it is supported by a recent randomized, controlled trial by Teele's group in Boston. Though conducted in the era of drug-resistant pneumococci, this study found that the AOM attack rate in infants younger than 1 year was cut in half by the dose of amoxicillin (20 mg/kg/d) used in older studies. Sulfisoxazole was not as effective, and the sample size was inadequate to determine if it was superior to placebo. Nonetheless, the widespread use of chemoprophylaxis is likely to lead to bacterial resistance in the community, and it can thus be recommended only for selected non-daycare-attending children. For example, children who have had three well-documented episodes within 6 months or four in 1 year may be candidates, as well as infants younger that 6 months who have had more than one episode. Prophylaxis for 3–4 months is still useful in the spring season, because the absence of URIs in summer may obviate the need for PE tube placement. It is also valuable for children with PE tubes who continue to experience AOM episodes.

A second method of prophylaxis is to educate parents about risk factors for recurrent disease. This is time-consuming, but valuable. Specific topics:

1. Smoking is a risk factor both for URI and for AOM, and primary care doctors can provide literature on smoking cessation programs and nicotine-containing gums or patches.
2. Breast-feeding protects children from AOM, but the mechanism is unknown. Some researchers believe that propping a bottle of milk in the crib increases AOM risk.
3. The pacifier has been implicated as a risk factor by a study done in Finland in 2000; after nurses had educated parents about the risk, children not given a pacifier continuously had a 29% lower rate of otitis media over the first 18 months of life.
4. Daycare is clearly a risk factor for AOM, but few working parents can hire a nanny. Alternatives to suggest include care by relatives or care of the child in a homecare setting with fewer children to expose the child to URIs.

Another method of prophylaxis being studied in Finland is xylitol, also known as birch sugar, found in plums, strawberries, and raspberries. It was first studied in Europe as a chewing gum to reduce dental caries, and was effective. Recently a double-blind study of chewing gum use in children with a mean age of 5 years found a 42% reduction in episodes of AOM. For children too young to chew gum safely, the same investigators studied a xylitol syrup given five times daily after meals or snacks, and found a 33% reduction. The main problem here is the frequency of dosing, which needs to be addressed before this therapy could be practical.

Surgical prevention of AOM is an effective, albeit expensive, alternative to antibiotic prophylaxis. A meta-analysis has shown that PE tubes reduce rates of AOM, but that adenoidectomy has only limited efficacy. Unfortunately, the rate of posttube otorrhea is 16%, and a small number of children will develop perforations after tube extrusion that require surgical repair. Adenoidectomy reduces the need for PE tube reinsertion and therefore will continue to play a role with the second insertion of PE tubes. The costs of the procedures and the possibility of long-term complications after tube extrusion have limited this method of prevention to children with long-standing problems.

## H. Vaccines for the Prevention of Otitis Media

With the increasing problems of antibiotic therapy and prophylaxis, the prevention of both viral and bacterial pathogens causing AOM has become an exciting area of research. Unfortunately, the currently available heptavalent vaccine (Prevnar) does not contain the majority of strains of pneumococci causing AOM and yielded only a 6% reduction in infections due to all causes. It did produce a 57% reduction in otitis media due to those serotypes found in the vaccine, and these stains include the serotypes most likely to be penicillin- and macrolide-resistant. The heptavalent vaccine also reduced PE tube placements by 20% compared with a control group in Kaiser of California and greatly reduced AOM incidence in children having six or more episodes per year. Furthermore, studies are showing a herd immunity effect on the older siblings of vaccinated children, which may further reduce drug-resistant serotype circulation. Now that the shortage has ended, the vaccine should be used as a single dose for children 2–5 years with a history of either recurrent AOM or OME with superimposed AOM episodes, with consideration of the 23-valent vaccine 8 weeks after the conjugate vaccine.

In recent studies, intranasal influenza vaccine reduced the number of influenza-associated cases of

AOM by 92%. For children older than 6 months with recurrent AOM, it seems prudent to recommend yearly influenza vaccine, although this is not yet an official recommendation.

Vaccines currently being studied in animals that hold promise for AOM prevention include a respiratory syncytial virus vaccine and a nontypeable *H influenzae* vaccine. Pregnant women in the third trimester may have their antibody levels raised by a heptavalent pneumococcal vaccine. This may raise antibody levels in the offspring. A recent study showed that low cord blood levels of two common pneumococcal serotypes is a risk factor for AOM and OME, so this passive route is a logical next step.

Dagan R et al: Bacteriologic and clinical efficacy of amoxicillin–clavulanate versus azithromycin in acute otitis media. Pediatr Infect Dis J 2000;19:95 [PMID: 10693993].

Dagan R et al: Bacteriologic and clinical efficacy of high-dose amoxicillin/clavulanate (90/6.4 mg/kg/day) in children with acute otitis media, including penicillin-resistant *Streptococcus pneumoniae*. Pediatr Infect Dis J 2001;20:829 [PMID: 11734759].

Dowell SF et al: Acute otitis media: Management and surveillance in an era of pneumococcal resistance—A report from the Drug-Resistant *Streptococcus pneumoniae* Therapeutic Working Group. Pediatr Infect Dis J 1999;18:1 [PMID: 9951971].

Heikkinen T et al: Prevalence of various respiratory viruses in the middle ear during acute otitis media. N Engl J Med 1999; 340:260 [PMID: 9920949].

Johnson CE, Belman S: The role of antibiotic therapy of acute otitis media in promoting drug resistance. Paediatr Drugs 2001; 3:639 [PMID: 11688595].

Klein JO et al:. Otitis media: A preventable disease? Proceedings of an International Symposium organized by the Marcel Merieux Foundation, Veyrier-du-Lac, France, February 13–16, 2000. Pediatr Infect Dis J 2001;20:473 [PMID: 11368103].

Leibovitz E, Dagan R: Otitis media therapy and drug resistance—Part 1: Management principles. Infect Med 2001;18:212.

Rosenfeld RM: Surgical prevention of otitis media. Vaccine 2000 (Suppl 1);S134 [PMID: 11163477].

Schrag SJ et al: Effect of short-course, high-dose amoxicillin therapy on resistant pneumococcal carriage: A randomized trial. JAMA 2001;286:49 [PMID: 11434826].

Shriberg LD et al: Otitis media, fluctuant hearing loss, and speech language outcomes: A preliminary structural equation model. J Speech Lang Hear Res 2000;43:100 [PMID: 10668655].

Takata GS et al: Evidence assessment of management of acute otitis media. Pediatrics 2001;108:239 [PMID: 11483783].

### Websites

American Academy of Pediatrics (www.aap.org/otitismedia/www/). This is a website on diagnosis and treatment of acute otitis media, written for the American Academy of Pediatrics. It features video clips of tympanic membranes being insufflated, to help clinicians learn normal landmarks and pathologic states. It is designed for all learners in medicine or nursing.

Centers for Disease Control: Appropriate Antibiotic Use (www.cdc.gov/antibiotresistance/files). This is a Centers for Disease Control and Prevention site with excellent advice for clinicians on (1) distinguishing OME from AOM, (2) careful antibiotic use for respiratory infections, and (3) patient education material on these two topics.

(www.resistanceimpactondemand.com). This site contains three lectures on treatment of otitis media, study design pitfalls, and pneumococcal drug resistance. Audio and video of the speakers accompanies each slide.

(www.pedisurg.com/pteducent/otitis_media.htm). Information for parents on AOM and PE tubes, with graphics.

The Ear Treatment Group at the University of Texas Medical Branch (www.atc.utmb.edu/aom/home.htm). This is an interactive site for medical students, residents, and physicians to learn about otitis media and to test their knowledge. The site contains links to other otitis-media-related resources as well as parent educational material.

## Management of Otitis Media with Residual and Persistent Effusions

OME has been treated primarily to avoid any prolonged conductive hearing loss. Available data show a causal relationship between severe sensorineural hearing loss and language delay, but not between conductive hearing loss due to OME and language delay. Studies looking at middle ear effusion (MEE) and its effects of language development do not show differences at age 3. But auditory processing disorders are not testable until age 5–7 years, so final results of these studies are still pending. Two thirds of children with AOM have an MEE or high negative middle ear pressure 2 weeks after diagnosis and one third at 1 month after diagnosis regardless of antibiotic therapy. The management options for otitis media with residual effusion at 6 weeks to 4 months include observation and corticosteroid therapy. Corticosteroid (prednisone, 1 mg/kg/d) can be administered for 7 days. Unvaccinated children with no clear history of varicella infection who have been exposed in the preceding month should not receive prednisone because of the potential risk of disseminated varicella-zoster viral disease. Short courses of prednisone increase appetite and cause fluid retention, occasional vomiting, and, rarely, marked behavioral changes.

If the patient clears the persistent MEE unilaterally or bilaterally, the physician should follow the patient monthly. Because of the increase in antibiotic resistance, the use of prophylaxis, even intermittently, must be restricted to carefully selected patients. The guideline recommendation developed by the Agency for Health Care Policy and Research for the management of OME is that ventilating tubes should be placed after the effusion has persisted for 4 months and is accompanied by a bilateral hearing impairment of 20 dB or greater. Earlier placement of ventilating tubes should depend on the child's developmental and behavioral status as well as on parental preference. The value of ventilating tubes for treating unilateral effusions in otherwise healthy children is unclear.

Children with otitis media and persistent effusion have an increased incidence of cholesteatoma, adhesive otitis, retraction pockets, membrane atrophy, and persistent membrane perforation. As there is no way to identify the small proportion of candidate children for whom insertion of ventilating tubes will prevent the damage, close follow-up of abnormal ears may be best accomplished by an otolaryngologist.

Berman S: Management of otitis media and functional outcomes related to language, behavior, and attention: Is it time to change our approach? Pediatrics 2001;107:1175 [PMID: 11331703].

Paradise JL et al: Effect of early or delayed insertion of tympanostomy tubes for persistent otitis media on developmental outcomes at the age of three years. N Engl J Med 2001;344: 1179 [PMID: 11309632].

Paradise JL et al: Language, speech sound production, and cognition in three-year-old children in relation to otitis media in their first three years of life. Pediatrics 2000;105:1119 [PMID: 10890473].

### 3. Mastoiditis

Mastoiditis is a spectrum of disease that ranges from inflammation of the mastoid periosteum to bony destruction of the mastoid air system (coalescent mastoiditis) or abscess development. Infection of the periosteum of the mastoid bone is a rare complication of AOM in the postantibiotic era. Mastoiditis can occur in any age group, but more than 60% of the patients are younger than age 2 years. The most common pathogens are *Streptococcus pneumonia* and *S pyogenes,* with *Staphylococcus aureus* and *H influenzae* occasionally seen. Rarely gram-negative bacilli and anaerobes are isolated. Antibiotics may affect the incidence and morbidity of acute mastoiditis. In the Netherlands, where only 31% of AOM patients receive antibiotics, the incidence of acute mastoiditis is 4.2 per 100,000 people-years. In the United States, where more than 96% of patients with AOM receive antibiotics, the incidence of acute mastoiditis is 2 per 100,000 people-years. The higher antibiotic usage in the United States correlates with a higher rate of resistant organisms and more adverse drug interactions. Moreover, despite the routine use of antibiotics, the incidence of acute mastoiditis has been rising in some cities. The pattern change may be secondary to the emergence of resistant *S pneumoniae.*

### Clinical Findings

The principal complaints of patients with mastoiditis are usually postauricular pain, fever, and outwardly dis-

placed pinna. On examination, the mastoid area often appears swollen and reddened. In the late stage, it may be fluctuant. The earliest finding is severe tenderness on mastoid palpation.

AOM, by otoscopy, is almost always present. Late findings are a pinna that is pushed forward by postauricular swelling and an ear canal that is narrowed in the posterosuperior wall because of pressure from the mastoid abscess. In infants younger than age 1 year, the swelling occurs superior to the ear and pushes the pinna downward rather than outward. In the acute phase, diffuse inflammatory clouding of the mastoid cells occurs, as in every case of AOM. In more severe cases, bony destruction and resorption of the mastoid air cells may occur. The best way to determine the extent of disease is by computed tomography (CT) scan.

Meningitis is a complication of acute mastoiditis and should be suspected when a child has associated high fever, stiff neck, severe headache, or other meningeal signs. Lumbar puncture should be performed for diagnosis. Brain abscess occurs in 2% of patients and may be associated with persistent headaches, recurring fever, or changes in sensorium. Facial palsy, cavernous sinus thrombosis, and thrombophlebitis may be encountered.

Treatment for noncoalescent mastoiditis is typically myringotomy, with or without tube placement, in order to obtain material for culture. Hospitalization for intravenous therapy follows. Reasonable initial therapy is ceftriaxone plus nafcillin or clindamycin until culture results are returned. If clinical improvement does not occur after 24–48 hours of intravenous or intramuscular therapy, or if any signs or symptoms of intracranial complications exist, immediate surgery to drain the mastoid abscess is indicated. The primary management for coalescent mastoiditis is cortical mastoidectomy. A recent review from the University of Texas–Southwestern revealed that 39% of patients required a mastoidectomy. After significant clinical improvement is achieved with parenteral therapy, oral antibiotics are begun and should be continued for 3 weeks.

### 4. Otitis Media with Complications

Complications of otitis media may involve damage to the middle ear structures, such as tympanosclerosis, retraction pockets, adhesions, ossicular erosion, cholesteatoma, perforations, and intratemporal and intracranial injury.

#### A. TYMPANOSCLEROSIS

A white plaque-like appearance on the TM is caused by chronic inflammation or trauma that produces granulation tissue and hyalinization. The appearance of a small defect in the posterosuperior area of the pars tensa or in the pars flaccida suggests a retraction pocket. Retraction pockets occur when chronic inflammation and negative pressure in the middle ear space produce atrophy and atelectasis of the TM.

Continued inflammation can cause adhesions between the retraction pocket and the ossicles. This condition, referred to as adhesive otitis, predisposes to formation of a cholesteatoma or fixation and erosion of the ossicles (Figure 17–5). Erosion of the ossicles results from osteitis and compromise of the blood supply. Ossicular discontinuity may produce a maximal hearing loss with a 50-dB threshold. A tympanogram with very high compliance suggests ossicular discontinuity.

## B. Cholesteatoma

A greasy-looking mass or pearly white debris seen in a retraction pocket or perforation suggests a cholesteatoma, whether or not there is discharge (see Figure 17–5). A perforation is usually painless. If infection is absent, the middle ear cavity generally contains normal mucosa. If infection is superimposed, serous or purulent drainage will be seen, and the middle ear cavity may contain granulation tissue or even polyps. Persistent or recurrent otorrhea following appropriate medical management should make one suspect a cholesteatoma.

## C. Tympanic Membrane Perforation

Occasionally, an episode of AOM is associated with otorrhea. An aural discharge indicates that the TM has perforated. Most likely the perforation will heal spontaneously. If the perforation has not healed within 3 months, surgical intervention will be necessary. A

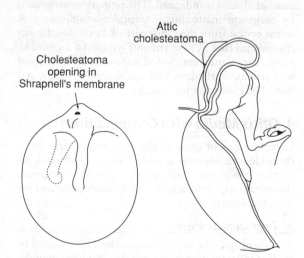

**Figure 17–5.** Attic cholesteatoma, formed from an indrawing of an attic retraction pocket.

Attic cholesteatoma

Cholesteatoma opening in Shrapnell's membrane

conductive hearing loss is usually present, depending on the size and location of the perforation. The site of perforation is important. Central perforations surrounded by intact TM are usually relatively safe from chloesteatoma formation. With a peripheral perforation, especially in the pars flaccida, the perforation extends to the canal wall without any intervening TM. Peripheral perforations create a risk for cholesteatoma because the ear canal epithelium may invade the perforation.

Most perforations with AOM heal within 2 weeks. When perforations fail to heal after 3–6 months, surgical repair may be needed. Repair of the defect in the TM is generally delayed until the child is older and eustachian tube function has improved. Procedures include paper patch, fat myringoplasty, and tympanoplasty. Tympanoplasty is generally deferred until age 7–9 years. In otherwise healthy children without any craniofacial anomalies, some surgeons repair the perforated TM earlier if the contralateral nonperforated drum remains free of infection and effusion for 1 year. This policy does not guarantee success. The age of the child when repair is performed is the more probable indicator of success. Occasionally, a perforation is closed in a child of younger age if recurrent otorrhea is thought to be secondary to water contamination or nasopharyngeal reflux. Earlier closure of the perforation will seal the middle ear space and reestablish the air cushion provided by the mastoid air system. An older child is more likely to have a successful outcome from closure of the perforation. Water activities should be limited to surface swimming, preferably with the use of an ear mold. Diving, jumping into the water, and underwater swimming should be prohibited.

## D. Facial Nerve Paralysis

The facial nerve crosses the middle ear as it courses through the temporal bone to its exit at the stylomastoid foramen. Occasionally, the nerve is incompletely encased in bone, which makes it susceptible to inflammation during an episode of AOM. The acute onset of a facial nerve paralysis is not idiopathic Bell palsy until all other causes have been excluded. If middle ear fluid is present, a prompt myringotomy is indicated. Placement of a ventilation tube will allow for prolonged ventilation. CT is indicated if a cholesteatoma is suspected or acute coalescent mastoiditis is present.

## E. Chronic Suppurative Otitis Media

Chronic suppurative otitis media is present when persistent otorrhea occurs in a child with tympanostomy tubes or TM perforations. Occasionally, it is an accompanying sign of cholesteatoma. Visualization of the TM, meticulous cleaning with culture of the drainage, and appropriate antimicrobial therapy are keys to management of cases not related to cholesteatoma. The successful treatment of chronic suppurative otitis usually requires therapy with an antibiotic that covers *Pseudomonas* and anaerobes. Oral quinolone antibiotics effective against *Pseudomonas* infection are not yet approved for use in growing children. Recent studies suggest that topical quinolones for 14 days may be effective. It is very important to clean the ear canal by suction to allow penetration of drops, and it is often useful to culture the secretions. An ear wick should be inserted and drops placed on the wick several times daily. The child should be seen in 7 days, the wick removed, and suction repeated if necessary. When a cholesteatoma is associated with chronic suppurative otitis media, medical therapy is not effective (see Figure 17–5). If the discharge does not respond to 2 weeks of aggressive therapy, mastoiditis, cholesteatoma, tuberculosis, or fungal infection should be suspected. Serious central nervous system (CNS) complications such as extradural abscess, subdural abscess, brain abscess, meningitis, labyrinthitis, or lateral sinus thrombophlebitis can occur with extension of this process. Therefore, patients with facial palsy, vertigo, or other CNS signs should be immediately referred to an otolaryngologist.

Bluestone CD: Clinical course, complications and sequelae of acute otitis media. Pediatr Infect Dis J 2000;19:S37 [PMID: 10821471].

Ghaffar FA et al: Acute mastoiditis in children: A seventeen-year experience in Dallas, Texas. Pediatr Infect Dis J 2001;20: 376 [PMID: 11332661].

Spratley J et al: Acute mastoiditis in children: Review of the current status. Int J Pediatr Otorhinolaryngol 2000;56:33 [PMID: 11074113].

Van Zuijlen DA et al: National differences in incidence of acute mastoiditis: Relationship to prescribing patterns of antibiotics for acute otitis media? Pediatr Infect Dis J 2001;20:140 [PMID: 11224830].

Zapalac JS et al: Suppurative complications of acute otitis media in the era of antibiotic resistance. Arch Otolaryngol Head Neck Surg 2002;128(6):660 [PMID: 12049560].

**Website**

(www.entnet.org). This is the official website of the American Academy of Otolarngology and Head and Neck Surgery. The site contains patient information, clinical indications for common surgical procedures, and links to other ENT sites.

## ACUTE TRAUMA TO THE MIDDLE EAR

Head injuries, a blow to the ear canal, sudden impact with water, blast injuries, or the insertion of pointed instruments into the ear canal can lead to perforation of the TM or hematoma of the middle ear. One study reported that 50% of serious penetrating wounds of the TM were due to parental use of a cotton-tipped swab.

Treatment of middle ear hematomas consists mainly of watchful waiting. Antibiotics are not necessary unless signs of infection appear. The prognosis for unimpaired hearing depends on whether the ossicles are dislocated or fractured in the process. The patient needs to be followed with audiometry until hearing has returned to normal.

Traumatic perforations of the TM often do not heal spontaneously, in which case the patient should be referred to an otolaryngologist. Perforations caused by a foreign body must be attended to immediately, especially if accompanied by vertigo.

## EAR CANAL FOREIGN BODY

Numerous objects can be inserted into the ear canal by a child. If the object is large, wedged into place, or difficult to remove with available instruments, the patient should be referred to an otolaryngologist early rather than risk traumatizing the ear canal and causing edema that will require removal under anesthesia. An emergency condition exists if the foreign body is a disk-type battery used in clocks, watches, and hearing aids. An electric current is generated in the moist canal, and a severe burn with resulting scarring can occur in less than 4 hours.

## HEMATOMA OF THE PINNA

Trauma to the ear can result in a hematoma between the perichondrium and cartilage. The hematoma appears as a boggy purple swelling of the upper half of the ear. If this is not treated, it can cause pressure necrosis of the underlying cartilage and result in "cauliflower ear." To prevent this cosmetic deformity, physicians should refer patients to an otolaryngologist for aspiration and application of a carefully molded pressure dressing. Recurrent or persistent hematoma of the ear may require surgical drainage.

## CONGENITAL EAR MALFORMATIONS

Agenesis of the external ear canal results in conductive hearing loss that requires evaluation in the first month of life by hearing specialists and an otolaryngologist.

"Lop ears," folded down or protruding ears (so-called Dumbo ears), are a source of much teasing and ridicule. In the past, surgical correction at age 5 or 6 years was the only answer. Taping the ears into a correct anatomic position is very effective if performed in the first 72–96 hours of life. Tape is applied over a molding of wax and continued for 2 weeks. Another alternative for the ear that can be molded solely by finger pressure into a normal configuration is an incisionless otoplasty, which can be performed at a much earlier age and is associated with little postoperative morbidity. Because no cartilage destruction is associated with this technique, future growth is unaffected.

An ear is low-set if the upper pole is below eye level. This condition is often associated with renal malformations (eg, Potter syndrome), and renal ultrasound examination is suggested.

Preauricular tags, ectopic cartilage, fistulas, sinuses, and cysts require surgical correction, mainly for cosmetic reasons. Children exhibiting any of these findings should have their hearing tested. Most preauricular pits cause no symptoms. If one should become infected, the patient should receive antibiotic therapy and be referred to an otolaryngologist for eventual excision.

Fritsch MH: Incisionless otoplasty. Laryngoscope 1995;105 (5 pt 3 Suppl 70) (entire issue) [PMID: 7760682].

Yotsuyanagi T et al: Nonsurgical treatment of various auricular deformities. Clin Plast Surg 2002;29(2):327 [PMID: 12120687].

## DETECTION & MANAGEMENT OF HEARING DEFICITS

Hearing deficits are classified as conductive, sensorineural, or mixed. Conductive hearing loss results from blockage of the transmission of sound waves from the external auditory canal to the inner ear and is characterized by normal bone conduction and reduced air conduction hearing. In children, conductive losses are most often caused by MEE. Sensorineural hearing loss occurs when the auditory nerve or cochlear hair cells are damaged. Mixed hearing loss is characterized by components of both conductive and sensorineural loss. The criteria for children are more stringent than for adults because children are in the process of learning language. In children, a hearing loss of 15–30 dB is considered mild, 31–50 dB moderate, 51–80 dB severe, and 81–100 dB profound.

### Conductive Hearing Loss

By far the most important cause of conductive hearing loss during childhood is otitis media and its sequelae such as MEE. Other causes include atresia, stenosis, or collapse of the ear canal; furuncle, cerumen, or foreign body in the ear; aural discharge; bony growths; otitis externa; perichondritis; and middle ear anomalies (eg, stapes fixation, ossicular malformation).

The average hearing loss due to MEE (whether serous, purulent, or mucoid) is 27–31 dB, the equivalent of a mild hearing loss. This loss may be intermittent in nature and may occur in one or both ears.

The American Academy of Pediatrics recommends that hearing be assessed and language skills monitored in children who have frequently recurring AOM or MEE persisting longer than 3 months. The effects of hearing loss may be insidious and not discernible until the explosive phase of expressive language development occurs between ages 16 and 24 months; therefore, the optimal time for screening language in young children is between 18 and 24 months. An acceptable tool for language screening at this time is the Early Language Milestone Scale. Children age 3, 4, and 5 years with recurring OME should also be screened for language delays.

To diminish the likelihood of communication disorder, the physician should inform the parents of a child with middle ear disease that the child's hearing may not be normal and should instruct the parents to (1) turn off sources of background noise (eg, televisions, radios, dishwashers) when speaking to the child, (2) focus on the child's face and gain his or her direct attention before speaking, (3) speak slightly louder than usual, and (4) have the teacher place the child in the front of the classroom.

### Sensorineural Hearing Loss

Sensorineural hearing loss arises from a lesion in the cochlear structures of the inner ear or in the neural fibers of the auditory nerve (cranial nerve VIII). Most sensorineural losses in children are congenital, with an estimated incidence of 2.0–3.0 per 1000 live births. Causes can be classified as either congenital or postnatal and, within each classification, as genetic or nongenetic. Approximately two thirds of genetic hearing loss is autosomal recessive and is not associated with a known syndrome. Mutations in the Connexin 26 (*Cx26*) gene have been found to account for approximately 20% of all childhood deafness. In older children, one should suspect congenital hearing loss if the hearing is normal in the low and high frequencies, but poor in the middle frequencies ("cookie bite" or U-shaped audiogram). Clues that a patient may have a syndrome associated with the hearing loss and should be referred to a geneticist include the following physical exam findings: asymmetrical face, skin tags, abnormal eye exam, widely spaced eyes, preauricular pits, abnormal ear appearance, café au lait spots, white forelock, sinus tracts in the neck, abnormal digits, and thyromegaly. One should consider screening of first-degree relatives if idiopathic sensorineural hearing loss is present. If a first-degree relative also has a sensorineural loss, the hearing loss is most likely genetic.

A common congenital genetic cause is inner ear dysplasia. Postnatal onset of sensorineural hearing loss often occurs with associated genetic abnormalities (eg,

Alport syndrome and Klippel–Feil syndrome). Nongenetic causes of congenital hearing loss include prenatal infections, teratogenic drugs, and perinatal injuries. Congenital syphilis is responsible for delayed-onset sensorineural hearing loss (usually after age 2 years). Common postnatal nongenetic causes are infections, trauma, ototoxic drugs, metabolic disorders, neoplastic diseases, and autoimmune diseases. A major factor in hearing loss in premature infants is hypoxia. A difficult delivery or an Apgar score of 6 or less is associated with an increased risk of hearing loss. Neonates with a history of persistent pulmonary hypertension or children who have been on ECMO are at an increased risk for late-onset hearing loss and should be followed closely. Before the introduction of *H influenzae* type B vaccine, meningitis was the most common cause of acquired hearing loss, with deafness occurring in about 10% of children who had bacterial meningitis. Pneumococcal and other bacterial meningitides still remain an indication to screen for hearing loss.

In the past, the effect of unilateral deafness on school performance was thought to be insignificant. Studies now show that more than one third of affected children fail one or more grades in school. Therefore, merely recommending preferential classroom seating for these children is no longer sufficient; they should be referred for full evaluation of their hearing needs.

Acquisition of language skills is affected more severely by bilateral than by unilateral sensorineural hearing loss. The earlier the hearing loss occurs, the graver the consequences for language development; thus, the earlier a sensorineural loss is detected and treated (by sound amplification and language habilitation), the better the chances of a good outcome. The mild, fluctuating hearing loss associated with OME is much less likely to cause language problems, presumably because it is intermittent and may often be unilateral. (See Otitis Media with Effusion section.)

## Screening for Hearing Deficits

Screening procedures are established for early detection and diagnosis of hearing deficits. Infants at high risk for hearing loss are best tested by auditory brainstem response (ABR) screening or evoked otoacoustic emission (OAE) testing, preferably before discharge from the hospital. Many states now mandate universal newborn hearing screening by physiologic test procedures. All universal newborn hearing screening programs are using either ABR or OAE as the screening test. The procedures listed in the following sections are intended to serve as a guide, and confirmation of sensorineural hearing loss is dependent on audiologic testing.

### A. Screening of Newborns (See Chapter 1.)

### B. Screening of Infants

Hearing screening for infants (29 days to 2 years) is recommended if one of the following risk criteria is identified: (1) concerns regarding hearing, speech, language, or developmental delay; (2) bacterial meningitis; (3) neonatal risk factors (see Chapter 1); (4) head trauma; (5) ototoxic drug use; (6) neurodegenerative disorders; and (7) childhood infectious diseases (eg, mumps, measles).

In the past, the parents' report of their infant's behavior was considered an adequate assessment of hearing. However, a deaf infant's behavior can appear normal and mislead the parents as well as the professional, especially if the infant has autosomal recessive deafness and is the firstborn child of carrier parents. The following office screening techniques should identify gross hearing losses but may not detect less severe losses due to otitis media:

**1. Birth to 4 months**—In response to a sudden loud sound (70 dB or more) produced by a horn, clacker, or special electronic device, the infant should show a startle reflex or blink the eyes.

**2. 4 months to 2 years**—While the infant is distracted with a toy or bright object, a noisemaker is sounded softly outside the field of vision at the child's waist level. Normal responses are as follows: at 4 months, there is widening of the eyes, interruption of other activity, and perhaps a slight turning of the head in the direction of the sound; at 6 months, the head turns toward the sound; at 9 months or older, the child is usually able to locate a sound originating from below as well as turn to the appropriate side; after 1 year, the child is able to locate sound whether it comes from below or above.

After responses to soft sounds are noted, a loud horn or clacker should be used to produce an eye blink or startle reflex. This latter maneuver is necessary because deaf children are often visually alert and able to scan the environment so actively that their scanning can be mistaken for an appropriate response to the softer noise test. A deaf child will not blink in response to the loud sound. Consonant sounds such as "mama," "dada," and "baba" should be present in speech by age 11 months. Children who fail to respond appropriately should be referred for audiologic assessment.

### C. Screening of Older Children

When children reach age 3 years, their hearing can be tested by earphones and pure tone audiometry. The test frequencies for screening are 1000 Hz, 2000 Hz, and 4000 Hz, with the same tone presented at each frequency. Normally, the screening level is 20 dB. If a soundproof room is not available, the screening may be done at 25 dB. If the child does not respond at any one of the test frequencies in either ear, the test should be repeated within 1 week. Failure on rescreening requires referral for audiologic evaluation.

High-risk categories in older children include those with osteogenesis imperfecta and conditions associated with deafness, such as Waardenburg, Hurler, Alport, Treacher Collins, Klippel–Feil, and fetal alcohol syndromes. Children with these disorders should always receive audiologic evaluation. In addition, before any child is labeled as having mental retardation, autism, or severe behavior problems, the adequacy of the child's hearing must be determined. If a developmental speech delay is diagnosed, the child's hearing should be tested as the first step in evaluating the language problem.

## Referral

In addition to the referrals for audiologic testing mentioned in the preceding section, a child with confirmed hearing loss should be referred to an otolaryngologist for evaluation and further treatment. Any child failing the language screen should be referred to a speech pathologist for language evaluation. Home language enrichment programs for children with mild language delays can be directed by the physician or by a speech pathologist. Programs for the deaf child vary from aural to total communication; the latter includes elements of aural programs plus signing. Each program should be scrutinized thoroughly for its relevance to the deaf child's age and hearing level.

## Prevention

Appropriate care may treat or prevent conditions causing hearing deficits. Aminoglycosides and diuretics, especially in combination, are potentially ototoxic and should be used judiciously and monitored carefully, especially in premature infants and in patients with renal insufficiency. Reduction of repeated exposure to loud noise in the child's environment—loud music, firecrackers, or shots from guns or cap pistols—may help prevent high-frequency hearing losses.

Avraham KB: Inherited connexin mutations associated with hearing loss. Cell Commun Adhes 2001;8(4–6):419 [PMID: 12064629]

Downs MP, Yoshinaga-Itano C: The efficacy of early identification and intervention for children with hearing impairment. Pediatr Clin North Am 1999;46:79 [PMID: 10079791].

Grundfast KM et al: Genetics and molecular biology of deafness. Update. Otolaryngol Clin North Am 2000;33:1367 [PMID: 11449793].

# ■ II. THE NOSE & PARANASAL SINUSES

## ACUTE VIRAL RHINITIS (Common Cold; see also Chapter 36.)

The common cold is the most common pediatric infectious disease, and the incidence is higher in early childhood than in any other period of life. Children younger than age 5 years have 6–12 colds per year, of which 30% are caused by rhinoviruses, 15% influenza or parainfluenza, 10% coronavirus, and 5% enterovirus.

## Clinical Findings

The patient usually experiences a sudden onset of clear or mucoid rhinorrhea, nasal congestion, and fever. Mild sore throat and cough may develop. Although the fever is usually low grade in older children, in the first 5 or 6 years of life it can be as high as 40.6°C without superinfection. The nose, throat, and TM can appear red and inflamed. Figure 17–6 shows the duration of cough, sore throat, and rhinorrhea in adults with rhinovirus-proven infections. Note that one quarter are still symptomatic at 14 days, although they may be improving.

## Treatment

An algorithm for the management of acute nasal congestion and sinusitis is presented in Figure 17–7. Treatment for the common cold should be purely symptomatic; however, a recent study showed that 44% of children younger than age 18 years seen by physicians were given an antibiotic prescription. Acetaminophen or ibuprofen is helpful for fever, sore throat, or muscle aches. A stuffy, congested nose can be treated with normal saline nose drops (mix ½ tsp table salt with 6 oz of water), 3 drops in each nostril. After several minutes, a suction bulb can be used to remove the secretions if the infant is unable to blow his or her nose. If this procedure fails after several attempts and the stuffy nose still interferes with feeding or sleep, consider long-acting xylometazoline or oxymetazoline 0.05% nose drops twice daily. Drops should be used only when the nose is congested and discontinued within 4 days to prevent rebound chemical rhinitis.

Antihistamines are not effective in relieving cold symptoms. In rhinoviral colds, increased levels of histamine are not observed. Antibiotics do not prevent superinfection and should not be used. Cough suppression at night is the number one goal of many parents; however, the effectiveness of dextromethorphan is un-

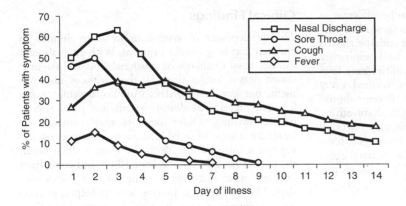

**Figure 17–6.** Duration of symptoms in the common cold in adults. (From Gwaltney JM: JAMA 1967;202:158.)

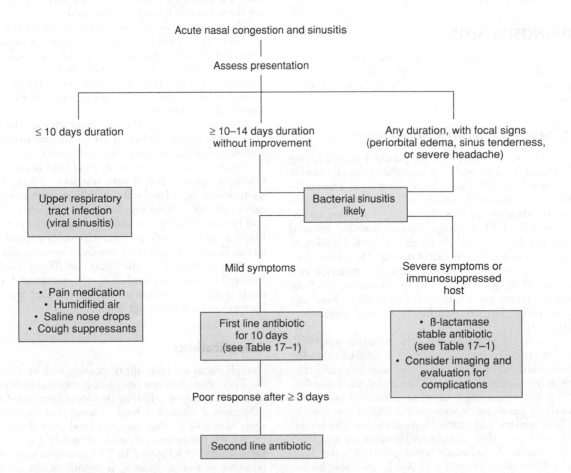

**Figure 17–7.** Algorithm for acute nasal congestion and sinusitis.

clear. It is believed by most experts to be effective in adults and adolescents, but it has not been studied adequately in children with colds. Use of codeine should be discouraged because it has caused fatal respiratory distress. A cool mist vaporizer or humidifier may help the cough, but the device should be washed every 3 days or less, to prevent mold growth. Parents should be instructed that fast breathing or difficult breathing with retraction is a sign of lower respiratory infection such as bronchiolitis or pneumonia. Prolonged fever may indicate otitis media or sinusitis. An antiviral agent called pleconaril is being studied for URIs due to rhinovirus or enterovirus.

Clemens CJ et al: Is an antihistamine-decongestant combination effective in relieving symptoms of the common cold in preschool children? J Pediatr 1997;130:463 [PMID: 9063425].

Nyquist AC et al: Antibiotic prescribing for children with colds, upper respiratory tract infections, and bronchitis. JAMA 1998;279:875 [PMID: 9516004].

## RHINOSINUSITIS

The use of the term *sinusitis* versus *rhinosinusitis* has been debated. Rhinosinusitis implies that the nasal and sinus mucosa are involved in similar and concurrent inflammatory processes.

## 1. Acute Bacterial Rhinosinusitis

Acute bacterial infection of the paranasal sinuses lasting less than 30 days and in which the symptoms resolve completely is called acute bacterial sinusitis. The maxillary and ethmoidal sinuses are most commonly involved when mucociliary clearance and drainage are impaired by a URI or allergic rhinitis. Both the ethmoid and maxillary sinuses are present at birth, forming in the third to fourth gestational month. The sphenoid sinuses pneumatize as an extension of a posterior ethmoid cell by age 5 years, and the frontal sinuses form from an anterior ethmoid cell appearing about age 7–8 years. Frontal sinusitis is unusual before age 10 years.

A combination of anatomic, mucosal, microbial, and immune pathogenic processes is believed to underlie sinusitis in children. Both viral and bacterial infections have integral roles in the pathogenesis of sinusitis. Viral URIs commonly cause sinus mucosal injury and swelling, resulting in osteomeatal obstruction, loss of ciliary activity, and mucous hypersecretion. The bacterial pathogens that cause acute sinusitis are usually *S pneumoniae, H influenzae* (nontypable), *M catarrhalis,* and β-hemolytic streptococci. Rarely, anaerobic bacterial infections can cause fulminant frontal sinusitis.

## Clinical Findings

The development of symptoms in acute sinusitis in children may be gradual or sudden. With gradual-onset disease, nasal discharge or postnasal drip and daytime cough persist longer than 10 days without improvement, but less than 30 days. Additional symptoms: a low-grade fever, malodorous breath, and painless periorbital swelling. Older patients may complain of headache, a sense of facial fullness, or facial pain overlying the involved sinus. With the more sudden onset, the patient has a fever of at least 102°F and concurrent purulent nasal discharge present for 3–4 consecutive days. The physical examination is rarely helpful in making a diagnosis of acute bacterial sinusitis, as the findings will be nearly the same as those in a child with viral rhinosinusitis. Occasionally percussion tenderness overlying the sinus is present, but this is a finding typical only of the older child and is unreliable when compared with antral irrigation results. Transillumination of the sinuses is difficult to perform and not very helpful unless the sinuses are grossly asymmetrical.

The physician should consider sinus aspiration by an otolaryngologist for diagnostic purposes in patients with complications and in immunocompromised patients. Gram stain or culture of nasal discharge does not correlate with cultures of sinus aspirates. If the patient is hospitalized because of complications, a blood culture should be obtained.

Imaging studies of the paranasal sinuses during acute illness are not indicated except for evaluation of complications. In the past, plain radiography was used to diagnose sinusitis when an air–fluid level or mucosal thickening greater than 4 mm was seen. Today, CT scans should be ordered only in children with complications or lack of resolution following adequate antibiotic therapy. Findings consistent with sinusitis may be found in asymptomatic patients with colds or nasal allergies. Because of the lack of specificity between abnormal CTs or plain films, the Sinus and Allergy Health Partnership (see references) does not recommend any imaging study to diagnose uncomplicated cases of acute bacterial sinusitis in any age group.

## Complications

Complications are most apt to develop with ethmoiditis. These complications represent a continuum beginning with preseptal cellulitis, then postseptal cellulitis, subperiosteal abscess, orbital abscess, and cavernous sinus thrombosis. They are associated with decreased extraocular movement, proptosis, chemosis, and altered visual acuity (see Chapter 15). The most common complication of frontal sinusitis is osteitis of the frontal bone (Pott puffy tumor). Intracranial extension leads to meningitis and to epidural, subdural, and brain abscesses. The most common maxillary complication is cellulitis of the cheek. Rarely, osteomyelitis of the maxilla can develop. In a series of children admitted for severe sinusitis, 17% had intracranial abscesses identified on CT scanning. In this and other studies, male adolescents predominated, for unknown reasons. Interestingly, only 1 of 13 children had a history of a previous sinus infection. No information is available on the rate of complications in ambulatory sinusitis patients, but the severity of the complications suggests that the patient should be carefully followed while receiving treatment.

## Treatment

A meta-analysis of five randomized controlled trials suggested a modest benefit of antibiotics in reducing sinus symptoms; however, approximately six children required therapy to achieve one additional cure. Despite limited proof of efficacy, antibiotic treatment is recommended for most children with acute and subacute sinusitis because bacterial pathogens are recoverable from the majority of affected sinuses. Patients with evidence of invasive infection or any CNS complications should be hospitalized immediately. Intravenous therapy with nafcillin or clindamycin plus a third-generation cephalosporin such as cefotaxime should be initiated until culture results become available. For uncomplicated sinus infections, oral antibiotics for 10 days is appropriate. Antibiotic treatment should continue for another week if the patient has improved but is not totally asymptomatic. Amoxicillin at 90 mg/kg/d can be used if the patient is older than 2 years old, not in daycare, has not had recent antibiotic therapy, and has sinusitis that is mild to moderate in severity. The majority of children, therefore, will need to be treated with high-dose amoxicillin–clavulanate ES-600 (amoxicillin, 90 mg/kg/d, and clavulanate, 6.4 mg/kg/d). Alternative therapy (eg, cefdinir, cefuroxime, or cefpodoxime) is recommended for children intolerant of amoxicillin. Resistance to any bacteriostatic antibiotic such as trimethoprim–sulfamethoxazole and erythromycin–sulfisoxazole is great enough that these medications are no longer recommended unless the patient is allergic to both penicillin and cephalosporin. Clindamycin is another possible choice, particularly in older patients, but it is not effective against gram-negative organisms such as H influenzae. Failure to improve after 48 hours suggests a resistant organism or potential complication. [See the section on unresponsive AOM for antibiotic recommendations (Table 17–2), which are also appropriate for sinusitis.]

Topical decongestants and oral combinations are frequently used in acute sinusitis to promote drainage. Their effectiveness has not been proved, and concern has been raised about potential adverse effects related to impaired ciliary function, decreased blood flow to the mucosa, and reduced diffusion of antibiotic into the sinuses. Patients with underlying allergic rhinitis may benefit from intranasal cromolyn or corticosteroid nasal spray. Vasoconstrictor nose drops and spray are associated with rebound edema if used for more than 4 days.

The patient may require acetaminophen, ibuprofen, or even codeine to permit sleep until drainage is achieved. The application of ice over the sinus may help to relieve pain.

Clinical Practice Guideline: Management of sinusitis: American Academy of Pediatrics. Pediatrics 2001;108:798 [PMID: 11533355].

Garbutt JM et al: A randomized, placebo-controlled trial of antimicrobial treatment for children with clinically diagnosed acute sinusitis. Pediatrics 2001;107:619 [PMID: 11335733].

Morris P: Antibiotics for persistent nasal discharge (rhinosinusitis) in children. Cochrane Database Syst Rev 2000;3:CD001094 [PMID: 10908484].

McAlister WH et al: Sinusitis in the pediatric population: American College of Radiology. ACR appropriateness criteria. Radiology 2000;215 (Suppl):811 [PMID: 11037504].

Nash D, Wald E: Sinusitis. Pediatr Rev 2001;22:111 [PMID: 11283323].

Sinus and Allergy Health Partnership: Antimicrobial treatment guidelines for acute bacterial rhinosinusitis. Otolaryngol Head Neck Surg 2004;13:1 [PMID: 14726904].

Sinus and Allergy Health Partnership: Antimicrobial treatment guidelines for acute bacterial rhinosinusitis. Executive summary. Otolaryngol Head Neck Surg 2000;123:1 [PMID: 10887345].

## 2. Recurrent or Chronic Sinusitis

Recurrent acute bacterial sinusitis is now defined as successive episodes of bacterial infections of the sinuses, each lasting less than 30 days and separated by intervals of at least 10 days, during which the patient is asymptomatic. Chronic sinusitis is now defined as episodes of inflammation of the paranasal sinuses lasting more than 90 days. Although recent meta-analysis evaluations have resulted in recommendations for acute sinusitis, there is a paucity of data for the treatment of recurrent or chronic sinusitis. Important factors to consider include allergies, anatomic variations, and disorders in host immunity. Mucosal inflammation leading to obstruction is most commonly caused by allergic rhinitis and occasionally by nonallergic rhinitis. Gastroesophageal reflux has also been found to be associated with chronic sinusitis, and its treatment may result in dramatic improvements in sinus symptoms. Rarely, chronic sinusitis is caused by anatomic variations, such as septal deviation, polyp, or foreign body. Allergic polyps are unusual in children younger than age 10 years and therefore indicate a work-up for cystic fibrosis. In cases of chronic or recurrent pyogenic pansinusitis, poor host resistance (eg, an immune defect, Kartagener syndrome, or cystic fibrosis)—though rare—must be ruled out by immunoglobulin studies, microscopic studies of respiratory cilia, and a sweat chloride test. Anaerobic and staphylococcal organisms are often responsible for chronic sinusitis. Evaluation by an allergist and an otolaryngologist may be useful in determining the underlying causes.

## Medical Treatment

Antibiotic therapy is similar to that used for acute sinusitis, but the duration is longer. Antimicrobial choice should include drugs effective against staphylococcal organisms. Adjuvant therapies such as saline nasal irrigations, decongestants, antihistamines, and topical intranasal steroids may be helpful depending on the underlying cause.

## Surgical Treatment

### A. ANTRAL LAVAGE

Antral lavage, generally regarded as a diagnostic procedure, may have some therapeutic value. An aspirate or a sample irrigated from the maxillary sinus is retrieved either with a spinal needle or a curved-tip instrument under anesthesia. In the very young child, this may be the only procedure that should be performed.

### B. ENDOSCOPIC SINUS SURGERY

No data are available comparing the outcome of this procedure with traditional surgical drainage procedures. There are large variations in the reported uses of this procedure by otolaryngologists, especially in younger patients.

### C. EXTERNAL DRAINAGE

External drainage procedures are reserved for complications arising from ethmoid and frontal sinusitis.

Jailwala JA, Shaker R: Oral and pharyngeal complications of gastroesophageal reflux disease: Globus, dental erosions, and chronic sinusitis. J Clin Gastroenterol 2000;30 (3 Suppl): S35 [PMID: 10777170].

Jiang RS, Hsu CY: Functional endoscopic sinus surgery in children and adults. Ann Otol Rhinol Laryngol 2000;109:1113 [PMID: 11130821].

Nostrant TT, Rabine JC: Diagnosis and management of supraesophageal complications of reflux disease. Curr Gastroenterol Rep 2000;2(3):210 [PMID: 10957932].

Phipps CD et al: Gastroesophageal reflux contributing to chronic sinus disease in children: A prospective analysis. Arch Otolaryngol Head Neck Surg 2000;126:831 [PMID: 10888994].

Suskind DL et al: Gastroesophageal reflux and pediatric otolaryngologic disease: The role of antireflux surgery. Arch Otolaryngol Head Neck Surg 2001;127:511 [PMID: 11346425].

## CHOANAL ATRESIA

Choanal atresia occurs in approximately 1 in 7000 live births. The female-to-male ratio is 2:1, and unilateral to bilateral is also 2:1. Bilateral atresia results in severe respiratory distress at birth and requires immediate placement of an oral airway. Unilateral atresia usually appears later as a unilateral chronic nasal discharge that can be confused with chronic sinusitis. Diagnosis may be suspected if a 6 Fr catheter cannot be passed through the nose and is confirmed by axial CT scan. CHARGE (coloboma, heart disease, atresia chonae, retarded growth and retarded development and/or CNS anomalies, genital hypoplasia, and ear anomalies and/or deafness) association (see Chapter 33) or other congenital anomalies are present in 50% of patients. An oral airway should be used when a newborn has been diagnosed with bilateral choanal atresia until more definitive treatment by an otolaryngologist has been accomplished.

Keller JL, Kacker A: Choanal atresia, CHARGE association, and congenital nasal stenosis. Otolaryngol Clin North Am 2000;33:1343 [PMID: 11449791].

## RECURRENT RHINITIS

Recurrent rhinitis is frequently seen in the office practice of pediatrics. The child is brought in with the chief complaint of having "one cold after another," "constant colds," or "always being sick." Approximately two thirds of these children have recurrent colds, and the remainder have either allergic rhinitis or recurrent sinusitis.

### Allergic Rhinitis

Allergic rhinitis has significant morbidity and may contribute to the development of sinusitis and asthma exacerbations. Symptoms of frequent sneezing, rubbing of the nose, and clear drainage interfere with concentration at school. Nighttime nasal congestion interferes with sleep and causes daytime somnolence and hyperactivity. On physical examination the nasal turbinates are swollen, but may be red or pale pink. Treatment with nasal steroids is effective in decreasing the airway obstruction and rhinorrhea. Sneezing and clear drainage are controlled with nonsedating antihistamines. Ipratropium can be used as an adjunctive therapy.

Pullerits T et al: Comparison of a nasal glucocorticoid, antileukotriene, and a combination of antileukotriene and antihistamine in the treatment of seasonal allergic rhinitis. J Allergy Clin Immunol 2002;109(6):949 [PMID: 12063523].

The allergy report: http://www.aaaai.org/ar/working_vol1/073.asp.

## Vasomotor Rhinitis

Some children react to sudden changes in environmental temperature with prolonged congestion and rhinorrhea. Air pollution (especially tobacco smoke) may be a factor. Oral decongestants or nasal steroids can be used to give symptomatic relief.

## EPISTAXIS

The nose is an extremely vascular structure. In most cases, epistaxis (nosebleed) is due to mild trauma to the anterior portion of the nasal septum (Kiesselbach area), usually due to vigorous nose rubbing, nose blowing, or nose picking. If a patient has been using a nasal steroid spray, check the patient's technique to make sure he or she is directing the nozzle at the lateral canthus of the eye and not the septum. If this does not reduce the nosebleeds, then the steroid spray should be discontinued. Examination of the Kiesselbach area usually reveals a red, raw surface with fresh clots or old crusts. Also look for telangiectasia, hemangiomas, or varicosities.

Less than 5% of epistaxis is caused by a bleeding disorder such as von Willebrand disease. Patients need a hematologic work-up if any of the following is present: a family history of a bleeding disorder; a medical history of easy bleeding, particularly with circumcision or dental extraction; spontaneous bleeding at any site; bleeding that lasts for over 30 minutes or blood that will not clot with direct pressure by the physician; onset before age 2 years; or a drop in hematocrit due to epistaxis. High blood pressure may rarely predispose to prolonged nosebleeds.

A nasopharyngeal angiofibroma may be manifested by recurrent epistaxis. Adolescent boys are affected almost exclusively. CT scan of the nasal cavity and nasopharynx is diagnostic.

## Treatment

The following approach can be carried out in the office or offered as phone advice: The patient should sit up and lean forward so as not to swallow the blood. Swallowed blood may cause nausea, and hematemesis alarms the family. The nasal cavity should be cleared of clots by gentle blowing. The soft part of the nose is pinched firmly enough to prevent arterial blood flow, with pressure over the bleeding site being maintained for 5 minutes by the clock. If bleeding continues, the bleeding site needs to be visualized. A small piece of gelatin sponge (Gelfoam) or collagen sponge (Surgicel) can be inserted over the bleeding site and held in place by the parent.

Friability of the nasal vessels can be decreased with daily application of water-based ointment by cotton-tipped applicator. The lubricant is applied daily until 5 days have passed without a nosebleed, then weekly for 1 month. Twice daily nasal saline irrigation and humidification of the patient's bedroom may also be helpful. Aspirin and ibuprofen should be avoided, as should vigorous blowing of the nose.

## NASAL INFECTION

A nasal furuncle is an infection of a hair follicle in the anterior nares. Hair plucking or nose picking can provide a route of entry. The most common organism is *S aureus.* The diagnosis is made by finding an exquisitely tender, firm, red lump in the anterior nares. Treatment includes dicloxacillin or cephalexin orally for 5 days to prevent spread. The lesion should be gently incised and drained as soon as it points, usually with a needle. Topical bacitracin ointment may be of additional value. Because this lesion is in the drainage area of the cavernous sinus, the patient should be followed closely until healing is complete. Parents should be advised never to pick or squeeze a furuncle in this location—and neither should the physician. Associated cellulitis or spread requires hospitalization for administration of intravenous antibiotics.

A nasal septal abscess usually follows nasal trauma or a nasal furuncle. Examination reveals a fluctuant gray septal swelling, usually bilateral. The possible complications are the same as for nasal septum hematoma (see following discussion). In addition, spread of the infection to the CNS is possible. Treatment consists of immediate hospitalization and incision and drainage by an otolaryngologist.

## NASAL TRAUMA

Newborn infants rarely present with subluxation of the quadrangular cartilage of the septum. In this disorder, the top of the nose deviates to one side, the inferior septal border deviates to the other side, the columella leans, and the nasal tip is unstable. This disorder must be distinguished from the more common transient flattening of the nose caused by the birth process. In the past, physicians were encouraged to reduce all subluxations in the nursery. Otolaryngologists are more likely to perform the reduction under anesthesia for more difficult cases.

Most blows to the nose result in swallowing of blood and hematoma formation without fracture. A persistent nosebleed after trauma, crepitus or instability of the bones in the nasal bridge, and marked deviation of the nose to one side indicate fracture. However, septal injury can be ruled out only by careful intranasal examination, not radiologically. Patients with suspected nasal fractures should be referred to an otolaryngologist for definitive therapy. Resetting of the nasal fracture can be postponed up to 1 week without resulting in permanent deformity.

After nasal trauma, it is essential to examine the inside of the nose with a nasal speculum. Hematoma of the nasal septum imposes a considerable risk of pressure necrosis and resorption of the cartilage, leading to septal perforation or a saddle-back nose in adulthood. This diagnosis is confirmed by the abrupt onset of nasal obstruction following trauma and the presence of a boggy, widened nasal septum. The normal nasal septum is only 2–4 mm thick, and the back end of a cotton swab may be helpful for palpation.

Treatment consists of prompt referral to an otolaryngologist for evacuation of the hematoma and packing of the nose.

## FOREIGN BODIES IN THE NOSE

The most common foreign bodies in the nose are seeds or beads. If the diagnosis is delayed, unilateral rhinorrhea, foul smell, halitosis, bleeding, or nasal obstruction may occur. The leading cause of halitosis in children is a nasal foreign body, and not dental disease as in adults.

There are many ways to remove nasal foreign bodies. The obvious first maneuver is vigorous nose blowing if the child is old enough. The next step in removal requires topical anesthesia, nasal decongestion, good lighting, correct instrumentation, and physical restraint. Topical tetracaine or lidocaine can be used in young children. Nasal decongestion can be achieved by topical pseudoephedrine or oxymetazoline. When the child is properly restrained, most nasal foreign bodies can be removed using a pair of alligator forceps through an operating head otoscope. If the object seems unlikely to be removed on the first attempt, is wedged in, or is quite large, the patient should be referred to an otolaryngologist rather than worsening the situation through futile attempts at removal.

Because the nose is a moist cavity, the electrical current generated by disk-type batteries—such as those used in clocks, watches, and hearing aids—can cause necrosis of mucosa and cartilage destruction in less than 4 hours. This constitutes a true foreign body emergency.

Kelley PE: Foreign bodies in the nose and pharynx. In Burg FD et al (eds): *Gellis and Kagan's Current Pediatric Therapy,* 16th ed. WB Saunders, 1999.

# III. THE THROAT & ORAL CAVITY

## ACUTE STOMATITIS

### Recurrent Aphthous Stomatitis

Also referred to as canker sores, these small ulcers (3–10 mm) are found on the insides of the lips or in the anterior mouth; rarely they may appear on the tonsils or palate. There is usually no associated fever and no cervical adenopathy. The ulcers may be painful and last 1–2 weeks. They may recur numerous times throughout life. The cause is unknown, although an allergic or autoimmune basis is suspected.

Treatment consists of coating the lesions with betamethasone valerate ointment twice daily, because unlike other topical steroids, it adheres to the mucosa. Pain can also be reduced by eating a bland diet, avoiding salty or acidic foods and juices, and giving acetaminophen or ibuprofen at bedtime.

Other less common causes of recurrent aphthous ulcers include Behçet disease, familial Mediterranean fever, and the fever, aphthous stomatitis, pharyngitis, and cervical adenopathy syndrome (FAPA) syndrome. A diagnosis of Behçet disease requires two of the following: genital ulcers, uveitis, and erythema nodosum-like lesions. Patients with Mediterranean fever have a positive family history, serosal involvement, and fever. FAPA syndrome was first described in 1987, and its cause is unknown. It usually begins before a child is 5 years of age and continues through adolescence, then resolves. It recurs at 4- to 6-week intervals, and an episode may be dramatically improved with prednisone bursts, but recurrences continue. In one case report it resolved totally with a 6-month course of cimetidine, suggesting an immune etiology. FAPA may also resolve with tonsillectomy (see Tonsillectomy section), and an otolaryngology referral is appropriate. The ulcers in all of these syndromes respond to betamethasone valerate application.

Dahn KA, Glode MP, Chan KH: Periodic fever and pharyngitis in young children: A new disease for the otolaryngologist? Arch Otolaryngol Head Neck Surg 2000;126:1146 [PMID: 10979131].

### Herpes Simplex Gingivostomatitis (see also Chapter 36)

Children having their first encounter with the herpes simplex virus develop 10 or more small ulcers (1–3 mm) of the buccal mucosa, anterior pillars, inner lips, tongue, and especially the gingiva. The lesions are often associated with fever lasting up to 7 days, tender cervical nodes, and generalized inflammation of the mouth. Affected children are commonly younger than 3 years of age. Gingivostomatitis lasts 7–10 days. Treatment is symptomatic, as described earlier for recurrent aphthous stomatitis, with the exception that corticosteroids are contraindicated because they may cause spread of the infection. If seen early in the course, the physician should prescribe oral acyclovir suspension (200 mg/5 mL), 20 mg/kg/dose, 4 times daily for 5 days. The patient must be followed closely because dehydration occasionally develops, requiring hospitalization. Herpetic laryngotracheitis is a rare complication.

## Thrush (see also Chapter 39)

Oral candidiasis mainly affects infants and occasionally older children in a debilitated state. *Candida albicans* is a saprophyte that normally is not invasive unless the mouth is abraded or the patient is immunocompromised. The use of broad-spectrum antibiotics and systemic or inhaled steroids may be contributing factors. The symptoms include soreness of the mouth and refusal of feedings. Lesions consist of white curd-like plaques predominantly on the buccal mucosa. These plaques cannot be washed away after a water feeding.

Specific treatment consists of nystatin oral suspension, 2 mL four times daily for 1 week, or miconazole gel. Treatment should be preceded by attempts to remove large plaques with a moistened cotton-tipped applicator or piece of gauze, or half the nystatin may be rubbed on the lesions with an applicator. Gentian violet is probably also effective, but stains clothing and skin.

## Traumatic Oral Ulcers

Mechanical trauma most commonly occurs on the buccal mucosa secondary to accidentally biting with the molars. Thermal trauma, from very hot foods, can also cause ulcerative lesions. Chemical ulcers can be produced by mucosal contact with aspirin, caustics, and the like. Oral ulcers can also occur with leukemia or on a recurrent basis with cyclic neutropenia. These lesions usually need no treatment. The pain subsides in 2 or 3 days.

## ACUTE VIRAL PHARYNGITIS & TONSILLITIS

Figure 17–8 is an algorithm for the management of a sore throat.

Over 90% of cases of sore throat and fever in children are due to viral infections. Most children develop associated rhinorrhea and mild cough. The findings seldom give any clue to the particular viral agent, but six types of viral pharyngitis are sufficiently distinctive to support an educated guess about the specific cause (see Chapter 36).

## Clinical Findings

### A. INFECTIOUS MONONUCLEOSIS

The findings are exudative tonsillitis, generalized cervical adenitis, and fever, usually in a patient older than 5 years of age. A palpable spleen or axillary adenopathy increases the likelihood of the diagnosis. The presence of more than 10% atypical lymphocytes on a peripheral blood smear or a positive mononucleosis spot test supports the diagnosis, although these tests are often falsely negative in children younger than age 5 years. Epstein–Barr virus serology showing an elevated IgM-capsid antibody is definitive.

### B. HERPANGINA

Herpangina ulcers, 2–3 mm in size and surrounded by a halo, are found on the anterior pillars, the soft palate, and the uvula. No ulcers are present in the anterior mouth as there are in herpes simplex. Herpangina is caused by several members of the coxsackie A group of viruses, and a patient may have several bouts of herpangina.

### C. LYMPHONODULAR PHARYNGITIS

The classic finding is small, yellow-white nodules in the same distribution as the small ulcers in herpangina. In this condition, which is caused by coxsackievirus A10, the nodules do not ulcerate.

### D. HAND, FOOT, AND MOUTH DISEASE

This entity is caused by coxsackieviruses A5, A9, A10, and A16. Ulcers occur on the tongue and oral mucosa. Vesicles, which usually do not ulcerate, are found on the palms, soles, interdigital areas, and buttocks.

### E. PHARYNGOCONJUNCTIVAL FEVER

This disorder is caused by an adenovirus and often is epidemic. Exudative tonsillitis, conjunctivitis, lymphadenopathy, and fever are the main findings, and treatment is symptomatic.

## ACUTE BACTERIAL PHARYNGITIS

Approximately 10% of children with sore throat and fever have a group A streptococcal infection. Less common causes of bacterial pharyngitis are *Mycoplasma pneumoniae, Chlamydia pneumoniae,* groups C and G streptococci, and *Arcanobacterium hemolyticum.* Of the five, *M pneumoniae* is by far the most common and may cause over one third of all pharyngitis cases in adolescents and adults.

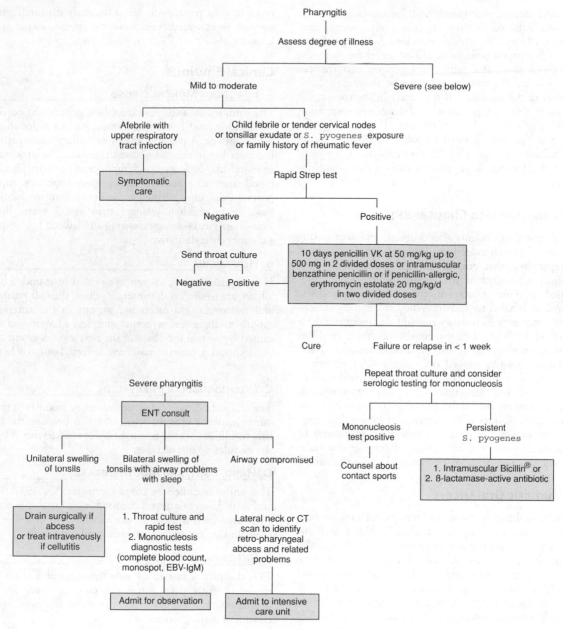

*Figure 17–8.* Algorithm for pharyngitis.

Untreated streptococcal pharyngitis can result in acute rheumatic fever, glomerulonephritis, and suppurative complications (eg, cervical adenitis, peritonsillar abscess, otitis media, cellulitis, and septicemia). Vesicles and ulcers are suggestive of viral infection, whereas tender anterior cervical nodes, petechiae, a beefy-red uvula, and a tonsillar exudate suggest streptococcal infection;

the only way to make a definitive diagnosis is by throat culture or rapid antigen test. Rapid antigen tests are very specific, but have a sensitivity of 85–95%. Therefore, a positive test indicates *S pyogenes* infection, but a negative result requires confirmation with culture.

The physician should treat cases of suspected or proven group A streptococcal infection with a 10-day course of oral penicillin V potassium, a cephalosporin, or intramuscularly injected penicillin G benzathine (Table 17–3). Penicillin VK is equally effective if given in two or three divided doses, except in adolescents, for whom three doses are recommended, but is not effective once daily. Amoxicillin, azithromycin, and cefadroxil may be given once daily. Cephalexin given in four divided doses is inexpensive, but it has never been studied with fewer daily doses. Penicillin-allergic patients should be given erythromycin estolate in two or three divided doses, not the poorly absorbed ethylsuccinate preparation, which causes vomiting and abdominal cramping. The treatment failure rate after 10 days of penicillin VK administered three times daily varies from 6% to 23%. The small differences between the cure rates of penicillin and cephalosporins reported in the literature may represent eradication of the carrier state rather than treatment failure. Causes of treatment failure include unrecognized carriers, poor compliance, acquisition of a different strain, inactivation of penicillin by β-lactamase produced by throat flora, or the development of tolerance by *S pyogenes*. Approximately 5% of *S pyogenes* are resistant to erythromycin. Trimethoprim–sulfamethoxazole is not an effective antibiotic against *S pyogenes*. Children should receive 24 hours of therapy before returning to school.

If the child has a history of recurrent streptococcal infection, the physician should document the absence of *S pyogenes* in an asymptomatic patient following a course of therapy. If compliance or the adequacy of antibiotic dosage was questionable, the infection may be treated with intramuscular penicillin; otherwise, an antibiotic effective against β-lactamase-producing organisms (amoxicillin plus clavulanate, a cephalosporin, or a macrolide) may be used. If this therapy fails to eradicate the organism, a course of clindamycin for 10 days should be considered.

In general, the carrier state is harmless, self-limited (2–6 months), and not contagious. An attempt to eradicate the carrier state is warranted only if the patient or another family member has frequent streptococcal infections or when a family member or patient has a history of rheumatic fever or glomerulonephritis.

Treatment should be considered for carriers who live in closed or semiclosed community settings. If the patient has had three or more documented infections within 6 months, daily penicillin prophylaxis may be given during the winter season. Patients may be referred for tonsillectomy if they continue to have frequent episodes or if persistently enlarged tonsils cause chronic upper airway obstruction. "Frequent" is defined as seven episodes in 1 year, five per year for 2 years, or three per year for 3 years.

**Table 17–3.** Treatment of group A streptococcal pharyngitis.

| Drug | Dosage | Maximum Adult Dose | Formulations | Comments |
|---|---|---|---|---|
| Penicillin VK | 250 mg bid for 10 days, 500 mg bid or tid for adolescents & adults | 1000 mg | 250 mg/tsp; 250 mg tablets and 500 mg tablets | Preferred by American Heart Association (AHA) |
| Amoxicillin[a] | 750 mg once daily for 10 days in patients older than age 3 years | 750 mg | 250 mg/tsp; 250 mg tablets | For poorly compliant patients |
| IM Benzathine penicillin | If < 27 kg, 600,000 U; if > 27 kg, 1.2 million U | | | If preferred by parent. AHA endorsed |
| **For penicillin-allergic patients** | | | | |
| Erythromycin estolate (250/5) | 20 mg/kg bid for 10 days | 250 mg bid | 250 mg/tsp; 250 mg tablets | Preferred by AHA |
| Zithromax | 12 mg/kg/d for 5 days (not the otitis media dose) | 500 mg on day 1 and 250 mg for 4 days more | 15 ml of 100/5 mL; 15 ml of 200/5 mL; 30 ml of 200/5 mL | Expensive. For poorly compliant patients |
| First-generation cephalosporins | Varies with agent | | | These agents should not be used to treat patients with immediate-type hypersensitivity to β-lactam antibiotics |

[a]Preferred by some doctors for younger children because of taste.

Bisno AL et al: Practice guidelines for the diagnosis and management of group A Streptococcal pharyngitis. Clin Infect Dis 2002;35:113 [PMID: 12087516].

Lan AJ, Colford JM: The impact of dosing frequency on the efficacy of 10-day penicillin or amoxicillin therapy for Streptococcal tonsillopharyngitis: A meta-analysis. Pediatrics electronic pages 2000;105:e19 [PMID: 10654979].

## PERITONSILLAR CELLULITIS OR ABSCESS (QUINSY)

Tonsillar infection occasionally penetrates the tonsillar capsule, spreads to the surrounding tissues, and causes peritonsillar cellulitis. If untreated, necrosis occurs and a tonsillar abscess forms. This can occur at any age. The most common cause is β-hemolytic streptococcal infection. Other pathogens are group D streptococci, β-hemolytic streptococci, *S pneumoniae,* and anaerobes.

The patient complains of a severe sore throat even before the physical findings become marked. A high fever is usually present, and the process is almost always unilateral. The tonsil bulges medially, and the anterior tonsillar pillar is prominent. The soft palate and uvula on the involved side are edematous and displaced toward the uninvolved side. In cases of abscess formation, trismus, ear pain, dysphagia, and, eventually, drooling occur. The most serious complication of inadequately treated peritonsillar abscess is a lateral pharyngeal abscess. This causes fullness and tenderness of the lateral neck as well as torticollis. Without intervention, the lateral pharyngeal abscess threatens life by airway obstruction or carotid artery erosion. If airway symptoms are present, an immediate otolaryngology consultation is indicated.

It is often difficult to differentiate peritonsillar cellulitis from abscess. In some children, it is possible to aspirate the peritonsillar space to diagnose and treat an abscess. However, it is reasonable to admit a child for 12–24 hours of intravenous antimicrobial therapy, because aggressive treatment in early cases of peritonsillar cellulitis usually prevents suppuration. Therapy with penicillin or clindamycin is appropriate. Failure to respond to therapy during the first 12–24 hours indicates a high probability of abscess formation. An otolaryngologist should be consulted for incision and drainage or for aspiration under local anesthesia.

Recurrent peritonsillar abscesses are so uncommon (7%) that routine tonsillectomy for a single bout is not indicated unless other tonsillectomy indications exist. Hospitalized patients can be discharged on oral antibiotics when fever has resolved for 24 hours and dysphagia has improved.

Herzon FS, Nicklaus P: Pediatric peritonsillar abscess: Management guidelines. Curr Probl Pediatr 1996;26:270 [PMID: 8899288].

## RETROPHARYNGEAL ABSCESS

Retropharyngeal nodes drain the adenoids, nasopharynx, and paranasal sinuses and can become infected. The most common causes are β-hemolytic streptococci and *S aureus.* If this pyogenic adenitis goes untreated, a retropharyngeal abscess forms. The process occurs most commonly during the first 2 years of life. Beyond this age, retropharyngeal abscess usually results from superinfection of a penetrating injury of the posterior wall of the oropharynx.

The diagnosis of retropharyngeal abscess should be strongly suspected in an infant with fever, respiratory symptoms, and neck hyperextension. Dysphagia, drooling, dyspnea, and gurgling respirations are also found and are due to impingement by the abscess. Prominent swelling on one side of the posterior pharyngeal wall confirms the diagnosis. Swelling usually stops at the midline because a medial raphe divides the prevertebral space. Lateral neck soft tissue films show the retropharyngeal space to be wider than the C4 vertebral body.

Although retropharyngeal abscess is a surgical emergency, frequently it cannot be distinguished from retropharyngeal adenitis. Immediate hospitalization and intravenous antimicrobial therapy with a semisynthetic penicillin or clindamycin is the first step for most cases. Immediate surgical drainage is required when a definite abscess is seen radiographically or when the airway is compromised markedly. In most instances, a period of 12–24 hours of antimicrobial therapy will help to differentiate the two entities. In the child with adenitis, fever will decrease and oral intake will increase. A child with retropharyngeal abscess will continue to deteriorate. A surgeon should incise and drain the abscess under general anesthesia to prevent its extension.

## LUDWIG ANGINA

Ludwig angina is a rapidly progressive cellulitis of the submandibular space that can cause airway obstruction and death. The submandibular space extends from the mucous membrane of the floor of the mouth to the muscular and fascial attachments of the hyoid bone. This infection is encountered infrequently in infants and children. The initiating factor in over 50% of cases is dental disease, including abscesses and extraction. Some patients have a history of lacerations and injuries to the floor of the mouth. Group A streptococcus is the most common organism identified, but other pathogens cause the infection.

The manifestations are fever and tender swelling of the floor of the mouth. The tongue can become enlarged as well as tender and erythematous. Upward displacement of the tongue may cause dysphagia, drooling, and airway obstruction.

Treatment consists of giving high doses of intravenous clindamycin or ampicillin plus nafcillin until the results of cultures and sensitivity tests are available. Because the most common cause of death in Ludwig angina is sudden airway obstruction, the patient must be monitored closely in the intensive care unit and intubation provided for progressive respiratory distress. An otolaryngologist should be consulted to identify and perform a drainage procedure.

Britt JC et al: Ludwig's angina in the pediatric population: Report of a case and review of the literature. Int J Pediatr Otorhinolaryngol 2000;52:79.

## ACUTE CERVICAL ADENITIS

Local infections of the ear, nose, and throat can spread to a regional node and cause a secondary inflammation. The typical case involves a large, unilateral, solitary, anterior cervical node. About 70% of these cases are due to β-hemolytic streptococcal infection, 20% to staphylococci, and the remainder to viruses, atypical mycobacteria, and *Bartonella henselae*. Surgeons report a higher incidence of staphylococcal infection, but they see a greater proportion of atypical cases that have failed to respond to penicillin therapy and thus require incision and drainage. The most common antecedent infection is pharyngitis. Other entry sites for cervical adenitis include a periapical dental abscess (usually producing a submandibular adenitis), facial impetigo (infected cuts or bug bites), infected acne, and otitis externa (usually producing a preauricular adenitis).

The initial evaluation of cervical adenitis should generally include a group A streptococcal diagnostic test, a complete blood count with differential (looking for atypical lymphocytes), and a purified protein derivative skin test (PPD), looking for nontuberculous mycobacteria. If no cause is found, a mononucleosis test is useful. Early treatment with antibiotics prevents many cases of pyogenic adenitis from progressing to suppuration. However, once fluctuation occurs, antibiotic therapy alone is often insufficient. When fluctuation is present, needle aspiration may promote resolution. If needle aspiration is done, the pus should be sent for a Gram stain, aerobic and anaerobic culture, an acid-fast stain for *Mycobacteria,* and an acid-fast smear and tuberculosis culture. If needle aspiration is not effective, a surgeon should incise and drain the abscess. Hospitalization is required only if the patient is toxic, dehydrated, dysphagic, or dyspneic.

Cat-scratch disease is frequently implicated in cases of chronic cervical adenopathy. The diagnosis is aided by the finding of a primary papule on the face. In over 90% of patients, cat scratches are present or there is a history of contact with kittens. The node is usually only mildly tender, but may suppurate and drain. About one third of children have fever and malaise, and, rarely, neurologic sequelae and prolonged fever occur. Cat-scratch disease, caused by *B henselae,* can be diagnosed by serologic testing available at commercial laboratories, but testing is not always confirmatory. Blood should be drawn 2–8 weeks after onset of symptoms. Because most nodes caused by this pathogen spontaneously resorb within 1–3 months, the benefit of antibiotics is controversial. In a placebo-controlled trial, azithromycin for 5 days caused a more rapid decrease in node size. Other drugs likely to be effective include rifampin, trimethoprim–sulfamethoxazole, erythromycin, clarithromycin, doxycycline, ciprofloxacin, and gentamicin.

Cervical lymphadenitis can be caused by nontuberculous mycobacterial species or *Mycobacterium avium* complex. The adenitis is usually unilateral and indolent, but may involve several adjacent nodes. A characteristic violaceous appearance may develop over a prolonged period of time without systemic signs or much local pain. Atypical mycobacterial infections are often associated with PPD skin reactions less then 10 mm.

Once the diagnosis is suspected due to a positive PPD, a chest radiograph should be done and all family members tested for tuberculosis. The node should not be incised and drained, because that may lead to a draining sinus tract. Instead, a complete excision of all nodes should be done by an experienced surgeon. Nodes may recur, usually within 3 months of surgery. In such cases, a newer macrolide in combination with a second drug (rifampin or ethambutol) is given for 3–6 months.

## Differential Diagnosis

### A. NEOPLASMS AND CERVICAL NODES

Malignant tumors usually are not suspected until the adenopathy persists despite treatment. Classically, the nodes are painless, nontender, and firm to hard in consistency. They may be fixed to underlying tissues. These nodes may occur as a single node, as unilateral multiple nodes in a chain, as bilateral cervical nodes, or as generalized adenopathy. Common malignancies that may present in the neck include Hodgkin disease, non-Hodgkin lymphoma, rhabdomyosarcoma, and thyroid carcinoma.

### B. IMITATORS OF ADENITIS

Several structures in the neck can become infected and resemble a node. The first three masses are of congenital origin and are listed in order of frequency.

**1. Thyroglossal duct cyst**—When superinfected, this congenital malformation can become acutely swollen.

Helpful findings are the fact that it is in the midline, located between the hyoid bone and suprasternal notch, and moves upward when the tongue is stuck out or during swallowing. Occasionally, the cyst develops a sinus tract and opening just lateral to the midline.

**2. Branchial cleft cyst**—When superinfected, this malformation can become a tender mass 3–5 cm in diameter. Aids to diagnosis are the fact that the mass is located along the anterior border of the sternocleidomastoid muscle and is smooth and fluctuant. Occasionally it is attached to the overlying skin by a small dimple or a draining sinus tract.

**3. Lymphatic malformation (cystic hygroma)**—Most of these lymphatic cysts are located in the posterior triangle just above the clavicle. The mass is soft and compressible and can be transilluminated. Over 60% of hygromas are noted at birth, and the remainder are usually seen by the time the child is age 2 years. If cysts become large enough, they can compromise the patient's ability to swallow and breath.

**4. Parotitis**—The most common pitfall in differential diagnosis of cervical adenopathy is mistaking parotitis for adenitis. However, a swollen parotid crosses the angle of the jaw, is associated with preauricular percussion tenderness, and is bilateral in 70% of cases. There may be a history of exposure to mumps, but in the United States other viruses are now the main cause. An amylase level will be elevated in parotitis.

**5. Ranula**—A ranula is a cyst in the floor of the mouth caused by obstruction of the ducts of the sublingual gland. A plunging ranula extends below the mylohyoid muscle and can appear as a neck mass.

**6. Sternocleidomastoid muscle hematoma**—This cervical mass is noted at age 2–4 weeks. On close examination, it is found to be part of the muscle body and not movable. An associated torticollis usually confirms the diagnosis.

Maltezou HC et al: Nontuberculous mycobacterial lymphadenitis in children. Pediatr Infect Dis J 1999;18:968 [PMID: 10571431].

Peters TR, Edwards KM: Cervical lymphadenopathy and adenitis. Pediatr Rev 2000;21:399 [PMID: 11121496].

## SNORING, MOUTH BREATHING, & UPPER AIRWAY OBSTRUCTION

In April 2002, the American Academy of Pediatrics published a Clinical Practice Guideline for the diagnosis and management of uncomplicated childhood obstructive sleep apnea syndrome (OSAS). The guideline emphasizes that pediatricians should screen all children for snoring and that complex high-risk patients should be referred to a specialist.

When parents report that their child has nightly snoring and is a mouth breather even during the day, one should be suspicious of obstructive sleep apnea (OSA). Figure 17–9 is an algorithm for management of these complaints. The adenoids can be assessed by mirror examination, endoscopy, or radiographic studies. Either adenoid hypertrophy or nasal obstruction can be assumed when a child has hyponasal speech. The consonants "m," "n," and "ng" rely on the palate not touching the posterior pharyngeal wall. By having a child repeat the word "banana" or "ninety-nine" with the nose open or pinched closed, one may assess the nasal and nasopharyngeal airways. If the voice does not change with occlusion of the nostrils, then either adenoid or nasal obstruction is present.

Although nasal obstruction is usually due to allergic rhinitis and can be diagnosed by a careful allergy history, there are other, less common causes. Nasal polyps appear as glistening, gray to pink, jelly-like masses that are prominent just inside the anterior nares and occur singly or in clusters. They occur in cystic fibrosis and severe allergic rhinitis. Persistent mouth-breathing may also rarely be due to a nasopharyngeal tumor, or to a meningocele herniated into the nasal cavity. For male patients, if unilateral nasal obstruction and epistaxis occur frequently, juvenile angiofibroma should be suspected. If allergic rhinitis is the suspected cause of snoring, a trial of intranasal corticosteroid spray is indicated. If enlarged tonsils (Figure 17–10) or adenoids are present, a referral to an otolaryngologist or a pediatric sleep laboratory is in order.

### Diagnosis

The gold standard for diagnosis of OSA is a polysomnogram. A patient's history and clinical examination cannot predict the presence or severity of OSA. An overnight oximetry study is a poor screening test for OSA. The test may detect those patients with severe disease but miss the milder cases. OSA is part of a spectrum of disorders that occur during sleep. A milder form of OSA is upper airway resistance syndrome. Patients with this syndrome have an otherwise normal polysomnogram with the only evidence of obstruction being increased respiratory effort. The criteria for diagnosing OSA differ between children and adults. An obstructive event occurs when airflow stops despite persistence of respiratory effort. A hypopnea is counted when airflow and respiratory effort decrease with an associated oxygen desaturation or arousal. Normative values are just being established. An investigation of sleep-disordered breathing in children between the ages of 6 and 11 years is the first study to evaluate clinical relevance using full polysomnograms. The study demonstrated that a respiratory disturbance index (RDI) of at least

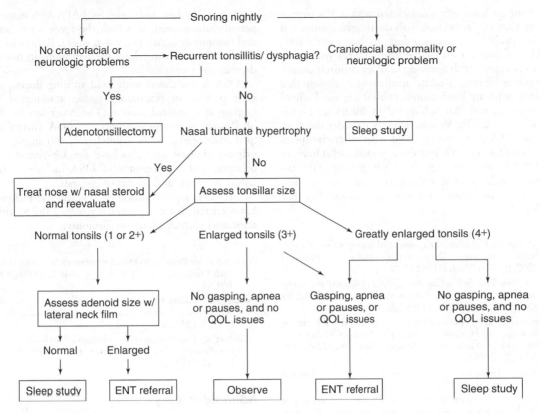

**Figure 17–9.** Algorithm for snoring. QOL = quality of life.

**Figure 17–10.** A grading scale for tonsil size that ranges from 0 to 4. With grade 0 the tonsils are small and contained within the tonsillar fossa; in grade 4 the tonsils are so large they almost touch ("kissing"). (Reprinted, with permission, from Brodksy L: Modern assessment of tonsils and adenoids. Pediatr Clin North Am 1989;36(6):1551.)

one event an hour when associated with a 3% oxygen desaturation was associated with daytime sleepiness and learning problems. If oxygen desaturations were absent, an RDI of five was associated with clinical symptoms. The importance of diagnosing OSA in children cannot be underestimated. Recent studies have shown that teenagers who are loud snorers exhibit impaired school performance, and that behavioral problems are associated with OSA. One should strongly consider the diagnosis of OSA in a snoring child who otherwise meets the criteria for ADHD. For those patients who have severe OSA by polysomnogram with large oxygen desaturations, obtain a chest radiograph and electrocardiogram to make sure that cor pulmonale has not developed.

Clinical Practice Guideline: Diagnosis and management of childhood obstructive sleep apnea syndrome. Pediatrics 2002;109:704 [PMID: 11927718].

Gozal D, Pope DW Jr: Snoring during early childhood and academic performance at ages thirteen to fourteen years. Pediatrics 2001;107:1394 [PMID: 11389268].

Goodwin JL et al: Symptoms related to sleep-disordered breathing in white and Hispanic children: The Tucson Children's Assessment of Sleep Apnea Study. Chest 2003;124(1):196 [PMID: 12853523].

Marcus CL: Sleep-disordered breathing in children. Am J Respir Crit Care Med 2001;164:16 [PMID: 11435234].

Schechter MS, Technical report: Diagnosis and management of childhood obstructive sleep apnea syndrome. Pediatrics 2002;109:e69 [PMID: 11927742]

### Websites

Information for Health Care Professionals (http://sleepapnea.org/promemb.html)

National Sleep Foundation (http://www.sleepfoundation.org/)

# TONSILLECTOMY & ADENOIDECTOMY
## Tonsillectomy

A tonsillectomy with or without adenoidectomy is typically performed for either hypertrophy or recurrent infections. Adenotonsillar hypertrophy may produce upper airway obstruction, dysphagia, or dental malocclusion. Rarely, the size may produce pulmonary hypertension or cor pulmonale. Recurrent infections are present when a child has seven or more documented *S pyogenes* infections in 1 year, five per year for 2 years, or three per year for 3 years. A tonsillectomy is reasonable if fewer infections are present but the child has missed multiple school days or has a complicated course. Recurrent peritonsillar abscesses and persistent streptococcal carrier state are other indications as well as unilateral tonsil hypertrophy that appears neoplastic.

A possible new indication is FAPA syndrome (see previous discussion), in which the fever is predictable and commonly occurs every 4–8 weeks. Removal of the tonsils was shown to relieve the symptoms in five children in one recent study.

OSA is associated with loud snoring during sleep with periods of respiratory pauses terminated with gasping and agitated arousal. The American Academy of Pediatrics technical report on OSA (http://www.pediatrics.org/cgi/content/full/109/4/e69) suggests that primary snoring may also have developmental consequences. Other symptoms of OSA include ADHD, failure to thrive, and nocturnal enuresis.

Recently, a proliferation of new surgical techniques has occurred that can potentially reduce the morbidity associated with an adenotonsillectomy.

Dahn KA et al: Periodic fever and pharyngitis in young children. Arch Otolaryngol Head Neck Surg 2000;126:1146 [PMID: 10979131].

Derkay CS, Maddern BR: Innovative techniques for adenotonsillar surgery in children Laryngoscope 2002;112(8 Pt 2):2 [PMID: 12172227]

Sood S et al: Effectiveness of the ultrasonic harmonic scalpel for tonsillectomy. Ear Nose Throat J 2001;80(8):514; 518 [PMID: 11523467]

## Adenoidectomy

The adenoids, composed of lymphoid tissue in the nasopharynx, are a component of the Waldeyer ring of lymphoid tissue with the palatine tonsils and lingual tonsils. Enlargement of the adenoids with or without infection can obstruct the upper airway, alter normal orofacial growth, and interfere with speech, swallowing, or eustachian tube function. Most children with prolonged mouth breathing eventually develop dental malocclusion and what has been termed an adenoidal facies. The face is pinched and the maxilla narrowed because the molding pressures of the orbicularis oris and buccinator muscles are unopposed by the tongue. The role of hypertrophy and chronic infection in the pathogenesis of sinusitis is unclear, but adenoidectomy has been shown to be effective in some patients with chronic rhinosinusitis.

Indications for adenoidectomy with or without tonsillectomy include pulmonary conditions such as chronic hypoxia related to upper airway obstruction, hypopnea, or obstructive sleep apnea; orofacial conditions such as mandibular growth abnormalities, dental malocclusion, and swallowing disorders; speech abnormalities; persistent middle ear effusion; recurrent and chronic otitis media; and chronic sinusitis. Chronic adenoiditis can seed the sinuses and cause the ongoing sinus disease.

Coyte PC et al: The role of adjuvant adenoidectomy and tonsillectomy in the outcome of the insertion of tympanostomy tubes. N Engl J Med 2001;344:1188 [PMID: 11390633].

## Complications of Tonsillectomy & Adenoidectomy

The reported mortality rates associated with tonsillectomy & adenoidectomy (T&A) now approximate that of general anesthesia alone. The rate of hemorrhage varies between 0.1% and 8.1% depending on the definition of hemorrhage; the rate of postoperative transfusion is 0.04%. Other complications include hypernasal speech (< 0.01%), and more rarely nasopharyngeal stenosis, atlantoaxial subluxation, mandible condyle fracture, and psychologic trauma.

## Contraindications to Tonsillectomy & Adenoidectomy

### A. SHORT PALATE

Adenoids should not be removed completely in a child with a cleft palate or submucous cleft palate because of the risk of aggravating the velopharyngeal incompetence and causing hypernasal speech and nasal regurgitation. A superior or partial adenoidectomy can be performed in a child with marked obstructive sleep apnea who has a submucous cleft palate or ongoing conductive hearing loss from middle ear effusion.

### B. BLEEDING DISORDER

If a chronic bleeding disorder is present, it must be diagnosed and treated before T&A.

### C. ACUTE TONSILLITIS

An elective T&A can often be postponed until acute tonsillitis is resolved. Urgent tonsillectomy may be required for tonsillitis unresponsive to medical therapy.

# DISORDERS OF THE LIPS

## Labial Sucking Tubercle

A small baby may present with a small callus in the mid-upper lip. It usually is asymptomatic and disappears after cup feeding is initiated.

## Cheilitis

Dry, cracked, scaling lips are usually caused by sun or wind exposure. Contact dermatitis from mouthpieces or various woodwind or brass instruments has also been reported. Licking the lips accentuates the process, and the patient should be warned of this. Liberal use of lip balms gives excellent results.

## Inclusion Cyst

Inclusion (retention) cysts are due to the obstruction of mucous glands or other mucous membrane structures. In the newborn, they occur on the hard palate or gums and are called Epstein pearls. These small cysts resolve spontaneously in 1–2 months. In older children, inclusion cysts usually occur on the palate, uvula, or tonsillar pillars. They appear as taut yellow sacs varying in size from 2 mm to 10 mm. Inclusion cysts that do not resolve spontaneously should undergo incision and drainage. Occasionally a mucous cyst on the lower lip (mucocele) requires drainage for cosmetic reasons. Minor salivary glands are present at this site. Blockage of the outflow of the individual gland initiates the development.

# DISORDERS OF THE TONGUE

## Geographic Tongue (Benign Migratory Glossitis)

This condition of unknown cause occurs in 1–2% of the population with no age, sex, or racial predilection and is characterized by irregularly shaped areas on the tongue devoid of papillae and surrounded by parakeratotic reddish borders. The pattern changes as alternating regeneration and desquamation occurs. The lesions are generally asymptomatic and require no treatment.

## Fissured Tongue (Scrotal Tongue)

This condition is marked by numerous irregular fissures on the dorsum of the tongue. It occurs in approximately 1% of the population and is usually a dominant trait. It is also frequently seen in children with trisomy 21 and other mentally delayed patients who have the habit of chewing on a protruded tongue.

## Coated Tongue (Furry Tongue)

The tongue normally becomes coated if mastication is impaired and the patient is taking a liquid or soft diet. Mouth breathing, fever, or dehydration can accentuate the process.

## Macroglossia

Tongue hypertrophy and protrusion may be a clue to Beckwith–Wiedemann syndrome, glycogen storage disease, cretinism, Hurler syndrome, lymphangioma, or hemangioma. Tongue reduction procedures should be considered in otherwise healthy subjects when macroglossia affects airway patency, eating, dental development, and normal mandibular growth. In trisomy

21, the normal-sized tongue protrudes because the patient's oral cavity is small.

Bezerra S, Costa I: Oral conditions in children from birth to 5 years: The findings of a children's dental program. J Clin Ped Dent 2000;25(1):79 [PMID: 11314357].

## HALITOSIS

Bad breath is usually due to acute stomatitis, pharyngitis, sinusitis, a nasal foreign body, or dental hygiene problems. In older children and adolescents, halitosis can be a manifestation of chronic sinusitis, gastric bezoar, bronchiectasis, or lung abscess. The presence of orthodontic devices or dentures can cause halitosis if good dental hygiene is not maintained. Halitosis can also be caused by decaying food particles embedded in cryptic tonsils. In adolescents, tobacco use is a common cause. Mouthwashes and chewable breath fresheners give limited improvement. Treatment of the underlying cause is indicated, and a dental referral may be in order.

Amir E et al: Halitosis in children. J Pediatr 1999;134(3):338 [PMID: 10064672].

## SALIVARY GLAND DISORDERS

### Parotitis

A first episode of parotitis may safely be considered to be of viral origin, unless fluctuance is present. The leading cause was mumps until adoption of vaccination; now the leading viruses are parainfluenza and Epstein–Barr virus. HIV should be considered if the child is known to be at risk.

### Suppurative Parotitis

Suppurative parotitis is an uncommon clinical disorder occurring chiefly in newborns and debilitated elderly patients. The parotid gland is swollen, tender, and often reddened and is usually a unilateral process. The diagnosis is made by expression of purulent material from the Stensen duct. The material should be smeared and cultured. Fever and leukocytosis may be present.

Treatment includes hospitalization and intravenous nafcillin because the most common causative organism is *S aureus.*

### Recurrent Idiopathic Parotitis

Some children experience repeated episodes of parotid swelling that last 1–2 weeks and then resolve spontaneously, or can become infected and require antibiotics for resolution. There is usually pain and often no fever. The process is most often unilateral, suggesting some sort of obstructive process, but can be associated with Sjögren syndrome, another autoimmune process, HIV infection, or a calculus in the parotid duct. Serum amylase levels are normal, which speaks against a diagnosis of viral parotitis. Many episodes may occur from age 2 years on. The problem may resolve spontaneously at puberty.

Treatment includes analgesics if pain is present and an antistaphylococcal antibiotic for prophylaxis of infection and quicker resolution at the onset of symptoms. A second attack of parotid swelling without fever should result in referral to an otolaryngologist to make the diagnosis.

Huisman TA et al: MRI of chronic recurrent parotitis in childhood. J Comput Assist Tomogr 2001;25:269 [PMID: 11242227].

### Tumors of the Parotid Gland

Mixed tumors, hemangiomas, sarcoidosis, and leukemia can be manifested in the parotid gland as a hard or persistent mass. A cystic mass or multiple cystic masses may represent an HIV infection. Work-up may require consultation with oncology, infectious diseases, hematology, and otolaryngology.

### Ranula

A ranula is a retention cyst of a sublingual salivary gland. It occurs on the floor of the mouth to one side of the lingual frenulum. Ranula has been described as resembling a frog's belly because it is thin-walled and contains a clear bluish fluid. Referral to an otolaryngologist for excision of the cyst and associated sublingual gland is the treatment of choice.

## CONGENITAL ORAL MALFORMATIONS

### Tongue-Tie (Ankyloglossia)

The tightness of the lingual frenulum varies greatly among normal people. A short frenulum prevents both protrusion and elevation of the tongue. Puckering of the midline of the tongue occurring with tongue movement is noted on physical examination.

When mild, treatment consists of reassurance. If the tongue cannot protrude past the teeth or alveolar ridge or move between the gums and cheek, referral to an otolaryngologist for evaluation is indicated. Frenulectomy may be recommended if there is a question of suckling difficulties, dental health (related to the inability to clear food from around the teeth), or articulation problems.

Messner AH, Lalakea ML: Ankyloglossia: Controversies in management. Int J Pediatr Otorhinolaryngol 2000;54:123 [PMID: 10967382].

Messner AH et al: Ankyloglossia: Incidence and associated feeding difficulties. Arch Otolaryngol Head Neck Surg 2000;126:36 [PMID: 10628708].

## Torus Palatini

Hard midline masses on the palate are called *torus palatini*. They are bony protrusions that form at suture lines of bone. Usually they are asymptomatic and require no therapy. They can be surgically reduced if necessary.

## Cleft Lip & Cleft Palate (see Chapter 33)

## Submucous Cleft Palate

A bifid uvula is present in 3% of healthy children. However, a close association exists (as high as 75%) between bifid uvula and submucous cleft palate. A submucous cleft can be diagnosed by noting a translucent zone in the middle of the soft palate. Palpation of the hard palate reveals absence of the posterior bony protrusion. Affected children have a 40% risk of developing persistent middle ear effusion. They are at risk also of incomplete closure of the palate, resulting in hypernasal speech. During feeding, some of these infants experience nasal regurgitation of food. Children with submucous cleft palate causing abnormal speech or nasal regurgitation of food require referral for surgical repair.

## High-Arched Palate

A high-arched palate is usually a genetic trait of no consequence. It also occurs in children who are chronic mouth breathers and in premature infants who undergo prolonged oral intubation. Some rare causes of high-arched palate are congenital disorders such as Marfan syndrome, Treacher Collins syndrome, and Ehlers–Danlos syndrome.

## Robin Sequence (Pierre Robin)

This group of congenital malformation is characterized by the triad of micrognathia, cleft palate, and glossoptosis. Affected children present as emergencies in the newborn period because of infringement on the airway by the tongue. The main objective of treatment is to prevent asphyxia until the mandible becomes large enough to accommodate the tongue. In some cases, this objective can be achieved by leaving the child in a prone position while unattended. In more severe cases, a tracheostomy is required. The child requires close observation and careful feeding until the problem is outgrown.

# Respiratory Tract & Mediastinum  18

Gwendolyn S. Kerby, MD, Gary L. Larsen, MD, Frank J. Accurso, MD, Robin R. Deterding, MD, Vivek Balasubramaniam, MD, & Scott D. Sagel, MD

## ■ RESPIRATORY TRACT

Pediatric pulmonary diseases account for almost 50% of deaths in children younger than age 1 year and about 20% of all hospitalizations of children younger than age 15 years. Approximately 7% of children have some sort of chronic disorder of the lower respiratory system. Understanding the pathophysiology of many pediatric pulmonary diseases requires an appreciation of the normal growth and development of the lung.

## GROWTH & DEVELOPMENT

The lung has its origins from an outpouching of the foregut during the fourth week of gestation. The development of the lung is divided into five overlapping stages. The first stage is the embryonic stage (3–7 weeks' gestation) during which the primitive lung bud undergoes asymmetrical branching and then subsequent dichotomous branching, leading to the development of the conducting airways. This stage of lung development is dependent on a complex crosstalk of various growth factors originating in both the pulmonary epithelium and the splanchnic mesenchyme. This stage also sees the development of the large pulmonary arteries from the sixth aortic arch and the pulmonary veins as outgrowths of the left atrium. Abnormalities during this stage result in congenital abnormalities such as lung aplasia, tracheoesophageal fistula, and congenital pulmonary cysts. The embryonic stage overlaps with the next stage: the pseudoglandular stage (5–17 weeks' gestation). During this stage the lung has a glandular appearance and witnesses the completion of the conducting airways (bronchi and bronchioles). The respiratory epithelium of these airways begins to differentiate, and the presence of cartilage, smooth muscle cells, and mucus glands are first seen. In addition, the pleuroperitoneal cavity divides into two distinct compartments. Abnormalities during this stage lead to pulmonary sequestration, cystic adenomatoid malformation, and congenital diaphragmatic hernia. The next stage witnesses the delineation of the pulmonary acinus: the canalicular stage (16–26 weeks' gestation). During this stage alveolar type II cell differentiate, the pulmonary capillary network develops, and the alveolar type I cells closely approximate with the developing capillary network. Abnormalities of development during this stage include neonatal respiratory distress syndrome and lung hypoplasia. The next stage is the saccular stage (26–36 weeks' gestation), during which further branching of the terminal saccules takes place as well as a thinning of the interstitium and fusion of the type I cell and capillary basement membrane in preparation for the lungs' function as a gas-exchange organ. The final stage of lung development is the alveolar stage (36 weeks's gestation to 3–8 years of age). Controversy surrounds the length of this stage of lung development. This stage witnesses secondary septal formation, further sprouting of the capillary network, and the development of true alveoli. Abnormalities during this stage lead to lung hypoplasia and can result in the development of bronchopulmonary dysplasia.

At birth, the lung assumes the gas-exchanging function served by the placenta in utero, placing immediate stress on all components of the respiratory system. Abnormalities in the lung, respiratory muscles, chest wall, airway, respiratory controller, or pulmonary circulation may therefore be present at birth. Survival after delivery depends, for example, on the development of the surfactant system to maintain airway stability and allow gas exchange. Immaturity of the surfactant system, often seen in infants born at less than 35 weeks' gestational age, can result in severe respiratory morbidity in the immediate neonatal period as well as subsequent chronic lung disease. A lethal form of lung disease has recently been recognized in infants homozygous for abnormalities in the surfactant protein B gene. Persistent pulmonary hypertension of the newborn—failure of the normal transition to a low-resistance pulmonary circulation at birth—can complicate a number of neonatal respiratory diseases. There is mounting evidence that abnormalities during fetal and neonatal growth and development of the lung have long-standing effects into adulthood, such as reduced gas exchange, exercise intolerance, asthma, and an increased risk of COPD.

Barker DJ: The intrauterine origins of cardiovascular and obstructive lung disease in adult life: The Marc Daniels Lecture 1990. J R Coll Physicians Lond 1991;25(2):129 [PMID: 2066923].

Bogue CW: Genetic and molecular basis of airway and lung development. In Haddad GG et al: *Basic Mechanisms of Pediatric Respiratory Disease.* BC Decker, 2002

Burri P: Structural aspects of prenatal and postnatal development and growth of the lung. In McDonald JA (ed): *Lung Growth and Development.* BC Dekker, 1997.

# DIAGNOSTIC AIDS

## PHYSICAL EXAMINATION OF THE RESPIRATORY TRACT

Assessing the rate, depth, ease, symmetry, and rhythm of respiration is critical to the detection of pulmonary disease. In young children, an elevated respiratory rate may be an initial indicator of pneumonia. Attention should be paid to tracheal position and thoracic configuration. Auscultation should assess the quality of breath sounds and detect the presence of abnormal sounds such as fine or coarse crackles, wheezing, or rhonchi. In older patients, unilateral crackles are the most valuable examination finding in pneumonia. Extrapulmonary manifestations of pulmonary disease include growth failure, altered mental status (from hypoxemia or hypercapnia), cyanosis, clubbing, and osteoarthropathy. In a study of children with respiratory illnesses, abnormalities of attentiveness, consolability, respiratory effort, color, and movement had a good diagnostic accuracy in detecting hypoxemia. Evidence of cor pulmonale (loud pulmonic component of the second heart sound, hepatomegaly, elevated neck veins, and, rarely, peripheral edema) signifies advanced lung disease.

Respiratory disorders can be secondary to disease in other systems. It is therefore important to look for other conditions such as congenital heart disease (murmur, gallop), neuromuscular disease (muscle wasting, scoliosis), immunodeficiency (rash, diarrhea), and autoimmune disease or occult malignancy (arthritis, hepatosplenomegaly).

Palafox M et al: Diagnostic value of tachypnea in pneumonia defined radiologically. Arch Dis Child 2000;82:41 [PMID: 10630911].

Wipf JE et al: Diagnosing pneumonia by physical examination: Relevant or relic? Arch Intern Med 1999; 159:1082 [PMID: 10335685].

## PULMONARY FUNCTION TESTS

Lung function tests can help to differentiate obstructive from restrictive lung diseases, measure disease severity, define precipitants of symptoms, and evaluate response to therapy. They can help define the risks of anesthesia and surgery and assist in the planning of respiratory care in the postoperative period. However, the range of normal values for a test may be wide, and the predicted normal values change dramatically with growth. For this reason, serial determinations of lung function are often more informative than a single determination. Patient cooperation is essential for almost all physiologic assessments. Most children are not able to perform the necessary maneuvers before age 5 years. Lung functions in infants and toddlers are available at specialized centers. Despite these problems, tests of lung function are valuable in the care of children.

Spirometers are available on which forced vital capacity can be recorded either as a volume–time tracing (spirogram) or a flow–volume curve. The patient inhales maximally, holds his or her breath for a short period, and then exhales as fast as possible for at least 3 seconds. The tracing produced by the exhalation shows forced vital capacity (FVC), which is the total amount of air that is exhaled from maximum inspiration, and the forced expiratory volume (FEV) in the first second of the exhalation ($FEV_1$). The maximum midexpiratory flow rate (MMEF, or $FEF_{25-75\%}$), is the mean flow rate during the middle portion of the FVC maneuver. The $FEV_1/FVC$ ratio is calculated from these absolute values; a ratio greater than 0.85 in children and young adults shows unlimited normal airflow.

These basic tests of lung function differentiate obstructive from restrictive processes. Examples of obstructive processes include asthma, chronic bronchitis, and cystic fibrosis (CF); restrictive problems include chest wall deformities that limit lung expansion and interstitial processes due to collagen–vascular diseases, hypersensitivity pneumonitis, and interstitial fibrosis. Classically, diseases that obstruct airflow decrease the $FEV_1$ more than the FVC, so that the $FEV_1/FVC$ ratio is low. In restrictive problems, however, the decreases in the $FEV_1$ and FVC are proportionate; thus, the ratio of $FEV_1$ to FVC is either normal or high. Clinical suspicion of a restrictive disease is usually an indication for referral to a specialist for evaluation.

The peak expiratory flow rate (PEFR), the maximal flow recorded during an FVC maneuver, can be assessed by handheld devices. The records of the PEFR can be helpful in following the course of pulmonary disorders that are difficult to control and require multiple medications (eg, asthma). These devices can also be used to give patients with poor perception of their disease an awareness of a decrease in lung function, thus facilitating earlier treatment.

Blonshine SB: Pediatric pulmonary function testing. Respir Care Clin North Am 2000;6:27 [PMID: 10639555].

Evans SE, Scanlon PD: Current practice in pulmonary function testing. Mayo Clin Proc 2003;78:758 [PMID: 12934788].

Sly PD et al: Lung function in cooperative patients. In Taussig LM, Landau LI (eds): *Pediatric Respiratory Medicine.* Mosby, 1999.

## ASSESSMENT OF OXYGENATION AND VENTILATION

Arterial blood gas determination defines the balance between respiration at the tissue level and that in the lungs. Assessment of blood gases is essential in critically ill children and may be used also for determining the severity of lung involvement in chronic conditions. Blood gas measurements are affected by abnormalities of respiratory control, gas exchange, respiratory mechanics, and the circulation. In pediatrics, hypoxia (low $PaO_2$) most commonly results from mismatching of ventilation and perfusion. Hypercapnia (elevated $PaCO_2$) results from inadequate alveolar ventilation, ie, inability to clear the $CO_2$ produced. This is termed *hypoventilation.* Causes include decreased central respiratory drive, paralysis of respiratory muscles, and low tidal volume breathing as seen in restrictive lung diseases, severe scoliosis, or chest wall trauma. Table 18–1 gives normal values for arterial pH, $PaO_2$, and $PaCO_2$ at sea level and at 5000 feet.

Exhaled or end-tidal $CO_2$ monitoring can be used to estimate arterial $CO_2$ content. It is used to monitor alveolar ventilation and is most accurate in patients without significant lung disease, particularly those with a good match of ventilation and perfusion and without airway obstruction. Exhaled or end-tidal $CO_2$ use has increased to confirm endotracheal tube placement and ensure endotracheal rather than esophageal intubation. This assessment is accurate in children who weigh more than 2 kg and have a perfusing rhythm. Exhaled $CO_2$ can be monitored by attaching a $CO_2$ detector to an endotracheal tube or to a nasal cannula. Qualitative $CO_2$ monitors use a chemical detector in a strip of paper that changes color when $CO_2$ is present. Capnography devices are quantitative and measure the concentration of $CO_2$ by infrared absorption detectors. These display continuous exhaled $CO_2$ concentration as a waveform and with a digital display of end-tidal $CO_2$.

Transcutaneous gas monitoring is a noninvasive assessment of $PaO_2$ and $PaCO_2$ using electrodes that measure gas tension at the skin surface. Transcutaneous monitoring can underestimate the $PaO_2$ and overestimate the $PaCO_2$ unless skin perfusion is maximal. Thus heating of the skin site is required, and cardiac function should be stable.

Pulse oximetry (measuring light absorption by transilluminating the skin) is the most reliable and easiest form of noninvasive monitoring of oxygenation. Oxygenated hemoglobin absorbs red light at certain wavelengths. Measurement during a systolic pulse allows estimation of arterial oxygen saturation as the machine corrects for the light absorbed at the tissue level between pulses. No heating of the skin is necessary. Values of oxygen saturation are reliable as low as 80%. The pulse oximeter has reduced reliability during conditions causing reduced arterial pulsation such as hypothermia, hypotension, or infusion of vasoconstrictor drugs. Carbon monoxide bound by hemoglobin results in higher than actual oxygen saturation readings.

Hay WW Jr: Pulse oximetry: As good as it gets? J Perinatol 2000;20:181 [PMID: 10802844].

Hazinski MF (ed): *Pediatric Advanced Life Support Provider Manual.* American Heart Association and the American Academy of Pediatrics, 2002.

Soubani AO: Noninvasive monitoring of oxygen and carbon dioxide. Am J Emerg Med 2001;19:141 [PMID: 11239260].

Tobias JD, Meyer DJ: Noninvasive monitoring of carbon dioxide during respiratory failure in toddlers and infants: End-tidal versus transcutaneous carbon dioxide. Anesth Analg 1997;85:55 [PMID: 9212122].

## CULTURE OF MATERIAL FROM THE RESPIRATORY TRACT

Expectorated sputum is rarely available from patients younger than age 8 years. In older children, a Gram-stained smear of sputum showing significant numbers of organisms within neutrophils may identify a pathogen. Bacterial stains and cultures of nasopharyngeal secretions are frequently misleading.

Cultures from the lower respiratory tract can be obtained invasively by tracheal aspiration through an endotracheal tube or rigid bronchoscope, or by performing a bronchoalveolar lavage through a flexible bronchoscope. Sputum induction, performed by inhaling aerosolized hypertonic saline, is a relatively safe noninvasive means of obtaining lower airway secretions. Where thoracoscopic lung biopsy by a skilled operator is unavailable, lung puncture directed to an area of consolidation by computed tomography (CT) scan or fluoroscopy may be the best approach for a child who deteriorates after initial antibiotic therapy or who

***Table 18–1.*** Normal arterial blood gas values on room air.

|  | pH | $PaO_2$ (mm Hg) | $PaCO_2$ (mm Hg) |
|---|---|---|---|
| Sea level | 7.38–7.42 | 85–95 | 36–42 |
| 5000 feet | 7.36–7.40 | 65–75 | 35–40 |

is critically ill or immunocompromised. However, pneumothorax may result. Open-lung biopsy, though a major intervention, should be considered in the worsening or critically ill child when other approaches are unsuccessful. In skilled hands, thoracoscopic lung biopsy may avoid open biopsy and its potential complications. Thoracentesis should be performed when pleural fluid is present. Blood glucose and lactate dehydrogenase should be drawn simultaneously for comparison with pleural fluid levels. Blood cultures must be obtained in children with acute pneumonia.

Specimens obtained by invasive means should be tested for viruses, *Mycoplasma pneumoniae, Chlamydia, Legionella pneumophila, Bordetella pertussis,* fungi, *Pneumocystis jiroveci* (formerly *Pneumocystis carinii*), acid-fast bacteria, and anaerobes or other bacteria. Rapid diagnostic techniques such as immunofluorescent antibody and enzyme-linked immunosorbent assay (ELISA) are best. Counterimmunoelectrophoresis of pleural fluid, serum, or concentrated urine may help identify disease due to *Streptococcus pneumoniae* or *Haemophilus influenzae.* Because these tests can be performed quickly, they may obviate further, more invasive studies.

Wiersma HE et al: Sputum induction for the diagnosis of pulmonary tuberculosis. Arch Dis Child Apr 2000;82:305 [PMID: 10991758].

Wood RE: Diagnostic and therapeutic procedures in pediatric pulmonary patients. In Taussig LM, Landau LI (eds): *Pediatric Respiratory Medicine.* Mosby, 1999.

## IMAGING OF THE RESPIRATORY TRACT

The plain chest radiograph remains the foundation for investigating the pediatric thorax. Both frontal and lateral views should be obtained. The radiograph is useful for evaluating air trapping caused by airway obstruction, volume loss caused by pneumonia, and interstitial problems such as pulmonary edema. Hyperaeration is best demonstrated in lateral views as flattening of the diaphragm. It is often seen because young children commonly develop small airway obstruction and asthma. Parenchymal changes may cause increased interstitial markings, consolidation, air bronchograms, or loss of diaphragm or heart contours. When pleural fluid is suspected, lateral decubitus radiographs may be helpful in determining the extent and mobility of the fluid. When a foreign body is suspected, forced expiratory radiographs may show focal air trapping and shift of the mediastinum to the contralateral side. Lateral neck radiographs can be useful in assessing the size of adenoids and tonsils and also in differentiating croup from epiglottitis, the latter being associated with the "thumbprint" sign.

Barium swallow is indicated for patients with suspected aspiration to detect swallowing dysfunction, tracheoesophageal fistula, gastroesophageal reflux, and achalasia. This technique is also important in detecting vascular rings and slings, because most of these abnormalities compress the esophagus. Airway fluoroscopy is another important tool for assessing both fixed airway obstruction (eg, tracheal stenosis) and dynamic airway obstruction (eg, tracheomalacia). Fluoroscopy or ultrasound of the diaphragm can detect paralysis by demonstrating paradoxic movement of the involved hemidiaphragm.

High-resolution CT scanning is useful to evaluate diffuse infiltrative lung disease, metastatic disease, mediastinal masses, and chest wall disease. Characteristic patterns seen in interstitial lung disease (eg, honeycombing in pulmonary fibrosis) or airway disease (eg, bronchiectasis) are often missed on chest radiographs. Magnetic resonance imaging (MRI) is useful for defining subtle or complex abnormalities and vascular rings. Ventilation–perfusion scans can provide information about regional ventilation and perfusion and can help detect vascular malformations and pulmonary emboli (rare in children). Pulmonary angiography is occasionally necessary to define the pulmonary vascular bed more precisely.

Cooper MI, Slovis TL: Imaging of the respiratory system. In Taussig LM, Landau LI (eds): *Pediatric Respiratory Medicine.* Mosby, 1999.

Harty MP et al: Current concepts on imaging of thoracic vascular abnormalities. Curr Opin Pediatr 2000;12(3):194 [PMID: 10836152].

Marchant JM et al: Application of chest high-resolution computer tomography in young children with cystic fibrosis. Pediatr Pulmonol 2001;31:24 [PMID: 11180671].

Williams HJ, Alton HM: Imaging of paediatric mediastinal abnormalities. Paediatr Respir Rev 2003;4(1):55 [PMID: 12615033].

## LARYNGOSCOPY & BRONCHOSCOPY

The indications for laryngoscopy include undiagnosed hoarseness, stridor, symptoms of obstructive sleep apnea, and laryngeal wheezing consistent with a diagnosis of vocal cord dysfunction; indications for bronchoscopy include wheezing, suspected foreign body, pneumonia, atelectasis, chronic cough, hemoptysis, and placement of an endotracheal tube and assessment of patency. In general, the more specific the indication, the higher the diagnostic yield.

Pediatric bronchoscopy instruments are of either the flexible fiberoptic or the rigid open tube type. Flexible bronchoscopy has the following advantages:

1. With sedation and topical anesthetics, the procedure can be done at the bedside.

2. Evaluation of the upper airway can be done with little risk in patients who are awake.

3. The distal airways of intubated patients can be examined without removing the endotracheal tube.

4. The instrument can be used as an obturator to intubate a patient with a difficult upper airway.

5. Endotracheal tube placement and patency can be checked.

6. Assessment of airway dynamics is generally better.

7. It is possible to examine more distal airways.

Improved digital optics has greatly enhanced the image quality. The advantages of using a rigid instrument are (1) easier removal of foreign bodies (so rigid bronchoscopy is preferred for suspected foreign body aspiration); and (2) better airway control, allowing the patient to be ventilated through the bronchoscope. In addition, this approach to the airway allows better assessment of the subglottic space for stenosis. The choice of procedures depends largely on the expertise available.

Bronchoalveolar lavage through a flexible bronchoscope is used to detect infection in immunocompetent and immunocompromised children. Aspiration and hemorrhage are also suspected in the presence of lipid and hemosiderin-laden macrophages, respectively. Surfactant protein analysis of lavage fluid can also be completed. Transbronchial biopsy is used to look for infection and rejection in transplant patients and to diagnose other conditions such as sarcoidosis.

Green CG et al: Technique. In Holinger LD et al (eds): *Pediatric Laryngology and Bronchoesophagology.* Lippincott-Raven, 1997.

Nicolai T: Pediatric bronchoscopy. Pediatr Pulmonol 2001;31: 150 [PMID: 11180692].

Schellhase DE: Pediatric flexible airway endoscopy. Curr Opin Pediatr 2002;14:327 [PMID: 12011674].

Tilles SA: Vocal cord dysfunction in children and adolescents. Curr Allergy Asthma Rep 2003;6:467 [PMID: 14531966].

# GENERAL THERAPY OF PEDIATRIC LUNG DISEASES

## OXYGEN THERAPY

Oxygen therapy in children with respiratory disease can reduce the work of breathing, resulting in fewer respiratory symptoms; relax the pulmonary vasculature, lessening the potential for pulmonary hypertension and congestive heart failure; and improve feeding. Patients breathing spontaneously can be treated by nasal cannula, head hood, or mask (including simple, rebreathing, nonrebreathing, or Venturi masks). The general goal of oxygen therapy is to achieve an arterial oxygen tension of 65–90 mm Hg or an oxygen saturation above 92%. The actual oxygen concentration achieved by nasal cannula or mask depends on the flow rate, the type of mask used, and the patient's age. Small changes in flow rate during oxygen administration by nasal cannula can lead to substantial changes in inspired oxygen concentration in young infants. The amount of oxygen required to correct hypoxemia may vary according to the child's activity. It is not unusual, for example, for an infant with chronic lung disease to require 0.75 L/min while awake but 1 L/min while asleep or feeding.

Although the head hood is an efficient device for delivery of oxygen in young infants, the nasal cannula is used more often because it allows the infant greater mobility. The cannula has nasal prongs that are inserted in the nares. Flow through the nasal cannula should generally not exceed 3 L/min to avoid excessive drying of the mucosa. Even at high flow rates, oxygen by nasal cannula rarely delivers inspired oxygen concentrations greater than 40–45%. In contrast, partial rebreathing and nonrebreathing masks or head hoods achieve inspired oxygen concentrations as high as 90–100%.

Because the physical findings of hypoxemia are subtle, the adequacy of oxygenation should be measured as the arterial oxygen tension, or oxygen saturation can be determined by oximetry. The advantages of the latter noninvasive method include the ability to obtain continuous measurements during various normal activities and to avoid artifacts caused by crying or breath holding during attempts at arterial puncture. For children with chronic cardiopulmonary disorders that may require supplemental oxygen therapy (eg, bronchopulmonary dysplasia or CF), frequent noninvasive assessments are essential to ensure the safety and adequacy of treatment.

Hazinski MF (ed): *Pediatric Advanced Life Support Provider Manual.* American Heart Association and the American Academy of Pediatrics, 2002.

Sivan Y et al: Assisted ventilatory support and oxygen treatment. In Taussig LM, Landau LI (eds): *Pediatric Respiratory Medicine.* Mosby, 1999.

## INHALATION OF BRONCHODILATORS

Airway obstruction that is at least partially reversed by a bronchodilator can be seen in CF, bronchiolitis, and bronchopulmonary dysplasia as well as in acute and chronic asthma.

The β-adrenergic agonists may be delivered by metered-dose inhaler (MDI), dry powder inhaler, or nebulizer. MDIs are convenient and best combined with valved holding chambers, especially for children who lack the ability to coordinate actuation of the MDI with inhalation. In contrast, the nebulizer is an effective method of delivering medication to infants and young children. Long-acting inhaled $\beta_2$-adrenergic agents that are relatively selective for the respiratory tract are described in Chapter 34. Inhaled bronchodilators are as effective as injected agents for treating acute episodes of airway obstruction and have fewer side effects. These drugs can be safely administered at home as long as both the physician and the family realize that a poor response may signify the need for corticosteroids to help restore $\beta$-adrenergic responsiveness.

Anticholinergic agents may also acutely decrease airway obstruction. Furthermore, they may yield a longer duration of bronchodilation than do many adrenergic agents. Selected patients may benefit from receiving both $\beta$-adrenergic and anticholinergic agents. In general, this class of drugs is most effective in the treatment of chronic bronchitis.

Everard ML, Le Souëf PN: Aerosol therapy and delivery systems. In Taussig LM, Landau LI (eds): *Pediatric Respiratory Medicine.* Mosby, 1999.

Kercsmar CM: Aerosol treatment of acute asthma. J Pediatr 2000;136:428 [PMID: 10753237].

Onhøj J et al: Lung deposition of inhaled drugs increases with age. Am J Respir Crit Care Med 2000;162:1819 [PMID: 11069819].

Rubin BK, Fink JB: The delivery of inhaled medication to the young child. Pediatr Clin North Am 2003;50:717 [PMID: 12877243].

## AIRWAY CLEARANCE THERAPY

Chest physical therapy, with postural drainage, percussion, and forced expiratory maneuvers, has been widely used to improve the clearance of lower airway secretions even though there is limited data on the efficacy of these techniques.

Children with CF have been shown to benefit from routine airway clearance. Many airway clearance techniques exist, but only a few long-term studies have compared the various options. The various techniques currently available include chest physiotherapy, autogenic drainage, positive expiratory pressure (PEP, Flutter, or Acapella), intrapulmonary percussive ventilation (IPV), or high-frequency chest compression (Vest). The decision on which technique to use should be based on the patient's age and preference after trying different approaches. Often bronchodilators or mucolytic medications are given prior to or during airway clearance therapy. Inhaled corticosteroids and inhaled antibiotics should be given after airway clearance therapy so that the airways are first cleared of secretions, allowing the medications to maximally penetrate into the lung.

McIlwaine PM et al: Long-term comparative trial of positive expiratory pressure versus oscillating positive expiratory pressure (flutter) physiotherapy in the treatment of cystic fibrosis. J Pediatr 2001;138(6):845 [PMID: 11391327].

van der Schans C et al: Chest physiotherapy compared to no chest physiotherapy for cystic fibrosis (Cochrane Review). In The Cochrane Library, Issue 3, 2003. Oxford: Update Software Ltd.

Wagener JS, Headley AA: Cystic fibrosis: Current trends in respiratory care. Respir Care 2003;48(3):234; discussion 246 [PMID: 12667274].

## AVOIDANCE OF ENVIRONMENTAL HAZARDS

All parents or other caregivers should be counseled about environmental hazards to the lung. The list of potential hazards includes small objects that may be aspirated, allergens that can precipitate respiratory symptoms in atopic children, and cigarette smoke.

The harmful effects of smoking in the home deserve special emphasis. Children from families where the parents and others smoke have decreased lung growth as well as decreased pulmonary function in comparison with children raised in smoke-free homes. Exposure of children to tobacco smoke also leads to an increased frequency of lower respiratory tract infections and an increased incidence of respiratory symptoms, including recurrent wheezing. Health care providers must increase their efforts to educate patients and their families about the hazards of smoking.

Chan-Yeung M, Dimich-Ward H: Respiratory health effects of exposure to environmental tobacco smoke. Respirology 2003;8:131 [PMID: 12753526].

Li Y-F et al: Effects of in utero and environmental tobacco smoke exposure on lung function in boys and girls with and without asthma. Am J Respir Crit Care Med 2000;162:2097 [PMID: 11112121].

Schwartz J et al: Respiratory effects of environmental tobacco smoke in a panel study of asthmatic and symptomatic children. Am J Respir Crit Care Med 2000;161:802 [PMID: 10712325].

## DISORDERS OF THE CONDUCTING AIRWAYS

The conducting airways (the nose, mouth, pharynx, larynx, trachea, bronchi, and bronchioles) direct inspired air to the gas-exchange units of the lung; they do not participate in gas exchange themselves. Airflow obstruction in the conducting airways occurs by (1) external compression (eg, vascular ring, tumor), (2) abnormalities of the airway structure itself (eg, congenital defects, thickening of an airway wall due to inflammation), or

(3) material in the airway lumen (eg, foreign body, mucus).

Airway obstruction can be fixed (airflow limited in both the inspiratory and the expiratory phases) or variable (airflow limited more in one phase of respiration than in the other). Variable obstruction is common in children because their airways are more compliant and susceptible to dynamic compression. With variable extrathoracic airway obstruction (eg, croup), airflow limitation is greater during inspiration, leading to inspiratory stridor. With variable intrathoracic obstruction (bronchomalacia), limitation is greater during expiration, producing expiratory wheezing. Thus determining the phase of respiration in which obstruction is greatest may be helpful in localizing the site of obstruction.

## EXTRATHORACIC AIRWAY OBSTRUCTION

Patients with abnormalities of the extrathoracic airway may present with snoring and other symptoms of obstructive apnea, hoarseness, brassy cough, or stridor. The course of the illness may be acute (eg, infectious croup), recurrent (eg, spasmodic croup), chronic (eg, subglottic stenosis), or progressive (eg, laryngeal papillomatosis). Significant risk factors are difficult delivery, ductal ligation, and intubation. Examination should determine if obstructive symptoms are present at rest or with agitation, if they are positional, or if they are related to sleep. The presence of agitation, air hunger, severe retractions, cyanosis, lethargy, or coma should alert the physician to a potentially life-threatening condition that may require immediate airway intervention. Helpful diagnostic studies in the evaluation of upper airway obstruction include chest and lateral neck radiographs, airway fluoroscopy, and barium swallow. In patients who have symptoms of severe chronic obstruction, an electrocardiogram (ECG) should be obtained to evaluate for right ventricular hypertrophy and pulmonary hypertension. Patients with obstructive sleep apnea should have polysomnography (measurements during sleep of the motion of the chest wall, airflow at the nose and mouth, heart rate, oxygen saturation, and selected electroencephalographic leads to stage sleep) to determine severity and to evaluate the need for tonsillectomy and adenoidectomy, oxygen, or continuous positive airway pressure (CPAP). In older children, pulmonary function tests can differentiate fixed from variable airflow obstruction and identify the site of variable obstruction. If noninvasive studies are unable to establish the cause, direct laryngoscopy and bronchoscopy remain the procedures of choice to establish the precise diagnosis. Treatment should be directed at relieving airway obstruction and correcting the underlying condition if possible.

Leung AK, Cho H: Diagnosis of stridor in children. Am Fam Physician 1999;60:2289 [PMID:10593320].

## INTRATHORACIC AIRWAY OBSTRUCTION

Intrathoracic airway obstruction usually causes expiratory wheezing. The history should include the following:

1. Age at onset
2. Precipitating factors (eg, exercise, upper respiratory illnesses, allergens, choking while eating)
3. Course—acute (bronchiolitis, foreign body), chronic (tracheomalacia, vascular ring), recurrent (reactive airways disease), or progressive (CF, bronchiolitis obliterans)
4. Presence and nature of cough
5. Production of sputum
6. Previous response to bronchodilators
7. Symptoms with positional changes (vascular rings)
8. Involvement of other organ systems (malabsorption in CF)

Physical examination should include growth measurements and vital signs. The examiner should look for cyanosis or pallor, barrel-shaped chest, retractions and use of accessory muscles, and clubbing. Auscultation should define the pattern and timing of respiration, detect the presence of crackles and wheezing, and determine whether findings are localized or generalized.

Routine tests include plain chest radiographs, a sweat test, and pulmonary function tests in older children. Other diagnostic studies are dictated by the history and physical findings. Treatment should be directed toward the primary cause of the obstruction but generally includes a trial of bronchodilators.

## CONGENITAL DISORDERS OF THE EXTRATHORACIC AIRWAY

### LARYNGOMALACIA

Laryngomalacia is a benign congenital disorder in which the cartilaginous support for the supraglottic structures is underdeveloped. It is the most common cause of persistent stridor in infants and usually is seen in the first 6 weeks of life. Stridor has been reported to be worse in the supine position, with increased activity, with upper respiratory infections, and during feeding; however, the clinical presentation can be variable. Patients may have slight oxygen desaturation during sleep.

Gastroesophageal reflux may also be associated with laryngomalacia requiring treatment. The condition usually improves with age and resolves by age 2 years, but in some cases symptoms persist for years. The diagnosis is established by direct laryngoscopy, which shows inspiratory collapse of an omega-shaped epiglottis (with or without long, redundant arytenoids). In mildly affected patients with a typical presentation (those without stridor at rest or retractions), this procedure may not be necessary. No treatment is usually needed. However, in patients with severe symptoms of airway obstruction associated with feeding difficulties, failure to thrive, obstructive sleep apnea, or severe dyspnea, surgical epiglottoplasty may be necessary.

Olney DR et al: Laryngomalacia and its treatment. Laryngoscope 1999;109:1770 [PMID: 10569405].

Toynton SC et al: Aryepiglottoplasty for laryngomalacia: 100 consecutive cases. J Laryngol Otol 2001;115:35 [PMID: 11233619].

## OTHER CONGENITAL PROBLEMS

Other rare congenital lesions of the larynx (laryngeal atresia, laryngeal web, laryngocele and cyst of the larynx, subglottic hemangioma, and laryngeal cleft) are best evaluated by direct laryngoscopy. Laryngeal atresia obviously presents immediately after birth with severe respiratory distress and is usually fatal. Laryngeal web, representing fusion of the anterior portion of the true vocal cords, is associated with hoarseness, aphonia, and stridor. Surgical correction may be necessary depending on the degree of airway obstruction.

Congenital cysts and laryngoceles are believed to have similar origin. Cysts are more superficial, whereas laryngoceles communicate with the interior of the larynx. Cysts are generally fluid-filled, whereas laryngoceles may be air- or fluid-filled. Airway obstruction is usually prominent and requires surgery or laser therapy.

Subglottic hemangiomas are seen in infancy with signs of upper airway obstruction and are often (but not always) associated with similar lesions of the skin. Although these lesions tend to regress spontaneously, airway obstruction may require laser surgical treatment or even tracheostomy.

Laryngeal cleft is a very rare condition resulting from failure of posterior cricoid fusion. Patients with this condition may have stridor but always aspirate severely, resulting in recurrent or chronic pneumonia and failure to thrive. Barium swallow is always positive for severe aspiration, but diagnosis can be very difficult even with direct laryngoscopy. Patients often require tracheostomy and gastrostomy, because surgical correction is not always successful.

Altman KW et al: Congenital airway abnormalities in patients requiring hospitalization. Arch Otolaryngol Head Neck Surg 1999;125:525 [PMID: 10326809].

Sichel JY et al: Management of congenital laryngeal malformations. Am J Otolaryngol 2000;21:22 [PMID: 10668673].

# ACQUIRED DISORDERS OF THE EXTRATHORACIC AIRWAY

## CROUP SYNDROME

Croup describes acute inflammatory diseases of the larynx, including viral croup (laryngotracheobronchitis), epiglottitis (supraglottitis), and bacterial tracheitis. These are the main entities in the differential diagnosis for patients presenting with acute stridor, although spasmodic croup, angioneurotic edema, laryngeal or esophageal foreign body, and retropharyngeal abscess should be considered as well.

### 1. Viral Croup

Viral croup generally affects younger children in the fall and early winter months and is most often caused by parainfluenza virus serotypes. Other organisms causing croup include respiratory syncytial virus (RSV), influenza virus, rubeola virus, adenovirus, and *Mycoplasma pneumoniae*. Although inflammation of the entire airway is usually present, edema formation in the subglottic space accounts for the predominant signs of upper airway obstruction.

### Clinical Findings

#### A. SYMPTOMS AND SIGNS

Usually a prodrome of upper respiratory tract symptoms is followed by a barking cough and stridor. Fever is usually absent or low-grade but may on occasion be as high as in patients with epiglottitis. Patients with mild disease may have stridor when agitated. As obstruction worsens, stridor occurs at rest, accompanied in severe cases by retractions, air hunger, and cyanosis. On examination, the presence of cough and the absence of drooling favor the diagnosis of viral croup over epiglottitis.

#### B. IMAGING

Lateral neck radiographs can be diagnostically helpful by showing subglottic narrowing and a normal epiglottis. This is not done routinely in the child with a classic presentation.

## Treatment

Treatment of viral croup is based on the symptoms. Mild croup, signified by a barking cough and no stridor at rest, requires supportive therapy with oral hydration and minimal handling. Mist therapy is used by some physicians, although clinical studies demonstrating its effectiveness are lacking. Conversely, patients with stridor at rest require active intervention. Oxygen should be administered to patients with oxygen desaturation. Nebulized racemic epinephrine (2.25% solution; 0.05 mL/kg to a maximum of 1.5 mL diluted in sterile saline) is commonly used because it has a rapid onset of action within 10–30 minutes. Both racemic epinephrine and epinephrine hydrochloride are effective in alleviating symptoms and decreasing the need for intubation. Once controversial, the efficacy of glucocorticoids in croup is now more firmly established. Dexamethasone, 0.6 mg/kg intramuscularly as one dose, improves symptoms, reduces the duration of hospitalizations and frequency of intubations, and permits earlier discharge from the emergency room. Oral dexamethasone appears equally effective, and limited data suggest that lower doses of oral dexamethasone (0.15 mg/kg) may be as effective as the higher dose. Inhaled budesonide (2–4 mg) also improves symptoms and decreases hospital stay. Onset of action occurs within 2 hours, and this agent may be as effective as dexamethasone; however, dexamethasone is still the most cost-effective steroid of choice. If symptoms resolve within 3 hours of glucocorticoids and nebulized epinephrine, patients can safely be discharged without fear of a sudden rebound in symptoms. If, however, recurrent nebulized epinephrine treatments are required or if respiratory distress persists, patients require hospitalization for close observation, supportive care, and nebulization treatments as needed. In patients with impending respiratory failure, an airway must be established (see following paragraph). Hospitalized patients with persistent symptoms over 3–4 days despite treatment should arouse suspicion of another cause of airway obstruction.

Patients with impending respiratory failure require an artificial airway. Intubation with an endotracheal tube of slightly smaller diameter than would ordinarily be used is reasonably safe. Extubation should be accomplished within 2–3 days to minimize the risk of laryngeal injury. If the patient fails extubation, tracheostomy may be required.

## Prognosis

Most children with viral croup have an uneventful course and improve within a few days. Some evidence suggests that patients with a history of croup associated with wheezing may have airway hyperreactivity, but it has not been determined if this was present prior to the croup episode or if the croup episode itself altered airway function. Recurrence of croup occurs in some instances, implying airway hyperreactivity.

Castro-Rodriguez JA et al: Relation of two different subtypes of croup before age three to wheezing, atopy, and pulmonary function during childhood: A prospective study. Pediatrics 2001;170:512 [PMID: 11230591].

Stroud RH, Friedman NR: An update on inflammatory disorders of the pediatric airway: Epiglottis, croup, and tracheitis. Am J Otolaryngol 2001;22:268 [PMID: 11264324].

Wright RB et al: New approaches to respiratory infections in children: Bronchiolitis and croup. Emerg Med Clin North Am 2002;20:93 [PMID: 11826639].

## 2. Epiglottitis

Epiglottitis is a true medical emergency. In published case series, it is almost always caused by *Haemophilus influenzae* type B, although other organisms such as nontypable *H influenzae, Streptococcus pneumoniae*, groups A and C *Streptococcus pyogenes, Neisseria meningitides,* and staphylococci have been implicated. Resulting inflammation and swelling of the supraglottic structures (epiglottis and arytenoids) can develop rapidly and lead to life-threatening upper airway obstruction. The incidence has decreased dramatically since *H influenzae* conjugate vaccine was introduced.

## Clinical Findings

### A. SYMPTOMS AND SIGNS

Typically, patients present with a sudden onset of fever, dysphagia, drooling, muffled voice, inspiratory retractions, cyanosis, and soft stridor. They often sit in the so-called sniffing dog position, which gives them the best airway possible under the circumstances. Progression to total airway obstruction may occur and result in respiratory arrest. The definitive diagnosis is made by direct inspection of the epiglottis, a procedure that should be done by an experienced airway specialist under controlled conditions (usually the operating room). The typical findings are cherry-red and swollen epiglottis and arytenoids.

### B. IMAGING

Diagnostically, lateral neck radiographs may be helpful in demonstrating a classic "thumbprint" sign. Obtaining radiographs, however, may delay important airway intervention.

## Treatment

Once the diagnosis of epiglottitis is made, endotracheal intubation must be performed immediately. Most anesthesiologists prefer general anesthesia (but not muscle relaxants) to facilitate intubation. After an airway is established, cultures of the blood and epiglottis should be obtained and the patient started on appropriate intravenous antibiotics to cover *H influenzae* (ceftriaxone sodium or equivalent cephalosporin). Extubation can usually be accomplished in 24–48 hours, when direct inspection shows significant reduction in the size of the epiglottis. Intravenous antibiotics should be continued for 2–3 days, followed by oral antibiotics to complete a 10-day course.

If a physician who has little experience in treating airway disorders and is located far from a pediatric care facility encounters a patient with epiglottitis, the following is recommended. Start the patient on oxygen and assemble all the airway equipment available. Manipulate the patient as little as possible, and allow the child to remain sitting up. Enlist the help of the most experienced airway person available, or call a transport team. Start an intravenous line and give antibiotics. If the patient obstructs completely and experiences respiratory arrest, attempt to establish an airway by any means possible: bag and mask ventilation, intubation, transtracheal ventilation with a large-bore angiocatheter attached to a 3-mm endotracheal tube adapter and resuscitation bag, or tracheostomy.

## Prognosis

Prompt recognition and appropriate treatment usually results in rapid resolution of swelling and inflammation. Recurrence is unusual.

Levy RJ, Helforr MA: Pediatric airway issues. Crit Care Clin 2000;16:489 [PMID: 10941587].

Rotta AT, Wiryawan B: Respiratory emergencies in children. Respir Care 2003;48:248 [PMID: 12667275].

## 3. Bacterial Tracheitis

Bacterial tracheitis (pseudomembranous croup) is a severe form of laryngotracheobronchitis. The organism most often isolated is *Staphylococcus aureus,* but organisms such as *H influenzae,* group A *Streptococcus pyogenes, Neisseria* species, *Moraxella catarrhalis,* and others have been reported. The disease probably represents localized mucosal invasion of bacteria in patients with primary viral croup, resulting in inflammatory edema, purulent secretions, and pseudomembranes. Although cultures of the tracheal secretions are frequently positive, blood cultures are almost always negative.

## Clinical Findings

### A. SYMPTOMS AND SIGNS

The early clinical picture is similar to that of viral croup. However, instead of gradual improvement, patients develop high fever, toxicity, and progressive upper airway obstruction that is unresponsive to standard croup therapy. The incidence of sudden respiratory arrest or progressive respiratory failure is high; in such instances, airway intervention is required. Findings of toxic shock and the acute respiratory distress syndrome (ARDS) may also be seen.

### B. LABORATORY FINDINGS

The white cell count is usually elevated, with left shift. Cultures of tracheal secretions usually demonstrate one of the causative organisms.

### C. DIAGNOSIS

Lateral neck radiographs show a normal epiglottis but often severe subglottic and tracheal narrowing. Irregularity of the contour of the proximal tracheal mucosa can frequently be seen radiographically. Bronchoscopy showing a normal epiglottis and the presence of copious purulent tracheal secretions confirm the diagnosis.

## Treatment

Suspected bacterial tracheitis should be managed in a fashion similar to that for epiglottitis. Because the incidence of respiratory arrest or progressive respiratory failure is high, intubation is usually necessary. Because these patients often have thick, purulent tracheal secretions, humidification, frequent suctioning, and intensive care monitoring are required to prevent endotracheal tube obstruction. Intravenous antibiotics to cover *Staphylococcus aureus, H influenzae,* and the other organisms are indicated. Because thick secretions persist for several days, the required period of intubation is longer for bacterial tracheitis than for epiglottitis. Despite the severity of this illness, the reported mortality rate is very low.

Rotta AT, Wiryawan B: Respiratory emergencies in children. Respir Care 2003;48:248 [PMID: 12667275].

Stroud RH, Friedman NR: An update on inflammatory disorders of the pediatric airway: Epiglottis, croup, and tracheitis. Am J Otolaryngol 2001;22:268 [PMID: 11464324].

Ward MA: Lower respiratory tract infections in adolescents. Adolesc Med 2000;11:251 [PMID: 10916123].

## VOCAL CORD PARALYSIS

Unilateral or bilateral vocal cord paralysis may be congenital or, more commonly, may result from injury to the recurrent laryngeal nerves. Risk factors for acquired paralysis include difficult delivery (especially face presentation), neck and thoracic surgery (eg, ductal ligation, repair of tracheoesophageal fistula), trauma, mediastinal masses, pulmonary hypertension, and central nervous system (CNS) disease (eg, Arnold–Chiari malformation). Patients usually present with varying degrees of hoarseness, aspiration, or high-pitched stridor. Unilateral cord paralysis is more likely to occur on the left because of the longer course of the left recurrent laryngeal nerve and its proximity to major thoracic structures. Patients with unilateral paralysis are usually hoarse but rarely have stridor. With bilateral cord paralysis, the closer to midline the cords are positioned, the greater the airway obstruction; the more lateral the cords are positioned, the greater the tendency to aspirate and experience hoarseness or aphonia. If partial function is preserved (paresis), the adductor muscles tend to operate better than the abductors, with a resultant high-pitched inspiratory stridor and normal voice. Airway intervention (intubation, tracheostomy) is rarely indicated in unilateral paralysis but is often necessary for bilateral paralysis. Recovery is related to the severity of nerve injury and the potential for healing.

de Jong AL et al: Vocal cord paralysis in infants and children. Otolaryngol Clin North Am 2000;33:131 [PMID: 10637348].

Portier F et al: Respiratory obstruction as a sign of brainstem dysfunction in infants with Chiari malformations. Int J Pediatr Otorhinolaryngol 2001;57:195 [PMID: 11223451].

## SUBGLOTTIC STENOSIS

Subglottic stenosis may be congenital or, more commonly, may result from endotracheal intubation. Neonates and infants are particularly vulnerable to subglottic injury from intubation: The subglottis is the narrowest part of an infant's airway, and the cricoid cartilage, which supports the subglottis, is the only cartilage that completely encircles the airway. The clinical presentation may vary from totally asymptomatic to the typical picture of severe upper airway obstruction. Patients with signs of stridor who repeatedly fail extubation are likely to have subglottic stenosis. Subglottic stenosis should also be suspected in children with multiple, prolonged, or severe episodes of croup. As with other conditions, diagnosis is made by direct laryngoscopy and bronchoscopy. Tracheostomy is often required when airway compromise is severe. Surgical intervention is ultimately required to correct the stenosis. Depending on the type of stenosis, a cricoid split in which the cricoid cartilage is surgically opened (better for acquired than for congenital lesions) may be tried. Laryngotracheal reconstruction in which a cartilage graft from another source (eg, rib) is used to expand the airway has become the standard procedure for symptomatic subglottic stenosis in children.

Cotton RT: Management of subglottic stenosis. Otolaryngol Clin North Am 2000;33:111 [PMID: 10637347].

Walner DL et al: Neonatal subglottic stenosis—incidence and trends. Laryngoscope 2001;111:48 [PMID: 11192899].

## LARYNGEAL TRAUMA

Injury to the larynx may result from external trauma, such as automobile accidents, snowmobile accidents (clothesline injury), and hanging; or internal trauma, such as noxious inhalation (burns and caustic substances) and intubation. External trauma can cause laryngeal fracture, which requires an emergency tracheostomy to prevent death. After appropriate airway intervention, attention should be directed to debridement and closure of lacerations. Reduction of laryngeal fractures should be performed as soon as the patient is stabilized.

Jewett BS et al: External laryngeal trauma: Analysis of 392 patients. Arch Otolaryngol Head Neck Surg 1999;125:87 [PMID: 10448735].

## LARYNGEAL PAPILLOMATOSIS

Papillomas of the larynx are benign, warty growths that are difficult to treat and are the most common laryngeal neoplasm in children. Human papillomaviruses 6, 11, and 16 have been implicated as causative agents. A substantial percentage of mothers of patients with laryngeal papillomas have a history of genital condylomas at the time of delivery, so the virus may be acquired during passage through an infected birth canal.

The age at onset is usually 2–4 years, but juvenile-onset recurrent respiratory papillomatosis is well documented. A younger age of onset may be a worse prognostic indicator. Patients usually develop hoarseness, voice changes, croupy cough, or stridor that can lead to life-threatening airway obstruction. Diagnosis is by direct laryngoscopy. The larynx was involved at the time of diagnosis in over 95% of patients, most of whom had only one site involved.

Treatment is directed toward relieving airway obstruction, usually by surgical removal of the lesions. Tracheostomy is necessary when life-threatening obstruction or respiratory arrest occurs. Various surgical procedures (laser, cup forceps, cryosurgery) have been used to remove papillomas, but recurrences are the rule, and frequent reoperation may be needed. The lesions occasionally spread down the trachea and bronchi, making surgical removal more difficult. The use of interferon therapy remains controversial. Fortunately, spontaneous remissions do occur, usually by puberty, so that the goal of therapy is to maintain an adequate airway until remission occurs.

Derkay CS: Recurrent respiratory papillomatosis. Laryngoscope 2001;111:57 [PMID: 11192901].

Reeves WC et al: National Registry for juvenile-onset recurrent respiratory papillomatosis. Arch Otolaryngol Head Neck Surg 2003;129:976 [PMID: 12975271].

# CONGENITAL DISORDERS OF THE INTRATHORACIC AIRWAYS

## MALACIA OF AIRWAYS

Tracheomalacia or bronchomalacia exists when the cartilaginous framework of the airway is inadequate to maintain airway patency. Because cartilage of the infant airway is normally soft, all infants may have some degree of dynamic collapse of a central airway when pressure outside the airway exceeds intraluminal pressure. In tracheomalacia, whether congenital or acquired, dynamic collapse leads to airway obstruction. The congenital variety may be isolated or associated with another developmental defect, such as tracheoesophageal fistula or vascular ring. It may be localized to part of the trachea or, more commonly, may involve the entire trachea as well as the remainder of the conducting airways. In severe cases, cartilage in the involved area may be missing or underdeveloped. The acquired variety has been associated with long-term ventilation of premature newborns that results in chronic tracheal injury.

Patients present with coarse wheezing, a prolonged expiratory phase, and a croupy cough, all of which increase with agitation and upper respiratory tract infections. Diagnosis can be made by cinefluoroscopy or bronchoscopy. Barium swallow may be indicated to rule out coexisting conditions. No treatment is usually indicated for the isolated condition, which generally improves over time. Coexisting lesions such as tracheoesophageal fistulas and vascular rings need primary repair. In severe cases of tracheomalacia, intubation or tracheostomy may be necessary, but this procedure alone is seldom satisfactory because airway collapse continues to exist below the tip of the artificial airway. CPAP through an artificial airway can sometimes stabilize the collapsing airway. When conventional therapy fails, surgical approaches to the problem (tracheopexy, aortopexy, placement of stents) may be considered.

Austin J, Ali T: Tracheomalacia and bronchomalacia in children: Pathophysiology, assessment, treatment and anaesthesia management. Paediatr Anaesth 2003;13:3 [PMID: 12535032].

Finder JD: Primary bronchomalacia in infants and children. J Pediatr 1997;130:59 [PMID: 9003852].

Masters IB et al: Series of laryngomalacia, tracheomalacia, and bronchomalacia disorders and their associations with other conditions in children. Pediatr Pulmonol 2002;34:189 [PMID: 12203847].

Paston F, Bye M: Tracheomalacia. Pediatr Rev 1996;17:328 [PMID: 8806208].

# VASCULAR RINGS & SLINGS

The most common vascular anomalies to compress the trachea or esophagus are a double aortic arch, right aortic arch with left ligamentum arteriosum or patent ductus arteriosus, pulmonary sling, anomalous innominate or left carotid artery, and aberrant right subclavian artery. All but the latter can cause tracheal compression and present in infancy with symptoms of chronic airway obstruction (stridor, coarse wheezing, and croupy cough). Symptoms are often worse in the supine position. Respiratory compromise is most severe with double aortic arch and may lead to apnea, respiratory arrest, or even death. Esophageal compression, present in all but anomalous innominate or carotid artery, may result in feeding difficulties, including dysphagia and vomiting. Barium swallow showing esophageal compression is the mainstay of diagnosis. An anomalous innominate or carotid artery is best diagnosed by cinefluoroscopy, MRI, or bronchoscopy.

Patients with significant symptoms require surgical correction, especially those with double aortic arch. Controversy exists about whether angiography is necessary to define the anatomy prior to surgery. Patients usually improve following correction but may have persistent but milder symptoms of airway obstruction due to associated tracheomalacia.

Krummel TM: Congenital malformations of the lower respiratory tract. In Chernick V, Boat TF (eds): *Kendig's Disorders of the Respiratory Tract in Children*, 6th ed. WB Saunders, 1998.

McLaughlin RB Jr et al: Vascular anomalies causing symptomatic tracheobronchial compression. Laryngoscope 1999;109:312 [PMID: 10890785].

Sebening C et al: Vascular tracheobronchial compression syndromes—Experience in surgical treatment and literature review. Thorac Cardiovasc Surg 2000;48:164 [PMID: 10903065].

# BRONCHOGENIC CYSTS

Bronchogenic cysts generally occur in the mid mediastinum (see Mediastinal Masses section) near the carina and adjacent to the major bronchi but can be found elsewhere in the lung. They range in size from 2 to 10 cm. Cyst walls are thick and may contain pus, mucus, or blood. These cysts develop from abnormal lung budding of the primitive foregut. They do not contain distal lung parenchyma and generally do not communicate with the airway.

Clinically, respiratory distress can appear acutely in early childhood or present as chronic wheezing, chronic cough, tachypnea, recurrent pneumonia, or stridor, depending on the location and size of the cysts and the degree of airway compression. On examination, the trachea may deviate from the midline, and the percussion noted over involved lobes may be hyperresonant. Breath sounds over such areas will also be decreased. The chest radiograph shows air trapping and hyperinflation of the affected lobes. Smaller lesions or those detected early may not be seen on chest radiographs or may appear spherical. Initial assessment of a suspected bronchogenic cyst usually includes barium swallow to look for a mass. This study also helps determine whether the lesion communicates with the gastrointestinal tract. CT scans or ultrasonography can differentiate solid versus cystic mediastinal masses and define the cyst's relationship to the rest of the lung.

Treatment is by surgical resection. Postoperatively, vigorous pulmonary physiotherapy is required to prevent complications (atelectasis, infection of lung distal to the site of resection of the cyst).

Ahrens B et al: Symptomatic bronchogenic cyst in a six-month-old infant: Case report and review of the literature. J Thorac Cardiovasc Surg 2001;122:1021 [PMID: 11689810].

Clements BS: Congenital malformations of the lungs and airways. In Taussig LM, Landau LI (eds): *Pediatric Respiratory Medicine.* Mosby, 1999.

McAdams HP et al: Bronchogenic cyst: Imaging features with clinical and histopathologic correlation. Radiology 2000;217: 441 [PMID: 11058643].

# ACQUIRED DISORDERS OF THE INTRATHORACIC AIRWAYS

## FOREIGN BODY ASPIRATION

Aspiration of a foreign body into the respiratory tract is rarely observed, so it is the abrupt onset of cough, choking, or wheezing—especially in children who have access to high-risk objects such as peanuts, hard candy, and small toys—that suggests the diagnosis. Children age 6 months to 4 years are at highest risk, and many deaths are caused by respiratory obstruction each year.

### 1. Foreign Bodies in the Upper Respiratory Tract

The diagnosis is established by acute onset of cyanosis and choking along with inability to vocalize or cough (complete obstruction) or with drooling and stridor (partial obstruction).

Foreign bodies that lodge in the esophagus may compress the airway and cause respiratory distress. More typically, the foreign body lodges in the supraglottic airway, triggering protective reflexes that result in laryngospasm. Onset is generally abrupt, with a history of the child's running with food in his or her mouth or playing with seeds, small coins, toys, and the

like. Poor child-proofing in the home and cases in which an older sibling feeds age-inappropriate foods (eg, peanuts, hard candy, carrot slices) to the younger child are typical. If the obstruction is only partial, coughing, stridor, and the ability to vocalize may persist. If complete, an inability to cough or vocalize (aphonia) and cyanosis with marked distress are observed. Without treatment, progressive cyanosis, loss of consciousness, seizures, bradycardia, and cardiopulmonary arrest follow.

### Treatment

The emergency treatment of upper airway obstruction due to foreign body aspiration is somewhat controversial. In general, it is recommended that if partial obstruction is present, children should be allowed to use their own cough reflex to extrude the foreign body. If after a brief observation period, the obstruction increases or the airway becomes completely obstructed, acute intervention is required. The American Academy of Pediatrics and the American Heart Association distinguish between children younger than and older than age 1 year. A choking infant younger than age 1 year should be placed face-down over the rescuer's arm, with the head positioned below the trunk. Five measured back blows are delivered rapidly between the infant's scapulas with the heel of the rescuer's hand. If obstruction persists, the infant should be rolled over and five rapid chest compressions performed (similar to cardiopulmonary resuscitation). This sequence is repeated until the obstruction is relieved. In children older than age 1 year, abdominal thrusts (Heimlich maneuver) may be performed, with special care in younger children because of concern about possible intraabdominal organ injury.

In both groups, blind probing of the airway to dislodge a foreign body is discouraged because of the risk of impaction. The airway may be opened by jaw thrust, and if the foreign body can be directly visualized, careful removal with the fingers or instruments (Magill forceps) can be attempted. Patients with persistent apnea and inability to achieve adequate ventilation may require emergency intubation, tracheostomy, or needle cricothyrotomy, depending on the setting and the rescuer's skills.

Friedman EM: Tracheobronchial foreign bodies. Otolaryngol Clin North Am 2000;33:179 [PMID: 10637351].

Hazinski MF (ed): *Pediatric Advanced Life Support Provider Manual.* American Heart Association and the American Academy of Pediatrics, 2002.

Halvorson DJ et al: Management of subglottic foreign bodies. Ann Otol Rhinol Laryngol 1996;105:541 [PMID: 8678431].

Walner DL et al: Utility of radiographs in the evaluation of pediatric upper airway obstruction. Ann Otol Rhinol Laryngol 1999;108:378 [PMID: 10214786].

## 2. Foreign Bodies in the Lower Respiratory Tract

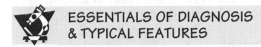

### ESSENTIALS OF DIAGNOSIS & TYPICAL FEATURES

- *Sudden onset of coughing, wheezing, or respiratory distress.*
- *Asymmetrical physical findings of decreased breath sounds or localized wheezing.*
- *Asymmetrical radiographic findings, especially with forced expiratory view.*

## Clinical Findings

### A. SYMPTOMS AND SIGNS

Respiratory symptoms and signs vary depending on the site of obstruction and the duration following the acute episode. For example, a large or central airway obstruction may cause marked distress. The acute cough or wheezing caused by a foreign body in the lower respiratory tract may diminish over time only to recur later and present as chronic cough or persistent wheezing. Foreign body aspiration should be suspected in children with chronic cough, persistent wheezing, or recurrent pneumonia. Long-standing foreign bodies may lead to bronchiectasis or lung abscess. Hearing asymmetrical breath sounds or localized wheezing also suggests a foreign body.

### B. IMAGING

Inspiratory and forced expiratory (obtained by manually compressing the abdomen during expiration) chest radiographs should be obtained if foreign body aspiration is suspected. The initial inspiratory view may show localized hyperinflation due to the ball-valve effect of the foreign body, causing distal air trapping. A positive forced expiratory study shows a mediastinal shift away from the affected side. If airway obstruction is complete, atelectasis and related volume loss will be the major radiologic findings. Chest fluoroscopy is an alternative approach for detecting air trapping and mediastinal shift.

## Treatment

If the imaging is positive or if, despite negative imaging, clinical suspicion persists, a bronchoscopy is indicated. Rigid bronchoscopy under general anesthesia is recommended. Flexible bronchoscopy may be helpful for follow-up evaluations (after the foreign object has been removed).

Children with suspected acute foreign body aspiration should be admitted to the hospital for evaluation and treatment. Chest postural drainage is no longer recommended because the foreign body may become dislodged and obstruct a major central airway. Bronchoscopy should not be delayed in children with respiratory distress but should be performed as soon as the diagnosis is made—even in children with more chronic symptoms. Following the removal of the foreign body, β-adrenergic nebulization treatments followed by chest physiotherapy are recommended to help clear related mucus or bronchospasm. Failure to identify a foreign body in the lower respiratory tract can result in bronchiectasis and lung abscess. This risk justifies an aggressive approach to suspected foreign bodies in suspicious cases.

Dunn GR et al: Management of suspected foreign body aspiration in children. Clin Otolaryngol 2002;27:384 [PMID: 12383302].

Rovin JD, Rodgers BM: Pediatric foreign body aspiration. Pediatr Rev 2000;21:86 [PMID: 10702322].

Skoulakis CE et al: Bronchoscopy for foreign body removal in children: A review and analysis of 210 cases. Int J Pediatr Otorhinolaryngol 2000;53:143 [PMID: 10906520].

## BRONCHITIS

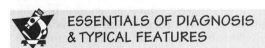

### ESSENTIALS OF DIAGNOSIS & TYPICAL FEATURES

- *Cough that usually progresses from dry to productive.*
- *Rhonchi heard on auscultation.*

## General Considerations

Bronchitis is inflammation of the major conducting airways within the lung and is unusual as an isolated entity in children. However, inflammation within this section of the airways commonly occurs in viral lower respiratory tract infections, on exposure to environmental irritants including tobacco smoke, and in association with other disease entities such as CF or primary ciliary dyskinesia. In adults, the diagnosis of chronic bronchitis is based on a history of at least 3 months of productive cough occurring for 2 or more years, but no generally acceptable criteria for this diagnosis exist in children.

## Clinical Findings

### A. Symptoms and Signs

Acute bronchitis usually begins as a nonproductive cough that may be associated with other features of an upper respiratory illness of viral origin. The longer the cough persists, the more likely it is to become productive. In general, children with uncomplicated acute bronchitis appear nontoxic, and fever, if present, is low-grade. Diffuse rhonchi are heard on auscultation. In uncomplicated acute bronchitis, mucus production decreases, and the cough disappears over a period of 7–10 days.

### B. Laboratory Findings

The white blood count is usually normal and, if elevated, may suggest a viral infection. Pulmonary function tests may reveal variable degrees of airway obstruction.

### C. Imaging

Radiographic examination of the chest may be normal or may show a mild increase in bronchovascular markings.

## Differential Diagnosis

Most attacks of acute bronchitis are caused by viral infections. Certain viral pathogens (eg, adenovirus) can produce a more severe clinical picture that resembles a pertussis-like illness. Bacteria that may produce disease in which bronchitis is a prominent symptom include *Bordetella pertussis, Mycobacterium tuberculosis, Corynebacterium diphtheriae,* and *Mycoplasma pneumoniae.*

Noninfectious diseases need to be considered in the evaluation of acute bronchitis that differs from the clinical picture described earlier and in cases of chronic or recurrent bronchitis. Asthma may present as a persistent cough with little or no wheezing. Sinus infections may provide a source of persistent irritation to the respiratory tract and lead to a chronic cough. CF, an immunodeficiency, or primary ciliary dyskinesia must also be considered if the bronchitis persists or recurs and if bronchiectasis is present or suspected. In the younger child, respiratory tract anomalies, foreign bodies, and recurrent aspiration must also be considered. Tobacco or marijuana smoking may contribute to this process in

older children. In patients of all ages, the potential role of irritants within the environment must also be evaluated.

## Complications

In otherwise healthy children, complications of acute bronchitis are extremely uncommon. If persistent, bronchiectasis, an irreversible dilatation and destruction of the bronchial walls, can result.

## Treatment

When bronchitis is secondary to an uncomplicated acute viral infection, supportive therapy is all that is necessary. Expectorants and cough suppressants, though commonly used, are seldom indicated. Avoidance of irritants during the viral infection may also decrease symptoms and morbidity. Antibiotics are indicated if a bacterial infection of the airway is suspected or proven.

Gonzales R, Sande MA: Uncomplicated acute bronchitis. Ann Intern Med 2000;133:981 [PMID: 11119400].

Loughlin GM: Bronchitis. In Chernick V, Boat TF (eds): *Kendig's Disorders of the Respiratory Tract in Children,* 6th ed. WB Saunders, 1998.

Meeks M, Bush A: Primary ciliary dyskinesia. Pediatr Pulmonol 2000;29:307 [PMID: 10738019].

## BRONCHIOLITIS

### ESSENTIALS OF DIAGNOSIS & TYPICAL FEATURES

- *Clinical syndrome characterized by coughing, tachypnea, labored breathing, and/or hypoxia.*
- *Irritability, poor feeding, vomiting.*
- *Wheezing and crackles on chest auscultation.*

Bronchiolitis is the most common serious acute respiratory illness in infants and young children. One to three percent of infants with bronchiolitis will require hospitalization, especially during the winter months. The typical presentation is acute onset of tachypnea, cough, rhinorrhea, and expiratory wheezing. Respiratory syncytial virus (RSV) is by far the most common pathogen; parainfluenza and influenza viruses, adenovirus, *Mycoplasma, Chlamydia, Ureaplasma,* and *Pneumocystis* are less common causes of bronchiolitis during early infancy. Major concerns include not only the acute effects of bronchiolitis but also the possible development of chronic airway hyperreactivity (asthma). Bronchiolitis due to RSV infection contributes substantially to morbidity and mortality in children with underlying medical disorders, including chronic lung disease of prematurity, CF, congenital heart disease, and immunodeficiency.

## Clinical Findings

### A. SYMPTOMS AND SIGNS

The usual course of RSV bronchiolitis is 1–2 days of fever, rhinorrhea, and cough, followed by wheezing, tachypnea, and respiratory distress. Typically the breathing pattern is shallow, with rapid respirations. Nasal flaring, cyanosis, retractions, and rales may be present, along with prolongation of the expiratory phase and wheezing, depending on the severity of illness. Some young infants present with apnea and few findings on auscultation but may subsequently develop rales, rhonchi, and expiratory wheezing.

### B. LABORATORY FINDINGS

The peripheral white blood cell count may be normal or may show a mild lymphocytosis.

### C. IMAGING

Chest radiographic findings typically include hyperinflation with mild interstitial infiltrates, but segmental atelectasis is common.

## Prevention & Treatment

The most effective prevention against RSV infection is to use proper hand-washing techniques and to reduce exposure to potential environmental risk factors. Major challenges have impeded the development of an RSV vaccine, but a licensed product may be expected in the near future. Prophylaxis with a monoclonal antibody (palivizumab or Synagis) has proven effective in reducing the rate of hospitalization in high-risk premature infants and those with chronic cardiopulmonary conditions.

Although most children with RSV bronchiolitis are readily treated as outpatients, hospitalization is frequently required in young infants (younger than 6 months of age) and in patients with hypoxemia on room air, a history of apnea, moderate tachypnea with feeding difficulties, marked respiratory distress with retractions, or underlying chronic cardiopulmonary disorders. Supportive strategies including frequent suctioning and providing adequate fluids to maintain hydration form the mainstays of treatment for bronchiolitis. If hypoxemia is present, supplemental oxygen should be administered. Although bronchodilators and corticosteroids may attenuate airway obstruction, their use remains controversial and empiric, and patients should be assessed individually to determine responsiveness.

In immunocompromised patients, especially bone marrow transplant recipients, a combination of RSV intravenous immune globulin (RSV-IVIG) and the antiviral ribavirin has been tried. Therapy for RSV, however, remains limited, controversial, and mostly supportive.

## Prognosis

The prognosis for the majority of infants with acute bronchiolitis is very good. With improved supportive care and prophylaxis with palivizumab, the mortality rate among high-risk infants has decreased substantially.

Paes BA: Current strategies in the prevention of respiratory syncytial virus disease. Paediatr Respir Rev 2003;4:21 [PMID: 12615029].

Schlesinger C, Koss MN: Bronchiolitis: Update 2001. Curr Opin Pulm Med 2002;8:112 [PMID: 11845006].

# BRONCHIECTASIS

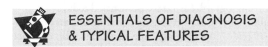

### ESSENTIALS OF DIAGNOSIS & TYPICAL FEATURES

- *Chronic cough with sputum production.*
- *Rhonchi and/or wheezes on chest auscultation.*
- *Diagnosis confirmed by high-resolution CT scan.*

## General Considerations

Bronchiectasis is the permanent dilatation of bronchi. The dilation may be regular, with the airway continuing to have a smooth outline (cylindric bronchiectasis); irregular, with areas of dilation and constriction (varicose bronchiectasis); or marked, with destruction of structural components of the airway wall (saccular or cystic bronchiectasis).

Bronchiectasis results from airway obstruction by retained mucus secretions or inflammation in response to chronic or repeated infection. It occurs either as a consequence of a preceding illness (severe pneumonia or foreign body aspiration) or as a manifestation of an underlying systemic disorder (CF or primary ciliary dyskinesia).

## Clinical Findings

### A. SYMPTOMS AND SIGNS

Persons with bronchiectasis will typically have chronic cough, purulent sputum, fever, and weight loss. Recurrent respiratory infections and dyspnea on exertion are also common. Some children present with recurrent fevers. Hemoptysis occurs less frequently in children than in adults with bronchiectasis. On physical examination, finger clubbing may be seen, and there may be evidence of sinusitis. Persistent moist rales, rhonchi, and decreased air entry are often noted over the bronchiectatic area when saccular changes are present.

### B. LABORATORY FINDINGS AND IMAGING

Cultures from the lower respiratory tract usually reveal normal oropharyngeal flora. These include *Streptococcus pneumoniae, Staphylococcus aureus,* and nontypable *H influenzae. Pseudomonas aeruginosa* can also be found in children with bronchiectasis, even in those without CF.

Chest radiographs may be mildly abnormal with slightly increased bronchovascular markings or areas of atelectasis, or they may demonstrate cystic changes in one or more areas of the lung. The extent of bronchiectasis is best defined by high-resolution CT scan of the lung, which often reveals far wider involvement of lung than expected from the plain chest radiograph. Contrast bronchography is rarely performed today.

Pulmonary function testing often reveals an obstructive pattern even in the absence of asthma, CF, or other disease processes leading to airway obstruction. Evaluation of lung function after use of a bronchodilator is helpful in assessing the benefit a patient may have from bronchodilators. Serial assessments of lung function help define the progression or resolution of the disease.

## Differential Diagnosis

Bronchiectasis has numerous causes. It can occur following severe respiratory tract infections by bacteria (*Bordetella pertussis*), viruses (adenovirus), or other organisms (*Mycobacterium tuberculosis*). Bronchiectasis is commonly seen in patients with CF, immunodeficiency, rheumatic conditions, and primary ciliary dyskinesia. Other diagnostic considerations include foreign body aspiration, chronic aspiration of gastric or oropharyngeal contents, and allergic bronchopulmonary aspergillosis.

And though uncommon, bronchiectasis may result from defective development of bronchial cartilage (Williams–Campbell syndrome) and developmental failure of elastic and muscular tissues of the trachea and bronchi (tracheobronchomegaly, or Mounier–Kuhn syndrome).

## Complications

Major concerns are severe pneumonia, hemoptysis, and cor pulmonale. Less frequent complications are abscesses of the lung, empyema, and bronchopleural fistula.

## Treatment

Aggressive antibiotic therapy during pulmonary exacerbations and routine airway clearance are mainstays of treatment. Inhaled mucolytic agents and bronchodilators may also be of benefit in individual patients.

Surgical removal of an area of lung affected with severe bronchiectasis is considered when the response to medical therapy is poor. Other indications for operation include severe localized disease, repeated hemoptysis, and recurrent pneumonia in one area of lung. If bronchiectasis is widespread, surgical resection offers little advantage.

## Prognosis

The prognosis depends on the underlying cause and severity of bronchiectasis, the extent of lung involvement, and the response to medical management. Good pulmonary hygiene and avoidance of infectious complications in the involved areas of lung may reverse cylindric bronchiectasis.

Barker AF: Bronchiectasis. N Engl J Med 2002;346:1383 [PMID: 11986413].

Chang AB et al: Non-CF bronchiectasis: Clinical and HRCT evaluation. Pediatr Pulmonol 2003;35:477 [PMID: 12746947].

# BRONCHIOLITIS OBLITERANS

Bronchiolitis obliterans is characterized by obstruction of bronchi and bronchioles by fibrous tissue. The disorder follows damage to the lower respiratory tract, such as inhalation of toxic gases, infections (adenovirus, influenza virus, rubeola virus, *Bordetella, Mycoplasma*), connective tissue diseases, transplantation, and aspiration. Bronchiolitis obliterans may also develop in children who have Stevens–Johnson syndrome with pulmonary involvement. Many cases of bronchiolitis obliterans are idiopathic. Adenovirus-induced bronchiolitis obliterans occurs more frequently in the Native-American population and in Polynesian children in New Zealand.

## Clinical Findings

### A. SYMPTOMS AND SIGNS

Bronchiolitis obliterans should be considered when persistent cough, wheezing, or sputum production is present after an episode of acute pneumonia. Prolonged rales or wheezing or persistent exercise intolerance following a pulmonary insult should also suggest this disease.

### B. LABORATORY FINDINGS AND IMAGING

Chest radiograph abnormalities include evidence of localized or generalized air trapping as well as (in some cases) nodular densities and alveolar opacification. Scattered areas of matched decreases in ventilation and perfusion are seen when the lung is scanned. Pulmonary angiograms reveal decreased vasculature in involved lung, and bronchograms show marked pruning of the bronchial tree. An assessment of lung function demonstrates an obstructive process that may be combined with evidence of restriction. Inhaled bronchodilators or corticosteroids provide little improvement in lung function.

## Differential Diagnosis

Poorly treated asthma, CF, and bronchopulmonary dysplasia must be considered in children with persistent airway obstruction. A trial of medications (including bronchodilators and corticosteroids) may help to determine the reversibility of the process when the primary differential is between asthma and bronchiolitis obliterans. Although the results of imaging and pulmonary function testing are very suggestive, the most definitive way to establish a diagnosis is by lung biopsy.

## Complications

Sequelae of bronchiolitis obliterans include persistent airway obstruction, recurrent wheezing, bronchiectasis, chronic atelectasis, recurrent pneumonia, and unilateral hyperlucent lung syndrome.

## Treatment

Supplemental oxygen should be given to patients with oxygen desaturation during normal activities or sleep. In addition, early treatment should be directed at preventing ongoing airway damage due to problems such as aspiration, which may be either the primary insult or an acquired problem secondary to marked hyperinflation. The effectiveness of other forms of treatment may be more difficult to evaluate. Oral and inhaled bronchodilators may reverse airway obstruction if the disease has a reactive component. Many children also receive at least one course of corticosteroid treatment in an attempt to reverse the obstruction or prevent ongoing damage. Antibiotics should be used as indicated for pneumonia.

## Prognosis

Prognosis may depend in part on the underlying cause as well as the age at which the insult occurred. The course varies from mild asthma-like symptoms to rapidly fatal deterioration despite therapy.

Kim CK et al: Bronchiolitis obliterans in the 1990s in Korea and the United States. Chest 2001;120:1101 [PMID: 11591545].

Mauad T, Dolhnikoff M; São Paulo Bronchiolitis Obliterans Study Group: Histology of childhood bronchiolitis obliterans. Pediatr Pulmonol 2002;33:466 [PMID: 12001281].

Zhang L et al: Clinical course of postinfectious bronchiolitis obliterans. Pediatr Pulmonol 2000;29:341 [PMID: 10790245].

# BRONCHOPULMONARY DYSPLASIA

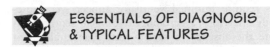

### ESSENTIALS OF DIAGNOSIS & TYPICAL FEATURES

- *Acute respiratory distress in first week of life.*
- *Required oxygen therapy or mechanical ventilation, with persistent oxygen requirement at 36 weeks' gestational age.*
- *Persistent respiratory abnormalities, including physical signs and radiographic findings.*

## General Considerations

Bronchopulmonary dysplasia (BPD) remains one of the most significant sequelae of acute respiratory distress in the neonatal intensive care unit, with an incidence of about 30% for infants with a birth weight of less than 1000 g. This disease was first characterized in 1967 when Northway and coworkers reported the clinical, radiologic, and pathologic findings in a group of premature newborns that required prolonged mechanical ventilation and oxygen therapy to treat hyaline membrane disease. The progression from acute hyaline membrane disease to chronic lung disease was divided into four stages: acute respiratory distress shortly after birth, usually hyaline membrane disease (stage I); clinical and radiographic worsening of the acute lung disease, often due to increased pulmonary blood flow secondary to a patent ductus arteriosus (stage II); and progressive signs of chronic lung disease (stages III and IV). The pathologic findings and clinical course of BPD in recent years have changed due to a combination of new therapies (surfactants, prenatal glucocorticoids, and different ventilation strategies) and increased survival of infants born at earlier gestational ages. Although the incidence of BPD has not changed, the severity of the lung disease has decreased. Pathologically this "new" BPD is characterized by a reduction in inflammation, decreased alveolar number, and a dysmorphic vascular structure.

A recent summary of a National Institutes of Health workshop on BPD proposes a definition of the disease that includes oxygen requirement for more than 28 days, a history of positive pressure ventilation or continuous positive airway pressure, and gestational age. The new definition accommodates several key observations regarding the disease, including: (1) Although most of these children were premature and had hyaline membrane disease, full-term newborns with such disorders as meconium aspiration or persistent pulmonary hypertension can also develop bronchopulmonary dysplasia; (2) some extremely preterm newborns require minimal ventilator support yet subsequently develop a prolonged oxygen requirement despite the absence of severe acute manifestations of respiratory failure; (3) newborns dying within the first weeks of life can already have the aggressive, fibroproliferative pathologic lesions that resemble bronchopulmonary dysplasia; and (4) physiologic abnormalities (increased airway resistance) and biochemical markers of lung injury (altered protease and antiprotease ratios, increased inflammatory cells and mediators), which may be predictive of bronchopulmonary dysplasia, are already present in the first week of life.

The precise mechanism that results in the development of BPD is unclear. The premature lung makes insufficient functional surfactant; furthermore, the antioxidant defense mechanisms are not sufficiently mature to protect the lung from the toxic oxygen metabolites generated from hyperoxia. Lungs destined to develop BPD show early inflammation and hypercellularity followed by healing with fibrosis. Thus abnormal lung mechanics due to structural immaturity, surfactant deficiency, atelectasis, and pulmonary edema—plus lung injury secondary to hyperoxia and mechanical ventilation—lead to further abnormalities of lung function, causing increases in ventilator and oxygen requirements and resulting in a vicious cycle that compounds the progression of lung injury. Excessive fluid administration, patent ductus arteriosus, pulmonary interstitial emphysema, pneumothorax, infection, pulmonary hypertension, and inflammatory stimuli secondary to lung injury or infection also play important roles in the pathogenesis of the disease. Although the exact mechanisms leading to chronic lung disease are not completely understood, bronchopulmonary dysplasia represents the consequences of lung injury caused by oxygen toxicity, barotrauma, and inflammation superimposed on a susceptible, generally immature lung.

## Differential Diagnosis

The radiologic appearance of BPD is changing, and severe chronic lung findings of fibrosis with infiltrate are less common. The changes in severe BPD necessitate ruling out meconium aspiration syndrome, congenital infection (eg, with cytomegalovirus [CMV] or *Ureaplasma*), cystic adenomatoid malformation, recurrent aspiration, pulmonary lymphangiectasia, total anomalous pulmonary venous return, overhydration, and idiopathic pulmonary fibrosis.

## Clinical Course & Treatment

The clinical course of infants with bronchopulmonary dysplasia ranges from a mild increased oxygen requirement that gradually resolves over a few months to more severe disease requiring chronic tracheostomy and mechanical ventilation for the first 2 years of life. In general, patients show slow, steady improvements in oxygen or ventilator requirements but can have frequent respiratory exacerbations leading to frequent and prolonged hospitalizations. Clinical management generally includes careful attention to growth, nutrition (caloric requirements of infants with oxygen dependence and respiratory distress are quite high), metabolic status, developmental and neurologic status, and related problems, along with the various cardiopulmonary abnormalities described in a later discussion.

Short courses of postnatal glucocorticoid therapy has been helpful in increasing the success of weaning from the ventilator. This therapy is controversial, however, because data show decreased alveolarization in preterm and postnatal animals given long courses of corticosteroids. Longer courses of postnatal glucocorticoids have been linked to an increased incidence of cerebral palsy. Inhaled glucocorticoids may help reduce the need for systemic steroids, but the overall incidence of bronchopulmonary dysplasia has not been affected. Early use of surfactant therapy increases the chance for survival without bronchopulmonary dysplasia and can decrease the overall mortality and reduce the need for ventilation. Thus early interventions are important prior to the development of bronchopulmonary dysplasia to decrease morbidity and mortality. Ongoing studies on the imbalance of proteolytic enzymes, elastolytic lung damage, and the role of specific antiinflammatory medications during the early development of bronchopulmonary dysplasia are needed.

Because increased airway resistance and bronchial hyperreactivity are common in affected infants, inhaled corticosteroids together with occasional use of β-adrenergic agonists are commonly part of the treatment plan. Part of the rationale for the use of corticosteroids is to decrease lung inflammation and enhance responsiveness to β-adrenergic drugs, as in the treatment of severe asthma. β-Adrenergic agonists followed by chest physiotherapy are often used for the thick secretions that may contribute to airway obstruction or recurrent atelectasis.

Although bronchial hyperreactivity in affected infants is well recognized, structural lesions (eg, subglottic stenosis, vocal cord paralysis, tracheal stenosis, tracheomalacia, bronchial stenosis, and granulomatous bronchial polyps) often contribute to airflow limitation. Children with significant stridor, sleep apnea, chronic wheezing, or excessive respiratory distress need diagnostic bronchoscopy. In addition, the contribution of gastroesophageal reflux and aspiration should be considered in the face of worsening chronic lung disease.

Infants often have recurrent pulmonary edema, which may be due to increased permeability of the injured pulmonary circulation or to increases in hydrostatic pressure if left ventricular dysfunction is present. Salt and water retention secondary to chronic hypoxemia, hypercapnia, or other stimuli may be present. Chronic or intermittent diuretic therapy is commonly used if rales or signs of persistent pulmonary edema are present and clinical studies show acute improvement in lung function. Unfortunately, diuretics often have adverse effects, including severe volume contraction, hypokalemia, alkalosis, and hyponatremia. Potassium and arginine chloride supplements are commonly required.

Infants with BPD are at risk of developing pulmonary hypertension, and in many of these children even mild hypoxemia can cause significant elevations of pulmonary arterial pressure. To minimize the harmful effects of hypoxemia, the $SaO_2$ should be kept above 93%, with care to avoid hyperoxia during retinal vascular development. Electrocardiographic and echocardiographic studies should be performed to monitor for the development of right ventricular hypertrophy. If hypertrophy persists or if it develops where it was not previously present, intermittent hypoxemia should be considered and further assessments of oxygenation pursued, especially while the infant sleeps. Even intermittent hypoxia contributes to the development or progression of pulmonary hypertension and cor pulmonale; therefore, noninvasive assessments of oxygenation must be made during all activities, including the infant's waking, sleeping, and feeding periods. Infants with a history of intubation can develop obstructive sleep apnea secondary to a high-arched palate or subglottic narrowing. Barium swallow, esophageal pH probe studies, bronchoscopy, and cardiac catheterization will diagnose unsuspected cardiac or pulmonary lesions that contribute to the underlying pathophysiology, such as aspiration, tracheomalacia, obstructive sleep apnea, and anatomic cardiac lesions. Long-term care should include monitoring for systemic hypertension and the development of left ventricular hypertrophy.

Nutritional problems in infants may be due to increased oxygen consumption, feeding difficulties, gastroesophageal reflux, and chronic hypoxemia. Hypercaloric formulas and gastrostomies are often required to ensure adequate intake while avoiding overhydration. Influenza vaccine is recommended. With the onset of acute wheezing secondary to suspected viral infection, rapid diagnostic testing for RSV infection may facilitate early treatment. Immune prophylaxis of RSV reduces the morbidity of bronchiolitis in infants with bronchopulmonary dysplasia.

For children who remain ventilator-dependent, attempts should be made to maintain $PaCO_2$ below 60 mm Hg—even when pH is normal—because of the potential adverse effects of hypercapnia on salt and water retention, cardiac function, and perhaps pulmonary vascular tone. Changes in ventilator settings in children with severe lung disease should be slow, because the effects of many of the changes may not be apparent for days. These signs may include poor feeding, irritability, weight loss, vomiting, increased retractions, wheezing, increased somnolence, and $CO_2$ retention. Medical staff should meet frequently with the parents to review progress and changes in treatment plans and thereby ease some of the family stresses involved in caring for a child who has a chronic disease. Patience, continued family support, attention to developmental issues, and speech and physical therapy help to improve the long-term outlook.

## Prognosis

Surfactant replacement therapy has had a significant effect on reducing morbidity and mortality from bronchopulmonary dysplasia. Infants of younger gestational age are surviving in greater numbers. Surprisingly, the effect of neonatal care has not decreased the incidence of bronchopulmonary dysplasia significantly, as half the survivors go on to develop this diagnosis. The disorder typically develops in the most immature infants, but the long-term outlook for most survivors is generally favorable. Long-term follow-up studies suggest that lung function may be altered for life. Hyperinflation and damage to small airways has been reported in children 10 years out from the first signs of bronchopulmonary dysplasia. In addition, these infants are at a higher risk for developing such sequelae as persistent airway hyperreactivity, exercise intolerance, pulmonary hypertension, increased risk for COPD, and perhaps abnormal lung growth. As smaller, more immature infants survive, abnormal neurodevelopmental outcomes become more likely. The incidence of cerebral palsy, hearing loss, vision abnormalities, spastic diplegia, and developmental delays is increased. Feeding abnormalities, behavior difficulties, and increased irritability have all been reported. Finally, children with bronchopulmonary dysplasia frequently develop airway obstruction, hyperreactive airways, and decreased oxygen saturation during exercise. This should be taken into account for children residing at higher altitudes. A focus on good nutrition, prophylaxis against respiratory pathogens and airway hyperreactivity, and attention to school performance continue to provide the best outcomes.

Abman SH: Bronchopulmonary dysplasia: "A vascular hypothesis." Am J Respir Crit Care Med 2001;164(10 Pt 1):1755 [PMID: 11734417].

Allen J et al; American Thoracic Society: Statement on the care of the child with chronic lung disease of infancy and childhood. Am J Respir Crit Care Med 2003;168(3):356 [PMID: 12888611].

Bancalari E et al: Bronchopulmonary dysplasia: Changes in pathogenesis, epidemiology and definition. Semin Neonatol 2003;8(1):63 [PMID: 12667831].

Charafeddine L et al: Atypical chronic lung disease patterns in neonates. Pediatrics 1999;103:759 [PMID: 10103299].

Cole CH: Inhaled glucocorticoid therapy in infants at risk for neonatal chronic lung disease. J Asthma 2000;37:533 [PMID: 11060660].

Gracey K et al: The changing face of bronchopulmonary dysplasia. Adv Neonatal Care 2002;2(6):327 [PMID: 12881945].

Jobe AH, Bancalari E: Bronchopulmonary dysplasia. Am J Respir Crit Care Med 2001;163:1723 [PMID: 11401896].

Jobe AH, Ikegami M: Prevention of bronchopulmonary dysplasia. Curr Opin Pediatr 2001;13:124 [PMID: 11317052].

Kresch MJ, Clive JM: Meta-analysis of surfactant replacement therapy of infants with birth weights less than 2000 grams. J Perinatol 1998;18:276 [PMID: 9730197].

Northway WH et al: Pulmonary disease following respiratory therapy of hyaline membrane disease: Bronchopulmonary dysplasia. N Engl J Med 1967;276:357 [PMID: 5334613].

Parker TA, Abman SH: The pulmonary circulation in bronchopulmonary dysplasia. Semin Neonatol 2003;8(1):51 [PMID: 12667830].

Saugstad OD: Bronchopulmonary dysplasia—Oxidative stress and antioxidants. Semin Neonatol 2003;8(1):39 [PMID: 12667829].

Speer CP: Inflammation and bronchopulmonary dysplasia. Semin Neonatol 2003;8(1):29 [PMID: 12667828].

# CYSTIC FIBROSIS

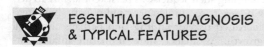

### ESSENTIALS OF DIAGNOSIS & TYPICAL FEATURES

- *Sweat chloride > 60 mmol/L.*
- *Mutated CFTR protein.*

- *Pulmonary, gastrointestinal, or hepatic dysfunction.*

## General Considerations

Cystic fibrosis is the most common lethal genetic disease in the United States, with an incidence of 1:3000–1:4000 among Caucasians. It is a major cause of pulmonary and gastrointestinal morbidity in children and a leading cause of death in early adulthood. Although CF is characterized by abnormalities in the hepatic, gastrointestinal, and male reproductive systems, lung disease is the major cause of morbidity and mortality. Almost all patients develop obstructive lung disease associated with chronic infection that leads to progressive loss of pulmonary function. The prognosis has improved steadily over the past 20 years, so that the median survival is now 33 years—perhaps because of antibiotics, better treatment of malabsorption, and development of a network of CF clinical care centers. The centers usually emphasize a multidisciplinary approach to patient care (www.cff.org).

The gene for CF is on the long arm of human chromosome 7 and codes for the cystic fibrosis transmembrane conductance regulator (CFTR) protein. CFTR functions as an ion channel and controls the movement of salt and water into and out of epithelial cells where it is expressed. Over 1000 mutations in the CF gene have been identified. The most common mutation, called delta F508, is a deletion of three base pairs at position 508 in the gene. These gene mutations lead to defects or deficiencies in CFTR, causing cells to produce abnormally thick mucus.

## Clinical Findings & Treatment

### A. CLINICAL PRESENTATIONS AND DIAGNOSIS

Approximately 15% of newborns with CF present at birth with meconium ileus, a severe intestinal obstruction resulting from inspissation of tenacious meconium in the terminal ileum. In the past, surgical removal of the meconium was common and often led to resection of bowel. Improved techniques of enema administration under radiologic observation have reduced the need for surgery.

Roughly 50% of patients with CF present in infancy with failure to thrive, respiratory compromise, or both. The age at presentation, however, can be variable; some patients are not diagnosed until adulthood. Newborn screening based on elevations of immunoreactive trypsinogen (IRT), a pancreatic enzyme precursor, in the blood is an alternative method of case identification.

In the presence of clinical symptoms such as meconium ileus, failure to thrive, or recurrent respiratory infections, or with elevated IRT levels, the diagnosis of CF is confirmed by a sweat chloride level above 60 mEq/L or by the presence of two known CF mutations. The most acceptable sweat testing procedure is the quantitative pilocarpine iontophoresis sweat test. Measurements of electrical conductivity alone can be unreliable.

## B. Gastrointestinal and Nutritional Findings and Treatment

Patients with untreated CF have abdominal distention and discomfort; bulky, greasy stools; and increased flatulence secondary to exocrine pancreatic insufficiency and malabsorption. Some infants present with hypoalbuminemia, anemia, edema, and hepatomegaly. Infants with severe protein–calorie malnutrition have particularly difficult courses, with high morbidity and mortality rates. Children and adults with CF are subject to intestinal blockage from inspissated stool. This so-called meconium ileus equivalent is now most often treated with cathartics and enemas and only rarely requires surgery. Persons with CF are more prone to intussusception (especially of the appendix) than are those without the disease.

The cornerstone of gastrointestinal treatment is pancreatic enzyme supplementation. Patients are required to take the enzyme capsules with each meal and with snacks. Newer enzyme preparations contain more lipase per capsule than older preparations; therefore, patients take fewer capsules, making administration easier. Occasionally, enzyme supplementation alone does not control the malabsorption, and antacids are added to the regimen.

Individuals with CF may have fat-soluble vitamin deficiency, hypoalbuminemia, and poor growth with decreased stores of body fat. In the past, fat-restricted diets were recommended. It is now recognized that persons with CF need all the calories they can take, and unrestricted diets are the norm in most centers. Moreover, caloric supplements, such as high-calorie commercial supplements or formulas or food modules (including Polycose and medium-chain triglycerides), are often added to the patient's diet. In patients who do not respond to oral supplementation, night-time nasogastric feeding or feeding by means of gastrostomy or jejunostomy has been tried. Although there is general agreement that quality of life is enhanced by improved nutrition, it is not known whether aggressive nutritional treatment increases longevity. The goals of nutritional treatment are to achieve normal height and weight. Patients may require many more calories than predicted because of stool loss of fat and protein and ongoing pulmonary infection and inflammation.

## C. Pulmonary Findings and Treatment

Infants with CF frequently have respiratory symptoms severe enough to require hospitalization. Cough, tachypnea, rales, and wheezing are common findings. RSV infection is associated with added morbidity in early infancy. Some patients develop cough only later in childhood or adolescence, but by adulthood almost all persons with CF have productive coughs. In more advanced disease, hemoptysis due to bronchiectasis, exercise limitation, and cor pulmonale may be present. Rales may be heard on physical examination. Clubbing also develops as the lung disease progresses.

Pulmonary function abnormalities initially show obstructive patterns with diminished flow rates and increased lung volumes. As the disease progresses, vital capacity is also affected. The incidence of airway reactivity in CF has been estimated to be 25–50%, several times the incidence in the general population. Initially, the airway is colonized with *Staphylococcus aureus,* but in most persons *Pseudomonas aeruginosa* eventually becomes the predominant pathogen. Acquisition of the characteristic mucoid *Pseudomonas* is associated with a more rapid decline in pulmonary function. In addition, infection with *Burkholderia cepacia* has been associated with rapid deterioration and death. Pathologically, the earliest lesions involve hyperplasia of the mucus glands of the bronchial epithelium and mucosal and submucosal cellular infiltrates. Bronchiolectasis and bronchiectasis throughout all lung fields usually follow.

Airway clearance therapy and aggressive antibiotic use form the mainstays of treatment for CF lung disease. Two evidence-based medications that are now routinely used in many persons with CF are inhaled recombinant human DNase (Pulmozyme) and inhaled tobramycin (TOBI). These therapies have been shown to maintain lung function and reduce the need for hospitalizations and intravenous antibiotics. Bronchodilators and antiinflammatory therapies are also frequently used.

Although corticosteroids have been shown to be effective in maintaining lung function in persons with CF, adverse effects, including glucose intolerance, frank diabetes, and decreased linear growth, have limited their use. Persons with CF derive hope from the range of agents being evaluated for restoring CFTR function. Gene therapy trials are also under way.

A subgroup of patients with CF have frequent pulmonary exacerbations characterized by difficult breathing, increased sputum production, decreased exercise tolerance, and diminished pulmonary function. These patients often benefit from hospital treatment, including intensified airway clearance therapy, intravenous antibiotics, bronchodilators, and concentrated efforts at nutritional rehabilitation. Increasingly, outpatient intravenous therapy is being used to shorten or eliminate the hospital stay.

### D. HEPATIC DISEASE

Although most patients with CF have cirrhosis at autopsy, only a small percentage develop portal hypertension. In these individuals, however, the clinical findings of the liver disease may be severe, with esophageal varices leading to life-threatening gastrointestinal bleeding and hypersplenism requiring splenic embolization.

### E. REPRODUCTIVE TRACT INVOLVEMENT

Failure of development of the vas deferens leaves more than 95% of males with CF infertile. CF is occasionally diagnosed through infertility evaluations in men with relatively mild involvement of the respiratory and gastrointestinal tracts. In general, women with CF are fertile, but pregnancy may place considerable stress on patients with limited pulmonary function.

## Prognosis

The rate of progression of lung involvement usually determines survival. Most patients now reach adulthood. Lung transplant for end-stage disease is an accepted treatment. In addition, new treatments, including gene therapy trials, are being developed based on improved understanding of the disease at the cellular and molecular levels.

Ratjen F, Doring G: Cystic fibrosis. Lancet 2003;361:681 [PMID: 12606185].

Welsh MJ et al: Cystic fibrosis. In Scriver CR et al (eds): *The Metabolic and Molecular Bases of Inherited Disease*, McGraw Hill, 2001, pp 521–588.

# CONGENITAL MALFORMATIONS OF THE LUNG

What follows is a brief description of selected congenital pulmonary malformations.

# PULMONARY AGENESIS & HYPOPLASIA

With unilateral pulmonary agenesis (complete absence of one lung), the trachea continues into a main bronchus and often has complete tracheal rings. The left lung is affected more often than the right. With compensatory postnatal growth, the remaining lung often herniates into the contralateral chest. Chest radi-ographs show a mediastinal shift toward the affected side, and vertebral abnormalities may be present. Absent or incomplete lung development may be associated with other congenital abnormalities, such as absence of one or both kidneys or fusion of ribs, and the outcome is primarily related to the severity of associated lesions. About 50% of patients survive; the mortality rate is higher with agenesis of the right lung than of the left lung. This difference is probably not related to the higher incidence of associated anomalies but rather to a greater shift in the mediastinum that leads to tracheal compression and distortion of vascular structures.

Pulmonary hypoplasia is incomplete development of one or both lungs, characterized by a reduction in alveolar number and a reduction in airway branches. Pulmonary hypoplasia is present in up to 10–15% of perinatal autopsies. The hypoplasia can be a result of an intrathoracic mass, resulting in lack of space for the lungs to grow; decreased size of the thorax; decreased fetal breathing movements; decreased blood flow to the lungs; or possibly a primary mesodermal defect affecting multiple organ systems. Congenital diaphragmatic hernia is the most common cause, with an incidence of 1:2200 births. Other causes include extralobar sequestration, diaphragmatic eventration or hypoplasia, thoracic neuroblastoma, fetal hydrops, and fetal hydrochylothorax. Chest cage abnormalities, diaphragmatic elevation, oligohydramnios, chromosomal abnormalities, severe musculoskeletal disorders, and cardiac lesions may also result in hypoplastic lungs. Postnatal factors may play important roles. For example, infants with advanced bronchopulmonary dysplasia can have pulmonary hypoplasia.

## Clinical Findings

### A. SYMPTOMS AND SIGNS

The clinical presentation is highly variable and is related to the severity of hypoplasia as well as associated abnormalities. Lung hypoplasia is often associated with pneumothorax. Some newborns present with perinatal stress, severe acute respiratory distress, and persistent pulmonary hypertension of the newborn secondary to primary pulmonary hypoplasia (without associated anomalies). Children with lesser degrees of hypoplasia may present with chronic cough, tachypnea, wheezing, and recurrent pneumonia.

### B. LABORATORY FINDINGS AND IMAGING

Chest radiographic findings include variable degrees of volume loss in a small hemithorax with mediastinal shift. Pulmonary agenesis should be suspected if tracheal deviation is evident on the chest radiograph. The chest CT scan is the optimal diagnostic imaging procedure if the chest radiograph is not definitive. Ventilation–perfusion scans, angiography, and bronchoscopy are often helpful in the evaluation, demonstrating decreased pulmonary vascularity or premature blunting of airways associated with the maldeveloped lung tissue. The degree of respiratory impairment is defined by analysis of arterial blood gases.

## Treatment & Prognosis

Treatment is supportive. The outcome is determined by the severity of underlying medical problems, the extent of the hypoplasia, and the degree of pulmonary hypertension.

Chinoy MR: Pulmonary hypoplasia and congenital diaphragmatic hernia: Advances in the pathogenetics and regulation of lung development. J Surg Res 2002;106(1):209 [PMID: 12127828].

Laudy JA, Wladimiroff JW: The fetal lung. 2: Pulmonary hypoplasia. Ultrasound Obstet Gynecol 2000;16(5):482 [PMID: 11169336].

Nowotny T et al: Right-sided pulmonary aplasia: Longitudinal lung function studies in two cases and comparison to results from term healthy neonates. Pediatr Pulmonol 1998;26:138 [PMID: 9727767].

Winn HN et al: Neonatal pulmonary hypoplasia and perinatal mortality in patients with midtrimester rupture of amniotic membranes—a critical analysis. Am J Obstet Gynecol 2000; 182.1630 [PMID. 10871491].

## PULMONARY SEQUESTRATION

Pulmonary sequestration is nonfunctional pulmonary tissue that does not communicate with the tracheobronchial tree and receives its blood supply from one or more anomalous systemic arteries. This abnormality originates during the embryonic period of lung development. It is classified as either extralobar or intralobar. Extralobar sequestration is a mass of pulmonary parenchyma anatomically separate from the normal lung, with a distinct pleural investment. Its blood supply derives from the systemic circulation (more typical), from pulmonary vessels, or from both. Rarely it communicates with the esophagus or stomach. Pathologically, extralobar sequestration appears as a solitary thoracic lesion near the diaphragm. Abdominal sites are rare. Size varies from 0.5 to 12 cm. The left side is involved in over 90% of cases. In contrast to intralobar sequestrations, venous drainage is usually through the systemic or portal venous system.

Histologic findings include uniformly dilated bronchioles, alveolar ducts, and alveoli. Occasionally the bronchial structure appears normal; however, often the cartilage in the wall is deficient, or no cartilage-containing structures can be found. Lymphangiectasia is sometimes found within the lesion. Extralobar sequestration can be associated with other anomalies, including bronchogenic cysts, heart defects, and diaphragmatic hernia, the latter occurring in over half of cases.

Intralobar sequestration is an isolated segment of lung within the normal pleural investment that often receives blood from one or more arteries arising from the aorta or its branches. Intralobar sequestration is usually found within the lower lobes (98%), two thirds are found on the left side, and it is rarely associated with other congenital anomalies (less than 2% versus 50% with extralobar sequestration). It rarely presents in the newborn period (unlike extralobar sequestration). Some researchers have hypothesized that intralobar sequestration is an acquired lesion secondary to chronic infection. Clinical presentation includes chronic cough, wheezing, or recurrent pneumonias. Rarely, patients with intralobar sequestration can present with hemoptysis. Diagnosis is often made by angiography, which shows large systemic arteries perfusing the lesion. Recently, spiral CT scans with contrast, or magnetic resonance angiography, have proven useful in identifying anomalous systemic arterial supply to the lung. Treatment is usually by surgical resection.

Alton H: Pulmonary vascular imaging. Paediatr Respir Rev 2001;2(3):227. [PMID: 12052324].

Blesovsky A: Pulmonary sequestration. A report of an unusual case and a review of the literature. Thorax 1967;22(4):351 [PMID: 6035799].

Conran RM, Stocker JT: Extralobar sequestration with frequently associated congenital cystic adenomatoid malformation, type 2: Report of 50 cases. Pediatr Dev Pathol 1999;2:454 [PMID: 10441623].

Halkic N et al: Pulmonary sequestration: A review of 26 cases. Eur J Cardiothorac Surg 1998;14(2):127 [PMID: 9754996].

Salmons S: Pulmonary sequestration. Neonatal Netw 2000;19(7): 27 [PMID: 11949021].

Zylak CJ et al: Developmental lung anomalies in the adult: Radiologic-pathologic correlation. Radiographics 2002;22 Spec No:S25 [PMID: 12376599].

## CONGENITAL LOBAR EMPHYSEMA

Patients with congenital lobar emphysema—also known as infantile lobar emphysema, congenital localized emphysema, unilobar obstructive emphysema, congenital hypertrophic lobar emphysema, or congenital lobar overinflation—present most commonly with severe neonatal respiratory distress or progressive respiratory impairment during the first year of life. Rarely the mild or intermittent nature of the symptoms in older children or young adults results in delayed diagnosis. Most patients are white males. Although the cause of congenital lobar emphysema is not well understood, some lesions show bronchial cartilaginous dysplasia due to abnormal orientation or distribution of the bronchial cartilage. This leads to expiratory collapse, producing obstruction and the symptoms outlined in the following discussion.

## Clinical Findings

### A. SYMPTOMS AND SIGNS

Clinical features include tachypnea, cyanosis, wheezing, retractions, and cough. Breath sounds are reduced on the affected side, perhaps with hyperresonance to percussion, mediastinal displacement, and bulging of the chest wall on the affected side.

### B. IMAGING

Radiologic findings include overdistention of the affected lobe (usually an upper or middle lobe; > 99%), with wide separation of bronchovascular markings, collapse of adjacent lung, shift of the mediastinum away from the affected side, and a depressed diaphragm on the affected side. The radiographic diagnosis may be confusing in the newborn because of retention of alveolar fluid in the affected lobe causing the appearance of a homogeneous density. Other diagnostic studies include chest radiograph with fluoroscopy, ventilation–perfusion study, and chest CT scan followed by bronchoscopy, angiography, and exploratory thoracotomy.

## Differential Diagnosis

The differential diagnosis of congenital lobar emphysema includes pneumothorax, pneumatocele, atelectasis with compensatory hyperinflation, diaphragmatic hernia, and congenital cystic adenomatoid malformation. The most common site of involvement is the left upper lobe (42%) or right middle lobe (35%). Evaluation must differentiate regional obstructive emphysema from lobar hyperinflation secondary to an uncomplicated ball-valve mechanism due to extrinsic compression from a mass (ie, bronchogenic cyst, tumor, lymphadenopathy, foreign body, pseudotumor or plasma cell granuloma, vascular compression) or intrinsic obstruction from a mucus plug due to infection and inflammation from various causes.

## Treatment

When respiratory distress is marked, a segmental or complete lobectomy is usually required. Less symptomatic older children may do equally well with or without lobectomy.

Al-Bassam A et al: Congenital cystic disease of the lung in infants and children (experience with 57 cases). Eur J Pediatr Surg 1999;9:364 [PMID: 10661844].

Babu R et al: Prenatal sonographic features of congenital lobar emphysema. Fetal Diagn Ther 2001;16(4):200 [PMID: 11399878].

Horak E et al: Congenital cystic lung disease: Diagnostic and therapeutic considerations. Clin Pediatr 2003;42(3):251 [PMID: 12739924].

Mandelbaum I et al: Congenital lobar obstructive emphysema: Report of eight cases and literature review. Ann Surg 1965;162(6):1075 [PMID: 5845589].

Ozcelik U et al: Congenital lobar emphysema: Evaluation and long-term follow-up of thirty cases at a single center. Pediatr Pulmonol 2003;35(5):384 [PMID: 12687596].

# CONGENITAL CYSTIC ADENOMATOID MALFORMATION

Patients with congenital cystic adenomatoid malformations (CAMs), which are unilateral hamartomatous lesions, generally present with marked respiratory distress within the first days of life. This disorder accounts for 95% of cases of congenital cystic lung disease.

Right and left lungs are involved with equal frequency. These lesions originate during the first 4–6 weeks of gestation during the embryonic period of lung development. These lesions appear as gland-like space-occupying masses or have an increase in terminal respiratory structures, forming intercommunicating cysts of various sizes, lined by cuboidal or ciliated pseudostratified columnar epithelium. They may have polypoid formations of mucosa, with focally increased elastic tissue in the cyst wall beneath the bronchial type of epithelium. Air passages appear malformed and tend to lack cartilage.

There are three types of such malformations. Type 1 is most common (55%) and consists of single or multiple large cysts (> 2 cm in diameter) with features of mature lung tissue. Type 1 is amenable to surgical resection. A mediastinal shift is evident on examination or chest radiograph in 80% of patients and can mimic infantile lobar emphysema. Approximately 75% of type 1 lesions are on the right side. A survival rate of 90% is generally reported.

Type 2 lesions (40% of cases) consist of multiple small cysts (< 2 cm) resembling dilated simple bronchioles and are often (60%) associated with other anomalies, especially renal agenesis or dysgenesis, cardiac malformations, and intestinal atresia. Approximately 60% of type 2 lesions are on the left side. Mediastinal shift is evident less often (10%) than in type 1, and the survival rate is worse (40%).

Type 3 lesions consist of small cysts (< 0.5 cm). They appear as a bulky, firm mass. The reported survival rate is 50%.

Recently, two additional types have been described: type 0, a malformation of the proximal tracheobronchial tree (incompatible with life), and type 4, a malformation of the distal acinus. Both types are extremely uncommon.

## Clinical Findings

### A. SYMPTOMS AND SIGNS

Clinically, respiratory distress is noted soon after birth. Expansion of the cysts occurs with the onset of breathing and produces compression of normal lung areas with mediastinal herniation. Breath sounds are decreased. With type 3 lesions, dullness to percussion may be present. Older patients can present with a spontaneous pneumothorax or with pneumonia-like symptoms.

### B. IMAGING

With type 1 lesions, chest radiograph shows an intrapulmonary mass of soft tissue density with scattered radiolucent areas of varying sizes and shapes, usually with a mediastinal shift and pulmonary herniation. Placement of a radiopaque feeding tube into the stomach helps in the differentiation from diaphragmatic hernia. Type 2 lesions appear similar except that the cysts are smaller. Type 3 lesions may appear as a solid homogeneous mass filling the hemithorax and causing a marked mediastinal shift. Differentiation from sequestration is not difficult because congenital cystic adenomatoid malformations have no systemic blood supply.

## Treatment

Treatment of types 1 and 3 lesions involves surgical removal of the affected lobe. Resection is often indicated because of the risk of infection and air trapping, since the malformation communicates with the tracheobronchial tree but mucous clearance is compromised. Because type 2 lesions are often associated with other severe anomalies, management may be more complex. Segmental resection is not feasible because smaller cysts may expand after removal of the more obviously affected area. CAMs have been reported to have malignant potential; therefore, expectant management with observation alone should proceed with caution. Recent development of intrauterine surgery for congenital malformations has led to promising results.

Breckenridge RL et al: Congenital cystic adenomatoid malformation of the lung. J Pediatr 1965;67(5):863 [PMID: 5845450].

Duncombe GJ et al: Prenatal diagnosis and management of congenital cystic adenomatoid malformation of the lung. Am J Obstet Gynecol 2002;187(4):950 [PMID: 12388984].

MacSweeney F et al: An assessment of the expanded classification of congenital cystic adenomatoid malformations and their relationship to malignant transformation. Am J Surg Pathol 2003;27(8):1139 [PMID: 12883247].

# ACQUIRED DISORDERS INVOLVING ALVEOLI
## BACTERIAL PNEUMONIA

 **ESSENTIALS OF DIAGNOSIS & TYPICAL FEATURES**

- *Fever, cough, dyspnea.*
- *Abnormal chest examination (rales or decreased breath sounds).*
- *Abnormal chest radiograph (infiltrates, hilar adenopathy, pleural effusion).*

## General Considerations

Bacterial pneumonia is inflammation of the lung classified according to the infecting organism. It usually develops when one or more of the defense mechanisms normally protecting the lung is inadequate. Patients with the following problems are particularly predisposed to this disease: aspiration, immunodeficiency or immunosuppression, congenital anomalies (intrapulmonary sequestration, tracheoesophageal fistula, cleft palate), abnormalities in clearance of mucus (CF, ciliary dysfunction, tracheomalacia, bronchiectasis), congestive heart failure, and perinatal contamination.

## Clinical Findings

### A. SYMPTOMS AND SIGNS

The bacterial pathogen, severity of the disease, and age of the patient may cause substantial variations in the presentation of acute bacterial pneumonia. Infants may have few or nonspecific findings on history and physical examination. Immunocompetent older patients may not be extremely ill. Some patients may present with fever only or only with signs of generalized toxicity. Others may have additional symptoms or signs of lower respiratory tract disease (respiratory distress, cough, sputum production), pneumonia (rales, decreased breath sounds, dullness to percussion, abnormal tactile or vocal fremitus), or pleural involvement (splinting, pain, friction rub, dullness to percussion). Some patients may have additional extrapulmonary findings, such as meningismus or abdominal pain, due to pneumonia itself. Others may have evidence of infection at other sites due to the same organism causing their pneumonia: meningitis, otitis media, sinusitis, pericarditis, epiglottitis, or abscesses.

### B. LABORATORY FINDINGS

Elevated white blood cell counts (> 15,000/µL) frequently accompany bacterial pneumonia. However, a low white blood count (< 5000/µL) can be an ominous finding in this disease.

### C. IMAGING

Chest radiographic findings (lateral and frontal views) define bacterial pneumonia. Patchy infiltrates, atelectasis, hilar adenopathy, or pleural effusion may be observed. Radiographs should be taken in the lateral decubitus position to identify pleural fluid. Complete lobar consolidation is not a common finding in infants and children. Severity of disease may not correlate with radiographic findings. Clinical resolution precedes resolution apparent on chest radiograph.

### D. SPECIAL EXAMINATIONS

Invasive diagnostic procedures (transtracheal aspiration, bronchial brushing or washing, lung puncture, or open or thoracoscopic lung biopsy) should be undertaken in critically ill patients when other means do not adequately identify the cause (see Culture of Material from the Respiratory Tract section).

## Differential Diagnosis

The differential diagnosis of pneumonia varies with the age and immunocompetence of the host. The spectrum of potential pathogens to be considered includes aerobic, anaerobic, and acid-fast bacteria as well as *Chlamydia trachomatis* and *C psittaci*, *Rickettsia quintana* (Q fever), *Pneumocystis jiroveci*, *Bordetella pertussis*, *Mycoplasma pneumoniae*, *Legionella pneumophila*, and respiratory viruses.

Noninfectious pulmonary disease (including gastric aspiration, foreign body aspiration, atelectasis, congenital malformations, congestive heart failure, malignant growths, tumors such as plasma cell granuloma, chronic interstitial lung diseases, and pulmonary hemosiderosis) should be considered in the differential diagnosis of localized or diffuse infiltrates. When effusions are present, additional noninfectious disorders such as collagen diseases, neoplasm, and pulmonary infarction should also be considered.

## Complications

Empyema may occur frequently with staphylococcal, pneumococcal and group A β-hemolytic streptococcal disease. Distal sites of infection—meningitis, otitis media, sinusitis (especially of the ethmoids), and septicemia—may be present, particularly with disease due to *S pneumoniae* or *H influenzae*. Certain immunocompromised patients, such as those who have undergone splenectomy or who have hemoglobin SS or SC disease or thalassemia, are especially prone to overwhelming sepsis with these organisms. Distal infection of the bones, joints, or other organs (eg, liver abscess) may occur in certain hosts with specific organisms.

## Treatment

Antimicrobial therapy should be guided by Gram stain of sputum, tracheobronchial secretions, or pleural fluid if available; radiographic findings; age and known or suspected immunocompetence of the host; and local epidemiologic information. Reasonable coverage for pneumonia in the sick, immunocompromised, or debilitated patient, pending the results of bronchoalveolar lavage or thoracoscopic biopsy, should include ceftazidime, clindamycin, vancomycin, erythromycin for *Legionella* and *Mycoplasma,* and possibly trimethoprim–sulfamethoxazole for *P jiroveci*. Depending on the circumstances and the level of illness, empiric antifungal or antiviral therapy may be considered. In specific circumstances such as aspiration due to neurologic impairment or in patients with tracheostomies, clindamycin is indicated, pending culture and sensitivity studies, owing to the likely presence of resistant anaerobes.

Less severe pneumonias can often be treated with oral antibiotics based on the patient's age and suspected organism. Lobar pneumonias presumed to be due to *S pneumoniae* can be treated initially with oral β-lactams, including cefuroxime axetil, amoxicillin, or amoxicillin–clavulanate. However, persistence or worsening of symptoms within 3–5 days suggests the presence of a resistant organism, and newer quinolones, clindamycin, or vancomycin may be required. When possible, therapy can be guided by the antibiotic sensitivity pattern of the organisms isolated.

Whether a child should be hospitalized depends on his or her age, the severity of illness, the suspected organism, and the anticipated reliability of compliance at home. Home treatment is adequate for most older children. With febrile pneumonias, infants generally—and toddlers often—require admission. Moderate to severe respiratory distress, apnea, hypoxemia, poor feeding, clinical deterioration on treatment, or associated complications (large effusions, empyema, or abscess) indicate the need for immediate hospitalization. Careful follow-up within 12 hours to 5 days is often indicated in those not admitted. Cefuroxime or a macrolide, depending on the clinical picture, may be appropriate initial therapy for patients in this category.

Additional therapeutic considerations include oxygen, humidification of inspired gases, hydration and electrolyte supplementation, and nutrition. Removal of pleural fluid for diagnostic purposes is indicated initially to guide antimicrobial therapy. Many feel that early chest tube drainage of empyema fluid due to *S aureus* is indicated. Empyema due to group A β-hemolytic streptococci, *S pneumoniae* or *H influenzae* can also necessitate chest tube drainage. Repeat pleural taps should be considered in the patient who has persistent high fever for more than 10 days in association with significant pleural effusions. The persistence of organisms in this fluid or the persistence of toxicity, malaise, anorexia, and wasting in the patient suggests the potential need for pleural decortication, a procedure that can be made less morbid by thoracoscopy in skilled hands.

Endotracheal intubation or mechanical ventilation may be indicated in patients with respiratory failure or in those too debilitated or overwhelmed to handle their secretions.

## Prognosis

For the immunocompetent host in whom bacterial pneumonia is adequately recognized and treated, the survival rate is high. For example, the mortality rate from uncomplicated pneumococcal pneumonia is less than 1%. If the patient survives the initial illness, persistently abnormal pulmonary function following empyema is surprisingly uncommon, even when treatment has been delayed or inappropriate.

McCracken GH Jr: Diagnosis and management of pneumonia in children. Pediatr Infect Dis J 2000;19:924 [PMID: 11001128].

McIntosh K: Community-acquired pneumonia in children. N Engl J Med 2002;346:429 [PMID: 11832532].

Owayed AF et al: Underlying causes of recurrent pneumonia in children. Arch Pediatr Adolesc Med 2000;154:190 [PMID: 10665608].

# VIRAL PNEUMONIA

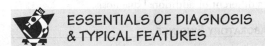

### ESSENTIALS OF DIAGNOSIS & TYPICAL FEATURES

- *Upper respiratory infection prodrome (fever, coryza, cough, hoarseness).*
- *Wheezing or rales.*
- *Myalgia, malaise, headache (older children).*

## General Considerations

Most pneumonias in children are caused by viruses. RSV, parainfluenza (1, 2, and 3) viruses, and influenza (A and B) viruses are responsible for more than 75% of cases. Severity of disease, height of fever, radiographic findings, and the characteristics of cough or lung sounds do not reliably differentiate viral from bacterial pneumonias. Furthermore, such infections may coexist. However, substantial pleural effusions, pneumatoceles, abscesses, lobar consolidation with lobar volume expansion, and "round" pneumonias are generally inconsistent with viral disease.

## Clinical Findings

### A. SYMPTOMS AND SIGNS

An upper respiratory infection frequently precedes the onset of lower respiratory disease due to viruses. Although wheezing or stridor may be prominent in viral disease, cough, signs of respiratory difficulty (retractions, grunting, nasal flaring), and physical findings (rales, decreased breath sounds) may not be distinguishable from those in bacterial pneumonia.

### B. LABORATORY FINDINGS

The peripheral white blood cell count can be normal or slightly elevated and is not useful in distinguishing viral from bacterial disease. A markedly elevated neutrophil count, however, indicates that viral disease is less likely.

Rapid viral diagnostic methods—such as fluorescent antibody tests or ELISA for RSV or other visuses—should be performed on nasopharyngeal secretions to confirm this diagnosis in high-risk patients and for epidemiology or infection control. Rapid diagnosis of RSV infection does not preclude the possibility of concomitant infection with other pathogens.

### C. IMAGING

Chest radiographs frequently show perihilar streaking, increased interstitial markings, peribronchial cuffing, or patchy bronchopneumonia. Lobar consolidation may occur, however, as in bacterial pneumonia. Patients with adenovirus disease may have severe necrotizing pneumonias, resulting in the development of pneumatoceles. Hyperinflation of the lungs may occur when involvement of the small airways is prominent.

## Differential Diagnosis

The differential diagnosis of viral pneumonia is the same as for bacterial pneumonia. Patients with prominent wheezing may have asthma, airway obstruction caused by foreign body aspiration, acute bacterial or viral tracheitis, or parasitic disease.

## Complications

Bronchiolitis obliterans or severe chronic respiratory failure may follow adenovirus pneumonia. Bronchiolitis or viral pneumonia may contribute to persistent reactive airway disease in some patients. Bronchiectasis, persistent interstitial lung diseases (fibrosis and desquamative interstitial pneumonitis), and unilateral hyperlucent lung (Swyer–James syndrome) may follow measles, adenovirus, and influenzal pneumonias. Viral pneumonia or laryngotracheobronchitis may predispose the patient to subsequent bacterial tracheitis or pneumonia as immediate sequelae. Plasma cell granuloma may develop as a rare sequel to viral or bacterial pneumonia.

## Treatment

General supportive care for viral pneumonia does not differ from that for bacterial pneumonia. Patients can be quite ill and should be hospitalized according to the level of their illness. Because bacterial disease often cannot be definitively excluded, antibiotics may be indicated.

Patients at risk for life-threatening RSV infections (eg, those with bronchopulmonary dysplasia or other severe pulmonary conditions, congenital heart disease, or significant immunocompromise) should be hospitalized and given ribavirin. Rapid viral diagnostic tests may be a useful guide for such therapy (see Bronchiolitis section regarding prevention). These high-risk patients should be immunized annually against influenza A and B viruses. Despite immunization, however, influenza can still occur. When available epidemiologic data indicate an active influenza A infection in the community, rimantadine, amantadine hydrochloride, or oseltamivir phosphate should be considered early for high-risk infants and children who appear to be infected. Children with suspected viral pneumonia should be placed in respiratory isolation.

## Prognosis

Although most children with viral pneumonia recover uneventfully, worsening reactive airway disease, abnormal pulmonary function or chest radiographs, persistent respiratory insufficiency, and even death may occur in high-risk patients such as newborns or those with underlying lung, cardiac, or immunodeficiency disease. Patients with adenovirus infection or those concomitantly infected with RSV and second pathogens such as influenza, adenovirus, CMV, or *P jiroveci* also have a poorer prognosis.

Faul JL et al: Influenza pneumonia in a paediatric lung transplant recipient. Transpl Int 2000;13:79 [PMID: 10743695].

Klig JE, Chen L. Lower respiratory infections in children. Curr Opin Pediatr 2003;15:121 [PMID: 12544283].

Shetty AK et al: Intravenous ribavirin therapy for adenovirus pneumonia. Pediatr Pulmonol 2000;29:69 [PMID: 10613789].

# CHLAMYDIAL PNEUMONIA

### ESSENTIALS OF DIAGNOSIS & TYPICAL FEATURES

- *Cough, tachypnea, rales, few wheezes, and no fever.*
- *Appropriate age: 2–12 weeks.*
- *Inclusion conjunctivitis, eosinophilia, and elevated immunoglobulins can be seen.*

## General Considerations

Pulmonary disease due to *C trachomatis* usually evolves gradually as the infection descends the respiratory tract. Infants may appear quite well despite the presence of significant pulmonary illness. Infant infections are now at epidemic proportions in urban environments worldwide. Other sexually transmitted organisms such as *Ureaplasma urealyticum* may also be widespread and contribute to lung disease in infants.

## Clinical Findings

### A. SYMPTOMS AND SIGNS

About 50% of patients with chlamydial pneumonia have active inclusion conjunctivitis or a history of it. Rhinopharyngitis with nasal discharge or otitis media may have occurred or may be currently present. Female patients may have vulvovaginitis.

Cough is usually present. It can have a staccato character and resemble the cough of pertussis. The infant is usually tachypneic. Scattered inspiratory rales are commonly heard, but wheezes rarely. Significant fever suggests a different or additional diagnosis.

### B. LABORATORY FINDINGS

Although patients may frequently be hypoxemic, $CO_2$ retention is not common. Peripheral blood eosinophilia (400 cells/$\mu$L) has been observed in about 75% of patients. Serum immunoglobulins are usually abnormal. IgM is virtually always elevated, IgG is high in many, and IgA is less frequently abnormal. *C trachomatis* can usually be identified in nasopharyngeal washings using fluorescent antibody or culture techniques.

### C. IMAGING

Chest radiographs may reveal diffuse interstitial and patchy alveolar infiltrates, peribronchial thickening, or focal consolidation. A small pleural reaction can be present. Despite the usual absence of wheezes, hyperexpansion is commonly present.

## Differential Diagnosis

Bacterial, viral, and fungal (*P jiroveci*) pneumonias should be considered. Premature infants and those with bronchopulmonary dysplasia may also have chlamydial pneumonia.

## Treatment

Erythromycin or sulfisoxazole therapy should be administered for 14 days. Hospitalization may be required for infants with significant respiratory distress, coughing paroxysms, or posttussive apnea. Oxygen therapy may be required for prolonged periods in some patients.

## Prognosis

An increased incidence of obstructive airway disease and abnormal pulmonary function tests may occur for at least 7–8 years following infection.

Hagiwara K et al: An epidemic of a pertussis-like illness caused by *Chlamydia pneumoniae*. Pediatr Infect Dis J 1999;18:271 [PMID: 10093951].

Jain S: Perinatally acquired *Chlamydia trachomatis* associated morbidity in young infants. J Matern Fetal Med 1999;8:130 [PMID: 10338068].

Principi N, Esposito S: Emerging role of *Mycoplasma pneumoniae* and *Chlamydia pneumoniae* in paediatric respiratory tract infections. Lancet Infect Dis 2001;1:334 [PMID: 11871806].

# MYCOPLASMAL PNEUMONIA

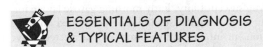

### ESSENTIALS OF DIAGNOSIS & TYPICAL FEATURES

- *Fever.*
- *Cough.*
- *Appropriate age: older than 5 years.*

## General Considerations

*M pneumoniae* is a common cause of symptomatic pneumonia in older children. Endemic and epidemic infection can occur. The incubation period is long (2–3 weeks), and the onset of symptoms is slow. Although the lung is the primary infection site, extrapulmonary complications sometimes occur.

## Clinical Findings

### A. SYMPTOMS AND SIGNS

Fever, cough, headache, and malaise are common symptoms as the illness evolves. Although cough is usually dry at the onset, sputum production may develop as the illness progresses. Sore throat, otitis media, otitis externa, and bullous myringitis may occur. Rales are frequently present on chest examination; decreased breath sounds or dullness to percussion over the involved area may be present.

### B. LABORATORY FINDINGS

The total and differential white blood cell counts are usually normal. The cold hemagglutinin titer can be determined and may be elevated during the acute presentation. A titer of 1:64 or higher supports the diagnosis. Acute and convalescent titers for *M pneumoniae* demonstrating a fourfold or greater rise in specific antibodies confirm the diagnosis.

### C. IMAGING

Chest radiographs usually demonstrate interstitial or bronchopneumonic infiltrates, frequently in the middle or lower lobes. Pleural effusions are extremely uncommon.

## Complications

Extrapulmonary involvement of the blood, CNS, skin, heart, or joints can occur. Direct Coombs-positive autoimmune hemolytic anemia, occasionally a life-threatening disorder, is the most common hematologic abnormality that can accompany *M pneumoniae* infection. Coagulation defects and thrombocytopenia can also occur. Cerebral infarction, meningoencephalitis, Guillain–Barré syndrome, cranial nerve involvement, and psychosis all have been described. A wide variety of skin rashes, including erythema multiforme and Stevens–Johnson syndrome, can occur. Myocarditis, pericarditis, and a rheumatic fever-like illness can also occur.

## Treatment

Antibiotic therapy with a macrolide for 7–10 days usually shortens the course of illness. Ciprofloxacin is a possible alternative. Supportive measures, including hydration, antipyretics, and bed rest, are helpful.

## Prognosis

In the absence of the less common extrapulmonary complications, the outlook for recovery is excellent. The extent to which *M pneumoniae* can initiate or exacerbate chronic lung disease is not well understood.

Hammerschlag MR: *Mycoplasma pneumoniae* infections. Curr Opin Infect Dis 2001;14:181 [PMID: 11979130].

Kim CK et al: Late abnormal findings on high-resolution computed tomography after *Mycoplasma pneumonia*. Pediatrics 2000;105:372 [PMID: 10654958].

# TUBERCULOSIS

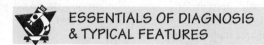

## ESSENTIALS OF DIAGNOSIS & TYPICAL FEATURES

- *Positive tuberculin skin test or anergic host.*
- *Positive culture for Mycobacterium tuberculosis.*

## General Considerations

There is a resurgence of tuberculosis in all age groups, including children. The clinical spectrum of tuberculosis includes a positive tuberculin skin test without evident disease, asymptomatic primary infection, the Ghon complex, bronchial obstruction with secondary collapse or obstructed airways, segmental lesions, calcified nodules, pleural effusions, progressive primary cavitating lesions, contiguous spread into adjacent thoracic structures, acute miliary tuberculosis, ARDS, overwhelming reactivation infection in the immunocompromised host, occult lymphohematogenous spread, and metastatic extrapulmonary involvement at almost any site. Symptoms of airway obstruction, sometimes with secondary bacterial pneumonia resulting from hilar adenopathy, are common presenting features in children.

## Clinical Findings

### A. SYMPTOMS AND SIGNS

The most important aspect of the history is contact with an individual with tuberculosis—often an elderly relative, a caregiver, or a person previously residing in a region where tuberculosis is endemic—or a history of travel to or residence in such an area. Homeless and extremely impoverished children are also at high risk, as are those in contact with high-risk adults (acquired immunodeficiency syndrome [AIDS] patients, residents or employees of correctional institutions or nursing homes, drug users, and health care workers). Once exposed, pediatric patients at risk for developing active disease include infants and those with malnutrition, AIDS, diabetes mellitus, or immunosuppression (cancer chemotherapy, corticosteroids). In suspected cases, the patient, immediate family, and suspected carriers should be tuberculin-tested. Spread is mainly respiratory, so isolated pulmonary parenchymal tuberculosis constitutes more than 95% of presenting cases. The primary focus (usually single) and associated nodal involvement may not be seen radiographically. Because healing—rather than progression—is the usual course in the uncompromised host, a positive tuberculin test may be the only manifestation. However, for patients born outside the United States, a positive test may indicate only a previous bacille Calmette–Guérin (BCG) immunization.

The tuberculous complications listed previously most often occur during the first year of infection. Thereafter, infection remains quiescent until adolescence, when reactivation of pulmonary tuberculosis is common. At any stage, chronic cough, anorexia, weight loss or failure to gain weight, and fever are useful clinical signs if present. Except in cases with complications or advanced disease, physical findings are few. Most children with pulmonary tuberculosis are asymptomatic.

### B. LABORATORY FINDINGS

A positive tuberculin skin test is defined as 10 mm or more of induration 48–72 hours after intradermal injection of 5 tuberculin units of purified protein derivative (PPD). Tine tests should not be used. Appropriate control skin tests, such as those for hypersensitivity to diphtheria–tetanus, mumps, or *Candida albicans,* should be applied at the same time PPD is applied. If the patient fails to respond to PPD and all of the controls, the possibility of tuberculosis is not excluded.

Anteroposterior and lateral chest radiographs should be obtained in all suspected cases. Culture for *M tuberculosis* is critical for proving the diagnosis and for defining drug susceptibility. Early morning gastric lavage following an overnight fast should be performed on three occasions in infants and children with suspected active pulmonary tuberculosis before treatment is started, when the severity of illness allows. Although stains for acid-fast bacilli on this material are of little value, this is the ideal culture site. Despite the increasing importance of isolating organisms because of multiple drug resistance, only 40% of children will yield positive cultures.

Sputum cultures from older children and adolescents are similarly useful. Stains and cultures of bronchial secretions are useful if bronchoscopy is performed as part of the patient's evaluation. When pleural effusions are present, pleural biopsy for cultures and histopathologic examination for granulomas or organisms provide diagnostic information. Meningeal involvement is a possibility in young children, and lumbar puncture should be considered in their initial evaluation.

## Differential Diagnosis

Fungal diseases that affect mainly the lungs, such as histoplasmosis, coccidioidomycosis, cryptococcosis, and North American blastomycosis, may resemble tuberculosis and in doubtful cases should be excluded by appropriate serologic studies. Atypical tuberculous organisms may involve the lungs, especially in the immunocompromised patient. Depending on the presentation, diagnoses such as lymphoreticular and other malignancies, collagen–vascular disorders, or other pulmonary infections may be considered.

## Complications

In addition to those complications listed in the General Considerations and Clinical Findings sections, lymphadenitis, meningitis, osteomyelitis, arthritis, enteritis, peritonitis, and renal, ocular, middle ear, and cutaneous disease may occur. The infant born to tuberculous parents is at great risk for developing illness. The possibility of life-threatening airway compromise must always be considered in patients with large mediastinal or hilar lesions.

## Treatment

Because the risk of hepatitis due to isoniazid is extremely low in children, this drug is indicated in those with a positive tuberculin skin test. This greatly reduces the risk of subsequent active disease and complications with minimal morbidity. Isoniazid plus rifampin treatment for 6 months, plus pyrazinamide during the first 2 months, is indicated when the chest radiograph is abnormal or when extrapulmonary disease is present. Without pyrazinamide, isoniazid plus rifampin must be given for 9 months. In general, the more severe tuberculous complications are treated with a larger number of drugs. Enforced, directly observed therapy (twice weekly or more often) is indicated when noncompliance is suspected. Recommendations for antituberculosis chemotherapy, based on disease stage, are continuously being updated. The most current edition of the AAP *Red Book* is a reliable source for these protocols.

Corticosteroids are used to control inflammation in selected patients with potentially life-threatening airway compression by lymph nodes, acute pericardial effusion, massive pleural effusion with mediastinal shift, or, perhaps, miliary tuberculosis with respiratory failure.

## Prognosis

In patients with an intact immune system, modern antituberculous therapy offers good potential for recovery. The outlook for patients with immunodeficiencies, organisms resistant to multiple drugs, poor drug compliance, or advanced complications is guarded. Organisms resistant to multiple drugs are increasingly common. Resistance emerges either because the physician prescribes an inadequate regimen or because the patient discontinues medications. When resistance to or intolerance of isoniazid and rifampin prevents their use, cure rates are 50% or less.

Smith KC: Tuberculosis in children. Curr Probl Pediatr 2001;31:1 [PMID: 11217659].

Starke JR: Diagnosis of tuberculosis in children. Pediatr Infect Dis J 2000;19:1095 [PMID: 11099094].

Starke JR: Directly observed therapy for tuberculosis in children. Pediatr Pulmonol 1999; (Suppl) 18:131 [PMID: 10093122].

# ASPIRATION PNEUMONIA

Patients whose anatomic defense mechanisms are impaired are at risk of aspiration pneumonia (Table 18–2). Acute disease is commonly caused by bacteria present in the mouth (especially gram-negative anaerobes). Chronic aspiration often causes recurrent bouts of acute febrile pneumonia. It may also lead to chronic focal infiltrates, atelectasis, illness resembling asthma or interstitial lung disease, or failure to thrive.

## Clinical Findings

### A. SYMPTOMS AND SIGNS

Acute onset of fever, cough, respiratory distress, or hypoxemia in a patient at risk suggests aspiration pneumonia. Chest physical findings, such as rales, rhonchi, or decreased breath sounds, may initially be limited to the lung region into which aspiration occurred. Although any region may be affected, the right side—especially the right upper lobe in the supine patient—is commonly affected. In patients with chronic aspiration,

***Table 18–2.*** Risk factors for aspiration pneumonia.

| |
|---|
| Seizures |
| Depressed sensorium |
| Recurrent gastroesophageal reflux, emesis, or gastrointestinal obstruction |
| Neuromuscular disorders with suck–swallow dysfunction |
| Anatomic abnormalities (laryngeal cleft, tracheoesophageal fistula, vocal cord paralysis) |
| Debilitating illnesses |
| Occult brainstem lesions |
| Near-drowning |
| Nasogastric, endotracheal, or tracheostomy tubes |
| Severe periodontal disease |

diffuse wheezing may occur. Generalized rales may also be present. Such patients may not develop acute febrile pneumonias.

### B. Laboratory Findings and Imaging

Chest radiographs may reveal lobar consolidation or atelectasis and focal or generalized alveolar or interstitial infiltrates. In some patients with chronic aspiration, perihilar infiltrates with or without bilateral air trapping may be seen.

In severely ill patients with acute febrile illnesses, a bacteriologic diagnosis should be made. In addition to blood cultures, cultures of tracheobronchial secretions and bronchoalveolar lavage or lung puncture specimens may be desirable (see Culture of Material from the Respiratory Tract section).

In patients with chronic aspiration pneumonitis, solid documentation of aspiration as the cause of illness may be elusive. Barium contrast studies may provide evidence of suck–swallow dysfunction, laryngeal cleft, occult tracheoesophageal fistula, or gastroesophageal reflux. Overnight or 24-hour esophageal pH probe studies may also help establish the latter. Although radionuclide scans are commonly used, the yield from such studies is disappointingly low. Rigid bronchoscopy in infants or flexible bronchoscopy in older children can be useful in more definitively excluding tracheoesophageal fistula and obtaining bronchoalveolar lavage specimens to search for lipid-laden macrophages, which can suggest chronic aspiration.

## Differential Diagnosis

In the acutely ill patient, bacterial and viral pneumonias should be considered. In the chronically ill patient, the differential diagnosis may include disorders causing recurrent pneumonia (eg, immunodeficiencies, ciliary dysfunction, foreign body), chronic wheezing, or interstitial lung disorders (see Interstitial Lung Disease section), depending on the presentation.

## Complications

Empyema or lung abscess may result from acute aspiration pneumonia. Chronic disease may result in bronchiectasis.

## Treatment

Antimicrobial therapy for acute aspiration pneumonia includes coverage for gram-negative anaerobic organisms. In general, clindamycin is appropriate initial coverage. However, in some hospital-acquired infections, additional coverage for multiply resistant *P aeruginosa*, streptococci, and other organisms may be required.

Treatment of recurrent and chronic aspiration pneumonia may include the following: surgical correction of anatomic abnormalities; improved oral hygiene; improved hydration; and inhaled bronchodilators, chest physical therapy, and suctioning. In patients with compromise of the CNS, exclusive feeding by gastrostomy and (in some) tracheostomy may be required to control airway secretions. Gastroesophageal reflux, often requiring surgical correction, is commonly present in such patients.

## Prognosis

The outlook is directly related to the disorder causing aspiration.

Brook I: Anaerobic infections in children. Microbes Infect 2002;4:1271 [PMID: 12467770].

Colombo JL, Hallberg TK: Pulmonary aspiration and lipid-laden macrophages: In search of gold (standards). Pediatr Pulmonol 1999;28:79 [PMID: 10423305].

Morton RE, Wheatley R, Minford J: Respiratory tract infection due to direct and reflux aspiration in children with severe neurodisability. Dev Med Child Neurol 1999; 41:329 [PMID: 10378759].

# PNEUMONIA IN THE IMMUNOCOMPROMISED HOST

Pneumonia in an immunocompromised host may be due to any common bacteria (streptococci, staphylococci, *M pneumoniae*) or less common pathogens such as *Toxoplasma gondii, P jiroveci, Aspergillus* species, *Mucor, Candida* species, *Cryptococcus neoformans,* gram-negative enteric and anaerobic bacteria, *Nocardia, Legionella pneumophila,* mycobacteria, and viruses (CMV, varicella-zoster, herpes simplex, influenza virus, RSV, adenovirus). Multiple organisms are commonly present.

## Clinical Findings

### A. Symptoms and Signs

Patients often present with subtle signs such as mild cough, tachypnea, or low-grade fever that can rapidly progress to high fever, respiratory distress, and hypoxemia. An obvious portal of infection, such as an intravascular catheter, may predispose to bacterial or fungal infection.

### B. Laboratory Findings and Imaging

Fungal, parasitic, or bacterial infection, especially with antibiotic-resistant bacteria, should be suspected in the neutropenic child. Cultures of peripheral blood, sputum, tracheobronchial secretions, urine, nasopharynx or sinuses, bone marrow, pleural fluid, biopsied lymph nodes, or skin lesions or cultures through intravascular catheters should be obtained as soon as infection is suspected.

Invasive methods are commonly required to make a diagnosis. Appropriate samples should be obtained soon after a patient with pneumonia fails to respond to initial treatment. The results of these procedures usually lead to important changes in empiric preoperative therapy. Sputum is often unavailable. Bronchoalveolar lavage frequently provides the diagnosis of one or more organisms and should be done early in evaluation. The combined use of a wash, brushing, and lavage has a high yield. In patients with rapidly advancing disease, lung biopsy becomes more urgent. The morbidity and mortality rates of this procedure can be reduced by a thoracoscopic approach by a skilled operator. Because of the multiplicity of organisms that may cause disease, a comprehensive set of studies should be done on lavage and biopsy material. These consist of rapid diagnostic studies, including fluorescent antibody studies for *Legionella*; rapid culture and antigen detection for viruses; Gram, acid-fast, and fungal stains; cytologic examination for viral inclusions; cultures for viruses, anaerobic and aerobic bacteria, fungi, mycobacteria, and *Legionella*; and rapid immunofluorescent studies for *P jiroveci*.

Chest radiographs may be useful. In *P jiroveci* pneumonia, dyspnea and hypoxemia may be marked despite minimal radiographic abnormalities.

## Differential Diagnosis

The organisms causing disease vary with the type of immunocompromise present. For example, the splenectomized patient may be overwhelmed by infection with *S pneumoniae* or *H influenzae*. The infant receiving adrenocorticotropic hormone therapy may be more likely to have *P jiroveci* infection. The febrile neutropenic child who has been receiving adequate doses of intravenous broad-spectrum antibiotics may have fungal disease. The key to diagnosis is to consider all possibilities of infection.

Depending on the form of immunocompromise, perhaps only one half to two thirds of new pulmonary infiltrates in such patients represent infection. The remainder are caused by pulmonary toxicity of radiation, oxygen, chemotherapy, or other drugs; pulmonary disorders, including hemorrhage, embolism, atelectasis, aspiration, or ARDS; recurrence or extension of primary malignant growths or immunologic disorders; transfusion reactions, leukostasis, or tumor cell lysis; or interstitial lung disease, such as lymphocytic interstitial pneumonitis with human immunodeficiency virus (HIV) infection.

## Complications

Respiratory failure, shock, multiple organ damage, disseminated infection, and death commonly occur in the infected immunocompromised host.

## Treatment

Broad-spectrum intravenous antibiotics are indicated early in febrile, neutropenic, or immunocompromised children. Trimethoprim–sulfamethoxazole (for *Pneumocystis*) and erythromycin (for *Legionella*) are also indicated early in the treatment of immunocompromised children before an organism is identified. Further therapy should be based on studies of specimens obtained from bronchoalveolar lavage or lung biopsy.

## Prognosis

Prognosis is based on the severity of the underlying immunocompromise, appropriate early diagnosis and treatment, and the infecting organisms.

Hansen K, Singer DB: Asplenic-hyposplenic overwhelming sepsis: Postsplenectomy sepsis revisited. Pediatr Dev Pathol 2001;4:105 [PMID: 11178626].

Labenne M et al: Blind protected specimen brush and bronchoalveolar lavage in ventilated children. Crit Care Med 1999;27:2537 [PMID: 10579277].

Neville K et al: Pneumonia in the immunocompromised pediatric cancer patient. Semin Respir Infect 2002;17:21 [PMID: 11891516].

Perez Mato S et al: Pulmonary infections in children with HIV infection. Semin Respir Infect 2002;17:33 [PMID: 11891517].

# HYPERSENSITIVITY PNEUMONIA

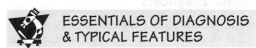

**ESSENTIALS OF DIAGNOSIS & TYPICAL FEATURES**

- *History of exposure (eg, birds, organic dusts, or molds).*
- *Interstitial infiltrates on chest radiograph or diffuse rales.*
- *Recurrent cough, fever, wheezing, or weight loss can occur.*

## General Considerations

Hypersensitivity pneumonitis, or extrinsic allergic alveolitis, is a T-cell–mediated disease involving the peripheral airways, interstitium, and alveoli. Both acute and chronic forms may occur. In children, the most common forms are brought on by exposure to domestic and occasionally wild birds or bird droppings (eg, pigeons, parakeets, parrots, doves). Inhalation of almost any organic dust, however (moldy hay, compost, logs or tree bark, sawdust, or aerosols from humidifiers), can cause disease. Methotrexate-induced hypersensitivity has also been described in a child with juvenile rheumatoid arthritis. A high level of suspicion and a thorough history are required for diagnosis.

## Clinical Findings

### SYMPTOMS AND SIGNS

Episodic cough and fever can occur with acute exposures. Chronic exposure results in weight loss, fatigue, dyspnea, cyanosis, and, ultimately, respiratory failure.

### B. LABORATORY FINDINGS

Acute exposure may be followed by polymorphonuclear leukocytosis with eosinophilia and evidence of airway obstruction on pulmonary function testing. Chronic disease results in a restrictive picture on lung function tests. Arterial blood gases may reveal hypoxemia with a decreased $PaCO_2$ and normal pH.

The serologic key to diagnosis is the finding of precipitins (precipitating IgG antibodies) to the organic dusts that contain avian proteins or fungal or bacterial antigens. Ideally, to identify avian proteins, the patient's sera should be tested with antigens from droppings of the suspected species of bird. However, exposure may invoke precipitins without causing disease.

## Differential Diagnosis

Patients with mainly acute symptoms must be differentiated from those with atopic asthma. Patients with chronic symptoms must be distinguished from those with collagen–vascular, immunologic, or primary interstitial pulmonary disorders.

## Complications

Prolonged exposure to offending antigens may result in pulmonary hypertension due to chronic hypoxemia, cor pulmonale, irreversible restrictive lung disease due to pulmonary fibrosis, or respiratory failure.

## Treatment

Complete elimination of exposure to the offending antigens is required. Corticosteroids may hasten recovery.

## Prognosis

With appropriate diagnosis and avoidance of offending antigens, the prognosis is excellent. A good prognosis, however, is dependent on early diagnosis before pulmonary damage is irreversible.

Fan LL: Hypersensitivity pneumonitis in children. Curr Opin Pediatr 2002;14:323 [PMID: 12011673].

Grech V et al: Pigeon breeder's lung in childhood: Varied clinical picture at presentation. Pediatr Pulmonol 2000;30: 145 [PMID: 10922137].

# INTERSTITIAL LUNG DISEASE

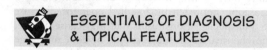

**ESSENTIALS OF DIAGNOSIS & TYPICAL FEATURES**

- *Tachypnea, dyspnea, retractions, or hypoxemia.*
- *Cough or rales.*
- *Bilateral pulmonary infiltrates.*

## General Considerations

Interstitial disorders in children are commonly caused by infection, immunodeficiency, aspiration, cardiac disease, or pulmonary vascular disease. Genetic causes such as SP-B and SP-C mutations are now also identified. Children are less likely than adults to have primary (idiopathic) pulmonary interstitial lung disorders (eg, desquamative, usual, or lymphocytic interstitial pneumonitis), hypersensitivity pneumonitis, or collagen–vascular diseases.

## Clinical Findings

### A. SYMPTOMS AND SIGNS

Children may present with a chronic dry cough or a history of dyspnea on exertion. The child with more advanced disease may have increased dyspnea, tachypnea, retractions, cyanosis, clubbing, failure to thrive, or weight loss. Physical examination may reveal these findings, and dry ("Velcro") rales may be present on chest auscultation, especially at the lung bases.

### B. LABORATORY FINDINGS AND IMAGING

Chest radiographs are normal in up to 10–15% of patients. More commonly, diffuse or perihilar bilateral reticular interstitial infiltrates are present. Nodular and reticulonodular diseases are uncommon in children except in HIV infection. Bilateral disease is the rule except in cases of infection and aspiration-related disorders, which may be unilateral.

On pulmonary function testing, interstitial disorders often show a restrictive pattern of decreased lung volumes, compliance, and diffusing capacity for carbon monoxide, whereas the $FEV_1/FVC$ ratio may be normal or increased. However, exercise-induced hypoxemia is often the earliest detectable abnormality of lung function. Blood gas abnormalities include hypoxemia, a low $PaCO_2$, and normal pH.

Many chronically ill patients can be investigated in a sequence of (1) serologic, (2) bronchoscopic, and (3) biopsy steps. Although bronchoalveolar lavage may be useful in identifying patients who have pulmonary hemosiderosis (hemosiderin-laden macrophages), aspiration (lipid-laden macrophages), and infectious disorders, lung biopsy is the most reliable method for definitive diagnosis.

During the initial phase, the following diagnostic studies may be considered: radiographs, barium swallow, pulmonary function tests, skin tests (see Tuberculosis section); complete blood count and erythrocyte sedimentation rate; sweat chloride test for CF; ECG or echocardiogram; serum immunoglobulins and other immunologic evaluations; sputum studies (see Pneumonia in the Immunocompromised Host section); and studies for Epstein–Barr virus, CMV, *M pneumoniae, Chlamydia, Pneumocystis,* and *U urealyticum.*

During the second phase, bronchoscopy should be performed to exclude anatomic abnormalities and obtain multiple bronchial biopsies or brushings to examine cilia. At the same procedure, bronchoalveolar lavage should be done for microbiologic and cytologic testing. In some instances, an SP-B protein analysis should also be performed. In patients with static or slowly progressing disease, one can then await results of bronchoscopic studies. In patients with acute, rapidly progressive disease, this stage should be combined with thoracoscopic biopsy. Special stains and cultures, immunofluorescence for immune complexes, and electron microscopy should be ordered. Genomic analysis of tissue or blood for SP-B and SP-C should be sought if clinically indicated. Although transbronchial biopsy may be useful in diagnosing a few disorders (eg, sarcoidosis), its overall usefulness in pediatrics is limited.

## Differential Diagnosis

Malignant disorders (histiocytosis X, disseminated carcinoma), congenital disorders (Gaucher disease, neurofibromatosis, tuberous sclerosis, familial interstitial lung disease), pulmonary hemosiderosis, pulmonary telangiectasia or lymphangiectasia, bronchiolitis obliterans, sarcoidosis, and ciliary dyskinesia should be con-

sidered in addition to the groups of disorders mentioned earlier.

## Complications

Respiratory failure or pulmonary hypertension with cor pulmonale may occur.

## Treatment

Therapy for interstitial lung disease due to infection, aspiration, or cardiac disorders should be directed toward the primary disorder. Most of the primary pulmonary interstitial disorders are treated initially with prednisone (2 mg/kg/d) for 6 weeks to 6 months depending on the severity of disease and the response. Many patients require even more protracted therapy with alternate-day prednisone. Chloroquine (5–10 mg/kg/d) may be useful in selected disorders such as desquamative interstitial pneumonitis. In refractory cases, azathioprine and cyclophosphamide may be tried. Pulse steroids given intravenously in doses of 10 to 30 mg/kg for 1 to 3 days have shown benefit in case reports of children with pulmonary fibrosis. Newer antifibrotic agents such as interferon gamma, being investigated in adult patients with interstitial pulmonary fibrosis, have not been tried in children to date. Addition of cytotoxic drugs (azathioprine, cyclophosphamide) has not been shown to be more beneficial than prednisone alone.

## Prognosis

The prognosis is guarded in children with interstitial lung disease due to collagen–vascular and primary pulmonary interstitial diseases, immunodeficiency diseases, surfactant protein mutations, and cancer.

Amin RS et al: Surfactant protein deficiency in familial interstitial lung disease. J Pediatr 2001;139:85 [PMID: 11445799].

Howenstine MS, Eigen H: Current concepts on interstitial lung disease in children. Curr Opin Pediatr 1999;11:200 [PMID: 10349096].

Whitsett JA: Genetic basis of familial interstitial lung disease. *Am J Respir Crit Care Med* 2002;165:1201 [PMID: 11991863].

# EOSINOPHILIC PNEUMONIA

### ESSENTIALS OF DIAGNOSIS & TYPICAL FEATURES

- *Pulmonary infiltrates, often migratory, seen on chest radiograph.*
- *Persistent cough; wheezes or rales on chest auscultation.*

• *Increased eosinophils in peripheral blood or in lung biopsy specimens.*

## General Considerations

A spectrum of diseases should be considered under this heading: (1) allergic bronchopulmonary helminthiosis (ABPH), (2) pulmonary eosinophilia with asthma (allergic bronchopulmonary aspergillosis and related disorders), (3) hypereosinophilic mucoid impaction, (4) bronchocentric granulomatosis, and (5) collagen–vascular disorders. The old term, Löffler syndrome (transient migratory pulmonary infiltrates and eosinophilia), is no longer used because most patients had undiagnosed ABPH, medication reactions (www.pneumotox. com), or allergic bronchopulmonary aspergillosis. Many of these disorders occur in children with personal or family histories of allergies or asthma. APBH may be related to hypersensitivity to migratory parasitic nematodes (*Ascaris, Strongyloides, Ancylostoma, Toxocara, Trichuris*) and larval forms of filariae (*Wuchereria bancrofti*). Allergic bronchopulmonary aspergillosis is related to hypersensitivity to the fungus *Aspergillus*. Hypersensitivity to other fungi has also been documented. Eosinophilic pneumonias are rare but can be associated with drug hypersensitivity, sarcoidosis, Hodgkin disease or other lymphomas, and bacterial infections, including brucellosis and those caused by *M tuberculosis* and atypical mycobacteria.

## Clinical Findings

### A. Symptoms and Signs

Cough, wheezing, and dyspnea are common presenting complaints. In ABPH, fever, malaise, sputum production, and, rarely, hemoptysis may be present. In allergic bronchopulmonary aspergillosis, patients may present all of these findings and occasionally produce brown mucus plugs. Anorexia, weight loss, night sweats, and clubbing can also occur.

### B. Laboratory Findings and Imaging

Elevated absolute peripheral blood eosinophil counts (3000/μL and often exceeding 50% of leukocytes) are present in APBH and allergic bronchopulmonary aspergillosis. Serum IgE levels as high as 1000–10,000 IU/mL are common. In allergic bronchopulmonary aspergillosis, the serum IgE concentration appears to correlate with activity of the disease. Stools should be examined for ova and parasites—often several times—to clarify the diagnosis. Isohemagglutinin titers are often markedly elevated in APBH.

In allergic bronchopulmonary aspergillosis and related disorders, patients may show central bronchiectasis on chest radiograph (so-called tramlines) or CT scan. Saccular proximal bronchiectasis of the upper lobes is pathognomonic. Although the chest radiograph may be normal, peribronchial haziness, focal or plate-like atelectasis, or patchy to massive consolidation can occur. Positive immediate skin tests, serum IgG precipitating antibodies, or IgE specific for the offending fungus is present.

## Differential Diagnosis

These disorders must be differentiated from exacerbations of asthma, CF, or other underlying lung disorders that cause infiltrates to appear on chest radiographs. Allergic bronchopulmonary aspergillosis can occur in patients with CF.

## Complications

Delayed recognition and treatment of allergic bronchopulmonary aspergillosis may cause progressive lung damage and bronchiectasis. Lesions of the conducting airways in bronchocentric granulomatosis can extend into adjacent lung parenchyma and pulmonary arteries, resulting in secondary vasculitis.

## Treatment

Therapy for the specific parasite causing ABPH should be given, and corticosteroids may be required when illness is severe. Treatment of disease due to microfilariae is both diagnostic and therapeutic. Allergic bronchopulmonary aspergillosis and related disorders are treated with prolonged courses of oral corticosteroids, bronchodilators, and chest physical therapy. In patients with CF, itraconazole may decrease steroid doses for those with allergic bronchopulmonary aspergillosis. Pulmonary vasculitis associated with collagen vascular disease usually is treated with high-dose steroids or cytotoxic agents.

Carroll JL, Sterni LM: Eosinophilic lung disorders and hypersensitivity pneumonitis. In Taussig LM, Landau LI (eds): *Pediatric Respiratory Medicine.* Mosby, 1999.

Nepomuceno IB et al: Allergic bronchopulmonary aspergillosis in cystic fibrosis: Role of atopy and response to itraconazole. Chest 1999;115:364 [PMID: 10027433].

Oermann CM et al: Pulmonary infiltrates with eosinophilia syndromes in children. J Pediatr 2000;136:351 [PMID: 10700692].

Wubbel C et al: Chronic eosinophilia pneumonia. Chest 2003; 123:1763 [PMID: 12740299].

# LUNG ABSCESS

Lung abscesses are most likely to occur in immunocompromised patients; in those with severe infections elsewhere (embolic spread); or in those with recurrent aspiration, malnutrition, or blunt chest trauma. Although organisms such as *S aureus, H influenzae, S pneumoniae,* and viridans streptococci more commonly affect the previously normal host, anaerobic and gram-negative organisms as well as *Nocardia, Legionella* species, and fungi (*Candida, Aspergillus*) should also be considered in the immunocompromised host.

## Clinical Findings

### A. SYMPTOMS AND SIGNS

High fever, malaise, and weight loss are often present. Symptoms and signs referable to the chest may or may not be present. In infants, evidence of respiratory distress can be present.

### B. LABORATORY FINDINGS AND IMAGING

Elevated peripheral white blood cell count with a neutrophil predominance or an elevated erythrocyte sedimentation rate may be present. Blood cultures are rarely positive except in the overwhelmed host.

Chest radiographs usually reveal single or multiple thick-walled lung cavities. Air–fluid levels can be present. Local compressive atelectasis, pleural thickening, or adenopathy may also occur. Chest CT scan may provide better localization and understanding of the lesions.

In patients producing sputum, stains and cultures may provide the diagnosis. Direct percutaneous aspiration of material for stains and cultures guided by fluoroscopy or ultrasonography should be considered in the severely compromised or ill.

## Differential Diagnosis

Loculated pyopneumothorax, an *Echinococcus* cyst, neoplasms, plasma cell granuloma, and infected congenital cysts and sequestrations should be considered.

## Complications

Although complications due to abscesses are now rare, mediastinal shift, tension pneumothorax, and spontaneous rupture can occur. Diagnostic maneuvers such as lung puncture may also cause complications (pneumothorax).

## Treatment

Because of the risks of lung puncture, uncomplicated abscesses are frequently conservatively treated in the uncompromised host with appropriate broad-spectrum antibiotics directed at *S aureus, H influenzae,* and streptococci. Additional coverage for anaerobic and gram-negative organisms should be provided for others. Prolonged therapy (3 weeks or more) may be required. Attempts to drain abscesses via bronchoscopy have caused life-threatening airway compromise. Surgical drainage or lobectomy is occasionally required, primarily in immunocompromised patients. However, such procedures may themselves cause life-threatening complications.

## Prognosis

Although radiographic resolution may be very slow, resolution occurs in most patients without risk factors for lower respiratory tract infections or loss of pulmonary function. In the immunocompromised host, the outlook depends on the underlying disorder.

Tan TQ et al: Pediatric lung abscess: Clinical management and outcome. Pediatr Infect Dis J 1995;14:51 [PMID: 7715991].

Wali SO et al: Percutaneous drainage of pyogenic lung abscess. Scand J Infect Dis 2002;34:673 [PMID: 12374359].

# PULMONARY TUMORS

Primary tumors of the airway and parenchyma of the lung are unusual in pediatrics. Most intrathoracic tumors occur in or close to the mediastinum (see Mediastinal Masses section). Other pulmonary tumors may be classified as benign, malignant, or metastatic. Benign pulmonary tumors include plasma cell granulomas, hamartomas, adenomas, papillomas, angiomas, leiomyomas, lipomas, and neurogenic tumors. The most common malignant tumor in children, a bronchogenic carcinoma, is also very rare. Other malignant tumors include fibrosarcomas and leiomyosarcomas. Metastatic tumors in childhood include Wilms tumor; hepatoblastoma; and osteogenic, chondrosarcoma, Ewing, reticulum cell, and soft tissue sarcomas. Lung tumors in children are more often metastatic than primary.

## Clinical Findings

### A. SYMPTOMS AND SIGNS

Symptoms, when they occur, may include pain, fever, cough, wheezing, weight loss, malaise, anemia, anorexia, and hemoptysis. On physical examination, signs of a pleural effusion, volume loss, or consolidation may be present if the tumor has led to significant airway obstruction.

### B. LABORATORY FINDINGS AND IMAGING

In addition to frontal and lateral chest radiographs, fluoroscopy, CT scans, and angiography may be helpful in defining and delineating the tumor. Sputum cultures and cytology, as well as tuberculin and fungal skin tests plus fungal serology, may be needed to exclude other conditions.

## Differential Diagnosis

The differential diagnosis includes acute, recurrent, or persistent viral and bacterial pneumonia, tuberculosis, and pulmonary infiltrates due to fungal infections. In infants, congenital malformations (pulmonary sequestration, cystic adenomatoid malformation) may also present as mass lesions.

## Treatment & Prognosis

The appropriate therapy and the response to therapy depend on the type and location of the tumor. Benign lesions may be cured with surgical resection, but the prognosis is more guarded with both primary and metastatic malignant lesions.

Brooks JW, Krummel TM: Tumors of the chest. In Chernick V, Boat TF (eds): *Kendig's Disorders of the Respiratory Tract in Children,* 6th ed. WB Saunders, 1998.

# DISEASES OF THE PULMONARY CIRCULATION

## PULMONARY HEMORRHAGE

Pulmonary hemorrhage is caused by a spectrum of disorders affecting the large and small airways and alveoli. It can occur as an acute or chronic process. Hemorrhage involving the alveoli is termed diffuse alveolar hemorrhage. If pulmonary hemorrhage is subacute or chronic, hemosiderin-laden macrophages are found in the sputum and tracheal or gastric aspirate. Many cases are secondary to infection (bacterial, mycobacterial, parasitic, viral, or fungal), lung abscess, bronchiectasis (CF or other causes), foreign body, coagulopathy (often with overwhelming sepsis), or elevated pulmonary venous pressure (secondary to congestive heart failure or anatomic heart lesions). Other causes include lung contusion from trauma, arteriovenous fistula, multiple telangiectasia, pulmonary sequestration, agenesis of a single pulmonary artery, and esophageal duplication or bronchogenic cyst. Rarer causes are tumors (eg, bronchial adenoma or left atrial myxoma) and pulmonary infarction secondary to pulmonary embolus.

Diffuse alveolar hemorrhage may be idiopathic or drug-related or may occur in Goodpasture syndrome, rapidly progressive glomerulonephritis, and systemic vasculitides (often associated with such collagen–vascular diseases as systemic lupus erythematosus, rheumatoid arthritis, Wegener granulomatosis, polyarteritis nodosa, Henoch–Schönlein purpura, and Behçet disease). Idiopathic pulmonary hemosiderosis refers to the accumulation of hemosiderin in the lung, especially the alveolar macrophage, as a result of chronic or recurrent hemorrhage (usually from pulmonary capillaries) that is not associated with the previously listed causes. Children and young adults are mainly affected, with the age at onset ranging from 6 months to 20 years. This group of disorders includes milk allergy in young infants (Heiner syndrome).

Several cases of pulmonary hemorrhage and pulmonary hemosiderosis have been reported in infants exposed to a toxigenic mold, *Stachybotrys chartarum,* and other fungi. This association was initially noted in Cleveland, Ohio. The infants were primarily African American, living in older homes, and often the homes had recent water damage. Environmental tobacco smoke was also frequently present in the environment. Other forms of hypersensitivity pneumonitis have also been reported to cause pulmonary bleeding.

## Clinical Findings

### A. SYMPTOMS AND SIGNS

Pulmonary hemorrhage has as many symptoms as it has causes. Large airway hemorrhage presents with hemoptysis and symptoms of the underlying cause, such as infection, foreign body, or bronchiectasis in CF. Hemoptysis from larger airways is often bright red or contains clots. Idiopathic pulmonary hemosiderosis usually presents with nonspecific respiratory symptoms (cough, tachypnea, retractions) with or without hemoptysis, poor growth, and fatigue. Some children or young adults may present with massive hemoptysis, marked respiratory distress, stridor, or a pneumonia-like syndrome. Fever, abdominal pain, digital clubbing, and chest pain may be reported. Jaundice and hepatosplenomegaly may be present with chronic bleeding. Physical examination often reveals decreased breath sounds, rales, rhonchi, or wheezing.

### B. LABORATORY FINDINGS AND IMAGING

Laboratory studies vary depending on the cause of hemorrhage. Following long-standing idiopathic pulmonary hemorrhage, iron deficiency anemia and heme-positive sputum are present. Nonspecific findings may include lymphocytosis and an elevated erythrocyte sedimentation rate. Peripheral eosinophilia is present in up to 25% of patients. Chest radiographs demonstrate a range of findings, from transient perihilar infiltrates to large, fluffy alveolar infiltrates with or without atelectasis and mediastinal adenopathy. Pulmonary function testing generally reveals restrictive impairment, with low lung volumes, poor compliance, and an increased diffusion capacity. Hemosiderin-laden macrophages are found in bronchial or gastric aspirates. The diagnostic usefulness of lung biopsy is controversial.

Diffuse alveolar hemorrhage with underlying systemic disease such as systemic lupus erythematosus, Wegener granulomatosis, and occasionally Goodpasture syndrome can occur with the histologic entity known as necrotizing pulmonary capillaritis. On lung biopsy the alveolar septa are infiltrated with neutrophils, and alveolar hemorrhage is acute or chronic. The septa can fill with edema or fibrinoid necrosis. Idiopathic pulmonary hemosiderosis may represent a mild form of capillaritis associated with alveolar hemorrhage. It might represent a process that waxes and wanes, and capillaritis may be focal or mild. Likewise, an immune-mediated process may cause idiopathic pulmonary hemosiderosis, although no serologic marker has yet been identified. Although capillaritis has been described without evidence of underlying systemic disease, the search for collagen–vascular disease, vasculitis, or pulmonary fibrosis should be exhaustive.

The investigation should include serologic studies such as antineutrophil cytoplasmic antibodies (c-ANCA) for Wegener granulomatosis, p- (perinuclear) or c-ANCA for microscopic polyangiitis, antinuclear antibodies for systemic lupus erythematosus, and antibasement membrane antibodies for Goodpasture syndrome. α1-Antitrypsin deficiency has been associated with vasculitides and should be considered.

Suspected cases of cow's milk-induced pulmonary hemosiderosis can be confirmed by laboratory findings that include high titers of serum precipitins to multiple constituents of cow's milk and positive intradermal skin tests to various cow's milk proteins. Improvement after an empiric trial of a diet free of cow's milk also supports the diagnosis.

## Differential Diagnosis

The search for the site of respiratory bleeding, underlying systemic illness, and cardiac or vascular abnormalities will help define the diagnosis. When gross hemoptysis is present, large airway bronchiectasis, epistaxis, foreign body, and arteriovenous or pulmonary malformations should be ruled out. MRI or CT-assisted angiography can localize abnormal or systemic arterial flow.

Alveolar bleeding with hemoptysis is often frothy and pink. The differential diagnosis includes the disorders causing diffuse alveolar hemorrhage listed earlier. In contrast to idiopathic pulmonary hemosiderosis, Goodpasture syndrome occurs in a slightly older age group (15–35 years), tends to have a more aggressive pulmonary course, and has renal involvement (crescentic proliferative glomerulonephritis and circulating antiglomerular basement membrane antibody). Wegener granulomatosis also has renal involvement (granulomatous glomerulitis with necrotizing vasculitis, but renal biopsy may be nonspecific) and other systemic manifestations, especially with upper and lower respiratory tract inflammation. Upper tract involvement includes sinusitis, rhinitis, recurrent epistaxis, otitis media, saddle nose deformity, and subglottic stenosis. Wegener granulomatosis may occur without renal involvement early in the course of the disease. The diagnosis can be made by biopsy or an elevated c-ANCA titer.

## Treatment

Therapy should be aimed at direct treatment of the underlying disease. Supportive measures, including iron therapy, supplemental oxygen, and blood transfusions, may be needed. A diet free of cow's milk should be tried in infants. Systemic corticosteroids have been used for various causes of diffuse alveolar hemorrhage and have been particularly successful in those secondary to collagen–vascular disorders and vasculitis. Case reports have been published on the variable effectiveness of steroids, chloroquine, cyclophosphamide, and azathioprine for idiopathic pulmonary hemosiderosis.

## Prognosis

The outcome of idiopathic pulmonary hemosiderosis is variable, characterized by a waxing and waning course of intermittent intrapulmonary bleeds and the gradual development of pulmonary fibrosis over time. The severity of the underlying renal disease contributes to the mortality rates associated with Goodpasture syndrome and Wegener granulomatosis. Diffuse alveolar hemorrhage is considered a lethal pulmonary complication of systemic lupus erythematosus.

Ben-Abraham R et al: Diffuse alveolar hemorrhage following allogeneic bone marrow transplantation in children. Chest 2003;124(2):660 [PMID: 12907557].

Etzel RA et al: Acute pulmonary hemorrhage in infants associated with exposure to *Stachybotrys atra* and other fungi. Arch Pediatr Adolesc Med 1998;152:757 [PMID: 9701134].

Etzel RA: *Stachybotrys.* Curr Opin Pediatr 2003;15(1):103 Review [PMID: 12544280].

Franks TJ, Koss MN: Pulmonary capillaritis. Curr Opin Pulm Med 2000;6(5):430. Review [PMID: 10958235].

Kiper N et al: Long-term clinical course of patients with idiopathic pulmonary hemosiderosis (1979–1994): Prolonged survival with low-dose corticosteroid therapy. Pediatr Pulmonol 1999;27:180 [PMID: 10213256].

Milman N, Pedersen FM: Idiopathic pulmonary haemosiderosis: Epidemiology, pathologic aspects, and diagnosis. Respir Med 1998;92:902 [PMID: 10070562].

Specks U: Diffuse alveolar hemorrhage syndromes. Curr Opin Rheumatol 2001;13:12 [PMID: 11148710].

Update: Pulmonary hemorrhage/hemosiderosis among infants–Cleveland, Ohio, 1993–1996. MMWR Morb Mortal Wkly Rep. 2000 Mar 10;49(9):180. Erratum in: MMWR Morb Mortal Wkly Rep 2000 Mar 17;49(10):213 [PMID: 11795499].

# PULMONARY EMBOLISM

Although pulmonary embolism is apparently rare in children, the incidence is probably underestimated because it is often not considered in the differential diagnosis of respiratory distress. It occurs most commonly in children with sickle cell anemia as part of the acute chest syndrome and with rheumatic fever, infective endocarditis, schistosomiasis, bone fracture, dehydration, polycythemia, nephrotic syndrome, atrial fibrillation, and other conditions. A recent report suggests that a majority of children with pulmonary emboli referred for hematology evaluation have coagulation regulatory protein abnormalities and antiphospholipid antibodies. Emboli may be single or multiple, large or small, with clinical signs and symptoms dependent on the severity of pulmonary vascular obstruction.

## Clinical Findings

### A. SYMPTOMS AND SIGNS

Pulmonary embolism usually presents clinically as an acute onset of dyspnea and tachypnea. Heart palpitations or a sense of impending doom may be reported.

Pleuritic chest pain and hemoptysis may be present (not common), along with splinting, cyanosis, and tachycardia. Massive emboli may be present with syncope and cardiac arrhythmias. Physical examination is usually normal (except for tachycardia and tachypnea) unless the embolism is associated with an underlying disorder. Mild hypoxemia, rales, focal wheezing, or a pleural friction rub may be found.

### B. LABORATORY FINDINGS AND IMAGING

Radiographic findings may be normal, but a peripheral infiltrate, small pleural effusion, or elevated hemidiaphragm can be present. If the emboli are massive, differential blood flow and pulmonary artery enlargement may be appreciated. The ECG is usually normal unless the pulmonary embolus is massive. Echocardiography is useful in detecting the presence of large proximal embolus. A negative D-dimer has a greater than 95% negative predictive value for an embolus. Ventilation–perfusion scans show localized areas of ventilation without perfusion. Spiral CT with contrast may be helpful, but

pulmonary angiography is the gold standard. Further evaluation may include Doppler ultrasound studies of the legs to search for deep venous thrombosis. Coagulation studies, including assessments of antithrombin III and protein C or S deficiencies or defective fibrinolysis, may be indicated. Antiphospholipid antibodies and other coagulation regulatory proteins (protein C and S, and factor V Leiden) should be checked as abnormalities have been demonstrated in 70% of the hematology referrals in one pediatric institution.

## Treatment

Acute treatment includes supplemental oxygen, sedation, and anticoagulation. Current recommendations include heparin administration to maintain an activated partial thromboplastin time that is one and one-half or more times the control value for the first 24 hours. Urokinase (2000–4000 U/kg for 36 hours) can be used to help dissolve the embolus. Tissue plasminogen activator (t-PA) is another option via central or peripheral administration. These therapies should be followed by warfarin therapy for at least 6 weeks with and INR of greater than 2. In patients with identifiable deep venous thrombosis of the lower extremities and significant pulmonary emboli (with hemodynamic compromise despite anticoagulation), inferior vena caval interruption may be necessary. Long-term prospective data regarding this latter therapy are lacking, however.

Bounameaux H: Review: ELISA D-dimer is sensitive but not specific in diagnosing pulmonary embolism in an ambulatory clinical setting. ACP J Club 2003;138(1):24 [PMID: 12511136].

Hyers TM: Management of venous thromboembolism: Past, present, and future. Arch Intern Med 2003;163(7):759 [PMID: 12695266].

Kearon C: Duration of therapy for acute venous thromboembolism. Clin Chest Med 2003;24(1):63 [PMID: 12685057].

Konstantinides S et al: Heparin plus alteplase compared with heparin alone in patients with submassive pulmonary embolism. N Engl J Med 2002;347(15):1143 [PMID: 12374874].

Remy-Jardin M et al: Pulmonary embolus imaging with multislice CT. Radiol Clin North Am 2003;41(3):507 [PMID: 12797603].

# PULMONARY EDEMA

Pulmonary edema is excessive accumulation of extravascular fluid in the lung. This occurs when fluid is filtered into the lungs faster than it can be removed, leading to changes in lung mechanics such as decreased lung compliance, worsening hypoxemia from ventilation–perfusion mismatch, bronchial compression, and, if advanced, decreased surfactant function. There are two basic types of pulmonary edema: increased pressure (cardiogenic or hydrostatic) and increased permeability (noncardiogenic or primary). Hydrostatic pulmonary edema is usually due to excessive increases in pulmonary venous pressure, which is most commonly due to congestive heart failure from multiple causes. In contrast, many lung diseases, especially ARDS, are characterized by the development of pulmonary edema secondary to changes in permeability due to injury to the alveolocapillary barrier. In these settings, pulmonary edema occurs independently of the elevations of pulmonary venous pressure.

## Clinical Findings

### A. SYMPTOMS AND SIGNS

Cyanosis, tachypnea, tachycardia, and respiratory distress are commonly present. Physical findings include rales, diminished breath sounds, and (in young infants) expiratory wheezing. More severe disease is characterized by progressive respiratory distress with marked retractions, dyspnea, and severe hypoxemia.

### B. IMAGING

Chest radiographic findings depend on the cause of the edema. Pulmonary vessels are prominent, often with diffuse interstitial or alveolar infiltrates. Heart size is usually normal in permeability edema but enlarged in hydrostatic edema.

## Treatment

Although specific therapy depends on the underlying cause, supplemental oxygen therapy and, if needed, ventilator support for respiratory failure are indicated. Diuretics, digoxin, and vasodilators may be indicated for congestive heart failure along with restriction of salt and water. Recommended interventions for permeability edema are reduction of vascular volume and maintenance of the lowest central venous or pulmonary arterial wedge pressure possible without sacrificing cardiac output or causing hypotension (see following discussion). β-Adrenergic agonists such as terbutaline have been shown to increase alveolar clearance of lung water, perhaps through the action of a sodium–potassium channel pump. Maintaining normal albumin levels and a hematocrit of greater than 30 maintains the filtration of lung liquid toward the capillaries, avoiding low oncotic pressure.

Cotter G et al: Pulmonary edema: New insight on pathogenesis and treatment. Curr Opin Cardiol 2001;16:159 [PMID: 11357010].

Redding GJ: Current concepts in adult respiratory distress syndrome in children. Curr Opin Pediatr 2001;13:261 [PMID: 11389362].

Van Kooy MA, Gargiulo RF: Postobstructive pulmonary edema. Am Fam Physician 2000;62:401 [PMID: 10929702].

# CONGENITAL PULMONARY LYMPHANGIECTASIA

Structurally, congenital pulmonary lymphangiectasia appears as dilated subpleural and interlobular lymphatic channels and may present as part of a generalized lymphangiectasis (in association with obstructive cardiovascular lesions—especially total anomalous pulmonary venous return) or as an isolated idiopathic lesion. Pathologically, the lung appears firm, bulky, and noncompressible, with prominent cystic lymphatics visible beneath the pleura. On cut section, dilated lymphatics are present near the hilum, along interlobular septa, around bronchovascular bundles, and beneath the pleura. Histologically, dilated lymphatics have a thin endothelial cell lining overlying a delicate network of elastin and collagen.

## Clinical Findings

Congenital pulmonary lymphangiectasia is a rare, usually fatal disease that generally presents as acute or persistent respiratory distress at birth. Although most patients do not survive the newborn period, some survive longer, and there are isolated case reports of its diagnosis later in childhood. It may be associated with features of Noonan syndrome, asplenia, total anomalous pulmonary venous return, septal defects, atrioventricular canal, hypoplastic left heart, aortic arch malformations, and renal malformations. Chylothorax has been reported. Chest radiographic findings include a ground-glass appearance, prominent interstitial markings suggesting lymphatic distention, diffuse hyperlucency of the pulmonary parenchyma, and hyperinflation with depression of the diaphragm.

## Prognosis

Although the onset of symptoms may be delayed for as long as the first few months of life, prolonged survival is extremely rare. Most deaths occur within weeks after birth. Rapid diagnosis is essential in order to expedite the option of pulmonary transplant.

Antonetti M et al: Congenital pulmonary lymphangiectasia: A case report of thoracic duct agenesis. Pediatr Pulmonol 2001;32:184 [PMID: 11477737].

Huber A et al: Congenital pulmonary lymphangiectasia. Pediatr Pulmonol 1991;10:310 [PMID: 1896243].

# DISORDERS OF THE CHEST WALL

## EVENTRATION OF THE DIAPHRAGM

Eventration of the diaphragm occurs when striated muscle is replaced with connective tissue and is demonstrated on radiograph by elevation of part or all of the diaphragm. This congenital disorder is thought to represent incomplete formation of the diaphragm in utero. When defects are small, there is no paradoxic movement of the diaphragm and little symptomatology. Small eventrations may be detected on a chest radiograph taken for another reason. When defects are large, there may or may not be paradoxic movement of the diaphragm, depending on the nature of the tissue replacing the normal diaphragm. The degree of respiratory distress depends in large part on the amount of paradoxic motion of the diaphragm. When the diaphragm moves upward during inspiration, instability of the inferior border of the chest wall increases the work of breathing and can lead to respiratory muscle fatigue. Treatment for respiratory distress is surgical plication, which stabilizes the diaphragm.

The differential diagnosis of eventration includes phrenic nerve injury and partial diaphragmatic hernia. The former can result from birth or other trauma and may also be seen following cardiac surgery. In most cases, only one phrenic nerve is involved. An elevated hemidiaphragm is noted on chest radiograph, and paradoxic motion of the diaphragm may be seen by fluoroscopy or ultrasonography. Patients often cannot be extubated or have persistent respiratory compromise, particularly with feeding. If symptoms persist for 2–4 weeks, the diaphragm is surgically plicated as described previously. Function returns to the diaphragm in about 50% of cases of phrenic nerve injury whether or not plication was performed. Recovery periods of up to 100 days have been reported in these cases.

Clements BS: Congenital malformations of the lungs and airways. In Taussig LM, Landau LI (eds): *Pediatric Respiratory Medicine.* Mosby, 1999.

de Vries TS et al: Surgical treatment of diaphragmatic eventration caused by phrenic nerve injury in the newborn. J Pediatr Surg 1998;33:602 [PMID: 9574760].

## SCOLIOSIS

Scoliosis—lateral curvature of the spine—can, if uncorrected, lead to severe restrictive lung disease and death from cor pulmonale. Most cases of idiopathic scoliosis occur in adolescent girls and are corrected before significant pulmonary impairment occurs. Congenital scoliosis of severe degree or with other major abnormalities carries a more guarded prognosis. Scoliosis may also occur in patients with progressive neuromuscular disease, such as Duchenne muscular dystrophy, and can be a major contributor to respiratory failure.

Dobbs MB, Weinstein SL: Infantile and juvenile scoliosis. Orthop Clin North Am 1999;30:331 [PMID: 10393759].

Jaskwhich D et al: Congenital scoliosis. Curr Opin Pediatr 2000;12:61 [PMID: 10676776].

Kearon C et al: Factors determining pulmonary function in adolescent idiopathic thoracic scoliosis. Am Rev Respir Dis 1993;148:288 [PMID: 8342890].

## PECTUS EXCAVATUM

Pectus excavatum is anterior depression of the chest wall that may be symmetrical or asymmetrical with respect to the midline. Reports of exercise testing and pulmonary function testing in patients with pectus excavatum are controversial as to whether this disorder causes physiologic limitations. Therefore, the decision to repair the deformity may be based on cosmetic or physiologic considerations. Care of patients following pectus excavatum repair requires mechanical ventilation and careful respiratory monitoring because of the weak chest wall following surgery.

Borowitz D et al: Pulmonary function and exercise response in patients with pectus excavatum after Nuss repair. J Pediatr Surg 2003;38:544 [PMID:12677562].

Fonkalsrud EW: Current management of pectus excavatum. World J Surg 2003;27:502 [PMID:12715210].

Malek MH et al: Ventilatory and cardiovascular responses to exercise in patients with pectus excavatum. Chest 2003;124:870 [PMID: 12970011].

## PECTUS CARINATUM

Pectus carinatum is a bowing out of the sternum, usually apparent at birth. The abnormality may be associated with systemic diseases such as the mucopolysaccharidoses. As with pectus excavatum, pulmonary function tests are not usually abnormal in the absence of other disorders. The decision to repair this deformity is based primarily on cosmetic grounds. Postoperative care similarly requires careful monitoring because of chest wall instability produced by the repair.

Robicek F: Surgical treatment of pectus carinatum. Chest Surg Clin North Am 2000;10:357 [PMID: 10803339].

Williams AM, Crabbe DC: Pectus deformities of the anterior chest wall. Paediatr Respir Rev 2003;4:237 [PMID: 12880759].

## NEUROMUSCULAR DISORDERS

Weakness of the respiratory and pharyngeal muscles leads to chronic or recurrent pneumonia secondary to aspiration and infection, atelectasis, hypoventilation, and respiratory failure in severe cases. Scoliosis, which frequently accompanies long-standing neuromuscular disorders, may further compromise respiratory function. Typical physical findings are a weak cough, decreased air exchange, rales, wheezing, and dullness to percussion. Signs of cor pulmonale (loud pulmonary component to the second heart sound, hepatomegaly, elevated neck veins) may be evident in advanced cases. Chest radiographs generally show small lung volumes. If chronic aspiration is present, increased interstitial infiltrates and areas of atelectasis or consolidation may be present. Arterial blood gases demonstrate hypoxemia in the early stages and compensated respiratory acidosis in the late stages. Typical pulmonary function abnormalities include low lung volumes and decreased inspiratory force generated against an occluded airway. Treatment is supportive and includes vigorous pulmonary toilet, antibiotics with infection, and oxygen to correct hypoxemia. Unfortunately, despite aggressive medical therapy, many neuromuscular conditions progress to respiratory failure and death. The decision to intubate and ventilate is a difficult one; it should be made only when there is real hope that deterioration, though acute, is potentially reversible or when chronic ventilation is wanted. Chronic mechanical ventilation using either noninvasive or invasive techniques is being used more frequently in patients with chronic respiratory insufficiency.

Birnkrant DJ: The assessment and management of the respiratory complications of pediatric neuromuscular diseases. Clin Pediatr 2002;41:301 [PMID: 12086195].

Chatwin M et al: Cough augmentation with mechanical insufflation/exsufflation in patients with neuromuscular weakness. Eur Respir J 2003;21:502 [PMID: 12662009].

Phillips MF et al: Changes in spirometry over time as a prognostic marker in patients with Duchenne muscular dystrophy. Am J Respir Crit Care Med 2001;164:2191 [PMID: 11751186].

Simonds AK: Nocturnal ventilation in neuromuscular disease—When and how? Monaldi Arch Chest Dis 2002;57:273 [PMID: 12814040].

# DISORDERS OF THE PLEURA & PLEURAL CAVITY

The visceral pleura covers the outer surface of the lungs, and the inner surface of the chest wall is the parietal pleura. Disease processes can lead to accumulation of air or fluid in the pleural space. Pleural effusions are classified as transudates or exudates. Transudates occur when there is imbalance between hydrostatic and oncotic pressure, so that fluid filtration exceeds reabsorption (eg, congestive heart failure). Exudates form as a result of inflammation of the pleural surface leading to

increased capillary permeability (eg, parapneumonic effusions). Other pleural effusions include chylothorax and hemothorax.

Thoracentesis is helpful in characterizing the fluid and providing definitive diagnosis. Recovered fluid is considered an exudate (as opposed to a transudate) if any of the following are found: a pleural fluid to serum protein ratio greater than 0.5, a pleural fluid to serum lactic dehydrogenase (LDH) ratio greater than 0.6, or a pleural fluid LDH greater than 200 units/L. Important additional studies on pleural fluid include cell count; pH and glucose; Gram, acid-fast, and fungal stains; cultures; counterimmunoelectrophoresis for specific organisms; and, occasionally, amylase concentration. Cytologic examination of pleural fluid should be performed to rule out leukemia or other neoplasm.

Hilliard TN et al: Management of parapneumonic effusion and empyema. Arch Dis Child 2003;88(10):915 [PMID: 14500314].

# PARAPNEUMONIC EFFUSION & EMPYEMA

Bacterial pneumonia is often accompanied by pleural effusion. Some of these effusions harbor infection, and others are inflammatory reactions to pneumonia. The nomenclature in this area is somewhat confusing. Some use the term *empyema* for grossly purulent fluid and *parapneumonic effusion* for nonpurulent fluid. It is clear, however, that some nonpurulent effusions will also contain organisms and represent either partially treated or early empyema. It is probably best to refer to all effusions associated with pneumonia as parapneumonic effusions, some of which are infected and some not.

The most common organism associated with empyema is *S pneumoniae*. Other common organisms include *H influenzae* and *S aureus*. Less common causes are group A streptococci, gram-negative organisms, anaerobic organisms, and *M pneumoniae*. Effusions associated with tuberculosis are almost always sterile and constitute an inflammatory reaction.

## Clinical Findings

### A. SYMPTOMS AND SIGNS

Patients usually present with typical signs of pneumonia, including fever, tachypnea, and cough. They may have chest pain, decreased breath sounds, and dullness to percussion on the affected side and may prefer to lie on the affected side. With large effusions, there may be tracheal deviation to the contralateral side.

## B. LABORATORY FINDINGS

The white blood cell count is often elevated, with left shift. Blood cultures are sometimes positive. The tuberculin skin test is positive in most cases of tuberculosis. Thoracentesis reveals findings consistent with an exudate. Cells in the pleural fluid are usually neutrophils in bacterial disease and lymphocytes in tuberculous effusions. In bacterial disease, pleural fluid pH and glucose are often low. pH less than 7.2 suggests active bacterial infection. The pH of the specimen should be determined in a blood gas syringe sent to the laboratory on ice. Extra heparin should not be used in the syringe since it can falsely lower the pH. Although in adults the presence of low pH and glucose necessitates aggressive and thorough drainage procedures, the prognostic significance of these findings in children is unknown. Gram stain, cultures, and counterimmunoelectrophoresis are often positive for the offending organism.

## C. IMAGING

The presence of pleural fluid is suggested by a homogeneous density on chest radiograph that obscures the underlying lung. Large effusions may cause a shift of the mediastinum to the contralateral side. Small effusions may only blunt the costophrenic angle. Lateral decubitus radiographs may help to detect freely movable fluid by demonstrating a layering-out effect. If the fluid is loculated, no such effect is perceived. Ultrasonography can be extremely valuable in localizing the fluid and detecting loculations, especially when thoracentesis is contemplated.

## Treatment & Prognosis

After initial thoracentesis and identification of the organism, appropriate intravenous antibiotics and adequate drainage of the fluid remain the mainstay of therapy. Although there is a trend toward managing smaller pneumococcal empyemas without a chest tube, most larger effusions require chest tube drainage. Often the empyema has been present for more than 7 days, increasing the chance for loculation of fluid. Aggressive management with drainage of pleural cavity fluid and release of adhesions is often sought in many institutions as a first line approach after thoracentesis, allowing the chest tube to be placed in the operating room under anesthesia. Some evidence suggests that thoracoscopically aided debridement may be beneficial in terms of morbidity and length of hospital stay. Early decortication using thoracoscopic techniques may reduce morbidity and the need for prolonged hospitalization.

The prognosis is related to the severity of disease but is generally excellent, with complete or nearly complete recovery expected in most instances.

Lewis RA, Feigin RD: Current issues in the diagnosis and management of pediatric empyema. Semin Pediatr Infect Dis 2002;13(4):280. Review [PMID: 12491234].

Quadri A, Thomson AH: Pleural fluids associated with chest infection. Paediatr Respir Rev 2002;3(4):349 [PMID: 12457606].

Rodgers BM: The role of thoracoscopy in pediatric surgical practice. Semin Pediatr Surg 2003;12(1):62 [PMID: 12520474].

# HEMOTHORAX

Accumulation of blood in the pleural space can be caused by surgical or accidental trauma, coagulation defects, and pleural or pulmonary tumors. With blunt trauma, hemopneumothorax may be present. Symptoms are related to blood loss and compression of underlying lung parenchyma. There is some risk of secondary infection, resulting in empyema. Drainage of a hemothorax is required when significant compromise of pulmonary function is present, as with hemopneumothorax. In uncomplicated cases, observation is indicated because blood is readily absorbed spontaneously from the pleural space.

Thoracoscopy with video assist has been used successfully in the management of hemothorax. Chest CT scan is helpful to select patients who may require surgery, as identification of blood and the volume of blood may be more predictive by this method than by chest radiograph.

Bliss D, Silen M: Pediatric thoracic trauma. Crit Care Med 2002;30 (11 Suppl):S409 [PMID: 12528782].

# CHYLOTHORAX

The accumulation of chyle in the pleural space usually results from accidental or surgical trauma to the thoracic duct. In the newborn, chylothorax can be congenital or secondary to birth trauma. This condition also occurs as a result of superior vena caval obstruction secondary to central venous lines and following Fontan procedures for tricuspid atresia. Symptoms of chylothorax are related to the amount of fluid accumulation and the degree of compromise of underlying pulmonary parenchyma. Thoracentesis reveals typical milky fluid (unless the patient has been fasting) containing chiefly T lymphocytes.

Treatment should be conservative because many chylothoraces resolve spontaneously. Oral feedings with medium-chain triglycerides reduce lymphatic flow through the thoracic duct. Drainage of chylous effusions should be performed only for respiratory compromise because the fluid often rapidly reaccumulates. Repeated or continuous drainage may lead to protein malnutrition and T-cell depletion, rendering the patient relatively immunocompromised. If reaccumulation of fluid persists, surgical ligation of the thoracic duct or sclerosis of the pleural space can be attempted, though the results may be less than satisfactory.

Beghetti M et al: Etiology and management of pediatric chylothorax. J Pediatr 2000;136:653 [PMID: 10802499].

Romero S: Nontraumatic chylothorax. Curr Opin Pulm Med 2000;6:287 [PMID: 10912634].

## PNEUMOTHORAX & RELATED AIR LEAK SYNDROMES

Pneumothorax can occur spontaneously in newborns and in older children or, more commonly, as a result of birth trauma, positive-pressure ventilation, underlying obstructive or restrictive lung disease, and rupture of a congenital or acquired lung cyst. Pneumothorax can also occur as an acute complication of tracheostomy. Air usually dissects from the alveolar spaces into the interstitial spaces of the lung. Migration to the visceral pleura ultimately leads to rupture into the pleural space. Associated conditions include pneumomediastinum, pneumopericardium, pneumoperitoneum, and subcutaneous emphysema. These conditions are more commonly associated with dissection of air into the interstitial spaces of the lung with retrograde dissection along the bronchovascular bundles toward the hilum.

### Clinical Findings

#### A. SYMPTOMS AND SIGNS

The clinical spectrum can vary from asymptomatic to severe respiratory distress. Associated symptoms include cyanosis, chest pain, and dyspnea. Physical examination may reveal decreased breath sounds and hyperresonance to percussion on the affected side with tracheal deviation to the opposite side. When pneumothorax is under tension, cardiac function may be compromised, resulting in hypotension or narrowing of the pulse pressure. Pneumopericardium is a life-threatening condition that presents with muffled heart tones and shock. Pneumomediastinum rarely causes symptoms by itself.

#### B. IMAGING

Chest radiographs usually demonstrate the presence of free air in the pleural space. If the pneumothorax is large and under tension, compressive atelectasis of the underlying lung and shift of the mediastinum to the opposite side may be demonstrated. Cross-table lateral and lateral decubitus radiographs can aid in the diagnosis of free air. Pneumopericardium is identified by the presence of air completely surrounding the heart, whereas in patients with pneumomediastinum, the heart and mediastinal structures may be outlined with air but the air does not involve the diaphragmatic cardiac border.

### Differential Diagnosis

Acute deterioration of a patient on a ventilator can be caused by tension pneumothorax, obstruction or dislodgment of the endotracheal tube, or ventilator failure. Radiographically, pneumothorax must be distinguished from diaphragmatic hernia, lung cysts, congenital lobar emphysema, and cystic adenomatoid malformation, but this task is usually not difficult.

### Treatment

Small or asymptomatic pneumothoraces usually do not require treatment and can be managed with close observation. Larger or symptomatic ones usually require drainage, although inhalation of 100% oxygen to wash out blood nitrogen can be tried.

Needle aspiration should be used to relieve tension acutely, followed by chest tube or pigtail catheter placement. Pneumopericardium requires immediate identification and, if clinically symptomatic, needle aspiration to prevent death, followed by pericardial tube placement.

In older patients with spontaneous pneumothorax, recurrences are common; sclerosing and surgical procedures are often required.

Damore DT, Dayan PS: Medical causes of pneumomediastinum in children. Clin Pediatr 2001;40:87 [PMID: 11261455].

Panitch HB et al: Abnormalities of the pleural space. In Taussig LM, Landau LI (eds): Pediatric Respiratory Medicine. Mosby, 1999.

## DISORDERS OF THE CONTROL OF BREATHING

### PEDIATRIC SLEEP APNEA

Sleep apnea has become recognized as a major public health problem in adults, with the risk of excessive daytime sleepiness, driving accidents, poor work performance, and effects on mental health. Pediatric sleep disorders are less commonly recognized because the presentation, risks, and outcome all differ from that in adults. Sleep apnea is defined as cessation of breathing and can be classified as central (the lack of effort to breathe) or obstructive (the attempt to breathe through an obstructed airway). Obstructive sleep apnea occurs in normal children with an incidence of about 2%, increasing in children with craniofacial abnormalities, neuropathies, or other medical problems. The incidence also increases when children are medicated with hypnotics, sedatives, or anticonvulsants. Central apnea, often seen in premature infants, may indicate abnormalities of the central control of breathing in the brainstem; however, with long-term obstructive sleep apnea, central components, or so-called mixed apnea, can develop.

The presentation of sleep apnea in children varies with age. It can present with life-threatening apnea in infants, hyperactivity and behavioral abnormalities in the sleep-deprived toddler, or with mood changes and sleepiness in the teenager. Unlike chronic snoring adults who tend to be obese, children with sleep apnea may present with failure to thrive, and a work-up of apnea is always indicated in these children. Another complication in childhood obstructive sleep apnea is the occurrence of partial obstruction, or hypopnea, which can cause long episodes of nighttime hypoventilation without arousal from sleep. This can also occur without clues such as snoring or noisy breathing. Sleep apnea should be suspected whenever a child presents with witnessed apnea, labored breathing, frequent nighttime arousals, failure to thrive, oxygen desaturation, life-threatening events, behavior abnormalities, obesity, or craniofacial abnormalities.

When sleep apnea is suspected, the polysomnogram is the diagnostic test of choice. This test measures sleep state with electroencephalographic leads, plus breathing rate, airflow at the nose, heart rate and rhythm, oxygen saturation, with other data including esophageal pH, end-tidal $CO_2$, body position, muscle activity, and optional additions. The test allows diagnosis of various forms of apnea, sleep fragmentation, or other sleep disorders of children.

First-line therapy for obstructive sleep apnea in children is adenotonsillectomy, which improves the clinical status of most children with normal craniofacial structure. Even children with underlying structural abnormalities of the face may benefit, although additional treatment with continuous positive airway pressure may be indicated. Additional therapy is also helpful for children with obstructive apnea and obesity, for whom adenotonsillectomy may be only partially beneficial. Central hypoventilation, either primary or secondary to long-standing obstructive apnea, requires treatment with positive airway pressure and a rated tidal volume. This can be accomplished with tracheostomy and ventilation, or noninvasively with bilevel positive airway pressure using a mask.

Because the differential diagnosis of sleepiness is quite varied among children, pediatric sleep disorder centers are the referral of choice for testing and initiation of therapy. Treatment of young or developmentally delayed children with apnea also presents several challenges.

Carroll JL: Obstructive sleep-disordered breathing in children: New controversies, new directions. Clin Chest Med 2003;24:261 [PMID:12800783].

Marcus CL: Sleep-disordered breathing in children. Am J Respir Crit Care Med 2001;164:16 [PMID: 11435234].

Schechter MS et al: Technical report: Diagnosis and management of childhood obstructive sleep apnea syndrome. Pediatrics 2002;109:e69 [PMID: 11927742].

Section on Pediatric Pulmonology, Subcommittee on Obstructive Sleep Apnea Syndrome. American Academy of Pediatrics: Clinical practice guideline: Diagnosis and management of childhood obstructive sleep apnea syndrome. Pediatrics 2002;109:704 [PMID: 11927718].

## APPARENT LIFE-THREATENING EVENTS IN INFANCY

Apparent life-threatening events (ALTEs) are characterized as being frightening to the observer and commonly include some combination of obstructive or central apnea, color change (usually cyanosis or pallor), a marked change in muscle tone (usually extreme limpness), choking, or gagging. The observer sometimes fears the infant has died. A substantial number of infants are brought to medical attention following ALTEs. The 50% of infants in whom no explanation for the episode can be found are said to have apnea of infancy. There is a relationship between apnea of infancy and sudden infant death syndrome (SIDS), with a small percentage of patients with apnea of infancy at risk for sudden death. In addition, only a small percentage of infants succumbing to SIDS have prior episodes of apnea.

The mechanism for ALTEs is unknown, but because they don't occur after infancy, immaturity is felt to play a major role. Indeed, classic studies on the nervous system, reflexes, and responses to apnea or hypoxia during sleep show profound cardiovascular compromise in infants during stimulation of the immature autonomic nervous system; adults would not be affected.

The following section describes an approach to the patient who has undergone an ALTE, taking note of the very broad differential diagnosis and uncertainties in both evaluation and treatment.

### Differential Diagnosis

Table 18–3 classifies disorders associated with ALTEs. A careful history is often the most helpful part of the evaluation. It is useful to determine whether the infant has been chronically ill or essentially well. A history of several days of poor feeding, temperature instability, or respiratory or gastrointestinal symptoms suggests an infectious process. Reports of "struggling to breathe" or "trying to breathe" imply airway obstruction. Association of the episodes with feeding implies discoordinated swallowing, gastroesophageal reflux, or airway obstruction. Episodes that typically follow crying may be related to breath-holding. Association of episodes with

***Table 18–3.*** Potential causes of apparent life-threatening events.

| | |
|---|---|
| Infectious | Viral: respiratory syncytial virus and other respiratory viruses |
| | Bacterial: sepsis, pertussis, chlamydia |
| Gastrointestinal | Gastroesophageal reflux with or without obstructive apnea |
| Respiratory | Airway abnormality; vascular rings, pulmonary slings, tracheomalacia |
| | Pneumonia |
| Neurologic | Seizure disorder |
| | Central nervous system infection: meningitis, encephalitis |
| | Vasovagal response |
| | Leigh encephalopathy |
| | Brain tumor |
| Cardiovascular | Congenital malformation |
| | Dysrhythmias |
| | Cardiomyopathy |
| Nonaccidental trauma | Battering |
| | Drug overdose |
| | Munchausen-by-proxy syndrome |
| No definable cause | Apnea of infancy |

sleeping may also suggest gastroesophageal reflux, apnea of infancy, or sleep-disordered breathing. Attempts should be made to determine the duration of the episode, but this is often difficult. It is helpful to role-play the episode with the family. Details regarding the measures taken to resuscitate the infant and the infant's recovery from the episode are often useful in determining severity.

The physical examination provides further direction in pursuing the diagnosis. Fever or hypothermia suggests infection. An altered state of consciousness implies a postictal state or drug overdose. Respiratory distress implies cardiac or pulmonary lesions.

Most patients are hospitalized for observation in order to reduce stress on the family and allow prompt completion of the evaluation. Laboratory evaluation includes a complete blood count for evidence of infection. Serum electrolytes are usually obtained. Elevations in serum bicarbonate suggest chronic hypoventilation, whereas decreases suggest acute acidosis, perhaps due to hypoxia during the episode. Chronic acidosis suggests an inherited metabolic disorder. The chest radiograph is examined for infiltrates suggesting acute infection or chronic aspiration and for cardiac size as a clue to intrinsic cardiac disease. Arterial blood gas studies provide an initial assessment of oxygenation and acid–base status, and low $PaO_2$ or elevated $PaCO_2$ (or both) implies cardiorespiratory disease. A significant base deficit suggests that the episode was accompanied by hypoxia or circulatory impairment. Oxygen saturation measurements in the hospital assess oxygenation status during different activities and are more comprehensive than a single blood gas sample.

Because apnea has been associated with respiratory infections, diagnostic studies for RSV and other viruses, pertussis, and *Chlamydia* may help with diagnosis. The apnea occurring with infection often precedes other physical findings. If the episode might have involved airway obstruction, the airway should be examined either directly, by fiberoptic bronchoscopy, or radiographically, by CT or barium swallow. Barium swallow is a useful tool to rule out the possibility of anatomic abnormalities such as vascular ring and tracheoesophageal fistula. This study may also demonstrate reflux and aspiration. If reflux is suspected, it should be documented by esophageal pH monitoring coupled with respiratory pattern recording. Most infants with reflux and apnea can be given medical antireflux treatment. Infants with reflux and repeated episodes of apnea may benefit from a surgical antireflux procedure.

ALTEs occur in the same age group as infants who die of sudden death (2–4 months is the peak age). Sleep-disordered breathing has been implicated as a possible cause of ALTEs and perhaps sudden death. Polysomnograms are used to determine abnormalities of cardiorespiratory function, sleep state, oxygen saturation, $CO_2$ retention, and seizure activity. This tool can be used in conjunction with pH monitoring to determine the contribution of reflux to apnea. Esophageal pressure manometry can be useful to detect subtle changes in respiratory effort related to partial obstructive breathing (hypopnea). Infants may be at more risk of adverse events from sleep-disordered breathing due to their immature nervous system.

There are several neurologic causes of ALTEs. Apnea as the sole manifestation of a seizure disorder is unusual but may occur. In cases of repeated episodes, 24-hour electroencephalographic monitoring may be helpful in detecting a seizure disorder. Leigh disease, a brainstem disorder characterized pathologically by neuronal dropout, may present with apneic episodes.

Apneic episodes have been linked to child abuse in several ways. Head injury following nonaccidental trauma may be first brought to medical attention because of apnea. Other signs of abuse are usually immediately apparent in such cases. Drug overdose, either accidental or intentional, may also present with apnea. Several series document that apneic episodes may be falsely reported by parents seeking attention (ie, Munchausen-by-proxy syndrome). Parents may physically interfere with a child's respiratory efforts, in which case pinch marks on the nares are sometimes found.

## Treatment

Therapy is directed at the underlying cause if one is found. After blood cultures are taken, antibiotics should be given to infants who appear toxic. Seizure disorders are treated with anticonvulsants. Vascular rings and pulmonary slings must be corrected surgically because of severe morbidity and high mortality rates when untreated.

The approach to care of infants with ALTEs where no definable cause can be ascertained is controversial. Home monitoring has been used in the past as treatment, but the efficacy of monitoring has not been demonstrated in controlled trials. With over 20 years of home monitoring, the sudden infant death rate did not change due to this intervention. Yet a rationale for the use of monitors is that infants at risk for subsequent severe episodes can be identified. Although monitors can detect apnea or bradycardia, they do not predict which children will have future ALTEs. Parents should be taught cardiopulmonary resuscitation prior to discharge. They should also be aware of the possibility of frequent false alarms. It must be noted that many parents cannot handle the stress associated with having a monitor in the home.

The decision to monitor these infants involves the participation of the family. Infants with severe initial episodes or repeated severe episodes are now thought to be at significant increased risk and should probably be monitored in the home. Episodes in these children are so severe that the parents want to know the infant's condition at all times. The decision to discontinue monitoring is usually based on the infant's ability to go several months without triggering the alarm.

Oxygen has been used as therapy for ALTEs for several reasons. First, it reduces periodic breathing of infancy, an immature pattern of breathing that can cause some degree of oxygen desaturation. Second, infants have small chest capacities with increased chest wall compliance that reduces lung volume. Oxygen can increase the baseline saturation, reducing the severity of desaturation with short apneas. Respiratory stimulants such as caffeine and aminophylline have been used in specific cases of central apnea or periodic breathing.

Brooks JG: Apnea of prematurity and apparent life-threatening events. In Taussig LM, Landau LI (eds): *Pediatric Respiratory Medicine.* Mosby, 1999.

Davies F, Gupta R: Apparent life threatening events in infants presenting to an emergency department. Emerg Med J 2002;19:11 [PMID: 11777863].

Farrell PA et al: SIDS, ALTE, apnea, and the use of home monitors. Pediatr Rev 2002;23:3 [PMID: 11773587].

Poets CF, Southhall DP: Sudden infant death syndrome and apparent life-threatening events. In Taussig LM, Landau LI (eds): *Pediatric Respiratory Medicine.* Mosby, 1999.

## SUDDEN INFANT DEATH SYNDROME

SIDS is defined as the sudden death of an infant younger than age 1 year that remains unexplained after a thorough case investigation, including performance of a complete autopsy, examination of the death scene, and review of the clinical history. The postmortem examination is an important feature of the definition because approximately 20% of cases of sudden death can be explained by autopsy findings. The incidence of SIDS in the United States has recently declined to less than 1:1000 live births. The part of the decline that has occurred since 1994 is likely due to alterations of risk factors (see following discussion).

Epidemiologic and pathologic data constitute most of what is known about SIDS. The number of deaths peaks between ages 2 and 4 months, and most deaths occur in infants a few weeks to 6 months of age. Most deaths occur between midnight and 8 AM, while the infant and often the caregiver are sleeping. In fact, the only unifying features of all SIDS cases are age and sleep. Previous studies showed a peak in SIDS during the respiratory virus season, but the association becomes weaker when the data are controlled for risk factors such as tobacco exposure. SIDS is more common among ethnic and racial minorities and socioeconomically disadvantaged populations. There is a 3:2 male predominance in most series. Other risk factors include low birth weight, teenage or drug-addicted mothers, maternal smoking, and a family history of SIDS. Most of these risk factors are associated with a two- to threefold elevation of incidence but are not specific enough to be useful in predicting which infants will die unexpectedly. Recent immunization is not a risk factor.

Since 1990, SIDS rates have declined more than 60% worldwide. Population studies in New Zealand and Europe identified risk factors, which when changed had a major effect on the incidence of SIDS. Since 1994 the AAP's "Back-to-Sleep" campaign has promoted education about SIDS risk factors in the United States. Modifiable risk factors include sleeping position, bottle feeding, maternal smoking, and infant overheating; sleeping position and smoke exposure may have the largest influence. The prone sleep position could contribute to SIDS through decreased arousal during sleep or during hypoxia, rebreathing of exhaled gases, or effects on the immature autonomic nervous system. The side position, often used in hospitals, also shows increased risk of SIDS compared with the supine position.

Maternal smoking, especially prenatal maternal smoking, increases the risk of SIDS. Investigations of tobacco effects on the autonomic nervous system of the developing fetus, pulmonary growth and function of the newborn, or its combination with viral infection all point to differences in SIDS compared with control subjects.

The most consistent pathologic findings are intrathoracic petechiae and mild inflammation and congestion of the respiratory tract. Subtler pathologic findings include brainstem gliosis, extramedullary hematopoiesis, and increases in periadrenal brown fat. These latter findings suggest that infants who succumb to SIDS have had intermittent or chronic hypoxia before death.

The mechanism or mechanisms of death in SIDS are unknown. For example, it is unknown whether the initiating event at the time of death is cessation of breathing, cardiac arrhythmia, or asystole. Suggested hypotheses have included upper airway obstruction, catecholamine excess, brainstem immaturity or injury, and increased fetal hemoglobin. It has been recognized that some infants who presented with apneic episodes subsequently died from SIDS; however, study of these infants and prospective studies of large numbers of newborns have indicated that most infants with apnea do not die from SIDS and that most infants with SIDS have no identifiable episodes of apnea (see Apparent Life-Threatening Events section).

A history of mild symptoms of upper respiratory infection before death is not uncommon, and SIDS victims are sometimes seen by physicians a day or so before death. When infants are discovered blue, cold, and motionless by parents or caregivers, they are most commonly taken to the emergency room, where resuscitation usually fails. Families must then be supported following the death. The National SIDS Resource Center (http://www.sidscenter.org/) provides information about psychosocial support groups and counseling for families of SIDS victims. The postmortem examination is essential for the diagnosis of SIDS and may help the family by excluding other possible causes of death. A death scene investigation is also important in determining the cause of sudden unexpected deaths in infancy.

The health care provider is instrumental in parental education regarding the modifiable risk factors for SIDS. Education includes promotion of the supine sleeping position, breast-feeding, avoidance of overheating, and smoking cessation (even prenatally). Hospitals should set an example by placing infants in the supine position. With education, the mortality rate, and perhaps the incidence of ALTEs, may continue to decline.

American Academy of Pediatrics Task Force on Infant Sleep Position and Sudden Infant Death Syndrome: Changing concepts of sudden infant death syndrome: Implications for infant sleeping environment and sleep position. Pediatrics 2000;105:650 [PMID: 10699127].

Committee on the Fetus and Newborn. American Academy of Pediatrics: Apnea, sudden infant death syndrome, and home monitoring. Pediatrics 2003;111:914 [PMID: 12671135].

Hunt CE: Sudden infant death syndrome and other causes of infant mortality: Diagnosis, mechanisms, and risk for recurrence in siblings. Am J Respir Crit Care Med 2001;164:346 [PMID: 11500332].

Nagler J: Sudden infant death syndrome. Curr Opin Pediatr 2002;14:247 [PMID: 11981299].

Ramanathan R et al: Cardiorespiratory events recorded on home monitors: Comparison of healthy infants with those at increased risk for SIDS. JAMA 2001;285:2199 [PMID: 11325321].

Toomey S, Bernstein H: Sudden infant death syndrome. Curr Opin Pediatr 2001;13:207 [PMID: 11317067].

# ■ MEDIASTINUM

## MEDIASTINITIS

Acute infection of the mediastinum in children is usually due to traumatic perforation of the esophagus. The trauma may be self-induced (foreign body, puncture injury to the pharynx with a sharp object) or iatrogenic (endoscopy, attempted endotracheal intubation). Vomiting can perforate the esophagus and lead to mediastinitis but this is rare. In addition, acute suppurative mediastinitis without trauma does occur but is unusual.

### Clinical Findings

#### A. SYMPTOMS AND SIGNS

The early symptoms and signs of acute mediastinitis may be vague and include the gradual onset of fever, chills, and dysphagia with substernal pain. Dyspnea and cough may also be present. Inspiration may be accompanied by discomfort due to stretching of inflamed mediastinal structures, leading to a pattern of spasmodic or halting inspiration. On physical examination, evidence of obstruction of venous return may be present, with substernal pain elicited on palpation of the structures of the thorax. In addition, subcutaneous emphysema may be appreciated in the thoracic and cervical areas.

#### B. LABORATORY FINDINGS AND IMAGING

The neutrophil and band count is usually high in mediastinitis. The chest radiograph may show widening of the upper mediastinum; the lateral view shows anterior displacement of the trachea and the esophagus. Mediastinal emphysema, pleural effusions, and pyopneumothorax may also be present.

## Differential Diagnosis

The differential diagnosis includes bacterial pneumonia, septicemia, and retropharyngeal abscesses.

## Complications

Untreated mediastinitis can progress rapidly to death from infection or tracheal obstruction. Mediastinal abscess is a possible complication.

## Treatment

Intravenous antibiotics should be given urgently. If significant tracheal obstruction is present, an airway must be provided. Drainage of abscesses in the mediastinum may also be indicated.

Kono T et al: CT findings of descending necrotizing mediastinitis via the carotid space ("Lincoln Highway"). Pediatr Radiol 2001;31:84 [PMID: 11214691].

Sztajnbok J et al: Descending suppurative mediastinitis: Nonsurgical approach to this unusual complication of retropharyngeal abscesses in childhood. Pediatr Emerg Care 1999;15:341 [PMID: 10532666].

# MEDIASTINAL MASSES

Mediastinal masses may present because of symptoms produced by pressure on the esophagus, airways, nerves, or vessels within the mediastinum or may be discovered on a routine chest radiograph. Once the mass is identified, localization to one of four mediastinal compartments aids in the differential diagnosis. The superior mediastinum is the area above the pericardium that is bordered inferiorly by an imaginary line from the manubrium to the fourth thoracic vertebra. The anterior mediastinum is bordered by the sternum anteriorly and the pericardium posteriorly, and the posterior mediastinum is defined by the pericardium and diaphragm anteriorly and the lower eight thoracic vertebrae posteriorly. The middle mediastinum is surrounded by these three compartments.

## Clinical Findings

### A. SYMPTOMS AND SIGNS

Respiratory symptoms, when present, are due to pressure on an airway (cough, wheezing) or an infection (unresolving pneumonia in one area of lung). Hemoptysis can also occur but is an unusual presenting symptom. Dysphagia may occur secondary to compression of the esophagus. Pressure on the recurrent laryngeal nerve can cause hoarseness due to paralysis of the left vocal cord. Superior vena caval obstruction can lead to dilation of neck vessels and other signs and symptoms of obstruction of venous return from the upper part of the body (superior mediastinal syndrome).

### B. LABORATORY FINDINGS AND IMAGING

The mass is initially defined by frontal and lateral chest radiographs together with thoracic CT scans and perhaps MRI. A barium swallow may also help define the extent of a mass. Other studies that may be required include angiography (to define the blood supply to large tumors), electrocardiography, echocardiography, ultrasound of the thorax, fungal and mycobacterial skin tests, and urinary catecholamine assays. MRI or myelography may be necessary in children suspected of having a neurogenic tumor in the posterior mediastinum.

## Differential Diagnosis

The differential diagnosis of mediastinal masses is determined by their location. Within the superior mediastinum, one may find cystic hygromas, vascular or neurogenic tumors, thymic masses, teratomas, intrathoracic thyroid tissue, and esophageal lesions. A mediastinal abscess may also be found in this region. Within the anterior mediastinum, thymic tissue (thymomas, hyperplasia, cysts) and teratomas, vascular tumors, and lymphatic tissue (lymphomas, reactive lymphadenopathy) give rise to masses. An intrathoracic thyroid and a pleuropericardial cyst may also be found in this region. Within the middle mediastinum one may again find lymphomas and hypertrophic lymph nodes, granulomas, bronchogenic or enterogenous cysts, metastases, and pericardial cysts. Abnormalities of the great vessels and aortic aneurysms may also present as masses in this compartment. Within the posterior mediastinum, neurogenic tumors, enterogenous cysts, thoracic meningoceles, or aortic aneurysms may be present.

In some series, more than 50% of mediastinal tumors occur in the posterior mediastinum and are mainly neurogenic tumors or enterogenous cysts. Most neurogenic tumors in children younger than age 4 years are malignant (neuroblastoma, neuroganglioblastoma), whereas a benign ganglioneuroma is the most common histologic type in older children. In the middle and anterior mediastinum, tumors of lymphatic origin (lymphomas) are the primary concern. Bulky anterior mediastinal tumors that compress the trachea and the great vessels can lead to a superior mediastinal syndrome, which presents a diagnostic problem because of anesthesia hazards. Definitive diagnosis in most instances relies on surgery to obtain the mass or a part of the mass for histologic examination. In cases of lymphoma, the scalene nodes may also contain tumor, and a biopsy should be performed in an attempt to establish a diagnosis.

## Treatment & Prognosis

The appropriate therapy and the response to therapy depend on the cause of the mediastinal mass.

Buckley JA et al: CT evaluation of mediastinal masses in children: Spectrum of disease with pathologic correlation. Crit Rev Diagn Imaging 1998;39:365 [PMID: 9791749].

Esposito G: Diagnosis of mediastinal masses and principles of surgical tactics and techniques for their treatment. Semin Pediatr Surg 1999;8:54 [PMID: 10344301].

Williams HJ, Alton HM: Imaging of paediatric mediastinal abnormalities. Paediatr Respir Rev 2003;4:55 [PMID: 12615033].

# Cardiovascular Diseases

# 19

*Anji T. Yetman, MD, Shelley D. Miyamoto, MD, Henry M. Sondheimer, MD*

Cardiovascular disease is a significant cause of death and chronic illness in childhood. In North America 8 in 1000 infants are born with a congenital heart defect. In addition, acquired heart disease, including Kawasaki disease, myocarditis, rheumatic heart disease, and others, remains a significant cause of pediatric morbidity and mortality. With advances in medical and surgical care, more than 85% of children with congenital heart defects will live into adulthood. It is therefore important that attention be paid not only to the diagnosis and treatment of congenital cardiac lesions but also to the prevention of secondary comorbidities, namely, hyperlipidemia and atherosclerosis. Maintenance pediatric health visits must focus on the diagnosis and prevention of hypercholesterolemia and hypertension. Counseling regarding the hazards of smoking and the benefits of regular exercise should be part of routine pediatric care. Subspecialty clinics designed to address the needs of the young adult with congenital heart disease will be needed to service this growing patient population. Previously rare clinical dilemmas, including the impact of pregnancy on congenital cardiac lesions, risks of anticoagulation during pregnancy, and vocational choices will need to be addressed.

## ■ DIAGNOSTIC EVALUATION

The presence of a heart murmur may suggest the possibility of heart disease. The murmur may be a functional or innocent one, however. Not all serious cardiovascular disorders are accompanied by an easily detectable murmur.

### Sequence of Evaluation

1. History
2. Physical examination
3. Electrocardiogram
4. Chest radiograph
5. Echocardiogram
6. Other ancillary studies, including cardiopulmonary stress testing, 24-hour Holter or other ambulatory ECG monitoring devices, cardiac catheterization,

angiocardiography, nuclear imaging studies, and cardiac magnetic resonance imaging (MRI)

## HISTORY

In obtaining a medical history from the family or the patient, one must keep in perspective the patient's age and activity level. Most congenital defects will lead to either decreased pulmonary blood flow or increased pulmonary blood flow with pulmonary congestion (see Table 19–10). Symptoms will vary according to the alteration in pulmonary blood flow (Table 19–1)

The presence of other cardiovascular symptoms such as palpitations and chest pain should also be determined by history in the older child, paying particular attention to the timing (rest or activity related), onset and termination (gradual vs sudden), and precipitating and relieving factors.

## PHYSICAL EXAMINATION

### General

The examination should begin with a careful inspection to note activity (agitation, lethargy), skin perfusion, and skin color. Heart rate, respiratory rate, blood pressure (in all four extremities), and oxygen saturation are required. Many congenital cardiac defects occur as part of a genetic syndrome (Table 19–2), and the overall assessment should include examination for dysmorphic features that may provide clues to the associated cardiac defect.

### 1. Cardiovascular Examination

#### Inspection & Palpation

The conformation of the chest should be noted by observing the supine patient from the end of the examining table. A left precordial bulge indicates long-standing cardiomegaly, which may be seen in association with dilated cardiomyopathy, or right or left heart obstructive lesions.

Palpation may reveal increased precordial activity, RV lift, or left-sided heave; a diffuse point of maximal impulse; or a thrill caused by a greater than grade III/VI murmur. Thrills are located where the murmur is most

**Table 19–1.** Symptoms of increased and decreased pulmonary blood flow.

| Decreased Pulmonary Blood Flow | Increased Pulmonary Blood Flow |
|---|---|
| *Infant/Toddler:* | |
| Cyanosis | Tachypnea with activity/feeds |
| Squatting | Diaphoresis |
| Loss of consciousness | Poor weight gain |
| *Older child:* | |
| Dizziness | Exercise intolerance |
| Syncope | Dyspnea on exertion, Diaphoresis |

intense and can sometimes be felt at the point of radiation. For example, a thrill in the suprasternal notch or carotid thrill is associated with aortic stenosis. In patients with severe pulmonary hypertension, palpable pulmonary closure is frequently noted at the upper left sternal border. A palpable fourth heart sound may be seen in association with a hypertrophied, noncompliant ventricle as in hypertrophic cardiomyopathy.

## Auscultation

### A. HEART SOUNDS

The first heart sound ($S_1$) is the sound of AV valve closure. It is best heard at the lower left sternal border and is usually medium-pitched. Although $S_1$ has multiple components, usually only one of these ($M_1$) is heard with a stethoscope.

The second heart sound ($S_2$) is the sound of semilunar valve closure. It is best heard along the mid and

**Table 19–2.** Cardiac defects in common syndromes.

| Genetic Syndrome | Commonly Associated Cardiac Defect |
|---|---|
| Down syndrome | AVSD |
| Turner's syndrome | Bicuspid aortic valve, coarctation |
| Noonan's syndrome | Dysplastic pulmonic valve, HCM |
| Williams–Beuren syndrome | Supravalval aortic stenosis, PPS |
| Marfan's syndrome | MVP, MR, dilated aortic root |
| Fetal alcohol syndrome | VSD, ASD |
| Maternal rubella | PDA, PPS |

AVSD = atrioventricvular septal defect; HCM = hypertrophic cardiomyopathy; MVP = mitral valve prolapse; MR = mitral regurgitation; VSD = ventricular septal defect; ASD = atrial septal defect; PDA = patent ductus arteriosus; PPS = peripheral pulmonary stenosis.

upper left sternal border. $S_2$ has two component sounds, $A_2$ and then $P_2$ (aortic and pulmonary valve closure). Splitting of $S_2$ varies with respiration, widening with inspiration and narrowing with expiration. It is best heard at the second left intercostal space at the sternal border. Abnormal splitting of $S_2$ may provide clues to the presence of cardiac disease (Table 19–3).

The third heart sound ($S_3$) is the sound of rapid filling of the LV. It occurs in early diastole, after $S_2$, and is medium- to low-pitched. When heard in healthy children, the sound diminishes or disappears when the position changes from supine to sitting or standing. It is usually intermittent. A persistent $S_3$ is often heard in the presence of a dilated LV caused by a cardiomyopathy or large left-to-right shunt.

The fourth heart sound ($S_4$) is associated with atrial contraction and increased atrial pressure and has a low pitch similar to that of $S_3$. It occurs just prior to $S_1$ and is not normally audible. It is heard in the presence of atrial contraction into a noncompliant ventricle as is present in hypertrophic or restrictive cardiomyopathy or a hypertrophied LV from other causes.

Ejection clicks are high-pitched and are usually related to dilated great vessels or valve abnormalities. They can be heard throughout ventricular systole and are classified as early, mid, or late. Early ejection clicks at the mid left sternal border are usually of pulmonary origin. Aortic clicks are typically best heard at the apex. In contrast to aortic clicks, pulmonic clicks vary with respiration, becoming louder during inspiration. A mid to late ejection click at the apex is most typically caused by mitral valve prolapse. Early clicks may also be heard with a closing ventricular septal defect (VSD).

### B. MURMURS

Murmurs are the most common cardiovascular finding leading to a cardiology referral. Innocent, or functional, heart murmurs are extremely common. Between 40% and 45% of children have an innocent murmur at some time during childhood.

**Table 19–3.** Abnormal splitting of $S_2$.

**Causes of wide split $S_2$**
RV volume overload: ASD, anomalous pulmonary venous return, PI
RV pressure overload: Pulmonary valve stenosis
Delayed RV conduction: RBBB
**Causes of narrow split $S_2$**
Pulmonary hypertension
Single semilunar valve (aortic atresia, pulmonary atresia, truncus arteriosus)

RV = right ventricle; ASD = atrial septal defect; PI = pulmonic insufficiency; RBBB = right bundle branch block.

**1. Characteristics**—All murmurs should be described based on the following characteristics:

**a. Location and radiation.** Where the murmur is best heard and where the sound extends.

**b. Relationship to cardiac cycle and duration.** Systolic ejection (immediately following S$_1$ with a crescendo/decrescendo change in intensity), pansystolic (occurring throughout most of systole and of constant intensity), diastolic, and continuous. The timing of the murmur provides valuable clues as to underlying pathology (Table 19–4).

**c. Intensity.** Classified as grade I, soft and heard with difficulty; grade II, soft but easily heard; grade III, loud but without a thrill; grade IV, loud and associated with a precordial thrill; grade V, loud, with thrill, and audible with the edge of the stethoscope; or grade VI, very loud and audible with the stethoscope off the chest.

**d. Quality.** Harsh, musical, or rough; high, medium, or low in pitch.

**e. Variation with position.** Audible when the patient is supine, sitting, standing, or squatting.

**2. Functional murmurs**—The six most common functional murmurs of childhood are:

**a. Newborn murmur.** Heard in the first few days of life, this murmur is at the lower left sternal border, without significant radiation. It has a soft, short, vibratory grade I–II/VI quality that often subsides when mild pressure is applied to the abdomen. It usually disappears by age 2–3 weeks.

**b. Functional murmur of peripheral arterial pulmonary stenosis.** This is frequently heard in newborns and is caused by the normal mild bending of the branches of the pulmonary artery. It is heard with equal intensity at the upper left sternal border, at the back, and in both axillae. It is a soft, short, high-pitched, grade I–II/VI systolic ejection murmur and usually disappears by age 4. This murmur must be differentiated from true peripheral pulmonary stenosis (Williams syn-

drome or rubella syndrome), coarctation of the thoracic aorta, valvular pulmonary stenosis, and atrial septal defect (ASD).

**c. Still murmur.** This is the most common innocent murmur of early childhood. It is most typically heard from age 2 years until preadolescence. Still's murmur is loudest midway between the apex and the lower left sternal border and often is transmitted to the remainder of the precordium. Still's murmur is a musical or vibratory, short, high-pitched, grade I–III early systolic murmur. It is loudest when the patient is in the supine position; it diminishes or disappears with inspiration, when the patient sits or stands, or during the Valsalva maneuver. Still's murmur will be louder in patients with fever or tachycardia.

**d. Pulmonary ejection murmur.** This is the most common innocent murmur in older children. It is heard throughout childhood from age 3 years onward. It is usually a soft, systolic ejection murmur, grade I–II in intensity and well localized to the upper left sternal border. The murmur becomes louder when the patient is supine or when cardiac output is increased and softens with standing or during the Valsalva maneuver. The pulmonary ejection murmur must be differentiated from other murmurs, such as those associated with pulmonary stenosis, coarctation of the aorta, ASD, and peripheral pulmonary artery stenosis.

**e. Venous hum.** This murmur is usually heard after age 2 years, is located in the left and right infraclavicular areas, and is usually louder on the right. It is a continuous musical hum of grade I–II intensity and it may be accentuated in diastole and with inspiration. This murmur is best heard with the child sitting. Turning the child's neck, placing him or her in a supine position, and compressing the jugular vein obliterates the venous hum. Venous hum is produced by turbulence at the confluence of the subclavian and jugular veins.

**f. Innominate or carotid bruit.** This murmur is more common in the older child and adolescent. It is heard in the right supraclavicular area. This is a long systolic ejection murmur, somewhat harsh and of grade

***Table 19–4.*** Pathologic murmurs.

| Systolic Ejection | Pansystolic | Diastolic | Continuous |
|---|---|---|---|
| Semilunar valve stenosis (AS/PS/truncal stenosis) ASD Coarctation | VSD AVVR (MR/TR) | Semilunar valve regurgitation (AI/PI/truncal insufficiency) AV valve stenosis (MS/TS) | Runoff lesions (PDA/AVM/aortopulmonary collaterals |

VSD = ventricular septal defect; AS/PS = aortic stenosis/pulmonic stenosis; MR/TR = mitral regurgitation/tricuspid regurgitation; AI/PI = aortic insufficiency/pulmonic insufficiency; PDA/AVM = patent ductus arteriosus/arteriovenous malformation; ASD = atrial septal defect; AV = atrioventricular; MS/TS = mitral stenosis/tricuspid stenosis.

II–III intensity. The bruit can be accentuated by light pressure on the carotid artery and must be differentiated from all types of aortic stenosis.

When functional murmurs are found in a child, the physician should assure the parents that these are normal heart sounds of the developing child and that they do not represent structural abnormality of the heart.

## 2. Extracardiac Examination

### Arterial Pulse

#### A. RATE AND RHYTHM

Cardiac rate and rhythm can vary greatly during infancy and childhood, so multiple determinations should be made. This caution is particularly important for infants (Table 19–5), whose heart rate varies with activity. In children, the rhythm may be regular, or there may be a phasic variation in the heart rate with respiration (sinus arrhythmia), which is normal.

#### B. QUALITY AND AMPLITUDE OF PULSE

The pulses of the upper and lower extremities should be compared. A bounding pulse is characteristic of run-off lesions, including patent ductus arteriosus (PDA), aortic regurgitation, arteriovenous malformation (AVM), or any condition with a low diastolic pressure (fever, anemia, septic shock). These conditions may also be associated with palpable palmar pulses, which otherwise are not normally present. Narrow or thready pulses are found in patients with reduced cardiac output as seen in cardiomyopathy, myocarditis, pericardial tamponade, or severe aortic stenosis. A reduction in pulse amplitude or blood pressure (> 10 mm Hg) with inspiration is referred to as pulsus paradoxus and is a telltale sign of pericardial tamponade. With inspiration, venous return is increased to the right side of the heart. Because of a fixed pericardial constraint, an increase in right heart volume must be accompanied by a reduction in left heart volume and thus a reduction in cardiac output during the inspiratory phase of respiration. The femoral pulse should be palpable and equal in amplitude and simultaneous with the brachial pulse. A

femoral pulse that is absent, or weak, or that is delayed in comparison with the brachial pulse, suggests coarctation of the aorta. An absent or diminished femoral pulse may be the only clue to the presence of this important clinical problem.

#### C. ARTERIAL BLOOD PRESSURE

Blood pressures should be obtained in the upper and lower extremities. Systolic pressure in the lower extremities should be greater than or equal to that in the upper extremities. The cuff must cover the same relative area of the arm and leg. Measurements should be repeated several times.

#### D. VENOUS PRESSURE & PULSE

The level of the distended jugular vein above the suprasternal notch, when the patient is placed at a 45-degree angle to the examination table, is a measure of venous pressure. Normally, one may observe the transition between collapsed and distended jugular vein approximately 1–2 cm above the notch. Although the venous pulse may not be helpful when examining infants and young children because of their short neck and increased subcutaneous tissue in this region, it may be a helpful adjunctive tool in the cardiac assessment of the older child.

#### E. EXTREMITIES

1. Cyanosis—Cyanosis is the result of an increased concentration (4–5 g/dL) of reduced hemoglobin in the blood. Bluish skin color is usually, but not always, a sign. Anemic patients may not appear blue, and patients with polycythemia may appear cyanotic, even though blood oxygen content is normal. Visible cyanosis accompanies low cardiac output, hypothermia, and systemic venous congestion, even in the presence of adequate oxygenation. Cyanosis should be judged only by the color of the mucous membranes (lips and nail beds). Bluish discoloration around the mouth (acrocyanosis) is a feature of skin that has not been exposed to sun, and it does not correlate with cyanosis.

2. Clubbing of fingers and toes—Clubbing implies the presence of fairly severe cyanotic congenital heart disease. It usually does not appear until after age 1 year. The first sign of clubbing is softening of the nail beds, followed by rounding of the fingernails and then by thickening and shininess of the terminal phalanx, with loss of creases.

Hypoxemia producing cyanosis is by far the most common cause of digital clubbing, but it also occurs in patients with infective endocarditis, chronic liver disease, inflammatory bowel diseases, chronic pulmonary insufficiency (PI), and lung abscess. Digital clubbing may be a benign genetic variant.

*Table 19–5.* Resting heart rates.

| Age | Low | High |
| --- | --- | --- |
| < 1 month | 80 | 160 |
| 1–3 months | 80 | 200 |
| 2–24 months | 70 | 120 |
| 2–10 years | 60 | 90 |
| 11–18 years | 40 | 90 |

**3. Edema**—Edema of dependent areas (lower extremities in the older child and the face and sacrum in the younger child) is characteristic of elevated right heart pressures, which may be seen with tricuspid valve pathology, or RV dysfunction from a variety of causes (right heart failure).

### F. ABDOMEN

Hepatomegaly is the cardinal sign of right heart failure in the infant and child. Presystolic pulsation of the liver may occur with right atrial hypertension and systolic pulsation with tricuspid insufficiency. Apparent hepatomegaly may also be seen in the child with pulmonary edema from lesions causing left-to-right shunting or left heart failure. Pulmonary congestion and associated lymphatic engorgement lead to lung hyperexpansion, pushing the liver further below the costal margin. Splenomegaly may be present in patients who have had long-standing congestive heart failure (CHF), and it is a characteristic feature of infective endocarditis. Ascites is also a feature of chronic right heart failure. Physical examination may be notable for shifting dullness or a fluid wave on abdominal examination.

Advani N et al: The diagnosis of innocent murmurs in childhood. Cardiol Young 2000;10(4):340 [PMID: 10950330].

Murphy DJ: The patient population and requirements for optimal care: Adult congenital heart disease. Prog Pediatr Cardiol 2003;17(1):1.

Williams CL et al: Cardiovascular health in childhood: A statement for health professionals. Circulation 2002;106(1):143 [PMID: 12093785].

## ELECTROCARDIOGRAPHY

The electrocardiogram (ECG) is an essential part of the evaluation of the cardiovascular system. A consistent approach to the ECG will allow for interpretation of even the most complex and initially confusing ECG recording. The heart rate should first be determined (Is it appropriate for the patient's age and state of well-being?), then the rhythm (Is the patient in a normal sinus rhythm or other rhythm as evidenced by a P wave with a consistent PR interval before every QRS complex?), and then the axis (Are the P and QRS axes normal for the patient's age?). Once this initial assessment of rate, rhythm, and axis is performed, attention can be directed toward assessment of chamber enlargement and finally to assessment of cardiac intervals and ST segments.

## Age-Related Variations

The ECG evolves with age and thus must be interpreted according to age-related norms. The rate gradually decreases and intervals increase with age. The dominance of ventricles changes from RV dominance in the newborn to LV dominance in the older infant, child, and adult. The normal ECG of the 1-week-old infant would be highly abnormal for a 1-year-old child, and the ECG of a 5-year-old child is abnormal for an adult.

## Electrocardiographic Interpretation

Figure 19–1 defines the events recorded by the ECG.

### A. RATE

The paper speed at which ECGs are normally obtained is 25 mm/s. Each small square is 1 mm, and each large square, 5 mm. Therefore, five large squares represent 1 second, one large square 0.2 second, and one small square 0.04 second. A common method of estimating the ventricular rate is to count the number of small squares between two QRS complexes (see following discussion) and to divide this number into 1500. If QRS complexes appear at a rate of one per 5 small squares, the ventricular rate is 300; if QRS complexes appear every 12 small squares, the ventricular rate is 125, and so on.

### B. RHYTHM

Sinus rhythm should always be present in normal children. In contrast to adults, premature atrial and ventricular contractions are uncommon during childhood.

### C. AXIS

P wave axis: The P wave is generated from atrial contraction beginning in the high right atrium at the site of the sinus node. The impulse proceeds leftward and inferiorly, thus leading to a positive deflection in all left-sided and inferior leads (II, III and aVF). Conversely, the P wave in patients in normal sinus rhythm should be negative in lead aVR.

QRS axis: The net voltage should be positive in leads I and aVF in children with a normal axis. In the young child, RV dominance may persist, leading to a negative net deflection in lead I. Several congenital cardiac lesions are associated with alterations in the normal QRS axis (Table 19–6)

### D. P WAVE

In the pediatric patient, the amplitude of the P wave is normally no greater than 2.5 mm or more than 0.08 second in duration. The P wave is usually best seen in leads II and $V_1$.

### E. PR INTERVAL

This interval is measured from the beginning of the P wave to the beginning of the QRS complex. It increases with age and with slower rates. The PR interval ranges from a minimum of 0.11 second in infants to a maximum of 0.18 second in older children with slow rates.

***Figure 19-1.*** Complexes and intervals of the ECG.

The PR interval is commonly prolonged in patients who have rheumatic heart disease and by digitalis.

### F. QRS COMPLEX

This represents ventricular depolarization, and its amplitude and direction of force (axis) reveal the relative size of (viable) ventricular mass in hypertrophy, hypoplasia, and infarction. Abnormal ventricular conduction (eg, right bundle branch block [RBBB], anterior fascicular block) is also revealed.

### G. QT INTERVAL

This interval is measured from the beginning of the QRS complex to the end of the T wave. The QT dura-

tion may be prolonged as a primary condition or secondarily due to drugs or electrolyte imbalances (Table 19–7) The normal QT duration is rate-related and must be corrected using the Bazett formula:

$$QTC = \frac{QT\ interval(s)}{\sqrt{R - R\ interval(s)}}$$

The normal QTc is less than 0.44 second or less than 0.46 second in postpubertal females.

### H. ST SEGMENT

This segment, lying between the end of the QRS complex and the beginning of the T wave, is affected by drugs, electrolyte imbalances, or myocardial injury.

### I. T WAVE

The T wave represents myocardial repolarization and is altered by electrolytes, myocardial hypertrophy, and ischemia.

### J. IMPRESSION

The ultimate impression of the ECG is derived from a systematic analysis of the features described earlier as

***Table 19-6.*** QRS axis deviation.

| Right Axis Deviation | Left Axis Deviation |
|---|---|
| Tetralogy of Fallot | Atrioventricular septal defect |
| Dextro transposition of the great arteries | Pulmonary atresia with intact ventricular septum |
| Total anomalous pulmonary venous return | Tricuspid atresia |
| Atrial septal defect | |

***Table 19–7.*** Causes of QT prolongation.*

**Cardiac Medications**
   **Antiarrhythmics:** IA (quinidine, procainamide, disopyra-
      mide) class III (amiodarone, sotalol)
   **Inotropic Agents:** dobutamine, dopamine, epinephrine,
      isoproterenol
**Noncardiac medications**
   **Antibiotics/Antivirals:** azithromycin, clarithromycin,
      levofloxacin, amantadine
   **Antipsychotics:** risperidol, thioridazine, lithium,
      haloperidol
   **Other:** albuterol, levalbuterol, ondansetron, phenytoin,
      pseudoephedrine
**Sedatives:** chloral hydrate, methadone
**Electrolyte disturbances:** hypokalemia, hypomagnesemia,
   hypocalcemia

*Partial list only

compared with expected normal values for the child's
age.

Al-Khatib SM et al: What clinicians should know about the QT interval. JAMA 2003;289(16):2120 [PMID: 12709470].

Benson DW Jr: The normal electrocardiogram. In Emmanouilides
   GC et al (eds): *Moss and Adams Heart Disease in Infants,
   Children, and Adolescents,* 5th ed. Williams & Wilkins, 1995.

Viskin S et al: Long QT syndrome caused by noncardiac drugs.
   Prog Cardiovasc Dis 2003;45(5):415 [PMID: 12704598].

## CHEST RADIOGRAPH

Evaluation of the chest radiograph for cardiac disease
should focus on: (1) position of the cardiac apex,
(2) position of the abdominal viscera, (3) cardiac size,
(4) cardiac configuration, and (5) character of the pulmonary vasculature.

A segmental approach is used when evaluating cardiac anatomy, either by chest radiograph or by echocardiography. The position of the cardiac apex should be
noted as either levocardia (apex points to the left), dextrocardia (cardiac apex to the right), or mesocardia (cardiac apex in the middle). The position of the liver and
stomach bubble should be noted as either in the normal
position (abdominal situs solitus), in reverse position
with stomach bubble on the right (abdominal situs inversus), or a variable stomach position with midline
liver (abdominal situs ambiguous). The heart appears
relatively large in normal newborns and decreases on
the chest radiograph with age. The heart size should be
less than 50% of the chest diameter in children older
than age 1 year. The cardiac configuration on chest radiograph may provide useful diagnostic information, as
certain cardiac lesions have a characteristic radiographic
appearance (Tables 19–8 and 19–9).

***Table 19–8.*** Radiographic changes with cardiac
chamber enlargement.

| Chamber Enlarged | Change in Cardiac Silhouette on Anteroposterior Film |
|---|---|
| Right ventricle | Apex of the heart is tipped upward |
| Left ventricle | Apex of the heart is tipped downward |
| Left atrium | Double shadow behind cardiac sil-houette |
|  | Increase in subcarinal angle |
| Right atrium | Prominence of right atrial border of the heart |

The pulmonary vasculature should be assessed in
every patient. The presence of increased or decreased
pulmonary blood flow provides a useful clue to cardiac
diagnosis, particularly in the cyanotic infant (Table
19–10)

The standard posteroanterior and left lateral chest
radiographs are used (Figure 19–2).

## Dextrocardia

Dextrocardia is a radiographic term used when the
heart is on the right side of the chest. When dextrocardia occurs with reversal of position of the other important organs of the chest and abdomen (eg, liver, lungs,
and spleen), the condition is called situs inversus totalis,
and the heart is usually completely normal. When dextrocardia occurs with otherwise normal organs (situs
solitus), the heart usually has severe defects.

***Table 19–9.*** Lesion-specific chest radiographic
findings.

| Diagnosis | Chest radiograph appearance |
|---|---|
| Dextrotransposition of the great arteries | Egg on a string |
| Tetralogy of Fallot | Boot-shaped heart |
| Unobstructed total anomalous pulmonary venous drainage | Snowman |
| Obstructed total anomalous pulmonary venous drainage | Small heart with congested lungs |
| Coarctation | Figure 3 sign + rib notching |

**Table 19–10.** Alterations in pulmonary blood flow in cyanotic cardiac lesions.

| Increased Pulmonary Blood Flow | Decreased Pulmonary Blood Flow |
| --- | --- |
| Total anomalous pulmonary venous return | Pulmonic stenosis |
| TA/large ventricular septal defect | Tricuspid atresia/restrictive ventricular septal defect |
| Complete transposition of great arteries | Tetralogy of Fallot |
| Truncus arteroisus | Pulmonary atresia with intact ventricular septum |
| | Hypoplastic left heart syndrome |

Rarely, the abdominal organs and lungs are neither in situs solitus nor situs inversus. These states are called situs ambiguous. The liver is central and anterior in the upper abdomen, with the stomach pushed posteriorly. Bilateral right-sidedness (asplenia syndrome) or bilateral left-sidedness (polysplenia syndrome) may occur, but, in virtually all cases of situs ambiguous, congenital heart disease is present.

Burrows PE et al: Imaging of the neonate with congenital heart disease. In Freedom RM (ed): *Neonatal Heart Disease.* Springer-Verlag, 1992.

## ECHOCARDIOGRAPHY

Echocardiography is a useful noninvasive method for diagnosing congenital heart defects and is used to further define anatomy, function, chamber size, vessel size, and valve abnormalities following cardiac examination, chest radiograph, and ECG. In most cases two-dimensional echocardiography is sufficient for the accurate diagnosis of congenital cardiac lesions, and no further testing is required prior to initial medical or surgical intervention. Two-dimensional echocardiography with Doppler ultrasonography (color, pulsed, or continuous-wave ultrasound measurements) is used to assess cardiac output, magnitude of regurgitant and stenotic lesions, diastolic LV relaxation, and pulmonary artery pressure. Stress echocardiography allows for quantification of ventricular systolic and diastolic function and assessment of myocardial wall motion abnormalities in patients after exercise or pharmacologic stress with dobutamine infusion.

Two-dimensional echocardiography should be performed with a systematic series of steps to define the intracardiac anatomy:

1. Position of the cardiac apex
2. Position of the abdominal vessels (inferior vena cava [IVC] and aorta)
3. Relationship between the atria and ventricles
4. Relationship between the ventricles and great vessels
5. Evaluation of intracardiac defects

The relationship between the atria and ventricles is noted. If the morphologic right atrium empties into a morphologic right ventricle (RV) and, similarly, the morphologic left atrium empties into a morphologic LV, atrioventricular concordance is present. If the atria correspond to the wrong ventricle (eg, right atrium emptying into LV), atrioventricular discordance is present. Other possible atrioventricular (AV) relationships include double-inlet LV (both atria empty into the LV), double-inlet RV, and atresia of a right or left AV valve with associated single inlet (eg, tricuspid atresia). Similarly, the relationship between the ventricles and great vessels is noted. Normally, the pulmonay artery (PA) arises from the RV and the aorta from the LV and ventriculoarterial concordance is present. If the relationships are reversed (ie, aorta from RV and PA from

Posteroanterior

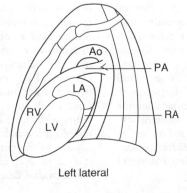
Left lateral

**Figure 19–2.** Position of cardiovascular structures in principal radiograph views. Ao = aorta, IVC = inferior vena cava, LA = left atrium, LA APP = left atrial appendage, LV = left ventricle, PA = pulmonary artery, RA = right atrium, RV = right ventricle, SVC = superior vena cava.

LV), then ventriculoarterial discordance is present (as in complete transposition of the great arteries [TGA]). Other possible ventriculoarterial relationships include double-outlet RV, double-outlet LV, and atresia of one outlet (eg, pulmonary or aortic atresia). If both AV discordance and ventriculoarterial discordance are present, the patient has what is referred to as congenitally corrected transposition.

Pahl E et al: The role of stress echocardiography in children. Echocardiography 2000;17(5):507 [PMID: 10979027].

Snider AR et al: *Echocardiography in Congenital Heart Disease.* Mosby, 1997.

## NUCLEAR CARDIOLOGY

Nuclear imaging may be used in patients with VSDs and other lesions with left-to-right shunting to noninvasively quantify the degree of shunting and thereby avoid cardiac catheterization.

Nuclear imaging may also be useful as an adjunct to cardiopulmonary exercise testing in assessing both fixed and reversible areas of myocardial ischemia. This testing is valuable in evaluating myocardial perfusion in patients with Kawasaki disease, repaired anomalous left coronary artery or other coronary anomalies, myocardial bridging in the setting of hypertrophic cardiomyopathy or chest pain in association with ECG changes with exercise.

## MAGNETIC RESONANCE IMAGING

MRI is a valuable tool in the evaluation and noninvasive follow-up of many congenital heart defects. It is particularly useful in imaging the vascular structures of the thorax, which are difficult to image by transthoracic echocardiogram. The addition of cardiac gated imaging allows dynamic evaluation of the structure and blood flow in the heart and great vessels. MRI is invaluable in the initial assessment and long-term follow-up of coarctation of the aorta, in following the progression of aortic dilation in patients with Marfan syndrome, in quantification of regurgitant lesions such as PI following repair of tetralogy of Fallot (ToF), and in quantification of ventricular function in patients whose echocardiographic images are inadequate. Because it allows the operator to move the heart and great vessels on the computer screen, three-dimensional MRI is an ideal method of noninvasive reconstruction of the entire heart and useful for both assessing intracardiac anatomy and analyzing great vessel anatomy and relationships. MRI combined with pharmacologic stress testing (dobutamine infusions) may allow for evaluation of cardiac reserve in patients who cannot undergo standard exercise testing because of size or disability.

Boxt LM, Rozenshtein A: MR imaging of congenital heart disease. Magn Reson Imaging Clin North Am 2003;11(1)27 [PMID: 12797509].

## Cardiopulmonary Stress Testing

Most children with heart disease are capable of normal activity, and data on cardiac function after exercise are essential to preventing the unnecessary restriction of activities. The response to exercise is valuable in determining the timing of, and need for, cardiovascular surgery as well as a useful objective outcome measure for the evaluation of medical and surgical interventions.

Bicycle ergometers or treadmills can be used to test children as young as age 5 years. The addition of a metabolic cart enables one to assess whether exercise impairment is secondary to cardiac limitation, pulmonary limitation, deconditioning, or lack of effort. Exercise variables include the ECG, blood pressure response to exercise, oxygen saturation, ventilation, maximal oxygen consumption, and peak work load attained. Cardiopulmonary stress testing is routine in children with congenital cardiac lesions to ascertain limitations, develop exercise prescriptions, assess the effect of therapies, and decide on the need for cardiac transplantation. Stress testing is also employed in children with structurally normal hearts to rule out cardiac or pulmonary pathology in children with chest pain, syncope, or shortness of breath on exertion. Significant stress ischemia or dysrhythmias warrant physical restrictions or appropriate therapy. Children with poor performance due to suboptimal conditioning benefit from a planned exercise program.

McManus A, Leung M: Maximizing the clinical use of exercise gaseous exchange testing in children with repaired cyanotic congenital heart defects: The development of an appropriate test strategy. Sports Med 2000;29(4)229 [PMID: 10783899].

## ARTERIAL BLOOD GASES

Quantitating the arterial $PO_2$ or $O_2$ saturation (eg, by pulse oximetry) during the administration of 100% oxygen is the most useful method of distinguishing cyanosis produced primarily by heart disease or by lung disease in sick infants. In cyanotic heart disease, $PaO_2$ increases very little when 100% oxygen is administered over the values obtained while breathing room air. However, $PaO_2$ usually increases very significantly when oxygen is administered to a patient who has lung disease. Table 19–11 illustrates the responses seen in patients with heart or lung disease during the hyperoxic test. Routine pulse oximetry has been advocated as an adjunct to the current newborn screening evaluation as it is a simple, cost-effective means of screening for major cardiac defects prior to hospital discharge.

*Table 19–11.* Examples of responses to 10 minutes of 100% oxygen in lung disease and heart disease.

|  | Lung Disease | | Heart Disease | |
|---|---|---|---|---|
|  | Room Air | 100% O₂ | Room Air | 100% O₂ |
| Color | Blue → | Pink | Blue → | Blue |
| Oximetry | 60% → | 99% | 60% → | 62% |
| Pao₂ (mm Hg) | 35 → | 120 | 35 → | 38 |

Koppel RI et al. Effectiveness of pulse oximetry screening for congenital heart disease in asymptomatic newborns. Pediatrics 2003;111:451 [PMID: 12612220].

# CARDIAC CATHETERIZATION & ANGIOCARDIOGRAPHY

Cardiac catheterization precisely defines the anatomic and physiologic abnormalities in simple and complex cardiac malformations. Cardiac catheterization, may be performed for diagnostic purposes when further anatomic or physiologic data are needed prior to a therapeutic decision or may be performed for therapeutic purposes when the cardiac condition can be palliated or treated in the catheterization laboratory.

## Therapeutic Cardiac Catheterization

Therapeutic procedures performed during cardiac catheterization include coil embolization of a PDA, balloon aortoplasty of aortic coarctation, balloon atrial septostomy, valvuloplasty of stenotic aortic or pulmonic valves, and placement of ASD and VSD devices. Cardiac catheterization is also performed to evaluate the effects of pharmaceutical therapy. An example of this use of catheterization is monitoring acute changes in pulmonary vascular resistance during the administration of nitric oxide or prostacyclin in a child with primary pulmonary hypertension. Electrophysiologic evaluation and ablation of abnormal electrical pathways in children can be performed by qualified personnel in the pediatric catheterization laboratory.

The risks of cardiac catheterization (morbidity and mortality) must be explained to the patient's family. Although the risks are very low for elective studies in older children (< 0.1%), the risk of major complications in distressed infants is about 2%. Interventional procedures such as balloon valvuloplasties increase these risks further.

## Cardiac Catheterization Data

Figure 19–3 shows oxygen saturation (in percent) and pressure (in mm Hg) values obtained at cardiac catheterization from the chambers and great arteries of the heart. These values are within the normal range for a child.

### A. OXYGEN CONTENT AND SATURATION; PULMONARY (Qₚ) AND SYSTEMIC (Qₛ) BLOOD FLOW (CARDIAC OUTPUT)

In most laboratories, left-to-right shunting is determined by changes of blood oxygen content or saturation during sampling through the right side of the heart. A significant increase in oxygen saturation between one right chamber and the other indicates the presence of a left-to-right shunt at the site of the increase. The oxygen saturation of the peripheral arterial blood should always be determined during cardiac catheterization. Normal arterial oxygen saturation is 95–97% at sea level and 92–94% at 5280 feet. Subnormal saturations suggest the presence of a right-to-left shunt, underventilation, or pulmonary disease.

*Figure 19–3.* Pressures (in mm Hg) and oxygen saturation (in percent) obtained by cardiac catheterization in a healthy child. 3 = mean pressure of 3 mm Hg in the right atrium, 5 = mean pressure of 5 mm Hg in the left atrium.

The size of a left-to-right shunt is usually expressed as a ratio of pulmonary to systemic blood flow ($Q_p/Q_s$) or as liters per minute as determined by the Fick principle:

$$\frac{\text{Cardiac output}}{\text{(L/min)}} = \frac{\text{Oxygen consumption (mL/min)}}{\text{Arteriovenous difference (mL/L)}}$$

## B. PRESSURES

Pressures should be determined in all chambers and major vessels entered. Pressures should be recorded as a catheter is pulled back from a distal chamber or vessel into a more proximal chamber. It is not normal for systolic pressure in the ventricles to exceed systolic pressure in the great arteries or mean diastolic pressure in the atria to exceed end-diastolic pressure in the ventricles. If a gradient in pressure exists, an obstruction is present, and the severity of the gradient is one criterion for the necessity of operative repair or catheter intervention. An RV systolic pressure of 100 mm Hg and a pulmonary artery systolic pressure of 20 mm Hg yield a gradient of 80 mm Hg. In this case, the patient would be classified as having severe pulmonary stenosis requiring balloon dilation of the pulmonic valve or surgery if valvuloplasty fails to reduce the gradient to less than 20 mm Hg.

## C. PULMONARY AND SYSTEMIC VASCULAR RESISTANCE

The vascular resistance is calculated from the following formula and reported in units or in dynes $\times$ cm$^{-5}$/m$^2$:

$$\text{Resistance} = \frac{\text{Pressure}}{\text{Flow}}$$

The pressure drop used to determine pulmonary vascular resistance is calculated by subtracting the mean pulmonary artery wedge or left atrial pressure from the mean pulmonary artery pressure. This pressure drop is divided by pulmonary blood flow per square meter of body surface area. (Pulmonary blood flow is determined by thermodilution or from the Fick principle, as noted earlier.) Similarly, systemic vascular resistance is determined by subtracting the mean central venous pressure from the mean systemic arterial pressure and dividing this pressure drop by systemic blood flow.

Normally, the pulmonary vascular resistance ranges from 1 to 3 units/m$^2$, or from 80 to 240 dynes $\times$ cm$^{-5}$/m$^2$. Systemic vascular resistance ranges from 15 to 20 units/m$^2$, or from 1200 to 1600 dynes $\times$ cm$^{-5}$/m$^2$. If pulmonary resistance is greater than 10 units or the ratio of pulmonary to systemic resistance is greater than 0.5, all other diagnostic findings should be reviewed carefully to confirm the presence of pulmonary hyper-

tension that is so severe as to render the patient inoperable.

Freedom RM et al: *Congenital Heart Disease: Textbook of Angiography.* Futura, 1997.

Simpson JM et al: Cardiac catheterization of low birth weight infants. Am J Cardiol 2001;87:1372 [PMID: 11397356].

# PERINATAL & NEONATAL CIRCULATION

At birth, two events occur that affect the cardiovascular and pulmonary system: (1) the umbilical cord is clamped, removing the placenta from the maternal circulation; and (2) breathing commences. As a result, marked changes in the circulation occur. During fetal life, the placenta offers low resistance to blood flow. In contrast, the pulmonary arterioles are markedly constricted and offer high resistance to the flow of blood into the lungs. Pulmonary vascular resistance is high in the fetus, and pulmonary blood flow accounts for only 7–10% of the combined in utero ventricular output. At birth, pulmonary blood flow dramatically increases 8- to 10-fold with a progressive fall in pulmonary vascular resistance and pressure. Mechanisms responsible for maintenance of high pulmonary vascular resistance include physical factors (lack of an air–liquid interface or ventilation), relative low oxygen tension, and perhaps vasoactive mediators such as elevated endothelin peptide levels or leukotrienes. Clamping the cord causes a sudden increase in resistance to flow in the systemic circuit. As the lung becomes the organ of respiration, the oxygen tension ($PO_2$) increases in the vicinity of the small pulmonary arterioles, resulting in a decrease in their constriction and thus a significant decrease in the pulmonary vascular resistance. Increased oxygen tension, rhythmic lung distention, and production of nitric oxide as well as prostacyclin likely play major roles in the fall in pulmonary vascular resistance at birth. The pulmonary vascular resistance shortly after birth falls below that of the systemic circuit, resulting in a change in blood flow across the ductus arteriosus to left to right.

Because of the changes in resistance, most of the RV outflow now passes into the lungs rather than through the ductus arteriosus into the descending aorta. In fact, functional closure of the ductus arteriosus begins to develop shortly after birth. The ductus arteriosus usually remains patent for 3–5 days. During the first hour after birth, a small right-to-left shunting is present (as in the fetus). However, after 1 hour, bidirectional shunting occurs, with the left-to-right direction predominating. In most cases, right-to-left shunting disappears completely by 8 hours. In patients with severe hypoxia (eg, in the syndrome of persistent pulmonary hypertension of the newborn), the pulmonary vascular resistance remains elevated, resulting in a continued right-to-left shunt. The cause of the functional closure of the ductus arteriosus is not completely known. Evidence indicates that the increased $PO_2$ of the arterial blood causes spasm of the ductus. Although flow through the ductus arteriosus usually is gone within 5 days, the vessel does not close anatomically for 7–14 days.

In fetal life, the foramen ovale serves as a one-way valve, permitting shunting of blood from the inferior vena cava through the right atrium into the left atrium. At birth, because of the changes in the pulmonary and systemic vascular resistance and the increase in the quantity of blood returning from the pulmonary veins to the left atrium, the left atrial pressure rises above that of the right atrium. This functionally closes the flap of the one-way valve, essentially preventing flow of blood across the septum. The foramen ovale remains patent in 10–15% of adults.

Persistent pulmonary hypertension is a clinical syndrome that occurs in full-term infants. The neonate develops tachypnea, cyanosis, and clinical evidence of pulmonary hypertension during the first 8 hours after delivery. These infants have massive right-to-left ductal or foramen shunting (or both) for 3–7 days because of high pulmonary vascular resistance. The clinical course is one of progressive hypoxia and acidosis, terminating in early death unless the pulmonary resistance can be lowered. Instituting appropriate means to increase alveolar $pO_2$—hyperventilation, alkalosis, paralysis, surfactant administration, high-frequency ventilation, and cardiac pressors—can usually reverse the resistance. Inhaled nitric oxide is a selective pulmonary vasodilator that produces a sustained improvement in oxygenation and reduces the use of extracorporeal membrane oxygenation. Postmortem findings include increased thickness of the pulmonary arteriolar media.

In the normal newborn, pulmonary vascular resistance and the pulmonary arterial pressure continue to fall during the first few months of life. This phenomenon results from the involution of the pulmonary arteriole from a relatively thick-walled, small-lumen vessel to a thin-walled, large-lumen vessel. Adult levels of pulmonary resistance and pressure are normally achieved by age 2 months. It is at this time typically that signs and symptoms of pulmonary overcirculation associated with moderate or large left-to-right shunting appear.

Fineman JR, Soifer SJ: The fetal and neonatal circulations. In Rudolph AR: *Congenital Diseases of the Heart: Clinical Physiologic Considerations,* 2nd ed. Futura, 2001.

# CONGESTIVE HEART FAILURE

Congestive heart failure (CHF) is the clinical condition in which the heart fails to meet the circulatory and metabolic needs of the body. Almost all infants who develop CHF from congenital heart lesions do so by age 6 months. Common causes of CHF include VSD, PDA, coarctation of the aorta, AV septal defect, large arteriovenous malformations (AVM), and chronic atrial tachyarrhythmias. CHF due to acquired cardiac conditions, such as myocarditis, may occur at any age. Patients present with symptoms of pulmonary congestion as noted in Table 19–1.

## Treatment

The therapy of CHF should be directed toward the underlying cause as well as the symptoms. Irrespective of the cause, neurohormonal activation occurs early when ventricular systolic dysfunction is present. Plasma catecholamine levels increase and account for the patient's symptoms. Increased plasma norepinephrine causes tachycardia and diaphoresis and indirectly, through activation of the renin–angiotensin system, causes peripheral vasoconstriction and salt and water retention. Increased metabolic demands cause increased caloric expenditure and failure to thrive. Inotropic agents, diuretics, afterload-reducing agents, and β-blockers may be used, together with supportive measures (oxygen, sedation, mechanical ventilation, and intravenous nutrition) in the treatment of the child with CHF.

## Inpatient Management of Congestive Heart Failure

Patients with cardiac decompensation may require hospital admission for initiation or augmentation of anticongestive therapies. Patients are routinely admitted to a cardiac intensive care unit where telemetry and invasive hemodynamic monitoring (arterial and central venous lines) are used to deliver and assess response to therapy. Table 19–12 demonstrates intravenous inotropic agents used to augment cardiac output and their relative effect on heart rate, systemic vascular resistance, and cardiac index. The drug used will depend in part on the cause of the CHF.

### A. Intravenous Inotropic Support

#### 1. Afterload reduction—

a. **Milrinone.** This selective phosphodiesterase inhibitor increases the level of cyclic adenosine monophosphate (cAMP), thereby improving the inotropic state of the heart. In addition to a dose-dependant increase in cardiac contractility, the drug is a systemic and pulmonary vasodilator and thus an effective agent in cases of right or left ventricular systolic dysfunction for increasing contractility and reducing afterload. Milrinone has been associated with a reduction in incidence of low cardiac output syndrome

***Table 19–12.*** Intravenous inotropic agents.

| Drug | Dose | Renal Perfusion | Heart Rate | Cardiac Index | SVR |
|---|---|---|---|---|---|
| Dopamine | 2–5 μg/kg/min | ↑via vasodilation | 0 | 0 | 0 |
| | 5–10 | ↑via ↑cardiac index | ↑ | ↑ | 0 |
| | >10 | ↓ | ↑ | ↑ | ↑ |
| Dobutamine | 2.5–10 μg/kg/min | ↑via ↑cardiac index | ↑ | ↑ | ↑↓ |
| Epinephrine | 0.2–2.0 μg/kg/min | ↓ | ↑ | ↑ | ↑ |
| Norepinephrine | 0.05–0.1 μg/kg/min | ↓ | 0 | ↑ | ↑↑ |
| Isoproterenol | 0.05–2.0 μg/kg/min | 0 | ↑↑ | ↑ | ↓↓ |

after cardiac surgery. The usual dosage range is 0.25–0.75 μg/kg/min.

**b. Nitroprusside.** This vasodilator acts directly on vascular smooth muscle, causing both venous and arterial vasodilation at dosages of 0.5–4.0 μg/kg/min. It is useful in the management of postoperative hypertension. Prolonged use should be carefully monitored as thiocyanate toxicity may occur.

**c. Nitroglycerin.** Nitroglycerin functions primarily as a dilator of venous capacitance vessels and causes a reduction of right and left atrial pressure. Systemic blood pressure may also fall, and reflex tachycardia may occur. Nitroglycerin is used to improve coronary blood flow and has been shown to be useful in the setting of low cardiac output following congenital heart surgery. Usual intravenous dosage range is 1–3 μg/kg/min.

**2. Extracorporeal membrane oxygenator (ECMO)—** Mechanical support devices including membrane oxygenators may be used in children with myocardial dysfunction following cardiac surgery or in children with refractory CHF secondary to cardiomyopathy or myocarditis. In all cases, mechanical support is used for a limited time while cardiac function improves, or as a bridge to cardiac transplantation. A cannula is placed in the right atrium, either through direct mediastinal cannulation, or through the internal jugular vein. An arterial catheter is placed either directly into the aorta or into an extrathoracic arterial site such as the common carotid artery. Flow from the venous return catheter passes through a membrane oxygenator and then is delivered back to the patient via the arterial catheter. Flow rates are adjusted to maintain adequate systemic perfusion, as judged by mean arterial blood pressure, acid–base status, end-organ function, and mixed venous oxygen saturation. The patient is monitored closely for return of cardiac contractility, and ECMO flows are adjusted accordingly. Risks are significant and include severe internal and external bleeding, infection, thrombosis, and pump failure.

## Outpatient Congestive Heart Failure Management

### A. MEDICATIONS

**1. Digitalis—**Digitalis is a primary drug for the treatment of CHF. The desired effect is improvement in myocardial performance (inotropic effect) with an associated decrease in systemic vascular resistance. The standard preparation used in pediatrics is digoxin, which may be administered intravenously, intramuscularly, or orally depending on how rapidly a therapeutic response is needed. The clinical urgency of the individual case dictates how quickly digitalization should be accomplished. Children require higher doses of digoxin on a per kilogram basis than adults, because of their superior renal function.

**a. Digitalization.** The routine schedule consists of giving one half of the total digitalizing dose initially, then one quarter of the total digitalizing dose at 6 and 12 hours of therapy (Table 19–13). Twenty-four hours after the last digitalizing dose, maintenance therapy is started.

Serum digoxin levels are not routinely monitored unless there are concerns regarding compliance or toxicity.

**b. Digitalis toxicity.** Any dysrhythmia that occurs during digitalis therapy should be attributed to the drug until proven otherwise. Ventricular bigeminy and first-, second-, or third-degree AV block are characteristic of digitalis toxicity. A trough level should be obtained if digitalis toxicity is suspected.

***Table 19–13.*** Digitalis dosing schedule.

| Age | Parenteral | Oral |
|---|---|---|
| Premature | 0.035 mg/kg | 0.04 mg/kg |
| 1 week to 2 years | 0.05 mg/kg | 0.06 mg/kg |
| < 1 week or > 2 years | 0.04 mg/kg | 0.05 mg/kg |

**c. Digitalis poisoning.** This is an acute emergency that must be treated without delay. Digitalis poisoning most commonly occurs in toddlers who have taken their parents' or grandparents' medications. The child's stomach should be emptied immediately even if several hours have passed since ingestion. Patients who have ingested massive amounts of digitalis should receive large doses of activated charcoal. Induction of vomiting or gastric lavage may be indicated but should not be performed if the patient is obtunded. In advanced heart block, atropine or temporary ventricular pacing may be beneficial. Digoxin immune Fab can be used to reverse potentially life-threatening intoxication. Antiarrhythmic agents may be useful.

**2. Diuretics**—Diuretics are almost always used in the treatment of CHF, either with or without digoxin.

**a. Furosemide.** This rapidly acting loop diuretic may be given intravenously or orally. Furosemide removes large amounts of potassium and chloride from the body, producing hypochloremic metabolic alkalosis when used chronically. Electrolytes should be monitored during long-term therapy.

**b. Thiazides** The thiazides are distal tubular diuretics used to complement furosemide in severe cases of CHF.

**c. Spironolactone** Spironolactone is a potassium-sparing aldosterone inhibitor diuretic. It is used frequently in conjunction with furosemide or thiazides for its enhanced diuretic function. Because it spares potassium, supplemental potassium may be avoided. Spironolactone may also be used as a neurohormonal antagonist with benefit in CHF irrespective of its diuretic effect. In adults with CHF, it has been associated with LV remodeling and improved life expectancy.

**d. Metolozone.** This potent oral loop diuretic is frequently used in patients who have become refractory to conventional doses of the other diuretics. Due to the marked diuresis that can be associated with this agent, electrolytes must be followed closely as even minor alterations in potassium may precipitate an arrhythmia in a patient with preexisting myocardial dysfunction.

**3. Afterload-reducing agents**—Oral afterload-reducing agents improve cardiac output by decreasing systemic vascular resistance. Angiotensin-converting enzyme (ACE) inhibitors (captopril, enalapril, lisinopril) are used in patients requiring long-term treatment. These agents, which block angiotensin II–mediated systemic vasoconstriction, are particularly useful in children with structurally normal hearts but reduced LV myocardial function (ie, myocarditis or dilated cardiomyopathies). These agents are also useful in ameliorating mitral and aortic insufficiency and have a role in controlling refractory CHF in patients with large left-to-right shunts in whom systemic vascular resistance is elevated.

**4. Fluid restriction**—Restricting fluids is a useful adjunct to medical therapy in children with CHF. When restricting fluids in infants and toddlers it is often necessary to fortify the formula and increase it caloric density in order to maintain adequate caloric intake at reduced volumes.

**5. Beta blockade**—β-blockers are a useful adjunctive therapy in children with refractory CHF already taking diuretics and ACE inhibitors. Carvedilol and other β-blockers, through their antirenin and anticatecholamine effects, decrease myocardial afterload and improve ventricular systolic function in some patients.

Azeka E et al: Delisting of infants and children from the heart transplantation waiting list after carvedilol treatment. J Am Coll Cardiol 2002;40(11):2034 [PMID: 12475466].

Fiser WP et al: Pediatric arteriovenous ECMO as a bridge to cardiac transplantation. J Heart Lung Transplant 2003;22(7): 770 [PMID: 12873545].

Hoffman TM et al: Efficacy and safety of milrinone in preventing low cardiac output syndrome in infants and children after corrective surgery for congenital heart disease. Circulation 2003;107(7):996 [PMID: 12600913].

# ■ CONGENITAL HEART DISEASE

Congenital heart disease occurs in 0.8% of North American and European populations, making this the most common category of congenital structural malformation. Curative or palliative surgical correction is now available for virtually all patients with congenital heart disease.

## Etiology

Congenital heart disease often has a genetic basis. The commonest abnormality now recognized is a microdeletion in the long arm of chromosome 22 (22q11) associated with the DiGeorge, Shprintzen, and conotruncal anomaly face syndromes. These children tend to have either interrupted aortic arch or conotruncal abnormalities such as ToF or double-outlet RV. Intrauterine factors such as maternal diabetes, alcohol consumption, progesterone use, viral infection, and other maternal teratogen exposure are associated with an increased incidence of malformations. These factors probably represent environmental triggers in persons susceptible or predisposed to congenital heart defects. Even acquired heart diseases, such as rheumatic fever, appear to be under strong genetic control. Atherosclerosis clearly occurs in families although in some circumstances it can also be influenced by diet, drugs, or lifestyle.

Genetic diagnosis may allow for a more accurate prediction of the risk of recurrence of a congenital heart disease in a subsequent pregnancy.

Boneva RS et al: Mortality associated with congenital heart defects in the United States, trends and racial disparities. Circulation 2001;103(19):2376 [PMID: 11352887].

# NONCYANOTIC CONGENITAL HEART DISEASE

## 1. Atrial Septal Defect of the Ostium Secundum Variety

 ESSENTIALS OF DIAGNOSIS & TYPICAL FEATURES

- RV heave.
- $S_2$ widely split and usually fixed.
- Grade I–III/VI ejection systolic murmur at the pulmonary area.
- Widely radiating systolic murmur mimicking peripheral pulmonary artery stenosis (common in infancy).
- Diastolic flow murmur at the lower left sternal border (if the shunt is significant in size).
- ECG with rsR' in lead $V_1$.

## General Considerations

An ASD is an opening in the atrial septum permitting the shunting of blood between the atria. There are three major types: (1) The ostium secundum type (discussed here) is the most common and is in the middle of the septum in the region of the foramen ovale. (2) The sinus venosus type is positioned high in the atrial septum, is the least common, and is frequently associated with partial anomalous pulmonary venous return. (3) The ostium primum type is low in position and is a form of AV septal defect. It is discussed in that section.

ASD of the ostium secundum variety occurs in approximately 10% of patients with congenital heart disease and is twice as common in females as in males. Diagnosis in infancy is becoming more common. Pulmonary hypertension and growth failure are uncommon but occur occasionally in infancy and childhood. After the third decade, pulmonary vascular disease may develop; left-to-right shunting then decreases, and

right-to-left shunting becomes the major clinical abnormality.

## Clinical Findings

### A. SYMPTOMS AND SIGNS

Infants with ASD rarely present with CHF. Children with ASDs most often have no cardiovascular symptoms. Some patients remain asymptomatic throughout life; others develop easy fatigability as older children or adults. Cyanosis does not occur unless pulmonary hypertension develops.

The peripheral pulses are normal and equal. The heart is usually hyperactive, with an RV heave felt best at the mid to lower left sternal border. No thrills are usually present. $S_2$ at the pulmonary area is widely split and often fixed. The pulmonary component is normal in intensity. A grade II–III/VI ejection-type systolic murmur is heard best at the left sternal border in the second intercostal space. This murmur is caused by increased flow across the pulmonic valve. No murmur is heard from the flow across the ASD. A middiastolic murmur can often be heard in the fourth intercostal space at the left sternal border. This murmur is caused by increased flow across the tricuspid valve during diastole. The presence of this murmur suggests a high flow with a pulmonary to systemic blood flow ratio greater than 2:1.

### B. IMAGING

Radiographs show cardiac enlargement. The main pulmonary artery may be dilated and pulmonary vascular markings increased owing to the increased pulmonary blood flow.

### C. ELECTROCARDIOGRAPHY

The usual ECG shows right axis deviation with a clockwise loop in the frontal plane. In the right precordial leads, a rsR' pattern is usually present.

### D. ECHOCARDIOGRAPHY

Echocardiography shows a dilated RV. Direct visualization of the ASD by two-dimensional echocardiography, plus demonstration of a left-to-right shunt through the defect by color-flow Doppler, confirms the diagnosis and has eliminated the need for cardiac catheterization prior to open-heart surgery or catheter closure of the defect. During the echocardiography evaluation, a careful assessment of the entry of all of the pulmonary veins into the left atrium is made to rule out associated anomalous pulmonary venous return.

### E. CARDIAC CATHETERIZATION

Oximetry reveals a significant increase in oxygen saturation at the atrial level. The pulmonary artery pressure is usually normal, as is pulmonary vascular resistance. The ratio of pulmonary to systemic blood flow may vary from 1.5:1 to 4:1. Cardiac catheterization is rarely needed for diagnostic purposes; however, placement of a device to close the ostium secundum ASD during cardiac catheterization is becoming increasingly common.

## Treatment

Surgical or catheterization laboratory closure with an interventional device is generally recommended for ostium secundum ASDs in which the ratio of pulmonary to systemic blood flow is greater than 2:1. Closure is performed electively in patients between ages 1 and 3 years. The mortality rate for surgical closure is less than 1%. When closure is performed by age 3 years, late complications of RV dysfunction and significant dysrhythmias are avoided. Early surgery is always indicated in infants with CHF or significant pulmonary hypertension. Surgical repair can now be safely performed via a "mini" median sternotomy or posterior thoracotomy approach. Many defects are amenable to nonoperative device closure in the cardiac catheterization laboratory, but the defect must have adequate tissue rims on either side on which to anchor the device.

## Course and Prognosis

Patients usually tolerate an ASD well in the first two decades of life. Occasionally a patient may never develop symptoms, but exercise intolerance is common in adulthood. Pulmonary hypertension and reversal of the shunt are rare late complications. Infective endocarditis is uncommon. Spontaneous closure occurs, most frequently in children with a defect originally estimated as less than 4 mm in diameter. Exercise tolerance and oxygen consumption in surgically corrected children are generally normal, and restriction of physical activity is unnecessary. Of all the forms of congenital heart disease, ostium secundum ASD is the most likely to present in middle to late adulthood, either with increased fatigue or with atrial tachyarrhythmias.

Fredriksen PM et al: Aerobic capacity in adults with various congenital heart diseases. Am J Cardiol 2001;87(3):310 [PMID: 11165966].

Lopez L et al: Echocardiographic considerations during deployment of the Helex Septal Occluder for closure of atrial septal defects. Cardiol Young 2003;13(3):290 [PMID: 12903878].

Roos-Hesselink JW et al: Excellent survival and low incidence of arrhythmias, stroke and heart failure long-term after surgical ASD closure at a young age: A prospective follow-up study of 21–33 years. Eur Heart J 2003;24(2):190 [PMID: 12573276].

Ryan WH et al: Safety and efficacy of minimally invasive atrial septal defect closure. Ann Thorac Surg 2003;75(5):1532 [PMID: 12735575].

## 2. Ventricular Septal Defect

### ESSENTIALS OF DIAGNOSIS & TYPICAL FEATURES

*Small- to moderate-sized left-to-right shunt without pulmonary hypertension:*

- *Acyanotic, relatively asymptomatic.*
- *Grade II–IV/VI pansystolic murmur, maximal along the lower left sternal border.*
- *$P_2$ not accentuated.*

*Large left-to-right shunt:*

- *Acyanotic.*
- *Easy fatigability.*
- *CHF in infancy (often).*
- *Hyperactive heart; biventricular enlargement.*
- *Grade II–IV/VI pansystolic murmur, maximal at the lower left sternal border.*
- *$P_2$ usually accentuated.*
- *Diastolic flow murmur at the apex.*

*Insignificant left-to-right shunt or bidirectional shunt with pulmonary hypertension:*

- *Quiet precordium with RV lift.*
- *Palpable $P_2$.*
- *Short ejection systolic murmur along the left sternal border; single accentuated $S_2$.*
- *Systemic arterial oxygen desaturation may be present; pulmonary arterial pressure and systemic arterial pressures are equal; little or no oxygen saturation increase at the RV level by catheterization.*

## General Considerations

Simple VSD is the most common congenital heart malformation, accounting for about 30% of all cases of congenital heart disease. Defects in the ventricular septum occur both in the membranous portion of the septum (most common) and in the muscular portion. VSDs follow one of four courses:

### A. SMALL, HEMODYNAMICALLY INSIGNIFICANT VENTRICULAR SEPTAL DEFECTS

Between 80% and 85% of all VSDs are small (< 3 mm in diameter) at birth, and will close spontaneously. In general, small defects in the muscular interventricular septum will close sooner than those in the membranous interventricular septum. In most cases, a small VSD never requires surgical closure. Fifty percent of small VSDs will close by age 2 years, and 90% will close by age 6 years. The remaining 10% will close during the school years, and parents should be told at the time of diagnosis and echocardiographic confirmation that all small VSDs will eventually close.

## B. Moderate Ventricular Septal Defects

Asymptomatic patients with moderate VSDs (3–5 mm in diameter) account for only 3–5% of children with VSDs. In general these children do not have CHF or pulmonary hypertension, the two indicators for surgical closure. In those who have cardiac catheterization, the ratio of pulmonary to systemic blood flow is usually less than 2:1, and serial cardiac catheterizations demonstrate that the shunts get progressively smaller. If there is neither CHF nor pulmonary hypertension, these defects can be followed until spontaneous closure.

## C. Large Ventricular Septal Defects with Normal Pulmonary Vascular Resistance

These defects are usually 6–10 mm in diameter. Unless they become markedly smaller within a few months after birth, they will require surgery. The timing of surgery depends on the clinical situation. Many infants with large VSDs and normal pulmonary vascular resistance will develop CHF and failure to thrive by age 3–6 months, and require correction at that time. In all cases, surgery before age 2 years is required so that the risk of pulmonary vascular disease can be minimized.

## D. Large Ventricular Septal Defects with Pulmonary Vascular Obstructive Disease

The vast majority of patients with inoperable pulmonary hypertension develop the condition progressively. The combined data of the multicenter National History Study indicate that almost all cases of irreversible pulmonary hypertension can be prevented by surgical repair of a large VSD before age 2 years.

## Clinical Findings

### A. Symptoms and Signs

Patients with small or moderate left-to-right shunts usually have no cardiovascular symptoms. Patients with large left-to-right shunts are usually ill early in infancy. Such patients have frequent upper and lower respiratory infections. They grow slowly and gain weight slowly. Dyspnea, exercise intolerance, and fatigue are common. CHF develops between 1 and 6 months. Patients who survive the first year usually improve, although easy fatigability may persist. With severe pulmonary hypertension (Eisenmenger syndrome), cyanosis is present.

**1. Small left-to-right shunt**—Usually no lifts, heaves, or thrills are present. The first sound at the apex is normal, and the second sound at the pulmonary area is split physiologically. The pulmonary component is normal. A grade II–IV/VI, medium- to high-pitched, harsh pansystolic murmur is heard best at the left sternal border in the third and fourth intercostal spaces. The murmur radiates over the entire precordium. No diastolic murmurs are heard.

**2. Moderate left-to-right shunt**—Slight prominence of the precordium is common. Moderate LV heave is evident. A systolic thrill may be palpable at the lower left sternal border between the third and fourth intercostal spaces. The second sound at the pulmonary area is most often split but may be single. A grade III–IV/VI, harsh pansystolic murmur is heard best at the lower left sternal border in the fourth intercostal space. A mitral diastolic flow murmur indicates that the pulmonary venous return is large and that the pulmonary-to-systemic blood flow ratio is at least 2:1.

**3. Large ventricular septal defects with pulmonary hypertension**—The precordium is prominent, and the sternum bulges. An LV thrust and an RV heave are palpable. $S_2$ may be felt at the pulmonary area. A thrill may be present at the lower left sternal border. $S_2$ is usually single or narrowly split, with accentuation of the pulmonary component. The murmur ranges from grade II to grade IV/VI and is usually harsh and pansystolic. Occasionally, when the defect is large, a murmur is difficult to hear. A diastolic flow murmur may be heard, depending on the size of the shunt.

### B. Imaging

Chest radiographic findings vary depending on the size of the shunt. In patients with small shunts, the radiograph may be normal. Patients with large shunts usually show significant cardiac enlargement involving both the left and right ventricles and the left atrium. The aorta is small to normal in size, and the main pulmonary artery segment is dilated. The pulmonary vascular markings are increased in patients with large shunts.

### C. Electrocardiography

The ECG is normal in patients with small left-to-right shunts. Left ventricular hypertrophy (LVH) usually occurs in patients with large left-to-right shunts and normal pulmonary vascular resistance (moderate-sized defects). Combined ventricular hypertrophy (both right and left) occurs in patients with pulmonary hypertension caused by increased flow, increased resistance, or both. Pure RV hypertrophy occurs in patients with pulmonary hypertension secondary to pulmonary vascular obstruction (Eisenmenger syndrome).

### D. Echocardiography

Two-dimensional echocardiography can reveal defects that are 2 mm or larger and often can be used to pinpoint the anatomic location of the defect. The addition of color-flow Doppler allows detection of even the smallest VSDs. Multiple defects can be detected by combining two-dimensional and color-flow imaging. Doppler can aid in the evaluation of VSDs by estimating the pressure difference between the left and right ventricles. A pressure difference greater than 50 mm Hg indicates the absence of severe pulmonary hypertension. The combination of excellent visualization of the VSD using echocardiography and Doppler plus the ability to estimate right-sided heart pressures by knowing the systemic blood pressure, and using the pressure drop by Doppler from the left to the right ventricle, allows many VSDs to be repaired surgically without cardiac catheterization and angiocardiography.

### E. Cardiac Catheterization and Angiocardiography

Cardiac catheterization and angiocardiography is rarely required for evaluation of an isolated VSD. The pulmonary artery pressure may vary from normal to systemic levels (equal to the aortic pressure). Left atrial pressure (pulmonary wedge pressure) may be normal to increased. Pulmonary vascular resistance varies from normal to markedly increased. Angiocardiographic examination defines the number, size, and location of the defects.

## Treatment

### A. Medical Management

Patients who develop CHF should receive vigorous treatment with anticongestive measures (see Congestive Heart Failure section). If the patient does not respond to vigorous anticongestive measures, or if he or she shows signs of progressive pulmonary hypertension, surgery is indicated without delay. Transcatheter closure of muscular VSDs is currently being used in selected cases.

### B. Surgical Treatment

The indications for surgical closure of a VSD are CHF combined with failure to thrive and pulmonary hypertension. Primary closure of the defect with a synthetic patch is used. The age at which elective surgery is performed has decreased in most pediatric cardiology centers; most defects are closed in infancy. Patients with cardiomegaly, poor growth, poor exercise tolerance, or other clinical abnormalities who have a significant shunt (> 2:1) without significant pulmonary hypertension typically undergo surgical repair at age 3–6 months. Patients with pulmonary artery pressures equal to systemic pressure (pulmonary hypertension) undergo surgical repair well before age 2 years to avoid pulmonary vascular disease. In most centers these children have surgery before age 1 year. As a result of this management, the incidence of VSD with pulmonary vascular disease and right-to-left shunting (Eisenmenger syndrome) has been virtually eliminated. In all cases of VSD, the surgical mortality rate is below 2%.

## Course & Prognosis

Significant late dysrhythmias are uncommon. Functional exercise capacity and oxygen consumption are usually normal, and physical restrictions are unnecessary. Adults with corrected defects have a normal quality of life. With complete VSD closure, antibiotic prophylaxis for bacterial endocarditis can be discontinued 6 months after surgery.

Thanopoulous B et al: Transcatheter closure of perimembranous ventricular septal defects with the Amplatzer asymmetric ventricular septal defect occluder: Preliminary experience in children. Heart 2003;89(8)918 [PMID: 12860872].

Thanopoulous B et al: Transcatheter closure of muscular ventricular septal defects with the Amplatzer ventricular septal defect occluder: Initial clinical applications in children. J Am Coll Cardiol 1999;33(5):1395 [PMID: 10193744].

## 3. Atrioventricular Septal Defect

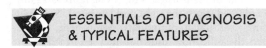

### ESSENTIALS OF DIAGNOSIS & TYPICAL FEATURES

- Murmur often inaudible in neonates.
- Loud pulmonary component of $S_2$.
- Common in infants with Down syndrome.
- ECG with left axis deviation.

## General Considerations

AV septal defect is a congenital cardiac abnormality resulting from incomplete fusion of the embryonic endocardial cushions. The endocardial cushions help to form the lower portion of the atrial septum, the membranous portion of the ventricular septum, and the septal leaflets of the tricuspid and mitral valves. These defects are not very common. They account for about 4% of all cases of congenital heart disease. Forty-five percent of children with Down syndrome have congenital heart disease. Of these, 20–25% have AV septal defects.

AV septal defects are divided into partial and complete forms. The complete form consists of a posterior-inlet VSD, an ostium primum ASD that is continuous with the ventricular defect, and a cleft in the anterior leaflet of the mitral valve. In the partial form, any one of these components may be present. The most common partial form of AV septal defect is the ostium primum type of ASD with a cleft in the mitral valve and little or no VSD.

The complete form results in large left-to-right shunts at both the ventricular and atrial levels, tricuspid and mitral regurgitation, and pulmonary hypertension, usually with some increase in pulmonary vascular resistance. When pulmonary hypertension is present, the shunts may be bidirectional. The hemodynamics in the partial form depend on the lesions present.

## Clinical Findings

### A. SYMPTOMS AND SIGNS

The clinical picture varies depending on the severity of the defect. In the partial form, patients may be clinically indistinguishable from children with ostium secundum ASDs. They are often asymptomatic. Patients with complete AV septal defect usually are severely affected. CHF often develops in infancy, and recurrent bouts of pneumonia are common.

In the neonate with the complete form, the murmur may be inaudible. After 4–6 weeks, a nonspecific systolic murmur develops. The murmur is usually not as harsh as that of an isolated VSD. The heart is significantly enlarged (both the right and left sides). $S_2$ is split, with an accentuated pulmonary component. A pronounced diastolic flow murmur may be heard at the apex and the lower left sternal border.

When severe pulmonary vascular obstructive disease is present, dominant RV enlargement usually occurs. $S_2$ can be palpated at the pulmonary area. No thrill is felt. $S_2$ is markedly accentuated and single. A nonspecific short systolic murmur is heard at the lower left sternal border. No diastolic flow murmurs are heard. Cyanosis is detectable in severe cases with predominant right-to-left shunts.

The physical findings in the incomplete form depend on the lesions. In the most common variety (ostium primum ASD with mitral regurgitation), the findings are similar to those of ostium secundum ASD with or without findings of mitral regurgitation.

### B. IMAGING

Cardiac enlargement is always present. In the complete form, all four chambers are enlarged. The pulmonary vascular markings are increased. In patients with pulmonary vascular obstructive disease, only the main pulmonary artery segment and its branches are prominent.

The peripheral pulmonary vascular markings are usually decreased.

### C. ELECTROCARDIOGRAPHY

In all forms of AV septal defect, left axis deviation with a counterclockwise loop in the frontal plane is present. The mean axis varies from approximately −30 to −90 degrees. Because left axis deviation is present in all patients with this condition, the ECG is an important diagnostic tool. Only 5% of isolated VSDs have this ECG abnormality. First-degree heart block is present in over 50% of patients. Right, left, or combined ventricular hypertrophy is present depending on the particular type of defect and the presence or absence of pulmonary hypertension.

### D. ECHOCARDIOGRAPHY

Echocardiography is the diagnostic technique of choice. The anatomy can be visualized directly by two-dimensional echocardiography, noting both AV valves to be at the same level. A primum ASD and an inlet VSD are present. AV valve regurgitation may be present. The LV outflow tract is elongated and has been likened to a "gooseneck." The LV outflow tract may be obstructed.

### E. CARDIAC CATHETERIZATION AND ANGIOCARDIOGRAPHY

Cardiac catheterization is not routinely used in the diagnostic assessment of AV septal defects but may be of value in assessing pulmonary artery pressures in the older infant with Down syndrome as this patient group is predisposed to early-onset pulmonary hypertension, which may prohibit surgical closure. If any anatomic questions still need to be answered, cardiac catheterization is of value. The results of cardiac catheterization vary with the type of defect. The catheter is easily passed across the atrial septum in its lowest portion and frequently enters the LV directly from the right atrium. This catheter course is a result of the very low ASD and the cleft in the mitral valve. Increased oxygen saturation in the RV or the right atrium identifies the level of the shunt. Angiocardiography reveals the characteristic gooseneck deformity of the LV outflow tract in the complete form.

## Treatment

Treatment consists of anticongestive measures; since spontaneous improvement does not occur, surgery is always required. In the partial form, surgery carries a low mortality rate (1–2%), but patients require ongoing follow-up because of the risk of late occurring LV outflow tract obstruction and mitral valve dysfunction. The complete form is associated with a somewhat higher mortality rate, but complete correction in the first year of life, prior to the onset of irreversible pulmonary hypertension, is obligatory. Patients with Down syndrome tend to have a lower incidence of associated mitral valve dysplasia and have a lesser risk of reoperation. Pulmonary artery banding procedures are rarely used for AV septal defects. Primary correction should be performed when the child is well and, if possible, weighs more than 5 kg. At corrective surgery, transesophageal echocardiography is useful in assessing the adequacy of repair in the operating room at the completion of cardiopulmonary bypass.

Al-Hay AA et al: Complete atrioventricular septal defect, Down syndrome and surgical outcome: Risk factors. Ann Thorac Surg 2003;75(2)412 [PMID: 12607648].

El-Najdawi EK et al: Operation for partial atrioventricular septal defect: A forty year review. J Thorac Cardiovasc Surg 2000;119(5):880 [PMID: 10788807].

# PATENT DUCTUS ARTERIOSUS

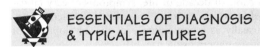

### ESSENTIALS OF DIAGNOSIS & TYPICAL FEATURES

- *Variable murmur, with active precordium and full pulses, in newborn premature infants.*
- *Continuous murmur and full pulses in older infants.*

## General Considerations

PDA is the persistence of the normal fetal vessel that joins the pulmonary artery to the aorta. It closes spontaneously in normal full-term infants at 3–5 days of age. It is a common abnormality, accounting for about 10% of all cases of congenital heart disease. The incidence of PDA is higher in infants born at high altitudes (over 10,000 ft). It is twice as common in females as in males. In preterm infants weighing less than 1500 g, the frequency of PDA ranges from 20 to 60%.

The defect occurs as an isolated abnormality, but associated lesions sometimes occur. Coarctation of the aorta and VSD are commonly associated with PDA. Even more important to recognize are those patients with murmurs of PDA but without readily apparent findings of other associated lesions who are being kept alive by the patent ductus (eg, a patient with PDA with unsuspected pulmonary atresia).

## Clinical Findings

### A. SYMPTOMS AND SIGNS

The clinical findings and the clinical course depend on the size of the shunt and the degree of pulmonary hypertension.

**1. Typical patent ductus arteriosus**—The pulses are bounding, and pulse pressure is widened. $S_1$ is normal. $S_2$ is usually narrowly split. Rarely, in large shunts, $S_2$ is paradoxically split; that is, $S_2$ closes on inspiration and splits on expiration. The paradoxical splitting is caused by the volume overload of the LV and the prolonged ejection of blood from this chamber.

The murmur is quite characteristic. It is a very rough "machinery" murmur that is maximal at the second intercostal space at the left sternal border and inferior to the left clavicle. It begins shortly after $S_1$, rises to a peak at $S_2$, and passes through the $S_2$ into diastole, where it becomes a decrescendo murmur and fades before the $S_1$. The murmur tends to radiate fairly well over the lung fields anteriorly but relatively poorly over the lung fields posteriorly. A diastolic flow murmur is often heard at the apex.

**2. Patent ductus arteriosus with pulmonary hypertension**—The physical findings depend on the cause of the pulmonary hypertension. If pulmonary hypertension is primarily the result of an increase in blood flow and only a slight increase in pulmonary vascular resistance, the physical findings are similar to those listed earlier. The significant difference is the presence of an accentuated pulmonary component of $S_2$. Bounding pulses and a loud continuous heart murmur are present. In patients with increased pulmonary vascular resistance, the findings are quite different. $S_2$ is single and accentuated, and no significant heart murmur is present. The pulses are normal rather than bounding.

**3. Patent ductus arteriosus in the premature neonate with associated respiratory distress syndrome**—A preterm neonate during or after respiratory distress syndrome may have a significant PDA that is difficult to detect by auscultation but which may still be clinically significant. A soft, nonspecific systolic murmur or no murmur is heard rather than the classic continuous murmur. Increase in peripheral pulses may be a helpful sign. Increasing oxygen requirement and increased need for respiratory support or CHF may be signs that a PDA is causing significant left-to-right shunting. The chest radiograph may show cardiomegaly. Echocardiography is always required to confirm the presence or absence of a PDA in the premature infant with lung disease.

### B. IMAGING

In simple PDA, the radiographic appearance depends on the size of the shunt. If the shunt is relatively small, the heart is not enlarged. If the shunt is large, both left atrial and LV enlargement may be present. The aorta and the main pulmonary artery segment may be prominent.

## C. ELECTROCARDIOGRAPHY

The ECG may be normal or may show LVH, depending on the size of the shunt. In patients with pulmonary hypertension caused by increased blood flow, biventricular hypertrophy usually occurs. In those with pulmonary vascular obstructive disease, pure right ventricular hypertrophy (RVH) occurs.

## D. ECHOCARDIOGRAPHY

Echocardiography provides direct visualization of the ductus and confirmation of the direction and degree of shunting. Preterm infants with a suspected PDA should have a complete echocardiographic evaluation to make a definitive diagnosis, assess the magnitude of the left-to-right shunt, and rule out associated, particularly ductal-dependent, lesions.

## E. CARDIAC CATHETERIZATION AND ANGIOCARDIOGRAPHY

Children with PDA never require a cardiac catheterization for diagnostic reasons. However, children with a small PDA routinely have the ductus closed in the catheterization laboratory. This is the sole indication for cardiac catheterization in PDA.

## Treatment

Treatment is surgical when the PDA is large, except in patients with pulmonary vascular obstructive disease. Patients with large left-to-right shunts and pulmonary hypertension should be operated on by age 1 year to prevent the development of progressive pulmonary vascular obstructive disease. A symptomatic PDA with normal pulmonary artery pressure can be safely coil-occluded during cardiac catheterization after the child has reached 5 kg.

Patients with nonreactive pulmonary vascular obstruction who have resistance greater than 10 units and a ratio of pulmonary-to-systemic resistance greater than 0.7 despite vasodilator therapy (eg, nitric oxide) should not be operated on. These patients are made worse by closure of the ductus, because the ductus serves as an escape route for their pulmonary hypertension.

Symptomatic PDA is a common problem in preterm infants. Indomethacin, a potent inhibitor of prostaglandin synthesis, is routinely used to close the PDA in premature infants. Indomethacin does not close the PDA of full-term infants or children. The success of indomethacin therapy is as high as 80–90% in premature infants with a birth weight over 1200 g, but

it is less successful in smaller infants. Indomethacin (0.1–0.3 mg/kg orally every 8–24 hours or 0.1–0.3 mg/kg parenterally every 12 hours) can be used if adequate renal, hematologic, and hepatic function is demonstrated. Management during indomethacin therapy includes fluid restriction with or without diuretics and close observation of the urinary output because of indomethacin's tendency to rapidly decrease renal function. If indomethacin is not successful and the ductus remains hemodynamically significant, surgical ligation should be performed without hesitation. If the ductus closes substantially so that it is no longer hemodynamically significant even with some residual flow from left to right, surgery is not needed, and a second course of indomethacin may complete ductal closure. Recent studies from Europe indicate that ibuprofen may be as effective as indomethacin for the medical closure of the preterm PDA.

## Course & Prognosis

Patients with simple PDA and small-to-moderate shunts usually do well without surgery. However, in the third or fourth decade of life, symptoms of easy fatigability, dyspnea on exertion, and exercise intolerance appear, usually as a consequence of the development of pulmonary hypertension or CHF.

Spontaneous closure of a PDA may occur up to age 1 year. This is especially true in preterm infants. After age 1 year, spontaneous closure is rare. Because infective endocarditis is a potential complication, closure by coil embolization or surgery is recommended if the defect persists beyond age 1 year.

The prognosis for patients with large shunts or pulmonary hypertension is not as good. Poor growth and development, frequent episodes of pneumonia, and the development of CHF occur in these children. Therefore, patients with PDA and large shunts who are beyond the newborn period should have immediate surgical ligation of their PDA.

Liang CD et al: Echocardiographic guidance for transcatheter coil occlusion of patent ductus arteriosus in the catheterization laboratory. J Am Soc Echocardiogr 2003;16(5):476 [PMID: 12724658]

Overmeire BV et al: A Comparison of ibuprofen and indomethacin for closure of patent ductus arteriosus. N Engl J Med 2000;343(10):674 [PMID: 10974130].

# MALFORMATIONS ASSOCIATED WITH OBSTRUCTION TO BLOOD FLOW ON THE RIGHT SIDE OF THE HEART

## 1. Valvular Pulmonary Stenosis with Intact Ventricular Septum

### ESSENTIALS OF DIAGNOSIS & TYPICAL FEATURES

- *No symptoms with mild and moderately severe cases.*
- *Cyanosis and a high incidence of right-sided CHF in very severe cases in infancy.*
- *RV lift; systolic ejection click at the pulmonary area in mild to moderately severe cases.*
- *$S_2$ widely split with soft to inaudible $P_2$; grade I–VI/VI obstructive systolic murmur, maximal at the pulmonary area.*
- *Dilated pulmonary artery on posteroanterior chest radiograph.*

## General Considerations

Pulmonic valve stenosis accounts for 10% of all cases of congenital heart disease. In the usual case, the cusps of the pulmonary valve are fused to form a membrane or diaphragm with a hole in the middle that varies from 2 to 10 mm in diameter. Occasionally, only two cusps may fuse, producing a bicuspid pulmonary valve. In the more severe cases, a secondary infundibular stenosis is present. The pulmonary valve annulus is usually small. Moderate to marked poststenotic dilation of the main and left pulmonary arteries is usually evident. Patent foramen ovale is fairly common.

Obstruction to blood flow across the pulmonary valve results in an increase in pressure developed by the RV to maintain an adequate output across that valve. Pressures greater than systemic are potentially life-threatening and are associated with critical obstruction. Because of the increased work required of the RV, severe RVH and eventual RV failure can occur. In contrast to patients with severe pulmonic valve stenosis, patients with this obstruction who also have a large VSD (ie, ToF) are not at risk for heart failure. In this situation, the septal defect limits the pressure developed in the RV to systemic pressure, making heart failure extremely uncommon.

When obstruction is severe and the ventricular septum is intact, a right-to-left shunt will often occur at the atrial level through a patent foramen ovale. Thus, patients with this condition may have cyanosis, which always indicates a severe degree of valvular obstruction.

## Clinical Findings

### A. SYMPTOMS AND SIGNS

The history varies with the severity of the obstruction. Patients with mild or even moderate valvular pulmonary stenosis are completely asymptomatic. Patients with more severe valvular obstruction may develop cyanosis very early—even as neonates. Hypoxemic spells characterized by a sudden onset of marked cyanosis and dyspnea occur, but are much less common than in ToF.

Patients with mild to moderate obstruction are acyanotic. These patients are usually well developed and well nourished. They are not prone to lung infections. The pulses are normal. Clubbing may occur in severe cases in which cyanosis has persisted for a long time. On examination of the heart, the precordium may be prominent. An RV heave can frequently be palpated. A systolic thrill is often palpated in the pulmonary area and occasionally in the suprasternal notch. $S_1$ is normal. In patients with mild to moderate stenosis, a prominent ejection click of pulmonary origin is heard best at the third left intercostal space. This click varies with respiration. It is much more prominent during expiration than inspiration. In patients with severe stenosis, the click tends to merge with $S_1$. $S_2$ also varies with the degree of stenosis. In mild valvular stenosis, $S_2$ is normal. In moderate degrees of obstruction, $S_2$ is more widely split and the pulmonary component is softer. In severe pulmonary stenosis, $S_2$ is single because the pulmonary component cannot be heard. An ejection-type, rough, obstructive systolic murmur is best heard at the second interspace at the left sternal border. It radiates very well to the back. With severe obstruction of the valve, the murmur is usually short and peaks in late systole. No diastolic murmurs are audible.

### B. IMAGING

In the mild form of pulmonary stenosis, the heart is normal in size. Poststenotic dilation of the main pulmonary artery segment and the left pulmonary artery often occurs. In moderate to severe cases, slight RV enlargement may occur, and poststenotic dilation of the main pulmonary artery may or may not be present. In cyanotic patients, the pulmonary vascular markings may be decreased.

### C. ELECTROCARDIOGRAPHY

Electrocardiography is usually normal in patients with mild obstruction. RVH is present in patients with moderate to severe valvular obstruction. In severe obstruction, RV hypertrophy and the RV strain pattern (deep inversion of the T wave) are seen in the right precordial leads. In the most severe form, right atrial hypertrophy is also present. Right axis deviation also occurs in the moderate to severe forms. Occasionally, the axis is as great as +180 degrees.

### D. ECHOCARDIOGRAPHY

The pulmonary valve may be unusually thickened with reduced valve leaflet excursion. The valve may bulge forward in systole. The transvalvular pressure gradient can be estimated accurately by Doppler echocardiography.

### E. CARDIAC CATHETERIZATION
### AND ANGIOCARDIOGRAPHY

Oxygen saturation or oxygen content does not increase in the right side of the heart. In more severe cases, a right-to-left shunt occurs at the atrial level. Pulmonary artery pressure is normal in milder cases and decreased in moderate to severe cases. RV pressure is always higher than pulmonary artery pressure. The gradient across the pulmonary valve varies from 10 to 200 mm Hg. In severe cases, the right atrial pressure is often elevated, with a predominant a wave. Cineangiocardiography after injection of contrast material into the RV shows thickening of the pulmonary valve and the very narrow opening of the pulmonary valve. This produces a jet of contrast from the RV into the pulmonary artery. Infundibular hypertrophy may be present. Diagnostic catheterization is rarely performed because pulmonic stenosis can be diagnosed easily using physical examination, the ECG, and echocardiography. Catheterization is performed only when balloon pulmonic valvotomy is planned.

### Treatment

Relief of pulmonic stenosis is recommended for children with RV systolic pressures greater than 60 mm Hg or higher than two thirds of systemic pressure. Immediate correction is indicated for patients with systemic or suprasystemic RV pressure. Percutaneous balloon valvuloplasty is the procedure of choice in most institutions. It appears to be as effective as surgery in relieving obstruction and causes less valve insufficiency. Surgery is needed to treat pulmonic valve stenosis only when balloon pulmonic valvuloplasty is unsuccessful.

### Course & Prognosis

Patients with mild pulmonary stenosis live normal lives. Those with stenosis of moderate severity rarely are symptomatic. Those with severe valvular obstruction may develop severe cyanosis and CHF in infancy.

After balloon pulmonic valvuloplasty or surgery, most patients have good voluntary maximum exercise capacity unless they have significant PI after valvuloplasty. Patients with isolated PI, a common occurrence after surgical pulmonary valvotomy, may be significantly limited in exercise performance. Severe PI leads to progressive RV dilation and dysfunction, which may precipitate ventricular arrhythmias or right heart failure in adulthood. Patients with severe PI may benefit from surgical placement of a pulmonic valve to restore RV outflow tract competence. If relief of valvular obstruction occurs before age 20 years, longevity is normal. Limitation of physical activity is unwarranted. The quality of life of adults with successfully treated pulmonary stenosis, and minimal PI is normal.

Yetman AT et al: Comparison of exercise performance in patients after pulmonary valvulotomy for pulmonary stenosis and tetralogy of Fallot. Am J Cardiol 2002;90(12) 1412 [PMID: 12480060].

## 2. Infundibular Pulmonary Stenosis Without Ventricular Septal Defect

Pure infundibular pulmonary stenosis is rare. One should suspect infundibular pulmonary stenosis when mild to moderate pulmonary stenosis, an intact ventricular septum, no audible pulmonary ejection click, and a murmur that is maximal in the third and fourth intercostal spaces rather than in the second intercostal space are present. The clinical picture is identical to that of pulmonic valve stenosis. Intervention, if indicated, is always surgical because this condition does not improve with balloon catheter dilation.

## 3. Distal Pulmonary Stenosis

### Supravalvular Pulmonary Stenosis

Supravalvular pulmonary stenosis, a relatively rare condition, is caused by narrowing of the main pulmonary artery. The clinical picture may be identical to that of valvular pulmonary stenosis, although the murmur is maximal in the first intercostal space at the left sternal border and in the suprasternal notch. No ejection click is audible. $S_2$ is usually narrowly split, and the pulmonary component is quite loud as a result of closure of the pulmonary valve under high pressure. The murmur radiates into the neck and over the lung fields. This condition occurs most often in children with Noonan syndrome.

### Peripheral Pulmonary Branch Stenosis

In peripheral pulmonary branch stenosis, multiple narrowings of the branches of the pulmonary artery occur at the bifurcation of the main pulmonary artery or in the periphery of the lung. Systolic murmurs may be heard over both lung fields, both anteriorly and posteriorly. Transient pulmonary branch stenosis murmurs of infancy are innocent. The three most common causes of significant pulmonary artery branch stenosis are Williams–Beuren syndrome, Alagille syndrome, and congenital rubella syndrome. Surgery is often unsuccessful. Transvenous balloon angioplasty is currently being used to treat this condition, with moderate success.

## 4. Other Congenital Right Heart Lesions

### Ebstein Malformation of the Tricuspid Valve

In the Ebstein malformation of the tricuspid valve, the tricuspid valve is displaced downward so that the septal leaflet of the valve is attached to the RV wall (inside the RV) rather than the to the tricuspid annulus. As a result, the upper portion of the RV is physiologically within the right atrium. The so-called atrialized portion of the RV is thin-walled and does not contribute to RV output. The portion of the ventricle below the displaced tricuspid valve is diminished in volume and represents the functioning RV. This is an uncommon condition.

### Clinical Findings

#### A. Symptoms & Signs

The degree of displacement of the tricuspid valve is variable, and the clinical significance of Ebstein malformation varies with this displacement. In the most extreme form, the septal leaflet is markedly displaced into the RV outflow tract, leading to significant reduction in antegrade flow to the pulmonary artery. Patients are cyanotic shortly after birth because of poor pulmonary artery flow. At the opposite extreme, symptoms may not develop until adulthood when tachyarrhythmias in association with right atrial dilatation or an associated reentrant pathway occur. These older patients typically have minimal displacement of the septal leaflet of the tricuspid valve.

#### B. Imaging

The chest radiograph usually shows cardiomegaly with prominence of the right heart border. The degree of cardiomegaly is influenced by the degree of tricuspid valve displacement and by the presence and size of the atrial level shunt. Massive cardiomegaly with a "wall to wall heart" occurs in the setting of severe displacement and a restrictive atrial level defect.

#### C. ECG

ECG may be normal but more typically shows right atrial enlargement. RBBB and LV enlargement may be found. A delta wave from coexisting Wolff–Parkinson–White syndrome (WPW) may be seen.

#### D. Echocardiography

Echocardiography is necessary to confirm the diagnosis and may aid in predicting outcome. The degree of displacement, the size of the right atrium, the presence of an associated atrial level shunt, and LV systolic function all affect outcome. The ratio of the atrialized area of the right heart to the area of the remainder of the heart is determined by echocardiography. The greater the ratio, the worse the prognosis.

#### E. Course and Prognosis

In cyanotic neonates, prostaglandin E infusion is used to maintain pulmonary blood flow until pulmonary vascular resistance decreases, facilitating antegrade pulmonary artery flow. If the patient remains significantly cyanotic, surgical intervention is required in the neonatal period.

Surgical repair consists of an annuloplasty to modify the level of the tricuspid orifice and diminish tricuspid insufficiency. The success rate of this procedure is highly variable. Late arrhythmias are common. Postoperative exercise tolerance increases but remains lower than that for age-related normals. If a significant Ebstein malformation is not treated, atrial tachyarrhythmias will frequently begin during adolescence.

### Absence of a Pulmonary Artery

Absence of a pulmonary artery (left or right) may be an isolated malformation or may occur in association with other congenital heart diseases. It occurs occasionally in patients with ToF.

### Absence of the Pulmonary Valve

Absence of the pulmonary valve is a rare abnormality usually associated with VSD. In about 50% of cases, infundibular pulmonary stenosis is also present (ToF with absent pulmonary valve).

Driscoll DJ et al: Spectrum of exercise intolerance in 45 patients with Ebstein's anomaly and observations on exercise tolerance in 11 patients after surgical repair. J Am Coll Cardiol 1988;11(4):831 [PMID: 3351151].

Yetman AT et al: Outcome in cyanotic neonates with Ebstein's anomaly. AJC 1998;81(6):1 [PMID: 9527086].

# MALFORMATIONS ASSOCIATED WITH OBSTRUCTION TO BLOOD FLOW ON THE LEFT SIDE OF THE HEART

## 1. Coarctation of the Aorta

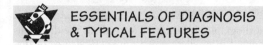

### ESSENTIALS OF DIAGNOSIS & TYPICAL FEATURES

- *Pulse lag in lower extremities.*
- *Systolic blood pressure of 20 mm Hg or greater in the upper than in the lower extremities.*
- *Blowing systolic murmur in the left axilla.*

## General Considerations

Coarctation is common, accounting for about 6% of all congenital heart disease. Three times as many males as females are affected. Many, though not all, affected females have 45 XO Turner syndrome. Coarctation usually occurs in the thoracic portion of the descending aorta distal to the takeoff of the left subclavian artery in the juxtaductal region. The abdominal aorta is rarely involved. The term "Shone syndrome" refers to multiple levels of left heart obstructive disease, including mitral stenosis, bicuspid aortic valve with or without aortic stenosis, tubular hypoplasia of the aortic isthmus, and coarctation of the aorta. The incidence of an associated bicuspid aortic valve with coarctation is 80–85%.

## Clinical Findings

### A. SYMPTOMS AND SIGNS

The cardinal physical finding is diminution or absence of femoral pulses. Infants with severe coarctation have equal upper and lower extremity pulses from birth to 2 days of age. Unequal pulses and clinical symptoms develop between 4 and 10 days of age as the ductus arteriosus closes. Approximately 40% of children with coarctation will present at this young age. Coarctation alone, or in combination with VSD, ASD, or other congenital cardiac anomalies, is the leading cause of CHF in the first month of life.

Coarctation presents more insidiously in the 60% of children with no symptoms in infancy. Their coarctation is diagnosed by a pulse discrepancy between the arms and legs on physical exam or by arm hypertension on blood pressure measurement. Normally, the systolic blood pressure in the upper extremities is slightly lower than in the lower extremities. The actual level of blood pressure in the arms may be elevated only moderately, even in severe coarctation, or it may be elevated significantly. In any case, the pulses in the legs are diminished or absent in affected infants. The left subclavian artery is occasionally involved in the coarctation, in which case the left brachial pulse is also weak. An ejection systolic murmur of grade II/VI intensity is often heard at the aortic area and the lower left sternal border along with an apical ejection click from the bicuspid aortic valve. The pathognomonic murmur of coarctation is heard in the left axilla and the left back. The murmur is usually systolic but may spill into diastole. If the coarctation is complicated by other malformations, murmurs associated with these other abnormalities will be audible.

### B. IMAGING

In the older child, radiographic findings may show a normal sized heart, although there is usually some evidence of LV enlargement. The aorta proximal to the coarctation is prominent. The aortic outline indents at the level of the coarctation. The poststenotic segment is dilated. This combination of abnormalities results in the "Figure 3" sign on chest radiograph. Notching or scalloping of the ribs caused by marked enlargement of the intercostal collaterals can be seen. MRI has become extremely useful for determining noninvasively the anatomy of the coarctation. In patients with a severe coarctation and associated CHF, marked cardiac enlargement and pulmonary venous congestion occur.

### C. ELECTROCARDIOGRAPHY

ECGs in older children may be normal or may show slight LVH. ECG usually shows RVH in infants with severe coarctation.

### D. ECHOCARDIOGRAPHY

Two-dimensional echocardiography and color-flow Doppler are used to visualize the coarctation directly, and continuous-wave Doppler may estimate the degree of obstruction. Diastolic run-off flow is found by continuous-wave Doppler if the obstruction is severe. If the ductus arteriosus is patent, echocardiography may not detect the coarctation. Associated lesions such as a bicuspid aortic valve or mitral abnormalities may suggest the presence of a coarctation. In the face of poor LV systolic function, the coarctation may be difficult to visualize. Flow velocities will not be obviously increased at the coarctation site due to reduced flow across the obstruction. A high index of suspicion of coarctation is required in such a patient.

## E. CARDIAC CATHETERIZATION AND ANGIOCARDIOGRAPHY

These studies demonstrate the position, anatomy, and severity of the coarctation and will assess the adequacy of collateral circulation. Cardiac catheterization and angiocardiography are rarely performed for infants or children with coarctation unless an interventional procedure to dilate the coarctation is planned.

## Treatment

Infants with coarctation of the aorta and CHF may present in extremus secondary to LV dysfunction and associated low cardiac output. Resuscitative measures should include initiation of prostaglandin infusion at a dose of 0.025–1.0 μg/kg/min to reopen the ductus arteriosus as well as initiation of inotropic support. Surgical repair should not be delayed by undue medical interventions. Once stabilized, the infant should undergo corrective repair. Some centers perform primary balloon dilation aortoplasty in infants with coarctation, but this is not universally standard. Infant surgery using either the modified end-to-end anastomosis technique or the left subclavian approach has a high success rate, but there is a significant incidence (20–30%) of recoarctation after repair. Fortunately, recurrent coarctation is highly amenable to balloon aortoplasty in the catheterization laboratory. Coarctation of the aorta in patients who do not have CHF in infancy is corrected electively. In elective coarctation repair, either surgery or primary balloon aortoplasty can be used. In the older patient, particularly when of adult size, aortic stent placement is effective.

## Course & Prognosis

Children with coarctation of the aorta who survive the neonatal period without developing CHF do quite well throughout childhood and adolescence. Fatal complications (eg, hypertensive encephalopathy, intracranial bleeding) occur uncommonly in childhood. Infective endocarditis (actually endarteritis in this condition) is rare before adolescence.

Children with coarctation corrected after age 5 years are at increased risk for systemic hypertension and myocardial dysfunction even with successful surgery. Careful exercise testing is mandatory for these children prior to their participation in athletic activities.

Hamdan MA et al: Endovascular stents for coarctation of the aorta: Initial results and intermediate-term follow-up. J Am Coll Cardiol 2001;38(5):1518 [PMID: 11691533].

Ovaert C et al. Balloon angioplasty of native coarctation: Clinical outcomes and predictors of success. J Am Coll Cardiol 2000;35(4):988 [PMID: 10732899].

# 2. Aortic Stenosis

### ESSENTIALS OF DIAGNOSIS & TYPICAL FEATURES

- *Systolic ejection murmur at the upper right sternal border.*
- *Thrill in the carotid arteries.*
- *Systolic click at the apex.*
- *Dilation of the ascending aorta on chest radiograph.*

## General Considerations

Aortic stenosis is an obstruction to the outflow from the LV at or near the aortic valve that causes a systolic pressure gradient of more than 10 mm Hg between the LV and the aorta. Aortic stenosis accounts for approximately 7% of all cases of congenital heart disease. Anatomically, congenital aortic stenosis is divided into three types:

### A. VALVULAR AORTIC STENOSIS (75%)

In critical aortic stenosis presenting in infancy, the aortic valve usually consists of a unicuspid diaphragm-like structure without well-defined commissures. Preschool and school-age children more commonly have a bicuspid aortic valve. Teenagers and young adults characteristically have a tricuspid valve with partially fused leaflets. This lesion is more common in males than in females.

### B. SUBVALVULAR AORTIC STENOSIS (23%)

In this condition, a membranous or fibrous ring occurs just below the aortic valve. The ring forms a diaphragm with a hole in the middle and results in obstruction to LV outflow. The aortic valve itself and the anterior leaflet of the mitral valve are often deformed.

### C. SUPRAVALVULAR AORTIC STENOSIS (1–2%)

In this type of aortic stenosis, constriction of the ascending aorta occurs just above the coronary arteries. This condition is often familial, and two different genetic patterns are associated, one with an abnormal facies and mental retardation (Williams–Beuren syndrome) and one with normal facies and without developmental delay.

## Clinical Findings

### A. Symptoms and Signs

Most patients with aortic stenosis have no cardiovascular symptoms. Except in the most severe cases, the patient may do well until the third to fifth decades of life, although some patients have mild exercise intolerance and fatigability. A small percentage of patients have significant symptoms (ie, dizziness and syncope) in the first decade. Sudden death, although uncommon, may occur in all forms of aortic stenosis, the greatest risk by far being in adolescents with hypertrophic cardiomyopathy.

Although isolated valvular aortic stenosis seldom causes symptoms in infancy, severe heart failure occasionally occurs when critical obstruction is present at birth. The response to medical management is poor; therefore, an aggressive approach using interventional catheterization or surgery is required. The physical findings vary depending on the anatomic type of lesion:

**1. Valvular aortic stenosis**—Affected patients are well developed and well nourished. The pulses are usually normal and equal throughout. If the stenosis is severe and a gradient of greater than 80 mm Hg exists, the pulses are diminished with a slow upstroke. Examination of the heart reveals an LV thrust at the apex. A systolic thrill at the right base, the suprasternal notch, and both carotid arteries accompanies moderate disease.

$S_1$ is normal. A prominent aortic ejection click is best heard at the apex. The click corresponds to the opening of the aortic valve at the conclusion of the isovolumic contraction phase of systole. It is separated from $S_1$ by a short but appreciable interval. It does not vary with respiration. $S_2$ at the pulmonary area is normal. The aortic component of $S_2$ is of good intensity. A grade III–V/VI, rough, medium- to high-pitched ejection-type systolic murmur is evident, loudest at the first and second intercostal spaces, and radiates well into the suprasternal notch and along the carotids. The murmur also radiates fairly well down the lower left sternal border and can be heard at the apex. The grade of the murmur correlates well with the severity of the stenosis.

**2. Discrete membranous subvalvular aortic stenosis**—The findings are essentially the same as those of valvular aortic stenosis except for the absence of a click. The murmur and thrill are usually somewhat more intense at the left sternal border in the third and fourth intercostal spaces than at the aortic area. Frequently, however, the murmur is equally intense at both areas. A diastolic murmur of aortic insufficiency is commonly heard after age 5 years.

**3. Supravalvular aortic stenosis**—The thrill and murmur are characteristically best heard in the suprasternal notch and along the carotids, although they are well transmitted over the aortic area and near the mid left sternal border. A difference in pulses and blood pressure between the right and left arms may be found, with the more prominent pulse and pressure in the right arm (Coanda effect).

### B. Imaging

In most cases the heart is not enlarged. The LV, however, is slightly prominent. In valvular aortic stenosis, dilation of the ascending aorta is frequently seen.

### C. Electrocardiography

Patients with mild aortic stenosis have normal ECGs. Patients with severe obstruction frequently demonstrate evidence of LVH and LV strain, but many do not. In about 25% of severe cases, the ECG is normal. Progressive increase in LVH on serial ECGs indicates a significant degree of obstruction. LV strain is an indication for surgery.

### D. Echocardiography

This has become a reliable noninvasive technique for the initial diagnosis and follow-up evaluation of all forms of aortic stenosis. Doppler accurately predicts the transvalvular gradient.

### E. Cardiac Catheterization and Angiocardiography

Left heart catheterization demonstrates the pressure differential between the LV and the aorta and the level at which the gradient exists. Echocardiography is now the standard method for following the severity of aortic valve stenosis, and cardiac catheterization is reserved for patients whose resting gradient has reached 60–80 mm Hg and in whom intervention is planned. For those with valvar aortic stenosis, balloon valvuloplasty is usually the first option. In subvalvular or supravalvular aortic stenosis, interventional catheterization is not useful and decisions must be made about surgical intervention.

## Treatment

Because operation offers less than a cure, surgical repair should be considered only in patients with symptoms, a large resting gradient (60–80 mm Hg) despite balloon angioplasty, or coexisting aortic insufficiency. In many cases, the gradient cannot be significantly diminished without producing aortic insufficiency. Percutaneous balloon valvuloplasty is now accepted as standard initial treatment. Patients who develop significant aortic insufficiency following the procedure will require surgical intervention to repair or replace the valve with either a prosthetic valve or with the patient's own pulmonic valve (Ross procedure). In the Ross procedure, an RV-to-PA conduit is used to replace the pulmonic valve. Discrete subvalvular aortic stenosis is usually surgically repaired at a lesser gradient because continued trauma to the aortic valve by the subvalvular jet may damage the valve and produce aortic insufficiency. Unfortunately, simple resection is followed by recurrence in more than 25% of patients with subvalvular aortic stenosis. All patients should have close follow-up, and those older than age 6 years should undergo yearly exercise testing. If exercise testing is normal, restriction of physical activity may not be necessary in patients with mild to moderate aortic stenosis.

## Course & Prognosis

All forms of LV outflow tract obstruction tend to be progressive. However, regression of the obstruction has been documented in a few patients with supravalvular obstruction. Pediatric patients with LV outflow tract obstruction—with the exception of those with critical aortic stenosis of infancy—are usually asymptomatic. Symptoms accompanying severe unoperated obstruction (angina, syncope, CHF) are all rare because of detection and surgical or catheter intervention. Preoperative or postoperative children whose obstruction is mild to moderate appear to have above-average oxygen consumption and maximum voluntary working capacity. Children in this category with normal heart size and normal resting and exercising ECG may safely participate in vigorous physical activity, including nonisometric competitive sports. Children with severe aortic stenosis may demonstrate ventricular dysrhythmias.

Mitchell BM et al. Serial exercise performance in children with surgically corrected congenital aortic stenosis. Pediatr Cardiol 2003;24(4):319 [PMID: 12632225].

Rao PS. Long-term follow-up results after balloon dilation of pulmonic stenosis, aortic stenosis and coarctation of the aorta: A review. Prog Cardiovasc Dis 1999;42(1):59 [PMID: 10505493].

## 3. Mitral Valve Prolapse

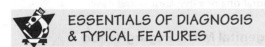

### ESSENTIALS OF DIAGNOSIS & TYPICAL FEATURES

- Midsystolic click best heard with the patient in the standing or squatting position.
- Occasional late systolic murmur.

## General Considerations

Mitral valve prolapse (MVP) is a common entity associated with abnormal auscultatory findings in older pedi-

atric patients. It is secondary to redundant valve tissue or abnormal tissue comprising the mitral valve apparatus. The mitral valve prolapses, moving posteriorly or superiorly into the left atrium during ventricular systole as the mitral valve returns to its closed position. A midsystolic click occurs at the time of this movement and is the clinical hallmark of this entity. Mitral insufficiency may occur late in systole, causing an atypical, short, late systolic murmur with variable radiation. MVP occurs in about 2% of thin adolescent females, a minority of whom have concomitant mitral insufficiency. Although MVP is most commonly an isolated lesion, it can occur in association with other conditions, namely Marfan syndrome and Ehlers–Danlos syndrome. These coexisting conditions should be ruled out by clinical examination.

## Clinical Findings

### A. SYMPTOMS AND SIGNS

The majority of patients with MVP are asymptomatic. Chest pain, palpitations, and dizziness may be reported, but it is unclear whether these symptoms are more common in affected patients than in the normal population. Significant dysrhythmias have been reported, including increased ventricular ectopy and nonsustained ventricular tachycardia. If significant associated mitral regurgitation is present, atrial arrhythmias may also occur. The standard approach to auscultation must be modified to diagnose MVP. Auscultation should be performed with the patient placed in various positions. Clicks, with or without systolic murmur, are elicited more commonly in the standing and squatting positions than in the supine and sitting positions. The systolic click occurs earlier in children than in adults; that is, it tends to be midsystolic rather than late systolic. Although it is usually heard at the apex, it may be audible at the left sternal border. A midsystolic or systolic murmur after the click implies mitral insufficiency and is much less common than isolated prolapse. The murmur is usually not typical of mitral insufficiency in that it is not pansystolic and radiates to the sternum rather than to the left axilla. Occasionally, a systolic "honk" is heard.

### B. IMAGING

In the rare case of significant mitral insufficiency, the left atrium may be enlarged. Left atrial enlargement may produce a "double shadow" seen best on the AP chest radiograph. In significant mitral regurgitation, the subcarinal angle will be increased to greater than 90 degrees. Most chest radiographs are normal, and their use is therefore largely unwarranted.

## C. ELECTROCARDIOGRAPHY

The ECG may be normal. Diffuse flattening or inversion of T waves may be seen in the precordial leads. U waves are prominent. Chest pain on exertion is rare and should be assessed with cardiopulmonary stress testing

## D. ECHOCARDIOGRAPHY

Significant posterior systolic movement of the mitral valve leaflets to the atrial side of the mitral annulus during systole is diagnostic. Echocardiography will assess the degree of myxomatous change of the mitral valve and the degree of associated mitral insufficiency.

## E. OTHER TESTING

Invasive procedures are rarely indicated. Holter monitoring or event recorders may be useful in establishing the presence of ventricular dysrhythmias in patients with palpitations.

## Treatment & Prognosis

Oral propranolol may be effective in treatment of coexisting arrhythmias. Prophylaxis for infectious endocarditis is indicated only in individuals with significant myxomatous change on echocardiography or with associated mitral insufficiency.

The natural course of this condition is largely unknown. Twenty years of observation indicate that isolated MVP in childhood is usually a benign entity. Surgery for clinically significant mitral insufficiency is very rarely needed.

Bobkowski W et al. A prospective study to determine the significance of ventricular late potentials in children with mitral valve prolapse. Cardiol Young 2002;12(4):333 [PMID: 12206555].

Freed LA et al: Prevalence and clinical outcome of mitral valve prolapse. N Engl J Med 1999;341(1):1 [PMID: 10387935].

## 4. Other Congenital Left Heart Valvular Lesions

## Congenital Mitral Stenosis

In congenital mitral stenosis, a rare disorder, the valve leaflets are thickened and fused to produce a diaphragm-like or funnel-like structure with a central opening. When mitral stenosis is seen in conjunction with other left-sided obstructive lesions, such as subaortic stenosis and coarctation of the aorta, the complex is known as Shone syndrome. Most patients develop symptoms early in life with symptoms such as tachypnea, dyspnea, and failure to thrive. Physical examination reveals an accentuated $S_1$ and a loud pulmonary closure sound. No opening snap can be heard. In most cases, a presystolic crescendo murmur is heard at the apex. Occasionally, only a middiastolic murmur can be heard. Rarely, no murmur at all is present. ECG shows right axis deviation, biatrial enlargement, and RVH. Radiograph reveals left atrial enlargement and frequently pulmonary venous congestion. Echocardiography shows abnormal mitral valve structures with reduced excursion and left atrial enlargement. Cardiac catheterization reveals an elevated pulmonary capillary wedge pressure and pulmonary hypertension.

Mitral valve repair or mitral valve replacement with a prosthetic mitral valve may be performed even in the young infant. Mitral valve repair is the preferred surgical option as mitral valve replacement is associated with a poor outcome in very young children.

## Cor Triatriatum

Cor triatriatum is a rare abnormality in which the pulmonary veins join together in their confluence but the confluence is not completely integrated into the left atrium. The chamber communicates with the left atrium through an opening of variable size. The physiologic consequences of this condition are similar to those of mitral stenosis. The clinical findings depend on the size of the opening, and the size and position of any associated atrial septal defect. If the opening is extremely small, symptoms develop very early in life. If the opening is larger, patients may be asymptomatic for a considerable time. Echocardiography reveals a linear density in the left atrium with a gradient between the pulmonary venous chamber and the left atrium proper. Cardiac catheterization may be needed if the diagnosis is in doubt. Finding a high pulmonary wedge pressure and a low left atrial pressure (if the catheter can be passed through the foramen ovale into the true left atrial chamber) confirms the diagnosis. Angiocardiographic studies will identify both the proximal and distal left atrium. Surgical repair is always required in the presence of an obstructive membrane, and long-term results are good. Coexisting mitral valve abnormalities may be noted, including a supravalval mitral ring or a dysplastic mitral valve.

## Congenital Mitral Regurgitation

Congenital mitral regurgitation is a relatively rare abnormality usually associated with other congenital heart lesions, such as congenitally corrected TGA, AV septal defect, and anomalous left coronary artery. Isolated congenital mitral regurgitation is very rare. It is sometimes present in patients with Marfan syndrome, usually associated with a myxomatous prolapsing mitral valve. Occasionally, congenital dilation of the valve ring occurs with an otherwise normal valve. In other cases, the chordae tendineae are malformed, resulting in mitral regurgitation.

## Congenital Aortic Regurgitation

Congenital aortic regurgitation is rare. The most common causes are bicuspid aortic valve, either uncomplicated or with coarctation of the aorta; VSD with aortic cusp prolapse and resultant aortic insufficiency; and fenestration of the aortic valve cusp (one or more holes in the cusp).

Eble BK et al: Mitral valve replacement in children: Predictors of long-term outcome. Ann Thorac Surg 2003;76(3):853 [PMID: 12963215].

## DISEASES OF THE AORTA

Aortic dilation and dissection may occur in childhood. Although the aorta may not be dilated at birth, the structural abnormality that predisposes to dilation is presumed to be congenital in origin. Patients at risk for progressive aortic dilation, and possible dissection, include those with isolated bicuspid aortic valve, Marfan syndrome, Turner syndrome, and type IV Ehlers–Danlos syndrome.

### Bicuspid Aortic Valve

Patients with bicuspid aortic valves have an increased incidence of aortic dilation and dissection, irrespective of the presence of aortic stenosis. Histologic examination demonstrates cystic medial degeneration of the aortic wall, probably as a result of smooth muscle cell apoptosis. Patients with isolated bicuspid aortic valve therefore require regular follow-up even in the absence of aortic insufficiency or aortic stenosis. Significant aortic root dilation requiring surgical intervention, in the absence of aortic stenosis, typically does not occur until adulthood.

### Marfan Syndrome

Marfan syndrome is an autosomal dominant disorder of connective tissue secondary to a mutation in the fibrillin-1 gene. The incidence of spontaneous mutations is 25%, and thus family history is not always helpful. Patients are diagnosed by the Ghent criteria and must have, at a minimum, major involvement of two body systems plus involvement of a third body system or a positive family history. Body systems that may be involved include cardiovascular, ocular, musculoskeletal, pulmonary, and integumentary. Cardiac manifestations include aortic root dilation and MVP, which may even be present at birth. Patients are at risk for aortic dilation and dissection and are restricted from competitive athletics, contact sports, and isometric activities. Beta-blockers or ACE inhibitors are used to lower blood pressure and slow the rate of aortic dilation. Elective surgical intervention is performed in patients of adult size when the aortic root dimension reaches 50–55 mm. The ratio of actual to expected aortic root dimension is used to determine the need for surgery in the young child. Surgical options include replacement of the dilated aortic root with a composite valve graft (Bentall technique) or a David procedure, wherein the patient's own aortic valve is spared and a Dacron tube graft is used to replace the dilated ascending aorta. Although young age at diagnosis was previously thought to confer a poor prognosis, early diagnosis in association with close follow-up and early initiation of medical therapy has been associated with a favorable outcome in most patients. Ventricular dysrhythmias may contribute to the increased mortality seen in this patient group.

### Turner Syndrome

Cardiovascular abnormalities are common in patients with Turner syndrome. Patients are at risk for aortic dissection, typically during adulthood. Risk factors for aortic dissection are usually present and include hypertension irrespective of cause, aortic dilation, bicuspid aortic valve, and coarctation of the aorta. There have been rare reports of aortic dissection occurring in adult Turner syndrome patients in the absence of any risk factors. Patients with Turner syndrome require routine follow-up during adolescence and adulthood to monitor this potentially lethal complication.

Bonderman D et al: Mechanisms underlying aortic dilation in congenital aortic valve malformation. Circulation 1999;99(16):2138 [PMID: 10217654].

Bordeleau L et al: Aortic dissection and Turner's syndrome: A review of the literature. J Emerg Med 1998;16(4):593 [PMID: 9696176].

Yetman AT et al: Comparison of outcome of the Marfan's syndrome in patients diagnosed at < or > 6 years of age. Am J Cardiol 2003;91(1):102 [PMID: 12505586].

Yetman AT et al: Long-term outcome in patients with Marfan's syndrome: Is aortic dissection the only cause of sudden death? J Am Coll Cardiol 2003;41(2):329 [PMID: 12535830].

## CORONARY ARTERY ABNORMALITIES

A number of anomalies involve the origin, course, and distribution of the coronary arteries. The only abnormality seen with any regularity, which has disastrous consequences if unrecognized, is anomalous origin of the left coronary artery.

### 1. Anomalous Origin of the Left Coronary Artery

In this condition, the left coronary artery arises from the pulmonary artery rather than the aorta. In the neonatal period, while the pulmonary arterial pressure is relatively high, the perfusion of the left coronary artery is adequate and the child is asymptomatic. However, by age 2 months, the pulmonary arterial pressure falls, resulting in a progressive decrease in the myocardial perfusion supplied by the left coronary artery. Ischemia and infarction of the LV occur. These infants present at age 2–4 months with severe CHF due to LV dysfunction and mitral insufficiency. Immediate surgery is needed, after the child is stabilized with anticongestive therapy, to bring aortic flow into the left coronary system. The surgery is relatively high risk, especially if infarction of the papillary muscles supporting the mitral apparatus has occurred. Mitral valve replacement is sometimes needed.

## Clinical Findings

### A. SYMPTOMS AND SIGNS

Patients appear healthy at birth. Growth and development are relatively normal for a few months, although detailed questioning of the parents often discloses a history of intermittent episodes of abdominal pain, pallor, and sweating, especially during or after feeding. These episodes are often thought to be secondary to colic but in fact are anginal attacks similar to those seen in adults.

On physical examination, the patients are usually well developed and well nourished. The pulses are typically weak but equal throughout. A prominent left precordial bulge is present. The pansystolic murmur of mitral regurgitation is frequently present, although a murmur need not be present to make this diagnosis.

### B. IMAGING

Chest radiographs show cardiac enlargement and left atrial enlargement and may show pulmonary venous congestion.

### C. ELECTROCARDIOGRAPHY

The ECG is very helpful. There are T wave inversions in leads I and aVL. The precordial leads show T wave inversions from $V_4$ to $V_7$. Deep, and often wide, Q waves are present in leads I, aVL, and sometimes in $V_4$–$V_6$. These findings of myocardial infarction are similar to those in adults.

### D. ECHOCARDIOGRAPHY

The diagnosis can be made with two-dimensional techniques by visualizing a single large right coronary artery arising from the aorta in infants with severe LV dysfunction and mitral insufficiency. The anomalous left coronary artery may be seen arising from the main pulmonary artery. The presence of flow reversal confirms the presence of an anomalous left coronary artery.

### E. CARDIAC CATHETERIZATION AND ANGIOCARDIOGRAPHY

A small left-to-right shunt (a result of the flow of blood from the right through the left coronary artery and into the pulmonary artery) can sometimes be detected. Cineangiocardiography after injection of contrast into the root of the aorta fails to show the origin of the left coronary artery. A large right coronary artery fills directly from the aorta, and the contrast material flows from the right coronary system via collaterals into the left coronary arteries and finally into the pulmonary artery.

## Treatment & Prognosis

Medical management with anticongestives and afterload reduction fails to correct the anatomic defect and should not delay surgical intervention. Early surgery is required to give a two coronary system. Simple ligation of the left coronary artery or subclavian to coronary artery anastomosis (without cardiopulmonary bypass) offer poor long-term results. Because survival after coronary surgery is highly dependent on the degree of mitral insufficiency, a decision must be made prior to bypass whether to leave or replace the mitral valve.

The prognosis is guarded. No therapeutic modality has been shown to be superior in follow-up studies of survivors.

Michielon G et al: Anomalous coronary artery origin from the pulmonary artery: Correlation between surgical timing and left ventricular function recovery. Ann Thorac Surg 2003;76(2):581 [PMID: 12902108].

## CYANOTIC CONGENITAL HEART DISEASE

### Tetralogy Of Fallot

### ESSENTIALS OF DIAGNOSIS & TYPICAL FEATURES

- *Cyanosis after the neonatal period.*
- *Hypoxemic spells during infancy.*
- *Right-sided aortic arch in 25% of patients.*
- *Systolic ejection murmur at the upper left sternal border.*

## General Considerations

In ToF, a VSD is present and obstruction to RV outflow occurs so that the intracardiac shunt is typically from right to left. This is the most common cyanotic lesion, accounting for 10% of all cases of congenital heart disease. The VSD is usually located in the membranous portion of the septum but may be surrounded completely by muscular tissue, and it is quite large. The obstruction to RV outflow may be primarily at the infundibular level (in 25–50% of cases), at the valvular level alone (rarely), or at both levels (most commonly). The primary embryologic abnormality is in the septation of the conus and truncus arteriosus with anterior deviation of the conus into the RV outflow tract, resulting in an enlarged overriding aorta and hypoplasia of the pulmonary outflow. Experimental lesions in specific loci of ectodermal (neural crest) tissue that migrate to the conus can reproduce the defects seen in ToF. The term "tetralogy" has been used to describe this combination of lesions, because RVH is always present and a varying degree of overriding of the aorta occurs in addition to the VSD and pulmonic and subpulmonic pulmonic stenosis. The overriding is caused by the anterior deviation of the conus, which brings the anterior wall of the aorta forward with it. A right-sided aortic arch is present in 25% of cases, and an ASD occurs in 15%.

Obstruction to RV outflow plus a large VSD results in a right-to-left shunt at the ventricular level and desaturation of the arterial blood. The degree of desaturation depends on the resistance to outflow from the RV, and the systemic vascular resistance. The greater the obstruction, and the lower the systemic vascular resistance, the greater the right-to-left shunting. Although the patient may be deeply cyanotic, the amount of pressure the RV can develop is limited to that of the systemic (aortic) pressure because the VSD is unrestrictive. The RV is usually able to maintain this level of pressure without developing heart failure. A high association between ToF and deletions in the long arm of chromosome 22 (22q11) has now been established, and as many as 15% of children with tetralogy appear to have this genetic abnormality.

## Clinical Findings

### A. Symptoms and Signs

The clinical findings vary depending on the degree of RV outflow obstruction. Patients with a mild degree of obstruction are only minimally cyanotic or may even be acyanotic. Those with maximal obstruction are deeply cyanotic from birth. Few children are asymptomatic. Most have cyanosis by age 4 months, and the cyanosis usually is progressive. Growth and development are not typically retarded, but easy fatigability and dyspnea on exertion are common. When these children learn to walk, they frequently squat suddenly to increase systemic vascular resistance to ward off cyanotic spells.

Hypoxemic spells, also called cyanotic spells or (Tet) tetralogy spells, are one of the hallmarks of severe ToF and are characterized by the following signs and symptoms: (1) sudden onset of cyanosis or deepening of cyanosis; (2) sudden onset of dyspnea; (3) alterations in consciousness, encompassing a spectrum from irritability to syncope; and (4) decrease in intensity or even disappearance of the systolic murmur. These episodes may begin in the neonatal period, but most commonly they start at age 4–6 months. Acute treatment of cyanotic spells consists of giving oxygen and placing the patient in the knee-chest position. Acidosis, if present, should be corrected with intravenous sodium bicarbonate. Morphine sulfate should be administered cautiously by a parenteral route in a dosage of 0.1 mg/kg. Propranolol, 0.1–0.2 mg/kg intravenously, is useful. Chronic (daily) prophylaxis of cyanotic spells with propranolol, 1 mg/kg orally every 4 hours while awake, remains controversial; however, in a significant number of patients, this regimen has prevented subsequent spells and made it possible to delay surgery. The degree of cyanosis in ToF is variable. The fingers and toes show varying degrees of clubbing depending on the age of the child and the severity of cyanosis.

On examination of the heart, an RV lift is palpable. $S_1$ is normal; occasionally, an ejection click is eveident at the apex that is aortic in origin. $S_2$ is predominantly aortic and single. A grade II–IV/VI, rough, ejection-type systolic murmur is present that is maximal at the left sternal border in the third intercostal space and that radiates well to the back.

### B. Laboratory Findings

The hemoglobin, hematocrit, and red blood cell count are usually elevated, depending on the degree of arterial oxygen desaturation.

### C. Imaging

Chest radiographs show a heart of normal size. Indeed, the radiograph is sometimes interpreted as entirely normal. However, the RV is hypertrophied, which is often shown in the posteroanterior projection by an upturning of the apex (boot-shaped heart). The main pulmonary artery segment is usually concave, and a right aortic arch is present in 25% of cases, with the aortic knob to the right of the trachea. The pulmonary vascular markings are usually decreased.

### D. Electrocardiography

The cardiac axis is to the right, ranging from +90 to +180 degrees. The P waves are usually normal, although evidence may indicate slight right atrial hypertrophy. RVH is always present, but RV strain patterns are rare.

### E. ECHOCARDIOGRAPHY

Two-dimensional imaging is diagnostic, revealing thickening of the RV wall, with overriding of the aorta and a large subaortic VSD. Furthermore, obstruction at the level of the infundibulum and pulmonary valve can be identified, and the size of the proximal pulmonary arteries can be measured. The anatomy of the coronary arteries may be visualized.

### F. CARDIAC CATHETERIZATION AND ANGIOCARDIOGRAPHY

Cardiac catheterization reveals the presence of a right-to-left shunt in most cases. Arterial desaturation of varying degrees is present. The right-to-left shunt occurs at the ventricular level. The RV pressure is at systemic levels, and the pressure tracing in the RV is identical to that of the LV. The pulmonary artery pressure is low. The pressure gradients may be noted at the valvular level or the infundibular level (or both).

Cineangiocardiography is helpful. Injection of contrast into the RV reveals the RV outflow obstruction and the right-to-left shunt at the ventricular level. The major indications for cardiac catheterization are to establish coronary artery and distal pulmonary artery anatomy. In addition, some patients may be palliated by balloon dilation of the RV outflow tract during infancy to improve the pulmonary blood flow, thereby delaying surgical intervention.

## Treatment

### A. PALLIATIVE TREATMENT

Palliative treatment is performed at some centers for small infants who have severe symptoms (severe cyanosis, frequent severe hypoxic spells) and in whom complete correction is deemed too risky. Medical (chronic oral β-blocking agents) or, more often, surgical (creation of a systemic arterial to pulmonary arterial anastomosis) palliation can be used. Balloon angioplasty is being used for palliation in some centers. In this procedure the pulmonic valve and the entire RV outflow tract are dilated in order to reduce RV outflow tract obstruction and improve pulmonary artery growth. The most common surgical palliation is the creation of a GoreTex shunt from the subclavian artery to the ipsilateral pulmonary artery (modified Blalock–Taussig shunt). This operation can be done with very low likelihood of mortality and with no significant distortion of the pulmonary arteries.

### B. TOTAL CORRECTION

The timing of open-heart surgery for repair of ToF ranges from birth to age 2 years, varying with the experience of each treatment center. The current surgical trend is toward earlier repair based on the severity of symptoms. Patients may be repaired in the neonatal period, although, if asymptomatic, surgery is deferred until 6–8 months of age. During surgery, the VSD is closed and the obstruction to RV outflow removed. The surgical death rate varies from 1% to 3%. The major limiting anatomic feature of total correction is the size of the pulmonary arteries.

## Course & Prognosis

Infants with the most severe form of ToF are usually deeply cyanotic at birth. Hypoxemic spells may occur during the neonatal period. Death is extremely rare during a severe hypoxemic spell. These children require early surgery, either a Blalock–Taussig shunt or primary correction.

All children with ToF require open-heart surgery. Complete repair before age 5 years usually results in fair to good function, although patients occasionally die as a result of ventricular dysrhythmias. A competent pulmonary valve without a dilated RV appears to diminish arrhythmias and enhance exercise performance.

Bacha EA et al: Long-term results after early primary repair of tetralogy of Fallot. J Thorac Cardiovasc Surg 2001;122:154 [PMID: 11436019].

Botto LD et al. A population-based study of the 22q11.2 deletion: Phenotype, incidence and contribution to major birth defects in the population. Pediatrics 2003;112(1 Pt 1):101 [PMID: 12837874].

Mulder TJ et al. A multicenter analysis of the choice of initial surgical procedure in tetralogy of Fallot. Pediatr Cardiol 2002; 23(6):580 [PMID: 12530488].

Therrien J et al: Impact of pulmonary valve replacement on arrhythmia propensity late after repair of tetralogy of Fallot. Circulation 2001;103(20):2489 [PMID: 11369690].

## PULMONARY ATRESIA WITH VENTRICULAR SEPTAL DEFECT

This condition consists of complete atresia of the pulmonary valve in association with VSD. Essentially, it is an extreme form of ToF. Because there is no antegrade flow from the RV into the pulmonary artery, the pulmonary blood flow must be derived either from a PDA or from aortopulmonary collateral arteries.

The clinical picture depends entirely on the size of the ductus and the collateral channels. If they are large, patients may be quite stable. If pulmonary blood flow is low, severe hypoxia results, and immediate palliation is required. Newborns are stabilized with intravenous prostaglandin $E_1$ (PGE$_1$) to maintain patency of the ductus arteriosus while being prepared for surgery. Once the child is stabilized, a decision must be made about whether to do a palliative Blalock–Taussig shunt or to proceed with primary correction. In most centers, a shunt is performed in the newborn period, with open-heart surgery planned for age 9–18 months.

Echocardiography or cardiac catheterization and angiocardiography are diagnostic. A corrective surgical procedure that has been successful in patients with adequate-sized pulmonary arteries consists of closing the VSD and inserting a homograft from the RV to the main pulmonary artery. Success depends on precise definition of pulmonary arterial and collateral blood supply to the lung and, if needed, prior unifocalization of segments with dual arterial blood supply into a single pulmonary arterial tree.

Mair DD, Puga FJ: Management of pulmonary atresia with ventricular septal defect. Curr Treat Options Cardiovasc Med 2003;5(5):409 [PMID: 12941209].

# PULMONARY ATRESIA WITH INTACT VENTRICULAR SEPTUM

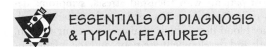

ESSENTIALS OF DIAGNOSIS & TYPICAL FEATURES

- Cyanosis at birth.
- Chest radiograph with a concave pulmonary artery segment and the apex tilted upward.

## General Considerations

In this uncommon condition, the pulmonary valve is atretic. The pulmonic annulus usually has a small diaphragm consisting of the fused valve cusps. The ventricular septum is intact. The main pulmonary artery segment is somewhat hypoplastic but almost always present. Although the RV is always reduced in size in this condition, the degree of reduction is variable. This factor is critical because some children with pulmonic atresia may have an adequate ventricle for ultimate "two-ventricular" repair; therefore, the assessment of the adequacy of the RV is important. The RV has three component parts (inlet, trabecular, and outlet), and the absence of any one of these three components makes the ultimate use of the RV extremely unlikely. Even with all three components, some RVs are inadequate.

Following birth, the pulmonary circulation is maintained by the PDA. Although a bronchial–pulmonary collateral network may be present, it is usually insufficient to maintain the pulmonary circulation. Accordingly, a continuous infusion of PGE$_1$ must be started as soon as possible after birth to maintain ductal patency.

## Clinical Findings

### A. SYMPTOMS AND SIGNS

Although patients may be normal at birth, they are usually cyanotic. Cyanosis progresses as the ductus arteriosus closes. A blowing systolic murmur resulting from the associated PDA may be heard at the pulmonary area. In addition, a pansystolic murmur is often heard at the lower left sternal border, because most of these children develop significant tricuspid insufficiency.

### B. IMAGING

The heart size may vary from small to markedly enlarged, depending on the degree of tricuspid insufficiency. With striking tricuspid insufficiency, right atrial enlargement may be massive and the cardiac silhouette may virtually fill the chest.

### C. ELECTROCARDIOGRAPHY

ECG reveals an axis that is leftward for age (45–90 degrees) in the frontal plane. Evidence for right atrial enlargement is usually striking. There is LV dominance for age with reduced RV forces.

### D. ECHOCARDIOGRAPHY

Echocardiography shows absence of the pulmonary valve, with varying degrees of hypoplasia of the RV cavity and tricuspid annulus. The severity of tricuspid regurgitation correlates with RV size.

### E. CARDIAC CATHETERIZATION AND ANGIOCARDIOGRAPHY

RV pressure is high and is almost always suprasystemic. A cineangiocardiogram in the RV reveals no filling of the pulmonary artery from the RV. It also demonstrates the size of the RV chamber, relative hypoplasia of the components of the tripartite RV, and the presence or absence of tricuspid regurgitation. Approximately 15% of children with pulmonic atresia and intact ventricular septum have sinusoids between the RV and the coronary arteries. The presence of these sinusoids indicates that the coronary circulation may depend on RV flow; this situation is associated with a high risk for sudden death.

## Treatment & Prognosis

As in pulmonary atresia with VSD, a PGE$_1$ infusion is used to stabilize the patient and maintain patency of the ductus until surgery can be performed. Surgery should be undertaken as soon as possible. A Rashkind balloon atrial septostomy is performed, depending on RV size, to open up the communication across the atrial septum. If the RV is tripartite and an eventual two-chamber repair is planned, the pulmonary valve plate is opened during cardiac catheterization in the newborn period to allow antegrade flow from the RV to the pulmonary artery and to encourage RV cavity growth. If the RV is inadequate, significant sinusoids are present, or the pulmonic valve cannot be opened successfully in the catheterization laboratory, an immediate Blalock–Taussig shunt is performed to establish pulmonary blood flow. Later in infancy, a communication between the RV and pulmonary artery can be created on bypass in an attempt to stimulate RV cavity growth. If RV dimensions or function are inadequate for a two-ventricular repair, a one-ventricular systemic venous to pulmonary artery palliation is indicated (Fontan procedure). Children with significant sinusoids receive a Blalock–Taussig shunt as immediate treatment, but they are often considered for cardiac transplantation if they are deemed at risk for coronary insufficiency and sudden death.

The prognosis in this condition remains guarded. Our overall experience strongly favors opening the atretic valve in the catheterization laboratory in the newborn period if possible. If this is impossible, a Blalock–Taussig shunt should be placed. Ultimate plans for a two-ventricular repair, a Fontan procedure, or cardiac transplantation depend on the anatomy.

Humpl T et al: Percutaneous balloon valvotomy in pulmonary atresia with intact ventricular septum: Impact on patient care. Circulation 2003;108(7):826 [PMID: 12885744].

Minnich LL et al: Usefulness of the preoperative tricuspid/mitral valve ratio for predicting outcome in pulmonary atresia with intact ventricular septum. Am J Cardiol 2000;85(11):1325 [PMID: 10831948].

Powell AJ et al: Outcome in infants with pulmonary atresia, intact ventricular septum, and right ventricular-dependent coronary circulation. Am J Cardiol 2000;86(11):1272 [PMID: 11090809].

# TRICUSPID ATRESIA

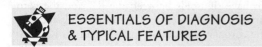

## ESSENTIALS OF DIAGNOSIS & TYPICAL FEATURES

- *Marked cyanosis present from birth.*
- *ECG with left axis deviation, right atrial enlargement, and LVH.*

## General Considerations

This relatively rare condition (< 1% of cases of congenital heart disease) is characterized by complete atresia of the tricuspid valve. As a result, no direct communica-

tion exists between the right atrium and the RV. Tricuspid atresia is divided into two types, depending on the relationship of the great vessels (Table 19–14).

Because no direct communication exists between the right atrium and the RV, the entire systemic venous return must flow through the atrial septum (either an ASD or patent foramen ovale) into the left atrium. Thus the left atrium receives both the systemic venous return and the pulmonary venous return. Complete mixing occurs in the left atrium, resulting in a greater or lesser degree of arterial desaturation.

As a result of the lack of direct communication, the development of the RV depends on the presence of a left-to-right shunt at the ventricular level. Therefore, severe hypoplasia of the RV occurs in those forms in which there is no VSD or in which the VSD is small.

## Clinical Findings

### A. SYMPTOMS AND SIGNS

In most patients with tricuspid atresia, symptoms develop early in infancy. Except in patients whose pulmonary blood flow is high, cyanosis is present at birth. Growth and development are poor, and the infant usually exhibits fatigability on feeding, tachypnea, dyspnea, anoxic spells, and evidence of right heart failure. Patients with marked increase in pulmonary blood flow—types 1(c) and 2(b)—may develop evidence of left heart failure as well.

Digital clubbing is present in older children. $S_1$ is normal. $S_2$ is most often single. A murmur is usually present, although it is variable. It ranges from grade II to grade III/VI in intensity and usually is a harsh blowing murmur heard best at the lower left sternal border.

**Table 19–14.** Tricuspid atresia.

| Type 1: Without transposition of the great arteries | Type 2: With transposition of the great arteries |
|---|---|
| (a) No ventricular septal defect; hypoplasia or atresia of the pulmonary artery; patent ductus arteriosus<br>(b) Small ventricular septal defect; pulmonary stenosis; hypoplastic pulmonary artery<br>(c) Large ventricular septal defect and no pulmonary stenosis; normal-sized pulmonary artery | (a) With ventricular septal defect and pulmonary stenosis<br>(b) With ventricular septal defect but without pulmonary stenosis |

## B. Imaging

Chest radiographic findings are variable. The heart is slightly to markedly enlarged. The main pulmonary artery segment is usually small or absent. The size of the right atrium varies from moderately to massively enlarged, depending on the size of the communication at the atrial level. The pulmonary vascular markings are usually decreased, although in types 1(c) and 2(b) they are increased.

## C. Electrocardiography

The ECG is usually helpful. It shows left axis deviation with a counterclockwise loop in the frontal plane. The P waves are tall and peaked, indicative of right atrial hypertrophy. LVH or LV dominance is found in almost all cases. RV forces on the ECG are usually low or absent.

## D. Echocardiography

M-mode and two-dimensional methods are diagnostic and show absence of the tricuspid valve, the relationship between the great arteries, and the size of the pulmonary arteries.

## E. Cardiac Catheterization and Angiocardiography

This technique reveals the large right-to-left shunt at the atrial level and desaturation of the left atrial blood. Because of the complete mixing in the left atrium, oxygen saturations in the LV, RV, pulmonary artery, and aorta are identical to the that in left atrium. The right atrial pressure is increased. LV and systemic pressures are normal. The catheter cannot be passed through the tricuspid valve from the right atrium to the RV. A balloon atrial septostomy is performed if a restrictive foramen ovale is present.

## Treatment & Prognosis

In infants with high pulmonary artery flow, conventional anticongestive therapy should be given until the infant begins to outgrow the VSD. Occasionally, a pulmonary artery band is needed to protect the pulmonary bed in preparation for a Fontan procedure. A Fontan procedure (connection of the systemic venous return to the pulmonary artery) is performed when increasing cyanosis occurs, typically at age 2–4 years.

In infants with diminished pulmonary blood flow, $PGE_1$ is infused until an aortopulmonary shunt can be performed. The Fontan procedure is frequently performed in stages; a Glenn procedure (superior vena cava to pulmonary artery anastomosis) is performed with concomitant ligation of the aortopulmonary shunt at age 3–9 months, and a completion Fontan procedure is performed at age 1–4 years.

The prognosis for all patients with tricuspid atresia depends on the achievement of a balance of pulmonary blood flow that permits adequate oxygenation of the tissues without producing CHF. The long-term prognosis for children treated by the Fontan procedure is unknown. In the short term, the best results for the Fontan procedure occur in children with low pulmonary artery pressures prior to open-heart surgery.

Fogel MA et al: Caval contribution to flow in the branch pulmonary arteries of Fontan patients with a novel application of magnetic resonance presaturation pulse. Circulation 1999; 99(9):1215 [PMID: 10069790].

Mair DD et al: The Fontan procedure for tricuspid atresia: Early and late results of a 25-year experience with 216 patients. J Am Coll Cardiol 2001;37(3):933 [PMID: 11693773].

# HYPOPLASTIC LEFT HEART SYNDROME

### ESSENTIALS OF DIAGNOSIS & TYPICAL FEATURES

- *Mild cyanosis at birth. Minimal auscultatory findings.*
- *Rapid onset of shock with ductal closure.*

## General Considerations

Hypoplastic left heart syndrome includes a number of conditions in which lesions of the left heart result in hypoplasia of the LV. The syndrome occurs in 1.4–3.8% of infants with congenital heart disease.

The most common lesions making up this syndrome are mitral atresia, aortic atresia, or both. Following birth, survival depends on a PDA because the antegrade flow into the systemic circulation is inadequate and the ductus arteriosus provides flow to the aorta. Children with hypoplastic left heart syndrome are usually stable at birth, but they deteriorate rapidly as the ductus starts to close later in the first week of life. Untreated, the average age at death is 5–7 days. In rare instances, the ductus will remain widely patent on its own, and children will survive for months without $PGE_1$ therapy.

## Clinical Findings

### A. Symptoms and Signs

Children with hypoplastic left heart syndrome appear stable at birth, because the ductus is widely patent. They deteriorate rapidly when the ductus starts to close with findings first of CHF, followed almost immediately by clinical shock with acidosis secondary to inadequate systemic perfusion.

## B. IMAGING

Chest radiographic findings at presentation are those of cardiac enlargement with severe pulmonary venous congestion.

## C. ELECTROCARDIOGRAPHY

The ECG demonstrates right axis deviation, right atrial hypertrophy, and RVH with relative paucity of LV forces and absence of a Q wave in lead $V_6$. A QR pattern is often seen in lead $V_1$.

## D. ECHOCARDIOGRAPHY

Echocardiography is diagnostic and eliminates the need for cardiac catheterization. A diminutive aorta and LV with an atretic mitral valve in the presence of a normal and easily definable tricuspid valve are diagnostic. The systemic circulation depends on the PDA. Color-flow Doppler imaging shows retrograde flow in the ascending aorta.

## Treatment & Prognosis

PGE$_1$ infusion is essential initially because systemic circulation depends on a PDA. Further management depends on balancing pulmonary and systemic blood flow because the RV provides both. Within a few days of birth, the pulmonary resistance falls, favoring pulmonary overcirculation and compromised systemic perfusion. Therapy must be directed to increasing pulmonary vascular tone using hypoxia or hypercapnic ventilation. We now use nitrogen to decrease the inspired oxygen content below 21%. This therapy, which must be carefully monitored, results in an increase in pulmonary arterial tone and systemic perfusion. Nitrogen is blended with room air, and the delivered $O_2$ content is monitored continuously. We typically start at 16–17% inspired oxygen with a goal of maintaining systemic $O_2$ saturation at 65–80% to balance the pulmonary and systemic blood flows.

Shortly after birth a decision must be made between several surgical options. In the Norwood procedure, the RV is used as the systemic ventricle while an aortopulmonary bypass is created for pulmonic flow. Alternatively, the child can be listed for orthotopic cardiac transplantation. Children who have a Norwood procedure (and subsequent Glenn anastomosis and completion Fontan procedure) or who are listed for receipt of a donor heart have a 50–60% chance for 5–year survival at the best centers. Although this is a major improvement over nonsurgical intervention, hypoplastic left heart syndrome remains one of the most challenging lesions in pediatric cardiology.

Mahle WT et al: Impact of prenatal diagnosis on survival and early neurologic morbidity in neonates with the hypoplastic left heart syndrome. Pediatrics 2001;107(6):1277 [PMID: 11389243].

Mosca RS et al: Early results of the Fontan procedure in one hundred consecutive patients with hypoplastic left heart syndrome. J Thorac Cardiovasc Surg 2000;119(6):1110 [PMID: 10838526].

Tworetzky W et al: Improved surgical outcome after fetal diagnosis of hypoplastic left heart syndrome. Circulation 2001;103(9): 1269 [PMID: 11238272].

# TRANSPOSITION OF THE GREAT ARTERIES

### ESSENTIALS OF DIAGNOSIS & TYPICAL FEATURES

- *Cyanotic newborn without respiratory distress.*
- *More common in males.*

## General Considerations

Transposition of the great arteries (d-TGA or complete TGA) is the second most common cyanotic congenital heart disease, accounting for 5% of all cases of congenital heart disease. The male-to-female ratio is 3:1. The disorder is caused by an embryologic abnormality in the spiral division of the truncus arteriosus, in which the aorta arises from the RV and the pulmonary artery from the LV. In 60% of cases only the two usual newborn cardiac connections (patent foramen ovale and PDA) are present, but VSDs, pulmonic stenosis, coarctation of the aorta, or aortic stenosis occurs in a significant number of patients. Left unrepaired, transposition is associated with a high incidence of early pulmonary vascular obstructive disease. TGA can be classified into two types (Table 19–15).

Because the aorta arises directly from the RV, survival would be impossible without mixing between the systemic and pulmonary circulations. Oxygenated blood from the pulmonary veins must reach the systemic arterial circuit. In patients with an intact ventricular septum, mixing occurs at the atrial and ductal levels. However, in most patients, these communications are small, and the ductus arteriosus closes shortly after birth. These patients are therefore severely cyanotic. Patients with a VSD may have better mixing and less cyanosis. Patients with a VSD and pulmonary stenosis

***Table 19–15.*** Complete (D) transposition of the great arteries.

| **Type 1:** With intact ventricular septum | **Type 2:** With ventricular septal defect |
|---|---|
| (a) Without pulmonary stenosis<br>(b) With pulmonary stenosis subvalvular or valvular (or both) | (a) With pulmonary stenosis<br>(b) With pulmonary vascular obstruction<br>(c) Without pulmonary vascular obstruction (normal pulmonary vascular resistance) |

(types 2[a] and 2[b]) are usually severely cyanotic because of the limited blood flow to the lungs. Patients with a VSD and normal pulmonary vascular resistance (type 2[c]) have the least cyanosis but often develop heart failure early because of high pulmonary blood flow.

## Clinical Findings

### A. SYMPTOMS AND SIGNS

Many of the neonates are large, some weighing 4 kg at birth, and most are severely cyanotic at birth. Infants with an intact ventricular septum are often quite striking in appearance because of their profound cyanosis (unresponsive to increasing the ambient $O_2$), the absence of a significant murmur, their lack of respiratory distress, and their large size. Only infants with a large VSD will be less cyanotic, and they usually have a prominent murmur. The findings on cardiovascular examination depend on the intracardiac defects. Patients with type 1(a) defects have only soft murmurs or none at all. $S_1$ is usually normal in these patients. $S_2$ is single and accentuated as the aortic valve is anterior. Patients with type 1(b) defects have loud obstructive systolic murmurs that are maximal at the second and third intercostal spaces and the left sternal border, radiating well to the first and second intercostal spaces. Patients with type 2(a) defects have a murmur of pulmonary stenosis (obstructive systolic murmur at the base of the heart, best heard to the right of the sternum). Those with type 2(c) defects have a systolic murmur along the lower sternal border and a mitral diastolic flow murmur at the apex.

### B. IMAGING

The chest radiograph in transposition is often nonspecific. Sometimes, however, there is an "egg on a string" appearance because the aorta is directly anterior to the main pulmonary artery, giving the image of a narrow mediastinum.

### C. ELECTROCARDIOGRAPHY

Because the newborn ECG normally has RV predominance, the ECG in transposition is of little help.

### D. ECHOCARDIOGRAPHY

Two-dimensional imaging and Doppler evaluation accurately describe the anatomy and physiology of transposition. The abnormal relationship of the great arteries is the hallmark of transposition on echocardiography. If clinically indicated, the balloon atrial septostomy may be performed with echocardiographic guidance.

### E. CARDIAC CATHETERIZATION AND ANGIOCARDIOGRAPHY

Cardiac catheterization is both diagnostic and therapeutic in this malformation. If complete transposition of the great arteries exists and if there are two well-developed ventricles, a Rashkind balloon atrial septostomy is performed to open the atrial septum unless a true ASD exists. The coronary anatomy is delineated by ascending aortography.

## Treatment

Early corrective surgery is recommended for transposition. The arterial switch operation (ASO) is performed at age 4–7 days. The arteries are switched in the anterior chest, and the coronaries are reimplanted into the neoaorta. Small associated VSDs may be left to close on their own, but large VSDs are always closed at this time. The atrial septum is also closed. The ASO has replaced the atrial switch procedures (Mustard and Senning operations), which were previously performed. Because the ASO must be performed while the LV musculature can still support systemic blood flow, it is rarely delayed beyond age 14 days in infants with an intact ventricular septum or small VSD. If a large, unrestrictive VSD is present that maintains LV pressure at systemic levels, corrective surgery can be delayed for a few months. Surgery should still be performed by age 3–4 months because of the high risk of early pulmonary vascular disease associated with transposition.

Survival after the ASO is now greater than 95% in major centers. In addition, the switch procedure greatly shortens the time that the child remains severely cyanotic before corrective surgery. Early relief of cyanosis may improve the developmental outcome for children with transposition. Finally, the switch procedure leaves the LV as the systemic ventricle. The older atrial corrective procedures (Senning and Mustard procedures) put the RV in this role, there was a significant incidence of late RV failure. Since the LV is designed for systemic pressures, late failure of the LV after the ASO has not been reported.

Bellinger DC et al: Developmental and neurological status of children at 4 years of age after heart surgery with hypothermic circulatory arrest or low flow cardiopulmonary bypass. Circulation 1999;100(5):526 [PMID: 10430767].

Singh TP et al: Assessment of progressive changes in exercise performance in patients with a systemic right ventricle following atrial switch repair. Pediatr Cardiol 2001;22(3):210 [PMID: 11343144].

Wernovsky G et al: Factors influencing early and late outcome of the arterial switch operation for transposition of the great arteries. J Thorac Cardiovasc Surg 1995;109(2):289 [PMID: 7583882].

# CONGENITALLY CORRECTED TRANSPOSITION OF THE GREAT ARTERIES

Congenitally corrected transposition of the great arteries (ccTGA or l-TGA) is a relatively uncommon form of congenital heart disease that may present with cyanosis depending on the presence of associated lesions. In ccTGA, both AV and VA discordance occurs, such that the right atrium connects to a morphologic LV, which supports the pulmonary artery. Conversely, the left atrium empties via a tricuspid valve, into a morphologic RV, which supports the aorta. Commonly associated lesions include VSDs and pulmonary stenosis. A dysplastic left-sided tricuspid valve is almost always present. Previously, surgical repair was directed at VSD closure and relief of pulmonary outflow tract obstruction. This surgical technique maintained the RV as the systemic ventricle supporting the aorta. It is now recognized that these patients have a reduced lifespan, and thus other surgical techniques have been advocated. The double-switch procedure is one such technique. In this procedure, an atrial level switch (Mustard or Senning technique) is performed, and an arterial switch operation then restores the morphologic LV to its position of systemic ventricle. In the absence of associated lesions, patients with ccTGA most often are undiagnosed until the adult years, when they present with either left-sided AV valve insufficiency or arrhythmias. Patients with ccTGA have an increased incidence of spontaneous complete heart block estimated at 1% per year with an overall frequency of 50%.

Graham TP et al: Long-term outcome in congenitally corrected transposition of the great arteries. J Am Coll Cardiol 2000; 36(1):255 [PMID: 10898443].

# DOUBLE-OUTLET RIGHT VENTRICLE

In this uncommon malformation, both great arteries arise from the RV. There is always a VSD that allows blood to flow from the LV. The presentation depends on the relationship of the VSD to the semilunar valves.

If the VSD is subaortic and no pulmonary stenosis is present, a large left-to-right shunt is present and the clinical picture resembles that of a large VSD. Early primary correction, with the VSD patch fashioned to the anterior aortic root, is very successful. If a subaortic VSD and pulmonic and subpulmonic stenosis are present, the physiology and the clinical management are the same as in ToF. However, if the VSD is subpulmonic (Taussig–Bing malformation), the presentation and management are analogous to those of an infant with transposition and an unrestrictive VSD.

In all forms of double-outlet RV, echocardiography with Doppler flow assessment is useful in clarifying the anatomy and physiology. Preoperative cardiac catheterization and angiocardiography are used if questions remain about the pulmonary or coronary arteries, or in children with the Taussig–Bing malformation who have severe cyanosis requiring balloon atrial septostomy for atrial mixing.

Dearani JA et al: Late follow-up of 1095 patients undergoing operation for complex congenital heart disease utilizing pulmonary ventricle to pulmonary artery conduits. Ann Thorac Surg 2003;75(2)399 [PMID: 12607647].

Sondheimer HM et al: Double outlet right ventricle: Clinical spectrum and prognosis. Am J Cardiol 1977;39(5):709 [PMID: 67796].

# TOTAL ANOMALOUS PULMONARY VENOUS RETURN WITH OR WITHOUT OBSTRUCTION

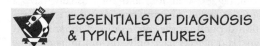

## ESSENTIALS OF DIAGNOSIS & TYPICAL FEATURES

- *Cyanosis.*
- *Systolic ejection murmur with lower left sternal border flow rumble and accentuated $P_2$.*
- *Right atrial and RVH.*
- *Abnormal pulmonary venous connection.*

## General Considerations

This malformation accounts for approximately 2% of all congenital heart lesions. The pulmonary venous blood drains into a confluence behind the left atrium, but the confluence is not connected to the left atrium. The pulmonary venous blood therefore finds another route to rejoin the circulation via the systemic veins. This leads to complete mixing at the level of the right atrium. The clinical presentation of total anomalous pulmonary venous return (TAPVR) depends on the method of return and whether that return to the systemic veins is unrestricted or restricted.

This malformation is classified by the site of entry of the pulmonary veins into the right side of the heart. Although the most common form of TAPVR is unobstructed via the left superior vena cava, three other distinct types exist:

> Type 1 (50%): Entry into the left superior vena cava (persistent anterior cardinal vein) or right superior vena cava, unobstructed or obstructed.
>
> Type 2 (20%): Entry into the right atrium directly or via the coronary sinus, unobstructed.
>
> Type 3 (20%): Entry below the diaphragm (usually into the portal vein), almost always obstructed.
>
> Type 4 (10%): Multiple sites of entry (mixed TAPVR).

Because the entire venous drainage from the body comes to the right atrium, a right-to-left shunt is always present at the atrial level. This may take the form of either an ASD or a patent foramen ovale. Occasionally the atrial septum is a restrictive foramen ovale, and a Rashkind procedure is needed at birth to allow filling of the left heart. Complete mixing of the systemic and pulmonary venous return occurs in the right atrium, so that the left atrial and the systemic arterial saturation levels approximately equal that of the right atrial saturation.

## Clinical Findings

### A. WITH UNOBSTRUCTED PULMONARY VENOUS RETURN

This large group includes all children (type 2) with pulmonary venous return to the right atrium and most children with supracardiac TAPVR. These patients tend to have a high total pulmonary flow typically present with cardiomegaly and early CHF rather than cyanosis. Oxygen saturations in the high 80s or low 90s are common. Most patients in this group have mild to moderate elevation of the pulmonary artery pressure owing to the elevated pulmonary blood flow. In most instances, the pressure does not reach systemic levels.

**1. Symptoms and signs**—These patients may have a history of mild cyanosis in the neonatal period and during early infancy. Thereafter, they do relatively well except for frequent respiratory infections. They are usually rather small and thin and resemble patients with very large ASDs.

Careful examination discloses duskiness of the nail beds and mucous membranes, but definite cyanosis and digital clubbing are usually absent. The arterial pulses are normal. An RV heave is palpable.

The pulmonary component of the second sound is usually increased. A grade II–III/VI ejection-type systolic murmur is heard at the pulmonary area. It radiates over the lung fields anteriorly and posteriorly. An early to middiastolic flow murmur is often heard at the lower left sternal border in the third and fourth intercostal spaces (tricuspid flow murmur).

**2. Imaging**—Chest radiography reveals cardiac enlargement primarily involving the right heart and pulmonary artery. Pulmonary vascular markings are markedly increased. A characteristic cardiac contour called a "snowman" or "figure of 8" is often seen when the anomalous veins drain via a persistent left superior vena cava to the innominate vein and then the right superior vena cava. This radiographic appearance is not present until approximately 3 months of age because it requires time for the vertical vein and innominate vein to dilate.

**3. Electrocardiography**—ECG shows right axis deviation and varying degrees of right atrial and right ventricular hypertrophy. A QR pattern is often evident over the right precordial leads.

**4. Echocardiography**—Demonstration by echocardiography of a chamber posterior to the left atrium is strongly suggestive of the diagnosis. However, echocardiographic discrimination between anomalies of pulmonary venous return and persistence of pulmonary fetal circulation can be challenging. The availability of two-dimensional echocardiography plus color-flow Doppler has increased the diagnostic accuracy.

### B. WITH OBSTRUCTED PULMONARY VENOUS RETURN

This group includes all patients with subdiaphragmatic TAPVR and a few of the patients in whom the venous drainage is into a systemic vein above the diaphragm.

**1. Symptoms and signs**—These infants usually present shortly after birth with severe cyanosis and require early corrective surgery. Cardiac examination discloses a striking RV impulse. $S_1$ is accentuated. $S_2$ is markedly accentuated and single. A grade I–III/VI ejection-type systolic murmur is frequently heard over the pulmonary area with radiation over the lung fields. Diastolic murmurs are uncommon. In many cases, no murmur is heard at all.

**2. Imaging**—In the most severe cases, the heart is small and pulmonary venous congestion is marked. In less severe cases, the heart size may be normal or slightly enlarged with slight pulmonary venous congestion.

**3. Electrocardiography**—The ECG shows right axis deviation, right atrial hypertrophy, and RVH.

**4. Echocardiography**—Echocardiography shows a combination of a small left atrium and LV and a vessel lying parallel and anterior to the descending aorta and to the left of the inferior vena cava. Color-flow Doppler echocardiography is useful in establishing the diagnosis and is often diagnostic. Right-to-left atrial shunting occurs.

**5. Cardiac catheterization and angiocardiography**—These procedures are diagnostic. Cardiac catheterization and cineangiocardiography demonstrate TAPVR and identify the site of entry of the anomalous veins. They also demonstrate the ratio of pulmonary to systemic blood flow and the degree of pulmonary hypertension and pulmonary vascular resistance.

## Treatment

Surgery is always required for TAPVR. If pulmonary venous return is obstructed, surgery must be performed during the immediate newborn period. In infants with unobstructed TAPVR, surgery is more elective and may be delayed for weeks to months. The timing of surgery can then be determined by the child's weight gain and the risk of pulmonary infection. If early surgery is not planned and the atrial septum is restrictive, a balloon atrial septostomy should be performed in the newborn period. The results of surgery are excellent.

## Course & Prognosis

Most children with TAPVR do very well after surgery. However, approximately 5% of surgical survivors develop late stenosis of the pulmonary veins. This devastating condition is difficult to treat either with interventional catheterization or surgery, and it has a very poor prognosis. Pulmonary vein stenosis, when it occurs, is most often seen in children who initially had obstructed total veins, but it occurs occasionally in children whose initial presentation was unobstructed. A new surgical technique involving sutureless in situ pericardial repair of the recurrent pulmonary venous obstruction holds great promise. By avoiding direct suturing at the pulmonary venous ostia, the chance of recurrent stenosis at the anastamotic site is lessened.

Lacour-Gayet F et al: Surgical management of progressive pulmonary venous obstruction after repair of total anomalous pulmonary venous connection. J Thorac Cardiovasc Surg 1999;117(4):679 [PMID: 10096962].

Monro JL et al. Reoperations and survival after primary repair of congenital heart defects in children. J Thorac Cardiovasc Surg 2003;126(2):511 [PMID: 12928652].

# TRUNCUS ARTERIOSUS

 **ESSENTIALS OF DIAGNOSIS & TYPICAL FEATURES**

- *Early CHF*
- *Mild or no cyanosis.*
- *Systolic ejection click.*

## General Considerations

Truncus arteriosus accounts for less than 1% of congenital heart malformations. A single great artery arises from the heart giving rise to the systemic, pulmonary, and coronary circulations. Truncus develops embryologically as a result of complete lack of formation of the spiral ridges that divide the primitive common truncus arteriosus into the aorta and the pulmonary artery. A high VSD is always present. The number of valve leaflets varies from two to six, and the valve may be sufficient, insufficient, or stenotic.

Although rare, truncus arteriosus is divided into four types by the anatomy of the pulmonary circulation:

Type 1 (48%): A main pulmonary artery arises from the base of the trunk just above the semilunar valve and runs parallel with the ascending aorta for a short time before dividing.

Type 2 (29%): Two pulmonary arteries arise side by side from the posterior aspect of the truncus.

Type 3 (11%): Two pulmonary arteries arise independently from either side of the trunk.

Type 4 (12%): No demonstrable main left and right pulmonary arteries are present. Pulmonary circulation is derived from bronchials arising from the descending thoracic aorta.

In this condition, blood leaves the heart through a single common exit. Therefore, the saturation of the blood in the pulmonary artery is the same as that in the systemic arteries. The degree of systemic arterial oxygen saturation depends on the ratio of pulmonary to systemic blood flow. If pulmonary vascular resistance is normal, the pulmonary blood flow is greater than the systemic blood flow and the saturation is relatively high. If pulmonary vascular resistance is elevated because of pulmonary vascular obstructive disease or very small pulmonary arteries, pulmonary blood flow is reduced and oxygen saturation is low. The systolic pressures are systemic in both ventricles.

## Clinical Findings

### A. SYMPTOMS AND SIGNS

The clinical picture depends on the degree of pulmonary blood flow.

**1. High pulmonary blood flow**—This is the most common presentation in truncus arteriosus. Patients with high pulmonary blood flow are usually acyanotic. Their clinical presentation resembles that of patients with large VSDs. Early CHF occurs. Examination of the heart reveals a hyperactive precordium. A systolic thrill is common at the lower left sternal border. $S_1$ is normal. A loud early systolic ejection click is commonly heard. $S_2$ is single and accentuated. A grade III–IV/VI pansystolic murmur is audible at the lower left sternal border. A diastolic flow murmur can often be heard at the apex (mitral flow murmur).

**2. Low pulmonary blood flow**—Patients with decreased pulmonary blood flow are cyanotic early and do poorly. The most common manifestations are growth retardation, easy fatigability, dyspnea on exertion, and CHF. The heart is not hyperactive. $S_1$ and $S_2$ are single and loud. A systolic grade II–IV/VI murmur is heard at the lower left sternal border. No diastolic flow murmur is heard. A continuous heart murmur is uncommon except in type 4, in which the large bronchial collateral vessels cause the continuous murmur. A loud systolic ejection click is commonly heard.

### B. IMAGING

The most common radiographic findings are a boot-shaped heart, absence of the main pulmonary artery segment, and a large aorta that has a right arch 30% of the time. The pulmonary vascular markings vary with the degree of pulmonary blood flow.

### C. ELECTROCARDIOGRAPHY

The axis is usually normal. RVH or combined ventricular hypertrophy is commonly present. LVH as an isolated finding is rare.

### D. ECHOCARDIOGRAPHY

A characteristic image shows override of a single great artery (similar to ToF). The origin of the pulmonary arteries and the degree of truncal valve abnormality can be seen. Color-flow Doppler can aid in the description of pulmonary flow and the function of the truncal valve, both of which are critical to management.

### E. ANGIOCARDIOGRAPHY

Cardiac catheterization is not routinely performed but may be of value in the older infant in whom pulmonary vascular disease must be ruled out. Injection of contrast material into either ventricle demonstrates the VSD and the single great artery arising from the heart. The exact type of truncus, however, is often best imaged from an injection in the truncal root itself. This will also allow for evaluation of truncal insufficiency.

## Treatment

Anticongestive measures are needed for patients with high pulmonary blood flow and congestive failure. Surgery is always required in this condition. Because of the severe CHF, surgery is usually performed in the neonatal period. The VSD is closed to allow LV egress to the truncal valve as in ToF. The pulmonary artery (type 1) or arteries (types 2–3) are separated from the truncus as a block, and a conduit is fashioned from the RV to the pulmonary circulation. The conduit may be valved or nonvalved, but most surgeons prefer a valved allograft for this repair. Children with type 4 truncus arteriosus are usually stable in infancy with adequate saturations and without CHF. This is fortunate, because their ultimate surgery depends on finding and joining together (unifocalizing) their pulmonary artery segments prior to attempted surgical correction.

## Course & Prognosis

Children with truncus types 1–3 with good surgical results do well. They almost always outgrow the RV to pulmonary conduit that is placed in infancy and require a revision of the conduit in later childhood. The rare child with type 4 truncus arteriosus will need staged preparation of the pulmonary arteries prior to corrective surgery. For children with types 1–3 truncus arteriosus the risk of early pulmonary vascular obstructive disease is high, and a decision to delay open-heart surgery beyond age 4–6 months, even if the child is clinically stable, must take this into account.

McElhinney DB et al: Reinterventions after repair of common arterial trunk in neonates and young infants. J Am Coll Cardiol 2000;35(5):1317 [PMID: 10758975].

# ■ ACQUIRED HEART DISEASE

## RHEUMATIC FEVER

Rheumatic fever still occurs regionally in the United States. Availability of penicillin, improvements in the standard of living and hygiene, and greater availability of medical care have greatly reduced the incidence of this disease since the 1950s. Acute rheumatic fever has had a resurgence in several regions of the United States (the Midwest in 1984 and the intermountain West since 1987). The character of the illness has changed, however. The reason for these regional epidemics is unknown. In both the Salt Lake City and Denver pediatric referral centers, 30–50 new cases are now seen each year.

Group A β-hemolytic streptococcal infection of the upper respiratory tract is the essential trigger that acts on predisposed individuals. The latest attempts to define host susceptibility implicate immune response (Ir) genes, which are present in approximately 15% of the population. The immune response triggered by colonization of the pharynx with group A streptococci consists of (1) sensitization of B lymphocytes by streptococcal antigens, (2) formation of antistreptococcal antibody, (3) formation of immune complexes that cross-react with cardiac sarcolemma antigens, and (4) myocardial and valvular inflammatory response.

The peak period of risk in the United States is age 5–15 years. The disease is slightly more common in girls and in African Americans, perhaps a reflection of socioeconomic factors. The annual death rate from rheumatic heart disease in school-age children (whites and nonwhites) recorded in the 1980s was less than 1:100,000.

The modified Jones criteria are used to diagnose acute rheumatic fever. Two major or one major and two minor manifestations (plus supporting evidence of streptococcal infection) are needed (Table 19–16).

***Table 19–16.*** Jones criteria (modified) for diagnosis of rheumatic fever.

---

**Major manifestations**
  Carditis
  Polyarthritis
  Sydenham's chorea
  Erythema marginatum
  Subcutaneous nodules
**Minor manifestations**
  *Clinical*
    Previous rheumatic fever or rheumatic heart disease
    Polyarthralgia
    Fever
  *Laboratory*
    Acute phase reaction: elevated erythrocyte sedimentation rate, C-reactive protein, leukocytosis
    Prolonged PR interval
**Plus**
Supporting evidence of preceding streptococcal infection, that is, increased titers of antistreptolysin O or other streptococcal antibodies, positive throat culture for group A *Streptococcus*

---

## Sydenham Chorea

Sydenham chorea is characterized by emotional instability and involuntary movements. These findings become progressively worse and may be accompanied by ataxia and slurring of speech. Muscular weakness becomes apparent following the onset of the involuntary movements. The attack of chorea is self-limiting, although it may last up to 3 months. Sometimes only one side is involved. Chorea may not be apparent for months to years after the acute episode of rheumatic fever.

## Polyarthritis

The large joints (knees, hips, wrists, elbows, shoulders) are most commonly involved. Joint swelling and associated limitation of movement should be present. Arthralgia alone is not a major criterion.

## Erythema Marginatum

A macular erythematous rash with a circinate border appears primarily on the trunk and the extremities. The face is usually spared.

## Subcutaneous Nodules

These usually occur only in severe cases, and then most commonly over the joints, scalp, and spinal column. They vary from a few millimeters to 2 cm in diameter and are nontender and freely movable under the skin.

## Essential Manifestation

Except in cases of rheumatic fever manifesting solely as Sydenham chorea or long-standing carditis, there should be clear evidence of a streptococcal infection such as scarlet fever, a positive throat culture for group A β-hemolytic *Streptococcus,* and increased antistreptolysin O or other streptococcal antibody titers. The antistreptolysin O titer is significantly higher in rheumatic fever than in uncomplicated streptococcal infections.

## Treatment & Prophylaxis

### A. TREATMENT OF THE ACUTE EPISODE

**1. Anti-infective therapy**—Eradication of the streptococcal infection is essential. Long-acting benzathine penicillin is the drug of choice. Depending on the age and weight of the patient, give a single intramuscular injection of 0.6–1.2 million units; alternatively, give penicillin V, 125–250 mg orally four times a day for 10 days. Erythromycin, 250 mg orally four times a day, may be substituted if the patient is allergic to penicillin.

**2. Anti-inflammatory agents—**

**a. Aspirin.** Currently, 30–60 mg/kg/d is given in four divided doses. This dosage is often more than sufficient to effect dramatic relief of the arthritis and fever. In general, higher dosages carry a greater risk of side effects, and there are no proven short- or long-term benefits of high doses to produce salicylate blood levels of 20–30 mg/dL. The duration of therapy must be tailored to meet the needs of the patient, but use of aspirin for 2–6 weeks, with reduction in dosage toward the end of the course, is usually sufficient. Other nonsteroidal antiinflammatory agents are commonly used because of the concerns about Reye syndrome, but they appear to be less effective.

**b. Corticosteroids.** Corticosteroids are rarely indicated. However, in the unusual patient with severe carditis and CHF, steroid therapy may be not only effective but also lifesaving. Corticosteroids may be given as follows: prednisone, 2 mg/kg/d orally for 2 weeks (or comparable doses of other corticosteroids); reduce prednisone to 1 mg/kg/d during the third week, and begin aspirin, 50 mg/kg/d; stop prednisone at the end of 3 weeks, and continue aspirin for 8 weeks or until the C-reactive protein is negative and the sedimentation rate is falling.

**3. Therapy of congestive heart failure**—See Congestive Heart Failure section.

**4. Bed rest and ambulation**—Bed rest is not required for patients with arthritis and mild carditis without CHF. Indoor activity followed by modified outdoor activity may be ordered when symptoms have disappeared but clinical and laboratory evidence of rheumatic activity remains. Modified bed rest for 2–6 weeks is generally adequate. Children should not return to school while there is clear evidence of rheumatic activity. Most acute episodes of rheumatic fever are managed on an outpatient basis.

**B. TREATMENT AFTER THE ACUTE EPISODE**

**1. Prevention**—The patient who has had a bout of rheumatic fever has a greatly increased risk of developing rheumatic fever after the next inadequately treated group A β-hemolytic streptococcal infection. Prevention is thus the most important aim for the physician to emphasize. The purpose of follow-up visits after the acute episode is not so much to evaluate the evolution of mitral or aortic insufficiency murmurs as to reinforce the physician's advice about the necessity for prophylaxis with regular long-acting benzathine penicillin. The physician should stress that protection is better with intramuscular than oral medication and that failure to comply with regular medication programs increases the risk for recurrence of rheumatic fever. If myocardial or valvular disease persists, antibacterial prophylaxis is a

lifelong commitment. More commonly with transient cardiac involvement, 3–5 years of therapy or discontinuance at adolescence is a practical and effective approach.

The following preventive regimens are in current use:

**a. Penicillin G. benzathine** 1.2 million units intramuscularly every 21–28 days, is the drug of choice.

**b. Sulfadiazine.** 500 mg daily as a single oral dose for patients weighing over 27 kg is the drug of second choice. Blood dyscrasias and a lesser effectiveness in reducing streptococcal infections make this drug less satisfactory than penicillin benzathine G.

**c. Penicillin V.** 250,000 units orally twice daily offers approximately the same protection afforded by sulfadiazine but is much less effective than intramuscular penicillin benzathine G (5.5 vs 0.4 streptococcal infections per 100 patient-years).

**d. Erythromycin.** 250 mg orally twice a day may be given to patients who are allergic to both penicillin and sulfonamides.

**2. Residual valvular damage**—Chronic CHF may follow a single severe episode of acute rheumatic carditis or, more commonly, may follow repeated episodes. In the United States, the typical manifestations of residual valvular damage in children are heart murmurs of mitral and aortic insufficiency. Murmurs are not accompanied by CHF in most children as long as repeated attacks are prevented.

Methods of managing CHF have been discussed previously. Children with severe valvular damage that cannot be managed adequately on a medical regimen must be considered for valve replacement before the myocardium is irreversibly damaged.

Ayoub EM: Resurgence of rheumatic fever in the United States: The changing picture of a preventable illness. Postgrad Med 1992;92(3):139 [PMID: 1518750].

Dajani AS et al: Guidelines for the diagnosis of rheumatic fever: Jones criteria, updated 1992. Circulation 1993;87(1):302.

Veasey LG: Time to take soundings in acute rheumatic fever? Lancet 2001;357(9273):1994 [PMID: 11438128].

# RHEUMATIC HEART DISEASE

## Mitral Insufficiency

Mitral insufficiency is the most common valvular residual of acute rheumatic carditis. There are reports from all over the world of silent mitral insufficiency with echocardiographic findings characteristic of acute rheumatic fever.

## Mitral Stenosis

Mitral stenosis after acute rheumatic fever is rarely encountered in the United States until 5–10 years after the first episode. Thus, mitral stenosis is much more commonly seen in adults than in children. Interventional cardiovascular balloon dilation of mitral stenosis is now being used in many patients prior to consideration of mitral valve replacement.

## Aortic Insufficiency

This early decrescendo diastolic murmur is occasionally encountered as the sole valvular manifestation of rheumatic carditis. It is the second most common valve affected in polyvalvular as well as in single valvular disease. It appears that the aortic valve is involved more often in males and in African Americans.

## Aortic Stenosis

Dominant aortic stenosis of rheumatic origin does not occur in pediatric patients. In one large study, the shortest length of time observed for a patient to develop dominant aortic stenosis secondary to rheumatic heart disease was 20 years.

## KAWASAKI DISEASE

Kawasaki disease was first described in Japan in 1967 and was initially called mucocutaneous lymph node syndrome. The cause of Kawasaki disease is unclear, and a specific diagnostic test does not exist. Eighty percent of affected patients are younger than age 5 years, and the male-to-female ratio is 1.5:1. The diagnostic criteria include fever for more than 5 days and at least four of the following features: (1) bilateral, painless, nonexudative conjunctivitis, (2) lip or oral cavity changes (eg, lip cracking and fissuring, strawberry tongue, inflammation of the oral mucosa), (3) cervical lymphadenopathy ($\geq$ 1.5 cm in diameter and usually unilateral), (4) polymorphous exanthema, and (5) extremity changes (redness and swelling of the hands and feet with subsequent desquamation). Clinical features not part of the diagnostic criteria, but frequently associated are shown in Table 19–17.

The potential for adverse cardiovascular effects is the most serious aspect of Kawasaki disease. Cardiovascular complications during the acute illness include myocarditis, pericarditis, valvular heart disease (usually mitral or aortic regurgitation), and coronary arteritis. Patients with fever but fewer than four of the diagnostic features can be diagnosed with atypical Kawasaki disease if they have coronary artery abnormalities.

Coronary artery lesions range from mild transient dilation of a coronary artery to large aneurysm forma-

**Table 19–17.** Noncardiac manifestations of Kawasaki disease.

| System | Associated Signs and Symptoms |
|---|---|
| Gastrointestinal | Vomiting, diarrhea, gallbladder hydrops, elevated transaminases |
| Blood | Elevated ESR or CRP, leukocytosis, hypoalbuminemia, mild anemia in acute phase and thrombocytosis in subacute phase (usually second to third week of illness) |
| Renal | Sterile pyuria, proteinuria |
| Respiratory | Cough, rhinorrhea, infiltrate on chest radiograph |
| Joint | Arthralgia and arthritis |
| Neurologic | Mononuclear pleocytosis of cerebrospinal fluid, irritability, facial palsy |

ERS = erythrocyte sedimentation rate; CRP = creatinine phosphokinase.

tion. Untreated patients have an approximately 25% risk of developing an aneurysm of the coronary arteries. Those at greatest risk of aneurysm formation are males, young children (< 6 months) and those not treated with intravenous immunoglobulin (IVIG).

Although the gold standard for diagnosing coronary artery aneurysms is angiography, two-dimensional echocardiography is highly sensitive and is the current standard screening test in children with Kawasaki disease. Fortunately, most coronary artery aneurysms resolve within 5 years of diagnosis. However, as aneurysms resolve, associated obstruction or stenosis (19% of all aneurysms) may develop, which may result in coronary ischemia. Giant aneurysms (> 8 mm) are much less likely to resolve, and nearly 50% eventually become stenotic. Of additional concern, acute thrombosis of an aneurysm can occur, resulting in a myocardial infarction, which is fatal in approximately 20% of cases.

The immediate management of Kawasaki disease consists of therapy with IVIG and high-dose aspirin. This therapy is effective in decreasing the incidence of coronary artery dilation and aneurysm formation. The currently recommended therapeutic regimen consists of 2 g/kg of IVIG administered over 10–12 hours and 80–100 mg/kg/d of aspirin in four divided doses until the patient is afebrile. In an effort to prevent acute thrombosis of coronary aneurysms, 3–5 mg/kg of aspirin daily is prescribed throughout the subacute phase of the illness (6–8 weeks) or until coronary artery abnormalities resolve. If fever recurs within 48–72 hours of the initial treatment course and no other source of the fever is detected, a repeat dose of IVIG is often recommended; however, the effectiveness of this approach has not been clearly demonstrated. Currently, corticosteroids are not felt to be effective in Kawasaki disease.

During the acute and subacute phases of the illness, patients should be monitored closely by serial electrocardiography, chest radiograph, and echocardiography. Selective coronary angiography is recommended in patients with evidence of myocardial ischemia. In 1994, the American Heart Association published guidelines for the long-term management of Kawasaki disease. The risk stratification and recommended follow-up can be reviewed in Table 19–18.

American Heart Association: Diagnostic guidelines for Kawasaki disease. Circulation 2001;103(2):335 [PMID: 11208699].

Burns JC et al: Intravenous gamma-globulin treatment and retreatment in Kawasaki disease. Pediatr Infect Dis J 1998;17(12): 1144 [PMID: 9877364].

McMorrow Tuohy AM et al: How many echocardiograms are necessary for follow-up evaluation of patients with Kawasaki disease? Am J Cardiol 2001;88(3):328 [PMID: 11472722].

## CARDIOMYOPATHY

As in adults, three patterns of cardiomyopathy are recognized in children: (1) dilated, (2) hypertrophic, and (3) restrictive.

## 1. Dilated Cardiomyopathy

The most frequent of the childhood cardiomyopathies occurs with an annual incidence of 4–8 cases per 100,000 population in the United States and Europe.

Although often idiopathic, known causes include acute or chronic myocarditis, long-standing untreated tachyarrhythmias, unrecognized left heart obstructive lesions, anthracycline toxicity, and genetic and metabolic diseases (including inborn errors of fatty acid oxidation and mitochondrial oxidative phosphorylation defects). Genetic causes include abnormalities of the dystrophin gene as in Duchenne and Becker muscular dystrophy.

## Clinical Findings

### A. SIGNS AND SYMPTOMS

As the heart dilates, cardiac output falls, and affected children exhibit signs and symptoms of CHF. The child experiences decreased exercise tolerance, failure to thrive, diaphoresis, and tachypnea. As the heart deteriorates, the pulses and perfusion become weaker, hepatomegaly and rales become prominent, and the cardiac examination shows a prominent gallop.

### B. IMAGING

The chest radiograph shows generalized cardiomegaly with or without pulmonary venous congestion.

### C. ELECTROCARDIOGRAPHY

Sinus tachycardia with ST-T segment changes are commonly seen on ECG. The criteria for right and left ventricular hypertrophy may also be met. One must ensure that a narrow complex tachycardia seen in this instance is in fact sinus tachycardia with a normal P wave axis as opposed to an atrial tachyarrhythmia that may be the underlying cause of the cardiomyopathy.

***Table 19–18.*** Long-term management in Kawasaki disease.

| Risk Level | Definition | Management Guidelines |
|---|---|---|
| I | No coronary artery changes at any stage of the illness | No ASA is needed beyond the subacute phase (6–8 weeks). No follow-up beyond the first year |
| II | Transient ectasia of coronary arteries during the acute phase | Same as above, or clinical follow-up ± ECG every 3–5 years |
| III | Single small to medium coronary aneurysm | ASA until abnormality resolves. Annual follow-up with ECG and echo if < 10 years old and every other year stress testing if > 10 years |
| IV | Giant aneurysm or multiple small to medium aneurysms without obstruction | Long term ASA ± warfarin. Annual follow-up with ECG, echo and stress testing (in those > 20 years) |
| V | Coronary artery obstruction | Long-term ASA ± warfarin ± calcium channel blocker to reduce myocardial oxygen consumption. Echo and ECG every 6 months. Stress testing and Holter exam annually |

ASA = acetyl salicylic acid; ECG = electrocardiogram; Echo = echocardiogram.

## D. ECHOCARDIOGRAPHY

The echocardiogram shows LV and left atrial enlargement with decreased LV shortening fraction. The calculated end diastolic and end-systolic dimensions are increased. With more advanced disease, mitral insufficiency will occur as the LV dilates.

## E. OTHER TESTING

Catheterization is most often done to obtain a biopsy evidence of myocarditis. In addition, polymerase chain reaction testing may be performed on biopsy specimens to detect the presence of viral genome remaining from an earlier bout of myocarditis. Finally, the biopsy can be analyzed by light and electron microscopy to look for metabolic causes of dilated cardiomyopathy. Skeletal muscle biopsy may also be helpful. Hemodynamic assessment during catheterization will assess the progression of the disease. The effect of drug therapy with afterload-reducing agents can be assessed in the catheterization laboratory prior to their clinical use.

Cardiopulmonary stress testing is a useful clinical tool in patients with cardiomyopathy for measuring the response to medical therapies as well as deciding on the appropriate timing of cardiac transplantation.

## Treatment & Prognosis

Patients with dilated cardiomyopathy may require in-hospital management of CHF (see section on Congestive Heart Failure). As outpatients they are treated with digoxin, diuretics, afterload-reducing agents, and fluid restriction. Once stabilized on these agents, some can be treated with carvedilol. Anticoagulants such as warfarin (Coumadin) may be used to prevent thrombus formation secondary to stagnant blood flow within the dilated, poorly contractile cardiac chambers. If arrhythmias occur, they require treatment. Antiarrhythmic agents that do not suppress myocardial contractility, such as digoxin and amiodarone, are preferred. Internal defibrillators are used in some patients with refractory arrhythmias in the setting of dilated cardiomyopathy. Specific therapy directed at the cause can have a dramatic effect; for instance, in some of the mitochondrial metabolic disorders. Treatment of carnitine deficiency may result in improved cardiac function. Antiarrhythmic therapy in patients with arrhythmia-induced cardiomyopathy is often curative. Ultimately, if medical management is unsuccessful, cardiac transplantation is considered.

## 2. Hypertrophic Cardiomyopathy

The most common cause of hypertrophic cardiomyopathy (HCM) is familial hypertrophic cardiomyopathy, which affects 1 in 500 individuals. It most com-

monly presents in the older child, adolescent, or adult although it may be seen as early as the neonatal period. Other causes of HCM seen in the neonatal and childhood period include glycogen storage disease, mitochondrial disorders, and other metabolic disorders.

## Familial Hypertrophic Cardiomyopathy

In the familial form, HCM is most commonly caused by a mutation in one of four genes that encode proteins of the cardiac sarcomere (the B-myosin heavy chain, cardiac troponin T, A-tropomyosin, and myosin-binding protein C genes).

## Clinical Findings

Patients may be asymptomatic, despite having significant hypertrophy, or may present with symptoms of inadequate coronary perfusion such as angina, syncope, or exercise intolerance. Patients may experience sudden cardiac death, often precipitated by sporting activities. Cardiac examination will demonstrate a left precordial bulge with a diffuse point of maximal impulse. An LV heave may be present. A palpable or audible $S_4$ may be present. If outflow tract obstruction is present, a systolic ejection murmur will be audible. A murmur may not be audible at rest but is easily provoked with minimal exercise. Although the older patient with HCM typically has disease primarily in the LV, RVH, either alone or in association with LVH, may be seen in the neonate. Affected neonates may be cyanotic if RV outflow tract obstruction is significant.

## A. ECHOCARDIOGRAPHY

The diagnosis of HCM is made in most cases by echocardiography, which demonstrates an asymmetrical septal hypertrophy. Younger patients may have concentric hypertrophy, making the diagnosis less obvious. Systolic anterior motion of the mitral valve leaflet may occur and may contribute to the degree of LV outflow tract obstruction. The mitral valve leaflet may become distorted with time, resulting in mitral insufficiency. LV outflow tract obstruction may be present at rest. Provokable outflow tract obstruction should be assessed with either amyl nitrate or monitored exercise. Systolic function is most often hypercontractile in the young child but may deteriorate over time, often in association with a change in morphology as hypertrophy develops into LV dilation. Diastolic function is often impaired. Patients are at risk for myocardial ischemia, possibly as a result of systolic compression of the intramyocardial septal perforators, myocardial bridging of epicardial coronary arteries, or an imbalance of coronary artery supply and demand due to the presence of massive myocardial hypertrophy.

## B. ELECTROCARDIOGRAPHY

The ECG may be normal, but more typically will demonstrate deep Q waves in the inferolateral leads (II, III, aVf, $V_5$, and $V_6$) secondary to depolarization of the hypertrophied septum. ST segment abnormalities may be seen in the same leads. Age-dependent criteria for LVH will often be met. Criteria for left atrial enlargement may be present.

## C. OTHER TESTING

Cardiopulmonary stress testing is a valuable tool in this patient population to ascertain the presence of provokable LV outflow tract obstruction, to assess for ischemia and arrhythmias, and to determine prognosis. A blunted blood pressure response and ventricular arrhythmias with exercise have both been associated with increased mortality in this patient group. Nuclear stress testing allows for assessment of myocardial perfusion defects.

## D. CARDIAC CATHETERIZATION

Cardiac catheterization should be performed in patients with HCM who have recurrent angina, syncope, resuscitated sudden death, or a worrisome stress test. Hemodynamic findings may include an elevated left atrial pressure secondary to impaired diastolic filling. If midcavitary LV outflow tract obstruction is present, an associated pressure gradient will be evident. Provocation of LV outflow tract obstruction with either rapid atrial pacing or isoproterenol may be sought. Angiography demonstrates a "ballerina slipper" configuration of the LV secondary to the midcavitary LV obliteration during systole. Coronary angiography should be performed to evaluate possible associated myocardial bridging, which may be an important source of myocardial ischemia in these patients. Angiography will show systolic obliteration, typically of the middle left anterior descending coronary artery.

## Treatment and Prognosis

The prognosis is variable and depends in part on the degree of hypertrophy, the degree of outflow tract obstruction, the particular genetic defect, and the presence of coronary compression. Patients are restricted from strenuous athletics. Patients with resting or latent LV outflow tract obstruction may be treated with either β-blockers or disopyramide with good, albeit temporary, relief of obstruction. Patients with a provokable LV outflow tract gradient above 60 mm Hg require additional treatment. Although dual-chamber pacing has been used in some children with good relief of obstruction, larger series demonstrate no significant improvement in obstruction. Surgical myectomy with resection of part of the hypertrophied septum has been used with

good results. Ethanol ablation is a technique being used with increasing frequency for the adult with HCM and LV outflow tract obstruction. This procedure, performed in the cardiac catheterization laboratory, involves the selective infiltration of ethanol in a coronary septal artery branch, thereby inducing a small myocardial infarction. This leads to a reduction in septal size and improvement of obstruction. The long-term effects of this procedure are unknown, and this procedure is not currently employed for pediatric patients. Surgical unroofing of a myocardial bridge may improve prognosis in those with myocardial ischemia secondary to epicardial coronary compression. Internal defibrillators are being placed in patients with documented ventricular arrhythmias, resuscitated sudden death, or a strong family history of HCM with associated sudden death.

## Glycogen Storage Disease of the Heart

At least 10 types of glycogen storage disease are recognized. The type that primarily involves the heart is Pompe disease (GSD IIa). The deficient enzyme (acid maltase) is necessary for hydrolysis of the outer branches of glycogen, and its absence results in marked deposition of glycogen within the myocardium. Cardiac glycogenosis is a rare heritable (autosomal recessive) disorder.

Affected infants are well at birth, but onset occurs by the sixth month of life. These children have a history of retardation of growth and development, feeding problems, poor weight gain, and CHF. Physical examination reveals generalized muscular weakness, a large tongue, cardiomegaly, and no significant heart murmurs. Chest radiographs reveal marked cardiomegaly with or without pulmonary venous congestion. The ECG shows a short PR interval with LVH with ST depression and T wave inversion over the left precordial leads. Echocardiography shows severe concentric LVH.

Children with this disease usually die before age 1 year. Death may be sudden or the result of progressive CHF.

## 3. Restrictive Cardiomyopathy

Restrictive cardiomyopathy is a rare entity in the pediatric population, accounting for less than 5% of all cases of cardiomyopathy.

## Clinical Findings

Patients present with signs of CHF as outlined previously. Physical examination is remarkable for a prominent $S_4$ and jugular venous distention.

## A. Electrocardiography

ECG demonstrates marked right and left atrial enlargement with normal ventricular voltages. ST/T wave abnormalities may be present.

## B. Echocardiography

The diagnosis may be confirmed echocardiographically, noting the presence of normal sized ventricles with massively dilated atrium. Due to infiltration of the ventricular myocardium, the LV becomes "restrictive," and atrial emptying is impaired.

## Course and Prognosis

The condition is usually idiopathic. Endocardial fibroelastosis, a histologic diagnosis, may be noted. The endocardium has marked milky white thickening, as do the subendocardial layers of the LV and left atrium. The mitral valve may be involved. Irrespective of cause, the prognosis is poor. Anticongestive therapy may be tried, but many patients will require cardiac transplantation.

Hauser M et al: Diagnosis of anthracycline-induced cardiomyopathy by exercise spiroergometry and stress echocardiography. Eur J Pediatr 2001;160(10):607 [PMID: 11686505].

Helton E et al: Metabolic aspects of myocardial disease and a role for L-carnitine in the treatment of childhood cardiomyopathy. Pediatrics 2000;105(6):1260 [PMID: 10835067].

Malcic I et al: Epidemiology of cardiomyopathies in children and adolescents: A retrospective study over the last 10 years. Cardiol Young 2002;12(3):253 [PMID: 12365172].

Nugent AW et al: Clinical, electrocardiographic, and histologic correlations in children with dilated cardiomyopathy. J Heart Lung Transplant 2001;20(11):1152 [PMID: 11704474].

Yetman AT et al: Myocardial bridging in children with hypertrophic cardiomyopathy—A risk factor for sudden death. N Engl J Med 1998;339(17):1201 [PMID: 9780340].

# MYOCARDITIS

The most common causes of myocarditis are adenovirus, coxsackie A and B, echovirus, and cytomegalovirus. In addition, the human immunodeficiency virus (HIV) causes myocarditis. Our ability to determine the cause of myocarditis has been enhanced greatly by the availability of polymerase chain reaction technology to replicate identifiable segments of viral genome from the myocardium of affected children.

## Clinical Findings

### A. Symptoms and Signs

The clinical picture usually falls into two separate patterns: (1) Onset of CHF is sudden in a newborn who has been in relatively good health 12–24 hours previously. This is a malignant form of the disease and is thought to be secondary to overwhelming viremia and tissue invasion of multiple organ systems, including the heart. (2) In the older child, the onset of cardiac findings tends to be more gradual. There is often a history of an upper respiratory tract infection or gastroenteritis within the month prior to the development of cardiac findings. This is a more insidious form of the disease and may have a late postinfectious or autoimmune component. However, clinical presentation can be acute or chronic in all ages and in all types of myocarditis.

In the newborn infant, the signs of CHF are usually apparent. The skin is pale and gray, and peripheral pallor may be present. The pulses are rapid, weak, and thready. Edema of the face and extremities may be present. Significant cardiomegaly is present, and the left and right ventricular impulses are weak. On auscultation, the heart sounds may be muffled and distant. $S_3$ and $S_4$ are common, resulting in a gallop rhythm. Murmurs are usually absent, although a murmur of tricuspid or mitral insufficiency can occasionally be heard. Moist rales are usually present at both lung bases. The liver is enlarged and frequently tender.

### B. Imaging

Generalized cardiomegaly can be seen on radiograph. Moderate to marked pulmonary venous congestion is evident. Pneumonia is commonly present.

### C. Electrocardiography

The ECG is variable. Classically, there is evidence of low voltage of the QRS throughout all frontal and precordial leads and depression of the ST segment and inversion of the T waves in leads I, III, and aVF and in the left precordial leads during the acute stage. Dysrhythmias are common, and AV and intraventricular conduction disturbances may be present. With the more benign form, or during the recovery phase of the malignant form, high-voltage QRS complexes are commonly seen and are indicative of LVH.

### D. Echocardiography

Echocardiography demonstrates four-chamber dilation with poor ventricular function and AV valve regurgitation.

### E. Myocardial Biopsy

A tissue diagnosis obtained from either myocardium or skeletal muscle is usually indicated in pediatric cardiomyopathy/myocarditis. Primary processes (metabolic disorders such as mitochondrial oxidation chain defects and glycogen storage disease, and muscular dystrophies such as Duchenne or Becker) can be differentiated from inflammatory diseases of the myocardium (myocarditis).

## Treatment

The use of digitalis in a rapidly deteriorating child with myocarditis is dangerous and should be undertaken with great caution as it may provoke ventricular dysrhythmias in this situation. The inpatient cardiac supports outlined previously are used in the treatment of these patients.

The administration of corticosteroids for myocarditis is controversial. If the patient's condition continues to deteriorate despite anticongestive measures, corticosteroids are commonly used, although conclusive data supporting their effectiveness in this condition are lacking. Other immunosuppressive agents, such as cyclosporine, are now being tried in viral myocarditis.

Subsequent to the successful use of intravenous immunoglobulin for children with Kawasaki disease, several trials have occurred using this product in presumed viral myocarditis. The therapeutic value of this treatment still remains unconfirmed in many practitioners' minds.

## Prognosis

The prognosis for a patient with myocarditis is related to the age at onset and to the patient's response to therapy. If the patient is younger than age 6 months or older than age 3 years and responds poorly to therapy, the prognosis is poor. Many patients recover clinically but have persistent LV dysfunction with cardiomegaly. It is possible that subclinical myocarditis in childhood is the pathophysiologic basis for some of the idiopathic dilated cardiomyopathies occurring later in life. Children with myocarditis whose ventricular function fails to return to normal are potential candidates for cardiac transplantation.

Baboonian C, McKenna W: Eradication of viral myocarditis: Is there hope? J Am Coll Cardiol 2003;42(3);473 [PMID: 12906975].

Bowles NE et al: Detection of viruses in myocardial tissues by polymerase chain reaction. Evidence of adenovirus as a common cause of myocarditis in children and adults. J Am Coll Cardiol 2003;42(3):466 [PMID: 12906974].

Liu PP, Mason JW: Advances in the understanding of myocarditis. Circulation 2001;104(9):1076 [PMID: 11524405].

# INFECTIVE ENDOCARDITIS

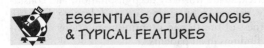

### ESSENTIALS OF DIAGNOSIS & TYPICAL FEATURES

- *Preexisting organic heart murmur.*
- *Persistent fever.*
- *Increasing symptoms of heart disease (ranging from easy fatigability to heart failure).*
- *Splenomegaly (70% of cases).*
- *Embolic phenomena (50% of cases).*
- *Leukocytosis, elevated erythrocyte sedimentation rate, hematuria, positive blood culture.*

## General Considerations

Bacterial or fungal infection of the endocardial surface of the heart or the intimal surface of certain arterial vessels (coarcted segment of aorta or ductus arteriosus) is a rare condition that usually occurs when a preexisting abnormality of the heart or great arteries is present. It may develop in a normal heart during the course of septicemia.

The frequency of infective endocarditis appears to be increasing owing to many factors, including (1) increased survival rates for children with congenital heart disease, (2) greater long-term use of central venous catheters, and (3) increased use of prosthetic material and valves. Pediatric patients without preexisting heart disease are also at increased risk for infective endocarditis owing to (1) increased survival rates for children with immune deficiencies, (2) greater long-term use of indwelling lines in critically ill newborns, and (3) increased incidence of intravenous drug abuse.

Patients at greatest risk include those with left-sided outflow obstruction or aorticopulmonary shunts and those with allograft, heterograft, or prosthetic cardiac valves. The actual cause of the episode of infective endocarditis can be identified approximately 30% of the time, and these include dental procedures, nonsterile surgical procedures, and cardiovascular surgery.

Organisms causing endocarditis include viridans streptococci (about 50% of cases), *Staphylococcus aureus* (about 30%), and fungal agents (about 10%).

## Clinical Findings

### A. HISTORY

Almost all patients with infective endocarditis have a history of heart disease. There may or may not be a history of infection or a surgical procedure (tooth extraction, tonsillectomy).

### B. SYMPTOMS, SIGNS, AND LABORATORY FINDINGS

Findings include changing murmurs, fever, positive blood culture, weight loss, cardiomegaly, elevated sedimentation rate, splenomegaly, petechiae, embolism, and leukocytosis. Other findings are hematuria, signs of CHF, clubbing, joint pains, and hepatomegaly. Vegetations are large enough to be seen by echocardiography in 70% of children with endocarditis.

## Prevention

Patients at risk for infective endocarditis should be given appropriate antibiotics before any type of dental work (tooth extraction, cleaning), before operations within the oropharynx, gastrointestinal tract, and genitourinary tract, and for body piercing and tattooing, which often are performed in less than sanitary conditions. Continuous antibiotic prophylaxis (as in the treatment of rheumatic fever) is not recommended in patients with congenital heart disease.

The following schedule is recommended: under 40 kg, 50 mg/kg of oral amoxicillin; over 40 kg, 2000 mg. This dose is to be given 1 hour prior to dental procedures. If the patient is allergic to amoxicillin, an alternative prophylactic antibiotic is used.

## Treatment

In a patient with known heart disease, the presence of an otherwise unexplained fever should alert the physician to the possibility of infective endocarditis. A positive blood culture or other major findings of infective endocarditis confirm the diagnosis. If a positive blood culture is obtained and the organism is identified, specific treatment should be begun immediately. Even if blood cultures are negative after 48 hours, it is advisable to begin antibiotic therapy (if other evidence of infective endocarditis is present), because most positive cultures are obtained within the first 48 hours. If CHF occurs and progresses unremittingly in the face of adequate antibiotic therapy, surgical excision of the infected area and prosthetic valve replacement must be considered.

## Course & Prognosis

The prognosis depends on how early in the course of the infectious process treatment is instituted. The prognosis is better in patients in whom the blood culture is positive. If CHF develops, the prognosis is poor. Embolization may occur during or after treatment from the vegetations themselves. Infective endocarditis is a serious condition and should be avoided if at all possible.

Dajani AS et al: Prevention of bacterial endocarditis: Recommendations by the American Heart Association. JAMA 1997; 277(22):1794 [PMID: 9178793].

Friedel JM et al. Infective endocarditis after oral body piercing. Cardiol Rev 2003;11(5):252 [PMID: 12943601].

# PERICARDITIS

## ESSENTIALS OF DIAGNOSIS & TYPICAL FEATURES

- *Retrosternal pain made worse by deep inspiration and decreased by leaning forward.*
- *Fever.*
- *Shortness of breath and grunting respirations are common.*
- *Pericardial friction rub.*
- *Tachycardia.*
- *Hepatomegaly and distention of the jugular veins.*
- *ECG with elevated ST segment.*

## General Considerations

Involvement of the pericardium rarely occurs as an isolated event. In most cases, pericardial disease occurs in association with a more generalized process. Common causes include rheumatic fever, viral pericarditis, purulent pericarditis, rheumatoid arthritis, uremia, and tuberculosis. Pericarditis after cardiac surgery (postpericardiotomy syndrome) is a common condition in pediatric cardiology, most commonly seen after surgical closure of an ASD.

In the pediatric age group, pericardial disease usually takes the form of acute pericarditis. In most cases, fluid effuses into the pericardial cavity. The consequences of such effusion depend on the amount, type, and speed of fluid accumulation. Under certain circumstances, serious compression of the heart occurs, which can lead to cardiac tamponade. Unless the pericardial fluid is evacuated in this situation, death may occur.

## Clinical Findings

### A. Symptoms and Signs

The symptoms depend to a great extent on the cause of the pericarditis. Pain is common. It is usually sharp and stabbing, located in the mid chest and in the shoulder and neck, made worse by deep inspiration, and considerably decreased by sitting up and leaning forward. Shortness of breath and grunting respirations are common findings in all patients.

The physical findings depend on whether a significant amount of effusion is present: (1) In the absence of significant accumulation of fluid, the pulses are normal.

The heart has a characteristic scratchy, high-pitched friction rub. The rub is often systolic and diastolic and can be located at any point between the apex and the left sternal border. The location and timing vary considerably from time to time. The heart sounds are usually normal, and the heart is not enlarged to percussion. (2) If considerable pericardial fluid has accumulated, the cardiovascular findings are different. The heart is enlarged to percussion, but on auscultation it is very quiet. Heart sounds are distant and muffled. A friction rub may not be present. In the absence of cardiac tamponade, the peripheral, venous, and arterial pulses are normal.

Cardiac tamponade is characterized by distention of the jugular veins, tachycardia, enlargement of the liver, peripheral edema, and pulses paradoxus in which the systolic pressure drops by more than 10 mm Hg during inspiration. This finding is best determined with the use of a manual blood pressure cuff. At this point, the patient is critically ill and has all the symptoms and signs suggestive of right-sided CHF.

Not all patients with marked cardiac compression demonstrate all of these findings. If the patient appears critically ill and pericarditis and effusion are evident, treatment should be instituted even though all the clinical signs of cardiac tamponade are not present.

## B. IMAGING

In pericarditis without significant effusion, chest radiographic findings are normal. With pericardial effusion, the cardiac silhouette is enlarged, often in the shape of a water bottle.

## C. ELECTROCARDIOGRAPHY

A number of ECG abnormalities occur in patients with pericarditis. Low voltage is commonly seen in patients with significant pericardial effusion. The ST segment is commonly elevated during the first week of involvement. The T wave is usually upright during this time. Following this, the ST segment is normal and the T wave becomes flattened.

## D. ECHOCARDIOGRAPHY

Echocardiography is essential in the diagnosis and management of pericarditis. Serial echo studies allow the cardiologist a direct noninvasive estimate of the volume of fluid and its changes over time. In addition, echocardiography will demonstrate cardiac tamponade by compression of the atria by the pericardial effusion.

## Treatment

Treatment depends on the cause of pericarditis. Cardiac tamponade resulting from any cause must be treated by evacuation of the fluid. If there are findings of impending circulatory collapse, an immediate pericardiocentesis is performed. If pericardiocentesis is unsuccessful, a surgical pericardiectomy is required. Diuretics are to be avoided in the patient with cardiac tamponade because they reduce ventricular preload, which can exacerbate the degree of cardiac compression.

## Prognosis

The prognosis depends to a great extent on the cause of the pericardial disease. Cardiac tamponade from any cause results in death unless the fluid is evacuated.

## SPECIFIC DISEASES INVOLVING THE PERICARDIUM

### Acute Rheumatic Fever

When pericarditis occurs during the course of acute rheumatic fever, it is almost always associated with involvement of the myocardium and the endocardium (pancarditis). Thus heart murmurs are almost always present. The pericarditis is usually of the serofibrinous variety and is usually not associated with a significant pericardial effusion. The treatment of the pericardial effusion is accomplished by the therapy for the acute rheumatic fever.

### Viral Pericarditis

Viral pericarditis occurs in children and young adults. The most common cause is coxsackie virus B. Influenza virus has also been implicated. There is usually a history of a protracted upper respiratory tract infection. The pericardial effusion may last for several weeks. Cardiac tamponade is rare. Constrictive pericarditis can occur as a sequela of viral pericarditis.

### Purulent Pericarditis

The most common causes of purulent pericarditis are pneumococci, streptococci, staphylococci, and *Haemophilus influenzae*. This disorder is always secondary to infection elsewhere, although occasionally the primary site is unknown. In addition to demonstrating signs of cardiac compression, patients are septic and run extremely high fevers. The purulent fluid accumulating within the pericardial sac is usually quite thick and filled with polymorphonuclear leukocytes. Although antibiotics will sterilize the pericardial fluid, pericardial tamponade commonly develops, and surgical excision of the pericardium is frequently necessary. Acutely, pericardiocentesis may be lifesaving if there are findings of tamponade on presentation. The wide use of the *H influenzae* vaccine in recent years has significantly reduced the incidence of this condition.

## Postpericardiotomy Syndrome

Postpericardiotomy syndrome is characterized by fever, chest pain, friction rub, and elevation of the ST segment noted on ECG 1–2 weeks after open-heart surgery. The syndrome appears to be an autoimmune disease with high titers of antiheart antibody and with detectable evidence of fresh or reactivated viral illness. The syndrome is often self-limited and responds well to short courses of aspirin or corticosteroid therapy. Rarely, it lasts for months to years and may require pericardiocentesis or pericardiectomy.

Cakir O et al: Purulent pericarditis in childhood: Ten years of experience. J Pediatr Surg 2002;37(10):1404 [PMID: 12378443].

Roodpeyma S, Sadeghian N: Acute pericarditis in childhood: A 10-year experience. Pediatr Cardiol 2000;21(4):363 [PMID: 10865014].

# HYPERTENSION

Blood pressure should be determined at every pediatric visit beginning at age 3 years. Because this is now being done, systemic hypertension has become more widely recognized as a pediatric problem. Pediatric standards for blood pressure have been published. Blood pressures in children must be obtained when the child is relaxed, and an appropriate-size cuff must always be used. The widest cuff that fits between the axilla and the antecubital fossa is used in each case. Most children age 10–11 years need a standard adult-size cuff (bladder width of 12 cm), and many high school students need a large adult-size cuff (width of 16 cm) or leg cuff (width of 18 cm). The 95th percentile value for blood pressure (Table 19–19) is similar for both sexes and all three ethnic groups. Blood pressure varies more with altitude and body weight than with sex or ethnic origin. If the blood pressure taken in a quiet atmosphere and sitting position exceeds the 95th percentile for systolic, diastolic muffle, or diastolic disappearance pressures, it should be repeated several times over a 2- to 4-week interval. If it is elevated persistently, an evaluation for the cause of the hypertension should be undertaken. Although most hypertension in children is essential, there is a higher incidence of treatable conditions within pediatrics than in adult medicine, such as coarctation of the aorta, renal artery stenosis, chronic renal disease, and pheochromocytoma. Over-the-counter and recreational drug use may be important causative or contributing factors. Pediatricians must look for these conditions when a child presents with hypertension. If no secondary cause is found, and the hypertension is deemed essential, anti-

**Table 19–19.** The 95th percentile value for blood pressure (mm Hg) taken in the sitting position.[a]

|  | Sea Level | | | 10,000 ft | | |
|---|---|---|---|---|---|---|
|  | S | Dm | Dd | S | Dm | Dd |
| 5 |  |  |  | 92 | 72 | 62 |
| 6 | 106 | 64 | 60 | 96 | 74 | 66 |
| 7 | 108 | 72 | 66 | 98 | 76 | 70 |
| 8 | 110 | 76 | 70 | 104 | 80 | 70 |
| 9 | 114 | 80 | 76 | 106 | 80 | 70 |
| 10 | 118 | 82 | 76 | 108 | 80 | 70 |
| 11 | 124 | 82 | 78 | 108 | 80 | 72 |
| 12 | 128 | 84 | 78 | 108 | 80 | 72 |
| 13 | 132 | 84 | 80 | 116 | 84 | 76 |
| 14 | 136 | 86 | 80 | 120 | 84 | 76 |
| 15 | 140 | 88 | 80 | 120 | 84 | 80 |
| 16 | 140 | 90 | 80 | 120 | 84 | 80 |
| 17 | 140 | 92 | 80 | 122 | 84 | 80 |
| 18 | 140 | 92 | 80 | 130 | 84 | 80 |

[a]Blood pressures: S = systolic (Korotkoff sound 1; onset of tapping), Dm = diastolic muffling (Korotkoff sound 4), Dd = diastolic disappearance (Korotkoff sound 5).

hypertensive therapy should be initiated in addition to nutritional and exercise counseling when applicable. Beta-blockers or ACE inhibitors are the usual first-line medical therapies for essential hypertension in children.

Gifford RW et al: The fifth report of the Joint National Committee on detection, evaluation, and treatment of high blood pressure. Arch Intern Med 1993;153(2):154 [PMID: 8422206].

Gillman MW et al: Identifying children at high risk for the development of essential hypertension. J Pediatr 1993;122(6):837 [PMID: 8501557].

# ATHEROSCLEROSIS AS A PEDIATRIC PROBLEM

Awareness of the importance of coronary artery risk factors in general—and atherosclerosis in particular—has risen dramatically in the general population since the mid 1970s. Although coronary artery disease is still the leading cause of death in the United States, the age-adjusted incidence of death from ischemic heart disease has been decreasing since that time as a result of an improved diet, decreased smoking, awareness and treatment of hypertension, and an increase in physical activity. During this period, a large number of serum samples from the pediatric population have been collected and analyzed for lipids, and epidemiologic studies have been performed to determine the relationship of lipid levels to coronary heart disease. The level of serum lipids in childhood usually remains the same through adolescence. Biochemical abnormalities in the lipid profile appear early in childhood and correlate with higher risk for coronary artery disease in adulthood. High-density lipoprotein (HDL) has been identified as an antiatherogenic factor. The most common lipid profile referred to treatment centers has changed to a high triglyceride level, modest elevation of low-density lipoprotein (LDL), and low HDL level associated with obesity, insulin resistance, and prediabetes.

The concept of routine universal pediatric screening after age 3 years remains controversial. The National Cholesterol Education Program recommends selective screening in children with high-risk family members, defined as a parent with a total cholesterol over 240 mg/dL or a parent or grandparent with early-onset cardiovascular disease. When children have LDL levels greater than 130 mg/dL on two successive tests, dietary lifestyle counseling is appropriate. Dietary modification may decrease cholesterol levels by 5–20%. If the patient is unresponsive to diet change and at extreme risk (ie, a LDL level > 160 mg/dL, an HDL level < 35 mg/dL, and a history of cardiovascular disease in a first-degree relative at an age younger than 40 years), drug therapy may be indicated. Cholestyramine, a bile exchange resin, has had moderate success, but compliance is poor in children because of the drug's unpalatability. Niacin and the HMG-CoA reductase inhibitors are also used in the pediatric population and have had encouraging preliminary results.

De Jongh S et al: Efficacy and safety of statin therapy in children with familial hypercholesterolemia: A randomized double-blind placebo-controlled trial with Simvastatin. Circulation 2002;106(17):2231 [PMID: 12390953].

Gidding SS: Preventive pediatric cardiology: Tobacco, cholesterol, obesity, and physical activity. Pediatr Clin North Am 1999; 46(2):253 [PMID: 10218073].

# PRIMARY PULMONARY HYPERTENSION

 ESSENTIALS OF DIAGNOSIS & TYPICAL FEATURES

- *Often subtle with symptoms of dyspnea, fatigue, chest pain, and syncope.*
- *Exclusion of all causes of secondary pulmonary hypertension.*
- *Rare, progressive, and often fatal disease without treatment.*
- *ECG with RVH.*
- *Loud pulmonary component of $S_2$.*

## General Considerations

Unexplained or primary pulmonary hypertension (PPH) in children is a rare disease with an estimated overall incidence of 1–2 persons per million worldwide. Pulmonary hypertension is defined as a mean pulmonary pressure that is greater than 25 mm Hg at rest or greater than 30 mm Hg during exercise. PPH is a diagnosis of exclusion of all other causes of pulmonary hypertension. Secondary pulmonary hypertension is most commonly associated with congenital heart disease, pulmonary parenchymal disease, causes of chronic hypoxia (upper airway obstruction), thrombosis, liver disease, and collagen vascular disease. The diagnosis of PPH is difficult to make in the early stages because of its subtle manifestations. Most patients with PPH are young adults, predominantly women; however, the sex incidence is equal in children. Familial PPH occurs in 6% of affected individuals. The locus for familial PPH is found on chromosome 2 (2q33) and is caused by abnormalities in the transforming growth factor beta family, specifically bone morphogenetic protein receptor II. Without treatment, the median survival is 2.5 years.

## Clinical Findings

### A. SYMPTOMS AND SIGNS

The clinical picture varies depending on the severity of the pulmonary hypertension. Initial symptoms may be brought on by strenuous exercise or competitive sports, and syncope may be the first symptom. Dyspnea on exertion is present in most patients; syncope occurs in approximately one third of patients. Palpitations or chest pain may occur with exercise. As the disease progresses, patients have signs of low cardiac output and right heart failure. Right heart failure may be manifested by an increase in hepatomegaly with peripheral edema and a gallop rhythm on examination. Murmurs of pulmonary regurgitation and tricuspid regurgitation are common. An $S_3$ is occasionally heard with advanced right heart failure.

### B. IMAGING

The chest radiograph typically shows an enlarged heart with a prominent pulmonary artery and dilated proximal right and left pulmonary arteries. The peripheral pulmonary vascular markings may be normal or diminished.

### C. ELECTROCARDIOGRAPHY

The ECG usually shows right atrial enlargement with RVH and right axis deviation.

### D. ECHOCARDIOGRAPHY

The echocardiogram is an important diagnostic tool for excluding causes of congenital heart disease. It frequently shows RVH and dilation. The tricuspid and pulmonary insufficiency jets may be used to estimate pulmonary artery systolic and diastolic pressures.

### E. CARDIAC CATHETERIZATION AND ANGIOCARDIOGRAPHY

Cardiac catheterization has an increased risk in children with pulmonary hypertension and should be performed with great caution. The procedure is done first to rule out cardiac causes of pulmonary hypertension and then to define treatment strategies. Patients who have a pulmonary vascular bed that is reactive to short-acting vasodilator agents (nitric oxide, adenosine, prostacyclin) may receive treatment with calcium channel blockers. In contrast, patients who have a pulmonary vascular bed that does not improve with these short-acting agents often receive prostacyclin therapy. Angiography may show a marked decrease in the number of small pulmonary arteries with tortuous vessels.

## Treatment

The goal of therapy is to reduce pulmonary artery pressure and increase cardiac output. The cardiac catheterization data are used to define the treatment plan. Patients who have shown a response to pulmonary vasodilators are given calcium channel blockers such as nifedipine or diltiazem. Patients who are unreactive to these vasodilators in the catheterization laboratory initially receive prostacyclin therapy. Patients with severe, unreactive pulmonary hypertension may be considered for lung transplantation. Common therapies include warfarin to prevent thromboembolic events. This approach is beneficial in adults. Digoxin and diuretics may be used if signs of right heart failure are present. Receptor antagonists to the potent vasoconstrictor peptide endothelin show great promise in the treatment of pulmonary hypertension.

Survival rates of greater than 90% have been reported using chronic oral calcium channel blockade in patients who responded acutely to vasodilator testing. In patients in whom calcium channel blockade fails, or in those who do not respond acutely to vasodilator therapy, intravenous prostacyclin has been used with a 5-year survival rate of greater than 80%.

Archer S, Rich S: Primary pulmonary hypertension. Circulation 2000;102(22):2781 [PMID: 11094047].

Deng Z et al: Familial primary pulmonary hypertension (gene PPH I) is caused by mutations in the bone morphogenentic protein receptor II gene. Am J Hum Genet 2000;67(3):737 [PMID: 10903931].

Ivy DD: Diagnosis and treatment of severe pediatric pulmonary hypertension. Cardiol Rev 2001;9(4):227 [PMID: 11405903].

# CHEST PAIN

## Overview

Chest pain is a common complaint of pediatric patients, accounting for 6 in 1000 visits to urban emergency rooms and urgent care clinics. Although children with chest pain are commonly referred for cardiac evaluation, chest pain in children is rarely due to cardiac pathology. Other possible causes of chest pain include musculoskeletal pain, esophagitis/gastritis, and functional pain.

## Approach to the Work-up

A detailed history and physical exam should guide the pediatrician through an appropriate work-up of chest pain. (A known medical history of cardiac or respiratory disease will of course provide additional guidance.) Rarely is there a need for laboratory tests or further evaluation by a specialist. The duration, location, intensity, frequency, and radiation of the pain should be documented, and possible triggering events preceding the pain should be explored. For instance, chest pain following exertion may lead to a more elaborate evaluation for a cardiac disorder. Or the timing of the pain in relation to meals may suggest a gastrointestinal cause. The patient should also be asked about how pain relief is achieved. A social history to reveal psychosocial stressors and cigarette smoke exposure may assist in determining the cause. On physical exam, attention must be placed on the vital signs, general appearance of the child, the chest wall musculature, cardiac, pulmonary, and abdominal exam findings, and quality of peripheral pulses. Attempts should be made to reproduce the pain by direct palpation and through forced resistance applied to the patient's upper extremities. If the pain is reproduced, it is almost always musculoskeletal in origin.

## Clinical Considerations

Cardiac disease is a rare cause of chest pain, but if misdiagnosed it may be life-threatening. Myocardial infarction rarely occurs in healthy children. Children with underlying illnesses such as diabetes mellitus, chronic anemia, or an anomalous left coronary artery may be at increased risk for ischemia. It is also important to ask the family specifically about a history of Kawasaki disease, treated or untreated. These children are at risk for cardiac sequelae including myocardial infarct secondary to thrombosis of their coronary aneurysms, cardiac arrhythmias, or sudden death. More than 50% of children and adolescents who exhibit sequelae from Kawasaki disease arrive at the emergency department with chest pain.

Other cardiac causes of chest pain include arrhythmias. The most common arrhythmia in children is supraventricular tachycardia (SVT), but atrial flutter and premature ventricular contractions (PVCs) may also be associated with chest pain in children. Other structural lesions that cause chest pain include aortic stenosis, pulmonary stenosis, and mitral valve prolapse. Structural cardiac lesions are usually detected prior to the child's emergency room visit. They are accompanied by significant findings on cardiac exam. Of children diagnosed with mitral valve prolapse, 31% will complain of chest pain, caused by papillary muscle ischemia. Other cardiac lesions that cause chest pain include dilated cardiomyopathy, hypertrophic obstructive cardiomyopathy, myocarditis, rheumatic fever, aortic dissection, and pericarditis. Pain from hypertrophic obstructive cardiomyopathy may be associated with exertion.

Noncardiac chest pain may be due to a respiratory illness—for example, reactive airway disease, pneumonia, pneumothorax, or pulmonary embolism. Gastrointestinal causes of chest pain include reflux, esophagitis, and foreign body. The most common cause of chest pain (30% of children) is inflammation of musculoskeletal structures of the chest wall. Costochondritis involves inflammation of the costochondral or costosternal junctions and is usually unilateral. Chest wall pain is more common in girls and is reproducible on examination.

After a complete history and physical are obtained, the information gathered can guide the examiner to the appropriate diagnosis or, if necessary, the appropriate laboratory tests to be ordered. In most cases, additional tests are not necessary. If a cardiac origin is suspected, a pediatric cardiologist should be consulted. Positive cardiac findings on initial evaluation should be followed with a combination of the following: an ECG, chest radiograph, echocardiogram, Holter monitor, and serum troponin and creatinine kinase assays.

# ■ CARDIAC TRANSPLANTATION

Cardiac transplantation has developed into an effective therapeutic modality for end-stage inflammatory cardiac diseases such as myocarditis and cardiomyopathies. In addition, transplantation has become a common final therapeutic pathway for many structural cardiac defects associated with cardiomyopathic changes. Cardiac damage from either long-standing congenital disease or surgery can also lead to transplantation. Approximately 300 pediatric cardiac transplant procedures are performed annually in the United States. The current estimated half-life for children undergoing cardiac transplantation in the 1980s and early 1990s is approximately 15 years. This is a rapidly developing field, and the most recent data indicate an improved prognosis.

Cardiac transplantation is the paradigm of an inflammatory disease of the transplanted myocardium. Because the donor and the recipient are not matched for histocompatibility antigens, the potential for graft rejection by the host immune system is always present. Long-term immunosuppressive medications are required to control this inflammatory process. The mainstay for immunosuppressive agents in cardiac transplant recipients remains cyclosporin A. Cyclosporine is usually well tolerated but has been associated with the potential for renal dysfunction, hypertension, and probably an increased risk of malignancy. In addition, adolescent patients are affected by the visible side effects of hirsutism and gingival hyperplasia. In the current era, the therapeutic blood levels of cyclosporine have been reduced, and most of these side effects occur less frequently. Graft rejection can be triggered by lack of compliance, infection, and other issues, which are not well understood. Although the greatest risk of rejection is in the first 3 months after transplant, a low risk persists even years after the transplant procedure.

Unlike other inflammatory diseases of the myocardium, the process of graft rejection is fairly well understood. The T lymphocyte is the predominant effector cell, which receives antigen presentation, predominantly from tissue histiocytes and macrophages. These cells present antigens to the T-cell receptor in a cradle. Because the donor antigens are new to the host, a population of T lymphocytes can react to these antigens. This process is in contrast to the presentation of host antigens, which do not have T lymphocytes that are programmed to respond. The process of elimination of self-responding T lymphocytes takes place largely in the thymus in utero. However, a process of acquired tolerance, even to the foreign antigens of the donor, may also involve the thymus and peripheral sites. Because the default mechanism for the immune system is to not react to an antigen, with the passage of time and under the influence of immunosuppression, the host becomes less and less responsive to donor antigens posttransplant.

The population of pediatric patients with a heart transplant in the United States is approximately 3000 and growing; thus the major medical challenge is surveillance and treatment of graft rejection.

## Clinical Findings

### A. SYMPTOMS AND SIGNS

Transplant recipients undergoing the process of graft rejection are usually asymptomatic in the early stages. With progression they may develop tachycardia, tachypnea, elevated central venous pressure, and a gallop rhythm. These findings are similar to what would be expected with CHF. As low cardiac output progresses, nausea and vomiting may ensue, followed by altered mental status, and finally peripheral circulatory collapse.

### B. Imaging

Chest radiographs often show cardiac enlargement and increased pulmonary vascular markings.

### C. Electrocardiography

Abnormalities in conduction can be present, although the most typical finding is a decrease in QRS voltage. Arrhythmias, both atrial and ventricular, can be evidence of rejection.

### D. Echocardiography

Echocardiography is a sensitive surveillance tool for graft rejection. Changes in ventricular compliance and function are typical and become progressive with increasing duration of the rejection episode. Valval insufficiency may also indicate rejection. A new pericardial effusion can also indicate inflammation due to the rejection process.

### E. Cardiac Catheterization and Endomyocardial Biopsy

The hemodynamic measurements can be relatively normal with mild rejection, but with progression the pulmonary capillary wedge pressure increases, indicating decreasing ventricular compliance. Often this is a global process, and the RV filling pressures or central venous pressure may also be elevated. The endomyocardial biopsy has remained the mainstay of tissue diagnosis for graft rejection. The appearance of infiltrating lymphocytes with myocellular damage is the hallmark of graft rejection. Occasionally patients may have only a sparse lymphocytic infiltration despite profound myocardial performance abnormalities. Presumably, the depression in the myocardial function in the absence of lymphocytes is related to inflammatory mediators such as tumor necrosis factor and the various interleukins.

## Treatment

The treatment for graft rejection depends on reversing the immunologic inflammatory cascade. High-dose corticosteroids are the first line of treatment. These can stabilize or reverse most rejection episodes. Occasionally additional therapy in the form of antithymocyte biologic preparations such as antithymocyte globulin or OKT-3 (a murine monoclonal antibody to the CD3 T-lymphocyte epitope) is needed to reverse the rejection process. Most rejection episodes can be treated effectively if diagnosed promptly. A high index of suspicion

must be maintained whenever a patient has a history of cardiac transplantation. Usually graft function will return to the baseline state, although severe rejection episodes can result in graft loss and patient death even with optimal therapy.

## Course & Prognosis

The clinical course of cardiac transplantation in pediatric patients is usually quite good. Despite the chronic immunosuppression, the risk of infection is low beyond the early posttransplant period. Most children seem to tolerate environmental pathogens quite readily. Overwhelming infection is uncommon. Noncompliance with lifetime immunosuppression, especially among adolescents, is of great concern. Several recent studies have identified noncompliance as the leading cause of late death after transplantation. Posttransplant lymphoproliferative disorder, a syndrome related to Epstein–Barr virus infection, can result in a Burkitt-like lymphoma that will usually respond to a reduction in immunosuppression. Most children are not physically limited, and they do not require restrictions related to the cardiovascular system. Because the heart is denervated, patients may exhibit a blunted response to exercise at the onset. The greatest concern over the long term following heart transplantation is related to a syndrome of accelerated coronary atherosclerosis. This premature form of atherosclerosis is unlike typical adult coronary disease in that it progresses quite rapidly. The insult to the coronary endothelium is immune-mediated and can cause coronary obliteration. If the process is recognized and treated, its late appearance may mimic the more typical adult atherosclerotic disease. This observation has led some researchers to suggest that adult atherosclerotic disease is largely an inflammatory process, perhaps initiated by environmental pathogens.

Overall, despite the concerns of immunosuppression and the risk of late rejection and graft atherosclerosis, the majority of pediatric patients enjoy physiologic rehabilitation following cardiac transplantation with a 60–70% 10-year survival. Newer, more specific, and more effective immunosuppressive agents are currently being tried in clinical studies or are being evaluated in preclinical studies, making the future almost certainly better for children after cardiac transplantation. Donor availability remains a major limitation to the expansion of indications for cardiac transplantation.

Boucek MM et al: The Registry of the International Society of Heart and Lung Transplantation: Sixth official pediatric report—2003. J Heart Lung Transplant 2001;20(6):39 [PMID: 12821161].

Moran AM et al: Non-invasive assessment of rejection in pediatric transplant patients: Serologic and echocardiographic prediction of biopsy-proven myocardial rejection. J Heart Lung Transplant 2000;19(8):756 [PMID: 10967269].

Mulla NF et al: Late rejection is a predictor of transplant coronary artery disease in children. J Am Coll Cardiol 2001; 37(1):243 [PMID: 11153746].

# ■ DISORDERS OF RATE & RHYTHM

The recognition and treatment of cardiac arrhythmias have improved markedly since the 1980s. Better monitoring has increased the awareness and detection of rhythm disturbances. There is also a true rise in the incidence of arrhythmias. More children are now surviving cardiac surgery and acute carditis and live chronically with altered hemodynamics, physiology, and structural changes. These changes over time will create altered conduction and new arrhythmias.

The advent of invasive electrophysiology with recordings from the endocardium has greatly improved our understanding of the conduction system. Now, with cardiac ablation techniques, we can offer these children a "cure" rather than lifelong antiarrhythmia treatment.

## Sinus Arrhythmia

It is normal to have phasic variation in the heart rate (sinus arrhythmia). Typically, the sinus rate varies with the respiratory cycle, whereas P-QRS-T intervals remain normal. Marked sinus arrhythmia is defined as a greater than 100% variation in heart rate. It may occur in association with respiratory distress or increased intracranial pressure, or it may be present in normal children. It alone never requires treatment; however, it may be associated with sinus node dysfunction or autonomic nervous system dysfunction.

## Sinus Bradycardia

Depending on the patient's age, sinus bradycardia is defined as either (1) a heart rate below the normal limit for age (neonates to 6 years, 60 beats/min; 7–11 years, 45 beats/min; older than 12 years, 40 beats/min) or (2) a heart rate inappropriately slow for the functional status of the patient (chronotropic incompetence). In critically ill patients, common causes of sinus bradycardia include hypoxia, central nervous system damage, and iatrogenic medication side effects. Only symptomatic bradycardia (syncope, low cardiac output, or ex-

ercise intolerance) requires treatment (atropine or cardiac pacing).

## Sinus Tachycardia

The heart rate normally accelerates in response to stress (eg, fever, hypovolemia, anemia, CHF). Although sinus tachycardia in the normal heart is well tolerated, symptomatic tachycardia with decreased cardiac output is more ominous and warrants evaluation for associated structural heart disease or true tachyarrhythmias. Treatment may be indicated for correction of the underlying cause of sinus tachycardia (eg, transfusion for anemia, correction of hypovolemia or fever).

# PREMATURE ATRIAL CONTRACTIONS

Premature atrial contractions are triggered by an ectopic focus in the atrium. They are one of the most common premature beats occurring in the pediatric population, particularly during the fetal and newborn periods. They may be conducted (followed by a QRS) or nonconducted (not followed by a QRS as the beat has occurred so early that the AV node is still refractory) (Figure 19–4). A less-than-compensatory pause usually occurs until the next normal sinus beat. Depending on the ectopic focus of the premature contraction, the frontal plane vector of the P wave may be normal (+30–90 degrees) or abnormal. As an isolated finding, premature atrial contractions are benign and require no treatment. They may need to be suppressed with antiarrhythmic agents when they trigger tachyarrhythmias or produce bradycardia secondary to nonconduction.

# PREMATURE JUNCTIONAL CONTRACTIONS

Premature junctional contractions arise within the AV node or the bundle of His. Most often, they induce a normal QRS complex with no preceding P wave. When conducted aberrantly to the ventricles, they cannot be distinguished from PVCs except by invasive electrophysiologic study. Premature junctional contractions are usually benign and require no specific therapy.

# PREMATURE VENTRICULAR CONTRACTIONS

PVCs may originate in either ventricle and are characterized by an abnormal QRS of over 80 ms duration in newborns and 120 ms in adolescents and adults (Figure 19–5). PVCs originating from a single ectopic focus all have the same configuration; those of multifocal origin show varying configurations. The consecutive occur-

***Figure 19–4.*** Lead II rhythm strip with premature atrial contractions. Beats 1, 3, 7, and 8 are conducted to the ventricles, whereas beats 2, 4, 5, and 6 are not.

Lead V₅

***Figure 19–5.*** Lead V₅ rhythm strip with unifocal premature ventricular contractions in a bigeminy pattern. The arrow shows a ventricular couplet.

rence of two PVCs is referred to as a ventricular couplet and of three or more as ventricular tachycardia.

Most unifocal PVCs in otherwise normal patients are benign. The significance of the PVCs can be confirmed by having the patient exercise. As the heart rate increases, benign premature contractions usually disappear. If exercise results in an increase or coupling of contractions, underlying disease may be present. Multifocal PVCs are always abnormal and may be more dangerous. They may be associated with drug overdose (tricyclic antidepressants, digoxin toxicity), electrolyte imbalance, myocarditis, or hypoxia. Treatment is directed at correcting the underlying disorder.

## SINUS NODE DYSFUNCTION

Sinus node dysfunction, or sick sinus syndrome, is a clinical syndrome of inappropriate sinus nodal function and rate. The abnormality may be a true anatomic defect of the sinus node or its surrounding tissue, or it may be an abnormality of autonomic input. It is defined as one or more of the following:

1. Sinus bradycardia
2. Marked sinus arrhythmia
3. Chronotropic incompetence
4. Sinus pause or arrest
5. Sinoatrial exit block
6. Combined bradyarrhythmias and tachyarrhythmias
7. Sinus node reentry
8. Atrial muscle reentry tachycardia.

It is usually associated with postoperative repair of congenital heart disease (most commonly the Mustard or Senning repair for complete transposition of the great arteries or the Fontan procedure), but it is also seen in unoperated congenital heart disease, in acquired heart diseases, and in normal hearts. In some cases the disorder is inherited. Symptoms usually manifest between ages 2 and 17 years and consist of episodes of syncope, presyncope, or disorientation. Some patients may experience palpitations, pallor, or exercise intolerance.

The evaluation of sinus node dysfunction involves both surface ECG and invasive electrophysiologic testing. Exercise testing, and ambulatory monitoring help define any arrhythmias and correlate rhythm changes with symptoms.

Treatment for sinus node dysfunction is indicated only in symptomatic patients. Asymptomatic patients can just be observed for the onset of exercise intolerance or syncope because there is little chance of sudden death prior to the onset of symptoms. Bradyarrhyth-mias are treated with vagolytic (atropine) or adrenergic (aminophylline) agents or permanent cardiac pacemakers. Antiarrhythmic treatment of tachyarrhythmias often produces or enhances bradycardia, thus requiring permanent cardiac pacing. In selected cases, a pacemaker is inserted prophylactically prior to the initiation of antiarrhythmic medications.

The prognosis is excellent when appropriate treatment is provided, with total morbidity and mortality rates nearly equal to those of the underlying heart disease. However, in severe cases, if left untreated, sinus node dysfunction may become chronic and may even lead to sudden death.

Miller MS et al: Neonatal bradycardia. Prog Pediatr Cardiol 2000;11:19 [PMID: 10822186].

## SUPRAVENTRICULAR TACHYCARDIA

SVT, also known as paroxysmal SVT or paroxysmal atrial tachycardia, is defined as an abnormal arrhythmia mechanism arising above or within the bundle of His. The mode of presentation depends on the tachycardia rate, the presence of underlying cardiac structural or functional abnormalities, coexisting illness and the patient's age. Tachycardia may be poorly tolerated in a child who has preexisting CHF or an underlying systemic disease such as anemia or sepsis, or it may go unnoticed in an otherwise healthy child. Incessant tachycardia in an otherwise healthy individual, albeit slow (120–150 beats/min), may cause myocardial dysfunction and CHF if left untreated. The mechanisms of tachycardia can be divided into three groups: reentry, enhanced automaticity, and triggered dysrhythmias.

Reentry is conduction through two or more pathways, creating a sustained repetitive circular loop. The circuit can be confined to the atrium (intraatrial reentry, a form of atrial flutter) (Figure 19–6). It may be confined within the AV node (AV nodal reentrant tachycardia), or it may encompass an accessory connection between atria and ventricle (atrioventricular tachycardia). The arrhythmia circuit includes conduction through the normal pathway (ie, the AV node) as well as the accessory AV connection. If during tachycardia the electrical impulse travels antegrade (from atria to ventricle) through the AV node and retrograde (from ventricle to atria) back up the accessory pathway, orthodromic reciprocating tachycardia is present. If during tachycardia the electrical impulse travels antegrade through the accessory pathway and retrograde up through the AV node, then antidromic reciprocating tachycardia is present. WPW syndrome is a subclass of reentrant tachycardia in which, during sinus rhythm, the impulse travels antegrade down the accessory connection, bypassing the AV node and creating ventricu-

***Figure 19–6.*** Leads aVF (F) and $V_1$, showing atrial flutter with "sawtooth" atrial flutter waves.

lar preexcitation (early eccentric activation of the ventricle with a short PR interval and slurred upstroke of the QRS, a delta wave) (Figure 19–7). Reentrant tachycardia represents approximately 80% of pediatric arrhythmias, has a wide range of rates, and may or may not demonstrate P waves. Reentrant tachycardia initiates and terminates abruptly. Most patients with WPW have otherwise structurally normal hearts. WPW however has been noted to occur with increased frequency in association with the following congenital cardiac lesions: tricuspid atresia, Ebstein anomaly of the tricuspid valve, HCM, and ccTGA.

Enhanced automaticity (also known as automatic or ectopic tachycardia) is created when a focus of cardiac tissue develops an abnormally fast spontaneous rate of depolarization. These arrhythmias represent approximately 20% of childhood arrhythmias and are usually under autonomic influence. ECG demonstrates a normal QRS complex preceded by an abnormal P wave (Figure 19–8). Junctional ectopic tachycardia does not have a P wave preceding the QRS waves and may be associated with AV dissociation or 1:1 retrograde conduction. Ectopic tachycardias demonstrate a gradual onset and offset and may be paroxysmal or incessant. When

they are incessant, they are usually associated with CHF and a clinical picture of dilated cardiomyopathy.

Triggered dysrhythmia is extremely rare. It is caused by enhanced afterdepolarizations of the action potential that reach the takeoff potential. These tachycardias are usually associated with diseased atrial myocardium, are triggered by premature atrial contractions or sinus tachycardia, initiate and terminate abruptly, and mimic intraatrial reentry (atrial flutter). However, they can be distinguished from atrial flutter: they terminate with the administration of adenosine, while atrial flutter does not (see section on Artial Flutter & Fibrillation).

## Clinical Findings

### A. SYMPTOMS AND SIGNS

Clinical presentation varies with the patient's age. Infants tend to turn pale and mottled with onset of tachycardia and may become irritable. With long duration of tachycardia, symptoms of CHF develop. Heart rates can be from 240 to 300 beats/min. Older children may complain of dizziness, palpitations, fatigue, and chest pain. Heart rates usually range from 240 beats/min in

***Figure 19–7.*** Leads I and II with spontaneous intermittent ventricular preexcitation (Wolff–Parkinson–White syndrome).

***Figure 19–8.*** Lead II rhythm strip of ectopic atrial tachycardia. The tracing demonstrates a variable rate with a maximum of 260 beats/min, an abnormal P wave, and a gradual termination.

the younger child to 150–180 beats/min in the teenager. CHF is less common in children than in infants. Tachycardia may be associated with either congenital heart defects, as mentioned earlier, or acquired conditions such as cardiomyopathies and myocarditis.

### B. IMAGING

Findings on chest radiograph are normal during the early course of tachycardia. If CHF is present, the heart is enlarged and pulmonary venous congestion is evident.

### C. ELECTROCARDIOGRAPHY

ECG is the most important tool in the diagnosis of SVT.

1. The heart rate is rapid and out of proportion to the patient's physical status (ie, a rate of 140 beats/min with an abnormal P wave while quiet and asleep).

2. The rhythm is extremely regular. There is little variation in the rate throughout the entire tracing.

3. P waves may or may not be present. If they are present, the PR interval and appearance do not vary. P waves may be difficult to find because they are superimposed on the preceding T wave. Furthermore, if the abnormal focus is located within the AV node, the P waves will not be seen.

4. The QRS complex is usually the same as during normal sinus rhythm. However, the QRS complex is occasionally widened (SVT with aberrant ventricular conduction), in which case the condition may be difficult to differentiate from ventricular tachycardia.

### Treatment

#### A. ACUTE TREATMENT

During initial episodes of SVT, patients require close monitoring. Correction of acidosis and electrolyte abnormalities is also indicated.

**1. Vagal maneuvers**—The "diving reflex," produced by placing an ice bag on the nasal bridge for 20 seconds (for infants) or by immersing the face in ice water (for children or adolescents), will increase parasympathetic tone and terminate some tachycardias. The Valsalva maneuver, which can be performed by older compliant children, may also terminate SVT.

**2. Adenosine**—Adenosine transiently blocks AV conduction and terminates tachycardias that incorporate the AV node.

Adenosine does not convert tachycardias whose mechanism is confined to the atria (atrial ectopic tachycardia, intraatrial reentry). However, it serves as a diagnostic tool in these arrhythmias by demonstrating continuation of the atrial tachycardia during AV block, implying that AV node conduction is not a crucial element of the tachycardia circuit. The dose is 50–250 μg/kg by rapid intravenous bolus. It is antagonized by aminophylline and should be used with caution in patients with sinus node dysfunction or asthma.

**3. Transesophageal atrial pacing**—Atrial overdrive pacing and termination can be performed from a bipolar electrode-tipped catheter positioned in the esophagus adjacent to the left atrium. Overdrive pacing at rates approximately 30% faster than the tachycardia rate will interrupt the tachycardia circuit and restore sinus rhythm.

**4. Direct current cardioversion**—Direct current (DC) cardioversion (0.5–2 synchronized J/kg) should be used immediately when a patient presents in cardiovascular collapse.

## B. Chronic Treatment

**1. Digitalis**—Digoxin is still frequently used for long-term treatment and maintenance of sinus rhythm. The doses used are the same as those for CHF. Conversion should be accomplished within 8–12 hours. In some patients digoxin can accelerate conduction over an accessory pathway, and in those children digitalis products are contraindicated. Patients with an accessory pathway (eg, those with WPW syndrome) often have primary atrial tachycardias (atrial flutter or fibrillation, atrial ectopic tachycardias), and with enhanced conduction in the accessory pathway these primary atrial tachycardias can transmit to the ventricles, causing ventricular fibrillation. Therefore, an evaluation of the effect of digoxin on the accessory pathway should be performed in the electrophysiology lab before chronic digoxin use in patients with WPW syndrome.

**2. Beta-adrenergic blocking agents**—Propranolol decreases sinus heart rate and AV nodal conduction. It is effective in the treatment of both reentrant and ectopic arrhythmias in doses ranging from 1 to 4 mg/kg/d. Long-acting β-blockers, such as atenolol and nadolol, are used because they have fewer central nervous system side effects than propranolol and may be given only once or twice a day.

**3. Calcium channel antagonists**—Verapamil and other calcium channel blockers markedly prolong conduction through the AV node and are effective in interrupting and preventing reentrant tachycardias that incorporate the AV node. They are ineffective in terminating atrial tachycardias but may be useful in controlling the ventricular response by producing AV blockade. Verapamil comes in short- and long-acting preparations; the dose is 3–5 mg/kg/d. It may cause myocardial dysfunction and is contraindicated in infants.

**4. Other drugs**—Recently introduced antiarrhythmic medications (eg, flecainide, propafenone, sotalol, and amiodarone) have increased pharmacologic actions and are extremely effective. However, these drugs also have serious side effects, including proarrhythmia (production of arrhythmias) and sudden death, and should be used only under the direction of a pediatric cardiologist.

**5. Radiofrequency ablation**—This is a nonsurgical transvascular catheter technique that will desiccate an arrhythmia focus or accessory pathway and permanently "cure" an arrhythmia. The immediate success rate is approximately 90%, with a rate of recurrence of 10%. The risk of developing complete heart block is approximately 2–10% when applying burns in the vicinity of the AV node/His bundle. The procedure can be performed in infants or adults. In children younger than age 4 years, the risks are higher, and the procedure should be reserved for those whose arrhythmias are refractory to medical management. In well-tolerated SVTs that respond to vagal maneuvers, no further treatment is necessary. However, the high success rate, low complication and recurrence rates, and the elimination of the need for chronic antiarrhythmic medications have made radiofrequency ablation the primary treatment option in most pediatric cardiovascular centers.

## Prognosis

SVT has an excellent prognosis. When it occurs in early infancy, 90% will respond to initial treatment. Approximately 30% will recur at an average age of 8 years.

Basson CT: A molecular basis for Wolff–Parkinson–White syndrome. N Engl J Med 2001;344(24):1861 [PMID: 11407351].

Dubin AM et al: Radiofrequency catheter ablation: Indications and complications. Pediatr Cardiol 2000;21(6):551 [PMID: 11050279].

Moak JP: Supraventricular tachycardia in the neonate and infant. Prog Pediatr Cardiol 2000;11(1):25 [PMID: 10822187].

## ATRIAL FLUTTER & FIBRILLATION

Atrial flutter and fibrillation are rare in children and are most often associated with organic heart disease—particularly postoperative congenital heart disease and sinus node dysfunction. Atrial flutter can occur in infancy and can mimic SVT. The atrial rate is usually greater than 240 beats/min and often more than 300 beats/min. The ventricular rate depends on the rate of AV conduction and is usually slower than the atrial rate.

## Treatment & Prognosis

Transesophageal atrial pacing is the treatment of choice to terminate atrial flutter. When it is not successful, antiarrhythmic medications (eg, digoxin, sotalol, and amiodarone) may succeed; however, DC cardioversion is frequently necessary.

The prognosis in neonates without structural heart disease is excellent, and after conversion these patients may need no further treatment.

## POSTOPERATIVE INCISIONAL INTRAATRIAL REENTRY

Improved surgical survival for patients with congenital heart disease has created a new, increasingly prevalent, chronic arrhythmia: incisional intraatrial reentry, or postoperative atrial flutter. In these tachycardias, electrically isolated corridors of atrial myocardium (eg, the tricuspid valve–inferior vena cava isthmus, or the region between an atrial incision and the crista terminalis) act as pathways for sustained reentrant circuits of electrical activity. These tachycardias are chronic, medically refractory, and clinically incapacitating. Electromagnetic mapping permits precise localization of these corridors. Long linear radiofrequency or surgical lesions are then used to interrupt the reentrant circuits.

Delacretaz E et al: Multiple atrial macro-reentry circuits in adults with repaired congenital heart disease: Entrainment mapping combined with three-dimensional electroanatomic mapping. J Am Coll Cardiol 2001;37(6):1665 [PMID: 11345382].

Van Hare GF: Intra-atrial reentry tachycardia in pediatric patients. Prog Pediatr Cardiol 2001;13(1):41 [PMID: 11413057].

## VENTRICULAR TACHYCARDIA

Ventricular tachycardia is uncommon in childhood (Figure 19–9). It is usually associated with underlying abnormalities of the myocardium (myocarditis, cardiomyopathy, myocardial tumors, postoperative congenital heart disease) or toxicity (hypoxia, electrolyte imbalance, drug toxicity). Sustained tachycardia is generally an unstable situation and, if left untreated, will usually degenerate into ventricular fibrillation.

Accelerated idioventricular rhythm is a sustained ventricular tachycardia occurring in neonates with normal hearts. The rate is within 10% of the preceding sinus rate, and it is a self-limiting arrhythmia that requires no treatment.

Acute termination of ventricular tachycardia involves restoration of the normal myocardium when possible (correct electrolyte imbalance, drug toxicity, and so on) and DC cardioversion (1–4 J/kg), cardioversion with lidocaine (1 mg/kg), or both. Chronic suppression of ventricular arrhythmias with antiarrhythmic drugs has many side effects (including proarrhythmia and death), and it must be initiated in the hospital under the direction of a pediatric cardiologist.

Alexander ME et al: Ventricular arrhythmias: When to worry. Pediatr Cardiol 2000;21(6):532 [PMID: 11050277].

Batra A et al: Ventricular arrhythmias. Prog Pediatr Cardiol 2000;11(1):39 [PMID: 10822188].

## LONG QT SYNDROME

The congenital long QT syndromes (types 1–6) in children are arrhythmic disorders in which ventricular re-

***Figure 19–9.*** Twelve-lead ECG from a child with imipramine toxicity and ventricular tachycardia.

polarization is irregular and prolonged (QTc > 0.44 seconds, or 0.46 seconds in postpubertal females). Some myocardial ion channelopathies predispose patients to "torsade de pointes" (multifocal ventricular tachycardia) and manifest as syncope, seizures, or sudden death in response to exercise. If untreated, they account for a very high mortality rate (5%/year). They are inherited genetically in an autosomal dominant or recessive pattern (the latter being associated with congenital deafness, the Jervell–Lange–Nielsen syndrome). Or they may arise spontaneously. Treatment with β-blockade and exercise limitation is only partially successful. In recurrent, medically refractory cases, implantable cardioverter defibrillators are necessary to prevent sudden death. Congenital long QT syndrome has now been demonstrated to be one of the causes of SIDS. The *SCN5A* gene has been isolated from a child who died from SIDS.

Acquired long QT syndrome—resulting from altered ventricular repolarization secondary to myocardial toxins, ischemia, or inflammation—also predisposes a patient to ventricular arrhythmias. Numerous medications as outlined previously can also cause QT prolongation. ECGs are recommended before therapy (for a baseline measurement) and after steady state is achieved. Another drug capable of prolonging the QT interval, cisapride (used for gastroesophageal reflux), has now been removed from the US market.

Gutgesell H et al: Cardiovascular monitoring of children and adolescents receiving psychotropic drugs. A statement for healthcare professionals from the Committee on Congenital Cardiac Defects, Counsel on Cardiovascular Diseases in the Young-American Heart Association. Circulation 1999;99(7):979 [PMID: 10027824].

Kimbrough J et al: Clinical implications for affected parents and siblings of probands with long QT syndrome. Circulation 2001;104(5):557 [PMID: 11479253].

Li H et al: Current concepts in long QT syndrome. Pediatr Cardiol 2000;21(6):542 [PMID: 11050278].

Moss AJ et al: Effectiveness and limitations of β-blocker therapy in congenital long QT syndrome. Circulation 2000;101(6):616 [PMID: 10673253].

Wedekind H et al: De novo mutation in the SCN5A gene associated with early onset of sudden infant death. Circulation 2001;104(10):1158 [PMID: 11535573].

Zhang L et al: Spectrum of ST-T wave patterns and repolarization parameters in congenital long QT syndrome ECG findings identify genotypes. Circulation 2000;102(23):2849 [PMID: 11104743].

## SUDDEN DEATH

Hypertrophic cardiomyopathy (the most common cause of sudden death in young athletes) and other cardiomyopathies (dilated cardiomyopathies, restrictive cardiomyopathy, or arrhythmogenic RV dysplasia) may be hereditary and should be looked for in patients with resuscitated cardiac arrest or family members of those who have died suddenly. Congenital structural anomalies of the coronary arteries are the second most common cause of sudden death in young athletes. These anomalies are not hereditary. The coronary arteries need to be evaluated in survivors of sudden death events. Arrhythmias in patients with postoperative congenital heart disease are important causes of morbidity and mortality and may present as sudden death events. All survivors of cardiac arrest require thorough evaluation for arrhythmias, including invasive electrophysiology. Episodes of seizures, syncope, and presyncope in congenital heart disease patients should be evaluated for the possibilities of arrhythmias, and they may also require thorough electrophysiologic evaluation and treatment.

When a child dies suddenly and unexpectedly, or is resuscitated from cardiac arrest that had no apparent cause, it is necessary to conduct a detailed family history looking for seizures, syncope, or early sudden death. Family members should be examined with an arrhythmia screen, physical examination, ECG, and echocardiography to detect arrhythmias or cardiomyopathies.

Corrado D et al: Right bundle branch block, right precordial ST-segment elevation, and sudden death in young people. Circulation 2001;103(5):710 [PMID: 11156883].

Gatzoulis MA et al: Risk factors for arrhythmia and sudden cardiac death later after repair of tetralogy of Fallot: A Multicentre Study. Lancet 2000;356(9234):975 [PMID: 11041398].

## HEART BLOCK

### 1. First-Degree Heart Block

First-degree heart block is an ECG diagnosis of prolongation of the PR interval. The block does not in itself cause problems, but it is frequently associated with congenital heart defects such as AV septal defects, ccTGA, and with diseases such as rheumatic carditis. The PR interval may also be prolonged as a result of digoxin therapy.

### 2. Second-Degree Heart Block

Mobitz type I (Wenckebach) heart block is recognized by progressive prolongation of the PR interval until there is no QRS following a P wave (Figure 19–10). Mobitz type I heart block occurs in normal hearts at rest and is usually benign. In Mobitz type II heart block, there is no progressive lengthening of the PR interval before the dropped beat (Figure 19–11). Mobitz type II heart block is frequently associated with organic heart disease, and a complete evaluation is necessary.

Lead I

***Figure 19–10.*** Lead I rhythm strip with Mobitz type I (Wenckebach) second-degree heart block. There is progressive lengthening of the PR interval prior to the nonconducted P wave (*arrows*).

### 3. Complete Heart Block

In complete heart block, the atria and ventricles beat independently. Ventricular rates can range from 40 to 80 beats/min, whereas atrial rates are faster (Figure 19–12).

Congenital complete heart block, the most common form of complete heart block, has a very high association with maternal systemic lupus erythematosus. Serologic screening should be performed in the mother of an infant with complete heart block even if she has no symptoms of collagen vascular disease. Congenital complete heart block is also associated with congenitally corrected transposition of the great vessels and AV septal defect. Acquired complete heart block may be secondary to acute myocarditis, drug toxicity, electrolyte imbalance, hypoxia, and cardiac surgery.

### Clinical Findings

Prenatal bradycardia is frequently noted in infants with congenital complete heart block, and emergent delivery is required if hydrops fetalis develops. Postnatal adaptation largely depends on the heart rate; infants with heart rates lower than 55 beats/min are at significantly greater risk for low cardiac output, CHF, and death. Wide QRS complexes and a rapid atrial rate are also poor prognostic signs. Most patients have an innocent flow murmur from increased stroke volume. In symptomatic patients, the heart can be quite enlarged, and pulmonary edema may be present. In older patients, syncope can be the presenting symptom, or heart block may be found unexpectedly on routine physical examination. Complete cardiac evaluation, including echocardiography and Holter monitoring, is necessary

Lead III

***Figure 19–11.*** Lead III rhythm strip with Mobitz type II second-degree heart block. There is a consistent PR interval with occasional loss of AV conduction (*arrow*).

***Figure 19–12.*** Twelve-lead ECG and lead II rhythm strip of complete heart block. The atrial rate is 150 beats/min, and the ventricular rate is 60 beats/min.

to assess the patient for ventricular dysfunction and to relate any symptoms to concurrent arrhythmias.

## Treatment

In patients thought to be at risk for syncope, CHF, or sudden death, the treatment of choice for complete heart block is insertion of a permanent pacemaker. Until permanent pacing can be instituted, patients can be assisted temporarily by infusions of isoproterenol or by temporary transcutaneous pacemakers.

Eronen M et al: Short and long-term outcome of children with congenital complete heart block diagnosed in utero or as a newborn. Pediatrics 2000;106(1 Pt 1):86 [PMID: 10878154].

Moak JP et al: Congenital heart block: Development of late-onset cardiomyopathy, a previously underappreciated sequela. J Am Coll Cardiol 2001;37(1):238 [PMID: 11153745].

## SYNCOPE (Fainting)

Syncope is a sudden transient loss of consciousness that resolves spontaneously. The common form of syncope (simple fainting) occurs in 15% of children and is a disorder of control of heart rate and blood pressure by the autonomic nervous system that causes hypotension or bradycardia. It is often associated with rapid rising and postural hypotension, prolonged standing, or hypovolemia. Patients exhibit vagal symptoms such as pallor, nausea, or diaphoresis. Syncope, also known as autonomic dysfunction, can be evaluated with head-up tilt table testing. The patient is placed supine on a tilt table, and then—under constant heart rate and blood pressure monitoring—is tilted to the upright position. If symptoms develop, they can be classified as vasodepressor (hypotension), cardioinhibitory (bradycardia), or mixed.

Syncope is usually self-limited (lasting approximately 6 months to 2 years) and can be controlled with dietary salt and volume loading to prevent hypovolemia. In refractory cases, medications to manipulate the autonomic nervous system have been useful. Flurocortisone (0.1 mg/kg/d) is a mineralocorticoid that causes renal salt resorption and thus increases intravascular volume. Beta-blockade (atenolol, 0.5 to 2.0 mg/kg/d) can inhibit the catecholamine surge and help prevent the rebound bradycardia and hypotension. Vagolytic agents (disopyramide 2.5 mg/kg qid) help control hypervagotonia, and the selective serotonin reuptake inhibitors have also been effective in alleviating symptoms. Syncope that occurs during exercise or stress or is associated with a positive family history is a warning sign that a serious underlying dysrhythmia may be present, calling for further investigation.

Johnsrude CL: Current approach to pediatric syncope. Pediatr Cardiol 2000;21(6):522 [PMID: 11050276].

# Gastrointestinal Tract

*Judith M. Sondheimer, MD*

## EVALUATION OF THE CHILD WITH VOMITING

Assessment of the child with recurrent episodes of vomiting should start with a complete history, physical examination, and description of the vomitus (Table 20–1). Emesis of gastric contents is characteristic of gastric outlet obstruction, central nervous system masses or infection, peptic disease, urinary tract infection, otitis or sinusitis, metabolic diseases (especially those causing acidosis), rumination, and psychogenic vomiting. Gastroesophageal (GE) reflux should be suspected in a healthy child with effortless postprandial spitting. An upper gastrointestinal (GI) series is essential to rule out anatomic causes in young infants. A urinalysis and culture will rule out urinary tract infection or urinary obstruction, which may cause vomiting, especially in young infants. Serum electrolytes should be measured as abnormalities of sodium, potassium, magnesium and calcium may also cause vomiting by interfering with normal motor functions of the GI tract. Increased intracranial pressure may cause vomiting. The decision to obtain radiographs and scans of the central nervous system, chest, or sinuses is based on a specific indication from the history or physical examination.

The child who vomits bile-stained material may have small intestinal obstruction and should be examined immediately. Bile staining may be gold or green in color. The history and physical examination are the essential starting points and should include duration of vomiting, the presence of blood in the vomitus, the presence of abdominal pain or distention, the character of the stools, and the presence of fever. Pain localized to the right lower quadrant suggests appendicitis. Midline or diffuse abdominal pain suggests pancreatitis or generalized peritonitis. Abdominal distention suggests intestinal obstruction. Viral and bacterial gastroenteritis are associated with diarrhea and may produce generalized ileus with bilious vomiting. Gallbladder disease is uncommon in childhood but should be suspected in children with a family or personal history of hemolytic disorders, hypercholesterolemia, or primary medical conditions promoting gallstones. The presence of mucus and blood in the stool should arouse suspicion of intestinal intussusception or bacterial or toxic colitis. Three-way radiographs of the abdomen are a first diagnostic step in localizing the site of intestinal obstruction.

The evaluation of bloody vomitus should start with confirmation that the material vomited is indeed blood. Numerous causes must be considered, including swallowed maternal blood in newborns, oropharyngeal lesions, nosebleed, peptic disease, bleeding disorders, foreign bodies, and esophageal varices. Mallory–Weiss tear of the mucosa of the GE junction is common after prolonged vomiting. Careful assessment of the cardiovascular stability of the child is essential before extensive evaluation is initiated. Passage of a nasogastric tube will help determine whether bleeding is ongoing. The hematocrit should be measured. If further diagnostic investigation is desired, the most productive test is upper intestinal endoscopy.

## GASTROESOPHAGEAL REFLUX

Postprandial regurgitation is the most common symptom of GE reflux in young infants. Regurgitation ranges from effortless spitting to forceful vomiting. Although usually a harmless condition of young infants, severe GE reflux may cause failure to thrive, esophagitis with hematemesis, occult blood loss, anemia, esophageal stricture, and inflammatory esophageal polyps. Aspiration pneumonia, chronic cough, wheezing, and asthma-like attacks are reported. Dysphagia, colic after feedings, and neck contortions (Sandifer syndrome) may occur. Ruminative behavior is sometimes a symptom. Apneic spells in young infants, especially occurring with position change after feeding, may be caused by GE reflux. GE reflux is common in neurologically impaired children. The underlying cause of GE reflux is unknown, but the facilitating mechanism appears to be spontaneous relaxation of the lower esophageal sphincter rather than a chronically weak or immature sphincter.

GE reflux is a clinical diagnosis in thriving infants younger than age 6 months. An upper GI series is important to rule out anatomic causes of vomiting, but is not an accurate test for GE reflux because of the 30% false-positive rate. Prolonged monitoring of esophageal pH is a more sensitive test if the symptoms are not typical. Esophageal intraluminal impedance monitoring is a pH-independent means to detect fluid movement in

***Table 20–1.*** Causes of vomiting and regurgitation.

| GASTROINTESTINAL TRACT DISORDERS | |
| --- | --- |
| **Esophagus** | **Intestine and colon** |
| Achalasia | Atresia and stenosis |
| Gastroesophageal | Meconium ileus |
| reflux (chalasia) | Malrotation, volvulus |
| Hiatal hernia | Duplication |
| Esophagitis | Intussusception |
| Atresia with or without | Foreign body |
| fistula | Polyposis |
| Congenital vascular or | Soy or cow's milk protein |
| mucosal rings, webs | intolerance |
| Stenosis | Gluten enteropathy |
| Duplication and divertic- | Food allergy |
| ulum | Hirschsprung disease |
| Foreign body | Chronic intestinal pseudo- |
| Periesophageal mass | obstruction |
| **Stomach** | Appendicitis |
| Hypertrophic pyloric | Inflammatory bowel disease |
| stenosis | Gastroenteritis, infections |
| Pylorospasm | **Other abdominal organs** |
| Diaphragmatic hernia | Hepatitis |
| Peptic disease and | Gallstones |
| gastritis | Pancreatitis |
| Antral web | Peritonitis |
| **Duodenum** | |
| Annular pancreas | |
| Duodenitis and ulcer | |
| Malrotation | |
| Mesenteric bands | |
| Superior mesenteric | |
| artery syndrome | |

| EXTRAGASTROINTESTINAL TRACT DISORDERS | |
| --- | --- |
| Sepsis | Adrenal insufficiency |
| Pneumonia | Renal tubular acidosis |
| Otitis media | Inborn errors |
| Urinary tract infection | Urea cycle disorders |
| Meningitis | Phenylketonuria |
| Subdural effusion | Maple syrup urine |
| Hydrocephalus | disease |
| Brain tumor | Organic acidemia |
| Reye syndrome | Galactosemia |
| Rumination | Fructose intolerance |
| Intoxications | Tyrosinosis |
| Alcohol | Scleroderma |
| Aspirin | Epidermolysis bullosa |
| Acetaminophen | |

the esophagus. It may be a more accurate method to detect and describe pathologic reflux once standards have been clarified in children. Esophageal and gastric scintiscanning is sometimes helpful in identifying pulmonary aspiration. Esophagoscopy is not diagnostic, but esophagitis can be identified.

## Treatment & Prognosis

In 85% of infants with GE reflux, the condition is self-limited, disappearing between ages 6 and 12 months, coincident with assumption of erect posture and initiation of solid feedings. Regurgitation may be reduced by offering small feedings at frequent intervals or by thickening feedings with rice cereal (2–3 tsp/oz of formula). Prethickened antireflux formulas are available. Histamine (H2)-receptor antagonists (ranitidine, 5 mg/kg/d in two doses) and proton pump inhibitors (eg, omeprazole, 0.5–1 mg/kg/d in one dose) are effective in controlling esophagitis and often reduce pain secondary to reflux. Prokinetic agents such as metoclopramide (0.1 mg/kg before meals) hasten gastric emptying and improve esophageal motor function, but studies have not supported their efficacy in controlling symptoms.

Antireflux surgery is indicated if reflux causes (1) persistent vomiting with failure to thrive, (2) esophagitis or esophageal stricture, and (3) apneic spells or chronic pulmonary disease unresponsive to 2–3 months of medical therapy. Children older than age 18 months, children with large hiatal hernias, and neurologically handicapped children respond less well to medical therapy.

Rudolph CD et al: Guidelines for evaluation and treatment of gastroesophageal reflux in infants and children: Recommendations of the North American Society for Pediatric Gastroenterology and Nutrition. J Pediatr Gastroenterol Nutr 2001;23(Suppl):1.

## ACHALASIA OF THE ESOPHAGUS

Esophageal achalasia is characterized by failure of relaxation of the lower esophageal sphincter in response to swallowing and abnormal, nonperistaltic motor activity in the esophageal body.

## Clinical Findings

### A. SYMPTOMS AND SIGNS

Achalasia is uncommon in children younger than age 5 years. Typical symptoms include retrosternal pain and episodes of food "sticking" in the throat or upper chest. Patients eat slowly and often drink large amounts of fluid with meals. Dysphagia is relieved by repeated forceful swallowing or by vomiting. Familial cases have been described in patients with Allgrove syndrome (alacrima, adrenal insufficiency, and achalasia) and in patients with familial dysautonomia. Chronic cough, wheezing, recurrent pneumonitis, anemia, and weight loss may occur.

### B. IMAGING AND MANOMETRIC STUDIES

The barium esophagagram shows a dilated esophagus with a short, tapered "beak" at the distal end. In infants, esophageal dilation may not be present. Cinefluoroscopy may show very disordered esophageal peristalsis. Esophageal manometry may show high resting pressure in the lower esophageal sphincter, failure of the sphincter to relax with swallowing, and abnormal or absent esophageal peristalsis. The cause is unknown. Decrease in neuronal nitric oxide synthetase (nNOS) in the area of the lower esophageal sphincter causes a local deficiency of nitric oxide, preventing normal sphincter relaxation. It is unclear whether the lack of nNOS is secondary or primary to achalasia. In acquired achalasia associated with Chagas' disease, nNOS is also reduced, and ganglion cells may be decreased or absent in the muscular esophagus near the lower esophageal sphincter.

### Differential Diagnosis

Congenital esophageal stricture, esophageal webs, peptic stricture secondary to chronic reflux, and esophageal masses may mimic esophageal achalasia. Intestinal pseudo-obstruction, multiple endocrine neoplasia IIb, systemic amyloidosis, and postvagotomy syndrome also cause esophageal dysmotility and symptoms similar to achalasia.

### Treatment & Prognosis

Pneumatic dilation of the lower esophageal sphincter is of value in most cases and can be repeated if symptoms recur. Botulinum toxin injected into the lower esophageal sphincter may be effective temporarily. More definitive results can be achieved by surgically splitting the lower esophageal sphincter muscle (Heller myotomy), a procedure that can be performed laparoscopically or thoracoscopically. Because of the shorter duration of esophageal obstruction in children, the prognosis for return of some normal esophageal motor function after surgery is better in pediatric patients than in adults.

Hussain SZ et al: A review of achalasia in 33 children. Dig Dis Sci 2002;47:2538 [PMID: 12452392].

## CAUSTIC BURNS OF THE ESOPHAGUS

Ingestion of caustic solids or liquids (pH > 12.0) may produce esophageal lesions ranging from superficial inflammation to coagulative necrosis with ulceration, perforation, and mediastinitis (or peritonitis if the stomach is involved). The severity of the oral or laryngeal lesions after ingestion does not correlate well with the degree of esophageal injury. Esophageal or laryngeal obstruction secondary to edema and exudate formation occurs within 24 hours. Pain may be severe. Strictures of the esophagus may develop quickly, or gradually over several months. Esophageal strictures develop in areas of anatomic narrowing such as the thoracic inlet, the GE junction, and at the point where the left bronchus crosses the esophagus. Stricture occurs only with full-thickness esophageal necrosis. Short circumferential strictures may occur, or the entire esophagus may become twisted and narrowed. Shortening of the esophagus may lead to hiatal hernia.

The lips, mouth, and airway should be carefully examined in any child with suspected alkali ingestion. Drooling is common. Oral lesions are especially common with solid agents. Vomiting should not be induced. Give intravenous corticosteroids (eg, methylprednisolone, 1–2 mg/kg/d) immediately to reduce oral cavity swelling and laryngeal edema. Intravenous fluids may be necessary if dysphagia is present. Esophagoscopy should be done within 24–48 hours after ingestion.

Treatment may be stopped if only first-degree burns are present. Corticosteroids may be beneficial in first- and second-degree burns, but are not likely to prevent stricture formation from third-degree burns. Repeated esophageal dilations may be necessary as a stricture develops but are not performed acutely. When radiographs show erosion into the mediastinum or peritoneum, antibiotics are mandatory. Intraluminal esophageal stenting may be beneficial during early management. Surgical replacement of the esophagus with a segment of colon or with a gastric tube may be necessary if dilation fails to control stricture.

Although other ingestants (eg, bleach, detergents, acids) may cause esophageal irritation, it is rare for any but the strongest acids and detergents to produce full-thickness necrosis and stricture.

Del Rosario JF, Orenstein SR: Common pediatric esophageal disorders. Gastroenterologist 1998;6:104.

## HIATAL HERNIA

Hiatal hernias are classified as (1) paraesophageal, in which the esophagus and GE junction are normally placed with the gastric cardia herniated beside the esophagus through the diaphragmatic hiatus; or (2) sliding, in which the GE junction and a portion of the proximal stomach are herniated through the esophageal hiatus. Paraesophageal hernia is rare in childhood and presents with pain, esophageal obstruction, or respiratory compromise. The most common situation in which a paraesophageal hernia occurs is in patients with previous fundoplication. Sliding hernia is common in children. GE reflux may accompany sliding hiatal hernia, although many cause no symptoms. Surgical correction of paraesophageal or hiatus hernia is indicated if symptoms persist in spite of medical treatment.

# PYLORIC STENOSIS

The cause of postnatal pyloric circular muscle hypertrophy leading to gastric outlet obstruction is unknown. The incidence is 1–8:1000 births, with a 4:1 male predominance. A positive family history is present in 13% of patients. Recent studies suggest that erythromycin therapy may be associated with development of pyloric stenosis in infants younger than 30 days.

## Clinical Findings

### A. SYMPTOMS AND SIGNS

Vomiting usually begins between ages 2 and 4 weeks and rapidly becomes projectile after every feeding; vomiting starts at birth in about 10% of cases. Onset of symptoms may be delayed in premature infants. The vomitus is rarely bilious but may be blood-streaked. The infant is hungry and nurses avidly. Constipation, dehydration, weight loss, fretfulness, and finally apathy occur. The upper abdomen may be distended after feeding, and prominent gastric peristaltic waves from left to right may be seen. An olive-sized mass can be felt on deep palpation in the right upper abdomen, especially after the child has vomited.

### B. LABORATORY FINDINGS

Hypochloremic alkalosis with potassium depletion occurs. Hemoconcentration is reflected by elevated hemoglobin and hematocrit values. Elevated unconjugated bilirubin occurs in 2–5% of cases.

### C. IMAGING

An upper GI series reveals gastric retention of contrast and an elongated narrowed pyloric channel with a double tract of barium. Many normal infants have some delay in gastric emptying during upper GI series due to pylorospasm. This by itself is insufficient to make a diagnosis of pyloric stenosis. The enlarged pyloric muscle causes characteristic semilunar impressions on the gastric antrum. Ultrasonography shows a hypoechoic ring with a hyperdense center. Thickness of circular muscle is greater than 4 mm in pyloric stenosis.

## Treatment & Prognosis

Pyloromyotomy is the treatment of choice and consists of incision down to the mucosa along the pyloric length. The procedure can be performed laparoscopically. To prevent complications during surgery, it is imperative first to resolve hydration and electrolyte abnormalities even if it takes 24–48 hours.

The outlook is excellent following surgery. Patients often vomit postoperatively as a consequence of gastritis, esophagitis, or associated GE reflux. The postoperative barium radiograph remains abnormal despite relief of symptoms.

Fugimoto T et al: Laparoscopic extramucosal pyloromyotomy versus open pyloromyotomy for infantile hypertrophic pyloric stenosis: Which is better? J Pediatr Surg 1999;34:370.

Mahon BE et al: Maternal and infant use of erythromycin and other macrolide antibiotics as risk factors for infantile hypertrophic pyloric stenosis. J Pediatr 2001;139:380.

# PEPTIC DISEASE

Peptic ulcers occur at any age but are more common between ages 12 and 18 years. Boys are affected more frequently than girls. Most ulcers in childhood are secondary to underlying illness, toxin, or a drug causing breakdown in normal mucosal defense, permitting acid peptic digestion of gastric or duodenal mucosa. Causes include (1) reduced mucosal protective mechanisms (aspirin, nonsteroidal anti-inflammatory drugs [NSAIDs], hypoxia); (2) reduced metabolic activity of the mucosal cell, which allows for diffusion of hydrogen ions into the mucosa (hypoxia, hypotension); (3) increased secretion of acid or pepsin (increased parietal cell mass, increased postprandial secretion of gastrin, increased vagal tone); (4) reflux of bile from duodenum to stomach; and (5) decreased neutralizing activity in duodenal secretions.

A close association exists between *Helicobacter pylori* infection of the gastric antrum and nodular antral gastritis, duodenal ulcer, and gastric ulcer. There is no evidence that *H pylori* infection causes recurrent abdominal pain of childhood or dyspepsia without gastritis. *H pylori* antibody positivity is found in 10–20% of healthy North American children. It tends to increase with age. The prevalence is higher in areas with poor sanitation and contaminated water supply and is higher in families with an antibody-positive member. Diagnosis of *H pylori* infection is made by seeing organisms in gastric antral tissue, testing antral tissue for bacterial urease activity, or using the urease breath test. Serum antibody positivity does not prove active *H pylori* infection.

## Clinical Findings

### A. SYMPTOMS AND SIGNS

In children younger than age 6 years, vomiting and upper GI bleeding are the most common manifestations of peptic ulcer disease. Older children are more likely to complain of abdominal pain. Acute *H pylori* infection with gastritis is characterized by vomiting and often by hematemesis. Large ulcers in the pyloric channel may cause gastric outlet obstruction. Acute illnesses responsible for secondary ulcers include central nervous system disease, burns, sepsis, and multiorgan system failure. Chronic conditions such as pulmonary insufficiency, Crohn disease, hepatic cirrhosis, and rheumatoid arthritis are associated with peptic disease. Upper GI bleeding requiring transfusion is more commonly seen in secondary ulcers, particularly following ingestion of aspirin, alcohol, and NSAIDs, than in primary ulcer disease. Ulcers may occur throughout the upper GI tract secondary to NSAIDs. The use of specific cyclooxygenase-2 (COX-2) inhibitors (celecoxib [Celebrex], rofecoxib [Vioxx]) instead of the standard NSAIDs and aspirin—which inhibit both COX-1 and COX-2 enzymes—may result in a decrease in NSAID-associated complications. COX-1 regulates the production of thromboxane from arachidonic acid and thus decreases platelet aggregation with a resultant increase in bleeding tendency. COX-2, an inducible enzyme present in many tissues, regulates prostaglandin synthesis. COX-2 inhibition has a purer anti-inflammatory and analgesic effect with a reduced tendency to produce GI complications.

### B. IMAGING AND ENDOSCOPY

An upper GI radiograph may show an ulcer crater. Soft signs of peptic disease, such as duodenal spasticity and irregularity, which are suggestive of ulcer in adults, are often seen in healthy children and are not reliable indicators of peptic disease. Upper intestinal endoscopy is the most accurate diagnostic test for peptic disease. It also allows for identification of other causes of peptic symptoms such as esophagitis, eosinophilic enteropathy, and celiac disease.

## Treatment

Acid suppression or neutralization is the mainstay of peptic ulcer therapy. Liquid antacids are usually unacceptable to children in the volumes needed to neutralize gastric acid. H2-receptor antagonists and proton pump inhibitors are more effective and usually produce endoscopic healing in 4–8 weeks. Bland "ulcer diets" are not indicated in children. Foods that cause pain should be avoided. Caffeine should be avoided because it increases gastric acid secretion. Aspirin and NSAIDs should not be used.

Treatment of the peptic disease associated with *H pylori* infection requires eradication of the organism. The optimal therapeutic regimen is still undetermined. The combination of amoxicillin, metronidazole, and bismuth subsalicylate for 10–14 days and omeprazole and amoxicillin, are both effective. Clarithromycin for 7 days with a proton pump inhibitor for 6 weeks is also effective.

Chang HY et al: Knowledge, attitudes and practice styles of North American pediatric gastroenterologists: *Helicobacter pylori* infection. J Pediatr Gastroenterol Nutr 2003;36:235 [PMID: 1254860].

Czinn S et al: Research agenda for pediatric gastroenterology, hepatology and nutrition: Acid peptic diseases: Report of the North American Society for Gastroenterology, Hepatology, and Nutrition for the Children's Digestive Health and Nutrition Foundation. J Pediatr Gastroenterol Nutr 2003; 35(Suppl 3) 250.

McCarthy DM: Nonsteroidal anti-inflammatory drugs: Reducing the risks to the gastrointestinal tract. Clin Perspect Gastroenterol 1999;2:219.

Suerbaum S, Michetti P: *Helicobacter pylori* infection. N Engl J Med 2002;347:1175 [PMID: 12374879].

## CONGENITAL DIAPHRAGMATIC HERNIA

Diaphragmatic hernia may be secondary to a posterolateral defect in the diaphragm (foramen of Bochdalek) or, in about 5% of cases, to a retrosternal defect (foramen of Morgagni). It represents failure of division of the thoracic and abdominal cavities at the 8th to 10th week of fetal life. All degrees of protrusion of the abdominal viscera through the diaphragmatic opening may occur. Eighty percent of posterolateral defects involve the left diaphragm. In eventration of the diaphragm, a leaf of the diaphragm with hypoplastic muscular elements balloons into the chest and leads to similar but milder symptoms.

Mild to severe respiratory distress is usually present at birth. The abdomen may be scaphoid because of displacement of the viscera. Breath sounds in the affected hemithorax are absent, with displacement of the point of maximal cardiac impulse. Thirty percent of newborn infants with diaphragmatic hernia die, mostly from pulmonary insufficiency. The lung on the affected side and also on the contralateral side may be hypoplastic, with decreased generations of airways, lymphatics, and pulmonary vessels. Pulmonary hypertension is present. Other complications include mediastinal shift with vascular kinking, pulmonary infection, prematurity, cardiac anomalies, and intestinal malrotation. Extracorporeal membrane oxygenation may decrease the early postoperative mortality rate in patients with poor lung compliance. Inhaled nitric oxide reduces pulmonary vascular hypertension, and it was hoped that its use might improve the outcome in patients with diaphragmatic hernia. Results in controlled trials have thus far been disappointing. Occasionally, a diaphragmatic hernia is first identified in an older infant or child by an incidental radiograph or routine physical examination. These children usually have a more favorable prognosis than diaphragmatic hernias identified at birth.

## CONGENITAL DUODENAL OBSTRUCTION

Extrinsic duodenal obstruction is usually due to congenital peritoneal bands associated with intestinal malrotation, annular pancreas, or duodenal duplication. Intrinsic obstruction is a result of stenosis, mucosal diaphragm (so-called wind sock deformity), or duodenal atresia. The duodenal lumen may be obliterated by a membrane or completely interrupted with a fibrous cord between the two segments. Atresia is more often distal than proximal to the ampulla of Vater.

### Clinical Findings

#### A. ATRESIA

A history of polyhydramnios is common. Vomiting (usually bile-stained) and epigastric distention begin within a few hours of birth. Meconium may be passed normally. Duodenal atresia is commonly associated with other congenital anomalies (30%), including esophageal atresia, other intestinal atresias, and cardiac and renal anomalies. Prematurity (25–50%) and Down syndrome (20–30%) are associated conditions. Abdominal radiographs show gaseous distention of the stomach and proximal duodenum (the "double-bubble" radiologic sign). With protracted vomiting, less air may be in the stomach. Absence of gas distal to the obstruction suggests atresia or an extrinsic obstruction severe enough to completely occlude the lumen, whereas air scattered over the lower abdomen may indicate a partial duodenal obstruction. A barium enema may be helpful in determining the presence of malrotation or atresia lower in the GI tract.

#### B. DUODENAL STENOSIS

Obvious symptoms of duodenal obstruction may be delayed for weeks or years. Although the stenotic area is usually beyond the ampulla of Vater, the vomitus does not always contain bile.

### Treatment & Prognosis

Duodenoduodenostomy is performed to bypass stenosis or atresia. Thorough exploration is necessary to ensure that no additional anomalies are present lower in the GI tract. The mortality rate is significantly increased in infants with prematurity, Down syndrome, and associated congenital anomalies. Duodenal dilation and hypomotility resulting from antenatal obstruction may cause functional obstructive symptoms even after surgical treatment.

## CONGENITAL INTESTINAL ATRESIAS & STENOSES

Excluding anal anomalies, intestinal atresia and stenosis account for one third of all cases of neonatal intestinal obstruction. Antenatal ultrasound can identify intestinal atresia in utero, and polyhydramnios occurs in most affected pregnancies. Prematurity and other congenital anomalies may be present. The localization and relative incidence of atresias and stenoses are listed in Table 20–2.

Failure to pass meconium, bile-stained vomiting, and abdominal distention usually begin in the first 48 hours of life. Atresias, stenoses, and obstructing membranes may affect multiple sites. The small intestine may be shortened significantly. Radiographic features include dilated loops of small bowel and absence of colonic gas. Barium enema reveals narrow-caliber microcolon if the atresia is in the lower small bowel. In over 10% of cases of intestinal atresia, the mesentery is absent, and the superior mesenteric artery cannot be identified beyond the origin of the right colic and ileocolic arteries. The ileum coils around one of these two arteries, giving rise to the so-called Christmas tree de-

**Table 20–2.** Localization and relative frequency of congenital gastrointestinal atresias and stenoses.

| | Area Involved | Type of Lesion | Relative Frequency |
|---|---|---|---|
| Pylorus | | Atresia; web or diaphragm | 1% |
| Duodenum | 80% are distal to the ampulla of Vater | Atresia, stenosis; web or diaphragm | 45% |
| Jejunoileal | Proximal jejunum and distal ileum | Atresia (multiple in 6–29%); stenosis | 50% |
| Colon | Left colon and rectum | Atresia (usually associated with atresias of the small bowel) | 5–9% |

formity. The tenuous blood supply often compromises surgical anastomoses. The differential diagnosis includes Hirschsprung disease, paralytic ileus secondary to sepsis, gastroenteritis or pneumonia, midgut volvulus, and meconium ileus. Surgery is mandatory. Postoperative complications include short bowel syndrome and hypomotility secondary to antenatal obstruction and proximal bowel dilation.

## ANNULAR PANCREAS

Annular pancreas results when rotation and fusion of the dorsal and ventral pancreatic anlagen is incomplete. The condition presents with symptoms of partial or complete duodenal obstruction. Down syndrome and congenital anomalies of the GI tract occur frequently. Polyhydramnios is common. Clinical manifestations can develop late in childhood when the obstruction is less than complete. Treatment consists of duodenoduodenostomy or duodenojejunostomy without operative dissection or division of the pancreatic annulus.

## INTESTINAL MALROTATION WITH OR WITHOUT VOLVULUS

The midgut, which extends from the duodenojejunal junction to the mid transverse colon, is supplied by the superior mesenteric artery, which runs in the root of the mesentery. During gestation, the midgut elongates into the umbilical sac, returning to the intra-abdominal position during the tenth week of gestation. The root of the mesentery rotates in a counterclockwise direction during retraction. This causes the colon to cross the abdominal cavity ventrally; the cecum to move from the left to the right lower quadrant, and the duodenum to cross dorsally and become partly retroperitoneal. When this rotation is incomplete, the dorsal fixation of the mesentery is defective and shortened, so that the bowel from the ligament of Treitz to the mid transverse colon may twist, causing a volvulus around the narrow mesenteric root and occluding the superior mesenteric artery.

### Clinical Findings

#### A. SYMPTOMS AND SIGNS

Malrotation accounts for 10% of neonatal intestinal obstructions. Most infants present with recurrent bile-stained vomiting or acute small-bowel obstruction in the first 3 weeks of life. Intrauterine volvulus has been reported. The neonate may present with ascites. Later in life signs of intermittent intestinal obstruction, malabsorption, protein-losing enteropathy, or diarrhea may be present. Associated congenital anomalies, especially cardiac manifestations, occur in over 25% of symptomatic patients.

#### B. IMAGING

An upper GI series shows the duodenojejunal junction on the right side of the spine along with the jejunal loops. The diagnosis of malrotation can be further confirmed by barium enema, which may demonstrate a mobile cecum located in the midline, right upper quadrant, or left abdomen.

### Treatment & Prognosis

The surgical treatment of malrotation is the Ladd procedure, in which the duodenum is mobilized and the short mesenteric root is extended. Midgut volvulus is a surgical emergency. Bowel necrosis results from occlusion of the superior mesenteric artery. When necrosis is extensive, it is recommended that a first operation include only reduction of the volvulus with lysis of mesenteric bands. Resection of necrotic bowel should be delayed if possible until a second-look operation 24–48 hours later can be undertaken in the hope that more bowel can be salvaged. The prognosis is guarded if perforation, peritonitis, or extensive intestinal necrosis is present. Treatment of malrotation discovered in children older than age 12 months is uncertain. Because volvulus can occur at any age, surgical repair is usually recommended, even in asymptomatic children. Laparoscopic repair of malrotation is possible but may be technically difficult and is never performed in the presence of volvulus.

### Complications

If bowel necrosis is extensive, the infant with malrotation and volvulus may be left with an intestine of insufficient length to support normal absorption and growth—the so-called short bowel syndrome. Estimates of the small-bowel length of a newborn range from 150 to 300 cm. The commonly accepted definition of neonatal short bowel syndrome is less than 50% of the small intestinal length remaining after resection. In these patients, it is almost certain that intravenous nutrition will be required for months to years to support growth. The most common causes of short bowel syndrome in the newborn vary with the patient referral patterns of the institution, but include necrotizing enterocolitis (45%), intestinal atresias (23%), gastroschisis (15%), volvulus (15%), and, less commonly, entities such as congenital short bowel and extensive Hirschsprung disease. Although the remaining intestine does not experience a compensatory increase in length, if nutrition can be maintained, the enterocytes will proliferate on lengthened villi, and over time, the intestine will elongate in proportion to the child's increasing height and eventually may be sufficient for the patient's nutritional needs. Achieving independence from intravenous nutrition becomes less likely when the remaining intestine measures less than 30 cm. The presence of an intact colon is a factor improving the chances of independence from intravenous nutrition. Liver failure, a consequence of intravenous nutrition and recurrent infection, among other causes, is the most common cause of death in patients with short bowel syndrome. The mortality rate among all infants with short bowel syndrome is about 10–15%.

Adzick NS, Nance ML: Pediatric surgery: First of two parts. N Engl J Med 2000;342:1651.

Adzick NS, Nance ML: Pediatric surgery: Second of two parts. N Engl J Med 2000;342:1726.

Andorsky DJ et al: Nutritional and other post operative management of neonates with short bowel syndrome correlates with clinical outcomes. J Pediatr 2001;139:27.

Sigalet DL: Short bowel syndrome in infants and children, an overview. Semin Pediatr Surg 2001;10:49.

# MECKEL DIVERTICULUM & OMPHALOMESENTERIC DUCT REMNANTS

## 1. Meckel Diverticulum

Meckel diverticulum is the most common of the omphalomesenteric duct remnants. It is usually found on the antimesenteric border of the mid to distal ileum. It is present in 1.5% of the population but rarely causes symptoms. In addition to the ileal mucosa, diverticula may contain gastric, pancreatic, jejunal, or colonic mucosa. Familial cases have been reported. Complications occur three times more frequently in males than in females and in 50–60% of cases within the first 2 years of life. Acid secreted by heterotopic gastric tissue causes ulceration and bleeding from adjacent ileal mucosa.

### Clinical Findings

#### A. SYMPTOMS AND SIGNS

In 40–60% of symptomatic patients, painless passage of maroon or melanotic blood per rectum occurs. Acute bleeding may cause shock. Occult bleeding is less common. Intestinal obstruction occurs in 25% of symptomatic patients as a result of ileocolonic intussusception. Intestinal volvulus may occur around a fibrous remnant of the vitelline duct extending from the tip of the diverticulum to the abdominal wall. In some patients, entrapment of a bowel loop under a band running between the diverticulum and the base of the mesentery occurs. The diverticulum may be trapped in an inguinal hernia (Littre hernia). Diverticulitis occurs in 10–20% of symptomatic patients and is clinically indistinguishable from acute appendicitis. Perforation and general-

ized peritonitis may occur. Chronic recurrent abdominal pain may rarely be the only symptom.

#### B. IMAGING

Diagnosis of Meckel diverticulum is seldom made on barium radiograph. Radionuclide imaging uses $^{99m}$Tc pertechnetate, which is taken up by the heterotopic gastric mucosa in the diverticulum. Stimulation of $^{99m}$Tc pertechnetate uptake and retention of radionuclide by the heterotopic gastric mucosa by pentagastrin or cimetidine can reduce the number of false-negative results. Angiography or tagged red cell scan may be useful when bleeding is brisk.

### Treatment & Prognosis

Treatment is surgical. At laparoscopy or laparotomy, the ileum proximal and distal to the diverticulum may reveal ulcerations and heterotopic tissue adjacent to the neck of the diverticulum. The prognosis for Meckel diverticulum is good. Marked hemorrhage may occur but is rarely exsanguinating.

## 2. Other Remnants of the Omphalomesenteric Duct

Fecal discharge from the umbilicus is evidence of a patent omphalomesenteric duct. The duct may be completely closed, causing a fibrous cord joining ileum and umbilicus and potentially the origin of a volvulus. A mucoid umbilical discharge may be indicative of a mucocele, which can protrude through the umbilicus and be mistaken for an umbilical granuloma because it is firm and bright red. In all cases, surgical excision of the omphalomesenteric remnant is indicated.

# DUPLICATIONS OF THE GASTROINTESTINAL TRACT

Duplications are congenital anomalies of the GI tract. They are fluid-filled, spherical, or tubular structures found anywhere along the GI tract, most commonly in the ileum. Duplications usually contain fluid and sometimes blood if necrosis has taken place. Most duplications do not communicate with the intestinal lumen but are attached to the mesenteric side of the gut and share a common muscular coat. The epithelial lining of the duplication is usually of the same type as that from which it originates. Some duplications (neuroenteric cysts) are attached to the spinal cord and are associated with hemivertebrae and anterior or posterior spina bifida.

Symptoms of vomiting, abdominal distention, colicky pain, rectal bleeding, partial or total intestinal obstruction, or an abdominal mass may start in infancy.

Diarrhea and malabsorption may result from bacterial overgrowth in communicating duplications. Physical examination reveals a rounded, smooth, movable mass, and radiographic films of the abdomen show a noncalcified mass displacing the intestines or stomach. Scanning with $^{99m}$Tc pertechnetate is useful in duplications containing gastric mucosa. Involvement of the terminal small bowel can give rise to an intussusception. Prompt surgical treatment is indicated.

# CONGENITAL AGANGLIONIC MEGACOLON (HIRSCHSPRUNG DISEASE)

Hirschsprung disease results from an absence of ganglion cells in the mucosal and muscular layers of the colon. Neural crest cells fail to migrate to the mesodermal layers, possibly mediated by abnormalities in endorgan cell surface receptors or local deficiency of nitric oxide synthesis. The rectum alone (30%) or the rectosigmoid (44%) is usually affected. The entire colon is aganglionic in 8% of patients. Segmental aganglionosis is very rare and may be an acquired lesion. The aganglionic segment is of normal caliber or slightly narrowed, with dilation of the normal colon proximal to the aganglionic segment. The mucosa of the dilated colonic segment may become thin and inflamed (enterocolitis), resulting in diarrhea, bleeding, and protein loss.

A familial pattern has been described, particularly in total colonic aganglionosis. The disease is four times more common in boys than in girls, and 10–15% of patients have Down syndrome. Mutations in the *ret* proto-oncogene are recognized in a significant proportion of familial and sporadic cases.

## Clinical Findings

### A. SYMPTOMS AND SIGNS

Failure of the newborn to pass meconium—followed by vomiting, abdominal distention, and reluctance to feed—suggests the diagnosis of Hirschsprung disease. Infants of diabetic mothers may demonstrate symptoms of apparent intestinal obstruction and failure to pass meconium at birth. In this setting, small left colon syndrome should be suspected. Meglumine diatrizoate (Gastrograffin) enema is both diagnostic and therapeutic as it reveals a meconium plug in the left colon, which is often passed during the diagnostic radiograph. The left colon is narrow but usually functional. In a small proportion of these patients, Hirschsprung disease may later be found. In some patients with Hirschsprung disease, symptoms of distention and vomiting appear later. Bouts of enterocolitis manifested

by fever, explosive diarrhea, and prostration are reported in about 50% of newborns with this disease. These episodes may lead to acute inflammatory and ischemic changes in the colon, with perforation (especially cecal) and sepsis. In later infancy, alternating obstipation and diarrhea predominate. The older child is more likely to present with constipation. The stools are foul-smelling and ribbon-like, the abdomen enlarged, and the veins prominent; peristaltic patterns are readily visible, and fecal masses are palpable. Intermittent bouts of intestinal obstruction due to fecal impaction, hypochromic anemia, hypoproteinemia, and failure to thrive are common. Encopresis occurs rarely.

On digital examination, the anal canal and rectum are devoid of fecal material despite fecal impaction obvious on abdominal examination or radiograph. If the aganglionic segment is short, there may be a gush of flatus and stool as the finger is withdrawn.

### B. LABORATORY FINDINGS

Ganglion cells are absent in both the submucosal and muscular layers of the involved bowel. Special stains may show nerve trunk hypertrophy and increased acetylcholinesterase activity. Ganglionated bowel above the aganglionic segment may be characterized by abnormal location and proliferation of ganglion cells. This finding—intestinal neuronal dysplasia—is sometimes associated with motor dysfunction that may result in poor motor function of the unresected intestine. A family history of Hirschsprung disease may be present in 5% of patients.

### C. IMAGING

Radiographic examination of the abdomen may reveal dilated proximal colon and absence of gas in the pelvic colon. A barium enema using a catheter with the tip inserted barely beyond the anal sphincter usually demonstrates the narrowed segment distally with a sharp transition to proximal dilated colon. A transition zone may not be seen in neonates since the normal proximal bowel has not had time to become dilated. Retention of barium for 24–48 hours is not diagnostic of Hirschsprung disease, because it also occurs in retentive constipation. Retention of barium for 24 hours is a more reliable sign in neonates.

### D. SPECIAL EXAMINATIONS

Failure of reflex relaxation of the internal anal sphincter muscle after balloon distention of the rectum occurs in all patients with Hirschsprung disease, regardless of the length of the aganglionic segment. In occasional patients, a nonrelaxing internal anal sphincter is the only abnormality. This condition is often called "ultrashort segment Hirschsprung disease."

## Differential Diagnosis

Hirschsprung disease accounts for 15–20% of cases of neonatal intestinal obstruction. In childhood, this disease must be differentiated from retentive constipation. In older infants and children it can be confused with celiac disease because of the striking abdominal distention and failure to thrive.

## Treatment

Treatment is surgical. Initially, diverting colostomy (or ileostomy) is performed proximal to the aganglionic segment. Resection of the aganglionic segment may be postponed until the infant is at least age 6 months. At the time of definitive surgery, the transition zone between ganglionated and nonganglionated bowel is identified. Aganglionic bowel is resected, and a pull-through of ganglionated bowel to the preanal rectal remnant is made. Several surgical techniques, including laparoscopic pull-through, are in use. In children with ultrashort segment disease, an internal anal sphincter myotomy or botulinum toxin injection of the internal anal sphincter may suffice to control symptoms.

## Prognosis

Complications following surgery include chronic constipation, fecal incontinence, anastomotic breakdown, or anastomotic stricture. Postoperative obstruction may result from inadvertent retention of a distal aganglionic colon segment or postoperative destruction of ganglion cells secondary to vascular impairment. Neuronal dysplasia of the remaining bowel may result in a pseudo-obstruction syndrome. Enterocolitis occurs postoperatively in 15% of patients.

Kubota M et al: External anal sphincter dysfunction and postoperative bowel habits in patients with Hirschsprung's disease. J Pediatr Surg 1997;32:22.

Wartiovaara K et al: Hirschsprung's disease genes and the development of the enteric nervous system. Ann Med 1998;30:66.

# CHYLOUS ASCITES

In the neonate, chylous ascites may be due to congenital infection or developmental abnormality of the lymphatic system (intestinal lymphangiectasia). If the thoracic duct is involved, chylothorax may be present. Later in life, chylous ascites may result from congenital lymphangiectasia, retroperitoneal or lymphatic tumors, peritoneal bands, abdominal trauma, or infection, or it may occur after cardiac or abdominal surgery. It may be associated with intestinal malrotation.

## Clinical Findings

### A. SYMPTOMS AND SIGNS

In both congenital and acquired lymphatic obstruction, chylous ascites, diarrhea, and failure to thrive are noted. The abdomen is distended, with a fluid wave and shifting dullness. Unilateral or generalized peripheral edema may be present.

### B. LABORATORY FINDINGS

Laboratory findings include hypoalbuminemia, hypogammaglobulinemia, and lymphopenia. Ascitic fluid contains lymphocytes and has the biochemical composition of chyle if the patient has just been fed; otherwise, it is indistinguishable from ascites secondary to cirrhosis.

## Differential Diagnosis

Chylous ascites must be differentiated from ascites due to liver failure and, in the older child, from constrictive pericarditis and neoplastic, infectious, or inflammatory diseases causing lymphatic obstruction.

## Complications & Sequelae

Chylous ascites from intestinal lymphatic obstruction is associated with fat malabsorption protein loss. Chronic intestinal loss of albumin and γ-globulin may lead to edema and increase the risk of infection. Rapidly accumulating chylous ascites may cause respiratory complications. The primary infections and malignancies causing chylous ascites may be life-rhreatening.

## Treatment & Prognosis

Little can be done to correct congenital abnormalities due to hypoplasia, aplasia, or ectasia of the lymphatics. Treatment is supportive, consisting mainly of a very high protein diet and careful attention to infections. Shunting of peritoneal fluid into the venous system is sometimes effective. A fat-free diet supplemented with medium-chain triglycerides decreases the formation of chylous ascitic fluid. Total parenteral nutrition may be necessary. In the neonate, congenital chylous ascites may spontaneously disappear following one or more paracenteses and a medium-chain triglyceride diet.

Chye JK et al: Neonatal chylosis ascites: Report of 3 cases and review of the literature. Pediatr Surg Int 1997;12:296.

# CONGENITAL ANORECTAL ANOMALIES

Anorectal anomalies occur once in every 3000–4000 births, and most types are more common in males. Inspection of the perianal area is an essential part of the newborn physical examination.

## Classification & Presentation

### A. ANTERIOR DISPLACEMENT OF THE ANUS

This anomaly is more common in girls than boys. It may be associated with a posterior rectal shelf and usually is characterized by constipation and straining with stool. The diagnosis of an anteriorly displaced anus depends on finding the anus located close to the base of the scrotum or vaginal fourchette. If the center of the anus is located less than 33% of the total distance from vaginal fourchette (or base of scrotum) to coccyx, there is a high likelihood of difficulty with defecation.

### B. ANAL STENOSIS

In anal stenosis, the anal aperture may be very small and filled with a dot of meconium. Defecation is difficult, and there may be ribbon-like stools, passage of blood and mucus per rectum, fecal impaction, and abdominal distention. This malformation accounts for about 10% of cases of anorectal anomalies. This anomaly may not be apparent at birth and may be discovered on rectal examination of the infant who is straining at stool.

### C. IMPERFORATE ANAL MEMBRANE

The infant with an imperforate anal membrane fails to pass meconium, and a greenish bulging membrane is seen in the anal aperture. After excision, bowel and sphincter function are normal.

### D. ANAL AGENESIS

In the child with anal agenesis, an anal dimple is present, and stimulation of the perianal area leads to puckering, indicating that the external sphincter is present. If no associated rectoperineal fistula is present, intestinal obstruction occurs. Fistulas may also be vulvar in the female and urethral in the male.

### E. ANORECTAL AGENESIS

Anorectal agenesis accounts for 75% of total anorectal anomalies. Fistulas are almost invariably present. In the female, they may be vaginal or may enter a urogenital sinus, which is a common passageway for the urethra and vagina. In the male, fistulas are rectovesical or rectourethral. Associated major congenital malformations are common. Sacral defects and absence of internal and external anal sphincters are common.

## Radiologic Findings

Careful radiologic evaluation is indicated immediately so that the anal anomaly and the extent of associated anomalies of the bowel and the urogenital tract can be identified.

## Treatment & Prognosis

Dilation of the anus should be undertaken in cases of anal stenosis. Treatment for imperforate anal membrane consists of excision of the membrane and dilation. Diverting colostomy is necessary in anorectal agenesis. In patients with anal agenesis and a visible perineal fistula of sufficient size to pass meconium, surgery can be deferred. Males without a visible fistula may have a urethral fistula, and diverting colostomy is recommended.

Of the patients with low imperforate anus, 80–90% are continent after surgery; of those with high imperforate anus, only 30% achieve continence. Gracilis muscle transplants may improve continence. Levatorplasty may also be used as a secondary operation following surgery for anorectal agenesis. Antegrade continence enema procedures may allow for continence in children without anal sphincter function by facilitating irrigation of the colon via a cecostomy or appendicostomy.

Endo M et al: Analysis of 1992 patients with anorectal malformations over the past two decades in Japan. J Pediatr Surg 1999;34:435.

## ACUTE ABDOMEN

Entities causing acute abdomen are shown in Table 20–3. Some of the specific entities are discussed in subsequent sections. Reaching a speedy and accurate diagnosis in the patient with an acute abdomen is critical and requires skill in physical diagnosis, intimate acquaintance with the characteristic symptoms of a large number of conditions, and the judicious selection of laboratory and radiologic tests.

Gauderer MW: Acute abdomen. When to operate immediately and when to observe. Semin Pediatr Surg 1997;6:74.

## PERITONITIS

Primary bacterial peritonitis accounts for less than 2% of pediatric cases of peritonitis. The most common organisms responsible are *Escherichia coli,* other enteric organisms, hemolytic streptococci, and pneumococci. Primary peritonitis occurs in patients with splenectomy, splenic dysfunction, or ascites (nephrotic syndrome, advanced liver disease, kwashiorkor). It occurs also in infants with pyelonephritis or pneumonia. Secondary peritonitis is associated with peritoneal dialysis, penetrating abdominal trauma, or a ruptured viscus. The organisms associated with secondary peritonitis vary depending on the cause. In association with peri-

**Table 20–3.** Etiologic classification of acute abdomen.

| Mechanical Obstruction | | Inflammatory Diseases and Infections | | | |
|---|---|---|---|---|---|
| Intraluminal Obstruction | Extraluminal Obstruction | Gastrointestinal Disease | Paralytic Ileus | Blunt Trauma | Miscellaneous |
| Foreign body | Hernia | Appendicitis | Sepsis | Accident | Lead poisoning |
| Bezoar | Intussusception | Crohn disease | Pneumonia | Battered child | Sickle cell crisis |
| Fecalith | Volvulus | Ulcerative colitis | Pyelonephritis | syndrome | Familial Mediterra- |
| Gallstone | Duplication | Henoch–Schönlein | Peritonitis | | nean fever |
| Parasites | Stenosis | purpura and other | Pancreatitis | | Porphyria |
| Distal intestinal obstruc- | Tumor | causes of vasculi- | Cholecystitis | | Diabetic acidosis |
| tion syndrome of | Mesenteric cyst | tis | Renal and gall- | | Addisonian crisis |
| cystic fibrosis | | | bladder stones | | |
| Tumor | Superior mesenteric | Peptic ulcer | Pelvic inflammation | | Torsion of testis |
| Fecaloma | artery syndrome | Meckel's diverticuli- | Lymphadenitis due | | Torsion of ovarian |
| | Pyloric stenosis | tis | to viral or bacterial | | pedicle |
| | | Acute gastroenteritis | infection | | |
| | | Pseudomembranous | | | |
| | | enterocolitis | | | |

Reproduced, with permission, from Roy CC, Morin CL, Weber AM: Gastrointestinal emergency problems in paediatric practice. Clin Gastroenterol 1981;10:225.

toneal dialysis, organisms not commonly pathogenic such as *Staphylococcus epidermidis* and *Candida* may be the cause of secondary peritonitis. Multiple enteric organisms may be isolated after penetrating abdominal injury or bowel perforation. Intra-abdominal abscesses may form in pelvic, subhepatic, or subphrenic areas, but such localization of infection is less common in young infants than in adults.

Symptoms include severe abdominal pain, fever, nausea, and vomiting. Respirations are shallow. The abdomen is tender, rigid, and distended, with involuntary guarding. Bowel sounds may be absent. Diarrhea is fairly common in primary peritonitis and less so in secondary peritonitis.

The leukocyte count is high initially (> 20,000/µL), with a predominance of immature forms, and later may fall to neutropenic levels, especially in primary peritonitis. Bacterial peritonitis should be suspected if paracentesis fluid contains more than 500 leukocytes/µL or more than 32 mg/dL of lactate; if it has a pH less than 7.34; or if the pH is over 0.1 pH unit less than arterial blood pH. Diagnosis is made by Gram stain and culture, preferably of 5–10 mL of fluid for optimal yield. The blood culture is often positive in primary peritonitis.

Antibiotic treatment and supportive therapy for dehydration, shock, and acidosis are indicated. Surgical treatment of the underlying cause of secondary peritonitis is critical. Removal of infected peritoneal dialysis catheters in patients with secondary peritonitis is sometimes necessary and almost always required if *Candida* infection is present.

# ACUTE APPENDICITIS

Acute appendicitis is the most common indication for emergency abdominal surgery in childhood. The frequency increases with age and peaks between 15 and 30 years. Obstruction of the appendix by fecaliths (25%) or parasites is a predisposing factor.

The incidence of perforation is high (40%) in infants and children. To avoid delay in diagnosis, it is important to maintain close communication with parents, perform a thorough physical examination and sequential examinations of the abdomen at frequent intervals over several hours, and interpret correctly the evolving symptoms and signs.

## Clinical Findings

### A. SYMPTOMS AND SIGNS

The typical child with appendicitis has fever and periumbilical abdominal pain, which then localizes to the right lower quadrant, accompanied by signs of peritoneal irritation. Anorexia, vomiting, constipation, and diarrhea also occur. The clinical picture is often atypical and includes generalized pain and tenderness around the umbilicus without leukocytosis. Rectal examination should always be done and may reveal localized mass or tenderness. Because many conditions give rise to symptoms mimicking appendicitis and because physical findings are often inconclusive, it is important to perform repeated examinations of the abdomen over several hours. In children younger than age 2 years, the pain of appendicitis is poorly localized, and perforation before surgery is common.

## B. LABORATORY FINDINGS

White blood cell counts are seldom higher than 15,000/μL. Pyuria, fecal leukocytes, and guaiac-positive stool are occasionally found.

## C. IMAGING

A radiopaque fecalith is reportedly present in two thirds of cases of ruptured appendix. A positive diagnosis of nonperforated appendicitis cannot be made by barium enema. In experienced hands, ultrasonography of the acutely inflamed appendix shows a noncompressible, thickened appendix in 93% of cases. A localized fluid collection adjacent to or surrounding the appendix may also be seen. Abdominal computed tomography scan after instillation of rectal contrast with thin cuts in the area of the appendix may be diagnostic. Indium-labeled white blood cell scan may localize to an inflamed appendix. Enlarged mesenteric lymph nodes are a nondiagnostic finding.

## Differential Diagnosis

The presence of intrathoracic infection (eg, pneumonia) or urinary tract infection should be kept in mind, along with other medical and surgical conditions leading to acute abdomen (see Table 20–3).

## Treatment & Prognosis

Exploratory laparotomy or laparoscopy is indicated whenever the diagnosis of appendicitis cannot be ruled out after a period of close observation. Postoperative antibiotic therapy is reserved for patients with gangrenous or perforated appendix. A single intraoperative dose of cefoxitin or cefotetan is recommended for all patients to prevent postoperative complications. The mortality rate is less than 1% during childhood despite the high incidence of perforation. In uncomplicated nonruptured appendicitis, laparoscopic approach is associated with a shortened hospital stay.

Mason JD: The evaluation of acute abdominal pain in children. Emerg Med Clin North Am 1996;14:629.

# INTUSSUSCEPTION

Intussusception is the most frequent cause of intestinal obstruction in the first 2 years of life. It is three times more common in males than in females. In most cases (85%) the cause is not apparent, although polyps, Meckel diverticulum, Henoch–Schönlein purpura, lymphoma, lipoma, parasites, foreign bodies, and viral enteritis with hypertrophy of Peyer patches are predisposing factors. Intussusception of the small intestine occurs in patients with celiac disease and cystic fibrosis—related to the bulk of stool in the terminal ileum. Henoch–Schönlein purpura may also cause isolated small-bowel intussusception. In children older than age 6 years, lymphoma is the most common cause. Intermittent small-bowel intussusception is a rare cause of recurrent abdominal pain.

The usual ileocolic intussusception starts just proximal to the ileocecal valve and extends for varying distances into the colon. Swelling, hemorrhage, incarceration, and necrosis of the intussuscepted bowel may occur. Intestinal perforation and peritonitis occur as a result of impairment of venous return.

## Clinical Findings

Characteristically, a thriving infant age 3–12 months develops recurring paroxysms of abdominal pain with screaming and drawing up of the knees. Vomiting and diarrhea occur soon afterward (90% of cases), and bloody bowel movements with mucus appear within the next 12 hours (50%). The child is characteristically lethargic between paroxysms. Prostration and fever supervene. The abdomen is tender and becomes distended. On palpation, a sausage-shaped mass may be found, usually in the upper mid abdomen. An intussusception can persist for several days if obstruction is not complete, and patients may present with separate attacks of enterocolitis. In older children, sudden attacks of abdominal pain may be related to chronic recurrent intussusception with spontaneous reduction. In July 1999, the American Academy of Pediatrics recommended suspending oral rotavirus immunization in the United States because of an increased occurrence of intussusception among young infants in the weeks following oral immunization.

## Treatment

### A. CONSERVATIVE MEASURES

Barium enema and air enema are both diagnostic and therapeutic. Reduction by barium enema should not be attempted if signs of strangulated bowel, perforation, or severe toxicity are present. Air insufflation of the colon under fluoroscopic guidance is a safe alternative to barium enema with excellent diagnostic sensitivity and specificity without the risk of contaminating the abdominal cavity with barium. Great care must be taken in performing either air or barium enema because ischemic damage to the colon secondary to vascular compromise increases the risk of perforation.

### B. SURGICAL MEASURES

In extremely ill patients and in patients who have evidence of bowel perforation or in whom hydrostatic or pneumatic reduction has been unsuccessful (25%), surgery is required. Surgery has the advantage of identifying any lead point such as a Meckel diverticulum. Surgical reduction of intussusception is associated with a lower recurrence rate than pneumatic reduction.

## Prognosis

The prognosis relates directly to the duration of the intussusception before reduction. The mortality rate with treatment is 1–2%. The patient should be observed carefully after hydrostatic or pneumatic reduction because intussusception recurs within 24 hours in 3–4% of patients.

Eshel G et al: Intussusception: A nine year survey. J Pediatr Gastroenterol Nutr 1997;24:253.

## FOREIGN BODIES IN THE ALIMENTARY TRACT

Most foreign bodies pass through the GI tract without difficulty, although objects longer than 5 cm may have difficulty negotiating the ligament of Treitz. Ingested foreign bodies tend to lodge in areas of natural constriction—valleculae, thoracic inlet, GE junction, pylorus, ligament of Treitz, and ileocecal junction. Foreign bodies lodged in the esophagus for more than 24 hours require removal. Smooth foreign bodies in the stomach, such as buttons or coins, may be watched without attempting removal for up to several months if the child is free of symptoms. Straight pins, screws, and nails generally pass without incident. Removal of open safety pins or wooden toothpicks is recommended. Disk-shaped batteries lodged in the esophagus should be removed immediately. Disk-shaped batteries in the stomach will generally pass uneventfully. The use of balanced electrolyte lavage solutions containing polyethylene glycol may help the passage of small, smooth foreign bodies lodged in the stomach or intestine. Lavage is especially useful in hastening the passage of disk-shaped batteries or ingested tablets that may be toxic. Failure of a smooth foreign body to exit the stomach suggests the possibility of gastric outlet obstruction.

Esophagogastroscopy will permit the removal of most foreign bodies lodged in the esophagus and stomach. A Foley catheter may be used to dislodge smooth, round esophageal foreign bodies in healthy children with no previous esophageal disease. The catheter is introduced into the esophagus, and the balloon at the distal end is inflated below the foreign body. Careful withdrawal of the catheter under fluoroscopic observation will bring the foreign body into the mouth, where it can be extracted. Only an experienced radiologist should attempt this maneuver.

## ANAL FISSURE

Anal fissure is a slit-like tear in the squamous epithelium of the anus, usually secondary to the passage of large, hard fecal masses. Anal stenosis, anal crypt abscess, and trauma can be contributory factors. Sexual abuse must be considered in children with large, irregular, or multiple anal fissures. Anal fissures may be the presenting sign of Crohn disease in older children.

The infant or child with anal fissure typically cries with defecation and will try to hold back stools. Sparse, bright red bleeding is seen on the outside of the stool or on the toilet tissue following defecation. The fissure can often be seen if the patient is examined in a knee-chest position with the buttocks spread apart. When a fissure cannot be identified, it is essential to rule out other causes of rectal bleeding such as juvenile polyp, perianal inflammation (due to group A streptococcal infection), or inflammatory bowel disease. Anal fissures should be treated promptly to break the constipation → fissure → retention → constipation cycle. A stool softener should be given. Anal dilation relieves sphincter spasm. Warm sitz baths after defecation may be helpful. In rare cases, silver nitrate cauterization or surgery is indicated. Anal surgery should be avoided in patients with Crohn disease because of the high risk of recurrence and progression after surgery.

## INGUINAL HERNIA

A peritoneal sac precedes the testicle as it descends from the genital ridge to the scrotum. The lower portion of this sac envelops the testis to form the tunica vaginalis, and the remainder normally atrophies by the time of birth. In some cases, peritoneal fluid may become trapped in the tunica vaginalis of the testis (noncommunicating hydrocele). If the processus vaginalis remains open, peritoneal fluid or an abdominal structure may be forced into it (indirect inguinal hernia).

Most inguinal hernias are of the indirect type and occur more frequently (9:1) in boys than in girls. Hernias may be present at birth or may appear at any age thereafter. The incidence in premature male infants is close to 5%. Inguinal hernia is reported in 30% of male infants weighing 1000 g or less.

### Clinical Findings

No symptoms are associated with an empty processus vaginalis. In most cases, a hernia is a painless inguinal swelling of variable size. The mother of the infant with an inguinal hernia may be the only person to see the mass, as it may retract when the infant is active, cold, frightened, or agitated from the physical examination. There may be a history of inguinal fullness associated with coughing or long periods of standing, or there may be a firm, globular, and tender swelling, sometimes associated with vomiting and abdominal distention. In some instances, a herniated loop of intestine may become partially obstructed, leading to pain and partial intestinal obstruction. Rarely, bowel becomes trapped in the hernia sac, and complete intestinal obstruction occurs. Gangrene of the hernia contents or testis may occur. In girls, the ovary may prolapse into the hernia sac. Inspection of the two inguinal areas may reveal a characteristic bulging or mass. Infants should be observed for evidence of swelling after crying, and older children after bearing down. A suggestive history is often the only criterion for diagnosis, along with the "silk glove" feel of the rubbing together of the two walls of the empty hernia sac.

## Differential Diagnosis

Inguinal lymph nodes may be mistaken for a hernia. Nodes are usually multiple with more discrete borders. A hydrocele of the cord should transilluminate. An undescended testis is usually mobile in the canal and is associated with absence of the gonad in the scrotum.

## Treatment

Manual reduction of incarcerated inguinal hernias can be attempted after the sedated infant is placed in the Trendelenburg position with an ice bag on the affected side. Manual reduction is contraindicated if incarceration has been present for more than 12 hours or if bloody stools are noted. Surgery is usually indicated if a hernia has ever incarcerated. Hydroceles frequently resolve by age 2 years. Controversy remains about exploration of the opposite side. Exploration of the unaffected groin can document the patency of the processus vaginalis, but patency does not always mean that herniation will occur, especially in patients older than age 1 year, in whom the risk of contralateral hernia is about 10%. Incarceration of an inguinal hernia is more likely to occur in boys and in children younger than 10 months of age.

Gahukamble DB, Khamage AS: Early vs delayed repair of reduced incarcerated inguinal hernias in the pediatric population. J Pediatr Surg 1996;31:1218 [PMID: 8887087].

Nicholls E: Inguinal scrotal problems in children. Practitioner 2003;247:226.

## UMBILICAL HERNIA

Umbilical hernias are more common in premature than in full-term infants and more common in black than in white infants. Small bowel may incarcerate in small-diameter umbilical hernias. Most umbilical hernias regress spontaneously if the fascial defect has a diameter of less than 1 cm. Large defects and smaller hernias persisting after age 4 years should be treated surgically. Reducing the hernia and strapping the skin over the abdominal wall defect does not accelerate the healing process.

# TUMORS OF THE GASTROINTESTINAL TRACT

## 1. Juvenile Polyps

Juvenile polyps are usually pedunculated and solitary. The head of the polyp is composed of hyperplastic glandular and vascular elements, often with cystic transformation. Juvenile polyps are benign, and 80% occur in the rectosigmoid. Their incidence is highest between ages 3 and 5 years, and they are rare before age 1 year and, because of autoamputation, after age 15 years. They are more frequent in boys. The painless passage of small amounts of bright red blood on a normal or constipated stool is the most frequent manifestation. Abdominal pain is rare, but a juvenile polyp can be the lead point for an intussusception. Low-lying polyps may prolapse during defecation.

Rarely, many juvenile polyps may be present in the colon, causing anemia, diarrhea, and protein loss. A few cases of generalized juvenile polyposis involving the stomach, small bowel, and colon have been reported. These cases are associated with a slightly increased risk of cancer.

Colonoscopy is both diagnostic and therapeutic when polyps are suspected. After removal of the polyp by electrocautery, nothing further should be done if histologic findings confirm the diagnosis. There is a slight risk of developing further juvenile polyps.

Other polyposis syndromes are summarized in Table 20–4.

## 2. Cancers of the Esophagus, Small Intestine, & Colon

Esophageal cancer is rare in childhood. Cysts, leiomyomas, and hamartomas predominate. Caustic injury of the esophagus increases the risk of squamous cell carcinoma as a very long term complication. Chronic peptic esophagitis is associated with Barrett esophagus, a precancerous lesion. Simple GE reflux in infancy without esophagitis is not a risk for cancer of the esophagus.

The most common gastric or small-bowel cancer in children is lymphoma or lymphosarcoma. Intermittent abdominal pain, abdominal mass, intussusception, or a celiac-like picture may be present. Carcinoid tumors are

**Table 20–4.** Gastrointestinal polyposis syndromes.

| | Location | Number | Histology | Extraintestinal Findings | Malignant Potential | Recommended Therapy |
|---|---|---|---|---|---|---|
| Juvenile polyps | Colon | Single (70%) Several (30%) | Hyperplastic, hamartomatous | None | None | Remove polyp for continuous bleeding or prolapse. |
| Familial juvenile polyposis coli[a] | Colon | More than ten | Hyperplastic with focal adenomatous change | None | 10–25%; higher if familial | Remove all polyps. Consider colectomy if very numerous or adenomatous. |
| Generalized juvenile polyposis[a] | Stomach, small bowel, colon | Multiple | Hyperplastic with focal adenomatous change | Hydrocephaly, cardiac lesions, mesenteric lymph-angioma, malrotation | 10–25% | Colectomy and close surveillance. |
| Familial adenomatous polyposis[a] | Colon; less commonly, stomach and small bowel | Multiple | Adenomatous | None | 95–100% | Colectomy by age 18 years. |
| Peutz–Jeghers syndrome[a] | Small bowel, stomach, colon | Multiple | Hamartomatous | Pigmented cutaneous and oral macules; ovarian cysts and tumors; bony exostoses | 2–3% | Remove accessible polyps or those causing obstruction or bleeding. |
| Gardner's syndrome | Colon; less commonly, stomach and small bowel | Multiple | Adenomatous | Cysts, tumors, and desmoids of skin and bone; ampullary tumors; other tumors; retinal pigmen-tations can be a screening tool in families | 95–100% | Colectomy by age 18 years. Upper tract surveillance. |
| Cronkhite–Canada syndrome | Stomach, colon; less commonly, esophagus and small bowel | Multiple | Hamartomatous | Alopecia; onychodystrophy; hyperpigmentation | Rare | None. |
| Turcot's syndrome[b] | Colon | Multiple | Adenomatous | Thyroid and brain tumors are the usual presen-tation | Possible | Central nervous system screening most important |

[a] Autosomal dominant.
[b] Autosomal recessive.

usually benign and most often an incidental finding in the appendix following appendectomy. Metastasis is rare. The carcinoid syndrome (flushing, sweating, hypertension, diarrhea and vomiting), associated with serotonin secretion, only occurs with metastatic carcinoid tumors.

Adenocarcinoma of the colon is rare in pediatric patients. The transverse colon and rectosigmoid are the two most commonly affected sites. The low 5-year survival rate relates to the nonspecificity of presenting complaints and the large percentage of undifferentiated types. Children with a family history of colon cancer, chronic ulcerative colitis, or familial polyposis syndromes are at greater risk.

### 3. Mesenteric Cysts

These rare tumors may be small or large and single or multiloculated. Invariably thin-walled, they contain serous, chylous, or hemorrhagic fluid. They are commonly located in the mesentery of the small intestine but may also be seen in the mesocolon. Most mesenteric cysts cause no symptoms. Traction on the mesentery may lead to colicky abdominal pain, which can be mild and recurrent but may appear acutely with vomiting. Volvulus may occur around a cyst, and hemorrhage into a cyst may be mild or hemodynamically significant. A rounded mass can occasionally be palpated or seen on radiograph to displace adjacent intestine. Abdominal ultrasonography is usually diagnostic. Surgical removal is indicated.

### 4. Intestinal Hemangioma

Hemangiomas of the bowel may cause acute or chronic blood loss. They may also cause intestinal obstruction via intussusception, local stricture, or intramural hematoma formation. Thrombocytopenia and consumptive coagulopathy are occasional complications. Some lesions are telangiectasias (Rendu–Osler–Weber syndrome), and others are capillary hemangiomas. The largest group are cavernous hemangiomas, which are composed of large, thin-walled vessels arising from the submucosal vascular plexus. They may protrude into the lumen as polypoid lesions or may invade the intestine from mucosa to serosa.

## ACUTE INFECTIOUS DIARRHEA (Gastroenteritis)

Viruses are the most common cause of acute gastroenteritis in developing and developed countries. Bacterial and parasitic enteric infections are discussed in Chapters 38 and 39. Of the viral agents causing enteric infection, rotavirus, a 67-nm double-stranded RNA virus

with at least eight serotypic variants, is the most common. As with most viral pathogens, rotavirus affects the small intestine, causing voluminous watery diarrhea without leukocytes or blood. In the United States, rotavirus affects mainly infants between ages 3 and 15 months. Peak incidence in the United States is in the winter months. Sporadic cases occur at other times. The virus is transmitted via the fecal–oral route and survives for hours on hands and for days on environmental fomites.

### Diagnosis & Treatment of Rotavirus Infections

The incubation period for rotavirus is 24–48 hours. Vomiting is the first symptom in 80–90% of patients, followed within 24 hours by low-grade fever and voluminous watery diarrhea. Diarrhea usually lasts 4–8 days but may last longer in young infants or immunocompromised patients. The white blood cell count is rarely elevated. The stool sodium level is usually less than 40 mEq/L. Thus, as patients become dehydrated from unreplaced fecal water loss, they may become hypernatremic. The stool does not contain blood or white cells. Metabolic acidosis results from bicarbonate loss in the stool, ketosis from poor intake, and lactic acidemia from hypotension and hypoperfusion.

Replacement of fluid and electrolyte deficits and ongoing losses is critical, especially in small infants. (Oral and intravenous therapy are discussed in Chapter 42.) The use of oral rehydration fluid is appropriate in most cases. The use of clear liquids or hypocaloric (dilute formula) diets for more than 48 hours is not advisable in uncomplicated viral gastroenteritis because starvation depresses digestive function and prolongs diarrhea.

Intestinal lactase levels are reduced during rotavirus infection. Brief use of a lactose-free diet is associated with a shorter period of diarrhea but is not critical to successful recovery in most healthy infants. Reduced fat intake during recovery may reduce nausea and vomiting.

Antidiarrheal medications are ineffective (kaolin–pectin combinations) or even dangerous (loperamide, tincture of opium, diphenoxylate with atropine). Bismuth subsalicylate preparations may reduce stool volume but are not critical to recovery. Oral immunoglobulin or specific antiviral agents have occasionally been useful in limiting duration of disease in immunocompromised patients.

Specific identification of rotavirus is not required in every case, especially in outbreaks. Rotavirus antigens can be identified in stool. False positives (which may actually be nonpathogenic rotavirus) are seen in neonates. Some immunity is imparted by the first episode of rotavirus infection. Serum antibodies are present, but their role in prevention of subsequent attacks is unclear. Repeat infections occur but are usually less severe. Prevention of rotavirus is mainly by good hygiene and prevention of fecal–oral contamination. In July 1999, the American Academy of Pediatrics recommended suspending the use of oral rotavirus vaccine in the United States despite an approximately 75% protection rate of vaccinated infants because of its association with intussusception in the first 3 weeks following vaccine administration.

## Diagnosis & Treatment of Other Viral Infections

Other viral pathogens in stool have been identified by electron microscopy, special viral cultures, or enzyme-linked immunoassays in infants with diarrhea. Depending on the geographic location, enteric adenoviruses (serotypes 40 and 41) or caliciviruses are the next most common viral pathogens in infants. The symptoms of enteric adenovirus infection are similar to those produced from rotavirus, but infection is not seasonal and duration of illness may be longer. The Norwalk agent, a calicivirus, is a small RNA virus that causes chiefly vomiting but also some diarrhea in older children and adults, usually in common source outbreaks (perhaps water-borne). The duration of symptoms is short, usually 24–48 hours. Other potentially pathogenic viruses include astroviruses, corona-like viruses, and other small round viruses. Cytomegalovirus rarely causes diarrhea in immunocompetent children but may cause erosive colitis or enteritis in immunocompromised hosts. Cytomegalovirus enteritis is particularly common after bone marrow transplantation and in late stages of HIV infection.

Caeiro JP et al: Etiology of outpatient pediatric nondysenteric diarrhea: A multicenter study in the United States. Pediatr Infect Dis J 1999;18:94.

# CHRONIC DIARRHEA

It is difficult to define chronic diarrhea because normal bowel habits vary greatly. Some infants normally have 5–8 soft small stools daily. A gradual or sudden increase in the number and volume of stools (> 15 g/kg/d) combined with an increase in fluidity should raise a suspicion that an organic cause of chronic diarrhea is present.

Diarrhea may result from any of the following pathogenetic mechanisms: (1) interruption of normal cell transport processes for water, electrolytes, or nutrients; (2) decrease in the surface area available for absorption, which may be due to shortening of the bowel or mucosal disease; (3) increase in intestinal motility;

(4) increase in unabsorbable osmotically active molecules in the intestinal lumen; (5) increase in intestinal permeability, leading to increased loss of water and electrolytes; and (6) stimulation of enterocyte secretion by toxins or cytokines.

## Noninfectious Causes of Diarrhea

### A. ANTIBIOTIC THERAPY

Diarrhea is reported in up to 60% of children receiving antibiotics. Eradication of normal gut flora and overgrowth of other organisms may cause diarrhea. Most antibiotic-associated diarrhea is watery in nature, is not associated with systemic symptoms, and decreases when antibiotic therapy is stopped. Pseudomembranous colitis, caused by the toxins produced by *Clostridium difficile,* occurs in 0.2–10% of patients taking antibiotics, especially clindamycin, cephalosporins, and amoxicillin. Patients develop fever, tenesmus, and abdominal pain with diarrhea, which contains leukocytes and sometimes gross blood up to 8 weeks after antibiotic exposure. Treatment with oral metronidazole (30 mg/kg/d) or oral vancomycin (30–50 mg/kg/d) for 7 days is recommended. Vancomycin is many times more expensive than metronidazole and no more efficacious. Relapse occurs after treatment in 10–50% of patients because of exsporulation of residual spores in the colon. Retreatment with the same antibiotic regimen is usually effective, but multiple relapses are possible.

### B. EXTRAINTESTINAL INFECTIONS

Infections of the urinary tract and upper respiratory tract (especially otitis media) are at times associated with diarrhea. The mechanism remains obscure. Antibiotic treatment of the primary infection, toxins released by infecting organisms, and local irritation of the rectum (in patients with bladder infection) may play a role.

### C. MALNUTRITION

Malnutrition is associated with an increased frequency of enteral infections. Decreased bile acid synthesis, pancreatic enzyme output, and disaccharidase activity; altered motility; and changes in the intestinal flora all may cause diarrhea. Severely malnourished children are at higher risk of enteric infections because of depressed immune functions, both cellular and humoral.

### D. DIET

Overfeeding may cause diarrhea, especially in young infants. Relative deficiency of pancreatic amylase in young infants may produce diarrhea after starchy foods. Fruit juices, especially those high in fructose or sorbitol, produce osmotic diarrhea because these osmotically active sugars are poorly absorbed by the immature gut.

Intestinal irritants (spices and foods high in fiber) and histamine-containing or histamine-releasing foods (eg, citrus fruits, tomatoes, certain cheeses, red wines, and scromboid fish) also cause diarrhea.

### E. ALLERGIC DIARRHEA

Diarrhea caused by allergy to dietary proteins is a frequently entertained but rarely authenticated diagnostic entity. Protein allergy is more common in infants younger than age 12 months, who may experience mild to severe colitis. A personal or family history of atopy is common in infants with enteric protein allergy. Older children may develop a celiac-like syndrome with flattening of small-bowel villi, steatorrhea, hypoproteinemia, occult blood loss, and chronic diarrhea. Skin testing is not reliable. Double-blind oral challenge with the suspected food under careful observation is necessary to confirm intestinal protein allergy. Mild diarrhea with blood and mucus may occur in thriving young infants receiving either breast milk or formula. In the breast-fed infant, maternal avoidance of milk protein may be effective in reducing the signs of colitis. Feeding a protein hydrolysate formula may also reduce symptoms. Because allergic colitis in young infants is self-limited, the condition does not absolutely require treatment if the infant is thriving and the colitic symptoms are not severe. Colonoscopy is not required for diagnosis, but rectal biopsies usually show mild lymphonodular hyperplasia, mucosal edema, and slight eosinophilia. In infants, the condition usually disappears after 12 months. Allergies to fish, peanuts, and eggs are more likely to be lifelong. Multiple food allergy (more than three) is rare.

Khan S, Orenstein S: Eosinophilic gastroenteritis: Epidemiology, diagnosis and management. *Paed Drugs* 2002;4:563.

### F. CHRONIC NONSPECIFIC DIARRHEA

Chronic nonspecific diarrhea is the most common cause of loose stools in thriving children. The typical patient is a healthy child age 6–20 months who was a colicky baby and who has three to six loose mucoid stools per day during the waking hours. The diarrhea worsens with a low-residue, low-fat, or high-carbohydrate diet and during periods of stress and infection. It clears spontaneously at about age 3½ years (usually coincident with toilet training). No organic disease is discoverable. Possible causes include abnormalities of bile acid absorption in the terminal ileum, incomplete carbohydrate absorption (excessive fruit juice ingestion seems to worsen the condition or in some cases appears to be the primary cause), and abnormal motor function. A high familial incidence of functional bowel disease is observed. Stool tests for blood, white cells, fat, parasites, and bacterial pathogens are negative.

The following measures are helpful: institution of a slightly high-fat (about 40% of total calories), low-carbohydrate, high-fiber diet; avoidance of between-meal snacks; and avoidance of chilled fluids, especially fruit juices. It may be helpful to give loperamide, 0.1–0.2 mg/kg/d in two or three divided doses; cholestyramine, 2–4 g in divided doses; or psyllium agents, 1–2 tsp twice daily.

### G. SECRETORY DIARRHEA

Certain malignancies of childhood, including neuroblastoma, ganglioneuroma, metastatic carcinoid, and GI neuroendocrine tumors such as pancreatic VIPoma or gastrinoma, may secrete substances such as gastrin and vasoactive interstinal polypeptide that promote small-intestine secretion of water and electrolytes. These children present with large volume, watery diarrhea that does not cease when they discontinue oral feedings. Fat malabsorption is not characteristic. The serum potassium level is often low because of losses in diarrhea. The hallmark of the diarrhea is that, unlike osmotic and infectious viral diarrheas, the sodium content of the stool water is high, usually between 90 and 140 mEq/L of stool. Other specific signs and symptoms are associated with specific tumors. Neuroblastoma and ganglioneuroma lead to elevations in urinary homovanillic acid and vanillylmandelic acid. Metastatic carcinoid is associated with characteristic flushing and sweating. Gastrinoma may be associated with multiple duodenal ulcers (Zollinger–Ellison syndrome). In all secretory diarrheas, a careful radiologic search for a tumor mass is indicated. Bacterial overgrowth of the small bowel in patients with short bowel, cancer chemotherapy, or anatomic abnormalities may lead to the production of enterotoxins, which can promote a secretory diarrhea without the presence of tumor. Cholera is the best known bacterial secretory diarrhea. Its enterotoxin stimulates cyclic adenosine monophosphate in the enterocyte, which promotes salt and water secretion.

## THE MALABSORPTION SYNDROMES

Malabsorption of ingested food has many causes (Table 20–5). Shortening of the small bowel (usually via surgical resection) and mucosal damage (celiac disease) both reduce surface area. Impaired motility of the small intestine may interfere with normal propulsive movements and mixing of food with pancreatic and biliary secretions. Anaerobic bacteria proliferate under these conditions and impair fat absorption by deconjugation of bile acids (intestinal pseudo-obstruction, postoperative blind loop syndrome). Impaired intestinal lymphatic (congenital lymphangiectasis) or venous drainage also causes malabsorption. Diseases reducing pancreatic exocrine function (cystic fibrosis, Shwach-

***Table 20–5.*** Malabsorption syndromes.

**Intraluminal phase abnormalities**
  Acid hypersecretion; Zollinger–Ellison syndrome
  Gastric resection
  Exocrine pancreatic insufficiency
    Cystic fibrosis
    Chronic pancreatitis
    Pancreatic pseudocysts
    Schwachman syndrome
    Enterokinase deficiency
    Lipase and colipase deficiency
    Malnutrition
  Decreased conjugated bile acids
    Liver production and excretion
      Neonatal hepatitis
      Biliary atresia: intrahepatic and extrahepatic
      Acute and chronic active hepatitis
      Disease of the biliary tract
      Cirrhosis
      Fat malabsorption in the premature infant
    Intestinal malabsorption of bile acids
      Short bowel syndrome
      Bacterial overgrowth
        Blind loop
        Fistula
        Strictures, regional enteritis
        Scleroderma, intestinal pseudo-obstruction
**Intestinal phase abnormalities**
  Mucosal diseases
    Infections, bacterial or viral
    Infections, parasitic
      *Giardia lamblia*
      Fish tapeworm
      Hookworm
      *Cryptosporidium*
    Malnutrition
      Marasmus
      Kwashiorkor
  Dermatitis herpetiformis
  Folic acid deficiency
  Drugs: methotrexate, antibiotics
  Crohn disease
  Cow's milk and soy protein intolerance
  Secondary disaccharidase deficiency
  Secondary monosaccharide intolerance
  Hirschsprung disease with enterocolitis
  Tropical sprue
  Celiac disease
  Radiation enteritis
  Lymphoma

**Intestinal phase abnormalities (cont'd)**
  Circulatory disturbances
    Cirrhosis
    Congestive heart failure
  Abnormal structure of gastrointestinal tract
    Dumping syndrome after gastrectomy
    Malrotation
    Stenosis of jejunum or ileum
    Small bowel resection; short bowel syndrome
    Polyposis
  Selective inborn absorptive defects
    Congenital malabsorption of folic acid
    Selective malabsorption of vitamin $B_{12}$
    Cystinuria, methionine malabsorption
    Hartnup disease, blue diaper syndrome
    Glucose–galactose malabsorption
    Primary disaccharidase deficiency
    Acrodermatitis enteropathica
    Abetalipoproteinemia
    Congenital chloridorrhea
    Primary hypomagnesemia
    Hereditary fructose intolerance
    Familial hypophosphatemic rickets
  Endocrine diseases
    Diabetes mellitus
    Addison disease
    Hyperthyroidism
    Hypoparathyroidism, pseudohypoparathyroidism
    Neuroblastoma, ganglioneuroma
**Vascular and lymphatic disorders**
  Whipple disease
  Intestinal lymphangiectasis
  Congestive heart failure
  Regional enteritis with lymphangiectasis
  Lymphoma
  Abetalipoproteinemia
**Miscellaneous**
  Renal insufficiency
  Carcinoid, mastocytosis
  Immune deficiency disorders
  Familial dysautonomia
  Collagen–vascular disease
  Wolman disease
  Histiocytosis X

man syndrome) or the production and flow of biliary secretions cause nutrient malabsorption. Malabsorption of specific nutrients may be genetically determined (disaccharidase deficiency, glucose–galactose malabsorption, and abetalipoproteinemia).

## Clinical Findings

GI symptoms such as diarrhea, vomiting, anorexia, abdominal pain, failure to thrive, and abdominal distension are common. Observation of the stools for abnormal color, consistency, bulkiness, odor, mucus, and blood is important. Microscopic examination of stools for neutral fat and fatty acids is helpful because most malabsorption syndromes involve some fat malabsorption. Pancreatic insufficiency is associated with neutral fat in the stool. Fatty acids are the major fatty material found in the stool of patients with mucosal disease (celiac disease) and liver disease.

Quantitative assessment of fat absorption requires measurement of fat excreted in the feces as a proportion of fat intake for a defined period. Excretion of 5% of ingested fat is normal for a child older than age 1 year; 10–15% is normal in a younger infant. Prothrombin time and serum carotene, vitamin E, and vitamin D levels may be depressed by long-standing fat malabsorption. Accurate assessment of protein absorption is difficult and requires isotopic labeling of amino acids. Loss of serum proteins across the intestinal mucosa can be estimated by measurement of fecal $\alpha_1$-antitrypsin. Malabsorption of complex carbohydrate is rarely measured. Disaccharide or monosaccharide malabsorption is estimated by reduction in stool pH, increased breath hydrogen after ingestion of carbohydrate, or decreased intestinal mucosal disaccharidase activity.

Other tests that may suggest a specific cause of malabsorption in a child include sweat chloride concentration (cystic fibrosis), intestinal mucosal biopsy (eg, celiac disease, intestinal lymphangiectasia, giardiasis, inflammatory bowel disease), liver and gallbladder function tests, and pancreatic secretion of enzymes after stimulation with secretin and cholecystokinin. Some of the most common disorders associated with malabsorption in pediatric patients are detailed in the following sections.

## 1. Protein-Losing Enteropathies

Loss of plasma proteins into the GI tract occurs in association with inflammatory conditions of the intestine, intestinal graft-versus-host disease, acute and chronic intestinal infections, venous or lymphatic obstruction or malformations, and malignant infiltration of the intestine or its lymphatics and vasculature.

## Clinical Findings

Signs and symptoms are mainly those related to hypoproteinemia, and in some instances to malabsorption. Edema, ascites, poor weight gain, and, depending on the underlying condition, signs of specific vitamin and mineral deficiencies may all be present. Serum albumin and globulins may be decreased. Fecal $\alpha_1$-antitrypsin, a marker for protein loss, is elevated (> 3 mg/g dry weight stool; slightly higher in breast-fed infants). Disorders associated with protein-losing enteropathy are listed in Table 20–6.

## Differential Diagnosis

Hypoalbuminemia may be due to an increased catabolic rate or may be associated with poor protein intake, impaired hepatic protein synthesis, or congenital malformations of lymphatics outside the GI tract. Proteinuria associated with nephritis and nephrotic syndrome may also cause hypoalbuminemia.

**Table 20–6.** Disorders associated with protein-losing enteropathy.

**Vascular obstruction**
Congestive heart failure
Constrictive pericarditis
Atrial septal defect
Primary myocardial disease
Increased right atrial pressure[a]

**Stomach**
Giant hypertrophic gastritis (Ménétrier disease), often secondary to cytomegalovirus infection
Polyps
Gastritis secondary to *Helicobacter pylori* infection

**Small intestine**
Celiac disease
Intestinal lymphangiectasia
Blind loop syndrome
Abetalipoproteinemia
Chronic mucosal ischemia (eg, from chronic volvulus or radiation enteritis)
Allergic enteropathy
Malrotation
Inflammatory bowel disease

**Colon**
Ulcerative colitis
Hirschsprung disease
Pseudomembranous colitis
Polyposis syndromes
Villous adenoma
Solitary rectal ulcer

[a]Children who undergo Fontan procedure for tricuspid atresia are especially prone.

## Treatment

Albumin infusions, diuretics, and a high-protein/low-fat diet may control symptoms. Treatment must be directed toward identifying and treating the underlying cause of GI protein loss if possible.

## 2. Celiac Disease (Gluten Enteropathy)

Celiac disease results from intestinal sensitivity to the gliadin fraction of glutens from wheat, rye, barley, and (possibly) oats. Most pediatric cases present during the second year of life, but the age at onset and the severity are both variable. Up-to-date estimates of disease frequency are being revised with the widespread use of sensitive screening tests such as the tissue transglutaminase and endomysial antibodies. Screening with antigliadin antibodies is no longer recommended because of the high frequency of false-positive tests. It is estimated that the frequency of celiac disease in the United States is around 1:300, a figure approaching the high incidence reported in the past from European countries. It is thought that intestinal damage and villous atrophy result from a cell-mediated immune response initiated by exposure to a polypeptide fragment of gliadin, the alcohol-soluble fraction of gluten. Ten percent of first-degree relatives may be affected. The inheritance is probably polygenic, but it might result from a single gene in combination with an environmental precipitant such as intestinal viral infection. The increased incidence of celiac disease in children with type I diabetes mellitus, IgA deficiency, and Down syndrome is consistent with possible immunologic factors in the development of celiac disease. Individuals with HLA-DR4 and perhaps DR3 tissue type are at higher risk.

## Clinical Findings

### A. Symptoms and Signs

**1. Diarrhea**—Affected children present with digestive disturbances starting at age 6–12 months—the age at which grains are first fed. Initially, the diarrhea may be intermittent; subsequently it is continuous, with bulky, pale, frothy, greasy, foul-smelling stools. During celiac crises, dehydration, shock, and acidosis occur. In cases in which anorexia is severe (about 10%), diarrhea may be absent.

**2. Constipation, vomiting, and abdominal pain**—This triad of symptoms may occasionally dominate the clinical picture and suggest a diagnosis of intestinal obstruction. Constipation generally results from a combination of anorexia, dehydration, muscle weakness, and bulky stools.

**3. Failure to thrive**—The onset of diarrhea is usually accompanied by loss of appetite, failure to gain weight, and irritability. Weight loss is most marked in the limbs and buttocks. The abdomen becomes distended secondary to gas and fluid in the intestinal tract. Short stature and delayed puberty are characteristic in older children and may be the only symptoms.

**4. Anemia and vitamin deficiencies**—Anemia usually responds to iron supplementation and is rarely megaloblastic. Anemia is more likely to be the presenting problem of adult patients with celiac disease. Deficiencies in fat-soluble vitamins are common. Rickets can be seen when growth has not been completely halted by the disease. Osteomalacia is more common, however, and pathologic fractures may occur. Hypoprothrombinemia secondary to vitamin K malabsorption can cause easy bleeding.

**5. Silent celiac disease**—Serologic screening among pediatric patients with nonspecific GI complaints, growth failure, conditions linked to celiac disease (type 1 diabetes, thyroid disease, vitiligo, IgA deficiency, Down syndrome), and family members of celiac patients is widespread. The therapy for a symptom-free child with positive serology is unclear. Intestinal biopsy specimens from children with positive serology are very often abnormal and consistent with celiac disease. In these patients, the prudent response is to recommend a gluten-free diet. In patients with positive serology but normal intestinal biopsies, careful follow-up without diet therapy is the most appropriate current recommendation.

### B. Laboratory Findings

**1. Fat content of stools**—A 3-day collection of stools usually reveals excessive fecal fat excretion. A normal child will excrete 5–10% of ingested fats. The patient with untreated celiac disease will excrete more than 15% of daily fat intake. Anorexia may be so severe that steatorrhea may not be present in 10–25% of patients until normal intake is established.

**2. Impaired carbohydrate absorption**—A low oral glucose tolerance curve is seen. Absorption of D-xylose is impaired, with blood levels lower than 20 mg/dL 60 minutes after ingestion.

**3. Hypoproteinemia**—Hypoalbuminemia can be severe enough to lead to edema. There is evidence of increased protein loss in the gut lumen and poor hepatic synthesis secondary to malnutrition.

### C. Imaging

A small-bowel series shows a malabsorptive pattern characterized by segmentation, clumping of the barium column, and hypersecretion. These changes are nonspecific and can be found in patients with other malabsorption states (see Table 20–5).

### D. BIOPSY FINDINGS

Intestinal biopsy is the most reliable test for celiac disease. Under the dissecting microscope, the jejunal mucosa lacks the slender, finger-like projections that characterize normal villi. Under the light microscope, the florid celiac mucosa has shortened or absent villi, lengthened crypts of Lieberkühn, intense plasma cell infiltration of the lamina propria, and numerous intraepithelial lymphocytes.

### E. SEROLOGIC TESTS

The false-positive rate for the IgG antigliadin antibody is 10% among healthy individuals. The false-positive rate for IgA antigliadin antibodies is lower. Endomysial or tissue transglutaminase antibody assays have greater than 95% sensitivity and slightly less specificity for the diagnosis. Because both of these antibodies are of the IgA class, screening for them in a patient who is IgA-deficient may yield a falsely negative result. The best available serologic screening test, therefore, is a quantitative IgA level with a transglutaminase antibody assay.

## Differential Diagnosis

The differential diagnosis includes disorders that cause malabsorption. Strict adherence to two diagnostic criteria is essential—the characteristic small-bowel microscopic changes and clinical improvement on a gluten-free diet. Repeated mucosal biopsies to prove histologic recovery on gluten-free diet and relapse on gluten challenge are not critical to the diagnosis in typical patients.

## Treatment

### A. DIET

Treatment consists of dietary gluten restriction for life. All sources of wheat, rye, and barley must be eliminated during the initial treatment. Some patients may be able to tolerate oats in the diet, but this should be tested only after recovery has occurred. Lactose is poorly tolerated in the acute stage because extensive mucosal damage causes secondary disaccharidase deficiency. Normal amounts of fat are advisable. Supplemental calories, vitamins, and minerals are indicated in the acute phase. Clinical improvement is usually evident within a week, and histologic repair is complete after 3–12 months. Tissue transglutaminase titers may decrease on a gluten-free diet, but usually do not disappear.

### B. CORTICOSTEROIDS

Corticosteroids can hasten clinical improvement but are indicated only in very ill patients with signs and symptoms of celiac crisis (profound anorexia, malnutrition, diarrhea, edema, abdominal distention, and hypokalemia).

## Prognosis

Clinical and histologic recovery is the rule but may be slow. Malignant lymphoma of the small bowel occurs with increased frequency in adults with long-standing disease. Dietary treatment seems to decrease the risk of this complication.

Cerf-Bensussan N: Coeliac disease: An update on facts and questions based on the 10th international symposium on coeliac disease. J Pediatr Gastroenterol Nutr 2003;37:412.

Fasano A et al: The prevalence of celiac disease in at risk and not at risk groups in the United States: A multicenter study. Arch Int Med 2003;163:286.

## *3. Disaccharidase Deficiency*

Starches and the disaccharides sucrose and lactose are quantitatively the most important dietary carbohydrates. The dietary disaccharides and oligosaccharide products of pancreatic amylase action on starch require hydrolysis by intestinal brush border disaccharidases before significant absorption can take place. Disaccharidase levels are higher in the jejunum and in the proximal ileum than in the distal ileum and duodenum.

In primary disaccharidase deficiency, a single enzyme is affected, disaccharide intolerance is likely to persist, intestinal histologic findings are normal, and a family history is common.

Because disaccharidases are located on the luminal surface of intestinal enterocytes, they are susceptible to mucosal damage. Many conditions cause secondary disaccharidase deficiency, with lactase usually most severely depressed. Histologic examination reveals changes compatible with the underlying disorder.

## Clinical Findings

### A. PRIMARY (CONGENITAL)

**1. Lactase deficiency**—Congenital lactase deficiency is rare. The ingestion of lactose results in diarrhea, gassy distention, and abdominal pain. The stools are frothy, with a pH below 4.5, owing to the presence of organic acids. Vomiting is common. Severe malnutrition may occur. Reducing substances are present in the stools. The blood glucose fails to rise more than 10 mg/dL after ingestion of 1 g/kg of lactose. A rise in breath hydrogen after oral administration of lactose (from hydrogen produced by normal colon flora during fermentation of unabsorbed carbohydrate) is also diagnostic.

Patients respond to a reduction of dietary lactose. Tolerance for dietary starch and sucrose is normal. Lactase extracted from *Aspergillus* and *Kluyvera* species (Lactaid) can be added to milk products or taken with meals to enhance lactose hydrolysis. Although all human racial groups are lactase-sufficient at birth, genetically determined lactase deficiency may develop after age 3 to 5 years in some groups. Certain racial groups are more likely to develop lactase deficiency. In Asians, genetic lactase deficiency develops in virtually 100% of individuals. In Africans, the incidence in most tribes is over 80%. In African Americans, the incidence is about 70%, and among European Americans, the incidence is between 30 and 60%.

**2. Sucrase and isomaltase deficiency**—This is a combined defect that is inherited as an autosomal recessive trait. Ten percent of Alaskan natives are affected. The condition is rare in other groups. Abdominal distention, failure to thrive, and chronic diarrhea may be the presenting symptoms. Distaste for and avoidance of sucrose occurs even in young infants.

Because sucrose is not a reducing sugar, tests for reducing substances in the stool may be negative unless the sucrose in the stool is hydrolyzed by colon bacteria. A sucrose tolerance test (1 g/kg) is likely to be abnormal. Breath hydrogen will be elevated after ingestion of sucrose. Treatment of primary sucrase–isomaltase deficiency requires elimination of most sucrose. A preparation of yeast sucrase taken with meals is also effective.

### B. SECONDARY (ACQUIRED)

**1. Secondary lactase deficiency**—The most common mechanism by which secondary lactase deficiency occurs is small intestinal injury due to viral infection. This condition is usually self-limited, lasting days or, at most, weeks after recovery from infection. Celiac disease, giardiasis, malnutrition, abetalipoproteinemia, immunoglobulin deficiencies, and intestinal mucosal injury secondary to radiation and cancer chemotherapy all can decrease intestinal lactase activity.

**2. Secondary sucrase deficiency**—Intestinal mucosal damage tends to lower the levels of all disaccharidases. Signs of sucrose intolerance are usually masked by the more striking symptoms of lactose intolerance. Infectious diarrhea is the most common cause of secondary sucrose intolerance.

### Prognosis

Primary disaccharidase deficiency is a lifelong defect. However, in both lactase and sucrase deficiencies, tolerance for the disaccharide may increase with age. The prognosis in the secondary or acquired forms of disaccharidase deficiency depends on the underlying illness.

Baudon JJ et al: Sucrase-isomaltase deficiency: Changing pattern over 2 decades. J Pediatr Gastroenterol Nutr 1996;22:284 [PMID: 8708882].

Treem WR et al: Saccharosidase therapy for congenital sucrase isomaltase deficiency. J Pediatr Gastroenterol Nutr 1999;28: 137.

## 4. Glucose–Galactose Malabsorption

Glucose–galactose malabsorption is a rare disorder in which the sodium–glucose transport protein is defective. The gene has been localized to the long arm of chromosome 22. Transport of glucose in the intestinal epithelium and renal tubular epithelium is severely impaired. Diarrhea begins with the first feedings, accompanied by reducing sugar in the stool and acidosis. Small-bowel histologic findings are normal. Glycosuria and aminoaciduria may occur. The glucose tolerance test is flat. Fructose is well tolerated. The diarrhea subsides promptly on withdrawal of glucose and galactose from the diet. The acquired form of glucose–galactose malabsorption occurs mainly in infants younger than age 6 months, usually following acute viral or bacterial enteritis.

In the congenital disease, exclusion of glucose and galactose from the diet is mandatory. A satisfactory formula is one with a carbohydrate-free base plus added fructose. The prognosis is good if the disease is diagnosed early, because tolerance for glucose and galactose improves with age. In secondary monosaccharide intolerance, prolonged parenteral nutrition may be required until intestinal transport mechanisms for monosaccharides return.

Wright EM: Glucose–galactose malabsorption. Am J Physiol 1998;275:G879.

## 5. Intestinal Lymphangiectasia

This form of protein-losing enteropathy results from a congenital ectasia of the bowel lymphatic system, often associated with abnormalities of the lymphatics in the extremities. Obstruction of lymphatic drainage of the intestine leads to rupture of the intestinal lacteals with leakage of lymph into the lumen of the bowel. Fat loss may be significant and lead to steatorrhea. Chronic loss of lymphocytes and immunoglobulins increases the susceptibility to infections.

### Clinical Findings

Peripheral edema, diarrhea, abdominal distention, lymphedematous extremities, chylous effusions, and repeated infections are common. Laboratory findings are low serum albumin, decreased immunoglobulin levels, lymphocytopenia, and anemia. Fecal fat loss is increased. Serum calcium and magnesium are frequently depressed as these cations are lost in complex with unabsorbed fatty acids. Lymphocytes may be seen in large numbers on a stool smear. Fecal $\alpha_1$-antitrypsin is elevated. Radiographic studies reveal an edematous small-bowel mucosal pattern, and biopsy reveals dilated lacteals in the villi and lamina propria. If only the lymphatics of the deeper layers of bowel or intestinal mesenterics are involved, laparotomy may be necessary to establish the diagnosis.

## Differential Diagnosis

Other causes of protein-losing enteropathy must be considered, although an associated lymphedematous extremity strongly favors this diagnosis.

## Treatment & Prognosis

A very high protein diet (up to 6–7 g/kg/d may be needed) enriched with medium-chain triglycerides as a fat source may allow for adequate nutrition and growth in patients with intestinal mucosal lymphangiectasia. Vitamin and calcium supplements should be given. Antibiotics are used for specific infections. Total parenteral nutrition is helpful on a temporary basis. Surgery is needed when the lesion is localized to a small area of the bowel or in cases of constrictive pericarditis or obstructing tumors. Intravenous albumin and immune globulin may also be used to control symptoms. The prognosis is not favorable, although remission may occur with age. Malignant degeneration of the abnormal lymphatics may occur, and intestinal lymphoma of the B-cell type may be a long-term complication of intestinal lymphangiectasia.

## 6. Cow's Milk Protein Intolerance

Milk protein intolerance is more common in males than females and in young infants with a family history of atopy. The estimated prevalence is 0.5–1%. Colic, vomiting, and diarrhea are the major symptoms. Stools often contain blood and mucus. Sigmoidoscopic examination reveals a superficial colitis, often with edema, a mild eosinophilic infiltrate, and lymphonodular hyperplasia. Pneumatosis intestinalis may be present on radiograph. Viral gastroenteritis sometimes precedes the onset of symptoms. Less commonly, milk protein may induce eosinophilic gastroenteritis with protein-losing enteropathy, hypoalbuminemia, and hypogammaglobulinemia. A celiac-like syndrome with villous atrophy, malabsorption, hypoalbuminemia, occult blood in the stool, and anemia can occur in older children. IgE-mediated anaphylactic shock is a rare but potentially life-threatening manifestation of milk protein sensitivity in infancy. If the symptoms suggest an anaphylactic response to milk or any other protein, food challenge should be performed only in a setting in which resuscitation can be carried out.

Infants who are solely breast-fed can also develop blood-streaked stools and a sigmoidoscopic picture similar to that of formula-fed infants with milk protein sensitivity. Tiny amounts of intact allergen passed in breast milk may be the cause, but other environmental allergens may play a role. Elimination of whole milk from the mother's diet sometimes resolves bloody diarrhea. A switch to a protein hydrolysate formula almost always results in improvement. Because the blood loss and diarrhea in these breast-fed infants are rarely severe, it is not essential that breast feeding be stopped. If symptoms are severe or prolonged, however, a trial of semielemental formula is recommended. The colitic pattern of milk protein sensitivity and colitis in breast-fed infants usually clears spontaneously by age 6–12 months.

Early reports that patients with milk protein allergy have a 30% incidence of sensitivity to soy protein, with similar symptoms, have not been uniformly confirmed.

## 7. Immunologic Deficiency States with Diarrhea or Malabsorption

Diarrhea is common in immune deficiency states, but the cause is often obscure. Between 50% and 60% of patients with idiopathic acquired hypogammaglobulinemia have steatorrhea and intestinal villous atrophy. Lymphonodular hyperplasia is a common feature in this group of patients. Patients with congenital or Bruton-type agammaglobulinemia usually have diarrhea and abnormal intestinal morphology. Patients with isolated IgA deficiency may also present with chronic diarrhea, a celiac-like picture, lymphoid nodular hyperplasia, and giardiasis. Patients with isolated cellular immunity defects, combined cellular and humoral immune incompetence, and HIV infection may have severe chronic diarrhea leading to malnutrition. The cause of diarrhea may be common bacterial, viral, fungal, or parasitic pathogens, organisms usually considered nonpathogenic (*Blastocystis hominis, Candida*); or unusual organisms (cytomegalovirus, *Cryptosporidium, Isospora belli, Mycobacterium* species, microsporidia, and algal organisms such as cyanobacteria). Often the cause is not found. The incidence of disaccharidase deficiency is high. Chronic granulomatous disease may be associated with intestinal symptoms suggestive of chronic inflammatory bowel disease. A rectal biopsy may reveal the presence of typical macrophages.

Treatment must be directed toward correction of the immunologic defect. Specific treatments are available or are being developed for many of the unusual pathogens causing diarrhea in the immunocompromised host. Thus a vigorous diagnostic search for specific pathogens is warranted in these individuals.

## 8. Pancreatic Insufficiency

The most common cause of pancreatic exocrine insufficiency in childhood is cystic fibrosis. Decreased secretion of pancreatic digestive enzymes is caused by obstruction of the exocrine ducts by thick secretions, which destroys the pancreatic acinar cells. This destruction of acinar cells may occur antenatally. Some genotypes of cystic fibrosis have partially or completely preserved pancreatic exocrine function. Other conditions associated with exocrine pancreatic insufficiency are discussed in Chapter 21.

## 9. Other Genetic Disorders Causing Malabsorption

### A. A-β-Lipoproteinemia

A-β-lipoproteinemia is an autosomal recessive condition in which the secretion of triglyceride-rich lipoproteins from the small intestine (chylomicrons) and liver (very low density lipoproteins) is abnormal. Profound steatosis of the intestinal enterocytes (and hepatocytes) and severe fat malabsorption occur. Deficiencies of fat-soluble vitamins occur over time, with neurologic complications of vitamin E deficiency and atypical retinitis pigmentosa. The serum cholesterol level is very low, and the red cell membrane lipids are abnormal, causing acanthosis of the red blood cells, which sometimes is the key to diagnosing this rare condition.

### B. Acrodermatitis Enteropathica

Acrodermatitis enteropathica is an autosomal recessive condition in which the intestine has a selective inability to absorb zinc. The condition usually becomes clinically obvious at the time of weaning and is characterized by rash on the extremities, rashes around the body orifices, eczema, profound failure to thrive, steatorrhea, diarrhea, and immune deficiency. Zinc supplementation by mouth results in rapid improvement.

## CONSTIPATION

Constipation is passage of bulky or hard stool at infrequent intervals. Retention of feces in the rectum results in encopresis (involuntary fecal leakage) in 60% of affected children. Organic causes of constipation are listed in Table 20–7. Most constipation in childhood is not organic but a result of voluntary or involuntary retentive behavior.

## Clinical Findings

Normal infants younger than age 3 months often grunt, strain, and turn red in the face while passing normal stools. This pattern may be viewed erroneously as constipation. Failure to appreciate this normal developmental pattern may lead to the unwise use of laxatives or enemas. Infants and children may gradually develop the ability to ignore the sensation of rectal fullness and retain stool. Many factors promote and reinforce this behavior, which results in impaction of the rectum and overflow incontinence or encopresis: painful defecation; skeletal muscle weakness; psychological issues, especially those relating to control and authority; modesty and distaste for school bathrooms; medications; and others listed in Table 20–7. The dilated rectum becomes less sensitive to dilation, thus perpetuating the problem, regardless of the original cause. As many as 1–2% of healthy primary school children have retentive constipation. The ratio of males to females is 4:1 in some studies.

## Differential Diagnosis

Features distinguishing retentive constipation from Hirschsprung disease are summarized in Table 20–8.

## Treatment of Retentive Constipation

Increased intake of fluids and high-residue foods such as bran, whole wheat, fruits, and vegetables may be sufficient therapy in mild constipation. It should be noted that the most likely response to increased fluid intake in normally hydrated children is increased urination with little effect on defecation. The use of a barley malt extract (Maltsupex), 1–2 tsp added to feedings two or three times daily, is helpful in small infants. Polyethylene glycol solution is also a safe softener. Stool softeners such as dioctyl sodium sulfosuccinate, 5–10 mg/kg/d, prevent excessive drying of the stool but are less effective in children with voluntary stool retention. Cathartics such as standardized extract of senna fruit (eg, Senokot syrup), 1–2 tsp twice daily depending on age, can be used for short periods.

If encopresis is present, treatment should start with relieving fecal impaction. An effective stool softener should be given as a maintenance medication in doses sufficient to induce two or three loose bowel movements per day. Such medications include mineral oil (2–3 mL/kg/d), a nonabsorbable osmotic agent such as polyethylene glycol (Miralax, 1 gm/kg/d), and milk of magnesia (1–2 mL/kg/d). After several weeks to months of regular loose stools, the stool softener can be tapered and stopped. Mineral oil should not be given to non-ambulatory infants, physically handicapped or bed-

**Table 20–7.** Causes of constipation.

| | |
|---|---|
| Functional or retentive causes | Abnormalities of myenteric ganglion cells |
|   Dietary causes |   Hirschsprung disease |
|     Undernutrition, dehydration |   Waardenburg syndrome |
|     Excessive milk intake |   Multiple endocrine neoplasia IIa |
|     Lack of bulk | Hypo- and hyperganglionosis |
|   Cathartic abuse |   von Recklinghausen disease |
|   Drugs |   Multiple endocrine neoplasia IIb |
|     Narcotics |   Intestinal neuronal dysplasia |
|     Antihistamines |   Chronic intestinal pseudo-obstruction |
|     Some antidepressants | Spinal cord defects |
|     Vincristine | Metabolic and endocrine disorders |
|   Structural defects of gastrointestinal tract |   Hypothyroidism |
|     Anus and rectum |   Hyperparathyroidism |
|       Fissure, hemorrhoids, abscess |   Renal tubular acidosis |
|       Anterior ectopic anus |   Diabetes insipidus (dehydration) |
|       Anal and rectal stenosis |   Vitamin D intoxication (hypercalcemia) |
|       Presacral teratoma |   Idiopathic hypercalcemia |
|     Small bowel and colon | Skeletal muscle weakness or incoordination |
|       Tumor, stricture |   Cerebral palsy |
|       Chronic volvulus |   Muscular dystrophy/myotonia |
|       Intussusception | |
|   Smooth muscle diseases | |
|     Scleroderma and dermatomyositis | |
|     Systemic lupus erythematosus | |
|     Chronic intestinal pseudo-obstruction | |

Modified and reproduced, with permission, from Silverman A, Roy CC: *Pediatric Clinical Gastroenterology*, 3rd ed. Mosby, 1983.

**Table 20–8.** Differentiation of retentive constipation and Hirschsprung disease.

| | Retentive Constipation | Hirschsprung Disease |
|---|---|---|
| Onset | 2–3 years | At birth |
| Abdominal distention | Rare | Present |
| Nutrition and growth | Normal | Poor |
| Soiling and retentive behavior | Intermittent or constant | Rare |
| Rectal examination | Ampulla full | Ampulla may be empty |
| Rectal biopsy | Ganglion cells present | Ganglion cells absent |
| Rectal manometry | Normal rectoanal reflex | Nonrelaxation of internal anal sphincter after rectal distention |
| Barium enema | Distended rectum | Narrow distal segment with proximal megacolon |

bound children, or those with GE reflux. Aspiration of mineral oil may cause lipid pneumonia. Stool softeners help extinguish the tendency to retention and the establishment of a regular bowel habit by making defecation quick, easy, and painless. Recurrence of encopresis should be treated promptly with a short course of stimulant laxatives or an enema. A multiple vitamin is recommended while mineral oil is administered. Psychiatric consultation may be indicated for patients with resistant symptoms or severe emotional disturbances.

## GASTROINTESTINAL BLEEDING

Vomiting blood and passing blood per rectum are alarming symptoms. The history is the key to identifying the bleeding source. The following questions should be answered:

1. Is it really blood, and is it coming from the GI tract? A number of substances simulate hematochezia or melena (Table 20–9). The presence of blood should be confirmed chemically. Genitourinary problems, coughing, tonsillitis, lost teeth, or epistaxis may cause what appears to be

**Table 20–9.** Pitfalls in the diagnosis of gastrointestinal bleeding in children.

| |
|---|
| **Exogenous blood** |
|     Maternal blood[a] |
|     Epistaxis |
|     Uncooked meat |
| **Pseudoblood** |
|     Medications in red syrup |
|     Red Kool-Aid, fruit punch, red gelatin |
|     Tomato skin |
|     Tomato juice |
|     Cranberry juice |
|     Beets |
|     Peach skin |
|     Red diaper syndrome[b] |
|     Red cherries |
| **Black stools** |
|     Iron preparations[c,d] |
|     Pepto-Bismol |
|     Grape juice |
|     Purple grapes |
|     Spinach |
|     Chocolate |

[a]From cracked nipples in a breast-fed baby.
[b]Red pigmentation of soiled diapers due to *Serratia marcescens* in stool.
[c]Ferrous sulfate and ferrous gluconate with guaiac and orthotolidine-based tests.
[d]High false-positive rate with orthotolidine-based tests.
Modified and reproduced, with permission, from Treem WR: Gastrointestinal bleeding in children. Gastrointest Endosc Clin North Am 1994;4:75.

GI bleeding. An adolescent female may be experiencing menarche.

2. How much blood is there and what is its color and character? Table 20–10 lists the sites of GI bleeding predicted by the appearance of the blood in the stools. Table 20–11 lists causes of rectal bleeding.

3. Is the child acutely or chronically ill? The physical examination should be thorough. Physical signs of portal hypertension, intestinal obstruction, or coagulopathy are particularly important. The nasal passages should be inspected for signs of recent epistaxis, the vagina for menstrual blood, and the anus for fissures and hemorrhoids.

A systolic blood pressure below 100 mm Hg and a pulse rate above 100 beats/min in an older child suggest at least a 20% reduction of blood volume. A pulse rate increase of 20 beats/min or a drop in systolic blood pressure greater than 10 mm Hg when the patient sits up is also a sensitive index of significant volume depletion.

4. Is the child still bleeding? Serial determinations of vital signs and hematocrit are essential to assess ongoing bleeding. Detection of blood in the gastric aspirate confirms a bleeding site proximal to the ligament of Treitz. However, its absence does not rule out the duodenum as the source. Testing the stool for occult blood will help in monitoring ongoing loss of blood.

### Treatment

If a hemorrhagic diathesis is detected, vitamin K should be given intravenously. In severe bleeding, the need for volume replacement is monitored by measurement of central venous pressure. In less severe cases, vital signs, serial hematocrits, and gastric aspirates are sufficient.

If blood is recovered from the gastric aspirate, gastric lavage with saline should be performed until only a blood-tinged return is obtained. Upper intestinal endoscopy is then done to identify the bleeding site. Endoscopy is superior to barium contrast study for lesions such as esophageal varices, stress ulcers, and gastritis. Colonoscopy may identify the source of bright red rectal bleeding but should be performed as an emergency only if the extent of bleeding warrants immediate inves-

**Table 20–10.** Identification of sites of gastrointestinal bleeding.

| Symptom or Sign | Location of Bleeding Lesion |
|---|---|
| Effortless bright red blood from the mouth | Nasopharyngeal or oral lesions; tonsillitis; esophageal varices; lacerations of esophageal or gastric mucosa (Mallory–Weiss syndrome) |
| Vomiting of bright red blood or of "coffee grounds" | Lesion proximal to ligament of Treitz |
| Melanotic stool | Lesion proximal to ligament of Treitz, upper small bowel. Blood loss in excess of 50–100 mL/24 h |
| Bright red or dark red blood in stools | Lesion in the ileum or colon. (Massive upper gastrointestinal bleeding may also be associated with bright red blood in stool.) |
| Streak of blood on outside of a stool | Lesion in the rectal ampulla or anal canal |

***Table 20–11.*** Differential diagnosis of gastrointestinal bleeding in children by symptoms and age at presentation.

| | Infant | Child (2–12 years) | Adolescent (> 12 years) |
|---|---|---|---|
| Hematemesis | Swallowed maternal blood<br>Peptic esophagitis<br>Mallory–Weiss tear<br>Gastritis<br>Gastric ulcer<br>Duodenal ulcer<br>Gastric, duodenal ulcer | Epistaxis<br>Peptic esophagitis<br>Caustic ingestion<br>Mallory–Weiss tear<br>Esophageal varices<br>Gastritis<br>Gastric ulcer<br>Duodenal ulcer<br>Hereditary hemorrhagic telangiectasia<br>Hemobilia<br>Henoch–Schönlein purpura | Esophageal ulcer<br>Peptic esophagitis<br>Mallory–Weiss tear<br>Esophageal varices<br>Gastric ulcer<br>Gastritis<br>Duodenal ulcer<br>Hereditary hemorrhagic telangiectasia<br>Hemobilia<br>Henoch–Schönlein purpura |
| Painless melena | Duodenal ulcer<br>Duodenal duplication<br>Ileal duplication<br>Meckel diverticulum<br>Gastric heterotopia[a] | Duodenal ulcer<br>Duodenal duplication<br>Ileal duplication<br>Meckel diverticulum<br>Gastric heterotopia[a] | Duodenal ulcer<br>Leiomyoma (sarcoma) |
| Melena with pain, obstruction, peritonitis, perforation | Necrotizing enterocolitis<br>Intussusception[b]<br>Volvulus | Duodenal ulcer<br>Hemobilia[c]<br>Intussusception[b]<br>Volvulus<br>Ileal ulcer (isolated) | Duodenal ulcer<br>Hemobilia[c]<br>Crohn disease (ileal ulcer) |
| Hematochezia with diarrhea, crampy abdominal pain | Infectious colitis<br>Pseudomembranous colitis<br>Eosinophilic colitis<br>Hirschsprung enterocolitis | Infectious colitis<br>Pseudomembranous colitis<br>Granulomatous (Crohn) colitis<br>Hemolytic–uremic syndrome<br>Henoch–Schönlein purpura<br>Lymphonodular hyperplasia | Infectious colitis<br>Pseudomembranous colitis<br>Granulomatous (Crohn) colitis<br>Hemolytic–uremic syndrome<br>Henoch–Schönlein purpura |
| Hematochezia without diarrhea or abdominal pain | Anal fissure<br>Eosinophilic colitis<br>Rectal gastric mucosa<br>   heterotopia<br>Colonic hemangiomas | Anal fissure<br>Solitary rectal ulcer<br>Juvenile polyp<br>Lymphonodular hyperplasia | Anal fissure<br>Hemorrhoid<br>Solitary rectal ulcer<br>Colonic arteriovenous malformation |

[a]Ectopic gastric tissue in jejunum or ileum without Meckel diverticulum.
[b]Classically, "currant jelly" stool.
[c]Hemobilia often accompanied by vomiting, right upper quadrant pain.
Reproduced, with permission, from Treem WR: Gastrointestinal bleeding in children. Gastrointest Endosc Clin North Am 1994;4:75.

tigation and if plain abdominal radiographs show no signs of intestinal obstruction. Colonoscopy on an un-prepped colon is often inadequate for making a diagnosis.

Small- or large-bowel lesions that bleed briskly (> 0.5 mL/min) may be localized by angiography or radionuclide scanning following injection of labeled red cells.

Persistent vascular bleeding (varices, vascular anomalies) may be relieved temporarily using intravenous vasopressin, 20 units/1.73 $m^2$ over a 20-minute period, or intravenous octreotide, 25–30 $\mu$ g/$m^2$/h (preferable because of fewer adverse effects). Sustained infusion of octreotide may be used for up to 48 hours if needed. Bleeding from esophageal varices may be stopped by temporary compression with a Sengstaken–Blakemore tube. Sclerotherapy or banding of bleeding varices is the treatment of choice.

If gastric decompression, acid suppressive therapy, and transfusion are ineffective in stopping ulcer bleeding, laser therapy, local injection of epinephrine, electrocautery, or emergency surgery may be necessary.

Fox VL: Gastrointestinal bleeding in infants and children. Gastrointest Clin North Am 2000;29:37.

# RECURRENT ABDOMINAL PAIN

About 10% of healthy school children between ages 5 and 15 years will at some time experience recurrent episodes of abdominal pain severe enough to interfere with normal activities. An organic cause can be found in fewer than 10% of patients.

## Clinical Findings

### A. SYMPTOMS AND SIGNS

Attacks of abdominal pain are characteristically of variable duration and intensity. It is not rare for the child or parent to report that the pain is constant, all day every day. Although the pain is usually located in the periumbilical area, location far from the umbilicus does not rule out recurrent abdominal pain. Pain may occur both day and night. Weight loss is rare. Pain may be associated with dramatic reactions—frantic crying, clutching the abdomen, doubling over. Parents may be alarmed, and children are often taken to emergency departments, where the evaluation is negative for an abdominal crisis. School attendance may suffer, and enjoyable family events may be disrupted. The pain may be associated with pallor, nausea, vomiting, and slight temperature elevation.

The pain usually bears little relationship to bowel habits and physical activity. However, some patients have a constellation of symptoms strongly suggesting irritable bowel syndrome—bloating, postprandial pain, lower abdominal discomfort, and erratic stool habits with a sensation of obstipation or incomplete evacuation of stool. A precipitating or stressful situation in the child's life at the time the pains began can sometimes be elicited. School phobia may be a precipitant. A history of functional GI complaints is often found in family members.

A thorough physical examination is essential and usually normal. Complaints of abdominal tenderness elicited during palpation sometimes seem out of proportion to visible signs of distress.

### B. LABORATORY FINDINGS

Complete blood count, sedimentation rate, urinalysis, and stool test for occult blood usually suffice. In the adolescent female patient, ultrasound of the abdomen may be helpful to detect gallbladder or ovarian pathology. If the pain is atypical, further testing suggested by symptoms and family history should be done.

## Differential Diagnosis

Abdominal pain secondary to disorders of the urinary tract and extra-abdominal sources are listed in Table 20–3. Pinworms, mesenteric lymphadenitis, and chronic appendicitis are improbable causes of recurrent abdominal pain. Lactose intolerance usually causes abdominal distention, gas, and diarrhea with milk ingestion. At times, however, abdominal discomfort may be the only symptom. Abdominal migraine and abdominal epilepsy are rare conditions with an episodic character often associated with vomiting. The incidence of peptic gastritis, esophagitis, duodenitis, and ulcer disease is probably underappreciated. Upper intestinal endoscopy may be useful.

## Treatment & Prognosis

Treatment consists of reassurance based on a thorough physical appraisal and a sympathetic, age-appropriate explanation of the nature of functional pain. The concept of "visceral hyperalgesia" or increased pain signaling from physiologic stimuli such as gas, acid secretion, or stool is one that parents can understand and helps them to respond appropriately to the child's complaints. Reassurance without education is rarely helpful. Regular activity should be resumed, especially school attendance. Therapy for emotional problems is sometimes required, but drugs should be avoided. In older patients, and in those with what appears to be visceral hyperalgesia, amitriptyline in low doses may occasionally be helpful. Antispasmodic medications are rarely helpful and should be reserved for patients with more typical irritable bowel complaints.

Hyams JS, Hyman PE: Recurrent abdominal pain and the biopsychosocial model of medical practice. J Pediatr 1998;133:472.

Hyams JS et al: Abdominal pain and irritable bowel syndrome in adolescents: A community based study. J Pediatr 1996; 129:220.

Van Ginkel R et al: Alterations in rectal sensitivity and motility in childhood irritable bowel syndrome. Gastroenterology 2001; 120:31.

# INFLAMMATORY BOWEL DISEASE

Crohn disease and ulcerative colitis are the two major idiopathic inflammatory bowel diseases of children. They share many features resulting from bowel inflammation, such as diarrhea, pain, fever, and blood loss, but they differ in important aspects, such as distribution of disease, histologic findings, incidence and type of extraintestinal symptoms, response to medications and surgery, and prognosis. A comparison of these two conditions is shown in Table 20–12. The cause is unknown but is probably a result of inappropriate activation of the mucosal immune system fueled by the presence of normal luminal flora. The aberrant response appears to be facilitated by defects in the barrier function of the intestinal epithelium as well. The single

***Table 20–12.*** Features of Crohn's disease and ulcerative colitis.

| | Crohn's Disease | Ulcerative Colitis |
|---|---|---|
| Age at onset | 10–20 years | 10–20 years |
| Incidence | 4–6 per 100,000 | 3–15 per 100,000 |
| Area of bowel affected | Oropharynx, esophagus, and stomach, rare; small bowel only, 25–30%; colon and anus only, 25%; ileocolitis, 40%; diffuse disease, 5% | Total colon, 90%; proctitis, 10% |
| Distribution | Segmental; disease-free skip areas common | Continuous; distal to proximal |
| Pathology | Full-thickness, acute, and chronic inflammation; noncaseating granulomas (50%), extraintestinal fistulas, abscesses, stricture, and fibrosis may be present | Superficial, acute inflammation of mucosa with microscopic crypt abscess |
| Radiographic findings | Segmental lesions; thickened, circular folds, cobblestone appearance of bowel wall secondary to longitudinal ulcers and transverse fissures; fixation and separation of loops; narrowed lumen; "string sign"; fistulas | Superficial colitis; loss of haustra; shortened colon and pseudopolyps (islands of normal tissue surrounded by denuded mucosa) are late findings |
| Intestinal symptoms | Abdominal pain, diarrhea (usually loose with blood if colon involved), perianal disease, enteroenteric or enterocutaneous fistula, abscess, anorexia | Abdominal pain, bloody diarrhea, urgency, and tenesmus |
| Extraintestinal symptoms<br>  Arthritis/arthralgia | 15% | 9% |
| Fever | 40–50% | 40–50% |
| Stomatitis | 9% | 2% |
| Weight loss | 90% (mean 5.7 kg) | 68% (mean 4.1 kg) |
| Delayed growth and sexual development | 30% | 5–10% |
| Uveitis, conjunctivitis | 15% (in Crohn colitis) | 4% |
| Sclerosing cholangitis | — | 4% |
| Renal stones | 6% (oxalate) | 6% (urate) |
| Pyoderma gangrenosum | 1–3% | 5% |
| Erythema nodosum | 8–15% | 4% |
| Laboratory findings | High erythrocyte sedimentation rate; microcytic anemia; low serum iron and total iron-binding capacity; increased fecal protein loss; low serum albumin; antineutrophil cytoplasmic antibodies present in 10–20%; *Saccharomyces cerevisiae* antibodies positive in 60%. | High erythrocyte sedimentation rate; microcytic anemia, high white blood cell count with left shift; antineutrophil cytoplasmic antibodies present in 80% |

Reproduced, with permission, from Kirschner BS: Inflammatory bowel disease in children. Pediatr Clin North Am 1988;35:189.

greatest risk factor for inflammatory bowel disease is a positive family history (found in 15–30% of inflammatory bowel disease patients). Monozygotic twins have a 37% concordance for Crohn disease and a 10% concordance for ulcerative colitis. Recent genetic studies have identified an inflammatory bowel disease susceptibility gene on chromosome 16 (*CARD15*), the product of which is involved in the activation of the nuclear factor NFκB and also in the responsiveness to bacterial lipopolysaccharides. More genetic loci are being identified, giving some hope that basic immune mechanisms of Crohn disease and perhaps ulcerative colitis will be soon discovered. There is no indication that emotional factors are a primary cause of these diseases.

## Diagnostic Testing

### A. CROHN DISEASE

Because Crohn disease can occur at any location in the GI tract from the mouth to the anus, a complete evaluation is required. Upper and lower endoscopy allows investigation of mouth, esophagus, duodenum, colon, and terminal ileum. Biopsy specimens from all these areas may reveal the typical histologic findings. Barium radiograph of the small intestine is still the best way to look for small-bowel disease, but capsule video endoscopy may soon be a more uniformly available means to study the small intestine. Computed tomographic scan and magnetic resonance imaging of the small bowel can show mucosal and mural edema but are not specific enough to confirm a diagnosis. Serum antibodies to *Saccharomyces cerevisiae* are present in 40–60% of patients with Crohn disease. This may be helpful for screening if positive, but it is not sensitive or specific enough to be diagnostic. Fecal calprotectin is a neutrophil-associated protein, which, when elevated in stool, suggests the presence of an inflammatory process. It may be more useful for monitoring therapy in established Crohn disease than for diagnosis.

### B. ULCERATIVE COLITIS

Colonoscopy with mucosal biopsy is the best diagnostic test for ulcerative colitis. Nearly pathognomonic signs may be seen on barium enema, but the test is being replaced in most instances by colonoscopy. The perinuclear neutrophil cytoplasmic antigen is positive in 60–70% of patients with ulcerative colitis. Fecal calprotectin is high in patients with active disease.

### C. INDETERMINATE COLITIS

This poorly defined entity is a diagnostic challenge and is generally a diagnosis of exclusion in patients in whom colonoscopic biopsy specimens do not seem typical of ulcerative colitis or Crohn disease. More experience is needed to determine whether this is indeed a separate

disease. These patients may have superficial Crohn colitis or may have ulcerative colitis with relative rectal sparing. The same group of medications are used for its treatment.

## Differential Diagnosis

### A. CROHN DISEASE

When extraintestinal symptoms predominate, Crohn disease can be mistaken for rheumatoid arthritis, systemic lupus erythematosus, or hypopituitarism. Frequently, the acute onset of ileocolitis is mistaken for acute appendicitis. Symptoms sometimes suggest celiac disease, peptic ulcer, intestinal obstruction, intestinal lymphoma, anorexia nervosa, or growth failure from endocrine causes.

### B. ULCERATIVE COLITIS

In the acute stage, bacterial pathogens and toxins causing colitis must be ruled out. These include *Shigella, Salmonella, Yersinia, Campylobacter, Entamoeba histolytica,* enteroinvasive *Escherichia coli* (*E coli* 0157), *Aeromonas hydrophila,* and *Clostridium difficile.* Mild ulcerative colitis sometimes mimics irritable bowel symptoms. Crohn disease of the colon is an important differential possibility.

## Complications (See Table 20–12.)

### A. CROHN DISEASE

Intestinal obstruction, fistula, and abscess formation are common. Perforation and hemorrhage are rare. Malnutrition is caused by anorexia and compounded by malabsorption, protein-losing enteropathy, disaccharidase deficiency, and diarrhea induced by bile salts. Systemic complications include perianal disease, pyoderma gangrenosum, arthritis, amyloidosis, and growth retardation. The risk of colon cancer is increased in patients with Crohn colitis, although not to the extent seen in ulcerative colitis.

### B. ULCERATIVE COLITIS

Arthritis, uveitis, pyoderma gangrenosum, and malnutrition all occur. Growth failure and delayed puberty are less common than in Crohn disease. Liver disease (chronic active hepatitis, sclerosing cholangitis) is more common. In patients with pancolitis, carcinoma of the colon occurs with an incidence of 1–2% per year after the first 10 years of disease. Cancer risk is a function of disease duration and not age at onset. The mortality rate from colon cancer is high because the usual signs (occult blood in stool, pain, and abnormal radiologic findings) are not specific and may be ignored in a patient with colitis. Routine cancer screening via colonoscopy, with multiple biopsies and evaluation of specimens by histology for metaplasia and by flow cytometry for aneuploidy, is recommended in pediatric patients after 10 years of pancolitis. Dysplasia that persists in absence of inflammation is an indication for colectomy, as is aneuploidy in multiple biopsies.

## Treatment

### A. MEDICAL TREATMENT

Medical treatment for Crohn disease and ulcerative colitis is similar and includes anti-inflammatory, antidiarrheal, and antibiotic medication. No medical therapy has proved uniformly effective.

**1. Diet**—A high-protein, high-carbohydrate diet with normal amounts of fat is recommended. Decreased amounts of fiber may help decrease symptoms in those with colitis or with partial intestinal obstruction. Lactose is poorly tolerated when disease is active. The main concern should be ensuring adequate caloric intake. Restrictive or bland diets are counterproductive because they usually result in poor intake. Vitamin and iron supplements are recommended. Zinc levels are often low in patients with Crohn disease and should be supplemented. Supplemental calories in the form of liquid diets are well tolerated. Total parenteral nutrition for periods of 4–6 weeks may induce remission of symptoms and stimulate linear growth and sexual development. Enteral administration of low-residue or elemental liquid diets is widely used outside of the United States to induce remission in patients with Crohn disease. It is less effective in ulcerative colitis. Home programs of both enteral and parenteral nutritional support have been especially effective in patients with intractable symptoms or growth failure.

**2. Nonabsorbable salicylate derivatives**—Sulfasalazine is effective in mild cases of ulcerative colitis and perhaps in cases of Crohn disease of the colon. It prevents relapse of ulcerative colitis once remission is induced. The drug is not absorbed in the small intestine. It is hydrolyzed by colon flora into sulfapyridine and 5-aminosalicylate. The sulfonamide moiety is probably inactive but is responsible for the allergic side effects of the drug. The salicylate moiety probably has local anti-inflammatory activity in the colon. Side effects are common, including skin rash, nausea, headache, and abdominal pain. More rarely, serum sickness, hemolytic anemia, aplastic anemia, and pancreatitis occur. Response to therapy may be slow. Sulfasalazine inhibits folic acid absorption, and supplemental folic acid is required.

The recommended dosage is 2–3 g/d in three divided doses for children over age 10 years or 50 mg/kg/d for younger children. Half of this dosage is used as a maintenance medication for well-controlled ulcerative colitis. Salicylate polymers for both oral and rectal use (olsalazine, mesalamine) are available. A variety of pH-sensitive tablet coatings and microencapsulation allow release of these products at specific locations in the GI tract, thereby improving their efficacy. They are no more effective than sulfasalazine but can be tolerated by sulfonamide-sensitive patients and have fewer side effects.

**3. Corticosteroids**—With more severe inflammatory bowel disease, corticosteroids are used. Methylprednisolone, 2 mg/kg/d, or hydrocortisone, 10 mg/kg/d, may be given intravenously when disease is severe. Prednisone, 1–2 mg/kg/d orally in two or three divided doses, is given for 6–8 weeks, followed by a gradual tapering. Alternate-day steroids are associated with fewer side effects as the dosage of drug is tapered. There is no evidence that corticosteroids prevent relapses. Prednisone is often given in conjunction with sulfasalazine. The patient's varicella immunity should be confirmed by history or antibody screen and the parents counseled appropriately as to risk and therapy after varicella exposure. Serum titers against *E histolytica* and stool examination for amebic parasites must be checked before starting therapy with corticosteroids, because amebic colitis may become generalized with steroid therapy. Hydrocortisone in the form of enema or foam can be instilled into the rectum in patients with tenesmus or ulcerative proctitis. Budesonide, which has "one pass metabolism" in the liver, is available in both oral and rectal preparations. These preparations are most useful for treatment of rectal disease (enemas and suppositories) and right-sided colon disease (oral) and in appropriate doses have fewer corticoid side effects.

**4. Azathioprine**—Azathioprine (Imuran), 1–2 mg/kg/d orally, or 6-mercaptopurine can be used when a high maintenance dose of corticosteroids is necessary to keep the inflammatory bowel disease under control (especially in Crohn disease). The optimal dose of 6-mercaptopurine depends on the patient's ability to metabolize the compound. Positive results of this therapy may be delayed weeks to months. Side effects include pancreatitis, hepatotoxicity, and bone marrow suppression. Metabolites of azathioprine should be monitored to avoid over- and underdosing in patients with variable metabolizing capacity. Genetic testing is available to identify individuals with diminished ability to metabolize azathioprine.

**5. Metronidazole**—This drug is used in treating Crohn disease in patients with perianal disease. Disease tends to recur when the drug is discontinued. It may also be effective in treating Crohn disease of the colon. The dosage of metronidazole is 15–30 mg/kg/d in three divided doses. Peripheral neuropathy may be a side effect with prolonged use. Ciprofloxacin may have similar therapeutic effects.

**6. Cyclosporine**—This powerful immunosuppressant is effective in severe, steroid-resistant ulcerative colitis, but because of side effects and rapid relapse after discontinuation, it is usually used to buy time in severely affected patients for whom surgical treatment is planned but who are too ill to tolerate surgery immediately.

**7. Methotrexate**—There has been recent encouraging experience with both oral and subcutaneous methotrexate in treating Crohn disease. Liver toxicity is a risk with prolonged use.

**8. Anticytokines**—Tumor necrosis factor alpha (TNF-α) is a proinflammatory cytokine produced in monocytes, macrophages, and activated T cells, which among other functions stimulates the production of proinflammatory cytokines such as interleukins IL-1, IL-6, IL-8, and granulocyte–macrophage colony-stimulating factor. TNF-α levels are increased in intestinal mucosa of Crohn disease patients. Administration of a chimeric human–mouse antibody to TNF-α (infliximab) has been effective in the treatment of Crohn disease, especially in patients with resistant perianal disease. Relapse is common within 3 months of first treatment, and most patients require repeated intravenous infusions of the medication at intervals ranging from 4 to 12 weeks in order to remain in remission. Anaphylactic reactions to this medication have been reported, and infusions should be carried out in a setting where emergency resuscitation is available. Humanizing the antibody and the concomitant use of azathioprine seem to decrease the incidence of severe allergic reactions. Treatment with the anti-inflammatory cytokine IL-10 is in the developmental stage for patients with Crohn disease. Anticytokine therapy is less effective in ulcerative colitis.

**9. Thalidomide**—Thalidomide has been used in patients with inflammatory bowel disease, especially those with oral and vaginal ulcers secondary to Crohn disease. The mechanism of its therapeutic action may be via its prevention of TNF secretion or its antiangiogenic activity. This medication must be used under strict supervision in postpubescent female patients because of the risk of teratogenesis.

## B. SURGICAL TREATMENT

**1. Crohn disease**—Crohn disease is not cured by surgery. However, 70% of patients eventually require surgery to relieve obstruction, drain abscess, relieve intractable symptoms, or encourage growth and sexual maturation. Newer treatment may decrease this figure. The relapse rate 6 years after surgery is 60%. Recurrence usually occurs at the site of anastomosis, most likely within 2 years. The rate of recurrence may be less in disease limited to the colon. Surgery performed to correct growth retardation must be performed before puberty.

**2. Ulcerative colitis**—Surgery is curative and is recommended for those with uncontrolled hemorrhage, toxic megacolon, unrelenting pain and diarrhea, growth failure, high-grade mucosal dysplasia, or malignant tumors. There are now several surgical approaches (ileoanal anastomosis, Koch-type continent ileostomy) that allow a near-normal lifestyle after colectomy. Liver disease associated with ulcerative colitis (sclerosing cholangitis) is not improved by colectomy.

## Prognosis

### A. CROHN DISEASE

Although the mortality rate is low (2% in the first 7 years), morbidity is high. The disease is progressive in most cases. Over 50% of patients experience symptoms that affect the quality of life. About 20% have severe disabling disease, and 20% have so few symptoms that they describe themselves as healthy.

### B. ULCERATIVE COLITIS

The prognosis is good. About 5% of patients present with toxic megacolon—massive colonic dilation secondary to full-thickness enterocolitis accompanied by shock and fever—and require immediate colectomy. Seventy-five percent have a relapsing and remitting course. Between 25% and 40% require colectomy—especially those with pancolitis, anemia, and hypoalbuminemia at the time of presentation.

Baldassano R et al: Infliximab (Remicade) therapy in treatment of pediatric Crohn's disease. Am J Gastroenterol 2003;98:833.

Bariol C et al: Early studies on the safety and effectiveness of thalidomide for symptomatic inflammatory bowel disease. J Gastroenterol Hepatol 2002;217:135 .

Bonen DK, Cho J: The genetics of inflammatory bowel disease. Gastroenterology 2003;124:521.

Markowitz J et al: A multi center trial of 6 MP and prednisone in children with newly diagnosed Crohn's disease. Gastroenterology 2000;119:895.

Ogata H, Hibi T: Cytokine and anticytokine therapies for inflammatory bowel disease. Cur Phar Des 2003;9:1108.

Tamboli CP et al: Fecal calprotectin in Crohn's disease. Gastroenterology 2003;124:1972.

## REFERENCES

### Websites

NASPGHAN@NASPGNHAN.ORG

The website for the North American Society for Pediatric Gastroenterology, Hepatology and Nutrition has an excellent selection of educational materials on many pediatric gastroenterologic conditions with parent information and recommendations for evaluation and therapy.

### General References

Silverman A, Roy CC: *Pediatric Clinical Gastroenterology,* 4th ed. Mosby, 1995.

Suchy FJ (ed): *Liver Disease in Children,* 2nd ed. Mosby, 2000.

Walker WA et al (eds): *Pediatric Gastrointestinal Disease,* 4th ed. BC Decker, 2003.

Wyllie R, Hyams JS (eds): *Pediatric Gastrointestinal Disease.* WB Saunders, 1993.

# Liver & Pancreas

*Ronald J. Sokol, MD, & Michael R. Narkewicz, MD*

## ■ LIVER

### PROLONGED NEONATAL CHOLESTATIC JAUNDICE

The main clinical features of disorders causing prolonged neonatal cholestasis are (1) elevated serum conjugated bilirubin fraction (> 2 mg/dL or > 20% of total bilirubin), (2) elevated serum bile acids (> 10 μmol/L), (3) variably acholic stools, (4) dark urine, and (5) hepatomegaly.

Prolonged neonatal cholestasis (conditions with decreased bile flow) has intrahepatic and extrahepatic causes. Specific clinical clues (Table 21–1) distinguish these two major categories of jaundice in 85% of cases. Histologic examination of tissue obtained by percutaneous liver biopsy increases the accuracy of differentiation to 95% (Table 21–2).

### INTRAHEPATIC CHOLESTASIS

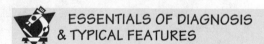

### ESSENTIALS OF DIAGNOSIS & TYPICAL FEATURES

- *Elevated total and conjugated bilirubin.*
- *Hepatomegaly and dark urine.*
- *Patency of extrahepatic biliary tree.*

### General Considerations

Intrahepatic cholestasis is characterized by hepatocyte dysfunction and patency of the extrahepatic biliary system. A specific cause can be identified in about 25% of cases. Patency of the extrahepatic biliary tract is suggested by pigmented stools and lack of bile duct proliferation on liver biopsy. It can be confirmed least invasively by hepatobiliary scintigraphy using technetium-99m ($^{99m}$Tc)-diethyliminodiacetic acid (diethyl-IDA [DIDA]). Radioactivity in the bowel within 4–24 hours is evidence of bile duct patency. Finding

bilirubin in duodenal aspirates also confirms patency. Patency can also be determined by cholangiography carried out intraoperatively, percutaneously by transhepatic cholecystography, or endoscopic retrograde cholangiopancreatography (ERCP) using a pediatric-size side-viewing endoscope.

### 1. Perinatal or Neonatal Hepatitis Resulting from Infection

This diagnosis is considered in infants with jaundice, hepatomegaly, vomiting, lethargy, fever, and petechiae. It is important to identify perinatally acquired viral, bacterial, or protozoal infections (Table 21–3). Infection may occur transplacentally, by ascent through the cervix into amniotic fluid, from swallowed contaminated fluids (maternal blood, urine) during delivery, from blood transfusions administered in the early neonatal period, or from breast milk or environmental sources. Infectious agents associated with neonatal intrahepatic cholestasis include herpes simplex virus (HSV), varicella virus, enteroviruses (coxsackievirus and echovirus), cytomegalovirus (CMV), rubella virus, adenovirus, parvovirus, human herpesvirus (HHV) type 6, hepatitis B virus (HBV), human immunodeficiency virus (HIV), *Treponema pallidum,* and *Toxoplasma gondii.* Although hepatitis C may be transmitted vertically, it rarely causes neonatal cholestasis. The degree of liver cell injury caused by these agents is variable, ranging from massive hepatic necrosis (herpes simplex, enteroviruses) to focal necrosis and mild inflammation (CMV, HBV). Serum bilirubin, bile acids, alanine aminotransferase (ALT), aspartate aminotransferase (AST), and alkaline phosphatase are elevated. The infant is jaundiced and generally appears ill.

### Clinical Findings

#### A. SYMPTOMS AND SIGNS

Clinical symptoms usually appear in the first 2 weeks of life but may appear as late as age 2–3 months. Jaundice may be noted in the first 24 hours or may develop later. Loss of appetite, poor sucking reflex, lethargy, and vomiting are frequent. Stools may be normal to pale in color but are seldom acholic. Dark urine stains the diaper. Hepatomegaly is present, and the liver has a uni-

**Table 21–1.** Characteristic clinical features of intrahepatic and extrahepatic neonatal cholestasis.

| Intrahepatic | Extrahepatic |
|---|---|
| Preterm infant, small for gestational age, appears ill; hepatosplenomegaly, other organ or system involvement; incomplete cholestasis (stools with some color); associated cause identified (infections, metabolic, familial, etc) | Full-term infant, seems well; hepatomegaly (firm to hard); complete cholestasis (acholic stools); polysplenia syndrome, equal right and left hepatic lobes |

form firm consistency. Splenomegaly is variably present. Macular, papular, vesicular, or petechial rashes may occur. In less severe cases, failure to thrive may be the major complaint. Unusual presentations include liver failure, hypoproteinemia, anasarca (nonhemolytic hydrops), and hemorrhagic disease of the newborn.

**B. Diagnostic Studies**

Neutropenia, thrombocytopenia, and signs of mild hemolysis are common. Mixed hyperbilirubinemia, elevated aminotransferases with near-normal alkaline phosphatase, prolongation of clotting studies, mild acidosis, and elevated cord serum IgM suggest congenital infection. Nasopharyngeal washings and urine, stool, and cerebrospinal fluid (CSF) should be cultured for virus. Specific IgM antibody and nucleic acid tests may be useful, as are long-bone radiographs to determine the presence of "celery stalking" in the metaphyseal regions of the humeri, femurs, and tibias. When indicated, computed tomography (CT) and magnetic reso-

**Table 21–2.** Characteristic histologic features of intrahepatic and extrahepatic neonatal cholestasis.

| | Intrahepatic | Extrahepatic |
|---|---|---|
| Giant cells | +++ | + |
| Lobules | Disarray | Normal |
| Portal reaction | Inflammation/minimal fibrosis | Fibrosis |
| Neoductular proliferation | Rare | Marked |
| Other | Steatosis, extramedullary hematopoiesis | Portal bile duct plugging, bile lakes |

nance imaging scans can identify intracranial calcifications (especially CMV and toxoplasmosis). Hepatobiliary scintigraphy shows decreased hepatic clearance of the circulating isotope with excretion into the gut. Careful ophthalmologic examination may be useful for diagnosis of HSV, CMV, toxoplasmosis, and rubella.

A percutaneous liver biopsy is useful in distinguishing intrahepatic from extrahepatic cholestasis, but may not identify a specific infectious agent (see Table 21–2). However, typical inclusions of CMV in hepatocytes or bile duct epithelial cells, the presence of intranuclear acidophilic inclusions of herpes simplex, or positive immunohistochemical stains for several viruses can be diagnostic. Variable degrees of lobular disarray characterized by focal necrosis, multinucleated giant-cell transformation, and ballooned pale hepatocytes with loss of cord-like arrangement of liver cells are usual. Intrahepatocytic and canalicular cholestasis may be prominent. Portal changes are not striking, but modest neoductular proliferation and mild fibrosis may occur. Viral cultures or polymerase chain reaction (PCR) testing of biopsy material may be helpful.

**Differential Diagnosis**

Great care must be taken to distinguish infectious causes of intrahepatic cholestasis from genetic or metabolic disorders because the clinical presentations are similar. Galactosemia, congenital fructose intolerance, and tyrosinemia must be investigated promptly, because specific dietary therapy is available. $\alpha_1$-Antitrypsin deficiency, cystic fibrosis, and neonatal iron storage disease must also be considered. Specific physical features may be helpful when considering Alagille or Zellweger syndrome. Idiopathic neonatal hepatitis may be indistinguishable from infectious causes.

Patients with intrahepatic cholestasis frequently appear ill, whereas infants with extrahepatic cholestasis do not appear ill, have stools that are usually completely acholic, and have an enlarged, firm liver. Histologic findings are shown in Table 21–2.

**Treatment**

Most forms of viral neonatal hepatitis are treated symptomatically. However, infections with HSV, varicella, CMV, parvovirus, adenovirus, and toxoplasmosis have specific treatments. Fluids and adequate calories are encouraged. Intravenous dextrose is needed if feedings are not well tolerated. The consequences of cholestasis are treated as indicated (Table 21–4). Vitamin K orally or by injection and vitamins D and E orally should be provided. Choleretics (cholestyramine or ursodeoxycholic acid [UDCA]) are used if cholestasis persists. Corticosteroids are contraindicated. Penicillin for sus-

***Table 21–3.*** Infectious causes of neonatal hepatitis.

| Infectious Agent | Diagnostic Tests | Specimens | Treatment |
|---|---|---|---|
| Cytomegalovirus | Culture and PCR, liver histology, IgM/[a]IgG | Urine, blood, liver | ?Ganciclovir (Foscarnet)[b] |
| Herpes simplex | PCR and culture, liver histology, Ag (skin) | Liver, blood, eye, throat, rectal, CSF, skin | Acyclovir |
| Rubella | Culture, IgM/[a]IgG | Liver, blood, urine | Supportive |
| Varicella | Culture, PCR, Ag (skin) | Skin, blood, CSF, liver | Acyclovir (Foscarnet)[b] |
| Parvovirus | Serum IgM/[a]IgG, PCR | Blood | Supportive, ? IVIG |
| Enteroviruses | Culture and PCR | Blood, urine, CSF, throat, rectal, liver | Pleconaril (investigative) |
| Adenovirus | Culture and PCR | Nasal/throat, rectal, blood, liver, urine | Cidofovir, ?IVIG |
| Hepatitis B virus (HBV) | HBsAg, HBcAg IgM | Serum | Supportive for acute infection |
| Hepatitis C virus (HCV) | HCV PCR, HCV-IgG | Serum | Supportive for acute infection |
| *Treponema pallidum* | Serology; dark-field exam | Serum, CSF | Penicillin |
| *Toxoplasma gondii* | IgM/[a]IgG, PCR, culture | Serum, liver | Pyrimethamine and sulfadiazine with folinic acid |
| *Mycobacterium tuberculosis* | PPD, chest radiograph, liver tissue histologic stains and culture, gastric aspirate stain and culture | Serum, liver, gastric aspirate | INH, pyrazinamide, rifampin and streptomycin |

[a]IgG = positive indicates maternal infection and transfer of antibody transplacentally; negative indicates unlikelihood of infection in mother and infant.

IVIG = intravenous gamma globulin, PCR = polymerase chain reactin test for viral DNA or RNA, Ag = viral antigen testing, INH = isoniazid, CSF = cerebrospinal fluid, HBsAg = hepatitis B surface antigen, HBC – hepatitis B core antigen, PPD = purified protein derivative.

[b]Use for resistant viruses.

pected syphilis or antibiotics for bacterial hepatitis need to be administered promptly.

## Prognosis

Multiple organ involvement is commonly associated with neonatal infectious hepatitis and has a poor outcome. Death from hepatic or cardiac failure, intractable acidosis, or intracranial hemorrhage may occur, especially in herpesvirus or enterovirus infection and occasionally in CMV or rubella infection. HBV may rarely cause fulminant neonatal viral hepatitis; most infected infants become asymptomatic carriers of hepatitis B. Persistent liver disease results in mild chronic hepatitis, portal fibrosis, or cirrhosis. Chronic cholestasis, although rare following infections, may lead to dental enamel hypoplasia, failure to thrive, biliary rickets, severe pruritus, and xanthoma.

## Specific Infectious Agents

### A. NEONATAL HEPATITIS B VIRUS DISEASE

Infection with HBV may occur at any time during perinatal life, but the risk is higher when acute maternal disease occurs during the last trimester of pregnancy. However, most cases of neonatal disease are acquired from mothers who are asymptomatic carriers of hepatitis B. Although HBV has been found in most body fluids, including breast milk, neonatal transmission occurs occasionally transplacentally and primarily from exposure to maternal blood at delivery. In chronic hepatitis B surface antigen (HBsAg) carrier mothers, fetal and infant acquisition risk is greatest if the mother (1) is also hepatitis B envelope antigen (HBeAg)-positive and hepatitis B envelope antibody (HBeAb)-negative, (2) has detectable levels of serum-specific hepatitis B DNA polymerase, or (3) has high serum levels of hepatitis B core antibody (HBcAb). These findings are

*Table 21–4.* Treatment of complications of chronic cholestatic liver disease.

| Indication | Treatment | Dose | Toxicity |
|---|---|---|---|
| Intrahepatic cholestasis | Phenobarbital | 3–10 mg/kg/d | Drowsiness, irritability, interference with vitamin D metabolism |
| | Cholestyramine/colestipol hydrochloride | 250–500 mg/kg/d | Constipation, acidosis, binding of drugs, increased steatorrhea |
| | Ursodeoxycholic acid | 15–20 mg/kg/d | Transient increase in pruritus |
| Pruritus | Phenobarbital or cholestyramine/colestipol (or both) | Same as above | |
| | Antihistamines: diphenhydramine hydrochloride hydroxyzine | 5–10 mg/kg/d 2–5 mg/kg/d | Drowsiness |
| | Ultraviolet light B | Exposure as needed | Skin burn |
| | Carbamazepine | 20–40 mg/kg/d | Hepatotoxicity, marrow suppression, fluid retention |
| | Rifampin | 10 mg/kg/d | Hepatotoxicity, marrow suppression |
| | Ursodeoxycholic acid | 15–20 mg/kg/d | Transient increase in pruritus |
| Steatorrhea | Formula containing medium-chain triglycerides (eg, Pregestimil) | 120–150 calories/kg/d for infants | Expensive |
| | Oil supplement containing medium-chain triglycerides | 1–2 mL/kg/d | Diarrhea, aspiration |
| Malabsorption of fat-soluble vitamins | Vitamin A | 10,000–25,000 units/d | Hepatitis, pseudotumor cerebri, bone lesions |
| | Vitamin D | 800–5000 units/d | Hypercalcemia, hypercalciuria |
| | 25-Hydroxycholecalciferol (vitamin D) | 3–5 µg/kg/d | Hypercalcemia, hypercalciuria |
| | 1,25-Dihydroxycholecalciferol (vitamin D) | 0.05–0.2 µg/kg/d | Hypercalcemia, hypercalciuria |
| | Vitamin E (oral) | 25–200 IU/kg/d | Potentiation of vitamin K deficiency |
| | Vitamin E (oral, TPGS[a]) | 15–25 IU/kg/d | Potentiation of vitamin K deficiency |
| | Vitamin E (intramuscular) | 1–2 mg/kg/d | Muscle calcifications |
| | Vitamin K (oral) | 2.5 mg twice per week to 5 mg/d | |
| | Vitamin K (intramuscular) | 2–5 mg each 4 wk | |
| Malabsorption of other nutrients | Multiple vitamin | 1–2 times the standard dose | |
| | Calcium | 25–100 mg/kg/d | Hypercalcemia, hypercalciuria |
| | Phosphorus | 25–50 mg/kg/d | Gastrointestinal intolerance |
| | Zinc | 1 mg/kg/d | Interference with copper and iron absorption |

[a]D-α-Tocopheryl polyethylene glycol-1000 succinate.

markers for circulating infectious virus; however, hepatitis B can be transmitted even if HBsAg is the only marker present.

Neonatal liver disease resulting from HBV is extremely variable. The infant has a 70–90% chance of acquiring HBV at birth from an HBsAg-positive mother if nothing is done to prevent infection. Most infected infants become prolonged asymptomatic carriers of HBV. Fulminant hepatic necrosis has rarely been reported. In such cases, progressive jaundice, stupor, shrinking liver size, and coagulation abnormalities dominate the clinical picture. Respiratory, circulatory, and renal failure usually follow. Histologically, the liver shows massive hepatocyte necrosis, collapse of the reticulum framework, minimal inflammation, and occasional pseudoacinar structures. Survival is rare but is associated with reasonable repair of liver architecture.

In less severe cases, focal hepatocyte necrosis occurs with a mild portal inflammatory response. Cholestasis is intracellular and canalicular. Chronic active hepatitis may be present for many years, with serologic evidence of persisting antigenemia (HBsAg) and mildly elevated serum aminotransferases. Chronic active hepatitis may rarely progress to cirrhosis within 1–2 years. Most infected infants have only mild evidence, if any, of liver injury.

To prevent perinatal transmission, all infants of mothers who are HBsAg-positive (regardless of HBeAg status) should receive hepatitis B immunoglobulin (HBIG) and hepatitis B vaccine within the first 24 hours after birth and vaccine again at ages 1 and 6 months (see Chapter 9). This prevents HBV infection in 85–95% of infants. HBIG can provide some protection when given as late as 72 hours after birth. If not given at birth it can be administered as late as 7 days postpartum as long as the infant has received vaccine.

### B. NEONATAL BACTERIAL HEPATITIS

Most bacterial liver infections in newborns are acquired by transplacental invasion from amnionitis with ascending spread from maternal vaginal or cervical infection. Onset is abrupt, usually within 48–72 hours after delivery, with signs of sepsis and often shock. Jaundice appears early and is of the mixed type. The liver enlarges rapidly, and the histologic picture is that of diffuse hepatitis with or without microabscess. The most common organisms involved are *Escherichia coli, Listeria monocytogenes,* and group B streptococci. Isolated neonatal liver abscess caused by *E coli* or *Staphylococcus aureus* is often associated with omphalitis or umbilical vein catheterization. Bacterial hepatitis and neonatal liver abscesses require specific antibiotics in large doses and, rarely, surgical or radiologic interventional drainage. Deaths are common, but survivors show no long-term consequences of liver disease.

### C. NEONATAL JAUNDICE WITH URINARY TRACT INFECTION

Jaundice in affected infants—usually males—typically appears between the second and fourth weeks of life. This disorder causes lethargy, fever, poor appetite, jaundice, and hepatomegaly. Except for mixed hyperbilirubinemia, other liver function tests (LFTs) are mildly abnormal. Leukocytosis is present, and infection is confirmed by culture. The mechanism for the liver impairment is the toxic action of bacterial products (endotoxins) and inflammatory cytokines.

Treatment of the infection leads to prompt resolution of the cholestasis without hepatic sequelae. Metabolic liver diseases, such as galactosemia and tyrosinemia, may present with gram-negative bacterial urinary tract infection and must be considered.

Broderick AL, Jonas MM: Hepatitis B in children. Semin Liver Dis 2003;23(1):59 [PMID: 12616451].

Kane MA: Hepatitis viruses and the neonate. Clin Perinatol 1997; 24:181 [PMID: 9099509].

Kesson AM: Management of neonatal herpes simplex virus infection. Paediatr Drugs 2001;3:81 [PMID: 11269641].

Rosenthal P: Neonatal hepatitis and congenital infections. In Suchy FJ et al (eds): *Liver Disease in Children.* Lippincott, Williams & Wilkins, 2001:239.

## 2. Intrahepatic Cholestasis Resulting from Inborn Errors of Metabolism, Familial & "Toxic" Causes

These cholestatic syndromes caused by specific enzyme deficiencies, other genetic disorders, or certain precipitants associated with neonatal liver disease feature intrahepatic cholestasis (ie, jaundice, hepatomegaly, and normal to completely acholic stools). Some of the specific clinical conditions have characteristic clinical signs.

### Enzyme Deficiencies & Other Inherited Disorders

Early specific diagnosis is important because dietary or pharmacologic treatment may be available (Table 21–5). Reversal of liver disease and clinical symptoms is prompt and permanent in several disorders as long as the diet is maintained. As with other inborn errors of metabolism, parents of the affected infant should be offered genetic counseling. For some disorders, prenatal genetic diagnosis is available.

Cholestasis caused by metabolic diseases such as galactosemia, fructose intolerance, and tyrosinemia may be accompanied by vomiting, lethargy, poor feeding, and irritability. Hepatomegaly is a constant finding. The infants often appear septic; gram-negative bacteria can be cultured from blood in 25–50% of cases, espe-

***Table 21–5.*** Metabolic and genetic causes of neonatal cholestasis.

| Disease | Inborn Error | Hepatic Pathology | Diagnostic Studies |
|---|---|---|---|
| Galactosemia | Galactose-1-phosphate uridylyltransferase | Cholestasis, steatosis, necrosis, pseudoacini, fibrosis | Galactose-1-phosphate uridylyltransferase assay of red blood cells |
| Fructose intolerance | Fructose-1-phosphate aldolase | Steatosis, necrosis, pseudoacini, fibrosis | Liver fructose-1-phosphate aldolase assay or leukocyte DNA analysis |
| Tyrosinemia | Fumarylacetoacetase | Necrosis, steatosis, pseudoacini, portal fibrosis | Urinary succinylacetone, fumarylacetoacetase assay of red blood cells |
| Cystic fibrosis | Cystic fibrosis transmembrane conductance regulator gene | Cholestasis, neoductular proliferation, excess bile duct mucus, portal fibrosis | Sweat test and leukocyte DNA analysis |
| Hypopituitarism | Deficient production of pituitary hormones | Cholestasis, giant cells | Thyroxine, TSH, cortisol levels |
| $\alpha_1$-Antitrypsin deficiency | Abnormal $\alpha_1$-antitrypsin molecule (Pi ZZ phenotype) | Giant cells, cholestasis, steatosis, neoductular proliferation, fibrosis, PAS-diastase-resistant cytoplasmic granules | Serum $\alpha_1$-antitrypsin phenotype |
| Gaucher disease | $\beta$-Glucosidase | Cholestasis, cytoplasmic inclusions in Kupffer's cells (foam cells) | $\beta$-Glucosidase assay in leukocytes |
| Niemann–Pick disease | Lysosomal sphingomyelinase | Cholestasis, cytoplasmic inclusions in Kupffer's cells | Sphingomyelinase assay of leukocytes or liver or fibroblasts (type C); leukocyte DNA analysis |
| Glycogen storage disease type IV | Branching enzyme | Fibrosis, cirrhosis, PAS-diastase-resistant cytoplasmic inclusions | Branching enzyme analysis of leukocytes or liver |
| Neonatal hemochromatosis | Unknown | Giant cells, portal fibrosis, hemosiderosis, cirrhosis | Histology, iron stains |
| Peroxisomal disorders (eg, Zellweger's syndrome) | Deficient peroxisomal enzymes or assembly | Cholestasis, necrosis, fibrosis, cirrhosis, hemosiderosis | Plasma very long chain fatty acids, qualitative bile acids, plasmalogen, pipecolic acid, liver electron microscopy |
| Abnormalities in bile acid metabolism | Several enzyme deficiencies defined | Cholestasis, necrosis, giant cells | Urine, serum, duodenal fluid analyzed for bile acids by fast atom bombardment-mass spectroscopy |
| Byler's disease (familial progressive intrahepatic cholestasis) | *FIC-1* and BSEP genes | Cholestasis, necrosis, giant cells, fibrosis | Histology, family history, normal cholesterol, low or normal $\gamma$-glutamyl transpeptidase, DNA analysis |
| MDR$_3$ deficiency | MDR$_3$ gene | Cholestasis, bile duct proliferation, portal fibrosis | Bile phospholipid level, DNA analysis |
| Alagille's syndrome (syndromic paucity of interlobular bile ducts) | *Jagged 1* gene mutations | Cholestasis, paucity of interlobular bile ducts, increased copper levels | Three or more clinical features, liver histology, DNA analysis |

TSH = thyroid-stimulating hormone, PAS = periodic acid-Schiff.

cially in patients with galactosemia. Neonatal screening for galactosemia usually detects the disorder before cholestasis develops. Other inherited conditions associated with neonatal intrahepatic cholestasis are outlined in Table 21–5. Treatment of these disorders is discussed in Chapter 32.

## "Toxic" Causes of Neonatal Cholestasis

### A. Neonatal Ischemic–Hypoxic Conditions

Perinatal events that result in hypoperfusion of the gastrointestinal system are sometimes followed in 1–2 weeks by cholestasis. This occurs in premature infants with respiratory distress, severe hypoxia, hypoglycemia, shock, and acidosis. When these perinatal conditions develop in association with gastrointestinal lesions such as ruptured omphalocele, gastroschisis, or necrotizing enterocolitis, a subsequent cholestatic picture is common (25–50% of cases). Liver function studies reveal mixed hyperbilirubinemia, elevated alkaline phosphatase and γ-glutamyl transpeptidase (GGT) values, and variable elevation of the aminotransferases. Stools are seldom persistently acholic.

Choleretics (cholestyramine or UDCA), introduction of enteral feedings as soon as possible, and nutritional support are the mainstays of treatment until the cholestasis resolves (see Table 21–4). In some cases, this resolution may take 3–6 months. As long as no severe intestinal problem is present (eg, short gut syndrome), complete resolution of the hepatic abnormalities is the rule. But portal fibrosis with periportal scarring is occasionally found on follow-up biopsy.

### B. Prolonged Parenteral Nutrition

Cholestasis may develop after 1–2 weeks in premature newborns receiving total parenteral nutrition (TPN). Even full-term infants with significant intestinal disease, resections, or dysmotility may develop TPN-related cholestasis. Contributing factors may include toxicity of intravenous amino acids, diminished stimulation of bile flow from prolonged absence of feedings, translocation of intestinal bacteria and their cell wall products, missing nutrients or antioxidants, photooxidation of amino acids, infusion of lipid hydroperoxides, and the "physiologic cholestatic" propensity of the premature infant. Histology of the liver may resemble that of extrahepatic biliary obstruction. Early introduction of feedings has reduced the frequency of this disorder. The prognosis is generally good. Occasional cases of cirrhosis, liver failure, and hepatoma may develop, particularly in infants with intestinal resections or anomalies.

### C. Inspissated Bile Syndrome

This syndrome is the result of accumulation of bile in canaliculi and in the small- and medium-size bile ducts in hemolytic disease of the newborn (Rh, ABO) and in some infants receiving TPN. The same mechanisms may cause intrinsic obstruction of the common duct. An ischemia–reperfusion injury may also contribute to cholestasis in Rh incompatibility. In extreme hemolysis, the cholestasis may be seemingly complete, with acholic stools. Levels of bilirubin may reach 40 mg/dL, primarily conjugated. If inspissation of bile occurs within the extrahepatic biliary tree, differentiation from biliary atresia may be difficult. A trial of choleretics is indicated. Once stools show a return to normal color or $^{99m}$Tc-DIDA scanning shows biliary excretion into the duodenum, patency of the extrahepatic biliary tree is ensured. Although most cases improve slowly over 2–6 months, persistence of complete cholestasis for more than 2 weeks requires further studies (ultrasonography, DIDA scanning, liver biopsy) with possible cholangiographic or magnetic resonance imaging of the extrahepatic biliary tree. Irrigation of the common bile duct is sometimes necessary to dislodge the obstructing inspissated biliary material.

Andorsky DJ et al: Nutritional and other postoperative management of neonates with short bowel syndrome correlates with clinical outcomes. J Pediatr 2001;139:27 [PMID: 11445790].

Colomb V et al: Role of lipid emulsions in cholestasis associated with long-term parenteral nutrition in children. J Parenter Ent Nutr 2000;24:345 [PMID: 11071594].

Heubi JE et al: Tauroursodeoxycholic acid (TUDCA) in the prevention of total parenteral nutrition-associated liver disease. J Pediatr 2002;141(2):237 [PMID: 12183720].

Teitelbaum DH, Tracy T: Parenteral nutrition-associated cholestasis. Semin Pediatr Surg 2001;10:72 [PMID: 11329608].

Weinberger B et al: Association of lipid peroxidation with hepatocellular injury in preterm infants. Crit Care 2002;6:521 [PMID: 12493074]

## 3. Idiopathic Neonatal Hepatitis (Giant-Cell Hepatitis)

This type of cholestatic jaundice of unknown cause presents with features of cholestasis and a typical liver biopsy appearance; it accounts for 25–50% of cases of neonatal intrahepatic cholestasis. The degree of cholestasis is variable, and the disorder may be indistinguishable from extrahepatic causes in 10% of cases. Viral infections, $\alpha_1$-antitrypsin deficiency, Alagille syndrome, Niemann–Pick type C disease (NPC), progressive familial intrahepatic cholestasis (PFIC), and bile acid synthesis defects may present in a similar clinical and histologic manner. However, in PFIC and bile acid synthesis defects the γ-glutamyl transpeptidase levels are normal or low. Electron microscopy of the liver biopsy may help distinguish NPC and PFIC.

Intrauterine growth retardation, prematurity, poor feeding, emesis, poor growth, and partially or intermittently acholic stools are characteristic of intrahepatic cholestasis. Patients with neonatal lupus erythematosus may present with giant-cell hepatitis; however, thrombocytopenia, skin rash, or congenital heart block is usually also present.

In cases of suspected idiopathic neonatal hepatitis (absence of infectious, metabolic, and toxic causes), patency of the biliary tree should be verified to exclude extrahepatic surgical disorders. DIDA scanning and ultrasonography may be helpful in this regard. Some clinicians have used the enteral string test during DIDA scanning to confirm bile duct patency. Liver biopsy findings are usually diagnostic after age 6–8 weeks (see Table 21–2) but may be misleading before age 6 weeks. Failure to detect patency of the biliary tree, nondiagnostic liver biopsy findings, or persisting complete cholestasis (acholic stools) are indications for minilaparotomy and intraoperative cholangiography performed by an experienced surgeon, ERCP, percutaneous cholecystography, or magnetic resonance cholangiopancreatography (MRCP). Occasionally, a small but patent (hypoplastic) extrahepatic biliary tree is demonstrated and is probably the result rather than the cause of diminished bile flow; surgical reconstruction of hypoplastic biliary trees should not be attempted.

Once a patent extrahepatic tree is confirmed, therapy should include choleretics, a special formula with medium-chain triglycerides (Pregestimil, Alimentum), and supplemental fat-soluble vitamins in water-miscible form (see Table 21–4). This therapy is continued as long as significant cholestasis remains (conjugated bilirubin > 1 mg/dL). Fat-soluble vitamin levels should be monitored while supplements are given and at least once after their discontinuation.

Eighty percent of patients recover without significant hepatic fibrosis. However, in 20% of cases with this presentation, the patient has PFIC and is likely to progress to cirrhosis. In general, failure to resolve the cholestatic picture by age 6–12 months is associated with progressive liver disease and evolving cirrhosis. This may occur with either normal or diminished numbers of interlobular bile ducts (paucity of interlobular ducts). Liver transplantation has been successful when signs of hepatic decompensation are noted (rising bilirubin, coagulopathy, intractable ascites).

Arora NK et al: Hepatic technetium-99m-mebrofenin iminodiacetate scans and serum gamma-glutamyl transpeptidase levels interpreted in series to differentiate between extrahepatic biliary atresia and neonatal hepatitis. Acta Paediatr 2001;90(9): 975 [PMID: 11683209].

McKiernan PJ: Neonatal cholestasis. Semin Neonatol 2002;7(2): 153 [PMID: 12208100].

Yerushalmi B et al: Niemann–Pick disease type C in neonatal cholestasis at a North American Center. J Pediatr Gastroenterol Nutr 2002;35(1):44 [PMID: 12142809].

## 4. Paucity of Interlobular Bile Ducts

Forms of intrahepatic cholestasis caused by decreased numbers of interlobular bile ducts (< 0.5 bile ducts per portal tract) may be classified according to whether they are associated with other malformations. The gene (*Jagged 1*) for the syndromic form, Alagille syndrome (arteriohepatic dysplasia), is located on chromosome 20p and codes for a ligand of the notch receptor, although the pathogenesis is not understood. Alagille syndrome is sometimes recognized by identification of the characteristic facies, which becomes more obvious with age. The forehead is prominent, as is the nasal bridge. The eyes are set deep and sometimes widely apart (hypertelorism), The chin is small and slightly pointed and projects forward. The ears are prominent. The stool color varies with the severity of cholestasis. Pruritus begins by age 3–6 months. Firm, smooth hepatomegaly may be present. Cardiac murmurs are present in 95% of patients, and butterfly vertebrae (incomplete fusion of the vertebral body or anterior arch) are present in 50%. Xanthomas develop later in the disease. Occasionally, early cholestasis is mild and not recognized.

Direct hyperbilirubinemia may be mild to severe (2–15 mg/dL). Serum alkaline phosphatase, GGT, and cholesterol are markedly elevated, especially early in life. Serum bile acids are always elevated. Aminotransferases are mildly increased, but clotting factors and other liver proteins are usually normal.

The cardiovascular abnormalities include peripheral and valvular pulmonary stenoses (most common), atrial septal defect, coarctation of the aorta, and tetralogy of Fallot. Up to 15% of patients develop intracranial hemorrhage early in childhood.

Eye abnormalities (posterior embryotoxon) and renal abnormalities (dysplastic kidneys, renal tubular ectasia, single kidney, hematuria) can also be present. Growth retardation with normal to increased levels of growth hormone is common. Although variable, the intelligence quotient is frequently low. Hypogonadism with micropenis may be present. A weak, high-pitched voice may develop. Neurologic disorders resulting from vitamin E deficiency (areflexia, ataxia, ophthalmoplegia) eventually develop in many children.

In the nonsyndromic form, paucity of interlobular bile ducts occurs in the absence of the extrahepatic malformations. Paucity of interlobular bile ducts may also occur in $\alpha_1$-antitrypsin deficiency, Zellweger syndrome, in association with lymphedema (Aagenaes' syndrome), PFIC, cystic fibrosis, CMV or rubella infection, and inborn errors of bile acid metabolism.

High doses (250 mg/kg/d) of cholestyramine may control pruritus, lower cholesterol, and clear xanthomas. Ursodeoxycholic therapy (15–25 mg/kg/d) appears to be more effective and less toxic than cholestyramine. Nutritional therapy to prevent wasting and deficiencies of fat-soluble vitamins is of particular importance because of the severity of cholestasis (see Table 21–4).

Prognosis is more favorable in the syndromic than in the nonsyndromic varieties. In the former, only 30–40% of patients have severe complications of disease, whereas over 70% of patients with nonsyndromic varieties progress to cirrhosis. Many of this latter group may have PFIC. In Alagille syndrome, cholestasis may improve by age 2–4 years, with minimal residual hepatic fibrosis. Survival into adulthood despite raised serum bile acids, aminotransferases, and alkaline phosphatase occurs in about 50% of cases. Several patients have developed hepatocellular carcinoma. Hypogonadism has been noted; however, fertility is not obviously affected. Cardiovascular anomalies may shorten life expectancy. Some patients have persistent, severe cholestasis, rendering their quality of life poor; liver transplantation has been performed under these circumstances.

Emerick KM et al: Features of Alagille syndrome in 92 patients: Frequency and relation to prognosis. Hepatology 1999;29: 822 [PMID: 10051485].

Lykavieris P et al: Bleeding tendency in children with Alagille syndrome. Pediatrics 2003;111(1):167 [PMID: 12509572].

McElhinney DB et al: Analysis of cardiovascular phenotype and genotype–phenotype correlation in individuals with a JAG1 mutation and/or Alagille's syndrome. Circulation 2002;106(20):2567 [PMID: 12417653]

## PROGRESSIVE FAMILIAL INTRAHEPATIC CHOLESTASIS (Byler Disease)

PFIC is a group of disorders presenting as pruritus, diarrhea, jaundice, and failure to thrive in the first 6–12 months of life. PFIC type I (Byler disease), caused by mutations in the *FIC1* gene, is associated with low to normal serum levels of GGT and cholesterol and elevated levels of bilirubin, aminotransferases, and bile acids. Diarrhea is common. Liver biopsy results are similar to those found with giant-cell hepatitis but sometimes with a paucity of interlobular bile ducts and centrolobular fibrosis that progresses to cirrhosis. Electron microscopy shows diagnostic granular "Byler bile" in canaliculi.

Treatment includes administration of UDCA, partial biliary diversion if the condition is unresponsive to UDCA, and liver transplantation. PFIC type II is caused by mutations in the bile salt export pump (*BSEP*) gene, which codes for an adenosine triphosphate (ATP)-dependent canalicular bile salt transport protein. Clinically and biochemically, patients are similar to PFIC type I patients, as are their liver histology and treatment options. PFIC type III is caused by mutations in the *MDR₃* (multiple drug resistance protein type 3) gene, which encodes a canalicular protein that pumps phospholipid into bile. Serum GGT and bile acid levels are elevated, bile duct proliferation and portal tract fibrosis are seen in liver biopsies, and bile phospholipid levels are low. Treatment is similar to that for other forms of PFIC. Bile acid synthesis defects are clinically similar to those in PFIC I and PFIC II, with low serum levels of GGT and cholesterol; however, the serum level of total bile acids is low and urine bile acid analysis may identify a defect.

Jacquemin E: Progressive familial intrahepatic cholestasis: Genetic basis and treatment. Clin Liver Dis 2000;4(4):753 [PMID: 11232355].

Melter M et al: Progressive familial intrahepatic cholestasis: Partial biliary diversion normalizes serum lipids and improves growth in noncirrhotic patients. Am J Gastroenterol 2000; 95(12):3522 [PMID: 11151888].

## EXTRAHEPATIC NEONATAL CHOLESTASIS

Extrahepatic neonatal cholestasis is characterized by complete and persistent cholestasis (acholic stools) in the first 3 months of life; lack of patency of the extrahepatic biliary tree proved by intraoperative, percutaneous, or endoscopic cholangiography; firm to hard hepatomegaly; and typical features on histologic examination of liver biopsy tissue (see Table 21–2). Causes include biliary atresia, choledochal cyst, spontaneous perforation of the extrahepatic ducts, and intrinsic obstruction of the common duct.

### 1. Biliary Atresia

Biliary atresia is the progressive fibroinflammatory obliteration of the lumen of all, or part of, the extrahepatic biliary tree presenting within the first 3 months of life. In European Americans, biliary atresia occurs in 1:10,000–1:15,000 births, and the incidence in both sexes is equal. In Asian Americans, the incidence is higher, and the disorder is twice as common in girls. The abnormality found most commonly is complete atresia of all extrahepatic biliary structures. There appear to be at least two types of biliary atresia: the perinatal form (80% of cases) and the fetal–embryonic form (20% of cases). In the perinatal form, meconium and first-passed stools are usually normal in color, suggesting early patency of the ducts. Evidence obtained from surgically removed remnants of the extrahepatic biliary tree suggests an inflammatory or sclerosing cholangiopathy. Although an infectious cause seems reasonable, no agent has been consistently found in such cases. A role for reovirus type 3 and rotavirus group C has been suggested. Certain histocompatibility locus antigen (HLA) types may predispose to biliary atresia. In the fetal–embryonic type, the bile duct presumably developed abnormally and is associated with other nonhepatic congenital anomalies. The strongest association of biliary atresia is with the polysplenia syndrome (situs inversus, preduodenal portal vein, interruption of the inferior vena cava, polysplenia, midline liver).

Jaundice may be noted in the newborn period but is more often delayed until age 2–3 weeks. The urine stains the diaper; and the stools are often pale yellow, buff-colored, gray, or acholic. Seepage of bilirubin products across the intestinal mucosa may give some yellow coloration to the stools. Hepatomegaly is common, and the liver may feel firm to hard; splenomegaly develops later. Pruritus, digital clubbing, xanthomas, and a rachitic rosary may be noted in older patients. By age 2–6 months, the growth curves reveal poor weight gain. Late in the course, ascites and bleeding complications occur.

No single laboratory test will consistently differentiate biliary atresia from other causes of complete obstructive jaundice. A study of hepatic 2,6-dimethyliminodiacetic acid (HIDA) excretion performed early in the course of disease and after pretreatment with phenobarbital (3–5 mg/kg/d for 5–7 days) helps to distinguish intrahepatic from extrahepatic causes of cholestasis, though it is not diagnostic. MRCP shows promise as an imaging study to define biliary atresia. Although biliary atresia is suggested by persistent elevation of serum γ-glutamyl transpeptidase or alkaline phosphatase levels, high cholesterol levels, and prolonged prothrombin times, these findings have also been reported in severe neonatal hepatitis, $\alpha_1$-antitrypsin deficiency, and bile duct paucity. Furthermore, these tests will not differentiate the location of the obstruction within the extrahepatic system. Generally, the aminotransferases are elevated only modestly in biliary atresia. Serum proteins and blood clotting factors are not affected early in the disease. Routine chest radiograph may reveal abnormalities suggestive of polysplenia syndrome. Ultrasonography of the biliary system should be performed to ascertain the presence of choledochal cyst and intra-abdominal anomalies. Liver biopsy specimens can differentiate intrahepatic causes of cholestasis from biliary atresia in over 90% of cases (see Table 21–2).

The major diagnostic dilemma is distinguishing between this entity and neonatal hepatitis, bile duct paucity, metabolic liver disease (particularly $\alpha_1$-anti-

trypsin deficiency), choledochal cyst, or intrinsic bile duct obstruction (stones, bile plugs). Although spontaneous perforation of extrahepatic bile ducts leads to jaundice and acholic stools, the infants are usually quite ill with chemical peritonitis from biliary ascites, and hepatomegaly is not found.

If the diagnosis of biliary atresia cannot be excluded by the diagnostic evaluation before age 60 days, surgical exploration is necessary. Laparotomy must include liver biopsy and an operative cholangiogram if a gallbladder is present. The presence of yellow bile in the gallbladder implies patency of the proximal extrahepatic duct system. Radiographic visualization of cholangiographic contrast in the duodenum excludes obstruction to the distal extrahepatic ducts.

In the absence of surgical correction, the following eventually develop: failure to thrive, marked pruritus, portal hypertension, hypersplenism, bleeding diathesis, rickets, ascites, and cyanosis. Bronchitis and pneumonia are common. Eventually, hepatic failure and death occur, almost always by age 18–24 months.

Except for the occasional example of correctable biliary atresia, in which choledochojejunostomy is feasible, the standard procedure is hepatoportoenterostomy (Kasai procedure). Occasionally, portocholecystostomy (gallbladder Kasai procedure) may be performed if the gallbladder is present and the passage from it to the duodenum is patent. These procedures are best done in specialized centers where experienced surgical, pediatric, and nursing personnel are available. Surgery should be performed as early as possible (before 60 days of life); the Kasai procedure should generally not be undertaken in infants older than age 4 months, because the likelihood of bile drainage at this age is very low. Orthotopic liver transplantation is now indicated for patients who do not undergo the Kasai procedure, who fail to drain bile after the Kasai procedure, or who progress to end-stage biliary cirrhosis despite surgical treatment. The 5-year survival rate following transplantation is 70–85%.

Whether or not the Kasai procedure is performed, supportive medical treatment measures consist of vitamin and caloric support (vitamins A, D, K, and E and formulas containing medium-chain triglycerides [Pregestimil or Alimentum]) (see Table 21–4). Bacterial infections (eg, ascending cholangitis) should be treated promptly with broad-spectrum antibiotics, and signs of bleeding tendency should be corrected with intramuscular vitamin K. Ascites can be managed initially with reduced sodium intake and spironolactone. Choleretics and bile acid-binding products (cholestyramine, aluminum hydroxide gel) are of little use. The value of UDCA remains to be determined.

When bile flow is sustained, the 10-year survival rate is 25–35%. Death is usually caused by liver failure, sepsis, acidosis, or respiratory failure secondary to intractable ascites. Esophageal variceal hemorrhage develops in 40% of patients. Surprisingly, terminal hemorrhage is unusual. Liver transplantation has dramatically changed the outlook for these patients.

Larrosa-Haro A et al: Duodenal tube test in the diagnosis of biliary atresia. J Pediatr Gastroenterol Nutr 2001;32:311 [PMID: 11345182].

Meyers RL et al: High-dose steroids, ursodeoxycholic acid, and chronic intravenous antibiotics improve bile flow after Kasai procedure in infants with biliary atresia. J Pediatr Surg 2003;38(3):406 [PMID: 12632357].

Miga D et al: Survival after first esophageal variceal hemorrhage in patients with biliary atresia. J Pediatr 2001;139:291 [PMID: 11487759].

Nio M et al: Japanese Biliary Atresia Registry: Five- and 10-year survival rates after surgery for biliary atresia: A report from the Japanese Biliary Atresia Registry. J Pediatr Surg 2003; 38(7):997 [PMID: 12861525].

Ohi R: Biliary atresia: A surgical perspective. Clin Liver Dis 2001;4:779 [PMID: 11232357].

Sokol RJ et al: Pathogenesis and outcome of biliary atresia: Current concepts. J Pediatr Gastroenterol Nutr 2003;37:4 [PMID: 12827000].

Sokol RJ, Mack C: Etiopathogenesis of biliary atresia. Semin Liver Dis 2001;21:517 [PMID: 11745039].

## 2. Choledochal Cyst

Choledochal cysts cause 2–5% of cases of extrahepatic neonatal cholestasis; the incidence is fourfold higher in girls and higher in patients of Asian descent. In most cases, the clinical manifestations, basic laboratory findings, and histopathologic features on liver biopsy are indistinguishable from those associated with biliary atresia. Neonatal symptomatic cysts are usually associated with atresia of the distal common duct—accounting for the diagnostic dilemma—and may simply be part of the spectrum of biliary atresia. However, a palpable subhepatic mass and a positive ultrasound scan promptly resolve the diagnostic question. Discovery of such a mass eliminates the need for other studies. Immediate operation is indicated once abnormalities in clotting factors have been corrected and bacterial cholangitis, if present, has been treated with intravenous antibiotics. In older children, choledochal cyst presents as recurrent episodes of obstructive jaundice, pancreatitis, or right upper quadrant abdominal pain and vomiting, or as a right abdominal mass.

Excision of the cyst and choledocho–Roux-en-Y jejunal anastomosis are recommended. In some cases, because of technical problems, only the mucosa of the cyst can be removed with jejunal anastomosis to the proximal bile duct. Anastomosis of cyst to jejunum or duodenum is not recommended.

The prognosis depends on the presence or absence of associated evidence of atresia and the appearance of the intrahepatic ducts. If atresia is found, the prognosis is similar to that described in the preceding section. If an isolated extrahepatic cyst is encountered, the outcome is generally excellent, with resolution of the jaundice and return to normal liver architecture. However, bouts of ascending cholangitis, particularly if intrahepatic cysts are present, or obstruction of the anastomotic site may occur. The risk of biliary carcinoma developing within the cyst is about 5–15% at adulthood; therefore, cystectomy or excision of cyst mucosa should be undertaken whenever possible.

Bismuth H, Krissat J: Choledochal cyst malignancies. Ann Oncol 1999;10:94 [PMID: 10436795].

He X et al: Congenital choledochal cyst—Report of 56 cases. Chin Med Sci J 2000;15(1):52 [PMID: 12899402].

Mackenzie TC et al: The management of prenatally diagnosed choledochal cysts. J Pediatr Surg 2001;36:1241 [PMID: 11479866].

## 3. Spontaneous Perforation of the Extrahepatic Bile Ducts

The sudden appearance of obstructive jaundice, acholic stools, and abdominal enlargement with ascites in a sick newborn is suggestive of this condition. The liver is usually normal in size, and a yellow-green discoloration can often be discerned under the umbilicus or in the scrotum. In 24% of cases, stones or sludge obstructs the common bile duct. DIDA scan or ERCP shows leakage from the biliary tree, and ultrasonography confirms ascites or fluid around the bile duct.

Treatment is surgical. Simple drainage, without attempts at oversewing the perforation, is sufficient in primary perforations. A diversion anastomosis is constructed in cases associated with choledochal cyst or stenosis. The prognosis is generally good.

Chardot C et al: Spontaneous perforation of the biliary tract in infancy: A series of 11 cases. Eur J Pediatr Surg 1996;6:341 [PMID: 9007467].

Xanthakos SA et al: Spontaneous perforation of the bile duct in infancy: A rare but important cause of irritability and abdominal distension. J Pediatr Gastroenterol Nutr 2003;36(2): 287 [PMID: 12548069].

## OTHER NEONATAL HYPERBILIRUBINEMIC CONDITIONS (Noncholestatic Nonhemolytic)

This group of disorders associated with hyperbilirubinemia is of two types: (1) unconjugated hyperbilirubinemia, consisting of breast milk jaundice,

Lucey–Driscoll syndrome, congenital hypothyroidism, upper intestinal obstruction, Gilbert disease, Crigler–Najjar syndrome, and drug-induced hyperbilirubinemia; and (2) conjugated noncholestatic hyperbilirubinemia, consisting of Dubin–Johnson syndrome and Rotor syndrome.

## 1. Unconjugated Hyperbilirubinemia

### Breast Milk Jaundice

Persistent elevation of the indirect bilirubin fraction may occur in up to 36% of breast-fed infants. Enhanced β-glucuronidase activity in breast milk as the cause for increased absorption of unconjugated bilirubin is controversial. The increased enterohepatic shunting of unconjugated bilirubin exceeds the normal conjugating capacity in the liver of these infants. The mutation for Gilbert syndrome predisposes to breast milk jaundice and to more prolonged jaundice.

Hyperbilirubinemia does not usually exceed 20 mg/dL, with most cases in the range of 10–15 mg/dL. In patients whose bilirubin levels are above 4–5 mg/dL, the jaundice is noticeable by the fifth to seventh day of breast-feeding. It may accentuate the underlying physiologic jaundice—especially early, when total fluid intake may be less than optimal. Except for jaundice, the physical examination is usually normal; urine does not stain the diaper, and the stools are golden yellow.

The jaundice peaks by the third week of life and clears before age 3 months in almost all infants, even when breast-feedings are continued. All infants who remain jaundiced past age 2 weeks should have measurements of conjugated bilirubin to exclude hepatobiliary disease.

Kernicterus has never been reported in association with this condition. In special situations, breast-feeding may be discontinued temporarily and replaced by formula feedings for 2–3 days until serum bilirubin decreases by 2–8 mg/dL. Cow's milk formulas inhibit the intestinal reabsorption of unconjugated bilirubin. When breast-feeding is reinstituted, the serum bilirubin may increase slightly but not to the previous level. Phototherapy is not indicated in the healthy full-term infant with this condition.

Kreamer BL et al: A novel inhibitor of beta-glucuronidase: L-Aspartic acid. Pediatr Res 2001 Oct;50(4):460 [PMID: 11568288].

Mauro Y et al: Prolonged unconjugated hyperbilirubinemia associated with breast milk and mutations of the bilirubin uridine diphosphate-glucuronosyl transferase gene. Pediatrics 2000; 106:E59 [PMID: 11061796].

Monaghan G et al: Gilbert's syndrome is a contributory factor in prolonged unconjugated hyperbilirubinemia of the newborn. J Pediatr 1999;134:441 [PMID: 10190918].

### Congenital Hypothyroidism

Although the differential diagnosis of indirect hyperbilirubinemia should always include congenital hypothyroidism, the diagnosis may be obvious from other clinical and physical clues or from the newborn screening results. The jaundice clears quickly with replacement thyroid hormone therapy, although the mechanism is unclear.

Labrune P et al: Bilirubin uridine diphosphate glucuronosyltransferase hepatic activity in jaundice associated with congenital hypothyroidism. J Pediatr Gastroenterol Nutr 1992;14:79 [PMID: 1573516].

### Upper Intestinal Obstruction

The association of indirect hyperbilirubinemia with high intestinal obstruction (eg, duodenal atresia, annular pancreas, pyloric stenosis) in the newborn has been observed repeatedly; the mechanism is unknown. Diminished levels of hepatic glucuronyl transferase have been found on liver biopsy in pyloric stenosis, and genetic studies suggest that this indirect hyperbilirubinemia is an early sign of Gilbert syndrome.

Treatment is that of the underlying obstructive condition (usually surgical). Jaundice disappears once adequate nutrition is achieved.

Trioche P et al: Jaundice with hypertrophic pyloric stenosis is an early manifestation of Gilbert's syndrome. Arch Dis Child 1999;81:301 [PMID: 10490432].

### Gilbert Syndrome

Gilbert syndrome is a common form (3–7% of the population) of familial hyperbilirubinemia associated with a partial reduction of hepatic bilirubin uridine diphosphate (UDP) glucuronyl transferase activity and perhaps an abnormality in the function or amount of one or more hepatocyte membrane protein carriers. Accelerated jaundice of the newborn, breast milk jaundice, and jaundice with intestinal obstruction may be present in affected infants. During puberty and beyond, mild fluctuating jaundice, especially with illness, and vague constitutional symptoms are common. Shortened red blood cell survival time in some patients is thought to be caused by reduced activity of enzymes involved in heme biosynthesis (protoporphyrinogen oxidase). Subsidence of hyperbilirubinemia has been achieved in patients by administration of phenobarbital (5–8 mg/kg/d), although this therapy is not justified.

The disease is inherited as an autosomal recessive abnormality of the promoter region of UDP-glucuronyl transferase-1; however, another factor is necessary for disease expression. The homozygous (16%) and heterozygous states (40%) are common. Males are affected more often than females (4:1). Serum unconjugated bilirubin is generally less than 3–6 mg/dL, although rare cases may exceed 8 mg/dL. The findings on liver biopsy and most other LFTs are normal except for prolonged indocyanine green and bromosulfophthalein (BSP) retention. An increase of 1.4 mg/dL or more in the level of unconjugated bilirubin after a 2-day fast (300 kcal/d) is consistent with the diagnosis of Gilbert syndrome. Genetic testing is available but rarely needed. No treatment is necessary.

Bancroft JD et al: Gilbert syndrome accelerates development of neonatal jaundice. J Pediatr 1998;132:656 [PMID: 9580766].

Ulgenalp A et al: Analyses of polymorphism for UGT1*1 exon 1 promoter in neonates with pathologic and prolonged jaundice. Biol Neonate 2003;83(4):258 [PMID: 12743455].

Vajro P et al: Unusual presentation of Gilbert's syndrome in pediatric recipients of liver transplantation. J Pediatr Gastroenterol Nutr 2000;31:238 [PMID: 10997365].

## Crigler–Najjar Syndrome

Infants with type I Crigler–Najjar syndrome usually develop rapid severe elevation of unconjugated bilirubin (> 30–40 mg/dL) with neurologic consequences (kernicterus). Consanguinity is often present. Prompt recognition of this entity and treatment with exchange transfusions are required, followed by phototherapy. Some patients have no neurologic signs until adolescence or early adulthood, at which time deterioration may occur suddenly. For diagnosis of this condition it is useful to obtain a duodenal bile specimen, which characteristically will be colorless and contain a predominance of unconjugated bilirubin, small amounts of monoconjugates, and only traces of diconjugated bilirubin. Phenobarbital administration in these patients does not significantly alter these findings, nor does it lower serum bilirubin levels. The glucuronyl transferase deficiency is inherited in an autosomal recessive pattern. A combination of phototherapy and cholestyramine may keep bilirubin levels below 25 mg/dL. The use of tin protoporphyrin or tin mesoporphyrin remains experimental. Liver transplantation is curative and may prevent kernicterus if performed early. An auxiliary orthotopic transplantation also relieves the jaundice while the patient retains native liver. Hepatocyte transplantation is experimental.

A milder form (type II) with both autosomal dominant and recessive inheritance is rarely associated with neurologic complications. Hyperbilirubinemia is less severe, and the bile is pigmented and contains bilirubin mono- and diglucuronide. Patients with this form respond to phenobarbital with lowering of serum bilirubin levels. An increased proportion of monoconjugated and diconjugated bilirubin in the bile follows phenobarbital treatment.

Liver biopsy findings and LFTs are consistently normal in both types.

Kadakol A et al: Genetic lesions of bilirubin uridine-diphosphoglucuronate glucuronosyltransferase (UGT1A1) causing Crigler–Najjar and Gilbert syndromes: Correlation of genotype to phenotype. Hum Mutat 2000;16:297 [PMID: 11013440].

Schauer R et al: Treatment of Crigler–Najjar type 1 disease: Relevance of early liver transplantation. J Pediatr Surg 2003;38(8):1227 [PMID: 12891498].

Strom SC et al: Hepatocyte transplantation for the treatment of human disease. Semin Liver Dis 1999;19:39 [PMID: 10349682].

## Drug-Induced Hyperbilirubinemia

Vitamin $K_3$ (menadiol) may elevate indirect bilirubin levels by causing hemolysis. Vitamin $K_1$ (phytonadione) can be used safely in neonates. Rifampin and antiretroviral protease inhibitors may cause unconjugated hyperbilirubinemia. Other drugs (eg, ceftriaxone, sulfonamides) may displace bilirubin from albumin, potentially increasing the risk of kernicterus—especially in the sick premature infant.

## 2. Conjugated Noncholestatic Hyperbilirubinemia (Dubin–Johnson Syndrome & Rotor Syndrome)

These diagnoses are suspected when persistent or recurrent conjugated hyperbilirubinemia and jaundice occur and liver function tests are normal. The basic defect in Dubin–Johnson syndrome affects the multiple organic anion transport protein ($MRP_2$) of the bile canaliculus, causing impaired hepatocyte excretion of conjugated bilirubin into bile. A variable degree of impairment in uptake and conjugation complicates the clinical picture. Transmission is autosomal recessive, so a positive family history is occasionally obtained. In Rotor syndrome, the defect lies in hepatic uptake and storage of bilirubin. Bile acids are metabolized normally, so that cholestasis does not occur. Bilirubin values range from 2 to 5 mg/dL, and other LFTs are normal.

In Rotor syndrome, the liver is normal; in Dubin–Johnson syndrome, it is darkly pigmented on gross inspection and may be enlarged. Microscopic examination reveals numerous dark-brown pigment granules consisting of polymers of epinephrine metabolites, especially in the centrilobular regions. However, the amount of pigment varies within families, and some jaundiced family members may have no demonstrable pigmentation in the liver. Otherwise, the liver is histologically normal. Oral cholecystography fails to visualize the gallbladder in Dubin–Johnson syndrome but is normal in Rotor syndrome. Differences in the excretion patterns of BSP, in results of DIDA cholescintigraphy, in urinary coproporphyrin I and III levels, and in the serum pattern of monoglucuronide and diglucuronide conjugates of bilirubin can help distinguish between these two conditions.

The prognosis is excellent, and no treatment is needed.

Kaplan M et al: Bilirubin genetics for the nongeneticist: Hereditary defects of neonatal bilirubin conjugation. Pediatrics 2003;111(4 Pt 1):886 [PMID: 12671128].

Regev RH et al: Treatment of severe cholestasis in neonatal Dubin–Johnson syndrome with ursodeoxycholic acid. J Perinat Med 2002;30(2):185 [PMID: 12012642].

## HEPATITIS A

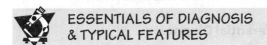

### ESSENTIALS OF DIAGNOSIS & TYPICAL FEATURES

- *Gastrointestinal upset (anorexia, vomiting, diarrhea).*
- *Jaundice.*
- *Liver tenderness and enlargement.*
- *Abnormal LFTs.*
- *Local epidemic of the hepatitis A infection.*
- *Positive Anti-HAV IgM antibody.*

## General Considerations

Hepatitis A virus (HAV) infection occurs in both epidemic and sporadic fashion (Table 21–6). Transmission by the fecal–oral route explains epidemic outbreaks from contaminated food or water supplies, including by food handlers. Viral particles 27 nm in diameter have been found in stools during the acute phase of hepatitis A infection and are similar in appearance to the enteroviruses. Sporadic cases usually result from contact with an affected individual. Transmission through blood products obtained during the viremic phase is a rare event, although it has occurred in a newborn nursery. The overt form of the disease is easily recognized by the clinical manifestations. However, two thirds of children are asymptomatic, and two thirds of symptomatic children are anicteric. Lifelong immunity to HAV follows infection. In developing countries, most children are exposed to HAV by age 10 years, while only 20% are exposed by age 20 years in developed countries.

***Table 21–6.*** Hepatitis viruses.

| | HAV | HBV | HCV | HDV | HEV |
|---|---|---|---|---|---|
| Type of virus | Enterovirus (RNA) | Hepadnavirus (DNA) | Flavivirus (RNA) | Incomplete (RNA) | Calicivirus (RNA) |
| Transmission routes | Fecal–oral | Parenteral, sexual, vertical | Parenteral, sexual, vertical | Parenteral, sexual | Fecal-oral |
| Incubation period (days) | 15–40 | 50–150 | 30–150 | 20–90 | 14–65 |
| Diagnostic test | Anti-HAV IgM | HBsAg, anti-HBc IgM | Anti-HCV, PCR–RNA test | Anti-HDV | Anti-HEV |
| Mortality rate (acute) | 0.1–0.2% | 0.5–2% | 1–2% | 2–20% | 1–2% (in pregnant women, 20%) |
| Carrier state | No | Yes | Yes | Yes | No |
| Vaccine available | Yes | Yes | No | Yes (HBV) | No |
| Treatment | None | Interferon-α or lamivudine | Interferon-α plus ribavirin Pegylated interferon (adults) | Treatment for HBV | None |

PCR = polymerase chain reaction; HAV = hepatitis A virus; HBsAg = hepatitis B surface antigen; HBc = hepatitis B core; HDV = hepatitis D (delta) virus; HBV = hepatitis B virus.

Antibody to HAV appears within 1–4 weeks of clinical symptoms. Although the great majority of children with infectious hepatitis are asymptomatic or have mild disease and recover completely, some will develop fulminant hepatitis.

---

**HEPATITIS VIRUS ABBREVIATIONS**

| | |
|---|---|
| **HAV** | Hepatitis A virus |
| **Anti-HAV IgM** | IgM antibody to HAV |
| **HBV** | Hepatitis B virus |
| **HBsAg** | HBV surface antigen |
| **HBcAg** | HBV core antigen |
| **HBeAg** | HBV envelope antigen |
| **Anti-HBs** | Antibody to HBsAg |
| **Anti-HBc** | Antibody to HBcAg |
| **Anti-HBc IgM** | IgM antibody to HBcAg |
| **Anti-HBe** | Antibody to HBeAg |
| **HCV** | Hepatitis C virus |
| **Anti-HCV** | Antibody to HCV |
| **HDV** | Hepatitis D (delta) virus |
| **Anti-HDV** | Antibody to HDV |
| **HEV** | Hepatitis E virus |
| **Anti-HEV** | Antibody to HEV |
| **NANBNC** | Non-A, non-B, non-C hepatitis virus |

---

## Clinical Findings

### A. HISTORY

Features of the patient's history elicit direct exposure to a previously jaundiced individual, consumption of seafood or contaminated water, or recent travel to an area of endemic infection. Following an incubation period of 15–40 days, the initial nonspecific symptoms usually precede the development of jaundice by 5–10 days.

### B. SYMPTOMS AND SIGNS

Fever, anorexia, vomiting, headache, and abdominal pain are the usual symptoms. Darkening of the urine precedes jaundice, which peaks in 1–2 weeks and then begins to subside. The stools may become light or clay-colored during this time. Clinical improvement can occur as jaundice develops. Tender hepatomegaly and jaundice are typically present; splenomegaly is variable.

### C. LABORATORY FINDINGS

Aminotransferases and conjugated and unconjugated bilirubin levels are elevated. The leukocyte count is normal to low; the sedimentation rate is elevated. Serum proteins are generally normal, but an elevation of the γ-globulin fraction (> 2.5 g/dL) can occur and indicates a worse prognosis. Hypoalbuminemia, hypo-glycemia, and marked prolongation of prothrombin time are serious prognostic findings. Diagnosis is made by serology. A positive anti-HAV IgM indicates acute disease, whereas IgG anti-HAV persists after recovery.

Percutaneous liver biopsy is rarely indicated but may be performed safely in most children provided that the partial thromboplastin time and platelet count are normal and the prothrombin time is prolonged less than 4–5 seconds. The presence of ascites may increase the risk of percutaneous liver biopsy. "Balloon cells" and acidophilic bodies are characteristic histologic findings. Liver cell necrosis may be diffuse or focal, with accompanying infiltration of inflammatory cells containing polymorphonuclear leukocytes, lymphocytes, macrophages, and plasma cells, particularly in portal areas. Some bile duct proliferation may be seen in the perilobular portal areas alongside areas of bile stasis. Regenerative liver cells and proliferation of reticuloendothelial cells are present. Occasionally massive hepatocyte necrosis occurs, portending a bad prognosis.

## Differential Diagnosis

Before jaundice appears, the symptoms are those of a nonspecific viral enteritis. Other diseases with somewhat similar onset include pancreatitis, infectious mononucleosis, leptospirosis, drug-induced hepatitis, Wilson disease, autoimmune hepatitis, and, most often, other hepatitis viruses. Acquired CMV disease may also mimic HAV, although lymphadenopathy is usually present in the former.

## Prevention

Some attempt at isolation of the patient during initial phases of illness is indicated, although most patients with hepatitis A are noninfectious by the time the disease becomes overt. Stool, diapers, and other fecally stained clothing should be handled with care for 1 week after the appearance of jaundice.

Passive–active immunization of exposed susceptible persons can be achieved by giving standard immune globulin, 0.02–0.04 mL/kg intramuscularly. Illness is prevented in 80–90% of individuals if immune globulin is given within 1–2 weeks of exposure. Individuals traveling to endemic disease areas should receive HAV vaccine or 0.02–0.06 mL/kg of immune globulin as prophylaxis if there is insufficient time (< 2 weeks) for the initial dose of vaccine. All children older than age 2 years with chronic liver diseases should receive two doses of HAV vaccine 6 months apart. It is currently recommended that universal childhood immunization for HAV be implemented in states in the United States with 20 or more cases per 100,000 population per year, and in local areas with a high prevalence.

## Treatment

There are no specific measures. Sedatives and corticosteroids should be avoided. At the start of the illness, a light diet is preferable. During the icteric phase, lower-fat foods may diminish gastrointestinal symptoms but do not affect overall outcome. Drugs and elective surgery should be avoided.

## Prognosis

Ninety-nine percent of children recover without sequelae. In rare cases of fulminant hepatitis, the patient may die in 5 days or may survive as long as 1–2 months without liver transplantation. The prognosis is poor if the signs and symptoms of hepatic coma develop, with deepening of jaundice and development of ascites; orthotopic liver transplantation is indicated under these circumstances. Incomplete resolution leads to prolonged hepatitis or chronic cholestatic hepatitis but not to cirrhosis. Rare cases of aplastic anemia following acute infectious hepatitis have been reported. A benign relapse of symptoms may occur in 10–15% of cases after 6–10 weeks of apparent resolution.

Advisory Committee on Immunization Practices: Prevention of hepatitis A through active or passive immunization: Recommendation of the Advisory Committee on Immunization Practices (ACIP). MMWR 1999;48:1 [PMID: 10543657].

Jacobs R et al: The cost-effectiveness of adolescent hepatitis A vaccination in states with the high disease rates. Arch Pediatr Adolesc Med 2000;154:763 [PMID: 10922291].

Demicheli V, Tiberti D: The effectiveness and safety of hepatitis A vaccine: A systematic review. Vaccine 2003;21(19–20): 2242 [PMID: 12744850].

# HEPATITIS B

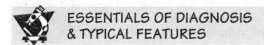

### ESSENTIALS OF DIAGNOSIS & TYPICAL FEATURES

- *Gastrointestinal upset, anorexia, vomiting, diarrhea.*
- *Jaundice, tender hepatomegaly, abnormal LFTs.*
- *Serologic evidence of hepatitis B disease: HBsAg, HBeAg, anti-HBc IgM.*
- *History of parenteral, sexual, or household exposure or maternal HBsAg carriage.*

## General Considerations

In contrast to hepatitis A, hepatitis B virus (HBV) infection has a longer incubation period of 21–135 days (see Table 21–5). The disease is caused by a DNA virus that is usually acquired perinatally from a carrier mother, or later in life from blood products, shared needles, needle sticks, skin piercing, or tattoos; or through sexual transmission. Transmission via blood products has been almost eliminated by anti-HBc antibody donor-screening protocols. The complete HBV particle is composed of a core (28-nm particle) that is found in the nucleus of infected liver cells and a double outer shell (surface antigen). The surface antigen in blood is termed HBsAg. The antibody to it is anti-HBs. The core antigen is termed HBcAg and its antibody is anti-HBc. A specific anti-HBc IgM antibody occurs during primary viral replication.

Another important antigen–antibody system associated with HBV disease is the "e" (envelope) antigen system. HBeAg, a truncated soluble form of HBcAg, appears in the serum of infected patients early and correlates with active virus replication. Persistence of HBeAg is a marker of infectivity, whereas the appearance of anti-HBe generally implies termination of viral replication. However, HBV mutant viruses (precore mutant) may replicate with negative HBeAg tests for and positive tests for anti-HBe antibody. Other serologic markers indicating viral replication include the presence of DNA polymerase and circulating HBV DNA.

## Clinical Findings

### A. SYMPTOMS AND SIGNS

The symptoms are nonspecific, consisting only of slight fever (which may be absent) and mild gastrointestinal upset. Visible jaundice is usually the first significant finding. It is accompanied by darkening of the urine and pale or clay-colored stools. Hepatomegaly is present. Occasionally a symptom complex (caused by antigen–antibody complexes) of macular rash, urticarial lesions, and arthritis antedates the appearance of icterus. Occasionally, HBV infection presents as a glomerulonephritis or nephrotic syndrome. When acquired vertically at birth, chronic disease is frequently completely asymptomatic despite ongoing liver injury.

### B. LABORATORY FINDINGS

To diagnose acute HBV infection, the HBsAg and anti-HBc IgM are the only tests needed. To document recovery, immunity, or response to the HBV vaccine, the anti-HBs is useful. If HBsAg persists after 8 weeks in acute infections, it may signify a chronic infection, although chronic infection is defined as lasting 6 months or more. Vertical transmission to newborns is documented by positive HBsAg.

LFT results are similar to those discussed earlier for hepatitis A. Liver histology is similar for HAV and

HBV disease, although specific stains may detect HBcAg or HBsAg in the liver.

Renal involvement may be suspected on the basis of urinary findings suggesting glomerulonephritis or nephrotic syndrome.

## Differential Diagnosis

The differentiation between HAV and HBV disease is made easier by a history of parenteral exposure, an HBsAg-positive parent, or an unusually long period of incubation. HBV and hepatitis C virus (HCV) infection or EBV infection are differentiated serologically. The history may suggest a drug-induced hepatitis, especially if a serum sickness prodrome is reported. Autoimmune hepatitis, Wilson disease, hemochromatosis, nonalcoholic steatohepatitis, and $\alpha_1$-antitrypsin deficiency should also be considered.

Non-A non-B non-C (NANBNC) hepatitis is diagnosed when test results for the serologic markers of HAV, HBV, HCV and EBV are negative; drug-induced hepatitis if there is a history of drug exposure; autoimmune hepatitis if autoimmune markers are present; Wilson disease if ceruloplasmin levels are abnormal; hemochromatosis if transferrin saturation is high; $\alpha_1$-antitrypsin deficiency if serum concentration is decreased, and steatohepatitis if liver biopsy findings are suggestive.

## Prevention

Control of hepatitis B in the population is based on screening of blood donors and pregnant women, use of properly sterilized needles and surgical equipment, avoidance of sexual contact with carriers, and vaccination of all infants and adolescents, as well as household contacts, sexual partners, medical personnel, and those at high risk. Universal immunization of all infants born in the United States and of adolescents is now recommended, as it is in most other countries. When acquired vertically at birth, chronic disease is frequently asymptomatic despite ongoing liver injury or a benign carrier state. The vaccine is highly effective for preexposure prophylaxis (see Chapter 9). Postexposure administration of HBIG (0.06 mL/kg intramuscularly, given as soon as possible after exposure, up to 7 days) and initiation of vaccination are also effective.

## Treatment

Supportive measures such as bed rest and a nutritious diet are used during the active stage of disease. Corticosteroids are contraindicated. No other treatment is needed for acute HBV infection. For patients with progressive disease (chronic active hepatitis), there are two treatment options. Treatment with $\alpha$-interferon (5–6 million units/m$^2$ body surface area injected subcutaneously three times a week for 4–6 months) inhibits viral replication in 30–40% of patients, normalizes the ALT level, and leads to the disappearance of HBeAg and the appearance of anti-HBe. Side effects are common. Younger children may respond better than older children. Orally administered lamivudine therapy (3 mg/kg/day up to 100 mg per day for 12 months) leads to a successful response in 25% of treated children, with minimal side effects. However, resistant organisms can emerge. Asymptomatic HBsAg carriers (normal serum ALT, no hepatomegaly) do not respond to either therapy. Liver transplantation is successful in acute fulminant hepatitis B; however, reinfection is common following liver transplantation for chronic hepatitis B. Chronic HBIG therapy or lamivudine therapy reduces recurrence after transplantation.

## Prognosis

The prognosis is good, although fulminant hepatitis or chronic hepatitis and cirrhosis may supervene in up to 10% of patients. The course of the disease is variable, but jaundice seldom persists for more than 2 weeks. HBsAg disappears in 95% of cases at the time of clinical recovery. Persistent asymptomatic antigenemia may occur, particularly in children with vertical transmission, Down syndrome, or leukemia and in those undergoing chronic hemodialysis. Persistence of neonatally acquired HBsAg occurs in 70–90% of infants without immunoprophylaxis or vaccination, and the presence of e antigen in the HBsAg carrier indicates ongoing viral replication. If HBV infection is acquired later in childhood, HBV is cleared and recovery occurs in 90–95% of patients. Chronic hepatitis B disease predisposes the patient to development of hepatocellular carcinoma. Once chronic HBV infection is established, surveillance for development of hepatocellular carcinoma with hepatic ultrasonography and serum $\alpha$-fetoprotein is performed annually. Routine HBV vaccination of newborns in endemic countries has reduced the incidence of hepatocellular carcinoma in children.

Broderick AL, Jonas MM: Hepatitis B in children. Semin Liver Dis 2003;23(1):59 [PMID: 12616451].

Chang MH et al: Hepatitis B vaccination and hepatocellular carcinoma rates in boys and girls. JAMA 2000;284:3040 [PMID: 11122592].

Comanor L et al: Impact of chronic hepatitis B and interferon-alpha therapy on growth of children. J Viral Hepat 2001;8:139 [PMID: 11264734].

Jonas MM et al; International Pediatric Lamivudine Investigator Group: Clinical trial of lamivudine in children with chronic hepatitis B. N Engl J Med 200219;347(12):955 PMID: [12037150].

Schwarz KB: Pediatric issues in new therapies for hepatitis B and C. Curr Gastroenterol Rep 2003;5(3):233 [PMID: 12734046].

# HEPATITIS C

## General Considerations

Hepatitis C virus (HCV) virus is the most common cause of most non-B chronic hepatitis (90% of post-transfusion hepatitis cases) (see Table 21–6). Risk factors include illicit use of intravenous drugs (40%), occupational or sexual exposure (10%), and transfusions (10%); 30% of cases have no known risk factors. In children, most cases are associated with blood or blood product transfusions, transmission from an infected mother, or other household transmission. In the past, children with hemophilia or on chronic hemodialysis were at significant risk. The risk from transfused blood products has diminished greatly (from 1–2:100 to 1:100,000 units of blood) since the advent of blood testing for ALT and anti-HCV. HCV infection has been caused by contaminated immune serum globulin preparations. Vertical transmission from HCV-infected mothers occurs more commonly with mothers who are HIV-positive (10–20%) compared with those who are HIV-negative (5–6%). About 0.4% of adolescents and 1.5% of adults in the United States are infected. Infected infants have elevated ALT levels, but do not appear ill; long-term outcome is unknown. Transmission of the virus from breast milk is probably rare. HCV rarely causes fulminant hepatitis in children or adults in Western countries, but different serotypes do so in Asia.

HCV is a single-stranded RNA virus in the flavivirus family. At least seven genotypes of HCV exist. Several well-defined HCV antigens are the basis for serologic antibody tests. The third-generation enzyme-linked immunosorbent assay (ELISA) test for anti-HCV is highly accurate. Anti-HCV is generally present when symptoms occur; however, test results may be negative in the first few months of infection. HCV RNA, which can be detected in serum by PCR and branched-DNA test, indicates active infection.

## Clinical Findings

### A. SYMPTOMS AND SIGNS

The incubation period is 1–5 months, with insidious onset of symptoms. Many childhood cases, especially those acquired vertically, are asymptomatic despite development of chronic hepatitis. Flu-like prodromal symptoms and jaundice occur in less than 25% of cases. Hepatosplenomegaly may or may not be evident in chronic hepatitis. Ascites, clubbing, palmar erythema, or spider angiomas indicate progression to cirrhosis.

### B. LABORATORY FINDINGS

Fluctuating mild to moderate elevations of aminotransferases over long periods are characteristic of chronic HCV infection. Diagnosis is established by the presence of anti-HCV (second-generation ELISA) confirmed by the radioimmunoblot assay (RIBA) or HCV RNA by PCR. Anti-HCV is acquired passively at birth from infected mothers and cannot be used to confirm disease in the neonate for the first 15 months. HCV RNA testing should be performed in suspicious cases. Results of this test may be negative in the first month of life, but become positive by 4 months.

Percutaneous liver biopsy should be considered in chronic cases. Histologic examination shows portal triaditis with chronic inflammatory cells, occasional lymphocyte nodules in portal tracts, mild macrovesicular steatosis, and variable bridging necrosis, fibrosis, and cirrhosis. Cirrhosis in adults generally requires 10–30 years of chronic HCV infection, but it has occasionally developed sooner in children.

## Differential Diagnosis

HCV hepatitis should be distinguished from HAV, HBV, and NANBNC hepatitis by serologic testing. Other causes of cirrhosis in children should be considered in cases of chronic illness, such as Wilson disease or $\alpha_1$-antitrypsin deficiency. Chronic hepatitis may also be caused by drug reactions, autoimmune disease, or steatohepatitis.

## Treatment

Treatment of acute HCV hepatitis is supportive. Indications for treatment of chronic infection will be determined by current clinical trials. Chronic infection responds to interferon-$\alpha$ (3 million units/$m^2$ three times a week for 6–12 months) in 30–50% of cases. Relapses are common and appear to depend on genotype of the virus. Overall only 10–20% are sustained responders, and the response is poorer with infections with genotype 1a or 1b. Combined interferon plus ribavirin is more successful in adults and is being tested in children. Long-acting (pegylated) interferon (with or without ribavirin) is effective in adults and is being tested in children. End-stage liver disease secondary to HCV responds well to liver transplantation, although reinfection is common and gradually progressive. There is no vaccine, and no benefit from using immune globulin in infants born to infected mothers. Elective C-section of HCV-infected pregnant women with a high titer of circulating virus may lessen the likelihood for transmission.

## Prognosis

In adults, 70–80% of HCV cases develop chronic hepatitis, and cirrhosis develops in 20% of those with chronic infection for 10–30 years. Alcohol intake increases this risk. HCV is now the leading indication for liver transplantation in adults. A strong association exists between chronic HCV disease and the development of hepatocellular carcinoma after as little as 15 years. The outcome in children is less well defined, although cirrhosis may develop rapidly or after decades. About 50% of children infected by transfusion in the first few years of life develop chronic infection. Infants infected at birth often have concomitant HIV infection; their outcome is unknown at present. In adults, chronic HCV infection has been associated with mixed cryoglobulinemia, polyarteritis nodosa, a sicca-like syndrome, and membranoproliferative glomerulonephritis.

Alter MJ et al: The prevalence of hepatitis C virus infection in the United States 1988 through 1994. N Engl J Med 1999;19: 341 [PMID: 10451460].

Bortolotti F et al: An epidemiological survey of hepatitis C virus infection in Italian children in the decade 1990–1999. J Pediatr Gastroenterol Nutr 2001;32:562 [PMID: 11419517].

Di Ciommo V et al: Interferon alpha in the treatment of chronic hepatitis C in children: A meta-analysis. J Viral Hepat 2003; 10(3):210 [PMID: 12753340].

European Pediatric Hepatitis C Virus Network: Effects of mode of delivery and infant feeding on the risk of mother-to-child transmission of hepatitis C virus. BJOG 2001;108:371 [PMID: 11305543].

Gibb DM et al: Mother-to-child transmission of hepatitis C virus: Evidence for preventable peripartum transmission. Lancet 2000;356:904 [PMID: 11036896].

Resti M et al: Hepatitis C virus infection in children coinfected with HIV: Epidemiology and management. Paediatr Drugs 2002;4(9):571 [PMID: 12175272].

Schwarz KB, Balistreri W: Viral hepatitis. J Pediatr Gastroenterol Nutr 2002;35 (Suppl 1):S29 [PMID: 12151818].

## HEPATITIS D (Delta Agent)

### General Considerations

The hepatitis D virus (HDV) is a 35-nm defective virus that requires a coat of HBsAg to be infectious (see Table 21–6). HDV infection thus can occur only in the presence of HBV infection. In developing countries, transmission is by intimate contact; in Western countries, by parenteral exposure. HDV is rare in North America. HDV can infect simultaneously with HBV, causing acute hepatitis, or can superinfect a patient with chronic HBV infection, predisposing the individual to chronic hepatitis or fulminant hepatitis. In children, the association between chronic HDV coinfection with HBV and chronic hepatitis and cirrhosis is a strong. Vertical HDV transmission is rare. The diagnosis of HDV is made by anti-HDV IgM. Treatment is directed at therapy for HBV infection (eg, interferon-α) or for fulminant hepatic failure.

Dalekos GN et al: Interferon-alpha treatment of children with chronic hepatitis D virus infection: The Greek experience. Hepatogastroenterology 2001;47:1072.

Kelly D, Skidmore S: Hepatitis C–Z: Recent advances. Arch Dis Child 2002;86(5):339 [PMID: 11970925].

## HEPATITIS E

### General Considerations

Hepatitis E virus (HEV) infection is a cause of enterically transmitted, epidemic non-A, non-B hepatitis (see Table 21–6). It is rare in the United States. HEV is a calicivirus-like agent that is transmitted via the fecal–oral route. It occurs predominantly in developing countries in association with water-borne epidemics, and has only a 3% secondary attack rate in household contacts. Areas reporting epidemics include southeast Asia, China, the Indian subcontinent, the Middle East, northern and western Africa, Mexico, and Central America. Its clinical manifestations are similar to those of HAV infection except that symptomatic disease is rare in children, more common in adolescents and adults, and is associated with a high mortality (10–20%) in pregnant women, particularly in the third trimester. Diagnosis is established by detecting anti-HEV antibody. The outcome in nonpregnant individuals is benign, with no chronic hepatitis or chronic carrier state reported. There is no effective treatment.

Aggarwal R et al: Hepatitis E: An overview and recent advances in clinical and laboratory research. J Gastroenterol Hepatol 2000;15:9 [PMID: 10719741].

Arora NK et al: Hepatitis E infection in children: Study of an outbreak. J Gastroenterol Hepatol 1999;14:572 [PMID: 10385067].

Arora NK et al: Acute liver failure. Indian J Pediatr 2003;70(1): 73 [PMID: 12619956].

Piper-Jenks N et al: Risk of hepatitis E infection to travelers. J Travel Med 2000;7:1949 [PMID: 11003732].

## OTHER HEPATITIS VIRUSES

The recently discovered hepatitis G virus (HGV), also called the GB virus, is relatively common and parenterally and vertically transmitted, but it has not been shown to produce acute or chronic liver disease. Coinfection appears to improve the prognosis of HIV disease. TT virus is also commonly transmitted, but is not a significant cause of hepatitis.

Other undiscovered NANBNC viruses probably cause the majority of cases of fulminant hepatitis in children. Infection with these uncharacterized agents is associated with the development of aplastic anemia in a small proportion of patients recovering from hepatitis and in 15–20% of those undergoing liver transplantation for fulminant hepatitis. Parvovirus has been associated with fulminant hepatitis; the prognosis is relatively good in children.

Infectious mononucleosis (Epstein–Barr virus) is commonly associated with acute hepatitis. CMV, adenovirus, and leptospirosis are other infectious causes of acute hepatitis.

Howard CR: Hepatitis viruses: A Pandora's box? J Gastroenterol Hepatol 2002;17 (Suppl):S464-7 [PMID: 12534779].

Sokal EM et al: Acute parvovirus B19 infection associated with fulminant hepatitis of favorable prognosis in young children. Lancet 1998;352:1739 [PMID: 9848349].

Tillmann HL et al: Infection with GB virus C and reduced mortality among HIV-infected patients. N Engl J Med 2001;345: 715 [PMID: 11547740].

# FULMINANT HEPATIC FAILURE (Acute Massive Hepatic Necrosis, Acute Liver Failure)

## ESSENTIALS OF DIAGNOSIS & TYPICAL FEATURES

- *Acute hepatitis with deepening jaundice.*
- *Extreme elevation of AST and ALT.*
- *Prolonged prothrombin time.*
- *Encephalopathy and cerebral edema.*
- *Asterixis and fetor hepaticus.*

## General Considerations

Fulminant hepatic failure is defined as acute liver dysfunction resulting in hepatic coma and coagulopathy within 6 weeks after onset. Mortality is 60–80% in children (without liver transplantation). An unusually virulent infectious agent or peculiar host susceptibility is postulated in many cases. In the first few weeks of life, fulminant hepatic failure can be caused by herpes simplex, enteroviruses, adenovirus, galactosemia, fructose intolerance, tyrosinemia, neonatal iron storage disease, respiratory chain and fatty acid oxidation defects, familial erythrophagocytic histiocytosis, bile acid synthesis defects, and peroxisomal diseases. In older infants and children, HBV, NANBNC hepatitis, parvovirus, and HEV are sometimes causative. HAV rarely is responsible. Patients with immunologic deficiency diseases and those receiving immunosuppressive drugs are vulnerable to herpes viruses. In children with HIV infection, nucleoside analogues have triggered lactic acidosis and liver failure. In older children, Wilson dis-

ease, acute fatty liver of pregnancy, Reye syndrome, autoimmune hepatitis, drugs (eg, acetaminophen, anesthetic agents) or toxins (eg, poisonous mushrooms, herbs), leukemia, and cardiac dysfunction must also be considered.

## Clinical Findings

In some patients, the disease proceeds in a rapidly fulminant course with deepening jaundice, coagulopathy, hyperammonemia, ascites, a rapidly shrinking liver, and progressive coma. Terminally, AST and ALT, which were greatly elevated (2000–10,000 units/L), may improve at the time when the liver is getting smaller and undergoing massive necrosis and collapse. Some patients start with a course typical of benign hepatitis and then suddenly become severely ill during the second week of the disease. Fever, anorexia, vomiting, and abdominal pain may be noted, and worsening of LFTs parallels changes in sensorium or impending coma. Hyperreflexia and a positive extensor plantar response are seen. A characteristic breath odor (fetor hepaticus) is present. A generalized bleeding tendency occurs at this time. Impairment of renal function, manifested by either oliguria or anuria, is an ominous sign. The striking laboratory findings include elevated serum bilirubin levels (usually > 20 mg/dL), high AST and ALT (> 3000 units/L) that may decrease terminally, low serum albumin, hypoglycemia, and prolonged prothrombin time. Blood ammonia levels may be elevated, whereas blood urea nitrogen is often very low. Hyperpnea is frequent, and mixed respiratory alkalosis and metabolic acidosis are present.

## Differential Diagnosis

Infectious, metabolic, and drug/toxin causes are most common. Patients with Reye syndrome or urea cycle defects are typically anicteric. Wilson disease, autoimmune hepatitis, acute leukemia, cardiomyopathy, and Budd–Chiari syndrome should be considered. Acetaminophen, herbal remedies and other toxins (eg, "Ecstasy") need to be considered even if there is a negative history.

## Complications

The development and depth of hepatic coma determine the prognosis. Patients in grade 3 or 4 coma (unresponsiveness to verbal stimuli, decorticate or decerebrate function) rarely survive without transplantation, and may have residual CNS deficits. Cerebral edema, which usually accompanies coma, is frequently the cause of death. Extreme prolongation of prothrombin time or international normalized ratio (INR) predicts poor recovery. Acetaminophen overdose is the exception. Sepsis, hemorrhage, renal failure, or cardiorespiratory arrest is a common terminal event. The rare survivor without transplantation may have residual fibrosis or even cirrhosis.

## Treatment

Many regimens have been tried, but controlled evaluation of therapy remains difficult. Exchange transfusion (with fresh heparinized blood) temporarily repairs both the chemical and hematologic abnormalities. Plasmapheresis with plasma exchange, total body washout, charcoal hemoperfusion, and hemodialysis using a special high-permeability membrane have been used in the treatment of fulminant hepatic failure. Removal of circulating toxins may be of greater benefit to extrahepatic organ function (brain) than to the liver itself. Reversal of hepatic encephalopathy may follow any of these therapeutic modalities, but without improving the final prognosis. Extracorporeal hepatic support devices are in development. Orthotopic liver transplantation is successful in 60–85% of cases; however, patients in grade 4 coma may not always recover cerebral function. Therefore, patients in hepatic failure should be transferred early to centers where liver transplantation can be performed. Criteria for deciding when to perform transplantation are not firmly established; however, serum bilirubin over 20 mg/dL, prothrombin time over 30 seconds, and factor V levels less than 20% indicate a poor prognosis. Living related donors may be required for transplantation in a timely fashion. The prognosis is better for acetaminophen ingestion, particularly when *N*-acetylcysteine treatment is given.

Corticosteroids may be harmful, unless autoimmune hepatitis is the cause. Sterilization of the colon with oral antibiotics such as metronidazole, neomycin, or gentamicin is recommended. An alternative is acidification of the colon with lactulose, 1–2 mL/kg three or four times daily, which reduces blood ammonia levels and traps ammonia in the colon. Some centers use *N*-acetylcysteine in all patients.

Close monitoring of fluid and electrolytes is mandatory and requires a central venous line. Ten percent dextrose solutions should be infused (6–8 mg/kg/min) to maintain normal blood glucose. Diuretics, sedatives, and tranquilizers are to be used sparingly. Early signs of cerebral edema are treated with infusions of mannitol (0.5–1 g/kg).

Comatose patients are intubated, given mechanical ventilatory support, and monitored for signs of infection. Coagulopathy is treated with fresh-frozen plasma, other clotting factor concentrates, platelet infusions, or exchange transfusion. Plasmapheresis and hemodialysis may help maintain a patient while awaiting liver transplantation. Epidural monitoring for increased intracranial pressure in patients awaiting liver transplantation is advocated. Artificial hepatic support devices are being developed, although continuous venous–venous dialysis may be helpful. Prophylactic immune globulin, 0.02 mL/kg intramuscularly, should be given to close contacts of patients who have HAV infection.

## Prognosis

The overall prognosis remains poor without liver transplantation. Exchange transfusions or other modes of heroic therapy do not improve survival figures. The presence of nests of liver cells seen on liver biopsy amounting to more than 25% of the total cells and rising levels of clotting factors V and VII coupled with rising levels of serum α-fetoprotein may signify a more favorable prognosis for survival. The survival rate in patients who undergo liver transplantation (60–85%) exceeds that of those who do not (20–40%).

Church JA et al: Mitochondrial DNA depletion, near-fatal metabolic acidosis, and liver failure in an HIV-infected child treated with combination antiretroviral therapy. J Pediatr 2001;138:748 [PMID: 11343055].

Ee LC et al: Acute liver failure in children: A regional experience. J Paediatr Child Health 2003;39(2):107 [PMID: 12603798].

Kjaergard LL et al: Artificial and bioartificial support systems for acute and acute-on-chronic liver failure: A systematic review. JAMA 2003;289(2):217 [PMID: 12517233].

Ostapowicz G et al; U.S. Acute Liver Failure Study Group: Results of a prospective study of acute liver failure at 17 tertiary care centers in the United States. Ann Intern Med 2002; 137(12):947 [PMID: 12484709].

Singer AL et al: Role of plasmapheresis in the management of acute hepatic failure in children. Ann Surg 2001;234:418 [PMID: 11524594].

## AUTOIMMUNE HEPATITIS (LUPOID HEPATITIS)

### ESSENTIALS OF DIAGNOSIS & TYPICAL FEATURES

- *Acute or chronic hepatitis*
- *Hypergammaglobulinemia*
- *Positive ANA, ASMA, or anti-LKM*

## General Considerations

Autoimmune hepatitis (AIH) is most common in adolescent girls, although it occurs at all ages and in either sex. Chronic hepatitis may also follow HBV, HCV, and

HDV infections. Rarely, chronic hepatitis evolves from drug-induced hepatitis (eg, pemoline) or may develop in conjunction with such diseases as ulcerative colitis, Sjögren syndrome, or autoimmune hemolytic anemia. Wilson disease, $\alpha_1$-antitrypsin deficiency, and bile acid synthesis defects may also present as chronic hepatitis. A positive HBsAg test implicates HBV, and anti-HCV and anti-HDV suggest HCV and HDV, respectively. Positive antinuclear antibodies, smooth muscle antibodies (type I AIH) or liver–kidney microsomal (LKM) antibodies (type II AIH), elevated serum IgG, and systemic manifestations (eg, arthralgia, weight loss, acne, amenorrhea) are characteristic of AIH.

A genetic susceptibility to development of this entity is suggested by the increased incidence of the histocompatibility antigens HLA-A1 and HLA-B8. These histocompatibility antigens may be related to a defect in suppressor T-cell function noted in patients with chronic hepatitis. Increased autoimmune disease in families of patients and a high prevalence of seroimmunologic abnormalities in relatives have been noted. Occasionally patients have an "overlap syndrome" of AIH and primary sclerosing cholangitis.

## Clinical Findings

Fever, malaise, recurrent or persistent jaundice, skin rash, arthritis, amenorrhea, gynecomastia, acne, pleurisy, pericarditis, or ulcerative colitis may be found in the history of these patients, or asymptomatic hepatomegaly or splenomegaly may be found on examination. Occasionally patients present in acute liver failure. Cutaneous signs of chronic liver disease may be noted (eg, spider angiomas, liver palms, digital clubbing). Hepatosplenomegaly is frequently present.

LFTs reveal moderate elevations of serum bilirubin, AST, ALT, and serum alkaline phosphatase. Serum albumin may be low. Serum IgG levels are strikingly elevated (in the range of 2–6 g/dL). Low levels of C3 complement have been reported. Three subtypes have been described based on autoantibodies present: type 1: antismooth muscle (antiactin), type 2: anti-LKM (anticytochrome P-450), and type 3: antisoluble liver antigen.

Histologic examination of liver biopsy specimens shows loss of the lobular limiting plate, and interface hepatitis ("piecemeal" necrosis). Portal fibrosis, an inflammatory reaction of lymphocytes and plasma cells in the portal areas and perivascularly, and some bile duct and Kupffer cell proliferation and pseudolobule formation may be present. Cirrhosis may exist at diagnosis in up to 50% of patients.

## Differential Diagnosis

Laboratory and histologic findings differentiate other types of chronic hepatitis (eg, HBV, HCV, and HDV infection; steatohepatitis; Wilson disease; $\alpha_1$-antitrypsin deficiency; primary sclerosing cholangitis). Primary sclerosing cholangitis occasionally presents in a manner similar to AIH, including the presence of autoantibodies. Wilson disease and $\alpha_1$-antitrypsin deficiency must be excluded if HBV and HCV studies are negative. Drug-induced (isoniazid, methyldopa, pemoline) chronic hepatitis should be ruled out. In acute, severe viral hepatitis, histologic examination may also show an "aggressive" lesion early in the disease (< 3 months).

## Complications

Untreated disease that continues for months to years eventually results in postnecrotic cirrhosis, with complications of portal hypertension. Persistent malaise, fatigue, amenorrhea, and anorexia parallel disease activity. Bleeding from esophageal varices and development of ascites usually usher in hepatic failure.

## Treatment

Corticosteroids (prednisone, 2 mg/kg/d) decrease the mortality rate during the early active phase of the disease. Azathioprine, 1–2 mg/kg/d, is of value in decreasing the side effects of long-term corticosteroid therapy but should not be used alone during the induction phase of treatment. Steroids are reduced over a 6- to 12-month period, and azathioprine is continued for 1–2 years if AST and ALT are normal. Liver biopsy is performed before stopping azathioprine therapy; if inflammation persists, then azathioprine is continued. Relapses are treated similarly. Many patients require chronic azathioprine therapy. UCDA, cyclosporine, tacrolimus, or methotrexate may be helpful in poorly responsive cases. Use of mycophenolate mofetil instead of azathioprine is under study. Liver transplantation is indicated when disease progresses to decompensated cirrhosis despite therapy or in unresponsive cases presenting in acute liver failure. Steroid therapy may be life-saving in those presenting in acute liver failure.

## Prognosis

The overall prognosis for AIH is improved significantly with early therapy. Some studies report cures (normal histologic findings) in 15–20% of patients. Relapses (seen clinically and histologically) occur in 40–50% of patients after cessation of therapy; remissions follow repeat treatment. Survival for 10 years is common despite residual cirrhosis. Of children with AIH, 20–50% eventually require liver transplantation. Complications of portal hypertension (bleeding varices, ascites) require specific therapy. Liver transplantation is successful 70–90% of the time. Disease recurrence after transplantation occurs 10–50% of the time and is treated similarly to pretransplant disease.

Alvarez F, Schwarz K: Immune diseases of the liver and biliary tract. J Pediatr Gastroenterol Nutr 2002;35 (Suppl 1):S39 [PMID: 12151820].

Bahar RJ et al: Orthotopic liver transplantation for autoimmune hepatitis and cryptogenic chronic hepatitis in children. Transplantation 2001;72:829 [PMID: 11571445].

Czaja AJ: Treatment of autoimmune hepatitis. Semin Liver Dis 2002;22(4):365 [PMID: 12447708].

Mieli-Vergani G, Vergani D: Autoimmune liver disease in children. Ann Acad Med Singapore 2003;32(2):239 [PMID: 12772529].

## STEATOHEPATITIS

Patients with steatohepatitis present with asymptomatic soft hepatomegaly or mild to moderately elevated aminotransferases (2 to 10 times the upper limit of normal). ALT is frequently higher than AST. Alkaline phosphatase and GGT may be mildly elevated, but bilirubin is normal. Liver biopsy shows macrovesicular steatosis, mild portal inflammation, normal bile ducts, and variable degrees of portal fibrosis to cirrhosis. Ultrasonography or CT scanning indicates fat density in the liver. Most cases are associated with obesity or type II diabetes mellitus. One to three percent of adolescents may have steatohepatitis, based on the observation that 15–25% of American adolescents are overweight or obese and that roughly 10% of these will have steatohepatitis. Steatohepatitis is also associated with Wilson disease, hereditary fructose intolerance, tyrosinemia, HCV hepatitis, cystic fibrosis, fatty acid oxidation defects, kwashiorkor, Reye syndrome, respiratory chain defects, and toxic hepatopathy (ethanol and others). Treatment is weight reduction and exercise for obesity or treatment for the other causes. A pilot trial suggests that vitamin E may be of value. A similar entity, termed nonalcoholic steatohepatitis, occurs in adults. Cirrhosis and liver failure have been described in adults with this disease.

Lavine JE: Vitamin E treatment of nonalcoholic steatohepatitis in children: A pilot study. J Pediatr 2000;136:734 [PMID: 10839868].

Molleston JP et al: Obese children with steatohepatitis can develop cirrhosis in childhood. Am J Gastroenterol 2002;97(9):2460 [PMID: 12358273].

Neuschwander-Tetri BA, Caldwell SH: Nonalcoholic steatohepatitis: Summary of an AASLD Single Topic Conference. Hepatology 2003;37(5):1202 [PMID: 12717402].

Roberts EA: Nonalcoholic steatohepatitis in children. Curr Gastroenterol Rep 2003;5(3):253 [PMID: 12734049].

Strauss RS et al: Prevalence of abnormal serum transaminase values in overweight and obese adolescents. J Pediatr 2000;136:727 [PMID: 10839867].

## $\alpha_1$-ANTITRYPSIN DEFICIENCY LIVER DISEASE

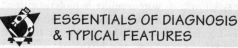

### ESSENTIALS OF DIAGNOSIS & TYPICAL FEATURES

- Serum $\alpha_1$-antitrypsin level less than 50–80 mg/dL.
- Identification of a specific protease inhibitor (Pi) system phenotype (ZZ, SZ).
- Detection of diastase-resistant glycoprotein deposits in periportal hepatocytes.
- Histologic evidence of liver disease.
- Family history of early-onset pulmonary disease or liver disease.

### General Considerations

The disease is caused by a deficiency in $\alpha_1$-antitrypsin, a protease inhibitor (Pi) system, predisposing patients to chronic liver disease and an early onset of pulmonary emphysema. It is most often associated with the Pi phenotype ZZ. The other phenotype associated with possible liver disease is SZ. Heterozygotes may have a slightly higher incidence of liver disease. The exact relationship between low levels of serum $\alpha_1$-antitrypsin and the development of liver disease is unclear. Emphysema develops because of a lack of inhibition of neutrophil elastase, which destroys pulmonary connective tissue. Although all patients with the ZZ genotype eventually have antitrypsin inclusions in hepatocytes, only about 10–20% develop significant liver disease. An associated abnormality in the microsomal disposal of accumulated aggregates may be necessary for the liver disease phenotype.

About 20% of affected individuals present with neonatal cholestasis. About 10% of individuals with $\alpha_1$-antitrypsin deficiency have or have had clinically significant liver injury by age 18 years. Very few children have significant pulmonary involvement. Most children are asymptomatic, with no laboratory or clinical evidence of liver disease.

### Clinical Findings

#### A. SYMPTOMS AND SIGNS

$\alpha_1$-Antitrypsin deficiency should be considered in all infants with neonatal cholestasis. Serum GGT is usually elevated. Jaundice, acholic stools, and malabsorption suggest neonatal hepatitis but are not pathognomonic of any one cause. Infants are often small for gestational age, and hepatosplenomegaly may be present. The family history may be positive for emphysema or cirrhosis.

In older children, hepatomegaly or physical findings suggestive of cirrhosis, especially in the face of a negative history of liver disease, should always lead one to consider $\alpha_1$-antitrypsin deficiency. Recurrent pulmonary disease (bronchitis, pneumonia) may be present in a few children.

### B. LABORATORY FINDINGS

Levels of the $\alpha_1$-globulin fraction may be less than 0.2 mg/dL on serum protein electrophoresis. $\alpha_1$-Antitrypsin levels are low (< 50–80 mg/dL) in homozygotes (ZZ). Specific Pi phenotyping should be done to confirm the diagnosis. LFTs often reflect underlying hepatic pathologic changes. Hyperbilirubinemia (mixed) and elevated aminotransferases, alkaline phosphatase, and GGT are present early. Hyperbilirubinemia generally resolves, while aminotransferase elevation may persist. Signs of cirrhosis and portal hypertension may develop.

Liver biopsy after age 6 months shows diastase-resistant, periodic acid-Schiff staining intracellular granules, with hyaline masses, particularly in periportal zones. These may be absent prior to age 6 months.

### Differential Diagnosis

In newborns, other specific causes of neonatal cholestasis need to be considered. In older children, other causes of insidious cirrhosis (eg, HBV or HCV infection, autoimmune hepatitis, Wilson disease, cystic fibrosis, hemochromatosis, glycogen storage disease) should be considered.

### Complications

Of all infants with Pi ZZ $\alpha_1$-antitrypsin deficiency, only 20% develop liver disease in childhood. The complications of portal hypertension, cirrhosis, and chronic cholestasis predominate in affected children. Occasionally, children develop paucity of interlobular bile ducts.

Early-onset pulmonary emphysema occurs in young adults (age 30–40 years), particularly in smokers. An increased susceptibility to hepatocellular carcinoma has been noted in cirrhosis associated with $\alpha_1$-antitrypsin deficiency.

### Treatment

There is no specific treatment for the liver disease of this disorder. Replacement of the protein by transfusion therapy is successful in preventing pulmonary disease in affected adults. The neonatal cholestatic condition is treated with choleretics, medium-chain triglyceride-containing formula, and water-miscible vitamins (see

Table 21–4). UCDA may reduce AST, ALT, and GGT, but its effect on outcome is unknown. Portal hypertension, esophageal bleeding, ascites, and other complications are treated as described elsewhere. Hepatitis A and B vaccines should be given to children with $\alpha_1$-antitrypsin deficiency. Genetic counseling is indicated whenever the diagnosis is made. Diagnosis by prenatal screening is possible. Liver transplantation cures the deficiency. Cigarette smoke exposure should be eliminated to help prevent pulmonary manifestations.

### Prognosis

Of those patients presenting with neonatal cholestasis, approximately 10–25% will need liver transplantation in the first 5 years of life, 15–25% during childhood or adolescence, and 50–75% will survive into adulthood with variable degrees of liver fibrosis. A correlation between histologic patterns and clinical course has been documented in the infantile form of the disease. Liver failure can be expected 5–15 years after development of cirrhosis. Recurrence or persistence of hyperbilirubinemia along with worsening coagulation studies indicates the need for evaluation for possible liver transplantation. Decompensated cirrhosis caused by this disease is an excellent indication for liver transplantation; the survival rate should reach 80–90%.

Francavilla R et al: Prognosis of alpha-1-antitrypsin deficiency-related liver disease in the era of paediatric liver transplantation. J Hepatol 2000;32:986 [PMID: 10898319].

Primahak RA, Tanner MS: Alpha-1 antitrypsin deficiency. Arch Dis Child 2001;85:2 [PMID: 11420185].

Piitulainen E, Sveger T: Respiratory symptoms and lung function in young adults with severe alpha(1)-antitrypsin deficiency (PiZZ). Thorax 2002;57(8):705 [PMID: 12149531].

Sveger T, Eriksson S: The liver in adolescents with α1-antitrypsin deficiency. Hepatology 1995;22:514 [PMID: 7635419].

Volpert D et al: Alpha 1-antitrypsin deficiency-associated liver disease progresses slowly in some children. J Pediatr Gastroenterol Nutr 2000;31:258 [PMID: 10997369].

## WILSON DISEASE (Hepatolenticular Degeneration)

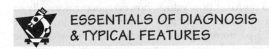

**ESSENTIALS OF DIAGNOSIS & TYPICAL FEATURES**

- *Acute or chronic liver disease.*
- *Deteriorating neurologic status.*
- *Kayser–Fleischer rings.*
- *Elevated liver copper.*

- *Abnormalities in levels of ceruloplasmin and serum and urine copper.*

## General Considerations

Wilson disease is caused by a mutation in the gene on chromosome 13 coding for a specific P-type ATPase involved in copper transport. This results in impaired bile excretion of copper and incorporation of copper into ceruloplasmin by the liver. The accumulated hepatic copper causes oxidant (free-radical) damage to the liver. Subsequently, copper accumulates in the basal ganglia and other tissues. The disease should be considered in all children older than 4 years old with evidence of liver disease (especially with hemolysis) or with suggestive neurologic signs. A family history is often present, and 25% of patients are identified by screening asymptomatic homozygous family members. The disease is autosomal recessive and occurs in 1:30,000 live births in all populations.

## Clinical Findings

### A. SYMPTOMS AND SIGNS

Hepatic involvement may be fulminant, present as an acute hepatitis, may masquerade as chronic liver disease, or may progress insidiously to postnecrotic cirrhosis. Findings include jaundice; hepatomegaly early in childhood; splenomegaly; Kayser–Fleischer rings; and later onset of neurologic manifestations such as tremor, dysarthria, and drooling beginning after age 10 years. Deterioration in school performance is often the earliest neurologic expression of disease. Psychiatric symptoms may also occur. The Kayser–Fleischer rings can sometimes be detected by unaided visual inspection as a brown band at the junction of the iris and cornea, but slitlamp examination is always necessary. Absence of Kayser–Fleischer rings does not exclude this diagnosis.

### B. LABORATORY FINDINGS

The laboratory diagnosis is sometimes difficult. Serum ceruloplasmin levels (measured by the oxidase method) are usually less than 20 mg/dL. (Normal values are 23–43 mg/dL.) Low values, however, occur normally in infants younger than age 3 months, and in at least 5–10% of homozygotes the levels may be within the lower end of the normal range (20–30 mg/dL), particularly if immunoassays are used for ceruloplasmin. Rare patients with higher ceruloplasmin levels have been reported. Serum copper levels are low, but the overlap with normal is too great for satisfactory discrimination. In acute fulminant Wilson disease, serum copper levels

are elevated markedly owing to hepatic necrosis and release of copper. The presence of anemia, hemolysis, very high serum bilirubin levels (> 20–30 mg/dL), and low alkaline phosphatase are characteristic of acute Wilson disease. Urine copper excretion in children older than age 3 years is normally less than 30 µg/d; in Wilson disease, it is greater than 150 µg/d. Finally, the tissue content of copper from a liver biopsy, normally less than 50 µg/g dry tissue, is greater than 250 µg/g in Wilson disease.

Glycosuria, aminoaciduria, and depressed serum uric acid levels have been reported. Hemolysis and gallstones may be present; bone lesions simulating those of osteochondritis dissecans have also been found.

The coarse nodular cirrhosis, steatosis, and glycogenated nuclei seen on liver biopsy may distinguish Wilson disease from other types of cirrhosis. Early in the disease, vacuolation of liver cells, steatosis, and lipofuscin granules can be seen, as well as Mallory bodies. The presence of Mallory bodies in a child is strongly suggestive of Wilson disease. Stains for copper may sometimes be negative despite high copper content in the liver. Therefore, liver copper levels must be determined biochemically on biopsy specimens. Electron microscopy findings may be helpful.

## Differential Diagnosis

During the icteric phase, acute viral hepatitis, $\alpha_1$-antitrypsin deficiency, autoimmune hepatitis, Indian childhood cirrhosis, and drug-induced hepatitis are the usual diagnostic possibilities. Later, other causes of cirrhosis and portal hypertension require consideration. Laboratory testing for serum ceruloplasmin, 24-hour urine copper excretion, liver copper concentration, and a slitlamp examination of the cornea will differentiate Wilson disease from the others. The radiocopper ceruloplasmin incorporation test is sometimes needed to differentiate Wilson disease with a normal ceruloplasmin level from other liver disease with increased liver and urine copper values. Urinary copper excretion during penicillamine challenge may help differentiate Wilson disease from other causes. Genetic testing may be necessary in confusing cases. Other copper storage diseases that occur in early childhood include Indian childhood cirrhosis, Tyrolean childhood cirrhosis, and idiopathic copper toxicosis. However, ceruloplasmin concentrations are normal in these conditions.

## Complications

Progressive liver disease, postnecrotic cirrhosis, hepatic coma, and death are common in the untreated patient. The complications of portal hypertension (variceal hemorrhage, ascites) are poorly tolerated by these patients. Progressive degenerating central nervous system disease and terminal aspiration pneumonia are common in untreated older people. Acute hemolytic disease may result in renal impairment and profound jaundice as part of the presentation of fulminant hepatitis.

## Treatment

Copper chelation with D-penicillamine or trientine hydrochloride, 1000–2000 mg/d orally, is the treatment of choice in all cases, whether or not the patient is symptomatic. It is best to begin with 250 mg/d and increase the dose weekly by 250 mg increments. The target dose is 20 mg/kg/d. Strict dietary restriction of copper intake is not practical. Supplementation with zinc acetate (25–50 mg orally, three times daily) may reduce copper absorption. Copper chelation is continued for life, although doses may be reduced transiently at the time of surgery or early in pregnancy. Vitamin $B_6$ (25 mg) is given daily while on penicillamine to prevent optic neuritis. In some countries, after a clinical response to penicillamine or trientine, zinc therapy is substituted and continued for life. Tetrathiomolybdate is being tested as an alternative therapy. Noncompliance with the drug regimen can lead to fulminant liver failure and death.

General treatment measures for acute hepatitis are as outlined for infectious hepatitis. Liver transplantation is indicated for all cases of acute fulminant disease, progressive hepatic decompensation despite several months of penicillamine, and severe progressive hepatic insufficiency in patients who unadvisedly discontinue penicillamine therapy.

## Prognosis

The prognosis of untreated Wilson disease is poor. Without transplantation, all patients with the fulminant presentation succumb. Copper chelation reduces hepatic copper content, reverses many of the liver lesions, and can stabilize the clinical course of established cirrhosis. Neurologic symptoms generally respond to therapy. All siblings should be immediately screened and homozygotes given treatment with copper chelation or zinc acetate therapy, even if asymptomatic. Genetic testing (haplotype analysis or genotyping) is available at a few centers for family members.

Brewer GJ et al: Treatment of Wilson's disease with zinc: XVI. Treatment during the pediatric years. J Lab Clin Med 2001; 137:191 [PMID: 11241029].

Loudianos G, Gitlin JD: Wilson's disease. Semin Liver Dis 2000; 20:353 [PMID: 11076401].

Roberts EA, Schilsky ML: A practice guideline on Wilson disease. Hepatology 2003;37(6):1475 [PMID: 12774027].

Scheinberg IH, Sternlieb I: *Wilson's Disease.* WB Saunders, 1984.

Sutcliffe RP et al: Liver transplantation for Wilson's disease: Long-term results and quality-of-life assessment. Transplantation 200315;75(7):1003 [PMID: 12698088].

Wilson DC et al: Severe hepatic Wilson's disease in preschool-aged children. J Pediatr 2000;137:719 [PMID: 11060541].

# REYE SYNDROME (Encephalopathy with Fatty Degeneration of the Viscera)

 **ESSENTIALS OF DIAGNOSIS & TYPICAL FEATURES**

- *Prodromal upper respiratory tract infection, influenza A or B illness, or varicella.*
- *Vomiting.*
- *Lethargy, drowsiness progressing to semicoma.*
- *Elevated AST, hyperammonemia, normal or slightly elevated bilirubin, prolonged prothrombin time.*
- *Microvesicular steatosis of the liver, kidneys, brain.*
- *Absence of other metabolic diseases.*

## General Considerations

The number of reported cases of Reye syndrome is decreasing, perhaps because of a decline in the use of salicylates among younger children, who seem to be at greater risk. Varicella, influenza A and B, echovirus 2, coxsackievirus A, and Epstein–Barr virus infection are associated. Salicylate use is associated with Reye syndrome. Many apparent cases are actually caused by defects in fatty acid oxidation and other newly discovered metabolic diseases.

The pathogenesis is thought to be damage to mitochondria caused by salicylate metabolites or some other toxin or chemical in the milieu of a viral infection or underlying polymorphism in mitochondrial function. Mitochondrial dysfunction leads to elevated short-chain fatty acids and hyperammonemia as well as directly to cerebral edema.

## Clinical Findings

### A. SYMPTOMS AND SIGNS

Varicella, influenza, or minor upper respiratory tract illness precedes the development of vomiting, irrational behavior, progressive stupor, and coma. Restlessness and convulsions may also occur. Striking physical findings are hyperpnea, irregular respirations, and dilated, sluggishly reacting pupils. Jaundice is minimal or absent. The liver may be normal or enlarged. Splenomegaly is absent. A positive Babinski sign, hyperreflexia, and decorticate and decerebrate posturing are consistent with increased intracranial pressure.

### B. LABORATORY FINDINGS

CSF is acellular, and CSF glucose may be low in younger patients who have hypoglycemia. CSF pressure is increased. Moderate to severe elevations of AST, ALT, and lactate dehydrogenase and normal serum bilirubin and alkaline phosphatase values are characteristic. The prothrombin time is usually prolonged, and the blood ammonia is elevated to varying degrees. A mixed respiratory alkalosis and metabolic acidosis is typical. Hyperaminoacidemia (glutamine, alanine, lysine) and hypocitrullinemia are present.

Histology of the liver shows diffuse microvesicular steatosis with minimal inflammatory changes. Glycogen is virtually absent from the hepatocytes in biopsy specimens taken before administration of hypertonic glucose. Mitochondria are large, pleomorphic, and have decreased matriceal density on electron microscopy.

The kidney changes include swelling and fatty degeneration of the proximal lobules.

### C. ELECTROENCEPHALOGRAPHY

The electroencephalogram shows diffuse slow wave activity.

## Differential Diagnosis

Differentiation of Reye syndrome from encephalitis, acute toxic encephalopathy, hepatic coma, or fulminant hepatitis can be made on clinical and laboratory grounds. A negative history and urine screen for ingestion of poisons and drugs, absence of cells in the CSF, and absence of jaundice favor a diagnosis of Reye syndrome. The fatty acid oxidation defects (eg, medium-chain acyl-CoA dehydrogenase deficiency) and other metabolic disorders may resemble Reye syndrome; gas chromatographic analysis of urine and serum acyl-carnitine levels will help differentiate them. Liver biopsy and electron microscopy can be diagnostic and are indicated in atypical cases.

## Treatment

Treatment in an intensive care unit is mainly supportive. If cerebral edema can be minimized, the liver makes a full recovery. Mechanical ventilation may become necessary if the patient reaches grade 3 coma (agitated delirium, combativeness). Intracranial pressure should be monitored directly and kept below 15–20 mm Hg, and systemic blood pressure should be kept high enough to maintain cerebral perfusion pressure above 45–50 mm Hg. Hyperventilation, mannitol infusions (0.5–1 g/kg every 4 hours), barbiturates, or ventricular drainage is used to lower intracranial pressure. Maintenance fluids using 10% glucose should be given at a rate sufficient to produce a urine flow of 1–1.5 mL/kg/h. Vitamin K, 3–5 mg intramuscularly, should be administered. Hypothermia and pentobarbital coma have been used to decrease body (brain) metabolic needs during the period of uncontrolled intracranial pressure.

## Prognosis

At least 70% of patients with Reye syndrome survive. The prognosis is related to the depth of coma and the peak ammonia level on admission. Because Reye syndrome is less common now, many patients are diagnosed only when in deep coma. All patients should be screened for fatty acid oxidation and other metabolic defects. Survivors should not be given aspirin.

Auret-Leca E et al: Incidence of Reye syndrome in France: A hospital-based survey. J Clin Epidemiol 2001;54:857 [PMID: 11470397].

Casteels-Van Daele M et al: Reye syndrome revisited: A descriptive term covering a group of heterogeneous disorders. Eur J Pediatr 2000;159:641 [PMID: 11014461].

da Silveira EB et al: Reye's syndrome in a 17-year-old male: Is this disease really disappearing? Dig Dis Sci 2002;47(9):1959 [PMID: 12353836].

Orlowski JP et al: Is aspirin a cause of Reye's syndrome? A case against. Drug Saf 2002;25(4):225 [PMID: 11994026].

## CIRRHOSIS

Cirrhosis is a histologically defined condition of the liver characterized by diffuse hepatocyte injury and regeneration, an increase in connective tissue (bridging fibrosis), and disorganization of the lobular and vascular architecture (regenerative nodules). It may be micronodular or macronodular in appearance. It is the vasculature distortion that leads to increased resistance to blood flow, producing portal hypertension and its consequences.

Many liver diseases may progress to cirrhosis. In children, the two most common forms of cirrhosis are postnecrotic and biliary—with different causes, symptomatology, and treatment requirements. Both forms can eventually lead to liver failure and death.

In the pediatric population, postnecrotic cirrhosis is often a result of acute or chronic liver disease (eg, idiopathic neonatal giant-cell hepatitis; viral hepatitis [HBV, HCV, or NANBNC hepatitis]; autoimmune or drug-induced hepatitis); or certain inborn errors of metabolism (see Table 21–5). Cirrhosis is an exceptional outcome of HAV infection and only follows massive hepatic necrosis. The evolution to cirrhosis may be insidious, with no recognized icteric phase, as in some cases of HBV or HCV infection, Wilson disease, hemochromatosis, or $\alpha_1$-antitrypsin deficiency. At the time of diagnosis of cirrhosis, the underlying liver disease may be active, with abnormal LFT results; or it may be quiescent, with normal LFTs. Most cases of biliary cirrhosis result from congenital abnormalities of the bile ducts (biliary atresia, choledochal cyst, common duct stenosis), tumors of the bile duct, Caroli disease, Byler disease, primary sclerosing cholangitis, paucity of the intrahepatic bile ducts, and cystic fibrosis.

Occasionally, cirrhosis may follow a hypersensitivity reaction to certain drugs such as phenytoin. Parasites (*Opisthorchis sinensis, Fasciola, Ascaris*) may be causative in children living in endemic areas.

## Clinical Findings

### A. SYMPTOMS AND SIGNS

General malaise, loss of appetite, failure to thrive, and nausea are frequent complaints, especially in anicteric varieties. Easy bruising may be reported. Jaundice may or may not be present. The first indication of underlying liver disease may be ascites, gastrointestinal hemorrhage, or hepatic encephalopathy. Variable hepatosplenomegaly, spider angiomas, warm skin, palmar erythema, or digital clubbing may be present. A small, shrunken liver may be detected by percussion over the right chest wall that reveals resonance rather than expected dullness. Most often, the liver is enlarged slightly, especially in the subxiphoid region, where it has a firm to hard quality and an irregular edge. Ascites may be detected as shifting dullness or a fluid wave. Gynecomastia may be noted in males. Digital clubbing occurs in 10–15% of cases. Pretibial edema often occurs, reflecting underlying hypoproteinemia. In adolescent girls, irregularities of menstruation and amenorrhea may be early complaints.

In biliary cirrhosis, patients often have jaundice, dark urine, pruritus, hepatomegaly, and sometimes xanthoma in addition to the previously mentioned clinical findings. Undernutrition and failure to thrive because of steatorrhea may be more apparent in this form of cirrhosis.

### B. LABORATORY FINDINGS

Mild abnormalities of aminotransferases (AST, ALT) are often present, with a decreased level of albumin and a variable increase in the level of γ-globulins. Prothrombin time is prolonged and may be unresponsive to vita-min K administration. Burr and target red cells may be noted on the peripheral blood smear. Anemia, thrombocytopenia, and leukopenia are present if hypersplenism exists. However, cirrhosis may be present despite normal blood tests.

In biliary cirrhosis, elevated conjugated bilirubin, bile acids, GGT, alkaline phosphatase, and cholesterol are common.

### C. IMAGING

Hepatic ultrasound or CT examination may demonstrate abnormal hepatic texture and nodules. In biliary cirrhosis, abnormalities of the biliary tree may be apparent by ultrasonography, CT, hepatobiliary scintigraphy, or cholangiography.

### D. PATHOLOGIC FINDINGS

Liver biopsy findings of regenerating nodules and surrounding fibrosis are hallmarks of cirrhosis. Pathologic features of biliary cirrhosis also include canalicular and hepatocyte cholestasis, as well as plugging of bile ducts. The interlobular bile ducts may be increased or decreased, depending on the cause and the stage of the disease process.

## Complications & Treatment

Major complications of cirrhosis in childhood include progressive nutritional disturbances and hormonal disturbances and the evolution of portal hypertension and its complications. Hepatocellular carcinoma occurs with increased frequency in the cirrhotic liver, especially in patients with the chronic form of hereditary tyrosinemia or after long-standing HBV or HCV disease. At present, there is no proven medical treatment for cirrhosis, but whenever a treatable condition is identified (eg, Wilson disease, galactosemia, congenital fructose intolerance) or an offending agent eliminated (HBV, HCV, drugs, toxins), disease progression can be altered; occasionally regression of fibrosis has been noted. Immunosuppressive treatment in autoimmune hepatitis can halt the progression of cirrhosis. Surgical correction of biliary tree abnormalities can stabilize the disease process or lead to a reversal in some situations. Children with cirrhosis should receive the hepatitis A and B vaccines. Liver transplantation may be appropriate in patients with cirrhosis whose disease is continuing to progress or in whom the complications of cirrhosis are no longer manageable.

## Prognosis

Postnecrotic cirrhosis has an unpredictable course. Without transplantation, affected patients may die from liver failure within 10–15 years. Patients with a rising bilirubin or a vitamin K-resistant coagulopathy along with diuretic refractory ascites usually survive less than 1–2 years. The terminal event in some patients may be generalized hemorrhage, sepsis, or cardiorespiratory arrest. For patients with biliary cirrhosis, the prognosis is similar, except for those with surgically corrected lesions that result in regression or stabilization of the underlying liver condition. With liver transplantation, the long-term survival rate is 70–80%.

Friedman SL: Hepatic fibrosis. In Schiff ER, Sorrell MF, Maddrey WC (eds): *Schiff's Diseases of the Liver*. Lippincott-Raven, 1999.

Hardy SC, Kleinman RE: Cirrhosis and chronic liver failure. In Suchy FJ, Sokol RJ, Balistreri WF (eds): *Liver Disease in Children*. Lippincott Williams & Wilkins, 2001.

Reddy SI, Grace ND: Liver imaging: A hepatologist's perspective. Clin Liver Dis 2002;6:297 [PMID: 11933595].

# PORTAL HYPERTENSION

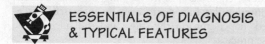

### ESSENTIALS OF DIAGNOSIS & TYPICAL FEATURES

- *Splenomegaly.*
- *Recurrent ascites.*
- *Variceal hemorrhage.*
- *Hypersplenism.*

## General Considerations

Portal hypertension is defined as an increase in the portal venous pressure to more than 5 mm Hg greater than the inferior vena caval pressure. Portal hypertension is most commonly a result of cirrhosis. However, portal hypertension without cirrhosis may be divided into prehepatic, suprahepatic, and intrahepatic causes. Although the specific lesions vary somewhat in their clinical signs and symptoms, the consequences of portal hypertension are common to all.

### A. PREHEPATIC PORTAL HYPERTENSION

Prehepatic portal hypertension from acquired abnormalities of the portal and splenic veins accounts for 5–8% of cases of gastrointestinal bleeding in children. A history of neonatal omphalitis, sepsis, dehydration, or umbilical vein catheterization is present in 30–50% of patients. Less common causes in older children include local trauma, peritonitis (pyelophlebitis), hypercoagulable states, and pancreatitis. Symptoms may occur before age 1 year, but in most cases the diagnosis is not

made until age 3–5 years. Patients with a positive neonatal history tend to be symptomatic earlier.

A variety of portal or splenic vein malformations, some of which may be congenital, have been described, including defects in valves and atretic segments. Cavernous transformation is probably the result of attempted collateralization around the thrombosed portal vein rather than a congenital malformation. The site of the venous obstruction may be anywhere from the hilum of the liver to the hilum of the spleen.

### B. SUPRAHEPATIC VEIN OCCLUSION OR THROMBOSIS (BUDD–CHIARI SYNDROME)

In most instances, no cause can be demonstrated. Suggested causes include endothelial injury to hepatic veins by bacterial endotoxins, which has been demonstrated experimentally. The occasional association of hepatic vein thrombosis in inflammatory bowel disease favors the presence of endogenous toxins traversing the liver. Allergic vasculitis leading to endophlebitis of the hepatic veins has been described occasionally. In addition, hepatic vein obstruction may be secondary to tumor, abdominal trauma, hyperthermia, or sepsis, or it may occur following the repair of an omphalocele or gastroschisis. Congenital vena caval bands, webs, a membrane, or strictures above the hepatic veins are sometimes causative. Hepatic vein thrombosis may be a complication of oral contraceptive medications. Underlying thrombotic conditions (deficiency of antithrombin III, protein C or protein S, factor V Leiden; antiphospholipid antibodies; or mutations of the prothrombin gene) should be evaluated.

### C. INTRAHEPATIC PORTAL HYPERTENSION

**1. Cirrhosis (see previous section).**

**2. Veno-occlusive disease (acute stage)**—This now occurs most frequently in bone marrow transplant patients. It may also develop after chemotherapy for acute leukemia, particularly with thioguanine. Additional causes include the ingestion of pyrrolizidine alkaloids ("bush tea") or other herbal teas and a familial form of the disease occurring in congenital immunodeficiency states.

The acute form of the disease generally occurs in the first month after bone marrow transplantation and is heralded by the triad of weight gain (ascites), tender hepatomegaly, and jaundice.

**3. Congenital hepatic fibrosis**—This is a rare autosomal recessive cause of intrahepatic presinusoidal portal hypertension (Table 21–7). Liver biopsy is generally diagnostic, demonstrating Meyenburg complexes. On angiography, the intrahepatic branches of the portal vein may be duplicated. Renal abnormalities (microcystic disease) are often associated with the hepatic lesion;

Table 21-7. Biliary tract diseases of childhood.

| | Acute Hydrops Transient Dilatation of Gallbladder[a,b] | Choledochal Cyst[c] (See Figure 20-1.) | Acalculous Cholecystitis[d] | Caroli Disease[e] (Idiopathic Intrahepatic Bile Duct Dilation) | Congenital Hepatic Fibrosis[f] |
|---|---|---|---|---|---|
| Predisposing or associated conditions | Premature infants with prolonged fasting or systemic illness. Hepatitis. Abnormalities of cystic duct. Kawasaki disease. Bacterial sepsis, EBV. | Congenital lesion. Female sex. Asians. Rarely with Caroli disease or congenital hepatic fibrosis. | Systemic illness, sepsis (Streptococcus, Salmonella, Klebsiella, etc), HIV infection. Gallbladder stasis, obstruction of cystic duct (stones, nodes, tumor). | Congenital lesion. Also found in congenital hepatic fibrosis or with choledochal cyst. Female sex. Autosomal-recessive polycystic kidney disease. | Familial (autosomal-recessive) 25% with autosomal-recessive polycystic kidney disease. Choledochal cyst. Caroli's disease. Meckel–Gruber, Ivemark's, or Jeune's syndrome. |
| Symptoms | Absent in premature infants. Vomiting, abdominal pain in older children. | Abdominal pain, vomiting, jaundice. | Acute severe abdominal pain, vomiting, fever. | Recurrent abdominal pain, vomiting. Fever, jaundice when cholangitis occurs. | Hematemesis, melena from bleeding esophageal varices. |
| Signs | Right upper quadrant abdominal mass. Tenderness in some. | Icterus, acholic stools, dark urine in neonatal period. Right upper quadrant abdominal mass or tenderness in older children. | Tenderness in mid and right upper abdomen. Occasional palpable mass in right upper quadrant. | Icterus, hepatomegaly. | Hepatosplenomegaly. |
| Laboratory abnormalities | Most are normal. Increased WBC count in sepsis (may be decreased in premature infants). Abnormal LFTs in hepatitis. | Conjugated hyperbilirubinemia, elevated GGT, slightly increased AST. Elevated pancreatic serum amylase if ampulla hepatopancreatica is involved. | Elevated WBC count, normal or slight abnormality of LFTs. | Abnormal LFTs. Increased WBC count with cholangitis. Urine abnormalities if associated with congenital hepatic fibrosis. | Low platelet and WBC count (hypersplenism), slight elevation of AST, GGT. Inability to concentrate urine. |
| Diagnostic studies most useful | Gallbladder ultrasonography. | Gallbladder ultrasonography hepatobiliary scintigraphy, ERCP, or MRCP. | Scintigraphy to confirm nonfunction of gallbladder. Ultrasonography or abdominal CT scan to rule out other neighboring disease. | Transhepatic cholangiography, ERCP, MRCP, scintigraphy, ultrasonography, intravenous pyelography. | Liver biopsy. Ultrasonography of the liver and kidneys. Upper endoscopy. |
| Treatment | Treatment of associated condition. Needle or tube cystostomy rarely required. Cholecystectomy seldom indicated. | Surgical resection and choledochojejunostomy | Broad-spectrum antibiotic coverage, then cholecystectomy or cholecystostomy drainage and definitive surgery 3–4 weeks later. | Antibiotics and surgical or endoscopic drainage for cholangitis. Liver transplantation for some. Lobectomy for localized disease. | Treatment of portal hypertension. Liver/kidney transplantation for some. |

(continued)

Table 21–7. Biliary tract diseases of childhood. (continued)

| | Acute Hydrops Transient Dilatation of Gallbladder[a,b] | Choledochal Cyst[c] (See Figure 20–1.) | Acalculous Cholecystitis[d] | Caroli Disease[e] (Idiopathic Intrahepatic Bile Duct Dilation) | Congenital Hepatic Fibrosis[f] |
|---|---|---|---|---|---|
| Complications | Perforation with bile peritonitis rare. | Progressive biliary cirrhosis. Increased incidence of cholangiocarcinoma. Cholangitis in some. | Perforation and bile peritonitis, sepsis, abscess or fistula formation. Pancreatitis. | Sepsis with episodes of cholangitis, biliary cirrhosis, portal hypertension. Intraductal stones. Cholangiocarcinoma. | Bleeding from varices. Splenic rupture, severe thrombocytopenia. Progressive renal failure. |
| Prognosis | Excellent with resolution of underlying condition. Consider cystic duct obstruction if disorder fails to resolve. | Depends on anatomic type of cyst, associated condition, and success of surgery. Liver transplantation required in some. | Good with early diagnosis and treatment. | Poor, with gradual deterioration of liver function. Multiple surgical drainage procedures expected. Liver transplantation should alter long-term prognosis. | Good in absence of serious renal involvement and with control of portal hypertension. Slightly increased risk of cholangiocarcinoma. |

Ultrasonography = liver and biliary tract scanning; scintigraphy = hepatobiliary scan using radiolabeled $^{99m}$technetium; AST = aspartate aminotransferase (SGOT); CT = computed tomography; ERCP = endoscopic retrograde cholangiopancreatography; GGT = γ-glutamyl transpeptidase; LFT = liver function tests; MRCP = magnetic resonance cholangiopancreatography; WBC = white blood count.

[a]Crankson S et al: Acute hydrops of the gallbladder in childhood. Eur J Pediatr 1992;151:318 [PMID 9788647].

[b]Zulian F et al: Acute surgical abdomen as presenting manifestation of Kawasaki disease. J Pediatr 2003;142:731 [PMID 12838207].

[c]deVries JS et al: Choledochal cysts: Age of presentation, symptoms and late complications related to Todani's classification. J Pediatr Surg 2002;37:36 [PMID 11781983].

[d]Imamoglu M et al: Acute acalculous cholecystitis in children: Diagnosis and treatment. J Pediatr Surg 2002;37:1568 [PMID 12407541].

[e]Levy AD et al: Careli's disease: Radiologic spectrum and pathologic correlation. Am J Roentgenol 2002;179:1053 [PMID 12239064].

[f]Perisic VN: Long term studies on congenital hepatic fibrosis in children. Acta Paediatr 1995;85:695 [PMID 7670259].

690

therefore, renal ultrasonography and urography should be routinely performed.

**4. Other rare causes**—Hepatoportal sclerosis (idiopathic portal hypertension, noncirrhotic portal fibrosis), noncirrhotic nodular transformation of the liver, and schistosomal hepatic fibrosis are also rare causes of intrahepatic presinusoidal portal hypertension.

## Clinical Findings

### A. Symptoms and Signs

For prehepatic portal hypertension, splenomegaly in an otherwise well child is the most constant physical sign. Recurrent episodes of abdominal distention resulting from ascites may also be noted. The usual presenting symptoms are hematemesis and melena.

The presence of prehepatic portal hypertension is suggested by the following: (1) an episode of severe infection in the newborn period or early infancy—especially omphalitis, sepsis, gastroenteritis, severe dehydration, or prolonged or difficult umbilical vein catheterizations; (2) no previous evidence of liver disease; (3) a history of well-being prior to onset or recognition of symptoms; and (4) normal liver size and tests with splenomegaly.

Most patients with suprahepatic portal hypertension present with abdominal pain, tender hepatomegaly of acute onset, and abdominal enlargement caused by ascites. Jaundice is present in only 25% of patients. Vomiting, hematemesis, and diarrhea are less common. Cutaneous signs of chronic liver disease are often absent, as the obstruction is usually acute. Distended superficial veins on the back and the anterior abdomen, along with dependent edema, are seen when inferior vena cava obstruction affects hepatic vein outflow. Absence of hepatojugular reflux (jugular distention when pressure is applied to the liver) is a helpful clinical sign.

The symptoms and signs of intrahepatic portal hypertension are generally those of cirrhosis (see section on Cirrhosis).

### B. Laboratory Findings and Imaging

Most other common causes of splenomegaly or hepatosplenomegaly may be excluded by proper laboratory tests. Cultures, Epstein–Barr virus titers, hepatitis serologies, blood smear examination, bone marrow studies, and LFTs may be necessary. In prehepatic portal hypertension, LFTs are generally normal. In Budd–Chiari syndrome and veno-occlusive disease, mild to moderate hyperbilirubinemia with modest elevations of aminotransferases and prothrombin time are often present. Hypersplenism with mild leukopenia and thrombocytopenia is often present. Upper endoscopy may reveal varices in symptomatic patients. When pos-

sible, confirmation of a normal liver is best obtained by liver biopsy.

Doppler-assisted ultrasound scanning of the liver, portal vein, splenic vein, inferior vena cava, and hepatic veins may assist in defining the vascular anatomy. In prehepatic portal hypertension, abnormalities of the portal or splenic vein may be apparent, whereas the hepatic veins are normal. When noncirrhotic portal hypertension is suspected, angiography often is diagnostic. Selective arteriography of the superior mesenteric artery is recommended prior to surgical shunting to determine the patency of the superior mesenteric vein.

For suprahepatic portal hypertension, an inferior venacavogram using catheters from above or below the suspected obstruction may reveal an intrinsic filling defect, an infiltrating tumor, or extrinsic compression of the inferior vena cava by an adjacent lesion. A large caudate lobe of the liver suggests Budd–Chiari syndrome. Care must be taken in interpreting extrinsic pressure defects of the subdiaphragmatic inferior vena cava if ascites is significant.

Simultaneous wedged hepatic vein pressure and hepatic venography are useful to demonstrate obstruction to major hepatic vein ostia and smaller vessels. In the absence of obstruction, reflux across the sinusoids into the portal vein branches can be accomplished. Pressures should also be taken from the right heart and supradiaphragmatic portion of the inferior vena cava to eliminate constrictive pericarditis and pulmonary hypertension from the differential diagnosis.

## Differential Diagnosis

All causes of splenomegaly must be included in the differential diagnosis. The most common ones are infections, immune thrombocytopenic purpura, blood dyscrasias, lipidosis, reticuloendotheliosis, cirrhosis of the liver, and cysts or hemangiomas of the spleen. When hematemesis or melena occurs, other causes of gastrointestinal bleeding are possible, such as gastric or duodenal ulcers, tumors, duplications, and inflammatory bowel disease.

Because ascites is almost always present in suprahepatic portal hypertension, cirrhosis resulting from any cause must be excluded. Other suprahepatic (cardiac, pulmonary) causes of portal hypertension must also be ruled out. Although ascites may occur in prehepatic portal hypertension, it is uncommon.

## Complications

The major manifestation and complication of portal hypertension is bleeding esophageal varices. Fatal exsanguination is uncommon, but hypovolemic shock or resulting anemia may require prompt treatment. Hypersplenism with leukopenia and thrombocytopenia occurs but seldom causes major symptoms. Rupture of the enlarged spleen secondary to trauma is always a threat. Retroperitoneal edema has been reported (Clatworthy sign).

Without treatment, complete and persistent hepatic vein obstruction leads to liver failure, coma, and death. A nonportal type of cirrhosis may develop in the chronic form of hepatic veno-occlusive disease in which small- and medium-sized hepatic veins are affected. Death from renal failure may occur in rare cases of congenital hepatic fibrosis.

## Treatment

Definitive treatment of noncirrhotic portal hypertension is generally lacking. In prehepatic portal hypertension, the experience with surgical portosystemic shunts is complicated by a lack of sustained patency in most children younger than age 10 years. Aggressive medical treatment of the complications of prehepatic portal hypertension is the preferred option. Some centers have reported good results with shunting procedures, and the mesorex shunt is preferred when possible. Veno-occlusive disease may be prevented somewhat by the prophylactic use of UCDA prior to conditioning for bone marrow transplantation. Withdrawal of the suspected offending agent, if possible, may increase the chance of recovery. For suprahepatic portal hypertension, efforts should be directed at determining the underlying cause and correction, if possible. Either surgical or angio-graphic relief of obstruction should be attempted if a defined obstruction of the vessels is apparent. Liver transplantation should be considered early in the course if direct correction is not possible. In most cases, management of portal hypertension is directed at management of the complications (Table 21–8).

## Prognosis

For prehepatic portal hypertension, the prognosis depends on the site of the block, the effectiveness of variceal eradication, the availability of suitable vessels for shunting procedures, and the experience of the surgeon. Each unsuccessful surgical procedure worsens the prognosis. In patients treated by medical means, bleeding episodes seem to diminish with adolescence.

The prognosis in patients treated by medical and supportive therapy may be better than in the surgically treated group, especially when surgery is performed at an early age. Portacaval encephalopathy is unusual after shunting except when protein intake is excessive, but neurologic outcome may be better in patients who receive a mesenterico-left portal bypass when compared with medical management alone.

The mortality rate of hepatic vein obstruction is very high (95%). In veno-occlusive disease, the prognosis is better, with complete recovery possible in 50% of acute forms and 5–10% of subacute forms.

Brown RS Jr, Lake JR: Transjugular intrahepatic portosystemic shunt as a form of treatment for portal hypertension: Indica-

**Table 21–8.** Treatment of complications of portal hypertension.

| Complication | Diagnosis | Treatment |
|---|---|---|
| Bleeding esophageal varices | Endoscopic verification of variceal bleeding | Endosclerosis or variceal band ligation. Octreotide, 30 µg/m²/h intravenous. Pediatric Sengstaken–Blakemore tube. Surgical variceal ligation, selective venous embolization, TIPS, OLT. Propranolol may be useful to prevent recurrent bleeding. |
| Ascites | Clinical examination (fluid wave, shifting dullness), abdominal ultrasonography | Sodium restriction (1–2 mEq/kg/d), spironolactone (3–5 mg/kg/d), furosemide (1–2 mg/kg/d), intravenous albumin (0.5–1 g/kg per dose), paracentesis, peritoneovenous (LeVeen) shunt, TIPS, surgical portosystemic shunt, OLT.[a] |
| Hepatic encephalopathy | Abnormal neurologic examination, elevated plasma ammonia | Protein restriction (0.5–1 g/kg/d), intravenous glucose (6–8 mg/kg/min), neomycin (2–4 g/m² BSA PO in 4 doses), lactulose (1 mL/kg per dose [up to 30 mL] every 4–6 h PO), plasmapheresis, hemodialysis, OLT.[a] |
| Hypersplenism | Low WBC count, platelets, and/or hemoglobin. Splenomegaly. | No intervention, partial splenic embolization, TIPS, surgical portosystemic shunt, OLT. Splenectomy may worsen variceal bleeding. |

[a]In order of sequential management.
TIPS = transjugular intrahepatic portosystemic shunt, OLT = orthotopic liver transplantation, BSA = body surface area, WBC = white blood cell.

tions and contraindications. Adv Intern Med 1997;42: 485 [PMID: 9048128].

Carreras E et al: Hepatic veno-occlusive disease after bone marrow transplant. Blood Rev 1993;7:43[PMID: 8467232].

Dhiman RK et al: Non-cirrhotic portal fibrosis (idiopathic portal hypertension): Experience with 151 patients and a review of the literature. J Gastroenterol Hepatol 2002;17:6 [PMID 11895549].

Dilawari JB et al: Hepatic outflow obstruction (Budd–Chiari syndrome): Experience with 177 patients and a review of the literature. Medicine 1994;73:21[PMID: 8309360].

Fuchs J et al: Mesenterico-left portal vein bypass in children with congenital extrahepatic portal vein thrombosis: A unique curative approach. J Pediatr Gastroenterol Nutr 2003;36:213 [PMID 12548056].

Hassall E: Nonsurgical treatments for portal hypertension in children. Gastrointest Endosc Clin North Am 1994;4:223 [PMID: 8137016].

McKiernan PJ: Treatment of variceal bleeding. Gastrointest Endosc Clin North Am 2001;11:789 [PMID 11689366].

Price MR et al: Management of esophageal varices in children by endoscopic variceal ligation. J Pediatr Surg 1996;31: 1056[PMID: 8863233].

Ryckman FC, Alonso MH: Causes and management of portal hypertension in the pediatric population. Clin Liver Dis 2001;5:789 [PMID 11565141].

Shun A et al: Portosystemic shunting for paediatric portal hypertension. J Pediatr Surg 1997;32:489[PMID: 9094025].

Vogelsang GB, Dalal J: Hepatic venoocclusive disease in blood and bone marrow transplantation in children: Incidence, risk factors and outcome. J Pediatr Hematol Oncol 2002;24:746 [PMID 12468908].

# BILIARY TRACT DISEASE

## 1. Cholelithiasis

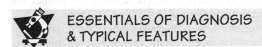

### ESSENTIALS OF DIAGNOSIS & TYPICAL FEATURES

- *Episodic right upper quadrant abdominal pain.*
- *Elevated bilirubin, alkaline phosphatase, and GGT*
- *Stones or sludge seen on abdominal ultrasound.*

## General Considerations

Gallstones may develop at all ages in the pediatric population and in utero. Gallstones may be divided into cholesterol stones, which contain more than 50% cholesterol, and pigment stones, black (sterile bile) and brown (infected bile). Pigment stones predominate in the first decade of life, while cholesterol stones account for up to 90% of gallstones in adolescence. For some patients, gallbladder dysfunction is associated with biliary sludge formation, which may evolve into "sludge balls" or tumefaction bile and then into gallstones. The process is reversible in many patients.

## Clinical Findings

### A. History

Most symptomatic gallstones are associated with acute or recurrent episodes of moderate to severe, sharp right upper quadrant or epigastric pain. The pain may radiate substernally or to the right shoulder. On rare occasions, the presentation may include a history of jaundice, back pain, or generalized abdominal discomfort, when it is associated with pancreatitis, suggesting stone impaction in the common duct or ampulla hepatopancreatica. Nausea and vomiting may occur during attacks. Pain episodes often occur postprandially, especially after ingestion of fatty foods. The groups at risk for gallstones include patients with known or suspected hemolytic disease; females; teenagers with prior pregnancy; obese individuals; certain racial or ethnic groups, particularly Native Americans (Pima Indians) and Hispanics; infants and children with ileal disease (Crohn disease) or prior ileal resection; and patients with cystic fibrosis or Wilson disease. Infants on prolonged parenteral hyperalimentation are at particular risk for gallstone formation. Other, less certain risk factors include a positive family history, use of birth control pills, and diabetes mellitus.

### B. Symptoms and Signs

During acute episodes of pain, tenderness is present in the right upper quadrant or epigastrium, with a positive inspiratory arrest (Murphy sign), usually without peritoneal signs. If present, scleral icterus is helpful. Evidence of underlying hemolytic disease in addition to icterus may include pallor (anemia), splenomegaly, tachycardia, and high-output cardiac murmur. Fever is unusual in uncomplicated cases.

### C. Laboratory Findings

Laboratory tests are usually normal unless calculi have lodged in the extrahepatic biliary system, in which case the serum bilirubin and GGT (or alkaline phosphatase) may be elevated. Amylase and lipase levels may be increased if stone obstruction occurs at the ampulla hepatopancreatica.

### D. Imaging

Ultrasound evaluation is the best imaging technique, showing abnormal intraluminal contents (stones, sludge) as well as anatomic alterations of the gallbladder or dilation of the biliary ductal system. The presence of an anechoic acoustic shadow differentiates calculi from intraluminal sludge or sludge balls. Ceftriaxone may cause similar findings. Plain abdominal radiographs will show calculi with a high calcium content in the region of the gallbladder in up to 15% of patients. Lack of visualization of the gallbladder with hepatobiliary scintigraphy suggests chronic cholecystitis. In selected cases, ERCP or MRCP may be helpful in defining subtle abnormalities of the bile ducts and locating intraductal stones.

## Differential Diagnosis

Other abnormal conditions of the biliary system with similar presentation are summarized in Table 21–7. Liver disease (hepatitis, abscess, tumor) can cause similar symptoms or signs. Peptic disease, reflux esophagitis, paraesophageal hiatal hernia, cardiac disease, and pneumomediastinum must be considered when the pain is epigastric or substernal in location. Renal or pancreatic disease is a possible explanation if the pain is localized to the right flank or mid back. Subcapsular or supracapsular lesions of the liver (abscess, tumor, hematoma) or right lower lobe infiltrate may also be a cause of nontraumatic right shoulder pain.

## Complications

Major problems are related to stone impaction in either the cystic or common duct and lead to stricture formation or perforation. Acute distention and subsequent perforation of the gallbladder may occur when gallstones cause obstruction of the cystic duct. Stones impacted at the level of the ampulla hepatopancreatica often cause gallstone pancreatitis.

## Treatment

Symptomatic cholelithiasis is best treated by either open or laparoscopic cholecystectomy. Intraoperative cholangiography via the cystic duct is required so that the physician can be certain the ductal system is free of retained stones. Calculi in the extrahepatic bile ducts may be removed by ERCP, sphincterotomy, and balloon extraction.

Gallstones developing in premature infants on total parenteral nutrition can be followed by ultrasound examination. Most of the infants are asymptomatic, and the stones will resolve in 3–36 months. Gallstone dissolution using cholelitholytics (UCDA) or mechanical means (lithotripsy) has not been approved for use in children. Asymptomatic gallstones do not usually require treatment, as less than 20% will eventually cause problems.

## Prognosis

The prognosis is excellent in uncomplicated cases that come to standard cholecystectomy.

Burch Bruch SW et al: The management of nonpigmented gallstones in children. J Pediatr Surg 2000;35:729 [PMID: 10813336].

Holcomb GW III et al; Laparoscopic cholecystectomy in children: Lessons learned from the first 100 patients. J Pediatr Surg 1999;34:1236 [PMID: 10466603].

Lobe, TE: Cholelithiasis and cholecystitis in children. Semin Pediatr Surg 2000;9:170 [PMID: 11112834].

Miltenburg DM et al: Changing indications for pediatric cholecystectomy. Pediatrics 2000;105:1250 [PMID: 10835065].

Zitsman JL: Current concepts in minimal access surgery for children. Pediatrics 2003;111:1239 [PMID: 12777537].

# 2. Primary Sclerosing Cholangitis

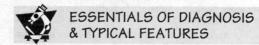

### ESSENTIALS OF DIAGNOSIS & TYPICAL FEATURES

- *Pruritus and jaundice.*
- *Elevated GGT.*
- *Associated with inflammatory bowel disease.*
- *Abnormal ERCP or MRCP.*

## General Considerations

Primary sclerosing cholangitis (PSC) is a progressive liver disease of unknown cause, characterized by chronic inflammation and fibrosis of the intra- or extrahepatic bile ducts (or both), with eventual obliteration of peripheral bile ducts, cholangiographic evidence of strictures, and dilation of all or parts of the biliary tree. PSC is more common in males with inflammatory bowel disease, particularly ulcerative colitis. It can also be seen with histiocytosis X, sicca syndromes, congenital and acquired immunodeficiency syndromes, and cystic fibrosis.

## Clinical Findings

### A. Symptoms and Signs

PSC often has an insidious onset. Clinical symptoms may include abdominal pain, fatigue, pruritus, and jaundice. Acholic stools and steatorrhea can occur. Physical findings include hepatomegaly, splenomegaly, and jaundice.

### B. Laboratory Findings

The earliest finding may be asymptomatic elevation of the GGT. Subsequent laboratory abnormalities include elevated levels of alkaline phosphatase and bile acids. Later, cholestatic jaundice and elevated AST and ALT may occur. Patients with associated inflammatory bowel disease often test positive for perinuclear anti-neutrophil cytoplasmic antibodies (pANCA). Other markers of autoimmune liver disease (antinuclear anti-bodies and antismooth muscle antibody) are often found but are not specific for PSC. Sclerosing cholangi-tis due to cryptosporidia is common in immunodefi-ciency syndromes.

#### C. RADIOLOGIC FINDINGS

Ultrasound may show dilated intrahepatic bile ducts behind strictures. ERCP or MRCP is the diagnostic study of choice, demonstrating irregularities of the bil-iary tree.

### Differential Diagnosis

The differential diagnosis includes infectious hepatitis, secondary cholangitis, autoimmune hepatitis, metabolic liver disease, cystic fibrosis, choledochal cyst, or other anomalies of the biliary tree, including Caroli disease and congenital hepatic fibrosis.

### Complications

Complications include secondary bacterial cholangitis, pancreatitis, biliary fibrosis, and cirrhosis. Progression to liver failure is common and the risk of cholangiocar-cinoma is higher in PSC.

### Treatment

No completely effective treatment is available. Patients with early disease may benefit from high-dose UCDA (20 mg/kg/d). Patients with autoimmune markers may benefit from treatment with corticosteroids and aza-thioprine. Antibiotic treatment of cholangitis and dila-tion and stenting of dominant bile duct strictures can reduce symptoms.

### Prognosis

The majority of patients will eventually require liver transplantation; however, the course of the disease may be 10–20 years.

Gilger MA et al: Efficacy of ursodeoxycholic acid in the treatment of primary sclerosing cholangitis in children. J Pediatr Gas-troenterol Nutr 2000;31:136 [PMID: 10941964].

Gregorio GV et al: Autoimmune hepatitis/sclerosing cholangitis overlap syndrome in childhood: A 16-year prospective study. Hepatology 2001;33:544 [PMID: 11230733].

Mieli-Vergani G, Vergani D: Sclerosing cholangitis in the paedi-atric patient. Best Pract Res Clin Gastroenterol 2001;15:681 [PMID: 11492976].

Wilschanske M et al: Primary sclerosing cholangitis in 32 children: Clinical, laboratory, and radiographic features, with survival analysis. Hepatology 1995;22:1415 [PMID: 7590657].

### 3. Other Biliary Tract Disorders

For a schematic representation of the various types of choledochal cysts, see Figure 21–1. For summary infor-mation on acute hydrops, choledochal cyst, acalculous cholecystitis, Caroli disease, and congenital hepatic fi-brosis, see Table 21–7.

## PYOGENIC & AMEBIC LIVER ABSCESS

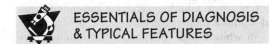

### ESSENTIALS OF DIAGNOSIS & TYPICAL FEATURES

- *Fever and painful enlarged liver.*
- *Ultrasound of liver demonstrating an abscess.*
- *Positive serum ameba antigen titer or positive bacterial culture of abscess fluid.*

| TYPE | | FINDINGS |
|---|---|---|
| I | | Spherical dilatation of the common duct |
| II | | Congenital diverticulum of the common bile duct |
| III | | Intraduodenal diverticulum of the common bile duct (choledochocele) |
| IVa | | Multiple intrahepatic communicating cysts (Caroli disease) |
| IVb | | Mixed extrahepatic and intrahepatic fusiform or cystic dilation (possibly variants of Caroli disease, congenital hepatic fibrosis) |

***Figure 21–1.*** Classification of cystic dilation of the bile ducts. Types I, II, and III are extrahepatic chole-dochal cysts. Type IVa is solely intrahepatic, and type IVb is both intrahepatic and extrahepatic. GB = gall-bladder; CBD = common bile duct.

## General Considerations

Pyogenic liver abscesses are often caused by intestinal bacteria seeded via the portal vein from infected viscera and occasionally from ascending cholangitis or gangrenous cholecystitis. Blood cultures are positive in up to 60% of patients. The resulting lesion tends to be solitary and located in the right hepatic lobe. Bacterial seeding may also occur from infected burns, pyodermas, and osteomyelitis. Unusual causes include omphalitis, subacute infective endocarditis, pyelonephritis, Crohn disease, and perinephric abscess. In immunocompromised patients, *S aureus,* gram-negative organisms, and fungi may seed the liver from the arterial system. Multiple pyogenic liver abscesses are associated with severe sepsis. Children receiving anti-inflammatory and immunosuppressive agents and children with defects in white blood cell function (chronic granulomatous disease) are prone to pyogenic hepatic abscesses, especially those caused by *S aureus.*

Amebic liver abscess is rare in children. An increased risk is associated with travel through areas of endemic infection (Mexico, Southeast Asia). *Entamoeba histolytica* invasion occurs via the large bowel, although a history of diarrhea (colitis-like picture) is not always obtained.

## Clinical Findings

With pyogenic liver abscess, nonspecific complaints of fever, chills, malaise, and abdominal pain are frequent. Weight loss is very common, especially in delayed diagnosis. A few patients have shaking chills and jaundice. The dominant complaint is a constant dull pain over an enlarged liver that is tender to palpation. An elevated hemidiaphragm with reduced or absent respiratory excursion may be demonstrated on physical examination and confirmed by fluoroscopy. Laboratory studies show leukocytosis and, at times, anemia. LFTs may be normal or reveal mild elevation of transaminases and alkaline phosphatase. Amebic liver abscesses are usually heralded by an acute illness with high fever, chills, and leukocytosis. Early in the course, liver tests may suggest mild hepatitis. An occasional prodrome may include cough, dyspnea, and shoulder pain as rupture of the abscess into the right chest occurs. Consolidation of the right lower lobe is common (10–30% of patients).

Ultrasound liver scan is the most useful diagnostic aid in evaluating pyogenic and amebic abscesses, detecting lesions as small as 1–2 cm. Nuclear scanning with gallium or technetium sulfur colloid or CT imaging may be useful in differentiating tumor or hydatid cyst.

The distinction between pyogenic and amebic abscesses is best made by indirect hemagglutination test (which is positive in more than 95% of patients with amebic liver disease) and the prompt response of the latter to antiamebic therapy (metronidazole). Examination of material obtained by needle aspiration of the abscess using ultrasound guidance is often diagnostic.

## Differential Diagnosis

Hepatitis, hepatoma, hydatid cyst, gallbladder disease, or biliary tract infections can mimic liver abscess. Subphrenic abscesses, empyema, and pneumonia may give a similar picture. Inflammatory disease of the intestines or of the biliary system may be complicated by liver abscess.

## Complications

Spontaneous rupture of the abscess may occur with extension of infection into the subphrenic space, thorax, peritoneal cavity, and, occasionally, the pericardium. Bronchopleural fistula with large sputum production and hemoptysis can develop in severe cases. Simultaneously, the amebic liver abscess may be secondarily infected with bacteria (in 10–20% of patients). Metastatic hematogenous spread to the lungs and the brain has been reported.

## Treatment

Ultrasound- or CT-guided percutaneous needle aspiration for aerobic and anaerobic culture with simultaneous placement of a catheter for drainage, combined with appropriate antibiotic therapy, is the treatment of choice for solitary pyogenic liver abscess. Multiple liver abscesses may also be treated successfully by this method. Surgical intervention may be indicated if rupture occurs outside the capsule of the liver or if enterohepatic fistulae are suspected.

Amebic abscesses in uncomplicated cases should be treated promptly with oral metronidazole, 35–50 mg/kg/d, in three divided doses for 10 days. Intravenous metronidazole can be used for patients unable to take oral medication. Failure to improve after 72 hours of drug therapy suggests superimposed bacterial infection or an incorrect diagnosis. At this point, needle aspiration or surgical drainage is indicated. Once oral feedings can be tolerated, a 20-day course of iodoquinol (30 mg/kg/d in three doses) is started as a luminal amebicide. Resolution of the abscess cavity occurs over 3–6 months.

## Prognosis

An unrecognized and untreated pyogenic liver abscess is universally fatal. With drainage and antibiotics, the cure rate is about 90%. Most amebic abscesses are cured with conservative medical management; the mortality rate is less than 3%. If extrahepatic complications occur (empyema, bronchopleural fistula, pericardial complications), 10–15% of patients will succumb.

Kumar A et al: Pyogenic liver abscess in children—South Indian experiences. J Pediatr Surg 1998;33:417 [PMID 9537550].

Moazam F, Nazir Z: Amebic liver abscess: Spare the knife but save the child. J Pediatr Surg 1998;33:119 [PMID: 9473115].

Rajak CL et al: Percutaneous drainage of liver abscesses: Needle aspiration versus catheter drainage. AJR Am J Roentgenol 1998;170:1035 [PMID 9530055].

Stanley SL: Amoebiasis. Lancet 2003;361:1025 [PMID 12700377].

# HEPATOMA

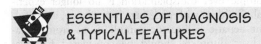

## ESSENTIALS OF DIAGNOSIS & TYPICAL FEATURES

- *Abdominal enlargement and pain, weight loss, anemia.*
- *Hepatomegaly with or without a definable mass.*
- *Mass lesion on imaging studies.*
- *Laparotomy and tissue biopsy.*

## General Considerations

Primary epithelial neoplasms of the liver represent 0.2–5.8% of all malignant conditions in children. After Wilms' tumor and neuroblastoma, hepatomas are the third most common intra-abdominal cancer. The incidence is higher in Southeast Asia, where childhood cirrhosis is more common. There are two basic morphologic types with certain clinical and prognostic differences. Hepatoblastoma predominates in male infants and children and accounts for 79% of liver cancer in children, with most cases appearing before age 5 years. There is an increased risk of hepatoblastoma in Beckwith–Wiedemann syndrome, hemihypertrophy, familial adenomatosis polyposis coli, and in premature or low-birth-weight infants. Most lesions are found in the right lobe of the liver. Pathologic differentiation from hepatocarcinoma may be difficult. Hepatocarcinoma, the other major malignant tumor of the liver, occurs more frequently after age 3 years. This type of neoplasm carries a poorer prognosis than hepatoblastoma and causes more abdominal discomfort. Patients with chronic HBV or HCV infection, cirrhosis, glycogen storage disease type I, tyrosinemia, or $\alpha_1$-antitrypsin deficiency have an increased risk for hepatocellular carcinoma. The late development of hepatoma in patients receiving androgens for treatment of Fanconi syndrome and aplastic anemia must also be kept in mind. The use of anabolic steroids by body-conscious adolescents poses a risk of hepatic neoplasia. An interesting aspect of primary epithelial neoplasms of the liver has been the increased incidence of associated anomalies and endocrine abnormalities. Virilization has been reported as a consequence of gonadotropin activity of the tumor. Feminization with bilateral gynecomastia may occur in association with high estradiol levels in the blood, the latter a consequence of increased aromatization of circulating androgens by the liver. Leydig cell hyperplasia without spermatogenesis is found on testicular biopsy. Hemihypertrophy, congenital absence of the kidney, macroglossia, and Meckel diverticulum have been found in association with hepatocarcinoma.

## Clinical Findings

A noticeable increase in abdominal girth with or without pain is the most constant feature of the history. A parent may note a bulge in the upper abdomen or report feeling a hard mass. Constitutional symptoms (eg, anorexia, fatigue, fever, chills) may be present. Teenage boys may complain of gynecomastia.

### A. SYMPTOMS AND SIGNS

Weight loss, pallor, and abdominal pain associated with a large abdomen are common. Physical examination reveals hepatomegaly with or without a definite tumor mass, usually to the right of the midline. In the absence of cirrhosis, signs of chronic liver disease are usually absent. However, evidence of virilization or feminization in prepubertal children may be noted.

### B. LABORATORY FINDINGS

Normal LFTs are the rule. Anemia frequently occurs, especially in cases of hepatoblastoma. Cystathioninuria has been reported. $\alpha$-Fetoprotein levels are often elevated, especially in hepatoblastoma. Estradiol levels are sometimes elevated. Final tissue diagnosis is best obtained at laparotomy, although ultrasound- or CT-guided needle biopsy of the liver mass can be used.

### C. IMAGING

Ultrasonography, CT, and MRI are useful for diagnosis and for following tumor response to therapy. A scintigraphic study of bone and lung and selective angiography are generally part of the preoperative work-up to evaluate metastatic disease.

## Differential Diagnosis

In the absence of a palpable mass, the differential diagnosis is that of hepatomegaly with or without anemia or jaundice. Hematologic and nutritional conditions should be ruled out, as well as HBV and HCV infection, $\alpha_1$-antitrypsin deficiency disease, lipid storage diseases, histiocytosis X, glycogen storage disease, tyrosinemia, congenital hepatic fibrosis, cysts, adenoma, focal nodular hyperplasia, inflammatory pseudotumor, and hemangiomas. If fever is present, hepatic abscess (pyogenic or amebic) must be considered. Veno-occlusive disease and hepatic vein thrombosis are rare possibilities. Tumors in the left lobe may be mistaken for pancreatic pseudocysts.

## Complications

Progressive enlargement of the tumor, abdominal discomfort, ascites, respiratory difficulty, and widespread metastases (especially to the lungs and the abdominal lymph nodes) are the rule. Rupture of the neoplastic liver and intraperitoneal hemorrhage have been reported. Progressive anemia and emaciation predispose the patient to an early septic death.

## Treatment

An aggressive surgical approach has resulted in the only long-term survivals. Complete resection of the lesion offers the only chance for cure. It appears that every isolated lung metastasis should also be surgically resected. Radiotherapy and chemotherapy have been disappointing in the treatment of primary liver neoplasms, although new combinations of drugs are continually being evaluated. These modalities are also used for initial cytoreduction of tumors found to be unresectable at the time of primary surgery. Second-look celiotomy has, in some cases, allowed resection of the tumor, resulting in a reduced mortality rate. Liver transplantation has been disappointing but continues to be performed in selected patients. The survival rate may be better for those patients in whom the tumor is incidental to another disorder (tyrosinemia, biliary atresia, cirrhosis). In HBV-endemic areas, childhood HBV vaccination has reduced the incidence of hepatocellular carcinoma.

## Prognosis

The survival rate if the tumor is completely removed is 90% for hepatoblastoma and 33% for hepatocellular carcinoma. Fibrolamellar oncocytic hepatocarcinoma has a more favorable prognosis. The overall survival and cure rate is less than 20%. If metastases are present, survival is reduced to 30% for hepatoblastoma.

Chang MH et al: Universal hepatitis B vaccination in Taiwan and the incidence of hepatocellular carcinoma in children. N Engl J Med 1997;336:1855 [PMID: 9197213].

Dower NA, Smith LJ: Liver transplantation for malignant liver tumors in children. Med Pediatr Oncol 2000;34:136 PMID 10657876.

Herzog CE et al: Childhood cancers: Hepatoblastoma. Oncologist 2000;5:445 [PMID 11110595].

Newman KD: Hepatic tumors in children. Semin Pediatr Surg 1997;6:38 [PMID:9117273 ].

Raney B: Hepatoblastoma in children: A review. J Pediatr Hematol Oncol 1997;19:418 [PMID: 9329462].

Reynolds M: Pediatric liver tumors. Semin Surg Oncol 1999;16: 159.

Stringer MD: Liver tumors. Semin Pediatr Surg 2000;9:196 [PMID 11112837].

# LIVER TRANSPLANTATION

Orthotopic liver transplantation is no longer experimental. Children with end-stage liver disease, acute fulminant hepatic failure, or complications from metabolic liver disorders should be considered for liver transplantation. Recent advances in immunosuppression (eg, cyclosporine and tacrolimus, use of monoclonal antibodies against T cells, introduction of mycophenolate mofetil and sirolimus), better candidate selection, improvements in surgical techniques, and experience in postoperative management have contributed to improved results.

The major indications for childhood transplantation are

1. A failed Kasai operation or decompensated cirrhosis caused by biliary atresia
2. $\alpha_1$-Antitrypsin deficiency
3. Posthepatitic (autoimmune chronic active hepatitis, hepatitis B or C disease) cirrhosis
4. Tyrosinemia
5. Crigler–Najjar syndrome type I
6. Wilson disease
7. Acute fulminant hepatic failure when recovery is unlikely
8. Primary sclerosing cholangitis
9. Hepatic-based malignancies
10. Cases in which the consequences of chronic cholestasis severely impair the patient's quality of life.

Children should be referred early for evaluation because the limiting factor for success is the small donor pool. Pared-down adult livers, organs from living related donors, and split adult donor livers are being used in children in many centers. Ten percent of recipients require retransplantation. In general, 75–85% of children survive at least 2–5 years after transplantation, with long-term survival expected to be comparable. Lifetime immunosuppression therapy using combinations of cyclosporine, tacrolimus, prednisone, or aza-thioprine, with its incumbent risks, is necessary to prevent rejection. The overall quality of life for children with a transplanted liver appears to be excellent. The lifelong risk of Epstein–Barr virus-induced lymphoproliferative disease is approximately 5% and is related to age and EBV exposure status at time of transplant and intensity of immunosuppression. Various protocols are being tested for prevention and treatment of lymphoproliferative disease.

Bucuvalas JC et al: Health-related quality of life in pediatric liver transplant recipients: A single-center study. Liver Transpl 2003;9(1):62 [PMID: 12514775].

Diem HV et al: Pediatric liver transplantation for biliary atresia: Results of primary grafts in 328 recipients. Transplantation 2003;75(10):1692 [PMID: 12777858].

Holmes RD, Sokol RJ: Epstein–Barr virus and post-transplant lymphoproliferative disease. Pediatr Transplant 2002;6(6):456 [PMID: 12453197].

Inomata Y et al: Living donor liver transplantation: An 8-year experience with 379 consecutive cases. Transplant Proc 1999;31: 381 [PMID: 10083152].

Krull K et al: Neurocognitive outcome in pediatric liver transplant recipients. Pediatr Transplant 2003;7(2):111 [PMID: 12654051]

Miller CM et al: One hundred nine living donor liver transplants in adults and children: A single center experience. Ann Surg 2001;234:301 [PMID: 11524583].

# ■ PANCREAS

## ACUTE PANCREATITIS

### ESSENTIALS OF DIAGNOSIS & TYPICAL FEATURES

- Epigastric abdominal pain radiating to the back.
- Nausea and vomiting.
- Elevated serum amylase and lipase.
- Evidence of pancreatic inflammation by CT or ultrasound.

## General Considerations

Most cases of acute pancreatitis are the result of drugs, viral infections, systemic diseases, abdominal trauma, or obstruction of pancreatic flow. More than 20% are idiopathic. Causes of pancreatic obstruction include stones, choledochal cyst, tumors of the duodenum, pancreas divisum, and ascariasis. Acute pancreatitis has been seen following treatment with sulfasalazine, thiazides, valproic acid, azathioprine, mercaptopurine, asparaginase, antiretroviral drugs (especially ddI), high-dose corticosteroids, and other drugs. It may also occur in cystic fibrosis, systemic lupus erythematosus, $\alpha_1$-antitrypsin deficiency, diabetes mellitus, Crohn disease, glycogen storage disease type I, hyperlipidemia types I and V, hyperparathyroidism, Henoch–Schönlein purpura, Reye syndrome, organic acidopathies, Kawasaki disease, or chronic renal failure; during rapid refeeding in cases of malnutrition; and in familial cases. Alcohol-induced pancreatitis should be considered in the teenage patient.

## Clinical Findings

### A. SYMPTOMS AND SIGNS

An acute onset of persistent (hours to days), moderate to severe upper abdominal and midabdominal pain occasionally referred to the back, and vomiting, is the common presenting picture. The abdomen is tender but not rigid, and bowel sounds are diminished, suggesting peritoneal irritation. Abdominal distention is common in infants and younger children. Jaundice is unusual. Ascites may be noted, and a left-sided pleural effusion is present in some patients. Periumbilical and flank bruising indicate hemorrhagic pancreatitis.

### B. LABORATORY FINDINGS

Leukocytosis and an elevated serum amylase (>3 times normal) should be expected early, except in infants younger than age 6 months who may have hypoamylasemia. Serum lipase is elevated and persists longer than serum amylase. The immunoreactive trypsinogen test may also be of value. Pancreatic amylase isoenzyme determination can help differentiate nonpancreatic causes (eg, salivary, intestinal, tubo-ovarian) of serum amylase elevation. Hyperglycemia (serum glucose > 300 mg/dL), hypocalcemia, falling hematocrit, rising blood urea nitrogen, hypoxemia, and acidosis may all occur in severe cases and imply a poor prognosis.

### C. IMAGING

Plain radiographic films of the abdomen may show a localized ileus (sentinel loop). Ultrasonography shows decreased echodensity of the gland in comparison with the left lobe of the liver. Pseudocyst formation can also be seen early in the course. CT scanning is better for detecting pancreatic phlegmon, or abscess formation. ERCP or MRCP may be useful in confirming patency of the main pancreatic duct in cases of abdominal trauma; in recurrent acute pancreatitis; or in revealing stones, ductal strictures, and pancreas divisum.

## Differential Diagnosis

Other causes of acute upper abdominal pain include lesions of the stomach, duodenum, liver, and biliary system; acute gastroenteritis or atypical appendicitis; pneumonia; volvulus; intussusception; and nonaccidental trauma.

## Complications

Complications early in the disease include shock, fluid and electrolyte disturbances, ileus, acute respiratory distress syndrome, and hypocalcemic tetany. Hypervolemia is seen between the third and fifth days, at which time renal tubular necrosis may occur. The gastrointestinal, neurologic, musculoskeletal, hepatobiliary, dermatologic, and hematologic systems may also be involved.

Later, 5–20% of patients develop a pseudocyst heralded by recurrence of abdominal pain and rise in the serum amylase. Up to 60–70% of these pseudocysts will resolve spontaneously. Infection, hemorrhage, rupture, or fistulization may occur. Phlegmon formation is common and may extend from the gland into the retroperitoneum or into the lesser sac. Most regress, but some require drainage. Infection in this inflammatory mass is a constant threat. Pancreatic abscess formation is rare (3–5%) and develops 2–3 weeks after the initial insult. Fever, leukocytosis, and pain suggest this complication; diagnosis is made by ultrasound or CT scanning.

Chronic pancreatitis, exocrine or endocrine pancreatic insufficiency, and pancreatic lithiasis are rare sequelae of acute pancreatitis.

## Treatment

Medical management includes rest, gastric suction, fluids, electrolyte replacement, and blood or colloid as needed. Pain should be controlled with opioids. Oxygen may be required if desaturation occurs. Acid suppression may be helpful. Nutrition is provided by the parenteral or enteral (jejunal) route. Broad-spectrum antibiotic coverage is useful only in necrotizing pancreatitis. Drugs known to produce acute pancreatitis should be discontinued.

Surgical treatment is reserved for traumatic disruption of the gland, intraductal stone, other anatomic obstructive lesions, and unresolved or infected pseudocysts or abscesses. Early endoscopic decompression of the biliary system reduces the morbidity associated with pancreatitis caused by obstruction of the common bile duct.

## Prognosis

In the pediatric age group, the prognosis is surprisingly good with conservative management. The mortality rate is 5–10% in patients treated by operation and 1% in those treated medically. The morbidity rate is high with surgery as a result of fistula formation.

Jackson WD: Pancreatitis: Etiology, diagnosis, and management. Curr Opin Pediatr 2001;13:447 [PMID: 11801891].

Pietzak MM, Thomas DW: Pancreatitis in childhood. Pediatr Rev 2000;21:406 [PMID: 11121497].

# CHRONIC PANCREATITIS

Chronic pancreatitis is differentiated from acute pancreatitis in that the pancreas remains structurally or functionally abnormal after an attack.

The causes are multiple and can be divided into toxic-metabolic (eg, alcohol, chronic renal failure, hypercalcemia), idiopathic, genetic, autoimmune, recurrent and severe acute pancreatitis, and obstructive pancreatitis (eg, pancreas divisum, choledochal cyst).

## Clinical Findings

The diagnosis often is delayed by the nonspecific symptoms and the lack of persistent laboratory abnormalities.

### A. Symptoms and Signs

There is usually a history of recurrent upper abdominal pain of variable severity but prolonged duration. Radiation of the pain into the back is a frequent complaint. Fever and vomiting are not common. Steatorrhea and symptoms of diabetes may develop later in the course, and malnutrition secondary to failure of pancreatic exocrine secretions may also occur.

### B. Laboratory Findings

Serum amylase and lipase levels are usually elevated during early acute attacks but are often normal later. Pancreatic insufficiency and reduced volume and bicarbonate response may be found at pancreatic stimulation testing or by determination of fecal pancreatic elastase 1. Mutations of the cationic trypsinogen gene, the pancreatic secretory trypsin inhibitor, and the cystic fibrosis transmembrane conductance regulator gene (CFTR) are associated with recurrent acute and chronic pancreatitis. Elevated blood glucose and glycohemoglobin levels and glycosuria frequently occur in protracted disease. Sweat chloride should be checked for cystic fibrosis and serum calcium for hyperparathyroidism.

### C. Imaging

Radiographs of the abdomen may show pancreatic calcifications in up to 30% of patients. Ultrasound or CT examination demonstrates pancreatic enlargement, ductal dilation, and calculi in up to 80%. CT is the initial imaging procedure of choice. ERCP can show ductal dilation, stones, strictures, or stenotic segments. The use of endoscopic ultrasound and MRCP in the diagnosis and staging of chronic pancreatitis is being evaluated.

## Differential Diagnosis

Other causes of recurrent abdominal pain must be considered. Specific causes of pancreatitis such as hyperparathyroidism; systemic lupus erythematosus; infectious disease; and ductal obstruction by tumors, stones, or helminths must be excluded by appropriate tests.

## Complications

Disabling abdominal pain, steatorrhea, nutritional deprivation, pancreatic pseudocysts, and diabetes are the most frequent long-term complications. Pancreatic carcinoma occurs more frequently in chronic pancreatitis, and in up to 40% of patients with hereditary pancreatitis by age 70.

## Treatment

Medical management of acute attacks is indicated (see Acute Pancreatitis section). If ductal obstruction is strongly suspected, endoscopic therapy (balloon dilation, stenting, stone removal, sphincterotomy) should be pursued. Relapses seem to occur in most patients. Orally ingested non–enteric-coated pancreatic enzymes at mealtime may reduce pain episodes in some patients. Antioxidant therapy is being investigated. Pseudocysts may be marsupialized to the surface or drained into the stomach or into a loop of jejunum if they fail to regress spontaneously. Experience in pediatric patients indicates that lateral pancreaticojejunostomy can reduce pain in patients with a dilated pancreatic duct and may prevent or delay progression of functional pancreatic impairment.

## Prognosis

In the absence of a correctable lesion, the prognosis is not good. Disabling episodes of pain, pancreatic insufficiency, diabetes, and pancreatic cancer may ensue. Narcotic addiction and suicide are risks in teenagers with disabling disease.

Etemad B, Whitcomb DC: Chronic pancreatitis: Diagnosis, classification, and new genetic developments. Gastroenterology 2001;120:682 [PMID: 11179244].

Witt H: Gene mutations in children with chronic pancreatitis. Pancreatology 2001;1:432 [PMID: 12120220].

## GASTROINTESTINAL & HEPATOBILIARY MANIFESTATIONS OF CYSTIC FIBROSIS

Cystic fibrosis is a disease with protean manifestations. Although pulmonary and pancreatic involvement dominate the clinical picture for most patients (see Chapter 18), a variety of other organs can be involved. Table 21–9 lists the important gastrointestinal, pancreatic, and hepatobiliary conditions that may affect cystic fibrosis patients along with their clinical findings, incidence, most useful diagnostic studies, and preferred treatment.

Diwakar V et al: Liver disease in children with cystic fibrosis. Paediatr Respir Rev 2001;2:340 [PMID: 12052306].

Dodge JA, Macpherson C: Colonic strictures in cystic fibrosis. J R Soc Med 1995;88(Suppl 25):3 [PMID: 7776325].

Ratjen F, Doring G: Cystic fibrosis. Lancet 2003;361:681 [PMID 12606185].

Riedel BD: Gastrointestinal manifestations of cystic fibrosis. Pediatr Ann 1997;26:235 [PMID: 9114442].

Sokol RJ, Durie PR: Recommendations for management of liver and biliary tract disease in cystic fibrosis: Cystic Fibrosis Foundation Hepatobiliary Disease Consensus Group. J Pediatr Gastroenterol Nutr 1999;28(Suppl 1):S1 [PMID: 9934970].

Taylor CJ, Aswani N: The pancreas in cystic fibrosis. Paediatr Respir Rev 2002;3:77 [PMID: 12065186].

## SYNDROMES WITH PANCREATIC EXOCRINE INSUFFICIENCY

Several syndromes are associated with exocrine pancreatic insufficiency. Clinically the patients present with a history of failure to thrive, diarrhea, fatty stools, and an absence of respiratory symptoms. Laboratory findings include a normal sweat chloride; low fecal pancreatic elastase 1; and low to absent pancreatic lipase, amylase, and trypsin levels on duodenal intubation. Each disorder has several associated clinical features that aid in the differential diagnosis. In Shwachman syndrome, pancreatic exocrine hypoplasia with widespread fatty replacement of the glandular acinar tissue is associated with neutropenia because of maturational arrest of the granulocyte series. Metaphyseal dysostosis and an elevated fetal hemoglobin are common, but immunoglobulin deficiency and hepatic dysfunction are also reported. CT examination of the pancreas demonstrates the widespread fatty replacement. Serum immunoreactive trypsinogen levels are extremely low.

Other associations of exocrine pancreatic insufficiency include (1) aplastic alae, aplasia cutis, deafness (Johanson–Blizzard syndrome); (2) sideroblastic anemia, developmental delay, seizures, and liver dysfunction (Pearson bone marrow pancreas syndrome);

**Table 21–9.** Gastrointestinal and hepatobiliary manifestations of cystic fibrosis.

| Organ | Condition | Symptoms | Age at Presentation | Incidence (%) | Diagnostic Evaluation | Management |
|---|---|---|---|---|---|---|
| Esophagus | Gastroesophageal reflux, esophagitis | Pyrosis, dysphagia, epigastric pain, hematemesis. | All ages | 10–20 | Endoscopy and biopsy, overnight pH study | H₂ blockers, antacids, carafate, PPIs, surgical antireflux procedure. |
| | Varices | Hematemesis, melena. | Childhood and adolescents | 3–10 | Endoscopy | Endosclerosis, band ligation, drugs (see text), TIPS liver transplantation. (see Table 21–8) |
| Stomach | Gastritis | Upper abdominal pain, vomiting, hematemesis. | School age and older | 10–25 | Endoscopy and biopsy | H₂ blockers, antacids, carafate, PPIs. |
| | Hiatal hernia | Reflux symptoms (see above), epigastric pain. | School age and older | 3–5 | Endoscopy; barium swallow | As above. Surgery in some. |
| Intestine | Meconium ileus | Abdominal distention, bilious emesis. | Neonate | 10–15 | Radiologic studies, plain abdominal films; contrast enema shows microcolon | Dislodgement of obstruction with Gastrografin enema. Surgery if unsuccessful or if case complicated by atresia, perforation, or volvulus. |
| | Distal intestinal obstruction syndrome | Abdominal pain, acute and recurrent; distention; occasional vomiting. | Any age, usually school age through adolescence | 10–15 | Palpable mass in right lower quadrant, radiologic studies | Gastrografin enema, intestinal lavage solution, diet, bulk laxatives, adjustment of pancreatic enzyme intake. |
| | Fibrosing colonopathy | As above. History of high enzyme dosage. | ≥3 years | < 1 | Barium enema or UGI/SBFT, abdominal ultrasound, or CT | Reduce pancreatic enzyme dose to < 2000 units of lipase/kg per dose if indicated. Surgical resection may be necessary. |
| | Intussusception | Acute, intermittent abdominal pain; distention; emesis. | Infants through adolescence | 1–3 | X-ray studies, barium enema | Reduction by barium or air enema or surgery if needed. Diet. Bulk laxatives. Adjustment of pancreatic enzyme intake. |
| | Rectal prolapse | Anal discomfort, rectal bleeding. | Infants and children to age 4–5 years | 15–25 | Visual mass protruding from anus | Manual reduction, adjustment of pancreatic enzyme dosage, reassurance as problem resolves by age 3–5 years. |

| System | Condition | Clinical features | Age | % | Diagnosis | Management |
|---|---|---|---|---|---|---|
| Intestine (cont'd) | Carbohydrate intolerance | Abdominal pain, flatulence, continued diarrhea with adequate replacement therapy. | Any age | 10–25 | Intestinal mucosal biopsy and disaccharidase analysis. Breath hydrogen after lactose load. | Reduce lactose intake; reduction of gastric hyperacidity if mucosa shows partial villous atrophy. Beware concurrent celiac disease or *Giardia* infection. |
| Pancreas | Total exocrine insufficiency | Diarrhea, steatorrhea, malnutrition, failure to thrive. Specific fat-soluble vitamin deficiency states. | Neonate through infancy | 85–90 | 72-h fecal fat evaluation, fecal pancreatic elastase | Pancreatic enzyme replacement, may need elemental formula, fat-soluble vitamin and vitamin E supplements. |
| | Pancreatic sufficiency (partial exocrine insufficiency) | Occasional diarrhea, mild growth delay. | Any age | 10–15 | 72-hour fecal fat evaluation, direct pancreatic function tests | Pancreatic enzyme replacement in selected patients. Fat-soluble vitamin supplements as indicated by biochemical evaluation. |
| | Pancreatitis | Recurrent abdominal pain, vomiting. | Older children through adolescence. Primarily in patients with partial pancreatic sufficiency. | 0.1 | Increased serum lipase and amylase, pancreatic provocative test, endoscopic pancreatogram | Addition of pancreatic enzymes to feeds, endoscopic removal of sludge or stones if present, endoscopic papillotomy. |
| | Diabetes | Weight loss, polyuria, polydipsia. | Older children through adolescence | 5–7 | Glucose tolerance test and insulin levels | Diet, insulin. |
| Liver | Steatosis | Hepatomegaly. | Neonates and infants, but can be seen at all ages | 20–60 | Liver biopsy | Improved nutrition, replacement of pancreatic enzymes and vitamins. |
| | Focal biliary cirrhosis | Hepatomegaly. | Infants and older patients. Prevalence increases with age. | 10–70 | Liver biopsy | As above. Taurine supplements (still experimental), ursodeoxycholic acid. |
| | Multilobular biliary cirrhosis | Hepatosplenomegaly, hematemesis from esophageal varices; hypersplenism, jaundice, ascites late in course. | School age through adolescence | 5–15 | Liver biopsy, endoscopy | Improved nutrition, ursodeoxycholic acid, endosclerosis or band ligation of varices, or partial splenic embolization, liver transplantation. |

(continued)

*Table 21-9.* Gastrointestinal and hepatobiliary manifestations of cystic fibrosis. (continued)

| Organ | Condition | Symptoms | Age at Presentation | Incidence (%) | Diagnostic Evaluation | Management |
|---|---|---|---|---|---|---|
| Liver (cont'd) | Neonatal jaundice | Cholestatic jaundice hepatomegaly; often seen with meconium ileus. | Neonates | 0.1–1 | Sweat chloride test, liver biopsy | Nutritional support, special formula with medium-chain triglyceride-containing oil, pancreatic enzyme replacement, vitamin supplements. |
| Gallbladder | Microgallbladder | None. | Congenital—present at any age | 30 | Ultrasound or hepatobiliary scintigraphy | None needed. |
| | Cholelithiasis | Recurrent abdominal pain, rarely jaundice. | School age through adolescence | 1–10 | Ultrasound | Surgery if symptomatic and low risk, trial of cholelitholytics in others. |
| Extrahepatic bile ducts | Intraluminal obstruction (sludge, stones, tumor) | Jaundice, hepatomegaly, abdominal pain. | Neonates, then older children through adolescence | Rare in neonates (< 0.1) | Ultrasound and hepatobiliary scintigraphy, endoscopic cholangiography | Surgery in neonates, endoscopic intervention in older patients or surgery. |
| | Extraluminal obstruction (intrapancreatic compression, tumor) | As above. | Older children to adults | Rare (< 1) | As above | Surgical biliary drainage procedure or biliary stent placement vs. balloon dilation endoscopically. |

PPI = proton pump inhibitor; CT = computed tomography; TIPS = transjugular intrahepatic portosystemic shunt; UGI/SBFT = upper gastrointestinal/small bowel follow-through radiologic series.

(3) duodenal atresia or stenosis; (4) malnutrition; and (5) pancreatic hypoplasia or agenesis.

The complications and sequelae of deficient pancreatic enzyme secretion are malnutrition, diarrhea, and growth failure. The degree of steatorrhea may lessen with age. Intragastric lipolysis primarily caused by lingual lipase may compensate in patients with low or absent pancreatic function. In Shwachman syndrome, the major sequela is short stature. Increased numbers of infections may result from chronic neutropenia. Neutrophil mobility is also impaired in many patients. In addition, an increased incidence of leukemia has been noted in these patients.

Pancreatic enzyme and fat-soluble vitamin replacement are required therapy in most patients. The prognosis appears to be good for those able to survive the increased number of bacterial infections early in life and those patients without severe associated defects.

Durie PR: Pancreatic aspects of cystic fibrosis and other inherited causes of pancreatic dysfunction. Med Clin North Am 2000; 84:609 [PMID: 10872418].

Dror Y, Freedman MH: Shwachman–Diamond syndrome. Br J Haematol 2002;118:701 [PMID: 12181037].

Rothbaum R et al: Shwachman–Diamond syndrome: Report from an international conference. J Pediatr 2002;141:266-70 [PMID: 12183725].

Sarles J, Guys JM, Sauniere JF: Pancreatic function and congenital duodenal abnormalities. J Pediatr Gastroenterol Nutr 1993; 16:284 [PMID 8492257].

Seneca S et al: Pearson marrow pancreas syndrome: A molecular study and clinical management. Clin Genet 1997;51:338 [PMID: 9212183].

Wright NM et al: Permanent neonatal diabetes mellitus and pancreatic exocrine insufficiency resulting from congenital pancreatic agenesis. Am J Dis Child 1993;147:607 [PMID: 8506821].

## ISOLATED EXOCRINE PANCREATIC ENZYME DEFECT

Normal premature infants and most newborns produce little, if any, pancreatic amylase following meals or exogenous hormonal stimulation. This temporary physiologic insufficiency may persist for the first 3–6 months of life and be responsible for diarrhea when complex carbohydrates (cereals) are introduced into the diet.

Congenital pancreatic lipase deficiency and congenital colipase deficiency are extremely rare disorders, causing diarrhea and variable malnutrition with malabsorption of dietary fat and fat-soluble vitamins. The sweat chloride level is normal, and neutropenia is absent. Treatment is oral replacement of pancreatic enzymes and a low-fat diet or formula containing medium-chain triglycerides.

***Table 21–10.*** Pancreatic tumors.

| | Age | Major Findings | Diagnosis | Treatment | Associated Conditions |
|---|---|---|---|---|---|
| Insulinoma | Any age | Hypoglycemia, seizures; high serum insulin; abdominal pain and mass infrequent | Ultrasound, CT scan, MRI, EUS | Surgery | |
| Adenocarcinoma | Any age | Epigastric pain, mass weight loss, anemia, biliary obstruction | Ultrasound, CT scan, MRI, EUS | Surgery | Chronic pancreatitis |
| Gastrinoma | Older than age 5–8 years | Male sex, gastric hypersecretion, peptic symptoms, multiple ulcers, gastrointestinal bleeding, anemia, diarrhea | Elevated fasting gastrin and postsecretin suppression test (> 300 pg/mL), CT scan, MRI, EUS laparotomy | $H_2$ blockers, omeprazole, surgical resection, total gastrectomy | Zollinger–Ellison syndrome, multiple endocrine neoplasia syndrome type I, neurofibromatosis |
| VIPoma | Any age | Secretory diarrhea, hypokalemia, weight loss | Elevated vasoactive intestinal polypeptide (VIP) levels; sometimes, elevated serum gastrin and pancreatic polypeptide | Surgery, octreotide | |
| Glucagonoma | Older patients | Necrolytic rash, diarrhea, anemia, thrombotic events | Elevated glucagon, gastrin, VIP | Surgery | |

CT = computed tomography, MRI = magnetic resonance imaging, EUS = endoscopic ultrasound.

Exocrine pancreatic insufficiency of proteolytic enzymes (eg, trypsinogen, trypsin, chymotrypsin) is caused by enterokinase deficiency, a duodenal mucosal enzyme required for activation of the pancreatic proenzymes. These patients present with malnutrition associated with hypoproteinemia and edema but are free of respiratory symptoms and have a normal sweat test. They respond to pancreatic enzyme replacement therapy and feeding formulas that contain a casein hydrolysate (eg, Nutramigen, Pregestimil).

Durie PR: Pancreatic aspects of cystic fibrosis and other inherited causes of pancreatic dysfunction. Med Clin North Am 2000; 84:609 [PMID: 10872418].

Mann NS, Mann SK: Enterokinase. Proc Soc Exp Biol Med 1994; 206:114 [PMID: 8208733].

McKenna LL: Pancreatic disorders in the newborn. Neonatal Netw 2000;19:13 [PMID: 11949098].

Stormon MO, Durie PR: Pathophysiologic basis of exocrine pancreatic dysfunction in childhood. J Pediatr Gastroenterol Nutr 2002;35:8 [PMID: 12142803].

## PANCREATIC TUMORS

Pancreatic tumors, whether benign or malignant, are rare lesions. They most often arise from ductal or acinar epithelium (malignant adenocarcinoma) or from islet (endocrine) components within the gland, such as the benign insulinoma (adenoma) derived from β cells. Other pancreatic tumors also originate from these pluripotential endocrine cells (gastrinoma, VIPoma,

glucagonoma). These malignant lesions produce diverse symptoms, because they release biologically active polypeptides from this ectopic location. The clinical features of these tumors are summarized in Table 21–10. The differential diagnosis of these abdominal tumors includes Wilms' tumor, neuroblastoma, and malignant lymphoma. In older children, endoscopic ultrasonography can aid in localizing these tumors.

Jaksic T et al: A 20-year review of pediatric pancreatic tumors. J Pediatr Surg 1992;27:1315 [PMID: 1328584].

Johnson PRV, Spitz L: Cysts and tumors of the pancreas. Semin Pediatr Surg 2000;9:209 [PMID 11112838].

Vossen S et al: Therapeutic management of rare malignant pancreatic tumors in children. World J Surg 1998;22:879 [PMID: 9673563].

## REFERENCES

Roy CC et al (eds): *Pediatric Clinical Gastroenterology*, 4th ed. Mosby-Year Book, 1995.

Sokol RJ, Feranchak AM: Genetic and metabolic basis of pediatric liver disease. Semin Liver Dis 2001;21:469.

Suchy FJ et al (eds): *Liver Disease in Children*, 2nd ed. Lippincott, Williams & Wilkins, 2001.

Walker WA et al (eds): *Pediatric Gastrointestinal Disease: Pathophysiology, Diagnosis, Management*, 2nd ed. Mosby-Year Book, 1996.

Wyllie R, Hyams JS (eds): *Pediatric Gastrointestinal Disease*. Saunders, 1999.

# Kidney & Urinary Tract

*Gary M. Lum, MD*

## ■ EVALUATION OF THE KIDNEY & URINARY TRACT

### HISTORY

When renal disease is suspected, the history should include

1. Family history of cystic disease, hereditary nephritis, deafness, dialysis, or renal transplantation
2. Preceding acute or chronic illnesses (eg, UTI, pharyngitis, impetigo, endocarditis)
3. Rashes or joint pains
4. Growth delay or failure to thrive
5. Polyuria, polydipsia, enuresis, urinary frequency, or dysuria
6. Documentation of hematuria, proteinuria, or discolored urine
7. Pain (abdominal, costovertebral angle, or flank) or trauma
8. Sudden weight gain or edema
9. Drug or toxin exposure

For the newborn or small infant, the physician should obtain birth history and information regarding prenatal ultrasonographic studies, birth asphyxia, Apgar scores, oligohydramnios, dysmorphic features, abdominal masses, voiding patterns, anomalous development, and umbilical artery catheterization.

### PHYSICAL EXAMINATION

Important aspects of the physical examination include the height, weight, skin lesions (café-au-lait or ash leaf spots), pallor, edema, or skeletal deformities. Anomalies of the ears, eyes, or external genitalia may be associated with renal disease. The blood pressure should be measured in a quiet setting. The cuff should cover two thirds of the child's upper arm, and peripheral pulses should be noted. An ultrasonic device is useful for measurements in infants. The abdomen should be palpated, with attention to the kidneys, abdominal masses, musculature, and the presence of ascites.

## LABORATORY EVALUATION OF RENAL FUNCTION

### Urinalysis

Commercially available dipsticks can be used to screen for the presence of red blood cells, hemoglobin, leukocytes, nitrites, and protein and to approximate pH. Positive results for blood should always be confirmed by microscopy, as should any suspicion of crystalluria. Significant proteinuria (> 150 mg/dL) detected by dipstick should be confirmed by quantitation either with a 24-hour collection or by the protein/creatinine ratio (see following section) of a random specimen.

### Serum Analysis

The standard indicators of renal function are serum levels of urea nitrogen and creatinine; their ratio is normally about 10:1. This ratio may increase when renal perfusion or urine flow is decreased, as in urinary tract obstruction or dehydration. Because serum urea nitrogen levels are more affected by these and other factors (eg, nitrogen intake, catabolism, use of corticosteroids) than are creatinine levels, the most reliable single indicator of glomerular function is the serum level of creatinine. For example, serum creatinine increasing from 0.5 mg/dL to 1.0 mg/dL represents a 50% decrease in glomerular filtration rate. Small children should have serum creatinine levels well under 0.8 mg/dL, and only larger adolescents should have levels exceeding 1 mg/dL. Less precise but nonetheless important indicators of the possible presence of renal disease are abnormalities of serum electrolytes, pH, calcium, phosphorus, magnesium, albumin, or complement.

### Measurement of Glomerular Filtration Rate

The endogenous creatinine clearance ($C_{cr}$) in milliliters per minute estimates the glomerular filtration rate (GFR). A 24-hour urine collection is usually obtained; however, in small children from whom collection is difficult, a 12-hour daytime specimen, collected when urine flow rate is greatest, is acceptable. The procedure for collecting a timed urine specimen should be explained carefully so that the parent or patient understands fully the rationale of (1) first emptying the bladder (discarding that urine) and noting the time; and (2) putting all urine subsequently voided into the collection receptacle, including the last void, 12 or 24 hours later. Reliability of the 24-hour collection can be checked by measuring the total 24-hour creatinine excretion in the specimen. Total daily creatinine excretion (creatinine index) should be in the range of 14–20 mg/kg. Creatinine indices on either side of this range suggest collections that were either inadequate or excessive. Calculation by the following formula requires measurements of plasma creatinine ($P_{cr}$) in mg/mL, urine creatinine ($U_{cr}$) in mg/mL, and urine volume (V) expressed as mL/min:

$$C_{Cr} = \frac{U_{Cr}\,V}{P_{Cr}}$$

Creatinine is a reflection of body muscle mass. Because accepted ranges of normal creatinine clearance are based on adult parameters, correction for size is needed to determine normal ranges in children. Clearance is corrected to a standard body surface area of 1.73 m$^2$ in the formula:

$$\text{"Corrected" } C_{Cr} = \frac{\text{Patient's } C_{Cr} \times 1.73\text{m}^2}{\text{Patient's body surface area}}$$

Although 80–125 mL/min/1.73 m$^2$ is the normal range for creatinine clearance, estimates at the lower end of this range may indicate problems.

A simple and tested formula for quick approximation of creatinine clearance incorporates use of the plasma creatinine level and the child's length in centimeters:

$$C_{Cr}\,(\text{mL}/\text{min}/1.73\text{m}^2) = \frac{0.55 \times \text{Height in cm}}{P_{Cr}\text{ in mg}/\text{dL}}$$

**Note:** Because this formula takes into account the body surface area, further correction is not necessary. Use 0.45 × length in centimeters for newborns and for infants younger than age 1 year. This method of calculation is not meant to detract from the importance of clearance determinations but is useful when a suspicious plasma creatinine needs to be checked.

## Urine Concentrating Ability

Inability to concentrate urine is associated with polyuria, polydipsia, or enuresis and is often the first sign of chronic renal failure. The first morning void should be concentrated. Evaluation of other abnormalities of urinary concentration or dilution is discussed later in the sections on specific disease entities, such as diabetes insipidus.

## Microhematuria or Isolated Proteinuria

In children with asymptomatic hematuria or proteinuria, the search for renal origins will yield the most results. Isolated proteinuria may reflect urologic abnormalities, benign excretion, or glomerular alterations. The presence of red cell casts suggests glomerulonephritis (GN), but the absence of casts does not rule out this disease. Anatomic abnormalities such as cystic disease may be a source of hematuria.

Benign hematuria, including benign familial hematuria, is diagnosed by exclusion. In this group are children whose hematuria is caused by asymptomatic hypercalciuria. Figure 22–1 suggests an approach to the renal work-up of hematuria. GN is discussed in more detail later in this chapter.

The association of proteinuria with hematuria is characteristic of more significant glomerular disease. Quantitation of the proteinuria is customarily accomplished by a time collection (eg, over a 24-hour period). However, an assessment of the degree of proteinuria may be made with the performance of the urine protein/creatinine ratio in a random urine sample. A protein-to-creatinine ratio of more than 0.2 is abnormal. A timed urine collection is performed as described previously for creatinine clearance. In the evaluation of asymptomatic proteinuria, orthostatic or postural proteinuria should be ruled out. The protein present in urine voided on arising in the morning is compared with that in urine formed in the upright position during the rest of the day. This can be accomplished more simply by comparing the protein/creatinine ratios. If the quantitation is accomplished by separation of the "upright" and "supine" portions of a 24-hour collection, if the upright collection contains 80–100% of the entire 24-hour measured protein, and if there are no other markers of renal disease, the diagnosis of benign postural proteinuria is acceptable.

An approach to the work-up of isolated proteinuria is shown in Figure 22–2. Note that corticosteroid therapy is indicated in the algorithm because this may be initiated prior to referral. Other renal lesions with proteinuric manifestations are discussed later in this chapter.

## Special Tests of Renal Function

Measurements of urinary sodium, creatinine, and osmolality are useful in differentiating prerenal causes of

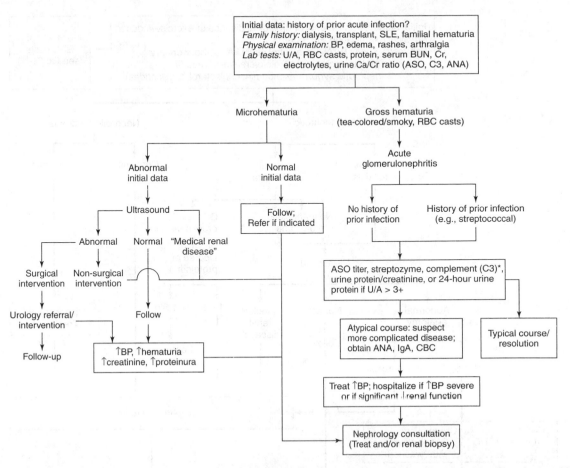

**Figure 22–1.** Approach to the renal work-up of hematuria. (Exclude UTI, lithiasis, trauma, bleeding disorders, sickle cell disease.) ANA = antinuclear antibody; ASO = antistreptolysin antibody; BP = blood pressure; BUN = blood urea nitrogen; C3 = complement; Ca = calcium; Cr = creatinine; GN = glomerulonephritis; IgA = immunoglobulin A; PSGN = poststreptococcal glomerulonephritis; RBC = red blood cell; SLE = systemic lupus erythematosus; U/A = urinalysis.

renal insufficiency from renal causes such as acute tubular necrosis. The physiologic response to decreased renal perfusion is decreased urinary output, increased urine osmolality, increased urinary solutes (eg, creatinine), and decreased urinary sodium (usually < 20 mEq/L). Prolonged underperfusion results in varying increases in the serum creatinine and blood urea nitrogen (BUN) concentrations, prompting the need to differentiate between this state and acute tubular necrosis (see Acute Renal Failure section).

The presence of certain substances in urine may suggest tubular dysfunction. For example, urine glucose should be less than 5 mg/dL. Hyperphosphaturia occurs with significant tubular abnormalities (eg, Fanconi syndrome). Measurement of the phosphate concentra-

tion of a 24-hour urine specimen and evaluation of tubular reabsorption of phosphorus (TRP) will help document renal tubular diseases as well as hyperparathyroid states. TRP (expressed as percentage of reabsorption) is calculated as follows:

$$TRP = 100 \left[ 1 - \frac{S_{Cr} \times U_{PO4}}{S_{PO4} \times U_{Cr}} \right]$$

where $S_{cr}$ = serum creatinine; $U_{cr}$ = urine creatinine; $S_{PO4}$ = serum phosphate; and $U_{PO4}$ = urine phosphate. All values for creatinine and phosphate are expressed in milligrams per deciliter for purposes of calculation. A

**Figure 22–2.** Approach to the work-up of isolated proteinuria. BP = blood pressure; Cr = creatinine; hpf = high-power field; RBC = red blood cell; U/A = urinalysis; VCUG = voiding cystourethrogram. *Complement is depressed in acute poststreptococcal glomerulonephritis, chronic glomerulonephritis, and lupus. Will normalize within a month in poststreptococcal glomerulonephritis.

TRP value of 80% or more is considered normal, although it depends somewhat on the value of $S_{PO4}$.

The urinary excretion of amino acids in generalized tubular disease reflects a quantitative increase rather than a qualitative change. Diseases affecting proximal tubular reabsorption of bicarbonate—including isolated renal tubular acidosis, Fanconi syndrome (which occurs in diseases such as cystinosis), and chronic renal failure—are discussed later in the chapter.

## LABORATORY EVALUATION OF IMMUNOLOGIC FUNCTION

Many parenchymal renal diseases are thought to have immune causation, although the mechanisms are largely unknown. Examples of mechanisms in the kidney include (1) deposition of circulating antigen–antibody complexes that are themselves injurious or incite injurious responses and (2) formation of antibody directed against the glomerular basement membrane itself (rare in children).

Total serum complement and the C3 and C4 complement components should be measured when immune-mediated renal injury or chronic GN is suspected. Where clinically indicated, antinuclear antibodies, hepatitis B surface antigen, and rheumatoid factor should be obtained. In rare cases the presence of cold-precipitable proteins (cryoglobulins), C3 "nephritic" factor, or antiglomerular basement membrane (anti-GBM) antibody may be helpful in determining a specific diagnosis. At some point in the workup, the diagnosis may be supported or confirmed by the description of renal histology.

## RADIOGRAPHIC EVALUATION

Renal ultrasonography is a useful noninvasive tool in the evaluation of renal parenchymal disease, urinary tract abnormalities, or renal blood flow. Excretory urography is used to assess the anatomy and function of the kidney, collecting system, and bladder. Radioisotope studies provide valuable information concerning renal anatomy, blood flow, and integrity and function of the glomerular, tubular, and collecting systems.

Evaluation of the lower urinary tract (voiding cystourethrography or cystoscopy) is indicated when vesicoureteral reflux or bladder outlet obstruction is suspected. Cystoscopy is rarely useful in the evaluation of asymptomatic hematuria or proteinuria in children.

Renal arteriography or venography is indicated to define vascular abnormalities (eg, renal artery stenosis) prior to surgical intervention. Less invasive measures such as ultrasonography and Doppler studies can demonstrate renal blood flow or thromboses.

## RENAL BIOPSY

Histologic information is valuable for diagnosis, treatment, and prognosis. Satisfactory evaluation of renal tissue requires examination by light, immunofluorescence, and electron microscopy.

When a biopsy is anticipated, a pediatric nephrologist should be consulted. In children, percutaneous renal biopsy with a biopsy needle is an acceptable low-risk procedure—avoiding the risks of general anesthesia—when performed by an experienced physician. A surgeon should perform the biopsy procedure if operative exposure of the kidney is necessary, if an increased risk factor (eg, bleeding disorder) is present, or if a "wedge" biopsy is preferred.

# ■ CONGENITAL ANOMALIES OF THE URINARY TRACT

## RENAL PARENCHYMAL ANOMALIES

About 10% of children have congenital anomalies of the genitourinary tract, which range in severity from asymptomatic to lethal. Some asymptomatic abnormalities may have significant complications. For example, patients with "horseshoe" kidney (kidneys fused in their lower poles) have a higher incidence of renal calculi. Unilateral agenesis is usually accompanied by compensatory hypertrophy of the contralateral kidney and thus should be compatible with normal renal function. Supernumerary and ectopic kidneys are usually of no significance. Abnormal genitourinary development can result in varying degrees of renal maldevelopment and function, of which complete renal agenesis is the most severe. When the agenesis is bilateral, it causes early death. Severe oligohydramnios is present and can result in pulmonary hypoplasia and peculiar (Potter) facies.

### Renal Dysgenesis

Renal dysgenesis represents a spectrum of anomalies. In simple hypoplasia, which may be unilateral or bilateral, the affected organs are smaller than normal. In the various forms of dysplasia, immature, undifferentiated renal tissue persists. In some of the dysplasias, the number of normal nephrons is insufficient to sustain life once the child reaches a critical body size. Such lack of renal tissue may not be readily discernible in the newborn period because the infant's urine production, though poor in concentration, may be adequate in volume. Often, the search for renal insufficiency is initiated only when growth fails or chronic renal failure develops.

Other forms of renal dysplasia include oligomeganephronia (characterized by the presence of only a few large glomeruli) and the cystic dysplasias (characterized by the presence of renal cysts). This group includes microcystic disease (congenital nephrosis). A simple cyst within a kidney may be clinically unimportant because it does not predispose to progressive polycystic development. An entire kidney lost to multicystic development with concomitant hypertrophy and normal function of the contralateral side may also be of little clinical consequence. Nonetheless, even a simple cyst could pose problems if it becomes a site for lithiasis, infection, or hematuria.

## Polycystic Kidney Disease

Autosomal recessive polycystic kidney disease (ARPKD) is increasingly diagnosed by prenatal ultrasound. In its most severe form the cystic kidneys are nonfunctional in utero, and, therefore, newborns can have Potter facies and other complications of oligohydramnios. In infancy and childhood, kidney enlargement by cysts may initially be recognized by abdominal palpation of the renal masses. Hypertension is an early problem. The rate of the progression of renal insufficiency varies, as does growth failure and other complications of chronic renal failure. Two genes (ADPKD-1 and ADPKD-2) account for 80% and 10% of cases of the autosomal dominant polycystic kidney disease, respectively. Susceptibility of members in ADPKD families is detected by gene linkage studies. Renal ultrasound identifies cysts in about 80% of affected children by age 5 years. Children with this diagnosis need close monitoring for the development and treatment of hypertension, and their families should be offered genetic counseling. Management of end-stage renal failure is by dialysis or renal transplantation.

Gabow PA: Utility of ultrasonography in the diagnosis of autosomal dominant polycystic kidney disease in children. J Am Soc Nephrol 1997;8:105.

Murcia NS, Sweeney WE Jr. Avner ED: New insights into the molecular pathophysiology of polycystic kidney disease. Kidney Int 1999;55:1187.

## Medullary Cystic Disease (Juvenile Nephronophthisis)

Medullary cystic disease is characterized by varying sizes of cysts in the renal medulla and is associated with tubular and interstitial nephritis. Children present with renal failure and signs of tubular dysfunction (decreased concentrating ability, Fanconi syndrome). This lesion should not be confused with medullary sponge kidney (renal tubular ectasia), a frequently asymptomatic disease occurring in adults.

# DISTAL URINARY TRACT ANOMALIES

Obstruction at the ureteropelvic junction may be the result of intrinsic muscle abnormalities, aberrant vessels, or fibrous bands. The lesion can cause hydronephrosis and usually presents as an abdominal mass in the newborn. Obstruction can occur in other parts of the ureter, especially at its entrance into the bladder, with resulting proximal hydroureter and hydronephrosis. Whether intrinsic or extrinsic, urinary tract obstruction should be relieved surgically as soon as possible to minimize damage to the kidneys.

Severe bladder malformations such as exstrophy are clinically obvious and provide a surgical challenge. More subtle—but urgent in terms of diagnosis—is obstruction of urine flow from vestigial posterior urethral valves. This anomaly, which occurs almost exclusively in males, usually presents as anuria or a poor voiding stream in the newborn period, with severe obstruction of urine flow. Ascites may occur, and the kidneys and bladder may be easily palpable. Surgical drainage of urine is urgently required to prevent irreversible damage, if possible.

## Complex Anomalies

Prune belly syndrome is an association of urinary tract anomalies with cryptorchidism and absent abdominal musculature. Although complex anomalies, especially renal dysplasia, usually cause early death or the need for dialysis or transplantation, some patients have lived into the third decade with varying degrees of renal insufficiency. Early urinary diversion is essential to sustain renal function. A renal biopsy at the time of this surgery may predict subsequent renal function.

Other complex malformations and external genital anomalies such as hypospadias are beyond the scope of this text. Overall, urologic abnormalities resulting in severe compromise and destruction of renal tissue provide therapeutic and management challenges aimed at preserving all remaining function and treating the complications of progressive chronic renal failure.

# ■ HEMATURIA & GLOMERULAR DISEASE

Children with painful hematuria should be investigated for urinary tract infection (UTI) or direct injury to the urinary tract. Dysuria commonly suggests cystitis or urethritis; back pain may support the presence of pyelonephritis; and colicky flank pain may mean the passage of a stone. Bright red blood or clots in the urine are associated with bleeding disorders, trauma, and arteriovenous malformations. Abdominal masses suggest the presence of urinary tract obstruction, cystic disease, or tumors involving the renal or perirenal structures.

Asymptomatic hematuria is a challenge because clinical and diagnostic data are required to decide whether to refer the child to a nephrologist. Figure 22–1 delineates the outpatient approach to renal hematuria. The concern regarding the differential diagnosis is the possible presence of glomerular disease.

# GLOMERULONEPHRITIS

## Poststreptococcal Glomerulonephritis

Acute poststreptococcal GN is the most common form of "postinfectious" GN. The epidemiologic relationship between certain strains of streptococci and GN is well recognized. Antigen–antibody complexes are formed in the bloodstream and deposited in the glomeruli. These deposited complexes may incite glomerular inflammation and activate the complement system.

The diagnosis of poststreptococcal disease is supported by a recent history (7–14 days previously) of group A β-hemolytic streptococcal infection. If a positive culture is not available, recent infection may be supported by an elevated antistreptolysin O titer or by high titers of other antistreptococcal antibodies. Other infections can cause similar glomerular injury; thus, "postinfection GN" may be a better term for this type of acute GN. In most cases recovery is expected and usually complete within weeks. In cases when the diagnosis is in some question, or in patients whose renal function progressively deteriorates, a renal biopsy should be performed.

The clinical presentation of GN is usually with gross hematuria (coffee-colored or tea-colored urine), with or without edema (eg, periorbital), which in mild cases occurs secondary to the alteration in glomerular function, resulting in sodium and water retention. Symptoms are usually nonspecific. In cases accompanied by hypertension (a common finding), headache may be present. Fever is uncommon. Severe glomerular injury (which usually occurs in severe, acute presentations of the more chronic or destructive forms of GN) may be accompanied by massive proteinuria (nephrotic syndrome), anasarca or ascites, and severe compromise of renal function.

Typical poststreptococcal GN has no specific treatment. Appropriate antibiotic therapy is indicated if an infection is still present. The disturbances in renal function and resulting hypertension may require close follow-up and management, with reduction in salt intake, treatment with diuretics, or antihypertensive drugs. In severe cases, with profound renal failure, hemodialysis or peritoneal dialysis may be necessary; corticosteroids may also be administered in an attempt to influence the course of the infection.

The acute abnormalities generally resolve in 2–3 weeks; serum complement (C3) may be normal as early as 3 days or as late as 30 days after onset. Although microscopic hematuria may persist for as long as a year, most children recover completely. Persistent deterioration in renal function, urinary abnormalities beyond 18 months, persistent hypocomplementemia, and nephrotic syndrome are ominous signs. If any one of these is present, a renal biopsy is indicated.

## IgA Nephropathy

When asymptomatic gross hematuria appears to accompany a minor acute febrile illness or other stressful occurrence, the diagnosis of IgA nephropathy may be entertained. In contrast to postinfection GN, in IgA nephropathy there is no evidence of prior infection, complement is not depressed, and serum immunoglobin A is elevated in 50% of all cases. Often there are no associated clinical factors. The gross hematuria resolves within days, and there are no serious sequelae in 85% of cases of IgA neprhopathy. Treatment is not indicated, and the prognosis is good in most cases. Prognosis is guarded, however, if severe proteinuria, hypertension, or renal insufficiency is present or ensues. In such instances, treatment is usually attempted. Although no treatment is universally accepted, corticosteroids and other immunosupressive drugs are used. Omega-3 fatty acids present in fish oils are thought to be helpful.

## Henoch–Schönlein Purpura

The diagnosis of Henoch–Schönlein purpura rests on the presence of a typical maculopapular rash found primarily, but not exclusively, on the dorsal surfaces of lower extremities and buttocks. Most children have abdominal pain and bloody diarrhea. Joint pain is common, and, depending on the extent of renal involvement, hypertension may be present. Joint and abdominal pain responds to treatment with corticosteroids. Renal involvement ranges from mild GN with microhematuria to severe GN and varying degrees of renal insufficiency. GN with massive proteinuria and renal insufficiency carries the worst prognosis. Twenty percent of such cases result in end-stage renal failure. There is no universally accepted treatment, but corticosteroids are often administered.

## Membranoproliferative Glomerulonephritis

The most common "chronic" form of GN occurring in children is membranoproliferative GN. The diagnosis is established from the histologic appearance of the glomeruli. The discussion of the various types of this form of GN is complex. Clinically, type II carries the worse prognosis, as end-stage renal failure develops in most cases. Type I more often responds to treatment with corticosteroids. C3 is depressed (in both types) and may be useful as a marker of response to treatment.

The various types of GN have similar manifestations. Table 22–1 lists the most commonly encountered entities in the differential diagnosis of GN in childhood and their clinical and histopathologic descriptions. Severe glomerular histopathologic and clinical entities, such as anti-GBM antibody disease (Good-

***Table 22–1.*** Glomerular diseases encountered in childhood.

| Entity | Clinical Course | Prognosis |
|---|---|---|
| **Postinfection glomerulonephritis.** Onset occurs 10–14 days after acute illness, commonly streptococcal. Characteristics include acute onset, tea-colored urine, mild to severe renal insufficiency, and edema. | Acute phase is usually over in 2 weeks. There is complete resolution in 95% of cases. Severity of renal failure and hypertension varies. Microhematuria may persist to 18 months. Hypocomplementemia resolves in 1–30 d. | Excellent. Chronic disease is rare. Severe proteinuria, atypical presentation or course, or persistent hypocomplementemia suggest another entity. |
| **Membranoproliferative glomerulonephritis.** Presentation ranges from mild microhematuria to acute GN syndrome. Diagnosis is made by renal biopsy. Etiology is unknown. Type I and type II are most common. Lesion is chronic. | Course can be mild to severe (rapid deterioration in renal function); may mimic postinfection GN. Proteinuria can be severe. Complement depression is intermittent to persistent. Hypertension is usually significant. | Type I may respond to corticosteroids. Type II (dense deposit disease) is less treatable; function decrease varies from immediate to as long as 15 y in 30–50% of untreated cases. |
| **IgA nephropathy.** Classic presentation consists of asymptomatic gross hematuria during acute unrelated illness, with microhematuria between episodes. There are occasional instances of acute GN syndrome. Etiology is unknown. Diagnosis is made by biopsy. | 90% of cases resolve in 1–5 y. Gross hematuric episodes resolve with recovery from acute illness. Severity of renal insufficiency and hypertension varies. Proteinuria occurs in more severe, atypical cases. | Generally good. Small percentage develop chronic renal failure. Proteinuria in the nephrotic range is a poor sign. There is no universally accepted medication. (Corticosteroids may be useful in severe cases.) |
| **Henoch–Schönlein purpura glomerulonephritis.** Degree of renal involvement varies. Asymptomatic microhematuria is most common, but GN syndrome can occur. Renal biopsy is recommended in severe cases; it can provide prognostic information. | Presentation varies with severity of renal lesion. In rare cases, may progress rapidly to serious renal failure. Hypertension varies. Proteinuria in the nephrotic range and severe decline in function can occur. | Overall, prognosis is good. Patients presenting with greater than 50% reduction in function or proteinuria exceeding 1 g/24 h may develop chronic renal failure. Severity of renal biopsy picture can best guide approach in such cases. There is no universally accepted medication. |
| **Glomerulonephritis of systemic lupus erythematosus (SLE).** Microhematuria and proteinuria are rarely first signs of this systemic disease. Renal involvement varies. GN often causes the most concern. | Renal involvement is mild to severe. Clinical complexity depends on degree of renal insufficiency and other systems involved. Hypertension is significant. Manifestations of the severity of the renal lesion guide therapeutic intervention. | Renal involvement accounts for most significant morbidity in SLE. Control of hypertension affects renal prognosis. Medication is guided by symptoms, serology, and renal lesion. End-stage renal failure can occur. |
| **Hereditary glomerulonephritis (eg, Alport syndrome).** Transmission is autosomal-dominant/X-linked, with family history marked by end-stage renal failure, especially in young males. Deafness and eye abnormalities are associated. | There is no acute syndrome. Females are generally less affected but are carriers. Hypertension and increasing proteinuria occur with advancing renal failure. There is no known treatment. | Progressive proteinuria and hypertension occur early, with gradual decline in renal function in those most severely affected. Disease progresses to end-stage renal failure in most males. |

pasture syndrome), Wegener granulomatosis, and idiopathic, rapidly progressive GN, may be considered in the differential diagnosis of acute GN. But these disorders are exceedingly rare in children.

## ACUTE INTERSTITIAL NEPHRITIS

Acute interstitial nephritis is characterized by diffuse or focal inflammation and edema of the renal interstitium

and secondary involvement of the tubules. It seems to be related most often to drugs (eg, β-lactam-containing antibiotics, such as methicillin).

Fever, rigor, abdominal or flank pain, and rashes may occur in drug-associated cases. Urinalysis should reveal leukocyturia and hematuria. Hansel staining of the urinary sediment is helpful in demonstrating the presence of eosinophils. The inflammation can be severe enough to cause significant deterioration of renal function. If the diagnosis is unclear from a history of drug or toxin exposure or the presence of eosinophils in the urine, a renal biopsy may be performed to demonstrate the characteristic tubular and interstitial inflammation. Immediate identification and removal of the causative agent is imperative and may be all that is necessary. Treatment with corticosteroids is helpful in cases with progressive renal insufficiency or nephrotic syndrome. Severe renal failure requires supportive dialysis.

## PROTEINURIA & RENAL DISEASE

Urine is not normally completely protein-free, but the average excretion is well below 150 mg/24 h. Small increases in urinary protein can accompany febrile illnesses or exertion and in some cases are produced while in the upright posture (discussed earlier).

An algorithm for investigation of isolated proteinuria is presented in Figure 22–2. In idiopathic nephrotic syndrome without associated features of GN, treatment with corticosteroids may be initiated as described later in this chapter. Nephrologic advice or follow-up should be sought, especially in difficult or frequently relapsing cases.

## CONGENITAL NEPHROSIS

Congenital nephrosis is a rare autosomal recessive disorder. The kidneys are pale and large and may show microcystic dilations (microcystic disease) of the proximal tubules and glomerular changes. The latter consist of proliferation, crescent formation, and thickening of capillary walls. The pathogenesis is not well understood.

Infants with congenital nephrosis commonly have low birth weight, a large placenta, wide cranial sutures, and delayed ossification. Mild edema may be seen after the first few weeks of life. Anasarca follows, and the abdomen can become greatly distended by ascites. Massive proteinuria associated with typical-appearing nephrotic syndrome and hyperlipidemia is the rule. Hematuria is common. If the patient lives long enough, progressive renal failure occurs. Most affected infants succumb to infections at the age of a few months.

Treatment prior to dialysis and transplantation has little to offer other than nutritional support and management of the chronic renal failure.

## IDIOPATHIC NEPHROTIC SYNDROME OF CHILDHOOD (Nil Disease, Lipoid Nephrosis, Minimal Change Disease)

Nephrotic syndrome is characterized by proteinuria, hypoproteinemia, edema, and hyperlipidemia. It may occur as a result of any form of glomerular disease and may rarely be associated with a variety of extrarenal conditions. In young children, the disease usually takes the form of idiopathic nephrotic syndrome of childhood (nil disease, lipoid nephrosis, minimal change disease), which has characteristic clinical and laboratory findings, but no well-understood cause.

### Clinical Findings

Affected patients are generally younger than age 6 years at the time of their first episode. Often following an influenza-like syndrome, periorbital swelling and perhaps oliguria are noticed. Within a few days, increasing edema—even anasarca—becomes evident. Other than vague malaise and occasionally abdominal pain, complaints are few. With significant "third spacing" of plasma volume, however, some children may present with hypotension. With marked edema, dyspnea due to pleural effusions may also occur.

Despite heavy proteinuria, the urine sediment is usually normal, although microscopic hematuria (< 20 RBC/high-power field) may be present. Plasma albumin levels are low, and lipid levels are increased. When azotemia occurs, it is usually secondary to intravascular volume depletion rather than to impairment of function.

Glomerular morphology is unremarkable except for fusion of foot processes of the glomerular basement membrane. This finding, however, is nonspecific and is associated with many proteinuric states. Changes in the glomerular mesangium may be minimal, with unremarkable findings on immunofluorescence and electron microscopic examination.

### Complications

Infections (eg, peritonitis) sometimes occur, and pneumococci are frequently the cause. Hypercoagulability may be present, and thromboembolic phenomena are commonly reported. Hypertension and varying degrees of renal insufficiency are often encountered. In cases of minimal-change disease (no significant glomerular lesions are demonstrated), hypertension can still be noted and renal insufficiency is primarily due to decreased renal perfusion.

### Treatment & Prognosis

As soon as the diagnosis of idiopathic nephrotic syndrome is made, corticosteroid treatment should be started. Prednisone, 2 mg/kg/d (maximum, 60 mg/d), is given as a single daily dose until the urine protein falls to trace or negative levels for a maximum of 8 weeks. The same dose is then administered on an alternate-day schedule for 6 weeks; thereafter, the dose is tapered gradually and discontinued over the ensuing 2 months. If remission is achieved, only to be followed by relapse, the treatment course may be repeated. If at any time the nephrosis becomes refractory to treatment or if three relapses occur within 1 year, renal biopsy may be considered. A renal biopsy is also often considered when there is little or no response to treatment. One should take into account that the histologic findings may not alter the treatment plan, which is more often influenced by the need to eliminate the nephrotic syndrome regardless of underlying renal histology.

Unless the edema is symptomatic (eg, respiratory compromise due to ascites), diuretics should be used with extreme care; patients may have decreased circulating volume and are also at risk for intravenous thrombosis. However, careful restoration of compromised circulating volume with intravenous albumin infusion and administration of diuretics is helpful in mobilizing edema. Infections (eg, acute peritonitis) should be treated promptly to reduce morbidity. Immunization with pneumoccocal vaccine is advised.

The initial response to corticosteroids is a guide to prognosis. A prompt remission lasting for over 1 year is almost always permanent. Failure to respond or early relapse usually heralds a prolonged series of relapses. This not only may indicate the presence of more serious nephropathy, but it presents a challenge in choosing future therapy. Chlorambucil or cyclophosphamide drug therapy is predictably successful only in children who respond to corticosteroids. Patients who do not respond to corticosteroids or who relapse frequently should be referred to a pediatric nephrologist. Intravenous solumedrol in more refractory cases has been shown to be helpful. In some cases, when the continued usage of corticostersoids alone is unsuccessful and raises concerns of toxicity, concomitant treatment with either cyclosporin A or tacrolimus appears to be helpful.

Chesney RW: The idiopathic nephrotic syndrome. Curr Opin Pediatr 1999;11:158.

## FOCAL GLOMERULAR SCLEROSIS

Focal glomerular sclerosis is one cause of corticosteroid-resistant or frequent relapsing nephrotic syndrome. The cause is unknown. The diagnosis is made by renal biopsy, which shows normal-appearing glomeruli as well as some partially or completely sclerosed glomeruli. The lesion has serious prognostic implications because as many as 15–20% of cases can progress to end-stage renal failure. The clinical response to corticosteroid treatment is variable. In difficult cases, cyclosporin A or tacrolimus has been used in addition to corticosteroids.

## MESANGIAL NEPHROPATHY (Mesangial Glomerulonephritis)

Mesangial nephropathy is another form of corticosteroid-resistant nephrotic syndrome. The renal biopsy shows a distinct increase in the mesangial matrix of the glomeruli. Very often the expanded mesangium contains deposits of IgM demonstrable on immunofluorescent staining. The cause is unknown. Corticosteroid therapy may induce remission, but relapses are common. Choices for treating this type of nephrotic syndrome are the same as noted earlier.

## MEMBRANOUS NEPHROPATHY (Membranous Glomerulonephritis)

Although largely idiopathic in nature, membranous nephropathy can be found in association with diseases such as hepatitis B antigenemia, systemic lupus erythematosus, congenital and secondary syphilis, and renal vein thrombosis; with immunologic disorders such as autoimmune thyroiditis; and with administration of drugs such as penicillamine. The pathogenesis is unknown, but the glomerular lesion is thought to be the result of prolonged deposition of circulating antigen–antibody complexes.

The onset of membranous nephropathy may be insidious or may resemble that of idiopathic nephrotic syndrome of childhood (see preceding section). It occurs more often in older children and adults. The proteinuria of membranous nephropathy responds little if at all to corticosteroid therapy. Low-dose corticosteroid therapy, however, has been shown to reduce or delay development of chronic renal insufficiency. The diagnosis is made by renal biopsy.

# ■ DISEASES OF THE RENAL VESSELS

## RENAL VEIN THROMBOSIS

In the newborn period, renal vein thrombosis may complicate sepsis or dehydration. It may be observed in an infant of a diabetic mother, or it may be the result of umbilical vein catheterization. It may result from any condition that produces a hypercoagulable state (eg, clotting factor deficiency, systemic lupus erythematosus, or thrombocytosis). Renal vein thrombosis is less common in older children and adolescents; it may develop following trauma or without any apparent predisposing factors. Nephrotic syndrome may either cause or result from renal vein thrombosis. Spontaneous renal vein thrombosis has been associated with membranous glomerulonephropathy.

## Clinical Findings

Renal vein thrombosis in newborns is generally characterized by the sudden development of an abdominal mass. If the thrombosis is bilateral, oliguria may be present; urine output may be normal with a unilateral thrombus. In older children, flank pain, sometimes with a palpable mass, is a common presentation.

No single laboratory test is diagnostic of renal vein thrombosis. Hematuria usually is present. Proteinuria is less constant. In the newborn, thrombocytopenia may be found; this is rare in older children. The diagnosis is made by ultrasonography and Doppler flow studies.

## Treatment

Anticoagulation with heparin is the treatment of choice both in newborns and in older children. In the newborn, a course of heparin combined with treatment of the underlying problem is usually all that is required. Management in other cases is less straightforward. The tendency for recurrence and embolization has led some to recommend long-term anticoagulation. If an underlying membranous GN is suspected, biopsy should be performed.

## Course & Prognosis

The mortality rate in newborns from renal vein thrombosis depends on the underlying cause. With unilateral thromboses, the prognosis for adequate renal function is good. Renal vein thrombosis may rarely recur in the same kidney or occur in the other kidney years after the original episode of thrombus formation. Extension into the vena cava, with pulmonary emboli, is possible.

## RENAL ARTERIAL DISEASE

Arterial disease (eg, fibromuscular hyperplasia and congenital stenosis) is a rare cause of hypertension in children. Although there are few clinical clues to underlying arterial lesions, arterial lesions should be suspected in children whose hypertension is severe, with onset at or before age 10 years, or associated with delayed visualization with nuclear medicine scan. The diagnosis is established by renal arteriography with selective renal vein renin measurements. Some of these lesions may be approached by transluminal angioplasty or surgery (see Renal Hypertension section), but repair may be technically impossible in many small children. Although thrombosis of renal arteries is rare, it should be considered in a patient experiencing acute onset of hypertension and hematuria in an appropriate setting (eg, in as-

sociation with hyperviscosity or umbilical artery catheterization). Early diagnosis and treatment (eg, heparin) provides the best chance of reestablishing renal blood flow.

## HEMOLYTIC–UREMIC SYNDROME

Hemolytic–uremic syndrome is the most common glomerular vascular cause of acute renal failure in childhood. It is usually the result of infection with Shiga-toxin-producing (also called verotoxin-producing) strains of *Shigella* or *Escherichia coli*. There are many serotypes, but the most common pathogen in the United States is *E coli* 0157:H7. Bloody diarrhea is the usual presenting complaint, followed by hemolysis and renal failure. Circulating verotoxin causes endothelial damage, which leads to platelet deposition, microvascular occlusion with subsequent hemolysis, and thrombocytopenia. Ingestion of undercooked ground beef or unpasteurized foods is a common cause. Such microvascular endothelial activation may also be triggered by some drugs (eg, cyclosporin A); by viruses (human immunodeficiency virus [HIV]); and by pneumococcal infections, in which bacterial neuraminidase exposes the Thomsen–Friedenrich antigen on red cells, platelets, and endothelial cells, thereby causing platelet aggregation, endothelial damage, and hemolysis. Rare cases are caused by predisposing genetic factors (eg, congenitally depressed C3 complement and factor H deficiency).

## Clinical Findings

The epidemic form begins with a prodrome of abdominal pain, diarrhea, and vomiting. Oliguria, pallor, and bleeding manifestations, principally gastrointestinal, occur next. Hypertension and seizures develop in some children—especially those who develop severe renal failure and fluid overload. There may also be significant direct involvement of the central nervous system (CNS).

Anemia is profound, and red blood cell fragments are seen on blood smears. A high reticulocyte count confirms the hemolytic nature of the anemia, but may not be noted in the presence of renal failure. Thrombocytopenia is profound, but other coagulation abnormalities are less consistent. Serum fibrin split products are often present, but fulminant disseminated intravascular coagulation is rare. Hematuria and proteinuria are often present. The serum complement level is normal except in those cases related to congenital predisposition.

## Complications

These usually result from renal failure. Neurologic problems, particularly seizures, may result from electrolyte abnormalities such as hyponatremia, hypertension, or from CNS vascular disease. Severe bleeding, transfusion requirements, and hospital-acquired infections must be anticipated.

## Treatment

Meticulous attention to fluid and electrolyte status is crucial. The use of antimotility agents and antibiotics is believed to worsen the disease. Antibiotics may up-regulate and cause the release of large amounts of bacterial Shiga toxin. Early dialysis improves the prognosis; the patient's size will usually dictate peritoneal dialysis as the technique of choice. Seizures usually respond to control of hypertension and electrolyte abnormalities. It has been suggested that the plasma in some cases lacks a prostacyclin-stimulating factor that is a potent inhibitor of platelet aggregation. Therefore, plasma infusion or plasmapheresis has been advocated in severe cases. Platelet inhibitors have also been tried, but the results have not been impressive, especially late in the disease. Nonetheless, it appears that using a platelet inhibitor early in the disease in an attempt to halt platelet consumption and microvascular occlusion may obviate the need for platelet transfusion and reduce the progression of renal failure. Red cell and platelet transfusions may be necessary; although the risk of volume overload is significant, it can be minimized by dialysis. Erythropoietin (epoetin alfa) treatment may reduce red cell transfusion needs. Although no therapy is universally accepted for patients with this syndrome, the strict control of hypertension and nutrition and the timely use of dialysis reduce morbidity and mortality. If renal failure is "nonoliguric," and thus output is sufficient to ensure against fluid overload and electrolyte abnormalities, management of renal failure without dialysis is possible.

## Course & Prognosis

Most commonly, children recover from the acute episode within 2–3 weeks. Some form of residual renal disease (including hypertension) occurs in about 30%, and end-stage renal failure in about 15%. Thus follow-up of children recovering from hemolytic–uremic syndrome should include serial determinations of renal function for 1–2 years and meticulous attention to blood pressure for 5 years. Mortality (about 3–5%) is of greatest concern in the early phase, primarily resulting from CNS complications.

Trachtman H, Christen E: Pathogenesis, treatment, and therapeutic trials in hemolytic uremic syndrome. Curr Opin Pediatr 1999;11:162.

# ■ RENAL FAILURE

## ACUTE RENAL FAILURE

Acute renal failure is the sudden inability to excrete urine of sufficient quantity or adequate composition to maintain body fluid homeostasis. The most common cause in children is dehydration. However, encountering signs of acute renal insufficiency in a hospitalized patient raises many other possibilities: impaired renal perfusion or renal ischemia, acute renal disease, renal vascular compromise, acute tubular necrosis, or obstructive uropathy. Table 22–2 lists such prerenal, renal, and postrenal causes.

## Clinical Findings

The hallmark of early renal failure is oliguria. Although an exact etiologic diagnosis may be unclear at the onset,

**Table 22–2.** Classification of renal failure.

**Prerenal**
　Dehydration due to gastroenteritis, malnutrition, or diarrhea
　Hemorrhage, aortic or renal vessel injury, trauma, cardiac disease and/or surgery, renal arterial thrombosis
　Diabetic acidosis
　Hypovolemia associated with capillary leak or nephrotic syndrome
　Shock
　Heart failure
**Renal**
　Hemolytic-uremic syndrome
　Acute glomerulonephritis
　Prolonged renal hypoperfusion
　Nephrotoxins
　Acute tubular necrosis or vascular nephropathy
　Renal (cortical) necrosis
　Intravascular coagulation—septic shock, hemorrhage
　Diseases of renal vessels
　Iatrogenic disorders
　Severe infections
　Drowning, especially fresh water
　Crystalluria: sulfonamide or uric acid
　Hyperuricacidemia from cancer treatment
　Hepatic failure
**Postrenal**
　Obstruction due to tumor, hematoma, posterior urethral valves, ureteropelvic junction stricture, ureterovesical junction stricture, ureterocele
　Stones
　Trauma to a solitary kidney or collecting system
　Renal vein thrombosis

classifying the oliguria as outlined in Table 22–2 is helpful in determining if any immediately reversible causes are present.

If the cause of an elevation in serum BUN and creatinine or oliguria is unclear, entities that can be quickly addressed and corrected (eg, volume depletion) should be considered first. Once normal renal perfusion is ensured and no clinical evidence for de novo renal disease is present, a diagnosis of acute tubular necrosis (vasomotor nephropathy, ischemic injury) may be entertained.

### A. PRERENAL CAUSES

The most common cause of decreased renal function in children is compromised renal perfusion. It is usually secondary to dehydration, although abnormalities of renal vasculature and poor cardiac performance may also be considered. Such causes should be sought and, if present, corrected to determine if true renal functional disturbances are present. Table 22–3 lists the urinary indices helpful in distinguishing these "prerenal" conditions from true renal parenchymal diseases, such as acute tubular necrosis.

### B. RENAL CAUSES

Causes of renal failure intrinsic to the kidney include acute glomerulonephritides, hemolytic–uremic syndrome, acute interstitial nephritis, and nephrotoxic injury. The diagnosis of acute tubular necrosis (vasomotor nephropathy)—which is reserved for those cases in which renal ischemic insult is believed to be the likely cause—should be considered when correction of prerenal or postrenal problems does not improve renal function.

### C. POSTRENAL CAUSES

Postrenal failure, usually found in newborns with urologic anatomic abnormalities, is accompanied by varying degrees of renal insufficiency. Obstruction of the bladder outlet, as in posterior urethral valves, should be relieved by insertion of a urethral catheter followed by surgical correction. Timely intervention may prevent irreversible renal injury and chronic renal failure. Delayed voiding in the newborn period, anuria, or poor urinary stream usually suggests obstruction. Ureteropelvic junctional obstruction usually presents as an abdominal mass.

## Complications

The clinical severity of the complications depends on the degree of renal functional impairment and oliguria. Common complications include (1) fluid overload (hypertension, congestive heart failure, pulmonary edema), (2) electrolyte disturbances (hyperkalemia), (3) metabolic acidosis, (4) hyperphosphatemia, and (5) uremia.

## Treatment

An indwelling bladder catheter is inserted to ascertain urine output. If urine volume is insignificant and renal failure is established, the catheter should be removed to minimize infection risks. Prerenal or postrenal factors should be excluded or rectified, and normal circulating volume established and maintained with appropriate fluids. Strict measurements of volume input and output must be maintained, and adjustments made to reduce input as reduction in output dictates. The patient's response is assessed by physical examination and measurement of urinary output. Measurement of central venous pressure may be indicated. If diuresis does not occur in response to these measures, furosemide (1–5 mg/kg, per dose, intravenously, maximum of 200 mg) may be used. The effective dose will depend on the amount of functional compromise (if < 50% function, initiate attempt at diuresis with maximum dose). If a response does not occur within 1 hour (ie, the urine output remains low [< 0.5 mL/kg/h]), the furosemide dose, if not already at maximum, should be increased up to 5 mg/kg. In some cases the addition of a long-acting thiazide diuretic, such as metolazone, may be useful. If no diuresis occurs with maximum dosing, further administration of diuretics will not be helpful.

If these maneuvers stimulate some urine flow but biochemical evidence of acute renal failure persists, the resulting nonoliguric acute renal failure should be more manageable. Fluid overload and dialysis may be averted. However, if the medications and nutrients required exceed the urinary output, dialysis is indicated. Institution of dialysis before the early complications of acute renal failure develop is likely to improve clinical management and outcome. It is important to adjust medication dosage according to the degree of renal function.

**Table 22–3.** Urine studies.

| Prerenal Failure | Acute Tubular Necrosis |
| --- | --- |
| Urine osmolality 50 mOsm/kg greater than plasma osmolality | Urine osmolality equal to or less than plasma osmolality |
| Urine sodium < 10 mEq/L | Urinary sodium > 20 mEq/L |
| Ratio of urine creatinine to plasma creatinine > 14:1 | Ratio of urine creatinine to plasma creatinine < 14:1 |
| Specific gravity > 1.020 | Specific gravity 1.012–1.018 |

## Acute Dialysis

### A. INDICATIONS FOR DIALYSIS

Immediate indications for dialysis are (1) severe hyperkalemia; (2) unrelenting metabolic acidosis (usually in a situation where fluid overload prevents sodium bicarbonate administration); (3) fluid overload with or without severe hypertension or congestive heart failure (a situation that would seriously compromise nutrition or drug administration); and (4) symptoms of uremia, usually manifested in children by CNS depression. The rate of rise of both urea nitrogen and creatinine levels may indicate the need for dialysis; it is generally accepted that the urea nitrogen level should not be allowed to exceed 100 mg/dL (keeping in mind nonrenal functional factors contributing to excessive BUN) in small children.

### B. METHODS OF DIALYSIS

The choice between peritoneal dialysis and hemodialysis may be dictated by their availability. Peritoneal dialysis is generally preferred in children because of the ease of performance and patient tolerance. Although peritoneal dialysis is technically less efficient than hemodialysis, hemodynamic stability and metabolic control can be better sustained because this technique can be applied on a relatively continuous basis. However, hemodialysis should be considered (1) if rapid removal of toxins is desired, (2) if the size of the patient makes hemodialysis less technically cumbersome and hemodynamically well tolerated, or (3) if impediments to efficient peritoneal dialysis are present (eg, ileus). Furthermore, if vascular access and usage of anticoagulation are not impediments, a slow, continuous hemodialytic process (continuous renal replacement treatment) may be applied, if the technical expertise is available.

### C. COMPLICATIONS OF DIALYSIS

Complications of peritoneal dialysis include peritonitis, volume depletion, and technical complications such as dialysate leakage and respiratory compromise from intraabdominal dialysate fluid. Peritonitis can be avoided by strict observance of aseptic technique. Peritoneal fluid cultures are obtained as clinically indicated. Dialysate can leak around the dialysis catheter or through tissue planes, causing dissection. Leakage is reduced by good catheter placement technique and appropriate intra-abdominal dialysate volumes. Technical problems causing abnormal flow of dialysate in and out of the peritoneal cavity require help from a nephrologist. Dialysis is useful in maintaining electrolyte balance. Potassium (absent from standard dialysis solutions) can be added to the dialysate as required. Phosphate is also absent because hyperphosphatemia is an expected problem in renal failure. Nonetheless, if phosphate intake is inade-

quate, hypophosphatemia must be addressed. High dextrose concentrations (maximum 4.25%) can correct fluid overload rapidly at the risk of causing hyperglycemia. Fluid removal may be increased with more frequent exchanges of the dialysate, but rapid osmotic transfer of water may result in hypernatremia.

Even in small infants, hemodialysis can rapidly correct major metabolic and electrolyte disturbances, as well as volume overload. The process is highly efficient, but the speed of the changes can cause problems such as hemodynamic instability. Anticoagulation is usually required. Careful monitoring of the appropriate biochemical parameters is important. Note that during or immediately following the procedure, blood sampling will produce misleading results because equilibration between extravascular compartments and the blood will not yet have been completed. Vascular access must be obtained and carefully monitored.

## Course & Prognosis

The period of severe oliguria, if it occurs, usually lasts about 10 days. Oliguria lasting longer than 3 weeks, or anuria, makes a diagnosis of acute tubular necrosis very unlikely and favors vascular injury, severe ischemia (cortical necrosis), GN, or obstruction. The diuretic phase begins with an increase in urinary output to passage of large volumes of isosthenuric urine containing sodium levels of 80–150 mEq/L. During the recovery phase, signs and symptoms subside rapidly, although polyuria may persist for several days or weeks. Urinary abnormalities usually disappear completely within a few months. If renal recovery does not ensue, arrangements are made for chronic dialysis and eventual renal transplantation.

## CHRONIC RENAL FAILURE

Chronic renal failure in children most commonly results from developmental abnormalities of the kidneys or urinary tract. The kidneys may develop poorly (dysgenesis) or not at all (agenesis). Cystic development may result in immediate or progressive insufficiency. Abnormal development of the urinary tract may not permit normal renal development. Obstructive uropathy or severe vesicoureteral reflux nephropathy, without (or despite) surgical intervention, continues to cause a significant amount of progressive renal insufficiency in children. In older children, the chronic glomerulonephritides and nephropathies, irreversible nephrotoxic injury, or hemolytic–uremic syndrome may also result in chronic renal failure.

When chronic renal failure is the result of an inadequate amount of normally functioning renal tissue, the inability to concentrate urine results in polyuria, polydipsia, or enuresis. Affected patients often fail to thrive. Without medical care, children with long-standing chronic renal failure may present with complications such as rickets or anemia.

Chronic renal failure may follow acute GN or develop with chronic GN in the absence of an obvious acute episode. Presentations range from hypertension to overt uremic symptoms. Growth failure depends on age at presentation and the rapidity of functional decline. Some of the chronic glomerulonephritides (eg, membranoproliferative GN) can progress unnoticed if subtle abnormalities of the urinary sediment are undetected or ignored. Any child with a history of chronic GN or significant renal injury needs close follow-up and monitoring of renal function. Angiotensin-converting enzyme (ACE) inhibitors decrease the glomerulosclerosis that follows glomerular injury and are often used to treat the associated hypertension.

## Complications

The kidney can compensate for gradual loss of functioning nephrons in progressive chronic renal failure until the GFR falls below 15 mL/min/1.73 m$^2$. Complications appear as compensatory power is lost. In children who have developmentally reduced function but are unable to concentrate the urine, polyuria and thus dehydration is more likely to be a problem than fluid overload. Output may be expected to gradually diminish with time as renal failure progresses to end stage; however, some children can continue to produce generous quantities of urine (but not of good quality) even though they require dialysis. Moreover, a salt-wasting state can occur. In contrast, children who develop chronic renal failure due to the glomerular disease or renal injury will characteristically retain sodium and water so that hypertension occurs relatively early.

Metabolic acidosis and growth retardation occur early in chronic renal failure. Disturbances in calcium, phosphorus, and vitamin D metabolism leading to renal osteodystrophy require prompt attention. Although renal compensation and increased parathyroid hormone can maintain a normal serum phosphate level early in the course, secondary hyperparathyroidism with resulting skeletal abnormalities will occur. This physiologic response to hyperphosphatemia can be reflected by an increase in serum alkaline phosphatase, but measurement of intact parathyroid hormone is more clinically specific.

Uremic symptoms occur late in chronic renal failure and include anorexia, nausea, and malaise. CNS features range from confusion, apathy, and lethargy to stupor and coma. Associated electrolyte abnormalities may precipitate seizures (more commonly, a result of untreated hypertension). Anemia (normochromic and normocytic from decreased renal erythropoietin synthesis) is usual. Platelet dysfunction and other abnormalities of the coagulation system may be present. Bleeding phenomena—especially gastrointestinal bleeding—may be a problem. Cardiovascular manifestations may be life-threatening. Uremic pericarditis, congestive heart failure, or hypertension may occur.

## Treatment

Treatment of chronic renal failure before dialysis is done to preserve remaining renal function and to avoid complications. Controlling hypertension (see Renal Hypertension section) and hyperphosphatemia and preventing UTI are important. Acidosis may be treated with sodium citrate solutions, as long as the added sodium will not aggravate hypertension. Sodium restriction is advisable when hypertension is present. Hyperphosphatemia is controlled by dietary restriction and dietary phosphate binders (eg, calcium carbonate). Vitamin D should be given to maintain normal serum calcium. When the BUN level exceeds approximately 50 mg/dL, or if the child is lethargic or anorexic, dietary protein should be restricted. Potassium restriction will be necessary as the GFR falls to a level where urinary output decreases sharply. Meanwhile, the diet must continue to provide the child's specific daily requirements.

Renal function must be monitored regularly (creatinine and BUN), and serum electrolytes, calcium, phosphorus, alkaline phosphatase, and hemoglobin and hematocrit levels must be checked. Results guide changes in fluid and dietary management as well as dosages of phosphate binder, citrate buffer, vitamin D, and blood pressure medications. Anemia may be treated with epoetin alfa. These treatment areas require careful monitoring to minimize symptoms while the child's need for chronic dialysis and transplantation continues to be assessed.

Care must be taken to avoid medications that aggravate hypertension; increase the body burden of sodium, potassium, or phosphate; or increase production of BUN. Successful management relies greatly on education of the patient and family.

Attention must also be directed toward the psychosocial needs of the patient and family during adjustment to chronic illness. The strategy for patient management—and the need for family education and adjustment—changes when a plan for chronic dialysis and possible renal transplantation is initiated. These changes may include a reduction in medications or dietary limitations, with the potential for improving growth. Some uremic children will grow significantly when given human recombinant growth hormone.

## Dialysis & Transplantation

The best tolerated treatment of end-stage renal disease in a child is a successful and uncomplicated renal transplant. The North American Pediatric Renal Transplant Collaborative Study reports a 1-year graft survival rate of living-related kidney transplants of 90%, with 85% at 2 years and 75% at 5 years. With cadaveric transplantation, percentages of graft survivals are 76%, 71%, and 62%, respectively. Overall, the mortality rate is 4% for recipients of living-related donors and 6.8% for recipients of cadaver organs. These percentages are affected by the increased mortality, reported to be as high as 75% in infants younger than age 1 year, primarily due to technical issues and complications of immunosuppression. Therefore, most transplantation centers are waiting until infants reach a body weight of about 15 kg. This body weight appears to be associated with a significantly improved survival rate. Adequate growth and well-being are directly related to acceptance of the graft, the degree of normal function, and the side effects of medications.

Great advances have also been made in peritoneal dialysis and hemodialysis, both in technique and in our understanding of the specialized approach required. Hemodialysis is now performed in major centers that devote their entire effort to the treatment of pediatric patients and is regarded as a reasonable long-range method of treating the older child with end-stage renal disease. The demonstrated feasibility of chronic peritoneal dialysis in children, however, has made it the primary choice of dialysis therapy, especially for small children. It is well accepted and can be performed in the home.

The best measure of the success of chronic dialysis in children is the level of physical and psychosocial rehabilitation achieved. Patients continue to participate in day-to-day activities and attend school. Although catch-up growth rarely occurs, patients can grow at an acceptable rate even though they may remain in the lower percentiles. Use of epoetin alfa, growth hormone, and better control of renal osteodystrophy contribute to improved outcome.

Neu AM, Warady BA: Dialysis and renal transplantation in infants with irreversible renal failure. Adv Ren Replace Ther 1996;3:48.

Warady BA et al: Optimal care of the pediatric end-stage renal disease patient on dialysis. Am J Kidney Dis 1999;33:567.

## RENAL HYPERTENSION

Hypertension in children is commonly of renal origin. It is anticipated as a complication of known renal parenchymal disease, but it may be found on routine physical examination in an otherwise normal child. Increased understanding of the roles of water and salt retention on the one hand and overactivity of the renin–angiotensin system on the other has done much to guide therapy; nevertheless, not all forms of hypertension can be explained by these two mechanisms.

The causes of renal hypertension in the newborn period include (1) congenital anomalies of the kidneys or renal vasculature, (2) obstruction of the urinary tract, (3) thrombosis of renal vasculature or kidneys, and (4) volume overload. Some instances of apparent paradoxic elevations of blood pressure have been reported in clinical situations in which chronic diuretic therapy is used, such as in bronchopulmonary dysplasia. Hypertensive infants should also be examined for renal, vascular, or aortic abnormalities (eg, thrombosis, neurofibromatosis, coarctation) as well as some endocrine disorders.

### Diagnosis

A child is normotensive if the average recorded systolic and diastolic blood pressures are lower than the 90th percentile for age and sex. The 90th percentile in the newborn period is approximately 85–90/55–65 mm Hg for both sexes. In the first year of life, the acceptable levels are 90–100/60–67 mm Hg. Incremental increases with growth occur, gradually approaching young adult ranges of 100–120/65–75 mm Hg in the late teens. Careful measurement of blood pressure includes ensuring correct cuff size and reliable equipment. The cuff should be wide enough to cover two thirds of the upper arm and should encircle the arm completely without causing an overlap in the inflatable bladder. Although an anxious child may have an elevation in blood pressure, abnormal readings must not be too hastily attributed to this cause. Repeat measurement is helpful, especially after the child has been consoled.

Routine laboratory studies include a complete blood count, urinalysis, and urine culture. Radiography and ultrasonography are used to study the anatomy of the urinary tract, the blood flow to the kidneys, and their function. A renal biopsy (which rarely reveals the cause of hypertension unless clinical evidence of renal disease is present) should always be undertaken with special care in the hypertensive patient and preferably after pressures have been controlled by therapy. Figure 22–3 presents a suggested approach to the outpatient work-up of hypertension.

### Treatment

#### A. TREATMENT OF ACUTE EMERGENT HYPERTENSION

A hypertensive emergency exists when CNS signs of hypertension appear, such as papilledema or encephalopathy. Retinal hemorrhages or exudates indicate a need for prompt and effective control. In children, however,

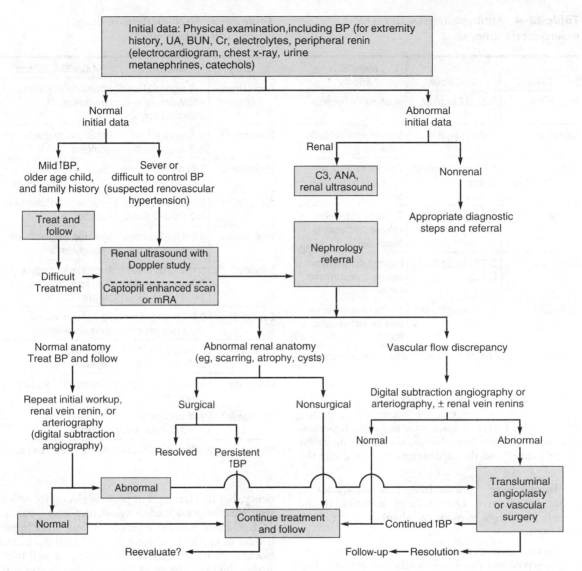

**Figure 22–3.** Approach to the outpatient work-up of hypertension. ANA = antinuclear antibody; BUN = blood urea nitrogen; Cr = creatinine.

end-organ abnormalities secondary to hypertension commonly are not present. Treatment varies with the clinical presentation. The primary classes of useful antihypertensive drugs are (1) diuretics, (2) α- and β-adrenergic blockers, (3) ACE inhibitors, (4) calcium channel blockers, and (5) vasodilators.

Whatever method is used to control emergent hypertension, medications for sustained control should also be initiated so that the effect will be maintained when the emergent measures are discontinued (Table 22–4). Acute elevations of blood pressure not exceeding

the 95th percentile for age may be treated with oral antihypertensives, aiming for progressive improvement and control within 48 hours.

**1. Sublingual nifedipine**—This calcium channel blocker is rapid acting, and, in appropriate doses, should not result in hypotensive blood pressure levels. The liquid from a 10-mg capsule can be drawn into a syringe and the dosage approximated. The exact dosage for children who weigh less than 10–30 kg is difficult to ascertain by this method, but 5 mg is a safe starting

**Table 22–4.** Antihypertensive drugs for emergent treatment.

| Drug | Oral Dose | Major Side Effects[a] |
|---|---|---|
| Nifedipine | 0.25–0.5 mg/kg/ SL | Flushing, tachycardia |
| Labetalol | 1–3 mg/kg/h IV | Secondary to β-blocking activity |
| Sodium nitroprusside | 0.5–10 mg/kg/min IV drip | Cyanide toxicity, sodium and water retention |
| Furosemide | 1–5 mg/kg IV | Secondary to severe volume contraction, hypokalemia |
| Diazoxide | 2–10 mg/kg IV bolus | Hyperglycemia, hyperuricemia, sodium and water retention |
| Hydralazine | 0.1–0.2 mg/kg IV | Sodium and water retention, tachycardia, flushing |

[a]Many more side effects than those listed have been reported.

**Table 22–5.** Antihypertensive drugs for ambulatory treatment.

| Drug | Oral Dose | Major Side Effects[a] |
|---|---|---|
| Hydrochloro-thiazide | 2–4 mg/kg/24 h as single dose or in 2 individual doses | Potassium depletion, hyperuricemia |
| Furosemide | 1–5 mg/kg/dose, 2–3 doses per day | Potassium and volume depletion |
| Hydralazine | 0.75 mg/kg/24 h in 4–6 divided doses | Lupus erythematosus, tachycardia, headache |
| Amlodipine | 0.2 to 0.5 mg/kg/d in 2 divided doses | Fatigue, headache, facial flushing |
| Propranolol | 0.2–5 mg/kg/dose, 2–3 doses per day | Syncope, cardiac failure, hypoglycemia |
| Minoxidil | 0.15 mg/kg/dose, 2–3 doses per day | Tachycardia, angina, fluid retention, hirsutism |
| Captopril | 0.3–2 mg/kg/dose, 2–3 doses per day | Rash, hyperkalemia, glomerulopathy |
| Enalapril | 0.2–0.5 mg/kg/d in 2 divided doses | Proteinuria, cough, hyperkalemia |
| Nifedipine | 0.5–1 mg/kg/d, 3 doses per day | Flushing, tachycardia |
| Verapamil | 3–7 mg/kg/d in 2 or 3 divided doses | AV conduction disturbance |

[a]Many more side effects than those listed have been reported.

point. Because the treatment is given for rising blood pressure, it is unlikely that the effects will be greater than desired. Larger children with malignant hypertension require 10 mg. In such cases, the capsule may simply be pierced and the medication squeezed under the patient's tongue.

**2. Intravenous hydralazine**—This vasodilator is sometimes effective. Dosage varies according to the severity of the hypertension and should begin at about 0.15 mg/kg.

**3. Sodium nitroprusside**—In an intensive care setting, this powerful vasodilator is very effective for reducing severely elevated blood pressure. Intravenous administration of 0.5–10 mg/kg/min will reduce blood pressure in seconds, and the dose must be monitored carefully. Metabolism of the drug results in thiocyanate; thus, with prolonged usage, levels of thiocyanate must be monitored, especially in renal insufficiency.

**4. Furosemide**—Administered at 1–5 mg/kg, intravenously, this diuretic will reduce blood volume and enhance the effectiveness of antihypertensive drugs.

## B. TREATMENT OF SUSTAINED HYPERTENSION

Several choices are available (Table 22–5). A single drug such as a β-blocker (unless contraindicated, eg, in reactive airway disease) may be adequate to treat mild hypertension. Diuretics are useful to treat renal insuffi-

ciency, but disadvantages of possible electrolyte imbalance must be considered. Single-drug therapy with an ACE inhibitor is useful, especially because most hypertension in children has renal causes. Calcium channel blockers are increasingly useful, and appear well tolerated in children. The use of the vasodilator type of antihypertensive drug requires concomitant administration of a diuretic to counter the effect of vasodilation on increasing renal sodium and water retention and a β-blocker to counter reflex tachycardia. Minoxidil, considered the most powerful of the orally administered vasodilators, can be extremely efficacious in the treatment of severe, sustained hypertension, but its effect is greatly offset by the other effects described. Hirsutism is a significant side effect. Hydralazine hydrochloride may still be the most common vasodilator in pediatric use—but, again, the necessity of using two additional drugs for maximum benefit keeps vasodilators in reserve for those severe situations calling for management with three or four drugs. The advice of a pediatric nephrologist should be sought.

Bartosh SM, Aronson AJ: Childhood hypertension. An update on etiology, diagnosis and treatment. Pediatr Clin North Am 1999;46:235.

# ■ INHERITED OR DEVELOPMENTAL DEFECTS OF THE URINARY TRACT

There are many developmental, hereditary, or metabolic defects of the kidneys and collecting system. The clinical consequences include metabolic abnormalities, failure to thrive, nephrolithiasis, renal glomerular or tubular dysfunction, and chronic renal failure. Table 22–6 lists some of the major entities; discussion of the rarer conditions is beyond the scope of this book.

## DISORDERS OF THE RENAL TUBULES

Three subtypes of renal tubular acidosis are well recognized: (1) the classic form, called type I or distal renal tubular acidosis; (2) the bicarbonate-wasting form, called type II or proximal renal tubular acidosis; and (3) type IV, or hyperkalemic renal tubular acidosis (rare in children), which is associated with hyporeninemic hypoaldosteronism. Type I and type II and their variants are encountered most frequently in children. Type III is a combination of types I and II.

**Table 22–6.** Inherited or developmental defects of the urinary tract.

| | |
|---|---|
| **Cystic diseases of genetic origin** | sis, Hurler syndrome, Niemann-Pick disease, familial metachromatic leukodystrophy, glycogenosis type I [von Gierke disease], glycogenosis type II [Pompe disease]) |
| Polycystic disease | |
|   Autosomal-recessive form (infantile) | |
|   Autosomal-dominant form (adult) | Hereditary amyloidosis (familial Mediterranean fever, heredofamilial urticaria with deafness and neuropathy, primary familial amyloidosis with polyneuropathy) |
|   Other syndromes that include either form | |
| Cortical cysts | |
|   Several syndromes are known to have various renal cystic manifestations, including "simple" cysts; may not have significant effect on renal functional status or be associated with progressive disease | **Hereditary renal diseases associated with tubular transport defects** |
| | Hartnup disease |
| | Fanconi's anemia |
| | Oculocerebrorenal syndrome of Lowe |
| Medullary cysts | Cystinosis (infantile, adolescent, adult types) |
|   Medullary sponge kidney | Wilson's disease |
|   Medullary cystic disease (nephronophthisis) | Galactosemia |
| Hereditary and familial cystic dysplasia | Hereditary fructose intolerance |
|   Congenital nephrosis | Renal tubular acidosis (many types) |
|   "Finnish" disease | Hereditary tyrosinemia |
| **Dysplastic renal diseases** | Renal glycosuria |
| Renal aplasia (unilateral, bilateral) | Vitamin D-resistant rickets |
| Renal hypoplasia (unilateral, bilateral, total, segmental) | Pseudohypoparathyroidism |
| Multicystic renal dysplasia (unilateral, bilateral, multilocular, postobstructive) | Vasopressin-resistant diabetes insipidus |
| | Hypouricemia |
| Familial and hereditary renal dysplasias | **Hereditary diseases associated with lithiasis** |
| Oligomeganephronia | Hyperoxaluria |
| **Hereditary diseases associated with nephritis** | L-Glyceric aciduria |
| Hereditary nephritis with deafness and ocular defects (Alport's syndrome) | Xanthinuria |
| | Lesch-Nyhan syndrome and variants, gout |
| Nail-patella syndrome | Nephropathy due to familial hyperparathyroidism |
| Familial hyperprolinemia | Cystinuria (types I, II, III) |
| Hereditary nephrotic syndrome | Glycinuria |
| Hereditary osteolysis with nephropathy | **Miscellaneous** |
| Hereditary nephritis with thoracic asphyxiant dystrophy syndrome | Hereditary intestinal vitamin $B_{12}$ malabsorption |
| | Total and partial lipodystrophy |
| **Hereditary diseases associated with intrarenal deposition of metabolites** | Sickle cell anemia |
| | Bartter syndrome |
| Angiokeratoma corporis diffusum (Fabry disease) | |
| Heredopathia atactica polyneuritiformis (Refsum disease) | |
| Various storage diseases (eg, $G_{M1}$ monosialogangliosido- | |

Primary tubular disorders in childhood, such as glycinuria, hypouricemia, or renal glycosuria, may result from a defect in a single tubular transport pathway (see Table 22–6).

## 1. Distal Renal Tubular Acidosis (Type I)

The most common form of distal renal tubular acidosis in childhood is the hereditary form. The clinical presentation is one of failure to thrive, anorexia, vomiting, and dehydration. Hyperchloremic metabolic acidosis occurs, with hypokalemia and a urinary pH exceeding 6.5. The acidosis is more severe in the presence of a bicarbonate "leak." This variant of distal renal tubular acidosis with bicarbonate wasting has been called type III, but for clinical purposes need not be considered as a distinct entity. Concomitant hypercalciuria may lead to rickets, nephrocalcinosis, nephrolithiasis, and renal failure.

Other situations that may be responsible for distal renal tubular acidosis are found in some of the entities listed in Table 22–6.

Distal renal tubular acidosis results from a defect in the distal nephron, in the tubular transport of hydrogen ion, or in the maintenance of a steep enough gradient for proper excretion of hydrogen ion. This defect can be accompanied by degrees of bicarbonate wasting.

The classic test for distal renal tubular acidosis is an acid load from $NH_4Cl$. The test is cumbersome and can produce severe acidosis. A clinical trial of alkali administration should be used to rule out proximal (type II) renal tubular acidosis. The dose of alkali required to achieve a normal plasma bicarbonate concentration in patients with distal renal tubular acidosis is low (seldom exceeding 2–3 mEq/kg/24 h)—in contrast to that required in proximal renal tubular acidosis (> 10 mEq/kg/24 h). Higher doses are needed, however, if distal renal tubular acidosis is accompanied by bicarbonate wasting. Correction of acidosis can result in reduced complications and improved growth.

Distal renal tubular acidosis is usually permanent, although it sometimes occurs as a secondary complication. If the defect is not caused by a greater tubular disorder and renal damage is prevented, the prognosis is good.

## 2. Proximal Renal Tubular Acidosis (Type II)

Proximal renal tubular acidosis is characterized by an alkaline urine pH, loss of bicarbonate in the urine, and mildly reduced serum bicarbonate concentrations. About 85–90% of bicarbonate reabsorption occurs in the proximal tubules. The lesion in proximal renal tubular acidosis is a lowering of the renal bicarbonate threshold, that is, the concentration of serum bicarbonate above which bicarbonate appears in the urine. With more severe acidosis, the concentration of serum bicarbonate drops and bicarbonate disappears from the urine; these changes reflect normal distal tubular acidification.

Proximal renal tubular acidosis is the most common type encountered in children. It is often an isolated defect, and in the newborn infant it can be considered an aspect of renal immaturity. Onset in infants is accompanied by failure to thrive, hyperchloremic acidosis, hypokalemia, and, rarely, nephrocalcinosis. Secondary forms result from reflux or obstructive uropathy and occur in association with other tubular disorders (see Table 22–6). Proximal renal tubular acidosis requires greater than 3 mEq/kg of alkali per day to correct the acidosis. Serum bicarbonate should be monitored weekly until a level of at least 20 mEq/L is attained.

Citrate solutions (eg, Bicitra, Polycitra) are somewhat more easily tolerated than sodium bicarbonate. Bicitra contains 1 mEq of $Na^+$ and citrate per milliliter. Polycitra contains 2 mEq per milliliter of citrate and 1 mEq each of $Na^+$ and $K^+$. The required daily dosage is given in three divided doses. Potassium supplementation may be required, because the added sodium load presented to the distal tubule may exaggerate potassium losses.

The prognosis is excellent in cases of isolated defects, especially when the problem is related to renal immaturity. Alkali therapy can usually be discontinued after several months to 2 years. Growth should be normal, and the gradual increase in the serum bicarbonate level to above 22 mEq/L heralds the presence of a raised bicarbonate threshold in the tubules. If the defect is part of a more complex tubular abnormality (Fanconi syndrome with attendant phosphaturia, glycosuria, and amino aciduria), the prognosis depends on the underlying disorder or syndrome.

## OCULOCEREBRORENAL SYNDROME (Lowe Syndrome)

Lowe syndrome results from a range of mutations in the *ORCL1* gene that codes for a Golgi apparatus phosphatase. Affected males have anomalies involving the eyes, brain, and kidneys. The physical stigmas and the degree of mental retardation are variable and depend on the location of the mutation. In addition to congenital cataracts and buphthalmos, the typical facies includes prominent epicanthal folds, frontal prominence, and a tendency to scaphocephaly. Muscle hypotonia is a prominent finding. The renal abnormalities are of tubule function and include hypophosphatemic rickets with low serum phosphorus levels, low to normal serum calcium levels, elevated serum alkaline phosphatase levels, renal tubular acidosis, and aminoaciduria. Treatment includes alkali therapy, phosphate replacement, and vitamin D. Antenatal diagnosis is possible.

Satre et al: Characterization of a germline mosaicism in families with Lowe syndrome, and identification of seven novel mutations in the ORCL1 gene. Am J Hum Genet 1999;65:68.

## CONGENITAL HYPOKALEMIC ALKALOSIS (Bartter Syndrome and Gitelman Syndrome)

Bartter syndrome is characterized by severe hypokalemic, hypochloremic metabolic alkalosis, extremely high levels of circulating renin and aldosterone, and a paradoxic absence of hypertension. On renal biopsy, a striking juxtaglomerular hyperplasia is seen.

A neonatal form of Bartter syndrome is thought to result from mutations in two genes affecting either $Na^+$–$K^+$ or $K^+$ transport. These patients have life-threatening episodes of fever and dehydration with hypercalciuria and early-onset nephrocalcinosis. Classic Bartter syndrome presenting in infancy with polyuria and growth retardation (but not nephrocalcinosis) is thought to result from mutations in a chloride channel gene. Gitelman syndrome occurs in older children and features episodes of muscle weakness, tetany, hypokalemia, and hypomagnesemia. These children have hypocalciuria.

Treatment with prostaglandin inhibitors and potassium-conserving diuretics (eg, amiloride combined with magnesium supplements) and potassium may be beneficial. Although the prognosis is guarded, a few patients seem to have less severe forms of the disease that are compatible with long survival times.

Rodriguez-Soriano J: Bartter's syndrome comes of age. Pediatrics 1999;103:663.

## CYSTINOSIS

Three types of cystinosis have been identified: adult, adolescent, and infantile. In children the adolescent type is characterized by cystine deposition and, if left untreated with phosphocysteamine (Cystagon), is accompanied by the development of the renal Fanconi syndrome and varying degrees of renal failure; growth is usually normal. The infantile type is both the most common and the most severe. Characteristically, children present in the first or second year of life with Fanconi syndrome and, without the metabolic benefit of Cystagon treatment, progress to end-stage renal failure.

Cystinosis results from mutations in the *CTNS* gene that codes for a cystine transporter. About 50% of patients share an identical deletion. Inheritance is autosomal recessive. Cystine is stored in cellular lysosomes in virtually all tissues. Eventually, cystine accumulation results in cell damage and cell death, particularly in the renal tubules. Renal failure between ages 6 and 12 years is common.

Whenever the diagnosis of cystinosis is suspected, slitlamp examination of the corneas by an ophthalmologist should be performed, because cystine crystal deposition causes an almost pathognomonic ground-glass "dazzle" appearance. Increased white cell cystine levels are diagnostic. Hypothyroidism is common.

Cystagon therapy is helpful in the treatment of cystinosis. Depending on the progression of chronic renal failure, management is directed toward all side effects of renal failure, with particular attention paid to the control of renal osteodystrophy. Dialysis and transplantation may be needed.

Anikster Y et al: Identification and detection of the common 65-kb deletion breakpoint in the nephropathic cystinosis gene. Mol Genet Metab 1999;66:111.

http://www.cystinosisfoundation.org

## PHOSPHATE-LOSING RENAL TUBULAR SYNDROMES & OTHER FORMS OF RICKETS

Recent investigation of the metabolic products of vitamin $D_3$ has done much to clarify the causes of various forms of rickets. Those forms due primarily to a lack of available calcium are described in Chapter 10. They include idiopathic hypercalciuria, in which there is excessive urinary calcium loss not responsive to reduction in calcium intake, lack of vitamin $D_3$ because of low dietary intake or from steatorrhea, and vitamin D dependency and azotemic rickets. In vitamin $D_3$ dependency, there is an inborn or acquired inability to synthesize 1,25-dihydroxycholecalciferol (the calcium transport stimulating factor, type I), or there may be end-organ insensitivity to this factor (type II). Treatment consists of giving supplementary calcium or vitamin D in appropriate doses.

Diseases associated with decreased availability of phosphorus also cause rickets. Excessive use of antacids may be responsible. Most commonly the defect is an inherited or acquired one in which a defect of phosphorus reabsorption is variably associated with other transport defects (eg, Fanconi syndrome). Certain generalized metabolic diseases—notably Wilson disease, galactosemia, fructose intolerance, and cystinosis—may cause similar tubular damage. Treatment of the primary type includes giving extra phosphorus. Acquired forms are treated in the same manner as the basic disease.

Familial hypophosphatemic vitamin D-resistant rickets is an example of a tubular nephropathy in which only phosphorus transport is affected. Most patients present during the second year of life, but some conditions have onset in the first 6 months.

Clinical features vary. Changes may be only biochemical, with a strikingly low serum phosphorus and an elevated alkaline phosphatase level. Muscle hypotonia may be severe; growth failure, bowing of the legs, and enlargement of the wrists, knees, and costochondral junctions are often associated with spinal deformities. Craniosynostosis has been described in infants with this disease. Pathologic fractures may be seen on radiograph as well as certain unique findings consisting of an irregular mosaic formation of the haversian system and trabecular "halos" of low-density bone.

In most cases, the serum phosphorus level is less than 2 mg/dL. The urinary calcium level is low, and the serum calcium level may be normal or slightly low. Serum levels of 1,25-dihydroxycholecalciferol are low, probably because high levels of phosphate in the tubule cell shut off the 1α-hydroxylase activity. Aminoaciduria is rare.

Treatment consists of giving 1–3 g of phosphorus daily, either as a buffered monosodium and disodium hydrogen phosphate solution at pH 7.4 or as Fleet's Phospho-Soda. Magnesium oxide, 10–15 mg/kg/d by mouth, may be of value. Supplementary calcitriol, up to 40 mg/kg/d, should be given if the serum calcium levels remain below normal.

Normal growth is never achieved unless every effort is made to keep the serum phosphorus level over 3 mg/dL.

Gregory MJ, Schwartz GJ: Diagnosis and treatment of renal tubular disorders. Semin Nephrol 1998;18:317.

## NEPHROGENIC DIABETES INSIPIDUS

In the normal kidney, the interstitial fluid of the papilla is hyperosmolar to the fluid in the collecting duct. The luminal cells have a specific receptor for antidiuretic hormone (ADH), which, acting via cyclic adenosine monophosphate, permits water to move across the cell membrane in response to the osmotic gradient. The congenital X-linked recessive form of nephrogenic diabetes insipidus results from mutations in the vasopressin receptor, *AVPR2*. Autosomal (recessive and dominant) forms of nephrogenic diabetes insipidus are caused by mutations of the *AQP2* gene that codes for a water channel protein, aquaporin-2. Genetic counseling and mutation testing are available.

The symptoms are limited to polyuria, polydipsia, and failure to thrive. In some children, particularly if the solute intake is unrestricted, adjustment to an elevated serum osmolality may develop. These children are particularly susceptible to episodes of dehydration, fever, vomiting, and convulsions.

Clinically, the diagnosis can be made on the basis of a history of polydipsia and polyuria that are not sensitive to the administration of vasopressin, desmopressin acetate, or lypressin. It is wise to confirm this diagnosis by performing a vasopressin test. Carefully monitored water restriction does not increase the tubular reabsorption of water (TcH$_2$O) to above 3 mL/min/m$^2$. Urine osmolality will remain lower than 450 mOsm/kg, whereas serum osmolality rises and total body weight falls. Before weight reduction greater than 5% occurs or before serum osmolality exceeds 320 mOsm/kg, vasopressin should be administered. Urine concentrating ability is impaired in a number of conditions—sickle cell anemia, pyelonephritis, potassium depletion, hypercalcemia, cystinosis and other renal tubular disorders and obstructive uropathy—and as a result of nephrotoxic drugs.

In infants, it is usually best to allow water as demanded and to restrict salt. Serum sodium levels should be evaluated at intervals to avoid hyperosmolality from inadvertent water restriction. In later childhood, sodium intake should continue to be restricted to 2–2.5 mEq/kg/24 h.

Treatment with hydrochlorothiazide is helpful, and many patients show improvement with administration of prostaglandin inhibitors such as indomethacin or tolmetin.

Wilden RS, Cogdell DE: Clinical utility of direct mutation testing for congenital nephrogenic diabetes insipidus in families. Pediatrics 1999;103:632.

## NEPHROLITHIASIS

Renal calculi in children may result from certain inborn errors of metabolism, such as cystine in cystinosis, glycine in hyperglycinuria, urates in Lesch–Nyhan syndrome, and oxalates in oxalosis. Stones may occur secondary to hypercalciuria in distal tubular acidosis, and large stones are quite often seen in children with spina bifida who have paralyzed lower limbs. Treatment is limited to that of the primary condition, if possible. Surgical removal of stones should be considered only for obstruction, intractable severe pain, and chronic infection.

### Cystinuria

Cystinuria, like Hartnup disease and a number of other disorders, is primarily an abnormality of amino acid transport across both the enteric and proximal renal tubular epithelium. There appear to be at least three biochemical types. In the first type, the bowel transport of basic amino acids and cystine is impaired, but transport of cysteine is not impaired. In the renal tubule, basic amino acids are again rejected by the tubule, but cystine absorption appears to be normal. The reasons for the cystinuria are, therefore, still obscure. Heterozygous individuals have no aminoaciduria. The second type is similar to the first except that heterozygous individuals excrete excess cystine and lysine in the urine, and cystine transport in the bowel is normal. In the third type, only the nephron is involved. The only clinical manifestations are related to stone formation: ureteral colic, dysuria, hematuria, proteinuria, and secondary UTI. Urinary excretion of cystine, lysine, arginine, and ornithine is increased.

The most reliable way to prevent stone formation is to maintain a constantly high free-water clearance. This involves generous fluid intake. Alkalinization of the urine is helpful. If these measures do not prevent significant renal lithiasis, the use of tiopronin (Thiloa) is recommended.

## Primary Hyperoxaluria

Oxalate production in humans is derived from the oxidative deamination of glycine to glyoxylate, from the serine-glycolate pathway, and from ascorbic acid. At least two enzymatic blocks have been described. Type 1 is a deficiency of liver-specific peroxisomal alanine:glyoxylate aminotransferase. Type 2 is glyoxylate reductase deficiency.

Excess oxalate combines with calcium to form insoluble deposits in the kidneys, lungs, and other tissues. The onset is during childhood. The joints are occasionally involved, but the main effect is on the kidneys, where progressive oxalate deposition leads to fibrosis and eventual renal failure.

Pyridoxine supplementation and a low-oxalate diet have been tried as therapy, but the overall prognosis is poor, and most patients succumb to uremia by early adulthood. Renal transplantation is not very successful because of destruction of the transplant kidney. However, encouraging results have been obtained with concomitant liver transplantation, correcting the metabolic defect.

Hyperoxaluria may also occur secondary to ileal disease or after ileal resection.

Broyer M et al: Management of oxalosis. Kidney Int 1996;53:593.

Cochat P: Primary hyperoxaluria type 1. Kidney Int 1999;55:2533.

# ■ URINARY TRACT INFECTIONS

UTI is common in children, but the frequency decreases with age. It is estimated that 8% of girls and 2% of boys will acquire UTIs in childhood. Girls older than age 6 months have UTIs far more commonly than boys, whereas uncircumcised boys younger than 3 months of age have more UTIs than girls. Circumcision reduces the likelihood of UTI in boys tenfold. The protective effect of circumcision is mediated by a reduction in the density of distal urethral and periurethral bacterial colonization. Similarly, the density of urethral and periurethral colonization with uropathogenic bacteria is correlated to the risk of UTI in girls.

Dysfunctional voiding, which is uncoordinated relaxation of the urethral sphincter during voiding leading to incomplete emptying of the bladder, may cause frequent UTI. Similarly, any condition that interferes with complete emptying of the bladder, such as constipation or a neurogenic bladder, is associated with an increased risk of UTI. Poor perineal hygiene, structural abnormalities of the urinary tract, catheterization, and instrumentation of the urinary tract are all associated with UTI. In sexually active teenagers, intercourse may introduce bacteria into the urethra and bladder, resulting in acute cystitis.

Most UTIs are ascending infections. Specific adhesins present on the fimbria of uropathogenic bacteria allow colonization of the uroepithelium in the urethra and bladder and increase the likelihood of UTI.

The inflammatory response to infection during pyelonephritis may result in renal parenchymal scars. It is hypothesized that renal parenchymal scars in infancy and childhood may contribute to hypertension, renal disease, and renal failure later in life. Unfortunately, long-term outcome studies of the natural history of pyelonephritis and the effect of medical intervention on the development of adult renal diseases are not available.

The organisms responsible for UTI are normal fecal flora, most commonly *E coli* (> 85%), *Klebsiella, Proteus,* other gram-negative bacteria, and, less frequently, *Enterococcus* or coagulase-negative staphylococci.

## A. SYMPTOMS AND SIGNS

Newborns and infants demonstrate nonspecific signs, including fever, hypothermia, jaundice, poor feeding, irritability, vomiting, failure to thrive, and sepsis. Strong, foul-smelling or cloudy urine may be noted. Preschool children may have abdominal or flank pain, vomiting, fever, urinary frequency, dysuria, urgency, or enuresis. School-age children commonly have classic signs of cystitis (frequency, dysuria, urgency) or pyelonephritis (fever, vomiting, flank pain). Costovertebral tenderness is unusual in young children, but may be demonstrated by school-age children.

Physical examination should include attention to blood pressure determination, abdominal exam, and a genitourinary exam. Urethritis, poor perineal hygiene, herpes simplex virus, or other genitourinary infections may be apparent on examination.

## B. LABORATORY TESTS

Collection of urine for urinalysis and culture is difficult in children due to frequent contamination of the sample. In toilet-trained, cooperative, older children, a midstream, clean-catch method is satisfactory. Although cleaning of the perineum does not improve specimen quality, straddling of the toilet to separate the labia in girls, retraction of the foreskin in boys, and collecting midstream urine significantly reduce contamination.

In infants and young children, bladder catheterization or suprapubic collection is necessary in most cases to avoid contaminated samples. Bagged urine specimens are helpful only if negative.

Screening urinalysis indicates pyuria (>5 WBC/hpf) in most children with UTI, but many children with pyuria do not have UTI. White cells may be present in urine from the urethra or vagina or be present because of a systemic infection. The leukocyte esterase test correlates well with the presence of pyuria, but has a similar false-positive rate. The detection of urinary nitrite by dipstick is highly correlated with urine culture positive for enteric organisms. Most young children (70%) with UTI have negative nitrite tests because they empty their bladder frequently, and several hours is required for bacteria to convert ingested nitrates to nitrite in the bladder. The sensitivity of nitrite detection is highest on a first morning void. Gram stain of unspun urine correlates well with culture recovery of $10^5$ cfu/mL or more, but is infrequently available outside of the hospital.

The gold standard for diagnosis remains the properly collected urine specimen. Specimens that are not immediately cultured should be refrigerated and kept cold during transport. Any growth is considered significant from a suprapubic culture. Quantitative recovery of $10^5$ cfu/mL or more is considered significant on clean-catch specimens, and $10^4$–$10^5$ is considered significant on catheterized specimens. Usually the recovery of multiple organisms indicates contamination; however, some contaminated specimens will yield only a single species.

Asymptomatic bacteriuria is detected in 0.5–1.0% of children who are screened with urine culture. Asymptomatic bacteriuria is believed to represent colonization of the urinary tract with nonuropathogenic bacteria. Treatment may increase the risk of symptomatic UTI by eliminating nonpathogenic colonization. Screening urine cultures in nonsymptomatic children are, therefore, generally discouraged. The treatment of children with fever, normal urinalysis, and significant growth on quantitative urine culture is controversial, because differentiating asymptomatic bacteriuria (eg, detected at the time of a febrile viral infection) from true UTI with no or minimal signs of inflammation in the urine can be difficult. Repeated urine cultures are often helpful in differentiating asymptomatic bacteriuria from contamination of the culture versus true UTI.

In children with pyelonephritis, a serum creatinine should be determined.

## C. TREATMENT

Management of UTI requires an assessment of toxicity, hydration, ability to tolerate oral intake, and signs of sepsis. Very young children (younger than 3 months) and children with dehydration, toxicity, or sepsis should be admitted to the hospital and treated with parenteral antimicrobials.

Older infants and children who are not seriously ill can be treated as outpatients. Initial antimicrobial therapy is based on prior history of infection and antimicrobial use, as well as location of the infection in the urinary tract. Uncomplicated cystitis can be treated with amoxicillin, trimethoprim–sulfamethoxazole, or a first-generation cephalosporin. Each of these antimicrobials is concentrated in the lower urinary tract, and high cure rates are common. There are significant differences in the rates of antimicrobial resistance, so knowledge of the rates in the local community is important. More seriously ill children are treated parenterally initially with a third-generation cephalosporin or parenteral aminoglycoside. The initial antimicrobial choice is adjusted after culture and susceptibility are known. For sexually mature teenagers, fluoroquinolones such as ciprofloxacin and levofloxacin given for 3 days for cystitis are usually cost-effective.

The recommended duration of antimicrobial therapy for uncomplicated cystitis is 7–10 days. Short-course therapy of cystitis is not recommended in children, because differentiating upper and lower tract disease may be difficult, and higher failure rates are reported in most studies of short-course therapy.

Acute pyelonephritis is usually treated for 10 days, although some very severe infections may require longer therapy. The duration of parenteral therapy in uncomplicated pyelonephritis is not well defined, but most children can complete therapy orally once symptomatic improvement has occurred. A repeat urine culture 24–48 hours after beginning therapy is not needed if the child is improving and doing well.

## D. RADIOLOGIC EVALUATION

Because congenital urologic abnormalities increase the risk of UTI, radiologic evaluation of first UTI has been routinely recommended. These recommendations usually include routine ultrasound of the kidneys and voiding cystourethrogram (VCUG). These recommendations are controversial because no good data are available to support the theory that the detection and management of vesicourethral reflux (VUR), the most commonly detected abnormality, improves the long-term renal health of most children.

VUR is a congenital abnormality present in about 1% of the population. VUR is graded using the international scale (I—reflux into ureter; II—reflux to the kidney; III—reflux to kidney with dilation of ureter only; IV—reflux with dilation of ureter and mild blunting of renal calyces; V—reflux with dilation of ureter and blunting of renal calyces). Reflux is detected in 30–50% of children 1 year of age and younger. The natural history of reflux is to improve, and 80% of reflux of grades I, II, or III will resolve or significantly improve within 3 years following detection.

VCUG should be done selectively on children with first UTI. Children with suspected urologic abnormality due to weak stream, dribbling, or perineal abnormalities should be studied with VCUG. Boys with first UTI should be studied to detect posterior urethral valves, an important congenital abnormality that requires surgery. Children older than 3 years who are otherwise healthy and growing well usually can be followed clinically and do not need VCUG with first UTI. The yield in sexually active teenagers is also very low.

Ultrasonographic examination of kidneys should be done in children with acute pyelonephritis who have not improved after 3–5 days of antimicrobial treatment adjusted for the susceptibility of the organism. The examination is done to detect renal or perirenal abscesses or obstruction of the kidney. The yield of routine ultrasound examination of first-time UTI in children who are improving on therapy is low in recent studies. Most obstructing lesions of the urinary system are detected prenatally by in utero ultrasound.

### E. FOLLOW-UP

Children with UTI should be followed with screening urinalysis 1 and 2 months after resolution of UTI. Dipstick nitrate determination can be used at home by parents on first morning voided urine in children with frequently recurring UTI.

### F. PROPHYLACTIC ANTIMICROBIALS

Selected children with frequently recurring UTI may benefit from prophylactic antimicrobials. In children with grades I–III, IV and V VUR, prophylactic antimicrobials may be beneficial in reducing UTI, as an alternative to surgical correction, or in the interval prior to surgical therapy. Many experts recommend surgical correction of higher grade reflux, particularly grade V. Trimethoprim–sulfamethoxazole and nitrofurantoin are approved for prophylaxis. Use of broader spectrum antimicrobials leads to colonization and infection with resistant strains.

Children with dysfunctional voiding generally do not benefit from prophylactic antimicrobials; rather, addressing the underlying dysfunctional voiding is most important.

In some children, erroneous diagnosis based on contaminated urine specimens leads to recovery of gram-negative rods with increasing antimicrobial resistance. Prophylactic antimicrobials are not helpful—catheterized or suprapubic urine specimens are often helpful in clarifying the underlying contamination.

Baker PC et al: The addition of ceftriaxone to oral therapy does not improve outcome in febrile children with urinary tract infections. Arch Pediatr Adolesc Med 2001;155(2):133 [PMID: 11177086].

Hoberman A et al: Imaging studies after a first febrile urinary tract infection in young children. N Engl J Med 2003;348(3): 195 [PMID: 12529459].

Huicho L et al: Meta analysis of urine screening tests for determining the risk of urinary tract infection in children. Pediatr Infect Dis J 2002;21(1):1 [PMID: 11791090].

Smellie JM et al: Outcome at 10 years of severe vesicoureteric reflux managed medically: Report of the international reflux study in children. J Pediatr 2001;139(5):656 [PMID: 11713442].

Subcommittee on Urinary Tract Infection, American Academy of Pediatrics: Practice parameter: The diagnosis, treatment, and evaluation of the initial urinary tract infection in febrile infants and young children. Pediatrics 1999;103(4):843 [PMID:10103321].

## REFERENCES

Barratt TM et al: *Pediatric Nephrology*, 5th ed. Lippincott Williams & Wilkins, 2003.

Webb N, Postlethwaite R: *Clinical Paediatric Nephrology*, 3rd ed. Oxford University Press, 2003.

# Neurologic & Muscular Disorders · 23

Paul G. Moe, MD, & Tim A. Benke, MD, PhD

## ◼ NEUROLOGIC ASSESSMENT & NEURODIAGNOSTIC PROCEDURES

### NEUROLOGIC HISTORY & EXAMINATION

Despite recent advances in neurodiagnostic testing and neuroimaging, a thorough history remains the most important tool in accurately diagnosing neurologic disorders. The chief complaint(s) and present illness should clearly delineate the temporal profile and sequence of neurologic symptoms. From a detailed history, the clinician will determine if the neurologic symptoms are acute or chronic, static or progressive, recurrent or monophasic, periodic or randomly intermittent, short or prolonged. The patient's description of his or her symptoms will provide clues as to the anatomic localization of the disturbance and possible pathogenic mechanisms. The history should also include what precipitates, palliates, or changes the symptoms.

The history and review of systems provide essential background information about the patient and may provide evidence for a more generalized disorder or for associated or predisposing conditions. Similarly, the family history and social history frequently provide clues for underlying genetic, hereditary, environmental, or psychological conditions that are the basis of the patient's complaints. The social history also provides insight into how the symptoms affect the child's and family's day-to-day living, school performance, and quality of life. A developmental history may provide the earliest clues of a degenerative disorder. Some developmental milestones are summarized in Table 23–1.

The physical examination should include the child's height, weight, head circumference, blood pressure, pulse rate, general appearance, and level of alertness and attentiveness. It is important to observe the child's spontaneous activity, behavior and responses to light, noise, and touch. Is the child abnormally irritable or demonstrating odd behavior for his or her age? Are there dysmorphic features of the face, head, ears, trunk, extremities, or digits? Are any discolored patches of skin such as hemangiomas, ash-leaf depigmented patches, or café au lait spots present? Is the fontanel open or closed, too big or too small? A more detailed mental status examination may be appropriate for school-age children (Table 23–2). The child should be observed for truncal sway or loss of balance (Romberg test). Testing for vibratory appreciation requires that the child be old enough to report whether he or she can feel the vibrations of a tuning fork applied to the digits or bony prominences. Muscle mass, consistency, tone, and strength should be assessed in all four limbs, across multiple joints, and in the neck and trunk. Muscle stretch reflexes can be elicited normally from infancy to adulthood at the biceps, triceps, knees, and ankles. The presence, absence, or asymmetry of automatic infantile movements and reflexes (automatisms) should be noted (see Table 23–1).

The examiner should then proceed with a systematic neurologic examination, including an assessment of cranial nerves II through XII, funduscopy, and testing of eye movements and pupillary light and near-vision reflexes. Cerebellar control of body and extremity posture, ambulation, and fine coordinated movements can usually be evaluated by watching the child walk, run, play with or reach for toys, sit, and stand still. Responses to light touch and mildly painful stimulation can be assessed by tickling or touching the child and lightly pinching toes or fingers and observing facial expression and withdrawal and avoidance movements. Position sensation can be assessed in older children by having them stand with eyes closed. The clinician should construct a differential diagnostic list of disorders that could account for the patient's symptoms and develop a systematic approach to neurodiagnostic testing and neuroimaging procedures.

### LUMBAR PUNCTURE

Spinal fluid is usually obtained by inserting a small-gauge needle (eg, No. 22) through the L3–L4 intervertebral space into the thecal sack while the patient is lying on his or her side. After an opening pressure is measured, a small amount of fluid is removed most frequently to examine for evidence of infection or inflammation (Table 23–3). Fluid is sent for red and white cell counts, for determination of the concentrations of

*Table 23–1.* Neurologic developmental milestones.

| | Birth | 3 Months | 6 Months | 9 Months | 12–15 Months | 24 Months |
|---|---|---|---|---|---|---|
| Motor | Flexor posture, lifts head prone, hands grasped | Sits: head forward, bobbing, lifts head supine, hands open, retains briefly | Rolls both ways, begins to sit alone, supports (erect), bounces | Creeps, pulls up standing, pincer grasp, sits well | Walks with one or both hands held, stands alone briefly, releases on command | Walks and runs well, walks downstairs, turns pages singly |
| Special senses | Regards (vision), may follow 45 degrees | Looks at hands, follows 90–180 degrees | Discriminates voices, localizes sounds | Picks up raisin, "bye-bye" | Localizes noises, localizes pain | Towers six or seven cubes, imitates scribble |
| Adaptive | Startles to sound, delayed nociceptive response | Smiles socially, vocalizes socially, follows vertically | Holds cube, palmar grasp, retrieves toy, transfers and rakes raisin | Bangs toys together, pat-a-cake | Assists in dressing, attempts spoon feeding, tries two-cube tower | Asks for toilet, pulls on garments, spoon-feeds well, parallel play |
| Language | Throaty noises | Coos, chuckles, vocal social response | Babbles (polysyllables), "mmm-mmm" | "Ma-ma, Da-da," one other "word" | Understands simple command, speaks one to three words | Speaks in phrases, names three to five pictures, pronouns: "I, me, you" |
| Reflex | Tonic neck, palmar grasp | Disappearing tonic neck, Moro reflex | Begins voluntary stepping | Parachute response | | |
| Automatisms | Moro reflex, sucks, roots, stepping, supporting, traction: head lag | Landau response, traction: no head lag | Neck righting, blinks to threat | | | |

*Table 23–2.* Mental status examination for school-age children.

**Orientation:** Time, place, situation, name, date, year.
**Memory:** Recent and remote, eg, "What did you have for lunch?" "What did you do on your birthday?" Remember (for 10 min): "Red flag, Washington's birthday, Christmas presents."
**Calculation:** Depends on educational background. Example: Subtract serial sevens.
**Proverbs:** Interpret: "Too many cooks spoil the broth." "A rolling stone gathers no moss."
**Situation:** "What would you do if you saw a fire?"
**Aphasia:** "What's this?" (chalk). "Stick out your tongue." "Put your right finger on your left ear." Sample speech, reading, and writing.

protein and glucose, and for viral and bacterial cultures. In some cases, additional information is obtained with special staining techniques for mycobacteria and fungus. Additional fluid may be sent for polymerase chain reaction (PCR) testing for specific viral agents, antibody titer determinations, cytopathologic study, lactate and pyruvate concentrations, and amino acid and neurotransmitter analysis. Lumbar puncture is imperative when bacterial meningitis is suspected. Caution must be exercised, however, when signs of increased intracranial pressure (eg, papilledema) or focal neurologic signs are present that might indicate a substantial risk of precipitating tentorial or tonsillar herniation.

## ELECTROENCEPHALOGRAPHY

Electroencephalography (EEG), a widely used noninvasive electrophysiologic method for recording cerebral activity, has its greatest clinical applicability in the

*Table 23–3.* Characteristics of cerebrospinal fluid in the normal child and in central nervous system infections and inflammatory conditions.

| Condition | Initial Pressure (mm H$_2$O) | Appearance | Cells/μL | Protein (mg/dL) | Glucose (mg/dL) | Other Tests | Comments |
|---|---|---|---|---|---|---|---|
| Normal | < 160 | Clear | 0–5 lymphocytes; first 3 months, 1–3 PMNs; neonates, up to 30 lymphocytes, 20–50 RBCs | 15–35 (lumbar), 5–15 (ventricular); up to 150 (lumbar) for short time after birth; to 6 months up to 65 | 50–80 (two thirds of blood glucose); may be increased after seizure | CSF-IgG index < 0.7[a]; LDH 2–27 units/L | CSF protein in first month may be up to 170 mg/dL in small-for-date or premature infants. No increase in WBCs due to seizure. |
| Bloody tap | Normal or low | Bloody (sometimes with clot) | One additional WBC/700 RBCs[b]; RBCs not crenated | One additional milligram per 800 RBCs[b] | Normal | RBC number should fall between first and third tubes; wait 5 min between tubes | Spin down fluid, supernatant will be clear and colorless.[c] |
| Bacterial meningitis, acute | 200–750+ | Opalescent to purulent | Up to thousands, mostly PMNs; early, few cells | Up to hundreds | Decreased; may be none | Smear and culture mandatory; LDH > 24 U/L; lactate, IL-8, TNF elevated, correlate with prognosis | Very early, glucose may be normal. PCR (meningo- and pneumococcus) plasma, CSF may aid diagnosis |
| Bacterial meningitis, partially treated | Usually increased | Clear or opalescent | Usually increased; PMNs usually predominate | Elevated | Normal or decreased | LDH usually > 24 U/L; PCR | Smear and culture may be negative if antibiotics have been in use. |
| Tuberculous meningitis | 150–750+ | Opalescent; fibrin web or pellicle | 250–500, mostly lymphocytes; early, more PMNs. | 45–500; parallels cell count; increases over time | Decreased; may be none | Smear for acid-fast organism; CSF culture and inoculation; PCR | Consider AIDS. |
| Fungal meningitis | Increased | Variable; often clear | 10–500; early, more PMNs; then mostly lymphocytes | Elevated and increasing | Decreased | India ink preparations, cryptococcal antigen, PCR, culture, inoculations, immunofluorescence tests | Often superimposed in patients who are debilitated or on immunosuppressive therapy. |
| Aseptic meningoencephalitis (viral meningitis, or parameningeal disease) | Normal or slightly increased | Clear unless cell count > 300/μL | None to a few hundred, mostly lymphocytes; PMNs predominate early | 20–125 | Normal; may be low in mumps, herpes, or other viral infections | CSF, stool, blood, throat washings for viral cultures; LDH < 28 U/L; PCR for HSV, CMV, EBV, enterovirus, etc. | Acute and convalescent antibody titers for some viruses. In mumps, up to 1000 lymphocytes; serum amylase often elevated. Rarely, a thousand cells present in enteroviral infection. |

734

| Condition | Pressure | Appearance | Cells | Protein | Glucose | Special tests | Notes |
|---|---|---|---|---|---|---|---|
| Parainfectious encephalomyelitis (ADEM) | 80–450, usually increased | Usually clear | 0–50+, mostly lymphocytes | 15–75 | Normal | CSF-IgG index may be increased; oligoclonal bands variable | No organisms. Fulminant cases resemble bacterial meningitis. |
| Polyneuritis | Normal and occasionally increased | Early: normal; late: xanthochromic if protein high | Normal; occasionally slight increase | Early: normal; late: 45–1500 | Normal | CSF-IgG index may be increased; oligoclonal bands variable | Try to find cause (viral infections, toxins, lupus, diabetes, etc). |
| Meningeal carcinomatosis | Often elevated | Clear to opalescent | Cytologic identification of tumor cells | Often mildly to moderately elevated | Often depressed | Cytology | Seen with leukemia, medulloblastoma, meningeal melanosis, histiocytosis X. *Notes:* May mimic meningitis. |
| Brain abscess | Normal or increased | Usually clear | 5–500 in 80%; mostly PMNs | Usually slightly increased | Normal; occasionally decreased | Imaging study of brain (MRI) | Cell count related to proximity to meninges; findings as in purulent meningitis if abscess perforates. |

[a] CSF-IgG index = CSF IgG/serum IgG ÷ CSF albumin/serum albumin.

[b] Many studies document pitfalls in using these ratios due to WBC lysis. Clinical judgment and repeat taps may be necessary to rule out meningitis in this situation.

[c] CSF WBC (predicted) = CSF RBC × (blood WBC/blood RBC). O:P ratio = observed CSF WBC ÷ predicted CSF WBC. Also, do WBC: RBC ratio. If O:P ratio ≤ 0.01, and WBC:RBC ratio ≤ 1:100, meningitis is absent.

PMN = polymorphonuclear neutrophil; CSF = cerebrospinal fluid; WBC = white blood cell; RBC = red blood cell; LDH = lactate dehydrogenase; AIDS = acquired immunodeficiency syndrome; PCR = polymerase chain reaction; HSV = herpes simplex virus; CMV = cytomegalovirus; EBV = Epstein–Barr virus; ADEM = acute disseminated encephalomyelitis; IL-8 = interleukin 8; TNF = tumor necrosis factor.

study of seizure disorders. Activation techniques to accentuate abnormalities or disclose latent abnormalities include photic stimulation, sustained hyperventilation for 3 minutes, and sleep deprivation, the last of which is an excellent, though less widely used, activation method.

EEG is also used in the evaluation of tumors, cerebrovascular accidents, neurodegenerative diseases, and other neurologic disorders causing brain dysfunction. Recordings over a 24-hour period or all-night recordings are invaluable in the diagnosis of sleep disturbances and narcolepsy. EEG with telemetry or simultaneous monitoring of behavior on videotape has great usefulness in selected cases. The EEG can be helpful in determining a possible cause or mechanism of coma and is frequently used to help determine whether coma is irreversible and brain death has occurred.

The limitations of EEG are considerable. In most cases, the duration of the actual tracing is about 45 minutes and reflects only surface cortical function. Many drugs, especially barbiturates and benzodiazepines, have considerable effects on the EEG and may confuse interpretation. Moreover, about 15% of nonepileptic individuals, especially children, may have an abnormal EEG. EEG findings such as those occasionally seen in migraine, learning disabilities, or behavior disorders are often nonspecific and do not reflect permanent brain damage. A major usefulness of EEG is to show epileptiform activity in children with seizure disorders. Sometimes the findings are diagnostic, as in the hypsarrhythmia EEG of infantile spasms or the prolonged 3/s spike-wave of absence seizures.

At present, computed tomography (CT) scans, evoked potentials, positron emission tomography (PET), regional cerebral blood flow studies, single-photon emission computed tomography (SPECT), and magnetic resonance imaging (MRI) supplement the EEG as a diagnostic and prognostic tool.

# EVOKED POTENTIALS

Cortical auditory, visual, or somatosensory evoked potentials (evoked responses) may be recorded from the scalp surface over the temporal, occipital, or frontoparietal cortex after repetitive stimulation of the retina by light flashes, the cochlea by sounds, or a nerve by galvanic stimuli of varying frequency and intensity, respectively. Computer averaging is used to recognize and enhance these responses while subtracting or suppressing the asynchronous background EEG activity. The presence or absence of evoked potential waves and their latencies (time from stimulus to wave peak or time between peaks) figures in the clinical interpretation.

The reproducible and quantifiable results obtained from brainstem auditory, pattern-shift visual, and short-latency somatosensory evoked potentials (see Short-Latency Somatosensory Evoked Potentials section) indicate the level of function of the relevant sensory pathway or system and identify the site of anatomic disruption. Although results of these tests alone are usually not diagnostic, the tests are noninvasive, sensitive, objective, and relatively inexpensive extensions of the clinical neurologic examination. Because the auditory and somatosensory tests and one type of visual test are completely passive, requiring only that the patient remain still, they are particularly useful in the evaluation of neonates, young children, and patients unable to cooperate. Knowledge of normal values and experience in testing are mandatory.

## Brainstem Auditory Evoked Potentials

A brief auditory stimulus (click) of varying intensity and frequency is delivered to the ear to activate the auditory nerve (nerve VIII) and sequentially activate the cochlear nucleus, tracts and nuclei of the lateral lemniscus, and inferior colliculus. Thus this technique assesses hearing and function of the brainstem auditory tracts.

Hearing in the neonate or uncooperative patient can be assessed objectively, making the technique particularly useful in high-risk infants and in mentally retarded or autistic patients. Brainstem auditory evoked potentials are used to judge brainstem dysfunction in sleep apnea, Arnold–Chiari malformation, and achondroplasia. Because high doses of anesthetic agents or barbiturates do not seriously affect results, the test is used to assess and monitor brainstem function of surgical patients (in the operating room) and those in hypoxic–ischemic coma or coma following head injury. Absence of evoked potential waves beyond the first wave from the auditory nerve usually signifies brain death. Brainstem auditory evoked potentials are also useful in the early evaluation of diseases affecting myelin, that is, the leukodystrophies and multiple sclerosis, although auditory evoked potentials are less valuable than visual evoked potentials in the evaluation of multiple sclerosis. Intrinsic brainstem gliomas can also be evaluated with auditory evoked potentials. They are sometimes useful in evaluation of hereditary ataxias, Wilson disease, and other degenerative disorders of the brainstem.

## Pattern-Shift Visual Evoked Potentials

The preferred stimulus is a shift (reversal) of a checkerboard pattern, and the response is a single wave (called P-100) generated in the striate and parastriate visual cortex. The absolute latency of P-100 (time from stimulus to wave peak) and the difference in latency between the two eyes are sensitive indicators of disease. The amplitude of response is affected by any process resulting in poor fixation on the stimulus screen or affecting visual acuity. Ability to focus on a checkerboard pattern is necessary. An LED (light-emitting diode), goggles, or bright flash stimulus can be used in younger and uncooperative children, but the norms are less standardized. Normal evoked potentials in infants age 6–7 months suggest that visual acuity is normal.

Clinical applications of the test include detection and monitoring of strabismus (eg, in amblyopia ex anopsia), optic neuritis, and lesions near the optic nerve and chiasm such as optic gliomas and craniopharyngiomas. Degenerative and immunologic diseases that affect visual transmission may be detected early and followed by serial evaluations. Examples of such diseases include adrenoleukodystrophy, Pelizaeus–Merzbacher disease, some spinocerebellar degenerations, sarcoidosis, and even multiple sclerosis. Flash visual evoked potentials are used to monitor function during surgery on the eyes or optic nerve, to assess cortical or hysterical blindness, and to evaluate patients with photosensitive epilepsy, who may have exaggerated responses.

## Short-Latency Somatosensory Evoked Potentials

Responses are commonly produced by electrical stimulation of peripheral sensory nerves, because this evokes potentials of greatest amplitude and clarity. Finger tapping and muscle stretching may also be used to stimulate somatosensory potentials. The function of this test is similar to that of the auditory test in closely correlating wave forms with function of the sensory pathways and permitting localization of conduction defects.

Short-latency somatosensory evoked potentials are used in the assessment of a wide variety of lesions of the peripheral nerve, root, spinal cord, and central nervous system (CNS) following trauma, neuropathies (eg, in diabetes mellitus or Guillain–Barré syndrome), myelodysplasias, cerebral palsy, and many other disorders. The procedure is often performed on an outpatient basis. One method is stimulation of the median nerve at the wrist with small (nonpainful) electrical shocks and recording of responses from the brachial plexus above the clavicle, the neck (cervical cord), and the opposite scalp area overlying the sensorimotor cortex. After stimulation from the knee (peroneal nerve) or ankle (tibial nerve), impulses are recorded from the lower lumbar spinal cord, cervical cord, and sensorimotor cortex. Such potentials are used to monitor spinal cord sensory functioning during surgery for scoliosis, myelodysplasias, tumors, and other lesions of the spinal cord or its blood vessels. The technique is also used in leukodystrophies involving peripheral nerves, in multiple sclerosis, and in the evaluation of hysteria and malingering (anesthetic limbs). In the diagnosis of coma

and brain death, somatosensory evoked potentials supplement the results of auditory evoked potentials.

# PEDIATRIC NEURORADIOLOGIC PROCEDURES

## Sedation for Procedures

Oral chloral hydrate, 30–60 mg/kg/dose, is safest. Many radiology departments, however, use intravenously administered agents because of the risks of vomiting and aspiration. One favorite is pentobarbital, 6 mg/kg for children weighing less than 15 kg and 5 mg/kg for larger children (up to a maximum of 200 mg) given intramuscularly or rectally (at least 20 minutes before a procedure) or 2–4 mg/kg given intravenously. Equipment to support blood pressure and respiration must be available. This dosage usually achieves sedation for up to 2 hours. If, however, sedation is inadequate 30 minutes after injection, and if the child's condition permits a second dose of pentobarbital, 2 mg/kg is given. General anesthesia may be indicated, especially if the child is to undergo surgery immediately on completion of a radiologic examination.

## Computed Tomography

CT scanning consists of a series of cross-sectional (axial) roentgenograms. Radiation exposure is approximately the same as that from a skull radiographic series. The images can be viewed on a television screen, as the scan is being done, and later examined on films. Both record variations in tissue density. CT scanning is of high sensitivity (88–96% of lesions larger than 1–2 cm can be seen) but low specificity (tumor, infection, or infarct may look the same).

The CT scan is often repeated after intravenous injection of iodized contrast for enhancement, which reflects the vascularity of a lesion or its surrounding tissues. Precautions should be taken to ensure that the patient is not sensitive to iodinated dyes and that allergic reactions can be managed promptly. Sufficient information is often obtained from a nonenhanced scan, thus reducing both cost and risk.

## Magnetic Resonance Imaging

MRI is a noninvasive technique that uses the magnetic properties of certain nuclei to produce diagnostically useful signals. Currently the technique is based on detecting the response (resonance) of hydrogen proton nuclei to applied radiofrequency electromagnetic radiation. These nuclei are abundant in the body and more sensitive to MRI than other nuclei. The strength of MRI signals varies with the relationship of water to protein and the amount of lipid in the tissue. The MRI image displayed provides high-resolution contrast of soft tissues. MRI can provide information about the histologic, physiologic, and biochemical status of tissues in addition to gross anatomic data.

MRI has been used to delineate brain tumors, edema, ischemic and hemorrhagic lesions, hydrocephalus, vascular disorders, inflammatory and infectious lesions, and degenerative processes. MRI can be used to study myelination and demyelination and, through the demonstration of changes in relaxation time, metabolic disorders of the brain, muscles, and glands. Because bone causes no artifact in the images, the posterior fossa and its contents can be studied far better using MRI than with CT scans. Even blood vessels and the cranial nerves can be imaged. In contrast, the inability of MRI to detect calcification limits its usefulness in the investigation of calcified lesions such as craniopharyngioma and leptomeningeal angiomatosis.

Magnetic resonance angiography (MRA) is a noninvasive (no arterial or venous puncture or dye injection) technique to show large extra- and intracranial blood vessels. It often replaces the more hazardous intra-arterial injection angiogram.

Perfusion imaging using a paramagnetic contrast agent is used in stroke patients to evaluate brain ischemic penumbra. Similarly, diffusion imaging (measuring random motion of water molecules) may show reduced diffusion in areas of cytoxic edema, useful in acute strokes, and toxic or metabolic brain injuries. The area of involvement often exceeds the T1 hypodense or T2 hyperdense stroke area, and possibly reflects recoverable tissue injury as compared with totally infarcted tissue, cell death, or apoptosis (programmed cell death) in the center of the stroke.

Another new MRI technique, proton MR spectroscopy, measures signals of increased cellular (neuronal?) activity, and oxidative metabolism: neuronal acetyl aspartate (NAA), phosphocreatinine (PCR), and phosphomonoester (PME) are increased. Ratios are often calculated to choline and $P_i$ (inorganic phosphate). Or increased lactate (anaerobic metabolism), choline, and creatinine, reflecting increased cell surface—as in gliosis or scarring—can be assessed in a chosen voxel or tiny area of interest. An epileptic focus in the medial temporal lobe is an example: an active seizure site might show increased metabolism. Sclerosis and gliosis ("scar") would show the converse.

Functional MRI (fMRI) can be performed at the same time as an ongoing regular MRI. Blood oxygenation changes in an area of interest (eg, an area of language acquisition) during rest and then during a verbal work paradigm can identify and lateralize the language cortex. A change in ratio of oxyhemoglobin to deoxyhemoglobin results in a detectable MRI signal.

## Positron Emission Tomography

PET is an imaging technique that measures the metabolic rate at a given site by CT scanning. For measurement of local cerebral metabolism, the radiolabeled substrate most frequently used has been intravenously administered fluorodeoxyglucose ($^{18}$F). Gray matter and white matter are clearly distinguishable; the skull and air- or fluid-filled cavities are least active metabolically.

PET has been used to study the cerebral metabolism of neonates and brain activation by visual or auditory stimuli. Pathologic states that have been studied include epilepsy, brain infarcts, brain tumors, and dementias. This functional test of brain metabolism is useful in preoperative evaluation for epilepsy surgery. The epileptogenic zone will often be hypermetabolic during seizures and hypoactive during the time between seizures. The information from PET scan complements EEG and MRI findings to aid in the decision about tissue removal. In infants with infantile spasms, PET scan has occasionally detected focal lesions, thereby leading to successful surgical removal. Clinical application is limited by the cost of the procedure and the clinician's need for access to a nearby cyclotron for preparation of the radiopharmaceuticals.

## Ultrasonography

Ultrasonography offers a pictorial display of the varying densities of tissues in a given anatomic region by recording the echoes of ultrasonic waves reflected from it. These waves, modulated by pulsations, are introduced into the tissue by means of a piezoelectric transducer. The many advantages of ultrasonography include the ability to assess a structure and its positioning quickly with easily portable equipment, without ionizing radiation, and at about one fourth the cost of CT scanning. Sedation is usually not necessary, and the procedure can be repeated as often as needed without risk to the patient. In brain imaging, B-mode and real-time sector scanners are usually used, permitting excellent detail in the coronal and sagittal planes. Contiguous structures can be studied by a continuous sweep and reviewed on videotape.

Ultrasonography has been used for in utero diagnosis of hydrocephalus and other anomalies. In neonates, the thin skull and the open anterior fontanelle have facilitated imaging of the brain, and ultrasonography is used to screen and follow infants of less than 32 weeks' gestation or weighing less than 1500 g for intracranial hemorrhage. Other uses in neonates include detection of hydrocephalus, major brain and spine malformations, and calcifications from intrauterine infection with cytomegalovirus (CMV) or *Toxoplasma*.

## Cerebral Angiography

Arteriography remains a useful procedure in the diagnosis of many cerebrovascular disorders, particularly in cerebrovascular accidents or in potentially operable vascular malformations. In some brain tumors, arteriography may be necessary to define the precise location or vascular bed, to differentiate among tumors, or to distinguish tumor from abscess or infarction. Noninvasive CTs, MRIs, and MRAs can diagnose many cases of static or flowing blood disorders (eg, sinus thromboses). If necessary, invasive arteriography is usually done via femoral artery–aorta catheterization.

## Myelography

Radiographic examination of the spine may be indicated in cases of spinal cord tumors or various forms of spinal dysraphism and in the rare instance of herniated disks in children. MRI has largely replaced sonography and CT.

Aydin K et al.: Utility of electroencephalography in the evaluation of common neurologic conditions in children. J Child Neurol 2003;18:394 [PMID: 128896973].

Dooley JM et al: The utility of the physical examination and investigations in the pediatric neurology consultation. Pediatr Neurol 2003;28:96 [PMID: 12699858].

Halsted HJ, Jones BV: Pediatric neuroimaging for the pediatrician. Pediatr Ann 2002;31:661 [PMID: 12389370].

Kim YO et al: Diagnostic capability of CSF ferritin in children with meningitis. Pediatr Neurol 2003;28:271 [PMID: 12849879].

Kleine TO et al: New and old diagnostic markers of meningitis in cerebrospinal fluid (CSF). Brain Res Bull 2003;61:287 [PMID: 12909299].

Krishnamoorthy KS et al: Diffusion-weighted imaging in neonatal cerebral infarction: Clinical utility and follow-up. J Child Neurol 2000;15:592 [PMID: 11019790].

Mazor SS et al: Interpretation of traumatic lumbar punctures: Who can go home? Pediatrics 2003;111:525 [PMID: 12612231].

Straussberg R et al: Absolute neutrophil count in aseptic and bacterial meningitis related to time of lumbar puncture. Pediatr Neurol 2003;28:365 [PMID: 12878298].

Tang RB et al: Interleukin-1 beta and tumor necrosis factor-alpha in cerebrospinal fluid of children with bacterial meningitis. Childs Nerv Syst 2001;17:453 [PMID: 11508533].

# ■ DISORDERS AFFECTING THE NERVOUS SYSTEM IN INFANTS & CHILDREN

## ALTERED STATES OF CONSCIOUSNESS

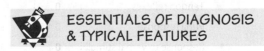

### ESSENTIALS OF DIAGNOSIS & TYPICAL FEATURES

- *Reduction or alteration in cognitive and affective mental functioning and in arousability or attentiveness.*
- *Acute onset.*

### General Considerations

Many terms are used to describe the continuum from full alertness to complete unresponsiveness and deep coma, including clouding, obtundation, somnolence or stupor, semicoma or light coma, and deep coma. Several scales have been used to grade the depth of unconsciousness (Table 23–4). The commonly used Glasgow Coma Scale is summarized in Table 11–5. Physicians should use one of these tables and provide further descriptions in case narratives. These descriptions help subsequent observers quantify unconsciousness and evaluate changes in the patient's condition.

The neurologic substrate for consciousness is the reticular activating system in the brainstem, up to and including the thalamus and paraventricular hypothalamus. Large lesions of the cortex, especially of the left hemisphere, can also cause coma. The term "locked-in syndrome" describes patients who are conscious but have no access to motor or verbal expression because of massive loss of motor function of the brainstem. Coma vigil refers to patients who seem comatose but have some spontaneous motor behavior, such as eye opening or eye tracking, almost always at a reflex level. Persistent vegetative state denotes a chronic condition in which there is preservation of the sleep–wake cycle but no awareness and no recovery of mental function.

### Emergency Measures

The clinician's first response is to ensure that the patient will survive. The ABCs of resuscitation are pertinent: Airway must be kept open with positioning or even endotracheal intubation. Breathing and adequate

**Table 23–4.** Gradation of coma.

| | Deep Coma | | Light Coma | | |
|---|---|---|---|---|---|
| | Grade 4 | Grade 3 | Grade 2 | Grade 1 | Stupor |
| Response to pain | 0 | + | Avoidance | Avoidance | Arousal unsustained |
| Tone/posture | Flaccid | Decerebrate | Variable | Variable | Normal |
| Tendon reflexes | 0 | +/– | + | + | + |
| Pupil response | 0 | + | + | + | + |
| Response to verbal stimuli | 0 | 0 | 0 | 0 | + |
| Other corneal reflex | 0 | + | + | + | + |
| Gag reflex | 0 | + | + | + | + |

air exchange can be assessed by auscultation; hand bag respiratory assistance with oxygen may be needed. Circulation must be ensured by assessing pulse and blood pressure. An intravenous line is always necessary. Fluids, plasma, blood, or even a dopamine drip (1–20 µg/kg/min) may be required in cases of hypotension. An extremely hypothermic or febrile child may require vigorous cooling or warming to save life. The assessment of vital signs may signal the diagnosis. Slow, insufficient respirations suggest poisoning by hypnotic drugs; apnea may indicate diphenoxylate hydrochloride poisoning. Rapid, deep respirations suggest acidosis, possibly metabolic, as with diabetic coma; toxic, such as that due to aspirin; or neurogenic, as in Reye syndrome. Hyperthermia may indicate infection or heat stroke; hypothermia may indicate cold exposure, ethanol poisoning, or hypoglycemia (especially in infancy).

The signs of impending brain herniation are another priority of the initial assessment. Bradycardia, high blood pressure, irregular breathing, increased extensor tone, and third nerve palsy with the eye deviated outward and the pupil dilated are possible signs of impending temporal lobe or brainstem herniation. These signs suggest a need for hyperventilation, reducing cerebral edema, prompt neurosurgical consultation, and possibly, in an infant with a bulging fontanelle, subdural or ventricular tap (or both). Initial intravenous fluids should contain glucose until further assessment disproves hypoglycemia as a cause.

A history obtained from parents or witnesses is desirable. Sometimes the only history will be obtained from ambulance attendants. An important point is whether the child is known to have a chronic illness, such as diabetes, hemophilia, epilepsy, or cystic fibrosis. Recent acute illness raises the possibility of coma caused by Reye syndrome or viral or bacterial meningitis. A combination of viral illness, especially varicella or influenza, followed by 1–3 days of intractable vomiting invariably precedes the coma of Reye syndrome. Trauma is a common cause of coma. Lack of a history of trauma, especially in infants, does not rule it out. Nonaccidental trauma or a fall not witnessed by caregivers may have occurred. In coma of unknown cause, poisoning is always a possibility. Absence of a history of ingestion of a toxic substance or of medication in the home does not rule out poisoning as a cause.

Often the history is obtained concurrently with a brief pediatric and neurologic screening examination. After the assessment of vital signs, the general examination proceeds with a trauma assessment. Palpation of the head and fontanelle, inspection of the ears for infection or hemorrhage, and a careful examination for neck stiffness are indicated. If circumstances suggest head or neck trauma, the head and neck must be immobilized so that any fracture or dislocation will not be aggravated. The skin must be inspected for petechiae or purpura that might suggest bacteremia, infection, bleeding disorder, or traumatic bruising. Examination of the chest, abdomen, and limbs is important to exclude enclosed hemorrhage or traumatic fractures.

Neurologic examination quantifies the stimulus response and depth of coma, such as responsiveness to verbal or painful stimuli. Examination of the pupils, optic fundi, and eye movements is important. Are the eye movements spontaneous, or is it necessary to do the doll's-eye maneuver (rotating the head rapidly to see whether the eyes follow)? Motor and sensory examinations assess reflex asymmetries, Babinski sign, and evidence of spontaneous posturing or posturing induced by noxious stimuli (eg, decorticate or decerebrate posturing).

If the cause of the coma is not obvious, emergency laboratory tests must be obtained. Table 23–5 lists some of the causes of coma in children. An immediate blood glucose (or Dextrostix), complete blood count, urine obtained by catheterization if necessary, pH and electrolytes (including bicarbonate), serum urea nitrogen, and aspartate aminotransferase (AST) are initial screens. Urine, blood, and even gastric contents must be saved for toxin screen if the underlying cause is not obvious. Spinal tap is often necessary to rule out CNS infection. Papilledema is a relative contraindication to lumbar puncture. Occasionally, blood culture is obtained, antibiotics started, and imaging study of the brain done prior to a diagnostic spinal tap. If meningitis is suspected and a tap is believed to be hazardous, antibiotics should be started and the diagnostic spinal puncture done later. Tests that are helpful in obscure cases of coma include $PO_2$, $PCO_2$, ammonia levels, serum and urine osmolality, porphyrins, lead levels, and urine and serum amino acids and urine organic acids.

If head trauma or increased pressure is suspected, an emergency CT scan or MRI is necessary. Bone windows on the former study or skull radiographs can be done at the same sitting. The absence of skull fracture does not rule out coma caused by closed head trauma. Injury that results from shaking a child is one example. In a child with an open fontanelle, a real-time ultrasound may be substituted for the other, more definitive imaging studies if there is good local expertise.

Rarely, an emergency EEG aids in diagnosing the cause of coma. A nonconvulsive status epilepticus or focal finding seen with herpes encephalitis (periodic lateralized epileptiform discharges) and focal slowing as seen with stroke or cerebritis are cases in which the EEG might be helpful. The EEG also may correlate with the stage of coma (eg, in Reye syndrome) and add prognostic information.

## Treatment

### A. GENERAL MEASURES

Vital signs must be monitored and maintained. Most emergency rooms and intensive care units have flow sheets that provide space for repeated monitoring of the coma; one of the coma scales (described earlier) can be a useful tool for this purpose. The patient's response to vocal or painful stimuli and orientation to time, place, and situation are monitored. Posture and movements of the limbs, either spontaneously or in response to pain, are serially noted. Pupillary size, equality, and reaction to light and movement of the eyes to the doll's-eye maneuver or ice-water calorics should be recorded. Intravenous fluids can be tailored to the situation, as for treatment of acidosis, shock, or hypovolemia. Nasogas-

tric suction is initially important. The bladder should be catheterized for monitoring urine output and for urinalysis.

### B. SEIZURES

An EEG should be ordered if seizures are suspected. If obvious motor seizures have occurred, treatment for status epilepticus is given with intravenous drugs (see section on Seizure Disorders). If brainstem herniation or increased pressure is possible, an intracranial monitor may be necessary. This procedure is described in more detail in Chapter 13. Initial treatment of impending herniation includes keeping the patient's head up (15–30 degrees) and providing hyperventilation. The use of mannitol, diuretics, corticosteroids, and drainage of cerebrospinal fluid (CSF) are more heroic measures covered in detail in Chapter 13.

## Prognosis

About 50% of children with nontraumatic causes of coma have a good outcome. In studies of adults assessed on admission or within the first days after the onset of coma, an analysis of multiple variables was most helpful in assessing prognosis. Abnormal neurophthalmologic signs (eg, the absence of pupillary reaction or of eye movement in response to the doll's-eye maneuver or ice water calorics and the absence of corneal responses) were unfavorable. Delay in the return of motor responses, tone, or eye opening was also unfavorable. In children, the assessment done on admission is about as predictive as one done in succeeding days. Approximately two thirds of outcomes can be successfully predicted at an early stage on the basis of coma severity, extraocular movements, pupillary reactions, motor patterns, blood pressure, temperature, and seizure type. Other characteristics, such as the need for assisted respiration, the presence of increased intracranial pressure, and the duration of coma, are not significantly predictive. Published reports suggest that an anoxic (in contrast to traumatic, metabolic, or toxic) coma, such as that caused by near drowning, has a much grimmer outlook.

## BRAIN DEATH

Many medical and law associations have endorsed the following definition of death: An individual who has sustained either (1) irreversible cessation of circulatory and respiratory functions or (2) irreversible cessation of all functions of the entire brain, including the brainstem, is dead. A determination of death must be made in accordance with accepted medical standards. Representatives from several pediatric and neurologic associations have endorsed the Guidelines for the Determina-

**Table 23–5.** Some causes of coma in childhood.

| Mechanism of Coma | Likely Cause | |
|---|---|---|
| | Newborn Infant | Older Child |
| Anoxia | | |
|   Asphyxia | Birth asphyxia | CO poisoning |
|   Respiratory obstruction | Meconium aspiration, infection (especially respiratory syncytial virus) | Croup, epiglottitis |
|   Severe anemia | Hydrops fetalis | Hemolysis, blood loss |
| Ischemia | | |
|   Cardiac | Shunting lesions, hypoplastic left heart | Shunting lesions, aortic stenosis, myocarditis |
|   Shock | Asphyxia, sepsis | Blood loss, infection |
| Head trauma | Birth contusion, hemorrhage, nonaccidental trauma | Falls, auto accidents, athletic injuries |
| Infection | Gram-negative meningitis, herpes encephalitis, sepsis | Bacterial meningitis, viral encephalitis, postinfectious encephalitis |
| Vascular | Intraventricular hemorrhage, sinus thrombosis | Arterial or venous occlusion with congenital heart disease |
| Neoplasm | "Unknown" | Brain stem glioma, increased pressure with posterior fossa tumors |
| Drugs | Maternal sedatives, injected analgesics | Overdose, many drugs |
| Epilepsy | Constant minor motor seizures; electrical seizure without motor manifestations | Constant minor motor seizures, petit mal status, postictal state; drugs given to stop seizures |
| Toxins | Maternal sedatives or injections | Arsenic, alcohol, drugs, pesticides |
| Hypoglycemia | Birth injury, diabetic progeny, toxemic progeny | Diabetes, "prediabetes," hypoglycemic agents |
| Increased intracranial pressure | Anoxic brain damage, hydrocephalus, metabolic disorders (urea cycle; amino-, organic acidurias) | Toxic encephalopathy, Reye syndrome, head trauma, tumor of posterior fossa |
| Hepatic causes | Hepatic failure, inborn metabolic errors in bilirubin conjugation | Hepatic failure |
| Renal causes | Hypoplastic kidneys | Nephritis, acute and chronic |
| Hypertensive encephalopathy | | Acute nephritis, vasculitis Reversible posterior leucoencephelopathy |
| Hypercapnia | Congenital lung anomalies, bronchopulmonary dysplasia | Cystic fibrosis |
| Electrolyte abnormalities | | |
|   Hypernatremia | Iatrogenic ($NaHCO_3$ use), salt poisoning | Diarrhea, dehydration |
|   Hyponatremia | Inappropriate antidiuretic hormone, adrenogenital syndrome, dialysis (iatrogenic) | Diarrhea, dehydration |
|   Severe acidosis | Septicemia, cold injury, metabolic errors | Infection, diabetic coma, poisoning (eg, aspirin) |
|   Hyperkalemia | Renal failure, adrenogenital syndrome | Poisoning (aspirin) |
| Purpuric | Disseminated intravascular coagulation, hemolytic-uremic syndrome | Disseminated intravascular coagulation, leukemia, thrombotic purpura (rare) |

Modified and reproduced, with permission, from Lewis J, Moe PG: The unconscious child. In: Conn H, Conn R (eds). *Current Diagnosis*, 5th ed. WB Saunders, 1977.

tion of Brain Death in Children. The criteria in full-term infants (ie, born at greater than 38 weeks' gestation) were applicable 1 week after the neurologic insult. Difficulties in assessing premature infants and full-term infants shortly after birth were acknowledged.

## Prerequisites

In assessment of brain death, the history is important. The physician must determine proximate causes to make sure no remediable or reversible conditions are present. Examples of such causes are metabolic conditions, toxic agents, sedative–hypnotic drugs, surgically remediable conditions, hypothermia, and paralytic agents.

## Physical Examination Criteria

(See also Chapter 13)

The following criteria are those established by the Task Force on Brain Death in Children:

**1. Coexistence of coma and apnea**—The patient must exhibit complete loss of consciousness, vocalization, and volitional activity.

**2. Absence of brainstem function**—As defined by the following: (a) Midposition or fully dilated pupils that do not respond to light. Drugs may influence and invalidate pupillary assessment. (b) Absence of spontaneous eye movements and those induced by side-to-side passive head movements (oculocephalic reflex) and ice water instillation in the external auditory canal (ice water calorics). (c) Absence of movement of bulbar musculature, including facial and oropharyngeal muscles. The corneal, gag, cough, sucking, and rooting reflexes are absent. (d) Absence of respiratory movements when the patient is off the respirator. Apnea testing using standardized methods can be performed but is done after other criteria are met.

**3. Temperature and blood pressure**—The patient must not be significantly hypothermic or hypotensive for age.

**4. Tone**—Tone is flaccid, and spontaneous or induced movements are absent, excluding spinal cord events such as reflex withdrawal or spinal myoclonus.

**5. General examination findings**—The examination should remain consistent with brain death throughout the observation and testing period.

## Confirmation

Apnea testing should be carried out at a $P_{CO_2}$ level greater than 60 mm Hg, and with normal oxygenation maintained throughout the test period. This level may be reached 3–15 minutes after taking the patient off the respirator. The recommended observation period to confirm brain death (repeated examinations) is 12–24 hours (longer in infants); reversible causes must be ruled out. If an irreversible cause is documented, laboratory testing is not essential. Helpful tests to support the clinical assertion of brain death include EEG and angiography. Electrocerebral silence on EEG should persist for 30 minutes, and drug concentrations must be insufficient to suppress EEG activity. Absence of intracerebral arterial blood flow can be confirmed by carotid angiography and cerebral radionuclide angiography. Persistence of dural sinus flow does not invalidate the diagnosis of brain death.

Cerebral evoked potentials, intracranial blood pulsations on ultrasound, and xenon-enhanced CT have not been sufficiently studied to be considered definitive in the diagnosis of brain death. In rare cases, preserved intracranial perfusion in the presence of EEG silence has been documented, and the converse has also been reported.

Alfonso I et al: Evaluation of the comatose full term neonate. Int Pediatr 1997;12:74.

Lazar NM et al: Bioethics for clinicians: 24. Brain death. CMAJ 2001;164:833 [PMID: 11276553].

Ruiz-Garcia M et al: Brain death in children: Clinical, neurophysiological and radioisotopic angiography findings in 125 patients. Childs Nerv Syst 2000;16:40 [PMID: 10672428].

Shewmon DA: Coma prognosis in children. Part II: Clinical application. J Clin Neurophysiol 2000;17:467 [PMID: 11085550].

Singhi P et al: Reversible brain lesions in childhood hypertension. Acta Paediatr 2002;91:1005 [PMID: 12412881].

Wijdicks EFM: Brain death worldwide: Accepted fact but no global consensus in diagnostic criteria. Neurology 2002;58:20 [PMID: 11781400].

Yager JY et al: Coma scales in pediatric practice. Am J Dis Child 1990;144:1088 [PMID: 2403089].

## SEIZURE DISORDERS (Epilepsies)

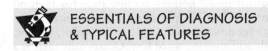

### ESSENTIALS OF DIAGNOSIS & TYPICAL FEATURES

- *Recurrent nonfebrile seizures.*
- *Often, interictal electroencephalographic changes.*

## General Considerations

A seizure is a sudden, transient disturbance of brain function, manifested by involuntary motor, sensory, autonomic, or psychic phenomena, alone or in any combination, often accompanied by alteration or loss of consciousness. A seizure may occur after a metabolic, traumatic, anoxic, or infectious insult to the brain.

Repeated seizures without evident cause justify the label of epilepsy. Seizures and epilepsy occur most commonly at the extremes of life. The incidence is highest in the newborn period and higher in childhood than in later life. Epilepsy in childhood often remits. Prevalence flattens out after age 10–15 years. The chance of having a second seizure after an initial unprovoked episode is 30%. The chance of remission from epilepsy in childhood is 50%. The recurrence rate after the withdrawal of drugs is about 30%. Factors adversely influencing recurrence include (1) difficulty in getting the seizures under control (ie, the number of seizures occurring before control is achieved), (2) neurologic dysfunction or mental retardation, (3) age at onset younger than 2 years, and (4) abnormal EEG at the time of discontinuing medication. The type of seizure also often determines prognosis.

Seizures are caused by any factor that disturbs brain function. Seizures and epilepsy are often classified as symptomatic (the cause is identified or presumed) or idiopathic (the cause is unknown or presumed to be genetic). The younger the infant or child, the more likely it is the cause can be identified. Idiopathic or genetic epilepsy most often appears between ages 4 and 16 years. A seizure disorder or epilepsy should not be considered idiopathic unless thorough history, examination, and laboratory tests have revealed no apparent cause.

## Clinical Findings

### A. SYMPTOMS AND SIGNS

The key to the diagnosis of epilepsy is the history. An aura sometimes precedes the seizure itself. The patient describes a feeling of fear, numbness or tingling in the fingers, or bright lights in one visual field. Sometimes the patient recalls nothing because there has been no aura or warning. The parent might report that the patient's eyes deviated to one side or that pallor, trismus, or body stiffening occurred first. Occasionally there is a prodrome. For example, the patient may experience a feeling of unwellness, a premonition that something is about to happen, or a recurrent thought for minutes or hours prior to the aura and seizure itself.

Minute details of the seizure can help determine the site of onset and aid in classification. Did the patient become extremely pale before falling? Was the patient able to respond to queries during the episode? Did the patient become completely unconscious? Did the patient fall stiffly or gradually slump to the floor? Was there an injury? How long did the stiffening or jerking last? Where in the body did the jerking take place?

Events after the seizure can be helpful in diagnosis. Was there loss of speech? Was the patient able to respond accurately before going to sleep? All the events prior to, during, and after the seizure can help to classify the seizure and, indeed, may help to determine if the event actually was an epileptic seizure or a pseudoseizure (a nonepileptic phenomenon mimicking a seizure). Classifying the seizure may aid in diagnosis or prognosis and may suggest appropriate laboratory tests and medications (Tables 23–6 and 23–7).

### B. STATUS EPILEPTICUS

Status epilepticus is a clinical or electrical seizure lasting at least 30 minutes, or a series of seizures without complete recovery over the same period of time. After 30 minutes of seizure activity, hypoxia and acidosis occur, with depletion of energy stores, cerebral edema, and structural damage. Eventually, high fever, hypotension, respiratory depression, and even death may occur. Status epilepticus is a medical emergency.

Status epilepticus is classified as (1) convulsive (the common tonic–clonic, or grand mal, status epilepticus) or (2) nonconvulsive (characterized by altered mental status or behavior with subtle or absent motor components). Absence status, or spike-wave stupor, and (very rare) partial complex status epilepticus are examples of the nonconvulsive type (Table 23–8). An EEG may be necessary to aid in diagnosing nonconvulsive status, because these patients sometimes appear merely stuporous and lack typical convulsive movements.

A child with status epilepticus may have a high fever with or without intracranial infection. Studies show that 25–75% of children with status epilepticus experience it as their initial seizure. Often it is a reflection of a remote insult (eg, anoxic or traumatic). Tumor, stroke, or head trauma, which are common causes of status epilepticus in adults, are uncommon causes in childhood. Fifty percent of cases are symptomatic of acute (25%) or chronic (25%) CNS disorders. Infection and metabolic disorders are the most common causes of status epilepticus in children. The cause is unknown in 50% of patients, but many of these patients will be febrile. Status epilepticus occurs most commonly in children age 5 years and younger (85%). The most common age is 1 year or younger (37%), and the distribution is even for each year thereafter (approximately 12% per year). For treatment options, see Table 23–9.

### C. FEBRILE SEIZURES

Criteria for febrile seizures are (1) ages 3 months to 5 years (most occur between ages 6 and 18 months), (2) fever of greater than 38.8°C, and (3) non-CNS infection. More than 90% of febrile seizures are generalized, last less than 5 minutes, and occur early in the illness causing the fever. Febrile seizures occur in 2–3%

*Table 23–6.* Seizures by age at onset, pattern, and preferred treatment.

| Age Group and Seizure Type | Age at Onset | Clinical Manifestations | Causative Factors | Electroencephalographic Pattern | Other Diagnostic Studies | Treatment and Comments (Anticonvulsants by Order of Choice) |
|---|---|---|---|---|---|---|
| Neonatal seizures | Birth to 2 wk | Often atypical; sudden limpness or tonic posturing, brief apnea, and cyanosis; odd cry; eyes rolling up; blinking or mouthing or chewing movements; nystagmus, twitchiness or clinic movements—focal, multifocal, or generalized. Some seizures are nonepileptic-decerebrate, or other posturings, release from forebrain inhibition; poor response to drugs. | Neurologic insults (hypoxia/ ischemia; intracranial hemorrhage) present more in first 3 d or after eighth day; metabolic disturbances alone between third and eighth days; hypoglycemia, hypocalcemia, hyper- and hyponatremia. Drug withdrawal. Pyridoxine dependency and other metabolic causes. CNS infections and structural abnormalities. | May correlate poorly with clinical seizures. Focal spikes or slow rhythms; multifocal discharges. Electroclinical dissociation may occur: EEG-electrical seizure without clinical manifestations and vice versa. | Lumbar puncture; CSF PCR for herpes, enterovirus; serum $Ca^{2+}$, $PO_4{}^{3-}$, glucose, $MG^{2+}$; BUN, amino acid screen, blood ammonia, organic acid screen, TOR-CHES[a] IgM. Ultrasound or CT scan for suspected intracranial hemorrhage and structural abnormalities | Phenobarbital, IV or IM; if seizures not controlled, add phenytoin IV (loading dose 20 mg/kg each). Diazepam 0.3 mg/kg. Treat underlying disorder. Seizures due to brain damage often resistant to anticonvulsants. When cause in doubt, stop protein feedings until enzyme deficiencies of urea cycle or amino acid metabolism ruled out. |
| West syndrome infantile spasms. (See also Lennox–Gastaut syndrome, below.) | 3–18 mos; occasionally up to 4 y | Sudden, usually symmetric adduction and flexion of limbs with concomitant flexion of head and trunk; also abduction and extensor movements like Moro reflex. Tendency for spasms to occur in clusters, on waking or falling asleep, or when fatigued, or may be noted particularly when the infant is being handled, is ill, or is otherwise irritable. Tendency to have own stereotyped pattern. | Pre- or perinatal brain damage or malformation in approximately one third; biochemical, infectious, degenerative causes in approximately one third; unknown in approximately one third. With early onset, pyridoxine deficiency, amino- or organic aciduria. Tuberous sclerosis in 5–10%. Chronic inflammatory brain disease, eg, TORCHES[a], homeobox gene mutations. | Hypsarrhythmia; chaotic high-voltage slow waves, random spikes, all leads (90%); other abnormalities in 10%. Rarely normal. EEG normalization usually early in course correlates with reduction of seizures; not helpful prognostically regarding mental development. | Funduscopic and skin examination, trial of pyridoxine. Amino and organic acid screen. Chronic inflammatory brain disease. TORCHES[a] screen, CT, or MRI scan should be done to (1) establish definite diagnosis, (2) aid in genetic counseling. SPECT or PET scan may identify focal lesion. | ACTH preferred (2–4 U/kg/d) IM Acthar gel once daily, then slow withdrawal. Some prefer oral corticosteroids. Clonazepam, valproic acid, vigabatrin, $B_6$ pyridoxine trial (Japan). In resistant cases, ketogenic or medium-chain triglyceride diet (see text). New drugs: zonisamide, topiramate, lamotrigine. Retardation of varying degree in approximately 90% of cases. Occasionally, surgical extirpation of focal lesion may be curative. |

*(continued)*

**Table 23–6.** Seizures by age at onset, pattern, and preferred treatment. (continued)

| Age Group and Seizure Type | Age at Onset | Clinical Manifestations | Causative Factors | Electroencephalographic Pattern | Other Diagnostic Studies | Treatment and Comments (Anticonvulsants by Order of Choice) |
|---|---|---|---|---|---|---|
| Febrile convulsions | 3 mos to 5 y (maximum 6–18 mos) Most common childhood seizure: incidence 2% | Usually generalized seizures, less than 15 mins; rarely focal in onset. May lead to status epilepticus. Latter usually benign. Recurrence risk of second febrile seizure 30%; 50% if under 1 y of age; recurrence risk is same after status. | Nonneurologic febrile illness (temperature rises to 39°C or higher); positive family history, day care, slow development, prolonged neonatal hospitalization are other risk factors. | Normal interictal EEG, especially when obtained 8–10 d after seizure. In older infants, 3/s generalized spike waves often seen. | Lumbar puncture in infants or whenever suspicion of meningitis exists. | Treat underlying illness, fever. Diazepam orally or rectally as needed, 0.3–0.5 mg/kg tid during illness or for prolonged (>5–15 mins) seizure. Prophylaxis with phenobarbital or valproic acid rarely needed: maybe with neurologic deficits; prolonged seizures, family anxiety. |
| Myoclonic-astatic (akinetic, atonic) seizures, formerly atypical absence. When mental retardation is presented, this is called Lennox–Gastaut syndrome. | Any time in childhood; normally 2–7 y | Shock-like violent contractions of one or more muscle groups, singly or irregularly repetitive; may fling patient suddenly to side, forward, or backward. Usually no or only brief loss of consciousness. Half of patients or more also have generalized grand mal seizures. | Multiple causes, usually resulting in diffuse neuronal damage. History of West's syndrome; prenatal or perinatal brain damage; viral meningoencephalitides; CNS degenerative disorders; lead or other encephalopathies; structural cerebral abnormalities; eg, migrational abnormalities. | Atypical slow (1–2.5 Hz) spike-wave complexes (petit mal variant) and bursts of high-voltage generalized spikes, often with diffusely slow background frequencies. See text. | As dictated by index of suspicion. Nerve conduction studies. Skin or conjunctival biopsy for electron microscopy, MRI scan, WBC lysosomal enzymes if metabolic degenerative disease suspected. | Difficult to treat. Valproic acid, clonazepam, ethosuximide. Felbamate. Diazepam. Ketogenic or medium-chain triglyceride diet. ACTH or corticosteroids as in West syndrome. Perhaps lamotrigine, topiramate, zonisomide. Protect head with helmet and chin padding. |
| Absence (petit mal). Also juvenile and myoclonic absence. | 3–15 y | Lapses of consciousness or vacant stares, lasting about 10 s, often in "clusters." Automatisms of face and hands; clonic activity in 30–45%. Often confused with complex partial seizures but no aura or postictal confusion. | Unknown. Genetic component: probably an autosomal dominant gene. | 3/s bilaterally synchronous, symmetric, high-voltage spikes and waves. EEG normalization correlates closely with control of seizures. | Hyperventilation when patient on inadequate or no medication often provokes attacks. CT scan is rarely of value. | Valproic acid or ethosuximide; with latter, add phenobarbital or valproate if major motor seizures. In resistant cases, ketogenic diet, lamotrigine, topiramate, acetazolamide. |

| Seizure type | Age at Onset | Clinical Features | Common Causes | EEG | Diagnostic Studies | Treatment |
|---|---|---|---|---|---|---|
| Simple partial or focal seizures (motor/sensory/jacksonian). | Any age | Seizure may involve any part of body; may spread in fixed pattern (jacksonian march), becoming generalized. In children, epileptogenic focus often "shifts," and epileptic manifestations may change concomitantly. | Often secondary to birth trauma, inflammatory process, vascular accidents, meningoencephalitis, etc. If seizures are coupled with new or progressive neurologic deficits, a structural lesion (eg, brain tumor) is likely | Focal spikes or slow waves in appropriate cortical region; sometimes diffusely abnormal or even normal. "Rolandic spikes" one typical (often benign) pattern. | If seizures are difficult to control or progressive deficits occur, neuroradiodiagnostic studies, particularly MRI brain scan, imperative (see text). | Carbamazepine, phenytoin. Valproic acid useful adjunct. Also used: lamotrigine, gabapentin, topiramate, and levetiracetam |
| Complex partial seizures (psychomotor, temporal lobe, or limbic seizures are older terms). | Any age | Aura may be a sensation of fear, eigastric discomfort, odd smell or taste (usually unpleasant), visual or auditory hallucination (either vague and "unformed" or well-formed image, words, music). Aura and seizure stereotyped for each patient. Seizure may consist of vague stare; facial, tongue, or swallowing movements and throaty sounds; or various complex automatisms. Unlike absences, complex partial seizures tend not to occur in clusters but singly and to last longer (1 min or more), followed by confusion. History of aura (eg, child running to adult from "vague fear") and of automatisms involving more than face and hands establish diagnosis. | As above. Temporal lobes especially sensitive to hypoxia; thus, this seizure type may be a sequela of birth trauma, febrile convulsions, etc. Also especially vulnerable to certain viral infections, especially herpes simplex. Remediable other causes are small cryptic tumors or vascular malformations. | As above, but occurring in temporal lobe and its connections, eg, frontotemporal, temporoparietal, temporo-occipital regions. | MRI when structural lesions suspected. PCR of cerebrospinal fluid in acute febrile situation for herpes; rarely, temporal lobe biopsy. Carotid amobarbital injection when lateralization of speech dominance in question and surgical extirpation of epileptogenic area is contemplated. | Carbamazepine, phenytoin. More than one drug may be necessary. Valproic acid may be useful. In cases uncontrolled by drugs and where a primary epileptogenic focus is identifiable, excision of anterior third of temporal lobe. Gabapentin, topiramate, lamotrigine, levetiracetam, and tiagabine (for > 16-year-olds). |

(continued)

*Table 23–6.* Seizures by age at onset, pattern, and preferred treatment. (continued)

| Age Group and Seizure Type | Age at Onset | Clinical Manifestations | Causative Factors | Electroencephalographic Pattern | Other Diagnostic Studies | Treatment and Comments (Anticonvulsants by Order of Choice) |
|---|---|---|---|---|---|---|
| Benign epilepsy of childhood (with centrotemporal or rolandic foci) | 5–16 y | Partial motor or generalized seizures. Similar seizure patterns may be observed in patients with focal cortical lesions. Usually nocturnal simple partial seizures of face, tongue, hand. | Seizure history or abnormal EEG findings in relatives of 40% of affected probands and 18–20% of parents and siblings, suggesting transmission by a single autosomal-dominant gene, possibly with age-dependent penetrance. | Centrotemporal spikes or sharp waves ("rolandic discharges") appearing paroxysmally against a normal EEG background. | Seldom need CT or MRI scan. | Carbamazepine or phenytoin. (See simple, complex partial seizures.) Often no medication is necessary, especially if seizure is exclusively nocturnal and infrequent. Lamotrigine, topiramate. |
| Juvenile myoclonic epilepsy (of Janz) | Late childhood and adolescence, peaking at 13 y | Mild myoclonic jerks of neck and shoulder flexor muscles after awakening. Intelligence usually normal. Often absence seizures, and GTCS as well. | 40% of relatives have myoclonias, especially in females; 15% have the abnormal EEG pattern with clinical attacks. | Interictal EEG shows variety of spike-and-wave sequences or 4- to 6-Hz multispike and wave complexes ("fast spikes") | Differentiate from progressive myoclonic encephalopathy of Unverricht-Lafora and other degenerative disorders by appropriate biopsies (muscles, liver, etc). | Valproic acid. Lamotrigine. topiramate ?Levetiracetam. |
| Generalized tonic–clonic seizures (grand mal) (GTCS) | Any age | Loss of consciousness; tonic–clonic movements, often preceded by vague aura or cry. Bladder and bowel incontinence in approximately 15%. Postictal confusion; sleep. Often mixed with or masking other seizure patterns. | Often unknown. Genetic component. May be seen with metabolic disturbances, trauma, infection, intoxication, degenerative disorders, brain tumors. | Bilaterally synchronous, symmetrical multiple high-voltage spikes, spikes and waves, mixed patterns. Often normal younger than age 4. | As above | Phenobarbital in infants; carbamazepine or valproic acid; phenytoin; topiramate, oxcarbazepine. Combinations may be necessary. |

<sup></sup>aTORCHES is a mnemonic formula for toxoplasmosis, rubella, cytomegalovirus, herpes simplex, and syphilis.

ACTH = adrenocorticotropic hormone; BUN = blood urea nitrogen; CNS = central nervous system; CT = computed tomography; EEG = electroencephalogram; IM = intramuscularly; IV = intravenously; MRI = magnetic resonance imaging; PCR = polymerase chain reaction; PET = positron emission tomography; SPECT = single photon emission computed tomography; WBC = white blood cell.

*Table 23–7.* Benign childhood epileptic syndromes.

| Syndrome | Characteristics |
|---|---|
| Benign idiopathic neonatal convulsions (BINC) | 6% of neonatal convulsions; 97% have onset on 3rd to 7th day of life (so-called 5th day fits); clonic; multifocal; usually brief; occasional status epilepticus |
| Benign familial neonatal convulsions (BFNC) | Autosomal-dominant; onset in 2–90 d; 20% have linkage to chromosome 20q13; clonic; 86% recover |
| Generalized tonic–clonic seizures (GTCS) | Age at onset, 3–11 y; may have family or personal history of febrile convulsions; 50% have 3/s spike-wave EEG; may have concurrent absence seizures |
| Childhood absence seizures | Incidence higher in girls than in boys; age at onset, 3–12 y (peak 6–7 years); 10–200 seizures per day; 3/s spike–wave EEG; 40% have GTCS; most remit at puberty |
| Juvenile absence seizures | Incidence higher in boys than in girls; age at onset, 10–12 y; uncommon; less frequent seizures; 3–4/s general spike–wave EEG; most have GTCS; some remit |
| Juvenile myoclonic epilepsy (Janz syndrome) | Age at onset, 12–18 y (average, 15 y); myoclonic jerks upper limbs, seldom fall; 4–6/s general spike–wave EEG; untreated, 90% have GTCS, mostly on waking; 20–30% have absence seizures; 25–40% are photosensitive; 10% remission rate |
| Benign epilepsy with centrotemporal spikes (BECTS); rolandic epilepsy | Autosomal-dominant; age at onset 3–13 y (most at 4–10 y); 80% have brief, 2–5 min sleep seizures only; usually simple partial seizures (face, tongue, cheek, hand) sensory or motor; occasionally have GTCS; bilateral spikes on EEG; may not need medication if seizures infrequent; remits at puberty |

EEG = electroencephalogram.

*Table 23–8.* Status epilepticus: clinical types.

**Generalized seizure (common)**
  Convulsive (tonic, clonic, myoclonic); 90%
  Nonconvulsive (absence, atypical absence, atonic); 10%
**Focal (partial) seizures (rare)**
  Simple partial
  Complex partial
**Neonatal**
  Many clinical varieties
  May be electrical (ie, on electroencephalogram) status only with no visible clinical findings; called electroclinical dissociation

febrile seizures have complex features, such as a duration of longer 15 minutes, more than one seizure in the same day, or focal features. Other adverse factors are an abnormal neurologic status preceding the seizures (eg, cerebral palsy or mental retardation), early onset of febrile seizure (before age 1 year), and a family history of epilepsy. Even with adverse factors, the risk of epilepsy after febrile seizures is low, in the range of 15–20%. Recurrent febrile seizures occur in 30–50% of cases but, in general, do not worsen the long-term outlook.

The child with a febrile seizure must be examined. Routine studies such as serum electrolytes, glucose, calcium, skull radiographs, or brain imaging studies are seldom helpful. A white count above 20,000/µL or an extreme left shift may correlate with bacteremia. Complete blood count and blood cultures may be appropriate studies. Serum sodium is often slightly low but not low enough to require treatment or to cause the seizure. Meningitis must be ruled out. Patients with bacterial meningitis can present with a fever and seizure. Signs of meningitis (eg, bulging fontanelle, stiff neck, stupor, and irritability) may all be absent, especially in a child younger than age 18 months.

After controlling the fever and stopping an ongoing seizure, the physician must decide whether to do a spinal tap. The fact that the child has had a previous febrile seizure does not rule out meningitis as the cause of the current episode. The younger the child, the more important the tap, because physical findings are less reliable in diagnosing meningitis. Although the yield is low, a tap should probably be done if the child is younger than age 2 years, if recovery is slow, if no other cause for the fever is found, or if close follow-up will not be possible. Occasionally observation in the emergency room for several hours obviates the need for a tap. A negative tap does not rule out the emergence of meningitis during the same febrile illness. Sometimes a second tap must be done.

of children. Acute respiratory illnesses are most commonly associated with febrile seizures. Gastroenteritis, especially when caused by *Shigella* or *Campylobacter,* and urinary tract infections are less common causes. Roseola infantum is a rare but classic cause. One study implicated viral causes in 86% of cases. Immunizations may be a cause.

Rarely status epilepticus may occur during a febrile seizure. Febrile seizures rarely (1–2.4%) lead to epilepsy or recurrent nonfebrile seizures in later childhood and adult life. The chance of later epilepsy is higher if the

***Table 23–9.*** Status epilepticus treatment.

---

1. ABCs
   a. Airway: Maintain oral airway; intubation may be necessary.
   b. Breathing: Oxygen.
   c. Circulation: Assess pulse, blood pressure; support with IV fluids, drugs. Monitor vital signs.
2. Start glucose-containing IV; evaluate serum glucose; electrolytes, $HCO_3^-$, CBC, BUN, anticonvulsant levels.
3. May need arterial blood gases, pH.
4. Give 50% glucose if dextrose low (1–2 mL/kg).
5. Begin IV drug therapy; goal is to control status epilepticus in 20–60 min.
   a. Diazepam 0.3–0.5 mg/kg over 1–5 min (20 mg maximum); may repeat in 5–20 min; or, lorazepam 0.05–0.2 mg/kg (less effective with repeated doses, longer-acting than diazepam). Midazolam IM or IV: 0.1–0.3 mg/kg; intranasally, 0.2 mg/kg.
   b. Phenytoin 10–20 mg/kg IV (not IM) over 5–20 min; 1000 mg maximum); monitor with blood pressure and ECG. Fosphenytoin may be given more rapidly—even IM—in the same dosage; order 10–20 mg/kg of "phenytoin equivalent."
   c. Phenobarbital 5–20 mg/kg (sometimes higher in newborns or refractory status in intubated patients).
6. Correct metabolic perturbations (eg, low-sodium, acidosis).
7. Other drug approaches in refractory status:
   a. Repeat phenytoin, phenobarbital (10 mg/kg). Monitor blood levels. Support respiration, blood pressure as necessary.
   b. Midazolam drip: 1-5 μg/kg/min (even to 20 kgm/min). Valproate sodium (Depacon), available as 100 mg/mL for IV use; give 15–30 mg/kg over 5–20 min.
   c. Pentobarb coma. Propofol. General anesthetic.
8. Consider underlying causes:
   a. Structural disorders or trauma. Consider CT scan.
   b. Infection: Spinal tap, blood culture, antibiotics.
   c. Metabolic disorders: Consider lactic acidosis, toxins, uremia. May need to evaluate medication levels, toxin screen, judicious fluid administration.
9. Give maintenance drug (if diazepam only was sufficient to halt status epilepticus): phenytoin 10 mg/kg, phenobarbital 5 mg/kg, daily dose IV (or by mouth) divided every 12 hours.

---

BUN = blood urea nitrogen; CBC = complete blood count; CT = computed tomography; ECG = electrocardiogram; IM = intramuscularly; IV = intravenously.

Prophylactic anticonvulsants are not required after the uncomplicated febrile seizure. If febrile seizures are complicated or prolonged, or if medical reassurance fails to relieve family anxiety, anticonvulsant prophylaxis may be indicated and can reduce the incidence of recurrent febrile or nonfebrile seizures. One remedy is to use diazepam at the first onset of fever for the duration of the febrile illness (0.5 mg/kg two or three times per day orally or rectally). Diastat is an expensive rectal diazepam preparation. Phenobarbital, 3–5 mg/kg/d as a single bedtime dose, is an inexpensive and safe prophylaxis. Often, increasing the dosage gradually (eg, starting with 2 mg/kg/d the first week, increasing to 3 mg/kg/d the second week, and so on) decreases side effects and noncompliance. A plasma phenobarbital level in the range of 15–40 mg/mL is desirable. Valproate sodium is more hazardous. In infants, the commonly used liquid suspension has a short half-life and causes more gastrointestinal upset than do the sprinkle capsules. The dosage is 15–60 mg/kg/d in two three or four divided doses. Precautionary laboratory studies are necessary. Phenytoin and carbamazepine have not shown effectiveness in the prophylaxis of febrile seizures (see Table 23–9). Measures to control fever such as sponging or tepid baths, antipyretics, and the administration of antibiotics for proven bacterial illness are reasonable but unproven to prevent recurrent febrile seizures.

Simple febrile seizures do not have any long-term adverse consequences. An EEG should be performed if the febrile seizure is complicated or unusual. In uncomplicated febrile seizures, the EEG is usually normal. About 22% of patients will show slowing or epileptiform abnormalities. Ideally the EEG should be done at least a week after the illness to avoid transient changes due to fever or the seizure itself. In older children, 3/s spike-wave discharge, suggestive of a genetic propensity to epilepsy, may occur. In the young infant, EEG findings seldom aid in assessing the chance of recurrence of febrile seizures or in long-term prognosis.

### D. LABORATORY FINDINGS AND IMAGING

Ordering of laboratory tests depends on the child's age, the severity and type of seizure, whether the child is ill or injured, and the clinician's suspicion about the underlying cause. Every case of suspected seizure disorder warrants an EEG. Other studies are used selectively. Seizures in early infancy are often symptomatic. Therefore, the younger the child, the more careful must be the laboratory assessment (Table 23–10).

Metabolic abnormalities are seldom found in the well child with seizures. Unless there is a high clinical suspicion of uremia, hyponatremia, or other serious conditions, laboratory tests are not necessary. Special studies may be necessary in unusual circumstances, for example, when hemolytic–uremic syndrome or lead poisoning is a suspected cause. CT scans are overused in patients with seizures. The youngster with a routine febrile seizure, a nonfebrile generalized seizure with normal examination and normal EEG, or an absence seizure does not need a CT or MRI scan. The yield in a child with normal neurologic examination and EEG is

**Table 23–10.** Laboratory studies after first seizure (nonneonatal).

| | |
|---|---|
| Well infant | EEG, calcium, BUN, or urinalysis, and perhaps CT or MRI. (Abnormal examination or focally abnormal EEG: do imaging study.) Rule out nonaccidental trauma. |
| Well older child | EEG; consider CT or MRI |
| Ill infant | Calcium, magnesium, CBC, BUN, glucose, electrolytes, blood culture, lumbar puncture, EEG, possibly CT or MRI |
| Ill older child | CBC, BUN, lumbar puncture, EEG, CT or MRI |
| Generalized tonic–clonic seizure | Calcium, glucose, CBC, BUN, electrolytes, lumbar puncture (may omit if afebrile, looks well) |
| Generalized absence | EEG only |
| Atypical absence | EEG, MRI: Consider studies for mental retardation: serum and urine amino and organic acids and chromosomes, including fragile X. If there is progressive worsening, consider lysosomal enzymes, lumbar puncture (protein, enzymes, IgG), long-chain fatty acids, skin or conjunctival biopsies. |
| Infantile spasms | See Atypical absence |
| Myoclonic progressive seizure with mental retardation | See Atypical absence |
| Focal | EEG. In cases of mental retardation, positive neurologic examination, EEG focal slow wave, or poorly controlled seizures, do MRI. In refractory cases, consider surgical evaluation. |

BUN = blood urea nitrogen; CBC = complete blood count; CT = computed tomography; EEG = electroencephalogram; MRI = magnetic resonance imaging.

less than 5%. Conversely, in children with symptomatic epileptic syndromes, the EEG will be abnormal in as many as 60–80% of patients. Examples include infantile spasms, Lennox–Gastaut syndrome, and progressive myoclonic epilepsy.

In focal seizures, children with benign rolandic epilepsy do not need a CT scan; it will invariably be normal. The yield with other focal seizures is 15–30%, with most of the findings unimportant in relation to diagnosis and prognosis (eg, a mildly dilated single ventricle, superficial atrophy). Nonetheless, an imaging study eases anxiety and rules out the remote possibility of tumor or vascular malformation. Other indications for MRI scan (the superior study) scan include difficulty in controlling seizures, progressive neurologic findings on serial examinations, worsening focal findings on the EEG, suspicion of increased pressure, and, of course, any case in which surgery is being considered. A previous normal scan does not rule out an emerging tumor; if the course is unsatisfactory, repeating the scan may be necessary. A neoplasm or other unexpected treatable lesion is found in a small number, perhaps 2–3%, of scans.

### E. ELECTROENCEPHALOGRAPHY

The limitations of EEG—even with epilepsy, for which it is most useful—are considerable. A seizure is a clinical phenomenon; an EEG showing epileptiform activity may confirm and even extend the clinical diagnosis, but it cannot make the diagnosis.

The EEG need not be abnormal in the epileptic child. Normal EEGs are seen following a first generalized seizure in one third of children younger than age 4 years. The initial EEG is normal in about 20% of older epileptic children and in about 10% of epileptic adults. These percentages are reduced when serial tracings are obtained. Focal spikes and generalized spike-wave discharges are seen in 30% of close nonepileptic relatives of patients with epilepsy.

**1. Diagnostic value**—The greatest value of the EEG in convulsive disorders is to help classify seizure types and select appropriate therapy (see Table 23–6). Petit mal absences and partial complex or psychomotor seizures are sometimes difficult to distinguish, especially when the physician must rely on the history and cannot observe the seizure. The differing EEG patterns of these seizures will then prove most helpful. Finding a mixed seizure EEG pattern in a child who clinically has only major motor seizures or only focal seizures will help the clinician select anticonvulsants effective for both seizure types identified by the EEG. The EEG may help in diagnosing neonatal seizures with minimal or atypical clinical manifestations; it may show hypsarrhythmia (high-amplitude spikes and slow waves with a disorganized background) in infantile spasms or 1–4/s slow spike-wave pattern of the Lennox–Gastaut syndrome. Both are expressions of diffuse brain dysfunction and generally of grave significance. The EEG may show focal slowing that, if constant, particularly when corresponding focal seizure manifestations and abnormal neurologic findings are present, will alert the physician to the presence of a structural lesion. In this case, brain imaging may establish the cause and help determine further investigation and treatment.

**2. Prognostic value**—A normal EEG following a first convulsion suggests (but does not guarantee) a favorable prognosis. Markedly abnormal EEGs may become normal with treatment (1) immediately following intravenous injection of 50 mg of vitamin $B_6$ in pyridoxine dependency or deficiency; (2) in infantile spasms and sometimes the Lennox–Gastaut syndrome (with the use of adrenocorticotropic hormone [ACTH] or corticosteroids); (3) in absence (appropriate anticonvulsants); and (4) in akinetic and other minor motor seizures, including the Lennox–Gastaut syndrome (ketogenic diet). If so, it is likely that seizure control will be achieved (although this offers no clues to the ultimate developmental status of the patient).

Electroencephalography should be repeated when the severity and frequency of seizures increase despite adequate anticonvulsant therapy, when the clinical seizure pattern changes significantly, or when progressive neurologic deficits develop. Emergence of new focal or diffuse slowing may indicate a progressive lesion. A normalized tracing may help confirm remission of absence seizures.

The EEG may be helpful in determining when to discontinue anticonvulsant therapy. The presence or absence of epileptiform activity on the EEG prior to withdrawal of anticonvulsants after a seizure-free period of several years on the medications has been shown to be correlated with the degree of risk of recurrence of seizures.

## Differential Diagnosis

It is extremely important to be accurate in the diagnosis of epilepsy and not to make the diagnosis without ample proof. To the layperson, epilepsy often has connotations of brain damage and limitation of activity. A person so diagnosed may be excluded from certain occupations in later life. It is often very difficult to change an inaccurate diagnosis of many years' standing. Some of the common nonepileptic events that mimic seizure disorder are listed in Table 23–11.

## Complications

Emotional disturbances—notably anxiety, depression, anger, and feelings of guilt and inadequacy—often occur not only in the patient but also in the parents of the child with seizures. The seizures, particularly the hallucinatory auras and psychomotor attacks, frequently set off in the prepubescent and adolescent patient fantasies (and sometimes obsessive ruminations) about dying and death that may become so strong that they lead to suicidal behavior. The limitations many school systems place on epileptic children add to the problem. Some children may react by acting out.

Pseudoretardation may occur in children with poorly controlled epilepsy because their seizures (or the subclinical paroxysms sustained) interfere with their learning ability. Anticonvulsants are less likely to cause such interference but may do so when given in toxic amounts. Phenobarbital is particularly implicated. True mental retardation is most commonly part of the same pathologic process that causes the seizures but may occasionally be worsened when seizures are frequent, prolonged, and accompanied by hypoxia.

Physical injuries, especially lacerations of the forehead and chin, are frequent in astatic or akinetic seizures (so-called drop attacks), necessitating protective headgear. In all other seizure disorders in childhood, injuries as a direct result of an attack are rare.

## Treatment

The ideal treatment of seizures is the correction of specific causes. However, even when a biochemical disorder, a tumor, meningitis, or another specific cause is being treated, anticonvulsant drugs are often still required.

### A. PRECAUTIONARY MANAGEMENT OF INDIVIDUAL BRIEF SEIZURES

Caregivers should be intstructed to protect the patient against self-injury and aspiration of vomitus; beyond that, no specific therapy is necessary. The less done to the patient during a brief seizure of less than 15 minutes, the better. Thrusting a spoon handle or tongue depressor into the clenched mouth of a convulsing patient or trying to restrain tonic–clonic movements may cause worse injuries than a bitten tongue or bruised limb. Mouth-to-mouth resuscitation is rarely necessary.

### B. GENERAL MANAGEMENT OF THE YOUNG EPILEPTIC PATIENT

**1. Education**—The patient and parents must be helped to understand the problem of seizures and their management. Many children—some even as young as age 3 years—are capable of cooperating with the physician in problems of seizure control.

All bottles containing antiepileptic drugs should be labeled. The parents should know the names and dosage of the anticonvulsants being administered.

Materials on epilepsy—including pamphlets, monographs, films, and videotapes suitable for children and teenagers, parents, teachers, and medical professionals—may be purchased through the Epilepsy Foundation of America, Materials Service Center, 4351 Garden City Drive, Landover, MD 20785. The Foundation's local chapter and other community organizations are eager to provide guidance and other services. Support groups exist in many cities for older chil-

*Table 23–11.* Nonepileptic paroxysmal events.

**Breath-holding attacks**

Age 6 mo to 3 y. Always precipitated by trauma and fright. Cyanosis; sometimes stiffening, tonic (or jerking-clonic) convulsion (anoxic seizure). Patient may sleep following attack. Family history positive in 30%. Electroencephalogram (EEG) normal. Treatment is interpretation and reassurance.

**Infantile syncope (pallid breath holding)**

No external precipitant (perhaps internal pain, cramp, or fear?). Pallor may be followed by seizure (anoxic–ischemic). Vagally (heart-slowing) mediated, like adult syncope. EEG normal; may see cardiac slowing with vagal stimulation (cold cloth on face) during EEG.

**Tics or Tourette syndrome**

Simple or complex stereotyped (the same time after time) jerks or movements, coughs, grunts, sniffs. Worse at repose or with stress. May be suppressed during physician visit. Family history often positive. EEG negative. Nonanticonvulsant drugs may benefit.

**Night terrors, sleep talking, walking, "sit-ups"**

Age 3–10. Usually occur in first sleep cycle (30–90 min after going to sleep), with crying, screaming, and "autonomic discharge" (pupils dilated, perspiring, etc). Lasts minutes. Child goes back to sleep and has no recall of event next day. Sleep studies (polysomnogram and EEG) are normal. Disappears with maturation. Sleep talking and walking and short "sit-ups" in bed are fragmentary arousals. If a spell is recorded, EEG shows arousal from deep sleep, but the behavior seems wakeful. The youngster needs to be protected from injury and gradually settled down and taken back to bed.

**Nightmares**

Nightmares or vivid dreams occur in subsequent cycles of sleep, often in the early morning hours, and generally are partially recalled the next day. The bizarre and frightening behavior may sometimes be confused with complex partial seizures. These occur during REM (rapid eye movement) sleep; epilepsy usually does not occur during that phase of sleep. In extreme or difficult cases, an all-night sleep EEG may help to differentiate seizures from nightmares.

**Migraine**

One variant of migraine can be associated with an acute confusional state. There may be the usual migraine prodrome with spots before the eyes, dizziness, visual field defects, and then agitated confusion. A history of other, more typical migraine with severe headache and vomiting but without confusion may aid in the diagnosis. The severe headache with vomiting as the youngster comes out of the spell may aid in distinguishing the attack from epilepsy. Other seizure manifestations are practically never seen, eg, tonic–clonic movements, falling, and complete loss of consciousness. The EEG in migraine is usually normal and seldom has epileptiform abnormalities often seen in patients with epilepsy. Lastly, migraine and epilepsy are sometimes linked: migraine-caused ischemia on the brain surface sometimes leads to later epilepsy.

**Benign nocturnal myoclonus**

Common in infants and may last even up to school age. Focal or generalized jerks (the latter also called hypnic or sleep jerks) may persist from onset of sleep on and off all night. A video record for physician review can aid in diagnosis. EEG taken during jerks is normal, proving that these jerks are not epilepsy. Treatment is reassurance.

**Shuddering**

Shuddering or shivering attacks can occur in infancy and be a forerunner of essential tremor in later life. Often, the family history is positive for tremor. The shivering may be very frequent. EEG is normal. There is no clouding or loss of consciousness.

**Gastroesophageal reflux**

Seen more commonly in children with cerebral palsy or brain damage; reflux of acid gastric contents may cause pain that cannot be described by the child. At times, there may be unusual posturings (dystonic or other) of the head and neck or trunk, an apparent attempt to stretch the esophagus or close the opening. There is no loss of consciousness, but there may be eye rolling, apnea, occasional vomiting that may simulate a seizure. An upper gastrointestinal series, cine of swallowing, sometimes even an EEG (which is always normal) may be necessary to distinguish this from seizures.

**Masturbation**

Rarely in infants, repetitive rocking or rubbing motions may simulate seizures. The youngster may look out of contact, be poorly responsive to the environment, and have autonomic expressions (eg, perspiration, dilated pupils) that may be confused with seizures. Observation by a skilled individual, sometimes even in a hospital situation, may be necessary to distinguish this from seizures. EEG is of course normal between or during attacks. Interpretation and reassurance are the only necessary treatment.

**Conversion reaction/pseudoseizures**

As many as 50% of patients with pseudoseizures have epilepsy. Episodes may be writhing, intercourse-like movements, tonic episodes, bizarre jerking and thrashing around, or even apparently sudden unresponsiveness. Often, there is ongoing psychological trauma. Often, but not invariably, the patients are developmentally delayed. The spells must often be seen or recorded on videotape in a controlled situation to distinguish them from epilepsy. A normal EEG during a spell is a key diagnostic feature. Often, the spells are so bizarre that they are easily distinguished. Sometimes, pseudoseizures can be precipitated by suggestion with injection of normal saline in a controlled situation. Combativeness is common; self-injury and incontinence rare.

**Temper tantrums and rage attacks**

These are sometimes confused with epilepsy. The youngster is often amnesic or at least claims amnesia for events during the spell. The attacks are usually precipitated by frustration or anger and are often directed either verbally

*(continued)*

***Table 23–11.*** Nonepileptic paroxysmal events. (continued)

or physically and subside with behavior modification and isolation. EEGs are generally normal but unfortunately seldom obtained during an attack. Anterior temporal leads may be helpful in ruling out temporal or lateral frontal abnormalities, the latter sometimes seen in partial complex seizures. Improvement of the attacks with psychotherapy, milieu therapy, or behavioral modification helps rule out epilepsy.

**Benign paroxysmal vertigo**

These are brief attacks of vertigo in which the youngster often appears frightened and pale and clutches the parent. The attacks last 5–30 s. Sometimes, nystagmus is identified. There is no loss of consciousness. Usually, the child is well and returns to play immediately afterward. The attacks may occur in clusters, then disappear for months. Attacks are usually seen in infants and preschoolers age 2–5. EEG is normal. If caloric tests can be obtained (often very difficult

in this age group), abnormalities with hypofunction of one side are sometimes seen. Medications are usually not desirable or necessary.

**Staring spells**

Teachers often make referral for absence or petit mal seizures in youngsters who stare or seem preoccupied at school. Helpful in the history is the lack of these spells at home, eg, before breakfast, a common time for absence seizures. A lack of other epilepsy in the child or family history often is helpful. Sometimes, these children have difficulties with school and a cognitive or learning disability. The child can generally be brought out of this spell by a firm command. An EEG is sometimes necessary to confirm that absence seizures are not occurring. A 24-hour ambulatory EEG to record attacks during the child's everyday school activities is occasionally necessary.

---

dren and adolescents and for their parents and others concerned.

**2. Privileges and precautions in daily life**—Encourage normal living within reasonable bounds. Children should engage in physical activities appropriate to their age and social group. After seizure control is established, swimming is generally permissible with a buddy system or adequate lifeguard coverage. High diving and high climbing should not be permitted. Physical training and sports are usually to be welcomed rather than restricted. Driving is discussed in the next section.

Loss of sleep should be avoided. Emotional disturbances may need to be treated. Alcohol intake should be avoided because it may precipitate seizures. Prompt attention should be given to infections. Further neurologic disturbances should be brought to the physician's attention promptly.

Although every effort should be made to control seizures, this must not interfere with a child's ability to function. Sometimes a child is better off having an occasional mild seizure than being so heavily sedated that function at home, in school, or at play is impaired. Therapy and medication adjustment often require much art and fortitude on the physician's part. Some patients with infrequent seizures, especially if only nocturnal partial seizures (eg, Rolandic seizures) may not need anticonvulsant medications.

**3. Driving**—Driving becomes important to most young people at age 15 or 16 years. Restrictions vary from state to state. In most states, a learner's permit or driver's license will be issued to an epileptic individual if he or she has been under a physician's care and free of seizures for at least 1 year, provided that the treatment

or basic neurologic problem does not interfere with the ability to drive. A guide to this and other legal matters pertaining to persons with epilepsy is published by the Epilepsy Foundation of America, whose legal department may be able to provide additional information (see reference at the end of this section).

**4. Pregnancy**—In the pregnant teenager with epilepsy, the possibility of teratogenic effects of anticonvulsants, such as facial clefts (two to three times increased risk), must be weighed against the risks from seizures. Such malformations occur in the infants of about 2.5% of mothers with untreated epilepsy.

**C. PRINCIPLES OF ANTICONVULSANT THERAPY**

**1. Drug selection**—Treat with the drug appropriate to the clinical situation, as outlined in Table 23–12.

**2. Treatment strategy**—Start with one drug in conventional dosage, and increase the dosage until seizures are controlled. If seizures are not controlled on the tolerated maximal dosage of one major anticonvulsant, gradually switch to another before using two-drug therapy. The dosages and usually effective blood levels are listed in Table 23–12. Individual variations must be expected. The therapeutic range may also vary somewhat with the method used to determine levels.

**3. Counseling**—Advise the parents and the patient that the prolonged use of anticonvulsant drugs will not produce significant or permanent mental slowing (although the underlying cause of the seizures might) and that prevention of seizures for 1–2 years substantially reduces the chances of recurrence. Advise them also that anticonvulsants are given to prevent further seizures and that they should be taken as prescribed.

**Table 23–12.** Guide to pediatric anticonvulsant drug therapy.[a]

| Drug | Average Total Dosage (mg/kg/d) | Steady State | Effective Blood Levels[b] | Side Effects and Precautions | Directions and Remarks |
|---|---|---|---|---|---|
| **Primary anticonvulsant** | | | | | |
| Carbamazepine (Tegretol) (Carbatrol, Tegretol XR are sustained release formulations) | 15–25 mg/kg/d in 2–4 divided doses | 3–6 d | 4–12 µg/mL (> 15) | Dizziness, ataxia, diplopia, drowsiness, nausea, rash. *Rare:* hepatotoxicity, bone marrow depression, dystonia, inappropriate ADH secretion, bizarre behaviors, tics. | Monitor CBC, platelet count, liver function tests periodically. Blood effects usually early and transient. *Drug interactions:* ↑ by fluoxetine, propoxyphene, erythromycin, cimetidine; ↓ by felbamate, phenobarbital, phenytoin. |
| Valproic acid (Depakene, Depakote) (Depacon) | 15–60 mg/kg/d in 2–4 divided doses | 2–4 d | 50–120 µg/mL (> 140) | Weight gain, occasional gastric discomfort, constipation. Tremor, hair loss in 5%. *Rare:* hepatotoxicity, hyperammonemia, leukopenia, polycystic ovaries (more toxic in infants younger than 2 years) | For prophylaxis in febrile convulsions, see text. Monitor CBC, platelets, liver function tests closely in first 6 months, then periodically. Can be given rectally (suspension: 250 mg/5 mL). Depacon is an IV preparation, 100 mg/mL. *Drug interactions:* ↓ by phenobarbital, phenytoin, carbamazepine, ↑ by lamotrigine felbamate. |
| Phenytoin (Dilantin) | 5–10 mg/kg/d in 1 or 2 doses | 5–10 d | 5–20 µg/mL (>25) | Gum hypertrophy, hirsutism, ataxia, nystagmus, diplopia, rash, anorexia, nausea, osteomalacia. *Rare:* macrocytic anemia, lymph node involvement, exfoliative dermatitis, peripheral neuropathy. | Good dental hygiene reduces gum hyperplasia. May aggravate absence and myoclonic seizures. Poorly absorbed by neonatal gut. Use 50 mg Infant tabs in infants (may be crushed to adjust dosage). Suspension not recommended. *Drug interactions:* ↑ by felbamate; ↓ by carbamazepine, phenobarbital, antacids. |
| Phenobarbital | 3–5 mg/kg/d as single daily dose | 10–21 d | 15–40 µg/mL (> 45) | Irritability and overactivity in many children; sedative effects in others. Mild ataxia, depression, skin rash. May interfere with learning. | Overall, the safest drug. Bitter taste. Higher blood levels sometimes required and tolerated in severe chronic epileptics. Useful in neonatal seizures and status epilepticus. Valproate increases unbound phenobarbital levels. |
| Primidone (Mysoline) | 10–25 mg/kg/d in 3 or 4 divided doses | 1–5 d | 4–12 µg/mL (> 15) | Drowsiness, ataxia, vertigo, anorexia, nausea, vomiting, rash. (Like phenobarbital.) | Start slowly with 25–35% of expected maintenance dose; increase every other day until full dose reached. |
| Ethosuximide (Zarontin) | 10–40 mg/kg/d in 1 or 2 doses | 5–6 d | 40–100 µg/mL (> 150) | Nausea, gastric discomfort, hiccups, blood dyscrasias. | May aggravate generalized seizures. Combine with valproic acid in refractory absence seizures. |
| Clonazepam (Klonopin) | 0.01–0.1 mg/kg/dose 1–2 times/day | 5–10 d | 15–80 ng/mL (> 80) | Drowsiness (> 50%): soporific effects greatest drawback. Behavior problems in 25%. Slurred speech, ataxia, salivation. | Start slowly with 25% of expected maintenance dosage; increase every 2 or 3 d. Useful with refractory minor motor seizures (astatic, myoclonic, infantile spasms; absences). Tolerance may occur. |

*(continued)*

***Table 23–12.*** Guide to pediatric anticonvulsant drug therapy.[a] (continued)

| Drug | Average Total Dosage (mg/kg/d) | Steady State | Effective Blood Levels[b] | Side Effects and Precautions | Directions and Remarks |
|------|-------------------------------|--------------|---------------------------|------------------------------|-------------------------|
| **Adjunctive or secondary drug** | | | | | |
| Acetazolamide (Diamox) | 5–20 mg/kg/d in 2 or 3 divided doses | 1–2 d | 10–14 µg/mL | Anorexia; numbness and tingling. Urinary frequency, so do not give in evening. Renal stones. | Supplement to other medications, especially in absence and complex partial seizures. Also in females 4 days prior to and in the first 2 or 3 days of menstrual period for catamenial seizures. |
| Levetiracetam (Keppra) | 10–20 mg/kg/d. To maximal 40–60 over 2–6 weeks | 1–3 d | 20–40 µg/mL | Somnolence, dizziness, headache, asthenia. *Rare:* decWBC | Complex partial seizures, myoclonic. Little effect on other drugs. |
| Oxcarbazepine (Trileptal) | 8–10 mg/kg/d initial, 20–50 mg/kg/d maint in 2 doses | 1–3d | MHD (breakdown product) 12–30 µg/mL | Dizziness, fatigue, somnolence, nausea, ataxia, headache, hyponatremia, rash | Partial, generalized seizures. Little effect on other drug levels. No need for lab (CBC, LFTs). |
| Felbamate (Felbatol) | 15–45 mg/kg/d in 3 or 4 divided doses | 5–7 d | 22–137 µg/mL | Anorexia, vomiting, insomnia, headache, somnolence. Rash in 1%. Aplastic anemia and hepatic failure are significant hazards. | A dangerous drug. Used in children with Lennox–Gastaut syndrome; in adults with complex partial seizures. Obtain informed consent. *Drug interactions:* ↓ by phenytoin, carbamazepine. |
| Vigabatrin (Sabril) | 20–100 mg/kg/d in 2–3 divided doses | Not known | Not known | Drowsiness, confusion, weight gain, retinal changes, visual loss | Infantile spasms, especially tuberous sclerosis. Add-on drug for partial seizures. Not licensed by FDA in United States as of 1999 |
| Gabapentin (Neurontin) > 12 years | 30–60 mg/kg/d in 3 divided doses (900–4800 mg total per day) | 1–2 d | 12–25 µg/mL | Drowsiness, dizziness, ataxia. | Add-on drug for partial seizures; no effect on other anticonvulsant drug levels. |
| Topiramate (Topomax) | Start 0.5–1 mg/kg/d to 10 mg/kg/d) in 2 divided doses (maximum, 400 mg/d) | Not known | 8–25 µg/mL | Somnolence, slowed mentation, dizziness, language problems, kidney stones (rarely, metabolic acidosis, anorexia). | Adjunctive drug for complex partial seizures. Minimal effect on other drug levels. Lennox–Gastaut, West syndrome. Broad-spectrum drug. |
| Tiagabine (Gabitril) | 0.1–1.5 mg/kg/d in 2 divided doses | 1–2 d | 20–70 µg/mL | Dizziness, tremor, abnormal thinking | Adjunctive drug for partial seizures. |
| Zonisamide (Zonegran) | 1–2 mg/kg/d to maximum 8–12 mg/kg/d in 1 or 2 divided doses | 5–7 d | 20–30 µg/mL | Drowsiness, anorexia, GI symptoms, weight loss, behavior changes, renal stones (0.2–2%), hypohidrosis. Rash | Effects in multi seizure types. A sulfonamide (don't use if allergic to sulfa drugs). Hazard: oligohydrosis-fever syndrome. Widely used in Japan. |

*(continued)*

***Table 23–12.*** Guide to pediatric anticonvulsant drug therapy.[a] (continued)

| Drug | Average Total Dosage (mg/kg/d) | Steady State | Effective Blood Levels[b] | Side Effects and Precautions | Directions and Remarks |
|---|---|---|---|---|---|
| Lamotrigine (Lamictal) | 5–15 mg/kg/d in 2 divided doses (1–5 mg/kg if taking valproic acid); 5–400 mg/d total | 8–15 d | 10–20 µg/mL | Dizziness, headaches, diplopia, ataxia, nausea. Rash in 5–10%. 1% Stevens–Johnson usually in first 4–8 wk. | Add-on drug for children older than 16 y with complex partial seizures, Lennox–Gastaut syndrome, absence seizures. Valproate increases drug half-life. Increase dose slowly over 2 mos. |
| **Treatment of status epilepticus**[a] | | | | | |
| Diazepam (Valium) | 0.3 mg/kg IV. Repeat dose: 0.1–0.3 mg/kg IV. | | | Administer slowly. Monitor pulse and blood pressure. May cause respiratory depression in presence of phenobarbital. | May need to be repeated every 3–4 h. Follow with phenytoin or phenobarbital for long-range control. **Note:** Intramuscular administration for status epilepticus ineffective. |
| Phenobarbital | 5–20 mg/kg IV initially. Repeat dose: 5–10 mg/kg IV. | | | See above. | Rule out pyridoxine deficiency. In neonatal seizures, load with 15–20 mg/kg IV. |
| Phenytoin (Dilantin); (Fosphenytoin newer, safer) | 10–20 mg/kg IV initially. Repeat dose: 5–10 mg/kg IV. | | | Administer IV over a 5-min period. Administer fosphenytoin IM only if no IV access. Monitor blood levels. | Adjunct in neonatal seizures (20 mg/kg IV) if phenobarbital alone fails. Fosphenytoin, new safe preparation. Same dose. May give rapidly IV, over 5 min. |
| Lorazepam (Ativan) | 0.05–0.2 mg/kg IV. May repeat. | | | Mild respiratory depression. | May be more effective than diazepam. Longer-acting. |
| Midazolam (Versed) | 0.1–0.3 mg/kg IM or IV; 0.2 mg/kg as nasal spray. IV drip 1–5++ µg/kg/min | | | See other benzodiazepines. | Short-acting. |
| Valproate sodium (Depacon) | 5–60 mg/kg IV (20 mg/min). Depacon rapid injection form (see Table 23–9) | | | Administer slowly. Dizziness, nausea, and injection-site pain. | Half-life 16 h. Useful when child can't take valproate orally, or for status epilepticus |

[a]Treatment of infantile spasms: See text regarding use of corticotropin or corticosteroids. See also clonazepam or valproic acid, especially with recurrences. ADH = antidiuretic hormone; CBC = complete blood count; IM = intramuscularly; IV = intravenously; MHD = mono hydroxy metabolite; LFT = liver function tests.
[b]In parentheses are shown the levels at which clinical toxicity becomes manifest in monotherapy.
[c]General anesthesia if other measures fail.

Changes in medications or dosages should not be made without the physician's knowledge. Unsupervised sudden withdrawal of anticonvulsant drugs may precipitate severe seizures or even status epilepticus. Anticonvulsants must be kept where they cannot be ingested by small children or suicidal patients.

**4. Follow-up**—Check the patient at intervals, depending on the underlying cause of the seizures, the degree of control, and the toxic properties of the anticonvulsant drug or drugs used. Blood counts and liver function tests must be obtained periodically in the case of some anticonvulsants, as indicated in Table 23–12. Periodic neurologic reevaluation is important. Repeat EEGs are not needed to achieve seizure control. Indications for repeat EEGs are discussed earlier.

**5. Long-term management**—Continue anticonvulsant treatment until the patient is free of seizures for at least 1–2 years or, in some cases, until the patient reaches adolescence. In about 75% of patients, seizures may not recur. Variables such as younger age at onset, normal EEG, and ease of controlling seizures carry a favorable prognosis, whereas later onset, epileptiform spikes on EEG, difficulty in controlling the seizures, polytherapy, generalized tonic–clonic or myoclonic seizures, and an abnormal neurologic examination are associated with a higher risk of recurrence.

**6. Withdrawal of treatment**—In general, there is no need to withdraw anticonvulsants before taking an EEG. Discontinue anticonvulsants gradually. If it becomes necessary to withdraw anticonvulsants abruptly, the patient should be under close medical surveillance. If seizures recur during or after withdrawal, anticonvulsant therapy should be reinstituted and again maintained for at least 1–2 years.

**D. BLOOD LEVELS OF ANTIEPILEPTIC DRUGS**

**1. General comments**—Most anticonvulsants take two or three times the length of their half-life to reach the steady states indicated in Table 23–12. This must be considered when blood levels are assessed after anticonvulsants are started or dosages are changed. Individuals vary in their metabolism and their particular pharmacokinetic characteristics. These and external factors, including, for example, food intake or illness, also affect the blood level. Thus the level reached on a milligram per kilogram basis varies among patients. Experience and clinical research in the determination of antiepileptic blood levels have shown that there is some correlation between (1) drug dose and blood level, (2) blood level and therapeutic effect, and (3) blood level and some toxic effects.

**2. Effective levels**—The ranges given in Table 23–12 are those within which seizure control without toxicity will be achieved in most patients. The level for any given individual will vary not only with metabolic makeup (including biochemical defects) but also with the nature and severity of the seizures and their underlying cause, and with other medications being taken, among other factors. Seizure control may be achieved at lower levels in some patients, and higher levels may be reached without toxicity in others. When control is achieved at a lower level, the dosage should not be increased merely to get the level into the therapeutic range. Likewise, toxic side effects will be experienced at different levels even within the therapeutic range. Lowering the dosage usually resolves the problem, but sometimes the drug must be withdrawn or another added (or both). Some serious toxic effects, including allergic reactions and bone marrow or liver toxicity, are independent of dosage.

**3. Interaction of antiepileptic drugs**—Blood levels of anticonvulsants may be affected by other drugs. Individual variations occur; adjustment of dosages may be required. (See Table 23–12.)

**4. Indications for determination of blood levels**—Drug blood levels should be measured after a new drug is introduced and seizure control without toxicity is achieved to determine the effective level for that patient. Blood level monitoring is useful also when expected control on a "usual" dosage has not been achieved either with a single drug or after adding another, when seizures recur in a patient with previously well-controlled seizures, or when control is poor in a patient taking anticonvulsants who is being seen for the first time. A low level may indicate inadequate dosage, drug interaction, or noncompliance with the prescribed regimen. A high level may indicate slowed metabolism or excretion or drug interaction.

Blood levels are mandatory when signs and symptoms of toxicity are present, especially when more than one drug is being used or when the dosage of a single drug has been changed. Blood levels may be the only means of detecting intoxication in a comatose patient or very young child. Toxic levels also occur with drug abuse and liver or renal disease. Blood levels of anticonvulsants are unnecessary when the patient's seizure control is satisfactory and he or she is free of toxic signs or symptoms.

**E. SIDE EFFECTS OF ANTIEPILEPTIC DRUGS**

(See also Table 23–12.)

**1. Allergic reactions**—Serious allergic reactions usually necessitate discontinuance of a drug. However, not every rash in a child receiving an anticonvulsant is drug-related. If a useful antiepileptic drug is discontinued and the rash disappears, restarting the drug in a smaller dosage may be warranted to see if the rash recurs.

**2. Drug toxicity**—Signs of drug toxicity often disappear when the daily dosage is reduced by 25–30%.

**3. Avoiding sedation**—The sedative effect of many of the anticonvulsants may be avoided by slowly working up to the usual therapeutic dose—for example, over 3–4 weeks for phenobarbital.

**4. Avoiding side effects**—Gingival hyperplasia secondary to phenytoin is best minimized through good dental hygiene but occasionally requires gingivectomy. This condition may recede within about 6 months after the drug is discontinued. The hypertrichosis associated with phenytoin does not regress when the drug is discontinued.

**F. ADRENOCORTICOTROPIC HORMONE AND CORTICOSTEROIDS**

**1. Indications**—These drugs are indicated for infantile spasms not due to causes amenable to specific therapy and in the Lennox–Gastaut syndrome, which cannot be controlled by anticonvulsant drugs. Duration of therapy is guided by cessation of clinical seizures and normalization of the EEG. ACTH or oral corticosteroids are usually continued in full doses for 2 weeks and then, if seizures have ceased, tapered over 1 week. Others use a total treatment period of about 2 months. If seizures recur, the dosage is increased to the last effective level and repeated for 2–4 weeks, or switching to or from prednisone is tried. Some clinicians keep the patient at this dosage for up to 6 months before attempting withdrawal. There is no strong evidence, however, that longer courses of treatment are more beneficial.

**2. Dosages—**

**a. ACTH gel**—Start with 2–4 units/kg/d intramuscularly in a single morning dose. Parents can be taught to give injections.

**b. Prednisone**—Start with 2–4 mg/kg/d orally in two or three divided doses.

**3. Precautions**—Give additional potassium, guard against infections, follow for possible hypertension, and discuss the cushingoid appearance and its disappearance. Do not withdraw oral corticosteroids suddenly. Side effects in some series occur in up to 40% of patients, especially with higher dosages than those listed here (used by some authorities). With long-term use, prophylaxis against *Pneumocystis* infection may be required.

## G. Ketogenic or Medium-Chain Triglyceride

# Diet in Treatment of Epilepsy

A ketogenic diet should be recommended in astatic and myoclonic seizures and absence seizures not responsive to drug therapy. It is occasionally recommended for infantile spasms that do not respond to ACTH or corticosteroids. Ketosis is induced by a diet high in fats and very limited in carbohydrates with sufficient protein for body maintenance and growth. The ratio of fat calories to carbohydrate calories may range from 2.5:1 up to 4:1. Adding medium-chain triglycerides to the diet induces ketosis more readily than does a high level of dietary fats and thus requires less carbohydrate restriction. The mechanism for the anticonvulsant action of the ketogenic diet is not understood. It is, however, the ketosis, not the acidosis, that raises the seizure threshold. The diet is most effective in children younger than age 8 years.

The ketogenic diet is difficult and expensive, tends to be monotonous, and depends on the caregiver's ability to weigh out the foods as well as on absolute adherence to the diet prescribed. Whether the ketosis is achieved by high-fat meals or by adding medium-chain triglycerides to the diet is often a matter of the physician's, the dietitian's, or the patient's preference. The result may also depend on which form of the diet is better tolerated. Full cooperation of all family members is required, including the patient if old enough. However, when seizure control is achieved by this method, the child is alert, he or she often needs no (or only small

amounts of) anticonvulsants, and parental and patient satisfaction is most gratifying.

## H. Surgery

In seizure disorders intractable to anticonvulsant therapy and primarily of focal origin, neurosurgery should be considered. Useful procedures, depending on the lesion, include corticectomy, hemispherectomy, anterior temporal lobectomy (for complex partial seizures), callosotomy (or commissurotomy), and stereotactic ablation. Vagal nerve stimulation with an implanted electrode is another new, expensive surgical approach for intractable epilepsy.

Avoli M et al: Generalized epileptic disorders: An update. Epilepsia 2001;42:445 [PMID: 11440339].

Berg AT et al: How long does it take for partial epilepsy to become intractable? Neurology 2003;60:186 [PMID: 12552028].

Berg AT et al: Neuroimaging in children with newly diagnosed epilepsy: A community based study. Pediatrics 2000;106:527 [PMID: 10969098].

Bourgeois BFD: .Chronic management of seizures in the syndromes of idiopathic generalized epilepsy. Epilepsia 2003;44:27 [PMID: 12752459].

Browne TR, Holmes GL: Epilepsy. N Engl J Med 2001;344:1145 [PMID: 11297707].

Buchhalter JR, Jarrar RG: Therapeutics in pediatric epilepsy, Part 2: Epilepsy surgery and vagus nerve stimulation. Mayo Clin Proc 2003;78:371 [PMID: 12630591].

Camfield P, Camfield C: Childhood epilepsy: What is the evidence for what we think and what we do? J Child Neurol 2003;18:272 [PMID: 12760431].

Capovilla G et al: Short-term nonhormonal and nonsteroid treatment in West syndrome. Epilepsia 2003;44:1085 [PMID: 12887441].

Claassen J et al: Treatment of refractory status epilepticus with pentobarbital, propofol, or midazolam: A systematic review. Epilepsia 2002;43:146 [PMID: 11903960].

Daulin M et al: Reduction of seizures with low-dose Clonazepam in children with epilepsy. Pediatr Neurol 2003;28:48 [PMID: 12657920].

DeViro DC: Metabolic determinants of infant epilepsy. J Child Neurol 2002;17 (Suppl 3):351.

Glauser TA, Pellock JM: Zonisamide in pediatric epilepsy: Review of the Japanese experience. J Child Neurol 2002;17:87 [PMID: 119952083].

Hancock E et al: The treatment of West syndrome: A Cochrane review of the literature to December 2000. Brain & Dev 2001;23:624 [PMID: 11701267].

Hawash KY, Rosman P: Do partial seizures predict an increased risk of seizure recurrence after antiepilepsy drugs are withdrawn? J Child Neurol 2003;18:331 [PMID: 12822817].

Hill A: Neonatal seizures. Pediatr Rev 2000;21:117 [PMID: 10756174].

Holmes G: Epilepsy surgery in children: When, why and how. Neurology 2002;58 (Suppl 7):$13 [PMID:12084863].

Holmes LB et al: The teratogenicity of anticonvulsant drugs. N Engl J Med 2001;344:1132 [PMID: 11297704].

Jarrar RG, Buchhalter JR: Therapeutics in pediatric epilepsy, Part 1: The new antiepileptic drugs and the ketogenic diet. Mayo Clin Proc. 2003;78:359 [PMID: 12630590].

Kanazawa O: Shuddering attacks—Report of four children. Pediatr Neurol 2000;23:421 [PMID: 11118798].

Knudsen JF et al: Oligohydrosis and fever in pediatric patients treated with zonisamide. Pediatr Neurol 2003;28:184 [PMID: 12770670].

Kossoff EH et al: Efficacy of the ketogenic diet for infantile spasms. Pediatrics 2002;109:780 [PMID: 11986436].

MacGregor DL: Vertigo. Pediatr Rev 2002;23:10 [PMID: 11773588].

Mulley JC et al: Channelopathies as a genetic cause of epilepsy. Curr Opin Neurol 2003;16:171 [PMID: 12644745].

Nordli DR et al: Experience with the ketogenic diet in infants. Pediatrics 2001;108:129 [PMID: 11433065].

Pavone P et al: Neuropsychological assessment in children with absence epilepsy. Neurology 2001;56:1047 [PMID: 11320177].

Philippi H et al: Topiramate and metabolic acidosis in infants and toddlers. Epilepsia 2002;43:744 [PMID: 12102678].

Prasad A et al: Evolving antiepileptic drug treatment in juvenile myoclonic epilepsy. Arch Neurol 2003;60:1100 [PMID: 12925366].

Sahin M, Riviello JJ: Prolonged treatment of refractory status epilepticus in a child. J Child Neurol 2001;16:147 [PMID: 11292225].

Sahin M et al: Prolonged treatment for acute symptomatic refractory status epilepticus. Neurology 2003;61:398 [PMID: 12913208].

Shinnar S, Glauser TA: Febrile Seizures. J Child Neurol 2002; 17:S44 [PMID: 11918463].

Shinnar S et al: Short-term outcomes of children with febrile status epilepticus. Epilepsia 2001;42:47 [PMID: 211207784].

Sinclair DB: Prednisone therapy in pediatric epilepsy. Pediatr Neurol 2003:28:194 [PMID: 12770672].

Singhi S et al: Continuous midazolam versus diazepam infusion for refractory convulsive status epilepticus. J Child Neurol 2002:17:106 [PMID: 11952069].

Snodgrass SR: Ambulatory management of children with epilepsy. Pediatr Ann 1999;28:246 [PMID: 10224618].

Snodgrass SR, Parks BR: Anticonvulsant blood levels: Historical review with a pediatric focus. J Child Neurol 2000; 15:734 [PMID: 11108507].

Stromme P et al: Infantile spasms, dystonia, and other X-linked phenotypes caused by mutations in Arista-less related homeobox gene, ARX. Brain Dev 2002;24:266 [PMID: 12142061].

Tromp SC et al: Relative influence of epileptic seizures and of epilepsy syndrome on cognitive function. J Child Neurol 2003;18:407 [PMID: 12886976].

Uneri A, Turkdogan D: Evaluation of vestibular functions in children with vertigo attacks. Arch Dis Child 2003;88:510 [PMID: 12765917].

Valente KD et al: The diagnostic role of short duration outpatient V-EEG monitoring in children. Pediatr Neurol 2003;28: 285 [PMID: 12829881].

VanNess PC: therapy for the epilepsies. Arch Neurol 2002;59:732 [PMID: 12020253].

Watemburg N, et al: Clinical experience with open-label Topiramate use in infants younger than 2 years of age. J Child Neruol 2003;18:258 [PMID: 12760428].

Wheless JW: Acute management of seizures in the syndromes of idiopathic generalized epilepsies. Epilepsia 2003;44 (Suppl 2):22 [PMID: 12752458].

Wirrell EC: Valproic acid-associated weight gain in older children and teens with epilepsy. Pediatr Neurol 2003;28:126 [PMID: 12699863].

Wong M, Trevathan E: Infantile spasms. Pediatr Neurol 2001;24: 89 [PMID: 11275456].

# SYNCOPE & FAINTING

Fainting is transient loss of consciousness and postural tone due to cerebral ischemia or anoxia. Up to 20–50% of children (age birth–20 years) will faint at some time. There may be a prodrome of dizziness, lightheadedness, nausea, so-called gray-out, sweating, and pallor. After falling, many children stiffen or have jerking motions when unconscious, a tonic–clonic, anoxic–ischemic seizure mimicking epilepsy. Watching or undergoing a venipuncture is a common precipitant of fainting, as is prolonged standing, fatigue, illness, overheating and sweating, dehydration, hunger, and athleticism with slow baseline pulse. The family history is positive for similar episodes in 90% of patients.

## Classification

Ninety-five percent of cases of syncope are of the vasovagal–vasodepressive or neurocardiogenic type (Table 23–13). Vasodilation, cardiac slowing, and hypotension

**Table 23–13.** Classification of syncope in childhood.

| |
|---|
| **Vasovagal, neurocardiogenic (neurally mediated)** |
|   Orthostatic |
|   Athleticism |
|   Pallid breath-holding |
|   Situational (stress, blood drawing) |
| **Cardiac** |
|   Obstructive |
|   Arrhythmia |
|   Prolonged QTc |
|   Hypercyanotic (eg, in tetralogy of Fallot) |
| **Nonsyncope mimicker** |
|   Migraine with confusion or stupor |
|   Seizure |
|   Hypoglycemia |
|   Hysteria |
|   Hyperventilation |
|   Vertigo |

cause transient (1–2 minutes) cerebral ischemia and result in the patient passing out. The patient arouses in 1–2 minutes, but full recovery may take an hour or more. Besides those already listed, rare precipitants include hair grooming, cough, micturition, neck stretching, and emotional stress. More ominous is cardiac syncope, which often occurs during exercise. Angina or palpitations may occur. An obstructive lesion such as aortic stenosis, cardiomyopathy, coronary disease, or dysrhythmia may be the cause. Other spells that may mimic syncope are listed in Table 23–13.

## Clinical Findings

### A. Symptoms and Signs

The work-up of fainting includes the history and a physical examination with emphasis on blood pressure and cardiac and neurologic features. In the adolescent, a blood pressure drop of more than 30 mm Hg after standing for 5–10 minutes or a baseline systolic pressure of less than 80 mm Hg suggests orthostasis.

### B. Laboratory Findings and Imaging

Hemoglobin should be checked if anemia is suggested by the history. Electrocardiography should be done. Consider Holter monitoring and echocardiography if cardiac causes seem likely. Tilt testing (though norms are vague) may have a role in frequent recurrent syncope to confirm a vasodepressive cause and avoid more expensive diagnostic investigations.

## Treatment

Treatment consists mostly of giving advice about the benign nature of fainting and about avoiding precipi-

tating situations. The patient should be cautioned to lie down if prodromal symptoms occur. Good hydration and reasonable salt intake are advisable. In some cases β-blockers and rarely fludrocortisone may have a role.

Kapoor WN: Syncope. N Engl J Med 2000;343:1856 [PMID: 11117979].

Narchi H: The child who passes out. Pediatr Rev 2000;21:384 [PMID: 11077022].

Sateriades ES et al: Incidence and prognosis of syncope. N Engl J Med 2002;347:878 [PMID: 12239256].

Willis J: Syncope. Pediatr Rev 2000;21:201 [PMID: 10854315].

## HEADACHES

Headache is one of the most common complaints in pediatric neurology clinics, accounting for 25–30% of all referrals. Epidemiologic studies indicate that headache occurs in 37% of children by age 7 years and in 69% of children by age 14 years. Migraine headache occurs in 5% and 15%, respectively, of children at these ages. Successful treatment requires an accurate diagnosis and proper classification of headache. Based on the patient's history, a simplified initial categorization as summarized in Table 23–14 can be made. A more exhaustive classification scheme has been developed by the International Headache Society and modified for use in children. Muscle contraction, tension headaches are common in older children and adolescents. They are frequently generalized over the head with a "hat band" pressure or squeezing quality. Although appetite may be diminished, nausea and vomiting are usually not present. Symptoms specifically referable to the CNS are absent. If this type of headache becomes very frequent (3 or more days per week) consideration should be given to

***Table 23–14.*** Differential features of headaches in children.

| | Muscle Contraction (Tension/Psychogenic) | Vascular (Migraine) | Traction and Inflammatory (Increased Intracranial Pressure) |
|---|---|---|---|
| Time course | Chronic, recurrent | Acute, paroxysmal, recurrent | Chronic or intermittent but increasingly frequent; progressive severity |
| Prodromes | No | Yes (sometimes in children) | No |
| Description | Diffuse, band-like, tight | Intense, pulsatile, unilateral in older child (70%); usually forehead in or behind one or both eyes. | Diffuse; more occipital with infratentorial mass, more frontal with supratentorial mass |
| Characteristic findings | Feelings of inadequacy, depression, or anxiety | Neurologic symptoms and signs usually transient | Positive neurologic signs, especially papilledema |
| Predisposing factors | Problems at home or school or socially (sexually) | Positive family history (75%); trivial head trauma may precipitate | No |

drug (analgesic) overuse or misuse, depression, or sleep disorder. The neurologic examination is normal, neuroimaging tests are generally not needed, and treatment is judicious use of ibuprofen with or without a limited trial of amitriptyline. If simple measures are not satisfactory, biofeedback may be useful.

Between 65% and 75% of children referred to neurology clinics for consultation regarding headaches have migraine. Many of these children are referred after they have seen ophthalmologists for "eye strain" or otolaryngologists to rule out sinusitis. Approximately 30% of children are referred after already undergoing one or more neuroimaging tests, the vast majority of which are normal.

## Clinical Findings

The diagnosis and proper classification of migraine depends primarily on a thorough and detailed history (Table 23–15). Migraine headaches are paroxysmal, recurrent events separated by symptom-free intervals in a child with normal growth and development and whose neurologic examination is normal. Migraine affects children of all ages but is difficult to diagnose before age 4 years. The family history is positive for vascular, migrainous headaches in 75% of patients. The headaches have a pulsatile quality and are located unilaterally or bilaterally in the frontal or temporal regions, or commonly in the retro-orbital and cheek regions. The headaches last from 2 to more than 24 hours. A nonspecific prodrome of decreased or increased appetite and change in mood and temperament may precede the headache by hours or days. Headaches may be triggered by specific foods, minor head injuries, sleep deprivation, or irregular eating patterns, but more often no precipitant can be identified. An aura such as visual scotomata is uncommon in children. The headache is frequently accompanied by nausea, vomiting, photophobia, sensitivity to sound, vertigo, lightheadedness, fatigue, and mood alterations. Occasionally children may have loss of speech, hemiparesis, ataxia, confusional states, and bizarre visual distortions (so-called Alice in Wonderland syndrome). Very young children may experience recurrent or cyclical vomiting, abdominal pain, or recurrent self-limited bouts of ataxia or vertigo as the early manifestations of migraine.

Occasionally the frequency of migraine may spontaneously increase and become almost daily, a condition referred to as transformed migraine. When this change in frequency happens, it should at least raise suspicion of medication overuse with development of rebound headache; successful treatment of which requires medication withdrawal for 6–12 weeks or longer.

In contrast to tension and migraine headaches, headaches caused by intracranial disorders or increased intracranial pressure rarely occur in children who are otherwise healthy and well and who have completely normal examinations.

Laboratory studies and neuroimaging tests are rarely needed if a thorough history has been taken and the neurologic examination is normal. If the progression of headache is atypical for migraine or tension-type headaches or if the neurologic examination is abnormal, an MRI scan should be considered. When papilledema is present but the MRI is normal, a lumbar puncture may be needed to diagnose pseudomotor cerebri.

## Treatment

Successful treatment of migraine is usually achieved with the systematic use of simple analgesics such as ibuprofen. The key to successful results is to take enough early enough to do the job. As soon as possible

**Table 23–15.** Proposed Revised IHS Classification

| Pediatric Migraine Without Aura (Common) | Pediatric Migraine With Aura[a] (Rare) |
|---|---|
| **Diagnostic Criteria** | **Diagnostic Criteria** |
| A. At least five attacks fulfilling B-D | A. At least two atacks fulfilling B |
| B. Headache attack lasting 1-48 hours | B. At least three of the following: |
| C. Headache has at least two of the following: |     1. One or more fully reversible aura aymptoms indicating focal cortical and/or brain stem dysfunction |
|     1. Bilateral location (frontal/temporal) or unilateral location |     2. At least one aura developing gradually over more than 4 minutes or 2 or more symptoms occurring in succession |
|     2. Pulsating quality |     3. No auras lasting more than 60 minutes |
|     3. Moderate to severe intensity |     4. Headache follows less than 60 minutes |
|     4. Aggravation by routine physical acitivity | |
| D. During headache, at least one of the following | |
|     1. Nausea and/or vomiting | |
|     2. Photophobia and/or phonophobia | |

[a]Idiopathic recurring disorder; headache usually lasts 1–48 hours.
IHS = International Headache Society.
Adapted from: Winner P et al: Classification of pediatric migraine: Proposed revisions of the IHS criteria. Headache 1995; 35:407.

after the headache starts, the child is given ibuprofen 10 mg/kg followed in 45 minutes by 5 mg/kg if needed. Additional doses of analgesics rarely provide additional benefit. The addition of 40–65 mg of caffeine, caffeine–ergotamine combinations, or 65 mg of isometheptene (Midrin) to ibuprofen may provide more reliable relief for some patients. Nausea and vomiting can be treated with metoclopramide (Reglan), taken 10–20 minutes before other medications. For frequently recurring migraine, prophylaxis with propranolol, amitriptyline, cyproheptadine, valproate, or calcium channel blockers should be considered. At this time experience with using triptan and dihydroergotamine (nasal spray) in children is limited, but some studies show sumatriptan, rizatriptan, naratriptan, and dihydroergotamine to be effective. Biofeedback, relaxation therapy, and other nonpharmacologic approaches to managing headache may be useful in children, and they provide an alternative method of treatment that avoids medication-related side effects.

Andrasik F et al: Brief neurologist-administered behavioral treatment of pediatric episodic tension-type headache. Neurology 2003;60:1215 [PMID: 12682344].

Hering-Hanit R et al: Successful withdrawal from analgesic abuse in a group of youngsters with chronic daily headache. J Child Neurol 2001;16:448 [PMID: 11417614].

Just U et al: Emotional and behavioral problems in children and adolescents with primary headache. Cephalalgia 2003; 23:206 [PMID: 12662188].

Lewis DW et al: Practice parameter: Evaluation of children and adolescents with recurrent headaches. Neurology 2002;59: 490 [PMID: 12196640].

Linder SL, Winner P: Pediatric headache. Med Clin North Am 2001;85:1037 [PMID: 11480257].

Medina LS et al: Children with headache suspected of having a brain tumor: A cost-effectiveness analysis of diagnostic strategies. Pediatrics 2001;108:255 [PMID: 11483785].

Millichap JG, Yee MM: The diet factor in pediatric and adolescent migraine. Pediatr Neurol 2003;28:9 [PMID: 12657413].

Powers SW et al: A pilot study of one-session biofeedback training in pediatric headache. Neurology 2001;56:133 [PMID: 11148256].

Wasiewski WW: Preventive therapy in pediatric migraine. J Child Neurol 2001;16:71 [PMID: 11292228].

Zwijnenburg PJG, et al: Alice in wonderland syndrome: A clinical presentation of frontal lobe epilepsy. Neuropediatrics 2002; 33:53 [PMID: 11930280].

# SLEEP DISORDERS

## 1. Sleep Apnea Syndrome in Older Children

Sleep apnea syndrome should be considered if there is a history of restless sleep with snoring or respiratory noise during sleep and frequent awakenings in an older child who shows poor school performance associated with excessive daytime sleepiness or irritability and hyperactivity. Children with these problems frequently have hypertrophied tonsils or adenoids, causing partial airway obstruction. Sleep apnea may be associated with facial dysmorphism; neuromuscular disorders with poor pharyngeal muscle control; and conditions with swelling of soft tissue in pharynx and neck such as myxedema, Hodgkin disease, and massive obesity (Pickwickian syndrome). Evaluation includes soft tissue radiographs of the lateral neck; chest radiograph; electrocardiogram (ECG) to rule out cardiomegaly, sinus dysrhythmias, and right-sided heart failure; arterial blood gas determinations while awake and during sleep; and polysomnography. Therapy is generally surgical, ranging from tonsillectomy and adenoidectomy when appropriate, to tracheostomy when medical measures fail.

## 2. Narcolepsy

Narcolepsy, a primary disorder of sleep, is characterized by chronic, excessive daytime sleeping that occurs regardless of activity or surroundings and is not relieved by increased sleep at night. Onset occurs as early as age 3 years. Of children with narcolepsy, 18% are younger than age 10, and 60% are between puberty and their late teens. Narcolepsy usually interferes severely with normal living. Months to years after onset, there may also be cataplexy (transient partial or total loss of muscle tone, often triggered by laughter, anger, or other emotional upsurge), hypnagogic hallucinations (visual or auditory), and sensations of paralysis on falling asleep. Studies have shown that rapid eye movement (REM) sleep, with loss of muscle tone and an EEG low-amplitude mixed frequency pattern, occurs soon after sleep onset in patients with cataplexy, whereas normal subjects experience 80–100 minutes or longer of non-REM (NREM) sleep before the initial REM period.

Recent research suggests absence of a hypothalamic neuropeptide, hypocretin (from autoimmune injury?), causes narcolepsy and cataplexy. Spinal fluid (but not plasma) levels of hypocretin-1 (also called orexin) are diagnostic (level will be nil or zero).

Narcolepsy is treated with a CNS stimulant (dextroamphetamine or long-acting methylphenidate is preferred). Cataplexy responds to venlafaxine, fluoxetine, or clomipramine. Modafinil is a new effective treatment for excessive daytime sleepiness. The condition persists throughout life.

## 3. Somnambulism

Somnambulism is one of a group of sleep disturbances known as disorders of arousal. The onset is abrupt, usually early in the night. It is characterized by coordinated activity (eg, walking, sometimes moving objects without seeming purpose) in a state of veiled consciousness. The episode is relatively brief and ceases spontaneously. There is poor recall of the event on waking in the morning. Somnambulism may be related to mental activities occurring in stages 3 and 4 of NREM sleep. Incidence has been estimated at only 2–3%, but up to 15% of cases are reported in children age 6–16 years. Boys are affected more often than girls, and many have recurrent episodes. Psychopathologic features are rarely demonstrated, but a strong association (30%) between childhood migraine and somnambulism has been noted. Episodes of somnambulism may be triggered in predisposed children by stresses, including febrile illnesses. No treatment of somnambulism is required, and it is not necessary to seek psychiatric consultation.

## 4. Night Terrors

Night terrors (pavor nocturnus) are a disorder of arousal from NREM sleep. Most cases occur in children age 3–8 years, and the disorder rarely occurs after adolescence. It is characterized by sudden (but only partial) waking, with the severely frightened child unable to be fully roused or comforted. Concomitant autonomic symptoms include rapid breathing, tachycardia, and perspiring. The child has no recall of any nightmare. Psychopathologic mechanisms are unclear, but falling asleep after watching scenes of violence on television or hearing frightening stories may play a role. Elimination of such causes and administration of a mild antianxiety agent such as chlordiazepoxide may be helpful. It is important to differentiate these episodes from complex partial (psychomotor) seizures. (See also Chapter 2.)

Guilleminault C, Pelayo R: Narcolepsy in children: A practical guide to its diagnosis, treatment and follow-up. Paediatr Drugs 2000;2:1. Review [PMID: 10937454].

Scammell TE: The neurobiology, diagnosis, and treatment of narcolepsy. Ann Neurol 2003;53:154 [PMID: 12557281].

Silber MH et al: Solving the mysteries of narcolepsy. Neurology 2001;56:1616 [PMID: 11425923].

Thiedke CC: Sleep disorders and sleep problems in childhood. Am Fam Physician 2001;63:277 [PMID: 11201693].

Tsukamoto H et al: Undetectable levels of CSF hypocretin-1 (orexin-A) in two prepubertal boys with narcolepsy. Neuropediatrics 2002;33:51 [PMID: 11930279].

## PSEUDOTUMOR CEREBRI

Pseudotumor cerebri is characterized by increased intracranial pressure in the absence of an identifiable intracranial mass or hydrocephalus. Manifestations of pseudotumor cerebri are those of increased intracranial

**Table 23–16.** Signs of increased intracranial pressure.

| |
|---|
| **Acute** |
| Macrocephaly |
| Excessive rate of head growth |
| Altered behavior |
| Decreased level of consciousness |
| Vomiting |
| Blurred vision |
| Double vision |
| Optic disk swelling |
| Abducens nerve paresis |
| **Chronic** |
| Macrocephaly |
| Growth impairment |
| Developmental delay |
| Optic atrophy |
| Visual field loss |

pressure as outlined in Table 23–16. The cause is usually unknown, but pseudotumor cerebri has been described in association with a variety of inflammatory, metabolic, toxic, and connective tissue disorders (Table 23–17). The diagnosis of pseudotumor cerebri is one of exclusion. CT or MRI scans of the head are needed to exclude hydrocephalus and intracranial masses. These studies demonstrate ventricles of small or normal size but no other structural abnormalities. Venus thrombo-

**Table 23–17.** Conditions associated with pseudotumor cerebri.

| |
|---|
| **Metabolic-toxic disorders** |
| Hypervitaminosis A |
| Hypovitaminosis A |
| Prolonged steroid therapy |
| Steroid withdrawal |
| Tetracycline therapy |
| Nalidixic acid therapy |
| Iron deficiency |
| Lead poisoning |
| Hypocalcemia |
| Hyperparathyroidism |
| Adrenal insufficiency |
| Lupus erythematosus |
| Chronic $CO_2$ retention |
| **Infectious and parainfectious disorders** |
| Chronic otitis media |
| Poliomyelitis |
| Guillain–Barré syndrome |
| **Dural sinus thrombosis** |
| **Minor head injury** |

sis, an underrecognized cause, must be ruled out by MRV (magnetic resonance venogram) or even injected venograms of cerebral sinuses. Lumbar puncture should be performed to document elevated CSF pressure. Examination of CSF reveals normal findings except for elevated pressure. In some inflammatory and connective tissue diseases, however, the CSF protein concentration may be increased.

Treatment of pseudotumor cerebri is aimed at correcting the identifiable predisposing condition. In addition, some patients may benefit from the use of furosemide or acetazolamide to decrease the volume and pressure of CSF within the CNS. These drugs may be used in combination with repeated lumbar punctures to remove CSF. If a program of repeated CSF removal and medical management is not successful or if central vision or visual field loss is detected despite these measures, lumboperitoneal shunt or another surgical decompression procedure may be necessary to prevent irreparable visual loss and damage to the optic nerves.

Friedman DI, Jacobson DM: Diagnostic criteria for idiopathic intracranial hypertension. Neurology 2002;59:1492 [PMID: 12455560].

Kesler A, Fattall-Valevski A: Idiopathic intracranial hypertension in the pediatric population. J Child Neurol 2002;17:745 [PMID: 12546428].

Mckiernan SP, Difazio M: Case 3. Diagnosis: Pseudotumor cerebri. Pediatr Rev 2001;22:211 [PMID: 11436223].

Salman MS et al: Idiopathic "benign" intracranial hypertension: Case series and review. J Child Neurol 2001;16:465 [PMID: 11453440].

# CEREBROVASCULAR DISEASE

Cerebrovascular disorders leading to vascular blockage, or stroke, occur with an age-related incidence in the pediatric population of approximately 28–93:100,000 per year in infancy and 1–8:100,000 per year in childhood. This excludes primary disorders involving vascular hemorrhage, whose incidence is greatest among premature infants. The initial approach to the patient should recognize that the timing of presentation represents a neurologic emergency, for which promptness in diagnosis can affect treatment considerations and outcome. Unfortunately, most pediatric stroke is not recognized until 24–36 hours after onset, when treatment considerations matter most. Following this, one should take into account the patient's age and any underlying systemic or neurologic illness. This should include a thorough history of prior illnesses, especially those associated with varicella (even in the prior 1–2 years), mycoplasma, human immunodeficiency virus (HIV), minor trauma to the head and neck, and familial clotting tendencies. A systematic search for evidence of cardiac, vascular, or hematologic disease and intracranial disorders should be undertaken (Table 23–18). Though most strokes are not associated with underlying systemic disorders, previously diagnosed congenital heart disease followed by hematologic and neoplastic disorders are the most common predisposing to stroke. In many instances the origin is multifactorial, necessitating a thorough investigation even when the cause may seem obvious. As a result, the cause of childhood stroke is often determined whereas in past studies up to 30% remained idiopathic. This is particularly important when considering that recurrence risk may be as high as 35%.

## Clinical Findings

### A. Symptoms and Signs

Manifestations of stroke in childhood vary according to the vascular distribution to the brain structure that is involved. Because many conditions leading to childhood stroke result in emboli, multifocal neurologic involvement is common. Children may present with acute hemiplegia similar to stroke in adults. Symptoms of unilateral weakness, sensory disturbance, dysarthria, and dysphagia may develop over a period of minutes, but at times progressive worsening of symptoms may evolve over several hours. Bilateral hemispheric involvement may lead to a depressed level of consciousness. The patient may also demonstrate disturbances of mood and behavior and experience focal or multifocal seizures. Physical examination of the patient is aimed not only at identifying the specific deficits related to impaired cerebral blood flow but also at seeking evidence for any predisposing disorder. Retinal hemorrhages, splinter hemorrhages in the nail beds, cardiac murmurs, and signs of trauma are especially important findings.

### B. Laboratory Findings

In the acute phase, certain investigations should be carried out emergently with consideration of treatment options. This should include complete blood count, erythrocyte sedimentation rate, basic chemistries, blood urea nitrogen, creatinine, prothrombin time/partial thromboplastin time, chest radiograph, ECG, urine toxicology, and imaging (see following section). Subsequent studies can be carried out systemically, with particular attention to disorders involving the heart, blood vessels, platelets, red cells, hemoglobin, and coagulation proteins. Additional laboratory tests for systemic disorders such as systemic lupus erythematosus and polyarteritis nodosa are usually indicated. Neonatal infarctions require pathological examination of the placenta.

Examination of CSF is indicated in patients with fever, nuchal rigidity, or obtundation when the diagnosis of intracranial infection requires exclusion. Lumbar

***Table 23–18.*** Etiologic risk factors for stroke in children.

---

**Cardiac disorders**
  Cyanotic heart disease
  Valvular disease
    Rheumatic
    Endocarditis
  Cardiomyopathy
  Cardiac dysrhythmia
**Vascular occlusive disorders**
  Arterial trauma (carotid dissections)
  Homocystinuria/homocysteinemia
  Vasculitis
    Meningitis
    Polyarteritis nodosa
    Systemic lupus erythematosus
    Drug abuse (amphetamines)
  Varicella
  *Mycoplasma*
  HIV
  Fibromuscular dysplasia
  Moyamoya disease
  Diabetes
  Nephrotic syndrome
  Systemic hypertension
  Dural sinus and cerebral venous thrombosis
  Cortical venous thrombosis
**Hematologic disorders**
  Iron deficiency anemia
  Polycythemia
  Thrombotic thrombocytopenia
  Thrombocytopenic purpura
  Hemoglobinopathies
    Sickle cell disease
  Coagulation defects
    Hemophilia
    Vitamin K deficiency
  Hypercoagulable states
    Prothrombin gene mutation
    Lipoprotein (a)
    Factor V Leiden
    Antiphospholipid antibodies
    Hypercholesterolemia
    Hypertriglyceridemia
    Factor VIII deficiency
    Pregnancy
    Systemic lupus erythematosus
    Use of oral contraceptives
    Antithrombin III deficiency
    Protein C and S deficiencies
  Leukemia
**Intracranial vascular anomalies**
  Arteriovenous malformation
  Arterial aneurysm
  Carotid-cavernous fistula

---

puncture, however, may be deferred until a neuroimaging scan excluding brain abscess or a space-occupying lesion that might contraindicate lumbar puncture has been obtained. In the absence of infection and frank intracranial subarachnoid hemorrhage, CSF examination is rarely helpful in defining the cause of the cerebrovascular disorder.

### C. IMAGING

CT and MRI scans of the brain are often helpful in defining the extent of cerebral involvement with ischemia or hemorrhage. CT scans, however, may be normal within the first 12–24 hours of an ischemic stroke and may need to be repeated several hours later. A CT scan early after the onset of neurologic deficits is valuable in excluding intracranial hemorrhage. This information may be helpful in the early stages of management and in the decision to treat with anticoagulants. State-of-the-art management of stroke in the adult population omits CT scanning but proceeds directly to urgent MRI, magnetic resonance angiography (MRA), and diffusion weighted imaging since these modalities are sensitive to acute stroke in the initial 3 hours when intravenous thrombolytics might be indicated. In consideration of venous occlusion either CT scan with contrast or MRV is indicated.

Except in cases where trauma resulting in arterial dissection is suspected, cerebral angiography (CA) is usually not urgently needed but may be needed to confirm disorders such as fibromuscular dysplasia and cerebral arteritis. If CA is done, all major vessels should be studied from the aortic arch. If evidence of fibromuscular dysplasia is present in the intracranial or extracranial vessels, renal arteriography is indicated. In studies where both MRA or CA have been used, nearly 80% of patients with ischemic stroke demonstrated a cerebrovascular abnormality.

When seizures are prominent, an EEG may be used as an adjunct in the patient's evaluation. An EEG and sequential EEG monitoring may help in patients with severely depressed consciousness.

ECG and echocardiography are useful both in the diagnostic approach to the patient and in ongoing monitoring and management, particularly when hypotension or cardiac arrhythmias complicate the clinical course.

## Differential Diagnosis

Patients with an acute onset of neurologic deficits must be evaluated for other disorders that can cause focal neurologic deficits. Hypoglycemia, prolonged focal seizures, a prolonged postictal paresis (Todd paralysis), meningitis, encephalitis, and brain abscess should all be considered. Migraine with focal neurologic deficits may be difficult to differentiate initially from ischemic stroke. Occasionally the onset of a neurodegenerative disorder (eg, adrenoleukodystrophy or mitochondrial disorder) may begin with the abrupt onset of seizures and focal neurologic deficits. The possibility of drug abuse (particularly cocaine) and other toxic exposures must be investigated diligently.

## Treatment

The initial management of stroke in a child is aimed at providing support for pulmonary, cardiovascular, and renal function. Appropriate fluid and electrolyte infusions should be started, and careful monitoring of heart rate and rhythm and blood pressure is required. Typically, maintenance fluids without added glucose are indicated to augment vascular volume. Specific treatment of stroke depends partly on the underlying pathogenesis and the specific predisposing disorder. Generally, aspirin 1–2 mg/kg daily is indicated to begin as soon as diagnosis is made. As clinical trials progress, aspirin use appears safe and has not been associated with Reye syndrome. In some situations, emergent heparinization for arterial dissection, emboli, and consumptive coagulopathies is indicated. In adults with cerebrovascular thrombosis, thrombolytic agents (tissue plasminogen activator) used systemically or delivered directly to a vascular thrombotic lesion using interventional radiologic techniques has been shown to improve outcome; although case reports exist, studies in children have not been completed. Exchange transfusion is indicated in cases of sickle cell disease.

Long-term management requires intensive rehabilitation efforts and therapy aimed at improving the child's language, educational, and psychologic performance. Length of treatment with various agents is still being studied and depends on etiology.

## Prognosis

The outcome of stroke in infants and children is variable. Roughly, 40% may have minimal deficits, 30% are moderately affected, and 30% are severely affected. Underlying predisposing conditions and the vascular territory involved all play a role in dictating the outcome for an individual patient. When the stroke involves extremely large portions of one hemisphere or large portions of both hemispheres and cerebral edema develops, the patient's level of consciousness may deteriorate rapidly, and death may occur within the first few days. Some patients may achieve almost complete recovery of neurologic function within several days if the cerebral territory is small. Seizures, either focal or generalized, may occur in 30–50% of patients at some point in the course of their cerebrovascular disorder.

Chronic problems with learning, behavior, and activity are common.

Delsing BJ et al: Early prognostic indicators of outcome in ischemic childhood stroke. Pediatr Neurol 2001;24:283 [PMID: 11377103].

deVeber, G: Stroke and the child's brain: An overview of epidemiology, syndromes and risk factors. Curr Opin Neurol 2002;15:133 [PMID: 11923625].

Gabis LV et al: Time lag to diagnosis of stroke in children. Pediatrics 2002;110:924 [PMID: 12415031].

Ganesan V et al: Investigation of risk factors in children with arterial ischemic stroke. Ann Neurol 2003;53:167 [PMID: 12557282].

Gordon AL et al: Functional outcome following stroke in children. J Child Neurol 2002;17:429 [PMID: 12174963].

Gruber A et al: Intra-arterial thrombolysis for the treatment of perioperative childhood cardioembolic stroke. Neurology 2000;54:1684 [PMID: 10762516].

Husson B et al: Magnetic resonance angiography in childhood arterial brain infarcts: A comparative study with contrast angiography. Stroke 2002;33:1280 [PMID: 11988604].

Nestoridi E et al: Arterial ischemic stroke in childhood: The role of plasma-phase risk factors. Curr Opin Neurol 2002;15:139 [PMID: 11923626].

Nowak-Gottl U et al: Antithrombotic drug treatment of pediatric patients with ischemic stroke. Pediatr Drugs 2003;5:167 [PMID: 12608881].

# CONGENITAL MALFORMATIONS OF THE NERVOUS SYSTEM

Malformations of the nervous system occur in 1–3% of living neonates and are present in 40% of infants who die. Developmental anomalies of the CNS may result from a variety of causes, including infectious, toxic, metabolic, and vascular insults that affect the fetus. The specific type of malformation that results from such insults, however, may depend more on the gestational period during which the insult occurs than on the specific cause. The period of induction, days 0–28 of gestation, is the period during which the neural plate appears and the neural tube forms and closes. Insults during this phase can result in a major absence of neural structures, such as anencephaly, or in a defect of neural tube closure, such as spina bifida, meningomyelocele, or encephalocele. Cellular proliferation and migration characterize neural development that occurs after 28 days' gestation. Lissencephaly, pachygyria, agyria, and agenesis of the corpus callosum may be the result of disruptions (genetic, toxic, infectious, or metabolic) that can occur during the period of cellular proliferation and migration.

## 1. Abnormalities of Neural Tube Closure

Defects of neural tube closure constitute some of the most common congenital malformations affecting the nervous system. Spina bifida with associated meningomyelocele or meningocele is commonly found in the lumbar region. Depending on the extent and severity of the involvement of the spinal cord and peripheral nerves, lower extremity weakness, bowel and bladder dysfunction, and hip dislocation may be present. Delivery via cesarean section followed by early surgical closure of meningoceles and meningomyeloceles is usually indicated. Additional treatment is necessary to manage chronic abnormalities of the urinary tract, orthopedic abnormalities such as kyphosis and scoliosis, and paresis of the lower extremities. Hydrocephalus associated with meningomyelocele usually requires ventriculoperitoneal shunting.

## Arnold–Chiari Malformations

Arnold–Chiari malformation type I consists of elongation and displacement of the caudal end of the brainstem into the spinal canal with protrusion of the cerebellar tonsils through the foramen magnum. In association with this hindbrain malformation, minor to moderate abnormalities of the base of the skull often occur, including basilar impression (platybasia) and small foramen magnum. Arnold–Chiari malformation type I may remain asymptomatic for years, but in older children and young adults it may cause progressive ataxia, paresis of the lower cranial nerves, and progressive vertigo. Posterior cervical laminectomy may be necessary to provide relief from cervical cord compression. Ventriculoperitoneal shunting is required for hydrocephalus.

Arnold–Chiari malformation type II consists of the malformations found in Arnold–Chiari type I plus an associated lumbar meningomyelocele. Hydrocephalus develops in approximately 90% of children with Arnold–Chiari malformation type II. These patients may also have aqueductal stenosis, hydromyelia or syringomyelia, and cortical dysplasias. The clinical manifestations of Arnold–Chiari malformation type II are most commonly caused by the associated hydrocephalus and meningomyelocele. In addition, dysfunction of the lower cranial nerves may be present. Up to 25% may have epilepsy, likely secondary to the cortical dysplasias. With the advent of "aggressive-selective" therapy, mortality is 14%; of survivors 74% are ambulatory and 73% have a normal IQ.

Arnold–Chiari malformation type III is characterized by occipital encephalocele, a closure defect of the rostral end of the neural tube. Hydrocephalus is extremely common with this malformation.

In general, the diagnosis of neural tube defects is obvious at the time of birth. Diagnosis may be strongly suspected prenatally on the basis of ultrasonographic findings and the presence of elevated α-fetoprotein in the amniotic fluid. All women of childbearing age should take prophylactic folate, which can prevent these defects and decrease the risk of recurrence by 70%.

## 2. Disorders of Cellular Proliferation and Migration

### Lissencephaly

Lissencephaly is a severe malformation of the brain characterized by an extremely smooth cortical surface with minimal sulcal and gyral development. Such a smooth surface is characteristic of fetal brain at the end of the first trimester. In addition, lissencephalic brains have a primitive cytoarchitectural construction with a four-layered cerebral mantle instead of the mature six-layered mantle. Pachygyria (thick gyri) and agyria (absence of gyri) may vary in an anterior to posterior gradient, which can be suggestive of the underlying genetic defect. Patients with lissencephaly usually have severe neurodevelopmental delay, microcephaly, and seizures (including infantile spasms); however, there is significant phenotypic heterogeneity, which can depend on the specific mutation. These disorders are autosomal recessive, except for the X-linked disorders. *LIS1* mutations on chromosome 17 are associated with dysmorphic features (Miller–Dieker syndrome). X-linked syndromes involving mutations in *DCX* (double cortin) and *ARX* (associated with ambiguous genitalia) affect males with lissencephaly and females with band heterotopias or agenesis of the corpus callosum. Lissencephaly in association with hydrocephalus, cerebellar malformations, and muscular dystrophy may occur in Walker–Warburg syndrome (*POMT1* mutation), Fukuyama muscular dystrophy (*fukutin* mutation), and muscle–eye–brain disease (*POMGnT1* mutation). It is particularly important to identify these syndromes not only because clinical tests are available but also because of their genetic implications. Lissencephaly may also be a component of Zellweger syndrome, a metabolic peroxisomal abnormality associated with the presence of elevated concentrations of very long-chain fatty acids in plasma. No specific treatment for lissencephaly is available and seizures are often difficult to control with standard medications.

MRI scans have helped to define a number of presumed migrational defects that are similar to but anatomically more restricted than lissencephaly. A distinctive example is bilateral perisylvian cortical dysplasia. Patients with this disorder have pseudobulbar palsy, variable cognitive deficits, facial diplegia, dysarthria, developmental delay, and epilepsy. Seizures are often difficult to control with antiepileptic drugs; some patients have benefited from corpus callosotomy. The cause of this syndrome is as yet unknown, though intrauterine cerebral ischemic injury has been postulated. Therapy is aimed at improving speech and oromotor functions and controlling seizures.

## Agenesis of the Corpus Callosum

Agenesis of the corpus callosum, once thought to be a rare cerebral malformation, is more frequently diagnosed with modern neuroimaging techniques. The cause of this malformation is unknown. Occasionally it appears to be inherited in either an autosomal dominant or recessive pattern. X-linked recessive patterns have also been described (*ARX* as mentioned earlier). Agenesis of the corpus callosum has been found in some patients with pyruvate dehydrogenase deficiency and in others with nonketotic hyperglycinemia. Most cases are sporadic. Maldevelopment of the corpus callosum may be partial or complete. No specific syndrome is typical of agenesis of the corpus callosum, although many patients have seizures, developmental delay, microcephaly, or mental retardation. Neurologic abnormalities may be related to microscopic cytoarchitectural abnormalities of the brain that occur in association with agenesis of the corpus callosum. The malformation may be found coincidentally by neuroimaging studies in otherwise normal patients and has been described as a coincidental finding at autopsy in neurologically normal individuals. A special form of agenesis of the corpus callosum occurs in Aicardi syndrome. In this X-linked disorder, agenesis of the corpus callosum is associated with other cystic intracerebral abnormalities, infantile spasms, mental retardation, lacunar chorioretinopathy, and vertebral body abnormalities.

## Dandy–Walker Malformation

Despite being described nearly a century ago, the exact definition of the Dandy–Walker malformation is in debate. Classically, it is characterized by aplasia of the vermis, cystic enlargement of the fourth ventricle, rostral displacement of the tentorium, and absence or atresia of the foramina of Magendie and Luschka. Although hydrocephalus is usually not present congenitally, it develops within the first few months of life. Ninety percent of patients who develop hydrocephalus do so by age 1 year. "Variants" have cerebellar hypoplasia without dilatation of the fourth ventricle and hydrocephalus and may suggest other subtle cortical abnormalities not classically present and could be confused with other disorders such as Joubert syndrome and its variants. On physical examination, a rounded protuberance or exaggeration of the cranial occiput often exists. In the absence of hydrocephalus and increased intracranial pressure, few physical findings may be present to suggest

neurologic dysfunction. An ataxic syndrome occurs in fewer than 20% of patients and is usually late in appearing. Many long-term neurologic deficits result directly from hydrocephalus. Diagnosis of Dandy–Walker malformation is confirmed by CT or MRI scanning of the head. Treatment is directed at the management of hydrocephalus.

## 3. Craniosynostosis

Craniosynostosis, or premature closure of cranial sutures, is usually sporadic and idiopathic. However, some patients have hereditary disorders, such as Apert syndrome and Crouzon disease, that are associated with abnormalities of the digits, extremities, and heart. Occasionally craniosynostosis may be associated with an underlying metabolic disturbance such as hyperthyroidism and hypophosphatasia. The most common form of craniosynostosis involves the sagittal suture and results in scaphocephaly, an elongation of the head in the anterior to posterior direction. Premature closure of the coronal sutures causes brachycephaly, an increase in cranial growth from left to right. Unless many or all cranial sutures close prematurely, intracranial volume will not be compromised, and the brain's growth will not be impaired. Closure of only one or a few sutures will not cause impaired brain growth or neurologic dysfunction. Management of craniosynostosis is directed at preserving normal skull shape and consists of excising the fused suture and applying material to the edge of the craniectomy to prevent reossification of the bone edges. The best cosmetic effect on the skull is achieved when surgery is done during the first 6 months of life.

## 4. Hydrocephalus

Hydrocephalus is characterized by an increased volume of CSF in association with progressive ventricular dilation. In communicating hydrocephalus, CSF circulates through the ventricular system and into the subarachnoid space without obstruction. In noncommunicating hydrocephalus, an obstruction blocks the flow of CSF within the ventricular system or blocks the egress of CSF from the ventricular system into the subarachnoid space. A wide variety of disorders, such as hemorrhage, infection, tumors, and congenital malformations, may play a causal role in the development of hydrocephalus. Attention to an X-linked inheritance pattern, the presence of radialized thumbs and aqueductal stenosis, is suggestive of X-linked hydrocephalus due to the clinically testable neural cell adhesion molecule (NCAM)–L1 deficiency.

Clinical features of hydrocephalus include macrocephaly, an excessive rate of head growth, irritability, vomiting, loss of appetite, impaired upgaze, impaired extraocular movements, hypertonia of the lower extremities, and generalized hyperreflexia. Without treatment, optic atrophy may occur. In infants, papilledema may not be present, whereas older children with closed cranial sutures can eventually develop swelling of the optic disk. Hydrocephalus can be diagnosed on the basis of the clinical course, findings on physical examination, and CT or MRI scan.

Treatment of hydrocephalus is directed at providing an alternative outlet for CSF from the intracranial compartment. The most common method is ventriculoperitoneal shunting. Other treatment should be directed, if possible, at the underlying cause of the hydrocephalus. For genetic testing, see www.genetests.org

Barkovich AJ et al: Radiologic classification of malformations of cortical development. Curr Opin Neurobiol 2001;12:145 [PMID: 11262727].

Kato M, Dobyns WB: Lissencephaly and the molecular basis of neuronal migration. Hum Mol Gen 2003;12:R89 [PMID: 12668601].

Leventer RJ et al: LIS1 missense mutations cause milder lissencephaly phenotypes including a child with normal IQ. Neurology 2001;57:416 [PMID: 11502906].

Patel S, Barkovich AJ: Analysis and classification of cerebellar malformations. AJNR Am J Neuroradiol 2002;23:1074 [PMID: 12169461].

Satran D et al: Cerebello–Oculo–Renal syndromes including Arima, Senior-Loken and COACH syndromes: More than just variants of Joubert Syndrome. Am J Med Genetics 1999;86:459 [PMID: 10508989].

# ABNORMAL HEAD SIZE

Bone plates of the skull have almost no intrinsic capacity to enlarge or grow. Unlike long bones, they depend on extrinsic forces to stimulate new bone formation at the suture lines. Although gravity and traction on bone by muscle and scalp probably stimulate some growth, the single most important stimulus for head growth during infancy and childhood is brain growth. Therefore, accurate assessment of head growth is one of the most important aspects of the neurologic examination of young children. A head circumference that is 2 SD above or below the mean for age requires investigation and explanation.

## 1. Microcephaly

A head circumference more than 2 SD below the mean for age and sex is by definition microcephaly. More important, however, than a single head circumference measurement is the rate or pattern of head growth through time. Head circumference measurements that progressively drop to lower percentiles with increasing age are indicative of a process or condition that has im-

paired the brain's capacity to grow. The causes of microcephaly are numerous. Some examples are listed in Table 23–19.

## Clinical Findings

### A. SYMPTOMS AND SIGNS

Microcephaly may be suspected in the full-term newborn and in infants up to age 6 months whose chest circumference exceeds the head circumference (unless the child is very obese). Microcephaly may be discovered when the child is examined because of delayed developmental milestones or neurologic problems, such as seizures or spasticity. There may be a marked backward slope of the forehead (as in familial microcephaly) with narrowing of the bitemporal diameter. The fontanelle may close earlier than expected, and sutures may be prominent.

### B. LABORATORY FINDINGS

Laboratory findings vary with the cause. Abnormal dermatoglyphics may be present when the injury occurred

**Table 23–19.** Microcephaly.

| Causes | Examples |
|---|---|
| Chromosomal | Trisomy 13, 18, 21 |
| Malformation | Lissencephaly, schizencephaly |
| Syndromes | Rubenstein–Taybi, Cornelia de Lange |
| Toxins | Alcohol, anticonvulsants (?), maternal phenylketonuria |
| Infections (intrauterine) | TORCHES[a] |
| Radiation | Maternal pelvis, first and second trimester |
| Placental insufficiency | Toxemia, infection |
| Familial | Autosomal-dominant, autosomal-recessive |
| Perinatal hypoxia, trauma | Birth asphyxia, injury |
| Infections (perinatal) | Bacterial meningitis (especially group B streptococci) Viral encephalitis (enterovirus herpes simplex) |
| Metabolic | Hypoglycemia, phenylketonuria, maple syrup urine disease |
| Degenerative disease | Tay–Sachs, Krabbe |

[a]TORCHES is a mnemonic formula for toxoplasmosis, rubella, cytomegalovirus, herpes simplex, and syphilis.

before 19 weeks' gestation. In the newborn, IgM antibody titers for toxoplasmosis, rubella, CMV, herpes simplex virus, and syphilis must be assessed. Elevated specific IgM titer is indicative of congenital infection. The urine culture for CMV will be positive at birth when this virus is the cause of microcephaly. Eye, cardiac, and bone abnormalities may also be clues to congenital infection. The child's serum and urine amino and organic acid determinations are occasionally diagnostic. The mother may require screening for phenylketonuria. Karyotyping, including for fragile X syndrome, should be considered.

### C. IMAGING

CT or MRI scans may aid in diagnosis and prognosis. These studies may demonstrate calcifications, malformations, or atrophic patterns that suggest specific congenital infections or genetic syndromes. Plain skull radiographs may show closed sutures, but these studies are of limited value in diagnosis and have been replaced by more sensitive and more informative scanning procedures. Genetic counseling should be offered to the family of any infant with significant microcephaly.

## Differential Diagnosis

Congenital craniosynostosis involving multiple sutures is easily differentiated by inspection of the head, history, identification of syndromes, hereditary pattern, and sometimes signs and symptoms of increased intracranial pressure. Common forms of craniosynostosis involving sagittal, coronal, and lambdoidal sutures are associated with abnormally shaped heads but do not cause microcephaly. Recognizing treatable causes of undergrowth of the brain such as hypopituitarism, hypothyroidism, and severe protein-calorie undernutrition is critical so that therapy can be initiated as early as possible.

## Treatment & Prognosis

Except for the treatable disorders already noted, treatment is usually supportive and directed at the multiple neurologic and sensory deficits, endocrine disturbances (eg, diabetes insipidus), and seizures. Many children but not all with microcephaly who are developmentally delayed, with head circumferences more than 2 SD below the mean, show variable degrees of mental retardation. The notable exceptions are found in cases of hypopituitarism (rare) or familial autosomal dominant microcephaly.

Mochida GH, Walsh CA: Molecular genetics of human microcephaly. Curr Opin Neurol 2001;14:151 [PMID: 11262728].

Vargas JE et al: Congenital microcephaly: Phenotypic features in a consecutive sample of newborn infants. J Pediatr 2001;139: 210 [PMID: 11487745].

Watemberg N et al: Significance of microcephaly among children with developmental disabilities. J Child Neurol 2002;17:117 [PMID: 11952071].

## 2. Macrocephaly

A head circumference more than 2 SD above the mean for age and sex denotes macrocephaly. Excessive head growth rate through time suggests increased intracranial pressure most likely caused by hydrocephalus, extra-axial fluid collections, or neoplasms. Macrocephaly with normal head growth rate suggests familial macrocephaly or true megalencephaly, as might occur in neurofibromatosis. Other causes and examples of macrocephaly are listed in Table 23–20.

**Table 23–20.** Macrocephaly.

| Causes | Examples |
|---|---|
| Pseudomacrocephaly, pseudohydrocephalus, catch-up growth crossing percentiles | Growing premature infant; recovery from malnutrition, congenital heart disease, postsurgical correction |
| Increased intracranial pressure | |
|   With dilated ventricles | Progressive hydrocephalus, subdural effusion |
|   With other mass | Arachnoid cyst, porencephalic cyst, brain tumor |
| Benign familial macrocephaly (idiopathic external hydrocephalus) | External hydrocephalus, benign enlargement of the subarachnoid spaces, benign subdural collections of infancy (synonyms) |
| Megalencephaly (large brain) | |
|   With neurocutaneous disorder | Neurofibromatosis, tuberous sclerosis, etc |
|   With gigantism | Sotos' syndrome |
|   With dwarfism | Achondroplasia |
|   Metabolic | Mucopolysaccharidoses |
|   Lysosomal | Metachromatic leukodystrophy |
|   Other leukodystrophy | Canavan spongy degeneration |
| Thickened skull | Fibrous dysplasia (bone), hemolytic anemia (marrow), sicklemia, thalassemia |

## Clinical Findings

Clinical and laboratory findings vary with the underlying process. In infants, transillumination of the skull with an intensely bright light in a completely darkened room may disclose subdural effusions, hydrocephalus, hydranencephaly, and cystic defects. A surgically or medically treatable condition must be ruled out. Thus the first decision is whether and when to perform an imaging study.

### A. Imaging Study Deferred

**1. Catch-up growth**—Catch-up growth may be evident, as it is in the thriving, neurologically intact premature infant whose rapid head enlargement is most marked in the first weeks of life, or the infant in the early phase of recovery from deprivation dwarfism. As the expected "normal" is reached, head growth slows and then resumes a normal growth pattern. If the fontanelle is open, cranial ultrasonography can assess ventricular size and diagnose or exclude hydrocephalus.

**2. Familial macrocephaly**—This condition may exist when another family member has an unusually large head with no signs or symptoms referable to such disorders as neurocutaneous dysplasias (especially neurofibromatosis) or cerebral gigantism (Sotos syndrome), or when there is no significant mental or neurologic abnormalities in the child.

### B. Imaging Study

CT or MRI scans (or ultrasonography, if the anterior fontanelle is open) are used to define any structural cause of macrocephaly and to identify an operable disorder. Even when the condition is untreatable (or does not require treatment), the information gained may permit more accurate diagnosis and prognosis, guide management and genetic counseling, and serve as a basis for comparison should future abnormal cranial growth or neurologic changes necessitate a repeat study. An imaging study is necessary if signs or symptoms of increased intracranial pressure are present (see Table 23–15).

Cutting LE et al: Megalencephaly in NF1. Neurology 2002;59:1388 [PMID: 12427889].

Piatt JH Jr: Monozygotic twins discordant for external hydrocephalus. Pediatr Neurosurg 2001;35:211 [PMID: 11694799].

Ravid S, Maytal J: External hydrocephalus: A probable cause for subdural hematoma in infancy. Pediatr Neurol 2003;28:139 [PMID: 12699866].

Suara RO et al: Benign subarachnoid space enlargement of infancy. J Natl Med Assoc 2001;93:70 [PMID: 12653385].

## NEUROCUTANEOUS DYSPLASIAS

Neurocutaneous dysplasias are diseases of the neuroectoderm and sometimes involve endoderm and mesoderm. Birthmarks and skin growths appearing later often suggest a need to look for brain, spinal cord, and eye disease. Hamartomas (histologically normal tissue growing abnormally rapidly or in aberrant sites) are common. The most common dysplasias are dominantly inherited. Benign and even malignant tumors may develop.

Dahan D et al: Neurocutaneous syndromes. Adolesc Med 2002;13:495 [PMID: 12270797].

Kandt RS: Tuberous sclerosis complex and neurofibromatosis type 1: The two most common neurocutaneous diseases. Neruol Clin 2002;20:941 [PMID: 12616676].

## 1. Neurofibromatosis (von Recklinghausen Disease)

### ESSENTIALS OF DIAGNOSIS & TYPICAL FEATURES

- More than six café au lait spots 5 mm in greatest diameter in prepubertal individuals and over 15 mm in greatest diameter in postpubertal individuals.
- Two or more neurofibromas of any type or one plexiform neurofibroma.
- Freckling in the axillary or inguinal regions.
- Optic glioma.
- Two or more Lisch nodules (iris hamartomas).
- Distinctive osseous lesions, such as sphenoid dysplasia or thinning of long bone with or without pseudarthroses.
- First-degree relative (parent, sibling, offspring) with neurofibromatosis type 1 by above criteria.

## General Considerations

Neurofibromatosis is a multisystem disorder with a prevalence of 1:4000. Fifty percent of cases are due to new mutations in the NF1 gene. Forty percent of patients will develop medical complications of the disorder in their lifetime.

## Clinical Findings

### A. Symptoms and Signs

The most common presenting symptoms are cognitive or psychomotor problems; 40% of patients have learning disabilities, and mental retardation occurs in 8%.

The family history is important in identifying dominant gene manifestations in parents. Parents should be examined in detail. The history should focus on lumps or masses causing disfigurement, functional problems, or pain. The clinician should ask about visual problems. Strabismus or amblyopia dictates a search for optic glioma, a common tumor in neurofibromatosis. Any progressive neurologic deficit calls for studies to rule out tumor of the spinal cord or CNS. Tumors of cranial nerve VIII virtually never occur in neurofibromatosis type 1 but are the rule in neurofibromatosis type 2, a rare autosomal dominant disease.

The physician should check blood pressure and examine the spine for scoliosis and the limbs for pseudarthroses. Head measurement often shows macrocephaly. Hearing and vision need to be assessed. The eye examination should include a check for proptosis and iris Lisch nodules. The optic disk should be examined for atrophy or papilledema. Short stature and precocious puberty are occasional findings. An examination for neurologic manifestations of tumors (eg, asymmetrical reflexes, spasticity) is important.

## B. LABORATORY FINDINGS

Laboratory tests are not likely to be of value in asymptomatic patients. Selected patients require brain MRI or CT scans with special cuts through the optic nerves to rule out optic glioma. Hypertension necessitates evaluation of renal arteries for dysplasia and stenosis. Cognitive and school achievement testing may be indicated. Scoliosis or limb abnormalities should be studied by appropriate roentgenograms such as an MRI scan of the spinal cord and roots.

## Differential Diagnosis

Patients with Albright syndrome often have larger café au lait spots with precocious puberty. One or two café au lait spots are often seen in normal children.

## Treatment

Genetic counseling is important. The risk to siblings is up to 50%. The disease may be progressive, with serious complications occasionally seen. Patients sometimes worsen during puberty or pregnancy. Genetic screening of family members is required. Annual or semiannual visits are important in the early detection of school problems or bony or neurologic abnormalities.

Multidisciplinary clinics at medical centers around the United States are excellent resources. Prenatal diagnosis is probably on the horizon, but the variability of manifestations (trivial to severe) will make therapeutic abortion an unlikely option. Chromosomal linkage studies are under way (chromosome 17q11.2). Infor-

mation for laypeople and physicians is available from the National Neurofibromatosis Foundation, Inc., 70 West 40th Street, New York, NY 10018.

Baser ME et al: Evaluation of clinical diagnostic criteria for neurofibromatosis 2. Neurology 2002;59:1759 [PMID: 12473765].

Friedman JM: Neurofibromatosis 1: Clinical manifestations and diagnostic criteria. J Child Neurol 2002;17:548 [PMID: 12403552].

Korf BR: Clinical features and pathobiology of neurofibromatosis 1. J Child Neurol 2002;17:573 [PMID: 12403555].

Lynch TM, Gutmann DH: Neurofibromatosis 1. Neurol Clin 2002;20:841 [PMID: 12432832].

Ruggieri M, Huson SM: The clinical and diagnostic implications of mosaicism in the neurofibromatosis. Neurology 2001;56:1433 [PMID: 11409413].

Tekin M et al: Café au lait spots: The pediatrician's perspective. Pediatr Rev 2001;22:82 [PMID: 11230626].

Vivarelli R et al: Epilepsy in neurofibromatosis 1. J Child Neurol 2003;18:338 [PMID: 12822818].

## 2. Tuberous Sclerosis (Bourneville Disease)

 **ESSENTIALS OF DIAGNOSIS & TYPICAL FEATURES**

- *Facial angiofibromas or subungual fibromas.*
- *Often hypomelanotic macules, gingival fibromas.*
- *Retinal hamartomas.*
- *Cortical tubers or subependymal glial nodules, often calcified.*
- *Renal angiomyolipomas.*

## General Considerations

Tuberous sclerosis is a dominantly inherited disease. Almost all patients have deletions on chromosome 9 (*TSC1* gene) or 16 (*TSC2* gene). The gene products hamartin and tuberin have tumor-suppressing effects. A triad of seizures, mental retardation, and adenoma sebaceum occurs in only 33% of patients. The disease was earlier thought to have a high rate of mutation. As a result of more sophisticated techniques such as MRI, parents formerly thought not to harbor the gene are now being diagnosed as asymptomatic carriers.

Like neurofibromatosis, tuberous sclerosis is associated with a wide variety of symptoms. The patient may be asymptomatic except for skin findings or may be devastated by severe infantile spasms in early infancy, by continuing epilepsy, and by mental retardation.

Seizures in early infancy correlate with later mental retardation.

## Clinical Findings

### A. SYMPTOMS AND SIGNS

**1. Dermatologic features**—Skin findings bring most patients to the physician's attention. Ninety-six percent of patients have one or more hypomelanotic macules, facial angiofibromas, ungual fibromas, or shagreen patches. Adenoma sebaceum, the facial skin hamartomas, may first appear in early childhood, often on the cheek, chin, and dry sites of the skin where acne is not usually seen. They often have a reddish hue. The off-white hypomelanotic macules are seen more easily in tanned or dark-skinned individuals than in those with lighter skin. The macules often are oval or "ash leaf" in shape and follow dermatomes. A Wood lamp (ultraviolet light) shows the macules more clearly, a great help in the light-skinned patient. In the scalp, poliosis (whitened hair) is the equivalent. In infancy, the presence of these macules accompanied by seizures is virtually diagnostic of the disease. Subungual or periungual fibromas are more common in the toes. Leathery, orange peel-like shagreen patches support the diagnosis. Café au lait spots are occasionally seen. Fibrous or raised plaques may resemble coalescent angiofibromas.

**2. Neurologic features**—Seizures are the most common presenting symptom. Five percent of patients with infantile spasms (a serious epileptic syndrome) have tuberous sclerosis. Thus any patient presenting with infantile spasms (and the parents as well) should be evaluated for this disorder. An imaging study of the CNS, such as a CT scan, may show calcified subependymal nodules; MRI may show dysmyelinating white matter lesions or cortical tubers. Virtually any kind of symptomatic seizure (eg, atypical absence, partial complex, and generalized tonic–clonic seizures) may occur.

**3. Mental retardation**—Mental retardation occurs in up to 50% of patients referred to tertiary care centers; the incidence is probably much lower in randomly selected patients. Patients with seizures are more prone to mental retardation or learning disabilities.

**4. Renal lesions**—Renal cysts or angiomyolipomas may be asymptomatic. Hematuria or obstruction of urine flow sometimes occurs; the latter requires operation. Ultrasonography of the kidneys should be done in any patient suspected of tuberous sclerosis, both to aid in diagnosis if lesions are found and to rule out renal obstructive disease.

**5. Cardiopulmonary involvement**—Rarely cystic lung disease may occur. Rhabdomyomas of the heart may be asymptomatic but can lead to outflow obstruc-tion, conduction difficulties, and death. Chest radiographs and echocardiograms can detect these rare manifestations. Cardiac rhabdomyoma may be detected on prenatal ultrasound examination.

**6. Eye involvement**—Retinal hamartomas are often near the disk.

**7. Skeletal involvement**—Findings sometimes helpful in diagnosis are cystic rarefactions of the bones of the fingers or toes.

### B. DIAGNOSTIC STUDIES

Plain radiographs may detect areas of thickening within the skull, spine, and pelvis, and cystic lesions in the hands and feet. Chest radiographs may show lung honeycombing. More helpful is CT scanning, which can show the virtually pathognomonic subependymal nodular calcifications and sometimes widened gyri or tubers and brain tumors. Contrast material may show the often classically located tumors near the foramen interventriculare. Hypomyelinated lesions may be seen with MRI. EEG is helpful in delineating the presence of seizure discharges.

## Treatment

Therapy is as indicated by underlying disease (eg, seizures and tumors of the brain, kidney, and heart). Skin lesions on the face may need dermabrasion or laser treatment. Genetic counseling emphasizes identification of the carrier. The risk of appearance in offspring if either parent is a carrier is 50%. The patient should be seen annually for counseling and reexamination in childhood. Identification of the chromosomes (9,16; *TSCI* and *TSC2* genes) may in the future make intrauterine diagnosis possible.

Curatolo P et al: Tuberous sclerosis complex: A review of neurological aspects. Eur J Paediatr Neurol 2002;6:15 [PMID: 11993952].

Harris-Stith R, Elston DM: Tuberous sclerosis. Cutis 2002;69: 103 [PMID: 11868973].

Jozwiak S et al: Usefulness of diagnostic criteria of tuberous sclerosis complex in pediatric patients. J Child Neurol 2000;15: 652 [PMID: 11063078].

MacCollin M, Kwiatkowski D: Molecular genetic aspects of the phakomatoses: Tuberous sclerosis complex and neurofibromatosis 1. Curr Opin Neurol 2001;14:163 [PMID: 11262730].

Roach ES et al: Tuberous sclerosis complex consensus conference: Revised clinical diagnostic criteria. J Child Neurol 1998;13:624 [PMID: 9881533].

## 3. Encephalofacial Angiomatosis (Sturge–Weber Disease)

Sturge–Weber disease consists of a facial port wine nevus involving the upper part of the face (in the first division of cranial nerve V), a venous angioma of the meninges in the occipitoparietal regions, and choroidal angioma. The syndrome has been described without the facial nevus.

## Clinical Findings

In infancy, the eye may show congenital glaucoma, or buphthalmos, with a cloudy, enlarged cornea. In early stages, the facial nevus may be the only indication, with no findings in the brain even on radiologic studies. The characteristic cortical atrophy, calcifications of the cortex, and meningeal angiomatosis may appear with time, solidifying the diagnosis.

Physical examination may show focal seizures or hemiparesis on the side opposite the cerebral lesion. The facial nevus may be much more extensive than the first division of cranial nerve V; it can involve the lower face, mouth, lip, neck, and even torso. Hemiatrophy of the opposite limbs may occur. Mental handicap may result from poorly controlled seizures. Late-appearing glaucoma and, rarely, CNS hemorrhage occur.

Radiologic studies may show calcification of the cortex; CT scanning may show this much earlier than plain radiographic studies. MRI often shows underlying brain involvement.

The EEG often shows depression of voltage over the involved area in early stages; later, epileptiform abnormalities may be present focally.

## Treatment

Sturge–Weber disease is sporadic. Early control of seizures is important to avoid consequent developmental setback. If seizures do not occur, normal development can be anticipated. Careful examination of the newborn, with ophthalmologic assessment to detect early glaucoma, is indicated. Rarely, surgical removal of the involved meninges and the involved portion of the brain may be indicated, even hemispherectomy.

Chapieski L, Friedman A, Lachar D: Psychological functioning in children and adolescents with Sturge–Weber syndrome. J Child Neurol 2000;15:660 [PMID: 11063079].

Comi AM et al: Encephalofacial anigomatosis sparing the occipital lobe and without facial nevus: On the spectrum of Sturge–Weber syndrome variants? J Child Neurol 2003; 18:35 [PMID: 12661936].

Kossoff EH et al: Outcomes of 32 hemispherectomies for Sturge–Weber syndrome worldwide. Neurology 2002;59: 1735 [PMID: 12473761].

Pfund Z et al: Quantitative analysis of gray- and white-matter volumes and glucose metabolism in Sturge–Weber syndrome. J Child Neurol 2003;18:119 [PMID: 12693779].

Sujansky E, Conradi S: Sturge–Weber syndrome: Age of onset of seizures and glaucoma and the prognosis for affected children. J Child Neurol 1995;10:49 [PMID: 7769179].

## 4. Von Hippel–Lindau Disease (Retinocerebellar Angiomatosis)

Von Hippel–Lindau disease is a rare, dominantly inherited condition with retinal and cerebellar hemangioblastomas; cysts of the kidneys, pancreas, and epididymis; and sometimes renal cancers. The patient may present with ataxia, slurred speech, and nystagmus due to a hemangioblastoma of the cerebellum or with a medullary spinal cord cystic hemangioblastoma. Retinal detachment may occur from hemorrhage or exudate in the retinal vascular malformation. Rarely a pancreatic cyst or renal tumor may be the presenting symptom.

The diagnostic criteria for the disease are a retinal or cerebellar hemangioblastoma with or without a positive family history, intra-abdominal cyst, or renal cancer.

Choyke PL et al: Von Hippel–Lindau disease: Genetic, clinical, and imaging features. Radiology 1995;194:629 [PMID: 7862955].

Roach ES: Von Hippel–Lindau disease: How does one gene cause multiple tumors? Neurology 1999;53:7 [PMID: 10408528].

## CENTRAL NERVOUS SYSTEM DEGENERATIVE DISORDERS OF INFANCY & CHILDHOOD

The CNS degenerative disorders of infancy and childhood are characterized by arrest of psychomotor development and loss, usually progressive but at variable rates, of mental and motor functioning and often of vision as well. Seizures are common in some disorders. Symptoms and signs vary with age at onset and primary sites of involvement of specific types.

These disorders are fortunately rare. An early clinical pattern of decline often follows normal early development. Referral for sophisticated biochemical testing is usually necessary before a definitive diagnosis can be made (Tables 23–21 and 23–22).

DeLonlay P et al: A broad spectrum of clinical presentations in congenital disorders of glycosylation. I: A series of 26 cases. J Med Genet 2001;38:14 [PMID: 11134235].

Goebel H et al: Neurodegenerative diseases. Neuroimaging Clin North Am 2001;11:37 [PMID: 11331227].

Kaye EM: Update on genetic disorders affecting white matter. Pediatr Neurol 2001;24:11 [PMID: 11182276].

Kristjansdottir R, Uvebrant P, Wiklund LM: Clinical characteristics of children with cerebral white matter abnormalities. Europe J Paediatr Neurol 2000;4:17 [PMID: 10701100].

Shahbazian MD, Zoghbi HY: Molecular genetic of Rett syndrome and clinical spectrum of MECP2 mutations. Curr Opin Neurol 2001;14:171 [PMID: 11262731].

Vargas AP: Unusual early-onset Huntington's disease. J Child Neurol 2003;18:429 [PMID: 12886981].

**Table 23–21.** Central nervous system degenerative disorders of infancy.

| Disease | Enzyme Defect and Genetics | Onset | Early Manifestations | Vision and Hearing | Somatic Findings |
|---|---|---|---|---|---|
| **WHITE MATTER** | | | | | |
| Globoid (Krabbe) leukodystrophy | Recessive galacto-cerebroside β-galac-tosidase deficiency. Chromosome 14. | First 6 mos; late-onset form 2–6 y | Feeding difficulties. Shrill cry. Irritability. Arching of back. | Optic atrophy, mid-course to late. Hyper-acusis occasionally. | Head often small. Often under-weight. |
| Metachromatic leukodystrophy | Recessive. Arylsul-fatase A deficiency. 22q13. | Second year; less often, later childhood or adult | Incoordination, especially gait disturbance; then general regression. Reverse in juveniles. | Optic atrophy, usually late. Hearing normal. | Head enlarged late. No change in juvenile form. |
| Neuroaxonal dystrophy | Familial, (?) recessive. More common in girls than boys; defect unknown. | 6 mos to 2 y | Arrest of development and dementia. Loss of motor functions. Occasionally hypesthesia over trunk and legs. | Nystagmus occasional; optic atrophy, blindness; abnormal VER. | Early, may lie in "frog position." |
| Hallervorden–Spatz syndrome | Unknown; may be familial. | By age 10 y | Rigidity, dystonia, gait disturbance, tremor. | Optic atrophy. | None |
| Pelizaeus–Merzbacher disease | X-linked recessive; rare female. Proteo-lipid protein (myelin) decreased. Xq22 | (?) Birth to 2 y | Eye rolling often shortly after birth. Head bobbing. Slow loss of intellect. | Slowly developing optic atrophy. Hearing normal. Nystagmus. | Head and body normal |
| **DIFFUSE, BUT PRIMARILY GRAY MATTER** | | | | | |
| Poliodystrophy (Alpers's disease) | Occasionally familial, recessive. Possibly viral. Metabolic forms. | Infancy to adolescence | Variable: loss of intellect, seizures, incoordination. Vomiting, hepatic failure. | Cortical blindness and deafness | Head normal initially; may fail to grow |
| Tay–Sachs disease and G$_{M2}$ gangliosidosis variants: Sandhoff disease; juvenile; chronic-adult | Recessive. Hexo-saminidase deficiencies. Tay–Sachs (93% East European Jewish), hexosaminidase A deficiency. Sand-hoff-hexosaminidase A and B deficiency. Juvenile-partial hexosaminidase A | Tay–Sachs, and Sandhoff; 3–6 mos; others 2–6 y or later. | Variable: shrill cry, loss of vision, infantile spasms, arrest of development. In juvenile and chronic forms: motor difficulties; later, mental difficulties. | Cherry-red macula, early blindness. Hyper-acusis early. Strabis-mus in juvenile form, blindness late. | Head enlarged late. Liver occasionally enlarged. None in juvenile chronic forms. |
| Niemann–Pick disease and variants | 50% Jewish. Recessive. Sphingomyeli-nase deficiency in types A and C involving the CNS. | First 6 mos. In variants, later onset: often non-Jewish. | Slow development. Protruding belly. | Cherry-red macula in 35–50%. Blindness late. Deafness occasionally. | Head usually normal. Spleen enlarged more than liver. Occasional xanthomas of skin. |
| Infantile Gaucher disease (gluco-sylceramide lipi-dosis) | Recessive. Glucocere-brosidase deficiency. | First 6 mos; rarely, late infancy | Stridor or hoarse cry; retraction; feeding difficulties | Occasional cherry-red macula. Convergent squint. Deafness occasionally. | Head usually normal. Liver and spleen equally enlarged. |

**Table 23–21.** Central nervous system degenerative disorders of infancy. (continued)

| Motor System | Seizures | Laboratory and Tissue Studies | Course |
|---|---|---|---|
| **WHITE MATTER** | | | |
| Early spasticity, occasionally preceded by hypotonia. Prolonged nerve conduction. | Early. Myoclonic and generalized, decerebrate posturing | CSF protein elevated; usually normal in late-onset forms. Sural nerve; nonspecific myelin breakdown. Enzyme deficiency in leukocytes, cultured skin fibroblasts. Demyelination, gliosis with low-signal CT scan, high-signal T$_2$-weighted MRI. | Rapid. Death usually by 1½–2 y. Late-onset cases may live 5–10 y. |
| Combined upper and lower motor neuron signs. Ataxia. Prolonged nerve conduction. | Infrequent, usually late and generalized | Metachromatic cells in urine: negative sulfatase A test. CSF protein elevated. Urine sulfatide increased. Sural nerve biopsy; metachromasia. Enzyme deficiency in leukocytes, cultured skin fibroblasts. Imaging: Same as globoid leukodystrophy. | Moderately slow. Death in infantile form by 3–8 y, in juvenile form by 10–15 y. |
| Combined upper and lower motor neuron lesions. Hypotonia, extrapyramidal manifestations. | Variable, but usually not a prominent feature | Denervation on EMG. Increased iron uptake in region of basal ganglia. Brain and sural nerve: axonal swellings or "spheroids" Cerebellar atrophy. Cause unknown. Conjunctival biopsy may yield nerves with "spheroids." | Progressive, with death early in second decade or earlier. |
| Extrapyramidal signs, dysarthria, increased deep tendon reflexes. | Variable, EEG may be abnormal | Seablue histiocytes in bone marrow. Iron deposits in basal ganglia on MRI. | Progressive mental/motor deterioration |
| Cerebellar signs early, hyperactive deep reflexes. Spasticity. | Usually only late | None specific. Brain biopsy: extensive demyelination with small perivascular islands of intact myelin. Exon abnormalities in PLP gene in 10–25%. | Very slow, often seemingly stationary. |
| **DIFFUSE, BUT PRIMARILY GRAY MATTER** | | | |
| Variable: incoordination, spasticity | Often initial manifestation: myoclinic, akinetic, and generalized | Nonspecific, CSF protein normal or slightly elevated. Extensive neuronal loss in cortex: may occur very late. Variably increased serum pryuvate, lactate; liver steatosis, cirrhosis late. | Usually rapid, with death within 1–3 y after onset. |
| Initially floppy. Eventual decerebrate rigidity. In juvenile and chronic forms: dysarthria, ataxia, spasticity. | Frequent, in mid-course and late. Infantile spasms and generalized | Blood smears: vacuolated lymphocytes; basophillic hypergranulation. Enzyme deficiencies in serum, leukocytes, culture skin fibroblasts. High-density thalami on CT scan, low-density white matter. | Moderately rapid. Death usually by 2–5 y. In juvenile form, 5–15 y. |
| Initially floppy. Eventually spastic. Occasionally extrapyramidal signs. Ataxia, dystonia. | Rare and late | Blood: vacuolated lymphocytes; increased lipids. X-rays: "mottled" lungs, decalcified bones. "Foam cells" in bone marrow, spleen, lymph nodes. WBC, fibroblast enzyme studies are diagnostic. | Moderately slow. Death usually by 3–5 y. |
| Opisthotonos early, followed rapidly by decerebrate rigidity | Rare and late | Anemia. Increased acid phosphatase. X-rays: thinned cortex, trabeculation of bones. "Gaucher cells" in bone marrow, spleen. Enzyme deficiency in leukocytes or cultured skin fibroblasts. | Very rapid |

*(continued)*

*Table 23–21.* Central nervous system degenerative disorders of infancy. (continued)

| Disease | Enzyme Defect and Genetics | Onset | Early Manifestations | Vision and Hearing | Somatic Findings |
|---|---|---|---|---|---|
| **DIFFUSE, BUT PRIMARILY GRAY MATTER** | | | | | |
| Lipogranulomatosis (Farber disease) | Ceramidase deficiency | Early in infancy | Hoarseness, irritability, restricted joint movements | Usually normal | Painful nodular swelling of joints; subcutaneous nodules |
| Generalized gangliosidosis and juvenile type ($G_{m1}$ gangliosidoses) | Recessive; β-galactosidase deficiency | First year; less often, second year | Arrest of development. Protruding belly. Coarse facies in infantile (generalized) form. | 50% "cherry-red spot." Hearing usually normal. In juvenile type. occasionally retinitis pigmentosa. | Head enlarged early; liver enlarged more than spleen |
| Subacute necrotizing encephalomyelopathy (Leigh disease) | Recessive or variable. May have deficiency of pyruvate carboxylase, pyruvate dehydrogenase, cytochrome enzymes. | Infancy to late childhood | Difficulties in feeding; feeble or absent cry; floppiness | Optic atrophy, often early. Roving eye movements. Ophthalmoplegia. | Head usually normal, occasionally small; cardiac and renal tubular dysfunction occasionally |
| Menkes disease (kinky hair disease) | X-linked recessive; defect in copper absorption | Infancy | Peculiar facies; secondary hair white, twisted, split; hypothermia | May show optic disk pallor and microcysts of pigment epithelium | Normal to small |
| Carbohydrate-deficient glycoprotein syndrome | Recessive glycoprotein abnormality; glycosolation faulty | Infancy | Failure to thrive, retardation | Strabismus Retinopathy | Dysmorphic facies. Prominent fat pads. |
| Abetalipoproteinemia (Bassen–Kornzweig disease) | Recessive; primary defect unknown | Early childhood | Diarrhea in infancy | Retinitis pigmentosa; late ophthalmoplegia | None |

Wisniewski KE et al: Neuronal ceroid lipofuscinoses: Classification and diagnosis. Adv Genet 2001;45:1 [PMID: 11332767].

# ATAXIAS OF CHILDHOOD

## 1. Acute Cerebellar Ataxia

Acute cerebellar ataxia occurs most commonly in children age 2–6 years. The onset is abrupt, and the evolution of symptoms is rapid. In about 50% of patients, a prodromal illness occurs with fever, respiratory or gastrointestinal symptoms, or an exanthem within 3 weeks of onset. Associated viral infections include varicella, rubeola, mumps, rubella, echovirus infections, poliomyelitis, infectious mononucleosis, and influenza. Bacterial infections such as scarlet fever and salmonellosis have also been incriminated.

## Clinical Findings

### A. SYMPTOMS AND SIGNS

Ataxia of the trunk and extremities may be so severe that the child exhibits a staggering, reeling gait and inability to sit without support or to reach for objects; or he or she may show only mild unsteadiness. Hypotonia, tremor of the extremities, and horizontal nystagmus may be present. Speech may be slurred. The child is frequently irritable, and vomiting may occur.

There are no clinical signs of increased intracranial pressure. Sensory and reflex testing usually shows no abnormalities.

### B. LABORATORY FINDINGS

CSF pressure and protein and glucose levels are normal; slight lymphocytosis ($\leq 30/mL$) may be present. At-

*Table 23–21.* Central nervous system degenerative disorders of infancy. (continued)

| Motor System | Seizures | Laboratory and Tissue Studies | Course |
|---|---|---|---|
| **DIFFUSE, BUT PRIMARILY GRAY MATTER** | | | |
| Psychomotor retardation and progressive paralysis | Usually none | Chest radiographs may show pulmonary infiltrates. Nodules: granulomatous lesions, resembling those in reticuloendotheliosis. Multiple infarcts on CNS imaging. | Rapid: death usually in 1–2 y. |
| Initially floppy, eventually spastic | Usually late | Blood: vacuolated lymphocytes. X-rays: dorsolumbar kyphosis, "beaking" of vertebrae. "Foam cells" similar to those in Niemann–Pick disease. | Very rapid. Death within a few years. Slower in juvenile type (to 10 y). |
| Flaccid and immobile; may become spastic. Spinocerebellar forms; ataxia. | Rare and late | Increased CSF and blood lactate and pyruvate. High-signal MRI $T_2$ foci in thalami; globus pallidus, subthalamic nuclei. | Usually rapid in infants, but may be slow with death after several years. Central hypoventilation a frequent cause of death. |
| Variable: floppy to spastic | Myoclonic infantile spasms, status epilepticus | Defective absorption of copper. Cerebral angiography shows elongated arteries. Hair shows pili torti, split shafts. Copper and ceruloplasmin low. | Moderately rapid. Death usually by 3–4 ys. |
| Variable hypotonia Neuropathy | Rare | Normal transferrin decreased. Carbohydrate-deficient transferrin increased. Liver steatosis. Cerebellar hypoplasia. | Cardiomyopathy, thrombosis |
| Ataxia, late extrapyramidal movement disorder | None | Abetalipoproteinemia: acanthocytosis, low serum vitamin E; cerebellar atrophy on imaging. | Progression arrested with vitamin E |

CSF = cerebrospinal fluid; CT = computed tomography; EEG = electroencephalogram; EMG = electromyelogram; MRI = magnetic resonance imaging; VER = visual evoked potential; WBC = white blood cell.

tempts should be made to identify the etiologic viral agent.

### C. IMAGING

CT scans are normal; MRI may show cerebellar postinfectious demyelinating lesions. The EEG may be normal or may show nonspecific slowing.

## Differential Diagnosis

Acute cerebellar ataxia must be differentiated from acute cerebellar syndromes due to phenytoin, phenobarbital, primidone, or lead intoxication. For phenytoin, the toxic level in serum is usually above 25 μg/mL; for phenobarbital, above 50 μg/mL; for primidone, above 14 μg/mL. (See Seizure Disorders section.) Papilledema, anemia, basophilic stippling of erythrocytes, proteinuria, typical radiographs, and elevated CSF protein are clinical clues to lead intoxication, which is confirmed by serum, urine, or hair lead levels. An occult neuroblastoma, usually seen with the polymyoclonus–opsoclonus syndrome (see following section) occasionally begins as acute cerebellar ataxia.

In rare cases, acute cerebellar ataxia may be the presenting sign of acute bacterial meningitis or may be mimicked by corticosteroid withdrawal, vasculitides such as in polyarteritis nodosa, trauma, the first attack of ataxia in a metabolic disorder such as Hartnup disease, or the onset of acute disseminated encephalomyelitis or of multiple sclerosis. The history and physical findings may differentiate these disturbances, but appropriate laboratory studies are often necessary.

*Table 23–22.* Central nervous system degenerative disorders of childhood.[a]

| Disease | Enzyme Defect and Genetics | Onset | Early Manifestations | Vision and Hearing | Motor System | Seizures | Laboratory and Tissue Studies | Course |
|---|---|---|---|---|---|---|---|---|
| Adrenoleukodystrophy and variants | X-linked recessive. Neonatal form recessive Xq28. Acyl-CoA synthetase deficiency. | 5–10 years May also present as newborn, adolescent or adult. | Impaired intellect; behavioral problems | Cortical blindness and deafness | Ataxia, spasticity; motor deficits may be asymmetrical or one-sided initially; adrenomyeloneuropathy in adults | Occasionally | Hyperpigmentation and adrenocortical insufficiency. ACTH elevated. Accumulation of very long chain fatty acids in plasma. | Fairly rapid. Death usually within 2–3 y after onset. |
| Neuronal ceroid lipofuscinosis (NCL; cerebromacular degeneration); infantile NCL (INCL); late infantile (LINCL); juvenile NCL (JNCL; Batten disease) | Recessive; multiple gene mutations, polymorphisms. (See Ref. Gene Reviews.) | 6–24 months INCL: 2–4 y LINCL; 4–8 y JNCL | Ataxia; visual difficulties; arrested intellectual development. Seizures | Pigmentary degeneration of macula; optic atrophy; ERG, VER abnormal | Ataxia; spasticity progressing to decerebrate rigidity | Often early; myoclonus and later generalized; refractory | Blood: vacuolated lymphocytes. Biopsy, EM of skin, conjunctiva; WBC: "curvilinear bodies, fingerprint profiles." Molecular testing of CLN1, CLN2, CLN3. Protein gene product testing for CLN1 and CLN2. | Moderately slow. Death in 3–8 y. |
| Subacute sclerosing panencephalitis (Dawson disease) | None. Measles "slow virus" infection. Also reported as result of rubella. | 3–22 years; rarely earlier or later | Impaired intellect; emotional lability; incoordination | Occasionally chorioretinitis or optic atrophy; hearing normal | Ataxia; slurred speech; occasionally involuntary movements; spasticity progressing to decerebrate rigidity | Myoclonic and akinetic seizures relatively early; later, focal and generalized | CSF protein normal to moderately elevated. High CSF IgG;[b] oligoclonal bands. Elevated CSF (and serum) measles (or rubella) antibody titers. Characteristic EEG. Brain biopsy: inclusion body encephalitis; culturing of measles virus, perhaps rubella virus. | Variable, death in months to years. Remissions of variable duration may occur. |

| Disease | Genetics | Age at onset | Clinical features | Ocular signs | Seizures | Laboratory | Course/Prognosis |
|---|---|---|---|---|---|---|---|
| Multiple sclerosis | None. Diagnosis difficult in childhood. | Adolescent; rare in childhood | Highly variable: may strike one or more sites of CNS; paresthesias common | Optic neuritis; diplopia, nystagmus at some time; vestibulocochlear nerves occasionally affected | Rare: focal or generalized | CSF may show slight pleocytosis, elevation of protein and gamma globulin,[b] oligoclonal bands present. CT scan may show areas of demyelination. Auditory, visual, and somatosensory evoked responses often show lesions in respective pathways. Changes in T-cell subsets. | Variable: complete remission possible. Recurrent attacks and involvement of multiple sites are prerequisites for diagnosis. |
| Cerebrotendinous xanthomatosis | ?Recessive. Abnormal accumulation of cholesterol. | Late childhood to adolescence | Xanthomas in tendons; mental deterioration | Cataracts; xanthelasma | Myoclonus | Xanthomas may appear in lungs. Xanthomas in tendons (especially Achilles). | Very slowly progressive into middle life. Replace deficient bile acid. |
| Huntington disease | Dominant. Chromosome 4p CAG repeat. | 10% childhood onset | Rigidity; dementia | Ophthalmoplegia late | 50% with major motor seizures | CT scan may show "butterfly" atrophy of caudate and putamen | Moderately rapid with death in 15 y |
| Refsum disease | Recessive. Phytanic acid oxidase deficiency. | 5–10 y | Ataxia; ichthyosis; cardiomyopathy | Retinitis pigmentosa; nystagmus | None | Serum phytanic acid elevated. Slow nerve conduction velocity. Elevated CSF protein. Peroxisomal disease. | Treat with low phytanic acid diet |

[a]For late infantile metachromatic leukodystrophy, Pelizaeus-Merzbacher disease, poliodystrophy, Gaucher's disease of later onset, and subacute necrotizing encephalomyelopathy, see Table 22–22.

[b]CSF γ-globulin (IgG) is considered elevated in children when > 9% of total protein (possibly even > 8.3%); definitively elevated when > 14%.

ACTH = adrenocorticotropic hormone; CSF = cerebrospinal fluid; CT = computed tomography; EEG = electroencephalogram; ERG = electroretinogram; VER = visual evoked response; CLN = ceroid lipofuscinosis.

For ataxias with more chronic onset and course, see the sections on spinocerebellar degeneration and the other degenerative disorders.

## Treatment & Prognosis

Treatment is supportive. The use of corticosteroids has no rational justification. Between 80% and 90% of children with acute cerebellar ataxia not secondary to drug toxicity recover without sequelae within 6–8 weeks. In the remainder, neurologic disturbances, including disorders of behavior and of learning, ataxia, abnormal eye movements, and speech impairment, may persist for months or years, and recovery may remain incomplete.

Go T: Intravenous immunoglobulin therapy for acute cerebellar ataxia. Acta Paediatr 2003;92:504 [PMID: 12801122].

Dinolfo E: Evaluation of ataxia. Pediatr Rev 2001;22:177 [PMID: 11331741].

Lamperti C et al: Cerebellar ataxia and coenzyme Q10 deficiency. Neurology 2003;60:1206 [PMID: 12682339].

Ryan MM, Engle EC: Acute ataxia I childhood. J Child Neurol 2003;18:309 [PMID: 12822814].

## 2. Polymyoclonia–Opsoclonus Syndrome of Childhood (Infantile Myoclonic Encephalopathy, "Dancing Eyes–Dancing Feet" Syndrome)

The symptoms and signs of this syndrome are at first similar to those of acute cerebellar ataxia. Often of sudden onset, polymyoclonus–opsoclonus syndrome is characterized by severe incoordination of the trunk and extremities with lightning-like jerking or flinging movements of a group of muscles, causing the child to be in constant motion while awake. Extraocular muscle involvement results in sudden irregular eye movements (opsoclonus). Irritability and vomiting are often present, but there is no depression of level of consciousness. This syndrome occurs in association with viral infections and tumors of neural crest origin among other disorders. Immunologic mechanisms have been postulated. Usually no signs of increased intracranial pressure are present. CSF may show normal or mildly increased protein levels. Special techniques show increased CSF levels of plasmacytes and abnormal immunoglobulins. The EEG may be slightly slow, but when performed together with EMG, it shows no evidence of association between cortical discharges and the muscle movements. An assiduous search must be made to rule out tumor of neural crest origin by chest radiographs and CT scan or ultrasound (or both) of the adrenal area as well as by assays of urinary catecholamine metabolites (vanillylmandelic acid and so on) and cystathionine.

The symptoms respond (often dramatically) to large doses of corticotropin. Plasmapheresis has been successful. When a neural crest (or other) tumor is found, surgical excision should be followed by irradiation and chemotherapy. Life span is determined by the biologic behavior of the tumor. The syndrome is usually self-limited but may be characterized by exacerbations and remissions. Even after removal of a neural crest tumor and without other evidence of its recurrence, symptoms may reappear. Mild mental retardation may be a sequela.

Krolczyk S: Opsoclonus: An early sign of neonatal herpes encephalitis. J Child Neurol 2003;18:356 [PMID: 12822821].

Pranzatelli MR et al: Screening for autoantibodies in children with opsoclonus–myoclonus-ataxia. Pediatr Neurol 2002;27:384 [PMID: 12504207].

Yiu VWY et al: Plasmapheresis as an effective treatment for opsoclonus–myoclonus syndrome. Pediatr Neurol 2001;24:72 [PMID: 11182286].

## 3. Spinocerebellar Degeneration Disorders

Spinocerebellar degeneration disorders may be hereditary or may occur in sporadic distribution. Hereditary disorders include Friedreich ataxia, dominant hereditary ataxia, and a group of miscellaneous diseases.

### Friedreich Ataxia

This is a recessive disorder characterized by onset of gait ataxia or scoliosis before puberty that becomes progressively worse. Reflexes, light touch, and position sensation are reduced. Dysarthria becomes progressively more severe. Cardiomyopathy usually develops, and diabetes mellitus occurs in 40% of patients, half of whom require insulin. Pes cavus typically is found. The GAA trinucleotide repeats on chromosome 9 can be used for laboratory diagnosis.

Treatment includes surgery for scoliosis and intervention as needed for cardiac disease and diabetes. Patients are usually confined to a wheelchair after age 20 years. Death occurs, usually from heart failure or dysrhythmias, in the third or fourth decade; some patients survive longer.

### Dominant Ataxia

These diseases (in the past known as olivopontocerebellar atrophy, Holmes ataxia, Marie ataxia, and the like) occur with varying manifestations, even among members of the same family. Ataxia occurs at onset, and progression continues with ophthalmoplegias (in some patients), extrapyramidal syndromes, polyneuropathy, and dementia. Several types have been found to be caused by CAG trinucleotide repeats. Levodopa may ameliorate rigidity and bradykinesia, but no other therapy is available. Only 10% of patients experience onset in childhood, and the course in these patients is often more rapid.

## Miscellaneous Hereditary Ataxias

Associated findings permit identification of these recessive disorders. These include ataxia–telangiectasia (telangiectasia, immune defects; see below); Wilson disease (Kayser–Fleischer rings); Refsum disease (ichthyosis, cardiomyopathy, retinitis pigmentosa, large nerves); Rett syndrome (regression to autism at age 7–18 months in girls, loss of use of hands, progressive failure of brain growth); and abetalipoproteinemia (infantile diarrhea, acanthocytosis, retinitis pigmentosa). Gluten sensitivity may cause ataxia. Patients with juvenile and chronic gangliosidoses and some hemolytic anemias and long-term survivors of Chédiak–Higashi disease may develop spinocerebellar degeneration. Idiopathic familial ataxia is called Behr syndrome. Neuropathies such as Charcot–Marie–Tooth disease produce ataxia.

Alper G, Narayanan V: Friedreich's ataxia. Pediatr Neurol 2003;2 8:335 [PMID: 12878293].

Babovic-Vuksanovic D et al: Spinocerebellar ataxia type 2 (SCA 2) in an infant with extreme CAG repeat expansion. Am J Med Genet 1998;79:383 [PMID: 9779806].

Hadjivassiliou M: Gluten ataxia I perspective: Epidemiology, genetic susceptibility and clinical characteristics. Brain 2003;126:685 [PMID: 12566288].

Macpherson J et al: Observation of an excess of fragile-X permutations in a population of males referred with spinocerebellar ataxia. Hum Genet 2003;112:619 [PMID: 12612802].

Parmeggiani A et al: Epilepsy, intelligence and psychiatric disorders in patients with cerebellar hypoplasia. J Child Neurol 2003;18:1 [PMID: 12661930].

Tranebjaerg L et al: Genome-wide homozygosity mapping localizes a gene for autosomal recessive non-progressive infantile ataxia to 20q11–q13. Hum Genet 2003;113:293 [PMID: 12811539].

## ATAXIA–TELANGIECTASIA (Louis-Bar Syndrome)

Ataxia–telangiectasia is a multisystem disorder inherited as an autosomal recessive trait. It is characterized by progressive ataxia; telangiectasia of the bulbar conjunctiva, external ears, nares, and (later) other body surfaces, appearing in the third to sixth year; and recurrent respiratory, sinus, and ear infections. Ocular dyspraxia, slurred speech, choreoathetosis, hypotonia and areflexia, and psychomotor and growth retardation may be present. Endocrinopathies are common. Nerve conduc-

tion velocities may be reduced. The entire nervous system may be affected in late stages of the disease. A spectrum of involvement may be seen in the same family. Immunodeficiencies of IgA and IgE are common (see Chapter 29), and the incidence of certain cancers is high. Elevated serum $\alpha$-fetoprotein is a screen for this disease.

Cabana MD et al: Consequences of the delayed diagnosis of ataxia–telangiectasia. Pediatrics 1998;102:98 [PMID: 9651420].

Crawford TO: Ataxia–telangiectasia. Semin Pediatr Neurol 1998;5:287 [PMID: 9874856].

Sandoval C, Swift M: Hodgkin disease in ataxia–telangiectasia patients with poor outcomes. Med Pediatr Oncol 2003;40: 162 [PMID: 12518345].

Tavani F et al: Ataxia–telangiectasia: The pattern of cerebellar atrophy on MRI. Neuroradiology 2003;45:315 [PMID: 12740724].

## EXTRAPYRAMIDAL DISORDERS

Extrapyramidal disorders are characterized by the presence in the waking state of one or more of the following features: dyskinesias, athetosis, ballismus, tremors, rigidity, and dystonias.

For the most part, the precise pathologic and anatomic localization of these disorders is not understood. Motor pathways synapsing in the striatum (putamen and caudate nucleus), globus pallidus, red nucleus, substantia nigra, and the body of Luys are involved; this system is modulated by pathways originating in the thalamus, cerebellum, and reticular formation.

## 1. Sydenham Postrheumatic Chorea

Sydenham chorea is characterized by an acute onset of choreiform movements and variable degrees of psychological disturbance. It is frequently associated with rheumatic endocarditis and arthritis. Although the disorder follows infections with group A β-hemolytic streptococci, the interval between infection and chorea may be greatly prolonged; throat cultures and antistreptolysin O (ASO) titers may therefore be negative. Chorea has also been associated with hypocalcemia; with vascular lupus erythematosus; and with toxic, viral, infectious, parainfectious, and degenerative encephalopathies.

### Clinical Findings

#### A. SYMPTOMS AND SIGNS

Chorea, or rapid involuntary movements of the limbs and face, is the hallmark physical finding. In addition to the jerky incoordinate movements, the following are noted: emotional lability, waxing and waning ("milkmaid's") grip, darting tongue, "spooning" of the extended hands and their tendency to pronate, and knee jerks slow to return from the extended to their prestimulus position ("hung up"). Seizures, while uncommon, may be masked by choreic jerks.

### B. LABORATORY FINDINGS

Anemia, leukocytosis, and an increased erythrocyte sedimentation rate may be present. The ASO titer may be elevated and C-reactive protein present. Throat culture is sometimes positive for group A-hemolytic streptococci.

ECG and echocardiography are often essential to detect cardiac involvement. Antineuronal antibodies are present in most patients but are not specific for this disease. Specialized radiologic procedures (MRI, SPECT) may show basal ganglia abnormalities.

### Differential Diagnosis

The diagnosis of Sydenham chorea is usually not difficult. Tics, drug-induced extrapyramidal syndromes, Huntington chorea, and hepatolenticular degeneration (Wilson disease), as well as other rare movement disorders, can usually be ruled out on historical and clinical grounds. Immunologic linkages among chorea, tics, and obsessive–compulsive disorder are being studied in pediatric patients. Other causes of chorea can be ruled out by laboratory tests, such as antinuclear antibody for lupus, thyroid screening tests, serum calcium for hypocalcemia, and immunologic tests for Epstein–Barr virus infection.

### Treatment

There is no specific treatment. Dopaminergic blockers such as haloperidol, 0.5 mg to 3–6 mg/d, and pimozide, 4–12 mg/d, have been used. Parkinsonian side effects such as rigidity and masked facies and, with high doses, tardive dyskinesia rarely occur in childhood. A variety of other drugs have been used with success in individual cases, such as the anticonvulsant sodium valproate, 50–60 mg/kg/d in divided doses; or prednisone, 0.5–2 mg/kg/d in divided doses. Emotional lability and depression sometimes warrant administration of antidepressants such as amitriptyline. All patients should be given antistreptococcal rheumatic fever prophylaxis, possibly through child-bearing age.

### Prognosis

Sydenham chorea is a self-limited disease that may last from a few weeks to months. Relapse of chorea may occur with nonspecific stress or illness—or with breakthrough streptococcus infections (if penicillin prophylaxis is not done). Two thirds of patients relapse one or more times, but the ultimate outcome does not appear to be worse in those with recurrences. In older studies, valvular heart disease occurs in about one third of patients, particularly if other rheumatic manifestations appear. Psychoneurotic disturbances occur in a significant percentage of patients.

Church AJ et al: Anti-basal ganglia antibodies in acute and persistent Sydenham's chorea. Neurology 2002;59:227 [PMID: 12316062].

Garvey MA, Giedd J, Swedo SE: PANDAS: The search for environmental triggers of pediatric neuropsychiatric disorders: Lessons from rheumatic fever. J Child Neurol 1998;13: 413 [PMID: 9733286].

Lee PH et al: Serial brain SPECT images in a case of Sydenham chorea. Arch Neurol 1999;56:237 [PMID: 10025430].

Murphy ML, Pichichero ME: Prospective identification and treatment of children with pediatric autoimmune neuropsychiatric disorder associated with group A streptococcal infection (PANDAS). Arch Pediatr Adolesc Med 2002;156: 356 [PMID: 11929370].

Pranzatelli MR: Movement disorders in childhood. Pediatr Rev 1996;17:388 [PMID: 8937171].

Schlaggar BL, Mink JW: Movement disorders in children. Pediatr Rev 2003;24:39 [PMID: 12563038].

## 2. Tics (Habit Spasms)

### Clinical Findings

Tics, or habit spasms, are quick repetitive but irregular movements, often stereotyped, and briefly suppressible. Coordination and muscle tone are not affected. A psychogenic basis is seldom discernible. Transient tics of childhood (12–24% incidence in school-age children) last from 1 month to 1 year and seldom need treatment. Many children with tics have a history of encephalopathic past events, neurologic soft signs, and school problems. Facial tics such as grimaces, twitches, and blinking predominate, but the trunk and extremities are often involved and twisting or flinging movements may be present. Vocal tics are less common.

Tourette syndrome is characterized by multiple fluctuating motor and vocal tics with no obvious cause lasting more than 1 year. Tics evolve slowly, new ones being added to or replacing old ones. Coprolalia and echolalia are relatively infrequent. Partial forms are common. The usual age at onset is 2–15 years, and the familial incidence is 35–50%. The disorder occurs in all ethnic groups. Tourette syndrome may be triggered by stimulants such as methylphenidate and dextroamphetamine. An imbalance of neurotransmitters, especially dopamine and serotonin, has been hypothesized.

In mild cases, tics are self-limited and, when disregarded, disappear. When attention is paid to one tic, it may disappear only to be replaced by another that is often worse. If the tic and its underlying anxiety or compulsive neuroses are severe, psychiatric evaluation and treatment are needed.

Important comorbidities are attention-deficit/hyperactivity disorder and obsessive–compulsive disorder. Learning disabilities, sleep difficulties, anxiety states, and mood swings are also common. Medications such as methylphenidate and dextroamphetamine should be carefully titrated to treat attention-deficit/hyperactivity disorder and avoid worsening tics. Fluoxetine and clomipramine may be useful for obsessive–compulsive disorder and rage episodes in patients with tics.

## Treatment

The most effective medications for treating Tourette syndrome are dopamine blockers; however, many pediatric patients can manage without drug treatment. Medications are generally reserved for patients with disabling symptoms; treatment may be relaxed or discontinued when the symptoms abate (Table 23–23). Nonpharmacologic treatment of Tourette syndrome includes education of patients, family members, and school personnel. In some cases, restructuring the school environment to prevent tension and teasing may be necessary. Supportive counseling, either at or outside school, should be provided. Medications usually do not eradicate the tics. The goal of treatment should be to reduce the tics to tolerable levels without inducing undesirable side effects. Medication dosage should be increased at weekly intervals until a satisfactory response is obtained. Often a single dose at bedtime is sufficient. The two neurolep-

**Table 23–23.** Medications for Tourette syndrome and tics.

| |
|---|
| **Dopamine blockers (many are antipsychotics)** |
|   Haloperidol (Haldol) |
|   Pimozide (Orap) |
|   Fluphenazine (Prolixin) |
|   Olanzapine (Zyprexa) |
|   Risperidone (Resperdal) |
| **Serotonergic drugs[a]** |
|   Fluoxetine (Prozac) |
|   Paroxetine (Paxil) |
|   Sertraline (Zoloft) |
|   Anafranil (Clomipromine) |
|   Fluvoxamine (Luvox) |
| **Noradrenergic drugs[b]** |
|   Clonidine (Catapres) |
|   Guanfacine (Tenex) |
| **Other** |
|   Clonazepam (Klonopin) |
|   Baclofen (Lioresal) |

[a]Useful for obsessive-compulsive disorder.
[b]Useful for attention-deficit/hyperactivity disorder.

tic agents used most often are pimozide and risperidone. Sleepiness and weight gain are the most common side effects; rare are prolonged QT interval (ECG), akathisia, and tardive dyskinesia. Clonidine, clonazepam, and calcium channel blockers have been used in individual patients with some success. Sometimes these agents are used in combination (eg, clonidine with pimozide).

Sydenham chorea is a well-documented pediatric autoimmune disorder associated with streptococcal infections (PANDAS). Patients with tic disorders occasionally have obsessive–compulsive disorder precipitated or exacerbated by streptococcal infections. Less definite (much less frequent) are tic flare-ups with streptococcal infection. Active prospective antibody (antineuronal and antistreptococcal) and clinical studies are in progress. Research centers have used experimental treatments (IVIG, plasmapharesis, steroids) in severe cases. At present, most patients with a tic do not worsen with group A streptococcal infections; with rare exceptions, penicillin prophylaxis is not generally necessary for the majority of patients with tic disorders.

Burd L et al: Long-term follow-up of an epidemiologically defined cohort of patients with Tourette syndrome. Neurology 2001;16:431 [PMID: 11417610].

Jankovic J: Tourette's syndrome. N Engl J Med 2001;345:1184 [PMID: 11642235].

Kossoff EH, Singer HS: Tourette syndrome: Clinical characteristics and current management strategies. Paediatr Drugs 2001;3:355 [PMID: 11393328].

Kurlan R et al: The behavioral spectrum of tic disorders: A community based study. Neurology 2002;59:414 [PMID: 12177376].

Leckman JF: Tourette's syndrome. Lancet 2002;360:1577 [PMID: 12443611].

Loiselle CR et al: Antistreptococcal, neuronal, and nuclear antibodies in Tourette syndrome. Pediatr Neurol 2003;28:119 [PMID: 12699862].

Murphy ML, Pichichero ME: Prospective identification and treatment of children with pediatric autoimmune neuropsychiatric disorder associated with a group A streptococcal infection (PANDAS). Arch Pediatr Adolesc Med 2002;156:356 [PMID: 11929370].

Singer HS et al: Baclofen treatment in Tourette syndrome: A double blind, placebo-controlled, crossover trial. Neurology 2001;56:599 [PMID:11245709].

Snider LA et al: Tics and problem behavior in school children: Prevalence, characterization, and associations. Pediatrics 2002;110:331 [PMID: 12165586].

Zinner SH: Tourette disorder. Pediatr Rev 2000;21:372 [PMID: 11077021].

## 3. Paroxysmal Dyskinesias/Chronic Dystonia

Sudden-onset, short-duration choreoathetosis or dystonia episodes occur in childhood. Most often these episodes are familial and genetic. Episodes may occur spontaneously or be set off by actions ("kinesiogenic," or movement-induced) such as rising from a chair, reaching for a glass, or walking. Sometimes only hard sustained exercise will induce the dyskinesia. (Nocturnal dyskinesia/dystonic episodes are currently thought to be frontal lobe seizures.)

The diagnosis is clinical. Onset is usually in childhood (1.5–14 years). The patient is alert and often disconcerted during an episode.

Episodes may last seconds to 5–20 minutes and occur several times daily or monthly. Laboratory work is normal. EEG is normal between or during an attack; brain imaging is normal. Inheritance is usually autosomal dominant. Anticonvulsants (eg, carbamazepine) usually prevent further attacks. Patients often grow out of this disease in one or two decades.

Nonkinesiogenic dyskinesia is often secondary to an identifiable brain lesion, less or not responsive to medications, and nongenetic.

Disorders of ion channels underlie many of the genetic cases; some cases are linked to epilepsy and hemiplegic migraine. Chromosome loci are known.

The diagnosis of chronic persistent dystonia (sometimes Ldopa-responsive) may be aided by spinal fluid neurotransmitter and genetic chromosome studies. Rarely, dyskinesia (e.g., dystonia) may be precipitated by fever. And, chorea (rarely) may be a benign life-long genetic disease.

Anca MH et al: Natural of Oppenheim's dystonia (DYT1) in Israel. J Child Neurol 2003;18:325 [PMID: 12822816].

Bandmann O, Wood NW: Dopa-response dystonia—The story so far. Neuropediatrics 2002;33:1 [PMID: 11930268].

Dooley JM et al: Fever-induced dystonia. Pediatr Neurol 2003;28:149 [PMID: 12699869].

Kleiner-Fisman G et al: Benign hereditary chorea: Clinical, genetic and pathological findings. Ann Neurol 2003;54:244 [PMID: 12891678].

MGrath TM, Dure LS: Paroxysmal dyskinesias in children. Curr Treat Options Neurol 2003;5:275 [PMID: 12791193].

Zorzi G et al: Paroxysmal dyskinesias in childhood. Pediatr Neurol 2003;28:168 [PMID: 12770667].

# ■ INFECTIONS & INFLAMMATORY DISORDERS OF THE CENTRAL NERVOUS SYSTEM

Infections of the CNS are among the most common neurologic disorders encountered by pediatricians. Although infections are among the CNS disorders most amenable to treatment, they also have a very high potential for causing catastrophic destruction of the nervous system. It is imperative for the clinician to recognize infections early in order to treat and prevent massive tissue destruction.

## Clinical Findings

### A. SYMPTOMS AND SIGNS

Patients with CNS infections, whether caused by bacteria, viruses, or other microorganisms, present with similar manifestations. Systemic signs of infection include fever; malaise; and impaired heart, lung, liver, or kidney function. General features suggesting CNS infection include headache, stiff neck, fever or hypothermia, changes in mental status (including hyperirritability evolving into lethargy and coma), seizures, and focal sensory and motor deficits. Meningeal irritation is manifested by the presence of Kernig and Brudzinski signs. In very young infants, signs of meningeal irritation may be absent, and temperature instability and hypothermia are often more prominent than fever. In young infants, a bulging fontanelle and an increased head circumference are common. Papilledema may eventually develop, particularly in older children and adolescents. Cranial nerve palsies may develop acutely or gradually during the course of neurologic infections. No specific clinical sign or symptom is reliable in distinguishing bacterial infections from infections caused by other microbes.

During the initial clinical assessment, conditions that predispose the patient to infection of the CNS should be sought. Infections involving the sinuses or other structures in the head and neck region can result in direct extension of infection into the intracranial compartment. Open head injuries, recent neurosurgical procedures, immunodeficiency, and the presence of a mechanical shunt may predispose to intracranial infection.

### B. LABORATORY FINDINGS

When CNS infections are suspected, blood should be obtained for a complete blood count, general chemistry panel, and culture. Most important, however, is obtaining CSF. In the absence of focal neurologic deficits or signs of increased intracranial pressure, CSF should be obtained immediately from any patient in whom serious CNS infection is suspected. When papilledema or focal motor signs are present, a lumbar puncture may be delayed until a neuroimaging procedure has been done to exclude brain abscess or other space-occupying lesion. It is generally safe to obtain spinal fluid from infants with nonfocal neurologic examination even if the fontanelle is bulging. Spinal fluid should be examined for the presence of red and white blood cells, protein concentration, glucose concentration, bacteria, and other microorganisms; a sample should be cultured. In addition, serologic, immunologic, and nucleic acid detection (PCR) tests may be performed on the spinal fluid in an attempt to identify the specific organism. As a general rule, spinal fluid that contains a high proportion of polymorphonuclear leukocytes, a high protein concentration, and a low glucose concentration strongly suggests bacterial infection (see Chapter 38). CSF containing predominantly lymphocytes, a high protein concentration, and a low glucose concentration suggests infection with mycobacteria, fungi, uncommon bacteria, and some viruses such as lymphocytic choriomeningitis virus, herpes simplex virus, mumps virus, and arboviruses (see Chapters 36 and 39). CSF that contains a high proportion of lymphocytes, normal or only slightly elevated protein concentration, and a normal glucose concentration is most suggestive of viral infections, although partially treated bacterial meningitis and parameningeal infections may also result in this type of CSF formula. Typical CSF findings in a variety of infectious and inflammatory disorders are shown in Table 23–3.

In some cases, brain biopsy may be needed to identify the presence of specific organisms and clarify the diagnosis. Herpes simplex virus infections can be confirmed using the PCR test to assay for herpes DNA in spinal fluid. This test has a 95% sensitivity and 99% specificity. Brain biopsy may be needed to detect the rare PCR-negative case of herpes simplex and various parasitic infections, brain tumors, and other structural abnormalities.

### C. IMAGING

Neuroimaging with CT and MRI scans may be helpful in demonstrating the presence of brain abscess, meningeal inflammation, or secondary problems such as venous and arterial infarctions, hemorrhages, and subdural effusions when these are expected. In addition, these procedures may identify sinus or other focal infections in the head or neck region that are related to the CNS infection. CT scanning may demonstrate bony abnormalities, such as basilar fractures.

EEGs may be helpful in the assessment of patients who have had seizures at the time of presentation. The changes are often nonspecific and characterized by generalized slowing. In some instances, such as herpes simplex virus infection, focal electronegative activity may be seen early in the course and may be one of the earliest laboratory abnormalities to suggest the diagnosis. EEGs may also show focal slowing over regions of abscesses. Unusual but characteristic electroencephalographic patterns are seen in some patients with subacute sclerosing panencephalitis.

## BACTERIAL MENINGITIS

Bacterial infections of the CNS may present acutely (symptoms evolving rapidly over 1–24 hours), suba-

cutely (symptoms evolving over 1–7 days), or chronically (symptoms evolving over more than 1 week). Diffuse bacterial infections involve the leptomeninges, superficial cortical structures, and blood vessels. Although the term "meningitis" is used to describe these infections, it should not be forgotten that the brain parenchyma is also inflamed and that blood vessel walls may be infiltrated by inflammatory cells that result in endothelial cell injury, vessel stenosis, and secondary ischemia and infarction.

Pathologically, the inflammatory process involves all intracranial structures to some degree. Acutely, this inflammatory process may result in cerebral edema or impaired CSF flow through and out of the ventricular system, resulting in hydrocephalus.

### Treatment

#### A. SPECIFIC MEASURES

(See also Chapter 35 and the *Haemophilus influenzae* Type B Infections section in Chapter 38.)

While awaiting the results of diagnostic tests, the physician should start broad-spectrum antibiotic coverage as noted in the following discussion. After specific organisms are identified, antibiotic therapy can be tailored based on antibiotic sensitivity patterns. Bacterial meningitis in children younger than age 3 months is treated initially with cefotaxime (or ceftriaxone if the child is older than age 1 month) and ampicillin; the latter agent is used to treat *Listeria* and enterococci infections, which rarely affect older children. Children older than age 3 months are given ceftriaxone, cefotaxime, or ampicillin plus gentamicin. If *Streptococcus pneumoniae* cannot be ruled out by the initial Gram stain, vancomycin or rifampin is added until cultures are reported, because penicillin-resistant pneumococci are common in the United States. Therapy may be narrowed when organism sensitivity allows. Duration of therapy is 7 days for meningococcal infections, 10 days for *H influenzae* or pneumococcal infection, and 14–21 days for other organisms. Slow clinical response or the occurrence of complications may prolong the need for therapy. Although therapy for 7 days has proved successful in many children with *H influenzae* infection, it cannot be recommended without further study if steroids are also used (see following discussion).

#### B. GENERAL AND SUPPORTIVE MEASURES

Children with bacterial meningitis are often systemically ill. The following complications should be looked for and treated aggressively: hypovolemia, hypoglycemia, hyponatremia, acidosis, septic shock, increased intracranial pressure, seizures, disseminated intravascular coagulation, and metastatic infection (eg, pericarditis, arthritis, pneumonia). Children should initially be monitored closely (cardiorespiratory monitor, strict fluid balance and frequent urine specific gravity assessment, daily weights, neurologic assessment every few hours), not fed until neurologically very stable, isolated until the organism is known, rehydrated with isotonic solutions until euvolemic, and then given intravenous fluids containing dextrose and sodium at no more than maintenance rate (assuming no unusual losses occur).

## Complications

Abnormalities of water and electrolyte balance result from either excessive or insufficient production of antidiuretic hormone and require careful monitoring and appropriate adjustments in fluid administration. Monitoring serum sodium every 8–12 hours during the first 1–2 days, and urine sodium if the inappropriate secretion of antidiuretic hormone is suspected, usually uncovers significant problems.

Seizures occur in up to 30% of children with bacterial meningitis. Seizures tend to be most common in neonates and less common in older children. Persistent focal seizures or focal seizures associated with focal neurologic deficits strongly suggest subdural effusion, abscess, or vascular lesions such as arterial infarct, cortical venous infarcts, or dural sinus thrombosis. Because generalized seizures in a metabolically compromised child may have severe sequelae, early recognition and therapy are critical; some practitioners prefer phenytoin for acute management because it is less sedating than phenobarbital.

Subdural effusions occur in as many as 50% of young children with *H influenzae* meningitis. Subdural effusions are often seen on CT scans of the head during the course of meningitis. They do not require treatment unless they are producing increased intracranial pressure or progressive mass effect. Although subdural effusions may be detected in children who have persistent fever, such effusions do not usually have to be sampled or drained if the infecting organism is *H influenzae, Meningococcus,* or *Pneumococcus.* These are usually sterilized with the standard treatment duration, and slowly waning fever during an otherwise uncomplicated recovery may be followed clinically. Under any other circumstance, however, aspiration of the fluid for documentation of sterilization or for relief of pressure should be considered.

Cerebral edema can participate in the production of increased intracranial pressure, requiring treatment with dexamethasone, osmotic agents, diuretics, or hyperventilation; continuous pressure monitoring may be needed.

Long-term sequelae of meningitis result from direct inflammatory destruction of brain cells, vascular injuries, or secondary gliosis. Focal motor and sensory deficits, visual impairment, hearing loss, seizures, hydrocephalus, and a variety of cranial nerve deficits can result from meningitis. Sensorineural hearing loss in *H influenzae* meningitis occurs in approximately 5–10% of patients during long-term follow-up. Recent studies have suggested that early addition of dexamethasone to the antibiotic regimen may modestly decrease the risk of hearing loss in some children with *H influenzae* meningitis (see Chapter 38).

In addition to the variety of disorders mentioned earlier in this section, some patients with meningitis have mental retardation and severe behavioral disorders that limit their function at school and later performance in life. Table 23–24 lists the overall mortality and morbidity figures for the most common organisms associated with acute bacterial meningitis in childhood.

## BRAIN ABSCESS

### Clinical Findings

Patients with brain abscess often appear to have systemic illness similar to patients with bacterial meningitis, but in addition they show signs of focal neurologic deficits,

**Table 23–24.** Outcome of acute bacterial meningitis by organism.

| Organism | Mortality (%) | Motor Handicap (%) | | Intellect (%) | |
|---|---|---|---|---|---|
| | | None | Severe | Normal | Severe Mental Retardation |
| *Escherichia coli,* other coliforms | 20–50 | 62 | 25 | 75 | 25 |
| *Haemophilus influenzae* | 5–10 | 87 | 3 | 82 | 5 |
| *Streptococcus pneumoniae* | 10–30 | 96 | 0 | 83 | 0 |
| *Neisseria meningitidis* | 5–10 | 100 | 0 | 93 | 0 |
| Group B streptococci | 20 | 85 | 10–15 | 100 | 0 |
| Overall total | 10–25 | 85 | 5 | 82 | 6 |

papilledema, and other evidence of increased intracranial pressure or a mass lesion. Symptoms may be present for a week or more; children with bacterial meningitis usually present within a few days. Conditions predisposing to development of brain abscess include penetrating head trauma; chronic infection of the middle ear, mastoid, or sinuses (especially the frontal sinus); chronic dental or pulmonary infection; cardiovascular lesions allowing right-to-left shunting of blood (including arteriovenous malformations); and endocarditis.

When brain abscess is strongly suspected, a neuroimaging procedure such as CT or MRI scans should be done prior to lumbar puncture. If a brain abscess is identified, lumbar puncture may be dangerous and rarely alters the choice of antibiotic or clinical management since the CSF abnormalities usually reflect only parameningeal inflammation. With spread from contagious septic foci, streptococci and anaerobic bacteria are most common. Staphylococci most often enter from trauma or from infections. Enteric organisms may form an abscess from chronic otitis. Unfortunately, cultures from a large number of brain abscesses remain negative.

The diagnosis of brain abscess is based primarily on a strong clinical suspicion and confirmed by a neuroimaging procedure. EEG changes are nonspecific but frequently demonstrate focal slowing in the region of brain abscess.

## Treatment

Initial therapy for infection from presumed contagious foci uses penicillin and metronidazole. Cefotaxime is a good alternative to penicillin, especially if enteric organisms are suspected. Enteric organisms are also often susceptible to trimethoprim–sulfamethoxazole. Suspicion of infection by staphylococci, or their recovery from an aspirate, should be treated with nafcillin or vancomycin. Treatment may include neurologic consultation and anticonvulsant and edema therapy if necessary. In their early stages, brain abscesses are areas of focal cerebritis and can be "cured" with antibiotic treatment alone. Well-developed abscesses require surgical drainage.

## Differential Diagnosis

Differential diagnosis of brain abscess includes any condition that produces focal neurologic deficits and increased intracranial pressure, such as neoplasms, subdural effusions, cerebral infarctions, and certain infections (herpes simplex, cysticercosis, and toxocariasis).

## Prognosis

The surgical mortality rate in the treatment of brain abscess is lower than 5%. Untreated cerebral abscesses lead to irreversible tissue destruction and may rupture into the ventricle, producing catastrophic deterioration in neurologic function and death. Because brain abscesses are often associated with systemic illness and systemic infections, the death rate is frequently high in these patients.

## VIRAL INFECTIONS

Viral infections of the CNS can involve primarily meninges (meningitis) (see Chapter 36) or cerebral parenchyma (encephalitis). All patients, however, have some degree of involvement of both the meninges and cerebral parenchyma (meningoencephalitis). Many viral infections are generalized and diffuse, but some viruses, notably herpes simplex and some arboviruses, characteristically cause prominent focal disease. Focal cerebral involvement is clearly evident on neuroimaging procedures. Some viruses have an affinity for specific CNS cell populations. Poliovirus and other enteroviruses can selectively infect anterior horn cells (poliomyelitis) and some intracranial motor neurons.

Although most viral infections of the nervous system have an acute or subacute course in childhood, chronic infections can occur. Subacute sclerosing panencephalitis, for example, represents a chronic indolent infection caused by measles virus and is characterized clinically by progressive neurodegeneration and seizures.

Inflammatory reactions within the nervous system may occur during the convalescent stage of systemic viral infections. Parainfectious or postinfectious inflammation of the CNS results in several well-recognized disorders: acute disseminated encephalomyelitis (25% of encephalitis), transverse myelitis, optic neuritis, polyneuritis, and Guillain–Barré syndrome.

Congenital viral infections can also affect the CNS. CMV, herpes simplex virus, and rubella virus are the most notable causes of viral brain injury in utero.

Treatment of CNS viral infections is usually limited to symptomatic and supportive measures, except for herpes simplex virus. Acyclovir is the treatment in suspected or proved cases of herpes simplex virus encephalitis. Acyclovir is also useful in some patients with varicella-zoster virus infections of the CNS. West Nile virus, new in the United States, is an arthropod-borne flavivirus. It is found in mosquitoes, birds, and horses, and accounts for 27% of hospitalized patients in New York (1991) with encephalitis and muscle weakness. Fourteen percent had encephalitis alone, and 6% had aseptic meningitis. CSF antibody studies and PCR (57% positive for viral RNA) were diagnostic aids. The infection is now endemic as far as the western United States, particularly in Colorado. Recent studies have suggested spread of the infection to mosquitoes further south along the Atlantic seaboard.

## Encephalopathy of HIV Infection

Neurologic syndromes associated directly with HIV infection include subacute encephalitis, meningitis, myelopathy, polyneuropathy, and myositis. In addition, secondary opportunistic infections of the CNS occur in patients with HIV-induced immunosuppression. Toxoplasma and CMV infections are particularly common. Progressive multifocal leukoencephalopathy, a secondary papillomavirus infection, and herpes simplex and varicella-zoster infections also occur frequently in patients with HIV infection. A variety of fungal (especially cryptococcal), mycobacterial, and bacterial infections have been described.

Neurologic abnormalities in these patients can also be the result of noninfectious neoplastic disorders. Primary CNS lymphoma and metastatic lymphoma to the nervous system are the most frequent neoplasms of the nervous system in these patients. See Chapters 29, 35, and 37 for diagnosis and management of HIV infection.

## OTHER INFECTIONS

A wide variety of other microorganisms, including *Toxoplasma,* mycobacteria, spirochetes, rickettsiae, amoebae, and mycoplasmas, can cause CNS infections. CNS involvement in these infections is usually secondary to systemic infection or other predisposing factors. Appropriate cultures and serologic testing are required to confirm infections by these organisms. Parenteral antimicrobial treatment for these infections is discussed in Chapter 35.

## NONINFECTIOUS INFLAMMATORY DISORDERS OF THE CENTRAL NERVOUS SYSTEM

The differential diagnosis of bacterial, viral, and other microbial infections of the CNS includes disorders that cause inflammation but for which no specific causal organism has been identified. Sarcoidosis, Behçet disease, systemic lupus erythematosus, other collagen–vascular disorders, and Kawasaki disease are examples. In these disorders, CNS inflammation usually occurs in association with characteristic systemic manifestations that allow proper diagnosis. Management of CNS involvement in these disorders is the same as the treatment of the systemic illness.

## OTHER PARAINFECTIOUS ENCEPHALOPATHIES

In association with systemic infections or other illnesses, CNS dysfunction may occur in the absence of direct CNS inflammation or infection. Reye syndrome is a prominent example of this type of encephalopathy that often occurs in association with varicella virus or other respiratory or systemic viral infections. In Reye syndrome, cerebral edema and cerebral dysfunction occur, but there is no evidence of any direct involvement of the nervous system by the associated microorganism or inflammation. Cerebral edema in Reye syndrome is accompanied by liver dysfunction and fatty infiltration of the liver. As a result of efforts to discourage use of aspirin in childhood febrile illnesses, the number of patients with Reye syndrome has markedly decreased. The precise relationship, however, between aspirin and Reye syndrome is unclear.

Aronin SI, Quagliarello VJ: New perspectives on pneumococcal meningitis. Hosp Pract (Off Ed):36:43,49,51 [PMID: 11220360].

De Tiege X et al: Herpes simplex encephalitis relapses in children. Neurology 2003;61:241 [PMID: 12874408].

Hunson JL et al: Clinical and neuroradiologic features of acute disseminated encephalomyelitis in children. Neurology 2001;56:1308 [PMID: 11376179].

Kimberlin DW et al: Natural history of neonatal herpes simplex virus infections in the acyclovir era. Pediatrics 2001;108:223 [PMID: 11484781].

Krshna Murthy SN et al: Acute disseminated encephalomyelitis in children. Pediatrics 2002;110:e21 [PMID: 12165620].

Nolan MA et al: Survival after pulmonary edema due to enterovirus 71 encephalitis. Neurology 2003;60:1651 [PMID: 12771257].

Redington JJ, Tyler KL: Viral infections of the nervous system, 2002. Arch Neurol 2002;59:712 [PMID: 12020250].

Sazgar M et al: Influenza B acute necrotizing encephalopathy: A case report and literature review. Pediatr Neurol 2003;28:396 [PMID: 12878304].

Sejvar JJ et al: Neurologic manifestations and outcome of west Nile virus infection. JAMA 2003;290:511 [PMID: 12876094].

Straussberg R et al: Improvement of atypical acute disseminated encephalomyelitis with steroids and intravenous immunoglobulins. Pediatr Neurol 2001;24:139 [PMID: 11275464].

Tenembaum S et al: Acute disseminated encephalomyelitis. Neurology 2002;59:1224 [PMID: 12391351].

Toth C et al: Neonatal herpes encephalitis: A case series and review of clinical presentations. Can J Neurol Sci 2003;30:36 [PMID: 12619782].

Tyler KL: West Nile virus encephalitis in America (editorial). N Engl J Med 2001;344:1858 [PMID: 11407349].

## SYNDROMES PRESENTING AS ACUTE FLACCID PARALYSIS

Flaccid paralysis evolving over hours or a few days suggests involvement of the lower motor neuron complex (see Floppy Infant Syndrome section). Anterior horn cells (spinal cord) may be involved by viral infection (paralytic poliomyelitis) or by paraviral or postviral immunologically mediated disease (acute transverse myelitis). The nerve trunks (polyneuritis) may be diseased as in Guillain–Barré syndrome or affected by toxins (diphtheria, porphyria). The neuromuscular junction may be blocked by tick toxin or botulinum toxin. The paralysis rarely will be due to metabolic (periodic paralysis) or inflammatory muscle disease (myositis). A lesion compressing the spinal cord must be ruled out.

## Clinical Findings

### A. Symptoms and Signs

Features assisting diagnosis are age, a history of preceding or waning illness, the presence (at time of paralysis) of fever, rapidity of progression, cranial nerve findings, and sensory findings (Table 23–25). The examination may show long tract findings (pyramidal tract), causing increased reflexes and a positive Babinski sign. The spinothalamic tract may be interrupted, causing loss of pain and temperature. Back pain, even tenderness to percussion, may occur, as well as bowel and bladder incontinence. Often the paralysis is ascending, symmetric, and painful (muscle tenderness or myalgia). Laboratory findings occasionally are diagnostic.

### B. Laboratory Findings (see Table 23–25)

Examination of CSF is helpful. Imaging studies of the spinal column (plain radiographs) and spinal cord (MRI, myelogram) are occasionally essential. Viral cultures (CSF, throat, stool) and titers aid in diagnosing poliomyelitis. A high sedimentation rate may suggest tumor or abscess; the presence of antinuclear antibody may suggest lupus arteritis.

EMG and nerve conduction velocity can be helpful in diagnosing polyneuropathy. Nerve conduction is usually slowed after 7–10 days. Findings in botulism and tick-bite paralysis can be specific and diagnostic. Rarely, elevation of muscle enzymes or even myoglobinuria may aid in diagnosis of myopathic paralysis. Porphyrin urine studies and heavy-metal assays (arsenic, thallium, lead) can reveal those rare toxic causes of polyneuropathic paralysis.

## Differential Diagnosis

The child who has been well and becomes paralyzed often has polyneuritis. Acute transverse myelitis sometimes occurs in an afebrile child. The child who is ill and febrile at the time of paralysis often has acute transverse myelitis or poliomyelitis. Acute epidural spinal cord abscess (or other compressive lesion) must be ruled out. Poliomyelitis is very rare in our immunized population. Paralysis due to tick bites occurs seasonally (spring and summer). The tick is usually found in the occipital hair. Removal is curative.

Paralysis due to botulinum toxin occurs most commonly younger than age 1 year (see Chapter 38). Intra-

venous drug abuse can lead to myelitis and paralysis. Furthermore, chronic myelopathy occurs with two human immunodeficiency virus infections: HTLV-I and HTLV-III (now called HIV-1).

## Complications

### A. Respiratory Paralysis

Early and careful attention to oxygenation is essential. Administration of oxygen, intubation, mechanical respiratory assistance, and careful suctioning of secretions may be required. Increasing anxiety and a rise in diastolic and systolic blood pressures are early signs of hypoxia. Cyanosis is a late sign. Deteriorating spirometric findings (forced expiratory volume in 1 second [$FEV_1$] and total vital capacity) may indicate the need for controlled intubation and respiratory support. Blood gases (usually late changes with increased $CO_2$, decreased $O_2$) can aid decisions.

### B. Infections

Pneumonia is common, especially in patients with respiratory paralysis. Antibiotic therapy is best guided by results of cultures. Bladder infections occur when an indwelling catheter is required because of bladder paralysis. Recovery from myelitis may be delayed by urinary tract infection.

### C. Autonomic Crisis

This may be a cause of death in Guillain–Barré syndrome. Strict attention to vital signs to detect and treat hypotension or hypertension and cardiac arrhythmias in an intensive care setting is advisable, at least early in the course and in severely ill patients.

## Treatment

Most of these syndromes have no specific treatment. Ticks causing paralysis must be removed. Other therapies include the use of erythromycin in *Mycoplasma* infections and botulism equine antitoxin in wound botulism. Recognized associated disorders (eg, endocrine, neoplastic, toxic) should be treated by appropriate means. Supportive care also involves pulmonary toilet, adequate fluids and nutrition, bladder and bowel care, prevention of decubiti, and, in many cases, psychiatric support.

### A. Corticosteroids

These agents are believed by most to be of no benefit in Guillain–Barré syndrome. Autonomic symptoms (eg, hypertension) in polyneuritis may require treatment.

### B. Plasmapheresis

Plasma exchange or intravenous IgG has been beneficial in severe cases of Guillain–Barré syndrome.

**Table 23–25.** Acute flaccid paralysis in children.

| | Poliomyelitis (Paralytic, Spinal, and Bulbar), With or Without Encephalitis | Landry-Guillain-Barré Syndrome ("Acute Idiopathic Polyneuritis") | Botulism | Tick-Bite Paralysis | Transverse Myelitis and Neuromyelitis Optica |
|---|---|---|---|---|---|
| Etiology | Poliovirus types I, II, and III; other enteroviruses; enteroviruses, eg EV71; vaccine strain polio virus (rare); West Nile virus: epidemic in birds. Mosquitoes infect horses, humans | Likely delayed hypersensitivity—with T-cell-mediated antiganglioside antibodies. Mycoplasmal and viral infections (EBV, CMV), *Campylobacter jejuni*, Hepatitis B. | *Clostridium botulinum* toxin. Block at neuromuscular junction. Under age 1, toxin synthesized in bowel by organisms in ingested dust or honey. At older ages toxin injected in food. Rarely from wound infection. | Probable interference with transmission of nerve impulse caused by toxin in tick saliva | Usually unknown; multiple viruses (herpes, EBV, varicella, hepatitis A) often postviral (see Guillain–Barré syndrome) |
| History | None, or inadequate polio immunization. Upper respiratory or gastrointestinal symptoms followed by brief respite. Bulbar paralysis more frequent after tonsillectomy. Often in epidemics, in summer and early fall. | Nonspecific respiratory or gastrointestinal symptoms in preceding 5–14 d common. Any season, though slightly lower incidence in summer. | Infancy: dusty environment (eg, construction area), honey. Older: food poisoning. Multiple cases hours to days after ingesting contaminated food. | Exposure to ticks (dog tick in eastern United States; wood ticks). Irritability 12–24 h before onset of a rapidly progressive ascending paralysis. | Rarely symptoms compatible with multiple sclerosis or optic neuritis. Progression from onset to paraplegia often rapid, usually without a history of bacterial infection. |
| Presenting complaints | Febrile at time of paralysis. Meningeal signs, muscle tenderness, and spasm. Asymmetrical weakness widespread or segmental (cervical, thoracic, lumbar). Bulbar symptoms early or before extremity weakness; anxiety; delirium. | Symmetrical weakness of lower extremities, which may ascend rapidly to arms, trunk, and face. Verbal child may complain of paresthesias. Fever uncommon. Facial weakness early. Miller–Fisher variant presents as ataxia and ophthalmoplegia (rare). | Infancy: constipation, poor suck and cry. "Floppy." Apnea. Lethargy. Choking (cause of SIDS?). Older: blurred vision, diplopia, ptosis, choking, weakness. | Rapid onset and progression of ascending flaccid paralysis; often accompanied by pain and paresthesias. Paralysis of upper extremities usually occurs on second day after onset. | Root and back pain in about one-third to one-half of cases. Sensory loss below level of lesion accompanying rapidly developing paralysis. Sphincter difficulties common. |
| Findings | Flaccid weakness, usually asymmetrical. Cord level: Lumbar: legs, lower abdomen Cervical: shoulder, arm, neck, diaphragm Bulbar: respiratory, lower cranial nerves Encephalopathy accompanies paralysis in West Nile. | Flaccid weakness, symmetric, usually greater proximally, but may be more distal or equal in distribution. Rarely cranial nerves IX–XI, III–VI. Miller–Fisher variant: ophthalmoplegia, ataxia. Bulbar involvement may occur. Slight distal impairment of position, vibration, touch; difficult to assess in young children. | Infants: Flaccid weakness. Alert. Eye, pupil, facial weakness. Deep tendon reflexes decreased. Absent suck, gag. Constipation. Older: paralysis accommodation, eye movements. Weak swallow. Respiratory paralysis. | Flaccid, symmetric paralysis. Cranial nerve and bulbar (respiratory) paralysis, ataxia, sphincter disturbances, and sensory deficits may occur. Some fever. Diagnosis rests on finding tick, which is especially likely to be on occipital scalp. | Paraplegia with areflexia below level of lesion early; later, may have hyperreflexia. Sensory loss below and hyperesthesia or normal sensation above level of lesion. Paralysis of bladder and rectum. Optic neuritis rarely may be present. |

*Table 23–25.* Acute flaccid paralysis in children. (continued)

| | Poliomyelitis (Paralytic, Spinal, and Bulbar), With or Without Encephalitis | Landry-Guillain-Barré Syndrome ("Acute Idiopathic Polyneuritis") | Botulism | Tick-Bite Paralysis | Transverse Myelitis and Neuromyelitis Optica |
|---|---|---|---|---|---|
| CSF | Pleocytosis (20–500+ cells) with PMN predominance in first few days, later monocytic preponderance. Protein frequently elevated (50–150 mg/dL). CSF IgM + in West Nile | Cytoalbuminologic dissociation; ten or fewer mononuclear cells with high protein after first week. Normal glucose. IgG may be elevated. West Nile will have cells; nerves can be involved in a myeloradiculitis | Normal | Normal | Usually no manometric block; CSF may show increased protein, pleocytosis with predominantly mononuclear cells, increased IgG |
| Electromyogram (EMG) | Denervation after 10–21 days. Nerve conduction normal. Amplitude reduced in West Nile | Nerve conduction velocities markedly decreased; may be normal early, or if axon only damage. | EMG distinctive: BSAP (brief small abundant potentials). | Nerve conduction slowed; returns rapidly to normal after removal of tick | Normal early. Denervation at level of lesion after 10–21 d. |
| Other studies | Virus in stool and throat. Serial serologic titers IgG, IgM in West Nile Hyponatremia 30% in West Nile. | Search for specific cause such as infection, intoxication, autoimmune disease. Antiganglioside antibodies to $GM_1$ (GQ1b in Miller–Fisher) | Infancy: stool culture, toxin. Rare serum toxin positive. Older: serum (or wound) toxin. | Leukocytosis, often with moderate eosinophilia | Normal spine x-rays do not exclude spinal epidural abscess. MRI to rule out cord-compressive lesions. Cord may be swollen in myelitis. |
| Course and prognosis | Paralysis usually maximal 3–5 d after onset. Transient bladder paralysis may occur. Outlook varies with extent and severity of involvement. **Note:** Mortality greatest from respiratory failure and superinfection. West Nile paralysis may be permanent | Course progressive over a few days to about 2 weeks. **Note:** Threat greatest from respiratory failure (10%), autonomic crises (eg, widely variable blood pressure, arrhythmia), and superinfection. Majority recover completely. Plasmapheresis may have a role. Intravenous IgG. Relapses occasionally occur. | Infancy: supportive. Penicillin. Botulism immune globulin intravenous (BIG-IV). Respiratory support, gavage feeding. Avoid aminoglycosides. Older: penicillin, antitoxin, prolonged respiratory support. Prognosis: excellent Fatality 3% | Total removal of tick is followed by rapid improvement and recovery. Otherwise, mortality rate due to respiratory paralysis is very high. | Large degree of functional recovery possible. Corticosteroids are of controversial benefit in shortening duration of acute attack or altering the overall course. |

CMV = cytomegalovirus; CSF = cerebrospinal fluid; EBV = Ebstein–Barr virus; PMN = polymorphonuclear neutrophil; SIDS = sudden infant death syndrome.

### C. PHYSICAL THERAPY

Rehabilitative measures are best instituted when acute symptoms have subsided and the patient is stable.

### D. ANTIBIOTICS

Appropriate antibiotics and drainage are required for epidural abscess.

Ahmed S et al: Guillain–Barré syndrome: An unusual presentation of West Nile virus infection. Neurology 2000;55:144 [PMID: 10891928].

Ammache Z et al: Childhood Guillain–Barré syndrome: Clinical and electrophysiologic features predictive of outcome. J Child Neurol 2001;16:477 [PMID: 11453442].

Cheng TL: Infant botulism. Pediatr Rev 2000;21:427 [PMID: 11121502].

Concepcion K: Guillain–Barré. Pediatr Rev 2001;22:22 [PMID: 11229324].

Defresne P et al: Acute transverse myelitis in children: Clinical course and prognostic factors. J Child Neurol 2003;18:401 [PMID: 12886975].

Graf WD et al: Outcome in severe pediatric Guillain–Barré syndrome after immunotherapy or supportive care. Neurology 1999;52:1494 [PMID: 10227643].

Green DM, Ropper AH: Mild Guillain–Barré syndrome. Arch Neurology 2001;58:1098 [PMID: 11448299].

Jeha LE et al: West Nile virus infection: A new acute paralytic illness. Neurology 2003;61:55 [PMID:12847156].

Mori M et al: Clinical features and prognosis of Miller–Fisher syndrome. Neurology 2001;56:1104 [PMID: 11320188].

MMWR, CDC: Infant botulism—New York City, 2001–2002. MMWR 2003;52:21 [PMID: 12608714].

Tekgul H et al: Outcome of axonal and demyelinating forms of Guillain–Barré syndrome in children. Pediatr Neurol 2003;28:295 [PMID: 12849884].

Vedanarayanan VV et al: Tick paralysis in children: Electrophysiology and possibility of misdiagnosis. Neurology 2002;59:1088 [PMID: 12370471].

Vriesendorp FJ et al: Prognostic factors of Guillain–Barré syndrome after intravenous immunoglobulin or plasma exchange. Neurology 1999;53:598 [PMID: 10449126].

# ◼ DISORDERS OF CHILDHOOD AFFECTING MUSCLES (Table 23–26)

## DIAGNOSTIC STUDIES

### Serum Enzymes

Creatine kinase reflects muscle damage or "leaks" from muscle into plasma. Blood should be drawn before EMG or muscle biopsy, which may lead to release of the enzyme. Corticosteroids may suppress levels despite very active muscle disease, for example, as in polymyositis.

### Electromyography

EMG is often helpful in grossly differentiating myopathic from neurogenic processes. Fibrillations occur in both. In the myopathies, very low spikes are more typical, and the motor unit action potentials seen during contraction characteristically are of short duration, are polyphasic, and are increased in number for the strength of the contraction (increased interference pattern). Neurogenic findings include decreased numbers of motor units, which may be polyphasic, larger than normal, or both. The interference pattern is decreased. In myotonic dystrophy, the EMG is characterized by prolonged discharge of electrical activity on movement of the probing needle (so-called dive bomber sound).

### Muscle Biopsy

Properly executed (by open biopsy or by using the Bergstrom muscle biopsy needle), this procedure is usually helpful. Histochemical techniques, histogram analysis of muscle fiber types and sizes, and electron microscopy are offering new classifications of the myopathies. Findings common to the muscular dystrophies include variation in the size and shape of muscle fibers, increase in connective tissue, interstitial infiltration of fatty tissue, degenerative changes in muscle fibers, and central location of nuclei.

Dystrophin is a normal intracellular plasma membrane protein in muscle, the gene product missing in Duchenne and Becker muscular dystrophies. Staining the muscle for dystrophin aids in differentiating Duchenne and Becker muscular dystrophies; dystrophin is absent in Duchenne muscular dystrophy and reduced in Becker muscular dystrophy. Electrophoresis can confirm whether the dystrophin is absent or present in small amounts and whether there is a qualitative difference from normal dystrophin, the latter two patterns being characteristic of Becker muscular dystrophy.

### Genetic Testing & Carrier Detection

Previously, detection of carriers for Duchenne muscular dystrophy (mothers and sisters of affected boys) rested on creatine kinase elevations (two thirds of patients will have this finding); physical findings of mild dystrophy (large calves, muscle weakness); abnormal muscle EMGs; or biopsy results. All are unreliable for diagnostic purposes.

DNA probes are now available for carrier detection and prenatal diagnosis of Duchenne and Becker muscular dystrophies. Deletions are often (60%) found on the short arm of the X chromosome; it is postulated that all patients and most mothers will show deletions when sufficient probes are developed to search the whole Duchenne genome (perhaps 4000 kb in length).

Amplification of DNA by the PCR test can detect the deletion. Moreover, this technique plus Southern blot analysis can detect abnormal DNA base repeats. For example, in myotonic dystrophy, a GCT triplet excess is currently the most sensitive test for that disease. The tests can be used for intrauterine diagnosis and prediction of whether the triplet is within the normal or mutant range. Thus, in many cases, the greater the number of repeats, the more severely involved the fetus or patient.

Mutations (especially deletions) of survivor motor neuron (SMN) and neuronal apoptosis inhibitory protein (NAIP) genes on chromosome 5q13 are present in 95% of patients with spinal muscular atrophy.

Finally, Kearns–Sayre progressive external ophthalmoplegia with retinopathy is inherited via maternal cytoplasmic mitochondria. Assay of mutations and deletions from blood or muscle samples are now commercially available.

Therapy for Duchenne muscular dystrophy continues to be frustrating. Prednisone in low doses has increased muscle strength and prolonged ambulation. Research emphasis is on gene therapy, but there is great difficulty in finding viral vectors able to carry the very large dystrophin gene into muscle cells.

Apkon SD: Osteoporosis in children who have disabilities. Phys Med Rehabil Clin North Am 2002;13:839 [PMID: 12465563].

Berven S, Bradford DS: Neuromuscular scoliosis: Causes of deformity and principles for evaluation and management. Semin Neurol 2002;22:167 [PMID: 12524562].

Bianchi ML et al: Bone mineral density and bone metabolism in Duchenne muscular dystrophy. Osteporos Int 2003;12:761 [PMID: 12897980].

Bonifati MD et al: A multicenter, double-blind, randomized trial of deflazacort versus prednisone in Duchenne muscular dystrophy. Muscle Nerve 2000;23:1344 [PMID: 10951436].

Bonnemann CG: Limb-girdle muscular dystrophies: An overview. J Child Neurology 1999;14:31 [PMID: 10223847].

Gendron NH, MacKenzie AE: Spinal muscular atrophy: Molecular pathophysiology. Curr Opin Neurol 1999;12:137 [PMID: 10226744].

Grewal PK, Hewitt JE: Glycosylation defects: A new mechanism for muscular dystrophy? Hum Mol Genet 2003; 12 Spec No 2:R259-64 [PMID: 12925572].

Kapsa R et al: Novel therapies for Duchenne muscular dystrophy. Lancet Neurol 2003;2:299 [PMID: 12849184].

Komura K et al: Effectiveness of creatine monohydrate in mitochondrial encephalomyopathies. Pediatr Neurol 2003;28:53 [PMID: 12657421].

Lois M et al: Beneficial effects of creatine supplementation in dystrophic patients. Muscle Nerve 2003;27:604 [PMID: 12707981].

Mathrew KD, Moore SA: Limb-girdle muscular dystrophy. Curr Neurol Neurosci Rep 2003;3:78 [PMID: 12507416].

Mendell JR: Congenital muscular dystrophy (editorial). Neurology 2001;56:993 [PMID: 11320168].

Mercuri E et al: Phenotypic spectrum associated with mutations in the fukutin-related protein gene. Ann Neurol 2003;53:537 [PMID: 12666124].

Muntoni F et al: Sixth International congenital muscular dystrophy workshop. Neuromuscul Disord 2002;12:69 [PMID: 11731288].

Muntoni F: Cardiac complications of childhood myopathies. J Child Neurol 2003;18:191 [PMID: 12731645].

Muntoni F et al: Defective glycosylation in muscular dystrophy. Lancet 2002;360:1419 [PMID: 12424008].

Palmucci L et al: Dystrophinopathy expressing as either cardiomyopathy or Becker dystrophy in the same family. Neurology 2000;54:529 [PMID: 10668737].

Roland EH: Muscular dystrophy. Pediatr Rev 2000;21:233 [PMID: 10878185].

Skuk D et al: Experimental and therapeutic approaches to muscular dystrophies. Curr Opin Neurol 2002;15:563 [PMID: 12352000].

Strober JB: Genetics of pediatric neuromuscular disease. Curr Opin Pediatr 2000 Dec;12(6):549 [PMID: 11106273].

Tubridy N et al: Congenital myopathies and congenital muscular dystrophies. Curr Opin Neurol 2001;14:575 [PMID: 11562568].

Zatz M et al: The 10 autosomal recessive limb-girdle muscular dystrophies. Neuromuscul Disord 2003;13:532 [PMID: 12921790].

Zhang W et al: Enzymatic diagnostic test for muscle-eye-brain type congenital muscular dystrophy using commercially available reagents. Clin Biochem 2003;36:339 [PMID: 12849864].

# BENIGN ACUTE CHILDHOOD MYOSITIS

Benign acute childhood myositis (myalgia cruris epidemica) is characterized by transient severe muscle pain and weakness affecting mainly the calves and occurring 1–2 days following an upper respiratory tract infection. Although symptoms involve mainly the gastrocnemius muscles, all skeletal muscles appear to be invaded directly by virus; recurrent episodes are due to different viral types. By seroconversion or isolation of the virus, acute myositis has been shown to be largely due to influenza types B and A and occasionally due to parainfluenza and adenovirus.

# MYASTHENIA GRAVIS

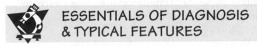

### ESSENTIALS OF DIAGNOSIS & TYPICAL FEATURES

- *Weakness, chiefly of muscles innervated by the brainstem, usually coming on or increasing with use (fatigue).*

***Table 23–26.*** Muscular dystrophies and myotonias of childhood.

| Disease | Genetic Pattern | Age at Onset | Early Manifestations | Involved Muscles | Reflexes |
|---|---|---|---|---|---|
| Muscular dystrophies Duchenne muscular dystrophy (pseudohypertrophic infantile) | X-linked recessive; autosomal-recessive unusual. 30–50% have no family history. | 2–6 y; rarely in infancy | Clumsiness, easy fatigability on walking, running, and climbing stairs. Walking on toes; waddling gait. Lordosis. (Climbing up on legs rising from supine position—Gower maneuver.) | Axial and proximal before distal. Pelvic girdle; pseudohypertrophy of gastrocnemius (90%), triceps brachii, and vastus lateralis. Shoulder girdle usually later, also articulation difficulties. Eventually cardiomyopathy (50%). | Knee jerks ± or 0; ankle jerks + to ++ |
| Becker muscular dystrophy (late onset) | X-linked recessive. (Allele at Xp21) | Childhood (usually later than in Duchenne) | Similar to Duchenne. | Similar to Duchenne | Similar to Duchenne |
| Limb-girdle muscular dystrophy<br><br>A. Pelvifemoral (Leyden–Möbius)<br>B. Scapulohumeral (Erb juvenile) | Autosomal-recessive in 60%; high sporadic incidence.<br>A. Relatively common<br>B. Rare | Variable; early childhood to adulthood | Weakness, with distribution according to type. Waddling gait, difficulty climbing stairs. Lordosis. | A. Pelvic girdle usually involved first and to greater extent. B. Shoulder girdle often asymmetric. Quadriceps and hamstrings may be weakest. | Usually present |
| Facioscapulohumeral muscular dystrophy (Landouzy–Déjérine) scapuloperoneal variant (rare) | Autosomal-dominant; sporadic cases not uncommon: Linkage to 4q35 | Usually late in childhood and adolescence; rare in infancy; not uncommon in 20s | Diminished facial movements with inability to close eyes, smile, or whistle. Face may be flat; unlined. Difficulty in raising arms over head. Lordosis. Tripping in scapuloperoneal type. | Facial muscles followed by shoulder girdle, with occasional spread to hips or distal legs (scapuloperoneal variant) | Present |
| Spinal muscular atrophy (SMA) Infantile SMA (Werdnig–Hoffman disease) | Autosomal-recessive | 0–2 y | Floppy infant | Pelvic and shoulder girdle. Tongue. Intercostals. Fingers and toes spared. | 0 or nearly so |
| Juvenile SMA (Kugelburg–Welander disease) | Autosomal-recessive | Onset after age 2 usually (age 5–15 typical) | Weakness. "Fasciculations" 50%. Rarely a cause of floppy infant. | Same | Same |
| Metabolic myopathies Carnitine deficiency (lipid storage myopathy) Primary (rare) Secondary: multiple forms | Genetics variable, often recessive | Infancy to adolescence | Fasting hypoglycemia and coma; less ketosis than expected. Myopathy. Cardiomyopathy. Fatty liver. Don't confuse with Reye, SIDS. | Weakness variable; may be precipitated by exercise (with resultant myoglobulinuria) or fasting | Normal to decreased |

| Muscle Biopsy Findings | Other Diagnostic Tests | Treatment | Prognosis |
|---|---|---|---|
| Degeneration and variation in fiber size; proliferation of connective tissue. Basophilia, phagocytosis. Poor differentiation of fiber types on ATPase reaction; deficiency of type IIB fibers. Dystrophin absent. | EMG myopathic. CK (4000–5000 IU) very high with decrease toward normal over the years. 60% have C-terminal Xp21 deletion on blood, amniotic fluid or chorionic villi. Positive test obviates need for muscle biopsy | Physical therapy, braces, wheelchair eventually, weight control. Prednisone, deflazacort improve motor function temporarily. Creatine, Some benefit. Gene transfer minidystrophin by viral vectors. Utrophin. | Ten percent show nonprogressive mental retardation. Osteoporosis, scoliosis common. Death from cardiac or respiratory failure 10–15 y after diagnosis with 75% of patients dead by age 20. |
| Similar to above, except type IIB fibers present. Reduced or abnormal size dystrophin. | Similar to above, although muscle enzymes may not be as elevated | As above. Wheelchair in late childhood or early adult life. | Slower progression than Duchenne's, with death usually in adulthood |
| Dystrophic muscle changes (see Duchenne). Dystrophin normal. Special stains for sarcoglycan (dystrophin associated glycoprotein–DAG deficiency. | EMG myopathic. CK variable; many severe cases have sarcoglycan deficiency (severe autosomal recessive type). Must exclude dystrophinopathy and SMA. | Physical therapy, weight control | Mildly progressive: spread from lower to upper limbs may take 15–20 y. Life expectancy mid to late adulthood. |
| Predominantly large fibers with scattered tiny atrophic fibers, "moth-eaten" and whorled fibers. Inflammatory response. Little or no fiber splitting, fibrosis, or type 1 fiber predominance. | EMG myopathic. Muscle enzymes usually normal. 4q35ter deletion. If blood test positive, biopsy unnecessary | Physical therapy where indicated. Wheelchair in 20%. Forty percent of biopsies show inflammation; steroids ineffective, however. | Very slowly progressive, often with plateaus, except in infantile form where there may be difficulties in walking by adolescence. Usually normal life span. |
| Small, group atrophy. Twin peak fiber size. Fiber type grouping. Minimal fibrosis. | EMG neuropathic. Nerve conduction, CSF, muscle enzymes normal. 90–95% have deletions or abnormalities in *SMN* (survival motor neuron) or other genes at band 5q13. | Supportive: respiratory care, positioning, secretion management. Genetic counseling. | 80–95% of patients 0–4 y die of pneumonia and respiratory failure. |
| Same | | Physical therapy, wheelchair positioning to avoid scoliosis. May walk, usually later lose this. | Fairly normal life expectancy. 4–40+ y. |
| Lipid droplets ± or ragged red fibers may be present. | Muscle biochemistry (carnitine, CPT enzyme). Urine organic acids (at time of illness). Plasma carnitine: deficiency may be in blood alone or blood and muscle. | Avoid fasting and mitochondrial toxins, eg, ASA, valproic acid. Carbohydrate. Treat acidosis. Carnitine orally. | Variable: occasionally fatal in infants. Progressive weakness, developmental delay, cardiomyopathy may occur. |

*(continued)*

***Table 23–26.*** Muscular dystrophies and myotonias of childhood. (continued)

| Disease | Genetic Pattern | Age at Onset | Early Manifestations | Involved Muscles | Reflexes |
|---------|-----------------|--------------|----------------------|------------------|----------|
| "Oculocraniosomatic syndrome" (ophthalmoplegia and "ragged reds"; progressive external ophthalmoplegia) Kearns–Sayre | Mitochondrial DNA deletion; other hereditary neurologic disorders may be found in patient or family | Variable; from infancy to adult life; most at about 10 y of age | Ptosis and limitation of eye movements; hearing and visual loss (retinitis pigmentosa); intellectual loss; cerebellar disturbance (ataxia) | Extraocular muscles, often asymmetric. Variable involvement of axial muscles; cardiac muscles, with conduction defect. | Depressed to ± or 0 |
| Myasthenia gravis Transient neonatal | Variable | At birth | Difficulty sucking, swallowing; trouble with secretions | Somatic and cranial muscles | Normal to decreased |
| Myasthenia gravis Persistent neonatal | Variable | Variable: birth, neonatal, infancy | Same as transient form. | Same as transient form. | Same as transient form. |
| Congenital myopathies Myotonic dystrophy (Neonatal onset) | Autosomal-dominant | At birth | Same as myasthenia. Ptosis. Facial diplegia. Arthrogyposis, club feet, thin ribs. | Cranial and somatic, pharyngeal. | Decreased to 0 |
| "Other" myopathies Central core Nemaline (rod body) Myotubular (centronuclear) | Dominant or rarely autosomal-recessive x-linked recessive in neonatal form | Severe variants present at birth; milder variants (more common) infancy, childhood | Severe variant, newborns with severe hypotonia and respiratory failure is rare. Later presentation—facial weakness, mild to moderate weakness, even "toe walking" only. | Similar to myotonic dystrophy | Decreased to 0 |
| Congenital muscular dystrophy (Fukayama) (FCMD) | Genetic; recessive. chromosome 9q31–33. fuKutin mutations | Birth to 9 mos. | Hypotonia, joint contractures, mental retardation. | Heterogenous. Facial (cranial) and somatic. Contracture common. | Variable |
| Congenital muscular dystrophy (occidental) | Unknown; usually not familial; merosin-deficient variant 6q2 Many variants (8) | Birth (or early infancy) | As above. Normal IQ. | Same (merosin negative may involve heart, nerves, and brain). | Same |
| Benign congenital hypotonia (Oppenheim) | Variable | Variable | Hypotonia only. Deep tendon reflexes positive. Laboratory tests, biopsy normal. | Somatic muscles (respiratory muscles spared) | Normal to decreased |
| Myotonias Myotonia congenita (Thomsen) | Autosomal-dominant (autosomal-recessive cases reported) | Early infancy to late childhood | Difficulty in relaxing muscles after contracting them, especially after sleep; aggravated by cold, excitement. | Hands especially; muscles may be diffusely enlarged, giving patient herculean appearance. | Normal |

| Muscle Biopsy Findings | Other Diagnostic Tests | Treatment | Prognosis |
|---|---|---|---|
| Mitochondrial abnormalities. "Ragged red" fibers. Changes in fiber size, usually due to type 2 fiber atrophy. | CK usually normal. ECG with conduction block. CSF protein elevated. Nerve conduction slowed. MRI of brain and brain stem auditory evoked response may be abnormal. Mitochondrial deletions. | Plastic retraction of eyelids. Cardiac support. Anticipate diabetes mellitus. Coenzyme Q? | Dysphagia may develop (50%) as well as generalized muscle weakness. Prognosis poor. In severe cases, spongy vacuolization of brain and brain stem. |
| Unnecessary | Edrophonium or neostigmine tests. Acetylcholine receptor (AChR) antibodies. Repetitive nerve stimulation, EMG. | Supportive. Anticholinergic drugs. | Usually transient (< 2 months) |
| Sophisticated end plate, nerve terminal ultrastructural studies may be necessary. | May be similar to above. AChR antibodies negative. | May not respond to ACh-ase drugs, steroids, or immunosuppressants | Variable, may have long-term severe course. |
| Generalized fiber hypertrophy, delay in maturation. Type I atrophy. Internal nuclei. | EMG myotonic in some (waning amplitude and pitch). Test mother. CK often normal. DNA testing (chromosome 19) for GCT repeat. | Supportive, even respiratory support. Genetic counseling. | Severely involved infant may improve dramatically over months; expect mental retardation in this same variant. |
| Distinctive diagnostic histochemistry, eg, "central cores," "nemaline rods," myotubes type II–I fibers of unequal size. | Myopathic EMG. | Supportive. Genetic counseling. | Variable. May shorten life. Death in infancy or severe handicap in severe neonatal form. Scoliosis prominent. |
| "Dystrophic" changes. Fibrosis. Necrotic fibers. Internal nuclei. ? regenerative fibers. | Myopathic EMG. CK increased. Positive CT, MRI scans: white matter low density, etc. | Supportive. | Physical and mental handicap lifelong. Virtually all are of Japanese ancestry. |
| Same. Evaluate for merosin (α-laminen-2 deficiency). | Brain imaging normal in pure form. Merosin-deficient form may have white matter abnormalities. | Supportive. | May improve, walk. Scoliosis. |
| Normal with sophisticated studies (histochemistry, electron microscopy, even metabolic studies). | Use of this diagnosis is shrinking with increasingly sophisticated biochemical (eg, cytochrome oxidase) studies. | Supportive | Good (by definition). (Few documented long-term studies.) |
| Nonspecific and minor changes; type IIB fibers may be absent. | EMG myotonic. | Usually none. Phenytoin, especially in cold weather, may improve muscle functioning. | Normal life expectancy, with only mild disability. |

*(continued)*

**Table 23–26.** Muscular dystrophies and myotonias of childhood. (continued)

| Disease | Genetic Pattern | Age at Onset | Early Manifestations | Involved Muscles | Reflexes |
|---|---|---|---|---|---|
| Myotonic dystrophy I (Steinert) (child-hood and adult form)<br>Myotonic dystrophy II [Proximal myotonic myopathy (PROMM)] | Autosomal-dominant | Late childhood to adolescence; neonatal and in-fantile forms in-creasingly recognized (see above) | Myotonia of grasp, tongue; worsened by cold, emotions. "Hatchet-face." Nasal voice. Weakness and easy fatigability. Mild to moderate mental retardation noted. | Wasting, weakness of facial muscles, (masti-cation); sternocleido-mastoids, hands. Myotonic phenomena: "bunching up" of muscles of tongue, thenar eminence, fin-ger extensors after tapping with percus-sion hammer. | In infantile form, marked hyporeflexia |

- *Positive response to neostigmine and edropho-nium.*
- *Acetylcholine receptor antibodies in serum (ex-cept in congenital form).*

## General Considerations

Myasthenia gravis is characterized by easy fatigability of muscles, particularly the extraocular muscles and those of mastication, swallowing, and respiration. In the neonatal period, however, or in early infancy, the weak-ness may be so constant and general that an affected in-fant may present nonspecifically as a "floppy infant." Girls are affected more frequently than boys. The age at onset is older than 10 years in 75% of patients, often shortly after menarche. If diagnosed before age 10 years, congenital myasthenia should be considered in retrospect. Thyrotoxicosis is found in almost 10% of affected female patients. The essential abnormality is a circulating antibody that binds to the acetylcholine re-ceptor protein and thus reduces the number of motor end plates for binding by acetylcholine.

## Clinical Findings

### A. SYMPTOMS AND SIGNS

**1. Neonatal (transient) myasthenia gravis**—This disorder occurs in 12% of infants born to myasthenic mothers. The condition is due to maternal acetyl-choline receptor antibody transferred across the pla-centa; a thymic factor in the infant may also be in-volved.

**2. Congenital (persistent) myasthenia gravis**—In this form of the disease, the mothers of the affected infants rarely have myasthenia gravis, but other relatives may. Sex distribution is equal. Symptoms are often subtle and not recognized initially. Differential diagnosis includes many other causes of the "floppy infant" syndrome, such as in-fant botulism, ocular myopathy, congenital ptosis, and Möbius syndrome (facial nuclear aplasia and other anom-alies). Congenital myasthenia gravis is not caused by re-ceptor antibodies and often responds poorly to therapy. It may result from a genetic abnormality of the acetyl-choline receptor protein, postsynaptic membrane struc-ture, or other myoneural transmission defects.

**3. Juvenile myasthenia gravis**—In this autoimmune form, the symptoms and signs are similar to those in adults. Receptor antibodies are usually present. The pa-tient may be first seen by an otolaryngologist or psychia-trist. The more prominent signs are difficulty in chew-ing, dysphagia, a nasal voice, ptosis, and ophthalmoplegia. Pathologic fatigability of limbs, chiefly involving the proximal limb and neck muscles, may be more prominent than the bulbar signs and may lead to an initial diagnosis of conversion hysteria, mus-cular dystrophy, or polymyositis. Weakness may be lim-ited to ocular muscles only. Associated disorders include autoimmune conditions, especially thyroid disease.

An acute fulminant form of myasthenia gravis has been reported in children age 2–10 years, who present with rapidly progressive respiratory difficulties. Bulbar paralysis may evolve within 24 hours. There is no his-tory of myasthenia. The differential diagnosis includes Guillain–Barré syndrome and bulbar poliomyelitis. Ad-ministration of anticholinesterase agents establishes the diagnosis and is lifesaving.

### B. LABORATORY FINDINGS

**1. Neostigmine test**—In newborns and very young infants, the neostigmine test may be preferable to the

**Table 23–26.**  (continued)

| Muscle Biopsy Findings | Other Diagnostic Tests | Treatment | Prognosis |
|---|---|---|---|
| Type I fiber atrophy, type II hypertrophy, sarcoplasmic masses, internal nuclei, phagocytosis, fibrosis, and cellular reaction. | EMG markedly myotonic. Glucose tolerance test, thyroid tests. ECG. Chest radiograph and pulmonary function tests. Immunoglobulins. PCR amplification of GCT repeat on chromosome 19q13 to distinguish normal from mutant alleles. CCTG repeat in zinc finger protein gene. | Procainamide, 250 mg tid orally, increased to tolerance; phenytoin 5–7 mg/kg/d orally. (Drugs usually little role.) | Frontal baldness, cataracts (85%), gonadal atrophy (85% of males), thyroid dysfunction, diabetes mellitus (20%). Cardiac conduction defects; impaired pulmonary function. Low IgG. Life expectancy decreased. Type II—slowly progressive weakening; good outlook |

ASA = acetyl salicyclic acid; CK = creatine kinase; CPT = carnitine palmityl transferase; CSF = cerebrospinal fluid; ECG = electrocardiogram; EMG = electromyogram; PCR = polymerase chain reaction; SIDS = sudden infant death syndrome.

edrophonium (Tensilon) test because the longer duration of its response permits better observation, especially of sucking and swallowing movements. The test dose of neostigmine is 0.02 mg/kg subcutaneously, usually given with atropine, 0.01 mg/kg subcutaneously. There is a delay of about 10 minutes before the effect may be manifest. The physician should be prepared to suction secretions.

**2. Edrophonium test**—Testing with edrophonium is used in older children who are capable of cooperating in certain tasks, such as raising and lowering their eyelids and squeezing a sphygmomanometer bulb or the examiner's hands. The test dose is 0.1–1 mL intravenously, depending on the size of the child. Maximum improvement occurs within 2 minutes.

**3. Other laboratory tests**—Serum acetylcholine receptor antibodies are often found in the neonatal and juvenile forms. Ophthalmologic tests of ocular motility with edrophonium are often positive in patients able to cooperate. In juveniles, thyroid studies are appropriate.

### C. ELECTRICAL STUDIES OF MUSCLE

Repetitive stimulation of a motor nerve at slow rates (3/s) with recording over the appropriate muscle reveals a progressive fall in amplitude of the muscle potential in myasthenic patients. A maximal stimulus must be given. At higher rates of stimulation (50/s), there may be a transient repair of this defect before the progressive decline is seen. If this study is negative, single-fiber EMG may be helpful diagnostically.

### D. IMAGING

Chest radiograph and CT scanning in older children may disclose benign thymus enlargement. Thymus tumors are rare in children.

## Treatment

### A. GENERAL AND SUPPORTIVE CARE

In the newborn or in a child in myasthenic or cholinergic crisis (see item 5 in the following section), suctioning of secretions is essential. Respiratory assistance may be required. Treatment should be conducted by physicians with experience in this disorder.

### B. ANTICHOLINESTERASE DRUG THERAPY

**1. Pyridostigmine bromide**—The dosage must be adjusted for each patient. A frequent starting dosage is 15–30 mg orally every 6 hours.

**2. Neostigmine**—Fifteen milligrams of neostigmine are roughly equivalent to 60 mg of pyridostigmine bromide. Neostigmine often causes gastric hypermotility with diarrhea, but it is the drug of choice in newborns, in whom prompt treatment may be lifesaving. It may be given parenterally.

**3. Atropine**—Atropine may be added on a maintenance basis to control mild cholinergic side effects such as hypersecretion, abdominal cramps, and nausea and vomiting.

**4. Immunologic intervention**—Such intervention is achieved primarily with prednisone. Plasmapheresis is effective in removing acetylcholine receptor antibody in severely affected patients.

**5. Myasthenic crisis**—Relatively sudden difficulties in swallowing and respiration may be observed in myasthenic patients. Edrophonium results in dramatic but brief improvement; this may make evaluation of the condition of the small child difficult. Suctioning, tracheostomy, respiratory assistance, and fluid and electrolyte maintenance may be required.

**6. Cholinergic crisis**—Cholinergic crisis may result from overdosage of anticholinesterase drugs. The resulting weakness may be similar to that of myasthenia, and the muscarinic effects (diarrhea, sweating, lacrimation, miosis, bradycardia, hypotension) are often absent or difficult to evaluate. The edrophonium test may help to determine whether the patient is receiving too little of the drug or is manifesting toxic symptoms due to overdosage. Improvement after the drugs are withdrawn suggests cholinergic crisis. A respirator should be available. The patient may require atropine and tracheostomy.

### C. SURGICAL MEASURES

Early thymectomy is beneficial in many patients whose disease is not confined to ocular symptoms; the effects may be delayed. Experienced surgical and postsurgical care are prerequisites.

## Prognosis

Neonatal (transient) myasthenia presents a great threat to life, primarily because of secretion aspiration. With proper treatment, the symptoms usually begin to disappear within a few days to 2–3 weeks, after which the child usually requires no further treatment. In the congenital (persistent) form, the symptoms may initially be as acute as in the transient variety. More commonly, however, they are relatively benign and constant, with gradual worsening as the child grows older. Fatal cases occur. In the juvenile form, patients may become resistant or unresponsive to anticholinesterase compounds and require corticosteroids or treatment in a hospital where respiratory assistance can be given. The overall prognosis for survival, for remission, and for improvement after therapy with prednisone and thymectomy is favorable. Death in myasthenic or cholinergic crisis may occur unless prompt treatment is given.

Gajdos P et al: Clinical trial of plasma exchange and high dose intravenous immunoglobulin in myasthenia gravis. Ann Neurol 1997;41:789 [PMID: 9668320].

Linduer A et al: Outcome in juvenile onset myasthenia gravis: A retrospective study with long-term follow-up of 79 patients. J Neurol 1997;244:515 [PMID: 9309559].

Sommer N et al: Ocular myasthenia gravis: Response to long-term immunosuppressive therapy. J Neurol Neurosurg Psychiatry 1997;62:156 [PMID: 9048716].

Tsao CY et al: Myasthenia gravis and associated autoimmune diseases in children. J Child Neurol 2000;15:767 [PMID: 11108515].

## PERIPHERAL NERVE PALSIES

## 1. Facial Weakness

Facial asymmetry may be present at birth or may develop later, either suddenly or gradually, unilaterally or bilaterally. Nuclear or peripheral involvement of the facial nerves results in sagging or drooping of the mouth and inability to close one or both eyes, particularly when newborns and infants cry. Inability to wrinkle the forehead may be demonstrated in infants and young children by getting them to follow a light moved vertically above the forehead. Loss of taste of the anterior two thirds of the tongue on the involved side may be demonstrated in cooperative children by age 4 or 5 years. Playing with a younger child and the judicious use of a tongue blade may enable the physician to note whether the child's face puckers up when something sour (eg, lemon juice) is applied with a swab to the anterior tongue. Ability to wrinkle the forehead is preserved, owing to bilateral innervation, in supranuclear facial paralysis.

Injuries to the facial nerve at birth occur in 0.25–6.5% of consecutive live births. Forceps delivery is the cause in some cases; in others, the side of the face affected may have abutted in utero against the sacral prominence. Often, no cause can be established.

Acquired peripheral facial weakness (Bell's palsy) of sudden onset and unknown cause is common in children. It often follows a viral illness (postinfectious) or physical trauma (eg, cold). It may be a presenting sign of tumor, Lyme disease, infectious mononucleosis, herpes simplex, or Guillain–Barré syndrome and is usually diagnosable by the history, physical examination, and appropriate laboratory tests.

Bilateral facial weakness in early life may be due to agenesis of the affected muscles or to nuclear causes (part of Möbius syndrome) or may even be familial. Myasthenia gravis, polyneuritis, and myotonic dystrophy must be considered.

Asymmetrical crying facies, in which one side of the lower lip depresses with crying (this is the normal side) and the other does not, is a common innocent form of autosomal dominant inherited congenital malformation. The defect in the parent (the asymmetry often improves with age) may be almost inapparent. EMG suggests congenital absence of the depressor anguli oris muscle of the lower lip. Forceps pressure is often erroneously incriminated as a cause of this innocent congenital anomaly. Occasionally other major (eg, cardiac septal defects) congenital defects accompany the palsy.

In the vast majority of cases of isolated peripheral facial palsy—both those present at birth and those acquired later—improvement begins within 1–2 weeks, and near or total recovery of function is observed within 2 months. Methylcellulose drops, 1%, should be instilled into the eyes to protect the cornea during the day; at night, the lid should be taped down with cellophane tape. Upward massage of the face for 5–10 minutes three or four times a day may help maintain muscle tone. Prednisone therapy likely does not aid recovery. Acyclovir (herpes antiviral agent) therapy may have a role in Bell's palsy.

In the few children with permanent and cosmetically disfiguring facial weakness, plastic surgical intervention at age 6 years or older may be of benefit. New procedures, such as attachment of facial muscles to the temporal muscle and transplantation of cranial nerve XI, are being developed.

Gimino V, Kamat B: Lyme disease. Pediatr Rev 2001;22:23,28.

Peitersen E: Bell's palsy: The spontaneous course of 2,500 peripheral facial nerve palsies of different etiologies. Acta Otolaryngol (Suppl) 2002;549:4 [PMID: 12482166].

Wilson C, Grant CC: Facial nerve palsy secondary to Epstein–Barr virus infection. Arch Pediatr Adolesc Med 1997;151:739 [PMID: 9232052].

## CHRONIC POLYNEUROPATHY

Polyneuropathy, usually insidious in onset and slowly progressive, occurs in children of any age. The presenting complaints are chiefly disturbances of gait and easy fatigability in walking or running and, slightly less often, weakness or clumsiness of the hands. Pain, tenderness, or paresthesias are mentioned less frequently. Neurologic examination discloses muscular weakness, greatest in the distal portions of the extremities, with steppage gait and depressed or absent deep tendon reflexes. Cranial nerves are sometimes affected. Sensory deficits occur in a stocking and glove distribution. The muscles may be tender, and trophic changes such as glassy or parchment skin and absent sweating may occur. Thickening of the ulnar and peroneal nerves may be felt. Pure sensory neuropathies show up as chronic trauma. That is, the patient does not feel minor trauma or burns, and thus allows trauma to occur.

Known causes include (1) toxins (lead, arsenic, mercurials, vincristine, and benzene); (2) systemic disorders (diabetes mellitus, chronic uremia, recurrent hypoglycemia, porphyria, polyarteritis nodosa, and lupus erythematosus); (3) inflammatory states (chronic or recurrent Guillain–Barré syndrome and neuritis associated with mumps or diphtheria); (4) hereditary, often degenerative conditions, which in some classifications include certain storage diseases, leukodystrophies, spinocerebellar degenerations with neurogenic components, and Bassen–Kornzweig syndrome; and (5) hereditary sensory or combined motor and sensory neuropathies (Table 23–27). Polyneuropathies associated with carcinomas, beriberi or other vitamin deficiencies, or excessive vitamin $B_6$ intake are not reported or are exceedingly rare in children.

The most common chronic neuropathy of insidious onset often has no identifiable cause. This chronic idiopathic neuropathy is assumed to be immunologically mediated and may have a relapsing course. Sometimes facial weakness occurs. CSF protein levels are elevated. Nerve conduction is slowed, and nerve biopsies are abnormal. Immunologic abnormalities are seldom demonstrated, although nerve biopsies may show round cell infiltration. Corticosteroids and other immunosuppressants may give long-term benefit.

Of the four defined hereditary sensory neuropathies, one rarer variant is familial dysautonomia, also called Riley–Day syndrome. Transmitted as an autosomal recessive trait and occurring mostly in Jewish children, this disorder has its onset in infancy. It is characterized by vomiting and difficulties in feeding that are due to abnormal esophageal motility, pulmonary infections, decreased or absent tearing, indifference to pain, diminished or absent tendon reflexes, absence of fungiform papillae of the tongue, emotional lability, abnormal temperature control with excessive sweating, labile blood pressure, abnormal intradermal histamine responses, and other evidences of autonomic dysfunction.

Rarely, a careful genetic history (pedigree) and examination and electrical testing (motor and sensory nerve conduction, EMG) of relatives are keys to diagnosis of hereditary neuropathy. This is the most common cause of chronic neuropathy in children. Other hereditary neuropathies may have ataxia as a prominent finding often overshadowing the neuropathy. Examples are Friedreich ataxia, dominant cerebellar ataxia, and Marinesco–Sjögren syndrome. Finally, some hereditary neuropathies are associated with identifiable and occasionally treatable metabolic errors. (see Table 23–22). These disorders are described in more detail in Chapter 32 (see also Table 23–21).

Laboratory diagnosis of chronic polyneuropathy is made by measurement of motor and sensory nerve conduction velocities. EMG may show a neurogenic polyphasic pattern. CSF protein levels are often elevated, sometimes with an increased IgG index. Nerve biopsy, with teasing of the fibers and staining for metachromasia, may demonstrate loss of myelin and, to a lesser degree, loss of axons and increased connective tissue or concentric lamellas (so-called onion skin appearance) around the nerve fiber. Muscle biopsy may show the pattern associated with denervation. Other laboratory studies directed toward specific causes mentioned above include screening for heavy metals and for metabolic, renal, or vascular disorders. Chronic lead intoxication, which rarely causes neuropathy in childhood, may escape detection until the child is given edetate calcium disodium and lead levels are determined in timed urine samples.

Therapy is directed at specific disorders whenever possible. Occasionally the weakness is profound and involves bulbar nerves, in which case tracheostomy and

***Table 23–27.*** Hereditary motor and sensory neuropathies; metabolic error unknown.

| Name | Prototype | Inheritance | Clinical Features | Nerve Biopsy |
|---|---|---|---|---|
| Sensory and auto-nomic neuropathy | Familial dysau-tonomia | Autosomal-recessive | See text | Decreased unmyelinated fibers posterior column and cord |
| HMSN I (if tremor is present, Roussy–Lévy syndrome) (60–90% of HMSN are type I) (CMT I) | "Classic" Charcot–Marie–Tooth (CMT) type I<br>(1) CMT 1A<br>(2) CMT 1B<br>(3) CMT 1C<br>(4) X-linked<br>(5) Type 4 | Autosomal-dominant<br><br>17p11.2<br>1g22<br>Connexin 32 | Onset 0–15 y. Weakness, atrophy of feet, calves (pes cavus, "stork legs"), hands. Sensory loss 0 or variable. Deep tendon reflexes 0. Motor nerve conduction velocities slowed. 10% have hyper-trophic (palpable) nerves. Type 1B is linked to Duffy blood group. | Segmental demyelination |
| HMSN II (10–30% of cases) (CMT 2) | Neuronal, axonal type 2 | Autosomal-dominant Multiple gene sites | Less severe; onset 10–y. Leg cramps, numbness, motor nerve conduction velocities normal or slightly slow. CSF protein often normal. | Axonal loss, secondary demyelination |
| HMSN III (CMT 3) | Hypertrophic CMT disease; Déjérine–Sottas disease | Autosomal-recessive (or AD, sporadic) | Onset in infancy. Severe. CSF protein increased. Very slow MNCV. Slowly progressive. | Hypertrophic ("onion bulb") interstitial changes |
| HMSN IV (CMT 4) | Refsum disease | Autosonal-recessive demyelinating, or axonal | Severe sensory, mild motor. Thick nerves. CSF protein elevated. Ichthyosis, retini-tis pigmentosa, ataxia, deaf-ness. Urine phytanic acid. | See HMSN III |
| HMSN V | CMT disease with spastic paraparesis | | Abnormal pyramidal tract findings. Rule out adreno-myelopathy. | Defined in pedigrees. Rule out adrenomyelopathy with long-chain fatty acids. |
| HNPP | Hereditary neuro-pathy with pressure palsies | Autosomal-dominant *PMP22* 17p11.2 deletion | Adolescent onset. Episodic numbness, peroneal palsy, carpal tunnel syndrome. | Occasional "tomaculous sausage" nerve formations. |

[1]CSF = cerebrospinal fluid; MNCV = motor nerve conduction velocity; HMSN = hereditary motor and sensory neuropathy; HNPP = heredi-tary neuropathy (with ability to) pressure palsies; PMP = peripheral myelin protein; MPZ/PO = myelin protein zero.

respiratory assistance are required. Corticosteroid ther-apy may be of considerable benefit in cases where the cause is unknown or neuropathy is considered to be due to chronic inflammation (this is not the case in acute Guillain–Barré syndrome). Prednisone is recom-mended, 1–2.5 mg/kg/d orally, with tapering to the lowest effective dose—discontinued if the process seems to be arresting and reinstituted when symptoms recur. Prednisone should probably not be used for treatment

of hereditary neuropathy. In all cases considered for corticosteroid therapy, the risks and benefits should be carefully weighed. When treatment is available, symp-toms regress and may disappear altogether over a period of months.

The long-term prognosis varies with the cause and the ability to offer specific therapy. In the corticoster-oid-dependent group, residual deficits and deaths within a few years are more frequent.

Burns TM et al: Current therapeutic strategies for patients with polyneuropathies secondary to inherited metabolic disorders. Mayo Clin Proc 2003;78:858 [PMID: 12839082].

Connolly AM: Chronic inflammatory demyelinating polyneuropathy in childhood. Pediatr Neurol 2001;24:177 [PMID: 11301217].

Donofrio PD: Immunotherapy of idiopathic inflammatory neuropathies. Muscle Nerve 2003;28:273 [PMID: 12929187].

Hughes R et al: Randomized controlled trial of intravenous immunoglobulin versus oral prednisone in chronic inflammatory demyelinating polyradiculoneuropathy. Ann Neurol 2001;50:195 [PMID: 11506402].

Ropper AH: Current treatments for CIDP. Neurology 2003;60 (Suppl 3):S16 [PMID: 12707418].

Sander HW, Hedley-Whyte ET: Case records of the Massachusetts General Hospital. Weekly clinicopathological exercises: Case 6-2003: A nine-year-old girl with progressive weakness and areflexia. N Engl J Med 2003;348:735 [PMID: 12594319].

# ■ MISCELLANEOUS NEUROMUSCULAR DISORDERS

## FLOPPY INFANT SYNDROME

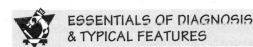

### ESSENTIALS OF DIAGNOSIS & TYPICAL FEATURES

- *In early infancy, decreased muscular activity, both spontaneous and in response to postural reflex testing and to passive motion.*
- *In young infants, "frog posture" or other unusual positions at rest.*
- *In older infants, delay in motor milestones.*

## General Considerations

In the young infant, ventral suspension (ie, supporting the infant with a hand under the chest) normally results in the infant's holding its head slightly up (45 degrees or less), the back straight or nearly so, the arms flexed at the elbows and slightly abducted, and the knees partly flexed. The "floppy" infant droops over the hand like an inverted U. The normal newborn attempts to keep the head in the same plane as the body when pulled up from supine to sitting by the hands (traction response). Marked head lag is characteristic of the floppy infant. Hyperextensibility of the joints is not a dependable criterion.

The usual reasons for seeking medical evaluation in older infants are delays in walking, running, or climbing stairs or motor difficulties and lack of endurance. Hypotonia or decreased motor activity is a frequent presenting complaint in neuromuscular disorders but may also accompany a variety of systemic conditions or may be due to certain disorders of connective tissue.

## 1. Paralytic Group

The hypotonic infant who is weak (appearing paralyzed) usually has a lesion of the lower motor neuron complex (Table 23–28). The child has significant lack of movement against gravity (eg, fails to kick the legs, hold up the arms, or attempt to stand when held) or in response to stimuli such as tickling or slight pain. Infantile progressive spinal muscular atrophy (Werdnig–Hoffman disease) is the most common cause. Neuropathy is rare. Botulism and myasthenia gravis (rare) are neuromuscular junction causes. Myotonic dystrophy and rare myopathies (eg, central core myopathy) are muscle disease entities.

In anterior horn cell or muscle disease, weakness is proximal (ie, in shoulders and hips); finger movement is preserved. Tendon reflexes are absent or depressed; strength (to noxious stimuli) is decreased (paralytic). Intelligence is preserved. Fine motor, language, and personal and social milestones are normal, as measured, for example, on a Denver Developmental Screening Test (DDST, or Denver II) (see Chapter 2).

## Myopathies

The congenital, relatively nonprogressive myopathies, muscular dystrophy, myotonic dystrophy, polymyositis, and periodic paralysis were discussed earlier in this chapter. Most cases of congenital or early infantile muscular dystrophy reported in the past probably represented congenital myopathies (see Table 23–28). Congenital muscular dystrophy, diagnosed by muscle biopsy, occurs in two forms: (1) a benign form, with gradual improvement in strength; and (2) a severe form, in which either weakness progresses rapidly and death occurs in the first months or year of life or severe disability is present with little or no progression but lifelong marked limitation of activity.

## Glycogenosis with Muscle Involvement

Glycogen storage diseases are described in Chapter 32. Patients with type II disease (Pompe disease, due to a deficiency of acid maltase) are most likely to present as floppy infants. Muscle cramps on exertion or easy fatigability, rather than floppiness in infancy, is the presenting complaint in type V disease (McArdle phosphorylase deficiency) or in the glycogenosis due to

***Table 23–28.*** Floppy infant: paralytic causes.

| Disease | Genetic | Early Manifestations |
|---|---|---|
| **IPSMA** (Infantile progressive spinal muscular atrophy) "Malignant" form | AR | In utero movements decreased by one third. Gradual weakness, delay in gross motor milestones. Weak cry. Abdominal breathing. Poor limb motion ("no kicking"). No deep tendon reflexes. Fasciculations of tongue. Normal personal-social behavior. |
| "Intermediate" form | AR | Onset under age 1 year usual. *Progression slower:* may be impossible to predict early course of IPSMA. Hand tremors common. |
| **Infantile botulism** | Acquired younger than age 1 y (mostly under 6 mos); botulism spore in stool makes toxin | Poor feeding. Constipation. Weak cry. Failure to thrive. Lethargy. Facial weakness, ptosis, ocular muscle palsy. Inability to suck, swallow. Apnea. Source: soil dust (outdoor construction workers or family gardeners may bring it home on clothes), honey. |
| **Myasthenia gravis** Neonatal transient | 12% of infants born from a myasthenia mother | Floppiness. Poor sucking and feeding; choking. Respiratory distress. Weak cry. |
| Congenital persistent | Mother normal. Rare AR (AD) | As above; may improve and later exacerbate. |
| **Myotonic dystrophy** | AD 99%—mother transmits gene | Polyhydramnios; failure of suck, respirations. Facial diplegia. Ptosis. Arthrogryposis. Thin ribs. Later, developmental delay. Examine mother for myotonia, physiognomy. |
| **Neonatal "rare myopathy," severe variant** Nemaline, central core, "minimal change," etc | AR, AD | Virtually all of the rare myopathies may have a severe (even fatal) neonatal or early infant form. Clinical features similar in infancy to infantile myotonic dystrophy. |
| **Congenital muscular dystrophy** Fukayama (FCMD) | Genetic | Early onset. Facial weakness. Joint contractures. Severe mental retardation. Seizures. Brain structural abnormalities. |
| Other | | Severe or benign. No mental retardation (see text). |
| **Infantile neuropathy** | HSMN most common cause | Demyelinating or axonal; a rare cause of floppy infant. Rule out mimicking IPSMA (deletion study). EMG, NCV are key studies. |
| **Benign congenital hypotonia** | Unknown cause | Diagnosis of exclusion. Family history variable. Mild to moderate hypotonia with weakness. (This term being used less with increasing genetic, microscopy advances) |

AD = autosomal dominant; AR = autosomal recessive; HSMN = hereditary sensory motor neuropathy; EMG = electromyelogram; NCV = nerve conduction velocity.

phosphofructokinase deficiency or phosphohexose isomerase inhibition.

## Myasthenia Gravis

Neonatal transient and congenital persistent myasthenia gravis, with patients presenting as paralytic floppy infants, is described earlier in this chapter.

## Arthrogryposis Multiplex (Congenital Deformities About Multiple Joints)

This symptom complex, sometimes associated with hypotonia, may be of neurogenic or myopathic origin (or both) and may be associated with a variety of other anomalies. Orthopedic aspects are discussed in Chapter 24.

## Spinal Cord Lesions

Severe limpness in newborns following breech extraction with stretching or actual tearing of the lower cervical to upper thoracic spinal cord is rarely seen today, owing to improved obstetric delivery. Klumpke lower brachial plexus paralysis may be present; the abdomen is usually exceedingly soft, and the lower extremities are flaccid. Urinary retention is present initially; later, the bladder may function autonomously. Myelography or MRI scanning may define the lesion. After a few weeks, spasticity of the lower limbs becomes obvious. Treatment is symptomatic and consists of bladder and skin care and eventual mobilization on crutches or in a wheelchair.

## 2. Nonparalytic Group

The nonparalytic hypotonic infant often has a damaged brain (Table 23–29). Deep tendon reflexes may be depressed or absent in this group. Brisk reflexes with hypotonia point to suprasegmental or general cerebral dysfunction. Intrauterine or perinatal insults to brain or spinal cord, while sometimes difficult to document, are major causes. (Occasionally, severe congenital myopathies presenting in the newborn period simulate nonparalytic hypotonia.) Persisting severe hypotonia is ominous. Tone will often vary. Spasticity and other forms of cerebral palsy may emerge; hypertonia and hypotonia may occur at varying times in the same infant. Choreoathetoid or ataxic movements and developmental delay can clarify the diagnosis. Reflexes are often increased; pathologic reflexes (Babinski, tonic neck) may persist or worsen.

The creatine kinase level and the EMG are usually normal. Prolonged nerve conduction velocities point to polyneuritis or leukodystrophy. Muscle biopsies, using special stains and histographic analysis, often show a remarkable reduction in size of type II fibers associated with decreased voluntary motor activity.

Limpness in the neonatal period and early infancy and subsequent delay in achieving motor milestones are the presenting features in a large number of children with a variety of CNS disorders, including mental retardation, as in trisomy 21. In many such cases, no specific diagnosis can be made. Close observation and scoring of motor patterns and adaptive behavior, as by the DDST, are helpful.

**Table 23–29.** Floppy infant: nonparalytic causes.

| | Causes | Manifestations |
|---|---|---|
| **Central nervous system disorders** | | |
| Atonic diplegia (prespastic diplegia) | Intrauterine, perinatal asphyxia, cord injury | Limpness, stupor; poor suck, cry, Moro reflex, grasp; later, irritability, increased tone and reflexes |
| Choreoathetosis | As above; kernicterus | Hypotonic early; movement disorder emerges later (6–18 mos) |
| Ataxic cerebral palsy | Same as choreoathetosis | Same as choreoathetosis |
| **Syndromes with hypotonia (CNS origin)** | | |
| Trisomy 21 | Genetic | All have hypotonia early |
| Prader–Willi syndrome | Genetic deletion 15q11 | Hypotonia, hypomentia, hypogonadism, obesity ("H$_3$O") |
| Marfan syndrome | Autosomal-dominant | Arachnodactyly |
| Dysautonomia | Autosomal-recessive | Respiratory infections, corneal anesthesia |
| Turner syndrome | 45X, or mosaic | Somatic stigmata (see Chapter 32) |
| **Degenerative disorders** | | |
| Tay–Sachs disease | Autosomal-recessive | Cherry-red spot on macula |
| Metachromatic leukodystrophy | Autosomal-recessive | Deep tendon reflexes increased early, polyneuropathy late; mental retardation |
| **Systemic diseases**[a] | | |
| Malnutrition | Deprivation, cystic fibrosis, celiac disease | |
| Chronic illness | Congenital heart disease; chronic pulmonary disease (eg, bronchopulmonary dysplasia); uremia, renal acidosis | |
| Metabolic disease | Hypercalcemia, Lowe disease | |
| Endocrinopathy | Hypothyroid | |

[a]See elsewhere in text for manifestations.

CDC MMWR: Infant botulism—New York City 2001–2002. JAMA 2003;52:21 [PMID: 12608714].

Castrodale V: The hypotonic infant: Case study of central core disease. Neonatal Netw 2003;22:53 [PMID: 12597091].

Dua T et al: Spectrum of floppy children in Indian scenario. Indian Pediatr 2001;38:1236 [PMID: 11721063].

Johnston HM: The floppy weak infant revisited. Brain Dev 2003;25:155 [PMID: 12689691].

Ogino S, Wilson RB: Genetic testing and risk assessment for spinal muscular atrophy (SMA). Hum Genet 2002;111:477 [PMID: 12436240].

Richer LP et al: Diagnostic profile of neonatal hypotonia: An 11-year study. Pediatr Neurol 2001;25:32 [PMID: 11483393].

Rick JR et al: Infantile botulism: An atypical case of an uncommon disease. Pediatrics 1999;103:1038 [PMID: 10224186].

Wilmshurst JM et al: Peripheral neuropathies of infancy. Dev Med Child Neurol 2003;45:408 [PMID: 12785442].

# CEREBRAL PALSY

The term "cerebral palsy" is a nonspecific term used to describe a chronic, static impairment of muscle tone, strength, coordination, or movements. The term implies that the condition is nonprogressive and originated from some type of cerebral insult or injury before birth, during delivery, or in the perinatal period. There is no implication in the use of this term about the child's intellect or whether other neurologic deficits or disorders (eg, blindness, deafness, epilepsy) exist. Some form of cerebral palsy occurs in about 0.2% of neonatal survivors. The fundamental course, severity, precise manifestations, and prognosis vary widely.

The most common forms of cerebral palsy (75% of cases) involve spasticity of the limbs. A variety of terms denote the specific limb or combination of limbs affected: monoplegia (one limb); hemiplegia (arm and leg on same side of body, but arm more affected than leg); diplegia (leg affected more than arms); paraplegia (both legs affected with arms unaffected); quadriplegia (all four limbs affected equally).

Ataxia is the second most common form of cerebral palsy, accounting for about 15% of cases. The ataxia frequently affects fine coordinated movements of the upper extremities, but may also involve lower extremities and trunk. An involuntary movement disorder usually in the form of choreoathetosis accounts for 5% of cases and persistent hypertonia without spasticity 1%.

Depending on the type and severity of the motor deficits, associated neurologic deficits or disorders may occur: seizure in up to 50%, mild mental retardation in 26%, and severe retardation in up to 27%. Disorders of language, speech, vision, hearing, and sensory perception are found in varying degrees and combinations.

The findings on physical examination are variable and are predominately those of spasticity, hyperreflexia, ataxia, and involuntary movements. Microcephaly is frequently present. In patients with hemiplegia, the affected arm and leg may be smaller and shorter than the unaffected limbs. Cataracts, retinopathy, and congenital heart defects may be indicative of congenital infections such as CMV and rubella.

Appropriate laboratory studies depend on the history and physical findings. MRI scans may be helpful in understanding the full extent of cerebral injury, and occasionally neuroimaging results suggest specific etiologies (eg, periventricular calcifications in congenital CMV infections). Other diagnostic tests that may be considered include IgG and IgM antibody determinations for specific infective agents; urine amino acids and organic acids; blood amino acids, lactate, pyruvate, and ammonia concentrations.

The determination that a child has cerebral palsy is based in part on excluding other neurologic disorders and following the child for a sufficient amount of time to ascertain the static, nonprogressive nature of the disorder.

Treatment and management are directed at assisting the child to attain maximal physical functioning and potential physical, occupational, and speech therapy; orthopedic monitoring and intervention and special educational assistance may all contribute to an improved outcome. Medications for spasticity and seizures are needed in many children. Also important is the general support of the parents and family with counseling, educational programs, and support groups.

The prognosis for patients with cerebral palsy depends greatly on the severity of the motor deficits and the degree of incapacity the patients ultimately experience. In severe cases, life span is greatly shortened to 10 years or less. Aspiration, pneumonia, or other intercurrent infections are the most common causes of death.

In contrast, patients with mild cerebral palsy may improve with age. Some patients experience resolution of their motor deficits by age 7 years. Many children with normal intellect have normal life spans and are able to lead productive, satisfying lives.

The cause is often obscure or multifactorial. No definite etiologic diagnosis is possible in over one third of cases. The incidence is high among infants small for gestational age. Intrauterine hypoxia is a frequent cause. Other known causes are intrauterine bleeding, infections, toxins, congenital malformations, obstetric complications (including birth hypoxia), neonatal infections, kernicterus, neonatal hypoglycemia, acidosis, and a small number of genetic syndromes.

Albright AL et al: Long-term intrathecal baclofen therapy for severe spasticity of cerebral origin. J Neurosurg 2003;98:291 [PMID: 12593613].

Awaad V et al: Functional assessment following intrathecal baclofen therapy in children with spastic cerebral palsy. J Child Neurol 2003;18:26 [PMID: 12661935].

Collet JP et al: Hyperbaric oxygen for children with cerebral palsy: A randomised multicentre trial. Lancet 2001;357:582 [PMID: 11558483]

Gibson CS et al: Antenatal causes of cerebral palsy: Associations between inherited thrombophilias, viral and bacterial infection, and inherited susceptibility to infection. Obstet Gynecol Surv 2003;58:209 [PMID: 12612461].

Perlman JM: Intrapartum hypoxic–ischemic cerebral injury and subsequent cerebral palsy: Medicolegal issues. Pediatrics 1997;99:851 [PMID: 9164779].

Petersen MC, Palmer FB: Advances in prevention and treatment of cerebral palsy. Ment Retard Dev Disabil Res Rev 2001;7:30 [PMID: 11241880].

Rosenbaum PL et al: Prognosis for gross motor function in cerebral palsy: Creation of motor development curves. JAMA 2002;288:1357 [PMID: 12234229].

Shevell MI et al: Etiologic yield of cerebral palsy: A contemporary case series. Pediatr Neurol 2003;28:352 [PMID: 12878296].

Singhi P et al: Epilepsy in children with cerebral palsy. J Child Neurol 2003;18:174 [PMID: 12731642].

### Internet References

Child Neurology Society

http://www.childneurologysociety.org

This site contains information about new developments, research and has practice parameters.

Child Neurology Foundation

http://www.childneurologyfoundation.org/index.html

Describes sites, resources, tests, related to child neurology.

E-Medicine

http://www.emedicine.com/neuro/PEDIATRIC NEUROLOGY.htm

This contains a list of various topics within pediatric neurology.

American Association of Child and Adolescent Psychiatry

http://www.aacp.org

Contains practice parameters and other information.

National Institute of Neurological Disorders and Stroke

http://www.ninds.nih.gov

Brief descriptions of neurological disorders.

Gene Tests

http://www.genetests.org

Lengthy descriptions of many of the genetic disorders.

Epilepsy Foundation of America

http://www.epilepsyfoundation.org

Describes epilepsy research and some basics about epilepsy

American Epilepsy Society

http://www.aesnet.org

Gives in formation about the society and general in formation about epilepsy. A good section on drugs given.

Neurofibromatosis Foundation

http://www.nf.org

Neurofibromatosis information

Tuberous Sclerosis Association

http://www.tsalliance.org

# Orthopedics

# 24

*Robert E. Eilert, MD*

Orthopedics is the medical discipline that deals with disorders of the neuromuscular and skeletal systems. Patients with orthopedic problems present with one or more of the following complaints: pain, loss of function, or deformity. Although review of the history reveals the patient's expectation, physical examination is the most important feature of orthopedic diagnosis.

## ■ DISTURBANCES OF PRENATAL ORIGIN

### CONGENITAL AMPUTATIONS AND LIMB DEFICIENCIES

Congenital amputations may be due to teratogens (eg, drugs or viruses), amniotic bands, or metabolic diseases (eg, diabetes in the mother). The incidence of multiple limb involvement is 30%.

Children with congenital limb deficiencies, such as absence of the femur, tibia, or fibula, also have a high incidence of associated congenital anomalies, including genitourinary and cardiac defects and cleft palate. A limb deficiency usually consists of partial absence of structures in the extremity along one side or the other. For example, in radial clubhand, the entire radius is absent, but the thumb may be either hypoplastic or completely absent; that is, the effect on structures distal to the amputation varies. Complex tissue defects are nearly always associated with longitudinal bone deficiency in that the associated nerves and muscles are not completely represented when a bone is absent.

Terminal amputations are treated by prosthesis, for example, to compensate for shortness of one leg. For certain types of severe anomalies, operative treatment is indicated to remove a portion of the malformed extremity (eg, foot) so that a prosthesis can be fitted early. An extension prosthesis fitted over the foot to equalize limb length is a reasonable nonsurgical alternative.

Lower extremity prostheses are best fitted between ages 12 and 15 months, when walking starts. They are consistently well accepted, because they are necessary for balancing and walking. For a unilateral upper extremity amputation, fitting the child with dummy-type prosthesis as early as age 6 months has the advantage of

instilling an accustomed pattern of proper length and bimanual manipulation. Although myoelectric prostheses have a technologic appeal, the majority of patients use the simplest construct in the long run.

Children quickly learn how to function with their prostheses and can lead active lives, even participating in sports with peers.

Kant P et al: Treatment of longitudinal deficiency affecting the femur: Comparing patient mobility and satisfaction outcomes of Syme amputation against extension prosthesis. J Pediatr Orthop 2003;23(2):236 [PMID: 12604957].

McCarthy JJ et al: Fibular hemimelia: Comparison of outcome measurements after amputation and lengthening. J Bone Joint Surg Am 2000;82-A(12):1732 [PMID: 11139646].

### DEFORMITIES OF THE EXTREMITIES

#### 1. Metatarsus Varus

Metatarsus varus is a common congenital foot deformity characterized by inward deviation of the forefoot. A vertical crease in the arch occurs when the deformity is more rigid. The angulation is at the level of the base of the fifth metatarsal, and this bone will be prominent. Most flexible deformities are secondary to intrauterine posture and usually resolve spontaneously. Several investigators have noticed that 10–15% of children with metatarsus varus have hip dysplasia; therefore, a careful hip examination is necessary. If the deformity is rigid and cannot be manipulated past the midline, it is worthwhile to use a cast changed at intervals of 2 weeks to correct the deformity. So-called corrective shoes do not live up to their name, although they can be used to maintain correction obtained by casting.

Lincoln TL, Suen PW: Common rotational variations in children. J Am Acad Orthop Surg 2003;11(5):312 [PMID: 14565753].

#### 2. Clubfoot (Talipes Equinovarus)

The diagnosis of classic talipes equinovarus, or clubfoot, requires three features: (1) plantar flexion of the foot at the ankle joint (equinus), (2) inversion deformity of the heel (varus), and (3) medial deviation of the forefoot (varus). The incidence of clubfoot is approximately 1:1000 live births. There are three major categories of clubfoot: (1) idiopathic, (2) neurogenic, and

(3) those associated with syndromes such as arthrogryposis and Larsen syndrome. Any infant with a clubfoot should be examined carefully for associated anomalies, especially of the spine. Idiopathic clubfeet may be hereditary.

Treatment consists of manipulation of the foot to stretch the contracted tissues on the medial and posterior aspects, followed by splinting to hold the correction. When this treatment is instituted shortly after birth, correction is rapid. When treatment is delayed, the foot tends to become more rigid within a matter of days. After full correction is obtained, a night brace is necessary for long-term maintenance of correction. Treatment by means of casting requires patience and experience, but fewer patients require surgery when attention is paid to details of the Ponsetti technique. If the foot is rigid and resistant to cast treatment, surgical release and correction are appropriate. Fifteen percent to 50% require a surgical release.

Colburn M, Williams M: Evaluation of the treatment of idiopathic clubfoot by using the Ponsetti method. J Foot Ankle Surg 2003;42(5):259 [PMID: 14566717].

Tredwell SJ et al: Review of the effect of early amniocentesis on foot deformity in the neonate. J Pediatr Orthop 2001;21:636 [PMID: 11521033].

## 3. Infantile Dysplasia of the Hip Joint

The definition of dysplasia is abnormal growth or development. Dysplasia of the hip encompasses a spectrum of conditions in which an abnormal relationship exists between the proximal femur and the acetabulum. In the most severe condition, the femoral head is not in contact with the acetabulum and is classified as a dislocated hip. A dislocatable hip is one in which the hip is within the acetabulum but can be dislocated with a provocative maneuver. A subluxatable hip is one in which the femoral head comes partially out of the joint with a provocative maneuver. Acetabular dysplasia is the term used to denote insufficient acetabular development on radiograph.

Congenital dislocation of the hip occurs in approximately 1:1000 live births. At birth, both the acetabulum and femur are underdeveloped. The dysplasia is progressive with growth unless the dislocation is corrected. If the dislocation is corrected in the first few days or weeks of life, the dysplasia is completely reversible and a normal hip will develop. As the child becomes older and the dislocation or subluxation persists, the deformity will worsen to the point where it will not be completely reversible, especially after the walking age. For this reason, it is important to diagnose the deformity early.

## Clinical Findings

The diagnosis of hip dislocation in the newborn depends on demonstrating instability of the joint by placing the infant on its back and obtaining complete relaxation by feeding with a bottle if necessary. The examiner's long finger is then placed over the greater trochanter and the thumb over the inner side of the thigh. Both hips are flexed 90 degrees and then slowly abducted from the midline, one hip at a time. With gentle pressure, an attempt is made to lift the greater trochanter forward. A feeling of slipping as the head relocates is a sign of instability (Ortolani sign). When the joint is more stable, the deformity must be provoked by applying slight pressure with the thumb on the medial side of the thigh as the thigh is adducted, thus slipping the hip posteriorly and eliciting a jerk as the hip dislocates (Barlow sign). The signs of instability are more reliable than a radiograph for diagnosing congenital dislocation of the hip in the newborn. Ultrasonography can be used but tends to result in overdiagnosis in the newborn. Asymmetrical skinfolds are present in about 40% of newborns and therefore are not particularly helpful.

After the first month of life, the signs of instability become less evident. Contractures begin to develop about the hip joint, limiting abduction to less than 90 degrees. It is important to hold the pelvis level to detect asymmetry of abduction. If the knees are at unequal heights when the hips and knees are flexed, the dislocated hip will be on the side with the lower knee. After the first 6 weeks of life, radiologic examination becomes more valuable, with lateral displacement of the femoral head being the most reliable sign. In mild cases, the only abnormality may be increased steepness of acetabular alignment, so that the acetabular angle is greater than 35 degrees.

If dysplasia of the hip has not been diagnosed during the first year of life and the child begins to walk, there will be a painless limp and a lurch to the affected side. When the child stands on the affected leg, a dip of the pelvis will be evident on the opposite side, owing to weakness of the gluteus medius muscle. This is called the Trendelenburg sign and accounts for the unusual swaying gait. In children with bilateral dislocations, the loss of abduction is almost symmetrical and may be deceiving. A radiograph of the pelvis is indicated in children with incomplete abduction in the first few months of life. As a child with bilateral dislocation of the hips begins to walk, the gait is waddling. The perineum is widened as a result of lateral displacement of the hips, and there is flexion contracture as a result of posterior displacement of the hips. This flexion contracture contributes to marked lumbar lordosis, and the greater trochanters are easily palpable in their elevated position. Treatment is still possible in the first 2 years of life, but the results are not nearly as effective as in children receiving treatment in the nursery.

## Treatment

Dislocation or dysplasia diagnosed in the first few weeks or months of life can easily be treated by splinting, with the hip maintained in flexion and abduction. Forced abduction is contraindicated, because this can lead to avascular necrosis of the femoral head. The use of double or triple diapers is never indicated because diapers are not adequate to obtain proper positioning of the hip. An orthopedic surgeon with experience managing the problem is best to supervise treatment of children requiring splints.

In the first 4 months of life, reduction can be obtained by simply flexing and abducting the hip; no other manipulation is usually necessary. In late cases, preoperative traction for 2–3 weeks relaxes soft tissues about the hip. Following traction in which the femur is brought down opposite the acetabulum, reduction can be easily achieved without force under general anesthesia. After reduction a hip spica is used for 6 months. If the reduction is not stable within a reasonable range of motion after closed reduction, open reduction is indicated. If reduction is done at an older age, operations to correct the deformities of the acetabulum and femur may be necessary as well as open reduction.

Committee on Quality Improvement, Subcommittee on Developmental Dysplasia of the Hip. American Academy of Pediatrics: Clinical practice guideline: Early detection of developmental dysplasia of the hip. Pediatrics 2000;105(4 Pt 1):896 [PMID: 10742345].

## 4. Torticollis

Wryneck deformities in infancy may be due either to injury to the sternocleidomastoid muscle during delivery or to disease affecting the cervical spine. When contracture of the sternocleidomastoid muscle causes torticollis, the chin is rotated to the side opposite to the affected muscle, and the head is tilted toward the side of the contracture. A mass felt in the midportion of the sternocleidomastoid muscle is not a true tumor but rather fibrous transformation within the muscle.

In most cases, passive stretching is effective. If the deformity has not been corrected by passive stretching within the first year of life, surgical release of the muscle origin and insertion will correct it. Excising the "tumor" of the sternocleidomastoid muscle creates an unsightly scar and is unnecessary. If the deformity is left untreated, a striking facial asymmetry will persist.

Torticollis is occasionally associated with congenital deformities of the cervical spine, and radiographs of the spine are indicated in all cases. In addition, there is a 20% incidence of hip dysplasia.

Acute torticollis may follow upper respiratory infection or mild trauma in children. Rotatory subluxation of the upper cervical spine requires computed tomography for accurate imaging. Traction or a cervical collar usually results in resolution of the symptoms within 1 or 2 days. Other causes of torticollis include spinal cord or cerebellar tumors, syringomyelia, and rheumatoid arthritis.

Fernandez Cornejo VJ et al: Inflammatory atlanto-axial subluxation (Grisel's syndrome) in children: Clinical diagnosis and management. Childs Nerv Syst 2003;19(5-6):342 [PMID: 12783261].

## GENERALIZED DISORDERS OF SKELETAL OR MESODERMAL TISSUES

### 1. Arthrogryposis Multiplex Congenita (Amyoplasia Congenita)

Arthrogryposis multiplex congenita consists of incomplete fibrous ankylosis (usually bilateral) of many or all joints of the body. Upper extremity contractures usually consist of adduction of the shoulders; extension of the elbows; flexion of the wrists; and stiff, straight fingers with poor muscle control of the thumbs. In the lower extremities, common deformities are dislocation of the hips, extension contractures of the knees, and severe club feet. The joints are fusiform and the joint capsules decreased in volume due to lack of movement during fetal development. Various investigations have attributed the basic defect to an abnormality of muscle or the lower motor neurons. Muscle development is poor, and muscles may be represented only by fibrous bands. Passive mobilization of joints is the early treatment. Prolonged casting for correction of deformities is contraindicated in these children because further stiffness results. Use of removable splints combined with vigorous therapy is the most effective conservative treatment. Surgical release of the affected joints is often necessary. The clubfoot associated with arthrogryposis is very stiff and nearly always requires an operation. Surgery about the knees, including capsulotomy, osteotomy, and tendon lengthening, is used to correct deformity. In the young child, a dislocated hip may be reduced operatively by the medial approach. Multiple operative procedures about the hip are contraindicated because further stiffness may be produced with consequent impairment of motion. Affected children are often able to walk if the dislocations and contractures are reduced surgically. The long-term prognosis for physical and vocational independence is guarded. These patients have normal intelligence, but they have such severe physical restrictions that gainful employment is hard to find.

Bernstein RM: Arthrogryposis and amyoplasia. J Am Acad Orthop Surg 2002;10(6):417 [PMID: 12470044].

## 2. Marfan Syndrome

Marfan syndrome is a connective tissue disorder characterized by unusually long fingers and toes (arachnodactyly); hypermobility of the joints; subluxation of the ocular lenses; other eye abnormalities including cataract, coloboma, megalocornea, strabismus, and nystagmus; a high-arched palate; a strong tendency to scoliosis; pectus carinatum; and thoracic aortic aneurysms due to weakness of the media of the vessels (see Chapter 33). Serum mucoproteins may be decreased, and urinary excretion of hydroxyproline increased. The condition is easily confused with homocystinuria, because the phenotypic presentation is identical. The two diseases are differentiated by detecting homocystine in the urine of patients with homocystinuria.

Treatment is usually supportive for associated problems such as flatfoot. Scoliosis may involve more vigorous treatment by bracing or spine fusion. The long-term prognosis has improved for patients because better treatment for their aortic aneurysms has been devised.

Aburawi EH et al: Marfan's syndrome: A review. Hosp Med 2001;62:153 [PMID: 11291465].

## 3. Klippel–Feil Syndrome

Klippel–Feil syndrome is characterized by failure of segmentation of some or all of the cervical vertebrae. Multiple congenital spinal anomalies may be present, with hemivertebrae and scoliosis. The neck is short and stiff, the hairline is low, and the ears are low-set. Common associated defects include congenital scoliosis, cervical rib, spina bifida, torticollis, web neck, high scapula, renal anomalies, and deafness. If there is evidence of abnormal renal function, renal ultrasound is indicated as well as a hearing test. Scoliotic deformities, if progressive, are an indication for spinal arthrodesis.

Guilde JT et al: The natural history of Klippel–Feil syndrome: Clinical roentgenographic and magnetic resonance imaging findings at adulthood. J Pediatr Orthop 1995;15:617 [PMID: 7593574].

## 4. Sprengel Deformity

Sprengel deformity is a congenital condition in which one or both scapulas are elevated and small. The child cannot raise the arm completely on the affected side,

and torticollis may be present. The deformity occurs alone or in association with Klippel–Feil syndrome. If the deformity is functionally limiting, the scapula may be surgically relocated lower in the thorax. Excision of the upper portion of the scapula improves cosmetic appearance but has little effect on function.

Williams MS: Developmental anomalies of the scapula—the "omo"st forgotten bone. Am J Med Genet 2003;120A(4):583 [PMID: 12884444].

## 5. Osteogenesis Imperfecta

Osteogenesis imperfecta is a rare genetic connective tissue disease characterized by multiple and recurrent fractures. The severe fetal type (osteogenesis imperfecta congenita) is characterized by multiple intrauterine or perinatal fractures. Moderately affected children have numerous fractures and are dwarfed as a result of bony deformities and growth retardation. Intelligence is not affected. The shafts of the long bones are reduced in cortical thickness, and wormian bones are present in the skull. Other features include blue scleras, thin skin, hyperextensibility of ligaments, otosclerosis with significant hearing loss, and hypoplastic and deformed teeth. In the tarda type, fractures begin to occur at variable times after the perinatal period, resulting in relatively fewer fractures and deformities. Affected patients are sometimes suspected of having suffered induced fractures, and the condition should be ruled out in any case of nonaccidental trauma.

Molecular genetic studies have identified more than 150 mutations of the *COL1A1* and *COL1A2* genes, which encode for type I procollagen. Parents without this mutation can be counseled that the likelihood of a second affected child is negligible.

Bisphosphonates show promise for decreasing the incidence of fractures. Surgical treatment involves correction of deformity of the long bones. Multiple intramedullary rods have been used to prevent deformity from poor healing of fractures. Patients are often confined to wheelchairs during adulthood.

Chevrel G, Meunier PJ: Osteogenesis imperfecta: Lifelong management is imperative and feasible. Joint Bone Spine 2001;68: 125 [PMID: 11324928].

## 6. Osteopetrosis (Osteitis Condensans Generalisata, Marble Bone Disease, Albers–Schönberg Disease)

Osteopetrosis is a rare disorder of osteoclastic resorption of bone, resulting in abnormally dense bones. The marrow spaces are reduced, resulting in anemia. There are two types: a milder autosomal dominant type and a more malignant autosomal recessive type. The findings may appear at any age. On radiologic examination, the bones show increased density, transverse bands in the shafts, clubbing of ends, and vertical striations of long bones. Thickening about the cranial foramina is present, and heterotopic calcification of soft tissues is possible.

The autosomal recessive form of osteopetrosis can be treated successfully by allogeneic bone marrow transplantation.

Armstrong DG et al: Orthopaedic management of osteopetrosis: Results of a survey and review of the literature. J Pediatr Orthop 1999;19:122 [PMID: 9890301].

## 7. Achondroplasia (Classic Chondrodystrophy)

Skeletal dysplasia is suspected based on abnormal stature, disproportion, dysmorphism, or deformity. Measurement of height is an excellent clinical screening tool. Achondroplasia is the most common form of short-limbed dwarfism. The upper arms and thighs are proportionately shorter than the forearms and legs. Findings frequently include bowing of the extremities, a waddling gait, limitation of motion of major joints, relaxation of the ligaments, short stubby fingers of almost equal length, frontal bossing, moderate hydrocephalus, depressed nasal bridge, and lumbar lordosis. Intelligence and sexual function are normal. The disorder is transmitted as an autosomal dominant trait, but 80% of cases result from a random mutation. Radiographs demonstrate short, thick tubular bones and irregular epiphysial plates. The ends of the bones are thick, with broadening and cupping. Epiphysial ossification may be delayed. Because the spinal canal is narrowed, a herniated disk in adulthood may lead to acute paraplegia. Growth hormone is given to some children with bone dysplasia. Limb lengthening is controversial, but possible.

Aldegheri R, Dall'Oca C: Limb lengthening in short stature patients. J Pediatr Orthop B 2001;10:238 [PMID: 11497369].

Kanaka-Gantenbein C: Present status of the use of growth hormone in short children with bone diseases (diseases of the skeleton). J Pediatr Endocrinol Metab 2001;14:17 [PMID: 11220700].

## 8. Osteochondrodystrophy (Morquio Disease)

Morquio disease is an autosomal recessive disorder of mucopolysaccharide storage. Skeletal abnormalities include shortening of the spine, kyphosis, scoliosis, shortened extremities, pectus carinatum, genu valgum, and a hypoplastic odontoid with atlantoaxial instability. The child generally appears normal at birth and begins to develop deformities between ages 1 and 4 years as a result of abnormal deposition of mucopolysaccharides.

Radiographs demonstrate wedge-shaped flattened vertebrae and irregular, malformed epiphyses. The ribs are broad and have been likened to canoe paddles. The lower extremities are more severely involved than the upper ones.

The major treatment issue revolves around the prevention of cervical myelopathy. Bone marrow transplantation has been successful in alleviating some of the symptoms.

Peters C, Steward CG: Hematopoietic cell transplantation for inherited metabolic diseases: An overview of outcomes and practice guidelines. Bone Marrow Transplant 2003;31(4):229 [PMID: 12621457].

# ■ GROWTH DISTURBANCES OF THE MUSCULOSKELETAL SYSTEM

## SCOLIOSIS

Scoliosis is characterized by lateral curvature of the spine associated with rotation of the involved vertebrae. Scoliosis is classified by its anatomic location, in either the thoracic or lumbar spine, with rare involvement of the cervical spine. The convexity of the curve is designated right or left. Thus a right thoracic scoliosis would denote a thoracic curve in which the convexity is to the right; which is the most common type of idiopathic curve. Posterior curvature of the spine (kyphosis) is normal in the thoracic area, although excessive curvature is pathologic. Anterior curvature of the spine, or lordosis, is normal in the lumbar and cervical spines. Idiopathic scoliosis generally begins at age 8 or 10 years and usually progresses during growth. In rare instances, infantile scoliosis may be seen in children age 2 years or younger.

Idiopathic scoliosis is about four or five times more common in girls. The disorder is usually asymptomatic in the adolescent years, but severe curvature can cause pain or loss of pulmonary function in later years. The screening examination for scoliosis is performed by having the patient bend forward 90 degrees with the hands joined in the midline. An abnormal finding consists of asymmetry of the height of the ribs or paravertebral muscles on one side, indicating rotation of the trunk associated with lateral curvature.

Diseases that may be associated with scoliosis include neurofibromatosis, Marfan syndrome, cerebral palsy, muscular dystrophy, poliomyelitis, and myelodysplasia.

Between 5% and 7% of cases of scoliosis are due to congenital vertebral anomalies such as a hemivertebra or unilateral vertebral bridge. These curves are more rigid than the more common idiopathic curve (see later discussion) and will often increase with growth, especially during adolescence. Eighty percent of cases of scoliosis are idiopathic. Because 30% of family members are also affected, siblings of an affected child should be examined.

Idiopathic infantile scoliosis, occurring in children age 2–4 years, is uncommon in the United States but more common in Great Britain. If the rib–vertebral angle of Mehta is less than 20 degrees, the curve will resolve spontaneously. If the angle is greater, the curve will progress. Sciatic scoliosis may result from pressure on the spinal cord or roots by infectious processes or herniation of the nucleus pulposus; the underlying cause must be sought. Secondary curvature will resolve as the primary problem is treated.

## Clinical Findings

### A. SYMPTOMS AND SIGNS

Scoliosis in adolescents does not cause significant pain. If a patient has significant pain, seek the underlying cause because the scoliosis is usually secondary to some other disorder such as a bone or spinal cord tumor. Deformity of the rib cage and asymmetry of the waistline are evident with curvatures of 30 degrees or more. A lesser curvature may be detected by the forward bending test described in the preceding section, which is designed to detect early abnormalities of rotation that may not be apparent when the patient is standing erect.

### B. IMAGING

The most valuable radiographs are those taken of the entire spine in the standing position in both the anteroposterior and lateral planes. Usually one primary curvature is evident with a compensatory curvature that develops to balance the body. At times two primary curvatures may be seen, usually in the right thoracic and left lumbar regions. Any left thoracic curvature should be suspected of being secondary to neurologic disease, prompting a more meticulous neurologic examination. If the curvatures of the spine are balanced (compensated), the head is centered over the center of the pelvis and the patient is "in balance." If the spinal alignment is uncompensated, the head will be displaced to one side, which produces an unsightly deformity. Rotation of the spine may be measured by scoliometer. This rotation is associated with a marked rib hump as the lateral curvature increases in severity. Deformity of the rib cage causes long-term problems when lung volumes are reduced.

## Treatment

Treatment of scoliosis depends on curve magnitude, skeletal maturity, and risk of progression. Curvatures of less than 20 degrees usually do not require treatment unless they show progression. Bracing is indicated for curvature of 20–40 degrees in a skeletally immature child. Treatment is indicated for any curvature that demonstrates progression on serial radiologic examination. Curvatures greater than 40 degrees are resistant to treatment by bracing. Thoracic curvatures greater than 60 degrees have been correlated with poor pulmonary function in adult life. Curvatures of such severity are an indication for surgical correction and posterior spinal fusion to maintain the correction. Curvatures of 40–60 degrees may also require spinal fusion if they are progressive, are causing decompensation of the spine, or cause unacceptable deformity.

Surgical fusion involves decortication of the bone over the laminas and spinous processes, with the addition of bone graft. Rods, hooks, or pedicle screws maintain postoperative correction, with activity restriction for several months until the bone fusion is solid. Treatment requires a team approach and is best done in centers with full support facilities.

## Prognosis

Compensated small curves that do not progress may be well tolerated throughout life, with minor deformity. Counsel the patients regarding the genetic transmission of scoliosis and caution that their children's backs should be examined as part of routine physicals. Large thoracic curvatures greater than 60 degrees are associated with shortened life span and may progress during adult life. Large lumbar curvatures may lead to subluxation of the vertebrae and premature arthritic degeneration of the spine, producing disabling pain in adulthood. Early detection allows for simple brace treatment.

Danielsson A, L Nachemson A: Back pain and function 22 years after brace treatment for adolescent idiopathic scoliosis: A case-control study—part I. Spine 2003;28(18):2078.

## SLIPPED CAPITAL FEMORAL EPIPHYSIS

Slipped capital femoral epiphysis is a condition caused by displacement of the proximal femoral epiphysis due to disruption of the growth plate. The head of the femur is usually displaced medially and posteriorly relative to the femoral neck. The condition occurs in adolescence and is most common in obese males. The cause is unclear, although some authorities have shown experimentally that the strength of the perichondrial ring stabilizing the epiphysial area is sufficiently weakened by hormonal changes during adolescence such that the overload of excessive body weight can produce a pathologic fracture through the growth plate. Hormonal studies in these children are usually normal, although slipped capital femoral epiphysis is associated with hypothyroidism.

The condition occasionally occurs acutely following a fall or direct trauma to the hip. More commonly, vague symptoms occur over a protracted period in an otherwise healthy child who presents with pain and limp. The pain can be referred into the thigh or the medial side of the knee. Examine the hip joint in any obese child complaining of knee pain! The consistent finding on physical examination is limitation of internal rotation of the hip. The diagnosis may be clearly apparent only in the lateral radiographic view.

Treatment is based on the same principles that govern treatment of any fracture of the femoral neck in that the head of the femur is internally fixed to the neck of the femur and the fracture line allowed to heal. Unfortunately, the severe complication of avascular necrosis occurs in 30% of these patients. There is a positive correlation between forceful reduction of the slip and avascular necrosis. In cases of acute slip, as evidenced by the absence of any callus formation about the growth plate, it may be possible to reduce the hip by gentle traction. In more chronic cases, a more expeditious procedure is to pin the slip as it lies. Remodeling of the fracture site often improves the position of the hip without further surgery.

The long-term prognosis is guarded because most of these patients continue to be overweight and overstress their hip joints. Follow-up studies have shown a high incidence of premature degenerative arthritis in this disease, even in those who do not develop avascular necrosis. The development of avascular necrosis almost guarantees a poor prognosis, because new bone does not readily replace the dead bone at this late stage of skeletal development. About 30% of patients have bilateral involvement, which may occur as late as 1 or 2 years after the primary episode.

Dobbs MB, Weinstein SL: Natural history and long-term outcomes of slipped capital femoral epiphysis. Instr Course Lect 2001;50:571.

## GENU VARUM & GENU VALGUM

Genu varum (bowleg) is normal from infancy through age 2 years. The alignment then changes to genu valgum (knock-knee) until about age 8 years, at which time adult alignment is attained. Criteria for referral to an orthopedist include persistent bowing beyond age 2 years, bowing that is increasing rather than decreasing, bowing of one leg only, and knock-knee associated with short stature.

Bracing may be appropriate. Rarely an osteotomy is necessary for a severe problem such as Blount disease (proximal tibial epiphysial dysplasia).

Zayer M: Long-term results after physiological genu varum. J Pediatr Orthop B 2000;9:271.

## TIBIAL TORSION

"Toeing in" in small children is a common parental concern. Tibial torsion is rotation of the leg between the knee and the ankle. Internal rotation amounts to about 20 degrees at birth but decreases to neutral rotation by age 16 months. The deformity is sometimes accentuated by laxity of the knee ligaments, allowing excessive internal rotation of the leg in small children. In children who have a persistent internal rotation of the tibia beyond age 16–18 months, the condition is often due to sleeping with feet turned in and can be reversed with an external rotation splint worn only at night.

Arazi M et al: Normal development of the tibiofemoral angle in children: A clinical study of 590 normal subjects from 3 to 17 years of age. J Pediatr Orthop 2001;21:264.

## FEMORAL ANTEVERSION

Toeing in beyond age 2 or 3 years is usually secondary to femoral anteversion, which is characterized by more internal rotation of the hip compared with external rotation. This femoral alignment follows a natural history of progressive decrease toward neutral during growth. Studies comparing the results of treatment with shoes or braces to the natural history have shown that little is gained by active treatment. Active external rotation exercises, such as skating or bicycle riding, can be encouraged. Osteotomy for rotational correction is rarely required. Children who have no external rotation of hip in extension are candidates for orthopedic consultation.

Lincoln TL, Suen PW: Common rotational variations in children. J Am Acad Orthop Surg 2003;11(5):312.

## COMMON FOOT PROBLEMS

When a child begins to stand and walk, the long arch of the foot is flat with a medial bulge over the inner border of the foot. The forefeet are mildly pronated or rotated inward, with a slight valgus alignment of the knees. As the child grows and joint laxity decreases, the long arch is better supported and more normal relationships occur in the lower extremities. (See also sections on Metatarsus Varus and Talipes Equinovarus.)

## 1. Flatfoot

Flatfoot is a normal condition in infants. If the heel cord is of normal length, full dorsiflexion is possible with the heel in the neutral position. As long as the heel cord is of normal length and a longitudinal arch is noted when the child is sitting in a non-weight-bearing position, the parents can be assured that a normal arch will probably develop. There is usually a familial incidence of relaxed flatfeet in children who have no apparent arch. In any child with a shortened heel cord or stiffness of the foot, other causes of flatfoot such as tarsal coalition or vertical talus should be ruled out by a complete orthopedic examination and radiograph.

In the child with an ordinary relaxed flatfoot, no active treatment is indicated unless calf or leg pain is present. In children who have leg pains attributable to flatfoot, a supportive shoe with scaphoid pad, such as a good-quality sports shoe, is useful. An orthotic that holds the heel in neutral and supports the arch may relieve discomfort if more support is needed. An arch insert should not be prescribed unless passive correction of the arch is easily accomplished; otherwise, the skin over the medial side of the foot will be irritated.

Song KM: Flexible flatfeet in pre-school children. J Pediatr Orthop 2002;22(1):134.

## 2. Talipes Calcaneovalgus

Talipes calcaneovalgus is characterized by excessive dorsiflexion at the ankle and eversion of the foot. It is often present at birth and is due to intrauterine position. Treatment consists of passive exercises, stretching the foot into plantar flexion. In rare instances, it may be necessary to use plaster casts to help with manipulation and positioning. Complete correction is the rule.

## 3. Cavus Foot

This deformity consists of an unusually high longitudinal arch of the foot. It may be hereditary or associated with neurologic conditions such as poliomyelitis, Charcot–Marie–Tooth disease, Friedreich ataxia, and diastematomyelia. There is usually an associated contracture of the toe extensor, producing a claw toe deformity in which the metatarsal phalangeal joints are hyperextended and the interphalangeal joints acutely flexed. Any child presenting with cavus feet should receive a careful neurologic examination and radiographs of the spine.

Conservative therapy is ineffective. In symptomatic cases, surgery may be necessary to lengthen the contracted extensor and flexor tendons and to release the plantar fascia and other tight plantar structures. The associated varus heel deformity causes more problems than the high arch.

Mosca VS: The cavus foot. J Pediatr Orthop 2001;21:423.

## 4. Bunions (Hallux Valgus)

Adolescents may present with lateral deviation of the great toe associated with a prominence over the head of the first metatarsal. This deformity is painful only with shoe wear and almost always can be relieved by fitting shoes that are wide enough in the toe. Surgery should be avoided in the adolescent, because further growth tends to cause recurrence of the deformity.

Talab YA: Hallux valgus in children: A 5–14-year follow-up study of 30 feet treated with a modified Mitchell osteotomy. Acta Orthop Scand 2002;73(2):195.

# ■ DEGENERATIVE PROBLEMS (ARTHRITIS, BURSITIS, & TENOSYNOVITIS)

Degenerative arthritis may follow childhood skeletal problems, such as infection, slipped capital femoral epiphysis, avascular necrosis, or trauma, or it may occur in association with hemophilia. Early effective treatment of these disorders can prevent arthritis. Degenerative changes in the soft tissues around joints may occur as a result of overuse syndrome in adolescent athletes. Young boys throwing excessive numbers of pitches, especially curve balls, may develop "little leaguer" elbow, consisting of degenerative changes around the humeral condyles associated with pain, swelling, and limitation of motion (see Chapter 25). In order to enforce the rest necessary for healing, a plaster cast may be necessary. A more reasonable preventive measure is to limit the number of pitches thrown by children.

Acute bursitis is uncommon in childhood, and other causes should be ruled out before this diagnosis is accepted.

Tenosynovitis is most common in the region of the knees and feet. Children taking dancing lessons, particularly toe dancing, may have pain around the flexor tendon sheaths in the toes or ankles. Rest is effective treatment. At the knee level, the patellar ligament may be irritated, with associated swelling in the infrapatellar fat pad. Synovitis in this area is usually due to overuse and is treated by rest and nonsteroidal anti-inflammatory drugs (NSAIDs). Corticosteroid injections are contraindicated.

# ■ TRAUMA

## SOFT TISSUE TRAUMA (Sprains, Strains, & Contusions)

A sprain is the stretching of a ligament, and a strain is a stretch of a muscle or tendon. Contusions are generally due to tissue compression, with damage to blood vessels within the tissue and the formation of hematoma.

A severe sprain is one in which the ligament is completely disrupted, resulting in instability of the joint. A mild or moderate sprain is one in which incomplete tearing of the ligament occurs but in which local pain and swelling results.

Mild or moderate sprains are treated by rest of the affected joint, with ice and elevation to prevent prolonged symptoms. By definition, mild or moderate sprain is not associated with instability of the joint.

If more severe trauma occurs, resulting in tearing of a ligament, instability of the joint may be demonstrated by gross examination or by stress testing with radiographic documentation. Such deformity of the joint may cause persistent instability resulting from inaccurate apposition of the ligament ends during healing. If instability is evident, surgical repair of the torn ligament may be indicated. If a muscle is torn at its tendinous insertion, it should be repaired.

The initial treatment of any sprain consists of ice, compression, and elevation. Splinting of the affected joint protects against further injury and relieves swelling and pain. Ibuprofen and other NSAIDs are useful for pain.

### 1. Ankle Sprains

The history will indicate that the injury was by either forceful inversion or eversion. The more common inversion injury results in tearing or injury to the lateral ligaments, whereas an eversion injury will injure the medial ligaments of the ankle. The injured ligaments may be identified by means of careful palpation for point tenderness around the ankle. The joint should be supported or immobilized at a right angle, which is the functional position. Adhesive taping may be effective but should be changed frequently to prevent blisters. Use of a posterior plaster splint or air splint produces joint rest, and the extremity can be protected by using crutches. Prolonged use of a plaster cast is usually not necessary, but the sprained ankle should be rested sufficiently to allow complete healing, which may take 3–6 weeks. Rehabilitation to include strengthening and restitution of kinesthetic sensation can prevent long-term disability.

McGuine TA et al: Balance as a predictor of ankle injuries in high school basketball players. Clin J Sport Med 2000;10:239.

Tabrizi P et al: Limited dorsiflexion predisposes to injuries of the ankle in children. J Bone Joint Surg Br 2000;82:1103.

### 2. Knee Sprains

Sprains of the collateral and cruciate ligaments are uncommon in children. These ligaments are so strong that it is more common to injure the epiphysial growth plates, which are the weakest structures in the region of the knees of children. In adolescence, however, the physes have started to close, and the knee joint is more like that of an adult, so that rupture of the anterior cruciate ligament can result from a hyperextension injury. If the injury produces avulsion of the tibial spine, open anatomic reduction is often required.

Effusion of the knee after trauma deserves referral to an orthopedic specialist. The differential diagnosis includes torn ligament, torn meniscus, and osteochondral fracture. Nontraumatic effusion should be evaluated for inflammatory conditions (eg, juvenile rheumatoid arthritis) or patellar malalignment.

Gabriel SE et al: Change in diagnosis among orthopedists compared to non-orthopedists in the management of acute knee injuries. J Rheumatol 2000;27:2412.

### 3. Internal Derangements of the Knee

Meniscal injuries are uncommon in children younger than age 12 years. Clicking or locking of the knee may occur in young children as a result of a discoid lateral meniscus, which is a rare congenital anomaly. As the child approaches adolescence, internal damage to the knee from a torsion weight-bearing injury may result in locking of the knee if tearing and displacement of a meniscus occurs. Osteochondral fractures secondary to osteochondritis dissecans may also present as internal derangements of the knee in adolescence. Posttraumatic synovitis may mimic a meniscal lesion. In any severe injury to the knee, epiphysial injury should be suspected; stress films will sometimes demonstrate separation of the distal femoral epiphysis in such cases. Epiphysial injury should be suspected whenever tenderness is present on both sides of the metaphysis of the femur after injury.

Smith AD: The skeletally immature knee: What's new in overuse injuries. Instr Course Lect 2003;52:691.

## 4. Back Sprains

Sprains of the ligaments and muscles of the back are unusual in children but may occur as a result of violent trauma from automobile accidents or athletic injuries. Back pain in a child may be the only symptom of significant disease and warrants clinical investigation. Inflammation, infection, renal disease, or tumors can cause back pain in children, and sprain should not be accepted as a routine diagnosis.

Balague F et al: Low-back pain in children. Lancet 2003;361 (9367):1403.

Wall EJ et al: Backpacks and back pain: Where's the epidemic? J Pediatr Orthop 2003;23(4):437.

## 5. Contusions

Contusion of muscle with hematoma formation produces the familiar "charley horse" injury. Treatment of such injuries is by application of ice, compression, and rest. Exercise should be avoided for 5–7 days. Local heat may hasten healing once the acute phase of tenderness and swelling is past.

## 6. Myositis Ossificans

Ossification within muscle occurs when there is sufficient trauma to cause a hematoma that later heals in the manner of a fracture. The injury is usually a contusion and occurs most commonly in the quadriceps of the thigh or the triceps of the arm. When a severe injury with hematoma is recognized, it is important to splint the extremity and avoid activity. If further trauma causes recurrent injury, ossification may reach spectacular proportions and resemble an osteosarcoma.

Disability is great, with local swelling and heat and extreme pain on the slightest motion of the adjacent joint. The limb should be rested, with the knee in extension or the elbow in 90 degrees of flexion, until the local reaction has subsided. After local heat and tenderness have decreased, gentle active exercises may be initiated. Passive stretching exercises are not indicated, because they may stimulate the ossification reaction. If surgery is necessary, it should not be attempted before 9 months to 1 year after injury, because it may restart the process and lead to an even more severe reaction.

## TRAUMATIC SUBLUXATIONS & DISLOCATIONS

Dislocation of a joint is always associated with severe damage to the ligaments and joint capsule. In contrast to fracture reduction, which may be safely postponed, dislocations must be reduced immediately. Dislocations can usually be reduced by gentle sustained traction. It often happens that no anesthetic is necessary for several hours after the injury, because of the protective anesthesia produced by the injury. Following reduction, the joint should be splinted for transportation of the patient.

The dislocated joint should be treated by immobilization for at least 3 weeks, followed by graduated active exercises through a full range of motion. Vigorous passive manipulation of the joint by a therapist may be harmful.

### 1. Subluxation of the Radial Head (Nursemaid Elbow)

Infants may sustain subluxation of the radial head as a result of being lifted or pulled by the hand. The child appears with the elbow fully pronated and painful. The usual complaint is that the child's elbow will not bend. Radiographic findings are normal, but there is point tenderness over the radial head. When the elbow is placed in full supination and slowly moved from full flexion to full extension, a click may be palpated at the level of the radial head. The relief of pain is remarkable, as the child usually stops crying immediately. The elbow may be immobilized in a sling for comfort for a day. Occasionally, symptoms last for several days, requiring more prolonged immobilization.

Pulled elbow may be a clue to battering. This should be considered during examination, especially if the problem is recurrent.

### 2. Recurrent Dislocation of the Patella

Recurrent dislocation of the patella is more common in loose-jointed individuals, especially adolescent girls. If the patella completely dislocates, it nearly always goes laterally. Pain is severe, and the patient is brought to the doctor with the knee slightly flexed and an obvious bony mass lateral to the knee joint associated with a flat area over the anterior knee. Radiologic examination confirms the diagnosis. The patella may be reduced by extending the knee and placing slight pressure on the patella while gentle traction is exerted on the leg. In subluxation of the patella, the symptoms may be more subtle, and the patient will complain that the knee "gives out" or "jumps out of place."

In the case of complete dislocation, the knee should be immobilized for 3–4 weeks, followed by a physical therapy program for strengthening the quadriceps muscle. Operation may be necessary to tighten the knee joint capsule if dislocation or subluxation is recurrent. In such instances, if the patella is not stabilized, repeated dislocation produces damage to the articular cartilage of the patellofemoral joint and premature degenerative arthritis.

Eilert RE: Congenital dislocation of the patella. Clin Orthop 2001;:22.

# FRACTURES

## 1. Epiphysial Separations

In children, epiphysial separations and fractures are more common than ligamentous injuries. This finding is based on the fact that the ligaments of the joints are generally stronger than the associated growth plates. In instances in which dislocation is suspected, a radiograph should be taken in order to rule out epiphysial fracture. Radiographs of the opposite extremity, especially for injuries around the elbow, may be valuable for comparison. Reduction of a fractured epiphysis should be done under anesthesia to align the growth plate with the least amount of force. Fractures across the growth plate may produce bony bridges that will cause premature cessation of growth or angular deformities of the extremity. Epiphysial fractures around the shoulder, wrist, and fingers can usually be treated by closed reduction, but fractures of the epiphyses around the elbow often require open reduction. In the lower extremity, accurate reduction of the epiphysial plate is necessary to prevent joint deformity if a joint surface is involved. If angular deformities result, corrective osteotomy may be necessary.

Peterson HA: Physeal fractures: Part 3. Classification. J Pediatr Orthop 1994;14:439 [PMID: 8077424].

## 2. Torus Fractures

Torus fractures consist of "buckling" of the cortex due to compression of the bone. They usually occur in the distal radius or ulna. Alignment is usually satisfactory, and simple immobilization for 3 weeks is sufficient.

## 3. Greenstick Fractures

Greenstick fractures involve frank disruption of the cortex on one side of the bone but no discernible cleavage plane on the opposite side. These fractures are angulated but not displaced, because the bone ends are not separated. Reduction is achieved by straightening the arm into normal alignment, and reduction is maintained by a snugly fitting plaster cast. It is necessary to get a radiograph of greenstick fractures again in a week to 10 days to make certain that the reduction has been maintained in the cast. A slight angular deformity can be corrected by remodeling of the bone. The farther the fracture is from the growing end of the bone, the longer the time required for remodeling. The fracture can be considered healed when no tenderness or local heat is present and when adequate bony callus is seen on radiograph.

## 4. Fracture of the Clavicle

Clavicular fractures are very common injuries in infants and children. The patient can be immobilized in a sling for comfort. The healing callus will be apparent when the fracture has consolidated, but this unsightly lump will generally resolve over a period of months to a year.

## 5. Supracondylar Fractures of the Humerus

Supracondylar fractures tend to occur in children age 3–6 years and are potentially dangerous because of the proximity to the brachial artery in the distal arm. They are usually associated with a significant amount of trauma, so that swelling may be severe. Most often, these fractures are treated by closed reduction and percutaneous pinning. Complications associated with supracondylar fractures include Volkmann ischemic contracture of the forearm due to vascular compromise and cubitus varus (decreased carrying angle) secondary to poor reduction. The so-called gunstock deformity of the elbow may be somewhat unsightly but does not usually interfere with joint function.

Gosens T, Bongers KJ: Neurovascular complications and functional outcome in displaced supracondylar fractures of the humerus in children. Injury 2003;34(4):267 [PMID: 12667778].

## 6. General Comments on Other Fractures in Children

Reduction of fractures in children is usually accomplished by simple traction and manipulation; open reduction is indicated if a satisfactory alignment is not obtained. Remodeling of the fracture callus usually produces an almost normal appearance of the bone over a matter of months. The younger the child, the more remodeling is possible. Angular deformities remodel reliably. Rotatory malalignment does not remodel.

The physician should be suspicious of child abuse whenever the age of a fracture does not match the history given or when the severity of the injury is more than the alleged accident would have produced. In suspected cases of battering where no fracture is present on the initial radiograph, a repeat radiograph 10 days later is in order. Bleeding beneath the periosteum will be calcified by 7–10 days, and the radiographic appearance is almost diagnostic of severe closed trauma characteristic of a battered child.

# ■ INFECTIONS OF THE BONES & JOINTS

## OSTEOMYELITIS

Osteomyelitis is an infectious process that usually starts in the spongy or medullary bone and then extends to involve compact or cortical bone. The lower extremities are most often affected, and there is commonly a history of trauma. Osteomyelitis may occur as a result of direct invasion from the outside through a penetrating wound (nail) or open fracture, but hematogenous spread of infection (eg, pyoderma or upper respiratory tract infection) from other infected areas is much more common. The most common infecting organism is *Staphylococcus aureus,* which has a tendency to infect the metaphyses of growing bones. Anatomically, circulation in the long bones is such that the arterial supply to the metaphysis just below the growth plate is close to end arteries, which turn sharply to end in venous sinusoids, causing a relative stasis. In the infant younger than age 1 year, there is direct vascular communication with the epiphysis across the growth plate, so that direct spread may occur from the metaphysis to the epiphysis and subsequently into the joint. In the older child, the growth plate provides an effective barrier, the epiphysis is usually not involved, and the infection spreads retrograde from the metaphysis into the diaphysis and, by rupture through the cortical bone, down along the diaphysis beneath the periosteum.

## 1. Exogenous Osteomyelitis

To avoid osteomyelitis by direct extension, all wounds must be carefully examined and cleansed. Osteomyelitis is a common occurrence from pressure sores in anesthetic areas, such as in patients with spina bifida. Cultures of the wound made at the time of exploration and debridement may be useful if signs of infection develop subsequently. Copious irrigation is necessary, and all nonviable skin, subcutaneous tissue, fascia, and muscle must be excised. In extensive or contaminated wounds, antibiotic coverage is indicated. Contaminated lacerations should be left open and secondary closure performed 3–5 days later. If at the time of delayed closure further necrotic tissue is present, it should be excised. Leaving the wound open allows the infection to stay at the surface rather than extend inward to the bone.

Puncture wounds are especially liable to lead to osteomyelitis and should be carefully debrided.

Initially, broad-spectrum antibiotics should be administered, but the final choice of antibiotics is directed by culture results. A tetanus toxoid booster may be indicated. Gas gangrene is best prevented by adequate debridement.

After exogenous osteomyelitis has become established, treatment becomes more complicated, requiring extensive surgical debridement and intravenous antibiotics.

## 2. Hematogenous Osteomyelitis

Hematogenous osteomyelitis is usually caused by pyogenic bacteria; 85% of cases are due to staphylococci. Streptococci are a less common cause of osteomyelitis. *Pseudomonas* organisms are common in cases of nail puncture wounds. Children with sickle cell anemia are especially prone to osteomyelitis caused by salmonellae.

### Clinical Findings

#### A. SYMPTOMS AND SIGNS

In infants, the manifestations of osteomyelitis may be subtle, presenting as irritability, diarrhea, or failure to feed properly; the temperature may be normal or slightly low; and the white blood count may be normal or only slightly elevated. There may be pseudoparalysis of the involved limb. In older children, the manifestations are more striking, with severe local tenderness and pain, often high fever, rapid pulse, and elevated white blood count and erythrocyte sedimentation rate (ESR). Osteomyelitis of a lower extremity often occurs around the knee joint in children age 7–10 years. Tenderness is most marked over the metaphysis of the bone where the process has its origin. For a child who refuses to bear weight, ostomyelitis is high in the differential diagnosis.

#### B. LABORATORY FINDINGS

Blood cultures are often positive early. The most significant test in infancy is the aspiration of pus. It is useful to needle the bone in the area of suspected infection and aspirate any fluid present. This fluid should be stained for organisms and cultured. Even edema fluid may be useful for determining the causative organism. Elevation of the ESR above 50 mm/h is typical for osteomyelitis. C reactive protein is elevated earlier than the ESR.

#### C. IMAGING

Nonspecific local swelling is the first radiographic finding. This is followed by elevation of the periosteum, with formation of new bone from the cambium layer of the periosteum occurring after 3–6 days. As the infection becomes chronic, areas of cortical bone are isolated by pus spreading down the medullary canal, causing rarefaction and demineralization of the bone. Such isolated pieces of cortex become ischemic and form sequestra (dead bone fragments). These radiographic findings are late but specific. Osteomyelitis should be diagnosed clinically before significant radiographic findings are present. Bone scan is sensitive but nonspecific and should be interpreted in the clinical context before radiographic findings become positive. Magnetic resonance imaging can demonstrate edema early or soft tissue thickening later.

## Treatment

### A. SPECIFIC MEASURES

Antibiotics should be started intravenously as soon as the diagnosis of osteomyelitis is made. Oral antibiotics are begun when tenderness, fever, the white cell count, and the ESR are all decreasing and the culture is positive. Agents that cover *S aureus* and *Streptococcus pyogenes* (eg, oxacillin, nafcillin, cefazolin, clindamycin) are appropriate for most cases. For specific recommendations and for possible *Pseudomonas* infection, see Chapter 38.

Chronic infections are treated for months. Following surgical debridement, *Pseudomonas* foot infections usually respond to 1–2 weeks of antibiotic treatment.

### B. GENERAL MEASURES

Splinting of the limb minimizes pain and decreases spread of the infection by lymphatic channels through the soft tissue. The splint should be removed periodically to allow active use of adjacent joints and prevent stiffening and muscle atrophy. In chronic osteomyelitis, splinting may be necessary to guard against fracture of the weakened bone.

### C. SURGICAL MEASURES

Aspiration of the metaphysis for culture and Gram stain is the most useful diagnostic measure in any case of suspected osteomyelitis. In the first 24–72 hours, it may be possible to treat osteomyelitis with antibiotics alone. If frank pus is aspirated from the bone, however, surgical drainage is indicated. If the infection has not shown a dramatic response within 24 hours, surgical drainage is also indicated. It is important that all devitalized soft tissue be removed and adequate exposure of the bone obtained to permit free drainage. Excessive amounts of bone should not be removed when draining acute osteomyelitis, because it will not be completely replaced by the normal healing process. Bone damage is limited by surgical drainage, whereas failure to evacuate pus in acute cases may lead to widespread damage.

## Prognosis

When osteomyelitis is diagnosed in the early clinical stages and prompt antibiotic therapy is begun, the prognosis is excellent. If the process has been unattended for a week to 10 days, there is almost always some permanent loss of bone structure, as well as the possibility of growth abnormality.

Song KM, Sloboda JF: Acute hematogenous osteomyelitis in children. J Am Acad Orthop Surg 2001;9:166 [PMID: 11421574].

# PYOGENIC ARTHRITIS

The source of pyogenic arthritis varies according to the child's age. In the infant, pyogenic arthritis often develops by spread from adjacent osteomyelitis. In the older child, it presents as an isolated infection, usually without bony involvement. In teenagers with pyogenic arthritis, an underlying systemic disease or an organism (eg, the gonococcus) that has an affinity for joints is usually the cause.

The infecting organism varies with age: group B streptococcus and *S aureus* in those younger than age 4 months; *Haemophilus influenzae* and *S aureus* in those age 4 months to 4 years; and *S aureus* and *S pyogenes* in older children and adolescents. *H influenzae* is now uncommon because of effective immunization. *Kingella kingae* is a gram-negative bacterium that occasionally causes pyarthrosis.

The initial effusion of the joint rapidly becomes purulent. An effusion of the joint may accompany osteomyelitis in the adjacent bone. A white cell count exceeding 100,000/$\mu$L in the joint fluid indicates a definite purulent infection. Generally, spread of infection is from the bone into the joint, but unattended pyogenic arthritis may also affect adjacent bone. The ESR is often above 50 mm/h.

## Clinical Findings

### A. SYMPTOMS AND SIGNS

In older children, the signs may be striking, with fever, malaise, vomiting, and restriction of motion. In infants, paralysis of the limb due to inflammatory neuritis may be evident. Infection of the hip joint in infants should be suspected if decreased abduction of the hip is present in an infant who is irritable or feeding poorly. A history of umbilical catheter treatment in the newborn nursery should alert the physician to the possibility of pyogenic arthritis of the hip.

## B. IMAGING

Early distention of the joint capsule is nonspecific and difficult to measure by radiograph. In the infant with unrecognized pyogenic arthritis, dislocation of the joint may follow within a few days as a result of distention of the capsule by pus. Later changes include destruction of the joint space, resorption of epiphysial cartilage, and erosion of the adjacent bone of the metaphysis. The bone scan shows increased flow and increased uptake about the joint.

## Treatment

Aspiration of the joint is the key to diagnosis. In the hip joint, pyogenic arthritis is most easily treated by surgical drainage because the joint is deep and difficult to aspirate and is also inaccessible to thorough cleaning through needle aspiration. Arthroscopic irrigation and debridement have been successful in treating pyogenic arthritis of the knee. If fever and clinical symptoms do not subside within 24 hours after treatment is begun, open surgical drainage is indicated. Antibiotics can be selected based on the child's age, results of the Gram stain, and culture of the aspirated pus. Reasonable empiric therapy in infants is nafcillin or oxacillin plus a third-generation cephalosporin. An antistaphylococcal agent alone is usually adequate for children older than age 5 years. For staphylococcal infections, 3 weeks of therapy is recommended; for other organisms, 2 weeks is usually sufficient. Oral therapy may be begun when clinical signs have improved markedly. It is not necessary to give intraarticular antibiotics, because good levels are achieved in the synovial fluid with parenteral administration.

## Prognosis

The prognosis for the patient with pyogenic arthritis is excellent if the joint is drained early, before damage to the articular cartilage has occurred. If infection is present for more than 24 hours, dissolution of the proteoglycans in the articular cartilage takes place, with subsequent arthrosis and fibrosis of the joint. Damage to the growth plate may also occur, especially within the hip joint, where the epiphysial plate is intracapsular.

Kothari NA et al: Imaging of musculoskeletal infections. Radiol Clin North Am 2001;39:653 [PMID: 11549164].

## TUBERCULOUS ARTHRITIS

Tuberculous arthritis is now a rare disease in the United States. Children in poor social circumstances, however, such as homeless families, are prone to tuberculous arthritis. Generally the infection may be ruled out by negative skin testing. The joints most commonly affected in children are the intervertebral disks, resulting in gibbus or dorsal angular deformity at the site of involvement.

Treatment is by local drainage of the abscess, followed by antituberculous therapy. Prolonged immobilization in a plaster cast or prolonged bed rest is necessary to promote healing. Spinal fusion may be required to preserve stability of the vertebral column.

Rasool MN: Osseous manifestations of tuberculosis in children. J Pediatr Orthop 2001;21:749 [PMID: 11675548].

## DISKITIS

Results of a study of 47 patients support the view that so-called diskitis is pyogenic infectious spondylitis in children and that supportive treatment and intravenous antibiotics are likely to lead to rapid relief of symptoms and signs without recurrence.

Brown R et al: Discitis in young children. J Bone Joint Surg Br 2001;83:106 [PMID: 11245515].

## TRANSIENT SYNOVITIS OF THE HIP

The most common cause of limping and pain in the hip in children in the United States is transitory synovitis, an acute inflammatory reaction that often follows an upper respiratory infection and is generally self-limited. In questionable cases, aspiration of the hip yields only yellowish fluid, ruling out pyogenic arthritis. Generally, however, toxic synovitis of the hip is not associated with elevation of the ESR, white blood count, or temperature above 38.3°C. It classically affects children age 3–10 years and is more common in boys than girls. There is limitation of motion of the hip joint, particularly internal rotation, and radiographic changes are nonspecific, with some swelling apparent in the soft tissues around the joint.

Treatment consists of bed rest and the use of traction with slight flexion of the hip. NSAIDs shorten the course of the disease, although even with no treatment, the disease usually runs its course in days. It is important to maintain radiographic follow-up because toxic synovitis may be the precursor of avascular necrosis of the femoral head (described in the next section) in a small percentage of patients. Radiographs can be obtained at 6 weeks, or earlier if either a persistent limp or pain is present.

Vila-Verde VM, da Silva KC: Bone age delay in Perthes disease and transient synovitis of the hip. Clin Orthop 2001;4:118 [PMID: 11302301].

# ■ VASCULAR LESIONS & AVASCULAR NECROSIS (Osteochondroses)

Osteochondrosis due to vascular lesions may affect various growth centers. Table 24–1 indicates the common sites and the typical ages at presentation.

In contrast to other body tissues that undergo infarction, bone removes necrotic tissue and replaces it with living bone in a process called creeping substitution. This replacement of necrotic bone may be so complete and so perfect that a completely normal bone results. Adequacy of replacement depends on the patient's age, the presence or absence of associated infection, the congruity of the involved joint, and other physiologic and mechanical factors.

Because of their rapid growth in relation to their blood supply, the secondary ossification centers in the epiphyses are subject to avascular necrosis. Despite the number of different names referring to avascular necrosis of the epiphyses, the process is identical, necrosis of bone followed by replacement (see Table 24–1).

Even though the pathologic and radiographic features of avascular necrosis of the epiphyses are well known, the cause is not generally agreed on. Necrosis may follow known causes such as trauma or infection, but idiopathic lesions usually develop during periods of rapid growth of the epiphyses.

## AVASCULAR NECROSIS OF THE PROXIMAL FEMUR (Legg–Calvé–Perthes Disease)

The vascular supply of the proximal femur is precarious, and when it is interrupted, necrosis results.

## Clinical Findings

### A. SYMPTOMS AND SIGNS

The highest incidence of Legg–Calvé–Perthes disease is between ages 4 and 8 years. Persistent pain is the most common symptom, and the patient may present with limp or limitation of motion.

### B. LABORATORY FINDINGS

Laboratory findings, including studies of joint aspirates, are normal.

### C. IMAGING

Radiographic findings correlate with the progression of the process and the extent of necrosis. The early finding

**Table 24–1.** The osteochondroses.

| Ossification Center | Eponym | Typical Age (years) |
|---|---|---|
| Capital femoral | Legg–Calvé–Perthes disease | 4–8 |
| Tarsal navicular | Köhler bone disease | 6 |
| Second metatarsal head | Freiberg disease | 12–14 |
| Vertebral ring | Scheuermann disease | 13–16 |
| Capitellum | Panner disease | 9–11 |
| Tibial tubercle | Osgood–Schlatter disease | 11–13 |
| Calcaneus | Sever disease | 8–9 |

is effusion of the joint associated with slight widening of the joint space and periarticular swelling. Decreased bone density in and around the joint is apparent after a few weeks. The necrotic ossification center appears more dense than the surrounding viable structures, and the femoral head is collapsed or narrowed.

As replacement of the necrotic ossification center occurs, rarefaction of the bone occurs in a patchwork fashion, producing alternating areas of rarefaction and relative density, referred to as "fragmentation" of the epiphysis.

In the hip, widening of the femoral head may occur associated with flattening, or coxa plana. If infarction has extended across the growth plate, a radiolucent lesion will be evident within the metaphysis. If the growth center of the femoral head has been damaged so that normal growth is arrested, shortening of the femoral neck results.

Eventually, complete replacement of the epiphysis develops as living bone replaces necrotic bone by creeping substitution. The final shape of the head depends on the extent of the necrosis and collapse of weakened bone.

## Differential Diagnosis

Differential diagnosis must include inflammation and infection and dysplasia. Transient synovitis of the hip may be distinguished from Legg–Calvé–Perthes disease by serial radiographs.

## Treatment

The principle of treatment is protection of the joint. If the joint is deeply seated within the acetabulum and normal joint motion is maintained, a reasonably good hip can result. Little benefit has been shown from bracing.

## Prognosis

The prognosis for complete replacement of the necrotic femoral head in a child is excellent, but the functional result depends on the amount of deformity that develops during the time the softened structure exists. In Legg–Calvé–Perthes disease, the prognosis depends on the completeness of involvement of the epiphysial center. In general, patients with metaphysial defects, those in whom the disease develops late in childhood, and those who have more complete involvement of the femoral head have a poorer prognosis.

Joseph B et al: Natural evolution of Perthes disease: A study of 610 children under 12 years of age at disease onset. J Pediatr Orthop 2003;23(5):590 [PMID: 12960621].

Hesse B, Kohler G: Does it always have to be Perthes' disease? What is epiphyseal dysplasia? Clin Orthop 2003(414):219 [PMID: 12966296].

## OSTEOCHONDRITIS DISSECANS

In osteochondritis dissecans, a wedge-shaped necrotic area of bone and cartilage develops adjacent to the articular surface. The fragment of bone may be broken off from the host bone and displaced into the joint as a loose body. If it remains attached, the necrotic fragment may be completely replaced by creeping substitution.

The pathologic process is the same as that described previously for avascular necrosing lesions of ossification centers. Because these lesions are adjacent to articular cartilage, however, joint damage may occur.

The most common sites of these lesions are the knee (medial femoral condyle), the elbow joint (capitellum), and the talus (superior lateral dome). Joint pain is the usual presenting complaint. However, local swelling or locking may be present, particularly if a fragment is free in the joint. Laboratory studies are normal.

Treatment consists of protection of the involved area from mechanical damage. If a fragment is free within the joint as a loose body, it must be removed. For some marginal lesions, it may be worthwhile to drill the necrotic fragment to encourage more rapid vascular ingrowth and replacement. If large areas of a weight-bearing joint are involved, secondary degenerative arthritis may result.

Wall E, Von Stein D: Juvenile osteochondritis dissecans. Orthop Clin North Am 2003;34(3):341 [PMID: 12974484].

# ◼ NEUROLOGIC DISORDERS INVOLVING THE MUSCULOSKELETAL SYSTEM

## ORTHOPEDIC ASPECTS OF CEREBRAL PALSY

Early physical therapy to encourage completion of the normal developmental patterns may benefit patients with cerebral palsy. The greatest gains from this therapy are obtained during the first few years of life, and therapy should not be continued when no improvement is apparent.

Bracing and splinting are of questionable benefit, although night splints may be useful in preventing equinus deformity of the feet or adduction contractures of the hips. Orthopedic surgery is useful for treating joint contractures that interfere with function. In general, muscle transfers are unpredictable in cerebral palsy, and most orthopedic procedures are directed at tendon lengthening or bony stabilization by osteotomy or arthrodesis.

Flexion and adduction of the hip due to hyperactivity of the adductors and flexors may produce a progressive paralytic dislocation of the hip, which can lead to pain and dysfunction. Treatment of this dislocation is difficult and unsatisfactory. The principal preventive measure is abduction bracing, but this must often be supplemented by release of the adductors and hip flexors in order to prevent dislocation. In severe cases, osteotomy of the femur may also be necessary to correct the bony deformities of femoral anteversion and coxa valga that are invariably present. Patients with a predominantly athetotic pattern are poor candidates for any surgical procedure or bracing.

Because it is difficult to predict the outcome of surgical procedures in cerebral palsy, the surgeon must examine patients on several occasions before any operative procedure is undertaken. Follow-up care by a physical therapist to maximize the anticipated long-term gains should be arranged before the operation.

Koman LA: Cerebral palsy: Past, present, and future. J South Orthop Assoc 2002;11(2):93 [PMID: 12741589].

## ORTHOPEDIC ASPECTS OF MYELODYSPLASIA

Patients born with spina bifida cystica (aperta) should be examined early by an orthopedic surgeon. The level of neurologic involvement determines the muscle imbalance that will be present and apt to produce deformity with growth. The involvement is often asymmetrical and tends to change during the first 12–18 months of life. Early closure of the sac is the rule, although there has been some hesitancy to provide treatment to all of these patients because of the extremely poor prognosis associated with congenital hydrocephalus, high levels of paralysis, and associated congenital anomalies. A high percentage of these children have hydrocephalus, which may be evident at birth or shortly thereafter, requiring shunting. Associated musculoskeletal problems may include clubfoot, congenital dislocation of the hip, arthrogryposis-type changes of the lower extremities, and congenital scoliosis. The most common lesions are at the level of L3–4 and tend to affect the hip joint, with progressive dislocation occurring during growth. Foot deformities may be in any direction and are complicated by the fact that sensation is generally absent. Spinal deformities develop in a high percentage of these children, with scoliosis present in approximately 40%. Ambulation may require long leg braces. Careful urologic follow-up must be obtained to prevent complications from bladder dysfunction.

In children who have a reasonable likelihood of walking, operative treatment consists of reduction of the hip and alignment of the feet in the weight-bearing position as well as stabilization of the scoliosis. In children who lack active quadriceps function and extensor power of the knee, the likelihood of ambulation is greatly decreased. In such patients, aggressive surgery in the hip region may result in stiffening of the joints, thus preventing sitting. Multiple foot operations are also contraindicated in these children.

The overall treatment of the child with spina bifida should be coordinated in a multidisciplinary clinic where various medial specialists work with therapists, social workers, and teachers to provide the best possible care.

Bartonek A, Saraste H: Factors influencing ambulation in myelomeningocele: A cross-sectional study. Dev Med Child Neurol 2001;43:253 [PMID: 11305403].

# NEOPLASIA OF THE MUSCULOSKELETAL SYSTEM

Neoplastic diseases of the musculoskeletal system are a serious problem because of the poor prognosis of malignant tumors arising in bone or other tissues derived from mesoderm. Fortunately, few of the benign lesions undergo malignant transformation. Accurate diagnosis depends on correlation of the clinical, radiograph, and microscopic findings. Complaints about the knee should be investigated for tumor, although the usual causes of knee pain are traumatic, infectious, or developmental in origin.

Miller SL, Hoffer FA: Malignant and benign bone tumors. Radiol Clin North Am 2001;39:673 [PMID: 11549165].

## Osteochondroma

Osteochondroma is the most common bone tumor in children. It usually presents as a pain-free mass. When present, pain is caused by adventitious bursitis or tendinitis due to irritation by the tumor. The lesion may be single or multiple. Pathologically, the lesion is a bone mass capped with cartilage. These masses tend to grow during childhood and adolescence in proportion to the child's growth.

On radiograph the tumors tend to be in the metaphysial region of long bones and may be pedunculated or sessile. The cortex of the underlying bone "flows" into the base of the tumor.

An osteochondroma should be excised if it interferes with function, is frequently traumatized, or is large enough to be deforming. The prognosis is excellent. Malignant transformation is very rare.

Bottner F et al: Surgical treatment of symptomatic osteochondroma: A three- to eight-year follow-up study. J Bone Joint Surg Br 2003;85(8):1161 [PMID: 14653600].

## Osteoid Osteoma

Osteoid osteoma classically produces night pain that can be relieved by aspirin. On physical examination there usually is tenderness over the lesion. An osteoid osteoma in the upper femur may cause pain referred to the knee.

On radiograph the lesion is a radiolucent nidus surrounded by dense osteosclerosis that may obscure the nidus. Bone scan shows intense uptake in the lesion.

Surgical incision of the nidus is curative and may be done using computed tomography imaging and minimally invasive technique. The prognosis is excellent, with no known cases of malignant transformation, although the lesion has a tendency to recur.

## Enchondroma

Enchondroma is usually a silent lesion unless it produces a pathologic fracture. On radiograph it is radiolucent, usually in a long bone. A speckled calcification may be present. The classic lesion looks as though someone dragged his or her fingernails through clay, making streaks in the bones. Enchondroma is treated by surgical curettage and bone grafting. The prognosis is excellent. Malignant transformation may occur but is very rare in childhood.

## Chondroblastoma

In chondroblastoma, the presenting complaint is pain around a joint. This neoplasm may produce a pathologic fracture. On radiograph the lesion is radiolucent and can perforate the epiphysial cartilage. Calcification is unusual, with little or no reactive bone. The lesion is treated by surgical curettage and bone grafting. The prognosis is excellent if complete curettage is performed. There is no known malignant transformation.

Masui F et al: Chondroblastoma: A study of 11 cases. Eur J Surg Oncol 2002;28(8):869 [PMID: 12477480].

## Nonossifying Fibroma

Nonossifying fibroma is also called benign cortical defect and is nearly always an incidental finding on radiograph. The most frequent sites are the distal femur and proximal tibia. Nonossifying fibroma is a radiolucent lesion eccentrically located in the bone. Usually a thin sclerotic border is evident. Multiple lesions may be present. No treatment is needed because these lesions heal as they ossify with maturation of the bone and growth.

## Osteosarcoma

In osteosarcoma, the presenting complaint is usually pain in a long bone, although functional loss, the mass of the tumor, or limp may be the complaint. Pathologic fracture is common. The malignant osseous tumor produces a destructive expanding and invasive lesion. A triangle may be adjacent to the tumor produced by elevated periosteum and subsequent tumor ossification. The lesion may contain calcification and violates the cortex of the bone. Femur, tibia, humerus, and other long bones are the sites usually affected.

Surgical excision (limb salvage) or amputation is indicated based on the extent of the tumor. The lesion is radioresistant and does not respond to chemotherapy. Adjuvant chemotherapy is routinely used prior to surgical excision. The prognosis is improving, with 30% 5-year survival rates being reported in modern series. Death usually occurs as a result of lung metastasis.

Smeland S et al; Scandinavian Sarcoma Group Osteosarcoma Study SSG VIII: Prognostic factors for outcome and the role of replacement salvage chemotherapy for poor histological responders. Eur J Cancer 2003;39(4):488 [PMID: 12751380].

## Ewing Sarcoma

In Ewing sarcoma, the presenting complaint is usually pain and tenderness. Fever and leukocytosis may also be present, which makes osteomyelitis the main differential diagnosis. The lesion may be multicentric. Ewing sarcoma is radiolucent and destroys the cortex, frequently in the diaphysial region. Reactive bone formation may occur about the lesion, seen as successive layers of so-called onion skin layering.

Treatment is with multiagent chemotherapy, radiation, and surgical resection. The prognosis is poor with large tumor size, pelvic lesions, and poor response to chemotherapy.

# ■ MISCELLANEOUS DISEASES OF BONE

## FIBROUS DYSPLASIA

Dysplastic fibrous tissue replacement of the medullary canal is accompanied by the formation of metaplastic bone in fibrous dysplasia. Three forms of the disease are recognized: monostotic, polyostotic, and polyostotic with endocrine disturbances (precocious puberty in females, hyperthyroidism, and hyperadrenalism [Albright syndrome]).

## Clinical Findings

### A. SYMPTOMS AND SIGNS

The lesion or lesions may be asymptomatic. Pain, if present, is probably due to pathologic fractures. In females, endocrine disturbances may be present in the polyostotic variety and associated with café au lait spots.

### B. LABORATORY FINDINGS

Laboratory findings are normal unless endocrine disturbances are present, in which case secretion of gonadotropic, thyroid, or adrenal hormones may be increased.

### C. IMAGING

The lesion begins centrally within the medullary canal, usually of a long bone, and expands slowly. Pathologic fracture may occur. If metaplastic bone predominates, the contents of the lesion will be of the density of bone. The disease is often asymmetrical, and limb length disturbances may occur as a result of stimulation of epiphysial cartilage growth. Marked deformity of the bone may result, and a shepherd's crook deformity of the upper femur is a classic feature of the disease.

## Differential Diagnosis

The differential diagnosis includes other fibrous lesions of bone as well as destructive lesions such as unicameral bone cyst, eosinophilic granuloma, aneurysmal bone cyst, nonossifying fibroma, enchondroma, and chondromyxoid fibroma.

## Treatment

If the lesion is small and asymptomatic, no treatment is needed. If the lesion is large and produces or threatens pathologic fracture, curettage and bone grafting are indicated.

## Prognosis

Unless the lesions impair epiphysial growth, the prognosis for patients with fibrous dysplasia is good. Lesions tend to enlarge during the growth period but are stable during adult life. Malignant transformation is rare.

## UNICAMERAL BONE CYST

Unicameral bone cyst occurs in the metaphysis of a long bone, usually in the femur or humerus. It begins within the medullary canal adjacent to the epiphysial cartilage. It probably results from some fault in enchondral ossification. The cyst is considered active as long as it abuts onto the metaphysial side of the epiphysial cartilage, and there is a risk of growth arrest with or without treatment.

When a border of normal bone exists between the cyst and the epiphysial cartilage, the cyst is inactive. The lesion is usually identified when a pathologic fracture occurs, producing pain. Laboratory findings are normal. On radiograph, the cyst is identified centrally within the medullary canal, producing expansion of the cortex and thinning over the widest portion of the cyst.

Treatment consists of curettage and bone grafting. The cyst may heal after a fracture.

Wilkins RM: Unicameral bone cysts. J Am Acad Orthop Surg 2000;8(4):217 [PMID: 10951110].

## ANEURYSMAL BONE CYST

Aneurysmal bone cyst is similar to unicameral bone cyst, but it contains blood rather than clear fluid. It usually occurs in a slightly eccentric position in the long bone, expanding the cortex of the bone but not breaking the cortex. Involvement of the flat bones of the pelvis is less common. On radiographs, the lesion appears somewhat larger than the width of the epiphysial cartilage. This feature distinguishes it from unicameral bone cyst.

Chromosomal abnormalities have been associated with aneurysmal bone cyst. The lesion may appear aggressive histologically, and it is important to differenti-

ate it from osteosarcoma or hemangioma. Treatment is by curettage and bone grafting. The prognosis is good.

Papagelopoulos PJ et al: Treatment of aneurysmal bone cysts of the pelvis and sacrum. J Bone Joint Surg Am 2001;83:1674 [PMID: 11701790].

Wyatt-Ashmead J et al: Primary aneurysmal bone cysts: 16q22 and/or 17p13 chromosome abnormalities. Pediatr Dev Pathol 2001;4:418 [PMID: 11441369].

## INFANTILE CORTICAL HYPEROSTOSIS (Caffey Syndrome)

Infantile cortical hyperostosis is a benign disease of unknown cause that has its onset before age 6 months and is characterized by irritability; fever; and nonsuppurating, tender, painful swellings. Swellings may involve almost any bone of the body and are frequently widespread. Classically, swellings of the mandible and clavicle occur in 50% of patients; swellings of the ulna, humerus, and ribs also occur. The disease is limited to the shafts of bones and does not involve subcutaneous tissues or joints. It is self-limited but may persist for weeks or months. Anemia, leukocytosis, an increased ESR, and elevation of the serum alkaline phosphatase concentration are usually present. Cortical hyperostosis is demonstrable by a typical radiographic appearance and may be diagnosed on physical examination by an experienced pediatrician.

Fortunately the disease appears to be decreasing in frequency. Indomethacin may be useful for treatment. The prognosis is good, and the disease usually terminates without deformity.

## GANGLION

A ganglion is a smooth, small cystic mass connected by a pedicle to the joint capsule, usually on the dorsum of the wrist. It may also occur in the tendon sheath over the flexor surfaces of the fingers. These ganglia can be excised if they interfere with function or cause persistent pain.

## BAKER CYST

A Baker cyst is a herniation of the synovium in the knee joint into the popliteal region. In children, the diagnosis may be made by aspiration of mucinous fluid, but the cyst nearly always disappears with time. Whereas Baker cysts may be indicative of intra-articular disease in the adult, they occur without internal derangement in children and rarely require excision.

Van Rhijn LW et al: Long-term follow-up of conservatively treated popliteal cysts in children. J Pediatr Orthop B 2000;9(1):62 [PMID: 10647115].

# Rehabilitation & Sports Medicine | 25

*Pamela E. Wilson, MD, & Dennis J. Matthews, MD*

The development of sports medicine as a unique discipline has grown since the 1980s in response to the expanding body of knowledge in the areas of exercise physiology, biomechanics, and musculoskeletal medicine. The boom in physical fitness and physical activity has generated a need for specialty training in these areas. With the current popularity of starting younger children in more structured athletics, it is essential that the pediatric general practitioner have an understanding of sports medicine.

## ■ BASIC PRINCIPLES

The basic unit of the musculoskeletal system is the muscle fiber, which can be classified as slow twitch, fast twitch, or of intermediate type. Slow twitch, or type I, fibers are smaller, are recruited in muscle contractions first, and are innervated by smaller motor neurons. Fast twitch, or type II, fibers make up white muscle and have a tendency to be larger. They are recruited when the body needs to produce rapid muscle tension. In general they produce more lactic acid than type I fibers. An intermediate type IIa fiber, called fast oxidative glycolytic or FOG, also exists. Untrained individuals have a 50:50 proportion of type I to type II fibers. Elite long-distance runners can have up to 90% type I fibers. This apparent adaptation raises the interesting question as to whether an athlete is genetically programmed or can develop adaptations to be successful in sports.

Exercise generates specific effects on the cardiorespiratory system that include increased $VO_2$ max (maximum amount of oxygen that can be consumed), increased cardiac output, reduced resting heart rate, and improved blood pressure responses.

Biomechanics, the study of movement and how the forces generated by the neuromuscular system translate into these movements, integrates principles of biology and physics. Through biomechanics we can understand the intricacies of movement and how these movements affect athletic performance and result in injuries.

## Types of Muscle Contraction

Dynamic contractions are those movements that result in motion of a limb or rotation around a joint axis. These contractions can be further divided into isotonic and isokinetic contractions. In an isotonic contraction, constant tension is generated during muscle contraction; in an isokinetic contraction, constant velocity is maintained during the contraction. Isotonic exercises can be further classified as detailed in the following sections:

### A. CONCENTRIC

In concentric exercises the force of a muscle contraction overcomes an external resistance, which results in shortening of the muscle. These muscles accelerate a distal segment in the kinetic chain and are therefore referred to as open-chain movements. An example of such an exercise is a biceps curl, during which the biceps is actively contracting or shortening to lift the weight.

### B. ECCENTRIC

In eccentric exercises, contractions increase muscle tension associated with lengthening of the muscle and are used to decelerate a distal segment in the kinetic chain. This type of exercise is exemplified by the squatting motion, in which the quadriceps are lengthening under tension to control downward motion. If the terminal segment in the chain is fixed, this type of movement is called closed kinetic chain movement.

### C. ISOMETRIC

In contrast to dynamic contractions, isometric contractions increase muscle tension without a change in length. An example of this type of exercise would be pushing against a wall. Tension is generated in the muscle, but no movement occurs.

Young JL, Press JM: The physiologic basis of sports rehabilitation. Phys Med Rehabil Clin North Am 1994;5:9.

## Strength Training

Strength is defined as the peak force that can be generated during a maximal single contraction. Strength training is therefore the use of progressive resistance to improve an athlete's ability to resist or exert force. This can be achieved by a variety of techniques, including body weight, free weight, and machine resistance. The benefits of weight training programs are improved performance, endurance, and muscular strength. These programs can be started in prepubescent athletes and, if designed appropriately, can be done safely with minimal risk for injury. Tanner staging (see Chapter 30) helps to define readiness for progression into more strenuous programs. Power lifting and weight lifting should be restricted to those athletes who have reached or passed Tanner stage V. Individuals at Tanner stage IV or less can safely participate in a strength training program that is specifically and carefully designed for younger athletes. These programs incorporate submaximal resistance with multiple repetitions. They can be generalized or sport-specific. Care should be taken to prevent injuries while using weight training equipment at home.

American Academy of Pediatrics: Strength training, weight and power lifting, and body building by children and adolescents. Pediatrics 1990;86:801 [PMID: 2235239].

Faigenbaum AD: Strength training for children and adolescents. Clin Sports Med 2000:19;4:593 [PMID: 11019731].

Jones CS, Christensen C, Young M: Weight training injury: A 20 year survey. Phys Sportsmed 2000;28:7:61.

# PREPARTICIPATION HISTORY & PHYSICAL EXAMINATION

The preparticipation medical examination is designed to evaluate children and screen for potential medical problems that could occur during athletic participation. The objectives of this evaluation are to establish baseline medical information, detect any medical condition that may limit athletic participation, evaluate the athlete for preventable injuries, meet the legal or insurance requirements of most states, assess the athlete's maturity, and make recommendations for necessary protective equipment. The ideal timing of this examination is in preseason, at least 4–6 weeks before training starts. This allows time for any needed interventions by the physician.

## Preparticipation History

The history is the most important part of the encounter. Many key elements need to be explored with the athlete. Several standardized forms are available, including the example in Figure 25–1. The history must include the following areas:

### A. CARDIOVASCULAR HISTORY

The physician should note any history of cardiac murmurs, chest pain at rest or with exertion, sycopal episodes or sudden fatigue, shortness of breath, or recent illnesses with chest pain. The family history should specifically ask about underlying cardiac diseases, including hypertrophic cardiomyopathy, prolonged QT syndrome, Marfan syndrome, arrhythmias, and sudden death in family members. These questions are necessary to identify potentially life-threatening cardiac lesions. The most common cause of sudden death in young athletes on the playing field is hypertrophic cardiomyopathy and congenital heart lesions.

### B. HISTORY OF HYPERTENSION

Any history of hypertension requires further investigation. The current guidelines for the diagnosis of hypertension are blood pressure over 130/75 mm Hg in a child younger than age 10 years or blood pressure over 140/85 mm Hg in a child age 10 years and older.

### C. HISTORY OF CHRONIC DISEASES

Diseases such as asthma or exercise-induced asthma, diabetes, renal disease, neurologic disorders, and hematologic diseases should be noted.

### D. MUSCULOSKELETAL LIMITATIONS AND PRIOR INJURIES

The physician should explore abnormal range of motion or prior injuries that may affect future performance.

### E. MENSTRUAL HISTORY IN FEMALES

The physician should pay particular attention to the so-called female athletic triad: amenorrhea, eating disorders, and osteoporosis.

### F. NUTRITIONAL ISSUES

The physician should record methods the athlete uses to maintain, gain, or lose weight.

### G. MEDICATION HISTORY

This information will provide data on current medications along with the opportunity to discuss the possible use of performance-enhancing supplements such as anabolic steroids, creatine, stimulants, and narcotics.

## Physical Examination

The physical examination should be focused on the needs of the athlete. It may be the only time that an athlete has contact with medical personnel and can be used to promote wellness along with screening for

**PREPARTICIPATION HISTORY**

Name_____DOB_____Age_____Sex (M or F)

Primary Physician_____Sports _____

Allergies (medications, latex, foods, bees, etc) _____

Medications (include prescription, nonprescription, supplements and vitamins) _____

_____

Answer questions by checking Yes (Y)/no (N)/don't know (? )

|  | Y | N | ? |
|---|---|---|---|
| **General Health** | | | |
| 1.  Have you had any injuries or illnesses? | | | |
| 2.  Have you ever been hospitalized? | | | |
| 3.  Do you think you are too thin or overweight? | | | |
| 4.  Have you ever used anything to gain or loss weight? | | | |
| 5.  Any problems exercising in the heat: heat cramps, heat exhaustion or heat stroke? | | | |
| 6.  Ever had frostbite? | | | |
| 7.  Any vision problems? | | | |
| 8.  Do you wear glasses, contact lens, or eye protection? | | | |
| 9.  Any dental appliances? | | | |
| 10. Have you had any surgeries? | | | |
| 11. Any organs missing? | | | |
| 12. Immunizations (tetanus/ hepatitis B) are they current? | | | |
| 13. Any concerns about participating in sports? | | | |
| **Cardiac/Respiratory History** | | | |
| 1.  Has any family member died suddenly, have heart disease before age 50 or other heart problems? | | | |
| 2.  Do you have any dizziness, chest pain, a racing heart, or shortness of breath with exercise? | | | |
| 3.  Have you ever passed out? | | | |
| 4.  Do you have a heart murmur, high blood pressure, or any heart condition? | | | |
| 5.  Can you exercise as much as your friends? | | | |
| 6.  Any history of asthma, problems breathing, coughing with exercise? | | | |
| **Neurologic History** | | | |
| 1.  Any history of a head injury/concussion: being knocked out, dazed, or having memory loss? | | | |
| 2.  Have you ever had a seizure or convulsion? | | | |
| 3.  Any nerve problems: stingers, burners, pinched nerves or numbness? | | | |
| 4.  Any problems with headaches? | | | |
| **Musculoskeletal History** | | | |
| 1.  Do you have a history of sprains, strains or fractures? | | | |
| 2.  Any hip, knee or ankle injuries? | | | |
| 3.  Any shoulder, elbow, wrist, hand or finger injuries? | | | |
| 4.  Any back or neck problems? | | | |
| 5.  Ever have to be in a splint, cast or use crutches? | | | |
| 6.  Do you use any special equipment when competing (braces, orthotics, pads etc) | | | |
| **Females Only** | | | |
| 1.  Any problems with menstruation: cramps, irregularity, etc. | | | |
| 2.  When was your last period? _____ | | | |

**COMMENT ON YES ANSWERS**

_____

_____

_____

_____

_____

_____

_____

*Figure 25–1.* Preparticipation history.

physical activity. Figure 25–2 is an example of a standardized physical examination form. The examination should include routine vital signs including blood pressure measurements obtained in the upper extremity. The cardiovascular examination should include palpation of pulses, auscultation for murmurs with the patient both sitting and standing, and evaluation of the effects of exercise on the individual. The musculoskeletal examination is used to determine strength, range of motion, flexibility, and previous injuries. Table 25–1 is a quick guide that can be used to screen for abnormalities in this area. The remainder of the examination should emphasize the following areas:

## A. SKIN

Are there any contagious lesions such as herpes or impetigo?

## B. VISUAL

Are there any visual problems? Is there any evidence of retinal problems? Are both eyes intact?

## C. ABDOMINAL

Is there any evidence of hepatosplenomegaly?

## D. GENITOURINARY

Is there any history of testicular abnormalities or hernia symptoms?

## E. NEUROLOGIC

Are there any problems with coordination, gait, or mental processing?

## F. SEXUAL MATURITY

What Tanner stage is this individual?

## Recommendations for Participation

After completing the medical examination (history and physical) the physician can make recommendations to the athlete on sports clearance. The options are unrestricted participation, limited participation, or no participation. The American Academy of Pediatrics (AAP) has a list of guidelines, which can be found on their Website. Table 25–2 shows considerations and recommendations for sports activities based on body systems.

American Academy of Pediatrics Committee on Sports Medicine and Fitness: Adolescents and anabolic steroids: A subject review. Pediatrics 1997;99:904 [PMID: 9190555].

Lively MW: Preparticipation physical examination: A collegiate experience. Clin J Sport Med 1999;9:3 [PMID: 10336045].

Myers A, Sickles T: Preparticipation sports examination. Prim Care 1998;25:225 [PMID: 9469925].

West RV: The female athlete. The triad of disordered eating, amenorrhea and osteoporosis. Sports Med 1998;26:63 [PMID: 9777680].

## REHABILITATION OF SPORTS INJURIES

Participation in sports can have tremendous benefits for the individual. It provides physical activity, acquisition of motor skills, and social opportunities. All sports participation, however, carries an inherent risk of injuries. These injuries are classified as either acute or chronic. Chronic injuries occur over time and are related to repetitive stress. These injuries develop in response to overuse, repeated microtrauma, and inadequate repair of injured tissue. Acute injuries, or macrotrauma, are one-time events that can cause alterations in biomechanics and physiology. In response to an acute injury the body responds in a predictable fashion. The first week is characterized by an acute inflammatory response. During this time initial vasoconstriction is followed by vasodilatation. Chemical mediators of inflammation are released and result in the classical physical findings of local swelling, warmth, pain, and loss of function. This phase is essential for injury healing. The next phase occurs over 2–4 weeks and involves repair and clean-up. Fibroblasts infiltrate and lay down new collagen. This allows for repair of the injured area.

The management of acute sports injuries is geared toward optimizing healing and restoring function. The goals of immediate care are to minimize the effects of the injury by reducing pain and swelling, to educate the athlete about the nature of the injury and how to take care of it, and to maintain the health of the rest of the body. The treatment for an acute injury is captured in the acronym PRICE:

- **P**rotect the injury from further damage (taping, splints, braces)
- **R**est the area
- **I**ce
- **C**ompression of the injury
- **E**levation immediately

The use of nonsteroidal anti-inflammatory agents reduces the inflammatory response and reduces discomfort. These medications may be used immediately after the injury. Glucocorticoids should be administered judiciously. If administered inappropriately they may prolong the acute phase of recovery. Therapeutic use of physical modalities, including early cold and later heat, hydrotherapy, massage, electrical stimulation, iontophoresis, and ultrasound, can enhance recovery in the acute phase.

The recovery phase can be lengthy and requires athlete participation. Initial treatment is focused on joint range of motion and flexibility. Range-of-motion exercises should follow a logical progression of starting with passive motion, then moving to active assistive, and finally to active movement. Active range of motion is ini-

# PREPARTICIPATION PHYSICAL EXAM

Name_____

Date of birth/age_____

Height_____Weight_____BP_____

Pulse R wrist_____L wrist_____other_____

Vision R 20/_____L 20/_____ (was it corrected  Y  or  N)

## GENERAL EXAM *(circle normal or abnormal and record results on the form)*

| | | |
|---|---|---|
| APPEARANCE | normal | |
| | abnormal_____ |
| HEENT | normal | |
| | abnormal_____ |
| LUNGS | normal | |
| | abnormal_____ |
| HEART | normal | |
| & PULSES | abnormal_____ |
| ABDOMEN | normal | |
| | abnormal_____ |
| GU | normal | |
| | abnormal_____ |
| SKIN & | normal | |
| LYMPH NODES | abnormal_____ |
| NEURO | normal | |
| | abnormal_____ |

## MUSCULOSKELETAL EXAM *(record ROM or instabilities if abnormal)*

| | | |
|---|---|---|
| NECK | normal | |
| | abnormal_____ |
| BACK | normal | |
| | abnormal_____ |
| SHOULDERS | normal | |
| | abnormal_____ |
| ELBOW & | normal | |
| WRIST | abnormal_____ |
| HANDS & | normal | |
| FINGERS | abnormal_____ |
| HIP | normal | |
| | abnormal_____ |
| KNEE | normal | |
| | abnormal_____ |
| ANKLE & | normal | |
| FOOT | abnormal_____ |

**Cleared for sports**:   YES or NO  If not cleared for sport **WHY?**_____

_____

**Further evaluation/rehab or/secondary clearance:**_____

_____

**Signature examinee:**_____**Date**_____

*Figure 25–2.* Preparticipation physical evaluation.

***Table 25–1.*** The screening sports exam.[a]

| | |
|---|---|
| General evaluation | Have person stand in front of the examiner and evaluate both front and back along with posture<br>Look at general body habitus<br>Look for asymmetry in muscle bulk, scars or unusual postures<br>Watch how the patient moves when instructed |
| Neck evaluation | Evaluate ROM by having person bend head forward (chin to chest), rotate from side to side, and laterally bend (ear to shoulder)<br>Observe for asymmetry, lack of motion or pain with movement |
| Shoulder and upper extremity evaluation | Observe clavicles, shoulder position, scapular position, elbow position, and fingers<br>ROM screening<br>  Fully abduct arms with palms in jumping jack position<br>  Internally and externally rotate shoulder<br>  Flex and extend wrist, pronate and supinate wrist, flex and extend fingers<br>Do the following manual muscle testing:<br>  Have person shrug shoulders (testing trapezius)<br>  Abduct to 90 degrees (testing deltoid)<br>  Flex elbow (testing biceps)<br>  Extend elbow over head (testing triceps)<br>  Test wrist flexion and extension<br>  Have person grasp fingers |
| Back evaluation | General inspection to look for scoliosis or kyphosis<br>ROM screening<br>  Bend forward touching toes with knees straight (spine flexion and hamstring range)<br>  Rotation, side bending, and spine extension |
| Gait and lower extremity evaluation | General observation while walking<br>Walk short distance normally (look at symmetry, heel-toe gait pattern, look at all joints involved in gait and leg lengths, any evidence of joint effusions or pain)<br>Have person toe-walk and heel-walk for short distance and check tandem walking (balance beam walking) |

[a]If any abnormalities are found, then a more focused evaluation is required.

tiated once normal joint range has been reestablished. Flexibility is sport-specific and aimed at reducing tight musculature. Strength training can begin early in this phase of rehabilitation. Initially only isometric exercises are encouraged. As recovery progresses and flexibility increases, isotonic and isokinetic exercises can be added to the program. These should be done at least three times per week. As the athlete approaches near-normal strength and is pain-free, the final maintenance phase can be introduced. During this phase the athlete will continue to build strength and work on endurance. The biomechanics of sport-specific activity needs to be analyzed and retraining incorporated into the exercise program. Generalized cardiovascular conditioning should continue during the entire rehabilitation treatment.

# ■ COMMON SPORTS MEDICINE ISSUES AND INJURIES

## INFECTIOUS DISEASES

Infectious diseases are common in both recreational and competitive athletes. These illnesses have an effect on basic physiologic function and athletic performance. Given this knowledge, physicians, parents, and coaches can adopt the common-sense guidelines listed in Table 25–3.

American Academy of Pediatrics Committee on Sports Medicine and Fitness: Human immunodeficiency virus (acquired immunodeficiency syndrome—AIDS virus) in the athletic setting. Pediatrics 1991;88:640 [PMID: 1881749].

## HEAD & NECK INJURIES

Head and neck injuries occur most commonly in contact and individual sports. The sports with the highest incidence of brain injury are football, bicycling, baseball, horseback riding, and golf. The treatment of these is controversial, with multiple guidelines being developed. Because young children have developing central nervous systems, injuries in these children should be treated conservatively.

**Concussion** is a temporary and immediate impairment of neurologic function and is classified by length of unconsciousness, posttraumatic amnesia (PTA), and confusion. Concussions are categorized as grade 1 (mild), grade 2 (moderate), or grade 3 (severe). Return-to-competition guidelines have been developed by several resources. Table 25–4 reviews guidelines for return to play.

***Table 25–2.*** Recommendations and considerations for paticipation in sports

| Disorders | Considerations and Recommendations | References |
|---|---|---|
| **Cardiac** | | |
| Anticoagulation treatment | Need to avoid all contact sports | |
| Aortic stenosis | Individualize treatment based on disease and systolic gradient<br>    Mild: < 20 mm Hg, all sports if asymptomatic.<br>    Moderate: limited sports.<br>    Severe: no competitive sports. | |
| Arrhythmias | Consult with cardiologist as WPW and long QT syndrome can have serious consequences. | |
| Congestive heart failure (CHF) | Screen patient with LVEF < 30 % for ischemia.<br>Use AHA risk stratification criteria to define exercise capacity. | Braith, 2002 |
| Heart implants | No jumping, swimming, or contact sports. | |
| Hypertrophic cardiomyopathy | Single most common cause of cardiac death in young athletes.<br>Athletes should not participate in sports except possibly low intensity forms (eg, golf, bowling).<br>Consult with cardiologist. | Maron, 2002a,b |
| Marfan syndrome | Aortic root dilation is associated with mitral valve prolapse and regurgitation.<br>Participate in sports with minimal physical demands. | Salim et al, 2001 |
| Mitral valve prolapse | Fairly common condition.<br>No restrictions unless there is a history of syncope, positive family history of sudden death, arrhythmias with exercise, or moderate regurgitation. | |
| Syncope | Unexplained syncopal episodes during exercise must be evaluated by ECG, echocardiograph, Holter, and tilt test prior to resumption of any activities. | Firoozi, 2002 |
| **Endocrine** | | |
| Diabetes type I | No restrictions to activity, however:<br>    Short-term exercise = no insulin changes.<br>    Vigorous exercise = 25% reduction in insulin with 15–30 g of carbohydrates before and every 30 min during exercise.<br>    Strenuous exercise = may require up to an 80% reduction in insulin with extra carbohydrates.<br>Generally monitor blood glucose closely. | Birrer et al, 2003<br>Draznin, 2000 |
| **Eye** | | |
| Detached retina | Do not participate in strenuous sports regardless of contact risk. | Moeller, 1996 |
| One eye | Consider avoiding contact sports although if patient does participate use of eye protection is a must. | Vinger, 2000 |
| **Gentiourinary** | | |
| One testicle | Need to wear protective cups in collision/contact sports. | |
| Solitary kidney | Advise not to participate in collision/contact sports. | Terrell, 1997 |
| **Hematologic** | | |
| Hemophilia | Avoid contact/collision sports. | |
| Sickle cell trait | No restrictions if disorder well under control.<br>Athletes should avoid dehydration and acclimate to altitude.<br>There is however a known association between exercise and sudden death. | |

*(continued)*

*Table 25–2.* Recommendations and considerations for paticipation in sports (continued)

| Disorders | Considerations and Recommendations | References |
|---|---|---|
| **Infectious Disease** | | |
| General considerations | Fevers; should not participate in activities with moderate fevers; exercise affects fluid balance, immune system function, and temperature regulation.<br>Intense exercise may worsen or prolong some viral illnesses. | Howe, 2003<br>Primos, 1996 |
| Enterovirus, coxsackie virus | Causes respiratory and GI symptoms but more importantly can cause myocarditis.<br>Anyone with systemic symptoms such as fever or myalgias should avoid strenuous exercise. | Primos, 1996 |
| Herpes simplex, impetigo, tinea corpora | Close contact is required for transmission; use commone sense guidelines.<br>For contact sports participation should not be allowed until lesions are crusted over or healed. | Moeller, 1996 |
| Infectious mononucleosis | Splenic rupture is most important consideration.<br>Risk of spleen rupture highest during second and third weeks of illness.<br>No athletic participation for a minimum of 21 days!<br>Splenic ultrasounds should be considered in decision making.<br>Too early a return to sports could cause EBV reactivation and relapse.<br>First week of return to activity should be noncontact.<br>Graded increases in intensity if fatigue tolerance is improved.<br>Return to full activity if: no abdominal pain, normal spleen and normal labs. | MacKnight, 2002 |
| Sinusitis | Similar considerations as cold (see below) except diving should be restricted until symptoms resolve. | |
| *Streptococcus* A | Restrict from activity until afebrile and on antibiotics for > 24 h | O'Kane, 2002 |
| Upper respiratory infections (including common cold) | "Neck check," with symptoms (fevers, myalgias, arthralgias, etc) above the neck participation can be allowed; however, if they migrate below that level activity should be limited. | Primos 1996 |
| **Neurologic** | | |
| Epiliepsy | Majority of sports are safe with good seizure control; contact sports are allowed with proper protection.<br>Definitely wear a helmet.<br>Fitness may reduce number of seizures.<br>Swimming and water sports should be supervised.<br>Sports such as free climbing, hang gliding, scuba not recommended. | Howard, 2004 |
| Herniated disk (with cord compression) | Avoid contact and collision sports. | |
| Muscle disease or myopathy | Exercise within physical limits.<br>Low to moderate intensity activity is appropriate for patients with slow progressive disorders.<br>Patients with disorder that are rapidly progressing should avoid high resistance and eccentric muscle activity.<br>Modification of exercise with intercurrent illness. | Tarnopolsky, 2002<br>Ansved, 2003 |
| Spinal stenosis | Avoid contact and colision sports. | |
| **Orthopedic** | | |
| Scoliosis | No restrictions unless severe. | |
| Spondylolisthesis | Grade 2 and above should avoid high-risk sports. | |
| Spondylolysis | Pars intrarticularis stress fracture.<br>No restrictions if pain-free. | |

*(continued)*

*Table 25–2.* Recommendations and considerations for paticipation in sports (continued)

| Disorders | Considerations and Recommendations | References |
|---|---|---|
| **Respiratory** | | |
| Asthma | No activity restrictions.<br>Use common sense about when to use medications. | Disabella et al. 1998 |
| Pneumothorax | Can occur in sports, expecially in males.<br>Increased risk for reoccurrence; should consider not participating in strenuous and contact sports. | |
| TB | Not allowed to participate because of exposure to other athletes. | |
| **Other** | | |
| Cerebral palsy | Full participation with modifications. | |
| Developmental disabilities | Athletes with developmental disabilities often have associated medical problems including diabetes, obesity, and hypokinesia. | Platt, 2001 |
| Downs syndrome | 10–20% have atlantoaxial instability.<br>All athletes need to be cleared with a lateral view radiograph including flexion and extension.<br>    If abnormal no contact sports should be allowed.<br>Evaluation of underlying congenital heart disorders should be considered in this population. | Platt, 2001<br>Winell, 2003 |
| Spinal cord injury/ spina bifida | Full participation.<br>Consider modification of equipment to accommodate activity and/or modification of activity to accommodate disability.<br>Consider how modification affects performance.<br>Beaware of thermoregulatory dysfunction, medications, and pressure areas. | |

**Second impact syndrome** is a rare but potentially deadly complication of head injuries. It occurs in athletes who have a second brain injury before recovering from a prior brain injury. It results in loss of vascular autoregulation and subsequent malignant cerebral edema.

**Cervical spine injuries** are fairly common but potentially serious. They can cause ligamentous injuries along with spinal cord injuries The most frequent neck injury is a cervical strain. Return to play is allowed when neck range of motion is full and pain-free, and strength is normal.

**Atlantoaxial instability** is common in children with Down syndrome because of underlying ligamentous laxity. Cervical neck films including the neck in flexion and extension evaluate the atlantodens interval. Normal is less than 2.5 mm, but up to 4.5 mm is acceptable in this population. Children with an interval greater than 4.5 mm should be restricted in activities.

American Academy of Neurology: Practice parameter: The management of concussion in sports (Summary statement). Report of the Quality standards subcommittee. Neurology 1997;48:581 [PMID: 9065530].

American Academy of Pediatrics Committee on Sports Medicine and Fitness: Atlantoaxial instability in Down syndrome: Subject review. Pediatrics 1995;96:151 [PMID: 7596705].

Cantu RC: Guidelines for return to contact sports after a cerebral concussion. Phys Sportsmed 1986;14:75.

Cole AJ et al: Cervical spine athletic injuries: A pain in the neck. Phys Med Rehabil Clin North Am 1994;5:37.

Colorado Medical Society: *Report of the Sports Medicine Committee: Guidelines for the Management of Concussion in Sports* (revised). Colorado Medical Society, 1991.

**Burners and stingers** are common injuries in contact sports, especially football. These types of cervical radiculopathies or brachial plexopathies occur when the head is laterally bent and the shoulder depressed. Symptoms include immediate burning pain and paresthesias down one arm, generally lasting only minutes. Weakness in the muscles of the upper trunk (supraspinatous, deltoid, and bicep) can persist for weeks. Work-up includes a thorough neurologic assessment. If symptoms persist, then a diagnostic evaluation should include cervical spine radiographs, magnetic resonance imaging (MRI) scans, and electromyography. The athlete can return to play once symptoms have resolved, neck and shoulder range of motion is pain-free,

***Table 25–3.*** Sports participation guidelines: infectious diseases.

Athletes with temperatures higher than 100°F should not participate in sporting activities.

Athletes who have had recent infectious mononucleosis can return to noncontact training at 3 wk as long as there is no splenic enlargement. They may return to contact sports after 4 wk and a normal abdominal examination.

Athletes with a streptococcal pharyngitis can resume activity once treatment has been initiated and they are afebrile.

If a localized herpes gladiatorum or impetigo lesion is present, no contact sports are allowed until the lesions have resolved. Athletes with herpes zoster have the same restrictions. There are no restrictions for athletes with common warts. Athletes with molluscum contagiosum can compete if the affected areas are covered. Athletes with furuncles cannot be involved in contact sports or swimming until the lesions are healed.

Athletes with HIV infection may compete in all types of sports. Universal precautions should be used with all athletes who have sustained injuries.

reflexes and strength are normal, and the Spurling's test is negative. Preventative strategies include always wearing protective gear, proper blocking and tackling techniques, and maintaining good neck and shoulder strength.

Feinberg JH: Burners and stingers. Phys Med Rehabil Clin North Am 2000;11:4:771 [PMID. 11092018].

## SPINE INJURIES

Injuries to the spine are fairly common even in the pediatric population. As children have become more competitive in sports, the number of reported injuries has increased. Sports with a fairly high incidence of back injuries are golf, gymnastics, football, dance, wrestling, and weight lifting. Pain lasting more than 2 weeks indicates a possible structural problem and needs to be investigated.

**Herniated discs** account for a small percentage of back injuries in children. These injuries are almost unheard of in preadolescence. Most injuries occur at the L4–5 and L5–S1 vertebrae. Symptoms include back and leg pain. Pain may be increased with activities such as bending, sitting, and coughing. Pain often radiates down the lower extremity in a radicular pattern. Evaluation comprises a physical and neurologic exam, including straight-leg testing, sensory testing, and checking reflexes. If symptoms persist, then the evaluation should include electromyographic, computed tomo-

graphic, and MRI scans. Treatment generally is conservative because most back injuries improve spontaneously. The athlete can rest the back for a short period and then begin on a structured exercise program of extension and isometrics followed by flexion exercises. If symptoms persist, then a short course of steroids may be indicated. Surgery is recommended only if neurologic compromise persists.

**Spondylolysis** is an injury to the pars interarticularis. Pars defects are present in 4–6 % of the population. Repetitive stress to this area results in fractures. The injury is common in gymnasts, dancers, and football players. Spondylolysis occurs at L5 in 85% of cases. Pain usually develops during an adolescent growth spurt. Back pain may radiate into the buttocks or thigh area. Extension of the spine increases pain. Evaluation includes an oblique radiographic view of the spine to look for the "Scottie dog sign." Treatment includes rest

***Table 25–4.*** Return-to-competition guidelines following concussion.

**Grade 1 or mild concussion**
No loss of consciousness (LOC)
PTA or confusion lasting less than 15 min
   *First Injury*
   • Remove from game
   • Return to play in 15 minutes if exam is normal
   *Second injury*
   • Return to play if asymptomatic after one week
**Grade 2 or moderate concussion**
No LOC
PTA or confusion lasting longer than 15 minutes
   *First Injury*
   • Remove from game
   • Hospital evaluation if symptoms persist for more than one hour
   • Return to play if asymptomatic after one week
   • CT or MRI if symptoms persist for more than 1 wk
   *Second Injury*
   • Return to play if asymptomatic after two weeks
   *Third Injury*
   • Out for season
**Grade 3 or severe concussion**
Any LOC
   *First Injury*
   • Transport to hospital for evaluation
   • With a brief LOC (seconds), return to play if asymptomatic after one week
   • With a longer LOC (minutes), return to play if asymptomatic after 2 wk
   *Second Injury*
   • No play for at least one month following absence of symptoms; consider ending season

from sporting activities, stretching of the hamstrings, stabilization exercises, lumbosacral bracing, and occasionally surgery.

If a bilateral pars injury occurs, then slippage of one vertebra over another (**spondylolisthesis**) can occur. These injuries are graded on a scale of 1 to 4 based on the percentage of slippage: grade 1, 0–25%; grade 2, 25–49%%; grade 3, 50–74%; and grade 4, 75–100%. Diagnosis is based on lateral radiographs, and treatment is symptomatic. Asymptomatic athletes with less than 30% slippage have no restrictions and are followed up on a routine basis. Slippage of 50% requires interventions of stretching hip flexors and hamstrings, along with bracing or surgery.

Drezner JA, Herring SA: Managing low back pain: Steps to optimize and hasten return to activity. Phys Sportsmed 1999; 272:37.

Letts M, McDonald P: Sports injuries to the pediatric spine. Spine: State of the Art Review 1990;4:49.

## SHOULDER INJURIES

In evaluating shoulder injuries it is necessary to look at both macro- and microtrauma. Fractures and dislocations account for most macrotrauma. The balance of other injuries are related to repetitive overuse and tissue failure. Rotator **cuff injuries** are common in athletics that require repetitive overhead motions (eg, gymnastics, and pitching in baseball). Muscle imbalances and injury cause the position of the humeral head to be abnormal which may cause impingement of the supraspinatous tendon under the acromial arch. Pain is usually reported in the anterior and lateral shoulder and is increased with overhead activities. Diagnostic work-up includes plain radiographs and an outlet view to look for anatomic variability. The rehabilitation of this injury is geared toward reduction of inflammation, improved flexibility, and strengthening of the scapular stabilizers and rotator cuff muscles. This is achieved by a progression of isometric followed by isotonic or isokinetic exercises. A biomechanics evaluation can assist in the recovery process by building sport-specific skills and eliminating substitution patterns.

Tytherleigh-Strong G et al: Rotator cuff disease. Curr Opin Rheumatol 2001;13;2:135 [PMID: 11224738].

## ELBOW & FOREARM INJURIES

Injuries in the forearm are quite common, with both chronic and acute causes (eg, the chronic overuse "little league elbow" and the frequent childhood fracture when falling on an outstretched arm).

## Medial Elbow Pain

Medial elbow pain can have multiple causes, but one of the most common is **medial epicondylitis,** an overuse injury caused by valgus stress at the elbow. **Little league elbow** consists of a group of abnormalities that develop in young baseball pitchers. These abnormalities are secondary to the biomechanical forces generated around the elbow during throwing. These forces can result in shearing, inflammation, traction, and abnormal bone development. Pitching can be divided into four phases: wind-up, cocking, acceleration, and follow-through. The acceleration phase is where most forces are generated.. The symptoms are primarily swelling, pain, performance difficulties, and weakness. The pain localizes to the medial epicondyle, which may be tender to palpation. Wrist flexion and pronation increase symptoms. The different phases of throwing should be analyzed to isolate when the pain appears. If pain is present in all phases this may indicate a severe injury. Work-up includes a series of elbow radiographs, including stress films and comparison films, to look for widening of the epiphysial lines, and MRI studies. Treatment of the acute injury includes rest. It is not uncommon for a player to be benched for up to 6 weeks. Competition can be resumed once the player is asymptomatic.

The key to treating this injury is prevention. Children should be properly conditioned and coached in correct throwing biomechanics. Guidelines are available for pitching limits in youth baseball. Little League limits 10- to 12-year-old children to six innings/week and 13- to 15-year-old children to nine innings/week. Limiting pitches per game has been outlined as shown in Table 25–5.

Other causes of medial elbow pain include ulnar collateral ligament injury, ulnar neuritis, apophysitis, and fractures.

***Table 25–5.*** Guidelines for pitching limits in youth baseball.

| Age (years) | Pitches/game[a] |
|---|---|
| 8–10 | 52 ± 15 |
| 11–12 | 68 ± 18 |
| 13–14 | 76 ± 16 |
| 15–16 | 91 ± 16 |
| 16–17 | 106 ± 16 |

[a]Based on 2 games/week.

## Lateral Elbow Pain

Lateral elbow pain can be the result of a few unique problems in growing athletes. **Panner disease** is also caused by valgus stress at the elbow. It is a focal process in the capitellum and occurs in players age 5–12 years. The child presents with dull aching in the lateral elbow that generally worsens when the child throws something. Swelling and reduced elbow extension are usually present. Radiographs show an abnormal capitellum with fragmentation and areas of sclerosis. Treatment is conservative, using rest, ice, and splinting. The child can return to play after the radiographs normalize.

The same type of pain in a 13- to 15-year-old athlete is usually **osteochondritis dissecans.** This injury is basically avascular necrosis of the capitellum, which can result in the formation of loose bodies. Radiographs are needed in the diagnosis and help to classify the injury into one of three categories. Treatment is based on the classification and can be either conservative or surgical in nature. The child should be seen by an orthopedic specialist.

**Lateral epicondylitis** is common in racquet sports, particularly tennis. It is an overuse of the extensor muscle in the forearm and causes pain in the lateral elbow. Pain is increased by wrist extension. Initial treatment is aimed at inflammation control. Stretching and strengthening of forearm muscles are the primary interventions during the subsequent phases. Stroke mechanics may need to be altered and a forearm brace used to decrease the forces in the extensor muscles.

## Posterior Elbow Pain

Posterior elbow pain is not very common. Causes include dislocations, fractures, triceps avulsions, and olecranon bursitis.

Abrams JS: Special shoulder problems in the throwing athlete: Pathology, diagnosis and nonoperative management. Clin Sports Med 1991;10:839 [PMID: 1934100].

Axe M: Recommendation for protecting youth baseball pitches. Sports Med Arthoscopy Rev 2001;9.

Chumbley EM et al: Evaluation of overuse elbow injuries. Am Fam Physician 2000;1:61:69 [PMID: 10695582].

Hall TJ: Osteochondritis dissecans of the elbow: Diagnosis, treatment and prevention. Phys Sportsmed 1999;272:75.

Johnson EW: Tennis elbow misconceptions and widespread mythology. Am J Phys Med Rehabil 2000;79:2:113 [PMID: 10744183].

# HAND & WRIST INJURIES

All hand and wrist injuries have the potential for long-term, often serious disability and deserve a thorough evaluation.

## 1. Hand Injuries

### Distal Phalanx Injuries

**Tuft injury** requires splinting for 6 weeks or until the patient is pain-free. If displacement is significant, then a K-wire can be used for reduction. **Nail bed injury** often requires splinting and drainage of subungual hematomas.

### Distal Interphalangeal Injuries

**Mallet finger** or **extensor tendon avulsion** occurs in ball-handling sports. The mechanism of injury is a force applied to an extended finger. Treatment is splinting in extension for 6 weeks for fractures and 8 weeks for tendon rupture.

### Thumb Injuries

**Gamekeeper's thumb** is an injury to the ulnar collateral ligament from forced abduction of the metacarpal phalangeal joint. It is a common skiing injury. If a radiograph shows an avulsed fragment is displaced less than 2 mm, a thumb spica cast can be used. If no fragment is apparent and less than 35 degrees of lateral joint space opening occurs, a spica cast is indicated for 6 weeks. Surgery is required for more serious injuries.

### Fractures

Boxer's fracture is a neck fracture of the fifth digit. These fractures can be treated by closed reduction and casting for 3 weeks. A displaced fracture requires open reduction and internal fixation.

## 2. Wrist Injuries

Most swollen wrists without evidence of instability can be splinted for several weeks. Radial and ulnar fractures must be ruled out because these are fairly common in children.

**Scaphoid fractures** are caused by a force applied to a hyperextended wrist. If evidence of snuff box tenderness and swelling is present, the wrist must be immobilized for 10 days and then reassessed, even if radiographs are normal. A nondisplaced fracture requires at least 6 weeks of immobilization in a thumb spica cast.

Geissler WB: Carpal fractures in athletes. Clin Sports Med 2001;1563:1961 [PMID: 11227704].

Krasin et al: Review of the current methods in the diagnosis and treatment of scaphoid fractures. Postgrad Med J 2001;77: 906:235 [PMID: 11264484].

Wang QC, Johnson BA: Fingertip injuries. Am Fam Physician 2000;1:61:69 [PMID: 11388710].

# HIP INJURIES

Because the pelvis and hip articulate with both the lower extremities and the spine, this is an area rich in ligaments, muscle attachments, and nerves. Injuries in young children are rare, but sprains and strains are common.

**Groin pull,** or **adductor strain,** is generally caused by forced abduction as in running, falling, twisting, or tackling. The associated pain is in the adductor muscle. Pain may arise with adduction or hip flexion, and tenderness may be present over the adductor tubercle. Treatment includes rest, ice, protection, and strengthening of the muscle when it heals.

**Quadriceps contusion** is caused by a direct macroinjury to the muscle, resulting in bruising, swelling, and pain. The anterior and lateral thigh regions are most commonly injured. If the muscle remains firm on examination after 2 weeks, then radiographs of the thigh should be done to rule out myositis ossificans. (**Myositis ossificans** is an abnormal deposition of calcium in the muscle that may be induced by aggressive stretching of the muscle too early in the clinical course.) Treatment is rest, ice, and protection for the first 24 hours. The knee should be kept in a fully flexed position. Two to three days after the injury, range-of-motion exercises may begin in both flexion and extension. Once 120 degrees of motion has been established and movement does not cause pain, the athlete may return to competitive activity.

**Hamstring strain** is very common in many sports. The mechanism of injury is forced extension of the knee. Examination reveals pain on palpation of the muscle. Pain also occurs with knee flexion against resistance. Treatment is rest, ice, and compression. The athlete can walk as soon as he or she can tolerate the activity. It is particularly important to stretch the hamstring because, as a two-joint muscle, it is more susceptible to injury than other types of muscle.

The bursa is a structure that allows for improved motion by reducing friction. When a bursa becomes inflamed, movement is painful and may be limited. Areas susceptible to bursal inflammation are the shoulder, elbow, patella, and hip. **Trochanteric bursitis,** causing pain when the hip is flexed, often results from reduced flexibility of the iliotibial band and gluteus medius tendons. It is best evaluated in a side-lying position, and pain is reproduced when the hip is actively flexed from a fully extended hip. Initial treatment is to alter the offending activity and then start a stretching program geared at the iliotibial band and hip abductors. Corticosteroid injections may be used after conservative treatment has failed.

Most **hip dislocations** are in the posterior direction. Athletes with this injury classically present with hip flexion, adduction, and internal rotation.

Hip dislocations in skeletally mature athletes are almost always associated with acetabular and femoral neck fracture. The preadolescent, skeletally immature competitor may have an isolated injury. This is a true on-field emergency, and the athlete should be transported to the nearest facility that has an orthopedic surgeon available. Severe bleeding, avascular necrosis, and nerve damage can result. Once reduction has been established in a noncomplicated case, protected weight bearing on crutches for 6 weeks is recommended, followed by another 6 weeks of range-of-motion and strengthening exercises. An athlete may return gradually to competition after 3 months when strength and motion are normal.

Femoral neck fractures (**stress fractures**) are generally the result of repetitive microtrauma. They commonly occur in track athletes who have increased their mileage. Athletes with this type of injury present with persistent pain in the groin and pain with internal and external rotation. Range of motion may be limited in hip flexion and internal rotation. If plain radiographs are negative, then a bone scan is indicated. Treatment is based on the type of fracture. A **transverse fracture** generally requires internal fixation to prevent femoral displacement from occurring and potentially causing avascular necrosis. A **compression fracture** is less likely to be displaced; treatment is conservative and involves resting the hip until it heals. Cardiovascular conditioning can be maintained easily through nonimpact exercises and activity.

Maffulli N: Lower limb injuries in children in sports. Clin Sports Med 2000;19:637 [PMID: 11019733].

# KNEE INJURIES

Knee injuries are one of the most common problems evaluated by any practitioner. The function of the knee is for mobility and stability. Knee movements include flexion, extension, rotation, rolling, and gliding. The knee is stabilized through a variety of ligaments, tendons, and the meniscus.

## Anterior Knee Pain

The most common knee compliant is anterior knee pain. This complaint can have multiple causes but should always include hip pathology as a possibility. Patellofemoral syndrome is a common cause of anterior knee pain. The differential diagnosis is quite extensive and requires a thorough examination.

**Patellofemoral overuse syndrome** occurs in runners and in athletes participating in sports with repetitive stress in the lower extremity. Classically, pain is located over the medial surface and under surface of the patella. It is associated with swelling and crepitus of the knee joint. The Q-angle often is increased. The Q-angle is measured by drawing a line from the anterior superior iliac spine down to the center of the patella and then through the tibial tubercle. The intersecting angle is the Q-angle. Normal is 14 degrees for males and 17 degrees for females. Q-angles greater than 20 degrees tend to track the patella laterally, changing the knee biomechanics.

**Plicae alares** are normal synovial folds in the knee joint. If they become thickened or fibrosed they can become entrapped. This happens with direct macrotrauma or repetitive microtrauma. The athlete complains of snapping or popping in the knee. The knee pain is worse with knee flexion, and activity intensifies symptoms. On examination the hamstrings may be tight. Physical findings include localized tenderness and occasionally popping palpable at 30–60 degrees of knee flexion.

**Tendonitis** of the patellar tendon is caused by overuse. The mechanism is repetitive loading of the quadriceps during running or jumping. **Osgood–Schlatter disease** occurs in the preteen and adolescent years. It is most common in boys age 12–15 years and in girls age 11–13 years. Pain usually is present at the tibial tubercle, and activities using eccentric quadriceps muscle movement aggravate the pain. The pain can become so extensive that routine activity must be curtailed. Radiographs may or may not show abnormalities. Type 1 disease has no findings, whereas type 2 shows evidence of fragmentation of the tibial tubercle. Many other conditions can cause anterior knee pain and need to be ruled out, including arthritis, complex regional pain syndrome, infections, and neoplasm. Finally, **chondromalacia patellae** is an arthroscopic diagnosis and should not be used as a clinical diagnosis.

## Treatment of Anterior Knee Pain

As with any acute injury, control of inflammation is essential. This begins with rest and ice. Alignment problems should be corrected with stretching and strengthening. Orthotics may need to be used for correction of foot deformities. Quadriceps strengthening begins with isometric exercises that progress to a concentric program. These include short-arc (the last 10 degrees of knee extension) contractions of the vastus medialis. In the last part of the therapy program, eccentric loading of the quadriceps can be incorporated. During this time the athlete should be working on endurance and cardiovascular conditioning. Knee bracing is controversial, and the major benefits are proprioceptive feedback and patellar tracking.

## Lateral Knee Pain

Lateral knee pain is most commonly associated with a tight iliotibial band, which can lead to **tendonitis** and

**bursitis.** Pain over the lateral femoral condyle is present along with a positive Ober test. The Ober test is done with the athlete in a side-lying position. The knee and hip are flexed to 90 degrees, then the hip is maximally abducted and extended. From this position the leg is allowed to drop by gravity while the knee is still controlled. It will not relax if the iliotibial band is tight. Treatment involves rest and stretching. Athletics should not be resumed until the patient is pain-free. This may take up to 6 weeks. Other sources of lateral knee pain are popliteus tendonitis and biceps tendonitis.

## Posterior Knee Pain

Posterior knee pain usually results from an injury to the gastrocnemius–soleus complex caused by overuse. It can also include a Baker cyst, tibial stress fracture, or tendonitis of the hamstring. Treatment is rest, ice, and strengthening exercises after symptoms have improved.

## Meniscal Injuries

The meniscus of the knee cushions forces in the knee joint, increases nutrient supply to the cartilage, and stabilizes the knee. Most injuries are related to directional changes on a weight-bearing extremity. **Medial meniscus injuries** have a history of tibial rotation in a weight-bearing position. This happens frequently in ball-handling sports. **Lateral meniscus injuries** occur with tibial rotation with a flexed knee. These injuries are uncommon in children younger than age 10 years. The athlete with such an injury has a history of knee pain, swelling, snapping, or locking, or may report a feeling of the knee giving way. Physical examination reveals joint line tenderness and a positive McMurray hyperflexion/rotation test. The diagnostic test of choice is MRI of the knee, although standard knee radiographs should be included. Arthrograms are still used by some practitioners. Treatment may be symptomatic for isolated injuries of the meniscus with no ligamentous involvement or mechanical blocks. . If surgery is needed, the athlete should not bear weight on the knee for 3 weeks. During this time, range-of-motion and strengthening exercises can be done.

## Medial & Lateral Collateral Ligament Injuries

The medial and lateral collateral ligaments are positioned along either side of the knee and act to stabilize it. They help to control varus and valgus stress applied to the knee joint. Excessive varus or valgus stress causes stretching of the ligament, producing tears. Medial injuries occur with a blow to the lateral aspect of the knee, as seen in a football tackle. The athlete may feel a pop or lose sensation along the medial aspect of the knee. The examination reveals an effusion and tenderness medially. A valgus stress test done in full extension and 20–30 degrees of flexion will reproduce pain. Diagnosis is made by routine and stress radiographs of the knee.

Treatment is almost always conservative. Initial injuries should be iced and elevated. A protective brace needs to be worn, and full knee motion in the brace can be done after 7 days. Weight bearing is allowed, and a strengthening program can be started. The athlete should use the brace until he or she is pain-free and has full range of motion. The use of a functional brace is often required when a player returns to competition. This is only temporary until the ligaments heal properly.

## Anterior Cruciate Ligament Injuries

The anterior cruciate ligament (ACL) has three bands and prevents anterior subluxation of the tibia. The ACL is injured by deceleration, twisting, and cutting motions. The mechanism of the injury involves force applied to the knee during hyperextension, with excessive valgus stress and forced external rotation of the femur on a fixed tibia. Evaluation of the knee begins with examining the noninjured knee. The Lachman test will provide information on knee stability in relation to the ACL. All other structures of the knee need to be examined to rule out concomitant injuries. Imaging of the knee includes plain radiographs along with MRI scan.

Treatment options include both conservative and surgical procedures. Conservative treatment includes bracing, strengthening, and restricting physical activity. The braces used today enhance proprioception and control terminal extension. Surgical repair is quite popular, and a patellar tendon graft is used frequently. Rehabilitation of the knee starts immediately after surgery. A continuous passive range-of-motion machine is used postoperatively. Partial weight bearing is allowed in a brace that is set in full extension as the quadriceps strengthen. After 2 weeks, partial weight bearing and walking are started. The goals of the subsequent program are continued strength, muscle reeducation, endurance, agility, and coordination.

## Posterior Cruciate Ligament Injuries

The posterior cruciate ligament (PCL) runs from the medial femoral condyle to the posterior tibial plateau and has two parts. Its main function is to prevent posterior tibial subluxation. This is an extremely rare injury and occurs when the individual falls on a flexed knee with the ankle in plantarflexion or with forced hy-

perflexion of the knee. The examination begins with the noninjured knee and proceeds to the injured side. Confirmatory testing includes the posterior drawer test done with the patient supine with the knee flexed to 90 degrees and the foot stabilized. Grading is based on the amount of translation. Grade 1 (mild) is translation up to 5 mm, grade 2 (moderate) is 5–10 mm, and grade 3 (severe) is greater than 10 mm. Diagnostic imaging includes plain radiographs and MRI scan.

Treatment can be determined as soon as the exact injury has been isolated. The use of surgical versus nonsurgical management is controversial. The use of braces and a progressive rehabilitation program have been used successfully in athletes with grade 1 and 2 injuries. Grade 3 injuries generally require surgery.

Andrish JT: Anterior cruciate ligament injuries in the skeletally immature patient. Am J Orthop 2001;30:2:103 [PMID: 11234936].

Beynnon BD et al: The effect of anterior cruciate ligament trauma and bracing on knee proprioception. Am J Sports Med 1999;27:150 [PMID: 10102093].

Evans NA et al: The natural history and tailored treatment of ACL injury. Phys Sportsmed 2001;29:19.

## FOOT & ANKLE INJURIES

Injuries in the lower leg, ankle, and foot are quite common in pediatric athletes. The types of injuries sustained tend to depend on the age group. Young children tend to have diaphysial injuries, in contrast to older children in rapid growth, who tend to have epiphysial and apophysial injuries. Perhaps the most common injury evaluated is the **ankle sprain.** When a ligament is overloaded, tearing occurs. These injuries are graded on a scale of 1 to 3. A grade 1 injury is a stretch without instability, grade 2 is a partial tear with some instability, and grade 3 is a total disruption of the ligament with instability of the joint. The ankle has three lateral ligaments (anterior talofibular, calcaneofibular, and posterior talofibular) and a medial deltoid ligament. Inversion of the foot generally damages the anterior talofibular ligament, whereas eversion injures the deltoid ligament. Physical examination often reveals swelling, bruising, and pain. The anterior drawer test is an easy to perform and reliable test of the anterior talofibular ligament. Other maneuvers include the talar tilt and valgus stress test. Diagnostic testing should be done when a bony injury is suspected. The adult Ottawa criteria do not pertain to patients younger than 18 year old. Tenderness over the malleoli, tenderness beyond ligament attachments, and excessive swelling are reasons to obtain radiographs.

Treatment of ankle injuries is imperative to ensure full recovery and should begin immediately after the injury. Phase 1 care involves immediate compressive wrapping and icing to control swelling and inflammation. Protected weight bearing is allowed in the early phase of rehabilitation. The second phase begins when the athlete can ambulate without pain. During this time ankle range of motion is emphasized, along with isometric contractions of the ankle dorsiflexors. Once 90% of strength has returned, active eccentric and concentric exercises can be added. Phase 3 is designed to increase strength, improve proprioception, and add ballistic activity. The "foot alphabet" and "tilt board" are excellent methods for improving ankle proprioception. This program may take up to 6 weeks before an athlete can return to full activity. The athlete should wear a protective brace for 3 to 4 months and continue to ice after exercising.

Plantar fasciitis is common problem that manifests itself as heel pain. It happens in runners who log more than 30 miles per week and in athletes who have tight Achilles tendons or poorly fitting shoes. It is common in people with cavus feet and in individuals who are overweight. The pain is worse on first standing up in the morning and taking a few steps. A bone spur is often found on examination. Treatment involves local massage, stretching of the gastrocsoleus, nonsteroidal anti-inflammatory drugs, arch supports, and local steroid injections. Runners may need to cut back on their weekly mileage until these measures eliminate pain.

Anderson SJ: Soccer: A case-based approach to ankle and knee injuries. Pediatr Ann 2000;29:3:178 [PMID: 10734652].

Aronen JG, Garrick JG: Sports-induced inflammation in the lower extremities. Hosp Pract (Off Ed) 1999;34:51 [PMID: 10047760].

Hockenbury RT, Sammarco J: Evaluation and treatment of ankle sprains: Clinical recommendations for a positive outcome. Phys Sportsmed 2001;29:2:57.

## PREVENTION

As in all activities most sports-related injuries can be prevented by the use of protective equipment, common sense, and proper training. Protective equipment should be properly fitted and maintained by an individual with training and instruction. Helmets should be used in football, baseball, hockey, bicycling, skiing, in-line skating, skateboarding, or any sport with risk for head injury. Eye protection should be used in sports that have a high incidence of eye injuries. Proper protective padding should be identified and used, including chest pads for catchers; shin guards in soccer; shoulder, arm, chest, and leg padding in hockey; and wrist and elbow protectors in skating. A few common-sense concepts should be addressed by coaches, parents, and

physicians in order to ensure the safety of children participating in sports. These include inspecting playing fields for potential hazards, adapting rules to the developmental level of the participants, and matching opponents equally.

The use of the preparticipation history and physical examination can identify potential problems and allow for prevention and early intervention. Proper training techniques reduce injuries by encouraging flexibility, promoting endurance, and teaching correct biomechanics. Sports education reinforces the concepts of fitness and a healthy lifestyle along with sport-specific training. Early identification of an injury allows the athlete to modify techniques and avoid micro- and macrotrauma. Once an injury has occurred, it needs to be identified properly and appropriate measures used to minimize inflammation. Rehabilitation of the injury starts as soon as it has been identified. Early and appropriate care offers the athlete an optimal chance for full recovery and return to full participation.

## REFERENCES

Ansved T: Muscular dystrophies: Influence of physical conditioning on the disease evolution. Curr Opin Clin Nutr Metab Care 2003;6(4):435 [PMID: 12806218].

Birrer RB, Sedaghat V: Exercise and diabetes mellitus: Optimizing performance who have type 1 diabetes. Phys Sportsmed 2003;31(5).

Braith RW: Exercise for those with chronic heart failure. Phys Sportsmed 2002;30(9).

Disabella V, Sherman C: Your guide to exercising with asthma. Phys Sportsmed 1998;26(6).

Draznin MB: Type 1 diabetes and sports participation: Strategies for training and competing safely. Phys Sportsmed 2000;28(12).

Firoozi S et al: Risk of competitive sport in young athletes with heart disease. Heart 2003;89(7):710 [PMID: 12807837].

Howard GM et al: Epilepsy and sports participation. Curr Sports Med Rep 2004;3(1):15.

Howe WB: Preventing infectious disease in sports. Phys Sportsmed 2003;31(2).

MacKnight JM: Infectious mononucleosis: Ensuring a safe return to sport. Phys Sportsmed 2002;30(1).

Maron BJ: Hypertrophic Cardiomyopathy: Practical Steps for Preventing Sudden Death. Phys Sportsmed 2002;30 (1).

Maron BJ: The young competitive athlete with cardiovascular abnormalities: Causes of sudden death, detection by preparticipation screening, and standards for disqualification. Card Electrophysiol Rev 2002;6(1-2):100 [PMID: 11984027].

Moeller JL: Contraindications to Athletic Participation: Spinal, Systemic, Dermatologic, Paired-Organ, and Other Issues. Phys Sportsmed 1996;24(9).

O'Kane JW: Upper respiratory infection. Phys Sportsmed 2002;30(9).

Platt LS: Medical and orthopaedic conditions in special olympics athletes. J Athl Train 2001;36(1):74.

Primos WA: Sports and exercise during acute illness: Recommending the right course for patients. Phys Sportsmed 1996;24(1).

Salim MA, Alpert BS: Sports and Marfan syndrome. Phys Sportsmed 2001;29(5).

Tarnopolsky MA: Metabolic myopathies and physical activity: When fatigue is more than simple exertion. Phys Sportsmed 2002;30(6).

Terrell T et al: Blunt trauma reveals a single kidney: A disqualification dilemma. Phys Sportsmed 1997;25 (11).

Vinger PF: A practical guide for sports eye protection. Phys Sportsmed 2000;28(6).

Winell J, Burke SW: Sports participation of children with Down syndrome. Orthop Clin North Am 2003;34(3):439 [PMID: 12974493].

# Rheumatic Diseases

**26**

*J. Roger Hollister, MD*

## JUVENILE RHEUMATOID ARTHRITIS (JUVENILE CHRONIC ARTHRITIS)

### ESSENTIALS OF DIAGNOSIS & TYPICAL FEATURES

- *Nonmigratory monarticular or polyarticular arthropathy, with a tendency to involve large joints or proximal interphalangeal joints and lasting more than 3 months.*
- *Systemic manifestations with fever, erythematous rashes, nodules, leukocytosis, and, occasionally, iridocyclitis, pleuritis, pericarditis, anemia, fatigue, and growth failure.*

## General Considerations

Patients with juvenile rheumatoid arthritis (JRA) have immunogenetic traits different from those of adults with rheumatoid arthritis. In JRA, human leukocyte antigen (HLA)-DR5 is associated with iritis and the production of antinuclear antibodies (ANA), whereas HLA-DR4 is found in seropositive, polyarticular disease. These traits may be important in the formation of antisuppressor cell antibodies, immune complex generation, and consequent chronic inflammatory disease. Genomics by microarray analysis show great promise in understanding the genetic predisposition to JRA. Tumor necrosis factor (TNF) may be the final common cytokine that perpetuates inflammation.

## Clinical Findings

### A. Symptoms and Signs

Three major clinical presentations in JRA provide clues to the prognosis and possible sequelae of the disease. In the acute febrile form, an evanescent salmon-pink macular rash, arthritis, hepatosplenomegaly, leukocytosis, and polyserositis characterize the constellation described by George Still. Patients with this form have episodic illness, and remission of the systemic features

can be expected within 1 year. They do not develop iridocyclitis.

The polyarticular pattern resembles the adult disease, with chronic pain and swelling of many joints in a symmetrical fashion. Both large and small joints are usually involved. Systemic features are less prominent, although low-grade fever, fatigue, rheumatoid nodules, and anemia may be present. Patients with this form tend to have long-standing arthritis, although the disease may wax and wane. Iridocyclitis occurs occasionally in this group. Older children may have a positive rheumatoid factor test.

The third pattern is characterized by pauciarticular disease, a chronic arthritis of a few joints—often the large weight-bearing joints—in an asymmetrical distribution. The synovitis is usually mild and may be painless. Systemic features are uncommon, but extra-articular involvement is severe, with inflammation in the eye. Up to 30% of children with pauciarticular JRA develop insidious, asymptomatic iridocyclitis, which may cause blindness if untreated. The activity of the eye disease does not correlate with that of the arthritis. Therefore, routine ophthalmologic screening with slitlamp examination must be performed at 3-month intervals if the ANA test is positive and at 6-month intervals if the ANA test is negative for 4 years after the onset of arthritis.

### B. Laboratory Findings

No completely reliable diagnostic test is available for JRA. Rheumatoid factor is positive in about 15% of patients, usually in patients with polyarticular disease whose onset occurs after age 8 years. ANA are most often present in pauciarticular disease with iridocyclitis and may be an indicator of this complication; they are also fairly common in the late-onset rheumatoid factor-positive group. A normal erythrocyte sedimentation rate (ESR) does not exclude the diagnosis.

Table 26–1 lists the general characteristics of joint fluid in various conditions. A positive Gram stain or culture is the only definitive test for infection. A leukocyte count over 2000/μL suggests inflammation due to infection, any of the collagen–vascular diseases, leukemia, or reactive arthritis. A very low glucose concentration (< 40 mg/dL) or very high polymorphonuclear leukocyte count (> 60,000/μL) is highly sugges-

**Table 26–1.** Joint fluid analysis.

| Disorder | Cells/µL | Glucose[a] |
|---|---|---|
| Trauma | More red cells than white cells; usually < 2000 white cells | Normal |
| Reactive arthritis | 3000–10,000 white cells, mostly mono-nuclears | Normal |
| Juvenile rheumatoid arthritis and other inflammatory arthritides | 5000–60,000 white cells, mostly neutrophils | Usually normal or slightly low |
| Septic arthritis | > 60,000 white cells, > 90% neutrophils | Low to normal |

[a]Normal value is 75% or more of serum glucose value.

tive of bacterial arthritis in a child. Chemical analysis of synovial fluid is otherwise of little diagnostic benefit.

### C. IMAGING

In the early stages of the disease, only soft tissue swelling and regional osteoporosis are seen. Magnetic resonance imaging (MRI) of involved joints may show joint damage earlier in the course of the disease than other imaging modalities.

### Differential Diagnosis

Table 26–2 lists the most common causes of limb pain in childhood. A few points of information may indicate the most likely diagnosis. For instance, orthopedic causes are due to increased physical activity, not major trauma. Reactive arthritides are suggested by a preceding viral infection, strep throat, or purpuric rash, and their course waxes and wanes over several days.

Monarticular arthritis is the most important disorder in the differential diagnosis to establish. Pain in the hip or lower extremity is a frequent symptom of childhood cancer, especially leukemia, neuroblastoma, and rhabdomyosarcoma. Infiltration of bone by tumor and actual joint effusion may be seen. Radiographs of the affected site and a careful examination of the blood smear for unusual cells and thrombocytopenia are necessary. A normal lactate dehydrogenase value is helpful in the exclusion of neoplastic disease. In doubtful cases, bone marrow examination is indicated.

Bacterial arthritis is usually acute and monarticular except for arthritis associated with gonorrhea, which may be associated with a migratory pattern. Fever, leukocytosis, and increased ESR with an acute process

in a single joint demand synovial fluid examination and culture to identify the pathogen.

The arthritis of rheumatic fever is migratory, transient, and often more painful than that of JRA. Rheumatic fever is rare in children younger than age 5 years. Evidence of rheumatic carditis should be sought. Evidence of recent streptococcal infection is essential to the diagnosis. The fever pattern in rheumatic fever is low grade and persistent compared with the spiking fever in the systemic form of JRA. Lyme arthri-

**Table 26–2.** Differential diagnosis of limb pain in children.

**Orthopedic**
  Stress fracture
  Overuse syndrome
  Chondromalacia patellae
  Osgood–Schlatter disease
  Slipped capital femoral epiphysis
  Legg–Calvé–Perthes disease
  Hypermobility syndrome
**Reactive arthritis**
  Schönlein–Henoch purpura
  Reactive arthritis following diarrhea
  Toxic synovitis of the hip
  Transient synovitis following viral infection
  Rheumatic fever
**Infections**
  Bacterial
    Lyme arthritis
    Osteomyelitis
    Septic arthritis
    Discitis
  Viral
    Parvovirus (in adolescents)
    Rubella
    Hepatitis B arthritis
**Collagen–vascular**
  Juvenile rheumatoid arthritis
  Spondyloarthropathy
  Systemic lupus erythematosus
  Dermatomyositis
**Neoplastic**
  Leukemia
  Lymphoma
  Neuroblastoma
  Reticuloendotheliosis
  Osteoid osteoma
  Bone tumors (benign or malignant)
**Syndromes of psycho-organic origin**
  Growing pains
  Fibromyalgia
  Reflex neurovascular dystrophy

tis resembles pauciarticular JRA, but the former occurs as discrete, recurrent episodes of arthritis lasting 2–6 weeks. A negative test for antibodies to *Borrelia burgdorferi* argues strongly against this diagnosis.

## Treatment

The objectives of therapy are to restore function, relieve pain, and maintain joint motion. In recent years, other nonsteroidal anti-inflammatory drugs (NSAIDs) have replaced salicylates in the medical treatment of JRA. Although their anti-inflammatory potency is not different from that of aspirin, their liquid form, decreased frequency of dosing, and diminished side effects appear to enhance compliance, cause fewer side effects, and justify their increased cost. Naproxen, 7.5 mg/kg twice daily; ibuprofen, 10 mg/kg four times daily; or diclofenac, 1 mg/kg given twice daily, may be used. If benefit occurs in the first 2 days, improvement will continue, with the maximum effect occurring at 6 weeks. Celecoxib and rofecoxib, two NSAIDs that are selective cyclo-oxygenase-2 (COX) inhibitors, show promise in relieving the gastrointestinal irritation seen with older NSAIDs which have both COX 1 and 2 activity. Dosages for children are under investigation. Range-of-motion and muscle-strengthening exercises should be taught and supervised by a therapist, and a home program should be instituted. Bed rest is to be avoided except in the most acute stages. Joint casting is almost never indicated.

Patients with JRA unresponsive to aspirin or other NSAIDS have a number of alternatives. Methotrexate is the second-line medication of choice. Symptomatic response usually occurs within 3–4 weeks. The low dosages used (5–10 mg/m$^2$/wk as a single dose) have been associated with few side effects. Stomatitis usually resolves with continued administration. Nausea may be prevented by splitting the dose. Hepatotoxicity, including fibrosis, has been reported. A complete blood count and liver function tests should be obtained at 2-month intervals. Liver biopsy may be performed if there are recurrent elevations of aminotransferases. Two new second-line agents are available for patients with progressive disease. Leflunomide is an antipyrimidine medication that is as effective as methotrexate. Side effects may include diarrhea and alopecia. Etanercept is a TNFα receptor construct that must be administered subcutaneously twice a week (0.4 mg/kg/dose). Infliximab, an anti-TNFα antibody, administered in combination with methotrexate, is another second-line treatment. Iridocyclitis should be treated by an ophthalmologist, and methotrexate may be used in difficult cases. Local corticosteroid injections into joints, synovectomy, or joint replacement may be indicated in selected patients.

## Prognosis

In the primarily articular forms of JRA, disease activity diminishes progressively with age and ceases by puberty in about 85% of patients. In a few instances, the disorder will persist into adult life. Problems after puberty relate primarily to residual joint damage. Presentation in the teen years usually presages adult disease. The children most liable to be handicapped permanently are those with unremitting synovitis, hip involvement, or positive rheumatoid factor tests.

Anthony KK, Schanberg LE: Pain in children with arthritis: A review of the current literature. Arthritis Rheum 2003;49:272.

Bowyer SL et al: Health status of patients with juvenile rheumatoid arthritis at 1 and 5 years after diagnosis. J Rheumatol 2003;30:394.

Flato B et al: Prognostic factors in juvenile rheumatoid arthritis: A case–control study revealing early predictors and outcomes after 14.9 years. J Rheumatol 2003;30:386.

Franco CA et al: Factors related to severe uveitis at diagnosis in children with juvenile idiopathic arthritis in a screening program. Am J Ophthalmol 2003;135:757.

Ilowite NT: Current treatment of juvenile rheumatoid arthritis. Pediatrics 2002;109:109.

Jarvis JN: Juvenile rheumatoid arthritis: A guide for pediatricians. Pediatr Ann 2002;31:437.

Lovell DJ et al: Long-term efficacy and safety of etanercept in children with polyarticular-course juvenile rheumatoid arthritis: Interim results from an ongoing multicenter, open-label, extended-treatment trial Arthritis Rheum 2003;48(1):218.

Patel H, Goldstein D: Pediatric uveitis. Pediatr Clin North Am 2003;50:125.

## SPONDYLOARTHROPATHY

Lower extremity arthritis, particularly in males older than age 10 years, suggests a form of spondyloarthropathy. Inflammation of tendinous insertions (enthesopathy) such as the tibial tubercle or the heel occurs in these diseases and not in JRA. Low back pain and sacroiliitis are quite specific for this form of arthritis. Carriage of HLA-B27 antigen occurs in 80% of patients with this disorder. No autoantibodies are found, but inflammatory indicators such as an elevated ESR or C-reactive protein are usually present. The episodes are usually intermittent, in contrast to the more chronic symptoms of JRA. Acute, not chronic, uveitis may occur.

The NSAIDs, particularly indomethacin (2–4 mg/kg/d) and naproxen (15 mg/kg/d), are more effective than salicylates in treating the spondyloarthropathies. Refractory cases may respond to methotrexate, etanercept, or infliximab. Local corticosteroid injections are contraindicated in Achilles tendinitis.

The disorder does not frequently progress to joint destruction or ankylosis in children as it does in adults.

Burgos-Vargas R: Juvenile onset spondyloarthropathies: Therapeutic aspects. Ann Rheum Dis 2002;61 (Suppl) 3:iii33.

# ENTEROPATHIC ARTHRITIS

Enteropathic arthritis comprises several syndromes, including Reiter syndrome, reactive arthritis, and the arthritis of inflammatory bowel disease and celiac disease. The unifying feature of these arthritides is the association of lower extremity arthritis with antecedent or concurrent gastrointestinal symptoms. Reactive arthritis after diarrhea caused by *Salmonella, Shigella, Yersinia,* or *Chlamydia* infection occurs in individuals who are HLA-B27-positive. The human gene product shares a six-amino acid homology with the cell wall of the provocative organism. Transvection experiments in which human HLA-B27 genes are inserted into rats and mice have supported the central role of the genetic predisposition in this form of arthritis. However, animals raised in a germ-free environment have less disease, emphasizing the role of enteric organisms in these spondyloarthropathies. In an analogous manner, the arthritis associated with Crohn disease and ulcerative colitis usually begins after or concurrent with active bowel disease. Other extraintestinal manifestations such as uveitis, stomatitis, hepatitis, and erythema nodosum may occur in these individuals.

Treatment for the musculoskeletal manifestations of inflammatory bowel disease includes controlling bowel disease and the use of NSAIDs, as in ankylosing spondylitis.

Baeten D et al: Immune linkages between inflammatory bowel disease and spondyloarthopathies. Curr Opin Rheumatol 2002;14:342.

# SYSTEMIC LUPUS ERYTHEMATOSUS

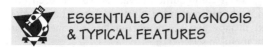

## ESSENTIALS OF DIAGNOSIS & TYPICAL FEATURES

- *Multisystem inflammatory disease of joints, serous linings, skin, kidneys, and the CNS.*
- *ANA must be present in active, untreated disease.*

## General Considerations

Systemic lupus erythematosus (SLE) is the prototype of immune complex diseases; its pathogenesis is related to the deposition in the tissue of circulating soluble immune complexes. The spectrum of symptoms appears to be due not to tissue-specific autoantibodies but rather to tissue damage by lymphocytes, neutrophils, and complement evoked by the deposition of antigen–antibody complexes. Many antigen–antibody systems are present in this disorder, but disease activity correlates best with DNA/anti-DNA complexes. Laboratory tests of these antibodies and complement components give an objective assessment of disease pathogenesis and response to therapy. Autoreactive T lymphocytes that have escaped clonal deletion and unregulated B-lymphocyte production of autoantibodies may initiate the disease. A genetic predisposition to lupus appears critical to causation of the disease.

## Clinical Findings

### A. SYMPTOMS AND SIGNS

SLE is more common in girls than boys (8:1). Disease onset most often occurs between ages 9 and 15 years. The symptoms depend on the organ involved with immune complex deposition.

**1. Joint symptoms**—Joint symptoms are the most common presenting feature. Nondeforming arthritis may involve any joint, often in a symmetrical manner. Myositis may also occur and is more painful than the inflammation in dermatomyositis.

**2. Systemic manifestations**—These include weakness, anorexia, fever, fatigue, and weight loss.

**3. Skin lesions**—Lesions include butterfly erythema and induration, small ulcerations in skin and mucous membranes, purpura, alopecia, and Raynaud phenomenon. The sun sensitivity of the dermal lesions may be striking.

**4. Polyserositis**—Polyserositis may include pleurisy with effusions, peritonitis, and pericarditis. Libman–Sacks endocarditis may occur in patients with antiphospholipid antibodies.

**5. Gastrointestinal findings**—Hepatosplenomegaly and lymphadenopathy may occur. Gastrointestinal presentations of SLE are unusual, with the exception of acute pancreatitis.

**6. Renal manifestations**—Renal SLE produces few symptoms at onset but is often progressive and is the leading cause of death among patients with SLE. Renal biopsy is indicated in patients who do not respond to corticosteroids or who cannot have corticosteroids tapered to a less-toxic, alternate-day regimen. The histologic pattern of diffuse proliferative nephritis requires the most aggressive treatment. Late complications are nephrosis and uremia. Control of hypertension is critical to maintaining renal function.

**7. Central nervous system (CNS)**—CNS involvement produces a variety of symptoms such as seizures; coma; hemiplegia; focal neuropathies; chorea; and behavior disturbances, including psychosis.

## B. LABORATORY FINDINGS

Leukopenia and anemia are frequently found with a low incidence of Coombs positivity. Thrombocytopenia and purpura may be early manifestations even in the absence of other organ involvement. The ESR is elevated, and hypergammaglobulinemia is often present. Renal involvement is indicated by the presence of red cells, white cells, red cell casts, and protein in the urine. The ANA test is invariably positive in patients with active untreated SLE, and a negative ANA test excludes the diagnosis. For patients with a positive ANA test, a profile identifying individual disease-specific antibodies should be ordered. Anticardiolipin antibody and the lupus anticoagulant are two autoantibodies that identify lupus patients at risk for thrombotic events.

In managing the disease, elevated titers of anti-DNA antibody and depressed levels of serum complement (C3) accurately reflect active disease, especially renal, CNS, and skin disease. A computed tomography or MRI scan may identify pathologic conditions of the brain in lupus cerebritis, such as infarction, vasculitis, or atrophy.

## Differential Diagnosis

SLE may simulate many inflammatory diseases such as rheumatic fever, rheumatoid arthritis, and viral infections. It is essential to review all organ systems carefully to establish a clinical pattern. Renal and CNS involvement is unique to SLE. A negative ANA test excludes the diagnosis of SLE. Tests yielding false-positive results are usually of low titer (1:320).

An overlap syndrome known as mixed connective tissue disease, with features of several collagen–vascular diseases, occurs in adults and children. The symptom complex is diverse and does not readily fit previous classifications. Arthritis, fever, skin tightening, Raynaud phenomenon, muscle weakness, and rashes are commonly present. Important factors in recognition of this disease entity are the relative infrequency of renal disease, which implies a better prognosis than SLE, and the corticosteroid responsiveness of symptoms, which distinguishes mixed connective tissue disease from scleroderma. The definition of the disease includes the presence of serum antibody to a ribonuclear protein. The initial ANA test is positive in very high titers. The ANA profile demonstrates the antibody to ribonuclear protein. Pulmonary disease in childhood produces major morbidity.

## Treatment

The treatment of SLE should be tailored to the organ system involved so that toxicities are minimized. Prednisone, 0.5–1 mg/kg/d orally, has significantly lowered the mortality rate in SLE and should be used in all patients with renal, cardiac, or CNS involvement. The dosage should be varied using clinical and laboratory parameters of disease activity, and the minimum amount necessary to control the disease should be used. Alternate-day regimens of corticosteroid are frequently possible. Skin manifestations, arthritis, and fatigue may be treated with antimalarials such as hydroxychloroquine, 5–7 mg/kg/d orally. Pleuritic pain or arthritis can usually be managed with NSAIDs.

If disease control is inadequate with prednisone or if the dose required produces intolerable side effects, an immunosuppressant should be added. Either azathioprine, 2–3 mg/kg/d orally, or cyclophosphamide, 0.5–1 g/m$^2$, administered intravenously once a month, has been most widely used. Recent studies indicate that mycophenolate mofetil may used in place of intravenous cyclophosphamide to induce remission or sustain remission after intravenous cyclophosphamide therapy. These drugs are ineffective during acute crises such as seizures. Thrombotic events due to clotting antibodies require long-term anticoagulation.

The toxicities of the regimens must be carefully considered. Growth failure, osteoporosis, Cushing syndrome, adrenal suppression, and aseptic necrosis are serious side effects of chronic use of prednisone. When high doses of corticosteroids are used (> 2 mg/kg/d), the risk of sepsis is real. Cyclophosphamide causes bladder epithelial dysplasia, hemorrhagic cystitis, and sterility. Azathioprine has been associated with liver damage, pancreatitis, and bone marrow suppression. Immunosuppressant treatment should be withheld if the total white count falls below 3000/$\mu$L or the neutrophil count below 1000/$\mu$L. Retinal damage from chloroquine derivatives has not been observed with recommended dosages. Intravenous pulse steroid therapy and plasmapheresis are treatments that may be useful in selected cases.

Amenorrhea may be a result of uncontrolled SLE but may also be a consequence of treatment with prednisone, cyclophosphamide, or azathioprine.

## Course & Prognosis

The prognosis in SLE relates to the severity of renal involvement or infectious complications of treatment. With improved diagnosis, milder cases are now identified. Nonetheless, the survival rate has improved from 51% at 5 years in 1954 to 90% today. The disease has a natural waxing and waning cycle, and periods of complete remission are not unusual.

Arbuckle MR et al: Development of autoantibodies before the clinical onset of systemic lupus erythematosus. N Engl J Med 2003;349:1526.

Bijl et al: Mycophenolate mofetil prevents a clinical relapse in patients with systemic lupus erythematosus at risk. Ann Rheumatol Dis 2003;62:534.

Boon SJ, McCurdy D: Childhood systemic lupus erythematosus. Pediatr Ann 2002;31:407.

Egner W: The use of laboratory tests in the diagnosis of SLE. J Clin Pathol 2000;53:424.

Greenberg SB: Infections in the immunocompromised rheumatologic patient. Crit Care Clin 2002;18:931.

Klein-Gitelman M et at: Systemic lupus erythematosus in childhood. Rheum Dis Clin North Am 2002;28:561.

# DERMATOMYOSITIS (POLYMYOSITIS)

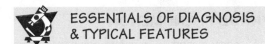

### ESSENTIALS OF DIAGNOSIS & TYPICAL FEATURES

- *Pathognomonic skin rash.*
- *Weakness of proximal muscles and occasionally of pharyngeal and laryngeal groups.*
- *Pathogenesis related to vasculitis.*

## General Considerations

Dermatomyositis, a rare inflammatory disease of muscle and skin in childhood, is uniquely responsive to corticosteroid treatment. The vasculitis in childhood dermatomyositis differs pathologically from the adult disease. Small arteries and veins are involved, with an exudate of neutrophils, lymphocytes, plasma cells, and histiocytes. The lesion progresses to intimal proliferation and thrombus formation. These vascular changes are found in the skin, muscle, kidney, retina, and gastrointestinal tract. Postinflammatory calcinosis is frequent.

The autoimmune pathogenesis of dermatomyositis has been difficult to unravel. Recent studies have shown that both cellular and humoral mechanisms may be involved. Lymphocytes from patients undergo blastogenesis in the presence of muscle tissue and release lymphotoxin, which destroys cultured fetal muscle cells. Biopsies studied with immunofluorescence techniques demonstrate immunoglobulin and complement in perivascular distribution. The putative antigen has not been identified, and results of viral studies have been negative.

## Clinical Findings

### A. SYMPTOMS AND SIGNS

The predominant symptom is proximal muscular weakness affecting pelvic and shoulder girdles. Tenderness, stiffness, and swelling may be found but are not striking. Neurologic findings, such as absence of tendon reflexes, are not seen until late in the disease. Pharyngeal and respiratory involvement can be life-threatening. Flexion contractures and muscle atrophy produce significant residual deformities. Calcinosis may follow the inflammation in muscle and skin.

The rash of dermatomyositis is very helpful in the diagnosis. Characteristically, the rash involves the upper eyelids and extensor surfaces of the knuckles, elbows, and knees with a distinctive heliotrope color that progresses to a scaling and atrophic appearance. Periorbital edema is not uncommon. Nail-fold capillary abnormalities are associated with poorer prognosis. None of the rashes associated with other childhood rheumatic diseases have these features of distribution. The severity of the rash frequently does not parallel that of the muscle disease.

### B. LABORATORY FINDINGS

Determination of muscle enzyme levels in blood is the most helpful tool in diagnosis and treatment. All enzymes, including serum aldolase, should be screened to detect an abnormality that reflects activity of the disease. In later years of the illness, MRI of weak muscles may show disease activity even when enzymes are normal. The ANA test may be positive. Electromyography is useful for distinguishing myopathic from neuropathic causes of muscle weakness. Muscle biopsy is indicated in doubtful cases of myositis without the pathognomonic rash.

## Treatment

Prednisone in high dosages (1–2 mg/kg/d orally) has been shown to speed recovery. The dosage should be maintained or increased until muscle enzymes have returned to normal. Functional recovery will lag somewhat behind laboratory improvement. With improvement, the dosage may be cut to a level that maintains disease control and normal muscle enzymes. Treatment must be continued for an average of 2 years. Methotrexate, 1 mg/kg/wk, is an effective, steroid-sparing treatment. Intravenous immune globulin or cyclosporine therapy is used in refractory cases. Physical therapy is critical to prevent or allay contractures.

## Course & Prognosis

Most children recover and discontinue medications in 1–3 years. Relapses may occur. Functional ability is very good in most patients. Myositis in childhood is not associated with an increased risk of cancer.

Mukamel M et al: New insight into calcinosis of juvenile dermatomyositis: A study of composition and treatment. J Pediatr 2001;138:763.

Pachman LM: Juvenile dermatomyositis: Immunogenetics, patho-physiology, and disease expression. Rheum Dis Clin North Am 2002;28:579.

Ramanan AV, Feldman BM: Clinical features and outcomes of ju-venile dermatomyositis and other childhood onset myositis syndromes. Rheum Dis Clin North Am 2002;28:833.

Rennebohm R: Juvenile dermatomyositis. Pediatr Ann 2002;31:426.

Trapani S, et al: Pulmonary involvement in juvenile dermatomyosi-tis: A two-year longitudinal study. Rheumatology 2001; 40:216.

## POLYARTERITIS NODOSA

Polyarteritis nodosa is a rare disease, but a significant number of cases have been reported in childhood and infancy. No single cause has been found, but evidence of a streptococcal trigger and poorly controlled par-vovirus infection have been found in some series.

Pathologically, the disease is a vasculitis of medium-sized arteries with fibrinoid degeneration in the media extending to the intima and adventitia. Neutrophils and eosinophils comprise the inflammatory reaction. Aneurysms may be palpated or seen radiographically. Thrombosis of diseased arteries may cause infarction in many organs. Fibrosis of vessels and surrounding tissues accompanies healing.

Symptoms arise from many organ systems, making diagnosis difficult. Unexplained fever, conjunctivitis, CNS involvement, and cardiac disease are more promi-nent in children than in adults. Many cases appear as acute myocarditis, and the peripheral neuropathy so common in adults with the disease is unusual in chil-dren. Diagnosis depends on biopsy-proved vasculitis or characteristic aneurysms on angiography.

The mortality rate is high, especially with cardiac in-volvement. Treatment usually consists of prednisone (1–1.5 mg/kg/d orally), immunosuppressants, and in-travenous immune globulin, but controlled studies on the efficacy of these therapies are not available.

Besbas N et al: Renal involvement in polyarteritis nodosa: Evalua-tion of 26 Turkish children. Pediatr Nephrol 2000;14:325.

Frankel SK et al: Vasculitis: Wegener granulomatosis, Churg-Strauss, microscopic polyangiitis, polyarteritis, Takayasu ar-teritis. Crit Care Clin 2002;18:855.

## SCLERODERMA

Fortunately, the most common forms of scleroderma in childhood are linear scleroderma and morphea, not sys-temic sclerosis. The skin disease begins with the appear-ance of indurated and depigmented patches (morphea) or streaks of skin on an extremity (linear scleroderma). As the linear form progresses over a 2- or 3-year period, subcutaneous tissue becomes atrophied and contrac-tures develop in affected joints. Physical therapy and treatment with methotrexate or vitamin D analogues may limit extension of the lesions but do not reverse previous damage. It is rare for the limited forms to progress to systemic sclerosis.

In systemic sclerosis, the dermal process is general-ized. Raynaud phenomenon is almost invariably pre-sent. Arthralgias, esophageal dysfunction, and renal dis-ease are present. Involvement of the lungs and kidneys may lead to rapid demise. The pathogenesis of systemic scleroderma is unknown and there are no effective ther-apies.

Murray KJ, Laxer RM: Scleroderma in children and adolescents. Rheum Dis Clin North Am 2002;28:603.

## RAYNAUD PHENOMENON

Raynaud phenomenon is an intermittent vasospastic disorder of fingers and sometimes the toes. As much as 10% of the adult population may have this disorder, and onset in childhood is not uncommon. The classic triphasic presentation is cold-induced pallor, then cyanosis, followed by hyperemia, but incomplete forms are common. In adults older than age 35 years who are ANA-positive, Raynaud phenomenon may be a harbin-ger of rheumatic disease. This progression is rarely seen in childhood. Evaluation should include a detailed his-tory with review of systems relevant to rheumatic dis-ease and examination for nail-fold capillary abnormali-ties. In the absence of positive findings, Raynaud phenomenon is likely to be idiopathic.

Treatment involves education about hand warming (eg, using mittens not gloves); the role of stress, which may be a precipitant; and in very symptomatic patients, treatment with calcium channel blockers such as nifedipine during winter months.

Nigrovic PA et al: Raynaud's phenomenon in children: A retro-spective review. Pediatrics 2003;111:715.

# ■ NONRHEUMATIC PAIN SYNDROMES

## 1. Reflex Sympathetic Dystrophy

Reflex sympathetic dystrophy is a painful condition that is frequently confused with arthritis. The preva-lence and recognition of the condition appear to be in-creasing. Severe extremity pain leading to nearly com-plete loss of function is the hallmark of the condition.

Evidence of autonomic dysfunction is demonstrated by color changes, temperature differences, and dyshidrosis in the affected extremity. Foot involvement is more common than hand involvement. A puffy swelling of the entire hand or foot is common. On examination, cutaneous hyperesthesia is evident to even the slightest touch. Results of laboratory tests are negative. Radiographic findings are normal except for the late development of osteoporosis. Bone scans are helpful and demonstrate either increased or decreased blood supply to the painful extremity.

The cause of this condition is unknown. Unlike adults, children only occasionally have a history of significant physical trauma at disease onset. How autonomic dysfunction causes severe somatic pain is unknown, but the feedback cycle does provide the basis for treatment. In mild cases, a program of rehabilitative physical therapy in combination with desensitization techniques will restore function and relieve pain. Patients with reflex sympathetic dystrophy who are unresponsive to therapy need family counseling and may respond to steroids or ganglionic blocks by local anesthesia. Long-term prognosis is good if recovery is rapid; recurrent episodes imply a less favorable prognosis.

Sherry D: An overview of amplified musculoskeletal pain syndromes. J Rheumatol 2000;27:44.

## 2. Fibromyalgia

Fibromyalgia is a diffuse pain syndrome in which patients experience pain all over their bodies without objective physical findings. Weather changes and fatigue exacerbate symptoms. A sleep disturbance, such as insomnia or prolonged periods of awakening at night, is an almost universal symptom. Patients should be carefully questioned about these symptoms. On examination, patients are normal except for pain during palpation of characteristic trigger points at the insertion of muscles, especially along the neck, spine, and pelvis.

Treatment consists of physical therapy and attention to relieving the sleep disorder. Low-dose antidepressant medication (amitriptyline, 25 mg) taken before sleep may produce a remarkable degree of pain relief. Physical therapy should emphasize a graded rehabilitative approach to stretching and exercise. Analgesics are often ineffective and should be avoided if possible to avoid habituation to narcotic medications.

The prognosis for young patients is unclear, and long-term strategies may be necessary to enable them to cope with the condition.

Schikler KN: Is it juvenile rheumatoid arthritis or fibromyalgia? Med Clin North Am 2000;84:967.

Worrel LM et al: Treating fibromyalgia with a brief interdisciplinary program: Initial outcomes and predictors of response. Mayo Clin Proc 2001;76:384.

## 3. Chronic Fatigue Syndrome

Since 1985, chronic fatigue syndrome has become an increasingly common diagnosis. The distinction between this apparent organic fatigue and fatigue associated with emotional causes is not easily made. Criteria have been developed by the National Institutes of Health to assist in classification. The fatigue should have a defined date of onset, and there is a long list of excludable diagnoses. Other clinical manifestations include low-grade fevers, sore throat, painful lymph nodes, and neuropsychiatric problems. Epstein–Barr virus infection does not account for all the patients described. Treatment is symptomatic and somewhat unsatisfactory.

Bell DS et al: Thirteen-year follow-up of children and adolescents with chronic fatigue syndrome. Pediatrics 2001;107:994.

Krilov LR, Fisher M: Chronic fatigue syndrome in youth: Maybe not so chronic after all. Contemp Ped 2002;19:61.

## HYPERMOBILITY SYNDROME

Ligamentous laxity, which previously was thought to occur only in Ehlers–Danlos syndrome or Down syndrome, is now recognized as a common cause of joint pain.

Children are now participating in a wide range of physically demanding sports and activities. Patients with hypermobility present with episodic joint pain and occasionally with swelling that lasts a few days after increased physical activity. Depending on the activity, almost any joint may be affected.

Physical examination may reveal joint swelling and tenderness, but the key to diagnosis is the demonstration of ligamentous laxity. Five criteria have been established: (1) passive opposition of the thumb to the flexor surface of the forearm; (2) passive hyperextension of the fingers so that they are parallel to the extensor surface of the forearm; (3) hyperextension of the elbow; (4) hyperextension of the knee (genu recurvatum); and (5) palms on floor with knees extended. Results of laboratory tests are normal. The pain associated with the syndrome is produced by improper joint alignment caused by laxity that is promoted by the stresses of vigorous exercise.

Treatment consists of a graded conditioning program designed to provide muscular support of the joints involved to compensate for the loose ligaments.

The prognosis is good, provided conditioning before activities is adequate.

Grahame R et al: The revised (Brighton 1998) criteria for the diagnosis of benign joint hypermobility syndrome (BJHS). J Rheumatol 2000;27:1777.

# REFERENCES

Cassidy JT, Petty RE: *Textbook of Pediatric Rheumatology,* 4th ed. WB Saunders, 2001.

Jacobs JC: *Pediatric Rheumatology for the Practitioner,* 2nd ed. Springer, 1993.

# Hematologic Disorders

*Daniel R. Ambruso, MD, Taru Hays, MD, Peter A. Lane, MD, & Rachelle Nuss, MD*

## NORMAL HEMATOLOGIC VALUES

The normal ranges for peripheral blood counts vary significantly with age. Normal neonates show a relative polycythemia with a hematocrit of 45–65%. The reticulocyte count at birth is relatively high at 2–8%. Within the first few days of life, erythrocyte production decreases, and the levels of hemoglobin and hematocrit fall to a nadir at about 6–8 weeks. During this period, known as physiologic anemia of infancy, normal infants have hemoglobins as low as 10 g/dL and hematocrits as low as 30%. Thereafter, the normal values for hemoglobin and hematocrit gradually increase until adult values are reached after puberty. Premature infants can reach a nadir hemoglobin level of 7–8 g/dL at 8–10 weeks.

Newborns have larger red cells than children and adults, with a mean corpuscular volume (MCV) at birth of more than 94 fL. The MCV subsequently falls to a nadir of 70–84 fL at about age 6 months. Thereafter, the normal MCV increases gradually until it reaches adult values after puberty.

The normal number of white blood cells is higher in infancy and early childhood than later in life. Neutrophils predominate in the differential white count at birth and in the older child. Lymphocytes predominate (up to 80%) between about ages 1 month and 6 years.

Normal values for the platelet count are 150,000–400,000/μL and vary little with age.

## ■ BONE MARROW FAILURE

Failure of the marrow to produce adequate numbers of circulating blood cells may be congenital or acquired and may cause pancytopenia (aplastic anemia) or involve only one cell line (single cytopenia). Constitutional and acquired aplastic anemias are discussed in this section and the more common single cytopenias in later sections. Bone marrow failure caused by malignancy or other infiltrative disease is discussed in Chapter 28. It is important to remember that many drugs and toxins may affect the marrow and cause single or multiple cytopenias.

Suspicion of bone marrow failure is warranted in children with pancytopenia and in children with single cytopenias who lack evidence of peripheral red cell, white cell, or platelet destruction. Macrocytosis often accompanies bone marrow failure. Many of the constitutional bone marrow disorders are associated with a variety of congenital anomalies.

Young NS, Maciejewski J: The pathophysiology of acquired aplastic anemia. N Engl J Med 1997;336:1365 [PMID: 9134878].

## CONSTITUTIONAL APLASTIC ANEMIA (Fanconi Anemia)

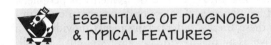

### ESSENTIALS OF DIAGNOSIS & TYPICAL FEATURES

- *Progressive pancytopenia.*
- *Macrocytosis.*
- *Multiple congenital anomalies.*
- *Increased chromosome breakage in peripheral blood lymphocytes.*

### General Considerations

Fanconi anemia is a syndrome characterized by defective DNA repair that is caused by a variety of genetic mutations. Inheritance is autosomal recessive, and the disease occurs in all ethnic groups. Hematologic manifestations usually begin with thrombocytopenia or neutropenia and subsequently progress over the course of months or years to pancytopenia. Typically the diagnosis is made between ages 2 and 10 years.

### Clinical Findings

#### A. SYMPTOMS AND SIGNS

Symptoms are determined principally by the degree of hematologic abnormality. Thrombocytopenia may cause purpura, petechiae, and bleeding; neutropenia may cause severe or recurrent infections; and anemia may cause weakness, fatigue, and pallor. Congenital anomalies are present in at least 50% of patients. The most common include abnormal pigmentation of the skin (generalized hyperpigmentation, café au lait or hypopigmented spots), short stature with delicate features, and skeletal malformations (hypoplasia, anomalies, or absence of the thumb and radius). More subtle anomalies include hypoplasia of the thenar eminence or a weak or absent radial pulse. Associated renal anomalies include aplasia, "horseshoe" kidney, and duplication of the collecting system. Other anomalies are microcephaly, microphthalmia, strabismus, ear anomalies, and hypogenitalism.

## B. LABORATORY FINDINGS

Thrombocytopenia or leukopenia typically occurs first, followed over the course of months to years by anemia and progression to severe aplastic anemia. Macrocytosis is virtually always present, is usually associated with anisocytosis and an elevation in fetal hemoglobin levels, and is an important diagnostic clue. The bone marrow reveals hypoplasia or aplasia. The diagnosis is confirmed by the demonstration of an increased number of chromosome breaks and rearrangements in peripheral blood lymphocytes. The use of diepoxybutane to stimulate these breaks and rearrangements provides for a sensitive assay that is virtually always positive in children with Fanconi anemia, even before the onset of hematologic abnormalities.

Specific molecular markers/genes called Fanc-A, B, C, and so on are found in different ethnic populations. These markers are identified in research laboratories and are not available as routine clinical tests.

## Differential Diagnosis

Because patients with Fanconi anemia frequently present with thrombocytopenia, the disorder must be differentiated from idiopathic thrombocytopenic purpura (ITP) and other more common causes of decreased platelets. In contrast to patients with ITP, those with Fanconi anemia usually exhibit a gradual fall in the platelet count, and counts less than 20,000/μL are often accompanied by neutropenia or anemia, along with phenotypical features. Fanconi anemia may also be manifested initially by pancytopenia, and must be differentiated from acquired aplastic anemia and other disorders such as acute leukemia. Examination of the bone marrow and chromosome studies of peripheral blood lymphocytes will usually distinguish between these disorders.

## Complications

The most important complications of Fanconi anemia are those related to thrombocytopenia and neutropenia. Endogenous endocrine dysfunction may include growth hormone deficiency, hypothyroidism, or impaired glucose metabolism. In addition, persons with Fanconi anemia have a significantly increased risk of developing malignancies, especially acute nonlymphocytic leukemia, solid tumors, and myelodysplastic syndromes. Death is usually the result of thrombocytopenic hemorrhage, overwhelming infection, or malignancy.

## Treatment

Attentive supportive care is a critical feature of management. Patients with neutropenia who develop fever require prompt evaluation and parenteral broad-spectrum antibiotics. Transfusions are important but should be used judiciously, especially in the management of thrombocytopenia, which frequently becomes refractory to platelet transfusions as a consequence of alloimmunization. Transfusions from family members should be discouraged because of the negative effect on the outcome of bone marrow transplantation. At least 50% of patients with Fanconi anemia respond, albeit incompletely, to oxymetholone, and many recommend institution of androgen therapy before transfusions are needed. However, oxymetholone is associated with hepatotoxicity, hepatic adenomas, and masculinization, which is particularly troublesome for female patients.

Successful bone marrow transplantation cures the aplastic anemia and is an important treatment option for children with Fanconi anemia who have a human leukocyte antigen (HLA)-identical sibling donor. Before transplantation the prospective donor must be screened for Fanconi anemia by testing his or her lymphocytes for chromosome breakage.

## Prognosis

Many patients succumb to bleeding, infection, or malignancy in adolescence or early adulthood. The long-term outlook for those undergoing successful bone marrow transplantation is uncertain, particularly with regard to the risk of subsequently developing malignancies.

Alter BP: Fanconi's anemia and malignancies. Am J Hematol 1996;3:99 [PMID: 8892734].

Butturini A et al: Hematologic abnormalities in Fanconi anemia: An international Fanconi anemia registry study. Blood 1994;84:1650 [PMID: 8068955].

Dufour C et al: Stem cell transplantation from HLA-matched related donor for Fanconi's anaemia: A retrospective review of the multicentric Italian experience on behalf of AIEOP-GITMO. Br J Haematol 2001;112:796 [PMID: 11260086].

Joenje H, Patel KJ: The emerging genetic and molecular basis of Fanconi anemia. Nat Rev Genet 2001;2:446 [PMID: 11389461].

# ACQUIRED APLASTIC ANEMIA

## ESSENTIALS OF DIAGNOSIS & TYPICAL FEATURES

- *Weakness and pallor.*
- *Petechiae, purpura, and bleeding.*
- *Frequent or severe infections.*
- *Pancytopenia with hypocellular bone marrow.*

## General Considerations

Acquired aplastic anemia is characterized by peripheral pancytopenia with a hypocellular bone marrow. Approximately 50% of the cases in childhood are idiopathic. Other cases are secondary to idiosyncratic reactions to drugs such as phenylbutazone, sulfonamides, nonsteroidal anti-inflammatories, and anticonvulsants. Toxic causes include exposure to benzene, insecticides, and heavy metals. Infectious causes include viral hepatitis (usually non-A, non-B, non-C), infectious mononucleosis, and human immunodeficiency virus (HIV). In immunocompromised children, aplastic anemia has been associated with human parvovirus B19. Immune mechanisms of marrow suppression are suspected in most cases.

## Clinical Findings

### A. SYMPTOMS AND SIGNS

Weakness, fatigue, and pallor result from anemia; petechiae, purpura, and bleeding occur because of thrombocytopenia; and fevers due to generalized or localized infections occur with neutropenia. Hepatosplenomegaly and significant lymphadenopathy are unusual.

### B. LABORATORY FINDINGS

Anemia is usually normocytic, with a low reticulocyte count. The white blood cell count is low, with a marked neutropenia. The platelet count is typically below $50,000/\mu L$ and frequently below $20,000/\mu L$. Bone marrow aspiration and biopsy show hypocellularity, often marked.

## Differential Diagnosis

Examination of the bone marrow usually excludes pancytopenia caused by peripheral destruction of blood cells or by infiltrative processes such as acute leukemia, storage diseases, and myelofibrosis. Many of these other conditions are associated with hepatosplenomegaly.

Preleukemic conditions also may present with pancytopenia and hypocellular bone marrows. Cytogenetic analysis of the marrow is helpful, because a clonal abnormality may predict the subsequent development of leukemia. Because some children with Fanconi anemia may not have apparent congenital anomalies, patients with newly diagnosed aplastic anemia should be studied for chromosome breaks and rearrangements in peripheral blood lymphocytes.

## Complications

Acquired aplastic anemia is characteristically complicated by infection and hemorrhage; these two complications are the leading causes of death. Other complications are those associated with therapy.

## Treatment

Comprehensive supportive care is most important in the management of acute acquired aplastic anemia. Febrile illnesses require prompt evaluation and usually parenteral antibiotics. Red blood cell transfusions alleviate symptoms of anemia. Platelet transfusions may be lifesaving, but they should be used sparingly because many patients eventually develop platelet alloantibodies and become refractory to platelet transfusions.

Bone marrow transplantation is generally considered the treatment of choice for severe aplastic anemia when an HLA-compatible sibling donor is available. Because the likelihood of success with transplantation is influenced adversely by multiple transfusions, HLA typing of family members should be undertaken as soon as the diagnosis of aplastic anemia is made. An increasing number of patients who lack HLA-matched siblings are able to find matched donors through the National Bone Marrow Registry.

The best alternative to bone marrow transplantation from an HLA-matched sibling donor is immunosuppression, usually with antithymocyte globulin (ATG) and cyclosporine. Responses are good. Most patients show hematologic improvement and become transfusion-independent.

## Prognosis

Children receiving early bone marrow transplantation from an HLA-identical sibling have a long-term survival rate of greater than 80%. Sustained, complete remissions may be seen in 65–80% of patients receiving immunosuppressive therapy. However, both therapies are associated with an increased risk of myelodysplastic syndromes, acute leukemia, and other malignancies in long-term survivors.

Fouladi M et al: Improved survival in severe acquired aplastic anemia of childhood. Bone Marrow Transplant 2000;26:1149 [PMID: 11149724].

Ohara A et al: Myelodysplastic syndrome and acute myelogenous leukemia as a late clonal complication in children with aplastic anemia. Blood 1997;90:1009 [PMID: 9242530].

Rosenfeld S et al: Antithymocyte globulin and cyclosporine for severe aplastic anemia: Association between hematologic response and long-term outcome. JAMA 2003;289:1130 [PMID: 12622583].

Rosenfeld SJ et al: Intensive immunosuppression with antithymocyte globulin and cyclosporine as treatment for severe aplastic anemia. Blood 1995;85:3058 [PMID: 7756640].

# ■ ANEMIAS

## APPROACH TO THE CHILD WITH ANEMIA

Anemia is a relatively common finding, and identifying the cause is important. Even though anemia in childhood has many causes, the correct diagnosis can usually be established with relatively little laboratory cost.

Frequently the cause is suggested by a careful history. The possibility of nutritional causes should be addressed by inquiry about dietary intake; growth and development; and symptoms of chronic disease, malabsorption, or blood loss. Hemolytic disease may be suggested by a history of jaundice (including neonatal jaundice) or by a family history of anemia, jaundice, gallbladder disease, splenomegaly, or splenectomy. The child's ethnic background may suggest the possibility of certain hemoglobinopathies or of deficiencies of red cell enzymes such as glucose-6-phosphate dehydrogenase (G6PD). The review of systems may reveal clues to a previously unsuspected systemic disease with which anemia may be associated. The patient's age is important because some causes of anemia are age-related. For example, patients with iron deficiency anemia and β-globin disorders present more commonly at ages 6–36 months than at other times in life.

The physical examination may also reveal clues to the cause of anemia. Poor growth may suggest chronic disease or hypothyroidism. Congenital anomalies may be associated with constitutional aplastic anemia (Fanconi anemia) or with congenital hypoplastic anemia (Diamond–Blackfan anemia). Other disorders may be suggested by the findings of petechiae or purpura (leukemia, aplastic anemia, hemolytic–uremic syndrome), jaundice (hemolysis or liver disease), generalized lymphadenopathy (leukemia, juvenile rheumatoid arthritis, HIV infection), splenomegaly (leukemia, sickle cell disease, hereditary spherocytosis, liver disease,

hypersplenism), or evidence of chronic or recurrent infections.

The initial laboratory evaluation of the anemic child consists of a complete blood count (CBC) with differential and platelet count, review of the peripheral blood smear, and a reticulocyte count. The algorithm in Figure 27–1 uses limited laboratory information, together with the history and physical examination, to reach a specific diagnosis or to focus additional laboratory investigations on a limited diagnostic category (eg, microcytic anemia, bone marrow failure, pure red cell aplasia, or hemolytic disease). This diagnostic scheme depends principally on the MCV to determine whether the anemia is microcytic, normocytic, or macrocytic, according to the percentile curves of Dallman and Siimes (Figure 27–2).

The incidence of iron deficiency in the United States has decreased significantly with improvements in infant nutrition. Still, iron deficiency is an important cause of microcytic anemia, especially at ages 6–24 months. A trial of therapeutic iron is appropriate in such children, provided the dietary history is compatible with iron deficiency and the physical examination or CBC count does not suggest an alternative cause for the anemia. If this is not the case or if a trial of therapeutic iron fails to correct the anemia and microcytosis, further laboratory evaluation is warranted.

Another key element of Figure 27–1 is the use of both the reticulocyte count and the peripheral blood smear to determine whether a normocytic or macrocytic anemia is due to hemolysis. Typically hemolytic disease is associated with an elevated reticulocyte count, but some children with chronic hemolysis initially present during a period of virus-induced aplasia when the reticulocyte count is not elevated. Thus review of the peripheral blood smear for evidence of hemolysis (eg, spherocytes, red cell fragmentation, sickle forms) is important in the evaluation of children with normocytic anemias and low reticulocyte counts. When hemolysis is suggested, the correct diagnosis may be suspected by specific abnormalities of red cell morphology or by clues from the history or physical examination. Autoimmune hemolysis is usually excluded by Coombs testing. Review of blood counts and the peripheral blood smears of the mother and father may suggest genetic disorders such as hereditary spherocytosis. Children with normocytic or macrocytic anemias, with relatively low reticulocyte counts and no evidence of hemolysis on the blood smear, usually have anemias caused by inadequate erythropoiesis in the bone marrow. The presence of neutropenia or thrombocytopenia in such children suggests the possibility of aplastic anemia, malignancy, or severe folate/vitamin $B_{12}$ deficiency, and usually dictates examination of the bone marrow.

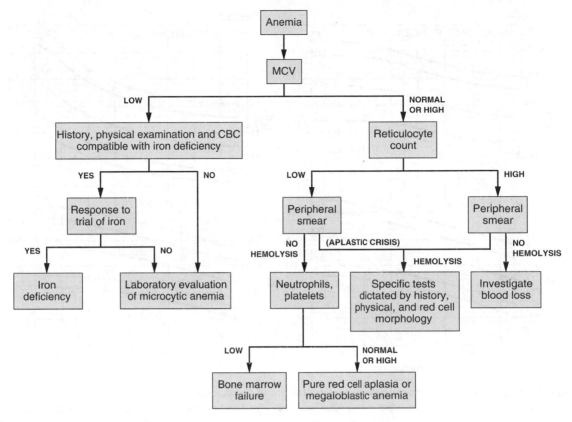

***Figure 27–1.*** Investigation of anemia.

Pure red cell aplasia may be congenital (Diamond–Blackfan anemia), acquired and transient (transient erythroblastopenia of childhood), a manifestation of a systemic disease such as renal disease or hypothyroidism, or due to malnutrition or mild deficiencies of folate or vitamin $B_{12}$.

Hermiston ML, Mentzer WC: A practical approach to the evaluation of the anemic child. Pediatr Clin North Am 2002;49:877 [PMID: 12430617].

## PURE RED CELL APLASIA

Infants and children with normocytic or macrocytic anemia, a low reticulocyte count, and normal or elevated numbers of neutrophils and platelets should be suspected of having pure red cell aplasia. Examination of the peripheral blood smear in such cases is important because signs of hemolytic disease suggest chronic hemolysis complicated by an aplastic crisis due to parvovirus infection. Appreciation of this phenomenon is important because chronic hemolytic disease may not

be diagnosed until the anemia is exacerbated by an episode of red cell aplasia that results in a rapidly falling hemoglobin level. In such cases, cardiovascular compromise and congestive heart failure may develop quickly.

## 1. Congenital Hypoplastic Anemia (Diamond–Blackfan Anemia)

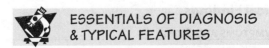

### ESSENTIALS OF DIAGNOSIS & TYPICAL FEATURES

- *Age: birth to 1 year.*
- *Macrocytic anemia with reticulocytopenia.*
- *Bone marrow with erythroid hypoplasia.*
- *Short stature or congenital anomalies in one third of patients.*

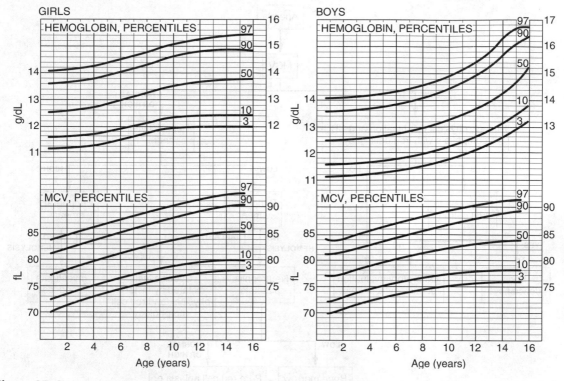

***Figure 27–2.*** Hemoglobin and red cell volume in infancy and childhood. (Reproduced, with permission, from Dallman PR, Siimes MA: Percentile curves for hemoglobin and red cell volume in infancy and childhood. J Pediatr 1979;94:26.)

## General Considerations

Diamond–Blackfan anemia is a relatively rare cause of anemia that usually presents in infancy or early childhood. Early diagnosis is important because treatment with corticosteroids results in increased erythropoiesis in about two thirds of patients, thus avoiding the difficulties and complications of long-term chronic transfusion therapy. The cause is unclear, and both autosomal dominant and autosomal recessive modes of inheritance have been reported.

## Clinical Findings

### A. SYMPTOMS AND SIGNS

Signs and symptoms are generally those of chronic anemia, such as pallor; congestive heart failure sometimes follows. Jaundice, splenomegaly, or other evidence of hemolysis is usually absent. Short stature or other congenital anomalies are present in one third of patients. A wide variety of anomalies have been described; those affecting the head, face, and thumbs are the most common.

### B. LABORATORY FINDINGS

Diamond–Blackfan anemia is characterized by severe anemia and marked reticulocytopenia. The neutrophil count is usually normal or slightly decreased, and the platelet count is normal or elevated. The bone marrow usually shows a marked decrease in erythroid precursors but is otherwise normal. In older children, fetal hemoglobin levels are usually increased and there is evidence of persistent fetal erythropoiesis, such as the presence of the i antigen on erythrocytes. In addition, the level of adenosine deaminase in erythrocytes is elevated.

## Differential Diagnosis

The principal differential diagnosis is transient erythroblastopenia of childhood. Children with Diamond–Blackfan anemia generally present at an earlier age, often have macrocytosis, and have evidence of fetal erythropoiesis and an elevated level of red cell adenosine deaminase. In addition, short stature and congenital anomalies, which occur in one third of patients with Diamond–Blackfan anemia, are not associated with transient erythroblastopenia. Lastly, transient erythroblastopenia of childhood usually resolves within 6–8 weeks of diagnosis, whereas Diamond–Blackfan anemia is generally a lifelong affliction. Other disorders associated with decreased red cell production such as renal failure, hypothyroidism, and the anemia of chronic disease need to be considered.

## Treatment

Oral corticosteroids should be initiated as soon as the diagnosis of Diamond–Blackfan anemia is made. Two thirds of patients will respond to prednisone, 2 mg/kg/d, and many of those who respond subsequently tolerate significant tapering of the dose. Patients who are unresponsive to prednisone require chronic red cell transfusion therapy, which inevitably causes transfusion-induced hemosiderosis and the need for chelation with parenteral deferoxamine. Bone marrow transplantation is an alternative therapy that should be considered for transfusion-dependent patients who have HLA-matched siblings. Hematopoietic growth factors have been used in some cases with limited success. Unpredictable, spontaneous remissions occur in up to 20% of patients.

## Prognosis

The prognosis for patients responsive to corticosteroids is generally good, particularly if remission is maintained with low doses of alternate-day prednisone. Patients dependent on transfusion are at risk for the complications of hemosiderosis, including death from congestive heart failure, cardiac arrhythmias, or hepatic failure. This remains a significant threat, particularly during adolescence, when compliance with nightly subcutaneous infusions of deferoxamine is often difficult to ensure.

Vlachos A et al: The Diamond–Blackfan Anemia Registry: Tool for investigating the epidemiology and biology of Diamond–Blackfan anemia. J Pediatr Hematol Oncol 2001;23:377 [PMID: 11563775].

Vlachos A et al: Hematopoietic stem cell transplantation for Diamond–Blackfan anemia: A report from the Diamond–Blackfan Anemia Registry. Bone Marrow Transplant 2001;27:381 [PMID: 11313667].

## 2. Transient Erythroblastopenia of Childhood

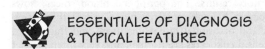

### ESSENTIALS OF DIAGNOSIS & TYPICAL FEATURES

- *Age: 6 months to 4 years.*
- *Normocytic anemia with reticulocytopenia.*
- *Absence of hepatosplenomegaly or lymphadenopathy.*
- *Erythroid precursors initially absent from bone marrow.*

## General Considerations

Transient erythroblastopenia of childhood is a relatively common cause of acquired anemia in early childhood. The disorder is suspected when a normocytic anemia is discovered during evaluation of pallor or when a CBC is obtained for another reason. Because the anemia is due to decreased red cell production, and thus develops slowly, the cardiovascular system has time to compensate. Therefore, children with hemoglobin levels as low as 4 or 5 g/dL may look remarkably well. The disorder is thought to be autoimmune in most cases, because IgG from some patients has been shown to suppress erythropoiesis in vitro.

## Clinical Findings

Pallor is the most common sign, and hepatosplenomegaly and lymphadenopathy are absent. The anemia is normocytic, and the peripheral blood smear shows no evidence of hemolysis. The platelet count is normal or elevated, and the neutrophil count is normal or, in some cases, decreased. Early in the course, no reticulocytes are identified. The Coombs test is negative, and there is no evidence of chronic renal disease, hypothyroidism, or other systemic disorder. Bone marrow examination shows severe erythroid hypoplasia initially; subsequently, erythroid hyperplasia develops along with reticulocytosis, and the anemia resolves.

## Differential Diagnosis

Transient erythroblastopenia of childhood must be differentiated from Diamond–Blackfan anemia, particularly in infants younger than age 1 year. In contrast to Diamond–Blackfan anemia, transient erythroblastopenia is not associated with macrocytosis, short stature, or congenital anomalies, or with evidence of fetal erythropoiesis prior to the phase of recovery. Also in contrast to Diamond–Blackfan anemia, transient erythroblastopenia is associated with normal levels of red cell adenosine deaminase. Transient erythroblastopenia of childhood must also be differentiated from chronic disorders associated with decreased red cell production, such as renal failure, hypothyroidism, and other chronic states of infection or inflammation. As with other single cytopenias, the possibility of malignancy (ie, leukemia) should always be considered, particularly if fever, bone pain, hepatosplenomegaly, or lymphadenopathy is present. In such cases, examination of the bone marrow is generally diagnostic. Confusion may sometimes arise when the anemia of transient erythroblastopenia is first identified during the early phase of recovery when the reticulocyte count is high. In such cases, the disorder may be confused with the anemia of acute blood loss or with hemolytic disease. In contrast to hemolytic disorders, transient erythroblastopenia of childhood is not associated with jaundice or peripheral destruction of red cells.

## Treatment & Prognosis

By definition, this is a transient disorder. Some children require red cell transfusions if cardiovascular compromise is present. Resolution of the anemia is heralded by an increase in the reticulocyte count, which generally occurs within 4–8 weeks of diagnosis. In contrast to other autoimmune disorders of childhood (eg, ITP, autoimmune hemolytic anemia), transient erythroblastopenia of childhood is not treated with corticosteroids.

Cherrick I et al: Transient erythroblastopenia of childhood: Prospective study of fifty patients. Am J Pediatr Hematol Oncol 1994;16:320 [PMID: 7978049].

Miller R, Berman B: Transient erythroblastopenia of childhood in infants < 6 months of age. Am J Pediatr Hematol Oncol 1994;16:246 [PMID: 8037344].

## NUTRITIONAL ANEMIAS

### 1. Iron Deficiency Anemia

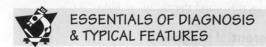

> ### ESSENTIALS OF DIAGNOSIS & TYPICAL FEATURES
>
> - *Pallor and fatigue.*
> - *Poor dietary intake of iron (ages 6–24 months).*
> - *Chronic blood loss (age > 2 years).*
> - *Microcytic hypochromic anemia.*

## General Considerations

Long considered the most common cause of anemia in pediatrics, the incidence of iron deficiency has decreased substantially due to improved nutrition and the increased availability of iron-fortified infant formulas and cereals. Thus the current approach to anemia in childhood must take into consideration a relatively greater likelihood of other causes.

Normal-term infants are born with sufficient iron stores to prevent iron deficiency for the first 4–5 months of life. Thereafter, enough iron needs to be absorbed to keep pace with the needs of rapid growth. For this reason, nutritional iron deficiency is most common between 6 and 24 months of life. A deficiency earlier than age 6 months may occur if iron stores at birth are reduced by prematurity, small birth weight, neonatal anemia, or perinatal blood loss or if there is subsequent iron loss due to hemorrhage. Iron-deficient children older than age 24 months should be evaluated for blood loss.

A significant body of evidence indicates that iron deficiency, in addition to causing anemia, has adverse effects on multiple organ systems. Thus, the importance of identifying and treating iron deficiency extends past the resolution of any symptoms directly attributable to a decreased hemoglobin concentration.

## Clinical Findings

### A. SYMPTOMS AND SIGNS

Symptoms and signs vary with the severity of the deficiency. Mild iron deficiency is usually asymptomatic. In infants with more severe iron deficiency, pallor, fatigue, irritability, and delayed motor development are common. Children whose iron deficiency is due in part to ingestion of unfortified cow's milk may be fat and flabby, with poor muscle tone. A history of pica is common.

### B. LABORATORY FINDINGS

The severity of anemia depends on the degree of iron deficiency, and the hemoglobin level may be as low as 3–4 g/dL in severe cases. Red cells are microcytic and hypochromic, with a low MCV and low mean corpuscular hemoglobin (MCH). The red blood cell distribution width (RDW) is typically elevated, even with mild iron deficiency. The reticulocyte count is usually normal or slightly elevated, but the reticulocyte index or absolute reticulocyte count is decreased. Iron studies show a decreased serum ferritin and a low serum iron, elevated total iron-binding capacity, and decreased transferrin saturation. These laboratory abnormalities are usually present with moderate to severe iron deficiency, but mild cases may be associated with variable laboratory results. The peripheral blood smear shows microcytic, hypochromic red blood cells with anisocytosis, and occasional target, teardrop, and fragmented red cells. Leukocytes are normal, and very often platelet count is increased with normal morphology.

The bone marrow examination is not helpful in the diagnosis of iron deficiency in infants and small children because little or no iron is stored as marrow hemosiderin at these ages.

## Differential Diagnosis

The differential diagnosis is that of microcytic, hypochromic anemia. The possibility of thalassemia ($\alpha$-thalassemia, $\beta$-thalassemia, hemoglobin E disorders) should be considered, especially in infants of African, Mediterranean, or Asian ethnic background. In contrast to infants with iron deficiency, those with thalassemia generally have an elevated number of erythrocytes (the index of the MCV divided by the red cell number is usually less than 13) and are less likely, in mild cases, to have an elevated RDW. Thalassemias are associated with normal or increased levels of serum iron and ferritin and with normal iron-binding capacity. The hemoglobin electrophoresis in $\beta$-thalassemia minor typically shows an elevation of hemoglobin $A_2$ levels, but coexistent iron deficiency may lower the percentage of hemoglobin $A_2$ into the normal range. Hemoglobin electrophoresis will also identify children with hemoglobin E, a cause of microcytosis common in Southeast Asians. In contrast, the hemoglobin electrophoresis in $\alpha$-thalassemia trait is normal. Lead poisoning has also been associated with microcytic anemia, but anemia with lead levels less than 40 mg/dL is often due to coexistent iron deficiency.

The anemia of chronic inflammation or infection is normocytic but in late stages may be microcytic. This anemia is usually suspected because of the presence of a chronic systemic disorder. The level of serum iron is low, but the iron-binding capacity is normal, and the serum ferritin level is elevated. Relatively mild infections, particularly during infancy, may cause transient anemia. As a result, caution should be exercised when the diagnosis of mild iron deficiency is entertained in infants and young children who have had recent viral or bacterial infections. Ideally, screening tests for anemia should not be obtained within 3–4 weeks of such infections.

## Treatment

The recommended oral dose of elemental iron is 4–6 mg/kg/d in three divided daily doses. Mild cases may be treated with 3 mg/kg/d given once daily before breakfast. Parenteral administration of iron is rarely necessary. Iron therapy results in an increased reticulocyte count within 3–5 days, which is maximal between 5 and 7 days. The hemoglobin level begins to increase thereafter. The rate of hemoglobin rise is inversely related to the hemoglobin level at diagnosis. In moderate to severe cases, an elevated reticulocyte count 1 week after initiation of therapy confirms the diagnosis and

documents compliance and response to therapy. When iron deficiency is the only cause of anemia, adequate treatment usually results in a resolution of the anemia within 4–6 weeks. Treatment is generally continued for a few additional months to replenish iron stores.

Buchanan GR: The tragedy of iron deficiency during infancy and early childhood. J Pediatr 1999;135:413 [PMID: 10518073].

Hermiston ML, Mentzer WC: A practical approach to the evaluation of the anemic child. Pediatr Clin North Am 2002; 49:877 [PMID: 12430617].

Kwiatkowski JL et al: Severe iron deficiency anemia in young children. J Pediatr 1999;135:514 [PMID: 10518088].

## 2. Megaloblastic Anemias

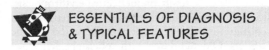

### ESSENTIALS OF DIAGNOSIS & TYPICAL FEATURES

- *Pallor and fatigue.*
- *Nutritional deficiency or intestinal malabsorption.*
- *Macrocytic anemia.*
- *Megaloblastic bone marrow changes.*

### General Considerations

Megaloblastic anemia is a macrocytic anemia caused by deficiency of cobalamin (vitamin $B_{12}$), folic acid, or both. Cobalamin deficiency due to dietary insufficiency may occur in infants who are breast-fed by mothers who are strict vegetarians or who have pernicious anemia. Intestinal malabsorption is the usual cause of cobalamin deficiency in pediatrics and occurs with Crohn disease, chronic pancreatitis, bacterial overgrowth of the small bowel, infection with the fish tapeworm (*Diphyllobothrium latum*), or after surgical resection of the terminal ileum. Deficiencies due to inborn errors of metabolism (transcobalamin II deficiency, methylmalonic aciduria) have also been described. Malabsorption of cobalamin due to deficiency of intrinsic factor (pernicious anemia) is rare in childhood.

Folic acid deficiency may be caused by inadequate dietary intake, malabsorption, increased folate requirements, or some combination of the three. Folate deficiency due to dietary deficiency alone is rare but occurs in severely malnourished infants and has been reported in infants fed goat's milk not fortified with folic acid. Folic acid is absorbed in the proximal small bowel, and deficiencies are encountered in malabsorptive syndromes such as celiac disease. Anticonvulsant medications (eg, phenytoin and phenobarbital) and cytotoxic drugs (eg, methotrexate) have also been associated with folate deficiency, caused by interference with folate absorption or metabolism. Finally, folic acid deficiency is more likely to develop in infants and children with increased requirements. This occurs during infancy because of rapid growth and also in children with chronic hemolytic anemia. Premature infants are particularly susceptible to the development of the deficiency because of low body stores of folate.

## Clinical Findings

### A. SYMPTOMS AND SIGNS

Infants with megaloblastic anemia may show pallor and mild jaundice as a result of ineffective erythropoiesis. Classically, the tongue is smooth and beefy red. Infants with cobalamin deficiency may be irritable and may be poor feeders. Older children with cobalamin deficiency may complain of paresthesias, weakness, or an unsteady gait and may show decreased vibratory sensation and proprioception on neurologic examination.

### B. LABORATORY FINDINGS

The laboratory findings of megaloblastic anemia include an elevated MCV and MCH. The peripheral blood smear shows numerous macro-ovalocytes with anisocytosis and poikilocytosis. Neutrophils are large and have hypersegmented nuclei. The white cell and platelet counts are normal with mild deficiencies, but may be decreased in more severe cases. Examination of the bone marrow typically shows erythroid hyperplasia with large erythroid and myeloid precursors. Nuclear maturation is delayed compared with cytoplasmic maturation, and erythropoiesis is ineffective. The serum indirect bilirubin concentration may be slightly elevated.

Children with cobalamin deficiency have a low serum vitamin $B_{12}$ level, but decreased levels of serum vitamin $B_{12}$ may also be found in about 30% of patients with folic acid deficiency. The level of red cell folate is a better reflection of folate stores than is the serum folic acid level. Serum levels of metabolic intermediates, methylmalonic acid, and homocysteine may help establish the correct diagnosis. Elevated methylmalonic acid levels are consistent with cobalamin deficiency, whereas elevated levels of homocysteine occur with both cobalamin and folate deficiency.

## Differential Diagnosis

Most macrocytic anemias in pediatrics are not megaloblastic. Other causes of an increased MCV include drug therapy (eg, anticonvulsants, anti-HIV nucleoside analogues), congenital heart disease, Down syndrome, an elevated reticulocyte count (hemolytic anemias), bone marrow failure syndromes (Fanconi anemia, Diamond–Blackfan anemia), liver disease, and hypothyroidism.

## Treatment

Treatment of cobalamin deficiency due to inadequate dietary intake is readily accomplished with oral supplementation. Most cases, however, are due to intestinal malabsorption and require parenteral treatment. In severe cases, parenteral therapy may induce life-threatening hypokalemia and require supplemental potassium. Folic acid deficiency is treated effectively with oral folic acid in most cases. Children at risk for the development of folic acid deficiencies, such as premature infants and those with chronic hemolysis, are often given folic acid prophylactically.

Graham SM et al: Long-term neurologic consequences of nutritional vitamin $B_{12}$ deficiency in infants. J Pediatr 1992;121: 710 [PMID: 1432418].

Pappo AS et al: Etiology of red blood cell macrocytosis during childhood: Impact of new diseases and therapies. Pediatrics 1992;89:1063 [PMID: 1534402].

Rosenblatt DS, Whitehead VM: Cobalamin and folate deficiency: Acquired and hereditary disorders in children. Semin Hematol 1999;36:19 [PMID: 9930566].

## ANEMIA OF CHRONIC DISORDERS

Anemia is a common manifestation of many chronic illnesses in children. In some instances, causes may be mixed. For example, children with chronic disorders involving intestinal malabsorption or blood loss may have anemia of chronic inflammation in combination with nutritional deficiencies of iron, folate, or cobalamin. In other settings, the anemia is due to dysfunction of a single organ (eg, renal failure, hypothyroidism), and correction of the underlying abnormality resolves the anemia.

## 1. Anemia of Chronic Inflammation

Anemia is frequently associated with chronic infections or inflammatory diseases. The anemia is usually mild to moderate in severity, with a hemoglobin level of 8–12 g/dL. In general, the severity of the anemia corresponds to the severity of the underlying disorder, and there may be microcytosis but not hypochromia. The reticulocyte count is low. The anemia is thought to be due to inflammatory cytokines that inhibit erythropoiesis and impair iron release by reticuloendothelial cells. Levels of erythropoetin are relatively low for the severity of the anemia. The serum iron concentration is low, but in contrast to iron deficiency, anemia of chronic inflammation is not associated with elevated iron-binding capacity and is associated with an elevated serum ferritin level. Treatment consists of correction of the underlying disorder, which, if controlled, generally results in improvement in hemoglobin level.

Ambruso DR: The anemias of chronic disease. In Gross S, Roath S (eds): *Hematology: A Problem Oriented Approach.* Williams & Wilkins, 1996, p 179.

Hagar W et al: Diseases of iron metabolism. Pediatr Clin North Am 2002;49:893 [PMID: 12430618].

## 2. Anemia of Chronic Renal Failure

Severe normocytic anemia occurs in most forms of renal disease that have progressed to renal insufficiency. Although white cell and platelet production remain normal, the bone marrow shows significant hypoplasia of the erythroid series and the reticulocyte count is low. The principal mechanism is deficiency of erythropoietin, a hormone produced in the kidney, but other factors may contribute to the anemia. In the presence of significant uremia, a component of hemolysis may also be present. In the past, treatment of the anemia of chronic renal failure depended on transfusions of packed red blood cells. However, recombinant human erythropoietin (epoetin alfa) corrects the anemia, and its use has largely eliminated the need for transfusions.

Brandt JR et al: Safety and efficacy of erythropoietin in children with chronic renal failure. Pediatr Nephrol 1999;13:143 [PMID: 10229004].

Seeherunvong W et al: Identification of poor responders to erythropoietin among children undergoing hemodialysis. J Pediatr 2001;138:710 [PMID: 11343048].

Yorgin PD et al: The clinical efficacy of higher hematocrit levels in children with chronic renal insufficiency and those undergoing dialysis. Semin Nephrol 2001;21:451 [PMID: 11559886].

## 3. Anemia of Hypothyroidism

Some patients with hypothyroidism develop significant anemia. Occasionally, anemia is detected before the diagnosis of the underlying disorder. A decreased growth velocity in an anemic child suggests hypothyroidism. The anemia is usually normocytic or macrocytic, but it is not megaloblastic and hence not due to deficiencies of cobalamin or folate. Replacement therapy with thyroid hormone is usually effective in correcting the anemia.

Cheu J-Y et al: Anemia in children and adolescents with hypothyroidism. Clin Pediatr 1981;20:696 [PMID: 7297010].

Franzese A et al: Anemia in infants with congenital hypothyroidism diagnosed by neonatal screening. J Endocrinol Invest 1996;19:613 [PMID: 8957746].

# CONGENITAL HEMOLYTIC ANEMIAS: RED CELL MEMBRANE DEFECTS

The congenital hemolytic anemias are usually divided into three categories: defects of the red cell membrane, hemoglobinopathies, and disorders of red cell metabolism. Hereditary spherocytosis and elliptocytosis are the most common red cell membrane disorders and are described here. The diagnosis is suggested by the peripheral blood smear, which shows characteristic red cell morphology (eg, spherocytes, elliptocytes). These disorders usually have an autosomal dominant inheritance, and the diagnosis may be suggested by a family history. The hemolysis is due to the deleterious effect of the membrane abnormality on red cell deformability. Decreased cell deformability leads to entrapment of the abnormally shaped red cells in the spleen. Many patients have splenomegaly, and splenectomy usually alleviates the hemolysis.

## 1. Hereditary Spherocytosis

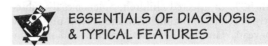

### ESSENTIALS OF DIAGNOSIS & TYPICAL FEATURES

- *Anemia and jaundice.*
- *Splenomegaly.*
- *Positive family history of anemia, jaundice, or gallstones.*
- *Spherocytosis with increased reticulocytes.*
- *Increased osmotic fragility.*
- *Negative direct antiglobulin test (DAT).*

### General Considerations

Hereditary spherocytosis is a relatively common inherited hemolytic anemia that occurs in all ethnic groups but is most common in persons of Northern European ancestry, in whom the incidence is about 1:5000. The disorder is a heterogeneous one, marked by variable degrees of anemia, jaundice, and splenomegaly. In some persons, the disorder is mild and there is no anemia because erythroid hyperplasia fully compensates for hemolysis. Severe cases are transfusion-dependent prior to splenectomy. The hallmark of hereditary spherocytosis is the presence of microspherocytes in the peripheral blood. The disease is inherited in an autosomal dominant fashion in about 75% of cases; the remainder is thought to be autosomal recessive or to be caused by new mutations.

Hereditary spherocytosis is usually the result of a partial deficiency of spectrin, an important structural protein of the red cell membrane skeleton. Spectrin deficiency weakens the attachment of the cell membrane to the underlying membrane skeleton and causes the red cell to lose membrane surface area. This process creates spherocytes that are poorly deformable and have a shortened life span because they are trapped in the microcirculation of the spleen and engulfed by splenic macrophages. The extreme heterogeneity of hereditary spherocytosis is related directly to variable degrees of spectrin deficiency. In general, children who inherit spherocytosis in an autosomal dominant fashion have lesser degrees of spectrin deficiency and mild or moderate hemolysis. In contrast, those with nondominant forms of spherocytosis tend to have greater deficiencies of spectrin and a more severe anemia.

## Clinical Findings

### A. SYMPTOMS AND SIGNS

Hemolysis causes significant neonatal hyperbilirubinemia in 50% of affected children. Splenomegaly subsequently develops in the majority and is often present by age 5 years. Jaundice is variably present and in many patients may be noted only during infection. Patients with significant chronic anemia may complain of pallor, fatigue, or malaise. Intermittent exacerbations of the anemia are caused by increased hemolysis or by aplastic crises and may be associated with severe weakness, fatigue, fever, abdominal pain, or even congestive heart failure.

### B. LABORATORY FINDINGS

Most patients have mild chronic hemolysis with hemoglobin levels of 9–12 g/dL. In some cases, the hemolysis is fully compensated and the hemoglobin level is in the normal range. Rare cases of severe disease require frequent transfusions. The anemia is usually normocytic and hyperchromic, and many patients have an elevated MCH concentration. The peripheral blood smear shows numerous microspherocytes and polychromasia. The reticulocyte count is elevated, often higher than might be expected for the degree of anemia. White blood cell and platelet counts are usually normal. The osmotic fragility is increased, particularly after incubation at 37°C for 24 hours. Serum bilirubin usually shows an elevation in the unconjugated fraction. DAT is negative.

## Differential Diagnosis

Spherocytes are frequently present in persons with immune hemolysis. Thus, in the newborn, hereditary spherocytosis must be distinguished from hemolytic disease caused by ABO or other blood type incompatibilities. Older patients with autoimmune hemolytic anemia frequently present with jaundice and splenomegaly and with spherocytes on the peripheral blood smear. The DAT is positive in most cases of immune hemolysis and negative in hereditary spherocytosis. Occasionally, the diagnosis is confused in patients with splenomegaly from other causes, especially when hypersplenism increases red cell destruction and when some spherocytes are noted on the blood smear. In such cases, the true cause of the splenomegaly may be suggested by signs or symptoms of portal hypertension or by laboratory evidence of chronic liver disease. In contrast to children with hereditary spherocytosis, those with hypersplenism typically have some degree of thrombocytopenia or neutropenia.

## Complications

Severe jaundice may occur in the neonatal period and, if not controlled by phototherapy, may occasionally require exchange transfusion. Splenectomy is associated with an increased risk of overwhelming bacterial infections, particularly with pneumococci. Gallstones occur in 60–70% of adults who have not undergone splenectomy and may form as early as age 5–10 years.

## Treatment

Supportive measures include the administration of folic acid to prevent the development of red cell hypoplasia due to folate deficiency. Acute exacerbations of anemia, due to increased rates of hemolysis or to aplastic crises due to infection with human parvovirus, may be severe enough to require red cell transfusions. Splenectomy is performed in many cases and always results in significant improvement. The procedure increases the survival of the spherocytic red cells and leads to complete correction of the anemia in most cases. Patients with more severe disease may show some degree of hemolysis after splenectomy. Except in unusually severe cases, the procedure should be postponed until the child is at least age 5 years because of the greater risk of postsplenectomy sepsis prior to this age. Alternatively, partial splenectomy may be considered for young children with severe hemolysis. All patients scheduled for splenectomy should be immunized with pneumococcal vaccine prior to the procedure, and some clinicians recommend penicillin prophylaxis afterward. The need for splenectomy in mild cases is somewhat controversial. Splenectomy in the middle childhood years prevents the subsequent development of cholelithiasis and eliminates the need for the activity restrictions recommended for children with splenomegaly. However, these benefits must be weighed against the risks of the surgical procedure and the subsequent lifelong risk of postsplenectomy sepsis.

## Prognosis

Splenectomy eliminates signs and symptoms in all but the most severe cases and reduces the risk of cholelithiasis. The abnormal red cell morphology and increased osmotic fragility persist without clinical consequence.

Delhommeau F et al: Natural history of hereditary spherocytosis during the first year of life. Blood 2000;95:393 [PMID: 10627440].

Hassoun H et al: Characterization of the underlying molecular defect in hereditary spherocytosis associated with spectrin deficiency. Blood 1997;90:398 [PMID: 9207476].

Michaels LA et al: Screening for hereditary spherocytosis by use of automated erythrocyte indexes. J Pediatr 1997;130:957 [PMID: 9202619].

Tchernia G et al: Initial assessment of the beneficial effect of partial splenectomy in hereditary spherocytosis. Blood 1993;81: 2014 [PMID: 8471763].

## 2. Hereditary Elliptocytosis

Hereditary elliptocytosis is a heterogeneous disorder that ranges in severity from an asymptomatic carrier state with normal red cell morphology to severe hemolytic anemia. Most affected persons have numerous elliptocytes on the peripheral blood smear but mild or no hemolysis. Those with hemolysis have an elevated reticulocyte count and may have jaundice and splenomegaly. These disorders are caused by mutations of red cell membrane skeletal proteins, and most have an autosomal dominant inheritance. Because most patients are asymptomatic, no treatment is indicated. Patients with significant degrees of hemolytic anemia may benefit from folate supplementation or from splenectomy.

Some infants with hereditary elliptocytosis present in the neonatal period with moderate to marked hemolysis and significant hyperbilirubinemia. This disorder has been termed "transient infantile poikilocytosis" because such infants exhibit bizarre erythrocyte morphology with elliptocytes, budding red cells, and small misshapen cells that defy description. The MCV is low, and the anemia may be severe enough to require red cell transfusions. Typically, one parent has hereditary elliptocytosis, usually mild or asymptomatic. The infant's hemolysis gradually abates during the first year of life, and the erythrocyte morphology subsequently becomes more typical of hereditary elliptocytosis.

Mentzer WC et al: Modulation of erythrocyte membrane mechanical stability by 2,3-diphosphoglycerate in the neonatal poikilocytosis/elliptocytosis syndrome. J Clin Invest 1987;79: 943 [PMID: 3818955].

Palek J, Sahr KE: Mutations of the red cell membrane proteins: From clinical evaluation to detection of the underlying genetic defect. Blood 1992;8:308 [PMID: 1627793].

## CONGENITAL HEMOLYTIC ANEMIAS: HEMOGLOBINOPATHIES

The hemoglobinopathies are an extremely heterogeneous group of congenital disorders that occur in many different ethnic groups. The relatively high frequency of these genetic variants is related to the malaria protection afforded to heterozygous individuals. The hemoglobinopathies are generally classified into two major groups. The first, the thalassemias, are caused by quantitative deficiencies in the production of globin chains. These quantitative defects in globin synthesis cause microcytic and hypochromic anemias. The second group of hemoglobinopathies are those caused by structural abnormalities of globin chains. The most important of these, hemoglobins S, C, and E, are all the result of point mutations and single amino acid substitutions in β-globin. Many, but not all, infants with hemoglobinopathies are identified by routine neonatal screening.

Figure 27–3 shows the normal developmental changes that occur in globin-chain production during gestation and the first year of life. At birth, the predominant hemoglobin is fetal hemoglobin (hemoglobin F), which is composed of two α-globin chains and two γ-globin chains. Subsequently, the production of γ-globin decreases and the production of β-globin increases so that adult hemoglobin (two α chains and two β chains) predominates after 2–4 months. Because α-globin chains are present in both fetal and adult hemoglobin, disorders of α-globin synthesis (α-thalassemia) are clinically manifest in the newborn as well as later in life. In contrast, patients with β-globin disorders such as β-thalassemia and sickle cell disease are generally asymptomatic during the first 3–4 months of age and present clinically after γ-chain production—and therefore fetal hemoglobin levels—have decreased substantially.

## 1. α-Thalassemia

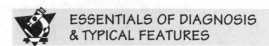

### ESSENTIALS OF DIAGNOSIS & TYPICAL FEATURES

- *African, Mediterranean, Middle Eastern, Chinese, or Southeast Asian ancestry.*
- *Microcytic, hypochromic anemia of variable severity.*

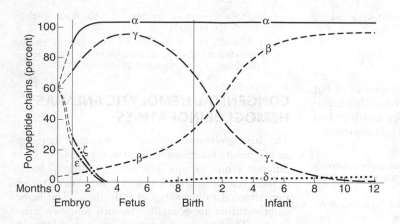

**Figure 27–3.** Changes in hemoglobin polypeptide chains during human development. (Reproduced, with permission, from Miller DR, Baehner RL: *Blood Diseases of Infancy and Childhood*, 6th ed. Mosby, 1989.)

• Hemoglobin Bart's detected by neonatal screening.

## General Considerations

Most of the α-thalassemia syndromes are the result of deletions of one or more of the α-globin genes on chromosome 16. Normal diploid cells have four α-globin genes; thus the variable severity of the α-thalassemia syndromes is related to the number of gene deletions (Table 27–1). The severity of the α-thalassemia syndromes varies among affected ethnic groups, depending on the genetic abnormalities prevalent in the population. In persons of African ancestry, α-thalassemia is usually caused by the deletion of only one of the two α-globin genes on each chromosome. Thus, in the African population, heterozygous individuals are silent carriers and homozygous individuals have α-tha-

lassemia trait. In Asians, deletions of one or of both α-globin genes on the same chromosome are common. Thus heterozygous individuals are either silent carriers or have α-thalassemia trait, and homozygous individuals or compound heterozygous individuals have α-thalassemia trait, hemoglobin H disease, or hydrops fetalis. Thus the presence of α-thalassemia in a child of Asian ancestry may have important implications for genetic counseling, whereas this is not usually the case in families of African ancestry.

## Clinical Findings

The clinical findings depend on the number of α-globin genes deleted. Table 27–1 summarizes the α-thalassemia syndromes.

Persons with three α-globin genes (one-gene deletion) are asymptomatic and have no hematologic abnormalities. Hemoglobin levels and MCV are normal. Hemoglobin electrophoresis in the neonatal period

**Table 27–1.** The α-thalassemias

| Usual Genotypes[a] | α Gene Number | Clinical Features | Hemoblobin Electrophoresis[b] Birth | > 6 mos |
|---|---|---|---|---|
| αα/αα | 4 | Normal | N | N |
| –α/αα | 3 | Silent carrier | 0–3% Hb Bart's | N |
| --/αα or -α/-α | 2 | α-thal trait | 2–10% Hb Bart's | N |
| --/-α | 1 | Hb H disease | 15–30% Hb Bart's | Hb H present |
| --/-- | 0 | Fetal hydrops | > 75% Hb Bart's | - |

[a]α indicates presence of α-globin gene, – indicates deletion of α-globin gene
[b]N = normal results, Hb = hemoglobin, Hb Bart's = $\gamma_4$, Hb H = $\beta_4$.

shows 0–3% Bart's hemoglobin, a variant hemoglobin composed of four γ-globin chains. Hemoglobin electrophoresis after the first few months of life is normal. Thus this condition is usually suspected only in the context of family studies or when a small amount of Bart's hemoglobin is detected by neonatal screening for hemoglobinopathies.

Persons with two α-globin genes (two-gene deletion) are typically asymptomatic. The MCV is usually less than 100 fL at birth. Hematologic studies in older infants and children show a normal or slightly decreased hemoglobin level with a low MCV and a slightly hypochromic blood smear with some target cells. The hemoglobin electrophoresis typically shows 2–10% Bart's hemoglobin in the neonatal period but is normal in older children and adults.

Persons with one α-globin gene (three-gene deletion) have a mild to moderately severe microcytic hemolytic anemia (hemoglobin level of 7–10 g/dL), which may be accompanied by hepatosplenomegaly and some bony abnormalities caused by the expanded medullary space. The reticulocyte count is elevated, and the red cells show marked hypochromia and microcytosis with significant poikilocytosis and some basophilic stippling. Hemoglobin electrophoresis in the neonatal period typically shows 15–30% Bart's hemoglobin. Later in life, hemoglobin H (composed of four β-globin chains) is present. Incubation of red cells with brilliant cresyl blue (hemoglobin H preparation) shows inclusion bodies formed by denatured hemoglobin H.

The deletion of all four α-globin genes causes severe intrauterine anemia and asphyxia and results in hydrops fetalis and fetal demise or neonatal death shortly after delivery. Extreme pallor and massive hepatosplenomegaly are present. Hemoglobin electrophoresis reveals a predominance of Bart's hemoglobin with a complete absence of normal fetal or adult hemoglobin.

### Differential Diagnosis

α-Thalassemia trait (two-gene deletion) must be differentiated from other mild microcytic anemias, including iron deficiency and β-thalassemia minor. In contrast to children with iron deficiency, those with α-thalassemia trait show normal or increased levels of ferritin and serum iron. In contrast to children with β-thalassemia minor, those with α-thalassemia trait have a normal hemoglobin electrophoresis after age 4–6 months. Finally, the history of a low MCV (96 fL) at birth or the presence of Bart's hemoglobin on the neonatal hemoglobinopathy screening test suggests α-thalassemia.

Children with hemoglobin H disease may have jaundice and splenomegaly, and the disorder must be differentiated from other hemolytic anemias. The key to the diagnosis is the decreased MCV and the marked hypochromia on the blood smear. With the exception of β-thalassemia, most other significant hemolytic disorders have a normal or elevated MCV and are not hypochromic. Infants with hydrops fetalis due to severe α-thalassemia must be distinguished from those with hydrops due to other causes of anemia such as isoimmunization.

### Complications

The principal complication of α-thalassemia trait is the needless administration of iron, given in the belief that a mild microcytic anemia is due to iron deficiency. Persons with hemoglobin H disease may have intermittent exacerbations of their anemia, which occasionally require blood transfusions. Splenomegaly may exacerbate the anemia and may require splenectomy. Women pregnant with hydropic α-thalassemia fetuses are subject to increased complications of pregnancy, particularly toxemia and postpartum hemorrhage.

### Treatment

Persons with α-thalassemia trait require no treatment. Those with hemoglobin H disease should receive supplemental folic acid and avoid the same oxidant drugs that cause hemolysis in persons with G6PD deficiency, because exposure to these drugs may exacerbate their anemia. The anemia may also be exacerbated during periods of infection, and transfusions may be required. Hypersplenism may develop later in childhood and require surgical splenectomy. Genetic counseling and prenatal diagnosis should be offered to families at risk for hydropic fetuses.

Chui DH, Waye JS: Hydrops fetalis caused by α-thalassemia: An emerging health care problem. Blood 1998;91:2213 [PMID: 9516118].

Lau Y-L et al: Prevalence and genotypes of α- and β-thalassemia carriers in Hong Kong—Implication for population screening. N Engl J Med 1997;336:1298 [PMID: 9113933].

Miller ST et al: A fast hemoglobin variant on newborn screening is associated with α-thalassemia trait. Clin Pediatr 1997;36:75 [PMID: 9118593].

## 2. β-Thalassemia

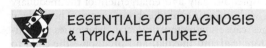

ESSENTIALS OF DIAGNOSIS & TYPICAL FEATURES

β-*Thalassemia minor:*

• *Normal neonatal screening test.*

• *African, Mediterranean, Middle Eastern, or Asian ancestry.*

- *Mild microcytic, hypochromic anemia.*
- *No response to iron therapy.*
- *Elevated level of hemoglobin A$_2$.*

*β-Thalassemia major:*

- *Neonatal screening shows hemoglobin F only.*
- *Mediterranean, Middle Eastern, or Asian ancestry.*
- *Severe microcytic, hypochromic anemia with marked hepatosplenomegaly.*

## General Considerations

In contrast to the four α-globin genes, only two β-globin genes are present in diploid cells, one on each chromosome 11. Some β-thalassemia genes produce no β-globin chains and are termed β$^0$-thalassemia. Other β-globin genes produce some β-globin but in diminished quantities and are termed β$^+$-thalassemia. Persons affected by β-thalassemia may be heterozygous or homozygous. Individuals heterozygous for most β-thalassemia genes have β-thalassemia minor. Homozygous individuals have β-thalassemia major (Cooley anemia), a severe transfusion-dependent anemia, or a condition known as thalassemia intermedia, which is more severe than thalassemia minor but is not generally transfusion dependent. β-Thalassemia major is the most common worldwide cause of transfusion-dependent anemia in childhood. In addition, β-thalassemia genes interact with genes for structural β-globin variants such as hemoglobin S and hemoglobin E to cause serious disease in compound heterozygous individuals. These disorders are discussed further in the sections dealing with sickle cell disease and with hemoglobin E disorders.

## Clinical Findings

### A. SYMPTOMS AND SIGNS

Persons with β-thalassemia minor are usually asymptomatic with a normal physical examination. Those with β-thalassemia major are normal at birth but develop significant anemia during the first year of life. If the disorder is not identified and treated with blood transfusions, such children grow poorly and develop massive hepatosplenomegaly and enlargement of the medullary space with thinning of the bony cortex. The skeletal changes cause characteristic facial deformities (prominent forehead and maxilla) and predispose the child to pathologic fractures.

### B. LABORATORY FINDINGS

Children with β-thalassemia minor have normal neonatal screening results but subsequently develop a decreased MCV with or without mild anemia. The peripheral blood smear typically shows hypochromia, target cells, and sometimes basophilic stippling. Hemoglobin electrophoresis performed after 6–12 months of age is usually diagnostic when levels of hemoglobin A$_2$, hemoglobin F, or both are elevated. β-Thalassemia major is often initially suspected when Hb A is absent on neonatal screening. Such infants are hematologically normal at birth but develop severe anemia after the first few months of life. The peripheral blood smear typically shows a severe hypochromic, microcytic anemia with marked anisocytosis and poikilocytosis. Target cells are prominent, and nucleated red blood cells often exceed the number of circulating white blood cells. The hemoglobin level usually falls to 5–6 g/dL or less, and the reticulocyte count is elevated but the reticulocyte index is normal to decreased. Platelet and white blood cell counts may be increased, and the serum bilirubin level is elevated. The bone marrow shows marked erythroid hyperplasia but is rarely needed for diagnosis. Hemoglobin electrophoresis shows only fetal hemoglobin and hemoglobin A$_2$ in children with homozygous β$^0$-thalassemia. Those with β$^+$-thalassemia genes make some hemoglobin A but have a marked increase in fetal hemoglobin and hemoglobin A$_2$ levels. The diagnosis of homozygous β-thalassemia may also be suggested by the finding of β-thalassemia minor in both parents.

## Differential Diagnosis

β-Thalassemia minor must be differentiated from other causes of mild microcytic, hypochromic anemias, principally iron deficiency and α-thalassemia. In contrast to patients with iron-deficiency anemia, those with β-thalassemia minor typically have an elevated number of red blood cells, and the index of the MCV divided by the red cell count is under 13. Generally, the finding of an elevated hemoglobin A$_2$ level is diagnostic; however, the A$_2$ level is lowered by coexistent iron deficiency, which may lead to some confusion. Thus, in children thought to be iron-deficient, hemoglobin electrophoresis with quantitation of hemoglobin A$_2$ is sometimes deferred until after a course of iron therapy.

β-Thalassemia major is rarely confused with other disorders. Hemoglobin electrophoresis and family studies readily distinguish it from hemoglobin E–β-thalassemia, which is the other important cause of transfusion-dependent thalassemia.

## Complications

The principal complication of β-thalassemia minor is the unnecessary use of iron therapy in a futile attempt to correct the microcytic anemia. Children with β-thalassemia major who are inadequately transfused experience poor growth and recurrent infections and may have hepatosplenomegaly, thinning of the cortical bone, and pathologic fractures. Without treatment, most children die within the first decade of life. The principal complications of β-thalassemia major in transfused children are hemosiderosis, splenomegaly, and hypersplenism. Transfusional hemosiderosis requires chelation therapy with deferoxamine to prevent cardiac, hepatic, and endocrine dysfunction. Noncompliance with chelation in adolescents and young adults may lead to death from congestive heart failure, cardiac arrhythmias, or hepatic failure. Even with adequate transfusions, many patients develop splenomegaly and some degree of hypersplenism. This may require surgical splenectomy because of the increasing transfusion requirements, but the procedure increases the risk of thrombosis and overwhelming septicemia.

## Treatment

β-Thalassemia minor requires no specific therapy but may have important genetic implications for the family. For patients with β-thalassemia major, two approaches to treatment are now available: chronic transfusion with iron chelation and stem cell transplantation. Programs of blood transfusion are generally targeted to maintain a nadir hemoglobin level of 9–10 g/dL. This approach gives increased vigor and well-being, improved growth, and fewer overall complications. However, maintenance of good health currently requires iron chelation with nightly subcutaneous infusion of deferoxamine. Small doses of supplemental ascorbic acid may enhance the efficacy of iron chelation. Newly developed oral iron chelators are under study. Patients who undergo splenectomy to reduce transfusion requirements, and hence iron loading, should receive pneumococcal vaccine prior to the procedure and prophylactic penicillin and urgent treatment of all febrile illness afterward.

Bone marrow or umbilical cord blood transplantation is an important therapeutic option for children with β-thalassemia major who have an HLA-identical sibling donor. The probability of hematologic cure is greater than 90% when transplantation is performed prior to the development of hepatomegaly or portal fibrosis.

Lucarelli G et al: Marrow transplantation in patients with thalassemia responsive to iron chelation therapy. N Engl J Med 1993;329:840 [PMID: 8355742].

Olivieri NF: Medical progress: The β-thalassemias. N Engl J Med 1999;34:99 [PMID: 10395635].

Olivieri NF, Brittenham GM: Iron-chelating therapy and the treatment of thalassemia. Blood 1997;89:739 [PMID: 9028304].

Olivieri NF et al: Survival in medically treated patients with homozygous β-thalassemia. N Engl J Med 1994;331:574 [PMID: 8047081].

## 3. Sickle Cell Disease

### ESSENTIALS OF DIAGNOSIS & TYPICAL FEATURES

- Neonatal screening test with hemoglobin FS, FSC, or FSA.
- African, Mediterranean, Middle Eastern, Indian, or Caribbean ancestry.
- Anemia, elevated reticulocyte count, jaundice.
- Recurrent episodes of musculoskeletal or abdominal pain.
- Hemoglobin electrophoresis with hemoglobins S and F; hemoglobins S and C; or hemoglobins S, A, and F with S > A.
- Splenomegaly in early childhood with later disappearance.
- High risk of bacterial sepsis.

### General Considerations

A high prevalence of sickle hemoglobin is found in persons of central African origin. It also occurs in other ethnic groups in Sicily, Italy, Greece, Turkey, Saudi Arabia, and India. Sickle cell anemia is caused by homozygosity for the sickle gene and is the most common form of sickle cell disease. Other clinically important sickling disorders are compound heterozygous conditions in which the sickle gene interacts with genes for hemoglobin C, $D_{Punjab}$, $O_{Arab}$, $C_{Harlem}$, or β-thalassemia.

Overall, sickle cell disease occurs in about one of every 400 African American infants. Eight percent of African Americans are heterozygous carriers of the sickle gene and are said to have sickle cell trait.

The protean clinical manifestations of sickle hemoglobinopathies can be linked directly or indirectly to the propensity of deoxygenated hemoglobin S to polymerize. Polymerization of sickle hemoglobin distorts erythrocyte morphology, decreases red cell deformability, causes a marked reduction in red cell life span, increases blood viscosity, and predisposes to episodes of vaso-occlusion.

Neonatal screening for sickle hemoglobinopathies is now routine in most of the United States. The identification of affected infants at birth, when combined with follow-up programs of parental education, comprehensive medical care, and prophylactic penicillin, markedly reduces morbidity and mortality in early childhood.

## Clinical Findings

### A. SYMPTOMS AND SIGNS

These are related to the hemolytic anemia and to tissue ischemia and organ dysfunction caused by vaso-occlusion. Children are normal at birth, and onset of symptoms is unusual before age 3–4 months because high levels of fetal hemoglobin inhibit sickling. A moderately severe hemolytic anemia may be present by age 1 year; causes pallor, fatigue, and jaundice; and predisposes to the development of gallstones during childhood and adolescence. Intense congestion of the spleen with sickled cells may cause splenomegaly in early childhood and results in functional asplenia as early as age 3 months. This places children at great risk for overwhelming infection with encapsulated bacteria, particularly pneumococci. Up to 30% of patients experience one or more episodes of acute splenic sequestration, characterized by sudden enlargement of the spleen with pooling of red cells, acute exacerbation of anemia, and, in severe cases, shock and death. Acute exacerbation of anemia also occurs with aplastic crises, usually caused by infection with human parvovirus, and other viruses.

Recurrent episodes of vaso-occlusion and tissue ischemia cause myriad acute and chronic problems. Dactylitis, or hand-and-foot syndrome, is the most common initial symptom of the disease and occurs in up to 50% of children before age 3 years. Recurrent episodes of ischemic pain, particularly abdominal and musculoskeletal pain, may occur throughout life. Strokes occur in about 8% of children and tend to be recurrent. The acute chest syndrome, characterized by fever, pleuritic chest pain, and acute pulmonary infiltrates with hypoxemia, is caused by pulmonary infection, infarction, or fat embolism from ischemic bone marrow. All tissues are susceptible to damage from vaso-occlusion, and multiple organ dysfunction is common by adulthood. Table 27–2 lists the common manifestations of sickle cell disease in children and adults.

### B. LABORATORY FINDINGS

Children with sickle cell anemia (homozygous sickle cell disease) generally show a baseline hemoglobin level of 7–10 g/dL. This value may fall to life-threatening levels at the time of a sequestration or aplastic crisis. The baseline reticulocyte count is elevated markedly. The anemia is usually normocytic or macrocytic, and the peripheral blood smear typically shows the characteristic sickle cells as well as numerous target cells. Patients with sickle β-thalassemia generally have a low MCV and hypochromia as well. Those with sickle β+-thalassemia tend to have lesser degrees of hemolysis and anemia. Persons with sickle hemoglobin C disease have fewer sickle forms and more target cells, and the hemo-

**Table 27–2.** Common clinical manifestations of sickle cell disease.

|  | Acute | Chronic |
|---|---|---|
| Children | Bacterial sepsis or meningitis[a]<br>Splenic sequestration[a]<br>Aplastic crisis<br>Vaso-occlusive events<br>  Dactylitis<br>  Bone infarction<br>  Acute chest syndrome[a]<br>  Stroke[a]<br>  Priapism | Functional asplenia<br>Delayed growth and development<br>Avascular necrosis of the hip<br>Hyposthenuria<br>Cholelithiasis |
| Adults | Bacterial sepsis[a]<br>Aplastic crisis<br>Vaso-occlusive events<br>  Bone infarction<br>  Acute chest syndrome[a]<br>  Stroke[a]<br>  Priapism<br>  Acute multiorgan failure syndrome[a] | Leg ulcers<br>Proliferative retinopathy<br>Avascular necrosis of the hip<br>Cholecystitis<br>Chronic organ failure[a]<br>  Liver<br>  Lung<br>  Kidney<br>Decreased fertility |

[a]Associated with significant mortality rate.

globin level may be normal or only slightly decreased because the rate of hemolysis is much less than in sickle cell anemia.

Most infants with sickle hemoglobinopathies born in the United States are now identified by neonatal screening. Results indicative of possible sickle cell disease require prompt confirmation with hemoglobin electrophoresis. Children with sickle cell anemia and with sickle β⁰-thalassemia have only hemoglobins S and F. Persons with sickle β+-thalassemia have a preponderance of hemoglobin S with a lesser amount of hemoglobin A. Persons with sickle hemoglobin C disease have equal amounts of hemoglobin S and hemoglobin C. The use of solubility tests to screen for the presence of sickle hemoglobin should be avoided because a negative result is frequently encountered in infants with sickle cell disease, and because a positive result in an older child does not differentiate sickle cell trait from sickle cell disease. Thus hemoglobin electrophoresis is always necessary to accurately identify a sickle disorder.

## Differential Diagnosis

Hemoglobin electrophoresis and sometimes hematologic studies of the parents are usually sufficient to confirm the correct diagnosis of a sickle cell disorder. Infants whose neonatal screening test shows only hemoglobins F and S occasionally have disorders other than sickle cell anemia or sickle $\beta^0$-thalassemia. The most important of these disorders is a compound heterozygous condition of sickle hemoglobin and pancellular hereditary persistence of fetal hemoglobin. Such children, when older, typically have 30% fetal hemoglobin and 70% hemoglobin S, but they do not have significant anemia nor are they subject to vaso-occlusive episodes.

## Complications

Repeated tissue ischemia and infarction causes damage to virtually every organ system. Table 27–2 lists the most important complications. Patients who require multiple transfusions are at risk for transfusional hemosiderosis and the development of red cell alloantibodies.

## Treatment

The cornerstone of treatment is enrollment in a program involving patient and family education, comprehensive outpatient care, and appropriate treatment of acute complications. Important to the success of such a program are psychosocial services, blood bank services, and the ready availability of baseline patient information in the setting in which acute illnesses are evaluated and treated. Management of sickle cell anemia and sickle $\beta^0$-thalassemia includes prophylactic penicillin, which should be initiated by age 2 months and continued at least until age 5 years. The routine use of penicillin prophylaxis in sickle hemoglobin C disease and sickle $\beta^+$-thalassemia is controversial. Pneumococcal conjugate and polysaccharide vaccine should be administered to all children who have sickle cell disease. Other routine immunizations, including yearly vaccination against influenza, should be provided. All illnesses associated with fever greater than 38.5°C should be evaluated promptly, bacterial cultures preformed, parenteral broad-spectrum antibiotics administered, and careful inpatient or outpatient observation conducted.

Treatment of painful vaso-occlusive episodes includes the maintenance of adequate hydration (with avoidance of overhydration), correction of acidosis if present, administration of adequate analgesia, maintenance of normal oxygen saturation, and the treatment of any associated infections.

Red cell transfusions play an important role in management. Transfusions are indicated to improve oxygen-carrying capacity during acute exacerbations of anemia, as occurs during episodes of splenic sequestration or aplastic crisis. Red cell transfusions are not indicated for the treatment of chronic steady-state anemia, which is usually well tolerated, or for uncomplicated episodes of vaso-occlusive pain. Simple or partial exchange transfusion to reduce the percentage of circulating sickle cells is indicated for some severe acute vaso-occlusive events and may be lifesaving. These events include stroke, moderate to severe acute chest syndrome, and acute life-threatening failure of other organs. Transfusions may also be used prior to high-risk procedures such as surgery with general anesthesia and arteriograms with ionic contrast materials. Some patients who develop severe vaso-occlusive complications may benefit from chronic transfusion therapy. The most common indication for this type of transfusion is stroke. Without transfusions, children with stroke have a 70–80% chance of recurrent stroke within a 2-year period. This risk of recurrent neurologic events is reduced markedly by the transfusion therapy.

Successful stem cell transplantation cures sickle cell disease, but to date its use has been limited because of the risks associated with the procedure, the inability to predict in young children the severity of future complications, and the paucity of HLA-identical sibling donors. Daily administration of oral hydroxyurea increases levels of fetal hemoglobin, decreases hemolysis, and reduces by 50% episodes of pain in severely affected adults with sickle cell anemia. The hematologic effects and short-term toxicity of hydroxyurea in children are similar to those in adults. Thus hydroxyurea is being used increasingly for selected children and adolescents who have frequent, severe complications.

## Prognosis

Early identification by neonatal screening of infants with sickle cell disease, combined with comprehensive care that includes prophylactic penicillin, has markedly reduced mortality in childhood. Most patients are now expected to live well into adulthood, but they eventually succumb to complications.

Academy of Pediatrics, Section on Hematology/Oncology and Committee on Genetics: Health supervision for children with sickle cell disease. Pediatrics 2002;109:526 [PMID: 11875155].

Kinney TR et al: Safety of hydroxyurea in children with sickle cell anemia: Results of the HUG-KIDS study, a phase I/II trial. Blood 1999;94:1550 [PMID: 10477679].

Lane PA: Sickle cell disease. Pediatr Clin North Am 1996;43: 639 [PMID: 8649903].

Ohene-Frempong K et al: Cerebrovascular accidents in sickle cell disease: Rates and risk factors. Blood 1998;91:288 [PMID: 9414296].

Steinberg MH: Drug therapy: Management of sickle cell disease. N Engl J Med 1999;340:1021 [PMID: 10099145].

Vichinsky EP et al: Causes and outcomes of the acute chest syndrome in sickle cell disease. N Engl J Med 2000;342: 1855 [PMID: 10861320].

Walters MC et al: Bone marrow transplantation for sickle cell disease. N Engl J Med 1996;335:369 [PMID: 8663884].

## 4. Sickle Cell Trait

Individuals who are heterozygous for the sickle gene are said to have sickle cell trait. This genetic carrier state occurs in 8% of African Americans and is more common in some areas of Africa and the Middle East. Infants with sickle cell trait are identified by neonatal screening results that show hemoglobins FAS. Accurate identification of older persons with sickle cell trait depends on hemoglobin electrophoresis, which typically shows about 60% hemoglobin A and about 40% hemoglobin S. No anemia or hemolysis is present, and the physical examination is normal. Persons with sickle cell trait are generally healthy, and most experience no illness attributable to the presence of sickle hemoglobin in their red cells. Life expectancy is normal.

Sickle trait erythrocytes are capable of sickling, particularly under conditions of significant hypoxemia, and a number of clinical abnormalities have been linked to this genetic carrier state. Exposure to environmental hypoxia (altitude > 3100 m [10,000 ft] above sea level) may precipitate splenic infarction. However, most persons with sickle cell trait who choose to visit such altitudes for skiing, hiking, or climbing do so without difficulty. Many develop some degree of hyposthenuria, and about 4% experience painless hematuria, usually microscopic but occasionally macroscopic. For the most part, these renal abnormalities are subclinical, and they do not progress to significant renal dysfunction. The incidence of bacteriuria and pyelonephritis may be increased during pregnancy, but overall rates of maternal and infant morbidity and mortality are not affected by the presence of sickle cell trait in the pregnant woman.

An epidemiologic study of army recruits in military basic training found a higher risk of sudden unexplained death following strenuous exertion in recruits with sickle cell trait than in those with normal hemoglobin. This study has raised concerns about exercise and exertion for persons with the trait. However, considerable evidence suggests that exercise is generally safe and that athletic performance is not adversely affected by sickle cell trait. Exercise tolerance is normal, and the incidence of sickle cell trait in black professional football players is similar to that of the general African American population, suggesting no barrier to achievement in such a physically demanding profession. Thus restrictions on athletic competition for children with sickle cell trait are not warranted. Sickle cell trait is most significant for its genetic implications.

American Academy of Pediatrics Committee on Sports Medicine: Recommendations for participation in competitive sports. Pediatrics 1988;81:737 [PMID: 3357741].

Kark JA et al: Sickle cell trait as a risk factor for sudden death in physical training. N Engl J Med 1987;317:781 [PMID: 3627196].

Nuss R et al: Cardiopulmonary function in men with sickle cell disease who reside at moderately high altitude. J Lab Clin Med 1993;122:382 [PMID: 8228552].

Pearson HA: Sickle cell trait and competitive athletics: Is there a risk? Pediatrics 1989;83:613 [PMID: 2928004].

## 5. Hemoglobin C Disorders

Hemoglobin C is detected by neonatal screening. Two percent of African Americans are heterozygous for hemoglobin C and are said to have hemoglobin C trait. Such individuals have no symptoms, anemia, or hemolysis, but the peripheral blood smear may show some target cells. Identification of persons with hemoglobin C trait is important for genetic counseling, particularly with regard to the possibility of sickle hemoglobin C disease in offspring.

Persons with homozygous hemoglobin C have a mild microcytic hemolytic anemia and may develop splenomegaly. The peripheral blood smear shows prominent target cells. As with other hemolytic anemias, complications of homozygous hemoglobin C include gallstones and aplastic crises.

Olson JF et al: Hemoglobin C disease in infancy and childhood. J Pediatr 1994;125:745 [PMID: 7965426].

## 6. Hemoglobin E Disorders

Hemoglobin E is the second most common hemoglobin variant worldwide, with a gene frequency greater than 10% in some areas of Thailand and Cambodia. In Southeast Asia, an estimated 30 million people have hemoglobin E trait. Persons heterozygous for hemoglobin E show hemoglobins FAE by neonatal screening and are asymptomatic and usually not anemic, but they may develop mild microcytosis. Persons homozygous for hemoglobin E are also asymptomatic but may have mild anemia; the peripheral blood smear shows microcytosis and some target cells.

Hemoglobin E is most important because of its interaction with $\beta$-thalassemia. Compound heterozygotes for hemoglobin E and $\beta^0$-thalassemia are normal at birth and, like infants with homozygous E, show hemoglobins FE on neonatal screening. Unlike homozygotes, they subsequently develop mild to severe microcytic hypochromic anemia. Such children may exhibit jaundice, hepatosplenomegaly, and poor growth if the disorder is not recognized and treated appropriately. In some cases, the anemia becomes severe enough to require lifelong transfusion therapy. In certain areas of the United States, hemoglobin E–$\beta^0$-thalassemia has become a more common cause of transfusion-dependent anemia than homozygous β-thalassemia.

Glader BE, Look KA: Hematologic disorders in children from Southeast Asia. Pediatr Clin North Am 1996;43:665 [PMID: 8649904].

Krishnamurti L et al: Coinheritance of α-thalassemia-1 and hemoglobin E/β⁰-thalassemia: Practical implications for neonatal screening and genetic counseling. J Pediatr 1998;132:863 [PMID: 9602201].

Weatherall DJ: Hemoglobin E–β⁰-thalassemia: An increasingly common disease with some diagnostic pitfalls. J Pediatr 1998;132:765 [PMID: 9602183].

## 7. Other Hemoglobinopathies

Hundreds of other human globin-chain variants have been identified and described. Some, such as hemoglobins D and G, are relatively common. Heterozygous individuals, who are frequently identified during the course of neonatal screening programs for hemoglobinopathies, are generally asymptomatic and usually have no anemia or hemolysis. The principal significance of most hemoglobin variants is the potential for disease in compound heterozygous individuals who also inherit a gene for β-thalassemia or sickle hemoglobin. For example, children who are compound heterozygous for hemoglobins S and D$_{Punjab}$ (D$_{Los Angeles}$) have sickle cell disease.

## CONGENITAL HEMOLYTIC ANEMIAS: DISORDERS OF RED CELL METABOLISM

Erythrocytes depend on the anaerobic metabolism of glucose for the maintenance of adenosine triphosphate (ATP) levels sufficient for homeostasis. Glycolysis also produces the 2,3-diphosphoglycerate (2,3-DPG) levels needed to modulate the oxygen affinity of hemoglobin. Glucose metabolism via the hexosemonophosphate shunt is necessary to generate sufficient reduced nicotinamide adenine dinucleotide phosphate (NADPH) and reduced glutathione to protect red cells against oxidant damage. Congenital deficiencies of many glycolytic pathway enzymes have been associated with hemolytic anemias. In general, the morphologic abnormalities present on the peripheral blood smear are nonspecific, and the inheritance of these disorders is autosomal recessive or X-linked. Thus the possibility of a red cell enzyme defect should be considered during the evaluation of a patient with a congenital hemolytic anemia when the peripheral blood smear does not show red cell morphology typical of membrane or hemoglobin defects (eg, spherocytes, sickle forms, target cells), when hemoglobin disorders are excluded by hemoglobin electrophoresis and by isopropanol precipitation tests, and when family studies do not suggest an autosomal domi-

nant disorder. The diagnosis is confirmed by finding a low level of the deficient enzyme.

The two most common disorders of erythrocyte metabolism are G6PD deficiency and pyruvate kinase deficiency.

## 1. Glucose-6-Phosphate Dehydrogenase (G6PD) Deficiency

### ESSENTIALS OF DIAGNOSIS & TYPICAL FEATURES

- *African, Mediterranean, or Asian ancestry.*
- *Neonatal hyperbilirubinemia.*
- *Sporadic hemolysis associated with infection or with ingestion of oxidant drugs or fava beans.*
- *X-linked inheritance.*

### General Considerations

Deficiency of G6PD is the most common red cell enzyme defect that causes hemolytic anemia. The disorder has X-linked recessive inheritance and occurs with high frequency among persons of African, Mediterranean, and Asian ancestry. Hundreds of different G6PD variants have been characterized. In most instances, the deficiency is due to enzyme instability; thus, older red cells are more deficient than younger ones. The consequence is the inability of erythrocytes to generate sufficient amounts of NADPH to maintain the levels of reduced glutathione necessary to protect the red cells against oxidant stress. Thus most persons with G6PD deficiency do not have a chronic hemolytic anemia but have episodic hemolysis at times of exposure to the oxidant stress of infection or of certain drugs or food substances. The severity of the disorder varies among ethnic groups; G6PD deficiency in persons of African ancestry usually is less severe than in other ethnic groups.

### Clinical Findings

#### A. SYMPTOMS AND SIGNS

Infants with G6PD deficiency may have significant hyperbilirubinemia and may require phototherapy or exchange transfusion to prevent kernicterus. The deficiency is an important cause of neonatal hyperbilirubinemia in infants of Mediterranean or Asian ancestry but less so in infants of African ancestry. Older children with G6PD deficiency are asymptomatic and appear

**Table 27–3.** Some common drugs and chemicals that can induce hemolytic anemia in persons with G6PD deficiency.

| | |
| --- | --- |
| Acetanilide | Niridazole |
| Doxorubicin | Nitrofurantoin |
| Furazolidone | Phenazopyridine |
| Methylene blue | Primaquine |
| Nalidixic acid | Sulfamethoxazole |

From Beutler E: Glucose-6-phosphate dehydrogenase deficiency. N Engl J Med 1991;324:171.

normal between episodes of hemolysis. Hemolytic episodes are often triggered by infection or by the ingestion of oxidant drugs such as antimalarial compounds and sulfonamide antibiotics (Table 27–3). Ingestion of fava beans may trigger hemolysis in children of Mediterranean or Asian ancestry but usually not in children of African ancestry. Episodes of hemolysis are associated with pallor, jaundice, hemoglobinuria, and sometimes cardiovascular compromise.

### B. LABORATORY FINDINGS

The hemoglobin, reticulocyte count, and peripheral blood smear are usually normal in the absence of oxidant stress. Episodes of hemolysis are associated with a variable fall in hemoglobin. "Bite" cells or blister cells may be seen, along with a few spherocytes. Hemoglobinuria is common, and the reticulocyte count increases within a few days. Heinz bodies may be demonstrated with appropriate stains. The diagnosis is confirmed by the finding of reduced levels of G6PD in erythrocytes. Because this enzyme is present in increased quantities in reticulocytes, the test is best performed at a time when the reticulocyte count is normal or near normal.

### Complications

Kernicterus is a risk for infants with significant neonatal hyperbilirubinemia. Episodes of acute hemolysis in older children may be life-threatening. Rare G6PD variants are associated with chronic hemolytic anemia; the clinical course of patients with such variants may be complicated by splenomegaly and by the formation of gallstones.

### Treatment

The most important treatment issue is avoidance of drugs known to be associated with hemolysis (see Table 27–3). For some patients of Mediterranean, Middle Eastern, or Asian ancestry, the consumption of fava beans must also be avoided. Infections should be

treated promptly and antibiotics given when appropriate. Most episodes of hemolysis are self-limiting, but red cell transfusions may be lifesaving when signs and symptoms indicate cardiovascular compromise.

Beutler E: G6PD deficiency. Blood 1994;84:3613 [PMID: 7949118].

Kaplan M et al: Conjugated bilirubin in neonates with glucose-6-phosphate dehydrogenase deficiency. J Pediatr 1996; 128:695 [PMID: 8627445].

Seidman DS et al: Role of hemolysis in neonatal jaundice associated with glucose-6-phosphate dehydrogenase deficiency. J Pediatr 1995;127:804 [PMID: 7472840].

## 2. Pyruvate Kinase Deficiency

Pyruvate kinase deficiency is an autosomal recessive disorder observed in all ethnic groups but is most common in northern Europeans. The deficiency is associated with a chronic hemolytic anemia of varying severity. Approximately one third of those affected present in the neonatal period with jaundice and hemolysis that require phototherapy or exchange transfusion. Occasionally, the disorder causes hydrops fetalis and neonatal death. In older children, the hemolysis may require red cell transfusions or be mild enough to go unnoticed for many years. Jaundice and splenomegaly frequently occur in the more severe cases. The diagnosis of pyruvate kinase deficiency is occasionally suggested by the presence of echinocytes on the peripheral blood smear, but these findings may be absent prior to splenectomy. The diagnosis depends on the demonstration of low levels of pyruvate kinase activity in red cells.

Treatment of pyruvate kinase depends on the severity of the hemolysis. Blood transfusions may be required for significant anemia, and splenectomy may be beneficial. The procedure does not cure the disorder but ameliorates the anemia and its symptoms. Characteristically, the reticulocyte count increases and echinocytes become more prevalent after splenectomy, despite the decreased hemolysis and increased hemoglobin level.

Gilsanz F et al: Fetal anaemia due to pyruvate kinase deficiency. Arch Dis Child 1993;69:523 [PMID: 8285758].

## ACQUIRED HEMOLYTIC ANEMIA
### 1. Autoimmune Hemolytic Anemia

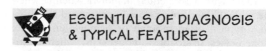

ESSENTIALS OF DIAGNOSIS & TYPICAL FEATURES

- *Pallor, fatigue, jaundice, and dark urine.*
- *Splenomegaly common.*

- Positive DAT.
- Reticulocytosis and spherocytosis.

## General Considerations

Acquired autoimmune hemolytic anemia is rare during the first 4 months of life but is one of the more common causes of acute anemia after the first year. It may arise as an isolated problem or may complicate an infection (hepatitis, upper respiratory tract infections, mononucleosis, cytomegalovirus [CMV] infection); systemic lupus erythematosus and other autoimmune syndromes; immunodeficiency states; or malignancies.

## Clinical Findings

### A. SYMPTOMS AND SIGNS

The disease usually has an acute onset, manifested by weakness, pallor, dark urine, and fatigue. Jaundice is a prominent finding, and splenomegaly is often present. Some cases are chronic and insidious in onset. Clinical evidence of an underlying disease may be present.

### B. LABORATORY FINDINGS

The anemia is normochromic and normocytic and may vary from mild to severe (hemoglobin concentration < 5 g/dL). The reticulocyte count is usually increased but occasionally may be normal or low. Spherocytes and nucleated red cells may be seen on the peripheral blood smear. Although leukocytosis and elevated platelet counts are a common finding, thrombocytopenia occasionally occurs. Other laboratory data consistent with hemolysis are present such as increased indirect and total bilirubin, lactic dehydrogenase, aspartate aminotransferase, and urinary urobilinogen. Intravascular hemolysis is indicated by hemoglobinemia or hemoglobinuria. Examination of bone marrow shows marked erythroid hyperplasia and hemophagocytosis, but is seldom required.

Serologic studies are helpful in defining pathophysiology, planning therapeutic strategies, and assessing prognosis (Table 27–4). In almost all cases, the direct and indirect antiglobulin (DAT and IAT) tests are positive. Further evaluation allows distinction into one of three syndromes. The presence of IgG on the patient's red blood cells, maximal in vitro antibody activity at 37°C, and either no antigen specificity or an Rh-like specificity constitute warm autoimmune hemolytic ane-

**Table 27–4.** Classification of autoimmune hemolytic anemia (AIHA) in children.

| Syndrome | Warm AIHA | Cold AIHA | Paroxysmal Cold Hemoglobinuria |
|---|---|---|---|
| Specific antiglobulin test<br>  IgG<br>  Complement | Strongly positive<br>Negative or mildly positive | Negative<br>Strongly positive | Negative<br>Strongly positive |
| Temperature at maximal reactivity (in vitro) | 37°C | 4 °C | 4 °C |
| Antigen specificity | May be panagglutinin or may have an Rh-like specificity | I or i | P |
| Other | . . . | . . . | Positive biphasic hemolysin test |
| Pathophysiology | Extravascular hemolysis, destruction by the RES (eg, spleen) | Intravascular hemolysis (may have extra-vascular component) | Intravascular hemolysis (may have extravascular component) |
| Prognosis | May be more chronic (> 3 months) with significant morbidity and mortality. May be associated with a primary disorder (lupus, immunodeficiency, etc) | Generally acute (< 3 months). Good prognosis: Often associated with infection. | Acute, self-limited. Associated with infection. |
| Therapy | Respond to RES blockade, including steroids (prednisone, 2 mg/kg/d), IVIG (1 g/kg/d for 2 days), or splenectomy | May not respond to RES blockade. Severe cases may benefit from plasmapheresis. | Usually self-limited. Symptomatic management. |

RES = reticuloendothelial system; IVIG = intravenous immune globulin.

mia with extravascular destruction by the reticuloendothelial system. In contrast, the detection of complement alone on red blood cells, optimal reactivity in vitro at 4°C, and I or i antigen specificity are diagnostic of cold autoimmune hemolytic anemia with intravascular hemolysis. Although these are relatively common (~10%) in normal individuals, clinically significant cold antibodies exhibit in vitro reactivity at 30°C or above.

Paroxysmal cold hemoglobinuria usually has a different cause. The laboratory evaluation is identical to cold autoimmune hemolytic anemia except for antigen specificity (P) and the exhibition of in vitro hemolysis. Almost always paroxysmal cold hemoglobinuria is associated with significant infections, such as *Mycoplasma*, Epstein–Barr virus (EBV), and CMV. Warm IgM antibodies are very rare.

## Differential Diagnosis

Autoimmune hemolytic anemia must be differentiated from other forms of congenital or acquired hemolytic anemias. The DAT discriminates antibody-mediated hemolysis from other causes, such as hereditary spherocytosis.

## Complications

The anemia may be very severe and result in cardiovascular collapse, requiring emergency management. The complications of the underlying disease such as disseminated lupus erythematosus or an immunodeficiency state may be present.

## Treatment

Medical management of the underlying disease is important in symptomatic cases. Defining the clinical syndrome provides a useful guide to treatment. Most patients with warm autoimmune hemolytic anemia (in which hemolysis is extravascular) respond to prednisone. After the initial treatment, the dose of corticosteroids may be decreased slowly. Patients may respond to 1 g of intravenous immune globulin (IVIG) per kilogram per day for 2 days, but fewer patients respond to IVIG than to prednisone. Although the rate of remission with splenectomy may be as high as 50%, particularly in warm autoimmune hemolytic anemia, this should be carefully considered in younger patients and withheld until other treatments have been tried. In severe cases unresponsive to more conventional therapy, immunosuppressive agents such as cyclophosphamide, azathioprine, busulfan, and cyclosporine may be tried alone or in combination with corticosteroids. In refrac-

tory cases, recent studies have documented responses to rituximab or bone marrow transplantation.

Patients with cold autoimmune hemolytic anemia and paroxysmal cold hemoglobinuria are less likely to respond to corticosteroids or IVIG. Because these syndromes are most apt to be associated with infections and have an acute, self-limited course, supportive care may be all that is required. Plasma exchange is effective in severe cold autoimmune (IgM) hemolytic anemia and may be helpful in severe cases because the offending antibody has only an intravascular distribution.

Supportive therapy is crucial. Patients with cold-reacting antibodies, particularly paroxysmal cold hemoglobinuria, should be kept in a warm environment. Transfusion may be necessary because of the complications of severe anemia but should be used only when there is no alternative. In most patients, crossmatch–compatible blood will not be found, and the least incompatible unit should be identified. Transfusion must be conducted carefully, beginning with a test dose (see Transfusion Medicine section). Identification of the patient's phenotype for minor red cell alloantigens may be helpful in avoiding alloimmunization or in providing appropriate transfusions if alloantibodies arise after initial transfusions. Patients with severe intravascular hemolysis may have associated disseminated intravascular coagulation (DIC), and heparin therapy should be considered in such cases.

## Prognosis

The outlook for autoimmune hemolytic anemia in childhood is usually good unless associated diseases are present (eg, congenital immunodeficiency, acquired immunodeficiency syndrome [AIDS], lupus erythematosus), in which case the hemolysis is likely to run a chronic course. In general, children with warm autoimmune hemolytic anemia are at greater risk for more severe and chronic disease with higher morbidity and mortality rates. Hemolysis and positive antiglobulin tests may continue for months or years. Patients with cold autoimmune hemolytic anemia or paroxysmal cold hemoglobinuria are more likely to have acute, self-limited disease (< 3 months). Paroxysmal cold hemoglobinuria is almost always associated with infection (eg, with *Mycoplasma* infection, CMV, EBV).

Petz LD, Garratty G: Unusual problems regarding autoimmune hemolytic anemias. In *Acquired Immune Hemolytic Anemias.* Churchill Livingstone, 1980.

Shirey RS et al: Prophylactic antigen-matched donor blood for patients with warm autoantibodies: An algorithm for transfusion management. Transfusion 2002;42:1435 [PMID: 12421216].

Zecca M et al: Rituximab for the treatment of refractory autoimmune hemolytic anemia in children. Blood 2003;101: 3857 [PMID: 12531800].

## 2. Nonimmune Acquired Hemolytic Anemia

Hepatic disease may alter the lipid composition of the red cell membrane. This usually results in the formation of target cells and is not associated with significant hemolysis. Occasionally, hepatocellular damage is associated with the formation of spur cells and brisk hemolytic anemia. Renal disease may also be associated with significant hemolysis; hemolytic–uremic syndrome is one example. In this disorder, hemolysis is associated with the presence, on the peripheral blood smear, of echinocytes, fragmented red cells, and spherocytes.

A microangiopathic hemolytic anemia with fragmented red cells and some spherocytes may be observed in a number of conditions associated with intravascular coagulation and fibrin deposition within vessels. This occurs with DIC such as may complicate severe infection, but it may also occur when the intravascular coagulation is localized, as with giant cavernous hemangiomas (Kasabach–Merritt syndrome). Fragmented red cells may also be seen with mechanical damage (eg, associated with artificial heart valves).

# ■ POLYCYTHEMIA & METHEMOGLOBINEMIA

## CONGENITAL ERYTHROCYTOSIS (FAMILIAL POLYCYTHEMIA)

In pediatrics, polycythemia is usually secondary to chronic hypoxemia. However, a number of families with congenital erythrocytosis have been described. The disorder differs from polycythemia vera in that only red blood cells are affected; the white blood cell and platelet counts are normal. It occurs as an autosomal dominant or recessive disorder. There are usually no physical findings except for plethora and splenomegaly. The hemoglobin level may be as high as 27 g/dL. Patients usually have no symptoms other than headache and lethargy. Studies in a number of families have revealed (1) an abnormal hemoglobin with increased oxygen affinity, (2) reduced red cell diphosphoglycerate, (3) autonomous increase in erythropoietin production, or (4) hypersensitivity of erythroid precursors to erythropoietin.

Treatment is not indicated unless symptoms are marked. Phlebotomy is the treatment of choice.

Juvonen E et al: Autosomal dominant erythrocytosis caused by increased sensitivity to erythropoietin. Blood 1991;78: 3066 [PMID: 1954391].

Sokol L et al: Primary familial polycythemia: A frameshift mutation in the erythropoietin receptor gene and increased sensitivity of erythroid progenitors to erythropoietin. Blood 1995;86:15 [PMID: 7795221].

## SECONDARY POLYCYTHEMIA

Secondary polycythemia occurs in response to hypoxemia. The most common cause of secondary polycythemia in children is cyanotic congenital heart disease. It also occurs in chronic pulmonary disease such as cystic fibrosis. Persons living at extremely high altitudes, as well as some with methemoglobinemia, develop polycythemia. It has on rare occasions been described without hypoxemia in association with renal tumors, brain tumors, Cushing disease, or hydronephrosis.

Polycythemia may occur in the neonatal period; it is particularly exaggerated in infants who are preterm or small for gestational age. In these infants, polycythemia is sometimes associated with other symptoms. It may occur in infants of diabetic mothers, in Down syndrome, and as a complication of congenital adrenal hyperplasia.

Iron deficiency may complicate polycythemia and aggravate the associated hyperviscosity. This complication should always be suspected when the MCV falls below the normal range. Coagulation and bleeding abnormalities, including thrombocytopenia, mild consumption coagulopathy, and elevated fibrinolytic activity, have also been described in severely polycythemic cardiac patients. Bleeding at surgery may be severe.

The ideal treatment of secondary polycythemia is correction of the underlying disorder. When this cannot be done, phlebotomy may be necessary to control symptoms. Iron sufficiency should be maintained. Adequate hydration of the patient and phlebotomy with plasma replacement may be indicated prior to major surgical procedures; these measures prevent the complications of thrombosis and hemorrhage. Isovolumetric exchange transfusion is the treatment of choice in severe cases.

Balcerzak SP, Bromberg PA: Secondary polycythemia. Semin Hematol 1975;12:353 [PMID: 1105791].

## METHEMOGLOBINEMIA

Methemoglobin is continuously formed at a slow rate by the oxidation of heme iron to the ferric state. Normally, it is enzymatically reduced back to hemoglobin. Methemoglobin is unable to transport oxygen and causes a shift in the dissociation curve of the residual oxyhemoglobin. Cyanosis is produced with methemo-globin levels of approximately 15% or greater. Levels of methemoglobin increase by several mechanisms.

## 1. Hemoglobin M

The designation M is given to several abnormal hemo-globins associated with methemoglobinemia. Affected individuals are heterozygous for the gene, which is transmitted as an autosomal dominant disorder. The different types of hemoglobin M result from different amino acid substitutions in α-globin or β-globin. He-moglobin electrophoresis at the usual pH will not al-ways demonstrate the abnormal hemoglobin, and iso-electric focusing may be needed. The patient has cyanosis but is otherwise usually asymptomatic. Exer-cise tolerance may be normal, and life expectancy is not affected. This type of methemoglobinemia does not re-spond to any form of therapy.

Vichinsky EP, Lubin BH: Unstable hemoglobins, hemoglobins with altered oxygen affinity, and M-hemoglobins. Pediatr Clin North Am 1980;27:421 [PMID: 7383714].

## 2. Congenital Methemoglobinemia Due to Enzyme Deficiencies

Congenital methemoglobinemia is caused most fre-quently by congenital deficiency of the reducing en-zyme diaphorase I (coenzyme factor I). It is transmitted as an autosomal recessive trait. Affected patients may have as high as 40% methemoglobin but usually have no symptoms, although a mild compensatory poly-cythemia may be present. Patients with methemoglo-binemia associated with a deficiency of diaphorase I re-spond readily to treatment with ascorbic acid and methylene blue (see following section), but treatment is not usually indicated.

## 3. Acquired Methemoglobinemia

A number of compounds activate the oxidation of he-moglobin from the ferrous to the ferric state, forming methemoglobin. These include the nitrites and nitrates (contaminated water), chlorates, and quinones. Drugs in this group are the aniline dyes, sulfonamides, ac-etanilid, phenacetin, bismuth subnitrate, and potassium chlorate. Poisoning with a drug or chemical containing one of these substances should be suspected in any in-fant or child who presents with sudden cyanosis. Methemoglobin levels in such cases may be extremely high and can produce anoxia, dyspnea, unconscious-ness, circulatory failure, and death. Young infants and newborns are more susceptible to acquired methemo-globinemia because their red cells have difficulty reduc-ing hemoglobin, probably because their NADH methe-moglobin reductase is transiently deficient. Infants with metabolic acidosis from diarrhea and dehydration or other causes may also develop methemoglobinemia.

Patients with the acquired form of methemoglobine-mia respond dramatically to methylene blue in a dose of 1–2 mg/kg intravenously. For infants and young chil-dren, a smaller dose (1–1.5 mg/kg) is recommended. Ascorbic acid administered orally or intravenously also reduces methemoglobin, but it acts more slowly.

Mansouri A, Lurie AA: Concise review: Methemoglobinemia. Am J Hematol 1993;42:7 [PMID: 8416301].

Osterhoudt KC et al: Rebound severe methemoglobinemia from ingestion of a nitroethane artificial-fingernail remover. J Pedi-atr 1995;126:819 [PMID: 7752015].

Sager S et al: Methemoglobinemia associated with acidosis of prob-able renal origin. J Pediatr 1995;126:59 [PMID: 7815226].

# ■ DISORDERS OF LEUKOCYTES

## NEUTROPENIA

**ESSENTIALS OF DIAGNOSIS & TYPICAL FEATURES**

- *Increased frequency of infections.*
- *Ulceration of oral mucosa and gingivitis.*
- *Normal numbers of red cells and platelets.*

## General Considerations

Neutropenia is an absolute neutrophil (granulocyte) count of less than 1500/μL in childhood, or below 1000/μL between ages 1 week and 2 years. During the first few days of life, an absolute neutrophil count of less than 3500 cells/μL may be considered neutropenia. Neutropenia results from absent or defective gran-ulocyte stem cells, ineffective or suppressed myeloid maturation, decreased production of hematopoietic cy-tokines (eg, granulocyte colony-stimulating factor [G-CSF], granulocyte-macrophage colony-stimulating factor [GM-CSF]), decreased marrow release, increased neutrophil destruction or consumption, or, in pseu-doneutropenia, from an increased neutrophil marginat-ing pool (Table 27–5).

The most severe types of congenital neutropenia in-clude reticular dysgenesis (congenital aleukocytosis), Kostmann syndrome (severe neutropenia with matura-

***Table 27–5.*** Classification of neutropenia of childhood.

---

**Congenital neutropenia with stem cell abnormalities**
    Reticular dysgenesis
    Cyclic neutropenia
**Congenital neutropenia with abnormalities of committed myeloid progenitor cells**
    Neutropenia with immunodeficiency disorders (T cells and B cells)
    Severe congenital neutropenia (Kostmann syndrome)
    Chronic idiopathic neutropenia of childhood
    Myelocathexis with dysmyelopoiesis
    Chédiak–Higashi syndrome
    Shwachman syndrome
    Cartilage-hair hypoplasia
    Dyskeratosis congenita
    Fanconi anemia
    Organic acidemias (eg, propionic, methylmalonic)
    Glycogenosis Ib
    Osteopetrosis
**Acquired neutropenias affecting stem cells**
    Malignancies (leukemia, lymphoma) and preleukemic disorders
    Drugs or toxic substances
    Ionizing radiation
    Aplastic anemia
**Acquired neutropenias affecting committed myeloid progenitors and/or survival of mature neutrophils**
    Ineffective granulopoiesis (vitamin $B_{12}$, folate, and copper deficiency)
    Infection
    Immune (neonatal alloimmune or autoimmune; autoimmune or chronic benign neutropenia of childhood)
    Hypersplenism

---

tion defect in the marrow progenitor cells), Shwachman syndrome (neutropenia with pancreatic insufficiency), neutropenia with immune deficiency states, cyclic neutropenia, and myelocathexis or dysgranulopoiesis. Genetic mutations for Chédiak–Higashi syndrome and Shwachman syndrome have recently been identified. Neutropenia may also be associated with storage and metabolic diseases and immunodeficiency states. The most common causes of neutropenia are viral infection or drugs resulting in decreased production in the marrow or increased destruction or both. Severe bacterial infections may be associated with neutropenia. Although rare, neonatal alloimmune neutropenia can be severe and associated with increased risk for infection. Autoimmune neutropenia in the mother can result in passive transfer of antibody to and neutropenia in the neonate. Malignancies, osteopetrosis, marrow failure syndromes, and hypersplenism are not usually associated with isolated neutropenia.

## Clinical Findings

### A. SYMPTOMS AND SIGNS

Acute severe bacterial or fungal infection is the most significant complication of neutropenia. Although the risk is increased when the absolute neutrophil count is less than 500/µL, the actual susceptibility is variable and depends on the cause of neutropenia, marrow reserves, and other factors. The most common types of infection include septicemia, cellulitis, skin abscesses, pneumonia, and perirectal abscesses. Sinusitis, aphthous ulcers, gingivitis, and periodontal disease also cause significant problems for these patients. In addition to local signs and symptoms, patients may have chills, fever, and malaise. In most cases, the spleen and liver are not enlarged. *Staphylococcus aureus* and gram-negative bacteria are the most common pathogens.

### B. LABORATORY FINDINGS

Neutrophils are absent or markedly reduced in the peripheral blood smear. In most forms of neutropenia or agranulocytosis, the monocytes and lymphocytes are normal and the red cells and platelets are not affected. The bone marrow usually shows a normal erythroid series, with adequate megakaryocytes but a marked reduction in the myeloid cells or a significant delay in maturation of this series. Total cellularity may be decreased.

In the evaluation of neutropenia (eg, persistent, intermittent, cyclic), careful attention should be paid to the duration and pattern of neutropenia, the types of infections and their frequency, and phenotypic abnormalities on physical examination. A careful family history and blood counts from the parents are useful. If an acquired cause, such as viral infection or drug, is not obvious and no other primary disease is present, white blood cell counts, white cell differential, and platelet and reticulocyte counts should be completed once or twice weekly for 4–6 weeks to determine the possibility of cyclic neutropenia. Bone marrow aspiration and biopsy are most important to characterize the morphologic features of myelopoiesis. Measuring the neutrophil counts in response to steroid infusion will document the marrow reserves. Tests for specific causes of neutropenia include measurement of neutrophil antibodies, immunoglobulin levels, antinuclear antibodies, and lymphocyte phenotyping to detect immunodeficiency states. Cultures of bone marrow are important for defining the numbers of stem cells and progenitors committed to the myeloid series or the presence of cytotoxic lymphocytes or humoral inhibitory factors. Cytokine levels in plasma or mononuclear cells can be measured directly. Some neutropenia disorders have abnormal neutrophil function. Recent studies have documented abnormalities in the elastase gene in severe congenital and cyclic neutropenias. Increased apoptosis in marrow precursors or circulating neutrophils has been described in several congenital disorders.

## Treatment

Identifiable toxic agents should be eliminated, or associated diseases (eg, infections) treated. Prophylactic antimicrobial therapy is not indicated for afebrile, asymptomatic patients. Recombinant G-CSF and GM-CSF will increase neutrophil counts in most patients. Patients may be started on 3–5 µg/kg/d of G-CSF (filgrastim) given subcutaneously or intravenously once a day. Depending on the counts, the dose may be increased or decreased. For patients with congenital neutropenia, the dose should be regulated to keep the absolute neutrophil count less than 10,000/µL. Some patients maintain adequate counts with G-CSF given 2–3 times/week.

## Prognosis

The prognosis varies greatly with the cause and severity of the neutropenia. In severe cases with persistent agranulocytosis, the prognosis is poor in spite of antibiotic therapy; in mild or cyclic forms of neutropenia, symptoms may be minimal and the prognosis for normal life expectancy excellent. Up to 50% of patients with Shwachman syndrome may develop aplastic anemia, myelodysplasia, or leukemia during their lifetime.

Patients with Kostmann syndrome also have a potential for leukemia. Recombinant hematopoietic hormones (ie, G-CSF) increase peripheral counts and decrease infectious complications.

Ambruso DR et al: Infectious and bleeding complications in patients with glycogenesis Ib. Am J Dis Child 1985;139: 691 [PMID: 3860000].

Ancliff PJ et al: Long-term follow-up of granulocyte colony-stimulating factor receptor mutations in patients with severe congenital neutropenia: Implications for leukaemogenesis and therapy. Br J Haematol 2003;120:685 [PMID: 12588357].

Ancliff PJ et al: Mutations in ELA2 gene encoding neutrophil elastase are present in most patients with sporadic severe congenital neutropenia but only in some patients with the familial form. Blood 2001;98:2645 [PMID: 11675333].

Dale DC et al: A randomized controlled phase III trial of recombinant human granulocyte colony-stimulating factor (filgrastim) for treatment of severe chronic neutropenia. Blood 1993;81:2496 [PMID: 8490166].

Dale DC et al: Mutations in the gene encoding neutrophil elastase in congenital and cyclic neutropenia. Blood 2000; 96:2317 [PMID: 11001877].

Kyono W, Coates TD: A practical approach to neutrophil disorders. Pediatr Clin North Am 2002;49:929 [PMID: 12430620].

# NEUTROPHILIA

Neutrophilia is an increase in the absolute neutrophil count in the peripheral blood to greater than 7500–8500 cells/µL for infants, children, and adults. To support the increased peripheral count, neutrophils may be mobilized from bone marrow storage or peripheral marginating pools. Neutrophilia occurs acutely in association with bacterial or viral infections, inflammatory diseases (eg, juvenile rheumatoid arthritis, inflammatory bowel disease, Kawasaki disease), surgical or functional asplenia, liver failure, diabetic ketoacidosis, azotemia, congenital disorders of neutrophil function (eg, chronic granulomatous disease and leukocyte adherence deficiency), and hemolysis. Drugs such as corticosteroids, lithium, and epinephrine increase the blood neutrophil count. Corticosteroids cause release of neutrophils from the marrow pool and inhibit egress from capillary beds and postpone apoptotic cell death. Epinephrine causes release of the marginating pool. Acute neutrophilia has been reported after stress such as from electric shock, trauma, burns, surgery, and emotional upset. Tumors involving the bone marrow, such as lymphomas, neuroblastomas, and rhabdomyosarcoma, may be associated with leukocytosis and the presence of immature myeloid cells in the peripheral blood. Infants with Down syndrome have defective regulation of proliferation and maturation of the myeloid series and may develop neutrophilia. At times this process may affect other cell lines and mimic myeloproliferative disorders or acute leukemia.

The neutrophilias must be distinguished from myeloproliferative disorders such as chronic myelogenous leukemia and juvenile chronic myelogenous leukemia. In general, abnormalities involving other cell lines, the appearance of immature cells on the blood smear, and the presence of hepatosplenomegaly are important differentiating characteristics.

# DISORDERS OF NEUTROPHIL FUNCTION

Neutrophils play a key role in host defenses. Circulating in capillary beds, they adhere to the vascular endothelium adjacent to sites of infection and inflammation. Moving between endothelial cells, the neutrophil migrates toward the offending agent. Contact with a microbe that is properly opsonized with complement or antibodies triggers ingestion, a process in which cytoplasmic streaming results in the formation of pseudopods that fuse around the invader, encasing it in a phagosome. During the ingestion phase, the oxidase enzyme system assembles and is activated, taking oxygen from the surrounding medium and reducing it to form toxic oxygen metabolites critical to microbicidal activity. Concurrently, granules from the two main classes (azurophil and specific) fuse and release their contents into the phagolysosome. The concentration of toxic oxygen metabolites (eg, hydrogen peroxide, hypochlorous acid, hydroxyl radical) and other compounds (eg, proteases, cationic proteins, cathepsins, defensins) increases dramatically, resulting in the death and dissolution of the microbe. Complex physiologic and biochemical processes subserve and control these functions. Defects in any of these processes may lead to inadequate cell function and an increased risk of infection.

## Classification

Table 27–6 summarizes congenital neutrophil function defects. Recently described is a syndrome of severe neutrophil dysfunction and severe infections associated with a mutation in a GTPase signaling molecule, Rac2. Other congenital or acquired causes of mild to moderate neutrophil dysfunction include metabolic defects (eg, glycogen storage disease, diabetes mellitus, renal disease, hypophosphatemia), viral infections, and certain drugs. Neutrophils from newborn infants have abnormal adherence, chemotaxis, and bactericidal activity. Cells from patients with thermal injury, trauma, and overwhelming infection have defects in cell motility and bactericidal activity similar to those seen in neonates.

## Clinical Findings

Recurrent bacterial or fungal infections are the hallmark of neutrophil dysfunction. Although many patients will have infection-free periods, episodes of pneumonia, sinusitis, cellulitis, cutaneous and mucosal infections (including perianal or peritonsillar abscesses), and lymphadenitis are frequent. As with neutropenia, aphthous ulcers of mucous membranes, severe gingivitis, and periodontal disease are also major complications. In general, *S aureus,* along with gram-negative organisms, is commonly isolated from infected sites; other organisms may be specifically associated with a defined neutrophil function defect. In some disorders, fungi account for an increasing number of infections. Deep or generalized infections such as osteomyelitis, liver abscesses, sepsis, meningitis, and necrotic or even gangrenous soft tissue lesions occur in specific syndromes (eg, leukocyte adherence deficiency or chronic granulomatous disease). Patients with severe neutrophil dysfunction may die in childhood from severe infections or associated complications. Table 27–6 summarizes pertinent laboratory findings.

## Treatment

The mainstays of management of these disorders remain the anticipation of infections and aggressive attempts to identify the foci and the causative agents. Surgical procedures to achieve these goals may be both diagnostic and therapeutic. Broad-spectrum antibiotics covering the range of possible organisms should be initiated without delay, switching to specific antimicrobial agents when the microbiologic diagnosis is made. When infections are unresponsive or they recur, granulocyte transfusions may be helpful.

Chronic management includes prophylactic antibiotics. Trimethoprim–sulfamethoxazole and other antibiotic compounds enhance the bactericidal activity of neutrophils from patients with chronic granulomatous disease. Some patients with Chédiak–Higashi syndrome improve clinically when given ascorbic acid. Recombinant γ-interferon has been shown to decrease the number and severity of infections in patients with chronic granulomatous disease. Demonstration of this activity with one patient group raises the possibility that cytokines, growth factors, and other biologic response modifiers may be helpful in other conditions in preventing recurrent infections. Bone marrow transplantation has been attempted in most major congenital neutrophil dysfunction syndromes, and reconstitution with normal cells and cell function has been documented. Combining genetic engineering with autologous bone marrow transplantation may provide a future strategy for curing these disorders.

***Table 27–6.*** Classification of congenital neutrophil function deficits.

| Disorder | Clinical Manifestations | Functional Defect | Biochemical Defect | Inheritance |
|---|---|---|---|---|
| Chédiak–Higashi syndrome | Oculocutaneous albinism, photophobia, nystagmus, ataxia. Recurrent infections of skin, respiratory tract, and mucous membranes with gram-positive and gram-negative organisms. Many die during lymphoproliferative phase with hepatomegaly, fever. This may be a viral-associated hemophagocytic syndrome secondary to Epstein–Barr virus infection. Older patients may develop degenerative CNS disease. | Neutropenia. Neutrophils, monocytes, lymphocytes, platelets, and all granule-containing cells have giant granules. Most significant defect is in chemotaxis. Also milder defects in microbicidal activity and degranulation. | Unknown. Alterations in membrane fusion with formation of giant granules. Other biochemical abnormalities in cAMP and cGMP, microtubule assembly. | Autosomal-recessive |
| Leukocyte adherence deficiency I | Recurrent soft tissue infections, including gingivitis, otitis, mucositis, periodontitis, skin infections. Delayed separation of the cord in newborn and problems with wound healing. | Neutrophilia. Diminished adherence to surfaces, leading to decreased chemotaxis. | Absence or partial deficiency of CD11/CD18 cell surface adhesive glycoproteins. | Autosomal-recessive |
| Leukocyte adherence deficiency II | Recurrent infections, mental retardation, craniofacial abnormalities, short stature. | Neutrophilia. Deficient "rolling" interaction with endothelial cells. Red cells have Bombay phenotype. | Deficient fucosyl transferase results in deficient sialyl Lewis X antigen, which interacts with P selectin on endothelial cell to establish neutrophil rolling, a prerequisite for adherence and diapedesis. | Autosomal-recessive |
| Chronic granulomatous disease | Recurrent purulent infections with catalase-positive bacteria and fungi. May involve skin, mucous membranes. Also develop deep infections (lymph nodes, lung, liver, bones) and sepsis | Neutrophilia. Neutrophils demonstrate deficient bactericidal activity but normal chemotaxis and ingestion. Defect in the oxidase enzyme system, resulting in absence or diminished production of oxygen metabolites toxic to microbes. | A number of molecular defects in oxidase components. Absent cytochrome b558 with decreased expression of either (1) or (2):<br><br>(1) gp91-phox<br><br>(2) p22-phox<br><br>Absent p47-phox or p67-phox (cytosolic components). | (1) X-linked (60–65% of cases).<br>(2) Autosomal recessive (< 5% of cases).<br>Autosomal-recessive (30% of cases). |
| Myeloperoxidase deficiency | Generally healthy. Fungal infections when deficiency associated with systemic diseases (eg, diabetes) | Diminished capacity to enhance hydrogen peroxide–mediated microbicidal activity. | Diminished or absent myeloperoxidase; posttranslational defect in processing protein. | Autosomal-recessive |
| Specific granule deficiency | Recurrent skin and deep tissue infections. | Decreased chemotaxis and bactericidal activity. | Failure to produce specific granules or their contents during myelopoiesis. | Autosomal-recessive |

## Prognosis

For mild to moderate defects, anticipation and conservative medical management ensure a reasonable outlook. For severe defects, excessive morbidity and significant mortality still exist. In some diseases, the development of noninfectious complications, such as the lymphoproliferative phase of Chédiak–Higashi syndrome or inflammatory syndromes in chronic granulomatous disease, may influence prognosis.

Ambruso DR et al: Human neutrophil immunodeficiency syndrome is associated with an inhibitory Rac2 mutation. Proc Natl Acad Sci U S A 2000;97:4654 [PMID: 10758162].

Etzioni A et al: Brief report: Recurrent severe infections caused by a novel leukocyte adhesion deficiency. N Engl J Med 1992;327:1789 [PMID: 1279426].

Kyono W, Coates TD: A practical approach to neutrophil disorders. Pediatr Clin North Am 2002;49:929 [PMID: 12430620].

## LYMPHOCYTOSIS

From the first week up to the fifth year of life, lymphocytes are the most numerous leukocytes in human blood. The ratio then reverses gradually to reach the adult pattern of neutrophil predominance. An absolute lymphocytosis in childhood is associated with acute or chronic viral infections, pertussis, syphilis, tuberculosis, and hyperthyroidism. Other noninfectious conditions, drugs, and hypersensitivity and serum sickness-like reactions cause lymphocytosis.

Fever, upper respiratory symptoms, gastrointestinal complaints, and rashes are clues in distinguishing infectious from noninfectious causes. The presence of enlarged liver, spleen, or lymph nodes is crucial to the differential diagnosis, which includes acute leukemia and lymphoma. Most cases of infectious mononucleosis are associated with hepatosplenomegaly or adenopathy. The absence of anemia and thrombocytopenia helps to differentiate these disorders. Evaluation of the morphology of lymphocytes on peripheral blood smear is crucial. Infectious causes, particularly infectious mononucleosis, are associated with atypical features in the lymphocytes such as basophilic cytoplasm, vacuoles, finer and less dense chromatin, and an indented nucleus. These features are distinct from the characteristic morphology associated with lymphoblastic leukemia. Lymphocytosis in childhood is most commonly associated with infections and resolves with recovery from the primary disease.

## EOSINOPHILIA

Eosinophilia in infants and children is an absolute eosinophil count greater than 300/µL. Marrow eosinophil production is stimulated by the cytokine interleukin-5. Allergies, particularly eczema, are the most common primary causes of eosinophilia in children. Eosinophilia also occurs in drug reactions, with tumors (Hodgkin and non-Hodgkin lymphomas and brain tumors), and with immunodeficiency and histiocytosis syndromes. Increased eosinophil counts are a prominent feature of many invasive parasitic infections. Gastrointestinal disorders such as chronic hepatitis, ulcerative colitis, Crohn disease, and milk precipitin disease may be associated with eosinophilia. Increased blood eosinophil counts have been identified in several families without association with any specific illness. Rare causes of eosinophilia include the hypereosinophilic syndrome, characterized by counts greater than 1500/µL and organ involvement and damage (hepatosplenomegaly, cardiomyopathy, pulmonary fibrosis, and central nervous system injury). This is a disorder of middle-aged adults and is rare in children. Eosinophilic leukemia has been described, but its existence as a distinct entity is controversial.

Eosinophils are sometimes the last type of mature myeloid cell to disappear after marrow ablative chemotherapy. Increased eosinophil counts are associated with graft versus host disease after bone marrow transplantation, and elevations are sometimes documented during rejection episodes in patients who have solid organ grafts.

# ■ BLEEDING DISORDERS

Bleeding disorders may occur as a result of (1) quantitative or qualitative abnormalities of platelets, (2) quantitative or qualitative abnormalities in plasma coagulation factors, (3) vascular abnormalities, or (4) accelerated fibrinolysis. The coagulation cascade and fibrinolytic system are shown in Figures 27–4 and 27–5.

For the bleeding patient, obtaining a detailed personal and family history is the most critical aspect of evaluation. The personal history should include bleeding complications associated with dental interventions, surgeries, suture placement and removal, and fractures. A history of mucosal bleeding is suggestive of a platelet disorder, von Willebrand disease, dysfibrinogenemia, or vasculitis. Bleeding into muscles and joints suggests a coagulation protein abnormality. A thorough physical examination should be performed with special attention to the skin, oral and nasal mucosa, liver, spleen, and joints. Excessive bleeding may be due to a congenital or acquired abnormality.

**Figure 27–4.** The procoagulant system and formation of a fibrin clot. Vascular injury initiates the coagulation process by exposure of tissue factor (TF); the dashed lines indicate thrombin actions in addition to clotting of fibrinogen. The finely dotted lines indicate the feedback activation of the VII-TF complex by Xa and Ixa. Abbreviations: HK = high-molecular-weight kininogen; PK = prekallikrein; $Ca^{2+}$ = calcium; PL = phospholipid. (Reproduced, with permission, from Goodnight SH, Hathaway WE [eds]: *Disorders of Hemostatis & Thrombosis: A Clinical Guide*, 2nd ed. McGraw-Hill, 2001.)

Screening tests to investigate patients for possible bleeding disorders should initially include the following:

1. Prothrombin time (PT) to screen for clotting activity of factors VII, X, II, V, and fibrinogen.
2. Activated partial thromboplastin time (aPTT) to screen for clotting activity of the following factors: high-molecular-weight kininogen (HMWK), prekallikrein (PK), XII, XI, IX, VIII, X, V, II, and fibrinogen.
3. Platelet count and size.
4. Functional assessment of vascular, platelet, von Willebrand factor interaction by platelet function analyzer-100 (PFA-100) or bleeding time, to screen for small vessel integrity, platelet function, and von Willebrand disease.

The following may be useful:

1. Thrombin time (TT) to measure the generation of fibrin following conversion of prothrombin to thrombin as well as the antithrombin effect of fibrin-split products or heparin.
2. Fibrinogen level. Additional tests to be performed in hospitalized patients include measurement of fibrin degradation products (FDP) and euglobulin lysis time (ELT), a measure of fibrinolysis.

Journeycake JM, Buchanan GR: Coagulation disorders. Pediatr Rev 2003;24:83 [PMID: 12612185].

**Figure 27–5.** The fibrinolytic system. Solid arrows indicate activation; dotted line arrows indicate inhibition. tPA = tissue plasminogen activator; uPA = urokinase; uPAR = cellular urokinase receptor; PAI = plasminogen activator inhibitor; FDP = fibrinogen–fibrin degradation products; MMP = matrix metalloproteinases; ECM = extracellular matrix; TAFI = thrombin activatable fibrinolysis inhibitor. (Reproduced, with permission, from Goodnight SH, Hathaway WE [eds]: *Disorders of Hemostatis & Thrombosis: A Clinical Guide*, 2nd ed. McGraw-Hill, 2001.

# ABNORMALITIES OF PLATELET NUMBER OR FUNCTION

## 1. Idiopathic Thrombocytopenic Purpura

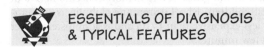

### ESSENTIALS OF DIAGNOSIS & TYPICAL FEATURES

- *Otherwise healthy child.*
- *Decreased platelet count.*
- *Petechiae, ecchymoses.*

## General Considerations

Acute idiopathic thrombocytopenic purpura (ITP) is the most common bleeding disorder of childhood. It occurs most frequently in children age 2–5 years and often follows infection with viruses such as rubella, varicella, measles, parvovirus, influenza, or EBV. Most patients recover spontaneously within a few months. Chronic ITP (> 6 months' duration) occurs in just 10–20% of patients with ITP. The thrombocytopenia results from immune clearance of platelets, which generally have IgM or IgG on their surface. The spleen plays a major role by forming antibodies and by sequestering damaged platelets.

## Clinical Findings

### A. SYMPTOMS AND SIGNS

Onset of ITP is usually acute, with the appearance of multiple ecchymoses. Petechiae are often present, especially on the lips and buccal mucosa, and epistaxis is common. No other physical findings are usually pre-

sent. Rarely, concurrent infection with EBV or CMV may cause hepatosplenomegaly or lymphadenopathy, simulating acute leukemia.

### B. LABORATORY FINDINGS

**1. Blood**—The platelet count is markedly reduced (usually < 50,000/μL and often < 10,000/μL), and platelets frequently are of larger size on peripheral blood smear, suggesting bone marrow response and increased production. The white blood count and differential count are normal. Anemia is not present unless hemorrhage has occurred.

**2. Bone marrow**—The number of megakaryocytes (which may be larger than normal) is increased. Erythroid and myeloid cellularity is normal.

**3. Other laboratory tests**—Because the PFA-100 and bleeding time are generally prolonged if the platelet count is less than 40,000/μL, these tests are not indicated. PTT and PT are normal and also not indicated. Platelet-associated IgG or IgM or both may be demonstrated on the platelets or in the serum.

## Differential Diagnosis

Table 27–7 lists common causes of thrombocytopenia. ITP is a diagnosis of exclusion. Bone marrow examination should be performed if the history is atypical, if abnormalities other than purpura and petechiae are present on physical examination, if other cell lines are affected on the CBC, or possibly if corticosteroid therapy is to be administered. Family history or the finding of predominantly giant platelets on the peripheral blood smear should be helpful in determining whether thrombocytopenia is hereditary.

## Complications

Severe hemorrhage and bleeding into vital organs are the feared complications of ITP. Intracranial hemorrhage is the most serious but rarely seen complication.

**Table 27–7.** Common causes of thrombocytopenia.

| Destruction | | | Decreased Production | |
|---|---|---|---|---|
| **Antibody-Mediated** | **Coagulopathy** | **Other** | **Congenital** | **Acquired** |
| Idiopathic thrombocytic purpura<br>Infection<br>Immunologic diseases | Disseminated intravascular coagulopathy<br>Sepsis<br>Necrotizing enterocolitis<br>Thrombosis<br>Cavernous hemangioma | Hemolytic—uremic syndrome<br>Thrombotic thrombocytopenic purpura<br>Hypersplenism<br>Respiratory distress syndrome<br>Wiskott–Aldrich syndrome | Fanconi anemia<br>Wiskott–Aldrich syndrome<br>Thrombocytopenia with absent radii<br>Metabolic disorders<br>Osteopetrosis | Aplastic anemia<br>Leukemia and other malignancies<br>Vitamin $B_{12}$ and folate deficiencies |

The most important risk factors for hemorrhage are a platelet count less than 10,000/μL and mean platelet volume less than 8 fL.

## Treatment

### A. GENERAL MEASURES

Most children require no therapy. Treatment should be given for bleeding, not just because the platelet count is low. Aspirin and aspirin-containing drugs should not be administered. Trauma should be avoided. Platelet transfusion should be avoided unless life-threatening bleeding is present and emergent splenectomy is to be pursued, when other therapies are ineffective, or when a procedure such as a craniotomy is necessary.

### B. CORTICOSTEROIDS

Patients with significant bleeding (ie, hematuria, hematochezia, epistaxis) or those with a platelet count of less than 10,000/μL may benefit from prednisone at 4 mg/kg orally per day for 3–5 days, decreasing to 2 mg/kg/d for a total of 14 days. The dosage is then tapered and stopped. No further prednisone is given regardless of the platelet count unless significant bleeding recurs, at which time prednisone is administered in the smallest dose that will give symptomatic relief (usually 2.5–5 mg twice daily). The patient is then followed up until spontaneous remission occurs or until the patient is a candidate for further therapy.

### C. INTRAVENOUS IMMUNE GLOBULIN

As an alternative or adjunct to corticosteroid treatment, IVIG may be given to raise the platelet count in both acute and chronic ITP of childhood. The platelet response to IVIG is comparable to the response to methylprednisolone (30 mg/kg/d for 7 days in acute ITP). IVIG may be effective even when the patient is resistant to corticosteroids; responses are prompt and may last for several weeks. Most patients receive 1 g/kg/d for 1–3 days. IVIG is the treatment of choice for severe, life-threatening bleeding. Platelets may be given simultaneously but are rapidly destroyed. IVIG-associated transient neurologic complications, including headache, nausea, and aseptic meningitis, occur in one third of patients. These symptoms mimic those of intracranial hemorrhage and can necessitate radiologic evaluation of the brain. A transient decrease in neutrophil number may also be seen.

### D. RHO(D) IMMUNE GLOBULIN

The intravenous preparation of anti-D immunoglobulin is a polyclonal immunoglobulin that binds to the D antigen on red blood cells, and the coated cells are cleared by the spleen as a result. The antibody-coated platelets are then not phagocytized. The drug is effective only in Rh-positive patients with a functional spleen. The time required for platelet increase is slightly longer than with steroids or IVIG. However, approximately 80% of children with acute or chronic ITP respond well. Coombs-positive hemolysis may occur transiently with an average hemoglobin concentration decrease of 0.8 g/dL. Severe hemolysis occurs in 5% of treated children. Rho(D) immune globulin is substantially less expensive than IVIG and is administered over just a few minutes.

### E. SPLENECTOMY

Most children with chronic ITP have platelet counts greater than 30,000/μL. Up to 70% of them recover to a platelet count greater than 100,000/μL without therapy within 1 year. For those who do not do so, corticosteroids, IVIG, and Rho(D) immune globulin are treatment options that are usually successful. Splenectomy produces permanent remission in 70–90% but should be considered only after persistence of significant thrombocytopenia for at least 1 year. Preoperative treatment with IVIG or Rho(D) immune globulin is indicated if the platelet count is decreased significantly. If the patient has been receiving corticosteroid therapy, the dose should be appropriately increased during and after surgery. Anticoagulant therapy is not indicated postoperatively, even though the platelet count may rise to 1 million/μL. The risk of overwhelming infection is increased after splenectomy, particularly in the young child. Therefore, the procedure should be postponed, if possible, until the child is at least age 5 years. Administration of pneumococcal and *Haemophilus influenzae* b vaccines at least 2 weeks prior to splenectomy is recommended. Meningococcal vaccine is controversial. Penicillin prophylaxis should be started postoperatively and continued for 1–3 years.

## Prognosis

Ninety percent of children with ITP will have a spontaneous remission. Features associated with the development of chronic ITP include female sex, age older than 10 years at presentation, a more insidious onset of bruising, and the presence of other autoantibodies. Teens with immune-mediated thrombocytopenia are at higher risk for chronic autoantibody diseases.

Bolton-Maggs PHB et al: The nontreatment of childhood ITP (or [The art of medicine consists of amusing the patient until nature cures the disease]). Semin Thromb Hemost 2001; 27:269 [PMID: 11446660].

Buchanan G, Adix L: Outcome measures and treatment endpoints other than platelet count in childhood idiopathic thrombocytopenic purpura. Semin Thromb Hemost 2001;27: 277 [PMID: 11446661].

DiPaola JA, Buchanan GR: Immune thrombocytopenic purpura. Pediatr Clin North Am 2002;49:911 [PMID: 12430619].

## 2. Thrombocytopenia in the Newborn

Thrombocytopenia is one of the most common causes of purpura in the newborn and should be considered and investigated in any newborn with petechiae or a significant bleeding tendency. A platelet count less than 150,000/μL establishes a diagnosis of thrombocytopenia. This occurs in approximately 0.9% of unselected neonates. A platelet count less than or equal to 50,000/μL occurs in 0.1–0.2% of otherwise well neonates. A number of specific entities may be responsible (see Table 27–7); however, one-half of such neonates have alloimmune thrombocytopenia. Infection and intravascular coagulation syndromes are the most common causes of thrombocytopenia in sick full-term newborns and in preterm newborns. In the well-appearing newborn, antibody-mediated thrombocytopenia (alloimmune or maternal autoimmune), viral syndrome, hyperviscosity, and major vessel thrombosis are frequent causes of thrombocytopenia. Management is directed toward alleviation of the specific cause.

### Thrombocytopenia Associated with Platelet Alloimmunization

Platelet alloimmunization occurs in one out of approximately 350 pregnancies. Unlike Rh incompatibility, 30–40% of affected neonates are first-born. Thrombocytopenia is progressive over the duration of the gestation and worse in subsequent pregnancies. Alloimmunization occurs when a platelet antigen of the infant differs from that of the mother and when the mother is sensitized by platelets that cross from the fetal to the maternal circulation. In Caucasians, alloimmune thrombocytopenia is most often due to HPA-1a incompatibility. Sensitization of a mother homozygous for human platelet antigen 1b against paternally acquired fetal HPA-1a antigen results in severe fetal thrombocytopenia in 1 in 1200 fetuses. Only 1 in 20 HPA-1a-positive fetuses of HPA-1a-negative mothers develop alloimmunization. The presence of antenatal platelet antibodies on more than one occasion persisting in the third trimester is predictive of severe neonatal thrombocytopenia. A weak or undetectable antibody does not exclude thrombocytopenia. Severe intracranial hemorrhage occurs in 10–30% of affected neonates as early as 20 weeks' gestation. Petechiae or other bleeding manifestations are usually present shortly after birth. The disease is self-limited, and the platelet count normalizes within 4 weeks.

If severe alloimmunization occurs, platelet concentrate from the mother will be more effective than random donor platelets in raising the platelet count. Type-matched platelets from a donor are also effective. IVIG infusions and steroids, which block the reticuloen-dothelial system, have also been successful in raising the platelet count. If alloimmunization is less severe, observation alone may be all that is required.

Intracranial hemorrhage in a previous child secondary to alloimmune thrombocytopenia is the worst risk factor for severe fetal thrombocytopenia in a subsequent pregnancy. Amniocentesis or chorionic villus sampling to obtain fetal DNA for platelet antigen typing is sometimes performed if the father is heterozygous for HPA-1a. If alloimmunization has occurred with a previous pregnancy, ultrasound examination of the fetal brain to detect hemorrhage should be obtained at 20 weeks' gestation and repeated regularly. Cordocentesis should be performed about 20 weeks' gestation with concentrated, irradiated, filtered, maternal platelets transfused to protect against fetal hemorrhage. If the fetal platelet count is less than 100,000/μL, IVIG should be administered to the mother weekly. Delivery by elective cesarean section is recommended if the fetal platelet count is less than 50,000/μL.

### Thrombocytopenia Associated with Idiopathic Thrombocytopenic Purpura in the Mother

Infants born to mothers with ITP or antiphospholipid antibodies may develop thrombocytopenia as a result of transfer of IgG antibody from the mother to the infant. Unfortunately, maternal platelet count, maternal antiplatelet antibody levels, and fetal scalp platelet counts are unreliable predictors of bleeding risk. Antenatal administration of prednisone is generally begun once maternal platelet count falls less than 50,000/μL. IVIG has been administered but is not well-studied.

Most neonates with thrombocytopenia secondary to passive transfer of maternal antibody do not bleed, and thus no specific treatment is indicated. The risk for intracranial hemorrhage is 0.2–2%. If petechiae or puncture wound bleeding ensues, a 1- to 2-week course of oral prednisone, 2 mg/kg/d, may be administered. If the platelet count remains consistently less than 20,000/μL or if severe hemorrhage is present, IVIG should be given. Platelet transfusions may not be helpful without prior removal of antibody by exchange transfusion. The platelet nadir is usually on the fourth to sixth day of life. Because the antiplatelet IgG may be passed through breast milk, the platelet count should be monitored. For infants with severe thrombocytopenia, full recovery may take 2–4 months.

### Neonatal Thrombocytopenia Associated with Infections

Thrombocytopenia is commonly associated with severe generalized infections during the newborn period. Between 50% and 75% of neonates with bacterial sepsis are thrombocytopenic. Intrauterine infections such as rubella, syphilis, toxoplasmosis, CMV, herpes simplex, enteroviruses, and parvovirus are often associated with thrombocytopenia.

In addition to specific treatment for the underlying disease, platelet transfusions may be indicated in severe cases. Platelet concentrates in doses of 10 mL/kg will raise the platelet count by about 75,000/µL.

## Thrombocytopenia Associated with Giant Hemangiomas (Kasabach–Merritt Syndrome)

A rare but important cause of thrombocytopenic purpura in the newborn is giant hemangioma. These lesions have a different histologic pattern from classic infantile hemangiomas. They are more appropriately termed "kaposiform hemangioendotheliomas," or "tufted angiomas." Platelet sequestration in the lesion results in peripheral depletion of platelets. The bone marrow usually shows megakaryocytic hyperplasia. The thrombocytopenia may be associated with hemolytic anemia and DIC and result in fatal hemorrhage. Treatment is indicated if a serious coagulopathy is present or if the lesion exerts pressure on a vital structure or is cosmetically unacceptable.

Surgery is usually contraindicated because of the risk of hemorrhage. Prednisone therapy has been associated with marked regression. Antiplatelet drugs and pentoxifylline may be helpful. If DIC is present, heparin or aminocaproic acid may be useful. Vascular embolization may be an option. Interferon-α has also been shown to be efficacious, but its use is controversial. When patients have been unresponsive to other treatment, chemotherapy has been given with some efficacy.

Bussel JB: Alloimmune thrombocytopenia in the fetus and neonate. Semin Thromb Hemost 2001;27:245 [PMID: 11446658].

Hall GW: Kasabach–Merritt syndrome: Pathogenesis and management. Br J Haematol 2001;112:851 [PMID: 11298580].

Modlin JF et al: Case 25-2003: A newborn boy with petechiae and thrombocytopenia. N Engl J Med 2003;349:691 [PMID: 12917307].

## 3. Disorders of Platelet Function

Platelet function has traditionally been screened by measurement of the bleeding time. If the bleeding time is prolonged, aggregation of platelets with agonists such as adenosine diphosphate, collagen, arachidonic acid, and ristocetin has been studied. Results are compared with those of a normal control subject. A relatively new instrument, the PFA-100, has become available for screening for platelet dysfunction and von Willebrand

disease, and may replace the bleeding time for this purpose. Platelet morphology is assessed with the light microscope and electron microscope.

Platelet dysfunction may be inherited or acquired, but acquired platelet dysfunction is more common. Persons with platelet function defects have skin and mucosal bleeding similar to that occurring in persons with thrombocytopenia. Platelet aggregation and degranulation studies are not uniformly predictive of the severity of clinical symptoms.

Persons with hereditary platelet dysfunction generally have a prolonged bleeding time with normal platelet number and morphology. The inherited disorders are due to defects in platelet–vessel interaction, platelet–platelet interaction, platelet granule defects, signal transduction, thromboxane and arachidonic acid pathway dysfunction, and platelet coagulant–protein interaction.

An example of a platelet–vessel wall dysfunction is Bernard–Soulier syndrome. In this condition the platelets are large and the platelet count slightly decreased. Because the platelets lack or have defective glycoprotein 1b on their surface they cannot adhere to the vessel wall von Willebrand factor (vWF). Glycoproteins V and IX may also be deficient. An example of platelet–platelet dysfunction is Glanzmann thromboasthenia. In this condition glycoprotein IIb–IIIa is deficient or defective so platelets cannot bind to fibrinogen to aggregate. Both conditions are rare and transmitted in an autosomal recessive pattern. Bleeding is treated with platelet concentrates.

Two examples of platelet granule defects are storage pool disease and Quebec platelet disorder. Persons with storage pool disease are missing adenosine dinucleotide phosphate and adenosine trinucleotide phosphate from the dense granules and are usually deficient in dense granules. The dense granules are also deficient in Hermansky–Pudlak, Chédiak–Higashi, and Wiskott–Aldrich syndromes. Deficient α-granules result in the gray platelet syndrome. Quebec platelet disorder is associated with abnormal proteolysis of α-granule proteins, deficiency of platelet α-granule multimerin, and marked impaired aggregation with epinephrine.

Signal transduction defects translate to primary degranulation defects. Platelet dysfunction may also result from abnormalities in the thromboxane and arachidonic acid pathways. Scott syndrome involves a defect in factor Va–Xa interaction on platelets. Platelet dysfunction may occur in persons with Down syndrome.

Acquired disorders of platelet function may occur secondary to uremia, cirrhosis, sepsis, myeloproliferative disorders, acyanotic congenital heart disease, and viral infections. Many pharmacologic agents decrease platelet function. The most common agents are aspirin, nonsteroidal anti-inflammatory agents, and synthetic penicillins.

## Treatment

Many individuals with hereditary and acquired platelet function defects will respond to therapy with desmopressin acetate. If this therapy is ineffective, treatment is with random donor platelets as discussed in the transfusion medicine section. Recombinant VIIa has variable efficacy.

Almeida AM et al: The use of recombinant factor VIIa in children with inherited platelet function disorders. Br J Haematol 2003;121:477 [PMID: 12716372].

Hayward CP: Inherited platelet disorders. Curr Opin Hematol 2003;10:362 [PMID: 12913791].

## INHERITED BLEEDING DISORDERS

Table 27–8 lists normal values for coagulation factors. The more common factor deficiencies are discussed in this section. All persons with bleeding disorders should avoid exposure to medications that inhibit platelet function. Participation in contact sports such as football and ice hockey should be considered in the context of the severity of the bleeding disorder.

## 1. Factor VIII Deficiency (Hemophilia A, Classic Hemophilia)

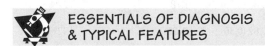

### ESSENTIALS OF DIAGNOSIS & TYPICAL FEATURES

- *Bruising, bleeding, and hemarthroses.*
- *Prolonged PTT.*
- *Reduced factor VIII activity.*

## General Considerations

Factor VIII activity is reported in units per milliliter, with 1 unit/mL equal to 100% of the factor activity found in 1 mL of normal plasma. The normal range for factor VIII activity is 50–150%. The disease occurs predominantly in males as an X-linked disorder. One third of cases are due to a new mutation. The incidence of factor VIII deficiency is 1:5000 male births.

## Clinical Findings

### A. SYMPTOMS AND SIGNS

Patients with severe factor VIII deficiency (< 1% circulating factor VIII activity) have frequent spontaneous bleeding episodes involving skin, mucous membranes, joints, muscles, and viscera. In contrast, patients with mild factor VIII deficiency (5–40% factor VIII activity) bleed only at times of trauma or surgery. Those with moderate factor VIII deficiency (1– < 5% factor VIII activity) have intermediate bleeding manifestations. The most crippling aspect of factor VIII deficiency is the tendency to develop recurrent hemarthroses that incite joint destruction.

### B. LABORATORY FINDINGS

Persons with factor VIII deficiency have a prolonged PTT. The bleeding time and PT are usually normal. The diagnosis is confirmed by finding decreased factor VIII activity with normal vWF activity. Cord blood can be assayed accurately to determine factor VIII activity.

In two thirds of families of hemophilic patients, the females are carriers and some are mildly symptomatic. Carriers of hemophilia can be detected by determination of the ratio of factor VIII activity to vWF antigen and by molecular genetic techniques.

## Complications

Intracranial hemorrhage is the leading disease-related cause of death among those with hemophilia. Up to 80% of intracranial hemorrhages are not trauma-associated. Hemarthroses begin early in childhood and, if recurrent, result in joint destruction. Large intramuscular hematomas can lead to a compartment syndrome with resultant muscle and nerve death. Each of these complications is more common in persons with severe hemophilia but may be experienced by persons with moderate or mild disease. A serious complication of hemophilia is the development of an acquired circulating antibody to factor VIII after treatment with factor VIII concentrate. Inhibitors or antibodies to factor VIII develop in 15–25% of severe factor VIII-deficient persons. The inhibitor is an antibody that may be amenable to desensitization and immunosuppressive therapy. Factor IX concentrate or activated prothrombin complex concentrates may be of help in stopping hemorrhage. Recombinant factor VIIa concentrate is an alternative.

Therapy-related complications have included infection with HIV and hepatitis B (until about 1985 in the United States) and hepatitis C (removed from most US preparations by 1990). By selecting donors seronegative for these infections and by heat- or chemically treating the factor concentrates to inactivate viruses, the risks of these infections have been eliminated. Safe concentrates are expensive and unobtainable in many parts of the world. Transmission of parvovirus and hepatitis A remains a problem, even with concentrates that have had viral inactivation. Immunization with hepatitis A and hepatitis B vaccines is recommended. Recombinant factor VIII concentrates are available but some contain pooled plasma-derived human albumin.

***Table 27–8.*** Physiologic alterations in measurements of the hemostatic system.

| Measurement | Normal Adults | Fetus (20 wk) | Preterm (25–32 wk) | Term Infant | Infant (6 mo) | Pregnancy (term) | Exercise (acute) | Aging (70–80 y) |
|---|---|---|---|---|---|---|---|---|
| **Platelets** | | | | | | | | |
| Count µL/$10^3$ | 250 | 107–297 | 293 | 332 | — | 260 | ↑18–40% | 225 |
| Size (fL) | 9.0 | 8.9 | 8.5 | 9.1 | — | 9.6 | ↑ | — |
| Aggregation ADP | N | + | ↓ | ↓ | — | ↑ | ↓15% | — |
| Collagen | N | ↓ | ↓ | ↓ | — | N | ↓60% | N |
| Ristocetin | N | — | ↑ | ↑ | — | — | ↓10% | — |
| BT (min) | 2–9 | — | 3.6±2 | 3.4±1.8 | — | 9.0±1.4 | — | 5.6 |
| **Procoagulant System** | | | | | | | | |
| PTT* | 1 | 4.0 | 3 | 1.3 | 1.1 | 1.1 | ↓15% | ↓ |
| PT* | 1.00 | 2.3 | 1.3 | 1.1 | 1 | 0.95 | N | — |
| TCT* | 1 | 2.4 | 1.3 | 1.1 | 1 | 0.92 | N | — |
| Fibrinogen mg/dL | 278 (0.61) | 96 (50) | 250 (100) | 240 (150) | 251 (160) | 450 (100) | ↓25% | ↑15% |
| II, U/mL | 1 (0.7) | 0.16 (0.10) | 0.32 (0.18) | 0.52 (0.25) | 0.88 (0.6) | 1.15 (0.68–1.9) | — | N |
| V, U/mL | 1.0 (0.6) | 0.32 (0.21) | 0.80 (0.43) | 1.00 (0.54) | 0.91 ( 0.55) | 0.85 (0.40–1.9) | — | N |
| VII, U/mL | 1.0 (0.6) | 0.27 (0.17) | 0.37 (0.24) | 0.57 (0.35) | 0.87 (0.50) | 1.17 (0.87–3.3) | ↑200% | ↑25% |
| VIIIc, U/mL | 1.0 (0.6) | 0.50 (0.23) | 0.75 (0.40) | 1.50 (0.55) | 0.90 (0.50) | 2.12 (0.8–6.0) | ↑250% | 1.50 |
| vWF, U/mL | 1.0 (0.6) | 0.65 (0.40) | 1.50 (0.90) | 1.60 (0.84) | 1.07 (0.60) | 1.7 | ↑75–200% | ↑ |
| IX, U/mL | 1.0 (0.5) | 0.10 (0.05) | 0.22 (0.17) | 0.35 (0.15) | 0.86 (0.36) | 0.81–2.15 | ↑25% | 1.0–1.40 |
| X, U/mL | 1.0 (0.6) | 0.19 (0.15) | 0.38 (0.20) | 0.45 (0.3) | 0.78 (0.38) | 1.30 | — | N |
| XI, U/mL | 1 (0.6) | 0.13 (0.08) | 0.2 (0.12) | 0.42 (0.20) | 0.86 (0.38) | 0.7 | — | N |
| XII, U/mL | 1.0 (0.6) | 0.15 (0.08) | 0.22 (0.09) | 0.44 (0.16) | 0.77 (0.39) | 1.3 (0.82) | — | ↑16% |
| XIII, U/mL | 1.04 (0.55) | 0.30 | 0.4 | 0.61 (0.36) | 1.04 (0.50) | 0.96 | — | — |
| PreK, U/mL | 1.12 (0.06) | 0.13 (0.08) | 0.26 (0.14) | 0.35 (0.16) | 0.86 (0.56) | 1.18 | — | ↑27% |
| HK, U/mL | 0.92 (0.48) | 0.15 (0.10) | 0.28 (0.20) | 0.64 (0.50) | 0.82 (0.36) | 1.6 | — | ↑32% |
| **Anticoagulant System** | | | | | | | | |
| AT-U/mL | 1.0 | 0.23 | 0.35 | 0.56 | 1.04 | 1.02 | ↑14% | N |
| $\alpha_2$MG, U/mL | 1.05 (0.79) | 0.18 (0.10) | — | 1.39 (0.95) | 1.91 (1.49) | 1.53 (0.85) | — | — |
| C1IN, U/mL | 1.01 | — | — | 0.72 | 1.41 | — | — | — |
| PC, U/mL | 1.0 | 0.10 | 0.29 | 0.50 | 0.59 | 0.99 | N | N |
| Total PS, U/mL | 1.0 (0.6) | 0.15 (0.11) | 0.17 (0.14) | 0.24 (0.1) | 0.87 (0.55) | 0.89 | — | N |
| Free, PS, U/mL | 1.0 (0.5) | 0.22 (0.13) | 0.28 (0.19) | 0.49 (0.33) | — | 0.25 | — | — |
| Heparin Cofactor II, U/mL | 1.01 (0.73) | 0.10 (0.06) | 0.25 (0.10) | 0.49 ( 0.33) | 0.97 (0.59) | — | — | ↓15% |
| TFPI, ng/mL | 73 | 21 | 20.6 | 38 | — | — | — | — |
| **Fibrinolytic System** | | | | | | | | |
| Plasminogen U/mL | 1.0 | 0.20 | 0.35 (0.20) | 0.37 (0.18) | 0.90 | 1.39 | ↓10% | N |
| t-PA, ng/mL | 4.9 | — | 8.48 | 9.6 | 2.8 | 4.9 | ↑300% | N |
| α2-AP, U/mL | 1.0 | 1.0 | 0.74 (0.5) | 0.83 (0.65) | 1.11 (0.83) | 0.95 | N | N |
| PAI-1, U/mL | 1.0 | — | 1.5 | 1.0 | 1.07 | 4.0 | ↓5% | N |
| Overall fibrinolysis | N | ↑ | ↑ | ↑ | — | ↓ | ↑ | ↓ |

Except as otherwise indicated values are mean ±2 SD or values in () are lower limits (–2SD or lower range); +, positive or present; ↓, decreased; ↑, increased; N, normal or no change; *, values as ratio or subject/mean of reference range; BT, bleeding time; TCT, thrombin clotting time: PreK, prekallikrein; HK, high molecular weight kininogen; PC, protein C; PS, protein S; t-PA, tissue plasminogen activator; PAI, plasminogen activator inhibitor; vWF, von Willebrand factor; AT, antithrombin; ADP, adenosine diphosphate; $\alpha_2$-AP, $\alpha_2$-antiplasmin; $\alpha_2$-MG, $\alpha_2$-macroglobulin; C1IN, C1 esterase inhibitor; TFPI, tissue factor pathway inhibitor. Overall fibrinolysis is measured by euglobulin lysis time.

Adapted with permission from Goodnight SH, Hathaway WE (eds): *Disorders of Hemostasis & Thrombosis: A Clinical Guide.* McGraw-Hill, 2001.

## Treatment

The aim of treatment is to correct the factor VIII activity to normal to prevent or stop bleeding. Some patients with mild factor VIII deficiency may respond to desmopressin; however, most patients require administration of factor VIII concentrates to achieve hemostasis. Factor VIII is available as concentrates from human plasma or as a recombinant protein. The in vivo half-life of factor VIII is generally 8–12 hours. Factor VIII must be prescribed in units rather than vials. Non-life-threatening hemorrhages are treated with about 20–30 units of factor VIII concentrate per kilogram of body weight. This dosage will increase factor VIII activity to 40–60%, respectively. Life-threatening hemorrhage is treated initially with approximately 50 units of factor VIII concentrate per kilogram of body weight, which will increase factor VIII activity by 100%. Subsequent doses are determined according to the situation. The dose given is determined by vial size. Excess factor VIII concentrate should always be infused rather than discarded. Monitoring the factor VIII activity may be warranted, depending on the situation. The majority of moderately to severely affected persons with hemophilia administer factor concentrate intravenously at home to treat routine bleeding episodes.

Hemarthroses are common in persons with hemophilia. Initial therapy is with 20–40 units of factor VIII concentrate per kilogram of body weight, with subsequent doses in accordance with joint status. Prophylaxis with infusions is likely to prevent the development of arthropathy. A prospective study comparing prophylaxis with multiple infusions at the time of an hemarthosis is ongoing.

## Prognosis

When care is coordinated through a hemophilia center where attention is given to the physical, emotional, social, and educational status of the child, the prognosis for good quality of life ensues.

Journeycake JM, Buchanan GR: Coagulation disorders. Pediatr Rev 2003;24:83 [PMID: 12612185].

Mannucci PM, Tuddenham EG: The hemophilias: From royal genes to gene therapy. N Engl J Med 2001;344:1773 [PMID: 11396445].

## 2. Factor IX Deficiency (Hemophilia B, Christmas Disease)

The mode of inheritance and clinical manifestations of factor IX deficiency are the same as those of factor VIII deficiency. Factor IX deficiency is 15–20% as prevalent as factor VIII deficiency. As in factor VIII deficiency, factor IX deficiency is associated with prolonged PTT, but PT and thrombin time are normal. Diagnosis is made by assaying factor IX activity, and severity is determined similarly to factor VIII deficiency.

Factor IX concentrate is the treatment product. Unlike factor VIII, about 50% of the administered dose of human-derived factor IX diffuses into the extravascular space. One unit of human-derived factor IX per kilogram is expected to increase the factor IX level by 1%. Recovery after recombinant factor IX concentrate is more variable. Factor IX has a half-life of 20–22 hours in vivo. Cryoprecipitates and factor VIII concentrates do not contain factor IX and should not be given. Virus-inactivating techniques for factor IX concentrates appear effective in eradicating HIV and hepatitis C. If recombinant factor IX concentrate is administered, strong consideration should be given to measuring a factor IX activity level to assess response because the individual response is highly variable. Only 1–3% of persons with factor IX deficiency form an inhibitor, but those who do may develop anaphylaxis when receiving factor IX concentrate. The prognosis for persons with factor IX deficiency is comparable to those with factor VIII deficiency. Gene therapy trials are ongoing.

Bolton Maggs PH, Pasi KJ: Haemophilias A and B. Lancet 2003;361:1801 [PMID: 12781551].

## 3. Factor XI Deficiency (Hemophilia C)

Factor XI deficiency is a genetic, autosomally transmitted bleeding diathesis of mild to moderate severity. Factor XI deficiency accounts for less than 5% of all hemophilia diseases. Homozygotes generally bleed at surgery or following severe trauma but rarely have spontaneous hemarthroses. In contrast to factor VIII and IX deficiency, factor XI activity is not predictive of risk for bleeding; bleeding may be seen in heterozygous individuals with factor XI activity as high as 60%. The aPTT may be normal. The PFA-100 may be prolonged with ADP and epinephrine or the bleeding time may be prolonged consistent with platelet dysfunction since some affected individuals will be deficient for platelet-associated as well as plasma factor XI. Intervention is usually required only at the time of surgery or trauma. Treatment is with desmopressin or fresh frozen plasma (FFP) to the extent volume expansion is tolerated, and sometimes with platelets. The prognosis for an average life span is excellent.

Bolton-Maggs PH: Factor XI deficiency and its management. Haemophilia 2000;6:100 [PMID: 10982275].

## 4. Other Inherited Bleeding Disorders

Other hereditary single clotting factor deficiencies are rare. Transmission is generally autosomal. Homozygous individuals with a deficiency or structural abnormality of prothrombin, factor V, factor VII, or factor X have excessive bleeding.

Persons with dysfibrinogenemia (abnormal fibrinogen) are usually asymptomatic but may develop recurrent venous thromboembolic episodes or have a bleeding tendency. Immunologic determinations of fibrinogen are normal, but the thrombin time and PT are often prolonged. Treatment is similar to that outlined for afibrinogenemia.

Afibrinogenemia resembles hemophilia clinically but has an autosomal recessive inheritance. The patients have mucosal bleeding and bleeding from small injuries and develop hematomas, ecchymoses, and hemarthroses. Fatal bleeding from the umbilical cord has been reported. The principal laboratory finding is prolongation of all of the usual clotting tests. Cryoprecipitate generally controls bleeding in persons with fibrinogen abnormalities.

Lak M et al: Bleeding and thrombosis in 55 patients with inherited afibrinogenaemia. Br J Haematol 1999;107:204 [PMID: 10520042].

# VON WILLEBRAND DISEASE

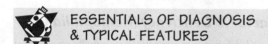

ESSENTIALS OF DIAGNOSIS & TYPICAL FEATURES

- *Easy bruising and epistaxis from early childhood.*
- *Menorrhagia*
- *Bleeding time usually prolonged; platelet count usually normal.*
- *Reduced activity or abnormal structure of von Willebrand factor.*

## General Considerations

Von Willebrand disease and its variants are due to abnormalities of vWF, a plasma protein that forms a multimeric complex in the blood that binds to factor VIII and also is a cofactor for platelet adhesion. Classic von Willebrand disease (type I) involves a partial quantitative deficiency of vWF. Type I comprises 70–80% of all von Willebrand disease. von Willebrand disease type II involves a qualitative abnormality of vWF. Type II disease accounts for less than 10% of von Willebrand disease. Persons with type III disease have virtually complete deficiency of vWF. Von Willebrand disease is the most common inherited bleeding disorder; 1% of

persons are affected, but only 10% of those affected are symptomatic. The disease is usually transmitted as an autosomal dominant trait. Acquired von Willebrand disease may develop in persons with hypothyroidism, Wilms tumor, cardiac disease, renal disease, or systemic lupus erythematosus and in those receiving valproic acid. It is most often due to development of an antibody.

## Clinical Findings

### A. SYMPTOMS AND SIGNS

A history of increased bruising and excessive epistaxis is usually present. Prolonged bleeding will also occur with lacerations or at surgery. Menorrhagia is often a problem.

### B. LABORATORY FINDINGS

The PTT may be prolonged. The PT is normal. A prolonged bleeding and PFA-100 time is usually present because vWF is involved in platelet binding to the blood vessel. Platelet number is decreased in types II and III. Factor VIII and vWF antigen are decreased in types I and III but may be normal in type II von Willebrand disease. vWF activity (ristocetin activity) is decreased in all types. Since vWF levels are dependent on blood type, blood type must be determined. Multimers must be assessed for classification into type.

## Treatment

The treatment to prevent or halt bleeding for most persons with von Willebrand disease types I and II is desmopressin acetate, which causes release of vWF from endothelial stores. It may be administered intravenously at a dose of 0.3 μg/kg diluted in at least 20–30 mL of normal saline and given over 20–30 minutes. A threefold to fivefold rise in plasma vWF is expected as it is released from endothelial stores. Efficacy is variable from patient to patient; factor VIII and vWF activity may be measured before and 60 minutes after infusion to assess response. A high-concentration desmopressin nasal spray (150 μg/spray) is an alternative, but the effect varies and response to intravenous desmopressin does not predict response to the nasal preparation. Low-concentration desmopressin spray used to treat enuresis and diabetes insipidus is ineffective. Because stored vWF release is limited, tachyphylaxis often occurs with desmopressin. Children under age 2 years are at increased risk for seizures secondary to desmopressin-induced hyponatremia. If further therapy is indicated, vWF-rich concentrate is recommended.

For persons with some subtypes of type II and all persons with type III disease, treatment is with vWF-enriched concentrate.

Antifibrinolytic drugs (eg, aminocaproic acid) may be useful for control of oral, nasal, or vaginal bleeding. Topical thrombin and fibrin glue may also be of benefit. Menorrhagia may abate with oral contraceptive therapy.

## Prognosis

Life expectancy is normal.

Castaman G et al: Von Willebrand's disease in the year 2003: Towards the complete identification of gene defects for correct diagnosis and treatment. Haematologica 2003;88:94 [PMID: 12551832].

# ACQUIRED BLEEDING DISORDERS

## 1. Disseminated Intravascular Coagulation (DIC)

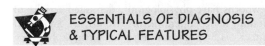

### ESSENTIALS OF DIAGNOSIS & TYPICAL FEATURES

- *Presence of disorder known to trigger disseminated intravascular coagulation.*
- *Evidence for activation of coagulation (prolonged PTT, PT, or thrombin time; FSP, decreased fibrinogen or platelets).*

## General Considerations

DIC is an acquired pathologic process characterized by tissue factor activation of the coagulation system. The primary mediator of DIC is interleukin-6. DIC leads to thrombin generation, intravascular fibrin deposition, and platelet consumption. Microthrombi, composed of fibrin and platelets, may produce ischemic tissue damage. The fibrinolytic system is frequently activated secondary to DIC, producing plasmin-mediated destruction of fibrin, fibrinogen, and other clotting factors (V, VIII). Degradation or split products of fibrin–fibrinogen are formed and function as anticoagulants and inhibitors of platelet function. DIC commonly accompanies disorders occurring in critically ill infants and children. Conditions known to trigger DIC include endothelial cell damage (endotoxin, virus), tissue destruction (necrosis, physical injuries), hypoxia (acidosis), ischemic and vascular changes (shock, hemangiomas), and release of tissue procoagulants (cancer, placental disorders).

## Clinical Findings

### A. SYMPTOMS AND SIGNS

Physical signs of DIC may include (1) diffuse bleeding tendency (hematuria, melena, purpura, petechiae, persistent oozing from needle punctures or other invasive procedures); (2) circulatory collapse, poor skin perfusion, early ischemic changes; and (3) evidence of thrombotic lesions (major vessel thrombosis, gangrene, purpura fulminans).

### B. LABORATORY FINDINGS

Tests that are most sensitive, easiest to perform, and best reflect the hemostatic capacity of the patient are the PT, PTT, platelet count, fibrinogen, and a test for fibrin–fibrinogen split products. A test that measures the cross-linked fibrin degradation byproducts called D-dimers may also be helpful in demonstrating activation of both coagulation and fibrinolysis. Often, the PT and PTT are prolonged and the platelet count and fibrinogen level are decreased. Levels of fibrin–fibrinogen split products and D-dimers are elevated. Often the level of physiologic inhibitors of coagulation, especially antithrombin III and protein C, are depressed and thrombosis may ensue.

The abnormalities associated with DIC may vary depending on the triggering event. Patients with infections may have predominantly thrombocytopenia, with only slight prolongation of the PTT and PT and mild elevation of fibrin–fibrinogen split products. Platelets may be consumed in bacterial sepsis without any other evidence of activated coagulation. In contrast, asphyxia may produce significant consumption of fibrinogen and elevated fibrin–fibrinogen split products without depression of platelets.

## Differential Diagnosis

Bleeding with liver disease, vitamin K deficiency, or uremia can mimic DIC. Patients with fulminant hepatitis or advanced cirrhosis often have evidence of both decreased production of liver-dependent coagulation factors and increased consumption of platelets and fibrinogen. Generally, factor VII activity is decreased markedly in liver disease compared to mild to moderate decreases in DIC. Factor VIII activity may be normal or even increased in liver disease compared to decreased activity in DIC.

## Treatment

### A. THERAPY FOR UNDERLYING DISORDER

The most important aspect of therapy is identification and treatment of the triggering event. If the event (eg, hypoxia, shock, sepsis) can be treated, often no other therapy is needed for the coagulopathy.

## B. Replacement Therapy

Replacement of depleted coagulation factors and platelets may be necessary in severe DIC. FFP replaces depleted coagulation factors; 10–15 mL/kg will raise clotting factor activities by about 10–15%. Fibrinogen (and factor VIII) can be given as cryoprecipitate also; one bag of cryoprecipitate per 3 kg in infants or one bag of cryoprecipitate per 6 kg in older children will raise the fibrinogen level by 75–100 mg/dL. Platelets are replaced with platelet concentrate; in the neonate, 10 mL of platelet concentrate per kilogram will raise the platelet count by 75,000–100,000/μL. In older children, one bag of platelet concentrate per 5–6 kg is the usual dose. An alternative formula is as follows: 1 unit/m$^2$ of platelet concentrate will increase the platelet count by about 20,000/μL. The minimal hemostatic goals in a bleeding patient are a platelet count greater than 40,000/μL, PT of less than 16 seconds, and fibrinogen over 100 mg/dL.

## C. Anticoagulant Therapy

Heparin is often given in hopes of interrupting the clotting process. The rationale for heparin therapy is to allow for more effective replacement therapy while the primary disease is being specifically treated, but there is no controlled trial to show that heparin is beneficial. The most effective and safest method of giving unfractionated heparin is by continuous intravenous administration. A loading dose of 50–100 units/kg is followed by 15–25 units/kg/h by continuous intravenous infusion. Heparin should be administered to achieve a therapeutic level between 0.4 and 0.7 unit/mL. Low-molecular-weight heparin is an alternative therapy that can be given subcutaneously twice a day; the therapeutic range is 0.5–1 unit/mL.

## D. Specific Factor Concentrates

Antithrombin concentrate may be of benefit. Protein C concentrate and activated protein C concentrate have been efficacious in the treatment of meningococcemia-associated DIC.

## 2. Liver Disease

The liver is the major synthetic site of prothrombin; fibrinogen; and factors HMWK, V, VII, IX, X, XI, XII, and XIII. It also produces plasminogen and three physiologic anticoagulants, antithrombin III, protein C, and protein S. α$_2$-Antiplasmin, which regulates fibrinolysis, is produced in the liver. Deficiency of factor V and the vitamin K-dependent factors (II, VII, IX, and X) is most often a result of decreased hepatic synthesis and is

manifested as PT prolongation. The PTT may also be prolonged. Extravascular loss and increased consumption of clotting factors may contribute to PT and PTT prolongation. The amount of fibrinogen may be decreased, or an abnormal fibrinogen (dysfibrinogen) containing excess sialic acid residues may be synthesized. Dysfibrinogenemia is associated with prolongation of thrombin time and reptilase time. Fibrin–fibrinogen degradation products and D-dimers may be present because of increased fibrinolysis. Thrombocytopenia secondary to hypersplenism and platelet aggregation abnormalities may occur. Treatment consists of replacement with FFP and platelets as needed. If liver disease is associated with fat malabsorption, vitamin K (1–5 mg) should be given. Desmopressin may shorten the bleeding time and PTT in patients with chronic liver disease. Recombinant VIIa also has been shown to be efficacious in advanced liver disease.

## 3. Vitamin K Deficiency

All newborns have physiologically depressed activity of the vitamin K-dependent factors (II, VII, IX, and X). If vitamin K is not administered at birth, a bleeding diathesis previously called hemorrhagic disease of the newborn, now termed vitamin K deficiency bleeding (VKDB), may develop. One of three patterns is seen:

1. Early VKDB of the newborn occurs within 24 hours of birth and is most often manifested by cephalhematoma, intracranial hemorrhage, or intra-abdominal bleeding. Although occasionally idiopathic, it is most often associated with maternal ingestion of drugs that interfere with vitamin K metabolism (eg, warfarin, phenytoin, isoniazid, rifampin). Early VKDB occurs in 6–12% of neonates born to mothers taking these medications but not receiving vitamin K supplementation. The disorder is often life threatening.

2. Classic VKDB of the newborn occurs at 24 hours to 7 days of age and usually is manifested as gastrointestinal, skin, or mucosal bleeding. Bleeding after circumcision may occur. Although occasionally associated with maternal drug usage, it most often occurs in well babies who do not receive vitamin K at birth and are solely breast-fed.

3. Late VKDB occurs on or after day 8 but rarely beyond age 3 months. Manifestations are intracranial, gastrointestinal, or skin bleeding. Usually it is secondary to chronic diarrhea, malabsorption syndromes, obstructive jaundice, or prolonged antibiotic therapy. It occurs almost exclusively in breast-fed infants.

4. Outside of the newborn period, vitamin K deficiency may occur as a consequence of malabsorp-

tion, fasting, alcoholism, or medications such as antibiotics, coumarins, megadose vitamin E, or salicylates.

The diagnosis of vitamin K deficiency is based on the history, physical examination, and laboratory results. The PT is markedly prolonged. The PTT may be prolonged. The thrombin time does not prolong until late in the course. Platelet counts are normal. The diagnosis is confirmed by a demonstration of noncarboxlyated proteins in vitamin K's absence in the plasma and by improvement following treatment with vitamin K. Intravenous or subcutaneous treatment with vitamin K should be given immediately and not withheld awaiting test results. Depending on the severity of bleeding, additional treatment with FFP prothrombin concentrate complex or recombinant VIIa may be indicated.

### 4. Uremia

Qualitative and quantitative platelet abnormalities are common hemostatic defects. Decreased activity of prothrombin and factors XII, XI, and IX secondary to increased urinary losses can result in prolongation of the PTT. vWF activity may also be decreased. Bleeding occurs in approximately 50% of patients with chronic renal failure. It is most often manifested as purpura, menorrhagia, or gastrointestinal bleeding. Bleeding time is the best predictor of bleeding risk. Bleeding may be managed with infusion of desmopressin, red blood cells, and FFP. Avoiding the development of severe anemia by administering erythropoietin prophylactically decreases the bleeding risk. Recombinant VIIa may be useful in refractory bleeding.

Dalton HJ: Recombinant activated protein C in pediatric sepsis. Pediatr Infect Dis J 2003;22:743 [PMID: 12913779].

Suzuki S et al: Vitamin K deficiency during perinatal and infantile period. Semin Thromb Hemost 2001;27:93 [PMID: 11372776].

## VASCULAR ABNORMALITIES ASSOCIATED WITH BLEEDING

### 1. Henoch–Schönlein Purpura (see Chapter 22) (Anaphylactoid Purpura)

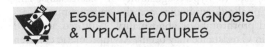

ESSENTIALS OF DIAGNOSIS & TYPICAL FEATURES

- *Purpuric cutaneous rash.*
- *Migratory polyarthritis or polyarthralgias.*

- *Colicky abdominal pain.*
- *Nephritis.*

## General Considerations

Henoch–Schönlein purpura, the most common small vessel vasculitis syndrome in children, occurs primarily in males age 2–7 years. Occurrence is highest in the spring and fall. Two thirds of affected children have a history of upper respiratory infection in the preceding 1–3 weeks.

Henoch–Schönlein purpura is characterized by vasculitis of the small vessels, particularly those of the skin, gastrointestinal tract, and kidney. The most common and earliest symptom is palpable purpura, which results from extravasation of erythrocytes into the tissue surrounding the involved venules. Serum IgA immune complexes are thought to trigger a leukocytoclastic vasculitis. Immune complexes are found in the kidney, intestine, and skin. Suspected though not proved inciting antigens include group A β-hemolytic streptococci and other bacteria, viruses, drugs, foods, and insect bites.

## Clinical Findings

### A. SYMPTOMS AND SIGNS

The skin rash is often urticarial initially and progresses to a macular–papular appearance, which transforms into a diagnostic symmetrical purpuric rash distributed on the ankles, buttocks, and elbows. Purpuric areas of a few millimeters in diameter are present and may progress to form larger hemorrhages (palpable purpura). Petechial lesions may occur, but most hemorrhages are slightly larger. The rash usually begins on the lower extremities and buttocks, but the entire body may be involved. New lesions can continue to appear for 2–4 weeks. Approximately two thirds of patients develop migratory polyarthralgias or polyarthritis, primarily of the ankles and knees. Edema of the hands, feet, scalp, and periorbital regions may occur. Abdominal colic—due to hemorrhage and edema primarily of the small intestine—occurs in about 50% of those affected. Between 25% and 50% of those affected develop renal involvement, with hematuria, proteinuria, or nephrotic syndrome. Some children develop hypertension. Hematuria alone is never the presenting complaint for Henoch–Schönlein purpura but usually manifests in the second to third week of illness. Renal involvement occurs more commonly in males than in females and in older patients than in younger ones. Testicular torsion may occur. Neurologic symptoms are possible.

## B. LABORATORY FINDINGS

The platelet count, platelet function tests, and bleeding time are usually normal, although the platelet count may even be elevated. Blood coagulation studies are normal. Urinalysis frequently reveals hematuria. Proteinuria may also be noted, but casts are uncommon. Stool analysis may be positive for blood even though melena is not observed. The antistreptolysin O (ASO) titer is frequently elevated and the throat culture positive for group A β-hemolytic streptococci. Serum IgA may be elevated.

## Differential Diagnosis

Henoch–Schönlein purpura, in contrast with thrombocytopenic purpura, causes a palpable rash and the platelet count is normal. The rash of septicemia (especially meningococcemia) may be similar to that of Henoch–Schönlein purpura, although the distribution tends to be more generalized with meningococcemia. The possibility of child abuse should be considered in any child presenting with purpura. Other vasculitides should also be considered.

## Complications

Intussusception of the small bowel may occur. About 5% of patients develop renal failure as a result of advancing proliferative glomerulonephritis with an associated mortality rate of 3%.

## Treatment

Generally, treatment is unwarranted. Corticosteroid therapy may provide symptomatic relief for severe gastrointestinal or joint manifestations but does not alter skin or renal manifestations. Aspirin is useful for the pain associated with arthritis. If culture for group A β-hemolytic streptococci is positive or if the ASO titer is elevated, penicillin should be given in full doses for 10 days.

## Prognosis

The prognosis for recovery is generally good, although symptoms frequently (25–50%) recur over a period of several months. In patients who develop renal manifestations, microscopic hematuria may persist for years. Progressive renal failure occurs in less than 5% of patients with Henoch–Schönlein purpura.

Cuttica RJ: Vasculitis in children: A diagnostic challenge. Curr Probl Pediatr 1997;27:309 [PMID: 9399074].

## 2. Other Vascular Disorders

Mild to life-threatening bleeding occurs with some types of Ehlers–Danlos syndrome—the most common collagen disorder (see Chapter 33). The Ehlers–Danlos syndromes are characterized by joint hypermobility, skin extensibility, bowel perforation, and often easy bruising. Despite easy bruising, coagulation abnormalities do not always occur. Reported abnormalities include deficiencies of coagulation factors VIII, IX, XI, and XIII as well as platelet dysfunction. Spontaneous rupture and dissection of aortic aneurysms have been reported in persons with specific types of Ehler–Danlos syndrome.

Beighton P et al: Ehlers–Danlos syndromes: Revised nosology. Villefranche, 1997. Am J Med Genet 1998;77:31 [PMID: 9557891].

# ■ THROMBOTIC DISORDERS

Thrombotic disorders are uncommon in children but are being recognized with increasing frequency. Multiple risk factors, both inherited and acquired, are usually present in children who develop a thromboembolic event. Conditions commonly associated with thrombosis during childhood are venous access devices and other implanted foreign bodies, malignancy, infection, trauma, collagen–vascular disease, surgery, renal disease, sickle cell anemia, cardiac disease, and immobilization.

Initial evaluation of the child who has a thrombosis must include a family history and definitive imaging study to delineate the type (venous versus arterial) and extent of the thrombosis. Laboratory evaluation is indicated to determine the presence of an underlying congenital or acquired hemostatic abnormality. Consultation with a pediatric hematologist is suggested to guide hemostatic evaluation because the normal ranges for some tests are age-dependent. A deficiency of the anticoagulant proteins, protein C, protein S, or antithrombin III may be congenital or acquired and associated with thrombosis. Activated protein C resistance due to the factor V Leiden mutation is the most common genetic hypercoagulable condition in Caucasians. A mutation in the prothrombin procoagulant protein also predisposes to hypercoagulability in Caucasians. Antiphospholipid antibodies are the most common acquired prothrombotic abnormality. Acquired activated protein C resistance may occur. Asymptomatic children with genetically transmitted prothrombotic risk factors or antiphospholipid antibodies generally do not receive prophylactic anticoagulation therapy. Children with an acute thrombosis should be treated according to published guidelines specifically designed for children. Heparin is generally administered, although site-directed and systemic administration of a fibrinolytic agent are other treatment options. Following acute therapy, warfarin is generally prescribed. The duration of warfarin therapy is dependent on the risk factors for a recurrent event.

## INHERITED DISORDERS

### 1. Protein C Deficiency

Protein C is a vitamin K-dependent protein that is normally activated by thrombin bound to thrombomodulin and inactivates activated factors V and VIII. In addition, it stimulates fibrinolysis. Two phenotypes of hereditary protein C deficiency exist. Heterozygous individuals with autosomal dominant protein C deficiency typically present with venous thromboembolism as young adults, but the disorder may manifest during childhood. Following a second event, lifelong warfarin therapy should be instituted.

Homozygous or compound heterozygous individuals generally present within the first 12 hours of life with purpura fulminans. Associated findings may include cerebral or retinal thrombosis resulting in blindness. Immediate treatment with FFP every 6–12 hours should be given. Heparin is generally administered simultaneously. Subsequent management requires chronic anticoagulation with warfarin compounds or infusion of protein C concentrate (not yet commercially available in the United States). The long-term outlook is unknown.

### 2. Protein S Deficiency

Protein S is a cofactor for protein C. Neonates with homozygous protein S deficiency have a course similar to protein C deficiency. Lifelong warfarin therapy is indicated for patients with a recurrent thrombotic event.

### 3. Antithrombin III Deficiency

Antithrombin III is the most important physiologic inhibitor of thrombin. In addition, it inhibits activated factors IX, X, XI, and XII. Antithrombin III deficiency is transmitted in an autosomal dominant pattern and is associated with venous thromboembolism. Symptoms before puberty are rare.

Availability of antithrombin III concentrate or replacement has been sporadic. Patients with recurrent venous thrombosis are maintained on lifelong warfarin.

### 4. Factor V Leiden Mutation

An amino acid substitution in the gene coding for factor V results in the production of factor V Leiden, a factor V variant that is resistant to inactivation by activated protein C. About 20% of unselected consecutive Caucasian adults with deep vein thrombosis and 40–60% of Caucasian adults from families with unexplained thrombophilia have been identified with this mutation. Venous thrombosis has been reported in children both heterozygous and homozygous for this mutation. This mutation also predisposes to ischemic stroke. Screening may be performed with an assay for activated protein C resistance. Confirmation is by genetic–molecular analysis.

### 5. Prothrombin Mutation

The 20210 glutamine to alanine mutation in the prothrombin gene is associated with a three-fold increased risk for venous thrombosis in Caucasians. Testing is by DNA analysis.

### 6. Other Inherited Disorders

Qualitative abnormalities of fibrinogen (dysfibrinogenemias) are usually inherited in an autosomal dominant manner. Most individuals with dysfibrinogenemia are asymptomatic. Some have problems with bleeding, and others develop venous or arterial thrombosis. This diagnosis is suggested by a prolonged thrombin time with a normal fibrinogen level. Whether dysfunction of the fibrinolytic system plays a role in the development of thrombosis is controversial. Hyperhomocystinemia can be an inherited or an acquired condition and is associated with an increased risk for both arterial and venous thromboses in adults. In children it is a risk factor for ischemic stroke. Elevated lipoprotein(a), a lipoprotein with homology to plasminogen, has been reported as an etiologic agent in childhood thrombosis. Lipoprotein(a) levels are genetically transmitted as an autosomal dominant trait.

## ACQUIRED DISORDERS

### 1. Antiphospholipid Antibodies

The development of antiphospholipid antibodies is the most common acquired blood protein abnormality associated with both venous and arterial thrombosis. Antiphospholipid antibodies include the lupus anticoagulant and the anticardiolipin antibody. The lupus anticoagulant is an immunoglobulin that inhibits in vitro phospholipid-dependent coagulation assays such as the aPTT and dilute Russell viper venom time. Anticardiolipin antibodies are detected by ELISA assays.

Both antibodies are associated with thrombosis. Although common in persons with collagen–vascular disorders such as systemic lupus erythematosus, they occur following drug exposure, infection, and lymphoproliferative diseases. They are also present in some well individuals.

Treatment for a thrombosis in a person found to have an antiphospholipid antibody is generally with heparin anticoagulation. Alternatives are local instillation of a fibrinolytic agent or systemic fibrinolysis. Anticoagulation with warfarin should be continued until the antiphospholipid antibody has resolved. The risk for recurrent thrombosis is high if anticoagulation is discontinued prematurely.

Jilma B et al: Antithrombotic therapy in special circumstances. II—In children, thrombophilia and miscellaneous conditions. BMJ 2003;326:93 [PMID: 12521976].

Manco-Johnson MJ et al: Laboratory testing for thrombophilia in pediatric patients. Thromb Haemost 2002;88:155 [PMID: 12152657].

Richardson MW et al: Thrombosis in children: Current perspective and distinct challenges. Thromb Haemost 2002;88:900 [PMID: 12529737].

Revel-Vilk S et al: Prothrombotic conditions in an unselected cohort of children with venous thromboembolic disease. J Thromb Haemost 2003;1:915 [PMID: 12871356].

# ■ SPLENIC ABNORMALITIES

## SPLENOMEGALY & HYPERSPLENISM

The differential diagnosis of splenomegaly includes the general categories of congestive splenomegaly, chronic infections, leukemia and lymphomas, hemolytic anemias, reticuloendothelioses, and storage diseases (Table 27–9).

Splenomegaly due to any cause may be associated with hypersplenism and the excessive destruction of circulating red cells, white cells, and platelets. The degree of cytopenia is variable and, when mild, requires no specific therapy. In other cases, the thrombocytopenia may cause life-threatening bleeding, particularly when the splenomegaly is secondary to portal hypertension and associated with esophageal varices or the consequence of a storage disease. In such cases, treatment with surgical splenectomy or with splenic embolization may be warranted. Although more commonly associated with acute enlargement, rupture of an enlarged spleen can be seen in more chronic conditions such as Gaucher disease.

Stone DL et al: Life threatening splenic hemorrhage in two patients with Gaucher's disease. Am J Hematol 2000;64:140 [PMID: 10814997].

## ASPLENIA & SPLENECTOMY

Children who lack normal splenic function are at risk for sepsis, meningitis, and pneumonia due to encapsulated bacteria such as pneumococci and *H influenzae.* Such infections are often fulminant and fatal because of inadequate antibody production and impaired phagocytosis of circulating bacteria.

Congenital asplenia is usually suspected when an infant is born with abnormalities of abdominal viscera and complex cyanotic congenital heart disease. Howell–Jolly bodies are usually present on the peripheral blood smear, and the absence of splenic tissue is confirmed by technetium radionuclide scanning. The prognosis depends on the underlying cardiac lesions, and many children die during the first few months. Prophylactic antibiotics, usually penicillin, and pneumococcal conjugate and polysaccharide vaccines are recommended.

The risk of overwhelming sepsis following surgical splenectomy is related to the child's age and to the underlying disorder. Because the risk is highest when the procedure is performed earlier in life, splenectomy is usually postponed until after age 5 years. The risk of postsplenectomy sepsis is also greater in children with malignancies, thalassemias, and reticuloendothelioses than in children whose splenectomy is performed for ITP, hereditary spherocytosis, or trauma. Prior to splenectomy, children should be immunized against *Pneumococcus, H influenzae,* and *Neisseria meningiditis.* Additional management should include penicillin prophylaxis and prompt evaluation for fever 38.8°C or above or signs of severe infection.

Children with sickle cell anemia develop functional asplenia during the first year of life, and overwhelming sepsis is the leading cause of early deaths in this disease. Prophylactic penicillin has been shown to reduce the incidence of sepsis by 84%.

Pickering L; American Academy of Pediatrics: Immunization in special circumstances. Red Book 2000;25:66.

# ■ TRANSFUSION MEDICINE

## DONOR SCREENING & BLOOD PROCESSING: RISK MANAGEMENT

Minimizing the risks of transfusion begins by asking the donor questions that will protect the recipient from transmission of infectious agents as well as other risks of

***Table 27–9.*** Causes of chronic splenomegaly in children.

| Cause | Associated Clinical Findings | Diagnostic Investigation |
|---|---|---|
| Congestive splenomegaly | History of umbilical vein catheter or neonatal omphalitis; signs of portal hypertension (varices, hemorrhoids, dilated abdominal wall veins); pancytopenia, history of hepatitis or jaundice | Complete blood count, platelet count, liver function tests, ultrasonography |
| Chronic infections | History of exposure to tuberculosis, histoplasmosis, coccidioidomycosis, other fungal disease; chronic sepsis (foreign body in bloodstream; subacute infective endocarditis) | Appropriate cultures and skin tests, ie, blood cultures; PPD, fungal serology and antigen tests; chest film; HIV serology |
| Infectious mononucleosis | Fever, fatigue, pharyngitis, rash, adenopathy, hepatomegaly | EBV antibody titers |
| Leukemia, lymphoma, Hodgkin disease | Evidence of systemic involvement with fever, bleeding tendencies, hepatomegaly, and lymphadenopathy; pancytopenia | Blood smear, bone marrow examination, chest film, gallium scan, LDH, uric acid |
| Hemolytic anemias | Anemia, jaundice; family history of anemia, jaundice, and gallbladder disease in young adults | Reticulocyte count, Coombs' test, blood smear, osmotic fragility test, hemoglobin electrophoresis |
| Reticuloendothelioses (histiocytosis X) | Chronic otitis media, seborrheic or petechial skin rashes, anemia, infections, lymphadenopathy, hepatomegaly, bone lesions | Skeletal x-rays for bone lesions; biopsy of bone, liver, bone marrow, or lymph node |
| Storage diseases | Family history of similar disorders, neurologic involvement, evidence of macular degeneration, hepatomegaly | Biopsy of liver or bone marrow in search for storage cells |
| Splenic cyst | Evidence of other infections (postinfectious cyst) or congenital anomalies; peculiar shape of spleen | Radionuclide scan, ultrasonography |
| Splenic hemangioma | Other hemangiomas, consumptive coagulopathy | Radionuclide scan, arteriography, platelet count, coagulation screen |

PPD = purified protein derivative; EBV = Epstein–Barr virus; LDH = lactic dehydrogenase; HIV = human immunodeficiency virus.

transfusions. In addition, information defining high-risk groups whose behavior increases the possible transmission of AIDS, hepatitis, and other diseases is provided, with the request that persons in these groups not donate blood.

Before blood components can be released for transfusion, donor blood is screened for antibodies to hepatitis B, hepatitis C, HIV-1 and HIV-2, and human T-cell lymphotropic virus (HTLV) I and II; and a serologic test for syphilis is performed. Testing for hepatitis B surface antigen and HIV p24 antigen is also performed. Screening donor blood for viral genome was mandated for HIV and HCV early in 2003. NAT testing for West Nile Virus was begun in 2003. Detection of other viral genomes may be expanded. The aminotransferases may be measured as surrogate tests for hepatitis (Table 27–10). Positive tests are repeated, and on their confirmation the unit in question is destroyed and the donor placed in a deferral category. Many of the screening tests used are very sensitive and have a high rate of false-positive results. As a result, confirmatory tests have been developed to check the initial screening results and separate the false-positives from the true-positives.

With these techniques, the risk of an infectious complication from blood components has been minimized (see Table 27–10), with the greatest risk being posttransfusion hepatitis (see sections on hepatitis C virus and non-A, non-B, non-C hepatitis in Chapter 21). Autologous donation is recognized by some centers as a safe alternative to homologous blood. Issues of

***Table 27–10.*** Transmission risks of infectious agents for which screening of blood products is routinely performed.

| Disease Entity | Transmission | Screening and Processing Procedures | Approximate Risk of Transmission |
|---|---|---|---|
| Syphilis | Low risk that fresh blood drawn during spirochetemia can transmit infection. Organism not able to survive behond 72 hours during storage at 4°C. | Donor history. RPR or VDRL. | < 1:100,000 |
| Hepatitis A | Units drawn during prodrome could transmit virus. Because of brief viremia during acute phase, absence of asymptomatic carrier phase, and failure to detect transmission in multiple transfused individuals, infection by this agent is unlikely. | Donor history. | 1:1,000,000 |
| Hepatitis B | Prolonged viremia during various phases of the disease and asymptomatic carrier state make HBV infection a significant risk of transfusion. Incidence has markedly decreased with screening strategies. | Donor history, education, and self-exclusion. Hepatitis B surface antigen (HBsAg). Surrogate tests for non-A, non-B hepatitis and screen for hepatitis C and retroviruses have helped screen out population at risk for transmitting hepatitis B virus. | 1:250,000–1:30,000 |
| Hepatitis C | Over two-thirds of cases of non-A, non-B posttransfusion hepatitis may be due to this agent. The virus has characteristics similar to those of HBV which are responsible for the risk from transfusion. Infection may lead to a significant incidence of cirrhosis and end-stage liver disease. | Donor history. Surrogate tests: ALT and hepatitis B core antibody (anti-HBc), anti-HCV. Nucleic acid testing for viral genome required. | 1:1,600,000 |
| Non-A, non-B, non-C hepatitis | Not a specific cause but a classification of agents other than HAV, HBV, HCV, Epstein-Barr virus, and cytomegalovirus, which can cause posttransfusion hepatitis. | Donor history. Surrogate tests: ALT and anti-HBc. | Undefined |
| Human immunodeficiency virus (HIV-1, HIV-2) infection | Cytotoxic retrovirus spread by sexual contact, parenteral (including transfusion) and vertical routes. Resultant destruction of CD4-positive cells leads to in clinical manifestations of AIDS. | Donor history, education, and self-exclusion. Anti-HIV by EIA, screening test. Western blot confirmatory. P[24] antigen testing. Nucleic acid testing for viral genome required. | 1:2,000,000–1:1,500,000 |
| Human T-cell lymphotropic virus I and II (HTLV-I and -II) infection | Retroviruses spread by sexual contact, parenteral (including transfusion) and vertical modes. Over years to decades, infection with HTLV-I may cause lymphoid malignancies or myelopathy. | Donor history. Anti-HTLV-I and -II by enzyme immunoassay screening test. Western blot confirmatory. | 1:600,000 |

ALT = alanine transaminase; HAV, HBV, HCV = hepatitis A virus, hepatitis B virus, hepatitis C virus; HTLV = human T-cell lymphotropic virus; RPR = rapid plasma reagin; VDRL = syphilis test; AIDS = acquired immunodeficiency syndrome.

donor size make the techniques of autologous donation difficult to apply to the pediatric population.

Primary CMV infections are significant complications of blood transfusion in transplant recipients, neonates, and immunodeficient individuals. Transmission of CMV can be avoided by using seronegative donors, apheresis platelet concentrates collected by techniques ensuring low numbers of residual white cells, or red cell or platelet products leukodepleted by filtering (white blood cell counts less than 5 million per packed red cell unit or apheresis platelet concentrate equivalent).

## STORAGE & PRESERVATION OF BLOOD & BLOOD COMPONENTS

Whole blood is routinely fractionated into packed red cells, platelets, and FFP or cryoprecipitate for most efficient use of all blood components. The storage conditions and biologic characteristics of the fractions are summarized in Table 27–11. The conditions provide the optimal environment to maintain appropriate recovery, survival, and function and are different for each blood component. For example, red cells undergo dramatic metabolic changes during their 35-day storage, with a decrease in 2,3-DPG during the second week of storage, a decrease in ATP, and a gradual loss of intracellular potassium into the plasma. Fortunately, these changes are reversed readily within hours to days after the red cells are transfused. However, in certain clinical conditions, these effects may define the type of components used. For example, blood less than 7–10 days old would be preferred for exchange transfusion or replacement of red cells in persons with cardiopulmonary disease to ensure adequate oxygen-carrying capacity. However, storage time is not an issue when administering transfusions to those with chronic anemia.

Under certain conditions in which excessive potassium load is a problem, one has the option of using blood less than 10 days old, making packed cells out of an older unit of whole blood, or washing blood stored as packed cells. Regardless of the blood's age, over 70% of the red cells will circulate after transfusion and approximate normal survival in the circulation.

Platelets can be stored at 22°C for a maximum of 5 days. At the extremes of storage, there should be at least a 60% recovery, a survival time that approximates turnover of fresh autologous platelets, and normalization of the bleeding time in proportion to the peak platelet count. Frozen components, red cells, FFP, and cryoprecipitate are outdated at 3 years, 1 year, and 1 year, respectively. Frozen red cells retain the same biochemical and functional characteristics as the day they were frozen. FFP contains 80% or more of all of the clotting factors of fresh plasma. Factor VIII and fibrinogen are concentrated in cryoprecipitate.

## PRETRANSFUSION TESTING

Both the donated blood and the recipient are tested for ABO and Rh(D) antigens and for autoantibodies or alloantibodies. The cross-match is required on any component that contains red cells. In the major cross-match, washed donor red cells are incubated with the serum from the patient, and agglutination is detected and graded. The antiglobulin phase of the test is then performed; Coombs reagent, which will detect the presence of IgG or complement on the surface of the red cells, is added to the mixture, and any possible reaction is evaluated. In the presence of a negative antibody screen in the recipient, a negative antiglobulin phase or immediate spin cross-match test confirms the compatibility of the blood. Further testing is required if the antibody screen or the cross-match is positive, and blood should not be given until the nature of the reactivity is delineated. An incompatible cross-match is evaluated first with a direct antiglobulin or Coombs test to detect IgG or complement on the surfaces of the recipient's red cells. The indirect antiglobulin test is also used to determine the presence of antibodies that will coat or activate complement on the surfaces of normal red cells.

## TRANSFUSION PRACTICE

### General Rules

Several rules should be observed in administering any blood component:

1. In final preparation of the component, no solutions should be added to the bag or tubing set except for normal saline (0.9% sodium chloride for injection, USP), ABO-compatible plasma, or other specifically approved expanders. Hypotonic solutions cause hemolysis of red cells, and, if these are transfused, a severe reaction will occur.

2. Transfusion products should be protected from contact with any calcium-containing solution (eg, lactated Ringer's); recalcification and reversal of the citrate effect will cause clotting of the blood component.

3. Blood components should not be warmed to a temperature greater than 37°C. If a component is incubated in a water bath, it should be enclosed in a watertight bag to prevent contamination of entry ports.

4. Whenever a blood bag is entered, the sterile integrity of the system is violated, and that unit

**Table 27–11.** Characteristics of blood and blood components.

| Component | Storage Conditions | Composition and Transfusion Characteristics | Indications | Risks and Precautions | Administration |
|---|---|---|---|---|---|
| Whole blood | 4°C for 35 d. RBC characteristics:<br>**Survival:** Recovery decreases during storage but is always > 70%. Cells that circulate approximate normal survival.<br>**Function:** 2,3-DPG levels fall to undetectable after second week of storage. This defect repaired within 24 h of transfusion.<br>**Electrolytes:** With storage, potassium increases in plasma. This rises to high levels after 2 wk of storage. | Contains RBCs and many plasma compounds of whole blood. Leukocytes and platelets lose activity or viability after a few days under these conditions. Procoagulant clotting factors (particularly VIII and V) deteriorate rapidly during storage. Each unit has about 500 mL volume and Hct 36–40%. | Oxygen carrying capacity (anemia). Volume replacement for blood loss (> 15–20%) or severe shock. | Must be ABO-identical and cross-match-compatible. Infectious diseases. Febrile or hemolytic transfusion reactions. Alloimmunization to red cell, white cell, or platelet antigens. | During acute blood loss, as rapidly as tolerated. In other settings, 2–4 h. 10 mL/kg will raise Hct by 5% and support volume. |
| Packed red cells | Same as for whole blood. Special rejuvenating solutions allow storage for 42 d. | Contains RBCs; plasma removed in preparation. Status of leukocytes, clotting factors, and platelets same as for whole blood. Hct about 70%, volume 200–250 mL. May request tighter pack to give Hct 80–90%. | Oxygen carrying capacity. Acute trauma or bleeding or situations requiring intensive cardiopulmonary support (Hct < 25–30%). Chronic anemia (Hct < 20%). | Same as for whole blood. | May be given as patient will tolerate based on cardiovascular status over 2–4 hours. Dose of 3 mL packed RBC/kg will raise the Hct by 3%. If cardiovascular status stable, give 10 mL/kg over 2–4 h. If unstable, use smaller volume or do packed RBC exchange. |

| Component | | | | |
|---|---|---|---|---|
| Washed or filtered red cells | When cells are washed, there is a 24-h outdate. Up to that time, they have the same characteristics as for packed red cells. | Same as for packed red cells | Same as packed red cells. Depending on technique used and extent of reduction of white blood cells, washed red cells may achieve the following:<br>• Avoid febrile reactions.<br>• Decrease the transmission of CMV.<br>• Decrease the incidence of alloimmunization to white cell antigens. | Same as whole blood. Removal of white cells diminishes the risk of febrile reactions. Filtration with high-efficiency white cell filters may decrease rate of alloimmunization to white cell antigens and transmission of CMV. | Same as for packed red cells. |
| Frozen red cells | Packed red cells frozen in 40% glycerol solution at less than −65°C. Stored 3 years. Retain the same biochemical characteristics, function, and capacity for survival as the day in storage they were frozen; when thawed, 24-h outdate. | Same as for packed red cells. | Same as packed red cells. Useful for avoiding febrile reactions, decreasing transmission of CMV, autologous blood donation, and developing an inventory of rare red cell blood groups. | Same as for whole blood. Risk of CMV transmission is at same level as using seronegative components. | Same as for packed red cells. |
| Fresh frozen plasma | Plasma from whole blood stored at under −18°C for up to 1 year | Contains > 80% of all procoagulant and anticoagulant plasma proteins | Replacement of plasma procoagulant and anticoagulant plasma proteins. May provide "other" factors, eg, treatment of TTP. | Need not be cross-matched; should be type-compatible. Volume overload, infectious diseases, allergic reactions. Solvent detergent–treated plasma or donor-retested plasma units have decreased risk for viral transmission. | As rapidly as tolerated by patient but not > 4 hours. Dose: 10–15 mL/kg will increase level of all clotting factors by 10–20%. |
| Cryoprecipitate | Produced by freezing fresh plasma to under −65°C, then allowing to thaw 18 hours at 4°C. After centrifugation, cryoprecipitable proteins are separated. May be stored at under −18°C for up to 1 y. | Contains factor VIII, fibrinogen, and fibronectin at concentrations greater than those of plasma. Also contains factor XIII. VIII > 80 IU/pack, fibrinogen 100–350 mg/pack. | Treatment of acquired or congenital deficiencies of VIII, von Willebrand factor, and fibrinogen. Useful in making biologic glues that contain fibrinogen. Commercial clotting factor concentrates are the treatment of choice for factor VIII deficiency and von Willebrand disease because sterilization procedures further reduce the risk of viral transmission. | Same as for fresh frozen plasma. ABO agglutinogens may also be concentrated and can give positive direct agglutination test if not type-specific | Cryoprecipitate can be given as a rapid infusion. Dose: ½ pack per kg body weight will increase factor VIII level by 80–100% and fibrinogen by 200–250 mg/dL. |

(continued)

**Table 27-11.** Characteristics of blood and blood components. (continued)

| Component | Storage Conditions | Composition and Transfusion Characteristics | Indications | Risks and Precautions | Administration |
|---|---|---|---|---|---|
| Platelet concentrates from whole blood donation | Separated from platelet-rich plasma and stored with gentle agitation at 22°C for 3–5 d. Containers currently in use are plastic and allow for gas exchange, diffusion of $CO_2$ helps keep pH > 6.00, a major factor in keeping platelets viable and functional. | Each unit contains about 5 × $10^{10}$ platelets. Survival: Although there may be some loss with storage, 60–70% recovery should be achieved, with stored platelets correcting the bleeding time in proportion to the peak counts reached. | Treatment of thrombocytopenia or platelet function defects. | No cross-match necessary. Should be ABO type-specific. Other risks as for whole blood. | Can be given as rapid transfusion or as defined by cardiovascular status, not more than 4 h. Dose: 10 mL/kg should increase platelet count by at least 50,000/μL. |
| Platelet concentrates by apheresis techniques | Same as random donor units | Platelet content is equivalent to 6–10 units of random donor concentrates. Depending on technique used, these may be relatively free of leukocytes, a product useful in avoiding alloimmunization. | As above, particularly useful in treating patients who have insufficient production in whom alloimmunization is a potential problem. | Same as above. | As above. |
| Granulocytes | Although they may be stored stationary at 20–24°C, transfuse as soon as possible after collection | Contains at least 1 × $10^{10}$ granulocytes but also platelets and red cells. When donors given 10 μg/kg G-CSF subcutaneously and 8 mg decadron orally 12–15 h before collection increases to > 5 × $10^{10}$ granulocytes. | Severely neutropenic individuals (< 500/μL) with poor marrow reserves and suspected bacterial or fungal infections not responding to 48–72 h of parenteral antibiotics. Also in patients with neutrophil dysfunction. | Same as for platelets. Pulmonary leukostasis reactions. Severe febrile reactions. | Given in an infusion over 2–4 h. Dose: 1 unit daily for newborns and infants, 1 × $10^9$ granulocytes per kg. |

CMV = cytomegalovirus; G-CSF = granulocyte colony-stimulating factor; Hct = hematocrit; RBC = red blood cell; TTP = thrombotic thrombocytopenic purpura.

should be discarded within 4 hours if left at room temperature or within 24 hours if the temperature is between 1°C and 4°C.

5. Transfusions of products containing red cells should not exceed 4 hours. Blood components in excess of what can be infused during this time period should be stored in the blood bank until needed.

6. Before transfusion, the blood component should be inspected visually for any unusual characteristics—such as the presence of flocculent material, hemolysis, or clumping of cells—and mixed thoroughly.

7. The unit and the recipient should be identified properly.

8. The administration set includes a standard 170–260 mm clot filter. Under certain clinical circumstances, an additional microaggregate filter may be used to eliminate small aggregates of fibrin, white cells, and platelets that will not be removed by the standard filter.

9. The patient should be observed during the entire transfusion but especially during the first 15 minutes. Any adverse symptoms or signs should be evaluated immediately and reactions to the transfusion reported promptly to the transfusion service.

10. When cross-match-incompatible red cells or whole blood unit(s) must be given to the patient (as with autoimmune hemolytic anemia), a test dose of 10% of the total volume (not to exceed 50 mL) should be administered over 15–20 minutes; the transfusion is then stopped and the patient evaluated for reaction. If no adverse effects are noted, the remainder of the volume can be infused carefully.

11. Blood for exchange transfusion in the newborn period may be cross-matched with either the infant's or the mother's serum. If the exchange is for hemolysis, 500 mL of whole blood stored for less than 7 days will be adequate. If replacement of clotting factors is a key issue, packed red cells (7 days old) reconstituted with FFP may be considered. Based on posttransfusion platelet counts, platelet transfusion may be considered. Other problems to be anticipated are acid–base derangements, hyponatremia, hyperkalemia, hypocalcemia, hypoglycemia, hypothermia, and hypervolemia or hypovolemia.

## Choice of Blood Component

Several principles should be considered when deciding on the need for blood transfusion. Indications for blood or blood components must be well defined, and the patient's medical condition, not just the laboratory results, should be the basis for the decision. Specific deficiencies exhibited by the patient (eg, oxygen-carrying capacity, thrombocytopenia) should be treated with appropriate blood components and the use of whole blood minimized. Information about specific blood components is summarized in Table 27–11.

### A. WHOLE BLOOD

Whole blood may be used in patients who require replacement of oxygen-carrying capacity and volume. More specifically, it should be considered when more than 15% of blood volume is lost. Doses vary depending on volume considerations (see Table 27–11). In acute situations, the transfusion may be completed rapidly to support blood volume.

### B. PACKED RED CELLS

Packed red cells (which include leukocyte-poor, filtered, or frozen deglycerolized products) prepared from whole blood by centrifugal techniques are the appropriate choice for almost all patients with deficient oxygen-carrying capacity. Exact indications will be defined by the clinical setting, the severity of the anemia, the acuity of the condition, and any other factors affecting oxygen transport.

### C. PLATELETS

The decision to transfuse platelets depends on the patient's clinical condition, the status of plasma phase coagulation, the platelet count, the cause of the thrombocytopenia, and the functional capacity of the patient's own platelets. With platelet counts less than 10,000–20,000/$\mu$L, the risk of severe, spontaneous bleeding is increased markedly, and—in the absence of antibody-mediated thrombocytopenia—transfusion should be considered. Under certain circumstances, especially with platelet dysfunction or treatment that inhibits the procoagulant system, transfusions at higher platelet counts may be necessary.

Transfused platelets are sequestered temporarily in the lungs and spleen before reaching their peak concentrations, 45–60 minutes after transfusion. A significant proportion of the transfused platelets never circulate but remain sequestered in the spleen. This phenomenon results in reduced recovery; only 60–70% of the transfused platelets are accounted for when peripheral platelet count increments are used as a measure of response.

In addition to cessation of bleeding, two variables indicate the effectiveness of platelet transfusions. The first is platelet recovery, as measured by the maximum number of platelets circulating in response to transfusion. The practical measure is the platelet count at

**Table 27–12.** Adverse events following transfusions.

| Event | Pathophysiology | Signs and Symptoms | Management |
|---|---|---|---|
| Acute hemolytic transfusion reaction | Preformed alloantibodies (most commonly to ABO) and occasionally autoantibodies cause rapid intravascular hemolysis of transfused cells with activation of clotting (DIC), activation of inflammatory mediators, and acute renal failure. | Fever, chills, nausea, chest pain, back pain, pain at transfusion site, hypotension, dyspnea, oliguria, dark urine. | The risk of this type of reaction overall is low (1:30,000), but the mortality rate is high (up to 40%). Stop the transfusion; maintain renal output with intravenous fluids and diuretics (furosemide or mannitol); treat DIC with heparin; and institute other appropriate supportive measures. |
| Delayed hemolytic transfusion reaction | Formation of alloantibodies after transfusion and resultant destruction of transfused red cells, usually by extravascular hemolysis. | Fever, jaundice, anemia. A small percentage may develop chronic hemolysis. | Detection, definition, and documentation (for future transfusions). Supportive care. Risk, 1:2500. |
| Febrile reactions | Usually caused by leukoagglutinins in recipient cytokines or other biologically active compounds. | Fever. May also involve chills. | Supportive. Consider leukocyte-poor products for future. Risk per transfusion, 1:200. |
| Allergic reactions | Most causes not identified. In IgA-deficient individuals, reaction occurs as a result of antibodies to IgA. | Itching, hives, occasionally chills and fever. In severe reactions, may see signs of anaphylaxis: dyspnea, pulmonary edema. | Mild to moderate reactions: diphenhydramine. More severe reactions: epinephrine subcutaneously and steroids intravenously. Risk for mild to moderate allergic reactions, 1:1000; severe anaphylactic reactions, 1:150,000. |
| Transfusion-related acute lung injury | Acute lung injury occurring within 4 h after transfusion. Two sets of factors interact to produce the syndrome. Patient factors: infection, surgery, cytokine therapy. Blood component factors: lipids, antibodies, cytokines. Two groups of factors interact during transfusion to result in lung injury indistinguishable from ARDS. | Tachypnea, dyspnea, hypoxia. Diffuse interstitial markings. Cardiac evaluation normal. | May consider younger products: packed red blood cells ≤ 2 weeks, platelets ≤ 3 days, washing components to prevent syndrome. Management: supportive care. Risk, 1:2000–1:3000 per transfusion. |
| Dilutional coagulopathy | Massive blood loss and transfusion with replacement with fluids or blood components and deficient clotting factors. | Bleeding. | Replacement of clotting factors or platelets with appropriate blood components. |
| Bacterial contamination | Contamination of units results in growth of bacteria or production of clinically significant levels of endotoxin. | Chills, high fever, hypotension, other symptoms of sepsis or endotoxemia. | Stop transfusion; make aggressive attempts to identify organism; provide vigorous supportive medical care including antibiotics |
| Graft-versus-host disease | Lymphocytes from donor transfused in an immunoincompetent host. | Syndrome can involve a variety of organs, usually skin, liver, gastrointestinal tract, and bone marrow. | Preventive management: irradiation (> 1500 cGy) of cellular blood components transfused to individuals with congenital or acquired immunodeficiency syndromes, intrauterine transfusion, very premature infants, and when donors are relatives of the recipient. |

*(continued)*

***Table 27–12.*** Adverse events following transfusions. (continued)

| Event | Pathophysiology | Signs and Symptoms | Management |
|---|---|---|---|
| Iron overload | There is no physiologic mechanism to excrete excess iron. Target organs include liver, heart, and endocrine organs. In patients receiving red cell transfusions over long periods of time, there is an increase in iron burden. | Signs and symptoms of dysfunctional organs affected by the iron. | Chronic administration of iron chelator such as deferoxamine. |

DIC = disseminated intravascular coagulation; ARDS = adult respiratory distress syndrome.

1 hour after transfusion. In the absence of immune or drastic nonimmune factors that markedly decrease platelet recovery, one would expect a 7000/μL increment for each random donor unit and a 40,000–70,000/μL increment for each single-donor apheresis unit in a large child or adolescent. For infants and small children, 10 mL/kg of platelets will increase the platelet count by at least 50,000/μL. The second variable is the survival of transfused platelets. Normally, transfused platelets have a half-life of 3–5 days. In the presence of immune or nonimmune destruction, the life span may be shortened to a few days or a few hours. Frequent platelet transfusions may be required to maintain adequate hemostasis.

A particularly troublesome outcome in patients receiving long-term platelet transfusions is the development of a refractory state characterized by poor (< 30%) recovery or no response to platelet transfusion (as measured at 1 hour). Most (70–90%) of these refractory states result from the development of alloantibodies directed against HLA antigens on the platelet. Platelets have class I HLA antigens, and the antibodies are primarily against HLA A or B determinants. A smaller proportion of these alloantibodies (10%) may be directed against platelet-specific alloantigens. The most effective approach to prevent HLA sensitization is to use leukocyte-depleted components (< 5 million leukocytes per unit of packed red cells or per apheresis or 6–10 random donor unit concentrates). For the alloimmunized, refractory patient, the best approach is to provide HLA-matched platelets for transfusion. Reports have suggested that platelet cross-matching procedures using HLA-matched or unmatched donors may be helpful in identifying platelet concentrates most likely to provide an adequate response.

## D. Fresh Frozen Plasma

The indication for FFP is replacement of plasma coagulation factors in clinical situations in which a deficiency of one or more clotting factors exists and associated bleeding manifestations are present. In some hereditary factor deficiencies such as factor VIII deficiency or von Willebrand disease, commercially prepared concentrates contain these factors in higher concentrations and, because of viral inactivation, impose less infectious risk and are more appropriate than plasma.

## E. Cryoprecipitate

This component may be used for acquired or congenital disorders of hypofibrinogenemia or afibrinogenemia. Although cryoprecipitate is a rich source for factor VIII or vWF, commercial concentrates that contain these factors are more appropriate (see preceding section). The dose given depends on the protein to be replaced. Cryoprecipitate can be given in a rapid transfusion over 30–60 minutes.

## F. Granulocytes

With better supportive care over the past 10 years, the need for granulocytes in neutropenic patients with severe bacterial infections has decreased. Indications still remain for severe bacterial infections unresponsive to vigorous medical therapy in either newborns or older children with bone marrow failure, or patients with neutrophil dysfunction. Newer mobilization schemes using G-CSF and steroids in donors result in granulocyte collections with at least $5 \times 10^{10}$ neutrophils. This may provide a better product for patients requiring granulocyte support.

## G. Apheresis Products and Procedures

Apheresis equipment allows one or more blood components to be collected from a donor while the rest are returned. Apheresis platelet concentrates, which have as many platelets as 6–10 units of platelet concentrates from whole blood donations, are one example; granulocytes another. Apheresis techniques can also be used to collect hematopoietic stem cells that have been mobilized into the blood by cytokines (G-CSF or GM-CSF) given alone or after chemotherapy. These stem cells are used for autologous bone marrow transplantation. Blood cell separators can be used for the collection of single-source plasma or removal of a blood component that is causing disease. Examples include red cell exchange in sickle cell disease and plasmapheresis in Goodpasture syndrome or in myasthenia gravis.

## Adverse Effects

The noninfectious complications of blood transfusions are outlined in Table 27–12. Most complications present a small but significant risk to the recipient.

Busch MP et al: Current and emerging infectious risks of blood transfusions. JAMA 2003;289:959 [PMID: 12597733].

Goodnough LT et al: Transfusion medicine. First of two parts—Blood transfusion. N Engl J Med 1999;340:438 [PMID: 9971869].

Goodnough LT et al: Transfusion medicine. Second of two parts—Blood conservation. N Engl J Med 1999;340:525 [PMID: 10021474].

National Institutes of Health Consensus Conference: Fresh frozen plasma: Indications and risks. JAMA 1985;253:551 [PMID: 3968788].

National Institutes of Health Consensus Conference: Platelet transfusion therapy. JAMA 1987;257:1777 [PMID: 3820494].

Silliman CC et al: Transfusion-related acute lung injury: Epidemiology and a prospective analysis of etiologic factors. Blood 2003;101:454 [PMID: 12393667].

Smith JW et al: Therapeutic apheresis: A summary of current indication categories endorsed by the AABB and the American Society for Apheresis. Transfusion 2003;43:820 [PMID: 12757535].

## REFERENCES

Goodnight SH, Hathaway WE: *Disorders of Hemostasis and Thrombosis: A Clinical Guide.* McGraw-Hill, 2001.

Petz LD, Garratty G: *Acquired Immune Hemolytic Anemias.* Churchill Livingstone, 1980.

Vichinsky E, Walters U, Feusner J (eds): Pediatric Hematology/Oncology, Part I, Pediatr Clin North Am 2002.

# Neoplastic Disease

*Edythe A. Albano, MD, Mylène Bassal, MDCM, Christopher C. Porter, MD, Brian S. Greffe, MD, Nicholas K. Foreman, MD, & Linda C. Stork, MD*

Each year approximately 150 out of every 1 million children younger than 20 years of age are diagnosed with cancer. For children between the ages of 1 and 20 years, cancer is the fourth leading cause of death, behind unintentional injuries, homicides, and suicides. However, combined-modality therapy, including surgery, chemotherapy, and radiation therapy, has improved survival dramatically, such that the overall 5-year survival rate of pediatric malignancies is now greater than 75%. It is estimated that by the year 2020, one in 600 adults will be a survivor of childhood cancer.

Because pediatric malignancies are rare, cooperative clinical trials have become the mainstay of treatment planning and therapeutic advances. The Children's Oncology Group (COG), representing the amalgamation of four prior pediatric cooperative groups (Children's Cancer Group, Pediatric Oncology Group, Intergroup Rhabdomyosarcoma Study Group, and the National Wilms Tumor Study Group), offers the most current therapeutic options and protocols and strives to answer important treatment questions in a timely manner. A child or adolescent newly diagnosed with cancer should be enrolled in a cooperative clinical trial whenever possible. Because many protocols are associated with significant toxicities, morbidity, and potential mortality, treatment of children with cancer should be supervised by a pediatric oncologist familiar with the hazards of treatment, preferably at a multidisciplinary pediatric cancer center.

Advances in molecular genetics, cell biology, and tumor immunology have contributed to the understanding of pediatric malignancies and their treatment. It is important that biopsy specimens of suspected malignancies be examined by a pathologist familiar with pediatric and adolescent cancers and with the role of ancillary studies. In addition to formalin-fixed tissue, fresh unfixed tissue is essential for metaphase chromosome analysis and electron microscopy. Molecular techniques can sometimes detect an aberrant gene product that is not detectable with routine cytogenetics, ensuring greater diagnostic accuracy and leading to appropriate therapy. The polymerase chain reaction (PCR) also aids in the detection of minimal residual disease. In addition, molecular techniques can determine whether a pathologic process is monoclonal (arising from a single cell and generally considered malignant) or polyclonal (arising from multiple cells and usually nonmalignant). Diverse rearrangements of the DNA of antigen receptor genes can characterize a benign process, whereas the cells of a lymphoma, for example, have uniform rearrangements.

Molecular techniques have also led to the characterization of oncogenes and tumor suppressor genes in human malignancies. An oncogene is one that causes malignant transformation or deregulated cell growth. For example, the proto-oncogene c-*myc* plays an important role in hematopoietic cell proliferation. It has been recognized at the site of three different translocations in Burkitt lymphomas: t(8;14), t(8;22), and t(2;8). A tumor suppressor gene (antioncogene) constrains cell proliferation; its absence can lead to unchecked cell growth. The retinoblastoma gene is the prototypical tumor suppressor gene. Inactivation of both copies of this gene in a cell leads to tumor formation.

Research in supportive care areas, such as prevention and management of infection, pain, and emesis, has improved the survival and quality of life for children undergoing cancer treatment. Long-term studies of childhood cancer survivors are yielding information that provides a rationale for modifying future treatment regimens to decrease morbidity.

Ries LAG et al: *SEER Cancer Statistics Review, 1975–2000,* http://seer.cancer.gov/csr/1975_2000, 2003.

# MAJOR PEDIATRIC NEOPLASTIC DISEASES

## ACUTE LYMPHOBLASTIC LEUKEMIA

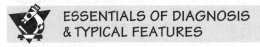

### ESSENTIALS OF DIAGNOSIS & TYPICAL FEATURES

- *Bone marrow aspirate or biopsy specimen shows more than 25% lymphoblasts.*
- *Pallor, petechiae, purpura (50%), bone pain (25%).*

- *Hepatosplenomegaly (60%), lymphadenopathy (50%).*
- *Single or multiple cytopenias: neutropenia, thrombocytopenia, anemia (99%).*
- *Leukopenia (15%) or leukocytosis (50%), often with lymphoblasts identifiable on blood smear.*
- *Diagnosis confirmed by bone marrow examination.*

## General Considerations

Acute lymphoblastic leukemia (ALL) is the most common malignancy of childhood, accounting for about 25% of all cancer diagnoses in patients younger than age 15 years. The worldwide incidence of ALL is about 1:25,000 children per year, including 3000 children per year in the United States. The peak age at onset is 4 years; 85% of patients are diagnosed between ages 2 and 10 years. Before the advent of chemotherapy, this disease was fatal, usually within 3–4 months, with virtually no survivors 1 year after diagnosis.

ALL results from uncontrolled proliferation of immature lymphocytes. Its cause is unknown, and genetic factors may play a role. Leukemia is defined by the presence of more than 25% malignant hematopoietic cells (blasts) on bone marrow aspirate. Leukemic blasts from the majority of cases of childhood ALL have an antigen on the cell surface called the common ALL antigen (CALLA). These blasts derive from B-cell precursors early in their development. Less commonly, lymphoblasts are of T-cell origin or of mature B-cell origin. Over 70% of children receiving aggressive combination chemotherapy and early presymptomatic treatment to the central nervous system (CNS) are now cured of ALL.

## Clinical Findings

### A. SYMPTOMS AND SIGNS

Presenting complaints of patients with ALL include those related to decreased bone marrow production of red blood cells (RBCs), white blood cells (WBCs), or platelets and to leukemic infiltration of extramedullary (outside bone marrow) sites. Intermittent fevers are common, as a result of either cytokines induced by the leukemia itself or infections secondary to leukopenia. About 25% of patients experience bone pain, especially in the pelvis, vertebral bodies, and legs. Physical examination at diagnosis ranges from virtually normal to highly abnormal. Signs related to bone marrow infiltration by leukemia include pallor, petechiae, and pur-

pura. Hepatomegaly or splenomegaly occurs in over 60% of patients. Lymphadenopathy is common, either localized or generalized to cervical, axillary, and inguinal regions. The testes may be unilaterally or bilaterally enlarged secondary to leukemic infiltration. Superior vena cava syndrome is caused by mediastinal adenopathy compressing the superior vena cava. A prominent venous pattern develops over the upper chest from collateral vein enlargement. The neck may feel full from venous engorgement. The face may appear plethoric, and the periorbital area may be edematous.

A mediastinal mass can cause tachypnea, orthopnea, and respiratory distress. Leukemic infiltration of cranial nerves may cause cranial nerve palsies with mild nuchal rigidity. The optic fundi may show exudates of leukemic infiltration and hemorrhage from thrombocytopenia. Anemia can cause a flow murmur, tachycardia, and, rarely, congestive heart failure. Bone and joint pain may be found on examination, particularly in the pelvis, lower spine, and femurs. Signs of infection may also be present.

### B. LABORATORY FINDINGS

A complete blood count (CBC) with differential is the most useful initial test because 95% of patients with ALL have a decrease in at least one cell type (single cytopenia): neutropenia, thrombocytopenia, or anemia. Most patients have decreases in at least two blood cell lines. The WBC count is low or normal ($\leq 10,000/\mu L$) in 50% of patients, but the differential shows neutropenia (absolute neutrophil count $< 1000/\mu L$) along with a small percentage of blasts amid normal lymphocytes. In 30% of patients the WBC count is between 10,000 and $50,000/\mu L$; in 20% of patients it is over $50,000/\mu L$, occasionally higher than $300,000/\mu L$. Blasts are usually readily identifiable on peripheral blood smears from patients with elevated WBC counts. Peripheral blood smears also show abnormalities in RBCs, such as tear drops. Most patients with ALL have decreased platelet counts ($< 150,000/\mu L$) and decreased hemoglobin ($< 11$ g/dL) at diagnosis. Fewer than 1% of patients diagnosed with ALL have entirely normal CBCs and peripheral blood smears but have bone pain that leads to bone marrow examination. Serum chemistries, particularly uric acid and lactate dehydrogenase (LDH), are often elevated at diagnosis as a result of cell breakdown. Serum phosphorus is occasionally elevated at diagnosis as well.

The diagnosis of ALL is made by bone marrow examination, which shows a homogeneous infiltration of leukemic blasts replacing normal marrow elements. The morphology of blasts on bone marrow aspirate can usually distinguish ALL from acute myeloid leukemia (AML). Lymphoblasts are typically small, with cell diameters of approximately two erythrocytes. Lymphoblasts have scant cytoplasm, usually without granules. The nucleus typically contains no nucleoli or one small, indistinct nucleolus. Immunophenotyping of ALL blasts by flow cytometry helps distinguish precursor B-cell ALL from T-cell ALL or AML. Histochemical stains specific for myeloblastic and monoblastic leukemias (myeloperoxidase and nonspecific esterase) distinguish ALL from AML. About 5% of patients present with CNS leukemia, which is defined as a cerebrospinal fluid (CSF) WBC count > 5/μL with blasts present on cytocentrifuged specimen.

### C. IMAGING

Chest radiograph may show mediastinal widening or an anterior mediastinal mass and tracheal compression secondary to lymphadenopathy or thymic infiltration, especially in T-cell ALL. Abdominal ultrasound may show kidney enlargement from leukemic infiltration or uric acid nephropathy as well as intra-abdominal adenopathy. Plain radiographs of the long bones and spine may show demineralization, periosteal elevation, growth arrest lines, or compression of vertebral bodies.

## Differential Diagnosis

The differential diagnosis, based on the history and physical examination, includes chronic infections by Epstein–Barr virus (EBV) and cytomegalovirus (CMV), causing lymphadenopathy, hepatosplenomegaly, fevers, and anemia. Prominent petechiae and purpura suggest a diagnosis of immune thrombocytopenic purpura (ITP). Significant pallor could be caused by transient erythroblastopenia of childhood (TEC), autoimmune hemolytic anemias, or aplastic anemia. Fevers and joint pains, with or without hepatosplenomegaly and lymphadenopathy, suggest juvenile rheumatoid arthritis (JRA). The diagnosis of leukemia usually becomes straightforward once the CBC reveals multiple cytopenias and leukemic blasts. Serum LDH levels may help distinguish JRA from leukemia. LDH is usually normal in JRA but often elevated in ALL patients presenting with bone pain. An elevated WBC count with lymphocytosis is typical of pertussis; however, in pertussis the lymphocytes are mature, and neutropenia is rarely associated.

## Treatment

### A. SPECIFIC THERAPY

Intensity of treatment is determined by specific prognostic features present at diagnosis or early in treatment. The majority of patients with ALL are enrolled in clinical trials designed by the Children's Oncology Group (COG) and approved by the National Cancer Institute (NCI). The first month of therapy consists of induction, at the end of which over 95% of patients exhibit remission on bone marrow aspirates. The drugs most commonly used in induction include oral prednisone or dexamethasone, intravenous vincristine and daunorubicin, intramuscular asparaginase, and intrathecal methotrexate. For T-cell ALL, intravenous cyclophosphamide may be added during induction.

Consolidation is the second phase of treatment, during which intrathecal chemotherapy and sometimes cranial radiation therapy are given to kill lymphoblasts "hiding" in the meninges.

Maintenance therapy includes daily oral mercaptopurine, weekly oral methotrexate, and, often, monthly pulses of intravenous vincristine and oral prednisone or dexamethasone. Intrathecal chemotherapy, either with methotrexate alone or combined with cytarabine and hydrocortisone, is usually given every 2–3 months. Several months of intensive chemotherapy, termed delayed intensification, is generally interposed early within the maintenance chemotherapy phase of treatment.

These drugs have significant potential side effects. Patients need to be monitored closely to prevent drug toxicities and to ensure early treatment of complications. The duration of treatment ranges between 2.2 years for girls and 3.2 years for boys. Treatment for ALL is tailored to prognostic, or risk, groups. A child age 1–9 years with a WBC count under 50,000/μL at diagnosis and without t(9;22) or t(4;11) is considered to be at "standard risk" and receives less intensive therapy than a "high-risk" patient who has a WBC count at diagnosis over 50,000/μL or is older than age 10 years. This risk-adapted treatment approach has significantly increased the cure rate among patients with less favorable prognostic features while minimizing treatment-related toxicities in those with favorable features. Bone marrow relapse is usually heralded by an abnormal CBC, either during treatment or for a few years thereafter.

The CNS and testes are sanctuary sites of extramedullary leukemia. Currently, about a third of all ALL relapses are isolated to these sanctuary sites. Systemic chemotherapy does not penetrate these tissues as well as it penetrates other organs. Thus, presymptomatic intrathecal chemotherapy is a critical part of ALL treatment, without which many more relapses would occur in the CNS, with or without bone marrow relapse. The majority of isolated CNS relapses are diagnosed in an asymptomatic child at the time of routine intrathecal injection, when CSF cell count and differential shows an elevated WBC with leukemic blasts. Occasionally, symptoms of CNS relapse develop: headache, nausea and vomiting, irritability, nuchal rigidity, photophobia, and cranial nerve palsies Previously, up to 15% of boys developed testicular relapse following completion of chemotherapy. The presentation of testicular relapse is usually unilateral painless testicular enlargement, without a distinct mass. The incidence of testicular relapse has decreased significantly as treatment for ALL has intensified. Routine follow-up of boys both on and off treatment includes physical examination of the testes.

Bone marrow transplantation, now called hematopoietic stem cell transplantation (HSCT), is rarely used as initial treatment for ALL, because most patients are cured with chemotherapy alone. Patients whose blasts contain certain chromosomal abnormalities, such as t(9;22) or hypodiploidy (< 44 chromosomes), and infants with t(4;11) may have a better cure rate with early HSCT from an HLA-DR-matched sibling donor, or perhaps a matched unrelated donor, than with intensive chemotherapy alone. HSCT cures about 50% of patients who relapse, provided that a second remission is achieved with chemotherapy before transplant. Children who relapse more than 1 year after completion of chemotherapy (late relapse) may be cured with intensive chemotherapy without HSCT. A number of new biologic agents, including tyrosine kinase inhibitors and immunotoxins, are currently in various stages of research and development. Some of these therapies may prove relevant for future treatment of poor risk or relapsed ALL.

## B. SUPPORTIVE CARE

Tumor lysis syndrome should be anticipated when treatment is started. Alkalinization of urine with intravenous sodium bicarbonate should be undertaken, and the patient should be hydrated and given oral allopurinol. If superior vena caval or superior mediastinal syndrome is present, general anesthesia is contraindicated temporarily. If hyperleukocytosis (WBC count > 100,000/μL) is accompanied by hyperviscosity and mental status changes, leukapheresis may be indicated to rapidly reduce the number of circulating blasts and minimize the potential thrombotic or hemorrhagic CNS complications. Severe anemia at diagnosis can usually be corrected with a number of small RBC transfusions and intravenous furosemide. Throughout the course of treatment, all transfused blood and platelet products should be irradiated to prevent graft-versus-host disease from the transfused lymphocytes. Whenever possible, blood products should be leukodepleted to minimize CMV transmission, transfusion reactions, and sensitization to platelets.

During the course of treatment, fever (temperature ≥ 38.3°C) and neutropenia (absolute neutrophil count < 500/μL) require treatment with empiric broad-spectrum antibiotics. Patients receiving ALL treatment must receive prophylaxis against *Pneumocystis jiroveci* (formerly *Pneumocystis carinii*). Trimethoprim–sul-

famethoxazole given twice each day on 2 or 3 consecutive days per week is the drug of choice. Patients nonimmune to varicella are at risk for very serious—even fatal—infection. Such patients should receive varicella-zoster immune globulin (VZIG) within 72 hours after exposure and treatment with intravenous acyclovir for active infection.

The treatment of a patient on chemotherapy for ALL is complex because of the infectious complications and potential toxicities of chemotherapy.

## Prognosis

Cure rates depend on specific prognostic features present at diagnosis. The two most important features are WBC count and age. Children age 2–9 years whose diagnostic WBC count is less than 50,000/μL have a higher rate of cure than other patients. The rapidity of response to induction treatment has prognostic significance as well, reflecting leukemic blast sensitivity to chemotherapy. Patients are categorized as rapid early responders (RER) or slow early responders (SER) based on the percentage of blasts present in bone marrow aspirates within 7–14 days after induction begins. More intensive treatment regimens are given to SERs than RERs to increase their chance of cure. Certain chromosomal abnormalities present in the leukemic blasts at diagnosis influence prognosis. Patients with t(9;22) generally have a very poor chance of cure even with intensive chemotherapy. Likewise, infants with t(4;11) have a poor chance of cure with conventional chemotherapy. In contrast, the 15% of patients whose blasts are hyperdiploid (containing over 50 chromosomes instead of the normal 46) with trisomies of chromosomes 4, 10, and 17 have a greater chance of cure than do children without these trisomies. About 25% of children with ALL have blasts that contain a gene rearrangement between chromosomes 12 and 21, called TEL-AML1, detected by molecular but not by cytogenetic techniques. Children with the TEL-AML1 rearrangement appear to have an excellent prognosis. Techniques based on leukemic blast immunophenotyping or immunoglobulin rearrangements have been developed to detect residual lymphoblasts in bone marrow, called minimal residual disease (MRD), at the end of induction and during remission. In future COG clinical trials, patients with levels of MRD above a certain threshold at the end of remission induction will receive intensified therapy, in an attempt to improve their outcome.

Arico M: Outcome of treatment in children with Philadelphia chromosome-positive acute lymphoblastic leukemia. N Engl J Med 2000;342:998 [PMID:10749961].

Bostrom BC: Dexamethasone versus prednisone and daily oral versus weekly intravenous mercaptopurine for patients with standard-risk acute lymphoblastic leukemia: A report from the Children's Cancer Group. Blood 2003:101:3809 [PMID: 12531809].

Gaynon PS: Children's Cancer Group trials in childhood acute lymphoblastic leukemia: 1983–1995. Leukemia 2000;14; 2223 [PMID: 11187913].

Loh ML: TEL/AML1-positive pediatric leukemia: Prognostic significance and therapeutic approaches. Curr Opin Hematol 2002:9;345 [PMID: 12042710].

Maloney KW: Long-term results of treatment studies for childhood acute lymphoblastic leukemia: Pediatric Oncology Group studies from 1986–1994. Leukemia 2000;14:2276 [PMID: 11187919].

# ACUTE MYELOID LEUKEMIA

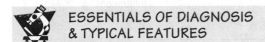

### ESSENTIALS OF DIAGNOSIS & TYPICAL FEATURES

- *Bone marrow aspirate or biopsy shows 20% or more leukemic blasts.*
- *Fatigue, bleeding, or infection.*
- *Adenopathy, hepatosplenomegaly, skin nodules (M4 and M5 subtypes).*
- *Cytopenias: neutropenia (69%), anemia (44%), thrombocytopenia (33%).*

## General Considerations

Approximately 500 new cases of acute myeloid leukemia (AML) occur per year in children and adolescents in the United States. Although AML accounts for only 25% of all leukemias in this age group, it is responsible for at least one third of deaths from leukemia in children and teenagers. Congenital conditions associated with an increased risk of AML include Diamond–Blackfan anemia, neurofibromatosis, Down syndrome, Wiskott–Aldrich, Kostmann, and Li–Fraumeni syndromes, as well as chromosomal instability syndromes such as Fanconi anemia. Acquired risk factors include exposure to ionizing radiation, cytotoxic chemotherapeutic agents, and benzenes. However, the vast majority of patients have no identifiable risk factors. Historically, the diagnosis of AML was based almost exclusively on morphology and immunohistochemical staining of the leukemic cells. AML has eight subtypes (M0–M7) according to the French–American–British (FAB) classification (Table 28–1). Immunophenotypic, cytogenetic, and molecular analyses are increasingly important in confirming the diagnosis of AML and subclassifying it into biologically distinct subtypes that have therapeutic and prognostic implications. Cytogenetic clonal abnormalities occur in 80% of patients with AML and are often predictive of outcome. Recently, the World Health Organization classified AML based on genetic, immunophenotypic, biologic, and clinical features, to more accurately characterize the distinct biologic and clinical behavior of the AML subtypes.

Aggressive induction therapy currently results in a 75–85% complete remission rate. However, long-term survival has improved only modestly to approximately 50%, despite the availability of a number of effective agents, improvements in supportive care, and increasingly intensive therapies.

## Clinical and Laboratory Findings

The clinical manifestations of AML commonly include anemia (44%), thrombocytopenia (33%), and neutropenia (69%). Symptoms may be few and innocuous or may be life-threatening. The median hemoglobin value at diagnosis is 7 g/dL, and platelets usually number fewer than 50,000/µL. Frequently the absolute neutrophil count is under 1000/µL, although the total WBC count is over 100,000/µL in 25% of patients at diagnosis.

Hyperleukocytosis may be associated with life-threatening complications. Venous stasis and sludging of blasts in small vessels cause hypoxia, hemorrhage, and infarction, most notably in the lung and CNS. This clinical picture is a medical emergency requiring rapid intervention, such as leukopheresis, to decrease the leukocyte count. CNS leukemia is present in 5–15% of patients at diagnosis, a higher rate of initial involvement than in ALL. Certain subtypes, such as M4 and M5, have a higher likelihood of meningeal infiltration than do other subtypes. Additionally, clinically significant coagulopathy may be present at diagnosis in patients with M3, M4, or M5 subtypes. This problem manifests as bleeding or an abnormal disseminated intravascular coagulation screen and should be at least partially corrected prior to initiation of treatment, which may transiently exacerbate the coagulopathy.

## Treatment

### A. SPECIFIC THERAPY

AML is less responsive to treatment than ALL and requires more intensive chemotherapy. Toxicities from therapy are common and likely to be life-threatening; therefore, treatment should be undertaken only at a tertiary pediatric oncology center.

**Table 28–1.** FAB subtypes of acute myeloid leukemia.

| FAB Classification | Common Name | Distribution in Childhood (Age) < 2 Years | > 2 Years | Cytogenetic Associations | Clinical Features |
|---|---|---|---|---|---|
| M0 | Acute myeloid leukemia, minimally-differentiated | | 1% | inv (3q26), t(3;3) | |
| M1 | Acute myeloblastic leukemia without maturation | 17% | 23% | | |
| M2 | Acute myeloblastic leukemia with maturation | | 26% | t(8;21) t(6;9); rare | Myeloblastomas or chloromas |
| M3 | Acute promyelocytic leukemia | | 4% | t(15;17); rarely, t(11;17) or (5;17) | Disseminated intravascular coagulation |
| M4 | Acute myelomonoblastic leukemia | 30% | 24% | 11q23, inv 3, t(3;3), t(6;9) | Hyperleukocytosis, CNS involvement, skin and gum infiltration |
| M4Eo | Acute myelomonoblastic leukemia with abnormal eosinophils | | | inv16, t(16;16) | |
| M5 | Acute monoblastic leukemia | 46% | 15% | 11q23, t(9;11), t(8;16) | Hyperleukocytosis, CNS involvement, skin and gum infiltration |
| M6 | Erythroleukemia | | 2% | | |
| M7 | Acute megakaryoblastic leukemia | 7% | 5% | t(1;22) | Down syndrome frequent (< 2 years of age) |

FAB = French–American–British classification; CNS = central nervous system.

Current AML protocols rely on intensive administration of anthracyclines, cytarabine, dexamethasone, 6-thiogunine, and etoposide for induction of remission. Studies have shown that intensively timed multiagent induction therapy results in significant improvement in outcome compared with standard timing for non-Down syndrome patients with AML. After remission is obtained those patients who have a matched sibling donor undergo allogeneic hematopoietic stem cell (HSC) transplantation while those patients without an appropriate related donor are treated with additional cycles of aggressive chemotherapy.

The biologic heterogeneity of AML is becoming increasingly important therapeutically. The M3 subtype, associated with t(15;17) demonstrated either cytogenetically or molecularly, is currently treated with all *trans*-retinoic acid (ATRA) in addition to chemotherapy with high-dose cytarabine and daunorubicin. ATRA leads to differentiation of promyelocytic leukemia cells and can induce remission, but cure requires conventional chemotherapy as well. The use of arsenic trioxide has also been investigated in the treatment of this subtype of AML with favorable results.

Another biologically distinct subtype of AML occurs in children with Down syndrome (DS), M7, or megakaryocytic AML.

Using less intensive treatment, remission induction rate and overall survival of these children are dramatically superior to non-DS children with AML. It are important that children with DS receive appropriate treatment specifically designed to be less intensive. Biologic agents are increasingly being studied in the treatment of AML. COG continues to collect data from a recent trial using interleukin-2 to stimulate the immune system against residual leukemia cells. The development and early success of antibody-targeted cytotoxic agents such as gemtuzumab ozogamicin (Mylotarg, a humanized anti-CD33 monoclonal antibody conjugated with calicheamicin) are encouraging in the quest for therapeutic agents that result in higher survival rates.

**B. Supportive Care**

Tumor lysis syndrome rarely occurs during induction treatment of AML, as opposed to high-risk ALL. Nevertheless, when the diagnostic WBC cell count is greater than 100,000 or significant adenopathy or organomegaly is present, one should alkalinize urine with intravenous sodium bicarbonate, maintain brisk urine output, and follow potassium, uric acid, and phosphorous lab values closely. Hyperleukocytosis (WBC > 100,000/µL) is a medical emergency and, in a symptomatic patient, requires rapid intervention such as leukapheresis to rapidly decrease the number of circulating blasts and thereby decrease hyperviscosity. Delaying transfusion of packed RBCs until the WBC can be decreased to below 100,000/µL avoids exacerbating hyperviscosity. It is also important to correct the coagulopathy commonly associated with M3, M4, or M5 subtypes prior to beginning induction chemotherapy. As with the treatment of ALL, all blood products should be irradiated and leukodepleted; pneumocystis prophylaxis must be administered during treatment and for several weeks afterward; and patients not immune to varicella must receive VZIG within 72 hours of exposure and prompt treatment with intravenous acyclovir for active infection.

Onset of fever (temperature ≥ 38.3°C) or chills associated with neutropenia requires prompt assessment, blood cultures from each lumen of a central venous line, other cultures such as throat or urine as appropriate, and prompt initiation of broad-spectrum intravenous antibiotics. Infections in this population of patients can rapidly become life-threatening. Because of the high incidence of invasive fungal infections, there should be a low threshold for initiating antifungal therapy. Filgrastim (granulocyte–colony-stimulating factor) is commonly used to stimulate granulocyte recovery during the treatment of AML and results in shorter periods of neutropenia and hospitalization. It must be stressed that the supportive care for this group of patients is as important as the leukemia-directed therapy and that this treatment should be carried out only at a tertiary pediatric cancer center.

## Prognosis

Published results from various centers show a 50–60% survival rate at 5 years following first remission for those patients that do not have matched sibling HSC donors. Patients with matched sibling donors fare slightly better, with 5-year survival rates of 60–70% after allogeneic HSC transplantation.

As treatment becomes more sophisticated, outcome is increasingly related to the subtype of AML. Currently, AML with t(8;21), t(15;17), or in children with DS has the most favorable prognosis, with 65–75% long-term survival using modern treatments. The least favorable outcome occurs in AML with monosomy 7 or 5, 7q, 5q–, or 11q23 cytogenetic abnormalities.

Alonzo TA et al: Impact of granulocyte colony-stimulating factor use during induction for acute myelogenous leukemia in chil-

dren: A report from the Children's Cancer Group. J Pediatr Hematol/Oncol 2002;24:627 [PMID: 12439034].

Sievers et al: Efficacy and safety of gemtuzumab ozogamicin in patients with CD33-positive acute myeloid leukemia in first relapse. J Clin Oncol 2001;19:3244 [PMID: 11432892].

Soignet SL et al: United States multicenter study of arsenic trioxide in relapsed acute promyelocytic leukemia. J Clin Oncol 2001;19:3852 [PMID: 11559723].

Vardiman JW et al: The World Health Organization (WHO) classification of the myeloid neoplasms. Blood 2002; 100:2292 [PMID: 12239137].

Woods WG et al: A comparison of allogeneic bone marrow transplantation, autologous bone marrow transplantation, and aggressive chemotherapy in children with acute myeloid leukemia in remission: A report from the Children's Cancer Group. Blood 2001;97:56 [PMID: 11133742].

# MYELOPROLIFERATIVE DISEASES

 **ESSENTIALS OF DIAGNOSIS & TYPICAL FEATURES**

- *Leukocytosis with predominance of immature cells.*
- *Often indolent course.*
- *Fever, bone pain, respiratory symptoms.*
- *Hepatosplenomegaly*

Myeloproliferative diseases in children are relatively rare. They are characterized by ineffective hematopoiesis that results in excessive peripheral blood counts. The three most important types are chronic myelogenous leukemia (CML), which accounts for less than 5% of the childhood leukemias, transient myeloproliferative disorder (TMD) in children with Down syndrome, and juvenile myelomonocytic leukemia (Table 28–2).

## 1. Chronic Myelogenous Leukemia

### General Considerations

CML with translocation of chromosomes 9 and 22 (the Philadelphia chromosome, Ph⁺) is identical to adult Ph⁺ CML. Translocation 9;22 results in the fusion of the *BCR* gene on chromosome 22 and the *ABL* gene on chromosome 9. The resulting fusion protein is a constitutively active tyrosine kinase that interacts with a variety of effector proteins and allows for deregulated cellular proliferation, decreased adherence of cells to the bone marrow extracellular matrix, and resistance to apoptosis. The disease usually progresses within 3 years to an accelerated phase and then to a blast crisis. It is generally accepted that Ph⁺ cells have an increased sus-

*Table 28–2.* Comparison of JMML, CML, and TMD

| | JMML | CML | TMD |
|---|---|---|---|
| Age at onset | <2 years old | >3 years old | <3 months old |
| Clinical presentation | Abrupt onset; exzematoid skin rash, marked lymphadeno-pathy, bleeding tendency, moderate hepatospleno-megaly, fever | Nonspecific constitutional complaints, massive spleno-megaly, variable hepato-megaly | DS features, often no or few symp-toms; or hepatosplenomegaly, res-piratory symptoms |
| Chromosomal alterations | Monosomy or del (7q) in 20% of patients | t(9;22) | Constitutional trisomy 21, but usu-ally no other abnormality |
| Laboratory features | Moderate leukocytosis (>10,000/µL), thrombocyto-penia, monocytosis (>1000/µL), elevated fetal hemoglobin, normal to dimin-ished leukocyte alkaline phosphatase, elevated muramidase | Marked leukocytosis (>100,000/µL), normal to elevated platelet count, de-creased to absent leukocyte alkaline phosphatase, usually normal muramidase | Variable leukocytosis, normal to high platelet count, large platelets, myeloblasts |

JMML = juvenile myelomonocytic leukemia; CML = chronic myelogenous leukemia; TMD = transient myeloproliferative disorder; DS = Down syndrome

ceptibility to the acquisition of additional molecular changes that lead to the accelerated and blast phases of disease.

## Clinical and Laboratory Findings

Patients with CML may present with nonspecific com-plaints similar to those of acute leukemia, including bone pain, fever, night sweats, and fatigue. Those pa-tients with a total WBC count of >100,000/µL may have symptoms of leukostasis, such as dyspnea, pri-apism, or neurologic abnormalities. Physical findings may include fever, pallor, ecchymoses, and he-patosplenomegaly. Anemia, thrombocytosis, and leuko-cytosis are frequent laboratory findings. The peripheral smear is usually diagnostic with a characteristic pre-dominance of myeloid cells in all stages of maturation and relatively few blasts.

## Treatment and Prognosis

Historically, hydroxyurea or busulfan has been used to reduce or eliminate Ph+ cells. However, HSC transplan-tation is the only consistently curative intervention. Re-ported survival rates for patients younger than age 20 years transplanted in the chronic phase from matched related donors are 70–80%. Unrelated stem cell transplants result in survival rates of 50–65%.

The understanding of the molecular mechanisms in-volved in the pathogenesis of CML has led to the ratio-nal design of molecularly targeted therapy. Imatinib mesylate (Gleevec) is a tyrosine kinase inhibitor that has had dramatic success in the treatment of CML, with most adults achieving cytogenetic remission. However, some patients are resistant to imatinib, and its role in the long-term management of children with CML awaits further studies.

## 2. Transient Myeloproliferative Disorder

### General Considerations

TMD is unique to patients with trisomy 21 or mo-saicism for trisomy 21. It is characterized by uncon-trolled proliferation of blasts, usually of megakaryocytic origin, during early infancy and spontaneous resolu-tion. The pathogenesis of this process is not well under-stood, although mutations in the *GATA1* gene have re-cently been implicated as initial events.

Although the true incidence is unknown, it is esti-mated to occur in up to 10% of patients with Down syndrome. Despite the fact that the process usually re-solves by 3 months of age, organ infiltration may cause significant morbidity and mortality.

### Clinical Findings, Treatment, and Prognosis

Patients can present with hydrops fetalis, pericardial or pleural effusions, or hepatic fibrosis. More frequently, they are asymptomatic or only minimally ill. Therefore, treatment is primarily supportive. Patients without symptoms are not treated, and those with organ dysfunction receive low doses of chemotherapy or leukopheresis (or both) to reduce peripheral blood blast counts. Although patients with TMD have apparent resolution of the process, approximately 30% go on to develop acute megakaryoblastic leukemia (AML M7) within 3 years.

## 3. Juvenile Myelomonocytic Leukemia

### Clinical and Laboratory Findings

Juvenile myelomonocytic leukemia (JMML), accounts for approximately one third of the myelodysplastic and myeloproliferative disorders in childhood. Patients with neurofibromatosis type 1 (NF-1) are at higher risk of JMML than the general population. It typically occurs in infants and very young children and is occasionally associated with monosomy 7 or a deletion of the long arm of chromosome 7.

### Clinical Findings, Treatment, and Prognosis

JMML patients present similarly to those with other hematopoietic malignancies, with lymphadenopathy, hepatosplenomegaly, skin rash, or respiratory symptoms. Patients may have stigmata of NF-1 with neurofibromas or café au lait spots. Laboratory findings include anemia, thrombocytopenia, leukocytosis with monocytosis, and elevated fetal hemoglobin.

The results of chemotherapy for children with JMML have been disappointing, with estimated survival rates of less than 30%. Approximately 40–45% of patients are projected to survive long term using HSC transplantation, although optimizing conditioning regimens and donor selection may improve these results.

Cwynarski K et al: Stem cell transplantation for chronic myeloid leukemia in children. Blood 2003;102:1224 [PMID: 12714525].

Goldman JM, Melo JV: Chronic myeloid leukemia—Advances in biology and new approaches to treatment. N Engl J Med 2003;349:1451 [PMID: 14534339].

Kantarjian H et al: Hematologic and cytogenetic responses to imatinib mesylate in chronic myelogenous leukemia. N Engl J Med 2002;346:645 [PMID: 11870241].

Maguire AM et al: Allogeneic bone marrow transplant improves outcome for juvenile myelomoncytic leukaemia. J Pediatr Child Health 2002;38:166 [PMID: 12030999].

Mundschau G et al: Mutagenesis of GATA1 is an initiating event in Down syndrome leukemogenesis. Blood 2003;101:4298 [PMID: 12560215].

Thornley I et al: Treating children with chronic myeloid leukemia in the imatinib era: A therapeutic dilemma? Med Pediatr Oncol 2003;41:115 [PMID: 12825214].

Woods WG et al: Prospective study of 90 children requiring treatment for juvenile myelomonocytic leukemia or myelodysplastic syndrome: A report from the Children's Cancer Group. J Clin Oncol 2002;20:434 [PMID: 11786571].

## BRAIN TUMORS

### ESSENTIALS OF DIAGNOSIS & TYPICAL FEATURES

- *Classic triad: morning headache, vomiting, and papilledema.*
- *Increasing head circumference, cranial nerve palsies, dysarthria, ataxia, hemiplegia, papilledema, hyperreflexia, macrocephaly, cracked pot sign.*
- *Seizures, personality change, blurred vision, diplopia, weakness, decreased coordination, precocious puberty.*

### General Considerations

The classic triad of morning headache, vomiting, and papilledema is present in less than 30% of children at presentation. School failure and personality changes are common in older children. Irritability, failure to thrive, and delayed development are common in very young children with brain tumors. Recent-onset head tilt can result from a posterior fossa tumor.

Brain tumors are the most common solid tumors of childhood, accounting for 1500–2000 new malignancies in children each year in the United States and for 25–30% of all childhood cancers. In general, children with brain tumors have a better prognosis than do adults. Favorable outcome occurs most commonly with low-grade and fully resectable tumors. Unfortunately, cranial irradiation in young children can have significant neuropsychological, intellectual, and endocrinologic sequelae.

Brain tumors in childhood are biologically and histologically heterogeneous, ranging from low-grade localized lesions to high-grade tumors with neuraxis dissemination. High-dose systemic chemotherapy is being used more frequently, especially in young children with high-grade tumors, in an effort to delay, decrease, or completely avoid cranial irradiation. Such intensive treatment may be accompanied by autologous HSCT or peripheral stem cell reconstitution.

The causes of pediatric brain tumors are unknown. The risk of developing astrocytomas is increased in children with neurofibromatosis or tuberous sclerosis. Several studies show that some childhood brain tumors occur in families with increased genetic susceptibility to childhood cancers in general, brain tumors, or leukemia and lymphoma. An excess of seizures has been observed in relatives of children with astrocytoma. Certain pediatric brain tumors such as ependymoma have been linked to polyomavirus, but the exact relationship is unknown. The risk of developing a brain tumor is increased in children who received cranial irradiation for treatment of meningeal leukemia.

Because pediatric brain tumors are rare, they are often misdiagnosed or diagnosed late; most pediatricians see no more than two children with brain tumors during their careers.

## Clinical Findings

### A. Symptoms and Signs

Clinical findings at presentation vary depending on the child's age and the tumor's location. Children younger than age 2 years more commonly have infratentorial tumors. Children with such tumors usually present with nonspecific symptoms such as vomiting, unsteadiness, lethargy, and irritability. Signs may be surprisingly few or may include macrocephaly, ataxia, hyperreflexia, and cranial nerve palsies. Because the head can expand in young children, papilledema is usually absent. Measuring head circumference and observing gait are essential in evaluating a child for possible brain tumor. Eye findings and apparent visual disturbances such as difficulty tracking can occur in association with optic pathway tumors such as optic glioma. Optic glioma occurring in a young child is often associated with neurofibromatosis.

Older children more commonly have supratentorial tumors, which are associated with headache, visual symptoms, seizures, and focal neurologic deficits. Initial presenting features are often nonspecific. School failure and personality changes are common. Vaguely described visual disturbance is often present, but the child must be directly asked. Headaches are common, but they often will not be predominantly in the morning. The headaches may be confused with migraine.

Older children with infratentorial tumors characteristically present with symptoms and signs of hydrocephalus, which include progressively worsening morning headache and vomiting, gait unsteadiness, double vision, and papilledema. Cerebellar astrocytomas enlarge slowly, and symptoms may worsen over several months. Morning vomiting may be the only symptom of posterior fossa ependymomas, which originate in the floor of the fourth ventricle near the vomiting center. Children with brainstem tumors may present with facial and extraocular muscle palsies, ataxia, and hemiparesis; hydrocephalus occurs in approximately 25% of these patients at diagnosis.

### B. Imaging and Staging

In addition to the tumor biopsy, neuraxis imaging studies are obtained to determine whether dissemination has occurred. It is unusual for brain tumors in children and adolescents to disseminate outside of the CNS.

Magnetic resonance imaging (MRI) has become the preferred diagnostic study for pediatric brain tumors. MRI provides better definition of the tumor and delineates indolent gliomas that may not be seen on computed tomography (CT) scan. In contrast, a CT scan can be done in less than 10 minutes—as opposed to the 30 minutes required for an MRI scan—and is still useful if an urgent diagnostic study is necessary or to detect calcification of a tumor. Both scans are generally done with and without contrast enhancement. Contrast enhances regions where the blood–brain barrier is disrupted. Postoperative scans to document the extent of tumor resection should be obtained within 48 hours after surgery to avoid postsurgical enhancement.

Imaging of the entire neuraxis and CSF cytologic examination should be part of the diagnostic evaluation for patients with tumors such as medulloblastoma, ependymoma, and pineal region tumors. Diagnosis of neuraxis drop metastases (tumor spread along the neuraxis) can be accomplished by gadolinium-enhanced MRI incorporating sagittal and axial views. MRI of the spine should be obtained preoperatively in all children with midline tumors of the fourth ventricle or cerebellum. A CSF sample should be obtained during the diagnostic surgery. Lumbar CSF is preferred over ventricular CSF for cytologic examination. Levels of biomarkers in the blood and CSF, such as human chorionic gonadotropin (HCG) and α-fetoprotein (AFP), may be helpful at diagnosis and in follow-up. HCG and AFP should be obtained from the blood preoperatively for all pineal and suprasellar tumors.

The neurosurgeon should discuss staging and sample collection with an oncologist before surgery in a child newly presenting with a scan suggestive of brain tumor.

### C. Classification

About 50% of the common pediatric brain tumors occur above the tentorium and 50% in the posterior fossa. In the very young child, posterior fossa tumors are more common. Most childhood brain tumors can be divided into two categories according to the cell of origin: (1) glial tumors such as astrocytomas and ependymomas or (2) nonglial tumors such as medulloblastoma and other primitive neuroectodermal tumors. Some tumors contain both glial and neural elements (eg, ganglioglioma). A group of less common CNS tumors do not fit into either category (ie, craniopharyngiomas, germ cell tumors, choroid plexus tumors, and meningiomas). Low-grade and high-grade tumors are found in most categories. Table 28–3 lists the locations and frequencies of the common pediatric brain tumors.

Astrocytoma is the most common brain tumor of childhood. Most are low-grade tumors found in the posterior fossa with a bland cellular morphology and few or no mitotic figures. Low-grade astrocytomas are in many cases curable by complete surgical excision alone. Chemotherapy is effective in low-grade astrocytomas.

Medulloblastoma and related primitive neuroectodermal tumors are the most common high-grade brain tumors in children. These tumors usually occur in the first decade of life, with a peak incidence between ages 5 and 10 years and a female-to-male ratio of 2.1:1.3. These tumors typically arise in the midline cerebellar vermis, with variable extension into the fourth ventricle. Reports of neuraxis dissemination at diagnosis range from 10% to 46% of patients. Prognostic factors are outlined in Table 28–4.

Brainstem tumors are third in frequency of occurrence in children. They are frequently of astrocytic origin and often are high-grade. Children with tumors that diffusely infiltrate the brainstem and involve primarily the pons have a long-term survival rate of less than 15%. Brainstem tumors that occur above or below the pons and grow in an eccentric or cystic manner

**Table 28–3.** Location and frequency of common pediatric brain tumors.

| Location | Frequency of Occurrence (%) |
|---|---|
| **Hemispheric** | **37** |
| Low-grade astrocytoma | 23 |
| High-grade astrocytoma | 11 |
| Other | 3 |
| **Posterior fossa** | **49** |
| Medulloblastoma | 15 |
| Cerebellar astrocytoma | 15 |
| Brainstem glioma | 15 |
| Ependymoma | 4 |
| **Midline** | **14** |
| Craniopharyngioma | 8 |
| Chiasmal glioma | 4 |
| Pineal region tumor | 2 |

**Table 28–4.** Prognostic factors in children with medulloblastoma.

| Factor | Favorable | Unfavorable |
|---|---|---|
| Extent of disease | Nondisseminated | Disseminated |
| Size of primary tumor after surgery | ≤ 3 cm (completely resected) | > 3 cm |
| Histologic features | Undifferentiated | Foci of glial, ependymal, or neuronal differentiation |
| Age | ≥ 4 years | < 4 years |

have a somewhat better outcome. Exophytic tumors in this location may be amenable to surgery. Generally, brainstem tumors are treated without a tissue diagnosis.

Other brain tumors such as ependymomas, germ cell tumors, choroid plexus tumors, and craniopharyngiomas are less common, and each is associated with unique diagnostic and therapeutic challenges.

## Treatment

### A. SUPPORTIVE CARE

Dexamethasone should be started prior to initial surgery (0.5–1 mg/kg initially, then 0.25–0.5 mg/kg/d in four divided doses). Anticonvulsants (usually phenytoin, 4–8 mg/kg/d) should be started if the child has had a seizure or if the surgical approach is likely to induce seizures. Because postoperative treatment of young children with high-grade brain tumors incorporates increasingly more intensive systemic chemotherapy, consideration should also be given to the use of prophylaxis for prevention of oral candidiasis and *Pneumocystis* infection. Dexamethasone and phenytoin potentially reduce the effectiveness of chemotherapy and should be discontinued as soon after surgery as possible.

Optimum care for the pediatric patient with a brain tumor requires a multidisciplinary team including subspecialists in pediatric neurosurgery, neuro-oncology, neurology, endocrinology, neuropsychology, radiation therapy, and rehabilitation medicine, as well as highly specialized nurses, social workers, and staff in physical therapy, occupational therapy, and speech and language science.

### B. SPECIFIC THERAPY

The goal of treatment is to eradicate the tumor with the least short- and long-term morbidity. Long-term neuropsychological morbidity becomes an especially important issue related to deficits caused by the tumor itself and the sequelae of treatment. Meticulous surgical removal of as much tumor as possible is generally the preferred initial approach. Technologic advances in the operating microscope, the ultrasonic tissue aspirator, and the $CO_2$ laser (which is less commonly used in pediatric brain tumor surgery); the accuracy of computerized stereotactic resection; and the availability of intraoperative monitoring techniques such as evoked potentials and electrocorticography have increased the feasibility and safety of surgical resection of many pediatric brain tumors. Second-look surgery after chemotherapy is increasingly being used when tumors are incompletely resected at initial surgery.

Radiation therapy for pediatric brain tumors is in a state of evolution. For tumors with a high probability of neuraxis dissemination (eg, medulloblastoma), craniospinal radiation is still standard therapy in children older than age 3 years. In others (eg, ependymoma), craniospinal radiation has been abandoned because neuraxis dissemination at first relapse is rare. Approaches to the delivery of radiation to minimize the adverse effects on normal brain tissue are being explored and include stereotactic radiation and the use of three-dimensional treatment planning.

Chemotherapy is effective in treating low-grade and malignant astrocytomas and medulloblastomas. A series of brain tumor protocols for children younger than age 3 years involved administering intensive chemotherapy after tumor resection and delaying or omitting radiation therapy. The results of these trials have generally been disappointing but have taught valuable lessons regarding the varying responses to chemotherapy of different tumor types. Future trials may give shorter courses of more intense chemotherapy followed by conformal radiotherapy. Conformal techniques allow the delivery of radiation to strictly defined fields and may limit side effects.

In older children with malignant glioma, the current approach would be surgical resection of the tumor and combined-modality treatment with irradiation and intensive chemotherapy. In patients with glioblastoma, the use of high-dose chemotherapy and autologous bone marrow or peripheral stem cell reconstitution is being studied. Initial results are promising, but the toxicity of such therapy remains a concern. Surgery is not indicated for diffuse brainstem gliomas. Traditional treatment of these tumors has been local irradiation. Hyperfractionation to increase the dose from the conventional 54 Gy to 72–78 Gy showed no apparent benefit in a recent CCG study. New approaches are needed for this prognostically poor tumor.

The treatment of low-grade astrocytomas is evolving. Increasing numbers of young children are receiving antitumor chemotherapeutic agents such as carboplatin and vincristine after incomplete resection of these tumors.

The role of irradiation after subtotal resection even in older children is being questioned. A CCG study is currently evaluating two different chemotherapy regimens in the treatment of progressive low-grade astrocytomas.

## Prognosis

Despite improvements in surgery and radiation therapy, the outlook for cure remains poor for children with high-grade glial tumors. For children with high-grade gliomas, an early CCG study showed a 45% progression-free survival rate for children who received radiation therapy and chemotherapy. A follow-up CCG study in which all patients had chemotherapy and radiation therapy showed a 5-year progression-free survival rate of 36%. There is a possibility of effective salvage therapy with high-dose chemotherapy for children who relapse. In addition, the extent of resection appeared to correlate positively with prognosis, with a 3-year progression-free survival rate of 17% for patients receiving biopsy only, 29–32% for patients receiving partial or subtotal resections, and 54% for those receiving 90% resections. Biologic factors that may affect survival are being increasingly recognized. The prognosis for diffuse pontine gliomas remains very poor, with no benefit from high-dose chemotherapy plus radiation versus radiation alone.

The 5- and even 10-year survival rate for low-grade astrocytomas of childhood is 60–90%. However, prognosis depends on both site and grade. A child with a pilocytic astrocytoma of the cerebellum has a considerably better prognosis than a child with a fibrillary astrocytoma of the cerebral cortex. For recurrent or progressive low-grade astrocytoma of childhood, relatively moderate chemotherapy may improve the likelihood of survival.

Conventional craniospinal irradiation for children with low-stage medulloblastoma results in survival rates of 60–90%. Ten-year survival rates are lower (40–60%). Chemotherapy allows a reduction in the craniospinal radiation dose while preserving survival rates for average-risk patients. However, even reduced-dose craniospinal radiation has an adverse effect on intellect, especially in children younger than 7 years of age. Five-year survival rates for high-risk medulloblastoma have been 25–40%, but recent trials suggest a dramatically improved prognosis for patients receiving intensive chemotherapy and radiation. Children with supratentorial primitive neuroectodermal tumors also benefit from the addition of chemotherapy to craniospinal radiation.

Major challenges remain in treating brain tumors in children younger than age 3 years and in treating brainstem gliomas and malignant gliomas. The increasing emphasis is on the quality of life of survivors, not just the survival rate.

Duffner PK et al: The treatment of malignant brain tumors in infants and very young children: An update of the pediatric oncology group experience. Neuro-Oncol 1999;1:152.

Merchant TE et al: Preliminary results from a Phase II trail of conformal radiation therapy for pediatric patients with localised low-grade astrocytoma and ependymoma. Int J Radiat Oncol Phys 2002;52:325.

Packer RJ et al: Long-term neurologic and neurosensory sequelae in adult survivors of a childhood brain tumor: Childhood cancer survivor study. J Clin Oncol 2003;21:3255.

Pollack IF et al: Association between chromosome 1p and 19q loss and outcome in pediatric malignant gliomas: Results from the CCG-945 cohort. Pediatr Neurosurg 2003;39:114.

# LYMPHOMAS AND LYMPHOPROLIFERATIVE DISORDERS

The term "lymphoma" refers to a malignant proliferation of lymphoid cells, usually in association with and arising from lymphoid tissues (ie, lymph nodes, thymus, spleen). In contrast, the term "leukemia" refers to a malignancy arising from the bone marrow, which may include lymphoid cells. Because lymphomas can involve the bone marrow, the distinction between the two can be confusing. The diagnosis of lymphoma is a common one among childhood cancers, accounting for 10–15% of all malignancies. The most common form is Hodgkin disease, which represents nearly half of all cases. The remaining subtypes, referred to collectively as non-Hodgkin lymphoma, are divided into four main groups: lymphoblastic, small non–cleaved-cell, large B-cell, and anaplastic large cell lymphomas.

In contrast to lymphomas, lymphoproliferative disorders (LPDs) are quite rare in the general population. Most are polyclonal, nonmalignant (though often life-threatening) accumulations of lymphocytes that occur when the immune system fails to control virally transformed lymphocytes. However, a malignant monoclonal proliferation can also arise. The transplant-associated LPDs arise in patients immunosuppressed to prevent solid organ or bone marrow transplant rejection. In highly selected populations, including liver and heart transplant patients, these disorders are a significant problem. Spontaneous LPDs occur in immunodeficient individuals and, less commonly, in immunocompetent persons.

## 1. Hodgkin Disease

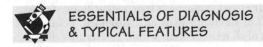

### ESSENTIALS OF DIAGNOSIS & TYPICAL FEATURES

- *Painless cervical (70–80%) or supraclavicular (25%) adenopathy; mediastinal mass (50%).*

- *Fatigue, anorexia, weight loss, fever, night sweats, pruritus, cough.*

## General Considerations

Children with Hodgkin disease have a better response to treatment than do adults, with a 75% overall survival rate at more than 20 years following diagnosis. Although adult therapies are applicable, the management of Hodgkin disease in children younger than age 18 years frequently differs. Because excellent disease control can result from several different therapeutic approaches, selection of staging procedures [radiographic, surgical, or other procedures to determine additional location(s) of disease] and treatment are often based on the potential long-term toxicity associated with the intervention.

Although Hodgkin disease represents 50% of the lymphomas of childhood, only 15% of all cases occur in children age 16 years or younger. Children younger than age 5 years account for 3% of childhood cases, whereas 60% of cases occur in the 10- to 16-year age group. There is a 4:1 male predominance in the first decade. Notably, in underdeveloped countries the age distribution is quite different, with a peak incidence in younger children.

Hodgkin disease is subdivided into four histologic groups, and the distribution in children parallels that of adults: lymphocyte-predominant (10–20%); nodular sclerosing (40–60%) (increases with age); mixed cellularity (20–40%); and lymphocyte-depleted (5–10%). Prognosis is independent of subclassification, with appropriate therapy based on stage (see Staging section).

## Clinical Findings

### A. SYMPTOMS AND SIGNS

Children with Hodgkin disease usually present with painless cervical adenopathy. The lymph nodes often feel firmer than inflammatory nodes and have a rubbery texture. They may be discrete or matted together and are not fixed to surrounding tissue. The growth rate is variable, and involved nodes may wax and wane in size over weeks to months.

As Hodgkin disease nearly always arises in lymph nodes and spreads to contiguous nodal groups, a detailed examination of all nodal sites is mandatory. Lymphadenopathy is common in children, so the decision to perform biopsy is often difficult or delayed for a prolonged period. Indications for consideration of early lymph node biopsy include lack of identifiable infection in the region drained by the enlarged node, a node greater than 2 cm in size, supraclavicular adenopathy or abnormal chest radiograph, and lymphadenopathy increasing in size after 2 weeks or failing to resolve within 4–8 weeks.

Constitutional symptoms occur in about one third of children at presentation. Symptoms of fever greater than 38°C, weight loss of 10%, and drenching night sweats are defined by the Ann Arbor staging criteria as B symptoms. The A designation refers to the absence of these symptoms. B symptoms are of prognostic value, and more aggressive therapy is usually required for cure. Generalized pruritus and pain with alcohol ingestion may also occur.

Half of patients have asymptomatic mediastinal disease (adenopathy or anterior mediastinal mass), although symptoms due to compression of vital structures in the thorax may occur. A chest radiograph should be obtained when lymphoma is being considered. The mediastinum must be evaluated thoroughly before any surgical procedure is undertaken to avoid airway obstruction or cardiovascular collapse during anesthesia and possible death. Splenomegaly or hepatomegaly is generally associated with advanced disease.

### B. LABORATORY FINDINGS

The CBC is usually normal, although anemia, neutrophilia, eosinophilia, and thrombocytosis may be present. The erythrocyte sedimentation rate and other acute-phase reactants are often elevated and can serve as markers of disease activity. Immunologic abnormalities occur, particularly in cell-mediated immunity, and anergy is common in advanced-stage disease at diagnosis. Autoantibody phenomena such as hemolytic anemia and an idiopathic thrombocytopenic purpura-like picture have been reported.

### C. STAGING

Staging of Hodgkin disease determines treatment and prognosis. The most common staging system is the Ann Arbor classification that describes extent of disease by I–IV and symptoms by an A or a B suffix (eg, stage IIIB). A systematic search for thoracic disease includes chest radiography and CT scan. Assessment of abdominal and pelvic disease is usually accomplished by CT scan. Bilateral bone marrow aspirates and biopsies are performed. Technetium bone scanning may show bony involvement and is usually reserved for patients with bone pain, as bone involvement is rare. Gallium scanning defines gallium-avid tumors and is most useful in evaluating residual mediastinal disease at the completion of treatment. Positron emission tomography is increasingly used in the staging and follow-up of patients with Hodgkin disease.

The staging laparotomy in pediatrics is rarely performed because almost all patients are given systemic chemotherapy rather than radiation. Although excellent disease control with radiation therapy can be achieved in laparotomy-staged children, this option must be weighed against the toxicities of high-dose, extended-field radiation in prepubertal children and the complications of laparotomy, including postsplenectomy sepsis. Reports linking splenectomy with secondary acute myelogenous leukemia following Hodgkin disease therapy are particularly disturbing.

### D. PATHOLOGY

The diagnosis of Hodgkin disease requires the presence of the Reed–Sternberg cell or its variants in tissue. When Reed–Sternberg cells are scanty the diagnosis becomes difficult. Reed–Sternberg cells are germinal-center B cells that have undergone malignant transformation. The molecular biology of Reed–Sternberg cell malignant transformation still remains to be elucidated, although it is interesting to note that nearly 20% of these tumors in developed countries are positive for EBV.

## Treatment & Prognosis

To achieve long-term disease-free survival while minimizing treatment toxicity, Hodgkin disease is increasingly treated by chemotherapy even in stage I and stage II disease—and less often by radiation therapy.

Several combinations of chemotherapeutic agents are effective, but the most commonly used are MOPP (mechlorethamine, vincristine, procarbazine, and prednisone) and ABVD (adriamycin [doxorubicin], bleomycin, vinblastine, and dacarbazine). These regimens are non–cross-resistant. When these schedules are alternated, exposure to an individual drug is decreased, and the toxicities associated with cumulative doses are minimized. The combination of cyclophosphamide, cytarabine, and etoposide is also being used increasingly.

Although risk-adapted chemotherapy alone is very effective in achieving cure, radiation continues to play a role in the treatment of childhood Hodgkin disease, because combined-modality therapy may increase the cure rate. The use of radiation therapy at the end of risk-adapted chemotherapy when no residual disease is present appears to improve short-term, event-free survival, but its benefit for long-term survival remains to be demonstrated.

Current treatment gives children with stage I and stage II Hodgkin disease at least a 90% disease-free likelihood of survival 5 years after diagnosis. Because two thirds of all relapses occur within 2 years after diagnosis and because relapse rarely occurs beyond 4 years, 5-year disease-free survival generally equates with cure. In more advanced disease (stage III and stage IV), 5-year event-free survival rates range from over 60% to 90%. With more patients being long-term survivors of Hodgkin disease, the risk of secondary malignancies, both leukemias and solid tumors, is becoming more apparent. The type of tumor depends on the treatments employed, but the risk is clearly greatest among those who are younger at diagnosis. Therefore, elucidating the optimal treatment strategy that minimizes such risk should be the goal of future studies.

Treatment of relapsed Hodgkin disease is usually successful and involves radiation therapy in combination with chemotherapy. An alternative is autologous or allogeneic hematopoietic stem cell transplant, which may improve survival rates.

Foss Abrahamsen A et al: Long-term risk of second malignancy after treatment of Hodgkin's disease: The influence of treatment, age and follow-up time. Ann Oncol 2002;13:1786 [PMID: 12419752].

Guay C et al: Prognostic value of PET using 18F-FDG in Hodgkin's disease for posttreatment evaluation. J Nucl Med 2003;44:1225 [PMID: 12902411].

Nachman JB et al: Randomized comparison of low-dose involved-field radiotherapy and no radiotherapy for children with Hodgkin's disease who achieve a complete response to chemotherapy. J Clin Oncol 2002;20:3765 [PMID: 12228196].

Sureda A et al: Autologous stem-cell transplantation for Hodgkin's disease: Results and prognostic factors in 494 patients from the Grupo Español de Linfomas Transplante Autologo de Médula Ósea Spanish Cooperative Group. J Clin Oncol 2001;19:1395 [PMID: 11230484].

## 2. Non-Hodgkin Lymphoma

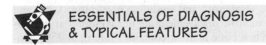

### ESSENTIALS OF DIAGNOSIS & TYPICAL FEATURES

- *Cough, dyspnea, orthopnea, swelling of the face, lymphadenopathy, mediastinal mass, pleural effusion.*
- *Abdominal pain, abdominal distention, vomiting, constipation, abdominal mass, ascites, hepatosplenomegaly.*
- *Adenopathy, fevers, neurologic deficit, skin lesions.*

### General Considerations

Non-Hodgkin lymphomas (NHLs) are a diverse group of cancers accounting for 5–10% of malignancies in children younger than age 15 years (about 500 new cases arise per year in the United States). The incidence of NHLs increases with age. Children age 15 years or younger account for only 3% of all cases of NHLs; it is uncommon before age 5 years. There is a male predominance of approximately 3:1. In equatorial Africa, NHLs cause almost 50% of pediatric malignancies.

Children with congenital or acquired immune deficiencies (eg, Wiskott–Aldrich syndrome, severe combined immunodeficiency syndrome, X-linked lymphoproliferative syndrome, HIV infection, immunosuppressive therapy following solid organ or marrow transplantation) have an increased risk of developing NHLs. It has been estimated that their risk is 100–10,000 times that of age-matched control subjects.

However, most children who develop NHL are immunologically normal. Animal models suggest a viral contribution to the pathogenesis of NHL, and there is evidence of viral involvement in human NHL as well. In equatorial Africa, 95% of Burkitt lymphomas contain DNA from the Epstein–Barr virus. But in North America, less than 20% of Burkitt tumors contain the EBV genome. The role of other viruses, such as human herpesviruses 6 and 8, disturbances in host immunologic defenses, chronic immunostimulation, and specific chromosomal rearrangements, is under investigation as potential triggers in the development of NHL.

Unlike adult NHL, virtually all childhood NHLs are rapidly proliferating, high-grade, diffuse malignancies. These tumors exhibit aggressive behavior but are usually very responsive to treatment. Nearly all pediatric NHLs are histologically classified into four main groups: lymphoblastic lymphoma (LL), small non–cleaved-cell lymphoma (Burkitt lymphoma [BL] and Burkitt-like lymphoma [BLL]), large B-cell lymphoma (LBCL), and anaplastic large cell lymphoma (ALCL) (Table 28–5). Malignant lymphoma cells often retain morphologic or immunohistochemical features similar to those of the lymphoid lineage cell from which they are derived. Cell membrane markers determined by immunophenotyping can therefore help clarify the origins of these cancers and serve as an adjunct to histologic classification. Typically, LL is associated with T-cell surface markers, whereas BL and BLL have a B-cell phenotype such as surface immunoglobulins. LBCL seems to arise from cells of the germinal center of lymph nodes and express B-cell markers. ALCL usually has T-cell or null-cell markers.

Recurrent cytogenetic abnormalities can be diagnostic in NHL. Burkitt lymphomas usually carry a translocation involving chromosomes 8 and 14 (or a variant thereof) that juxtaposes a highly active immunoglobulin promoter with the c-*myc* gene. Deregulation of the protein expressed by this gene promotes cellular proliferation. An analogous translocation occurs in LL, in-

***Table 28–5.*** Comparison of pediatric non-Hodgkin lymphomas.

| | Lymphoblastic Lymphoma | Small Noncleaved Cell Lymphoma (BL and BLL) | Large B-Cell Lymphoma | Anaplastic Large Cell Lymphoma |
|---|---|---|---|---|
| Incidence (%) | 30–40 | 35–50 | 10–15 | 10–15 |
| Histopathologic features | Indistinguishable from ALL lymphoblasts | Large nucleus with prominent nucleoli surrounded by very basophilic cytoplasm that contains lipid vacuoles | Large cells with cleaved or non-cleaved nuclei | Large pleomorphic cells |
| Immunophenotype | Immature T cell | B cell | B cell | T cell or null cell |
| Cytogenetic markers | Translocations involving chromosome 14q11 and chromosome 7; interstitial deletions of chromosome 1 | t(8;14), t(8;22), t(2;8) | Many | t(2;5) |
| Clinical presentation | Intrathoracic tumor, mediastinal mass (50–70%), lymphadenopathy above diaphragm (50–80%) | Intra-abdominal tumor (90%), jaw involvement (10–20% sporadic BL, 70% endemic BL), bone marrow involvement | Abdominal tumor most common; unusual sites: lung, face, brain, bone, testes, muscle | Lymphadenopathy, fever, weight loss, night sweats, extranodal sites including viscera and skin |
| Treatment | Similar to ALL therapy; 24 mos duration | Intensive administration of alkylating agents and methotrexate; CNS prophylaxis; 3–9 mos duration | Similar to therapy for BL/BLL | Similar to therapy for lymphoblastic lymphoma or BL/BLL |

ALL = acute lymphoblastic leukemia; BL = Burkitt lymphoma; BLL = Burkitt-like lymphoma.

volving the T-cell receptor promoter and the *TAL1* gene. Another translocation occurs in ALCL [t(2;5)] that fuses the *NMP* gene (a transcription factor) to the *ALK* gene (a tyrosine kinase), thereby creating a new gene product.

## Clinical Findings

### A. Symptoms and Signs

Childhood NHLs can arise in any site of lymphoid tissue, including lymph nodes, the Waldeyer ring, Peyer patches, thymus, liver, and spleen. Common extralymphatic sites include bone, bone marrow, CNS, skin, and testes. Signs and symptoms at presentation are determined by the location of lesions and the degree of dissemination. Because NHL usually progresses very rapidly, the duration of symptoms is quite brief, from days to a few weeks. Nevertheless, children present with a limited number of syndromes, most of which correlate with cell type.

Children with LL often present with symptoms of airway compression (cough, dyspnea, orthopnea) or superior vena cava obstruction (facial edema, chemosis, plethora, venous engorgement), which are a result of mediastinal disease. *These symptoms are a true emergency necessitating rapid diagnosis and treatment.* Pleural or pericardia effusions may further compromise the patient's respiratory and cardiovascular status. CNS and bone marrow involvement are not common at diagnosis. When bone marrow contains more than 25% lymphoblasts, patients are considered to have ALL.

Most patients with BL and BLL present with abdominal disease. Abdominal pain, distention, a right lower quadrant mass, or intussusception in a child older than age 5 years suggests the diagnosis of BL. Bone marrow involvement is common (≤ 65% of patients). BL is the most rapidly proliferating tumor known and has a high rate of spontaneous cell death as it outgrows its blood supply. Consequently, children presenting with massive abdominal disease frequently have metabolic abnormalities (hyperuricemia, hyperphosphatemia, and hyperkalemia) due to tumor lysis. These abnormalities can be aggravated if tumor infiltration of the kidney, urinary obstruction by tumor, or urate nephropathy interferes with renal function. Although similar histologically, numerous differences exist between cases of BL occurring in endemic areas of equatorial Africa and the sporadic cases of North America (Table 28–6).

**Table 28–6.** Comparison of endemic and sporadic[a] Burkitt lymphoma.

|  | Endemic | Sporadic |
|---|---|---|
| Incidence | 10 per 100,000 | 0.9 per 100,000 |
| Cytogenetics | Chromosome 8 breakpoint upstream of c-myc locus | Chromosome 8 breakpoint within c-myc locus |
| EBV association | ≥ 95% | ≤ 20% |
| Disease sites at presentation | Jaw (58%), abdomen (58%), CNS (19%), orbit (11%), marrow (7%) | Jaw (7%), abdomen (91%), CNS (14%), orbit (1%), marrow (20%) |

[a]EBV = Epstein–Barr virus; CNS = central nervous system.

Large cell lymphomas are similar clinically to the small non–cleaved-cell lymphomas, although unusual sites of involvement are quite common, particularly with ALCL. Skin lesions, focal neurologic deficits, and pleural or peritoneal effusions without an obvious associated mass are frequently seen.

### B. Diagnostic Evaluation

Diagnosis is made by biopsy of involved tissue with histology, immunophenotyping, and cytogenetic studies. If mediastinal disease is present, general anesthesia must be avoided if the airway or vena cava is compromised by tumor. In these cases samples of pleural or ascitic fluid, bone marrow, or peripheral nodes obtained under local anesthesia may confirm the diagnosis. Major abdominal surgery and intestinal resection should be avoided in patients with an abdominal mass that is likely to be BL, as the tumor will regress rapidly with the initiation of chemotherapy. Following the diagnosis of NHLs, studies should be obtained to determine the extent of disease. The rapid growth of these tumors and the associated life-threatening complications demand that studies be done expeditiously so that specific therapy is not delayed.

After a thorough physical examination, a CBC, liver and renal function tests, and a biochemical profile (electrolytes, calcium, phosphorus, uric acid) should be obtained. LDH reflects tumor burden and can serve as a marker of disease activity. Imaging studies should include a chest radiograph and chest CT scan if the plain radiographs are abnormal, an abdominal ultrasound or CT scan, and possibly a gallium scan. Bone marrow and CSF examinations are also essential.

## Treatment

### A. Supportive Care

The management of life-threatening problems at presentation is critical. The most common complications are superior mediastinal syndrome and acute tumor lysis syndrome. Patients with airway compromise require prompt initiation of specific therapy. Because of the risk of general anesthesia in these patients, it is occasionally necessary to initiate steroids or low-dose radiation until the mass is small enough for a biopsy to be undertaken safely. Response to steroids and radiation is usually prompt (12–24 hours).

Tumor lysis syndrome should be anticipated in all patients who have NHL with a large tumor burden. Maintaining a brisk urine output (> 5 mL/kg/h) with intravenous fluids and diuretics is the key to management. Allopurinol will reduce serum uric acid, and alkalinization of urine will increase its solubility. Because phosphate precipitates in alkaline urine, alkali administration should be discontinued if hyperphosphatemia occurs. Renal dialysis is occasionally necessary to control metabolic abnormalities. Every attempt should be made to correct or minimize metabolic abnormalities before initiating chemotherapy; however, this period of stabilization should not exceed 24–48 hours.

### B. Specific Therapy

Systemic chemotherapy is the bulwark of therapy for NHLs. All patients with NHL require intensive intrathecal chemotherapy for CNS prophylaxis. Surgical resection is not indicated unless the entire tumor can be resected safely, which is rare. Partial resection or debulking surgery has no role. Radiation therapy does not improve outcome, so its use is confined to exceptional circumstances.

Therapy for LL is generally based on treatment protocols designed for ALL and involves dose-intensive, multiagent chemotherapy. Moderately high-dose methotrexate is emerging as an important strategy for minimizing induction failures and CNS relapses. The duration of therapy in recent trials has ranged from 11 months to 2 years.

BL and BLL do not respond well to therapy based on ALL protocols. Protocols using alkylating agents and intermediate- to high-dose methotrexate administered intensively but for a relatively short time produce the highest cure rates. LBCL is treated similarly, whereas ALCL has been treated with BL and LL protocols.

Monoclonal antibodies such as rituximab (anti-CD20) allow for more targeted therapy of lymphomas and have been successful in improving outcomes in adults. Studies employing this type of therapy in children are underway in those with refractory or relapsed NHL.

## Prognosis

A major predictor of outcome in NHL is the extent of disease at diagnosis. Ninety percent of patients with localized disease can expect long-term, disease-free survival, and patients with extensive disease on both sides of the diaphragm, CNS involvement, or bone marrow involvement in addition to a primary site have a 70–80% failure-free survival rate. Relapses occur early in NHL; patients with LL rarely have recurrences after 30 months from diagnosis, whereas patients with BL and BLL very rarely have recurrences beyond 1 year. Patients who experience relapse may have a chance for cure by autologous or allogeneic HSCT.

Cairo MS et al: Burkitt and Burkitt-like lymphoma in children and adolescents: A review of the Children's Cancer Group experience. Br J Hematol 2003;120:660 [PMID: 12588354].

Cairo MS et al: Childhood and adolescent large-cell lymphoma (LCL): A review of the Children's Cancer Group experience. Am J Hematol 2002;72:53 [PMID: 12508269].

Coiffier B et al: CHOP chemotherapy plus rituximab compared with CHOP alone in elderly patients with diffuse large-B-cell lymphoma. N Engl J Med 2002;346:235 [PMID: 11807147].

Kobrinsky NL et al: Outcomes of treatment of children and adolescents with recurrent non-Hodgkin's lymphoma and Hodgkin's disease with dexamethasone, etoposide, cisplatin, cytarabine and L-asparaginase maintenance chemotherapy and transplantation. Children's Cancer Group Study CCG-5912. J Clin Oncol 2001;19:2390 [PMID: 11331317].

Williams DM et al: Anaplastic large cell lymphoma in childhood: Analysis of 72 patients treated on The United Kingdom Children's Cancer Study Group chemotherapy regimens. Br J Hematol 2002;117:812 [PMID: 12060115].

## 3. Lymphoproliferative Disorders

LPDs can be thought of as a part of a continuum with lymphomas. Whereas LPDs represent inappropriate, often polyclonal proliferations of nonmalignant lymphocytes, lymphomas represent the development of malignant clones, sometimes arising from recognized LPDs.

## Post-Transplantation Lymphoproliferative Disorders

Post-transplantation lymphoproliferative disorders (PTLDs) arise in patient populations that have received substantial immunosuppressive medications for solid organ or bone marrow transplantation. In these patients, reactivation of latent EBV infection in B cells drives a polyclonal proliferation of these cells that is fatal if not halted. Occasionally a true lymphoma develops, often bearing a chromosomal translocation.

LPDs are an increasingly common and significant complication of transplantation. The incidence of PTLD ranges from approximately 2% to 15% of trans-

plant recipients, depending on the organ transplanted and the immunosuppressive regimen.

Treatment of these disorders is a challenge for transplant physicians and oncologists. The initial treatment is reduction in immunosuppression, which allows the patient's own immune effector cells to destroy the virally transformed lymphocytes. However, this is only effective in approximately half of patients. For those patients who do not respond to reduced immune suppression, chemotherapy of various regimens may succeed. EBV LPDs in some transplant recipients may be prevented or experimentally treated by infusion of EBV-specific T cells or even unmanipulated donor leukocytes. Additionally, the use of anti-B-cell antibodies, such as anti-CD20 (rituximab), for the treatment of PTLDs has been promising in early trials.

## Spontaneous Lymphoproliferative Disease

Immunodeficiencies in which LPDs occur include Bloom syndrome, Chédiak–Higashi syndrome, ataxia–telangiectasia, Wiskott–Aldrich syndrome, X-linked lymphoproliferative syndrome, congenital T-cell immunodeficiencies, and HIV infection. Treatment depends on the circumstances, but unlike PTLD few therapeutic options are often available. Castleman disease is an LPD occurring in pediatric patients without any apparent immunodeficiency. The autoimmune lymphoproliferative syndrome (ALPS) is characterized by widespread lymphadenopathy with hepatosplenomegaly, and autoimmune phenomena. ALPS results from mutations in the Fas ligand pathway that is critical in regulation of apoptosis.

Collins MH et al: Post-transplant lymphoproliferative disease in children. Pediatr Transplant 2001;5:250 [PMID: 11472603].

Gross TG: Low dose chemotherapy for children with post-transplant lymphoproliferative disease. Recent Results Cancer Res 2002;159:96 [PMID: 11785850].

Hayashi RJ et al: Post-transplant lymphoproliferative disease in children: Correlation of histology to clinical behavior. J Pediatr Hematol Oncol 2001;23:14 [PMID: 11196263].

Orjuela M et al: A pilot study of chemoimmunotherapy (cyclophosphamide, prednisone, and rituximab) in patients with post-transplant lymphoproliferative disorder following solid organ transplantation. Clin Cancer Res 2003;9:3945S [PMID: 14506193].

## NEUROBLASTOMA

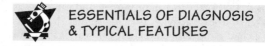

### ESSENTIALS OF DIAGNOSIS & TYPICAL FEATURES

- *Bone pain, abdominal pain, anorexia, weight loss, fatigue, fever, irritability.*

- *Abdominal mass (65%), adenopathy, proptosis, periorbital ecchymosis, skull masses, subcutaneous nodules, hepatomegaly, spinal cord compression.*

## General Considerations

Neuroblastoma (NB) arises from neural crest tissue of the sympathetic ganglia or adrenal medulla. It is composed of small, fairly uniform cells with little cytoplasm and hyperchromatic nuclei that may form rosette patterns. Pathologic diagnosis is not always easy, and NB must be differentiated from the other "small, round, blue cell" malignancies of childhood (Ewing sarcoma, rhabdomyosarcoma, peripheral neuroectodermal tumor, lymphoma).

NB accounts for 7–10% of pediatric malignancies and is the most common solid neoplasm outside the CNS. Fifty percent of NBs are diagnosed before age 2 years and 90% before age 5 years.

The biologic diversity of NB makes this a fascinating tumor for study. Spontaneous regression in stage 4-S disease (small primary, with metastases confined to liver, skin, or bone marrow in infants younger than age 1 year) and spontaneous or induced differentiation to a benign neoplasm are examples of the unique behavior of this tumor. Unfortunately NB is also an extremely malignant neoplasm, and the overall survival rate in advanced disease has changed little in 20 years despite significant advances in our understanding of this tumor at a cellular and molecular level.

## Clinical Findings

### A. SYMPTOMS AND SIGNS

Clinical manifestations vary with the primary site of metastatic disease and the neuroendocrine function of the tumor. Many children present with constitutional symptoms such as fever, weight loss, and irritability. Bone pain suggests metastatic disease, which is present in 70% of children older than age 1 year at diagnosis. Physical examination may reveal a firm, fixed, irregularly shaped mass that extends beyond the midline. The margins are often poorly defined. Although most children have an abdominal primary tumor (40% adrenal gland, 25% paraspinal ganglion), NB can arise wherever there is sympathetic tissue. In the posterior mediastinum, the tumor is usually asymptomatic and discovered on a chest radiograph obtained for other reasons. Patients with cervical NB present with a neck mass, which is often misdiagnosed as infection. Horner syndrome (unilateral ptosis, myosis, and anhydrosis) or heterochromia iridis (differently colored irises) may ac-

company cervical NB. Paraspinous tumors can extend through the spinal foramina, causing cord compression. Patients may present with paresis, paralysis, and bowel or bladder dysfunction.

The most common sites of metastases are bone, bone marrow, lymph nodes (regional as well as disseminated), liver, and subcutaneous tissue. NB has a predilection for metastasis to the skull, in particular the sphenoid bone and retrobulbar tissue. This causes periorbital ecchymosis and proptosis. Liver metastasis, particularly in the newborn, can be massive. Subcutaneous nodules are bluish in color and associated with an erythematous flush followed by blanching when compressed, probably secondary to catecholamine release.

NB may also be associated with unusual paraneoplastic manifestations. Examples include chronic watery diarrhea associated with tumor secretion of vasoactive intestinal peptides and opsoclonus–myoclonus (so-called dancing eyes/dancing feet syndrome). It is postulated that the neurologic manifestations are secondary to cross-reacting antibodies and often persist even after therapy.

### B. LABORATORY FINDINGS

Anemia is present in 60% of children with NB and can be due to chronic disease or marrow infiltration. Thrombocytopenia may be present. Thrombocytosis is a more common finding than thrombocytopenia, even with metastatic disease in the marrow. Urinary catecholamines (vanillylmandelic acid, homovanillic acid) are elevated in at least 90% of patients at diagnosis and should be measured prior to surgery. An elevated level of ferritin and LDH at diagnosis appears to have prognostic significance, especially when combined with age, stage, and tumor histology.

### C. IMAGING

Plain radiographs of the primary tumor may show stippled calcifications. CT scanning provides more information, including the extent of the primary tumor, its effects on surrounding structures, and the presence of liver and lymph node metastases. Classically, in tumors originating from the adrenal, the kidney is displaced inferolaterally, which helps to differentiate NB from Wilms tumor. MRI is useful in determining the presence of spinal cord involvement in tumors that appear to invade neural foramina.

Both skeletal survey and technetium bone scanning are obtained in the evaluation of bone metastases. NB may often be seen on bone scan because it takes up technetium. On plain radiographs, lesions are usually symmetrical and appear irregular and lytic, and periosteal reaction and pathologic fractures may also be seen. Metaiodobenzyl-guanidine (MIBG) scanning has been shown to be very sensitive for evaluating metastatic disease in NB, particularly for detecting bone and bone marrow metastases. Response to induction chemotherapy can also be evaluated by MIBG scanning and may be of prognostic significance.

## D. STAGING

Staging of NB is performed according to the International Neuroblastoma Staging System (INSS), which has been implemented worldwide. In addition to the radiographic evaluation, a tissue diagnosis must be established. Tumors are histologically classified as either favorable or unfavorable based on a modified Shimada system. In addition, bilateral bone marrow aspirates and biopsies must be performed to evaluate marrow involvement, even if the CBC is normal.

Molecular parameters are essential to supplement clinical staging and aid in treatment planning. Amplification of the *MYCN* proto-oncogene or its gene product can be detected in approximately 20% of NBs. It is a reliable marker of aggressive clinical behavior with rapid disease progression.. Tumor cell DNA content is also predictive of outcome. Hyperdiploidy is a favorable finding, whereas diploid DNA content is associated with a poorer outcome. Common cytogenetic abnormalities associated with high-risk features and adverse outcome include deletion of the short arm of chromosome 1 and gains of 17q genetic material

## Treatment & Prognosis

When deciding on a treatment plan, the COG uses a risk stratification system (low, intermediate, or high) based on INSS stage, age, *MYCN* status, histology, and DNA index. The mainstay of NB therapy is surgical resection coupled with chemotherapy. The usually massive size of the tumor often makes primary resection impossible. Under these circumstances, only a biopsy may be performed. Following chemotherapy, a second surgical procedure may allow for resection of the primary tumor. Radiation is sometimes also necessary. Effective chemotherapeutic agents in the treatment of NB include cyclophosphamide, doxorubicin, etoposide, cisplatin, vincristine, and topotecan. There is clear dose-response relationship in NB. About 80% of patients achieve complete or partial remission, although in advanced disease, remission is seldom durable.

For low-risk disease (stage 1, and 2), surgical resection alone may be sufficient to affect a cure. Infants younger than 1 year with stage 4 disease may need little if any therapy although chemotherapy may be initiated because of bulky disease causing mechanical complications. In intermediate-risk NB (subsets of patients with stage 3 and 4 disease) the primary treatment approach is surgical combined with chemotherapy. High-risk patients (the majority with stage 3 and 4 disease) require multimodal therapy, including surgery, radia-

tion, chemotherapy, and even autologous stem cell transplant. In a recent CCG study, autologous HSCT was unequivocally shown to improve survival rates in this group of patients.

Several clinical trials are under way in high-risk patients using radiolabeled MIBG and ch14.18 (a human–mouse monoclonal antibody specific for ganglioside GD2, the predominant antigen on NB cells) as well as interleukin-2 (IL-2) to eradicate minimal residual disease. A phase III randomized trial conducted by CCG has shown that the administration of *cis*-retinoic acid, a differentiating agent, can prolong disease-free survival in advanced-stage NB when administered in the setting of minimal residual disease after HSCT. Current phase I and II studies are underway using fenretinide (4-HPR), a synthetic retinoid.

For children with stage 1, 2, or 4-S disease, the 5-year survival rate is 70–90%. Infants younger than age 1 year who have stage 4 disease have a greater than 60% likelihood of long-term survival. Children older than age 1 year with stage 3 disease have an intermediate prognosis (approximately 40–70%), and those with stage 4 disease have a poor prognosis (5–50% survival 5 years from diagnosis).

Katzenstein HM et al: Treatment and outcome of 83 children with intraspinal neuroblastoma: The Pediatric Oncology Group experience. J Clin Oncol 2001;19:1047 [PMID: 11181668].

Reynolds CP et al: Retinoid therapy of high-risk neuroblastoma. Cancer Lett 2003;197:185 [PMID: 12880980].

Schwab M et al: Neuroblastoma: Biology and molecular and chromosomal pathology. Lancet Oncol 2003;4:472 [PMID: 12901961].

Shimada H et al: International neuroblastoma pathology classification for prognostic evaluation of patients with peripheral neuroblastic tumors: A report from the Children's Cancer Group. Cancer 2001;92:2451 [PMID: 11745303].

Weinstein JL et al: Advances in the diagnosis and treatment of neuroblastoma. Oncologist 2003;8:278 [PMID:12773750].

# WILMS TUMOR (NEPHROBLASTOMA)

## ESSENTIALS OF DIAGNOSIS & TYPICAL FEATURES

- *Asymptomatic abdominal mass or swelling (83%).*
- *Fever (23%), hematuria (21%).*
- *Hypertension (25%), genitourinary malformations (6%), aniridia, hemihypertrophy.*

## General Considerations

Approximately 460 new cases of Wilms tumor occur annually in the United States, representing 5–6% of cancers in children younger than age 15 years. After neuroblastoma, this is the second most common abdominal tumor in children. The tumor arises from kidney and is usually composed of three elements: blastema, epithelium, and stroma. The majority of Wilms tumors are of sporadic occurrence. However, in a few children, Wilms tumor occurs in the setting of associated malformations or syndromes, including aniridia, hemihypertrophy, genitourinary malformations (eg, cryptorchidism, hypospadias, gonadal dysgenesis, pseudohermaphroditism, horseshoe kidney), Beckwith–Wiedemann syndrome, Denys–Drash syndrome, and WAGR syndrome (Wilms tumor, aniridia, ambiguous genitalia, mental retardation). Although most patients with Wilms tumor are karyotypically normal, those with sporadic aniridia frequently have a constitutional deletion at the 11p13 locus. This deletion has also been found in the tumor cells of Wilms patients without aniridia who are karyotypically normal.

The median age at diagnosis is related both to gender and laterality, with bilateral tumors presenting at a younger age than unilateral tumors, and males being diagnosed earlier than females. Wilms tumor occurs most commonly between ages 2 and 5 years; it is unusual after age 6 years. The mean age at diagnosis is 4 years.

## Clinical Findings

### A. Symptoms and Signs

Most children with Wilms tumor present with increasing size of the abdomen or an asymptomatic abdominal mass incidentally discovered by a parent. The mass is usually smooth and firm, well demarcated, and rarely crosses the midline, though it can extend inferiorly into the pelvis. Gross hematuria is an uncommon presentation, although microscopic hematuria occurs in approximately 25% of patients.

### B. Laboratory Findings

The CBC is usually normal, but some patients have anemia secondary to hemorrhage into the tumor. Blood urea nitrogen and serum creatinine are usually normal. Urinalysis may show some blood or leukocytes.

### C. Imaging and Staging

Ultrasonography or CT of the abdomen should establish the presence of an intrarenal mass. It is also essential to evaluate the contralateral kidney for presence and function as well as synchronous Wilms tumor. The inferior vena cava needs to be evaluated by ultrasonography for the presence and extent of tumor propagation.

The liver should be imaged for the presence of metastatic disease. A plain chest radiograph (four views) or chest CT scans (or both) should be obtained to determine whether pulmonary metastases are present. Approximately 10% of patients will have metastatic disease at diagnosis. Of these, 80% will have pulmonary disease and 15% liver metastases. Bone and brain metastases are extremely uncommon and usually associated with more aggressive renal tumors, such as clear cell sarcoma or rhabdoid tumor; hence, bone scans and brain imaging are not routinely performed. The clinical stage is ultimately decided at surgery and confirmed by the pathologist.

## Treatment & Prognosis

In the United States, treatment of Wilms tumor begins with surgical exploration of the abdomen via an anterior surgical approach to allow for inspection and palpation of the contralateral kidney. The liver and lymph nodes are inspected and suspicious areas biopsied or excised. En bloc resection of tumor is performed. Every attempt is made to avoid tumor spillage at surgery. Because therapy is tailored to tumor stage, it is imperative that a surgeon familiar with the staging requirements perform the operation.

In addition to the staging, the histologic type has implications for therapy and prognosis. Favorable histology (FH; see later discussion) refers to the classic triphasic Wilms tumor and its variants. Unfavorable histology (UH) refers to the presence of diffuse anaplasia (extreme nuclear atypia) and is present in 5% of Wilms tumors. Only a few small foci of anaplasia in a Wilms tumor give a worse prognosis to patients with stage II, III, or IV tumors. Following excision and pathologic examination, the patient is assigned a stage that defines further therapy.

Although clear cell sarcoma of the kidney (CCSK) and rhabdoid tumor of the kidney were previously classified as UH Wilms tumor, they are no longer thought to be Wilms tumor variants, but rather separate renal malignancies.

Progress in the treatment of Wilms tumor stems from clinical trials by the National Wilms Tumor Study (NWTS) begun in 1969 that resulted in an overall cure rate of approximately 90%. NWTS-4 demonstrated that survival rates were improved by intensifying therapy during the initial treatment phase while shortening overall treatment duration (24 weeks vs 60 weeks of treatment). It is the first study of a pediatric population to evaluate the economic effect of two different treatment approaches.

Table 28–7 provides an overview of the current treatment recommendations in NWTS-5. Patients with stage III or IV Wilms tumor require radiation therapy

*Table 28–7.* Treatment of Wilms tumor

| Stage/Histologic Subtype | Treatment |
|---|---|
| I–II FH and I UH | 18 wk (dactinomycin and vincristine) |
| III–IV FH and II–IV focal anaplasia | 24 wk (dactinomycin, vincristine, and doxorubicin) with radiation |
| II–IV UH (diffuse anaplasia) | 24 wks (vincristine, doxorubicin, etoposide, and cyclophosphamide with radiation |

to the tumor bed and to sites of metastatic disease. Chemotherapy is optimally begun within 5 days after surgery, whereas radiation therapy should be started within 10 days. Stage V (bilateral Wilms tumor) disease dictates a different approach, consisting of bilateral renal biopsies followed by chemotherapy and second-look renal-sparing surgery. Radiation may also be necessary.

Using these approaches, 4-year overall survival rates through NWTS-4 are as follows: stage I FH, 96%; stage II–IV FH, 82–92%; stage I–III UH (diffuse anaplasia), 56–70%; stage IV UH, 17%. Patients with recurrent Wilms tumor have approximately a 50% salvage rate with surgery, radiation therapy, and chemotherapy (singly or in combination). HSCT is also being explored as a way to improve the chances of survival after relapse.

## Future Considerations

Although progress in the treatment of Wilms tumor has been extraordinary, important questions remain to be answered. Questions are being raised regarding the role of prenephrectomy chemotherapy in the treatment of Wilms tumor. Presurgical chemotherapy seems to decrease tumor rupture at resection but may unfavorably affect outcome by changing staging. Whether pulmonary radiation can be eliminated in metastatic pulmonary disease is also being investigated.

Blakely ML et al: Outcome of children with cystic partially differentiated nephroblastoma treated with or without chemotherapy. J Pediatr Surg 2003;38:897 [PMID: 12778388].

Green DM et al: Treatment with nephrectomy only for small, stage I/favorable histology Wilms' tumor: A report from the National Wilms' Tumor Study Group. J Clin Oncol 2001;19:3719 [PMID:11533093].

McLorie GA. Wilms' tumor (nephroblastoma). Curr Opin Urol 2001;11:567 [PMID:11734691].

Merguerian PA. Pediatric genitourinary tumors. Curr Opin Oncol 2003;15:222 [PMID:12778016]

# BONE TUMORS

Primary malignant bone tumors are uncommon in childhood. Osteosarcoma accounts for 60% of cases and occurs mostly in adolescents and young adults. Ewing sarcoma is the second most common malignant tumor of bony origin. Both tumors have a male predominance.

The cardinal signs of bone tumor are pain at the site of involvement, often following slight trauma; mass formation; and fracture through an area of cortical bone destruction.

## 1. Osteosarcoma

### General Considerations

Although osteosarcoma is the sixth most common malignancy in childhood, it ranks third among adolescents and young adults. This peak occurrence during the adolescent growth spurt suggests a causal relationship between rapid bone growth and malignant transformation. Further evidence for this relationship is found in epidemiologic data showing patients with osteosarcoma to be taller than their peers, osteosarcoma occurring most frequently at sites where the greatest increase in length and size of bone occurs, and osteosarcoma occurring at an earlier age in girls than boys, corresponding to their earlier growth spurt. The metaphyses of long tubular bones are primarily affected. The distal femur accounts for more than 40% of cases, with the proximal tibia, proximal humerus, and mid and proximal femur following in frequency.

### Clinical Findings

#### A. Symptoms and Signs

Pain over the involved area is the usual presenting symptom with or without an associated soft tissue mass. Systemic symptoms (fever, weight loss) are rare. Laboratory evaluation may reveal elevated serum alkaline phosphatase or LDH levels.

#### B. Imaging and Staging

Radiographic findings show permeative destruction of the normal bony trabecular pattern with indistinct margins. In addition, periosteal new bone formation and lifting of the bony cortex may create a Codman triangle. A soft tissue mass plus calcifications in a radial or sunburst pattern are frequently noted. MRI is more sensitive in defining the extent of the primary tumor and in many centers has replaced CT scanning. The most common sites of metastases are the lung (≤ 20%

of newly diagnosed cases) and the bone (10%). A CT scan of the chest and a bone scan are essential for detecting metastatic disease. Bone marrow aspirates and biopsies are not indicated.

Despite the rather characteristic radiographic appearance, a tissue sample is needed to confirm the diagnosis. Placement of the incision for biopsy is of critical importance. A misplaced incision could preclude a limb salvage procedure and necessitate amputation. The surgeon who will carry out the definitive surgical procedure should perform the biopsy. A staging system for osteosarcoma based on local tumor extent and presence or absence of distant metastasis has been proposed, but it has not been validated.

## Treatment and Prognosis

Historical studies showed that over 50% of patients receiving surgery alone developed pulmonary metastases within 6 months after surgery. This suggests the presence of micrometastatic disease at diagnosis. Adjuvant chemotherapy trials showed improved disease-free survival rates of 55–85% after 3–10 years of follow-up.

Osteosarcomas are highly radioresistant lesions; for this reason, radiation therapy has no role in its primary management. Chemotherapy is often administered prior to definitive surgery (neoadjuvant chemotherapy). This permits an early attack on micrometastatic disease and may also shrink the tumor, facilitating a limb salvage procedure. Preoperative chemotherapy also makes detailed histologic evaluation of tumor response to the chemotherapy agents possible. If the histologic response is poor (> 10% viable tumor tissue), postoperative chemotherapy can be changed accordingly. Chemotherapy may be administered intra-arterially or intravenously, although the benefits of intra-arterial chemotherapy are disputed. Agents having efficacy in the treatment of osteosarcoma include doxorubicin, cisplatin, high-dose methotrexate, and ifosfamide.

Definitive cure requires en bloc surgical resection of the tumor with a margin of uninvolved tissue. Amputation and limb salvage are equally effective in achieving local control of osteosarcoma. Contraindications to limb-sparing surgery include major involvement of the neurovascular bundle by tumor; immature skeletal age, particularly for lower extremity tumors; infection in the region of the tumor; inappropriate biopsy site; and extensive muscle involvement that would result in a poor functional outcome.

Postsurgical chemotherapy is generally continued until the patient has received 1 year of treatment. Relapses are unusual beyond 3 years, but late relapses do occur. Histologic response to neoadjuvant chemotherapy is an excellent predictor of outcome. Patients having 90% tumor necrosis have a 70–90% long-term, dis-

ease-free survival rate. Other favorable prognostic factors include distal skeletal lesions, longer duration of symptoms, age older than 20, female gender, and near-diploid tumor DNA index.

## 2. Ewing Sarcoma

### General Considerations

Ewing sarcoma accounts for only 10% of primary malignant bone tumors; fewer than 200 new cases occur each year in the United States. It is a disease primarily of white males, almost never affects blacks, and occurs mostly in the second decade of life. Ewing sarcoma is considered a "small, round, blue cell" malignancy. The differential diagnosis includes rhabdomyosarcoma, lymphoma, and neuroblastoma. Although most commonly a tumor of bone, it may also occur in soft tissue (extraosseous Ewing sarcoma or peripheral neuroectodermal tumor [PNET]).

### Clinical Findings

#### A. SYMPTOMS AND SIGNS

Pain at the site of the primary tumor is the most common presenting sign, with or without swelling and erythema. No specific laboratory findings are characteristic of Ewing sarcoma, but an elevated LDH may be present and is of prognostic significance.

#### B. IMAGING AND STAGING

The radiographic appearance of Ewing sarcoma overlaps with osteosarcoma, although Ewing sarcoma usually involves the diaphyses of long bones. The central axial skeleton gives rise to 40% of Ewing tumors. Evaluation of a patient diagnosed as having Ewing sarcoma should include CT scan or MRI (or both) of the primary lesion to define the extent of local disease as precisely as possible. This is imperative for planning future surgical procedures or radiation therapy. Metastatic disease is present in 25% of patients at diagnosis. The lung (38%), bone (particularly the spine) (31%), and bone marrow (11%) are the most common sites for metastasis. CT scan of the chest, bone scanning, and bilateral bone marrow aspirates and biopsies are all essential to the staging work-up.

A biopsy is essential in establishing the diagnosis. Histologically, Ewing sarcoma consists of sheets of undifferentiated cells with hyperchromatic nuclei, well-defined cell borders, and scanty cytoplasm. Necrosis is common. Electron microscopy, immunocytochemistry, and cytogenetics may be necessary to confirm the diagnosis. A generous tissue biopsy specimen is often necessary for diagnosis but should not delay starting chemotherapy.

A consistent cytogenetic abnormality, t(11;22), has been identified in Ewing sarcoma and PNET and is present in 85–90% of tumors. These tumors also express the proto-oncogene c-*myc,* which may be helpful in differentiating Ewing sarcoma from neuroblastoma, where it is not expressed.

Therapy usually commences with the administration of chemotherapy after biopsy and is followed by local control measures. Depending on many factors, including the primary site of the tumor and the response to chemotherapy, local control could be achieved by surgery, radiation therapy, or a combination of these methods. Following local control, chemotherapy continues for approximately 1 year. Effective treatment for Ewing sarcoma uses combinations of dactinomycin, vincristine, doxorubicin, cyclophosphamide, etoposide, and ifosfamide. Patients with small localized primary tumors have a 50–70% long-term, disease-free survival rate. For patients with metastatic disease and large pelvic primary tumors, survival is poor. Autologous HSCT is being investigated for the treatment of these high-risk patients.

Burdach S et al: High-dose therapy for patients with primary multifocal and early relapsed Ewing's tumors: Results of two consecutive regimens assessing the role of total-body irradiation. J Clin Oncol 2003;21:3072 [PMID:12915596].

Ferguson WS, Goorin AM: Current treatment of osteosarcoma. Cancer Invest 2001;19:292 [PMID:11338887].

Goorin et al: Phase II/III trial of etoposide and high-dose ifosphamide in newly diagnosed metastatic osteosarcoma: A Pediatric Oncology Group trial. J Clin Oncol 2002;20:426 [PMID:11786570].

Goorin AM et al: Presurgical chemotherapy compared with immediate surgery and adjuvant chemotherapy for nonmetastatic osteosarcoma: Pediatric Oncology Group Study POG-8651. J Clin Oncol 2003;15:1574 [PMID:12697883].

Petrilli AS et al: Use of amifostine in the therapy of osteosarcoma in children and adolescents. J Pediatr Hematol Oncol 2002;24:188 [PMID:11990304].

Rodriguez-Galindo C et al. Treatment of Ewing sarcoma family of tumors: Current status and outlook for the future. Med Pediatr Oncol 2003;40:276 [PMID:12652615].

# RHABDOMYOSARCOMA

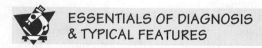

## ESSENTIALS OF DIAGNOSIS & TYPICAL FEATURES

- *Painless, progressively enlarging mass; proptosis; chronic drainage (nasal, aural, sinus, vaginal); cranial nerve palsies.*
- *Urinary obstruction, constipation, hematuria.*

## General Considerations

Rhabdomyosarcoma is the most common soft tissue sarcoma occurring in childhood and accounts for 10% of solid tumors in childhood. The peak incidence is at age 2–5 years; 70% of children are diagnosed before age 10 years. A second smaller peak is seen in adolescents with extremity tumors. Males are affected more commonly than females.

Arising from embryonic mesenchymal cells, rhabdomyosarcoma can occur anywhere in the body. When rhabdomyosarcoma imitates striated muscle and cross-striations are seen by light microscopy, the diagnosis is straightforward. Immunohistochemistry, electron microscopy, or chromosomal analysis is sometimes necessary to make the diagnosis. Rhabdomyosarcoma is further classified into subtypes based on pathologic features: embryonal (59%), of which botryoid is a variant; alveolar (21%); undifferentiated sarcoma (8%); pleomorphic, which is seen in adults (1%); and other (11%). These subtypes occur in characteristic locations and have different metastatic potentials and outcomes (Table 28–8).

Although the pathogenesis of rhabdomyosarcoma is unknown, in rare cases a genetic predisposition has been determined. Li–Fraumeni syndrome is an inherited mutation of the *p53* tumor suppressor gene that results in a high risk of bone and soft tissue sarcomas in childhood plus breast cancer and other malignant neoplasms before age 45 years. A characteristic chromosomal translocation [t(2;13)] has been described in alveolar rhabdomyosarcoma. A recent analysis from the Intergroup Rhabdomyosarcoma Study Group-IV (IRSG-IV) suggests that the gene fusion protein associated with this translocation is of poor prognostic significance.

## Clinical Findings

### A. SYMPTOMS AND SIGNS

The presenting symptoms and signs of rhabdomyosarcoma result from disturbances of normal body function due to tumor growth (see Table 28–8). For example, patients with orbital rhabdomyosarcoma present with proptosis, whereas patients with rhabdomyosarcoma of the bladder can present with hematuria, urinary obstruction, or a pelvic mass.

### B. IMAGING

A plain radiograph and a CT or MRI scan should be obtained to determine the extent of the primary tumor and to assess regional lymph nodes. A lung CT scan is obtained to rule out pulmonary metastasis, the most common site of metastatic disease at diagnosis. A skeletal survey and a bone scan are obtained to determine whether bony metastases are present. Bilateral bone

*Table 28–8.* Characteristics of rhabdomyosarcoma.

| Primary Site | Frequency (%) | Symptoms and Signs | Predominant Pathologic Subtype |
|---|---|---|---|
| **Head and neck** | **35** | | Embryonal |
| Orbit | 9 | Proptosis | |
| Parameningeal | 16 | Cranial nerve palsies; aural or sinus obstruction with or without drainage | |
| Other | 10 | Painless, progressively enlarging mass | |
| **Genitourinary** | **22** | | Embryonal (botryoid variant in bladder and vagina) |
| Bladder and prostate | 13 | Hematuria, urinary obstruction | |
| Vagina and uterus | 2 | Pelvic mass, vaginal discharge | |
| Paratesticular | 7 | Painless mass | |
| **Extremities** | **18** | Adolescents, swelling of affected body part | Alveolar (50%), undifferentiated |
| **Other** | **25** | Mass | Alveolar, undifferentiated |

marrow biopsies and aspirates are obtained to rule out bone marrow infiltration. Additional studies may be warranted in certain sites. For example, in parameningeal primaries, a lumbar puncture is performed to evaluate CSF for tumor cells.

## Treatment

Optimal management and treatment of rhabdomyosarcoma is complex and requires combined modality therapy. When feasible, the tumor should be excised, but this is not always possible because of the site of origin and size of tumor. When only partial tumor resection is feasible, the operative procedure is usually limited to biopsy and sampling of lymph nodes. The role of debulking of unresectable tumor is unclear. Chemotherapy can often convert an inoperable tumor to a resectable one. A second-look procedure to remove residual disease and confirm the clinical response to chemotherapy and radiation therapy is generally performed at about week 20 of therapy.

Radiation therapy is an effective method of local tumor control for both microscopic and gross residual disease. It is generally administered to all patients, the only exception being those with localized tumor that has been completely resected. All patients with rhabdomyosarcoma receive chemotherapy, even when the tumor is fully resected at diagnosis. The exact regimen and duration of chemotherapy are determined by primary site, group, and tumor node metastasis (TNM) classification. Vincristine, dactinomycin, and cyclophosphamide have shown the greatest efficacy in the treatment of rhabdomyosarcoma.

## Prognosis

The extent of tumor at diagnosis, the primary site, the pathologic subtype, and the response to treatment all influence the long-term, disease-free survival rate from the time of diagnosis. Children with localized disease at diagnosis have a 77% 3-year disease-free survival rate, whereas children with metastatic disease at presentation have a poorer outcome (3-year disease-free survival 39%).

Newer treatment strategies for high-risk patients include different drug combinations and dosing schedules with hematopoietic growth factor support, hyperfractionated radiation therapy, and autologous HSCT.

Breneman JC et al: Prognostic factors and clinical outcomes in children and adolescents with metastatic rhabdomyosarcoma—A report from the Intergroup Rhabdomyosarcoma Study IV. J Clin Oncol 2003;21:78 [PMID:12506174].

Crist WM et al: Inter-group Rhabdomyosarcoma Study—IV: Results for patients with non-metastatic disease. J Clin Oncol 2001;19:3091 [PMID:11408506].

Pappo AS et al: Treatment of localized nonorbital, nonparameningeal head and neck rhabdomyosarcoma: Lessons learned from intergroup rhabdomyosarcoma studies III and IV. J Clin Oncol 2003;21:638 [PMID:12586800].

Raney RB et al: Rhabdomyosarcoma and undifferentiated sarcoma in the first two decades of life: A selective review of intergroup rhabdomyosarcoma study group experience and rationale for inter-group rhabdomyosarcoma study V. J Pediatr Hematol Oncol 2001;23:215 [PMID:11846301].

Sorensen PHB et al: *PAX3-FKHR* and *PAX7-FKHR* gene fusions are prognostic indicators in alveolar rhabdomyosarcoma: A report from the Children's Oncology Group. J Clin Oncol 2002;20:2672. [PMID:12039929].

# RETINOBLASTOMA

## General Considerations

Retinoblastoma is a neuroectodermal malignancy arising from embryonic retinal cells that accounts for 3% of malignant disease in children younger than age 15 years. It is the most common intraocular tumor in pediatric patients and causes 5% of cases of childhood blindness. Two hundred to 300 new cases occur per year in the United States. This is a malignancy of early childhood, with 90% of the tumors diagnosed before age 5 years. Bilateral involvement occurs in 20–30% of children and typically is diagnosed at a younger age (median age 14 months) than unilateral disease (median age 23 months).

Retinoblastoma is the prototype of hereditary cancers due to a mutation in the retinoblastoma gene (*RB1*), which is located on the long arm of chromosome 13 (13q14). This gene is a tumor suppressor gene that normally controls cellular growth. When the gene is inactivated, as in retinoblastoma, cellular growth is uncontrolled. Uncontrolled cell growth leads to tumor formation. Inactivation of both *RB1* alleles within the same cell is required for tumor formation.

Retinoblastoma is known to arise in heritable and nonheritable forms. Based on the different clinical characteristics of the two forms, Knudson proposed a "two-hit" hypothesis for retinoblastoma tumor development. He postulated that two independent events were necessary for a cell to acquire tumor potential. Mutations at the *RB1* locus can be inherited or arise spontaneously. In heritable cases, the first mutation arises during gametogenesis, either spontaneously (90%) or through transmission from a parent (10%). This mutation is present in every retinal cell and in all other somatic and germ cells. Ninety percent of persons who carry this germline mutation will develop retinoblastoma. For tumor formation, the loss of the second *RB1* allele within a cell must occur; loss of only one allele is insufficient for tumor formation. The second mutation occurs in a somatic (retinal) cell. In nonheritable cases (60%), both mutations arise in a somatic cell after gametogenesis has taken place.

## Clinical Findings

### A. SYMPTOMS AND SIGNS

Children with retinoblastoma generally come to medical attention while the tumor is still confined to the globe. Although present at birth, retinoblastoma is not usually detected until it has grown to a considerable size. Leukocoria (white pupillary reflex) is the most common sign (found in 60% of patients). Parents may note an unusual appearance of the eye or asymmetry of the eyes in a photograph. The differential diagnosis of leukocoria includes *Toxocara canis* granuloma, astrocytic hamartoma, retinopathy of prematurity, Coats disease, and persistent hyperplastic primary vitreous. Strabismus (in 20% of patients) is seen when the tumor involves the macula and central vision is lost. Rarely (in 7% of patients), a painful red eye with glaucoma, a hyphema, or proptosis is the initial manifestation. A single focus or multiple foci of tumor may be seen in one or both eyes at diagnosis. Bilateral involvement occurs in 20–30% of children.

### B. EVALUATION

Suspected retinoblastoma requires a detailed ophthalmologic examination under general anesthesia. An ophthalmologist makes the diagnosis of retinoblastoma by the appearance of the tumor within the eye without pathologic confirmation. A white to creamy pink mass protruding into the vitreous matter suggests the diagnosis; intraocular calcifications and vitreous seeding are virtually pathognomonic of retinoblastoma. A CT scan of the orbits detects intraocular calcification, evaluates the optic nerve for tumor infiltration, and detects extraocular extension of tumor. A single focus or multiple foci of tumor may be seen in one or both eyes at diagnosis. Metastatic disease of the marrow and meninges can be ruled out with bilateral bone marrow aspirates and biopsies plus CSF cytology.

## Treatment

Each eye is treated according to the potential for useful vision, and every attempt is made to preserve vision. The choice of therapy depends on the size, location, and number of intraocular lesions. Absolute indications for enucleation include no vision, neovascular glaucoma, inability to examine the treated eye, and inability to control tumor growth with conservative treatment. External beam irradiation has been the mainstay of therapy. A total dose of 35–45 Gy is administered. However, many centers are investigating the role of systemic chemotherapy for the treatment of retinoblastoma confined to the globe in an effort to eliminate the need for external beam radiotherapy. Cryotherapy, photocoagulation, and radioactive plaques can be used for local tumor control. Patients with metastatic disease receive chemotherapy.

Children with retinoblastoma confined to the retina (whether unilateral or bilateral) have an excellent prognosis, with 5-year survival rates greater than 90%. Mortality is correlated directly with extent of optic nerve involvement, orbital extension of tumor, and massive choroid invasion. Patients who have disease in the optic nerve beyond the lamina cribrosa have only a 40% 5-year survival rate. Patients with meningeal or metastatic spread rarely survive, although intensive chemotherapy and autologous HSCT have produced long-term survivors.

Patients with the germline mutation (heritable form) have a significant risk of developing second primary tumors. Osteosarcomas account for 40% of such tumors. Second malignant neoplasms occur in both patients who have and those who have not received radiation therapy. The 30-year cumulative incidence for a second neoplasm is 35% in patients who received radiation therapy and 6% in those who did not receive radiation therapy. The risk continues to increase over time. Although radiation contributes to the risk, it is the presence of the retinoblastoma gene itself that is responsible for the development of nonocular tumors in these patients.

Antoneli CB et al: Extraocular retinoblastoma: A 13-year experience. Cancer 2003;15:1292 [PMID:12973854].

Brichard B et al: Combined chemotherapy and local treatment in the management of intraocular retinoblastoma. Med Pediatr Oncol 2002;38:411 [PMID:11984802].

Nahum MP et al: Long-term follow-up of children with retinoblastoma. Pediatr Hematol Oncol 2001;18:173 [PMID:11293284].

Rodriguez-Galindo C et al: Treatment of intraocular retinoblastoma with vincristine and carboplatin. J Clin Oncol 2003;15:2019 [PMID:12743157].

# HEPATIC TUMORS

Two thirds of liver masses found in childhood are malignant. Ninety percent of hepatic malignancies are either hepatoblastoma or hepatocellular carcinoma. Hepatoblastomas are somewhat more frequent than hepatocellular carcinomas (51% vs 39%). A comparison of the features of these hepatic malignancies is presented in Table 28–9. Of the benign tumors, 60% are hamartomas or vascular tumors such as hemangiomas.

Children with hepatic tumors usually come to medical attention because of an enlarging abdomen. Approximately 10% of hepatoblastomas are first discovered on routine examination. Anorexia, weight loss, vomiting, and abdominal pain are associated more commonly with hepatocellular carcinoma. Serum AFP is often elevated and is an excellent marker for response to treatment.

Imaging studies should include abdominal ultrasound, CT scan, or MRI. Malignant tumors have a diffuse hyperechoic pattern on ultrasonography, whereas benign tumors are usually poorly echoic. Vascular lesions contain areas with varying degrees of echogenicity. Ultrasound is also useful for imaging the hepatic veins, portal veins, and inferior vena cava. CT scanning and, in particular, MRI are important for defining the extent of tumor within the liver. CT scanning of the chest and bone scan should be obtained to evaluate for metastatic spread.

Because bone marrow involvement is extremely rare, bone marrow aspirates and biopsies are not indicated. The prognosis for children with hepatic malignancies depends on the tumor type and the resectability of the tumor. Complete resectability is essential for survival. Chemotherapy can decrease the size of most hepatoblastomas. Following biopsy of the lesion, neoadjuvant chemotherapy is administered prior to attempting complete surgical resection. Chemotherapy can often con-

**Table 28–9.** Comparison of hepatoblastoma and hepatocellular carcinoma in childhood.

| | Hepatoblastoma | Hepatocellular Carcinoma |
|---|---|---|
| Median age at presentation | 1 y (0–3 y) | 12 y (5–18 y) |
| Male-to-female ratio | 1.7:1 | 1.4:1 |
| Associated conditions | Hemihypertrophy, Beckwith–Wiedemann syndrome, prematurity, Gardner's syndrome | Hepatitis B virus infection, hereditary tyrosinemia, biliary cirrhosis, $\alpha_1$-antitrypsin deficiency |
| Pathologic features | Fetal or embryonal cells; mesenchymal component (30%) | Large pleomorphic tumor cells and tumor giant cells |
| Solitary hepatic lesion | 80% | 20–50% |
| Unique features at diagnosis | Osteopenia (20–30%), isosexual precocity (3%) | Hemoperitoneum, polycythemia |
| Laboratory features Hyperbilirubinemia Elevated AFP Abnormal liver function tests | 5% >90% 15–30% | 25% 50% 30–50% |

AFP = $\alpha$-fetoprotein.

vert an inoperable tumor to a completely resectable one and can also eradicate metastatic disease. Approximately 50–60% of hepatoblastomas are fully resectable, whereas only one third of hepatocellular carcinomas can be completely removed. Even with complete resection, only one third of patients with hepatocellular carcinoma are long-term survivors. A recent CCG/POG trial has shown cisplatin, fluorouracil, and vincristine to be as effective as but less toxic than cisplatin and doxorubicin in treating hepatoblastoma. Other drugs that have demonstrated benefit include fluorouracil and cyclophosphamide. Etoposide, carboplatin, and ifosfamide are under investigation. Radiation as well as liver transplantation is being investigated for patients whose tumors cannot be completely resected following chemotherapy.

Feusner J, Plaschkes J: Hepatoblastoma and low birth weight: A trend or chance observation? Med Pediatr Oncol 2002;39:508 [PMID:12228908].

Katzenstein HM et al: Hepatocellular carcinoma in children and adolescents: Results from the Pediatric Oncology Group and the Children's Cancer Group intergroup study. J Clin Oncol 2002;12:2789 [PMID:12065555].

Katzenstein HM et al: Treatment of unresectable and metastatic hepatoblastoma: A Pediatric Oncology Group Phase II study. J Clin Oncol 2002;20:3438 [PMID:12177104].

Malogolowkin MH et al: Feasibility and toxicity of chemoembolization for children with liver tumors. J Clin Oncol 2000;18:1279 [PMID:10715298].

Stocker JT: Hepatic tumors in children. Clin Liver Dis 2001;5:259 [PMID:11218918].

# LANGERHANS CELL HISTIOCYTOSIS

Langerhans cell histiocytosis (LCH; formerly called histiocytosis X) is a rare and poorly understood spectrum of disorders. It can occur as an isolated lesion or as widespread systemic disease involving virtually any body site. Eosinophilic granuloma, Hand–Schüller–Christian disease, and Letterer–Siwe disease are all syndromes encompassed by this disorder. LCH is not a true malignancy, but is a clonal, reactive proliferation of normal histiocytic cells, perhaps resulting from an immunoregulatory defect.

The distinctive pathologic feature is proliferation of histiocytic cells beyond what would be seen in a normal inflammatory process. Langerhans histiocytes have typical features: on light microscopy, the nuclei are deeply indented (coffee bean-shaped) and elongated, and the cytoplasm is pale, distinct, and abundant. Additional diagnostic characteristics include Birbeck granules on electron microscopy, expression of CD1 on the cell surface, and positive immunostaining for S-100 protein.

## Clinical Findings

Because LCH encompasses a broad spectrum of diseases, its presentation can be variable, from a single asymptomatic lesion to widely disseminated disease.

Patients with localized disease present primarily with lesions limited to bone. Occasionally found incidentally on radiographs obtained for other reasons, these lesions are well-demarcated and frequently found in the skull, clavicles, ribs, and vertebrae. These lesions can be painful. Patients can also present with localized disease of the skin, often as a diaper rash that does not resolve.

Bony lesions, fever, weight loss, otitis media, exophthalmos, and diabetes insipidus occur in a small number of children with the disease. Formerly called Hand–Schüller–Christian disease, this multifocal disease commonly presents with generalized symptoms and organ dysfunction.

Children with disseminated LCH (formerly called Letterer–Siwe disease) typically present before age 2 years with a seborrheic skin rash, fever, weight loss, lymphadenopathy, hepatosplenomegaly, and hematologic abnormalities.

Diagnosis is made with biopsy of the involved organ. The work-up should include a CBC, liver and kidney function tests, a skeletal survey or technetium bone scan, and a urinalysis with specific gravity to rule out diabetes insipidus.

## Treatment & Prognosis

The outcome of LCH is extremely variable, but the process usually resolves spontaneously. Isolated lesions may need no therapy at all. Intralesional corticosteroids, curettage, and low-dose radiation therapy are useful local treatment measures for symptomatic focal lesions. Patients with localized disease have an excellent prognosis.

Multifocal disease is often treated with systemic chemotherapy. Prednisone with vinblastine or etoposide can be given repeatedly or continuously until lesions heal; the drugs can then be reduced and finally stopped.

Multifocal disease is less predictable, but most cases resolve without sequelae. Age, degree of organ involvement, and response to therapy are the most important prognostic factors. Infants with disseminated disease tend to do poorly, with mortality rates approaching 50%. New treatment approaches for patients that do not respond to conventional chemotherapy have been evaluated in small studies. 2-Chlorodeoxyadenosine (2-CDA) has been used with some success. Therapeutic strategies targeting the dysregulated immune response using interferon-α or etanercept (anti-tumor necrosis factor-α) have also been reported.

Arceci RJ et al: Atypical cellular disorders. Hematology 2002;297: [PMID: 12446429].

Gadner H et al: A randomized trial of treatment for multisystem Langerhans' cell histiocytosis. J Pediatr 2001;138: 728 [PMID: 11343051].

Henter JI et al: Successful treatment of Langerhan's cell histiocytosis with etanercept. N Engl J Med 2001;345:1577 [PMID: 11794238].

Kiss C et al: Interferon-alpha therapy in children with malignant diseases: Clinical experience in twenty-four patients treated in a single pediatric oncology unit. Med Pediatr Oncol 2002;39:115 [PMID: 12116059].

Kusumakumary P, James FU: Permanent disabilities in childhood survivors of Langerhans' cell histiocytosis. Pediatr Hematol Oncol 2000;17:375 [PMID: 10914047].

Rodriquez-Galindo C et al: Treatment of children with Langerhans cell histiocytosis with 2-chlorodeoxyadenosine. Am J Hematol 2002;69:179 [PMID: 11891804].

Titgemeyer C et al: Pattern and course of single-system disease in Langerhans cell histiocytosis data from the DAL-HX 83- and 90 study. Med Pediatr Oncol 2001;37:108 [PMID: 11496348].

# ■ HEMATOPOIETIC STEM CELL TRANSPLANTATION

*Douglas K. Graham, MD, PhD, Roger H. Giller, MD, & Ralph R. Quinones, MD*

Hematopoietic stem cell transplantation (HSCT), often referred to as bone marrow transplantation, involves the intravenous infusion of hematopoietic stem cells to reestablish normal hematopoiesis following marrow ablative or subablative chemotherapy or radiation therapy. The first successful human HSCTs were performed in the 1960s in ALL patients who received supralethal total body irradiation (TBI). The technology associated with HSCT subsequently has been expanded to include transplants that are either autologous (infusion of the patient's own hematopoietic stem cells) or allogeneic (infusion of another individual's hematopoietic stem cells). Different hematopoietic stem cell sources for stem cell transplantation include bone marrow, peripheral blood, and umbilical cord blood.

Advantages of peripheral and umbilical cord blood have led to increased use of these stem cell sources in recent years. Peripheral blood progenitor cells offer more rapid hematologic recovery and less supportive care after transplantation than HSCTs. One drawback of this stem cell source in allogeneic HSCT may be heightened risk of graft versus host disease (GVHD). Umbilical cord blood provides an easily accessible, rich supply of hematopoietic stem cell precursors. Use of cord blood at times can be restricted due to limited cell doses available for large adolescent and adult patients. Registries of bone marrow and umbilical cord blood from unrelated individuals catalogue several million potential donors worldwide for patients who lack suitably matched allogeneic family member donors.

HSCT is now considered standard therapy for a variety of malignancies, hematopoietic disorders (aplastic anemia, hemoglobinopathies), storage diseases, and severe immunodeficiencies. Pediatric malignancies that are candidates for HSCT include ALL, AML, CML, juvenile myelomonocytic leukemia, Hodgkin disease and non-Hodgkin lymphoma, brain tumors, NB, and other solid tumors. In many of these instances, transplantation is recommended only in high-risk situations or when conventional treatment fails. For example, HSCT has been used in sickle cell patients with a history of stroke, recurrent acute chest syndrome, or recurrent painful crises. AML patients or ALL patients who have high-risk cytogenetic features such as monosomy 7 or the Philadelphia chromosome [t(9;22)] may be candidates for transplantation in the first clinical remission. In illnesses such as JMML, HSCT is used as primary therapy since no other curative treatment exists.

The rationale for HSCT in oncologic disorders is that much higher dose chemotherapy, often in combination with myeloablative TBI, may overcome cancer cell resistance and achieve optimal tumor cell kill. This strategy is feasible because marrow toxicity from high-dose chemotherapy is circumvented by hematopoietic rescue. In allogeneic HSCT, an additional benefit of graft versus tumor effect may occur in which the donor hematopoietic cells attack the noncompatible antigens in the malignant cells of the recipient. In patients with nonmalignant hematopoietic disorders or immunodeficiencies, HSCTs allow for replacement of defective hematopoietic or lymphoid cells. Patients with storage diseases such as Hurler disease receive HSCT to provide enzyme-making donor macrophages to populate host tissues.

A major challenge in performing allogeneic transplants is finding a closely HLA-matched sibling or unrelated donor. Also, sufficient host immunosuppression must be achieved to prevent allograft rejection and postengraftment GVHD. The primary obstacle in autologous transplantation is collecting sufficient hematopoietic progenitor cells that are not contaminated by tumor cells. Hematopoietic stem cells can be identified within the mononuclear cell subset by the CD34 cell surface marker. Anti-CD34 monoclonal antibodies are sometimes used to positively select and thus enrich the stem cell population. In addition, purging of tumor cells (negative selection) can be achieved by several methods, including pharmacologic agents, monoclonal antibodies, or cell culture techniques. Despite these advances, relapse of the original disease has been the greatest obstacle in autologous transplantation.

The selection of the most suitable donor for allogeneic transplant is critical since degree of compatibility is inversely correlated with risk for graft rejection and GVHD. The primary genes known to encode for allogeneic recognition reside within the major histocompatibility complex (MHC) located on chromosome 6. The MHC class I antigens include HLA-A, HLA-B, and HLA-C, and the important class II antigens include HLA-DR and HLA-DQ. Both class I and II antigens can mediate graft rejection or GVHD. The class I and class II antigens are transmitted as dominantly inherited mendelian traits, and each child expresses one set of paternal and one set of maternal HLA antigens. Thus, the probability of one child inheriting any specific combination is 25% (ie, the chance of a perfect match for a sibling allogeneic transplant is 1 in 4). HLA typing traditionally has been based on serologic or cellular (mixed lymphocyte culture) techniques to define cell surface antigens. More recently, molecular techniques such as restriction fraction length polymorphism (RFLP) and DNA sequencing have been employed to more precisely delineate genetic alleles which affect donor–recipient compatibility.

Transplantation has four major treatment phases: preparative therapy, lymphohematopoietic rescue, supportive care, and long-term follow-up. The preparative phase is designed to be both myeloablative and antineoplastic. In the allogeneic transplant recipient, the preparative treatment also provides the necessary immunosuppression for successful donor engraftment. Preparative regimens use one or more chemotherapy drugs, often in combination with TBI.

Preliminary clinical studies have shown that engraftment of allogeneic donor stem cells can be achieved in certain settings with immunosuppressive nonmyeloablative preparative regimens that are less toxic than traditional myeloablative regimens. In nonmyeloablative transplants, subsequent donor lymphocyte infusions (DLIs) can play an important role in enhancing donor engraftment and immune-mediated graft versus malignancy effect.

Lymphohematopoietic rescue is accomplished by the intravenous infusion of bone marrow, peripheral blood progenitor cells, or umbilical cord blood. Graft failure after allogeneic transplant is rare in patients receiving stem cells from genotypically identical donors but may be as high as 5–15% if the donor and patient are mismatched. Marrow processing prior to infusion may include removal of contaminating RBCs if an ABO incompatibility exists. T-cell depletion of the allograft is sometimes employed to reduce the risk of GVHD. In autologous transplant, tumor purging or stem cell enrichment procedures can be performed for selected indications.

Supportive care in the initial months after transplant includes transfusions of RBCs and platelets and infec-

tion prophylaxis and treatment. GVHD prophylaxis is necessary in allogeneic transplants. All blood products should be leukocyte-depleted to reduce the risk of CMV transmission. Some institutions also use CMV seronegative blood to help prevent CMV infection in selected patients. In addition, blood products are irradiated to prevent GVHD from any contaminating lymphocytes that remain in blood products. Successful engraftment usually occurs about 10–28 days following transplant. Peripheral blood stem cell transplant patients usually recover neutrophil counts earlier than patients receiving bone marrow or cord blood transplants. Platelet recovery generally occurs 6 or more weeks after HSCT. Hematopoietic growth factors such as granulocyte colony-stimulating factor or granulocyte/macrophage colony-stimulating factor may be used to hasten myeloid recovery.

The post-transplantation period can be complicated by bacterial, viral, fungal, and protozoal infections. Certain infections are typically seen at different time intervals after the transplant. The post-transplant period can be divided into an early phase (0–1 month), an intermediate phase (1–6 months), and a late phase (6–12 months) with respect to infectious risks. During the early phase when profound neutropenia and mucosal disruption occur, gram-negative and gram-positive bacteria from the patient's own aerodigestive tract flora are common culprits in bacteremia. Empiric antibiotic coverage and intravenous γ-globulin decrease the risk of gram-negative sepsis immediately following transplant. The presence of central venous catheters makes antibiotic coverage against gram-positive bacteria an important consideration in infection management. Reactivation of herpes simplex virus may occur in as many as 70% of seropositive patients due to the mucosal disruption and profound lymphopenia; thus, acyclovir prophylaxis is commonly employed. Fungal infections, particularly with *Candida* and *Aspergillus,* have made antifungal prophylaxis routine. In the intermediate post-HSCT phase (1–6 months after transplant), the patient often has reduced T-lymphocyte numbers and abnormal T-cell function and thus is susceptible to viral infections, including those from CMV, adenovirus, and respiratory syncytial virus. Prophylactic administration of acyclovir or ganciclovir helps reduce CMV and other herpesvirus (herpes simplex virus, varicella-zoster virus) infections in this post-transplant period. Protozoan infections such as *Pneumocystis jiroveci* pneumonia are also a risk in this intermediate phase. HSCT patients receive trimethoprim–sulfamethoxazole, dapsone, or pentamidine as prophylaxis against *Pneumocystis.* The late phase, 6–12 months after transplant, is characterized by infections from encapsulated bacteria such as *Pneumococcus* due to dysfunction of the reticuloendothelial system. Reactivation of varicella-zoster virus as shingles is also common. Patients on prolonged immunosuppressive treatment for chronic GVHD have increased and protracted risk of infections.

Despite the use of immunosuppressive agents, anti–T-cell antibodies, and T-cell depletion of the donor graft, approximately 20–70% of allogeneic HSCT patients experience some degree of acute GVHD. Factors influencing GVHD risk include the degree of HLA match, stem cell source, patient age, and donor sex. Acute GVHD occurs within the first 100 days after transplant. The first manifestation typically is a maculopapular skin rash. Skin biopsies reveal epidermal basal cell vacuolization and apoptosis as well as lymphoid infiltration. Intestinal involvement results in secretory diarrhea, and hepatic involvement leads to cholestatic jaundice. Chronic GVHD occurs after day 100 and may involve multiple organ systems. Sclerotic skin, malabsorption, progressive weight loss, keratoconjunctivitis sicca, oral muscositis, chronic lung disease, and cholestatic jaundice are common manifestations. Pathologic changes of the skin include fibrosis. Treatment for GVHD consists of further use of immunosuppressive agents.

Long-term follow-up of HSCT patients is essential. Patients are at risk for numerous complications, including pulmonary disease, cataracts, endocrine dysfunction affecting growth and fertility, cardiac dysfunction, avascular necrosis of bone, developmental delay, and secondary malignancies. Although HSCT has many challenges, it represents an important advance in curative treatment for a variety of serious pediatric illnesses.

Barker JN et al: Umbilical cord blood transplantation: Current state of the art. Curr Opin Oncol 2002;14:160 [PMID: 11880705].

Guinan EC et al: Principles of bone marrow and stem cell transplantation. In *Nathan and Oski's Hematology of Infancy and Childhood.* Nathan DG, Orkin SH (eds). WB Saunders, 2003.

Sanders JE: Bone marrow transplantation in pediatric oncology. In *Principles and Practice of Pediatric Oncology.* Pizzo PA, Poplack DG (eds). Lippincott Williams & Wilkins, 2002.

# ■ LATE EFFECTS OF PEDIATRIC CANCER THERAPY

Late effects of treatment by surgery, radiation, and chemotherapy have been identified in survivors of pediatric cancer. Current estimates are that 1 in every 900 adults younger than age 45 years is a pediatric cancer survivor. In some studies, up to 60% of survivors of pediatric cancer will have some disability secondary to treatment. Virtually any organ system can demonstrate sequelae related to previous cancer therapy. This has necessitated the creation of specialized oncology clinics whose function it is to identify and provide treatment to these patients.

The Childhood Cancer Survivor Study, a pediatric multi-institutional collaborative project, was designed to investigate the various aspects of late effects of pediatric cancer therapy in a cohort of over 14,000 survivors of childhood cancer.

## GROWTH COMPLICATIONS

Children who have received cranial irradiation are at highest risk of developing growth complications. Growth complications of cancer therapy in the pediatric survivor are generally secondary to direct damage to the pituitary gland, resulting in growth hormone deficiency. However, new evidence in children treated for ALL suggests that chemotherapy alone may result in an attenuation of linear growth without evidence of catch-up growth once therapy is discontinued. Up to 90% of patients who receive greater than 30 Gy of radiation to the CNS will show evidence of growth hormone deficiency within 2 years. Approximately 50% of children receiving 24 Gy will have growth hormone problems. The effects of cranial radiation appear to be age-related, with children younger than age 5 years at the time of therapy being particularly vulnerable. These patients usually benefit from growth hormone therapy. There is currently no evidence that such therapy causes a recurrence of cancer.

Spinal radiation inhibits vertebral body growth. In 30% of such individuals, standing heights may be less than the fifth percentile. Asymmetrical exposure of the spine to radiation may result in scoliosis.

Growth should be monitored closely, particularly in young survivors of childhood cancer. Follow-up studies should include height, weight, growth velocity, scoliosis examination, and, when indicated, growth hormone testing.

## ENDOCRINE COMPLICATIONS

Thyroid dysfunction, manifesting as hypothyroidism, is common in children who received TBI, cranial radiation, or local radiation therapy to the neck. Particularly at risk are children with brain tumors who received more than 3000 cGy and those who received more than 4000 cGy to the neck region. The average time to develop thyroid dysfunction is 12 months after exposure, but the range is wide. Therefore, individuals at risk should be monitored yearly for at least 7 years from the completion of therapy. Although signs and symptoms of hypothyroidism may be present, most patients will have a normal thyroxine level with an elevated thyroid-stimulating hormone level. These individuals should be given thyroid hormone replacement because persistent stimulation of the thyroid from an elevated thyroid-stimulating hormone level may predispose to thyroid nodules and carcinomas. In a recent report from the Childhood Cancer Survivor Study, thyroid cancer occurred at 18 times the expected rate for the general population in pediatric cancer survivors who received radiation to the neck region. Hyperthyroidism, although rare, also occurs in patients who have received neck irradiation.

Precocious puberty, delayed puberty, and infertility are all potential consequences of cancer therapy. Precocious puberty, more common in girls, is usually a result of cranial irradiation causing premature activation of the hypothalamic–pituitary axis. This results in premature closure of the epiphysis and decreased adult height. Luteinizing hormone analogue and growth hormone are used to halt early puberty and facilitate continued growth.

Gonadal dysfunction in males is usually the result of radiation to the testes. Patients who receive testicular radiation as part of their therapy for ALL, abdominal radiation for Hodgkin disease, or TBI for HSCT are at highest risk. Radiation damages both the germinal epithelium, producing azoospermia, and Leydig cells, causing low testosterone levels and delayed puberty. Alkylating agents such as ifosfamide and cyclophosphamide can also interfere with male gonadal function, resulting in oligo- or azoospermia, low testosterone levels, and abnormal follicle-stimulating hormone (FSH) and luteinizing hormone (LH) levels. Determination of testicular size, semen analysis, and measurement of testosterone, FSH, and LH levels will help identify abnormalities in patients at risk. When therapy is expected to result in gonadal dysfunction, pretherapy sperm banking should be offered to adolescent males.

Exposure of the ovaries to abdominal radiation may result in delayed puberty with a resultant increase in FSH and LH and a decrease in estrogen. Girls receiving TBI as preparation for HSCT and those receiving craniospinal radiation are at particularly high risk for delayed puberty as well as premature menopause. In patients at high risk for development of gonadal complications, a detailed menstrual history should be obtained, and LH, FSH, and estrogen levels should be monitored if indicated.

No studies to date have confirmed an increased risk of spontaneous abortions, stillbirths, premature births, congenital malformations, or genetic diseases in the offspring of childhood cancer survivors. Women who have received abdominal radiation may develop uterine vascular insufficiency or fibrosis of the abdominal and pelvic musculature or uterus, and their pregnancies should be considered high-risk.

## CARDIOPULMONARY COMPLICATIONS

Pulmonary dysfunction generally manifests as pulmonary fibrosis. Therapy-related factors known to cause pulmonary toxicities include certain chemotherapeutic agents, such as bleomycin, the nitrosoureas, and busulfan, as well as lung radiation or TBI. Pulmonary toxicity due to chemotherapy is related to the total cumulative dose received. Pulmonary function tests in patients with therapy-induced toxicity show restrictive lung disease, with decreased carbon monoxide diffusion and small lung volumes. Individuals exposed to these risk factors should be counseled to refrain from smoking and to give proper notification of the treatment history if they should require general anesthesia.

Cardiac complications usually result from exposure to anthracyclines (daunorubicin, doxorubicin, mitoxantrone), which destroy myocytes and lead to inadequate myocardial growth as the child ages and eventually result in congestive heart failure. The incidence of anthracycline cardiomyopathy increases in a dose-dependent fashion. At least 5% of patients who have received a cumulative dose of more than 550 mg/m$^2$ of anthracyclines experience cardiac dysfunction. In a recent study, complications from these agents appeared 6–19 years following administration of the drugs. Pregnant women who have received anthracyclines should be followed up closely for signs and symptoms of congestive heart failure, as peripartum cardiomyopathy has been reported.

Radiation therapy to the mediastinal region, which is common as part of therapy for Hodgkin disease, has been linked to an increased risk of coronary artery disease; chronic restrictive pericarditis may also occur in these patients.

Current recommendations include an exercise echocardiogram and electrocardiogram every 1–5 years, depending on the age at therapy, total cumulative dose received, and presence or absence of mediastinal irradiation. Selective monitoring with various modalities is indicated for those who were treated with anthracyclines when they were younger than age 4 years or received more than 500 mg/m$^2$ of these drugs. Measurement of serum levels of cardiac troponin-T or atrial natriuretic peptide may be useful in assessing early cardiotoxicity of anthracyclines.

## RENAL COMPLICATIONS

Long-term renal side effects stem from therapy with cisplatin, alkylating agents (ifosfamide and cyclophosphamide), or pelvic radiation. Patients who have received cisplatin may develop abnormal creatinine clearance, which may or may not be accompanied by abnormal serum creatinine levels, as well as persistent tubular dysfunction with hypomagnesemia. Alkylating agents can cause hemorrhagic cystitis, which may continue after chemotherapy has been terminated and has been associated with the development of bladder carcinoma. Ifosfamide can also cause Fanconi syndrome, which may result in clinical rickets if adequate phosphate replacement is not provided. Pelvic radiation may result in abnormal bladder function with dribbling, frequency, and enuresis.

Patients seen in long-term follow-up who have received nephrotoxic agents should be monitored with urinalysis, appropriate electrolyte profiles, and blood pressure. Urine collection for creatinine clearance or renal ultrasound may be indicated in individuals with suspected renal toxicity.

## NEUROPSYCHOLOGICAL COMPLICATIONS

Pediatric cancer survivors who have received cranial radiation for ALL or brain tumors appear to be at greatest risk for neuropsychological sequelae. The severity of cranial radiation effects varies among individual patients and depends on the dose and dose schedule, the size and location of the radiation field, the amount of time elapsed after treatment, the child's age at therapy, and the child's gender. Girls may be more susceptible than boys to CNS toxicity because of more rapid brain growth and development during childhood.

The main effects of CNS radiation appear to be related to attention capacities, ability with nonverbal tasks and mathematics, and short-term memory. Recent studies support the association between high-dose systemic methotrexate, triple intrathecal chemotherapy, and more recently, dexamethasone with more significant cognitive impairment.

Additionally, pediatric cancer patients have been reported as having more behavior problems and as being less socially competent than a sibling control group. Adolescent survivors of cancer demonstrate an increased sense of physical fragility and vulnerability manifested as hypochondriasis or phobic behaviors.

Finally, childhood cancer survivors are more likely to report symptoms of depression and somatic distress in adulthood. Pediatric cancer survivors may require ongoing counseling or other psychological interventions once they have completed therapy.

## SECOND MALIGNANCIES

Approximately 3–12% of children receiving cancer treatment will develop a new cancer within 20 years of their first diagnosis. This is a tenfold increased incidence when compared with age-matched control subjects. Particular risk factors include exposure to alkylating agents, epipodophyllotoxins (VP-16), and radiation therapy, primary diagnosis of retinoblastoma or Hodgkin disease, or the presence of an inherited genetic susceptibility syndrome (Li– Fraumeni syndrome or NF). In a recent report, the cumulative estimated incidence of second malignant neoplasms for the cohort of the Childhood Cancer Survivor Study was 3.2% at 20 years from diagnosis.

Second hematopoietic malignancies (acute myelogenous leukemia) occur as a result of therapy with epipodophyllotoxins or alkylating agents. It is unclear whether the schedule of drug administration and the total dose are related to the development of this secondary leukemia.

Children receiving radiation therapy are at risk for developing second malignancies, such as sarcomas, carcinomas, or brain tumors, in the field of radiation. A recent report examining the incidence of second neoplasms in a cohort of pediatric Hodgkin disease patients showed the cumulative risk of a second neoplasm to be as high as 8% at 15 years from diagnosis. The most common solid tumor was breast cancer (the majority located within the radiation field) followed by thyroid cancer. Girls age 10–16 years when they received radiation were at highest risk and had an actuarial incidence that approached 35% by age 40 years.

Friedman DL, Meadows AT: Late effects of childhood cancer therapy. Pediatr Clin N Am 2002;49:1083 [PMID:12430627].

Hudson MM et al: Health status of adult long-term survivors of childhood cancer: A report from the Childhood Cancer Survivor Study. J Am Med Assoc 2003;290:1583 [PMID:14506117].

Kimball-Dalton V et al: Height and weight in children treated for acute lymphoblastic leukemia: Relationship to CNS treatment. J Clin Oncol 2003;21:2953 [PMID:12885815].

Neglia IP et al: Second malignant neoplasms in five-year survivors of childhood cancer: Childhood Cancer Survivor Study. J Natl Cancer Inst 2001;93:618 [PMID:11309438].

Poutanen T et al: Long-term prospective follow-up of cardiac function after cardiotoxic therapy for malignancy in children. J Clin Oncol 2003;21:2349 [PMID:12805337].

Reiter-Purtill J et al: A controlled longitudinal study of the social functioning of children who completed treatment of cancer. J Pediatr Hematol Oncol 2003;25:467 [PMID:12794525].

Zebrack BJ et al: Psychological outcomes in long-term survivors of childhood leukemia, Hodgkin's disease, and non-Hodgkin's lymphoma: A report from the Childhood Cancer Survivor Study. Pediatr 2002;110:42 [PMID:12093945].

# Immunodeficiency

## Anthony R. Hayward, MD, PhD

Recurrent or severe infection is the most common symptom of immunodeficiency, but most children with frequent minor infections (particularly otitis and sinusitis) do not have an immunodeficiency that is definable by currently available tests. Host defenses against infection depend mainly on excluding pathogens at surfaces and then decontaminating these mechanically. Specific and nonspecific immune mechanisms are needed only after an organism gains access to the body. Specific immunity in this context consists of antibody- and cell-mediated immunity (CMI). Nonspecific immune mechanisms include mechanical barriers, complement, antibacterial peptides, phagocytes, and natural killer cells. Nonspecific mechanisms may be guided by specific responses, as when antibody directs killing by natural killer cells or promotes phagocytosis by opsonizing bacteria.

Before investigating a patient for a defined primary immunodeficiency (most of which are rare), one should exclude the more common conditions that increase local susceptibility to infection, such as allergic rhinitis (causing sinusitis), cystic fibrosis, and asthma as causing pneumonia and conditions that interfere with the integrity of the skin or the normal flora of mucous membranes (Table 29–1). Common causes of secondary immunodeficiency (human immunodeficiency virus [HIV] infection, malnutrition, drugs, protein loss) must also be excluded.

Chapel H et al: Primary immunodeficiency diseases: An update. Clin Exp Immunol 2003;132:9 [PMID: 12653830]

## ■ NONSPECIFIC FACTORS IN RESISTANCE TO INFECTION

### DEFECTS OF COMPLEMENT

Complement proteins are activated by certain lectins and bacterial proteins and also by surface-bound IgG or IgM antibodies. The split products of C3 and C5 activation attract neutrophils, and bound C3b opsonizes bacteria for phagocytosis by neutrophils. Deficiencies of individual classic pathway factors (C1–C9) occur as autosomal recessive traits and are rare. Deficiencies of fac-

tors 1q, 4, and 2 are associated with a 90, 75, and 20% risk of developing systemic lupus erythematosus, respectively. Chronic glomerulonephritis, dermatomyositis, and cutaneous vasculitis are also more common. Primary deficiency of C3 interferes with the opsonization of bacteria by the classic and alternative pathways of complement activation and results in recurrent bacterial infections. Deficiency of properdin (an alternative pathway factor) may also occasionally predispose to meningococcal infection. C5, C6, C7, C8, and C9 deficiencies are associated with dissemination of neisserial infections, increasing the risks for arthritis. Survivors of meningococcal meningitis should probably have their complement function screened with a hemolytic assay.

Colten HR: Navigating the maze of complement genetics: A guide for clinicians. Curr Allergy Asthma Rep 2002;2:379 [PMID: 12165203].

Walport MJ: Complement. First of two parts. N Engl J Med 2001;344:1058 [PMID: 11287977].

Walport MJ: Complement. Second of two parts. New Engl J Med 2001;344:1140 [PMID: 11297706].

Complement-activating lectins include mannan-binding lectin (MBL). About 7% of the population has MBL alleles associated with reduced function. Allelic variants in MBL have recently been associated with susceptibility to meningococcal meningitis. Susceptibility to other infections in infants with low MBL levels seems to decrease with age.

Ezekowitz RA: Role of the mannose-binding lectin in innate immunity. J Infect Dis 2003;187(Suppl 2):S335 [PMID: 12792848].

Hibberd ML et al: Association of variants of the gene for mannose-binding lectin with susceptibility to meningococcal disease: Meningococcal Research Group. Lancet 1999;353:1049 [PMID: 10199352].

Hereditary angioedema is a rare disorder that results from C1 esterase inhibitor deficiency in which susceptibility to infection is not increased. Transmission is autosomal dominant, and an acquired form associated with angiotensin-converting enzyme inhibitor treatment is being recognized more frequently. Persons with this disorder typically have recurrent episodes of edema lasting 48–72 hours and affecting the face or a limb.

**Table 29–1.** Host defense mechanisms and examples of nonspecific defects.

| Protection by | Defect |
|---|---|
| Intact skin | Burns, eczema, sinus tracks, indwelling catheters |
| Drainage | Auditory tube obstruction, cystic fibrosis, foreign body, urinary obstruction |
| Normal flora | Overgrowth of antibiotic-resistant organisms causing candidiasis or diarrhea |

Edema affecting the bowel can be very painful. Laryngeal edema is life-threatening and occurs in over 40% of patients. The diagnosis is suggested by decreased activity of whole complement, C4, and C2 and confirmed by direct assay of the C1 inhibitor. Symptomatic subjects have levels below 30%. The synthetic androgen danazol (50–200 mg/d) prevents attacks by increasing C1 inhibitor levels. C1-inhibitor concentrate is useful for the emergency treatment of acute edema. Liver tumors are a risk after many years of danazol treatment. Defects in other innate immune systems can cause autoinflammatory syndromes. Familial Mediterranean fever results from mutations in the pyrin protein gene and is characterized by episodes of fever and abdominal pain. Onset is generally in childhood, but substantial phenotypic variations occur, with the most severe forms leading to renal failure from amyloidosis in the teens. Related conditions and their pathogenesis likely result from failure to control the activation of inflammatory mediators such as interleukin-1 (IL-1). Mutations in cryopyrin causes a familial cold autoinflammatory syndrome.

Bork K et al: Clinical studies of sudden upper airway obstruction in patients with hereditary angioedema due to C1 esterase inhibitor deficiency. Arch Int Med 2003;163:1229 [PMID: 12767961].

## CELLULAR DEFECTS

Defects of neutrophil function comprise adhesion defects, chemotaxis defects, and defects of bacterial killing. They are summarized here in the context of the investigation of a child with recurrent infections and are fully described in Chapter 27. Patients with leukocyte adhesion defects present with infections ranging from progressive periumbilical necrosis with onset in infancy to recurrent surface infections starting in adult life. The severity of the clinical picture depends on the underlying defect. The infections are caused by a range of organisms and, although the neutrophil count is normal or high, relatively little pus is present. In childhood, the infections are often around body orifices, but they also involve the skin, esophagus, and respiratory tract. Death in childhood is common. Other patients with a milder phenotype have survived for 20 or more years. Diagnosis is by phenotyping blood mononuclear cells for LFA-1 or Mac-1; this approach can also be used for antenatal diagnosis. Chédiak–Higashi syndrome is caused by mutations of a lysosomal trafficking gene. The cells of affected individuals have giant lysosomes, impairing chemotaxis by neutrophils and interfering with the stimulation of T cells by lymphocytes and monocytes. Abnormal pigment handling gives a characteristic partial oculocutaneous albinism. Progressive local infections (without much pus formation) occur. Later the incidence of lymphoproliferative disease is high. Most other chemotaxis defects are probably secondary. A wide variety of other conditions also can be associated with depressed motility of phagocytic cells: burns; infections such as HIV, rubella, and influenza; metabolic and nutritional disorders, including diabetes mellitus; the hypophosphatemia associated with intravenous alimentation; and uremia. The association of impaired neutrophil chemotaxis with hyperimmunoglobulinemia E (IgE levels are usually > 2000 units/mL), recurrent staphylococcal abscesses of the skin, eczema, and otitis media is clinically recognizable and sometimes called Job syndrome. These patients can have impaired CMI, and the disorder also occurs in some patients with acquired immunodeficiency syndrome (AIDS). Treatment is symptomatic. Patients with bacterial killing defects (eg, chronic granulomatous disease) usually have staphylococcal infections in the first months of life and develop groin, cervical, or axillary abscesses requiring incision and drainage. Sometimes they are infected by *Serratia* or *Nocardia* species. The infections cause high neutrophil counts and fever and sometimes spread to cause osteomyelitis or lung or liver abscesses. Colitis, leading to diarrhea and slow growth, is common. The abscesses require drainage and appropriate antibiotics for lengthy courses (3 weeks or more). As underlying tissues become damaged, fungal and *Pseudomonas cepacia* infections become increasingly common. Neutrophil granule deficiency predisposes to recurrent pyogenic infections similar to chronic granulomatous disease. This defect is recognized by microscopy, and the molecular basis has recently been defined.

Neutropenia in the warts, hypogammaglobulinemia, and immunodeficiency (WHIM) syndrome occurs until infections stimulate the release of neutrophils from the marrow, so the response to antibiotics is good. Numbers of blood T and B cells vary: at least some of these patients have mutations of the *CXCR4* chemokine receptor gene that seem likely to contribute to their susceptibility to papillomavirus infections. Defects of monocyte–macrophage function occur in lysosomal storage diseases, but infections are only a minor component of their symptomatology. Natural killer (NK) cell defects are most commonly associated with severe herpesvirus infections such as the EBV-induced hemophagocytic lymphohistiocytosis (HLH) in Chédiak–Higashi and Griscelli syndromes. Disorders of granule traffic are responsible for some of these defects while defects in perforin or granzyme also impair NK cell function. A familial variety of HLH is now being reported, resulting from lack of NK cell surface receptors for IgG. Symptoms result from infection, most notably herpesvirus infections. About 20% of familial HLH cases result from deficiency of perforin—a pore-forming protein used by NK cells. Rarer are defects in the *SH2DIA* gene that cause the X-linked lymphoproliferative syndrome [q.v.]. The lymphohemophagocytic component is the result of cytokine secretion by T cells that undergo uncontrolled activation. Immunosuppression followed by bone marrow transplantation (BMT) using nonmyeloablative conditioning regimens may prove the best treatment for severe cellular defects. At least in chronic granulomatous disease, transplant treatment is easier before systemic fungal infections develop.

Hernandez PA et al: Mutations in the chemokine receptor CXCR4 are associated with the WHIM syndrome, a combined immunodeficiency disease. Nat Genet 2003;34:70 [PMID: 12692554].

Horwitz ME: Stem-cell transplantation for inherited immunodeficiency disorders. Pediatr Clin North Am 2000;47:1371 [PMID: 11131001].

Karim MA et al: Apparent genotype-phenotype correlation in childhood, adolescent, and adult Chédiak–Higashi syndrome. Am J Med Genet 2002;108:16 [PMID: 11857544].

# ■ DEFICIENCIES OF SPECIFIC IMMUNITY

Defects of specific immunity are broadly subdivided into those affecting predominantly antibody formation, those affecting cellular immunity, and those in which both mechanisms are impaired. The classification in Table 29–2 is based on combinations of clinical and laboratory results and includes only the most common of the 80 or so primary immunodeficiencies now known. Enormous advances are being made in identifying the mechanisms of immunodeficiencies with simple mendelian inheritance. Linkages are being mapped for some multifactorial conditions (common variable immunodeficiency, selective IgA deficiency).

**Table 29–2.** Classification of defects of specific immunity.

| | |
|---|---|
| Deficiency of immunoglobulin | Deficiency of all Igs = hypogammaglobulinemia<br>Congenital (sometimes with high IgM)<br>Acquired<br>Unclassified (common variable hypogammaglobulinemia)<br>Selective immunoglobulin deficiency<br>IgA deficiency<br>IgG subclass deficiencies<br>IgM deficiency<br>Antibody deficiency with immunoglobulins |
| Deficiency of cell-mediated immunity | Purine nucleoside phosphorylase<br>DiGeorge syndrome<br>Cartilage-hair hypoplasia<br>Unclassified (common variable immunodeficiency affecting cell-mediated immunity) |
| Deficiency of both antibody- and cell-mediated immunity | Severe combined immunodeficiency (various types)<br>Ataxia–telangiectasia<br>Wiskott–Aldrich syndrome |

Bonilla FA, Geha RS: Primary immunodeficiency diseases. J Allergy Clin Immunol 2003;111:S571 [PMID: 12592303].

Fischer A: Human primary immunodeficiency diseases: A perspective. Nat Immunol 2004;5:23 [PMID: 14699405].

Vihinen M et al: Primary immunodeficiency mutation databases. Adv Genet 2001;43:103 [PMID: 11037300].

# IMMUNOGLOBULIN & ANTIBODY DEFICIENCY SYNDROMES

## 1. Hypogammaglobulinemia Syndromes

Patients who do not make antibodies have low (hypogammaglobulinemia) or absent (agammaglobulinemia) levels of all immunoglobulin isotypes (IgG, IgA, IgM, IgE). They usually present with recurrent or severe bacterial infection of the respiratory tract (sinusitis, otitis, pneumonia) or skin (cellulitis, abscesses). Without antibiotic treatment, these infections tend to spread to cause septicemia and meningitis. There are several types of hypogammaglobulinemia (see Table 29–2), and in the congenital X-linked agammaglobulinemia infections usually start after age 4 months, when passively acquired maternal IgG levels have declined. *Haemophilus influenzae* and *Streptococcus pneumoniae* cause most of the infections, but following courses of antibiotics, deep tissue infections by *Mycoplasma* family members such as *Ureaplasma* become important. Inflammatory arthritis or persistent cellulitis may be due to opportunists such as *Helicobacter cinaedi* and *Flexispira rappini* that are difficult or impossible to culture and difficult to treat. Antibody-deficient patients have had severe infections with enteroviruses, particularly vaccine strains of poliovirus and echovirus 11. Although polioviruses typically caused paralysis, the echoviruses often caused a chronic encephalitis, optic atrophy, or convulsions. Intravenous replacement of IgG provides subjects with some protection because higher IgG levels are achieved. Active enteroviral infections are generally treated with pleconaril. Some boys have asymmetrical arthritis, mostly of the knee or ankle, at the time of diagnosis, which may resolve after adequate IgG replacement. These patients typically have little or no tonsillar and adenoidal tissue. The severity of infections varies, so the diagnosis may not be made for many years. Congenital X-linked agammaglobulinemia occurs in about 1:200,000 male births and results from mutations in the B-cell tyrosine kinase gene (*btk*). Patients have few if any B cells in their blood, though they have normal blood lymphocyte counts. Almost all have very low to undetectable levels of IgG, IgA, and IgM in blood. Molecular diagnosis and carrier detection are available. Occasional patients have impaired growth hormone production. Autosomal recessive congenital agammaglobulinemia is rare: the commonest result from defects of the μ heavy-chain gene, and these patients tend to have an earlier onset of infections and complications than the *btk*-deficient boys. Acquired types of hypogammaglobulinemia are more common and may develop at any age. The diagnosis of hypogammaglobulinemia is based on low serum immunoglobulin levels for age with absence of serum isohemagglutinins and of antibody response to immunization. Blood B cells should be measured to identify the subset of patients for whom a gene defect results in failure of B-cell production. Causes of secondary hypogammaglobulinemia (nephrotic syndrome, HIV infection, and protein-losing enteropathy) should be excluded by measuring serum albumin. Morphologic disorders or associated syndromes (as with the recently described primary antibody deficiency with spondyloepiphyseal and retinal dystrophy) may point to a specific diagnosis.

Conley ME: Early defects in B cell development. Curr Opin Allergy Clin Immunol 2002;2:517 [PMID: 14752335].

Lopez Granados E et al: Clinical and molecular analysis of patients with defects in μ heavy chain gene. J Clin Invest 2002;110:1029 [PMID: 12370281].

Roifman CM: Antibody deficiency, growth retardation, spondyloepiphyseal dysplasia and retinal dystrophy: A novel syndrome. Clin Genet 1999;55:103 [PMID: 10189087].

X-linked immunodeficiency with hyper-IgM (HIGM1) occurs in fewer than $1:10^6$ male births. Affected boys have low IgG and IgA levels. Their IgM levels may start in the normal range but can rise to 1000 mg/dL or more. In addition to infections, these children often have lymphadenopathy and episodes of autoimmune neutropenia. The disease results from mutation in the CD40 ligand gene so that the patient's T cells are unable to switch their B cells from making IgM to making IgG and IgA. CMI is also impaired, so these patients have *Pneumocystis jiroveci* (formerly *Pneumocystis carinii*) infections, cryptosporidiosis of the biliary tree and intestine, sclerosing cholangitis, and a high incidence of biliary tract carcinomas. The fraction of patients surviving beyond 25 years is so low that treatment by BMT is increasingly used. Children with autosomal recessive forms of hyper-IgM immunodeficiency have normal expression of CD40L and mutations in an activation-induced cytidine deaminase.

McLauchlin J et al: Polymerase chain reaction-based diagnosis of infection with *Cryptosporidium* in children with primary immunodeficiencies. Pediatr Infect Dis J 2003;22:329 [PMID: 11124791].

Notarangelo LD, Hayward AR: X-linked immunodeficiency with hyper-IgM (XHIM). Clin Exp Immunol 2000;120:399 [PMID: 10844515].

Quartier P et al: Clinical, immunologic and genetic analysis of 29 patients with autosomal recessive hyper-IgM syndrome due to Activation-Induced Cytidine Deaminase deficiency. Clin Immunol 2004;110:22 [PMID: 14962793].

Winkelstein JA et al: The X-linked hyper-IgM syndrome: Clinical and immunologic features of 79 patients. Medicine (Baltimore) 2003;82:373 [PMID: 14663287].

## Common Variable Immunodeficiency Syndromes

Patients with congenital or acquired antibody deficiency syndromes not classified elsewhere are often included in the group called common variable immunodeficiency syndromes (CVID), and they outnumber patients with all other types of antibody deficiency. Onset of the immunodeficiency may be at any age, and in populations of European heritage the incidence approaches 1:25,000. Susceptibility to common variable immunodeficiency and selective IgA deficiency is inherited and associated with certain HL-DR/DQ alleles, but the factors that precipitate expression of common variable immunodeficiency in susceptible individuals are unknown. The association with HLA-DR/DQ suggests an underlying autoimmune cause for CVID. Patients usually have B cells in their blood, but these do not differentiate normally. Infections follow the patterns described for other types of antibody deficiency, and lung damage leading to bronchiectasis in adult life is common. Some patients have remarkably few infections despite long-standing very low immunoglobulin levels. The laboratory findings vary. Low levels of one or more immunoglobulin classes are associated with different degrees of impairment of T-cell proliferative responses. Autoantibody formation, raised IgE levels, and positive immediate hypersensitivity skin reactions occur, as do neutropenia and thrombocytopenia. Patients with hypogammaglobulinemia, facial dysmorphism, mental retardation, or hypertelorism may have the immunodeficiency-chromosome instability-facial anomaly (ICF) syndrome that most commonly results from mutations in DNA methyltransferase 3B at 20q11.2. Their rather variable immunodeficiency most commonly comprises low IgA, and inheritance is autosomal recessive. Abnormal serum immunoglobulins occur also in the hypohidrotic or anhidrotic ectodermal dysplasia syndromes that result from abnormal signaling through the NF-κB molecule.

Doffinger R et al: X-linked anhidrotic ectodermal dysplasia with immunodeficiency is caused by impaired NF-kappaB signaling. Nat Genet 2000;27:277 [PMID: 11242109].

Kralovicova J et al: Fine-scale mapping at IGAD1 and genome-wide genetic linkage analysis implicate HLA-DQ/DR as a major susceptibility locus in selective IgA deficiency and common variable immunodeficiency. J Immunol 2003;170:2765 [PMID: 12594308].

Martinez-Garcia MA et al: Respiratory disorders in common variable immunodeficiency. Respir Med 2001;95:191 [PMID: 11266236].

Strober W, Chua K: Common variable immunodeficiency. Clin Rev Allergy Immunol 2000;19:157 [PMID: 11107500].

Wijmenga C et al: Genetic variation in ICF syndrome: Evidence for genetic heterogeneity. Hum Mutat 2000;16:509 [PMID: 11102980].

## Complications of Hypogammaglobulinemia

Many CVID patients have B-cell hyperplasia in the gut. About 10% of patients develop diarrhea and malabsorption that may be severe enough to resemble Crohn disease. Infection is the likeliest cause of the diarrhea, and efforts should be made to exclude treatable agents such as *Giardia lamblia* or *Cryptosporidium*. In adult life, the patients often develop gastric atrophy with achlorhydria, sometimes followed by pernicious anemia. Affected boys occasionally develop optic atrophy or ataxia, evolving slowly or rapidly into fatal encephalitis. Echoviruses have sometimes been isolated from their cerebrospinal fluid or brains at biopsy or autopsy. A smaller proportion develop a dermatomyositis-like syndrome, with prominent peripheral cyanosis and myopathy but little heliotrope coloration. It is thought that both of these complications are seen less com-

monly now that much higher immunoglobulin replacements are given. An increased rate of cancer in patients with antibody deficiency has been reported. The association is predominantly with lymphoreticular proliferation and may sometimes result from Epstein–Barr virus (EBV) infection. Lymphoreticular proliferations in hypogammaglobulinemic patients are not always malignant. The incidence of hepatitis C and G virus carriage is increased, owing in part to the presence of hepatitis C virus in batches of intravenous IgG through 1995. Patients should have their aminotransferase levels checked, and, if necessary, they should be tested for hepatitis C virus antigenemia. Many infected children fail to clear the virus, and about 25% progress to liver failure. The risk of hepatitis C virus has been virtually eliminated since more stringent viral inactivation steps have been introduced (eg, solvent detergent).

Bjoro K et al: The spectrum of hepatobiliary disease in primary hypogammaglobulinaemia. J Intern Med 1999;245:517 [PMID: 10363753].

Chapel HM et al: Five-year follow-up of patients with primary antibody deficiencies following an outbreak of acute hepatitis C. Clin Immunol 2001;99:320 [PMID: 11358426].

## Treatment of Hypogammaglobulinemia

Patients with hypogammaglobulinemia should have serum IgG replaced to protect against infection. IgG is usually given by intravenous infusions of specially prepared deaggregated IgG (200–600 mg/kg every 4 weeks). If intravenous treatment is very difficult in young children, they may be temporarily treated with intramuscular injections of IgG concentrate (0.6 mL/kg every 2–3 weeks). Some adults are treated more cheaply with subcutaneous infusions of the intramuscular IgG preparation, given overnight on several nights per week. The aim of treatment must be to avoid—or minimize progression of—chronic lung disease (bronchitis, bronchiectasis). Productive cough and purulent sputum or conjunctivitis must be taken seriously, and antibiotics given until radiologic and clinical resolution occur. *Mycoplasma* infections of the respiratory or urinary tract should be sought and treated with doxycycline or other appropriate antibiotics. Minor reactions to immunoglobulin infusions or injections are common, especially with the initial infusion. They include headache, back and limb pain, anxiety, and tightness of the chest. Signs are tachycardia, shivering, fever, and, in severe cases, shock. Reactions are frequent in some patients and rare in others; their occurrence is sporadic and not generally due to hypersensitivity (anti-IgA reactions may be an exception but are rare). Skin tests are not helpful. When indicated, immunoglobulin replacement should be maintained for life, and the severity of the reactions limited by premedication with acetaminophen, an antihistamine, or intravenous hydrocortisone immediately before the infusion. Alternative brands of IgG should be tried if reactions persist despite premedication. Intravenous IgG has been used extensively for inflammatory disorders ranging from asthma to autoimmunity. When benefit results, the mechanism may involve a suppression of inflammatory cytokine production.

Minegishi Y et al: Recent progress in the diagnosis and treatment of patients with defects in early B-cell development. Curr Opin Pediatr 1999;11:528 [PMID: 10590911].

Schwartz SA: Intravenous immunoglobulin treatment of immunodeficiency. Pediatr Clin North Am 2000;47:1355 [PMID: 11131000].

## 2. Other Types of Hypogammaglobulinemia

### Transient Hypogammaglobulinemia

Infants' IgG levels fall during the first 4–5 months of life, as maternal IgG is diluted and catabolized. The physiologic trough that occurs before the infant's IgG production attains adult levels is accentuated in premature and dysmature infants. IgG levels of 250–300 mg/dL lie within 2 standard deviations of the mean at age 3–4 months, and the diagnosis of transient hypogammaglobulinemia is often made in infants with infections and IgG levels in this range. Immunoglobulin levels should return to normal by age 30 months, and the diagnosis can only be made retrospectively. The only diagnostic laboratory findings are low IgG—with or without low IgA and IgM—and subsequent return to normal levels. Salivary IgA is generally detectable, and, despite the low immunoglobulin levels, antibody activity (isohemagglutinin or antidiphtheria or tetanus antibody) is present in serum. IgG antibody is generally made following immunization, and tests for cellular immunity are normal. Usually no treatment is required, other than appropriate antibiotics for bacterial infections, for infants who make antibody following immunization. Infants with severe infection and hypogammaglobulinemia could rationally be given IgG injections, since maternal antibody to the infecting organism will be rapidly depleted, but this is rarely necessary. The prognosis for affected infants is excellent provided they do not succumb to infection before normal immunity is achieved.

Kowalczyk D et al: Intracellular cytokine production by Th1/Th2 lymphocytes and monocytes of children with symptomatic transient hypogammaglobulinaemia of infancy (THI) and selective IgA deficiency (SIgAD). Clin Exp Immunol 2002;127:507 [PMID: 11966768].

## IgA Deficiency

This disorder, defined by a serum IgA less than 5 mg/dL, occurs in about 1:800 people of European heritage, making it the most common defect of specific immunity. Serum IgM and IgG are normal, as is IgG antibody production and CMI. Susceptibility is linked to the same HLA-DR/DQ alleles as common variable immunodeficiency (q.v.). Fifty percent or more of IgA-deficient subjects have no symptoms arising from the deficiency, perhaps because they can protect their mucosa adequately with IgG and IgM antibodies. Failure of antibody responses in the IgG4 and IgG2 subclasses is reported in many symptomatic patients, but there is no simple relationship with IgA levels. When symptoms are present, they are predominantly upper respiratory tract infections or diarrhea. There are also strong associations with inflammatory bowel disease, allergy (mainly respiratory and gut), and autoimmune disorders (thyroiditis, arthritis, vitiligo, thrombocytopenia, and diabetes). The selective lack of IgA antibody responses and the presence of normal antibody responses in other immunoglobulin classes distinguish IgA deficiency from unclassified variable immunodeficiency. IgA has a short half-life in serum, and replacement is impractical. It is conceivable but unproved that colostrum feeding could modify severe gut symptoms. Symptomatic IgA-deficient subjects who are also IgG2-deficient have sometimes been treated with IgG replacement. This approach has been both advocated and condemned on theoretical grounds but without controlled data to support the theories. A subset of IgA-deficient patients make antibodies to IgA, which are an important cause of transfusion reactions. Most IgA-deficient patients manage reasonably well with antibiotics only; atopic or autoimmune symptoms should be treated conventionally.

Aittoniemi J et al: The significance of IgG subclasses and mannan-binding lectin (MBL) for susceptibility to infection in apparently healthy adults with IgA deficiency. Clin Exp Immunol 1999;116:505 [PMID: 10361242].

Sundin U et al: Induction of unresponsiveness against IgA in IgA-deficient patients on subcutaneous immunoglobulin infusion therapy. Clin Exp Immunol 1998;112:341 [PMID: 9649200].

## 3. Other Selective Subclass Deficiencies

The possibility that deficiency of an IgG subclass might predispose to recurrent upper respiratory tract infections in patients who have normal serum immunoglobulin levels is not established, and the issue is confused by the absence of any prospective studies. The IgG heavy-chain genes on chromosome 11 (grouped with IgG1 close to IgG3 and IgG2 close to IgG4) are, with rare exceptions, normal in subclass deficiencies. Normally, IgG1 comprises over 60% of total IgG and IgG2 over 10%. IgG3 accounts for about 5%, and IgG4 may be undetectable in up to 20% of healthy persons. Serum levels are age-related. When IgG1 is deficient, IgG2 and IgG3 are generally low also, giving the clinical picture of hypogammaglobulinemia. IgG1 and IgG2 contain much of the antibody to capsular polysaccharides. IgG2 (and IgG4) deficiency is also associated with IgA deficiency. IgG3 deficiency is less common but has been incriminated in subjects with antibody deficiency syndromes who have normal total IgG or IgG1 subclass levels. Even in adults it has been difficult to establish a link between IgG subclass deficiencies and any consistent pattern of infections. IgG replacement should be reserved for patients with defects of antibody production; many patients are treated with antibiotics alone.

Selective deficiencies of IgM, IgE, and κ or λ light chains due to gene deletions may be symptomless and are very rare. Selective IgM deficiency is reported in Bloom syndrome and, in adults, predisposes to septicemia. Since IgM replacement is impractical on a long-term basis, reliance is placed mainly on antibiotics.

Lawton AR: IgG subclass deficiency and the day-care generation. Pediatr Infect Dis J 1999;18:462 [PMID: 10353521].

Pan Q, Hammarstrom L: Molecular basis of IgG subclass deficiency. Immunol Rev 2000;178:99 [PMID: 11213812].

## SELECTIVE DEFECTS OF CELL-MEDIATED IMMUNITY

### 1. Purine Nucleoside Phosphorylase Deficiency

Purine nucleoside phosphorylase deficiency causes a relatively selective CMI defect. It results in increased intracellular deoxyguanosine triphosphate, which inhibits ribonucleotide reductase and interferes with DNA synthesis, especially in T cells. T-cell help to B cells is not prevented, probably because it does not depend on cell division. The gene for purine nucleoside phosphorylase is on chromosome 14, and transmission is recessive. Presenting features may be neurologic (developmental retardation, behavior disorders, and spasticity), with immunodeficiency (severe varicella infection, anemia, and growth deficiency) developing later. The age at presentation has ranged from 6 months to 7 years. Investigations show low serum uric acid levels, lymphopenia, absent delayed hypersensitivity skin responses, and low or absent lymphocyte responses to mitogens. Serum immunoglobulins and antibody responses to injected antigens may be normal. Several patients developed an autoimmune hemolytic anemia. Diagnosis depends on enzyme measurement, and all patients with severely impaired cellular immunity who make immunoglobulin should probably be tested. Antenatal diagnosis is possible. It has been difficult to achieve stable engraftment following BMT.

Moallem HJ et al: Purine nucleoside phosphorylase deficiency: A new case report and identification of two novel mutations (Gly156A1a and Val217Ile), only one of which (Gly156A1a) is deleterious. Clin Immunol 2002;105:75 [PMID: 12483996].

### 2. Thymic Hypoplasia (DiGeorge Syndrome)

DiGeorge syndrome is one of the so-called CATCH 22 disorders (cardiac defects, abnormal facies, thymic hypoplasia, cleft palate, and hypocalcemia) caused by monosomy of the chromosome regions 22q11.2 and a haploinsufficiency of T-box1 genes. Microdeletions at 10p12–13 may cause a similar phenotype. Related syndromes are the velocardiofacial syndrome and isolated conotruncal cardiac disease. The incidence is about 1 per 3000 births, and the defective chromosome is usually inherited from the mother. The hypocalcemia results from lack of parathyroid glands, and the common major vessel abnormalities are truncus arteriosus, anomalous pulmonary venous drainage, and right-sided aortic arch. Clinically important issues include delayed speech acquisition and behavioral problems. The term "partial DiGeorge syndrome" is commonly applied to infants who have impaired rather than absent parathyroid or thymus function. Clinical presentation usually results from cardiac failure or, after 24–48 hours, from hypocalcemia, and the diagnosis is sometimes made during the course of cardiac surgery, when no thymus is found in the mediastinum. Postoperative hypocalcemia can be severe and persistent, requiring both calcium and vitamin D supplements. Despite receiving fresh blood transfusions during cardiopulmonary bypass, patients do not usually develop graft-versus-host disease (GVHD). Their susceptibility to infection varies—a few have died with septicemia, and some have had chronic candidiasis, but many appear to respond normally. This may reflect the tendency for the number of T cells in the patient's blood to rise spontaneously over the course of several years. The differential diagnosis includes hypocalcemia and a small or absent thymus on chest radiograph secondary to infection. A subset of patients with DiGeorge syndrome has severe problems with production of autoantibodies to red cells, white cells, and platelets. These patients may respond to intravenous IgG or to corticosteroids. Treatment of other DiGeorge features may require surgery for the cardiac defects and vitamin D and calcium to correct hypocalcemia. Blood for these patients should be irradiated. Grafting thymic hypoplasia patients with cultured thymus tissue is followed by the appearance of new, functional T cells in the blood and by resolution of infections. Infusion of HLA-matched sibling blood or marrow has been tried in a few patients who did not improve spontaneously and carries a risk for GVHD. Intrauterine ultrasound may lead to antenatal diagnosis of the congenital heart disease.

Chinen J et al: Long term assessment of T cell populations in diGeorge syndrome. J Allergy Clin Immunol 2003;111:573 [PMID: 12642839].

Guidelines on gamma irradiation of blood components for the prevention of transfusion-associated graft-versus-host disease: BCSH Blood Transfusion Task Force. Transfus Med 1996;6:261.

Heineman-de Boer JA et al: Behavior problems and personality aspects of 40 children with velo-cardio-facial syndrome. Genet Couns 1999;10:89 [PMID: 10191434].

Markert ML et al: Thymus transplantation in complete DiGeorge syndrome: Immunologic and safety evaluations in 12 patients. Blood 2003;102:1121 [PMID: 12702512].

Perez E, Sullivan KE: Chromosome 22g11.2 deletion syndrome (DiGeorge and velocardiofacial syndrome). Curr Opin Pediatr 2002;14:678 [PMID: 12436034].

## Other Defects of Cell-Mediated Immunity

Idiopathic CD4 lymphopenia is characterized by low CD4 counts with opportunistic infection but without HIV infection. Causes may include human herpesvirus 8 infections or a primary sensitivity of CD4 cells to death by apoptosis (or both). Many patients with cartilage-hair hypoplasia have a moderate degree of lymphopenia, low lymphocyte responses to mitogens, and higher than normal morbidity and mortality rates from pneumonias, herpesviruses, and *Candida* and poxvirus infections. About a third have abnormal IgG or IgA levels. They also have an increased incidence of lymphoma. The disorder results from mutation in the *RMRP* gene that encodes the RNA component of an RNase MRP complex. BMT can restore CMI but does not correct the cartilage abnormality. Short-limbed dwarfs who are immunodeficient should probably be tested for adenosine deaminase deficiency, which also is treatable. Other types of immunodeficiency affecting predominantly cellular immunity exist but are poorly classified. These are currently included in the so-called varied immunodeficiency group. Infections in affected individuals resemble those described earlier, with the frequent addition of chronic diarrhea and malabsorption and lung infections due to atypical mycobacteria, fungi, and *Pneumocystis jiroveci*. Treatment is experimental.

Elder ME: T-cell immunodeficiencies. Pediatr Clin North Am 2000;47:1253 [PMID: 11130995].

Fischer A et al: Bone marrow transplantation (BMT) in Europe for primary immunodeficiencies other than severe combined immunodeficiency: A report from the European Group for BMT and the European Group for Immunodeficiency. Blood 1994;83:1149.

Makitie O et al: Increased mortality in cartilage-hair hypoplasia. Arch Dis Child 2001;84:65.

Tanaka S et al:. Idiopathic CD4+ T-lymphocytopenia in a boy with Down syndrome: Report of a patient and a review of the literature. Eur J Pediatr 2004;163:122 [PMID: 14689305].

Torikai K: Idiopathic CD4+ T-lymphocytopenia. Intern Med 1997;36:759 [PMID: 9392344].

Yel L et al: Cartilage-hair hypoplasia syndrome. J Clin Immunol 1999;19:428 [PMID: 10634217].

## Defects Affecting Gamma Interferon

Almost all cells have IFNγ receptors that mediate host defense responses. Macrophage-derived IL-12 increases IFNγ production by T and NK cells that triggers Jak-1 and Stat3 messengers. Failure of any component of the IL-12 IL-12R IFNγ IFNRγ Jak–Stat pathway seems to increase susceptibility to mycobacterial or salmonella infection. Most reported patients have come from North Africa, and their infections have responded to extended courses of antibiotics.

Fieschi C, Casanova J-L: The role of interleukin-12 in human infectious diseases: Only a faint signature. Eur J Immunol 2003;33:1461 [PMID: 2778462].

Remus N et al: Impaired ?interferon gamma-mediated immunity and susceptibility to mycobacterial infection in childhood. Pediatr Res 2001;5:8 [PMID: 11420412].

## IMMUNE DYSREGULATION

### Autoimmune Lymphoproliferative Syndromes

Autoimmune lymphoproliferative syndromes (ALPS) result from mutations of genes coding for death pathways (CD95, CD95 ligand, or caspase 10) for lymphocytes. Symptoms result primarily from the associated autoimmune disorder (autoimmune hemolytic anemia, neutropenia, thrombocytopenia, and sometimes arthritis) and include frequent infections in some patients. Lymphadenopathy and splenomegaly developing in the first years of life are the principal clinical findings. An increase in the number of CD4⁻CD8⁻ (double negative) T cells in blood suggests the diagnosis, and different types of ALPS are distinguished by the response of lymphocytes to Fas-induced apoptosis. Patients are often heterozygous, and inheritance is mostly dominant. Prednisone controls the lymphadenopathy, and infections, when present, should be treated. The risk of

Hodgkin and non-Hodgkin lymphomas is increased. BMT can correct the disorder by replacing the defective lymphocyte precursors.

Mutations affecting an apoptosis-related protein, caspase 8, cause an ALPS variant syndrome in which the susceptibility to infection by herpes simplex virus also increases.

Rieux-Laucat F et al: Cell-death signaling and human disease. Curr Opin Immunol 2003;15:325 [PMID: 12787759].

The autoimmune polyendocrinopathy candidiasis ectodermal dysplasia (APECED) syndrome is caused by defects of the autoimmune regulator (AIRE) protein encoded at 21q22.3 and expressed in lymph nodes and spleen. Candidiasis has developed around 5 years of age, hypoparathyroidism around 10 years, followed by Addison disease. Other autoimmune diseases occur, including cytopenias, probably as a consequence of T-cell dysregulation. Affected children may die of septic shock if their Addison disease is not recognized. Boys with the immune dysregulation, polyendocrinopathy, enteropathy X-linked (IPEX) syndrome develop severe diarrhea with failure to thrive, insulin-dependent diabetes mellitus, or severe eczema in the first months of life and progress to develop autoimmune cytopenias, lymphadenopathy, splenomegaly, and alopecia or candidiasis. Many die before their first birthday, but a few long-term survivors have developed sarcoid, pemphigoid, or glomerulonephritis. The disorder results from mutations in the *FOXP3* gene that encodes a protein with transcriptional repressor function. Leukocyte counts including T-/B-cell numbers are generally normal, as are immunoglobulin levels prior to the development of protein loss from the gut. Immunosuppression has provided temporary improvements, but early BMT may be required.

Halonen M et al: APECED-causing mutations in AIRE reveal the functional domains of the protein. Hum Mutat 2004;23: 245 [PMID: 14974083].

Torgerson TR, Ochs HD: Immune dysregulation, polyendocrinopathy, enteropathy, X-linked syndrome: A model of immune dysregulation. Curr Opin Allergy Immunol 2002;2:481 [PMID: 14752330].

# ■ COMBINED IMMUNODEFICIENCY DISORDERS

Severe combined immunodeficiency disease (SCID) comprises a heterogeneous group of conditions that have in common a primary severe impairment of both antibody and CMI (Table 29–3). The term "SCID" is usually restricted to infants with congenital immunodeficiency, but equally severe defects can be caused by AIDS or lymphocyte loss. The heterogeneity of the congenital forms reflects the range of underlying defects that block the development or function of different subsets of lymphocytes, modulated by the varying degrees of engraftment with maternal lymphocytes that can occur during gestation or at birth. X-linked SCID (severe combined immunodeficiency-X1) results from mutations in the γ chain shared by the cell surface receptors for the cytokines IL-2, IL-4, IL-7, IL-9, and IL-15. It accounts for 40% of SCID cases and is described as the prototype. The SCID syndromes that result from mutations in the receptor for IL-7 and in Jak3, the intracellular signaling molecule for the cytokine receptors, are generally similar but with an autosomal recessive inheritance. These mutations vary in their interference with γ-chain receptor function, and this allows for a range of clinical severity in cytokine receptor X-linked SCID syndromes. Diarrhea, vomiting, and cough in the first 3 months of life are common symptoms. The

**Table 29–3.** Gene defects causing severe combined immunodeficiency (SCID).

| Gene | Phenotype |
|---|---|
| ADA deficiency | Lymphopenic; accounts for 25% of autosomal-recessive SCID |
| Cytokine γ chain receptor | Low T and NK cells, high B cells; accounts for most X-linked SCID |
| Zap-70 | Normal/low CD3 and CD4, absent CD8; low immunoglobulins; autosomal recessive inheritance |
| Jak3[a] | Absent CD3, low NK cells, normal B cells |
| P56lck[b] | Percentages of CD3 low to normal, CD4 low, CD8 normal; NK cells present |
| Whn[c] | Hairless, dystrophic nails, absent T cells |
| Artemis[d] | Absent T and B, Athabascan |

[a]Macchi P et al: Mutations of Jak-3 gene in patients with autosomal severe combined immune deficiency (SCID). Nature, 1995; 377:65.
[b]Goldman FD et al: Defective expression of p56lck in an infant with severe combined immunodeficiency. Clin Invest 1998; 102:421.
[c]Frank J et al. Exposing the human nude phenotype. Nature 1999; 398:473.
[d]Li L et al: A founder mutation in Artemis, an SNM1-like protein, causes SCID in Athabascan-speaking native Americans. J Immunol 2002;168:6323.

diarrhea causes growth deficiency and, although it may briefly remit after dietary changes, it recurs after a few days. The cough is usually persistent; it is often due to *P jiroveci* infection and can cause cyanosis. Skin rashes are common and frequently evanescent, except for rash following blood transfusion, which is due to GVHD (see section on graft-versus-host disease). A *Candida* diaper rash is usual. Findings initially include absence of tonsils or palpable lymph nodes; later, emaciation occurs. All patients with SCID have some degree of hypogammaglobulinemia and failure of antibody production (though maternal IgG is present in infants). Lymphopenia is inconstant, but, with rare exceptions, all have very low or absent T (CD3, CD4, and CD8) cells, with normal numbers of NK (CD16) cells. B lymphocytes (with surface IgM) are usually increased as a percentage but normal in number. In vitro lymphocyte responses to mitogens are generally absent. Antigen-specific responses (T cell or antibody) are difficult to test for in infancy because of uncertainty about prior experience and because the tests are generally too time-consuming for clinical purposes. Antenatal diagnosis is possible.

### Differential Diagnosis & Treatment

Diarrhea and hypogammaglobulinemia in infancy suggests SCID. The main differential is between severe varied immunodeficiency and a secondary immunodeficiency due to HIV infection or severe gastrointestinal disease with loss of protein and cells. Some CD3, CD4, and CD8 T cells are usually present in these secondary immunodeficiencies, with a weak lymphocyte response to phytohemagglutinin, and the serum albumin concentration may be low. Infants in whom the diagnosis of SCID is suspected should receive antibiotics for infection, trimethoprim–sulfamethoxazole for *Pneumocystis* prophylaxis, and IgG replacement. They should not be transfused with blood unless it has first been irradiated. Confirmation of the diagnosis usually requires specialist help and should include screening for SCID subtypes listed in Table 29–3. BMT offers the best hope for cure of SCID and other severe immunodeficiencies. If an HLA-matched sibling is available, the chance of success is high; the treatment can be given without depleting the marrow of T cells or immunosuppressing the recipient. Most SCID patients do not have HLA-matched donors and are given grafts of parental bone marrow from which the T cells are removed by lectins or monoclonal antibodies. Umbilical cord blood stem cells are increasingly used as a source. Pregraft suppression, with the attendant hazards of thrombocytopenia and neutropenia, may be required; reconstitution takes 4 months; but the overall rate of T-cell engraftment is approaching 80%. Reconstitution

for antibody responses occurs in only 50% even if B cells are produced. X-linked SCID was successfully treated by autologous transplants with stem cells transfected with cytokine receptor DNA, but the integration of the retroviral vectors resulted in some oligoclonal T-cell proliferations. The development of safer vectors is awaited.

Barker JN et al: Survival after transplantation of unrelated donor umbilical cord blood is comparable to that of human leukocyte antigen-matched unrelated donor bone marrow: Results of a matched-pair analysis. Blood 2001;97:2957 [PMID: 11342417].

Buckley RH et al: Hematopoietic stem-cell transplantation for the treatment of severe combined immunodeficiency. N Engl J Med 1999;340:508 [PMID: 10021471].

Hacein-Bey-Abina S et al: LMO2-associated clonal T cell proliferation in two patients after gene therapy for SCID-X1. Science 2003;302:415 [PMID: 14564000].

## VARIANTS OF SEVERE COMBINED IMMUNODEFICIENCY

### 1. Adenosine Deaminase Deficiency

Adenosine deaminase (ADA) converts adenosine and deoxyadenosine to inosine and deoxyinosine, respectively. Individuals homozygous for a null gene account for about 20% of cases of SCID. ADA deficiency impairs immunity through inhibition of ribonucleotide reductase by raised deoxy-ATP, so that T lymphocytes are prevented from dividing. DNA fragmentation, interference with methylation reactions, and aberrant receptor signaling also increase. Affected infants may be near-normal at birth (presumably because their mothers keep deoxyadenosine levels down in utero). Their cellular immunity fails first; they become lymphopenic and then become antibody-deficient, though they may continue to make immunoglobulin for months or years. Diagnosis is by assay of ADA in red cell lysates. A bone marrow transplant from a matched normal sibling is the ideal treatment (see section on HSCT in Chapter 28). Immune competence is also restored by weekly infusions of polyethylene glycol-stabilized ADA enzyme conjugate. Transfection of stem cells with a retroviral construct has been successful, but the development of safer vectors is awaited.

Aiuti A et al: Correction of ADA-SCID by stem cell gene therapy combined with nonmyeloablative conditioning. Science 2002;296:2410 [PMID: 14612670].

Hershfield MS: Adenosine deaminase deficiency: Clinical expression, molecular basis, and therapy. Semin Hematol 1998;35:291 [PMID: 9801258].

## 2. SCID with Leukopenia (Reticular Dysgenesis)

SCID with leukopenia occurs in infants with SCID who also have severe leukopenia, often with reduced numbers of granulocyte precursors in the marrow. Only about 20 cases have been reported. There is a familial trend, but the severity of the leukopenia varies and may result from deficiency of a cytokine.

Cham B et al: Neutropenia associated with primary immunodeficiency syndromes. Semin Hematol 2002;39:107 [PMID: 11957193 ].

## 3. SCID Due to DNA Repair Defects

SCID in a subset of patients results from failure to repair the breaks in DNA that lymphocytes need to make in the course of generating a receptor for antigen. NK cell numbers are normal though cultured fibroblasts are unusually sensitive to irradiation. Examples include the *Artemis* deficiency in the Na-dene American Indian population and the SCID with reticuloendotheliosis, or Omenn syndrome, caused by defects in *RAG1* and *RAG2* genes. Omenn syndrome patients have a severe eczematoid skin rash, lymphadenopathy, hepatosplenomegaly with diarrhea, and failure to thrive. Most of these patients have eosinophilia with high IgE and low IgG and IgM levels; blood B cells are low or absent. Blood T cells are low and the repertoire restricted. Many of the cells are activated and make IL-4 and IL-5. Some cases have been treated successfully by marrow ablation followed by transplantation. Other defects of DNA repair that interfere with T- and B-cell production include DNA-ligase deficiency: identical mutations in *RAG1* or *RAG2* genes leading to defective V(D)J recombinase activity can cause either T–B-SCID or Omenn syndrome.

## 4. SCID with Defective Expression of HLA Antigens

Deficiency of class II (HLA-DR, -DP, and -DQ) histocompatibility antigen expression is difficult to diagnose because affected patients generally make immunoglobulins and have low to normal numbers of B and T cells in their blood, together with positive responses to phytohemagglutinin stimulation. Their clinical symptoms are nevertheless those of SCID, and the T cells do not make antigen-specific responses, so the patients remain antibody-deficient. At least four complementation groups occur, and diagnosis is by testing blood lymphocytes for HLA-DR antigen expression. A number of affected families has been of North African descent. BMT for these children can be difficult. Defects of class

I histocompatibility antigen range from abnormalities of antigen transport inside the cell to abnormal or unstable expression of HLA-A or HLA-B at the cell surface. In general, these conditions are associated with milder degrees of immunodeficiency.

Gadola SD et al: TAP deficiency syndrome. Clin Exp Immunol 2000;121:173 [PMID: 10931128].

## 5. Other Combined Immunodeficiency Disorders

A poorly defined group of infants exists with more severe impairment of antibody and CMI than occurs in common variable immunodeficiency disease but who have more T cells than are usually seen in SCID. These patients have severe and protracted infections, mainly of the respiratory tract and gut. A subgroup with multiple intestinal atresias, hypogammaglobulinemia, and impaired CMI has recently been recognized; the mechanism for this association is unknown. Many have severe herpesviruses infections. Autoimmune neutropenia, anemia, and thrombocytopenia are common, as are allergies. Immune deficiency in some of these patients has been corrected by BMT.

Moore SW et al: Immune deficiency in familial duodenal atresia. J Pediatr Surg 1996;31:1733 [PMID: 8987005].

## 6. Nude/SCID phenotype

Mutations of forkhead/winged helix transcription factor causes thymic aplasia with congenital alopecia—a human equivalent of the nude mouse. One affected child was successfully treated with a marrow transplant from an HLA-matched sibling.

Pignata C: A lesson for unraveling complex aspects of novel immunodeficiencies from the human equivalent of the nude/SCID phenotype. J Hematotherapy Stem Cell Res 2002;11:409 [PMID: 11983112].

# ■ OTHER DISORDERS ASSOCIATED WITH IMMUNODEFICIENCY

## WISKOTT–ALDRICH SYNDROME

Patients with Wiskott–Aldrich syndrome have thrombocytopenia, eczema, and recurrent infection (originally draining ears). The syndrome results from mutation of the *WASP* gene at X11p. Inheritance is X-linked recessive; the incidence is about 4 per million male births. The mutated gene is for a protein involved in the rearrangement of actin. Common presenting symptoms are bloody diarrhea, cerebral hemorrhage, and septicemia followed by severe infections with polysaccharide-encapsulated bacteria. Symptoms can fluctuate over time so they depend only in part on the domains of the WAS protein that are inactivated by the mutation. The main causes of death in infancy are bleeding and infections, but with time lymphomas become increasingly common. Autoimmune syndromes, particularly thrombocytopenia, hemolysis, and vasculitis, occur in about 50% of patients by 5 years of age. Survival through the teens is rare in patients not receiving treatment, though partial syndromes are sometimes diagnosed in adults. A specific diagnosis should be easier now that the gene has been identified. Routine laboratory findings that suggest the diagnosis are a low platelet count, low or absent isohemagglutinins, and reduced antibody response to polysaccharides. IgM may be low; IgA and IgE are often high. BMT using the best-matched donor offers the best hope for long-term correction of the defect and is generally necessary for patients who develop autoimmune hemolytic anemia. Patients with increased susceptibility to infection are often given IgG replacement and trimethoprim–sulfamethoxazole for *Pneumocystis* prophylaxis. The platelet count generally rises following splenectomy, but this operation must be followed by antibiotic prophylaxis because of the increased risk of septicemia and sudden death.

Dupuis Girod S et al: Autoimmunity in Wiskott–Aldrich syndrome: Risk factors, clinical features, and outcome in a single-center cohort of 55 patients. Pediatrics 2003;111:e622 [PMID: 12728121].

Ochs HD: The Wiskott–Aldrich syndrome. Clin Rev Allergy Immunol 2001;20:61 [PMID: 11269229].

## ATAXIA–TELANGIECTASIA

Ataxia–telangiectasia is characterized by cerebellar ataxia (due to degeneration of Purkinje cells), usually developing between ages 2 and 5 years and followed by the appearance of telangiectasias, particularly on the conjunctiva and over exposed areas (ie, nose, ears, and shoulders). The ataxia–telangiectasia mutated (ATM) protein is kinase, encoded on chromosome 11, and required for cell cycle regulation and DNA repair. The Nijmegen breakage syndrome is probably a variant of ataxia–telangiectasia with more severe clinical features, including microcephaly and bird-like facies. Abnormal findings in ataxia–telangiectasia include raised serum α-fetoprotein levels (useful diagnostically), thymic hypoplasia, low or absent serum IgE, low IgA in 50%, abnormal carbohydrate tolerance, and defective ability to repair radiation-induced DNA fragmentation. Clinically, the most important symptom is progressive loss of motor coordination, followed by weakness. Respiratory tract infections and many types of malignancy (including carcinomas) are the major causes of death. About 10% of patients develop lymphomas, the majority of which are T–cell-derived. Many of the lymphomas have translocations or inversions at sites where T-cell receptor genes are normally rearranged. Radiotherapy has been followed by skin breakdown, presumably the result of the DNA repair defect. Heterozygotes number 0.5–5%, depending on geographic and ethnic factors, and have a small increase in risk for breast cancer.

Perlman S et al: Ataxia-telangiectasia: Diagnosis and treatment. Semin Pediatr Neurol 2003;10:173 [PMID: 14653405].

## CHRONIC MUCOCUTANEOUS CANDIDIASIS

This entity consists of chronic candidiasis affecting the skin or nails and mucous membranes not attributable to antibiotic treatment or another defined immunodeficiency disease. Involvement of the scalp and flexural creases is common, usually as erythema and scaling but occasionally as granulomas with skin hypertrophy. The recurrent candidiasis points to an underlying immunodeficiency, but the faulty mechanism has not been identified. Affected patients make anti-*Candida* antibodies, and their in vitro lymphocyte responses may be positive even when *Candida* skin tests are negative. Evidence for the complexity of this form of immunodeficiency includes the frequent association with endocrinopathy, sometimes autoimmune (affecting the parathyroids, thyroid, pituitary, or gonads), and, less commonly, increased susceptibility to staphylococcal infections with defective neutrophil mobility. Some control of the candidiasis can usually be achieved with continuous fluconazole treatment.

de Moraes-Vasconcelos D et al: Characterization of the cellular immune function of patients with chronic mucocutaneous candidiasis. Clin Exp Immunol 2001;123:247 [PMID: 11207655.

## X-LINKED LYMPHOPROLIFERATIVE SYNDROME

This term is applied to boys who develop bone marrow aplasia, hypogammaglobulinemia, or a lymphoproliferative syndrome following EBV infection. The defective gene encodes a signaling protein used by T lymphocytes and NK cells. Antenatal diagnosis is possible. Affected boys are immunologically normal prior to EBV infection, and during acute mononucleosis they make some antibody to the EBV. In most instances, the EBV infection results in a lethal lymphoproliferative syndrome characterized by liver failure, disseminated intravascular coagulation, and multiple monoclonal serum IgM bands. Acyclovir is sometimes beneficial, and treatment with IFNα and monoclonal anti-B-cell antibodies is being investigated. Only 10–20% of affected boys who are infected with EBV survive to develop hypogammaglobulinemia.

Benoit L et al: Defective NK cell activation in X-linked lymphoproliferative disease. J Immunol 2000;165:3549 [PMID: 11034354].

## GRAFT-VERSUS-HOST DISEASE

GVHD follows transfusion of immunocompetent but incompatible lymphocytes into a person incapable of rejecting them. It causes significant morbidity in about 30% of BMT recipients and causes death in infants with SCID. It has been reported in infants receiving transfusions from HLA homozygous donors, so blood products for infants should be irradiated. An erythematous macular and then bullous skin rash is variably followed by diarrhea, hepatitis, nephritis, pulmonary infiltrates, and fever, whereas marrow damage results in neutropenia and then thrombocytopenia. Many patients develop high IgE levels. The diagnosis is suspected on the basis of transplantation and a history of an unirradiated blood or blood product transfusion, usually into an immunodeficient patient, and is confirmed by skin or lip biopsy. Prophylaxis in transplant recipients is with corticosteroids and cyclosporine, and when the disease becomes severe it may be slowed by high-dose corticosteroids or at least temporarily halted by anti-T-cell antibodies (see Table 29–5). Chronic GVHD after allogeneic BMT causes scleroderma and bile duct destruction. The liver damage can be severe enough to require transplantation.

Henslee-Downey PJ: Mismatched bone marrow transplantation. Curr Opin Oncol 1995;7:115 [PMID: 7756375].

Takanashi M et al: Graft-versus-host disease associated with transfusions of HLA-matched, HLA-homozygous platelets. Transfusion 1995;35:535 [PMID: 7878725].

## BIOCHEMICAL DEFECTS SOMETIMES ASSOCIATED WITH IMMUNODEFICIENCY

Several primary errors of metabolism affect immunity adversely. Transcobalamin 2 deficiency causes a megaloblastic anemia with impaired bacterial killing by neutrophils and reduced serum immunoglobulins of all classes. Biotin-dependent decarboxylase deficiencies may be associated with convulsions, alopecia, candidiasis, low serum IgA, and a reduced number of T cells. Lymphopenia and impaired CMI are reported in hereditary orotic aciduria. Bloom syndrome, in which mutations in a DNA helicase result in excess sister chromatid exchanges, is associated principally with lymphoma and cancer, as well as life-threatening infections. Serum IgA and IgM are sometimes low, and lymphocytes respond abnormally in laboratory tests. A systematic listing of genetic disorders with immunodeficiency is given in the review by Ming and others.

Bloom syndrome:

http://www3.ncbi.nlm.nih.gov/entrez/dispomim.cgi?id=210900

Ming JE et al: Syndromic immunodeficiencies: Genetic syndromes associated with immune abnormalities. Crit Rev Clin Lab Sci 2003;40:587 [PMID: 14708957].

# ■ SECONDARY IMMUNODEFICIENCY

Secondary immunodeficiency is a common cause of pediatric illness. The mechanisms that may be impaired are summarized in Table 29–4, and the symptoms are generally those that would be anticipated from the combination of the primary disorder and the complicating immunodeficiency. Whenever possible, treatment should be directed at the primary disorder. Occasionally, immunologic methods may help; for example, postexposure varicella-zoster immune globulin may prevent varicella infection in patients with leukemia, and intravenous immune globulin replacement might provide added protection when antibody production is diminished. IgG replacement is unlikely to help when loss (as in nephrotic syndrome) is responsible for hypogammaglobulinemia.

Lee ML et al: Use of intravenous immunoglobulin to prevent or treat infections in persons with immune deficiency. Annu Rev Med 1997;48:93 [PMID: 9046948].

## POST-BONE MARROW TRANSPLANT IMMUNODEFICIENCY

In the months following a BMT, patients remain highly susceptible to herpesvirus, *P jiroveci,* and other fungal infections even when their blood leukocyte counts recover. They require prophylaxis with trimethoprim–sulfonamide, acyclovir, and intravenous immune globulin, and pulmonary symptoms (cough, impaired oxygenation) must be investigated promptly.

**Table 29–4.** Mechanisms of secondary immunodeficiency.

| Mechanism | Example |
|---|---|
| Loss | |
|   Immunoglobulin | Renal, in nephrotic syndrome |
|   Immunoglobulin | Skin, from burns |
|   Immunoglobulin and cells | Gut, in intestinal lymphangiectasia |
|   Phagocytes | Following splenectomy |
| Malnutrition | Kwashiorkor |
|   Zinc deficiency | Impaired cell-mediated immunity |
|   Copper and iron deficiency | Impaired neutrophil function |
| Drugs | Steroids, cancer chemotherapy |
| | Specific immunosuppressants |
| | Phenytoin → IgA deficiency |
| Infections | HIV, EBV, CMV, measles, rubella, hepatitis, malaria |

HIV = human immunodeficiency virus; EBV = Epstein–Barr virus; CMV = cytomegalovirus.

These problems arise partly from immunosuppression by cyclosporine and steroids that reduces GVHD, partly from delay in recovery of the B lymphocytes required for antibody responses, and, under some circumstances, because of cytokines given to boost neutrophil production.

Volpi I et al: Postgrafting administration of granulocyte colony-stimulating factor impairs functional immune recovery in recipients of human leukocyte antigen haplotype-mismatched hematopoietic transplants. Blood 2001;97:2514 [PMID: 11290617].

## THERAPEUTIC IMMUNOSUPPRESSION

Therapeutic immunosuppression is increasingly used in pediatrics for transplant recipients and for autoimmune disease. Corticosteroids at doses equivalent to 2 mg/kg of prednisolone per day interfere with cytokine production and cause lymphopenia by directing lymphocytes to the marrow; the effects of a single dose last about 24 hours. Much higher doses, equivalent to 20–30 mg/kg of prednisolone per day, are used in 3- to 5-day courses for treatment of life-threatening conditions or to evaluate the potential for more powerful immunosuppressive agents. Corticosteroids are satisfactory anti-inflammatory and immunosuppressive agents when they can be given on alternate days as a single morning dose (as is sometimes the case for systemic lupus erythematosus or autoimmune anemias). The use of higher doses of corticosteroids is limited by the growth arrest and severe cushingoid changes, which occur even in dosages of 2 mg/kg of prednisolone per day. Transplant recipients require additional powerful immunosuppressives such as cyclosporine or tacrolimus (FK506). Both bind to immunophilins to form a complex that reversibly inhibits calcineurin-dependent signaling in lymphocytes, blocking cytokine production and release. Immunosuppression achievable by both agents is limited by their nephrotoxicity; trough blood levels need to be monitored carefully, and drugs that affect their metabolism (erythromycin, theophylline) tracked. Tacrolimus is increasingly used because rejection episodes tend to be fewer, though a possible increase in post-transplant lymphoproliferative disease (PTLD) is a concern. Preventing organ rejection usually requires two drugs, such as cyclosporine with either mycophenolate mofetil (MMF) or azathioprine. MMF inhibits purine synthesis and is relatively specific for lymphocytes. It is usually taken by mouth, absorption is erratic, and blood levels must be checked. High cost is one reason why MMF has not replaced azathioprine, which causes much more general marrow suppression. Patient compliance with chronic antirejection medicines is a significant problem. Because MMF causes gastrointestinal disturbance, patients may not take it, and teenagers who have received organ transplants sometimes become depressed and stop taking all their medicines.

Sirolimus (rapamycin) inhibits T-cell activation and proliferation as well as antibody production. It is orally active and is generally combined with cyclosporine for treating transplant rejection. It has activity in chronic GVHD: Increases in cholesterol and triglycerides are adverse effects. Animal models suggest that the currently popular combinations of steroids and cyclosporine interfere with the acquisition of tolerance for grafts, and combinations of newer agents (rapamycin with monoclonal antibodies to the IL-2 receptor) are being evaluated clinically.

Severe organ rejection episodes, or GVHD, can be controlled acutely with antibodies to T lymphocytes such as antithymocyte globulin and monoclonal CD3 antibody. Both deplete T cells and clear antigen receptors off the T-cell surface. Some T cells are activated as well, causing a cytokine syndrome of fever, malaise, skin rash, and pulmonary edema. This syndrome is minimized by premedicating patients with an antihistamine, acetaminophen, corticosteroids, and even cyclosporine. Patients generally need to be tested for antihorse, antirabbit, or antimouse antibodies after treatment, and those who test positive should not receive the same preparation again.

Antimitotic agents (eg, cyclophosphamide, chlorambucil) and antimetabolites (methotrexate) that block lymphocyte proliferation are effective but toxic immunosuppressants. The range of licensed monoclonal antibodies with immunosuppressive or anticancer activities has increased greatly (Table 29–5). Immunosuppressive antibodies carry the risk of reactivation of latent herpesviruses (ie, cytomegalovirus, herpes simplex virus, varicella-zoster virus), although antiviral treatments have made these infections less life-threatening. EBV reactivation is hazardous if it results in a lymphoproliferative disease, which, when severe, is associated with marrow phagocytosis of red and white cells. The appearance of free EBV genome in the plasma probably provides the best advance warning of this dangerous complication. Testing serum for oligoclonal immunoglobulin bands may give some indication of the progression or regression of lymphoproliferative disease. The usual treatment strategy is to reduce the dosage of agents such as cyclosporine and tacrolimus while continuing immunosuppression with steroids. Rituximab may be useful too. Combined immunosuppression with agents having different modes of action tends to be much more potent, with a greater potential for opportunistic infections, than immunosuppression by single agents. The risk of infection is greatest when the neutrophil count is depressed by antimitotic agents at the same time that specific immunity is suppressed by corticosteroids and cyclosporine.

Davis JE, Moss DJ: Treatment options for post-transplant lymphoproliferative disorder and other Epstein–Barr virus-associated malignancies. Tissue Antigens 2004;63:285 [PMID: 15009802].

Dror Y et al: Lymphoproliferative disorders after organ transplantation in children. Transplantation 1999;67:990 [PMID: 10221483].

Kruithof E et al: Repeated infusions of infliximab, a chimeric anti-TNF monoclonal antibody, in patients with active spondyloarthropathy: A one-year follow up. Ann Rheum Dis 2002;61:207 [PMID: 11830424].

Vincenti F et al: Multicenter trial exploring calcineurin inhibitors avoidance in renal transplantation. Transplantation 2001;71:1282 [PMID: 11397963].

# ■ INVESTIGATION OF IMMUNODEFICIENCY

Physical and anatomic defects are the most common causes of recurrent infections, and if a single site is af-

**Table 29–5.** Monoclonal antibodies.

| Disorder Treated[a] | Antibody[b] | Comments/Adverse Reactions |
|---|---|---|
| Crohn disease, rheumatoid arthritis | Infliximab: tumor necrosis factor alpha | Single-dose infusions at 5 mg/kg. 28% of recipients had DNA antibodies and EBV reactivation. 5% severe infections include Tb reactivation and retropharyngeal abscesses |
| B-cell lymphomas, autoantibody production | Rituximab: CD20 | B-cell lymphopenia, tumor lysis, rare severe infusion reactions |
| Transplant rejection, graft-versus-host disease. | Daclizumab: IL-2R (Tac) | Appears well tolerated, usually given as 1–2 infusions |
| Graft-versus-host disease | Visilizumab: CD3 | Depletes T cells, EBV reactivation |
| Graft-versus-host disease. | ABX-CBL: CD147 (mouse IgM) | Myalgias reported |
| Non-Hodgkin lymphoma, chronic lymphocytic leukemia | Alemtuzumab: CD52 | T-cell activation and cytokine syndrome, lymphopenia |
| Transplant rejection | Muromonab-CD3 (OKT3) | T-cell activation, cytokine syndrome, lymphopenia, EBV reactivation |
| B-cell lymphomas | Epratuzumab: CD22 | Four treatments at weekly intervals, no effect on Ig levels |
| Psoriasis, asthma | Efalizumab: CD11a | Flu-like syndrome with headache after first injection |

[a]Experimental treatment included.
[b]These are humanized mouse antibodies unless otherwise indicated.

fected it should be searched for a local abnormality. The age at onset of infections is important because defects of phagocytes, C3, or cellular immunity becomes symptomatic in the first months of life, whereas maternal antibody protects infants with hypogammaglobulinemia for 3–6 months. Antibody, complement, and phagocyte defects predispose mainly to bacterial infections; diarrhea, superficial candidiasis, and severe herpesvirus infections are typical of cellular immunodeficiency. A simple protocol for testing these mechanisms is presented in Table 29–6, and the level of investigation should reflect the frequency and severity of infections. A complete blood count and quantitative immunoglobulin measurement will identify more than 90% of primary immunodeficiency syndromes.

Fleisher TA: Evaluation of the potentially immunodeficient patient. Adv Intern Med 1996;41:1 [PMID: 8903585].

## PHAGOCYTE FUNCTION

Tests of phagocytic cell function should first rule out neutropenia with white blood cell count and differential. A blood film is useful to exclude the Howell–Jolly bodies of asplenia and to look for normal lysosomal granules in neutrophils. Myeloperoxidase deficiency is excluded by histochemical stains available in most oncology laboratories. The respiratory burst and generation of bactericidal factors can be tested by nitroblue tetrazolium reduction, so this test screens for most types of chronic granulomatous disease (the most common bacterial killing defect) and for leukocyte glucose-6-phosphate dehydrogenase deficiency. Leukocyte adhesion molecules are screened by flow cytometry, although the difference in symptoms of these various phagocyte defects should dictate which tests are used. Chemotaxis can be measured in migration chambers in the laboratory and can also be assessed by migration of cells from abraded skin onto a sterile coverslip. Results of chemotaxis tests must be interpreted cautiously, because secondary and transient defects in chemotaxis are common. Quantitations of bacterial ingestion and microbicidal activity are mostly research procedures.

## COMPLEMENT

Deficiency of a classic pathway component can be excluded by a normal hemolytic complement titer, for which the patient's serum must be separated and frozen to –70°C within 30 minutes of collection. Alternative pathway function is tested by lysis of rabbit red blood cells. There is little point in measuring individual complement component levels if the hemolytic titer is normal—unless it is done to follow the activity of an immune complex-associated disease in which C4 and C3 may be low. The common form of opsonizing defect of yeast is now known to be due to allelic variants of mannan-binding protein.

Martin P et al: Inherited mannose-binding lectin deficiency as evidenced by genetic and immunologic analyses: Association with severe recurrent infections. Ann Allergy Asthma Immunol 2003;91:386 [[PMID: 14582818].

## ANTIBODIES & IMMUNOGLOBULINS

In patients who are not blood group AB, isohemagglutinins are the most easily tested naturally occurring antibodies. They are of the IgM class, become detectable by age 6 months, and reach adult levels about 1 year later. Tetanus and diphtheria antibody tests are widely available, as are antibodies to the 23-valent pneumococcal polysaccharide, rubella, and mumps. In practice, it is often easier to measure serum immunoglobulins as a screening procedure than to test for antibodies, but some patients with varied immunodeficiency syndromes and some infants with severely impaired CMI make immunoglobulin that does not have useful antibody activity. Properly performed immunoglobulin estimations are reproducible to ±10% for IgG and IgA

***Table 29–6.*** Hierarchy of tests for investigation of primary immunodeficiency.

| Test Level | Complement | Phagocytes | Antibody | CMI |
|---|---|---|---|---|
| Screening | CH$_{50}$ | Count, morphology | Ig measurement | Delayed hypersensitivity skin tests |
| First level | | NBT, LFA-1[a] | IHA,[b] TT | T-cell counts[c] |
| Second level | Factor assays | Killing and chemotaxis | Immunize | In vitro tests |

[a]Only when chronic granulomatous disease or LFA-1 deficiency is suspected.
[b]IHA = isohemagglutinins, after age 1; TT = tetanus toxoid.
[c]Identify all T cells with CD3, subsets with CD4, CD8. CD45RO for memory cells.
CMI = cell-mediated immunity.

*Table 29–7.* Blood lymphocyte phenotyping.

| Antigen | Cells Stained | Normal Range and Changes Seen Clinically |
|---------|---------------|------------------------------------------|
| CD2 | T, NK | 70–90%. Falls to 10–20% when T cells absent. |
| CD3 | All T | 55–85%. Falls when T-cell number reduced. Increases to 90% when B cells absent. |
| CD4 | HLA-D restricted T cells | 35–60%. Selectively reduced in HIV infections. Reduced with other T cells by steroids, defect of cell-mediated immunity. |
| CD5 | T cells, immature B cells | 55–85%. Falls when T-cell number reduced. Increased with immature B cells. |
| CD8 | HLA-A/B restricted T cells | 25–50%. Selectively increased in response to some viral infections. Reduced with other T-cell defects. |
| CD11 | Monocytes | Lacking in LFA-1 deficiency. |
| CD16 | NK cells | Increased by viral infections. |
| CD19 | B cells | Absent or low in congenital X-linked agammaglobulinemia and common variable immunodeficiency disease. Increased when T cells are lacking. |
| CD20 | B cells | Increased when T cells lacking. |
| CD25 | IL-2 receptor | Activated T cells. Increased in graft-versus-host disease. |
| CD45RO | T cells | Memory T cells, low in newborns. |
| CD56 | NK cells | Raised in active viral infections. |

NK = natural killer; HLA = human leukocyte antigen; LFA1 = leukocyte functional antigen-1.

and ±20% for IgM, so small changes are of no significance. Measurement of serum IgD is not generally of diagnostic value in pediatrics. Immunoglobulin concentrations are lower in infants than in adults, and laboratories may erroneously report normal children's values as low. Patients with very low immunoglobulins of all classes should have blood T- and B-cell counts as most boys with BTK deficiency lack B cells—as do the small number of patients with μ chain deficiency. Protein electrophoresis is valuable for identifying the monoclonal excesses seen in macroglobulinemia, in the oligoclonal gammopathy of EBV infections in X-linked lymphoproliferative syndrome, and in heavy-chain diseases. Serum albumin should be measured at least once in patients with hypogammaglobulinemia to exclude secondary deficiencies due to loss. IgG or IgA subclass measurements may be abnormal in patients with varied immunodeficiency syndromes, but they are rarely helpful.

## CELL-MEDIATED IMMUNITY

Positive delayed hypersensitivity skin tests give good evidence for antigen-specific T-cell immunity. Only a positive response is interpretable—particularly in infancy, when prior immunization may not have been adequate to elicit good skin responses.

Blood T- and B-lymphocyte counts are good screening tests for disorders of CMI. Only small volumes of blood are required, and results are rapidly available. Some of the more useful phenotypes—and common deviations from normal—are summarized in Table 29–7. When abnormalities are suspected, it is important to check absolute numbers of lymphocytes and their subsets. Tests of T-cell proliferation and cytokine production are useful for characterizing immunodeficiency detected by simpler tests, but they are not useful screening tests for children with recurrent infections.

Sorensen RU, Moore C: Antibody deficiency syndromes. Pediatr Clin North Am 2000;47:1225 [PMID: 11130994].

Wasserman RL, Sorensen RU: Evaluating children with respiratory tract infections: The role of immunization with bacterial polysaccharide vaccine. Pediatr Infect Dis J 1999;18:157 [PMID: 10048691].

# Endocrine Disorders

**30**

*Philip S. Zeitler, MD, PhD, Sharon H. Travers, MD, Jennifer Barker, MD, Kristen Nadeau, MD, & Michael S. Kappy, MD, PhD*

## ■ GENERAL CONCEPTS

One of the major functions of the endocrine system is to regulate enzymatic and other metabolic processes (eg, molecular transport) responsible for maintaining the equilibrium (homeostasis) of the internal environment to ensure survival of the individual. Other critical roles for the endocrine system are regulation of growth (in utero and postnatal), pubertal development and reproduction, energy production, blood pressure, and, to a lesser extent, behavior.

The classic concept that endocrine effects are the result of hormones secreted into the blood to reach a target cell has been updated to account for other ways in which hormonal effects occur. Specifically, some hormone systems involve the stimulation or inhibition (or both) of metabolic processes in neighboring (as opposed to distant) cells (eg, within the pancreatic islets or cartilage). This phenomenon is termed *paracrine*. Other hormone effects reflect the action of particular hormones on the same cells that produced them. This action is termed *autocrine*. The discoveries of local production of insulin, glucagon, atrial natriuretic hormone, and many other hormones in the brain and gut support the concept of paracrine and autocrine processes in these tissues.

Another significant discovery in endocrine physiology was an appreciation of the role of specific hormone receptors in target tissues, without which the hormonal effects could not occur. In the *complete* androgen insensitivity (resistance) syndrome, androgen receptors are absent, and the individual develops normal female external genitalia despite the presence of testes (usually intra-abdominal) and adequate testosterone production. Similarly, in nephrogenic diabetes insipidus or Albright hereditary osteodystrophy (pseudohypoparathyroidism), affected persons have abnormal antidiuretic hormone (ADH) or parathyroid hormone (PTH) receptor function and show the metabolic effects of diabetes insipidus or hypoparathyroidism (low serum calcium and high serum phosphate levels), despite more than adequate hormone secretion. Alternatively, autonomous (abnormal) activation of a hormone receptor leads to the effects of the hormone without its abnormal secretion. Examples of this phenomenon include McCune–Albright syndrome (precocious puberty and hyperthyroidism) and testotoxicosis (familial male precocious puberty).

## HORMONE TYPES

Three main structural types of hormones exist: peptides and proteins, steroids, and amines. The peptide hormones include the releasing factors secreted by the hypothalamus, the hormones of the anterior and posterior pituitary gland, pancreatic islet cells and parathyroid glands, insulin-like growth factor 1 (IGF-1) from the liver and other tissues, angiotensin II, atrial natriuretic hormone, and many local growth factors. Steroid hormones are secreted primarily by the adrenal cortex, the gonads, and the liver and kidney (active vitamin D). The amine hormones are secreted by the adrenal medulla (epinephrine) and the thyroid gland (triiodothyronine [$T_3$] and thyroxine [$T_4$]).

As a rule, the peptide hormones and epinephrine act more rapidly than the others and bind to specific receptors on the surface of their target cell. The metabolic effect of these hormones is usually stimulation or inhibition of the activity of pre-existing enzymes or transport proteins (post-translational effects). The steroid hormones and active vitamin D, in contrast, act more slowly and bind to specific cytoplasmic receptors within the target cell and subsequently to specific regions (genes) on nuclear DNA, where they direct a read-out of specific protein(s). Their metabolic effects are generally caused by stimulating or inhibiting the synthesis of new enzymes or transport proteins (transcriptional effects), thereby increasing or decreasing the amount rather than the activity of these proteins in the target cell.

Metabolic processes that must be regulated rapidly (eg, blood glucose or calcium homeostasis) are usually under the control of the peptide hormones and epinephrine, whereas those processes that may be regulated more slowly (eg, pubertal development, metabolic rate) are under the control of the steroid hormones and thyroid hormone (Table 30–1). The control of electrolyte homeostasis is intermediate and is regulated by a

***Table 30–1.*** Hormonal regulation of metabolic processes.

| First Level (Most Direct) | | | |
|---|---|---|---|
| **Metabolite or Other Parameter** | **Abnormality** | **Endocrine Gland** | **Hormone** |
| Glucose | Hyperglycemia | Pancreatic beta cell | Insulin |
| Glucose | Hypoglycemia | Pancreatic alpha cell | Glucagon |
| Glucose | Hypoglycemia | Adrenal medulla | Epinephrine |
| Calcium | Hypercalcemia | Thyroid C cell | Calcitonin (?) |
| Calcium | Hypocalcemia | Parathyroid | PTH |
| Sodium/plasma osmolality | Hypernatremia/hyperosmolality | Hypothalamus (posterior pituitary gland) | ADH |
| Plasma volume | Hypervolemia | Heart | ANH |
| **Second Level: Sodium and Potassium Balance** | | | |
| **Metabolite or Other Parameter** | **Abnormality** | **Endocrine Gland** | **Hormone** |
| Sodium/potassium | Hyponatremia | Kidney | Renin (an enzyme) |
| | Hyperkalemia | Liver and others | Angiotensin I |
| | Hypovolemia | Lung | Angiotensin II |
| | | Adrenal cortex | Aldosterone |
| **Third Level (Most Complex)** | | | |
| **Releasing Hormone** | **Tropic Hormone** | **Endocrine Gland** | **Endocrine Gland Hormone** |
| CRH | ACTH | Adrenal cortex | Cortisol |
| GHRH | GH | Liver | IGF-1 |
| GnRH | LH | Testis | Testosterone |
| GnRH | FSH/LH | Ovary | Estradiol/progesterone |
| TRH | TSH | Thyroid gland | $T_4$ (some $T_3$) |

ACTH = corticotropin; ADH = antidiuretic hormone; ANH = antinaturietic hormone; CRH = corticotropin-releasing hormone; FSH = follicle-stimulating hormone; GH = growth hormone; GHRH = growth hormone-releasing hormone; GnRH = gonadotropin-releasing hormone; IGF = insulin-like growth factor; LH = luteinizing hormone; PTH = parathyroid hormone; $T_3$ = triiodothyronine; $T_4$ = thyroxine; TRH = thyrotropin-releasing hormone; TSH = thyroid-stimulating hormone.

combination of peptide and steroid hormones (see Table 30–1).

## FEEDBACK CONTROL OF HORMONE SECRETION

Hormone secretion is regulated, for the most part, by feedback in response to changes in the internal environment as postulated by Claude Bernard in the nineteenth century (see Table 30–1). When the metabolic imbalance is corrected, stimulation of the hormone's secretion ceases and may even be inhibited. Overcorrection of the imbalance stimulates secretion of a counterbalancing hormone or hormones, so that the circulating concentrations of metabolites are kept within relatively narrow limits.

Hypothalamic–pituitary control of hormonal secretion is also regulated by feedback, so that end-organ failure (endocrine gland insufficiency) leading to decreased circulating concentrations of endocrine gland hormones results in increased secretion of hypothalamic releasing and pituitary hormones (see Table 30–1; Figure 30–1). If restoration of normal circulating concentrations of endocrine gland hormones occurs, feedback inhibition at the pituitary and hypothalamus results in cessation of the previously stimulated secretion of releasing and pituitary hormones and restoration of their circulating concentrations to normal.

Similarly, if autonomous endocrine gland hyperfunction is present (eg, McCune–Albright syndrome, Graves disease, adrenal tumor), the specific hypothalamic releasing and pituitary hormones are suppressed (see Figure 30–1). An understanding of the basic phenomenon of feedback control of hormonal secretion is fundamental to the understanding of endocrine disorders and their evaluation in children.

**Figure 30–1.** General scheme of the hypothalamus–pituitary–endocrine gland axis. Releasing hormones synthesized in the hypothalamus are secreted into the hypophysial portal circulation. Trophic hormones are secreted by the pituitary gland in response, and they in turn act on specific endocrine glands to stimulate the secretion of their respective hormones. The endocrine gland hormones exert their respective effects on various target tissues (end organs) and exert an indirect negative feedback (feedback inhibition) on their own secretion by acting at the level of the pituitary and hypothalamus. This system is characteristic of those hormones listed in Table 30–1 (third level).

# ■ DISTURBANCES OF GROWTH

Disturbances of growth and development are the most common presenting complaints in the pediatric endocrine clinic. It is critical to distinguish between normal and abnormal growth patterns, because deviation from a normal growth pattern can be the first or only manifestation of a wide variety of diseases. Determination of height velocity is the single most critical factor in evaluating the growth of a child, and a persistent increase or decrease in height percentiles between age 2 years and the onset of puberty should warrant further evaluation. It is a little more difficult to distinguish

normal from abnormal growth in the first 2 years of life, as infants will show catch-up or catch-down growth during this period. It is also important to evaluate a child's growth in the context of normal standards. The National Center for Health Statistics provides standard growth charts derived from growth data of North American children (see Chapter 1). Height and weight measurements should be plotted on these charts. Growth charts are also available for children with specific growth disturbances, such as Turner syndrome and Down syndrome.

## TARGET HEIGHT AND SKELETAL MATURATION

The growth and height potential of a child is determined largely by genetic factors. The target (midparental) height of a child can be determined by calculating the mean parental height and adding or subtracting 6.5 cm for boys and girls, respectively. Most children will achieve an adult height that is within 8 cm of their target height; consequently, this calculation is very helpful in evaluating a child's genetic growth potential. Another important parameter in determining growth potential is bone age, which is a measure of skeletal maturation. Beyond the neonatal period, a radiograph of the left hand and wrist is obtained and compared with the published standards of Greulich and Pyle. The extent of skeletal maturation can be used to predict a child's ultimate height potential because growth ceases when epiphyseal fusion is complete. A delayed bone age is not diagnostic of a specific disease but indicates that there is residual growth potential.

## SHORT STATURE

Short stature has many causes, and it is important to distinguish between normal variants of growth (familial short stature and constitutional growth delay) and pathologic conditions (Table 30–2). Pathologic short stature should be suspected in children who have an abnormal growth velocity (crossing major height percentiles on the growth curve) or in children who are significantly short for their family. Children with chronic illness or nutritional deficiencies may have poor linear growth, but this is typically associated with inadequate weight gain. In contrast, endocrine causes of short stature are usually associated with normal or excessive weight gain.

### Familial Short Stature and Constitutional Growth Delay

Children with familial short stature are typically born with normal weight and length. In the first 2 years of

***Table 30–2.*** Causes of short stature.

| | |
|---|---|
| **A. Genetic-familial short stature** | **D. Intrauterine growth retardation (*cont.*)** |
| **B. Constitutional growth delay** |    b. Drug use |
| **C. Endocrine disturbances** |    c. Malnutrition |

**A. Genetic-familial short stature**
**B. Constitutional growth delay**
**C. Endocrine disturbances**
  1. Growth hormone deficiency
    a. Hereditary—gene deletion
    b. Idiopathic—deficiency of growth hormone or growth hormone-releasing hormone (or both) with and without associated abnormalities of midline structures of the central nervous system
    c. Acquired
       Transient—eg, psychosocial short stature
       Organic—tumor, irradiation of the central nervous system, infection, or trauma
  2. Hypothyroidism
  3. Excess cortisol—Cushing disease and Cushing syndrome (including iatrogenic causes)
  4. Precocious puberty
  5. Diabetes mellitus (poorly controlled)
  6. Pseudohypoparathyroidism
  7. Rickets
**D. Intrauterine growth retardation**
  1. Intrinsic fetal abnormalities—chromosomal disorders
  2. Syndromes (eg, Russell–Silver, Noonan, Bloom, de Lange, Cockayne)
  3. Congenital infections
  4. Placental abnormalities
  5. Maternal abnormalities
    a. Hypertension/toxemia

**D. Intrauterine growth retardation (*cont.*)**
    b. Drug use
    c. Malnutrition
**E. Inborn errors of metabolism**
  1. Mucopolysaccharidosis
  2. Other storage diseases
**F. Intrinsic diseases of bone**
  1. Defects of growth of tubular bones or spine (eg, achondroplasia, metatropic dwarfism, diastrophic dwarfism, metaphyseal chondrodysplasia)
  2. Disorganized development of cartilage and fibrous components of the skeleton (eg, multiple cartilaginous exostoses, fibrous dysplasia with skin pigmentation)
  3. Abnormalities of density of cortical diaphyseal structure or metaphyseal modeling (eg, osteogenesis imperfecta congenita, osteopetrosis, tubular stenosis)
**G. Short stature associated with chromosomal defects**
  1. Autosomal (eg, Down syndrome, Prader–Willi syndrome)
  2. Sex chromosomal (eg, Turner syndrome-XO)
**H. Chronic systemic diseases, congenital defects, and cancers** (eg, chronic infection and infestation, inflammatory bowel disease, hepatic disease, cardiovascular disease, hematologic disease, central nervous system disease, pulmonary disease, renal disease, malnutrition, cancers, collagen vascular disease)
**I. Psychosocial short stature (deprivation dwarfism)**

life, however, they will have a deceleration in linear growth to reach their target percentile, which is determined largely by genetic factors. Once this target percentile is obtained, the child will have normal linear growth parallel to the growth curve. Skeletal maturation and the timing of puberty are consistent with chronologic age. Consequently, the height percentile the child has been following is maintained, and final height is short but appropriate for the family (Figure 30–2). For example, an infant boy of a mother who is 5'0" and father who is 5'5" may have a birth length at the fiftieth percentile. However, this child's length will probably change percentiles downward within the first 2 years of life to reach the fifth percentile. The calculated midparental height of this child is 5'5", which is at the fifth percentile for a full grown male. Consequently, the fifth percentile is an appropriate growth trajectory for this child.

Children with constitutional growth delay do not necessarily have short parents but have a growth pattern similar to those with familial short stature. The difference is that children with constitutional growth delay will have a delay in skeletal maturation and a delay in the onset of puberty. In these children, growth continues beyond the time the average child has stopped growing, and final height is appropriate for target height (Figure 30–3). There is often a history of other family members being so-called "late bloomers."

## Growth Hormone Deficiency

Human growth hormone (GH) is produced by the anterior pituitary gland under the stimulation of growth hormone-releasing hormone (GHRH) and the inhibition of somatostatin. GH is secreted in a pulsatile pattern in response to sleep, exercise, and hypoglycemia and has direct growth-promoting and metabolic effects (Figure 30–4). GH also promotes growth indirectly by stimulating the production of insulin-like growth factors, primarily IGF-1.

Growth hormone deficiency (GHD) is characterized by decreased growth velocity, delay in skeletal maturation, absence of other explanations for poor growth, and laboratory tests indicating subnormal GH secretion. GHD may be isolated or may occur with other pituitary hormone deficiencies. Identifiable causes of

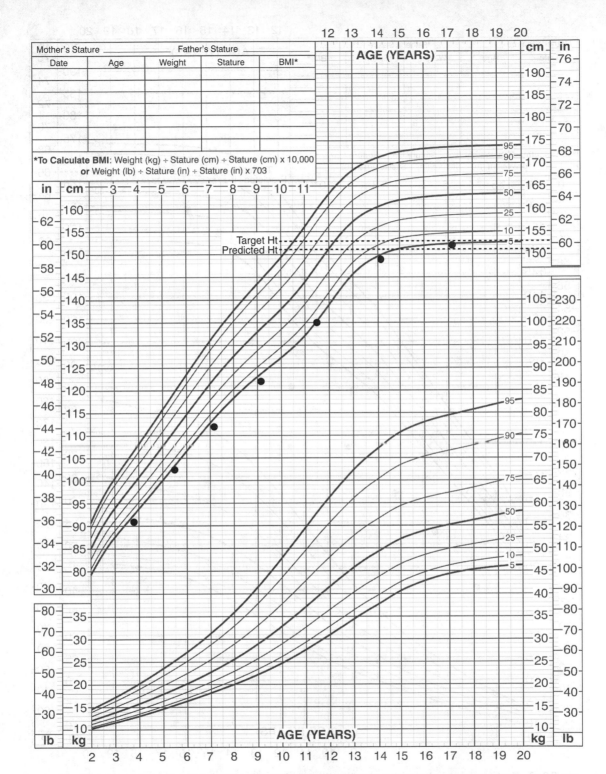

**Figure 30–2.** Typical pattern of growth in a child with familial short stature. After attaining an appropriate percentile during the first 2 years of life, the child will have normal linear growth parallel to the growth curve. Skeletal maturation and the timing of puberty are consistent with chronological age. The height percentile the child has been following is maintained, and final height is short but appropriate for the family.

965

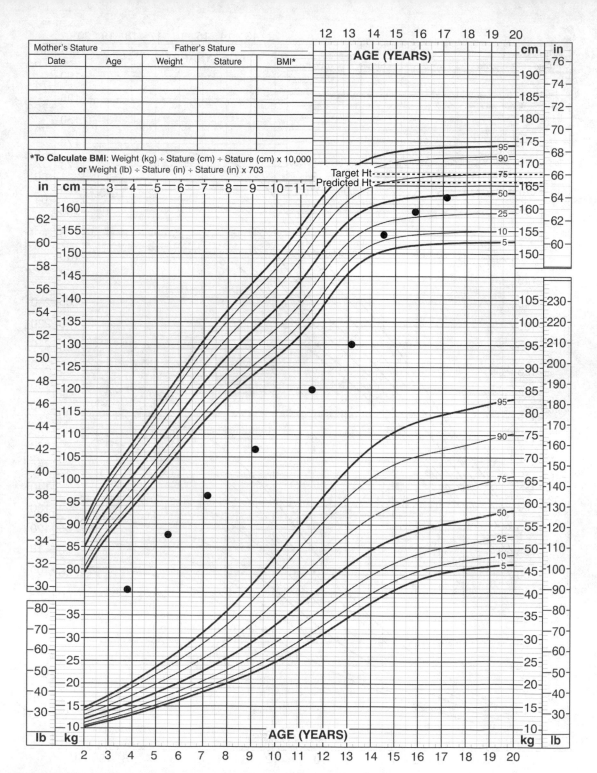

**Figure 30–3.** Typical pattern of growth in a child with constitutional growth delay. Growth slows during the first 2 years of life, similar to children with familial short stature. Subsequently the child will have normal linear growth parallel to the growth curve. However, skeletal maturation and the onset of puberty are delayed. Growth continues beyond the time the average child has stopped growing, and final height is appropriate for target height.

***Figure 30–4.*** The GHRH/GH/IGF-1 system. The effects of growth hormone (GH) on growth are partly due to its direct anabolic effects in muscle, liver, and bone. In addition, GH stimulates many tissues to produce insulin-like growth factor 1 (IGF-1) locally, which stimulates the growth of the tissue itself (paracrine effect of IGF-1). The action of GH on the liver results in the secretion of IGF-1 (circulating IGF-1), which stimulates growth in other tissues (endocrine effect of IGF-1). The action of growth hormone on the liver also enhances the secretion of IGF-binding protein-3 (IGFBP-3) and acid-labile subunit (ALS), which form a high-molecular-weight complex with IGF-1. The function of this complex is to transport IGF-1 to its target tissues, but the complex also serves as a reservoir and possible inhibitor of IGF-1 action. In various chronic illnesses, the direct metabolic effects of growth hormone are inhibited; the secretion of IGF-1 in response to GH is blunted, and in some cases IGFBP-3 systhesis is enhanced, resulting in marked inhibition in the growth of the child. (GHRH = growth hormone-releasing hormone.)

GHD may be congenital (septo-optic dysplasia, empty-sella syndrome), genetic (HGH or GHRH gene mutation), or acquired (craniopharyngioma, germinoma, histiocytosis, cranial irradiation). Idiopathic GHD, however, occurs more commonly than any of these recognized causes, with an incidence of approximately 1:4000 children. The GH insensitivity syndrome (Laron dwarfism) is caused by a mutation in the GH receptor. These children present in a manner similar to those with GHD, but children with Laron dwarfism may have a distinctive facial appearance.

Infants with GHD are of normal birth weight; birth length may be reduced slightly, suggesting that GH is not a major contributor to intrauterine growth. Classic HGH-deficient infants may present initially with hypoglycemia or evidence of other pituitary deficiencies such as central hypothyroidism or adrenal insufficiency. Gonadotropin and GH deficiency may be suspected in the newborn male who has a micropenis. Growth retardation may begin in infancy or may be delayed until later childhood. In children with acquired or idiopathic GHD, the primary manifestation is a subnormal growth velocity (Figure 30–5). Because GH promotes lipolysis, many GH-deficient children will also have truncal adiposity.

Laboratory tests to assess GH status may be difficult to interpret. Children with normal and short stature have a broad range of HGH secretion patterns, and significant overlap exists between test results of normal and GH-deficient children. Traditionally, provocative studies are performed using such agents as insulin-induced hypoglycemia, arginine, levodopa, clonidine, or glucagon. Serum concentrations of IGF-1 and IGF-binding protein 3 may give reasonable estimations of

**Figure 30–5.** Typical pattern of growth in a child with acquired growth hormone deficiency. Children with acquired growth hormone deficiency have an abnormal growth velocity and fail to maintain height percentile during childhood. Other phenotypic features (central adiposity, immaturity of facies) may be present. Children with congenital growth hormone deficiency will cross percentiles during the first 2 years of life, similar to the pattern seen in familial short stature and constitutional delay, but will fail to attain a steady height percentile subsequently.

GH secretion in the adequately nourished child (see Figure 30–4). When results of GH tests are equivocal, a trial of HGH treatment may be useful in determining whether an abnormally short child will benefit from GH. Currently the treatment of choice for GHD is recombinant HGH in a dose of 0.15–0.3 mg/kg/wk administered subcutaneously divided into six or seven equal once-daily doses.

GH therapy is FDA-approved for children with GHD and growth retardation associated with chronic renal failure, for girls with Turner syndrome, children with Prader–Willi syndrome, and children born small for gestational age (SGA) who fail to demonstrate "catch-up" growth by age 4. GH therapy has been recently approved for children with idiopathic short stature whose current height is more than 2.25 SD below the norm for age. Final height improvement may be 5–7 cm in this population. This indication has generated much controversy, and the role of GH in these children remains unclear. GH therapy is expensive, and indications other than these remain controversial. Reported side effects of recombinant GH therapy are uncommon but include benign intracranial hypertension and slipped capital femoral epiphysis. With early diagnosis and treatment, children with GHD reach normal or nearly normal adult height.

## Small for Gestational Age/Intrauterine Growth Restriction

Small-for-gestational-age (SGA) infants are those who have birth weights less than the tenth percentile for the population's birth weight/gestational age relationship. SGA infants include those who are constitutionally small and growing at their potential, as well as those with intrauterine growth retardation (IUGR). IUGR refers to a heterogeneous group of patients who fail to grow at a normal rate in utero. SGA/IUGR occurs secondary to poor maternal environment, intrinsic fetal abnormalities, congenital infections, or other forms of fetal malnutrition. Conditions secondary to intrinsic fetal abnormalities are often referred to as primordial short stature and include the Russell–Silver, Seckel, Noonan, Bloom, and Cockayne syndromes, and progeria. Many children with milder degrees of SGA/IUGR (except those with intrinsic fetal abnormalities) exhibit catch-up growth during their first 3 years of life. However, 15–20% will remain short throughout life, particularly those whose growth restriction in utero occurred over several months rather than just the last 2 or 3 months of gestation, as well as those born preterm with subsequent inadequate postnatal nutrition. Those children who do not show catch-up growth will have a normal growth velocity, although they will follow a lower height percentile than expected for the family. In most instances, skeletal maturation corresponds to chronologic age or is delayed only mildly—in contrast to the delay occurring in children with constitutional growth delay. GH therapy has been evaluated in SGA children, and short-term studies have shown increases in growth velocity. Consequently, growth hormone has recently been approved for treatment in these children.

## Disproportionate Short Stature

Skeletal dysplasias are disorders that result in disproportionate short stature. More than 200 different types of skeletal dysplasias may occur, either sporadically or genetically. Measurements of arm span and upper-to-lower body segment ratio are helpful in determining whether a child has normal body proportions. If disproportionate short stature is found, a skeletal survey may be useful because specific radiographic features characterize certain disorders. Because skeletal dysplasias are individually rare, the effect of GH on most types is largely unknown.

## Short Stature Associated with Syndromes

Short stature is associated with many syndromes, including Turner, Down, and Prader–Willi. Girls with Turner syndrome typically have such other typical features as micrognathia, webbed neck, low posterior hairline, edema of hands and feet, multiple pigmented nevi, and an increased carrying angle. In some girls with Turner syndrome, however, short stature is the only clinical manifestation. Consequently, any girl with unexplained short stature should have a chromosomal evaluation. Although girls with Turner syndrome are not classically GH-deficient, GH therapy has been shown to improve final height by an average of 6.0 cm. The duration of GH therapy is a significant predictor of long-term height gain; consequently, it is important that Turner syndrome be diagnosed early and GH started as soon as possible.

GH is also approved for growth failure associated with Prader–Willi syndrome, a syndrome in which many individuals are GH-deficient. GH improves growth as well as body composition and physical activity in these patients. A few fatalities have been reported in Prader–Willi children treated with GH. All of these children were severely obese or had a history of respiratory impairment, sleep apnea, or an unidentified respiratory infection. The role of GH, if any, in contributing to these deaths is unknown. As a precaution, it is recommended that all Prader–Willi patients be evaluated for upper airway obstruction and sleep apnea prior to initiation of GH therapy.

Children with Down syndrome should be evaluated for GHD only if their linear growth is abnormal compared with the Down syndrome growth chart.

## Psychosocial Short Stature (Psychosocial Dwarfism)

Psychosocial short stature is characterized by growth retardation in association with emotional deprivation. Undernutrition contributes to the growth retardation of some affected children. In addition to impaired growth, bizarre eating and drinking habits, bowel and bladder incontinence, social withdrawal, and delayed speech may occur. GH secretion in children with psychosocial short stature is diminished, but GH therapy is usually not beneficial. Foster home placement or a change in the psychological environment at home usually results in improved growth and normalization of GH secretion, personality, and eating behaviors.

## Diagnostic Approach to Short Stature

Laboratory investigation should be guided by information gained from the history and physical examination. Initial considerations should include size at birth, presence of dysmorphology, pattern of growth since birth, family pattern of growth, pubertal stage, body segment proportion, and psychological problems. In a child who has poor weight gain as the primary disturbance, history of chronic illness and nutritional assessment are indicated. The following laboratory tests may be useful:

1. Radiograph of left hand and wrist for bone age
2. Complete blood count (to detect chronic anemia, infection)
3. Erythrocyte sedimentation rate (often elevated in collagen–vascular disease, cancer, chronic infection, inflammatory bowel disease)
4. Urinalysis, blood urea nitrogen, and serum creatinine (occult renal disease)
5. Serum electrolytes, calcium, and phosphorus (renal tubular disease, metabolic bone disease)
6. Stool examination for fat, serum endomysial antibody (malabsorption, celiac disease)
7. Karyotype (in girls)
8. Thyroid function tests: free thyroxine ($FT_4$) and thyroid-stimulating hormone (TSH)
9. IGF-1 and IGF-binding protein 3 (IGFBP-3)

Carrel AL et al: Benefits of long-term GH therapy in Prader–Willi syndrome: A 4-year study. J Clin Endocrinol Metab 2002; 87:1581 [PMID: 11932286].

Fjellestad-Paulsen A et al: Three-year data from a comparative study with recombinant human growth hormone in the treatment of short stature in young children with intrauterine growth retardation. Acta Paediatr 1998;87:511 [PMID: 9641731].

Hintz RL et al: Effect of growth hormone treatment on adult height of children with idiopathic short stature: Genentech collaborative group. N Engl J Med 1999;340:502 [PMID: 10021470].

Hintz RL: Approaches to the diagnosis and management of growth failure. Pediatr Ann 2000;29:537 [PMID: 11016046].

## TALL STATURE

Although we typically think of growth disturbances in relation to short stature, potentially serious pathologic conditions may be associated with tall stature and excessive growth (Table 30–3). Excessive GH secretion is rare in children and is generally associated with a functioning pituitary adenoma. GH excess leads to gigantism if the epiphyses are open and to acromegaly if the epiphyses are closed. Affected children present with an accelerated growth velocity. The diagnosis is confirmed by demonstrating elevated GH and IGF-1 levels and failure of GH to suppress during a standard oral glucose tolerance test.

Constitutional tall stature may be a concern to adolescent girls. However, the upper limit of acceptable height in both sexes is increasing, and concerns about excessive growth for girls are becoming less frequent. When such concerns arise, the family history, growth curve, pubertal stage, and assessment of skeletal maturation allow assessment of predicted final adult height. Reassurance, counseling, and education may alleviate the family's concerns. In extremely rare instances in which the predicted height appears to be excessive and unacceptable, estrogen therapy may accelerate bone maturation and shorten the growth period.

Eugster EA: Gigantism. J Clin Endocrinol Metab 1999;84:4379 [PMID: 10599691].

Stewart PM: Current therapy for acromegaly: Trends. J Clin Endocrinol Metab 2000;11:128 [PMID: 10754533].

**Table 30–3.** Causes of tall stature.

**A. Constitutional (familial)**
**B. Endocrine causes**
   1. Growth hormone excess (pituitary gigantism)
   2. Precocious puberty
   3. Hypogonadism
**C. Nonendocrine causes**
   1. Klinfelter syndrome
   2. XYY males
   3. Marfan syndrome
   4. Cerebral gigantism (Soto syndrome)
   5. Homocystinuria

# THE POSTERIOR PITUITARY GLAND

The posterior pituitary (neurohypophysis) is an extension of the ventral hypothalamus. The two principal neurohormones of the posterior pituitary, oxytocin and arginine vasopressin (AVP), are synthesized in the supraoptic and paraventricular nuclei. After synthesis, these neurohormones are packaged in granules with specific neurophysins and transported via the axons to their storage site in the neurohypophysis. AVP is essential for fluid homeostasis; its primary action is on the kidney to cause antidiuresis. Oxytocin is primarily important during parturition and breast-feeding and is not discussed further here.

## Arginine Vasopressin (Antidiuretic Hormone)

Osmoreceptors in the anterolateral hypothalamus and baroreceptors in the cardiac atria regulate AVP release. The release of vasopressin is primarily influenced by serum osmolality and vascular volume. Disorders of vasopressin release and action include (1) central (neurogenic) diabetes insipidus (discussed in the following section), (2) nephrogenic diabetes insipidus (see Chapter 22), and (3) the syndrome of inappropriate antidiuretic hormone (SIADH) (see Chapter 42).

## CENTRAL DIABETES INSIPIDUS

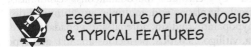

### ESSENTIALS OF DIAGNOSIS & TYPICAL FEATURES

- *Polydipsia and polyuria (> 2 L/m²/d).*
- *Urine specific gravity (< 1.010; osmolality < 300 mOsm/kg).*
- *Inability to concentrate urine after fluid restriction.*
- *Hyperosmolality of plasma.*
- *Subnormal plasma AVP concentration.*
- *Responsiveness to AVP administration.*

## General Considerations

Central diabetes insipidus, a result of vasopressin deficiency, is caused by defects in hypothalamic vasopressin synthesis, packaging, or transport along the neurohypophyseal tract to the posterior pituitary gland. Genetic causes of vasopressin deficiency are rare and include inherited mutations in the vasopressin structural gene, defects in the neurophysin protein, and the DIDMOAD syndrome (diabetes insipidus, diabetes mellitus, optic atrophy, and deafness). Midline brain abnormalities such as septo-optic dysplasia and holoprosencephaly may also be associated with central diabetes insipidus. Accidental or surgical trauma to the axons of the vasopressin-containing neurons can cause transient or permanent diabetes insipidus. In this situation, a triphasic pattern often results, in which transient diabetes insipidus occurs first as a consequence of edema in the hypothalamic–pituitary area. This is followed in 2–5 days by SIADH, caused by the unregulated release of vasopressin from the dying neurons. The third phase is permanent diabetes insipidus, which results if significant damage to the vasopressin neurons has occurred.

Hypothalamic tumors and infiltrative diseases are found in a significant number of children who present with diabetes insipidus. In patients with craniopharyngiomas, diabetes insipidus usually develops only after surgical intervention. This is in contrast to germinomas in which diabetes insipidus is often the presenting symptom. Germinomas may be undetectable by magnetic resonance imaging (MRI) for several years; consequently, children with unexplained diabetes insipidus should have regularly repeated MRI scans. Infiltrative diseases such as histiocytosis and lymphocytic hypophysitis also cause diabetes insipidus in children. In these conditions, as well as germinomas, MRI scans characteristically show thickening or a mass within the infundibular stalk.

## Clinical Findings

The onset of diabetes insipidus is often abrupt and is characterized by polyuria and intense thirst. The affected child typically has nocturia or enuresis and cannot go through the night without drinking water. Cold water is typically the preferred fluid. Dehydration may occur if fluid intake is not sufficient to keep up with urine losses or if concomitant damage has occurred to the normal thirst mechanism. In infants, symptoms may also include failure to thrive, vomiting, constipation, and unexplained fevers. It is especially difficult to recognize polyuria and polydipsia in a young infant on an ordinary feeding regimen, and the infant may present with severe dehydration, circulatory collapse, and convulsions. Familial diabetes insipidus may have a more insidious onset and a slowly progressive course.

Symptoms and signs of AVP deficiency may be absent in patients with panhypopituitarism due to the impaired excretion of free water that may accompany adrenal insufficiency. Treating these patients with glucocorticoids may unmask underlying polyuria and polydipsia.

## Diagnosis

The diagnosis of diabetes insipidus is confirmed when hypotonic urine accompanies hypertonic serum. Response to vasopressin or desmopressin indicates central rather than nephrogenic diabetes insipidus. In children with symptoms of increased thirst and urination, primary polydipsia must be distinguished from true diabetes insipidus. If the history reveals that the child can go through the night comfortably without drinking, screening tests can be obtained as an out patient. Oral intake of fluid is prohibited after midnight. A first morning void is obtained to determine urine osmolality, and sodium concentration, and a standard urinalysis is performed. A blood sample should be obtained within a few minutes of the urine collection and analyzed for osmolality, sodium, potassium, creatinine, and calcium levels. Children with primary polydipsia will produce appropriately concentrated urine. If screening results are unclear or if symptoms preclude safely withholding fluids at home, a water deprivation test performed in the hospital is indicated. During fluid deprivation, a serum osmolality of greater than 290 mOsm/kg associated with excretion of dilute urine (osmolality < 300 mOsm/kg) is suggestive of diabetes insipidus. Measurement of serum AVP concentration at the end of the test and the administration of parenteral AVP may help distinguish between central neurogenic and nephrogenic forms of diabetes insipidus. When the diagnosis of central diabetes insipidus is made, an MRI scan with contrast should be obtained to look for tumors or infiltrative processes. An absent posterior bright spot on MRI also correlates with AVP deficiency.

Decreased ability to concentrate urine may also occur with hypokalemia (eg, hyperaldosteronism), with various forms of hypercalcemia (including hypervitaminosis D), and with renal tubular abnormalities (eg, Fanconi syndrome).

## Treatment

### A. MEDICAL TREATMENT

The treatment of choice for partial and total diabetes insipidus is desmopressin acetate (DDAVP) administered orally or intranasally. The aim of therapy is to provide the child with antidiuresis and uninterrupted sleep during the night and allow for approximately 1 hour of diuresis before the next DDAVP dose. Treatment of diabetes insipidus in infants is more difficult because formula and breast milk have a large amount of free water; consequently, the risk of water overload with DDAVP therapy is great. For this reason, infants are often given extra free water, rather than DDAVP, to maintain normal hydration. Chlorothiazides, as prescribed for nephrogenic diabetes insipidus, may also be helpful in the infant with central diabetes insipidus.

### B. OTHER THERAPY

Specific therapy is directed toward specific causative diseases when they are identified. Radiation therapy, chemotherapy, or surgery may be indicated for germinomas, histiocytosis, and craniopharyngiomas.

Cheetham T, Baylis PH: Diabetes insipidus in children: Pathophysiology, diagnosis and management. Paediatr Drugs 2002;4:785 [PMID: 12431131].

Leger J et al: Thickened pituitary stalk on magnetic resonance imaging in children with central diabetes insipidus. J Clin Endocrinol Metab 1999;84:1954 [PMID: 10372693].

## AUTOIMMUNE POLYGLANDULAR SYNDROMES

Two autoimmune polyglandular syndromes (APS types 1 and 2) causing multiple endocrine deficiencies are distinguished by their clinical, laboratory, and epidemiologic characteristics. APS type 1 is also known as autoimmune polyendocrinopathy candidiasis ectodermal dystrophy (APECED). Inactivating mutations of the autoimmune regulator gene (AIRE) cause the disease. It is inherited as an autosomal recessive trait and therefore affects females and males equally. There is no HLA association. APS-1 typically presents in childhood. It is characterized by chronic mucocutaneous candidiasis, ectodermal dysplasia, and multiple autoimmune diseases: hypoparathyroidism, adrenal and gonadal failure, alopecia, vitiligo, hepatitis, pernicious anemia, and type 1 diabetes mellitus. Autoimmune thyroid disease is rare.

In contrast, APS-2, Schmidt syndrome, is a polygenic disorder highly influenced by HLA. Specifically it is associated with HLA DR3. It is defined by at least two of three autoimmune diseases: type 1 diabetes mellitus, Addison disease, or thyroid disease. Other autoimmune disease such as vitiligo, alopecia, hypogonadism, pernicious anemia, rheumatoid arthritis, celiac disease, and other autoimmune gastroenteropathies can also occur. There is a 2–3:1 female preponderance. Treatment is specific for each complication that occurs, and recognition of the associations of disorders in these syndromes may help to detect them early in their course.

Kumar PG et al: Population genetics and functions of the autoimmune regulatory (AIRE). Endocrinol Metab Clin North Am 2002;31:321 [PMID: 12092453].

Schatz DA, Winter WE: Autoimmune polyglandular syndrome II: Clinical syndrome and treatment. Endocrinol Metab Clin North Am 2002;31:339 [PMID: 12092454].

# ■ THE THYROID GLAND

## FETAL DEVELOPMENT OF THE THYROID

The thyroid is capable of hormone synthesis in the fourteenth week of gestation, when TSH is detected in the fetal serum and pituitary gland. TSH does not normally cross the placenta, but $T_4$ and $T_3$ cross in limited amounts. The fetal pituitary–thyroid axis functions largely independently of the maternal pituitary–thyroid axis. Antithyroid drugs, including propylthiouracil (PTU) and methimazole, freely cross the placenta, and goitrous hypothyroid newborns may be born to hyperthyroid mothers who undergo treatment during pregnancy.

Mothers who have thyroid-stimulating immunoglobulins (TSI) can transmit these antibodies transplacentally, causing thyrotoxicosis in newborns who may be born with goiter and exophthalmos. Because TSI may be present in the serum of controlled, previously hyperthyroid mothers—or even in women who have had surgical or radioiodine-induced removal of their thyroid glands—the possible transmission of TSI should be considered in all mothers who are or have been hyperthyroid. In addition, thyroid-binding inhibitory immunoglobulins (TBIIs) can cross the placenta, so that the newborn is also at risk for hypothyroidism. Both maternal TSI and TBII usually disappear from the infant's circulation by 6–8 weeks.

## Physiology

Pituitary TSH stimulates the thyroid gland to take up iodine and synthesize active thyroid hormones (ie, $T_3$, $T_4$). Active hormone produced in excess of physiologic needs is stored within the thyroid follicles as thyroglobulin. The release of active thyroid hormones into the circulation is regulated by a negative feedback mechanism involving pituitary TSH and free thyroid hormone (see Figure 30–1).

Most $T_3$ and $T_4$ circulates bound to thyroid hormone–binding globulin (TBG), albumin, and prealbumin, and less than 1% of $T_3$ and $T_4$ is free. $T_4$ is deiodinated in the tissues to either $T_3$ (active) or reverse $T_3$ (inactive), and the physiologic activity of thyroid hormone depends primarily on the amount of $FT_4$ presented to the cells. Receptors for $T_3$ are present on the cell surface, in the nucleus, in the cytosol, and on mitochondria.

At birth, the newborn's $T_4$ approximates that of the mother, but levels increase rapidly during the first 5 days of life in response to a TSH surge immediately following birth. TSH levels subsequently decrease to childhood levels by age 2–4 weeks. This physiologic neonatal TSH surge can cause falsely positive neonatal screens for hypothyroidism (ie, high TSH), because blood specimens for screening may be collected on the first day of life.

The total thyroxine ($TT_4$) level is low in hypothyroidism and may be reduced in premature infants (particularly those with sepsis or respiratory distress), subacute and chronic thyroiditis, hypopituitarism, nephrosis, cirrhosis, hypoproteinemia, malnutrition, and following therapy with $T_3$. Prolonged administration of high doses of adrenocorticosteroids—as well as of sulfonamides, testosterone, phenytoin, and salicylates—may also produce a decrease in the $TT_4$ level. However, since these effects are primarily on TBG levels, and not on thyroid function per se, TSH and $FT_4$ levels remain in the normal range. Total $T_3$ and $T_4$ levels are high in hyperthyroidism and may be elevated in acute forms of thyroiditis and hepatitis; in some types of inborn errors of thyroid hormone synthesis, release, or binding; following the administration of estrogens or clofibrate or during pregnancy; and following the administration of various iodine-containing globulins.

TBG levels are increased in pregnancy, after estrogen therapy (including oral contraceptives), occasionally as a genetic variation, in certain hepatic disorders, following administration of phenytoin or phenothiazines, and occasionally from an unknown cause. TBG levels are decreased in familial TBG deficiency; following the administration of glucocorticoids, androgens, or anabolic steroids; in nephrotic syndrome with marked hypoproteinemia; in some forms of hepatic disease; or as an idiopathic finding.

Because of the many "nonthyroidal" effects on $TT_4$, it is recommended that $FT_4$ be measured routinely in children suspected of having disorders of thyroid function.

## HYPOTHYROIDISM (Congenital & Acquired Hypothyroidism)

### ESSENTIALS OF DIAGNOSIS & TYPICAL FEATURES

- *Growth retardation, diminished physical activity, impaired tissue perfusion, constipation, thick tongue, poor muscle tone, hoarseness, anemia, and intellectual retardation. (These findings can arise in the first 2 months of life, but are absent in 75% of newborns with documented hypothyroidism.)*

- *Thyroid hormone concentrations low (TT₄, FT₄, and T₃ resin uptake [T₃RU]); TSH levels are elevated in primary hypothyroidism.*

**Note:** Most newborns with congenital hypothyroidism appear normal at birth and gain weight normally, even if not receiving treatment, for the first 3–4 months of life. Because congenital hypothyroidism must be treated as early as possible to avoid intellectual impairment, the diagnosis should be based on the newborn screening test and not on abnormal physical findings.

## General Considerations

Thyroid hormone deficiency may be either congenital or acquired (juvenile hypothyroidism). Although hypothyroidism in the newborn has many causes (Table 30–4), most cases are a result of hypoplasia or aplasia of the thyroid gland or failure of the gland to migrate into its normal anatomic location (ie, lingual or sublingual thyroid glands). Juvenile hypothyroidism, particularly if goiter is present, usually results from chronic lymphocytic (Hashimoto) thyroiditis (see later discussion).

Of the genetically determined enzymatic defects causing hypothyroidism (see Table 30–4), only Pendred syndrome (a defect in iodide organification with congenital nerve deafness) has distinguishing clinical features. In children who have enzymatic defects, thyroid enlargement is usually not present in the newborn period but occurs within the first two decades of life. Although thyroid function tests (including radioactive iodide uptake studies) may be helpful in diagnosis, final clarification of the defect generally requires chromatographic fractionation of iodinated compounds in the serum, urine, and thyroid tissue.

Cabbage, soybeans, aminosalicylic acid, thiourea derivatives, resorcinol, phenylbutazone, cobalt, and iodides have been reported to cause goiter and hypothy-

***Table 30–4.*** Causes of hypothyroidism.

| | |
|---|---|
| **A. Congenital (cretinism)**<br>  1. Aplasia, hypoplasia, or associated with maldescent of thyroid<br>    a. Embryonic defect of development<br>    b. Autoimmune disease (?)<br>  2. Familial iodine-induced goiter secondary to metabolic inborn errors<br>    a. Iodide transport defect (defect 1)<br>    b. Organification defect (defect 2)<br>      (1) Lack of iodine peroxidase<br>      (2) Lack of iodine transferase: Pendred syndrome, associated with congenital nerve deafness<br>    c. Coupling defect (defect 3)<br>    d. Iodotyrosine deiodinase defect (defect 4)<br>    e. Abnormal iodinated polypeptide (defects 5a and 5b)<br>      (1) Resulting from defect in intrathyroidal proteolysis of thyroglobulin<br>      (2) Abnormal plasma binding preventing use of T₄ by peripheral cells<br>    f. Inability of tissues to convert T₄ to T₃<br>  3. Maternal ingestion of medications during pregnancy<br>    a. Maternal radioiodine<br>    b. Goitrogens (propylthiouracil, methimazole)<br>    c. Iodides<br>  4. Iodide deficiency (endemic cretinism)<br>  5. Idiopathic | **B. Acquired (juvenile hypothyroidism)**<br>  1. Thyroidectomy or radioiodine therapy for<br>    a. Thyrotoxicosis<br>    b. Cancer<br>    c. Lingual thyroid<br>    d. Isolated midline thyroid<br>  2. Destruction by x-ray<br>  3. Thyrotropin deficiency<br>    a. Isolated<br>    b. Associated with other pituitary tropic hormone deficiencies<br>  4. TRH deficiency due to hypothalamic injury or disease<br>  5. Autoimmune disease (lymphocytic thyroiditis)<br>  6. Chronic infections<br>  7. Medications<br>    a. Iodides<br>      (1) Prolonged, excessive ingestion<br>      (2) Deficiency<br>    b. Cobalt<br>  8. Idiopathic |

T₃ = triiodothyronine; T₄ = thyroxine; TRH = thyrotropin-releasing hormone.

roidism during pregnancy. Because many of these agents cross the placenta freely, they should be used with great caution during pregnancy.

Several hundred patients with clinical and laboratory features of resistance to thyroid hormone have been described. These syndromes are generally familial and are classified on the basis of the site of the resistance (eg, generalized; pituitary or peripheral tissue).

## Clinical Findings

The severity of the findings in patients with thyroid deficiency depends on the age at onset and the degree of deficiency.

### A. Symptoms and Signs

Even with congenital absence of the thyroid gland, the first finding may not appear for several days or weeks. Consequently, any suspected abnormality in the results of the newborn screen should be investigated promptly. Findings include physical and mental sluggishness; pale, gray, cool, or mottled skin; nonpitting myxedema; constipation; large tongue; poor muscle tone giving rise to a protuberant abdomen, umbilical hernia and lumbar lordosis; hypothermia; bradycardia; diminished sweating (variable); decreased pulse pressure; hoarse voice or cry; delayed transient deafness; and a slow relaxation component of deep tendon reflexes (best appreciated in the ankles). Nasal obstruction and discharge and persistent jaundice may be present in the neonatal period.

The skin may be dry, thick, scaly, and coarse, with a yellowish tinge due to excessive deposition of carotene. The hair is dry, coarse, and brittle (variable) and may be excessive. Lateral thinning of the eyebrows may occur. The axillary and supraclavicular fat pads may be prominent in infants. Muscular hypertrophy (Kocher–Debré–Sémélaigne syndrome) is an unusual association with congenital hypothyroidism.

Growth changes include short stature; infantile skeletal proportions with relatively short extremities; infantile naso-orbital configuration (bridge of nose flat, broad, and underdeveloped; eyes seem to be widely spaced); delayed epiphyseal development; delayed closure of fontanelles; and retarded dental eruption. Treatment of acquired hypothyroidism may not result in the attainment of predicted adult target height. Metromenorrhagia may occur in older girls, and galactorrhea resulting from the stimulation of prolactin secretion or elevated thyrotropin-releasing hormone (TRH) has been reported.

In hypothyroidism resulting from enzymatic defects, ingestion of goitrogens, or chronic lymphocytic thyroiditis, the thyroid gland may be enlarged. Thyroid enlargement in children is usually symmetrical, and the gland is moderately firm and without nodularity. In chronic lymphocytic thyroiditis, however, the thyroid frequently has a cobblestone surface; size and shape are readily apparent on inspection in children. Slowing of mental responsiveness and retardation of development of the brain may occur in neonates and infants, and a coincidental congenital malformation of the brain is present in some patients.

### B. Laboratory Findings

$TT_4$ and $FT_4$ levels are decreased. Radioiodine uptake is below 10% (normal: 10–30%). The binding of $T_3$ by erythrocytes or resin in vitro ($T_3RU$ test) is lowered. With primary hypothyroidism, the serum TSH concentration is elevated. Normocytic anemia is common, but microcytic or macrocytic anemia may occur as a result of decreased iron, folate, and cobalamin absorption. Serum cholesterol and carotene are usually elevated in childhood but may be low or normal in infants. Cessation of therapy in previously treated hypothyroidism produces a marked rise in serum cholesterol levels in 6–8 weeks. Urinary creatinine excretion is decreased, and urinary hydroxyproline is low. Circulating autoantibodies to thyroid constituents may be present. Serum GH may be decreased, with subnormal HGH response to stimulation in children with severe primary hypothyroidism, as well as low IGF-1 or IGF binding protein 3 (or both).

### C. Imaging

Skeletal maturation (bone age) is delayed. Centers of ossification, especially of the hip, may show multiple small centers or a single stippled, porous, or fragmented center (epiphyseal dysgenesis). Vertebrae may show anterior beaking. Coxa vara and coxa plana may occur. Cardiomegaly is common.

## Screening Programs for Neonatal Hypothyroidism

Congenital hypothyroidism should by diagnosed by neonatal screening within 10 days of birth. It may be recognized clinically during the first month of life or may be so mild that it is unrecognized clinically for months. Adequate treatment started as soon as possible—but certainly before the end of the first month of life—improves the prognosis for intellectual performance later in life.

## Differential Diagnosis

The causes of primary hypothyroidism due to intrinsic defects of the thyroid gland must be differentiated from pituitary and hypothalamic failure with secondary thyroid insufficiency. TSH and $FT_4$ levels are the most useful tests and are usually sufficient in directing treatment or the need for further investigations.

Down syndrome, chondrodystrophy, generalized gangliosidosis, I-cell disease, Hurler and Hunter syndromes, and certain other causes of short stature and coarse features can all be readily distinguished from hypothyroidism by their clinical manifestations and by laboratory studies.

## Treatment

Levothyroxine is the drug of choice in a dosage of 75–100 μg/m$^2$/d as a single dose. In newborns and infants, the dose is 10–12 μg/kg. The hypothyroid patient may be very responsive to thyroid and may be sensitive to slight excesses of thyroid hormone. A dose of 0.0375 μg (37.5 μg) of levothyroxine is often recommended initially. Serum FT$_4$ concentrations should be used to monitor the adequacy of therapy initially, because the elevated TSH may not fall into the normal range for several days to weeks. Subsequently, elevations of serum TSH are sensitive early indicators of the need for increased medication (or increased compliance).

In the treatment of neonatal goiter with or without hypothyroidism resulting from drugs and goitrogens taken by the pregnant woman, temporary use of levothyroxine may be helpful in decreasing the size of the goiter.

Briet JM et al: Neonatal thyroxine supplementation in very preterm children. Pediatrics 2001;107:712 [PMID: 11335749].

Castanet M et al: Nineteen years of neonatal screening for congenital hypothyroidism. J Clin Endocrinol Metab 2001;86:2009 [PMID: 11344199].

Smallridge RC, Ladenson PW: Hypothyroisidm in pregnancy: Consequences to neonatal health. J Clin Endocrinol Metab 2001;86:2349 [PMID: 11397821].

Van Vliet G: Treatment of congenital hypothyroidism. Lancet 2001;358:86 [PMID: 11463405].

# THYROIDITIS

Chronic lymphocytic (Hashimoto) thyroiditis is perhaps the most common pediatric endocrinopathy, particularly in adolescent girls. Acute and subacute thyroiditis are rare in all age groups.

## 1. Acute Suppurative Thyroiditis

Acute thyroiditis is rare. Oropharyngeal organisms are thought to reach the thyroid via a patent foramen cecum and thyroglossal duct tract. The most common pathogens are group A streptococci, pneumococci, *Staphylococcus aureus,* and anaerobes. The patient is invariably toxic, and the thyroid gland is exquisitely tender. Pain may radiate to adjacent areas of the neck or to the ear or chest. No endocrine disturbance is consistently associated with this disorder. Specific antibiotic therapy should be administered.

## 2. Subacute Nonsuppurative Thyroiditis

Subacute thyroiditis (de Quervain thyroiditis) is rare in the United States. In most cases, the cause is a virus (mumps, influenza, echovirus, coxsackievirus, Epstein–Barr virus, or adenovirus). Presenting features are similar to those of acute thyroiditis: fever, malaise, sore throat, dysphagia, pain in the thyroid gland that may radiate to the ears, and mild and transient manifestations of hyperthyroidism. In contrast to acute thyroiditis, the onset of the subacute form is generally insidious. The thyroid gland is firm, and the enlargement may be confined to one lobe. Radioiodine uptake is usually reduced, but thyroid hormone levels in the blood are normal or elevated. The differentiation from bacterial thyroiditis is difficult, and antibiotic therapy is therefore recommended.

## 3. Chronic Lymphocytic Thyroiditis (Chronic Autoimmune Thyroiditis, Hashimoto Thyroiditis)

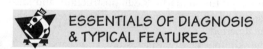

### ESSENTIALS OF DIAGNOSIS & TYPICAL FEATURES

- *Firm, freely movable, nontender, and diffusely enlarged goiter.*
- *Serum FT$_4$ concentrations are generally normal but may be elevated or decreased depending on the stage of the disease.*

## General Considerations

Chronic lymphocytic thyroiditis is occurring with increasing frequency in all age groups and currently is the most common cause of goiter and hypothyroidism in childhood. In children and adolescents, the incidence peaks between 8 and 15 years of age and occurs most commonly in females (4:1). The disease is the result of an autoimmune attack on the thyroid. Susceptibility to thyroid autoimmunity (and other endocrine autoimmune disorders) is associated with inheritance of certain histocompatibility alleles in APS type II (described earlier in this chapter).

## Clinical Findings

### A. SYMPTOMS AND SIGNS

The goiter is characteristically firm, freely movable, nontender, and symmetrical, with a pebbly consistency. Onset is usually insidious, and except for painless goiter, clinical manifestations are unusual. Occasionally a sensation of tracheal compression or fullness, hoarseness, and dysphagia are described by the patient. No local signs of inflammation or evidence of systemic infection are present.

### B. LABORATORY FINDINGS

Laboratory findings vary. Serum concentrations of $T_4$, $FT_4$, and $T_3RU$ are usually normal but may be elevated (hashitoxicosis) or depressed. Thyroid antibodies (antithyroglobulin, antithyroid peroxidase) are usually present, though titers are frequently low. A variety of abnormalities in radioactive iodide uptake studies have been described; thyroid scans usually show a diffuse or patchy pattern, and cold (nonfunctioning) nodules have been reported. Thyroid scans and uptake studies add little to the diagnosis. Surgical or needle biopsy is diagnostic but seldom indicated.

## Treatment

The treatment of chronic lymphocytic thyroiditis is controversial. Full therapeutic doses of thyroid hormone (levothyroxine, 75–100 $\mu g/m^2/d$) may decrease the size of the goiter within 3 months, but in controlled trials the efficacy of thyroid hormone therapy is unsupported in the euthyroid child. Hypothyroidism is believed to be a common end result of autoimmune thyroiditis in the second to third decades of life; consequently, patients with adolescent goiter require lifelong surveillance, and children with documented hypothyroidism should receive levothyroxine in full replacement doses.

## HYPERTHYROIDISM

### ESSENTIALS OF DIAGNOSIS & TYPICAL FEATURES

- *Nervousness, irritability, emotional lability, tremor, excessive appetite, weight loss; smooth, moist, warm skin; increased perspiration, and heat intolerance.*
- *Goiter, exophthalmos, tachycardia, widened pulse pressure (systolic hypertension).*
- *Thyroid function studies elevated (eg, $TT_4$, $FT_4$, $T_3RU$). TSH concentration suppressed.*

## General Considerations

Most cases of hyperthyroidism in children have an autoimmune cause. Hyperthyroidism occurs with certain diseases that have an autoimmune basis, and a familial pattern with a predilection for females supports a role for a heritable and autoimmune basis. IgG antibody to thyroid receptors (TSI) stimulates thyroid hormone production in one form of hyperthyroidism accompanied by exophthalmos (Graves disease). Transient congenital hyperthyroidism may occur in infants of thyrotoxic mothers and is potentially life-threatening. Hyperthyroidism may be associated with acute, subacute, or chronic thyroiditis; tumors of the thyroid; other tumors producing thyrotropin-like substances; and exogenous thyroid hormone excess.

## Clinical Findings

### A. SYMPTOMS AND SIGNS

Hyperthyroidism is four times more common in females than in males. The disease most frequently occurs in childhood between ages 12 and 14 years; only 2% of patients present before age 10 years. The course of hyperthyroidism tends to be cyclic, with spontaneous remissions and exacerbations. A deterioration in school performance is a common historical feature. Findings include weakness, dyspnea, dysphagia, amenorrhea, emotional instability, nervousness, marked variability in mood, personality disturbances, and (rarely) tremors and movements that may simulate chorea. The skin is warm and moist; the face is flushed. Palpitations, tachycardia, and systolic hypertension with increased pulse pressure are common. Proptosis and exophthalmos are common in hyperthyroid children. Goiter is present in more than 90% of cases and is characteristically diffuse and usually firm. A bruit and thrill may be present. Variable degrees of accelerated growth and development occur, and loss of weight is common despite polyphagia. In neonatal hyperthyroidism, hepatosplenomegaly and thrombocytopenia with antiplatelet antibodies are occasionally seen.

### B. LABORATORY FINDINGS

$TT_4$, $FT_4$, and $T_3RU$ are elevated except in rare cases in which only the serum $T_3$ is elevated ($T_3$ thyrotoxicosis). Radioiodine uptake is elevated and does not suppress with $T_3$ (liothyronine). The basal metabolic rate is elevated, and the serum cholesterol level is low. Antibodies to thyroglobulin are found in most patients. Circulating TSH concentrations measured by very sensitive assays are depressed, and TSI is often present in plasma.

### C. IMAGING

Skeletal maturation assessed radiographically is advanced in younger children. In newborns, accelerated bone maturation may be associated with subsequent premature closure of the cranial sutures. Long-standing hyperthyroidism is associated with osteoporosis.

## Differential Diagnosis

Although the well-established case of hyperthyroidism seldom presents a problem in diagnosis, the findings in the early stages of the disease may be confused with chorea or, more commonly, with euthyroid goiter. Typically the patient is an adolescent with a recent decline in school performance, nervousness, emotional lability, and increased perspiration. Repeated clinical and laboratory evaluations may be required to make the diagnosis. Disease states associated with hypermetabolism (severe anemia, leukemia, chronic infections, pheochromocytoma, and muscle-wasting disease) may resemble hyperthyroidism clinically but differ in the thyroid function studies.

## Treatment

The symptoms of hyperthyroidism can fluctuate and in some mild cases may not require treatment.

### A. GENERAL MEASURES

Bed rest is advisable only in severe cases, in preparation for surgery, or at the beginning of a medical regimen. The diet should be high in calories, carbohydrates, and vitamins (particularly vitamin $B_1$).

### B. MEDICAL TREATMENT

It takes 2–3 weeks to see a clinical response, and adequate control may take 2–3 months. The thyroid frequently increases in size as treatment is started but then usually decreases within several months.

**1. β-Adrenergic blocking agents**—These agents may be helpful in controlling symptoms of nervous instability and tachycardia and are indicated in severe disease with cardiovascular abnormalities (tachycardia, hypertension). In mild cases, β-blockade without other antithyroid treatment may be adequate. $β_1$-Specific agents (metoprolol, atenolol) are preferable to nonspecific agents, such as propanolol, due to their lower likelihood of exacerbating pulmonary bronchospasm, greater specificity for tachycardia, and additional effect in decreasing conversion of $T_4$ to $T_3$.

**2. Antithyroid agents (PTU, methimazole)**—These drugs interfere with thyroid hormone synthesis and, in large doses, with the peripheral conversion of $T_4$ to $T_3$. The correct dose must always be determined individually. Antithyroid agents are frequently used in the initial treatment of hyperthyroidism in children. Short-term therapy is occasionally successful, but treatment usually must be continued for at least 18–24 months.

The optimal dose of antithyroid agent for maintenance treatment remains somewhat unclear. Recent studies suggest that 10–15 mg/d of methimazole or 100–150 mg/d of PTU provide adequate long-term control in most patients with a minimum of side effects. If $T_4$ levels rise rapidly with reduction in drug dosage after 18–24 months of therapy, continued or alternative therapy, such as radioablation of the thyroid gland, will be necessary. Relapse occurs in 10–30% of patients, and severe cases may not respond to initial treatment.

**a. Initial dosage**—Treatment with methimazole is initiated with a dose of 15 mg/d in mild cases, 30 mg/d in moderate cases, and 45 mg/d in patients with severe symptoms and markedly elevated $FT_4$. Methimazole can be given once a day. PTU dosing is 10 times that for methimazole (150–450 mg/d) given in three divided doses 8 hours apart. Initial dosing is continued until $FT_4$ or $TT_4$, measured every 2 weeks, is clearly improving and signs and symptoms have subsided. Larger doses are rarely necessary.

**b. Maintenance**—Give methimazole 10–15 mg/d as a single dose or PTU 100–150 mg/d in two or three divided doses. Some authors recommend continuing the drug at higher levels until the euthyroid state is approached or reached and then, as the TSH level rises, adding thyroid hormone. This approach can simplify the management of some cases of Graves disease. However, the role of adjunctive thyroxine therapy in preventing recurrence of hyperthyroidism in Graves disease is not proven. Free $T_4$ and TSH levels should be monitored during antithyroid treatment to determine whether the patient is becoming hypothyroid; thyroid hormone is added when indicated to maintain normal TSH while the patient is receiving maintenance antithyroid therapy.

**c. Toxicity**—Granulocytopenia, fever, rash, and arthralgia may occur. The drug must be discontinued, and antibiotics and a short course of one of the adrenocorticosteroids should be prescribed if indicated.

**3. Iodide**—By itself, treatment with orally administered iodide usually produces a rapid but brief response. Because the efficacy of iodide is short-lived, it is generally recommended only for acute management. A progressive increase in dosage is often required for satisfactory control, and toxic reactions to iodide sometimes occur.

### C. RADIATION THERAPY

Radioactive iodide ($^{131}$I) ablation of the thyroid gland is used as definitive therapy for hyperthyroidism in children and adolescents that does not remit after 2 years or more of medical therapy or in situations in which compliance with medication is poor. Reports do not support the fear of an increased incidence of thyroid cancer or other neoplasms, particularly when an ablative dose of $^{131}I$ is used. Therapy with a β-adrenergic antagonist may be necessary for 1–2 months after ablation, until $FT_4$ is in the normal range. In most cases, thyroid hormone replacement is ultimately necessary.

## D. SURGICAL TREATMENT

Thyroidectomy is no longer considered a primary form of treatment. An exception would be in the case of a noncompliant pregnant female in whom radioiodine would be contraindicated because it crosses the placenta. The patient should be prepared first with bed rest, diet, and propranolol (as detailed earlier) and with iodide and PTU as follows: PTU should be given for 2–4 weeks. Iodide (as saturated solution of potassium iodide) is added 10–21 days before surgery is scheduled. Iodides act by blocking the effect of TSH on the thyroid, with a resulting decrease in iodine trapping and reduction of vascularity, and by inhibiting the release of hormone, thus reducing the possibility of thyroid storm. Give 1–10 drops daily for 10–21 days. Continue the drug for 1 week after surgery.

## Course & Prognosis

Improvement may rarely occur without therapy, but partial remissions and exacerbations may continue for several years. With medical treatment alone, prolonged remissions may be expected in one half to two thirds of patients in the first 2 years or so.

Cooper DS: Antithyroid drugs in the management of patients with Graves' disease: An evidence-based approach to therapeutic controversies. J Clin Endocrinol Metab 2003;88:3474 [PMID: 12915620].

Kadmon PM et al: Thryoid storm in a child following radioactive iodine therapy. J Clin Endocrinol Metab 2001;86:1865 [PMID: 11344172].

## Management of Congenital (Transient) Hyperthyroidism

Congenital hyperthyroidism has a significant death rate in the neonatal period, but the eventual prognosis in surviving infants is excellent. Temporary treatment of congenital hyperthyroidism may be necessary, in which case iodides appear to be the initial drug of choice, to be followed by PTU or methimazole. β-adrenergic antagonists may be necessary to control cardiac arrhythmias. Transection of an enlarged thyroid isthmus may be of value if respiratory distress due to tracheal compression is present.

Radetti G et al: Fetal and neonatal thyroid disorders. Minerva Pediatr 2002;54:383 [PMID: 12244277].

## CARCINOMA OF THE THYROID

Carcinoma of the thyroid is uncommon in childhood. The child usually presents with asymptomatic asymmetrical thyroid enlargement. Neck discomfort, dysphagia, voice changes, and respiratory difficulty are unusual but may occur. Fifty percent of children have metastatic disease, usually to regional lymph nodes, at the time of presentation. Pulmonary metastasis occurs in 5% of patients.

Thyroid function tests are usually normal. A technetium or iodine scan of the thyroid shows a so-called cold nodule and is the most definitive diagnostic test. Pulmonary metastases should be excluded by computed tomography (CT) scan of the chest.

Papillary carcinoma is the most common form in childhood, and the prognosis with treatment is relatively good (survival rate greater than 80% after 10–20 years). The treatment of choice is surgical excision of the entire gland and removal of all involved lymph nodes. If metastatic disease is not identified at surgery or by radioactive iodide scan postoperatively, replacement thyroid hormone is generally the only additional therapy required. Follow-up thyroid scans every 2–5 years are recommended.

Less common malignant tumors of the thyroid are follicular, medullary, and undifferentiated carcinomas, lymphomas, and sarcomas. Medullary carcinoma of the thyroid may be familial (autosomal dominant), usually occurring as a component of type 2 multiple endocrine neoplasia (MEN). This condition may be associated with excessive elaboration of gastrin and calcitonin, with pheochromocytoma, parathyroid hyperplasia, marfanoid habitus, and mucosal neuromas (MEN type 2b). The treatment and prognosis depend on the cell type present, but the outcome is generally less favorable.

Bentley AA et al: Evaluation and management of a solitary thyroid nodule in a child. Otolaryngol Clin North Am 2003;36: 117 [PMID: 12803013].

Hung W, Sarlis NJ: Current controversies in the management of pediatric patients with well-differentiated nonmedullary thyroid cancer: A review. Thyroid 2002;12:683 [PMID: 12225637].

# ■ DISORDERS OF CALCIUM HOMEOSTASIS

The parathyroid glands, kidney, liver, and small intestine tightly regulate serum calcium concentration. Parathyroid hormone (PTH) acts in concert with dietary vitamin D or with active vitamin D produced in the course of sun exposure and subsequent hydroxylation of precursors in the liver and kidney. Low calcium levels stimulate PTH release. PTH in turn acts on the bone to cause release of calcium and phosphorous and on the kidney to cause resorption of calcium and activation of the 1-hydroxylation of 25-hydroxylated vitamin D to 1,25-$(OH)_2$ vitamin D. 1,25-$(OH)_2$ vitamin D acts in the intestine to promote the absorption of calcium. Deficiencies or excesses of these agents, as well as abnormalities in their receptors or of vitamin D metabolism, lead to clinical disturbances described in the following section. Less important factors contributing to calcium homeostasis include calcitonin, magnesium, pyrophosphate, prostaglandins, and phosphate.

## HYPOCALCEMIC DISORDERS

A normal serum calcium concentration is 8.9–10.1 mg/dL or an ionized level of 1.2–1.4 mg/dL. Levels in newborns are slightly lower, whereas premature infants may have levels as low as 7 mg/dL. Because 50–60% of calcium in the serum is protein-bound, determination of an ionized calcium level may be helpful in conditions with low serum protein. Some laboratories report calcium levels in units of mEq/L. Units of mEq/L can be converted to mg/dL by multiplying the value by 2.

### ESSENTIALS OF DIAGNOSIS & TYPICAL FEATURES

- *Tetany with facial and extremity numbness, tingling, cramps, spontaneous muscle contractures, carpopedal spasm, positive Trousseau and Chvostek signs, loss of consciousness, convulsions.*
- *Diarrhea, photophobia, prolongation of electrical systole (QT interval), and laryngospasm.*
- *In hypoparathyroidism or pseudohypoparathyroidism—Defective nails and teeth, cataracts, and ectopic calcification in the subcutaneous tissues and basal ganglia.*

### General Considerations

Hypocalcemia is a consistent feature of conditions such as hypoparathyroidism, pseudohypoparathyroidism, transient tetany of the newborn, and severe vitamin D–deficiency rickets (milder rickets generally has normal calcium level), and may be present in rare disorders of vitamin D action. Hypocalcemia may also occur in other conditions such as malabsorption syndromes, chronic renal disease, hypophosphatemic rickets, tumor lysis syndrome, or rhabdomyolysis (Table 30–5).

Hypoparathyroidism may be idiopathic or may be a result of autoimmune damage. Table 30–6 summarizes the findings in various disorders of parathyroid hormone secretion or action. Autoimmune parathyroid destruction with subsequent hypoparathyroidism may be isolated, or associated with other autoimmune disorders in the APECED syndrome (APS-1).

Hypoparathyroidism may also result from congenital absence of the parathyroid glands, which can occur in DiGeorge syndrome. Other features of this disorder include congenital absence of the thymus (with resultant thymus-dependent immunologic deficiency) and cardiovascular anomalies. A monosomy in the q11 region of chromosome 22 is responsible for the majority of DiGeorge syndrome cases.

Autosomal dominant hypocalcemia is associated with a gain of function mutation in the calcium receptor. This causes a low PTH in the face of hypocalcemia and excessive loss of urinary calcium. Affected individuals present in childhood. A family history of hypocalcemia may provide a clue to differentiate this condition from other forms of hypoparathyroidism.

Hypoparathyroidism may develop following thyroidectomy, with either acute or insidious onset, and may be transient or permanent. Parathyroid deficiency following irradiation of the neck or the administration of therapeutic doses of radioactive iodine for carcinoma of the thyroid has been reported.

Transient neonatal hypoparathyroidism, also known as transient tetany of the newborn, is caused by a relative deficiency of PTH or hormone action (see Table 30–6). There are two forms of this condition. The early form occurs within the first 2 weeks of life in newborns with a history of birth asphyxia or in those born to mothers with diabetes mellitus or hyperparathyroidism. Hypomagnesemia may occur in the early form and augments the severity of hypocalcemia. The late form occurs after 2 weeks and has been associated with infant formulas high in phosphate.

Both tumor lysis syndrome and rhabdomyolysis can cause hypocalcemia. These conditions involve cellular destruction with liberation of large amounts of intracellular phosphate that subsequently complex with serum calcium.

Malabsorption states result in hypocalcemia by impairing absorption of calcium, vitamin D, and magnesium (see Table 30–6). Hypomagnesemia may cause or augment the severity of hypocalcemia by impairing the release of PTH. Magnesium may be lost from either the gastrointestinal tract or the kidney.

Rickets describes a characteristic radiographic picture. Radiographic evidence of rickets includes meta-

**Table 30–5.** Hypocalcemia associated with rickets and other disorders.

| Condition | Pathogenesis | Disease States/Inheritance | Clinical Features | Biochemical Findings | | | |
|---|---|---|---|---|---|---|---|
| | | | | Serum Calcium | Serum Phosphorus | Serum Alkaline Phosphatase | Other |
| Malabsorption | Impairment in intestinal absorption in any or all of the following: calcium, vitamin D, and magnesium | Cystic fibrosis, celiac disease, sprue, Shwachman syndrome | Failure to thrive, poor weight gain, steatorrhea, superimposed vitamin D deficiency rickets. | Low or normal | Low or normal | Variable, may be low with concomitant zinc deficiency | Potentially low magnesium levels, potentially low 25-OH vitamin D |
| Chronic renal insufficiency | Decreased renal phosphate excretion, decreased 1-hydroxylase activity | Obstruction, glomerulonephritis, dysplastic kidneys | Uremia, growth failure, acidosis | Low or normal | Elevated | Elevated or normal | Elevated PTH levels in longstanding cases, low 1,25-OH vitamin D |
| Rhabdomyolysis | Muscle damage with liberation of large amounts of intracellular phosphate | Crush injuries of muscles, Pompe disease, carnitine deficiency | Hypocalcemic tetany, cardiac arrhythmia, risk of renal failure | Low | Elevated | Normal | Myoglobinuria |
| Tumor lysis syndrome | Release of intracellular phosphate and potassium | Initiation of chemotherapy for ALL, Burkitt's lymphoma, or other malignancies | Hypocalcemic tetany, cardiac arrhythmia, risk of renal failure | Low | Elevated | Normal | Hyperkalemia, elevated uric acid |
| Vitamin D deficiency rickets | Deficient dietary vitamin D intake, vitamin D malabsorption, other risk factors include dark skin and lack of sunlight exposure | May cluster in families due to various risk factors | Characteristic skeletal changes appear early, poor growth, symptomatic hypocalcemia is a late finding | Normal until late in course | Low or normal | Elevated | Elevated PTH levels, low 25-OH vitamin D |
| Vitamin D refractory rickets type I | Mutation in 1-hydroxylase enzyme required for synthesis of fully active 1,25-OH vitamin D | Autosomal recessive inheritance | Skeletal changes of rickets, symptomatic hypocalcemia | Low | Low or normal | Elevated | Elevated PTH, low 1,25-OH vitamin D |
| Vitamin D refractory rickets type II | Mutation in 1,25-OH vitamin D receptor | Autosomal recessive inheritance | Severe skeletal changes of rickets, total alopecia, symptomatic hypocalcemia | Low | Low or normal | Elevated | Elevated PTH, elevated 1,25-OH vitamin D |
| Hypophosphatemic rickets | Excessive loss of phosphate in the urine, ? abnormal humoral factor | X-linked dominant | Skeletal changes primarily in the lower extremities—genu varum or valgus, short stature | Normal or low | Very low | Usually normal | Normal PTH levels, abnormally high urinary phosphate excretion |

PTH = parathyroid hormone; ALL = acute lymphoblastic leukemia.

981

**Table 30–6.** Disorders of parathyroid hormone secretion or action.

| Condition | Pathogenesis | Inheritance Pattern | Clinical Features | Biochemical Findings | | | |
|---|---|---|---|---|---|---|---|
| | | | | Serum Calcium | Serum Phosphorus | Serum Alkaline Phosphatase | Serum PTH |
| Isolated hypoparathyroidism | Trauma, surgical destruction, isolated autoimmune destruction, rare familial forms | None; reports in familial forms of inheritance as X-linked recessive, autosomal recessive, or autosomal dominant | Symptoms of hypocalcemia | Low | High | Normal/Low | Low |
| DiGeorge syndrome | Deletion in chromosome 22 | Majority represent new mutations | Symptoms of hypocalcemia, cardiac anomalies, immune disorder | Low | High | Normal/Low | Low |
| APS type I | Autoimmune destruction | Autosomal recessive | Mucocutaneous candidiasis, Addison disease, potential for autoimmune destruction in other endocrine glands | Low | High | Normal/Low | Low |
| PHP type IA | Mutation in stimulatory G protein; resistance to PTH action | Autosomal dominant | AHO phenotype, variable hypocalcemia, may have resistance to other hormones using G protein signaling | Low or normal | Elevated or normal | Variable | Elevated |
| PPHP | Mutation in stimulatory G protein | Autosomal dominant—frequently found within same families with PHP type IA | AHO phenotype, biochemical parameters are normal | Normal | Normal | Normal | Normal |
| Transient tetany of the newborn—early onset | Deficiency in PTH secretion and/or action | Sporadic—associated with difficult deliveries, infants of diabetic mothers, or maternal hyperparathyroidism | Onset of symptoms of hypocalcemia within 2 wk of birth | Low | Normal or low | Normal or low | Normal or low |
| Transient tetany of the newborn—late onset | Deficiency in PTH secretion and/or action | Sporadic—associated with infant formulas that had a high phosphate content | Onset of symptoms of hypocalcemia after 2 wk of age | Low | Normal or low | Normal or low | Normal or low |
| Autosomal dominant hypocalcemia | Gain of function mutation of calcium receptor | Autosomal dominant | Symptoms of hypocalcemia family history | Low | High | Normal/Low | Low |

PTH = parathyroid hormone; APS = autoimmune polyglandular syndrome; PHP = pseudohypoparathyroidism; PPHP = pseudopseudohypoparathyroidism; AHO = Albright hereditary osteodystrophy.

physeal cupping and irregularity. Vitamin D deficiency caused by lack of sunlight exposure or dietary deficiency is the most common cause of rickets. It is classically described in dark-skinned, breast-fed infants born in the winter months. However, occult vitamin D deficiency may be more common than initially recognized. This concern forms the basis for the recommendation by the American Association of Pediatrics that breast-fed infants receive vitamin D supplementation of 200 IU/d. Rickets can be caused by several defects in the metabolism of vitamin D (see Table 30–6). Less common causes of rickets include defects in vitamin D metabolism including liver disease (with impaired 25-hydroxylation of vitamin D), kidney disease (with impaired 1-hydroxylation of 25-(OH) vitamin D), an inherited deficiency of 1α-hydroxylase (vitamin D-dependent rickets type 1) or end-organ resistance to vitamin D (vitamin D-dependent rickets type 2).

Familial hypophosphatemic rickets (vitamin D-resistant rickets) has skeletal findings similar to those of vitamin D-related rickets; however, the basic defect in this condition is abnormal renal phosphate loss. Dietary deficiency of calcium may also be an important cause of rickets.

DeLucia MC et al: Nutritional rickets with normal circulating 25-hydroxyvitamin D: A call for reexamining the role of dietary calcium intake in North American infants. J Clin Endocrinol Metab 2003;88:3539 [PMID: 12915633].

Gartner LM, Greer FR: Prevention of rickets and vitamin D deficiency: New guidelines for vitamin D intake. Pediatrics 2003;111:908 [PMID: 12671133].

Jan de Beur SM, Levine MA: Molecular pathogenesis of hypophosphatemic rickets. J Clin Endocrinal Metab 2002;87:2467 [PMID: 12050201].

Marx SJ: Hyperparathyroid and hypoparathyroid disorders. N Engl J Med 2000;343:1863 [PMID: 11117980].

Mughal Z: Rickets in childhood. Semin Musculoskelet Radiol 2002;6:183 [PMID: 12541195].

Perez E, Sullivan KE: Chromosome 22q11.2 deletion syndrome (DiGeorge and velocardiofacial syndrome). Curr Opin Pediatr 2002;14:678 [PMID: 12436034].

## Clinical Findings

### A. SYMPTOMS AND SIGNS

Prolonged hypocalcemia causes tetany, photophobia, blepharospasm, and diarrhea. The symptoms of tetany include numbness, cramps, and twitchings of the extremities; carpopedal spasm and laryngospasm; a positive Chvostek sign (tapping of the face in front of the ear produces spasm of the facial muscles); unexplained bizarre behavior; irritability; loss of consciousness; convulsions; and retarded physical and mental development. Headache, vomiting, increased intracranial pressure, and papilledema may occur. In early infancy, respiratory distress may be the presenting finding.

### B. LABORATORY FINDINGS

Calcium levels may be low or normal (see Tables 30–5 and 30–6). Phosphate levels may be low, normal, or high depending on the cause of the hypocalcemia. Magnesium levels may also be low. PTH levels are elevated in the hypocalcemic conditions, with the notable exception of hypoparathyroidism. Markedly elevated serum PTH may be associated with pseudohypoparathyroidism (see following discussion). Measurement of urinary excretion of calcium and phosphate can assist in diagnosis and monitoring of therapy.

### C. IMAGING

Soft tissue and basal ganglia calcification may occur in idiopathic hypoparathyroidism and pseudohypoparathyroidism. A variety of skeletal changes are associated with rickets, including cupped and irregular appearance at the metaphysis of the long bones. Torsional deformities can result in genu varum (bowleg). Accentuation of the costochondral junction gives the rachitic rosary appearance seen on the chest wall.

## Differential Diagnosis

Tables 30–5 and 30–6 outline the features of disorders associated with hypocalcemia. An artifactually low total serum calcium level may be seen with low serum albumin, and measurement of ionized calcium is advised in these cases.

## Treatment

### A. ACUTE OR SEVERE TETANY

The objective of treatment is to correct hypocalcemia immediately by the administration of intravenous calcium. Calcium gluconate and calcium chloride 10 mg/kg are generally used for acute treatment. To avoid cardiac arrhythmia, intravenous calcium infusions should not exceed 50 mg/min. Cardiac monitoring should be performed during the infusion.

### B. MAINTENANCE MANAGEMENT OF HYPOPARATHYROIDISM OR CHRONIC HYPOCALCEMIA

The objective of treatment is to maintain the serum calcium and serum phosphate at approximately normal levels without excessive urinary calcium excretion.

**1. Diet**—In addition to a diet high in calcium, calcium supplements are generally required. A starting dosage of 50–75 mg of elemental calcium per kilogram of body weight per day divided in three to four doses is used as initial management and should be titrated based on serum calcium levels and urinary calcium excretion.

Therapy should be monitored to prevent hypercalcemia and its complications (see Monitoring section). Often, supplemental calcium can be decreased or discontinued after vitamin D therapy has reached its peak effect. Supplemental phosphate and activated vitamin D (calcitriol) are required in the treatment of hypophosphatemic rickets.

**2. Vitamin D supplementation**—A variety of vitamin D preparations are available for treatment. Ergocalciferol (vitamin $D_2$) and calcitriol (1,25-dihydroxyvitamin $D_3$) are used in the majority of cases. Ergocalciferol is the preferred agent for the treatment of vitamin D deficiency. Impaired metabolism of vitamin D to its active end product 1,25-$(OH)_2$ vitamin D or impaired function of PTH requires supplementation with calcitriol. Selection and dosage of a vitamin D supplement vary with the condition to be treated and the patient's response to therapy. As with calcium supplementation, monitoring of therapy is essential to avoid toxicity.

**3. Monitoring**—Dosages of calcium and vitamin D must be tailored for each patient. Monitoring serum calcium, urine calcium, and serum alkaline phosphatase levels at 1- to 3-month intervals is necessary to ensure adequacy of therapy and to prevent hypercalcemia and nephrocalcinosis.

Basic goals in monitoring therapy include the following: (1) maintenance of serum calcium and phosphorous concentrations within normal ranges; (2) normalization of alkaline phosphatase concentrations for age; (3) regression of skeletal changes, if present; and (4) maintenance of spot urine calcium to creatinine ratio between 0.1 and 0.3 (0.05–0.15 if calcium is measured in mEq/L).

Hypophosphatemic rickets is an exception, since the monitoring goals are somewhat different. Serum calcium and alkaline phosphatase should be maintained within normal limits; however, phosphorus levels should be corrected only to the low normal range. Monitoring of serum PTH level is necessary to ensure that secondary hyperparathyroidism does not develop from excessive phosphate treatment or inadequate calcitriol replacement.

Singh J et al: The investigation of hypocalcaemia and rickets. Arch Dis Child 2003;88:403 [PMID: 12716711].

## PSEUDOHYPOPARATHYROIDISM (Resistance to Parathyroid Hormone Action)

In pseudohypoparathyroidism (PHP), PTH production is adequate; however, target organs (renal tubule, bone, or both) fail to respond. This receptor resistance to PTH action is due to a heterozygous inactivating mutation in the stimulatory G protein subunit associated with the PTH receptor, which leads to impaired signaling. Resistance to other G protein-dependent hormones may also be present.

Several types of PHP have been identified, with variable biochemical and phenotypic features (see Table 30–6). PHP has biochemical abnormalities similar to hypoparathyroidism with hypocalcemia and hyperphosphatemia. However, PTH levels are elevated, suggesting resistance to the action of the hormone. It may be accompanied by a characteristic phenotype known as Albright osteodystrophy (AHO). The AHO phenotype includes short stature; round, full facies; irregularly shortened fourth metacarpal; a short, thick-set body; delayed and defective dentition; and mild mental retardation. Corneal and lenticular opacities and ectopic calcification of the basal ganglia and subcutaneous tissues may occur with or without abnormal serum calcium levels. Treatment is the same as that for hypoparathyroidism.

Pseudopseudohypoparathyroidism (PPHP) describes individuals with the AHO phenotype, but normal calcium homeostasis. PHP and PPHP can occur in the same cohort. Genomic imprinting is thought to be responsible for the differential phenotypic expression of disease. With heterozygous loss of maternal allele associated with PHP and heterozygous loss of paternal allele associated with PPHP.

Weinstein LS et al: Gs(alpha) mutations and imprinting defects in human disease. Ann NY Acad Sci 2002;968:173 [PMID: 12119276].

Wilson LC, Hall CH: Albright's hereditary osteodystrophy and pseudohypoparathyroidism. Semin Musculoskelet Radiol 2002;6:273 [PMID: 12541184].

## HYPERCALCEMIC STATES

Hypercalcemia is defined as a serum level greater than 11 mg/dL. Severe hypercalcemia is defined as a level above 13.5 mg/dL. Some laboratories report calcium levels in units of mEq/L. Units of mEq/L can be converted to mg/dL by multiplying the value by 2.

### ESSENTIALS OF DIAGNOSIS & TYPICAL FEATURES

- *Abdominal pain, polyuria, polydipsia, hypertension, nephrocalcinosis, failure to thrive, renal stones, intractable peptic ulcer, constipation, uremia, and pancreatitis.*

- *Bone pain and, rarely, pathologic fractures. Radiograph shows subperiosteal resorption, loss of the lamina dura of the teeth, renal parenchymal calcification or stones, and osteitis fibrosa cystica (brown tumors).*

- *Vague psychiatric symptoms, impaired concentration, altered mental status, mood swings, coma.*
- *Transient or mild hypercalcemia may be entirely asymptomatic; hypercalcemia and mild hyperparathyroidism noted frequently as incidental findings in routine laboratory screening.*

## General Considerations

More than 80% of hypercalcemic children or adolescents have either hyperparathyroidism or a malignant tumor as the underlying cause. Table 30–7 summarizes the differential diagnosis of childhood hypercalcemia.

Hyperparathyroidism is rare in childhood and may be primary or secondary. The most common cause of primary hyperparathyroidism is a parathyroid adenoma. Diffuse parathyroid hyperplasia or multiple adenomas have also been described in families. Familial hyperparathyroidism may be an isolated disease, or it may be associated with multiple endocrine neoplasia (MEN), usually type 1 and, rarely, type 2A. Hypercalcemia of malignancy can be associated with both solid and hematologic malignancies. Hypercalcemia of malignancy is caused by local destruction of bone by tumor infiltration. Another cause is the secretion of PTH-related protein (PTH-RP). PTH-RP is responsible for parathyroid hormone-like actions. With PTH-RP as the causative agent, calcium is elevated, PTH is suppressed, and PTH-RP is high. Chronic renal disease with impaired phosphate excretion is the most common secondary cause of hyperparathyroidism.

Hsu SC, Levine MA: Primary hyperparathyroidism in children and adolescents: The Johns Hopkins Children's Center experience 1984–2001. J Bone Miner Res 2002:17 (Suppl 2): N44 [PMID: 12412777].

Marx SJ et al: Hyperparathyroidism in hereditary syndromes: Special expressions and special managements. J Bone Miner Res 2002;17 (Suppl 2):N37 [PMID: 12412776].

***Table 30–7.*** Hypercalcemic states.

**A. Primary hyperparathyroidism**
1. Parathyroid hyperplasia
2. Parathyroid adenoma
3. Familial, including MEN types I and II
4. Ectopic PTH secretion

**B. Hypercalcemic states other than primary hyperparathyroidism associated with increased intestinal or renal absorption of calcium**
1. Hypervitaminosis D (including idiopathic hypercalcemia of infancy)
2. Familial hypocalciuric hypercalcemia
3. Lithium therapy
4. Sarcoidosis
5. Phosphate depletion
6. Aluminum intoxication

**C. Hypercalcemic states other than hyperparathyroidism associated with increased mobilization of bone minerals**
1. Hyperthyroidism
2. Immobilization
3. Thiazides
4. Vitamin A intoxication
5. Malignant neoplasms
    a. Ectopic PTH secretion or PTH-related protein
    b. Prostaglandin-secreting tumor and perhaps prostaglandin release from subcutaneous fat necrosis
    c. Tumors metastatic to bone
    d. Myeloma

MEN = multiple endocrine neoplasia; PTH = parathyroid hormone.

## Clinical Findings

### A. SYMPTOMS AND SIGNS

**1. Due to hypercalcemia**—Findings include hypotonicity and weakness of muscles; apathy, mood swings, and bizarre behavior; nausea, vomiting, abdominal pain, constipation, and weight loss; hyperextensibility of joints; and hypertension, cardiac irregularities, bradycardia, and shortening of the QT interval. Coma occurs rarely. Calcium deposits in the cornea or conjunctiva (band keratopathy) may occur and are detected by slit-lamp examination of the eye. Intractable peptic ulcer and pancreatitis occur in adults but rarely in children.

**2. Due to increased calcium and phosphate excretion**—Findings include loss of renal concentrating ability with polyuria, polydipsia, precipitation of calcium phosphate in the renal parenchyma or as urinary calculi, and progressive renal damage.

**3. Due to changes in the skeleton**—Findings may include bone pain, osteitis fibrosa cystica, subperiosteal absorption of the distal clavicles and phalanges, absence of lamina dura around the teeth, spontaneous fractures, and a moth-eaten appearance of the skull on radiograph. Later, there is generalized demineralization with a predilection for subperiosteal cortical bone.

### B. IMAGING

Bone changes may be subtle in children even when radiography shows nephrocalcinosis. Technetium sestamibi scintigraphy is now shown to be more promising than conventional procedures such as ultrasonography, CT, and MRI for localizing parathyroid tumors.

## Treatment

### A. SYMPTOMATIC

Initial management consists of vigorous hydration with normal saline and forced calcium diuresis using a loop diuretic such as furosemide (1 mg/kg given every 6 hours). In cases of inadequate response to initial intervention, interventions with glucocorticoids or calcitonin have been used. Bisphosphonates, standard agents for the management of acute hypercalcemia in adults, are being used with increasing frequency for cases of refractory pediatric hypercalcemia.

### B. CHRONIC

Treatment options vary depending on the condition. Removal of a parathyroid adenoma or subtotal removal of hyperplastic parathyroid glands will treat hyperparathyroidism. Postoperatively, hypocalcemia due to the rapid remineralization of chronically calcium-deprived bones may occur. A diet high in calcium and vitamin D is recommended immediately postoperatively and is continued until serum calcium concentrations are normal and stable. Treatment of secondary hyperparathyroidism from chronic renal disease is primarily directed at controlling serum phosphorus levels with phosphate binders. Pharmacologic doses of calcitriol are used to suppress PTH secretion.

Long-term therapy for hypercalcemia of malignancy is the treatment of the underlying disorder.

## Course & Prognosis

The prognosis following removal of a single adenoma is excellent. The prognosis following subtotal parathyroidectomy for diffuse hyperplasia or removal of multiple adenomas is usually good and depends on correction of the underlying defect. In patients with multiple sites of parathyroid adenoma or hyperplasia, MEN is likely, and other family members may be at risk. Genetic counseling and DNA analysis to determine the specific gene defect are indicated.

Allgrove J: Use of bisphosphonates in children and adolescents. J Pediatr Endocrinol Metab 2002;15(Suppl 3):921 [PMID: 12199351].

Mathur M et al: Treatment of acute lymphoblastic leukemia-induced extreme hypercalcemia with pamidronate and calcitonin. Pediatr Crit Care Med 2003;4(2):252 [PMID: 12749663].

## FAMILIAL HYPOCALCIURIC HYPERCALCEMIA (Familial Benign Hypercalcemia)

Familial hypocalciuric hypercalcemia is distinguished by low to normal urinary calcium excretion as a result of high renal reabsorption of calcium. PTH is normal or slightly elevated.

In most cases, the gene defect has been identified as a mutation in the membrane-bound calcium-sensing receptor expressed on parathyroid and renal tubule cells. It is inherited as an autosomal dominant trait with high penetrance. There is a low rate of new mutations. The majority of patients are asymptomatic, and treatment is unnecessary. A severe form of symptomatic neonatal hyperparathyroidism may occur in infants homozygous for the receptor mutation.

Heath DA: Familial hypocalciuric hypercalcemia. Rev Endocr Metab Disord 2000;1:291 [PMID: 11706743].

## HYPERVITAMINOSIS D

Vitamin D intoxication is almost always the result of ingestion of excessive amounts of vitamin D, some forms of which may be stored for months in adipose tissue.

Signs, symptoms, and treatment of vitamin D-induced hypercalcemia are the same as those in other hypercalcemic conditions.

Treatment depends on the stage of hypercalcemia. Severe hypercalcemia requires hospitalization and aggressive intervention. Due to the storage of vitamin D in the adipose tissue, several months of a low-calcium, low-vitamin D diet may be required.

## IDIOPATHIC HYPERCALCEMIA OF INFANCY (Williams Syndrome)

Williams syndrome is an uncommon disorder of infancy characterized in its classic form by elfin-appearing facies and hypercalcemia in infancy. Other features include failure to thrive, mental and motor retardation, cardiovascular abnormalities (primarily supravalvular aortic stenosis), irritability, purposeless movements, constipation, hypotonia, polyuria, polydipsia, and hypertension. A gregarious and affectionate personality is the rule in older children with the syndrome. Hypercalcemia may not appear until several months after birth. Treatment consists of rigid restriction of dietary calcium and vitamin D, and, in severe cases, moderate doses of glucocorticoids.

A defect in the metabolism of, or responsiveness to, vitamin D is postulated as the cause of Williams syndrome. Elastin deletions localized to chromosome 7 have been identified in over 90% of patients; thus, fluorescent in situ hybridization analysis may be the best initial diagnostic tool. The risk of hypercalcemia generally resolves by age 4, and dietary restrictions can be relaxed.

Morris CA, Mervis CB: Williams syndrome and related disorders. Annu Rev Genomics Hum Genet. 2000;1:461 [PMID: 11701637].

## IMMOBILIZATION HYPERCALCEMIA

Abrupt immobilization, particularly in a rapidly growing adolescent, is a risk factor for hypercalcemia. Hypercalcemia and hypercalciuria often appear 1–3 weeks after immobilization. Medical or dietary intervention may be required in severe cases.

## HYPOPHOSPHATASIA

Hypophosphatasia is an uncommon autosomal recessive condition characterized by a deficiency of alkaline phosphatase activity in serum, bone, and tissues. The deficiency of this enzyme leads to inadequate skeletal mineralization with clinical and radiographic features similar to rickets. Six different clinical forms have been identified. The perinatal form is characterized by severe skeletal deformity and death that occurs within a few days. The infantile form includes failure to thrive, hypotonia, and craniosynostosis. The childhood form has variable skeletal findings, reduced bone mineral density, and is associated with premature loss of deciduous teeth. Serum calcium levels may be elevated. The diagnosis of hypophosphatasia is made by demonstrating elevated levels of urinary phosphoethanolamine associated with low serum alkaline phosphatase.

Therapy is generally supportive. Children who survive the neonatal period may experience an improvement in severity of disease. Calcitonin may be of value for the temporary treatment of hypercalcemia.

Sato S, Matsuo N: Genetic analysis of hypophosphatasia. Acta Paediatr Jpn 1997;39:528 [PMID: 9316305].

Whyte MP: Hypophosphatasia and the role of alkaline phosphatase in skeletal mineralization. Endocr Rev 1994;15:439 [PMID: 7988481].

## ■ THE GONADS (Ovaries & Testes)

## DEVELOPMENT & PHYSIOLOGY

The fetal gonads develop from bipotential anlagen in the genital ridge. In addition to gonadal tissue, both müllerian and wolffian structures are present and have the potential to differentiate into components of the internal reproductive structures. Table 30–8 summarizes the male and female structures arising from müllerian and wolffian ducts. The Y chromosome, specifically the

**Table 30–8.** Sexual differentiation in the female and male.

| Internal Duct Derivatives | |
| --- | --- |
| Müllerian Duct Derivatives | Wolffian Duct Derivatives[a] |
| Fallopian tubes (oviducts) and fimbriae | Epididymis |
| | Vas deferens |
| Uterus | Seminal vesicles |
| Cervix | Ejaculatory duct |
| Vagina (posterior two thirds) | Prostatic urethra |

| External Genitalia Homologues | | |
| --- | --- | --- |
| Primitive Structure | Female Genitalia | Male Genitalia[b] |
| Undifferentiated gonad | Ovary | Testis |
| Genital tubercle | Clitoris | Glans penis |
| Genital swelling | Labia majora | Scrotum |
| Genital/urethral fold | Labia minora | Penile urethra/corpora |

[a]Normal wolffian duct development is dependent on the local production of testosterone by Leydig cells of the adjacent testis and on testosterone's diffusion into the surrounding embryonic tissues. Thus females with congenital adrenal hyperplasia who are virilized as the result of circulating androgens do not have wolffian duct development. Normal male development is also dependent on regression of müllerian duct derivatives through the local action of müllerian inhibiting factor elaborated by the Sertoli cells of the adjacent testis.

[b]The normal development of male external genitalia is dependent on an adequate circulating concentration of testosterone, which is then further converted to dihydrotestosterone in the target tissues through the action of the enzyme 5α-reductase. Significantly elevated circulating concentrations of other (adrenal) androgens, as in females with congenital adrenal hyperplasia, can virilize the genital tubercle, genital swelling, and genital/urethral folds along the lines of their male homologues, resulting in varying degrees of female pseudohermaphroditism (ambiguity) (see text).

SRY gene region of the chromosome, promotes testicular differentiation of the bipotential gonads. Once testicular differentiation has been determined, the fetal testis produces two substances critical for further male differentiation. Antimüllerian hormone (AMH) promotes the regression of müllerian structures, and the rising concentrations of testosterone stimulate growth of wolffian derivatives into male internal structures. Dihydrotestosterone (DHT), formed by 1α-reductase action on testosterone, is primarily responsible for virilization of the external genitalia. In the absence of both AMH and testosterone, differentiation into female internal and external genitalia occurs.

# AMBIGUOUS GENITIALIA IN THE NEWBORN

A variety of abnormalities in chromosomal allocation, gonadal differentiation, gonadal function, testosterone synthesis and action, or adrenal function can lead to aberrant development of internal and external genital structures. These abnormalities can be divided into four categories.

## A. ABNORMALITIES IN NORMAL GONADAL DIFFERENTIATION

These abnormalities usually result from an abnormality in the number of sex chromosomes. Klinefelter syndrome (see Chapter 32), with a 47,XXY karyotype, is associated with a male phenotype but with poorly functioning testes. Turner syndrome with a 45,XO karyotype (see Chapter 32) is associated with a female phenotype but with streak ovaries (gonadal dysgenesis) or premature ovarian failure. The phenotype is less severe if mosaicism or only partial absence of an X chromosome occurs. Mosaic forms of gonadal dysgenesis that contain a Y-bearing cell line have variable ambiguous internal and external phenotypes. Idiopathic testicular failure prior to completion of sexual differentiation results in ambiguous genitalia (incomplete virilization). True hermaphroditism, with the presence of both testicular and ovarian tissue, is rare and associated with external genitalia that range from fully masculine to almost completely feminine.

## B. ABNORMALITIES IN TESTOSTERONE SYNTHESIS OR ACTION

These disorders generally present as micropenis, genital ambiguity, or complete absence of male external genitalia in an XY individual (Figure 30–6). Testicular tissue is present and produces AMH; therefore, internal structures are wolffian. Disorders in this category include enzymatic defects in testosterone synthesis (such as 12-ketoreductase deficiency) or defects in conversion of testosterone to DHT ($5\alpha$-reductase deficiency). If the enzyme defect is incomplete, the external genitalia may masculinize at puberty when testosterone production increases. Since the gonads and adrenal gland share common enzymes of steroid hormone production, some of the enzymatic defects associated with male genital ambiguity may also affect production of cortisol and aldosterone, leading to cortisol deficiency and salt wasting. Defects in testosterone action result from absent or defective androgen receptors (androgen insensitivity) and, depending on the resultant degree of defect in androgen binding, the genital phenotype can range from relatively mild male ambiguity to complete female external development.

## C. DISORDERS OF ADRENAL ANDROGEN PRODUCTION

These disorders can cause genital ambiguity in both XY and XX individuals. Excessive adrenal androgen production secondary to an enzyme defect in cortisol synthesis (ie, congenital adrenal hyperplasia, described in a later section) is the cause of 95% of inappropriate virilization in 46,XX newborns. An enzyme defect in adrenal androgen, cortisol, and aldosterone production ($3\beta$HSD deficiency) is a rare cause of genital ambiguity in XY individuals.

## D. MISCELLANEOUS SYNDROMES

Various syndromes, such as VATER, WAGR, Denys–Drash, and Smith–Lemli–Opitz, have a wide variety of congenital anomalies, including genital ambiguity. Maternal exposure to androgens or androgen antagonists is a rare cause of genital ambiguity in newborns.

Gottlieb B et al: Androgen insensitivity. Am J Med Genet 1999; 89:210 .

Hiort O et al: Puberty in disorders of somatosexual differentiation. J Pediatr Endocrinol Metab 2003;16 (Suppl 2):297 [PMID: 12729408].

Hughes IA et al: Developmental aspects of androgen action. Mol Cell Endocrinol 2001;185:33 [PMID: 11738792].

Migeon CJ, Wisniewski AB: Human sex differentiation and its abnormalities. Best Pract Res Clin Obstet Gynaecol 2003;17:1 [PMID: 12758223].

# ABNORMALITIES IN FEMALE PUBERTAL DEVELOPMENT AND OVARIAN FUNCTION

## 1. Precocious Puberty in Girls

Puberty is considered precocious in girls if the onset of secondary sexual characteristics occurs before 7–8 years of age. Precocious puberty is thought to be more common in girls than in boys, but this may be the result of the inclusion, in published studies, of a large group of 6- to 8-year-old girls who have a benign, slowly progressing form that is probably a normal variant. The age of pubertal onset may also be advanced by obesity.

True (gonadotropin-releasing hormone [GnRH]-dependent) precocious puberty refers to early sexual maturation in response to hypothalamic–pituitary stimulation (GnRH, FSH, LH). In pseudoprecocity (ie, GnRH-independent precocity), the cause is elsewhere (eg, adrenal gland or ovary, or the result of exogenous estrogen). GnRH-dependent precocious puberty is always isosexual and may progress to the production of mature ova. In pseudoprecocity, sexual characteristics may be isosexual or heterosexual; secondary sexual characteristics develop, but the hypothalamic–pituitary gonadal axis (see Figure 30–1) does not mature, unless the

**Figure 30–6.** The corticosteroid hormone synthetic pathway. The pathways illustrated are present in differing amounts in the steroid-producing tissues: adrenal glands, ovaries, and testes. In the adrenal glands, mineralocorticoids from the zona glomerulosa, glucocorticoids from the zona fasciculata, and androgens (and estrogens) from the zona reticularis are produced. The major adrenal androgen is androstenedione, because the activity of 17-ketoreductase is relatively low. The adrenal gland does secrete some testosterone and estrogen, however. The pathways leading to the synthesis of mineralocorticoids and glucocorticoids are not present to any significant degree in the gonads; however, the testes and ovaries each produce both androgens and estrogens. Further metabolism of testosterone to dihydrotestosterone occurs in target tissues of the action of the enzyme 5α-reductase.

bone age is advanced sufficiently to stimulate central (GnRH-dependent) puberty.

## Clinical Findings

### A. SYMPTOMS AND SIGNS

Sexual development in girls usually starts with breast development, followed by pubic hair growth and menarche, but the order may vary. The interval between breast development and menarche can range from 1 to 6 years but is usually about 2 years. Girls with ovarian or adrenal tumors may have a palpable abdominal mass, also visualized by ultrasonography. A history of excessive mood changes and emotional lability is common. Children with precocious puberty usu-

ally have accelerated growth and may appear tall during childhood. However, because skeletal maturation (bone age) advances at a more rapid rate than linear growth (particularly in the female), final adult stature may be short.

### B. LABORATORY FINDINGS

In true precocious puberty, the basal serum concentrations of FSH and LH may still be in the prepubertal range. Thus documentation of the maturity of the hypothalamic–pituitary axis depends on demonstrating a pubertal LH response 30–40 minutes after stimulation with GnRH. In pseudoprecocity, basal serum FSH and LH are low, and the LH response to GnRH stimulation is suppressed as a result of feedback inhibition of the hypothalamic–pituitary axis by the autonomously secreted gonadal steroids (see Figure 30–1).

## C. Imaging

Determination of skeletal maturation at onset and then every 6–12 months is helpful in predicting the effect of precocity on adult height and may be used as one of several criteria to determine if treatment is warranted.

Abdominal and pelvic ultrasonography can usually identify an ovarian mass, follicular cyst, or adrenal mass greater than 5 mm in diameter. Serial examinations are useful in demonstrating significant changes. An MRI of the hypothalamic and pituitary regions can identify mass lesions and other structural abnormalities of the CNS. Because some of these lesions produce no clinical manifestations for prolonged periods, examinations should be performed periodically.

## Differential Diagnosis

In girls with precocious puberty, 90% have true precocious puberty (Table 30–9). Definable abnormalities on MRI scans are seen more commonly in younger children. With newer scanning techniques, static (presumably congenital) mass lesions in the hypothalamus,

**Table 30–9.** Causes of isosexual precocious pubertal development.

**A. True (GnRH-dependent) precocious puberty**
 1. Constitutional (idiopathic)
 2. Hypothalamic lesions (hamartomas, tumors, congenital malformations)
 3. Dysgerminomas
 4. Hydrocephalus
 5. CNS infections
 6. CNS trauma, irradiation
 7. Pineal tumors (rare)
 8. Neurofibromatosis with CNS involvement
 9. Tuberous sclerosis
 10. HCG-secreting tumors (eg, hepatoblastomas, choriocarcinomas)

**B. Pseudo (GnRH-independent)-precocious puberty**
 1. CAH in males
 2. Adrenal tumors
 3. McCune–Albright syndrome (polyostotic fibrous dysplasia)
 4. Familial Leydig cell hyperplasia (testotoxicosis)—males
 5. Gonadal tumors
 6. Exogenous estrogen—oral (contraceptive pills) or topical

CAH = congenital adrenal hyperplasia; CNS = central nervous system; GnRH = gonadotropin-releasing hormone; HCG = human chorionic gonadotropin.

including benign hypothalamic hamartomas, can be seen. The most common cause of pseudoprecocious puberty is McCune–Albright syndrome. Clinical manifestations of this disorder include polyostotic fibrous dysplasia, café au lait lesions with irregular borders, and autonomous hyperfunction of several endocrine glands, resulting in sexual precocity and other findings (eg, hyperthyroidism). Laboratory and radiographic findings helpful in differentiating true and pseudoprecocious puberty are discussed earlier.

Premature thelarche—benign early breast development—occurs most commonly between ages 12 and 36 months. It is often bilateral but may begin or remain as unilateral breast enlargement. In the absence of other signs of pubertal development (eg, accelerated growth rate or skeletal maturation, pubic hair, or vaginal mucosal maturation), no laboratory evaluation is necessary. Treatment consists of reassurance regarding the self-limited nature of this condition, but observation of the child at regular intervals (eg, twice a year) is also useful. Onset of thelarche after age 3 or in association with other signs of puberty requires more evaluation.

Premature adrenarche—benign early adrenal maturation—is manifested by gradual increase in pubic hair and body odor and, less commonly, axillary hair and acne. The average age at onset is 5–6 years. It is seen more commonly in obese girls. No increase in growth rate or skeletal maturation occurs, and no abnormal virilization (eg, clitoromegaly) is present. No treatment is required, though the possibility that premature adrenarche is a risk factor for later development of syndrome X is currently an area of investigation. Early adrenarche can also occur with undiagnosed CAH and may be associated with other signs of virilization.

## Treatment

In pseudoprecocious puberty, removal of the adrenal or ovarian tumor or correction of the adrenal enzyme disorder usually halts abnormal pubertal development. True precocious puberty can be treated with an analog of GnRH when bone age advancement indicates that adult height will be reduced or when precocious development is causing psychosocial stress. Some long-term outcomes (eg, fertility rate) have not been established. The analogs—given as a depot sustained-release preparation—interrupts the physiologic pulsatile effect of native GnRH on the pituitary. Down-regulation of the pituitary GnRH receptor also occurs, resulting in inhibition of pituitary LH secretion and release and the return of plasma estrogen concentrations to prepubertal values. If present initially, menses cease, secondary sexual development stabilizes or regresses, and linear growth and skeletal maturation slow to normal prepubertal rates.

In McCune–Albright syndrome, analogs of GnRH are not initially helpful. Therapy with antiestrogens (eg, tamoxifen) or agents that block estrogen synthesis (eg, ketoconazole or testolactone), or both, may be effective. Regardless of the cause of precocious puberty or the medical therapy selected, attention to the psychological needs of the patient and family is essential.

Biro FM et al: Impact of timing of pubertal maturation on growth in black and white female adolescents. J Pediatr 2001;138: 636 [PMID: 11343036].

de Sanctis C et al: Pubertal development in patients with Mc-Cune–Albright syndrome or pseudohypoparathyroidism. J Pediatr Endocrinol Metab 2003;16 (Suppl 2):293 [PMID: 12729407].

Gillis D, Schenker J: The evolving story of female puberty. Gynecol Endocrinol 2002;16:163 [PMID: 12012628].

Legro RS: Detection of insulin resistance and its treatment in adolescents with polycystic ovary syndrome. J Pediatr Endocrinol Metab 2002;15 (Suppl 5):1367 [PMID: 12510993].

Partsch CJ et al: Management and outcome of central precocious puberty. Clin Endocrinol (Oxf) 2002;56:129 [PMID: 11874402].

## 2. Amenorrhea

Primary amenorrhea is the absence of menarche in a female age 14 years or older or in a female of any age who is more than 3 years postpubertal maturation (Table 30–10). Secondary amenorrhea is cessation of established menses after an interval of time equal to at least 6 months postmenarche or three menstrual cycles. A history and physical examination (including pelvic examination) often identify possible causes of amenorrhea. The term "pseudoamenorrhea" is used when the patient is menstruating but has a genital tract obstruction that prevents release of menstrual blood. Sexual development is usually at Tanner state III or IV, and cyclic abdominal pain without menstruation is noted.

### Primary Amenorrhea

The most common cause of primary amenorrhea is physiologic or constitutional delay. However, Turner syndrome, chronic illness, and severe undernutrition or strenuous exercise also can lead to delay in onset of menses.

Turner syndrome (45,XO syndrome and its variants) should be considered in patients with short stature and sexual infantilism or adrenarche without normal pubertal progression. This is a form of hypergonadotropic hypogonadism in which serum concentrations of FSH and LH are elevated but plasma estrogen concentration is low after attainment of pubertal age owing to a total or relative lack of ovarian tissue. Skeletal maturation is usually delayed. The phenotypic

**Table 30–10.** Causes of amenorrhea.

**A. With obstruction of outflow tract**
1. Fusion or stenosis of labia, hymen (imperforate), vagina, or cervix
2. Müllerian agenesis (Mayer–Rokitansky–Küster–Hauser syndrome)
3. Postabortion infection, cesarean section, hysterectomy
4. Complete androgen resistance syndrome (46,XY female)

**B. Estrogen deficiency**
1. Primary ovarian insufficiency
   a. Gonadal agenesis
   b. Gonadal dysgenesis (Turner syndrome variants, true gonadal dysgenesis)
   c. Ovarian steroid biosynthesis deficiency (enzyme defects)
   d. Premature ovarian failure
      (1) Autoimmune disease
      (2) Infection, surgery, radiation, chemotherapy
2. Secondary/tertiary ovarian insufficiency
   a. Hypothalamic or pituitary tumor, infection, irradiation
   b. Kallman syndrome (GnRH/FSH/LH deficiency associated with anosmia)
   c. Eating disorders (eg, anorexia nervosa, bulimia)
   d. Excessive exercise (swimmers, runners, gymnasts)
   e. Chronic illness, malnutrition

**C. Androgen excess**
1. Polycystic ovary syndrome
2. Adrenal androgen excess (CAH, Cushing disease or syndrome)

**D. Ovarian tumors—granulosa-theca cell, and others**

CAH = congenital adrenal hyperplasia; FSH = follicle-stimulating hormone; GnRH = gonadotropin-releasing hormone; LH = luteinizing hormone.

features of Turner syndrome (described in Chapter 32) may be absent in 40–50% of girls with the syndrome. Current treatment for short stature includes HGH with or without anabolic steroids. Low doses of estrogens are added to the treatment regimen when breast development is desired, but usually at a later age than the average girl, to ensure that maximal height will be achieved. After 2–3 years of estrogen therapy, a combination of estrogen and progesterone in physiologic doses is indicated.

Mayer–Rokitansky–Küster–Hauser syndrome is characterized by congenital müllerian agenesis with normal ovaries, normal ovarian function, and normal breast development. Pelvic examination reveals an absent vagina and various uterine abnormalities with or without additional renal and skeletal anomalies. Full evaluation is necessary, including karyotype, renal ultrasonography, and laparoscopy. Therapy for this syndrome is surgical vaginoplasty.

Androgen insensitivity syndrome (androgen receptor defect) may be manifested as primary amenorrhea because the affected individual (46,XY) has functioning testes that produce müllerian-inhibiting hormone during fetal life. Thus no müllerian duct (oviduct, uterus) development occurs, but external sexual characteristics appear female.

The history should include whether and when puberty commenced, level of exercise, nutritional intake, presence of stressors, and the age of menarche for female relatives. A careful physical examination should note the percentage of ideal body weight for height and age, Tanner stage, vaginal patency, presence of a uterus (assessed through pelvic examination or ultrasonography), signs of virilization, excess body hair, or stigmata of Turner syndrome.

A bone age radiograph should be obtained. If the patient has not attained an age consistent with pubertal onset, further evaluation should focus on determining the cause of the delay. Laboratory studies should include a complete blood count, erythrocyte sedimentation rate, chemistry panel, and renal and liver function tests to screen for undiagnosed chronic medical illness. Tests for $FT_4$ and TSH can exclude hypothyroidism. Measurement of FSH and LH will not be helpful in this setting since prepubertal levels are normally low. Determination of a karyotype should be considered if short stature, stigmata of Turner syndrome, or genital abnormalities noted on exam or ultrasonography are present.

If the patient has attained a skeletal age consistent with onset of puberty and there are minimal or no signs of puberty on physical exam, determination of FSH and LH will distinguish between hypergonadotropic states (gonadal dysgenesis, Turner syndrome, premature ovarian failure) and hypogonatotropic states (anorexia, chronic disease, severe stress). If significant pubertal signs are present, the patient should be given a course of medroxyprogesterone, 10 mg/day orally for 10 days. If withdrawal bleeding occurs within 7 days of completion of the course, normal anatomy and adequate estrogen effect can be assumed. If the patient is obese, a work-up for the metabolic syndrome is indicated, and weight loss or insulin-sensitizing medications may restore menses. If no bleeding occurs, FSH, LH, and prolactin levels should be drawn.

## Secondary Amenorrhea (See Chapter 3, Adolescence.)

## OVARIAN TUMORS

Ovarian tumors are not rare in children. They may occur at any age and are usually large, benign, and uni-

lateral. They may be estrogen-producing. Ovarian tumors account for about 1% of cases of female sexual precocity. The most common estrogen-producing tumor is the granulosa cell tumor. Other tumors causing sexual precocity include thecomas, luteomas, mixed types, theca-lutein and follicular cysts, and ovarian tumors (teratomas, choriocarcinomas, and dysgerminomas). Ovarian tumors are usually palpated on rectal examination and are seen readily by ovarian ultrasonography. Treatment is surgical removal. Recurrences are uncommon.

## ABNORMALITIES IN MALE PUBERTAL DEVELOPMENT AND TESTICULAR FUNCTION

### 1. Precocious Puberty in Boys

Puberty is considered precocious in boys if secondary sexual characteristics appear before age 9 years. Precocious puberty appears to be much less common in boys than in girls. In boys presenting with sexual precocity, pseudoprecocious puberty is as common as true GnRH-dependent, precocious puberty. In addition, boys with true precocious puberty are more likely to have an identifiable pathologic process (eg, CNS abnormality) than are girls.

Two primary GnRH-independent forms of precocious puberty have been described in boys: McCune–Albright syndrome (described previously) and familial Leydig cell hyperplasia, or testotoxicosis, a condition in which a mutated LH receptor on the Leydig cell is autonomously activated, resulting in testicular production of testosterone despite prepubertal LH concentrations.

### Clinical Findings

#### A. SYMPTOMS AND SIGNS

In precocious development, increases in growth rate and growth of pubic hair are the common presenting signs. Testicular size may differentiate true precocity, in which the testes enlarge, from pseudoprecocity (most commonly due to congenital adrenal hyperplasia), in which the testes usually remain small. Some exceptions do occur—for example, testicular enlargement may occur in pseudoprecocity of long-standing due to secondary activation of central precocity from prolonged elevation of androgen levels. Tumors of the testis are associated with asymmetrical testicular enlargement.

#### B. LABORATORY FINDINGS

Basal serum LH and FSH concentrations are usually not in the pubertal range in boys with true sexual precocity, but the LH response to GnRH stimulation testing is pubertal (> 10 IU/L). Sexual precocity caused by congenital adrenal hyperplasia is usually associated with abnormal plasma concentrations of dehydroepiandrosterone (DHEA), androstenedione, 17-hydroxyprogesterone (in congenital adrenal hyperplasia due to 21-hydroxylase deficiency), 11-deoxycortisol (in congenital adrenal hyperplasia due to 11-hydroxylase deficiency), or a combination of these steroids (see Adrenal Cortex section). Serum HCG concentrations can identify the presence of an HCG-producing tumor (eg, CNS dysgerminoma, hepatoma) in boys who present with apparent true sexual precocity (ie, accompanied by testicular enlargement) but suppressed gonadotropins following LHRH.

### C. IMAGING

Diagnostic studies are similar to those used to evaluate sexual precocity in girls. Ultrasonography may be useful in detecting hepatic, presacral, and testicular tumors.

## Differential Diagnosis

The causes of isosexual precocity are outlined in Table 30–9. In boys, it is particularly important to differentiate pseudoprecocity from true sexual precocity. Seventy percent of boys with pseudoprecocious puberty have an adrenal enzyme abnormality (congenital adrenal hyperplasia). Of boys with true precocious puberty, 70% have benign CNS mass lesions. Premature adrenarche (described earlier) may occur in males as well as females.

## Treatment

Specific therapy should be provided whenever possible. Treatment of idiopathic true precocious puberty in boys is similar to that in girls (see previous discussion). Treatment of McCune–Albright syndrome or familial Leydig cell hyperplasia with agents that block steroid synthesis (eg, ketoconazole), with an antiandrogen (eg, spironolactone), or a combination of both has been successful.

de Roux N, Milgrom E: Inherited disorders of GnRH and gonadotropin receptors. Mol Cell Endocrinol 2001;179:83 [PMID: 11420132].

De Sanctis V et al: Etiology of central precocious puberty in males: The results of the Italian Study Group for Physiopathology of Puberty. J Pediatr Endocrinol Metab 2000;13:687 [PMID: 10969910].

Shinozaki H et al: Desensitization of Gs-coupled receptor signaling by constitutively active mutants of the human lutropin/choriogonadotropin receptor. J Clin Endocrinol Metab 2003;88: 1194 [PMID 12629106]

## 2. Delayed Puberty (Primary & Secondary Testicular Failure)

Lack of development of secondary sexual characteristics after age 15 years suggests abnormal testicular maturation. Although delay of puberty until age 15 years may be physiologically normal, boys generally become concerned if pubertal changes do not occur by then, and evaluation should be initiated at that time. Hypogonadism may be difficult to differentiate from constitutionally delayed adolescence. Although the latter may be associated with a delay in testicular function, normal puberty occurs at a later date.

Testicular failure or insufficiency may be primary, resulting from the absence, malfunction, or destruction of testicular tissue, or secondary, due to pituitary (or hypothalamic) insufficiency. Primary testicular failure may be due to anorchia, surgical castration, Klinefelter syndrome or other sex chromosome abnormalities, enzymatic defects in testosterone synthesis or action, or inflammation and destruction of the testes following infection (eg, mumps), autoimmune disorders, radiation, trauma, or tumor.

Secondary testicular failure may accompany panhypopituitarism, empty-sella syndrome, Kallmann syndrome (gonadotropin deficiency accompanied by anosmia), or isolated LH or FSH deficiencies. Destructive lesions in or near the anterior pituitary, especially craniopharyngiomas, gliomas, or infection, may also result in hypothalamic or pituitary dysfunction. Prader–Willi syndrome and Laurence–Moon syndrome (Bardet–Biedl syndrome) are frequently associated with LH and FSH deficiency secondary to GnRH deficiency. Miscellaneous causes of secondary testicular failure include chronic debilitating disease and hypothyroidism.

## Clinical Findings

### A. SYMPTOMS AND SIGNS

Physical examination may not be helpful in differentiating primary from secondary testicular insufficiency. Whereas cryptorchidism suggests primary testicular failure, hypothalamic or pituitary insufficiency as well as anatomic abnormalities may also lead to failure of testicular descent.

### B. LABORATORY FINDINGS

In primary testicular failure, the plasma testosterone concentration is low, whereas LH and FSH values are elevated into the castrate range in children who have attained a pubertal skeletal age. In secondary testicular failure, circulating concentrations of all three hormones are below the normal adult range. To establish the presence of the testes and their ability to respond to stimulation, chorionic gonadotropin (1500 units) is given intramuscularly on days 1, 3, and 5. The plasma testosterone should rise to above 200 mg/dL 24 hours after the final dose. A karyotype should be determined in primary testicular failure of unknown cause.

### C. IMAGING

Skeletal (epiphyseal) maturation is usually delayed. A cranial CT scan or MRI should be performed in cases of secondary testicular failure.

## Treatment

Specific therapy is indicated when the cause of testicular failure is known. Treatment with depot testosterone (eg, testosterone enanthate), beginning with 75–100 mg intramuscularly and increasing to 200 mg every 3–4 weeks, may be continued indefinitely. Specific therapy (pulsatile subcutaneous delivery of GnRH) may result in fertility in patients with hypothalamic–pituitary insufficiency.

Reiter EO, Lee PA: Delayed puberty. Adolesc Med 2002;13:101 [PMID: 11841958].

Silveira LF et al: Hypogonadotropic hypogonadism. Semin Reprod Med 2002;20:327 [PMID: 12536356].

Simon D: Puberty in chronically diseased patients. Horm Res 2002;57 (Suppl 2):53 [PMID: 12065928].

## 3. Cryptorchidism

Cryptorchidism (undescended testis) is a common disorder in children. It may be unilateral or bilateral and may be classified as ectopic or true cryptorchidism. Approximately 3% of full-term male newborns have an undescended testis at birth, with a higher proportion among premature infants. In over 50% of these patients, the testes descend by the third month; by age 1 year, 80% of all undescended testes are in the scrotum. Further descent may occur through puberty, the latter perhaps stimulated by endogenous gonadotropins.

Infertility and testicular malignancy risk must be considered in cases of cryptorchidism. The exact incidence of impairment in fertility is unknown and incidence figures vary in reported studies. However, histologic changes clearly occur as early as age 6 months in children with undescended testes. The reported malignancy rate in cryptorchidism is 48.9 per 100,000, which is 22 times higher than in the general population. In addition, 25% of tumors develop in the contralateral testis, indicating that abnormality of testicular development (dysgenesis) may be bilateral in unilateral cryptorchidism.

Ectopic testes are presumed to develop normally but are diverted as they descend through the inguinal canal. True cryptorchidism is thought in most cases to be the result of dysgenesis. Cryptorchid testes frequently have a short spermatic artery, poor blood supply, or both. Although early scrotal positioning of these testes will obviate further damage related to intra-abdominal loca-tion, the testes generally remain abnormal, spermatogenesis is rare, and the risk of malignant neoplasm is increased. These testes should probably be removed if spermatogenesis does not occur after a reasonable period of observation.

Cryptorchidism can occur in an isolated fashion or may be associated with other findings. Abnormalities in the hypothalamic–pituitary–gonadal axis predispose to cryptorchidism. Androgen biosynthesis or receptor defects may also predispose to cryptorchidism and undervirilization.

The diagnosis of bilateral cryptorchidism in an apparently male newborn should never be made until ruling out the possibility that the child is actually a fully virilized female with potentially fatal salt-losing congenital adrenal hyperplasia. (see Adrenal Cortex section).

## Clinical Findings

Plasma testosterone concentrations may be obtained after HCG stimulation to confirm the presence or absence of abdominal testes (see preceding section).

## Differential Diagnosis

In palpating the testis, the cremasteric reflex may be elicited, causing the testis to be retracted into the inguinal canal or abdomen (pseudocryptorchidism). To prevent retraction, the fingers first should be placed across the abdominal ring and the upper portion of the inguinal canal, obstructing ascent. Examination while the child is in the squatting position or in a warm bath is also helpful. No treatment for retractile testes is necessary, and the prognosis for testicular descent and competence is excellent.

## Treatment

### A. SURGICAL TREATMENT

The current recommendation for treatment of cryptorchidism is that surgical orchidopexy be performed by an experienced surgeon if no descent has occurred by 1 year of age.

### B. HORMONAL TREATMENT

Various treatment regimens have been used, ranging from 250 to 1000 IU given twice weekly for 5 weeks. Such therapy will generally cause descent of retractile testes, but is generally not successful in treating cryptorchidism. Androgen treatment (eg, depot testosterone) is indicated as replacement therapy in the male child who lacks functional testes beyond the normal age of puberty.

## 4. Gynecomastia

Adolescent gynecomastia is a common, self-limited finding in boys that can occurs in up to 75% of normal boys during puberty. Adolescent gynecomastia typically resolves within 2 years. Gynecomastia may sometimes occur as part of Klinefelter syndrome, or it may occur in boys who are taking drugs such as antidepressants or marijuana. Therapy, either medical (antiestrogens, aromatase inhibitors) or surgical, should be considered in cases that are prolonged or severe. This topic is discussed in more detail in Chapter 3.

## TESTICULAR TUMORS

The major primary malignant tumors of the testis are seminomas and teratomas. Seminomas are rare in childhood; they may be hormone-producing. The major hormone-producing tumor of the testis is the Leydig cell tumor. It is frequently associated with sexual precocity. Other testicular tumors (choriocarcinomas and dysgerminomas) have been reported in association with sexual precocity.

Treatment of testicular tumors is surgical removal; chemotherapy and radiation therapy are not used in childhood unless a high-grade malignancy or metastasis is present. The prognosis in patients with Leydig cell tumors is generally good.

## ■ ADRENAL CORTEX

The adult adrenal cortex displays relative regional specificity of terminal steroid production. The outermost zona glomerulosa is the predominant source of aldosterone, whereas the zona fasciculata makes cortisol, the major glucocorticoid, as well as small amounts of mineralocorticoids. The innermost zona reticularis produces mainly adrenal androgens and estrogens. During fetal life, a fetal zone, or provisional cortex, predominates. This fetal zone produces glucocorticoids, mineralocorticoids, androgens, and estrogens but is relatively deficient in 3β-ol dehydrogenase (see Figure 30–6). Therefore, placentally produced progesterone serves as the major precursor for the fetal adrenal production of cortisol and aldosterone.

The adrenal cortex produces cortisol under the control of pituitary corticotropin (ACTH) (see Figure 30–1 and Table 30–1), which is, in turn, regulated by corticotropin-releasing hormone (CRH), a hypothalamic peptide. The complex interaction of CNS influences on CRH secretion coupled with negative feedback of serum cortisol leads to a marked diurnal pattern of ACTH and cortisol release. ACTH concentrations are greatest during the early morning hours, display a smaller peak in the late afternoon, and are lowest during the night. The pattern of serum cortisol concentration closely follows this diurnal pattern with a lag of a few hours. In the absence of cortisol feedback, both CRH and ACTH display dramatic hypersecretion.

At the cellular level, glucocorticoids are critical for normal gene expression in a wide variety of cells. In excess, glucocorticoids are both catabolic and antianabolic; that is, they promote the release of amino acids from muscle and increase gluconeogenesis while decreasing incorporation of amino acids into muscle protein. They also antagonize insulin action and facilitate lipolysis. Glucocorticoids help maintain blood pressure through their supportive effect on peripheral vascular tone and by promoting sodium and water retention.

Mineralocorticoids (primarily aldosterone in humans) promote sodium retention and stimulate potassium excretion in the distal tubule. Although ACTH can stimulate aldosterone production, the predominant regulator of aldosterone secretion is the volume- and sodium-sensitive renin–angiotensin–aldosterone system. Elevations of serum potassium concentrations also directly influence aldosterone release from the cortex.

Androgen (DHEA and androstenedione) production by the zona reticularis is insignificant in prepubertal children. At the onset of puberty, androgen production increases and may be an important factor in the dynamics of puberty in both sexes. The adrenal gland is a major source of androgen in the pubertal and adult female.

## ADRENOCORTICAL INSUFFICIENCY (Adrenal Crisis, Addison Disease)

The leading causes of adrenal insufficiency today are hereditary enzymatic defects (congenital adrenal hyperplasia), loss of adrenal function due to autoimmune destruction of the glands (Addison disease), and central adrenal insufficiency following an intracranial neoplasm or its treatment, or congenital midline defects in association with optic nerve hypoplasia (Septo-optic dysplasia). A rare form of familial adrenal insufficiency can occur in association with cerebral sclerosis and spastic paraplegia (adrenoleukodystrophy). Autoimmune Addison disease may be familial and has been described in association with hypoparathyroidism, candidiasis, hypothyroidism, pernicious anemia, hypogonadism, and diabetes mellitus as one of the polyglandular autoimmune syndromes. The finding of circulating antibodies to adrenal tissue and other tissues involved in these conditions suggests that an autoimmune mechanism is the cause. Less commonly, the gland is destroyed by tumor, calcification, or hemorrhage (Waterhouse–Friederichsen syndrome). Adrenal disease secondary to opportunistic infections (fungal, tuberculous) is again being reported in adults who have acquired immunodeficiency syndrome. A similar relationship is likely in children. In children, central adrenal insufficiency due to a primary anterior pituitary tumor is rare. A temporary salt-losing disorder due to partial mineralocorticoid deficiency or renal underresponsiveness (pseudohypoaldosteronism) may occur during infancy or with pyelonephritis.

Any acute illness, surgery, trauma, or exposure to excessive heat may precipitate an adrenal crisis in patients with adrenal insufficiency. Patients with primary adrenal insufficiency are generally at greater risk for life-threatening crisis than patients with central ACTH deficiency. This is a consequence of intact mineralocorticoid secretion and low-level autonomous cortisol secretion in central ACTH deficiency.

## Clinical Findings

### A. SYMPTOMS AND SIGNS

**1. Acute form (adrenal crisis)**—Manifestations include nausea and vomiting, diarrhea, abdominal pain, dehydration, fever (which may be followed by hypothermia), weakness, hypotension, circulatory collapse, and confusion or coma. Increased pigmentation may be associated with primary adrenal insufficiency as a result of the melanocyte-stimulating activity of the hypersecreted parent molecule of ACTH.

**2. Chronic form**—Manifestations include fatigue, hypotension, weakness, failure to gain or loss of weight, increased appetite for salt (primary insufficiency), vomiting (which may become forceful and sometimes projectile), and dehydration. Diffuse tanning with increased pigmentation over pressure points, scars, and mucous membranes may be present in primary adrenal insufficiency. A small heart may be seen on chest radiograph.

### B. LABORATORY FINDINGS

**1. Suggestive of adrenocortical insufficiency**—In primary adrenal insufficiency, serum sodium and bicarbonate levels, $PaCO_2$, blood pH, and blood volume are decreased. Serum potassium and urea nitrogen levels are increased. Urinary sodium levels and the ratio of sodium to potassium are elevated for the degree of hyponatremia. In central adrenal insufficiency, serum sodium levels may be mildly decreased as a result of impaired water excretion. Eosinophilia and moderate lymphopenia may be present in either form of insufficiency.

**2. Confirmatory tests**—The following tests measure the functional capacity of the adrenal cortex:

**a. The ACTH (cosyntropin) stimulation test**—This is the most direct test of adrenal gland function. In primary adrenal insufficiency (ie, originating in the gland itself), plasma cortisol and aldosterone concentrations fail to increase significantly over baseline 60 minutes after an intravenous dose of ACTH (250 μg). To diagnose central adrenal insufficiency, a low dose of ACT is given (1 μg).

**b. Baseline serum ACTH concentrations**—These are elevated in primary adrenal failure and are low in central adrenal insufficiency.

**c. Urinary free cortisol and 17-hydroxycorticosteroid excretion**—These values are decreased.

**d. The CRH test**—This recently introduced test can be used to assess responsiveness of the entire hypothalamic–pituitary–adrenal axis. After administration of ovine CRH, serum concentrations of ACTH and cortisol can be measured over a period of 2 hours. Verification of the presence of an intact axis or localization of the site of impairment is possible with careful interpretation of these results.

## Differential Diagnosis

Acute adrenal insufficiency must be differentiated from severe acute infections, diabetic coma, various disturbances of the CNS, and acute poisoning. In the neonatal period, adrenal insufficiency may be clinically indistinguishable from respiratory distress, intracranial hemorrhage, or sepsis.

Chronic adrenocortical insufficiency must be differentiated from anorexia nervosa, certain muscular disorders (eg, myasthenia gravis), salt-losing nephritis, and chronic debilitating infections (eg, tuberculosis) and must be considered in cases of recurrent spontaneous hypoglycemia.

## Treatment

### A. ACUTE (ADRENAL CRISIS)

**1. Hydrocortisone sodium succinate**—Hydrocortisone sodium succinate, initially 50 mg/m$^2$ intravenously over 2–5 minutes or intramuscularly; thereafter, it is given intravenously, 12.5 mg/m$^2$, every 4–6 hours until stabilization is achieved and oral therapy can be tolerated.

**2. Fluids and electrolytes**—In primary adrenal insufficiency, 5–10% glucose in normal saline, 10–20 mL/kg intravenously, is given over the first hour and repeated if necessary to reestablish vascular volume. Normal saline is continued thereafter at one and one-half to two times the maintenance fluid requirements. In addition, intravenous boluses of glucose (10% glucose, 2 mL/kg) may be needed every 4–6 hours for hypoglycemia. In central adrenal insufficiency, routine fluid management is generally adequate following reinstatement of vascular volume and institution of cortisol replacement.

**3. Fludrocortisone**—When oral intake is tolerated, fludrocortisone, 0.05–0.15 mg daily, is started and continued as necessary every 12–24 hours for primary adrenal insufficiency.

**4. Inotropic agents**—Rarely, inotropic agents such as dopamine and dobutamine are needed. However, adequate cortisol replacement is critical because pressor agents may be ineffective in adrenal insufficiency.

**5. Waterhouse–Friderichsen syndrome with fulminant infections**—The use of adrenocorticosteroids and norepinephrine in the treatment or prophylaxis of fulminant infections remains controversial; corticosteroids may augment the generalized Shwartzman reaction in fatal cases of meningococcemia. However, corticosteroids should be considered in the presence of possible adrenal insufficiency, particularly with hypotension and circulatory collapse.

### B. Maintenance Therapy

Following initial stabilization, the most effective substitution therapy is hydrocortisone, combined with fludrocortisone in primary adrenal insufficiency. Overtreatment should be avoided because it may result in obesity, growth retardation, and other cushingoid features. Additional hydrocortisone, fludrocortisone, or sodium chloride, singly or in combination, may be necessary with acute illness, surgery, trauma, or other stress reactions.

Supportive adrenocortical therapy should be given whenever surgical operations are performed in patients who have at some time received prolonged therapy with adrenocorticosteroids (see below).

**1. Glucocorticoids**—A maintenance dosage of 8–10 mg/m$^2$/d of hydrocortisone (or equivalent) is given orally in two or three divided doses. For adrenal enzyme defects (see following section), this dosage may need to be increased to 18–22 mg/m$^2$/d to obtain adequate suppression of the adrenal axis, with two thirds given at night (the time of greatest axis suppressibility). The dosage of all glucocorticoids is increased to 30–50 mg/m$^2$/d during intercurrent illnesses or other times of stress.

**2. Mineralocorticoids**—In primary adrenal insufficiency, give fludrocortisone, 0.05–0.15 mg orally daily as a single dose or in two divided doses. Periodic monitoring of blood pressure is recommended to avoid overdosing.

**3. Salt**—The child should be given ready access to table salt. Frequent blood pressure determinations in the recumbent position should be made to ensure that hypertension is avoided. In the infant, supplementation of 3–5 mEq Na$^+$/kg/d by adding the injectable solution (4 mg/mL) to formula or breast milk is generally required until table foods are introduced.

### C. Corticosteroids in Patients with Adrenocortical Insufficiency Who Undergo Surgery

**1. Before operation**—Hydrocortisone sodium succinate, 30–50 mg/m$^2$/d intravenously, is given 1 hour before surgery.

**2. During operation**—Hydrocortisone sodium succinate, 25–100 mg intravenously, is administered with 5–10% glucose in saline throughout surgery.

**3. During recovery**—Hydrocortisone sodium succinate, 12.5 mg/m$^2$ intravenously, is given every 4–6 hours until oral doses are tolerated. The oral dose of three to five times the maintenance dose is continued until the acute stress is over, at which time the patient can be returned to the maintenance dose.

## Course & Prognosis

### A. Acute Adrenal Insufficiency

The course of acute adrenal insufficiency is rapid, and death may occur within a few hours, particularly in infants, unless adequate treatment is given. Spontaneous recovery is unlikely. Patients who have received long-term treatment with adrenocorticosteroids may exhibit adrenal collapse if they undergo surgery or other acute stress. Pharmacologic doses of glucocorticoids during these episodes may be needed throughout life.

In all forms of acute adrenal insufficiency, the patient should be observed carefully once the crisis has passed and evaluated with laboratory tests to assess the degree of permanent adrenal insufficiency.

### B. Chronic Adrenal Insufficiency

Adequately treated, chronic adrenocortical insufficiency is consistent with a relatively normal life.

Dattani MT, Robinson IC: HESX1 and septo-optic dysplasia. Rev Endocr Metab Disord 2002;3:289 [PMID: 12424431].

Devendra D, Eisenbarth GS: 17. Immunologic endocrine disorders. J Allergy Clin Immunol 2003;111(2 Suppl):S624 [PMID: 12592308].

Geffner ME: Hypopituitarism in childhood. Cancer Control 2002;9:212 [PMID: 12060819].

Thaler LM, Blevins LS Jr: The low dose (1-μg) adrenocorticotropin stimulation test in the evaluation of patients with suspected central adrenal insufficiency. J Clin Endocrinol Metab 1998;83:2726 [PMID: 9709938].

# CONGENITAL ADRENAL HYPERPLASIAS

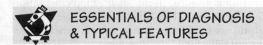

### ESSENTIALS OF DIAGNOSIS & TYPICAL FEATURES

- *Pseudohermaphroditism in females, with urogenital sinus, enlargement of the clitoris, or other evidence of virilization.*
- *Salt-losing crisis in infant males or isosexual precocity in older males with infantile testes.*
- *Increased linear growth in young children; advancement of skeletal maturation.*
- *Urinary and plasma androgen elevation; plasma 17-hydroxyprogesterone and urinary pregnanetriol concentrations increased in the common form; may be associated with electrolyte and water disturbances (hyponatremia, hyperkalemia, and metabolic acidosis), particularly in the newborn period.*

## General Considerations

Autosomal recessive enzyme defects involved in adrenal steroidogenesis have in common a defect in cortisol biosynthesis with resultant increased ACTH secretion during fetal life. ACTH excess subsequently results in adrenal hyperplasia with increased production of various adrenal hormone precursors, including androgens, and increased urinary excretion of their metabolites. Increased pigmentation, especially of the scrotum, labia majora, and nipples, frequently results from excessive ACTH secretion. Congenital adrenal hyperplasia (CAH) is most commonly (in > 80% of patients) the result of homozygous 21-hydroxylase (P450c21) deficiency (see Figure 30–6), an autosomal recessive disorder. In its severe form, excess adrenal androgen production beginning in the first trimester of fetal development results in virilization of the female infant and life-threatening hypovolemic, hyponatremic shock (adrenal crisis) in the newborn. Other enzyme defects that less commonly result in congenital adrenal hyperplasia include 20,22-desmolase, 3β-ol dehydrogenases, 18-hydroxylase-17,22-desmolase, and 11-hydroxylase deficiencies. The clinical syndromes associated with each of these defects can be predicted from Figure 30–6 and Table 30–11. All of these enzymes except 3β-ol dehydrogenase have been shown to be associated with the cy-

***Table 30–11.*** Clinical and laboratory findings in adrenal enzyme defects resulting in CAH.

| Enzyme Deficiency[a] | Urinary 17-Ketosteroids | Elevated Plasma Metabolite | Plasma Androgens | Aldosterone | Hypertension/ Salt Loss | External Genitalia |
|---|---|---|---|---|---|---|
| 20,22-Desmolase | ↓↓↓ | — | ↓↓↓ | ↓↓↓ | –/+ | Males: ambiguous<br>Females: normal |
| 3β-ol Dehydrogenase | ↑↑<br>(DHEA) | 17-OH pregnenolone (DHEA) | ↑<br>(DHEA) | ↓↓↓ | –/+ | Males: ambiguous<br>Females: possibly virilized |
| 17-Hydroxylase | ↓↓↓ | Progesterone | ↓↓ | Normal to ↑ | +/– | Males: ambiguous<br>Females: normal |
| 21-Hydroxylase[a] | ↑↑↑ | 17-OHP | ↑↑ | ↓↓ | –/+ | Males: normal<br>Females: virilized |
| 11-Hydroxylase | ↑↑ | 11-Deoxycortisol | ↑↑ | ↓↓<br>(↑ Deoxycorticosterone) | +/– | Males: normal<br>Females: virilized |
| 17,20-Desmolase | ↓↓↓ | 17-Hydroxysteroids (?) | ↓↓ | Normal | –/– | Males: ambiguous<br>Females: normal |

[a]Children with "simple virilizing (non–salt-wasting)" forms of 21-hydroxylase deficiency congenital adrenal hyperplasia (CAH) may have normal aldosterone production and serum electrolytes, but some children have normal aldosterone production and serum electrolytes at the expense of elevated plasma renin activity and are, by definition, compensated salt-wasters. These children usually receive mineralocorticoid as well as glucocorticoid treatment. Children with 21-hydroxylase deficiency CAH should therefore have documented normal plasma renin activity in addition to normal serum electrolytes before they are considered non–salt-wasters.

tochrome P-450 complex. A new enzyme nomenclature has been established, and it is given along with the older, more familiar nomenclature in Figure 30–6.

Studies of patients with 21-hydroxylase deficiency indicate that the clinical type (salt-wasting versus non–salt-wasting) is usually consistent within a family and that a close genetic linkage exists between the 21-hydroxylase gene and the HLA complex on chromosome 6. The latter finding has allowed more precise heterozygote detection and prenatal diagnosis. Population studies indicate that the defective gene is present in 1:250–1:100 people and that the incidence of the disorder is 1:15,000–1:5000. Evaluation of the hormone responses of unaffected family members following ACTH stimulation allows detection of the heterozygote with a certainty of 80–90%, and a combination of hormonal and HLA studies can increase the number of cases detected. HLA typing in combination with the measurement of 17-hydroxyprogesterone and androstenedione in amniotic fluid has been used in the prenatal diagnosis of 21-hydroxylase deficiency. Mass screening for this enzyme defect, using a microfilter paper technique to measure 17-hydroxyprogesterone, has been established in some US states.

Nonclassic presentations of 21-hydroxylase deficiency have been reported with increasing frequency. Affected persons have a normal phenotype at birth and develop evidence of virilization during later childhood, adolescence, or early adulthood. In these cases, previously referred to as late-onset or acquired enzyme deficiency, results of hormonal studies are characteristic of 21-hydroxylase deficiency. An asymptomatic form has also been identified in which individuals have none of the phenotypic features of the disorder but have hormonal study results identical to those of patients with nonclassic 21-hydroxylase deficiency. The nonclassic form appears to be less severe than the classic form. Because members of the same family may have classic, nonclassic, and asymptomatic forms, the disorders may be due to allelic variations of the same enzyme.

Male pseudohermaphroditism may occur in children with 17,20-desmolase deficiency because that enzyme is necessary for normal androgen biosynthesis (see Table 30–11).

## Clinical Findings

### A. Symptoms and Signs

**1. In females**—In the female with potentially normal ovaries and uterus, virilization occurs, and sexual development is therefore along heterosexual lines. The abnormality of the external genitalia may vary from mild enlargement of the clitoris to complete fusion of the labioscrotal folds, forming a scrotum, a penile urethra, a penile shaft, and enlargement of the clitoris to form a normal-sized glans (see Table 30–8). Signs of adrenal insufficiency (salt loss) may be present during the first days of life (typically in the first or second week). In rare cases, adrenal insufficiency does not occur for months or years. When the enzyme defect is milder, salt loss may not occur, and virilization predominates (simple virilizing form). In untreated, non–salt-losing 21-hydroxylase or 11-hydroxylase deficiency, growth rate and skeletal maturation are accelerated, and patients may become muscular. Pubic hair appears early (often before the second birthday); acne may be excessive; and the voice may deepen. Excessive pigmentation may develop. Final adult height is often compromised.

**2. In males**—In males, sexual development proceeds normally. The male infant usually appears normal at birth but may present with a salt-losing crisis in the first 2–4 weeks of life. In milder forms, salt-losing crises may not occur. In this circumstance, enlargement of the penis and increased pigmentation may be noted during the first few months. Other symptoms and signs are similar to those seen in females. The testes are soft and not enlarged except in the rare male in whom aberrant adrenal cells (adrenal rests) are present in the testes and produce unilateral or bilateral enlargement, often asymmetrical. In the rare isolated defect of 17,20-desmolase activity, ambiguous genitalia may be present because of the compromise in androgen production (see Figure 30–6).

### B. Laboratory Findings

**1. Blood and urine**—Hormonal studies are essential for accurate diagnosis. Findings characteristic of the enzyme deficiencies are shown in Table 30–11. With adrenal tumor, secretion of DHEA is greatly elevated, and determining plasma concentrations of DHEA sulfate may be useful in the differential diagnosis.

**2. Genetic studies**—Rapid chromosomal diagnosis should be obtained in any newborn with ambiguous genitalia.

### C. Imaging

Adrenal ultrasonography, CT scanning, and MRI may be useful in defining pelvic anatomy or enlarged adrenals or in localizing an adrenal tumor. Vaginograms using contrast material and pelvic ultrasonography may be helpful in delineating the internal anatomy in a newborn with ambiguous genitalia.

## Treatment

### A. Medical Treatment

Treatment goals in congenital adrenal hyperplasia consist of normalizing growth velocity and skeletal maturation using the smallest dose of glucocorticoid that will suppress adrenal function. The use of excessive amounts of glucocorticoids results in the undesirable side effects of Cushing syndrome. Mineralocorticoid replacement helps to sustain normal electrolyte homeostasis, although excessive mineralocorticoid dosing results in hypertension. (See Uses of Glucocorticoids & ACTH in Treatment of Nonendocrine Diseases section for a more complete discussion of the effects of pharmacologic glucocorticoid therapy.)

**1. Glucocorticoids**—Initially hydrocortisone given in a dosage of 30–50 mg/m²/d parenterally or orally suppresses abnormal adrenal steroidogenesis within 2 weeks. When adrenal suppression has been accomplished, as evidenced by normalization of serum 17-hydroxyprogesterone, the patients are placed on maintenance doses of 15–20 mg/m²/d in two or three divided doses. Between 50% and 60% of the daily dose should be given in the late evening to suppress the early morning ACTH rise. Dosage is adjusted to maintain normal growth rate and skeletal maturation. A variety of serum and urine androgens have been used to monitor adequacy of therapy, including 17-hydroxyprogesterone, androstenedione, and urinary pregnanetriol. However, none of these has been universally accepted. In adolescent females, normal menses are a sensitive index of the adequacy of therapy. Therapy should be continued throughout life in both males and females because of the possibility of malignant degeneration of the hyperplastic adrenal gland. In pregnant females who have congenital adrenal hyperplasia, adequate suppression of adrenal androgen secretion is critical to avoid virilization of the fetus, particularly a female fetus.

**2. Mineralocorticoids**—Fludrocortisone in a dose of 0.05–0.15 mg is given orally once a day or in two divided doses. Periodic monitoring of blood pressure and plasma renin is recommended to adjust dosing.

### B. SURGICAL TREATMENT

Consultation with a urologist experienced with female genital reconstruction is indicated in affected females as soon as possible during infancy.

## Course & Prognosis

When therapy is initiated in early infancy, abnormal metabolic effects and progression of masculinization can be avoided. Treatment with glucocorticoids permits normal growth, development, and sexual maturation. However, if not adequately controlled, congenital adrenal hyperplasia results in sexual precocity and masculinization throughout childhood. Affected individuals will be tall as children but short as adults because the rate of skeletal maturation is rapid with resultant pre-

mature closure of the epiphyses. If treatment is delayed or inadequate until somatic development is over 12–14 years as determined by skeletal maturation (bone age), true central sexual precocity may occur in males and females.

Patient education stressing lifelong therapy is important to ensure compliance in adolescence and later life.

Virilization and multiple surgical genital reconstructions are associated with a high risk of psychosexual disturbances in female patients. Ongoing psychological evaluation and support is a critical component of care.

When virilization of the patient (male or female) is caused by a tumor, the progression of signs and symptoms ceases after surgical removal; however, evidence of masculinization, particularly deepening of the voice, may persist.

Prenatal treatment of the mother with dexamethasone can eliminate or reduce virilization of female infants. However, this requires treatment of seven eighths of fetuses unnecessarily (only one quarter of offspring are affected with CAH and only half of these are females) and causes maternal side effects as well. Therefore, such treatment is still under investigation.

Eugster EA et al: Height outcome in congenital adrenal hyperplasia caused by 21-hydroxylase deficiency: A meta-analysis. J Pediatr 2001;138:26 [PMID: 11148508].

Hughes I: Congenital adrenal hyperplasia: Phenotype and genotype. J Pediatr Endocrinol Metab 2002;15 (Suppl 5):1329 [PMID: 12510987].

Hughes IA: Congenital adrenal hyperplasia: 21-Hydroxylase deficiency in the newborn and during infancy. Semin Reprod Med 2002;20:229 [PMID: 12428203].

Merke DP et al: NIH conference. Future directions in the study and management of congenital adrenal hyperplasia due to 21-hydroxylase deficiency. Ann Intern Med 2002;136:320 [PMID: 11848730].

# ADRENOCORTICAL HYPERFUNCTION (Cushing Disease, Cushing Syndrome)

### ESSENTIALS OF DIAGNOSIS & TYPICAL FEATURES

- *Truncal adiposity with thin extremities, moon facies, muscle wasting, weakness, plethora, easy bruising, purplish striae, decreased growth rate, delayed skeletal maturation.*
- *Hypertension, osteoporosis, glycosuria.*
- *Elevated serum and urine adrenocorticosteroids; low serum potassium levels; eosinopenia, lymphopenia.*

## General Considerations

Cushing syndrome is nonspecific. It may result from excessive secretion of adrenal steroids autonomously (adenoma or carcinoma), from excessive ACTH secretion from the pituitary (Cushing disease) or from ectopic sources, or from chronic exposure to pharmacologic doses of glucocorticoids.

In children younger than age 12 years, Cushing syndrome is usually iatrogenic (secondary to pharmacologic doses of ACTH or one of the glucocorticoids). It may rarely be due to an adrenal tumor, adrenal hyperplasia, an adenoma of the pituitary gland, or, even more rarely, an extrapituitary (ectopic) ACTH-producing tumor.

## Clinical Findings

### A. SYMPTOMS AND SIGNS

**1. Excess glucocorticoid**—Adiposity, most marked on the face, neck, and trunk (a fat pad in the interscapular area is characteristic); easy fatigability and weakness; plethoric facies; purplish striae; easy bruising; ecchymoses; hirsutism; osteoporosis; hypertension; diabetes mellitus (usually latent); pain in the back; muscle wasting and weakness; and marked retardation of growth and skeletal maturation.

**2. Excess mineralocorticoid**—Hypokalemia, mild hypernatremia with water retention, increased blood volume, edema, and hypertension.

**3. Excess androgen**—Hirsutism, acne, and varying degrees of virilization. Menstrual irregularities occur during puberty in older girls.

### B. LABORATORY FINDINGS

**1. Blood**—

a. **Plasma cortisol concentrations**—These are elevated, with loss of the normal diurnal variation in cortisol secretion. Determination of cortisol level between midnight and 2 AM may be a sensitive indicator of loss of variation.

b. **Serum chloride and potassium concentrations**—These values may be lowered. Serum sodium and bicarbonate concentrations may be elevated (metabolic alkalosis).

c. **Serum ACTH concentrations**—ACTH concentrations are slightly elevated with adrenal hyperplasia (Cushing disease), decreased in cases of adrenal tumor, and greatly increased with ACTH-producing pituitary or extrapituitary tumors.

d. **The leukocyte count**—This measurement shows polymorphonuclear leukocytosis with lymphopenia, and the eosinophil count is low. The erythrocyte count may be elevated.

**2. Saliva**

a. **Salivary cortisol**—This value is elevated and is a less invasive means by which to measure several samples (may be performed at home). A salivary cortisol obtained at midnight is a highly specific and sensitive test in adults, but has not yet been studied in children.

**3. Urine**—

a. **Urinary free cortisol excretion**—This value is elevated. This is currently considered the most useful initial diagnostic test.

b. **Urinary 17-hydroxycorticosteroid excretion (excretion products of the glucocorticoids)**—This value is elevated.

c. **Urinary 17-ketosteroid excretion**—This is usually elevated in association with adrenal tumors.

d. **Glycosuria**—This finding may be present.

**3. Response to dexamethasone suppression testing**—Adrenal function suppression is diminished after a small dose (0.5 mg) of dexamethasone; larger doses of dexamethasone cause suppression of adrenal activity when the disease is due to adrenal hyperplasia. Adenomas and adrenal carcinomas may rarely be suppressed by large doses of dexamethasone (4–16 mg/d in four divided doses).

**4. CRH test**—The CRH stimulation test may replace the high-dose dexamethasone test for differentiating pituitary and ectopic sources of ACTH excess.

### C. IMAGING

Pituitary imaging may demonstrate a pituitary adenoma. This can be used in conjunction with petrosal sinus blood sampling for localization of ACTH-secreting adenomas. Adrenal imaging (eg, CT scan) may demonstrate adenoma or bilateral hyperplasia. Radionuclide studies of the adrenals may be useful in complex cases. Osteoporosis (evident first in the spine and pelvis) with compression fractures may occur in advanced cases, and skeletal maturation is usually delayed.

## Differential Diagnosis

Children with exogenous obesity, particularly when accompanied by striae and hypertension, are frequently suspected of having Cushing syndrome. The child's height, growth rate, and skeletal maturation are helpful in differentiating the two, because children with Cushing syndrome have a poor growth rate, relatively short stature, and delayed skeletal maturation, whereas those with exogenous obesity usually have a normal or slightly increased growth rate, normal to tall stature, and advanced skeletal maturation. In addition, the color of the striae (purplish in Cushing syndrome, pink in obesity) and the distribution of the obesity assist in the differentiation. The urinary free cortisol excretion (mg/g creatinine) and salivary cortisol are normal in obesity.

## Treatment

In all cases of primary adrenal hyperfunction due to tumor, surgical removal, if possible, is indicated. ACTH should be given preoperatively and postoperatively to stimulate the nontumorous contralateral adrenal cortex, which is generally atrophied. Glucocorticoids should be administered parenterally in pharmacologic doses during and after surgery until the patient is stable. Supplemental oral glucocorticoids, potassium, salt, and mineralocorticoids may be necessary until the suppressed contralateral adrenal gland has recovered, sometimes over a period of several months. (See earlier discussion of corticosteroid administration in surgical patients.)

The use of mitotane, a DDT derivative that is toxic to the adrenal cortex, and aminoglutethimide, an inhibitor of steroid synthesis, has been suggested, but the efficacy of these agents in children with adrenal tumors has not been determined.

Adrenal hyperplasia resulting from a pituitary microadenoma may respond to pituitary surgery or irradiation.

## Prognosis

If the tumor is malignant, the prognosis is poor if it cannot be completely removed. If it is benign, cure is to be expected following proper preparation and surgery.

Morris D, Grossman A: The medical management of Cushing's syndrome. Ann N Y Acad Sci 2002;970:119 [PMID: 12381547].

Raff H, Findling JW: A physiologic approach to diagnosis of the Cushing syndrome. Ann Intern Med 2003;138:980 [PMID: 12809455].

Savage MO et al: Growth in disorders of adrenal hyperfunction. Horm Res 2002;58 (Suppl 1):39 [PMID: 12373013].

Yehuda R et al: Relationship between 24-hour urinary-free cortisol excretion and salivary cortisol levels sampled from awakening to bedtime in healthy subjects. Life Sci 2003;73:349 [PMID: 12757842].

## PRIMARY HYPERALDOSTERONISM

Primary hyperaldosteronism may be caused by a benign adrenal tumor or by adrenal hyperplasia. It is characterized by paresthesias, tetany, weakness, polyuria (nocturnal enuresis is common in young children), periodic paralysis, low serum potassium and elevated serum sodium levels, hypertension, metabolic alkalosis, and production of a large volume of alkaline urine with a low fixed specific gravity; the latter does not respond to vasopressin. Edema is rare. The glucose tolerance test is frequently abnormal. Plasma and urinary aldosterone are elevated, but other steroid levels are variable. Plasma renin activity is suppressed, in contrast to the secondary hyperaldosteronism due to renal vascular disease and Bartter syndrome. In patients with adrenal tumor, the administration of ACTH may further increase the excretion of aldosterone. Marked decrease of aldosterone-induced hypokalemia, alkalosis, hypochloremia, or hypernatremia after the administration of an aldosterone antagonist such as spironolactone may be of diagnostic value.

Treatment is with glucocorticoids or spironolactone, subtotal or total adrenalectomy for hyperplasia, and surgical removal if a tumor is present.

Ghose RP et al: Medical management of aldosterone-producing adenomas. Ann Intern Med 1999;131:105 [PMID: 10419425].

Young WF Jr: Minireview: Primary aldosteronism—Changing concepts in diagnosis and treatment. Endocrinology 2003; 144:2208 [PMID: 12746276].

## USES OF GLUCOCORTICOIDS & ACTH IN TREATMENT OF NONENDOCRINE DISEASES

Glucocorticoids are used for their anti-inflammatory and immunosuppressive properties in a variety of conditions in childhood. Pharmacologic doses are necessary to achieve these effects, and side effects are common. Numerous synthetic preparations possessing variable ratios of glucocorticoid to mineralocorticoid activity are available (Table 30–12).

## Actions

Glucocorticoids exert a direct or permissive effect on virtually every tissue of the body; major known effects include the following:

1. Gluconeogenesis in the liver
2. Stimulation of fat breakdown (lipolysis) and redistribution of body fat
3. Catabolism of protein with an increase in nitrogen and phosphorus excretion
4. Decrease in lymphoid and thymic tissue and a decreased cellular response to inflammation and hypersensitivity
5. Alteration of CNS excitation

***Table 30–12.*** Potency equivalents for adrenocorticosteroids.

| Adrenocorticosteroid | Trade Names | Potency/mg Compared with Cortisol (Glucocorticoid Effect) | Potency/mg Compared with Cortisol (Sodium-Retaining Effect) |
|---|---|---|---|
| **Glucocorticoids** | | | |
| Hydrocortisone (cortisol) | Cortef | 1 | 1 |
| Cortisone | Cortone Acetate | 0.8 | 1 |
| Prednisone | Meticorten, others | 4–5 | 0.4 |
| Methylprednisolone | Medrol, Meprolone | 5–6 | Minimal |
| Triamcinolone | Aristocort, Kenalog Kenacort, Atolone | 5–6 | Minimal |
| Dexamethasone | Decadron, others | 25–40 | Minimal |
| Betamethasone | Celestone | 25 | Minimal |
| **Mineralocorticoid** | | | |
| Fludrocortisone | Florinef | 15–20 | 300–400 |

6. Retardation of connective tissue mitosis and migration, decreased wound healing

7. Improved capillary tone and increased vascular compartment volume and pressure

## Uses

Glucocorticoids are used in physiologic doses to treat adrenal insufficiency (eg, Addison disease and congenital adrenal hyperplasia) and in pharmacologic doses to treat a wide variety of inflammatory and autoimmune malignant conditions in childhood. Corticosteroid use is contraindicated in active, questionably healed, or suspected tuberculosis. Corticosteroids should be used with extreme caution in the presence of herpes simplex infection of the eye, osteoporosis, peptic ulcer, active systemic infections, emotional instability, and thrombophlebitis.

## Side Effects of Therapy

When prolonged use of pharmacologic doses of glucocorticoids is necessary, clinical manifestations of Cushing syndrome are common. Side effects may occur with the use of synthetic exogenous agents by any route, including inhalation and topical administration (inflamed skin), or with the use of ACTH, which stimulates excessive production of endogenous corticosteroids. Use of a larger dose of glucocorticoids given once every 48 hours (alternate-day therapy) lessens the incidence and severity of some of the side effects (Table 30–13).

## Tapering of Pharmacologic Doses of Steroids

Prolonged use of pharmacologic doses of glucocorticoids results in suppression of ACTH secretion and consequent adrenal atrophy. Thus the abrupt discontinuation of glucocorticoids may result in adrenal insufficiency. Furthermore, ACTH secretion generally does not occur until the administered steroid has been given in subphysiologic doses (< 8 mg/m$^2$/d orally) for several weeks.

If pharmacologic glucocorticoid therapy has been given for less than 10–14 days, the drug can be discontinued abruptly (if the condition for which it was prescribed allows) because adrenal suppression will be short-lived. However, it is advisable to educate the patient and family about the signs and symptoms of adrenal insufficiency in case problems arise.

If tapering is necessary in treating the condition for which the glucocorticoid is prescribed, a reduction of 25–50% every 2–7 days is sufficiently rapid to permit observation of clinical symptomatology. Moreover, the use of an alternate-day schedule (ie, a single dose given every 48 hours) will allow for a 50% decrease in the total 2 days' dosage while providing the desired pharmacologic effect. If tapering is not necessary for the underlying disease, the dosage can be decreased safely to the physiologic range. However, although a rapid decrease in dose to the physiologic range will not lead to frank adrenal insufficiency (because adequate exogenous cortisol is being provided), some patients may experience a steroid withdrawal syndrome, characterized by malaise, fatigue, and loss of appetite. These symp-

***Table 30–13.*** Side effects of glucocorticoid use.

**A. Endocrine and metabolic effects**
  1. Hyperglycemia and glycosuria (chemical diabetes).
  2. Cushing syndrome.
  3. Persistent suppression of pituitary-adrenal responsiveness to stress with resultant hypoadrenocorticism.

**B. Effects on electrolytes and minerals**
  1. Marked retention of sodium and water, producing edema, increased blood volume, and hypertension (more common in endogenous hyperadrenal states).
  2. Potassium loss with symptoms of hypokalemia.
  3. Hypocalcemia, tetany.

**C. Effects on protein metabolism and skeletal maturation**
  1. Negative nitrogen balance, with loss of body protein and bone protein, resulting in osteoporosis, pathologic fractures, and aseptic bone necrosis.
  2. Suppression of growth, retarded skeletal maturation.
  3. Muscular weakness and wasting.
  4. Osteoporosis.

**D. Effects on the gastrointestinal tract**
  1. Excessive appetite and intake of food.
  2. Activation or production of peptic ulcer.
  3. Gastrointestinal bleeding from ulceration or from unknown cause (particularly in children with hepatic disease).
  4. Fatty liver with embolism, pancreatitis, nodular panniculitis.

**E. Lowering of resistance to infectious agents; silent infection; decreased inflammatory reaction**
  1. Susceptibility to fungal infections; intestinal parasitic infections.
  2. Activation of tuberculosis; false-negative tuberculin reaction.
  3. Stimulation of activity of herpes simplex virus.

**F. Neuropsychiatric effects**
  1. Euphoria, excitability, psychotic behavior, and status epilepticus with electroencephalographic changes.
  2. Increased intracranial pressure with pseudotumor cerebri syndrome.

**G. Hematologic and vascular effects**
  1. Bleeding into the skin as a result of increased capillary fragility.
  2. Thrombosis, thrombophlebitis, cerebral hemorrhage.

**H. Miscellaneous effects**
  1. Myocarditis, pleuritis, and arteritis following abrupt cessation of therapy.
  2. Cardiomegaly.
  3. Nephrosclerosis, proteinuria.
  4. Acne (in older children), hirsutism, amenorrhea, irregular menses.
  5. Posterior subcapsular cataracts; glaucoma.

toms may necessitate a two- or three-step decrease in dose to the physiologic range.

Once a physiologic equivalent dose (8–10 mg/m$^2$/d hydrocortisone or equivalent) is achieved and the patient's underlying disease is stable, the dose can be decreased to 4–5 mg/m$^2$/d given only in the morning. This will allow the adrenal axis to recover. After this dose has been given for 4–6 weeks, assessment of endogenous adrenal activity can be estimated by obtaining fasting plasma cortisol concentrations between 7 and 8 AM prior to the morning steroid dose or by a low-dose ACTH stimulation test (1 μg corsyntropin with cortisol measured 30 minutes after). When an alternate-day schedule is followed, plasma cortisol is measured the morning prior to treatment. A plasma cortisol concentration within the physiologic range (> 10 mg/dL) demonstrates return of basal physiologic adrenal rhythm. Exogenous steroids may then be discontinued safely, although it is advisable to continue to give the patient stress doses of glucocorticoids when appropriate until recovery of the response to stress has been documented.

After basal physiologic adrenal function returns, the adrenal reserve or capacity to respond to stress and infection can be estimated by the low-dose ACTH stimulation test, in which 1 μg of synthetic ACTH (cosyntropin) is administered intravenously. Plasma cortisol is measured prior to (zero time) and at 45–60 minutes after the infusion. A plasma cortisol concentration of greater than 18 mg/dL at 60 minutes indicates a satisfactory adrenal reserve.

Even if the results of testing are normal, patients who have received prolonged treatment with glucocorticoids may exhibit signs and symptoms of adrenal insufficiency during acute stress, infection, or surgery for months to years after treatment has been stopped. Careful monitoring and, when necessary, the use of stress doses of glucocorticoids should be considered during severe illnesses and surgery.

National Asthma Education and Prevention Program: Long-term management of asthma in children: Safety of inhaled corticosteroids. J Allergy Clin Immunol 2002;110(5 Suppl):S160 [PMID: 12542074].

Steelman J, Kappy M: Adrenal suppression and growth retardation from ocular corticosteroids. J Pediatr Ophthalmol Strabismus 2001;38:177 [PMID: 11386652].

Thaler LM, Blevins LS Jr: The low dose (1-microg) adrenocorticotropin stimulation test in the evaluation of patients with suspected central adrenal insufficiency. J Clin Endocrinol Metab 1998;83:2726 [PMID: 9709938].

## ADRENAL MEDULLA
## PHEOCHROMOCYTOMA

Pheochromocytoma is an uncommon tumor in childhood. Only 10% of the reported cases occur in pediatric patients. The tumor may be located wherever chromaffin tissue (eg, adrenal medulla, sympathetic ganglia, carotid body) is present. It may be multiple, familial (autosomal dominant, in which case a high prevalence of MEN exists), recurrent, and sometimes malignant.

Although the symptoms of pheochromocytoma may result from physical expansion of lesions into surrounding tissue (eg, spinal cord), they are generally caused by excessive secretion of epinephrine or norepinephrine. Attacks of anxiety, unexplained perspiration, and headaches should arouse suspicion. Other findings are palpitation and tachycardia, dizziness, weakness, nausea and vomiting, diarrhea, dilated pupils with blurring of vision, abdominal and precordial pain, hypertension (usually persistent), heat intolerance, and vasomotor instability (flushing, postural hypotension). The symptoms may be sustained, producing all of the previously mentioned findings plus papilledema, retinopathy, and enlargement of the heart. There is an increased incidence of pheochromocytomas in patients and families with neurofibromatosis and MEN type 2 (described earlier). Neuroblastomas, ganglioneuromas, and other neural tumors may secrete pressor amines and may occasionally simulate the symptoms and signs of pheochromocytoma. Carcinoid tumors may produce cardiovascular changes similar to those associated with pheochromocytoma.

Laboratory diagnosis is possible in over 90% of cases. Serum catecholamines are elevated, particularly while the patient is symptomatic, and urinary excretion of catecholamines parallels this elevation. Catecholamine levels are characteristically high enough to be diagnostic but may be limited to the period of a paroxysm. The 24-hour urine excretion of metanephrines and vanillylmandelic acid is increased. Testing of plasma free metanephrine levels is the gold standard for diagnosis. Provocative tests using histamine, tyramine, or glucagon and the phentolamine tests may be abnormal but are dangerous and are rarely necessary for diagnosis. Displacement of the kidney may be shown by intravenous urography, and the tumor may be identified by CT scans or MRI. Angiocatheterization with localized measurement of circulating concentrations of catecholamines may be helpful in localizing the tumor prior to surgery.

Surgical removal of the tumor is the treatment of choice; however, the procedure must be undertaken with great caution and with the patient properly stabilized because manipulation of the tumor may cause sudden, profound, potentially fatal changes in blood pressure. Oral phenoxybenzamine or intravenous phentolamine is used preoperatively. Profound hypotension may occur as the tumor is removed but may be controlled with an infusion of norepinephrine, which may have to be continued for 1–2 days.

Unless irreversible secondary vascular changes have occurred, complete relief of symptoms is to be expected after recovery from removal of a benign tumor. Without treatment, severe cardiac, renal, and cerebral damage may result.

Kinney MA et al: Perioperative management of pheochromocytoma. J Cardiothorac Vasc Anesth 2002;16:359 [PMID: 12073213].

Lenders JW et al: Biochemical diagnosis of pheochromocytoma: Which test is best? JAMA 2002;287:1427 [PMID: 11903030].

Newman KD, Ponsky T: The diagnosis and management of endocrine tumors causing hypertension in children. Ann N Y Acad Sci 2002;970:155 [PMID: 12381550].

Thakker RV: Multiple endocrine neoplasia type 1. Endocrinol Metab Clin North Am 2000;29:541 [PMID: 11033760].

# Diabetes Mellitus

## H. Peter Chase, MD, & George S. Eisenbarth, MD, PhD

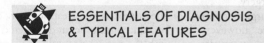

### ESSENTIALS OF DIAGNOSIS & TYPICAL FEATURES

- Polyuria, polydipsia, and weight loss.
- Hyperglycemia and glucosuria with or without ketonuria.

## General Considerations

**Type 1 diabetes** or immune-mediated diabetes (previously called juvenile diabetes or insulin-dependent diabetes mellitus [IDDM]) is the most common type of diabetes in people younger than age 40 years. It is associated with islet cell antibodies (immunologic markers), diminished insulin production, and being ketosis-prone.

**Type 2 diabetes** (non–insulin-dependent diabetes mellitus [NIDDM], non–immune-mediated) is the most common type in persons older than age 40 years; it is associated with being overweight, insensitivity to insulin, and not being prone to ketosis. Type 2 diabetes is increasing in frequency in children and is found in up to half of black and Hispanic children and in over two thirds of American Indian children who develop diabetes. It occurs most frequently in overweight teenagers.

**Maturity-onset diabetes of youth (MODY)** is much less common and comprises several forms of diabetes in children with identified genetic mutations (eg, mutations of glucokinase and hepatic nuclear factor 1 and 2 genes).

## Etiology

### A. TYPE 1 DIABETES

Type 1 diabetes results from immunologic damage to the insulin-producing β-cells of the pancreatic islets. This damage occurs gradually—over months or years in most people—and symptoms do not appear until about 90% of the pancreatic islets have been destroyed. The immunologic damage requires a genetic predisposition and is probably influenced by environmental factors.

The importance of genetics is shown by the fact that 35–50% of second identical twins develop diabetes after the first twin develops the disease. About 6% of siblings or offspring of persons with type 1 diabetes also develop diabetes (compared with a prevalence in the general population of 0.2–0.3%). The condition is more common in white children but occurs in all racial groups. There is an association with HLA-DR3 and HLA-DR4, and about 95% of white diabetic children have at least one of these HLA types. Forty percent have both HLA-DR3 and HLA-DR4 (one from each parent), compared with only 3% of the general population.

The importance of environmental factors is suggested because not all second identical twins develop diabetes. If the condition were purely genetic and had no random factors, the second twin would always develop the disease. Important environmental factors may be viral infections or factors in the diet. For example, 40% of infants with congenital rubella develop diabetes or an abnormal glucose tolerance test by age 20 years, and the incidence of diabetes is high in individuals after eating foods accidentally preserved with excessive nitrates. The early introduction of cow's milk has also been suggested as an environmental factor, but recent prospective studies have failed to confirm this association.

The immunologic basis of diabetes is demonstrated by the ability of cyclosporine, a potent immunosuppressive agent, to preserve islet tissue for 1–2 years when given to newly diagnosed patients. However, renal damage from cyclosporine precludes its use. White blood cells are found in the islets of newly diagnosed patients and may release toxic products (free radicals, interleukin-1, tumor necrosis factor) that injure the islets. Antibodies to islet cells (ICA), insulin, "64 K" or glutamic acid decarboxylase (GAD), ICA512 (IA-2), and other antibodies are present for months to years prior to diagnosis in the serum of over 90% of patients who will develop type 1 diabetes. These antibodies are probably the effect and not the cause of islet β-cell destruction.

### B. TYPE 2 DIABETES

Type 2 diabetes has a strong genetic component, although the defects inherited in different families vary. Obesity (particularly central) and lack of exercise are often major environmental contributing factors. Insulin insensitivity results from all of the above-mentioned circumstances. The prevalence is increased among females, which may be related to the association with polycystic ovary syndrome (PCOS). Acanthosis nigricans, a thickening and darkening of the skin over the posterior neck, armpits or elbows, may aid in the diagnosis of type 2 diabetes.

## Prevention

### A. TYPE 1 DIABETES

Many centers now screen for prediabetes using the previously mentioned antibody tests. Intervention trials on antibody-positive first-degree relatives have begun in an effort to try to prevent type 1 diabetes. European investigators conducted a double-blind study of nicotinamide, which did not show an effect. United States centers conducted randomized trials of both oral and injected insulin. Unfortunately, neither had an effect in preventing or delaying the onset of type 1 diabetes.

### B. TYPE 2 DIABETES

The prevention of type 2 diabetes was evaluated in a large study, the Diabetes Prevention Program (DPP). The study found that 30 minutes of exercise per day (5 days/week) and a low-fat diet reduced the risk for diabetes by 58%. Taking metformin (Glucophage) also reduced the risk for getting type 2 diabetes by 31%.

## Diagnosis

The classic symptoms of polyuria, polydipsia, and weight loss are now so well recognized that friends or family members often suspect the diagnosis of type 1 diabetes in affected individuals. Other cases may be detected by finding glucosuria on routine office urinalysis. Up to 50% of new cases of diabetes used to be diagnosed in patients presenting in coma, but most are now diagnosed before the individuals develop severe ketonuria, ketonemia, and secondary acidosis. Children often have a preceding minor illness, such as a flu-like episode. The check of a blood or urine glucose can be done in a few seconds and could be life-saving. No disease other than diabetes (mellitus or insipidus) presents with continued frequent urination in spite of a dry tongue. An oral glucose tolerance test is rarely necessary in children. A random blood glucose level above 300 mg/dL (16.6 mmol/L) or a fasting blood glucose above 200 mg/dL (11 mmol/L) is sufficient to make the diagnosis of diabetes. The 1997 revised guidelines for the diagnosis of diabetes (see references) are a fasting plasma glucose level over 126 mg/dL (7 mmol/L) or a plasma glucose level above 200 mg/dL (11.1 mmol/L) taken randomly (with symptoms of diabetes) or 2 hours

after an oral glucose load (1.75 g glucose/kg up to a maximum of 75 g). Confirmation of such abnormalities on more than one occasion is recommended as transient hyperglycemia can occur, particularly with illness. Impaired (not yet diabetic) fasting glucose values are 110–125 mg/dL (6.1–6.9 mmol/L) and impaired 2-hour values are 140–200 mg/dL (7.8–11.1 mmol/L). If the presentation is mild, hospitalization is usually not necessary.

Education about diabetes for all family members is essential for the home management of diabetes. The use of an educational book (see References *Understanding Diabetes*) can be very helpful to the family. All caregivers need to learn about diabetes, how to give insulin injections, perform home blood glucose monitoring, and handle acute complications. The stress imposed on the family around the time of initial diagnosis may lead to feelings of shock, denial, sadness, anger, fear, and guilt. Meeting with a counselor to express these feelings at the time of diagnosis helps with long-term adaptation.

## Treatment

Most children have type 1 diabetes. The five major variables in treatment are (1) insulin type and dosage, (2) diet, (3) exercise, (4) stress management, and (5) blood glucose and ketone monitoring. All must be considered to obtain safe and effective metabolic control. Although teenagers can be taught to perform many of the tasks of diabetes management, they do better when supportive—not overbearing—parents continue to be involved in management of their disease. Children younger than age 10 or 11 years cannot reliably administer insulin without adult supervision because they lack fine motor control and may not understand the importance of accurate dosage.

### A. INSULIN

Insulin functions (1) to allow glucose to pass into the cell, (2) to decrease the physiologic production of glucose, particularly in the liver, and (3) to turn off ketone production.

**1. Treatment of new-onset diabetes**—The greater the acidemia and ketone production, the greater the amount of insulin needed. If ketonemia is significant, the venous blood pH low (< 7.30), and the patient dehydrated, intravenous insulin and fluid therapy should be given (see Ketonuria, Ketonemia, and Ketoacidosis section). If the child is adequately hydrated and has a normal venous blood pH, one or two intramuscular or subcutaneous injections of 0.1–0.2 unit/kg of regular insulin—or preferably of insulin lispro (Humalog, [H]), or insulin aspart (NovoLog, [NL]) 1 hour apart will help shut down ketone production. If ketone production is insignificant or absent, this regimen is not necessary, and routine subcutaneous injections can be started.

When ketones are not present, the child is usually more sensitive to insulin, and a total daily dosage of 0.25–0.5 unit/kg/24 h (by subcutaneous injection) can be used. If ketones are or were present, the child usually does not produce as much insulin and will require 0.5–1 unit/kg of total insulin per 24 hours.

Children usually receive mixtures of a short-acting insulin (to cover food intake or high blood sugars) and a longer-acting insulin (to suppress endogenous hepatic glucose production). This is achieved by combining insulins of different formulations with the desired properties (Table 31–1). The dosages are adjusted with each injection during the first week. Most physicians begin newly diagnosed children with two injections per day of an intermediate-acting insulin (eg, NPH) and a short-acting insulin such as Humalog or NovoLog (H or NL). About two-thirds of the total dosage is usually given before breakfast and the remainder before dinner. If human regular insulin is used, the injections are given 30–60 minutes before meals; when using H or NL as the short-acting insulin, the injections are given just before eating. In young children who eat irregular amounts of food, it is often helpful to wait until after the meal to give the injection and decide on the appropriate dose of H or NL. Children younger than age 4 years usually need 1 or 2 units of short-acting insulin to cover meals, and the remainder of the dosage is NPH insulin. Children age 4–10 years may require up to 4 units of short-acting insulin to cover breakfast and dinner, whereas proportionately higher doses (usually 4–10 units) of H or NL or regular insulin are used for older children.

The onset of activity for H or NL is 10–15 minutes rather than the 30–60 minutes associated with regular insulin (see Table 31–1). It is not necessary to wait 30–60 minutes to eat after injection of H or NL. These insulins also peak sooner than regular insulin, and activity is gone within 4 hours. The shorter duration reduces the risk of later hypoglycemia.

A new 24-hour basal insulin, insulin glargine (Lantus), is now available, and many physicians initiate therapy with this insulin. It has an acidic pH and must be given alone in the syringe. It is given once daily in the morning, at dinner, or at bedtime depending on patient and family wishes. The Lantus dose is adjusted up or down depending on the morning fasting glucose levels. The most physiologic insulin regimen is then to add H/NL prior to each meal/snack. Children who are unable to consistently get H or NL at lunch can receive H/NL with NPH at breakfast. The main advantage of Lantus over two injections of NPH daily is that severe hypoglycemic episodes (particularly at night) are greatly reduced with its use.

**2. Continuing insulin dosage**—The total daily insulin dosage may need to be increased gradually to 1 unit/kg (especially if ketones are present at onset). When gluconeogenesis and glycolysis are suppressed by insulin, a honeymoon or grace period is a common phenomenon. This often occurs 1–4 weeks after diagnosis in over 50% of children and tends to last longer in older children.

In helping families with day-to-day dosing of regular insulin or H or NL , some physicians initially use sliding scales, more recently referred to as "thinking" scales, to emphasize that the family must always be thinking about food recently eaten, or to be eaten, and recent or forthcoming exercise in addition to the blood glucose level. Examples of thinking scales are given in *Understanding Diabetes* (see references).

After the appropriate dosage of intermediate (eg, NPH) or long-acting (Lantus) insulin is achieved, daily adjustments usually are not needed. However, small decreases may be made for heavy activity (eg, afternoon sports or overnight events). Many families gradually learn to make small (0.5–1 unit) weekly adjustments in insulin dosage based on home blood glucose testing. Understanding the onset, peak, and duration of insulin activity is essential (see Table 31–1).

Most children receive two to four injections of insulin daily. The most common combinations are mix-

***Table 31–1.*** Kinetics of insulin action.

| Type of Insulin | Begins Working | Main Effect | All Gone |
|---|---|---|---|
| **Short-acting** | | | |
| Regular | ½ h | 2–4 h | 6–9 h |
| Humalog or Novolog | 10–15 min | 30–80 min | 4 h |
| **Intermediate-acting** | | | |
| NPH | 2–4 h | 6–8 h | 12–15 h |
| Ultralente | 4–6 h | 8–15 h | 15–18 h |
| **Long-acting** | | | |
| Lantus | 1–2 h | 2–23 h | 24–26 h |
| **Premixed** | | | |
| Lente[a] | 1–2 h | 6–12 h | 15–18 h |
| NPH/ Regular | ½ h | Variable[b] | 12–15 h |
| 75/25[c] | 15 min | 1–8 h | 12–15 h |

[a]30% Semilente and 70% Ultralente.
[b]Available in various combinations to fit individual needs.
[c]A mixture of 75% NPH and 25% Humalog.
NPH = neutral protamine Hagedorn insulin.

tures of either H or NL or regular insulin and NPH insulin twice daily (see Table 31–1) or H or NL (or regular) insulin and NPH insulin in the morning and H/NL at dinner and NPH insulin at bedtime.

As noted earlier, when the more physiologic (closer to human insulin output) basal insulin, Lantus, is used, it must be given alone in the syringe or pen. When changing a patient from two shots/day of NPH insulin to Lantus, the total 24-hour dose of NPH is divided in half to use as the initial dose of Lantus. The Lantus dose is then increased or decreased 1 or 2 units every few days based on the fasting morning blood sugars. Common glucose level goals are 70–180 mg/dL (3.9–10 mmol/L) for preteens and 70–150 mg/dL (3.9–8.3 mmol/L) for teens. A short-acting insulin (H or NL) is then given prior to meals/snacks or a mixture of H or NL and NPH is given in the morning and H or NL at dinner. The dosages of H or NL may initially be based on a "thinking" scale (see previous discussion), and may later be based on carbohydrate-counting as the family becomes more knowledgeable (see Diet section).

Continuous subcutaneous insulin (insulin pump) therapy is now being used more often in children, particularly for emotionally mature teens who are willing to do frequent blood glucose monitoring and to count carbohydrates. Basal insulin doses (usually H/NL) to use are chosen by the physician, with bolus doses prior to meals selected by the patient (or an appropriate adult) depending on the carbohydrate content of the food to be eaten. Insulin pump therapy is discussed in depth in Chapter 26 of *Understanding Diabetes*.

The following constitutes intensive diabetes management: (1) three or more insulin injections per day, or insulin pump therapy; (2) four or more blood glucose determinations per day; (3) careful attention to dietary intake; and (4) frequent contact with the health care provider. This was shown in the Diabetes Control and Complications Trial (DCCT; see Diet section) to result in improved glucose control and to reduce the risk for retinal, renal, and neurologic complications of diabetes. All teenagers with suboptimal glucose control who are willing to comply should be considered for intensive diabetes management.

**3. Treatment of type 2 diabetes**—The treatment of type 2 diabetes in children varies with the severity of the disease. If the glyosylated hemoglobin ($HbA_{1c}$) is still normal (or near normal) and ketone levels are not moderately or significantly increased, modification of lifestyle (preferably for the entire family) is the first line of therapy. This must include reducing caloric intake and increasing exercise. If the $HbA_{1c}$ is mildly elevated (6.2–9.0%) and ketone levels are not moderately or significantly increased, an oral hypoglycemia agent can be tried. Metformin is usually tried along with modifica-

tion of lifestyle, starting with a dose of 250–500 mg once daily. If needed, and if gastrointestinal adaptation has occurred, the dose can be gradually increased to 1 g bid. If the presentation is more severe, with moderately or significantly increased urine ketone levels, or blood β-hydroxybutyrate (βOHB) > 1.0 mmol/L, the initial treatment is similar to that of type 1 diabetes (including intravenous or subcutaneous insulin). Oral hypoglycemic agents may be tried at a later date, particularly if weight loss has been successful.

## B. Diet

The mainstays of dietary treatment are discussed in detail in *Understanding Diabetes* (see References). The American Diabetes Association (ADA) no longer recommends any one diabetic diet or ADA diet. Instead, nutrition therapy for diabetics should be individualized, with consideration given to the patient's customary cultural eating habits and other lifestyle circumstances. Some families and children (particularly those with weight problems) find exchange diets helpful initially while they are learning food categories. Most centers now just use exchanges of carbohydrates, referred to below as carbohydrate-counting or "carb-counting."

The DCCT found that four nutrition factors contributed to better sugar control (lower $HbA_{1c}$ levels). These factors are (1) adherence to a meal plan, (2) avoidance of extra snacks, (3) avoidance of overtreatment of low blood sugars (hypoglycemia), and (4) prompt treatment of high blood sugars. Two other nutritional factors include adjusting insulin levels for meals and maintaining a consistent schedule of nighttime snacks. The DCCT popularized the carb-counting dietary plan in which the dosage of H/NL or regular insulin is altered with each injection to adjust for the amount of carbohydrate to be eaten and the amount of exercise contemplated. One carbohydrate choice is 15 g of glucose in the United States (10 g in Canada and the United Kingdom). A common formula is to use 1 unit of H/NL for each 15 g of carbohydrate eaten, although this ratio must be adjusted (using blood glucose levels 2 hours after meals) for each person.

## C. Exercise

Regular aerobic exercise—at least 30 minutes a day—is important for children with diabetes. Exercise fosters a sense of well-being; helps increase insulin sensitivity; and helps maintain proper weight, blood pressure, and blood fat levels. Exercise may also help maintain normal peripheral circulation in later years. It is particularly important for children with type 2 diabetes.

Hypoglycemia during exercise or in the 2–8 hours after exercise (delayed hypoglycemia) can be prevented by careful monitoring of blood sugar before, during, and after exercise; sometimes by reducing the dosage of the insulin active at the time of the exercise; and by providing extra snacks. Children using insulin pumps should reduce pre-exercise bolus insulin dosages as well as the basal dosages during the exercise. In general, the longer and more vigorous the activity, the greater the reduction in insulin dose before exercising. Extra snacks should also be eaten. Fifteen grams of glucose usually covers about 30 minutes of exercise. The use of drinks containing 5–10% dextrose, such as Gatorade, during the period of exercise is often beneficial.

### D. STRESS MANAGEMENT

Management of stress is important on a short-term basis because stress hormones increase blood glucose levels. Chronic emotional upsets may lead to missed injections or other compliance problems. When this happens, counseling for the family and child becomes an important part of diabetes management.

### E. BLOOD GLUCOSE MEASUREMENTS

All families must be able to monitor blood glucose levels three or four times daily—and more frequently in small infants or patients who have glucose control problems or intercurrent illnesses. Blood glucose levels can be monitored using any of the available meters, which generally have an accuracy of 90% or better. Target levels when no food has been eaten for 2 or more hours vary according to age (Table 31–2).

Blood glucose results should be recorded even if the meter has a memory feature. This allows the family to look for patterns and make changes in insulin dosage. If more than 50% of the values are above the desired range for age or more than 12% below the desired range, the insulin dosage usually needs to be adjusted. Some families are able to make these changes independently (particularly after the first year), whereas others need help from the health care provider. Children with diabetes should have clinic visits every 3 months. This provides an opportunity to adjust insulin dosages according to changes in growth and blood glucose levels

as well as to check for changes noted on physical examination (eg,, eyes, thyroid). Continuous subcutaneous glucose monitoring using the Continuous Glucose Monitoring System (CGMS) by MiniMed or the GlucoWatch by Cygnus may also be helpful in monitoring glucose trends.

## Laboratory Evaluations

In addition to home measurements of blood glucose and blood or urine ketone levels, $HbA_{1c}$ should be measured every 3 months. This test reflects the frequency of elevated blood glucose levels over the previous 3 months. Normal values vary among laboratories but are usually below 6.2% ($HbA_{1c}$) or below 8% (total glycosylated hemoglobin). The desired ranges are based on age. For the $HbA_{1c}$ method, these ranges are as follows: 12 years or older, less than 7.8%; 5–11 years, less than 8.0%; and younger than 5 years, 7.5–9%. Higher levels are allowed in younger children to reduce the risk of hypoglycemia because their brains are still developing and they may not relate symptoms of hypoglycemia to a need for treatment. Low $HbA_{1c}$ values are generally associated with a greater risk for hypoglycemia (see following section). Using either method, researchers found that longitudinal averages more than 33% above the upper limit of normal are associated with a higher risk for later renal and retinal complications. In the intensive treatment group of the DCCT, the lower $HbA_{1c}$ values resulted in a greater than 50% reductions in the retinal, renal, and neurologic complications of diabetes in pubertal patients.

Since atherosclerosis is the major cause of death in older patients with diabetes it is important to measure serum cholesterol, LDL, and HDL levels once yearly. Cholesterol levels should be below 200 mg/dL and LDL levels below 100 mg/dL in post-pubertal people with diabetes.

When puberty is reached and the individual has had diabetes for 3 years or longer, the urinary excretion of albumin should be measured (as microalbumin) in two separate urine samples once yearly (see Chronic Complications section). This can be done using timed overnight urine collections as teens are less likely to collect 24-hour specimens. Normal values differ with the methodology of the laboratory but are generally below 20 μg/min. People with type 2 diabetes should have this test done soon after diagnosis and then annually.

If the thyroid is enlarged (about 20% of patients with type 1 diabetes), the thyroid-stimulating hormone (TSH) level should be measured yearly. This is usually the first test to become abnormal in the autoimmune thyroiditis commonly associated with type 1 diabetes.

In recent years antiendomysial and transglutaminase antibodies, reliable predictors of celiac disease, have

***Table 31–2.*** Ideal glucose levels after 2 or more hours of fasting.[a]

| Age (years) | Glucose Level |
|---|---|
| ≤ 4 | 80–200 mg/dL (4.6–11 mmol/L) |
| 5–11 | 70–180 mg/dL (3.9–10 mmol/L) |
| ≥ 12 | 70–150 mg/dL (3.9–8.3 mmol/L) |

[a]At least half of the values must be below the upper limit to have a good $HbA_{1c}$ value. The values should also be below the upper limits for age when tested 2 h after a meal.

been shown to be more common in children with diabetes as well as in their siblings. Risk of celiac disease is associated with HLA-DR3 and is more frequent in children with diabetes (celiac disease occurring in about 5%). The celiac antibodies should be checked in diabetic children with poor growth (especially when not related to poor glucose control) or those who present with gastrointestinal symptoms. The 21-hydroxylase autoantibody, a marker of increased risk of Addison disease, is present in approximately 1.3% of patients with type 1 diabetes, although Addison disease is found in only 1 in 200.

Type 2 diabetes is not an autoimmune disease, and the islet antibody tests are negative. An elevated insulin or C-peptide level is also helpful, indicating that insulin production is normal or elevated.

A checklist of the physician's contributions to good diabetes care is presented in Table 31–3.

## Acute Complications

### A. HYPOGLYCEMIA

Hypoglycemia (or insulin reaction) is defined as a blood glucose level below 60 mg/dL (or 3.3 mmol/L). For preschool children, values below 70 mg/dL (3.9 mmol/L) should be cause for concern. The common symptoms of hypoglycemia are hunger, weakness,

***Table 31–3.*** Physician's checklist of good diabetes management.

| Variable | Frequency of Measurement | Tests and Values |
|---|---|---|
| Blood sugars | 3–4 times daily | See age-appropriate values. |
| Hemoglobin A$_{1c}$ | Every 3 mos | See age-appropriate values. |
| Urine micro-albumin | Annually after 3 y of diabetes (pubertal patients) | < 20 µg/min |
| Ophthalmology referral | Annually after 3 y of diabetes (10 y old or greater) | Retinal photographs |
| Signs of other endocrinopathy | Evaluate at least annually (eg, thyroid enlargement) | (eg: TSH: 0.5–5.0 IU/mL) |
| Blood lipid panel | Annually | eg: Cholesterol = <200 mg/dL; LDL = <100 |

TSH = thyroid-stimulating hormone.

shakiness, sweating, drowsiness (at an unusual time), headache, and behavioral changes. Children learn to recognize hypoglycemia at different ages but can often report "feeling funny" as young as age 4–5 years. If low blood sugar is not treated immediately with simple sugar, the hypoglycemia may result in loss of consciousness or convulsions. If hypoglycemia is left untreated for several hours, brain damage or death can occur.

Consistency in daily routine, correct insulin dosage, regular blood glucose monitoring, controlled snacking, compliance of patients and parents, and good education are all important in preventing severe hypoglycemia. In addition, insulin should not be injected prior to getting into a hot tub, bath, or shower. The heat will increase circulation to the skin and cause more rapid insulin uptake. The use of H/NL insulin and of Lantus insulin has also helped to reduce the occurrence of hypoglycemia.

The treatment of mild hypoglycemia involves giving 4 oz of juice, a sugar-containing soda drink, or milk, and waiting 10 minutes. If the blood glucose level is still below 60 mg/dL (3.3 mmol/L), the liquids are repeated. If the glucose level is above 60 mg/dL, solid foods are given. Moderate hypoglycemia, in which the person is conscious but incoherent, is treated by squeezing one-half tube of concentrated glucose (eg,, Insta-Glucose or cake frosting) between the gums and lips and stroking the throat to encourage swallowing.

In the DCCT study, 10% of patients with standard management and 25% of those with intensive insulin management—insulin pumps or three or more insulin shots per day—had one or more severe hypoglycemic reactions each year. Families are advised to have glucagon in the home and to treat hypoglycemia by giving subcutaneous or intramuscular injections of 0.3 mL (30 units in an insulin syringe) for children younger than age 5 years and 0.5 mL (50 units) to those older than age 5 years. Some patients (usually those who have had diabetes for more than 10 years) fail to recognize the symptoms of low blood sugar (hypoglycemic unawareness). For these individuals, glucose control must be liberalized to prevent severe hypoglycemic reactions. School personnel, sports coaches, and baby-sitters must be trained to recognize and treat hypoglycemia.

### B. KETONURIA, KETONEMIA, AND KETOACIDOSIS

Families must be educated to check blood or urine ketone levels during any illness (including vomiting even once) or any time a fasting blood glucose level is above 240 mg/dL (13.3 mmol/L), or a randomly measured glucose level is above 300 mg/dL (16.6 mmol/L). If moderate or significant ketonuria is detected, or the blood ketone (βOHB—using the Precision Xtra meter) is above 1.0 mmol/L, the health care provider must be called. Usually 10–20% of the total daily insulin dosage is given subcutaneously as H or NL (or regular) insulin every 2–3 hours until the elevated ketones are gone. This prevents ketonuria/ketonemia from progressing to ketoacidosis and allows most patients to receive treatment at home by telephone management. Juices and other fluids to help wash out the ketones and to prevent dehydration are encouraged, and suppositories of promethazine to prevent vomiting may be indicated. If deep breathing (Kussmaul respirations) or excessive weakness occurs, the patient should be evaluated promptly by a physician.

Acidosis (venous blood pH < 7.30) is now present in fewer than 25% of newly diagnosed children. Acidosis may also occur in those with known diabetes who do not check blood or urine ketone levels or fail to call the health care provider when ketones levels are elevated. Repeated episodes of ketoacidosis usually result from missed insulin injections and signify that counseling may be indicated, and that a responsible adult must take over the diabetes management. If, for any reason this is not possible, a change in the child's living situation may be necessary.

Treatment of diabetic ketoacidosis (DKA) is based on four physiologic principles: (1) restoration of fluid volume, (2) inhibition of lipolysis and return to glucose utilization, (3) replacement of body salts, and (4) correction of acidosis. Laboratory tests at the start of treatment should include venous blood pH, blood glucose, and an electrolyte panel. Mild DKA is defined as a venous blood pH of 7.2–7.3; moderate DKA, a pH of 7.10–7.19; and severe DKA, a pH below 7.10. Patients with severe DKA should be hospitalized in a pediatric intensive care unit, if available in the area. More severe cases may benefit from determination of osmolality, calcium and phosphorus, and blood urea nitrogen levels. Severe and moderate episodes of DKA generally require hourly determinations of serum glucose, electrolytes, and venous pH levels, whereas these parameters can be measured every 2 hours if the pH level is 7.20–7.30.

**1. Restoration of fluid volume**—Dehydration is judged by (1) acute loss of body weight (if a recent weight is known), (2) dryness of oral mucous membranes, (3) low blood pressure, and (4) tachycardia. Initial treatment is with physiologic saline (0.9%), 10–20 mL/kg during the first hour. If indicated by continued signs of dehydration, this is repeated during the second hour. The total volume of fluid in the first 4 hours of treatment should not exceed 40 mL/kg because of the danger of cerebral edema (see Management of Cerebral Edema section). Human albumin, 10 mL/kg of 5% solution, can be given over 30 minutes if the patient is in shock. After initial reexpansion, half-physiologic (0.45%) saline usually is given at

1.5 times maintenance. Maintenance fluids are as shown in Chapter 42.

**2. Inhibition of lipolysis and return to glucose utilization**—Insulin turns off fat breakdown and ketone formation. Regular insulin is usually given intravenously at a rate of 0.1 unit/kg/h. The insulin solution should be administered by pump and can be made by diluting 30 units of regular insulin in 150 mL of 0.9% saline (1 unit/5 mL). If the glucose level falls below 250 mg/dL (13.9 mmol/L), 5% dextrose is added to the intravenous fluids. If the glucose level continues to decrease below 120 mg/dL (6.6 mmol/L), 10% dextrose can be added. If necessary, the insulin dosage can be reduced to 0.05 unit/kg/h, but it should not be discontinued before the venous blood pH reaches 7.30. The half-life of intravenous insulin when discontinued is 6 minutes, whereas subcutaneous H or NL insulin takes 10–15 minutes, and regular insulin takes 30–60 minutes, to begin activity. Thus it is often better to continue intravenous insulin until subcutaneous insulin can begin acting.

**3. Replacement of body salts**—In patients with DKA, both sodium and potassium pass into the urine with the ketones and are depleted. Serum sodium concentrations may be falsely lowered by hyperglycemia, causing water to be drawn into the intravenous space, and by hyperlipidemia if fat replaces some of the water in the serum used for electrolyte analysis. Sodium is usually replaced adequately by the use of physiologic and half-physiologic saline in the rehydration fluids as discussed earlier.

Serum potassium levels may be elevated initially because of inability of potassium to stay in the cell in the presence of acidosis (even though total body potassium is low). Potassium should not be given until the serum potassium level is known to be low or normal and the pH is above 7.10. It is then usually given at a concentration of 40 mEq/L, with one half of the potassium (20 mEq/L) either as potassium acetate or potassium chloride and the other half as potassium phosphate (20 mEq/L). Hypocalcemia can occur if all of the potassium is given as the phosphate salt; hypophosphatemia occurs if none of the potassium is of the phosphate salt.

**4. Correction of acidosis**—Acidosis is corrected as the fluid volume and aerobic glycolysis are restored and as insulin is administered to inhibit ketogenesis. As noted earlier, measurement of the venous blood pH (identical to arterial blood pH) reveals the severity of acidosis. Bicarbonate is usually not given, even with severe DKA.

**5. Management of cerebral edema**—Some degree of cerebral edema has been shown by computed tomography scan to be common in DKA. Associated clinical symptoms are rare, unpredictable, and often associated with demise. Cerebral edema may be related to overhydration with hypotonic fluids, although the cause is not well understood. It is now recommended that no more than 40 mL/kg of fluids be given in the first 4 hours of treatment. Cerebral edema is more common with a pH lower than 7.1, a $PCO_2$ lower than 20 mm Hg, or when the serum sodium is noted to be falling rather than rising. Early neurologic signs may include headache, excessive drowsiness, and dilated pupils. Prompt initiation of therapy should include elevation of the head of the bed, hyperventilation, mannitol (1 g/kg over 30 minutes), and fluid restriction. If the cerebral edema is not recognized and treated early, over 50% of patients will die or have permanent brain damage.

## Chronic Complications

In the past, about 30–40% of persons with type 1 diabetes eventually developed renal failure or loss of vision. Factors that greatly reduce this likelihood are longitudinal $HbA_{1c}$ levels in a good range, maintenance of blood pressure below the 90th percentile for age, and abstinence from smoking or chewing tobacco. Annual retinal examinations and urine microalbumin measurements are important for children age 10 years or older who have had diabetes for 3 years or longer (see Laboratory Evaluations section). Data now show that the use of angiotensin-converting enzyme inhibitors may reverse or delay kidney damage when it is detected in the microalbuminuria stage (20–300 µg/min). Similarly, laser treatment to coagulate proliferating capillaries prevents bleeding and leakage of blood into the vitreous fluid or behind the retina. This treatment helps to prevent retinal detachment and to preserve useful vision for many people with proliferative diabetic retinopathy.

## REFERENCES

American Diabetes Association: Standards of medical care for patients with diabetes mellitus. Diabetes Care 2003;26(Suppl 1):S33.

American Diabetes Association: Type 2 diabetes in children and adolescents. Diabetes Care 2000;23:381.

Chase HP: *Understanding Diabetes,* 10th ed. SFI, 2002. (Available from Children's Diabetes Foundation, 777 Grant Street, Suite 302, Denver, CO 80203 for $18.00 [phone: 1-800-695-2873 or www.barbaradaviscenter.org]).

Chase HP et al: The impact of the Diabetes Control and Complications Trial and Humalog insulin on glycohemoglobin levels and severe hypoglycemia in type 1 diabetes. Diabetes Care 2001;24:430.

Chase HP et al: Continuous subcutaneous glucose monitoring in children with type 1 diabetes. Pediatrics 2001;107:222.

Chase HP et al: Use of the GlucoWatch Biographer in children with Type 1 diabetes. Pediatrics 2003;111:790.

Diabetes Control and Complications Trial Research Group, The effect of intensive treatment of diabetes on the development and progression of long-term complications in insulin-dependent diabetes mellitus. N Engl J Med 1993;329:977.

Glaser N et al: Risk factors for cerebral edema in children with diabetic ketoacidosis. N Engl J Med 2001;344:264.

Krane EJ et al: Subclinical brain swelling in children during treatment of diabetic ketoacidosis. N Engl J Med 1985;312:1147.

Mahoney CP et al: Risk factors for developing brain herniation during diabetic ketoacidosis. Pediatr Neurol 1999;21:721.

Maniatis AK et al: Continuous subcutaneous insulin infusion therapy for children and adolescents: An option for routine diabetes care. Pediatrics 2001;107:351.

Reduction in the incidence of type 2 diabetes with lifestyle intervention or metformin: Diabetes Prevention Program Research Group. N Engl J Med 2002;346:393.

Roberts MD et al: Diabetic ketoacidosis with intracerebral complications. Pediatric Diabetes 2001;2:109.

Report of the Expert Committee on the Diagnosis and Classification of Diabetes Mellitus. Diabetes Care 1997;20:1183.

Rutledge SK et al: Effectiveness of postprandial Humalog in toddlers with diabetes. Pediatrics 1997;100:968.

# Inborn Errors of Metabolism 32

Carol L. Greene, MD, Janet A. Thomas, MD, & Stephen I. Goodman, MD

Disorders in which defects of single genes cause clinically significant blocks in metabolic pathways are called inborn errors of metabolism. For many years after Garrod first described them in 1908, these conditions were thought rare. Because the number of recognized inborn errors has increased, they are now acknowledged to be important causes of disease in children. Many of these disorders can now be treated effectively. Even when treatment is not available, correct diagnosis permits parents to make informed decisions about future offspring.

The pathology is almost always due either to accumulation of enzyme substrate behind the metabolic block or to deficiency of the reaction product. In some cases, the accumulated enzyme substrate is diffusible and has an adverse effect on distant organs; in other cases, as in lysosomal storage diseases, the substrate primarily accumulates locally.

The clinical manifestations of inborn errors vary widely; both mild and severe forms of virtually every disorder occur, and many patients do not match the classic phenotype. Often this is because the mutations in different patients, even though in the same gene, are not identical.

Strategies used to treat inborn errors include avoiding enzyme substrate in the diet (eg, low-phenylalanine diet for phenylketonuria), removing accumulated substrate by pharmacologic means (eg, glycine therapy for isovaleric acidemia), supplementing an inadequately produced metabolite (eg, arginine administration for urea cycle disorders), providing additional coenzyme (eg, vitamin $B_{12}$ therapy for methylmalonic acidemia), and providing normal enzyme (eg, enzyme infusion in Gaucher disease or liver transplantation for Wilson disease). Gene replacement is a long-term goal, and various gene therapy trials are in progress. However, problems of delivery to target organs and control of gene action make this an unrealistic option at present for treating most of these disorders.

Inborn errors can become manifest at any time, affect virtually any organ system, and cause all but the most common pediatric problems. This chapter focuses first on when these conditions should be considered in the differential diagnosis of common pediatric problems. A few of the more important disorders are then discussed in greater detail.

## DIAGNOSIS

### SUSPECTING INBORN ERRORS

In general, inborn errors must be considered in the differential diagnosis of the critically ill newborn and of the child with seizures, mental retardation or developmental delay, recurrent vomiting, Reye-like syndromes, parenchymal liver disease, unusual odor, unexplained acidosis, hyperammonemia, and hypoglycemia. Inborn errors should be strongly suspected when (1) symptoms accompany changes in diet, (2) the child is developmentally slow or regresses, (3) the child has a history of food preferences or aversions, or (4) the family has a history of parental consanguinity or of problems that could be due to an inborn error, such as retardation or unexplained deaths in siblings, cousins, or other relatives.

Physical findings that should always arouse suspicion of an inborn error include alopecia or abnormal hair, retinal cherry-red spot or retinitis pigmentosa, cataracts or corneal opacity, hepatomegaly or splenomegaly, coarse features, skeletal changes (including gibbus), and ataxia. Features that may be important, in combination with a suspicious history, include failure to thrive, microcephaly, rash, jaundice, hypotonia, and hypertonia.

Finding an immediate cause of symptoms does not rule out an underlying inborn error. For example, renal tubular acidosis and cirrhosis may be due to an underlying inborn error. Some inborn errors predispose to infection, for example, gram-negative septicemia in patients with galactosemia. In other inborn errors, acute crises may be brought on by intercurrent infections. Manifestation of some inborn errors has been mistaken for nonaccidental trauma (eg, glutaric acidemia type I) or poisoning (eg, methylmalonic acidemia); in addition, children with inborn errors of metabolism may be at higher risk for child abuse or neglect because of the much greater irritability that some of these children often demonstrate.

### LABORATORY STUDIES

Table 32–1 lists common clinical and laboratory features of different groups of inborn errors. Table

***Table 32–1.*** Presenting clinical and laboratory features of inborn errors.[a]

| | Defects of Carbohydrate Metabolism | Defects of Amino Acid Metabolism[b] | Organic Acid Disorders[c] | Defects of Fatty Acid Oxidation | Defects of Purine Metabolism | Lysosomal Storage Diseases | Disorders of Peroxisomes |
|---|---|---|---|---|---|---|---|
| **Neurodevelopmental** | | | | | | | |
| Mental/developmental retardation | +++ | +++ | +++ | + | ++ | +++ | +++ |
| Developmental regression | – | – | + | – | | +++ | +++ |
| Acute encephalopathy | +++ | +++ | +++ | +++ | – | – | – |
| Seizures | ++ | +++ | +++ | + | – | +++ | ++ |
| Ataxia/movement disorder | – | + | ++ | | +++ | – | – |
| Hypotonia | ++ | ++ | ++ | +++ | – | + | +++ |
| Hypertonia | – | ++ | +++ | – | ++ | + | |
| Abnormal behavior | – | ++ | ++ | – | ++ | +++ | – |
| **Growth** | | | | | | | |
| Failure to thrive | +++ | +++ | +++ | + | – | + | |
| Short stature | ++ | – | + | – | – | ++ | – |
| Macrocephaly | – | – | + | – | – | +++ | ++ |
| Microcephaly | + | ++ | +++ | – | – | + | – |
| **General** | | | | | | | |
| Vomiting/anorexia | ++ | +++ | +++ | +++ | – | – | ++ |
| Food aversion or craving | ++ | +++ | +++ | | | | |
| Odor | – | ++ | ++ | – | – | – | – |
| Dysmorphic features | – | + | + | – | – | ++ | ++ |
| Congenital malformations | – | ++ | ++ | | – | – | ++ |
| **Organ-specific** | | | | | | | |
| Hepatomegaly | +++ | – | ++ | +++ | – | +++ | +++ |
| Liver disease/cirrhosis | ++ | + | – | + | – | – | + |
| Splenomegaly | – | – | – | – | – | ++ | + |
| Skeletal dysplasia | – | – | – | | | ++ | ++ |
| Cardiomyopathy | ++ | – | + | +++ | – | ++ | – |
| Tachypnea/hyperpnea | ++ | ++ | ++ | ++ | – | – | – |
| Rash | – | ++ | ++ | – | – | – | – |
| Alopecia or abnormal hair | – | + | ++ | | | | + |
| Cataracts or corneal opacity | ++ | – | – | – | – | ++ | – |
| Retinal abnormality | – | + | + | + | – | ++ | ++ |
| Frequent infections | ++ | – | ++ | – | ++ | | |
| Deafness | – | – | + | | | ++ | – |

*(continued)*

***Table 32–1.*** Presenting clinical and laboratory features of inborn errors.[a] (continued)

| | Defects of Carbohydrate Metabolism | Defects of Amino Acid Metabolism[b] | Organic Acid Disorders[c] | Defects of Fatty Acid Oxidation | Defects of Purine Metabolism | Lysosomal Storage Diseases | Disorders of Peroxisomes |
|---|---|---|---|---|---|---|---|
| **Laboratory** | | | | | | | |
| Hypoglycemia | +++ | + | ++ | ++ | – | – | – |
| Hyperammonemia | – | ++ | ++ | ++ | – | – | – |
| Metabolic acidosis | ++ | ++ | +++ | +++ | – | – | – |
| Respiratory alkalosis | – | ++ | – | – | – | – | – |
| Elevated lactate/pyruvate | ++ | – | +++ | ++ | – | – | – |
| Elevated liver enzymes | ++ | ++ | ++ | +++ | – | + | + |
| Neutropenia or thrombocytopenia | + | – | + | – | ++ | + | – |
| Ketosis | +++ | ++ | +++ | – | – | – | – |
| Hypoketosis | – | – | + | +++ | – | – | – |

[a]+++, most conditions in group; ++, some; +, one or few; –, not found.
[b]Includes disorders of urea cycle but not maple syrup urine disease.
[c]Includes maple syrup urine disease and disorders of pyruvate oxidation.

32–2 lists the most common laboratory tests used to diagnose these diseases and offers some comments about their use.

Laboratory studies are almost always needed for the diagnosis of inborn errors. Serum electrolytes and pH should be used to estimate anion gap as well as acid–base status. Analysis of serum lactate, pyruvate, and ammonia levels may be available in large hospitals. Amino acid and organic acid studies must be performed at specialized facilities to ensure adequate analysis and interpretation. An increasing number of inborn errors are diagnosed with DNA probes, although this method may require an extensive genealogic chart or knowledge of the precise mutation carried in the family.

The physician should know what conditions a test will detect and when it will detect them. For example, urine organic acids may be normal in patients with medium-chain acyl-CoA dehydrogenase deficiency or biotinidase deficiency; glycine may be elevated only in cerebrospinal fluid (CSF) in patients with glycine encephalopathy; and a result that is normal in one physiologic state may be abnormal in another. For instance, the urine of a hypoglycemic child should be positive for ketones; in such a child, a ketone-negative urine test may suggest the presence of a defect in fatty acid oxidation.

Samples used to diagnose metabolic disease may be obtained at autopsy. They may be analyzed directly or stored frozen until a particular analysis is justified by the results of postmortem examination, new clinical information, or new developments in the field. Studies of other family members may also help to establish the diagnosis in a deceased patient; these include demonstrating that the parents are heterozygous carriers of a particular disorder or showing that another sibling has the condition.

## COMMON CLINICAL SITUATIONS

### Mental Retardation

Many inborn errors can cause mental retardation without other distinguishing characteristics. Laboratory studies of serum and urine amino acids should be obtained for every patient who has nonspecific mental retardation. Urine screens for mucopolysacchariduria are useful because some mucopolysaccharidoses do not have specific physical findings. The presence of a high anion gap or renal tubular acidosis significantly increases the chance of finding an underlying inborn error.

### Acute Presentation in the Neonate

Acute metabolic disease in the newborn may be clinically indistinguishable from sepsis and is most often caused by disorders of protein or carbohydrate metabolism. Initial symptoms may be poor feeding or vomit-

**Table 32–2.** Obtaining and handling samples to diagnose inborn errors.

| Test | Comments |
|---|---|
| Acid-base status | Accurate estimation of anion gap must be possible. Samples for blood gases should be kept on ice and analyzed immediately. |
| Blood ammonia | Sample should be collected without a tourniquet, kept on ice, and analyzed immediately. |
| Blood lactic acid and pyruvic acid | Sample should be collected without a tourniquet, kept on ice, and analyzed immediately. Reduction of pyruvic acid to lactic acid must be prevented. Normal literature values are for the fasting, rested state. |
| Amino acids | Blood and urine should be examined. CSF glycine should be measured if non-ketotic hyperglycinemia is to be ruled out. Normal literature values are for the fasting state. Growth of bacteria in urine should be prevented. At autopsy: liver, kidney, or aqueous humor may be analyzed if urine is not available. |
| Organic acids | Urine preferred for analysis. At autopsy: liver, kidney, or aqueous humor may be analyzed if urine is not available. |
| Carnitine and acylcarnitine profile | Blood (plasma) may be analyzed for total, free, and esterified carnitine; normal values are for the healthy, nonfasted state. Acylcarnitine profile in blood may identify compounds esterified to carnitine, and urine and tissue studies may be needed for certain conditions. |
| Urine mucopoly-saccharides | Variations in urine concentration may cause errors in screening tests. Diagnosis requires knowing which mucopoly-saccharides are increased. Some patients with Morquio disease do not have abnormal mucopolysacchariduria. |
| Enzyme assays | Specific assays must be requested. Exposure to heat may cause loss of enzyme activity. Enzyme activity in whole blood may become normal after transfusion or vitamin therapy. Leukocyte or fibroblast pellets should be kept frozen prior to assays. Fibroblasts may be grown from skin biopsies taken up to 72 h after death. Tissues such as liver and kidney should be taken as soon as possible after death, frozen immediately, and kept at $-70°C$ until assayed. |

CSF = cerebrospinal fluid.

ing, altered mental status or tone, jitteriness or seizures, and jaundice. Acidosis or altered mental status out of proportion to systemic symptoms should increase suspicion of a metabolic disorder. Laboratory measurements should include the following: electrolytes, ammonia, glucose, urine pH, and urine ketones. Glycine in CSF should be measured if glycine encephalopathy is suspected. Serum and urine to be used for amino acid and organic acid analysis should be collected, before oral intake is stopped, and sent for analysis if indicated by the results of initial studies.

## Vomiting & Encephalopathy in the Infant or Older Child

Electrolytes, ammonia, glucose, urine pH, urine-reducing substances, and urine ketones should be measured in all patients who exhibit vomiting and encephalopathy, before any treatment affects the results. Samples for amino and organic acid analysis should be obtained early and frozen pending the results of initial studies. An inborn error is even more likely when the presentation is judged typical of Reye syndrome (ie, vomiting, encephalopathy, hepatomegaly), and amino acids and organic acids should be studied immediately. If hypoglycemia with inappropriately low urine or serum ketones is present, disorders of fatty acid oxidation should be considered.

## Hypoglycemia

Electrolytes, ammonia, uric acid, urine-reducing substances, and urine ketones should be measured, along with urinary organic acids. Ketone body production is usually not efficient in the neonate, and ketonuria in a hypoglycemic or acidotic neonate suggests an inborn error. In the older child, inappropriately low urine ketone levels suggest an inborn error of fatty acid oxidation.

## Hyperammonemia

Symptoms of hyperammonemia may appear and progress rapidly or insidiously. Decreased appetite and irritability usually appear first, with vomiting, lethargy, seizures, and coma appearing as ammonia levels increase. Tachypnea is caused by a direct effect on respiratory drive. Physical examination cannot exclude the presence of hyperammonemia, and serum ammonia should be measured whenever hyperammonemia is possible.

Severe hyperammonemia may be due to urea cycle disorders, organic acidemias, or carnitine–acylcarnitine translocase deficiency or, in the neonate, to transient hyperammonemia of the newborn. The cause can usually be ascertained by measuring citrulline, electrolytes, and carnitine and acylcarnitine esters in serum and measuring amino acids, organic acids, and orotic acid in urine. Respiratory alkalosis is usually present in transient hyperammonemia of the newborn and hyperammonemia due to a urea cycle defect, whereas metabolic acidosis is usually associated with hyperammonemia due to organic acidemia. Urine organic acid analysis will identify organic acidemia. Serum citrulline is usually low or undetectable in early urea cycle defects, normal or slightly high in transient hyperammonemia of the newborn, and very high in citrullinemia and argininosuccinic acidemia. Argininosuccinic acid is found in urine only in the last case. Of infants with early urea cycle defects, only those with hyperammonemia due to ornithine transcarbamoylase deficiency have increased urine orotic acid levels and (often) a family history of male newborn deaths consistent with X-linked inheritance. Infants with carnitine–acylcarnitine translocase deficiency often have low serum carnitine and elevated palmitoylcarnitine.

## Acidosis

Inborn errors may cause chronic or acute acidosis at any age and with or without an increased anion gap. Inborn errors are in the differential diagnosis of acidosis occurring with recurrent vomiting or hyperammonemia and when acidosis is out of proportion to the clinical status. Acidosis due to an inborn error is usually difficult to correct. The presence of renal tubular acidosis does not exclude an underlying inborn error.

Serum glucose and ammonia levels and urine pH and ketone levels should always be examined. Samples for amino acids and organic acids should be obtained at once and sent to the laboratory or saved in the freezer, depending on how strongly an inborn error is suspected. It is useful to test blood lactate and pyruvate levels in the chronically acidotic patient even if urine organic acid levels are normal. Lactate and pyruvate levels are difficult to interpret in the acutely ill patient, but in the absence of shock, high levels of lactic acid suggest primary lactic acidosis.

## ■ MANAGEMENT OF METABOLIC EMERGENCIES

Patients with severe acidosis, hypoglycemia, and hyperammonemia may be very ill; initially mild symptoms may worsen quickly, and coma and death may ensue within hours. With prompt and vigorous treatment, however, patients can recover completely, even from

deep coma. All oral intake should be stopped. Sufficient glucose should be given intravenously to avoid or minimize catabolism in a patient with a known inborn error who is at risk for crisis. Most conditions respond favorably to glucose administration, and few (eg, primary lactic acidosis due to pyruvate dehydrogenase deficiency) do not. Severe or increasing hyperammonemia should be treated pharmacologically or with dialysis, and severe acidosis should be treated with bicarbonate. More specific measures can be instituted when a diagnosis is established.

## ■ NEWBORN SCREENING

Criteria used to decide whether to screen newborns for a disorder include the disorder's frequency, the significance of consequences if it is not treated, the ability to avert or mitigate those consequences with therapy, the cost of screening and diagnostic tests, and the cost of treatment. All states in the United States screen newborns for phenylketonuria and hypothyroidism, and in most states newborns are screened for galactosemia. Other metabolic disorders for which newborns are frequently screened include maple syrup urine disease, homocystinuria due to cystathionine synthase deficiency, biotinidase deficiency, and, using tandem mass spectrometry, several disorders of amino acid, organic acid, and fatty acid metabolism.

Some screening tests measure a metabolite (eg, phenylalanine) that becomes abnormal only with time and exposure to diet, and in such instances the disease cannot be detected reliably until intake of the enzyme substrate has become established. Other tests (eg, for biotinidase deficiency) assay an enzyme and can be performed at any time; however, transfusions may cause false-negative results, and exposure of the sample to heat may cause false-positive results. Technologic advances extend the power of newborn screening but sometimes bring additional challenges. For example, although tandem mass spectrometry (MS-MS) is capable of detecting many more disorders in the newborn period, wider application is controversial because of the cost and the limitations of some treatments.

Screening tests are not diagnostic, and diagnostic tests must be undertaken when an abnormal screening result is obtained. Furthermore, because false-negative results occur, a normal newborn screening test does not rule out a condition.

The timing of newborn screening recommended by the American Academy of Pediatrics (AAP) is appropriate for the detection of phenylketonuria, but hypothyroidism, for instance, can be missed when screening is carried out at the same time. Early discharge of neonates causes significant problems with newborn screening, with both false-negative and false-positive results. Nevertheless, all babies should be screened before discharge from the hospital.

The appropriate response to an abnormal screening test depends on the condition for which screening is conducted and the predictive value of the screening test. For example, when screening for galactosemia using enzyme assay, complete absence of enzyme activity is highly predictive of classic galactosemia, and failure to treat may rapidly lead to death. In that case, treatment must be initiated immediately while diagnostic studies are pending. In PKU, however, a diet restricted in phenylalanine is harmful to the baby who proves to have had a false-positive screen, but an excellent outcome of therapy in the affected baby is well demonstrated so long as treatment is established within the first weeks of life. Therefore, initiation of treatment for PKU is contraindicated until diagnosis is confirmed. Physicians should combine current AAP recommendations and state laws and regulations to arrive at appropriate strategies for each hospital and practice.

American College of Medical Genetics/American Society of Human Genetics Test and Technology Transfer Committee Working Group: Tandem mass spectrometry in newborn screening. Genet Med 2000;2:267 [PMID: 11252712].

Buist NR et al: Metabolic evaluation of infantile epilepsy: Summary recommendations of the Amalfi Group. J Child Neurol 2002;17 (Suppl 3):3S98 [PMID: 12597059].

Carpenter KH, Wiley V: Application of tandem mass spectrometry to biochemical genetics and newborn screening. Clin Chim Acta 2002;322(1-2):1 [PMID: 12104075].

Carreiro-Lewandowski E: Newborn screening: An overview. Clin Lab Sci 2002;15(4):229 [PMID: 12776783].

Cederbaum S: Molecular diagnosis and inborn errors of metabolism: A practitioner's view. Genet Med 2000;2:345 [PMID: 11339655].

Clayton PT: Applications of mass spectrometry in the study of inborn errors of metabolism. J Inherit Metab Dis 2001;24:139 [PMID: 11405336].

Clayton PT: Inborn errors presenting with liver dysfunction. Semin Neonatol 2002;7(1):49 [PMID: 12069538].

Ellaway CJ et al: Clinical approach to inborn errors of metabolism presenting in the newborn period. J Paediatr Child Health 2002;38(5):511 [PMID: 12354271].

Jones PM, Bennett MJ: The changing face of newborn screening: Diagnosis of inborn errors of metabolism by tandem mass spectrometry. Clin Chim Acta 2002;324(1-2):121 [PMID: 12204433].

Korson MS: Advances in newborn screening for metabolic disorders: What the pediatrician needs to know. Pediatr Ann 2000; 29:294 [PMID: 10826324].

Leonard JV, Morris AA: Inborn errors of metabolism around time of birth. Lancet 2000;356:583 [PMID: 10950248].

Ogier de Baulny H: Management and emergency treatments of neonates with a suspicion of inborn errors of metabolism. Semin Neonatol 2002;7(1):17 [PMID: 12069535].

Pass KA et al: US newborn screening system guidelines II: Follow-up of children, diagnosis, management, and evaluation: Statement of the Council of Regional Networks for Genetic Services (CORN). J Pediatr 2000;137 (Suppl 4):S1.

Saudubray JM et al: Clinical approach to inherited metabolic disorders in neonates: An overview. Semin Neonatol 2002; 7(1):3 [PMID: 12069534].

Schulze A et al: Expanded newborn screening for inborn errors of metabolism by electrospray ionization-tandem mass spectrometry: Results, outcome, and implications. Pediatrics 2003:111(6):1399 [PMID: 12777559].

Velazquez A et al: Diagnosis of inborn errors of metabolism. Arch Med Res 2000;31:145 [PMID: 10880718].

# DISORDERS OF CARBOHYDRATE METABOLISM

## GLYCOGEN STORAGE DISEASES

Glycogen is a highly branched polymer of glucose that is stored in liver and muscle. Different enzyme defects affect its biosynthesis and degradation. The most common glycogenoses cause growth failure, hepatomegaly, and fasting hypoglycemia. The so-called hepatic forms of the disease include glucose-6-phosphatase (type I; von Gierke disease), debrancher enzyme (type III), hepatic phosphorylase (type VI), and phosphorylase kinase (type IX), which normally regulates hepatic phosphorylase activity. There are two forms of glucose-6-phosphatase deficiency: In one, the enzyme defect can be demonstrated in fresh or frozen liver; in the other, the defect can be demonstrated only in fresh tissue.

Forms of the disease affecting primarily muscle include acid maltase deficiency (type II; Pompe disease), which may occur in infancy and is associated with cardiomegaly and macroglossia, and muscle phosphorylase (type V) and phosphofructokinase (type VII) deficiencies, in which the most striking features are easy fatigability and muscle weakness and stiffness.

### Diagnosis

Precise diagnosis is by biochemical tests, such as responsiveness of blood glucose to fasting and glucagon, and enzyme assays on leukocytes, liver, or muscle. Disorders that can be diagnosed using red or white blood cells include deficiencies of debrancher enzyme (type III) and phosphorylase kinase (IX). Pompe disease can usually be diagnosed by assaying acid maltase in fibroblasts.

## Treatment

Treatment is designed to prevent hypoglycemia while avoiding storage of even more glycogen in the liver. In the most severe hepatic forms, this requires careful monitoring of specific diets, using restriction of free sugars and measured amounts of cornstarch, and good results have been reported following continuous night-time carbohydrate feeding.

Chou JY et al: Type I glycogen storage diseases: Disorders of the glucose-6-phosphatase complex. Curr Mol Med 2002;2(2): 121 [PMID: 11949931].

Janecke AR et al: Molecular genetics of type 1 glycogen storage disease. Mol Genet Metab 2001;73:117 [PMID: 11386847].

Kannourakis G: Glycogen storage disease. Semin Hematol 2002; 39(2):103 [PMID: 11957192].

Moses SW: Historical highlights and unsolved problems in glycogen storage disease type 1. Eur J Pediatr 2002;161 (Suppl 1):S2 [PMID: 12373565].

Rake JP et al: Guidelines for management of glycogen storage disease type I—European Study on Glycogen Storage Disease Type I (ESGSD I). Eur J Pediatr 2002;161 (Suppl 1): S112 [PMID: 12373584].

Tsujino S et al: Glycogen storage myopathies. Neurol Clin 2000;18:125 [PMID: 10658171].

Visser G et al: Consensus guidelines for management of glycogen storage disease type 1b—European Study on Glycogen Storage Disease Type 1. Eur J Pediatr 2002;161 (Suppl 1): S120 [PMID: 12373585].

## GALACTOSEMIA

Classic galactosemia is caused by almost total deficiency of galactose-1-phosphate uridyltransferase. Accumulation of galactose-1-phosphate in liver, brain, and renal tubules causes hepatic parenchymal disease, mental retardation, and renal Fanconi syndrome. Accumulation of galactitol (dulcitol) in the lens produces cataracts. With prompt institution of a galactose-free diet, the prognosis for survival without severe mental retardation and liver disease is excellent.

Onset of the severe form of the disease is accompanied by vomiting, jaundice, and hepatomegaly in the newborn period after milk feeding. Without treatment, death frequently occurs in the first month of life, often from *Escherichia coli* sepsis. Cataracts usually develop within 2 months in untreated cases, and hepatic cirrhosis is progressive. Survival is possible, but mental retardation is irreversible. Even when dietary restrictions are instituted early, patients with galactosemia are at increased risk for speech and language deficits and ovarian failure, and some patients develop progressive delay, tremor, and ataxia. Milder variants of galactosemia with better prognosis exist in all populations.

The disorder is inherited as an autosomal recessive trait with an incidence of approximately 1:40,000 live births. Because disease in infancy may be severe and diagnosed late, newborn screening is common. Screening is accomplished by demonstrating enzyme deficiency in red cells with the Beutler test or by demonstrating increased serum galactose. Prenatal diagnosis is possible if a specific DNA mutation in a family is known.

## Diagnosis

In infants receiving foods containing galactose, laboratory findings include galactosuria and hypergalactosemia together with proteinuria and aminoaciduria. Absence of urine-reducing substances does not exclude the diagnosis. When the diagnosis is suspected, galactose-1-phosphate uridyltransferase should be assayed in erythrocytes. Blood transfusions give false-negative results and sample deterioration false-positive results.

## Treatment

A galactose-free diet should be instituted as soon as the diagnosis is made. Compliance with the diet must be monitored because it is not a simple exclusion of milk and requires extensive knowledge about the galactose content of foods. Avoidance of galactose should be lifelong in severe cases, with appropriate calcium replacement. Heterozygous mothers may be advised to maintain a galactose-free diet during pregnancy.

Garden AS, Davidson DC: Recommendations for the management of galactosemia. Arch Dis Child 2000;82(3):266 [PMID: 10722417]

Guerrero NV et al: Risk factors for premature ovarian failure in females with galactosemia. J Pediatr 2000;137:833 [PMID: 11113841].

Liu G et al: Galactose metabolism and ovarian toxicity. Reprod Toxicol 2000;14:377 [PMID: 11020650].

Novelli G, Reichardt JK: Molecular basis of disorders of human galactose metabolism: Past, present, and future. Mol Genet Metab 2000;71:62 [PMID: 11001796].

Robertson A, Singh RH: Outcomes analysis of verbal dyspraxia in classic galactosemia. Genet Med 2000;2:142 [PMID: 11397328].

Shield JP et al: The relationship of genotype to cognitive outcome in galactosaemia. Arch Dis Child 2000;83:248 [PMID: 10952646].

Tyfield LA: Galactosaemia and allelic variation at the galactose-1-phosphate uridyltransferase gene: A complex relationship between genotype and phenotype. Eur J Pediatr 2000; 159 (Suppl 3):S207 [PMID: 11216901].

A patient/parent support group website with useful information for families: www.galactosemia.org

## HEREDITARY FRUCTOSE INTOLERANCE

Hereditary fructose intolerance is an autosomal recessive disorder in which deficient activity of fructose-

1-phosphate aldolase causes hypoglycemia and tissue accumulation of fructose-1-phosphate on fructose ingestion. Other abnormalities include failure to thrive, vomiting, jaundice, hepatomegaly, proteinuria, and generalized aminoaciduria. The untreated condition can progress to death as a result of liver failure.

## Diagnosis

The diagnosis is supported by the demonstration of fructosuria following an in-patient, closely monitored fructose load. The appearance of hypoglycemia and hypophosphatemia after fructose loading (200 mg/kg) is diagnostic, as is reduced activity of fructose-1-phosphate aldolase in the liver. Some patients may be diagnosed by identification of one of the common mutations on DNA analysis.

## Treatment

Treatment consists of eliminating fructose from the diet and is complicated by the fact that many proprietary drugs and vitamins are in a sucrose base. If the diet is relaxed, physical growth retardation may occur, but growth will resume when more stringent dietary restrictions are instituted. If the disorder is recognized early, the prospects for normal development are good. As affected individuals grow up, they may recognize the association of nausea and vomiting with fructose-containing foods and selectively avoid them.

Ali M et al: Hereditary fructose intolerance. J Med Genet 1998; 35:353 [PMID: 9610797].

## ■ PRIMARY LACTIC ACIDEMIAS & OTHER DISORDERS OF ENERGY METABOLISM

Primary lactic acidemia is a diagnosis being made with increasing frequency and may be one of the more common causes of static, progressive, or self-limited neurodevelopmental problems in children. The range of severity and prognosis in these disorders is illustrated by extremes. For example, defects in the mitochondrial respiratory chain, including complex IV deficiency, may cause Leigh disease, a fatal neurodegenerative disorder, whereas another manifestation of complex IV deficiency is benign-resolving congenital hypotonia. Lactic acidemia is said to be primary when it is due to a defect in the metabolism of pyruvic acid and secondary when a change in cellular redox potential favors the reduction of pyruvate to lactate (as in shock). Table

**Table 32–3.** Causes of primary lactic acidosis in childhood.

**Defects of the pyruvate dehydrogenase complex**
$E_1$ (pyruvate decarboxylase) deficiency
$E_2$ (dihydrolipoyl transacetylase) deficiency
$E_3$ (lipoamide dehydrogenase) deficiency
Pyruvate decarboxylase phosphate phosphatase deficiency
**Abnormalities of gluconeogenesis**
Pyruvate carboxylase deficiency
    Isolated
    Biotinidase deficiency
    Holocarboxylase synthetase deficiency
Fructose-1,6-diphosphatase deficiency
Glucose-6-phosphatase deficiency (von Gierke disease)
**Defects in mitochondrial respiratory chain**
Complex I deficiency
Complex IV deficiency (cytochrome C oxidase deficiency; frequent cause of Leigh disease)
ATPase deficiency (frequent cause of Leigh disease)
Other respiratory chain disorders

32–3 lists some causes of primary lactic acidosis. In general, such disorders may present at any age with neurologic findings and, when the defect is in gluconeogenesis, with hypoglycemia. Patients with a defect in the $E_1$ component of the pyruvate dehydrogenase complex often have central nervous system (CNS) malformations or mild facial dysmorphism. Recurrent altered mental status, recurrent ataxia, and recurrent acidosis are typical of many disturbances of pyruvate metabolism.

Patients with defects in the mitochondrial respiratory chain also may present with nonspecific findings such as hypotonia, failure to thrive, or renal tubular acidosis or with more specific features such as ophthalmoplegia or cardiomyopathy. Ragged red fibers and mitochondrial abnormalities may be noted on histologic examination of muscle. Thirteen of the more than 100 genes that control activity of the respiratory chain are part of the mitochondrial genome. Therefore, inheritance of defects in the respiratory chain may be mendelian or maternal.

## Diagnosis

Diagnosis of primary lactic acidemia may be based on (1) demonstration of significant elevations of lactic or pyruvic acid concentrations in the blood (in a fasting, resting, free-flowing sample) with absence of causes of secondary lactic acidemia; (2) elevated lactic or pyruvic acid in spinal fluid; or (3) demonstration of classic features of mitochondrial disorder, such as ragged red fibers in skeletal muscle biopsy. Primary lactic acidemia may be present even if the blood lactic acid concentration is normal, because lactate levels may vary according to the state of the patient (eg, resting versus active; fasting versus fed). Carefully controlled and monitored provocative testing such as fasting, challenge with carbohydrates, or exercise may identify affected individuals, and the specific responses to challenge may suggest both a diagnosis and possible treatment. Diagnostic tests of blood samples for enzyme activity (eg, biotinidase, pyruvate carboxylase) may be diagnostic, but enzyme analysis of fibroblasts or skeletal muscle is often required. For some clinical presentations, mitochondrial DNA analysis of blood or tissue may identify a diagnostic mutation. With many patients, the cause of lactic acidemia cannot yet be defined. In some instances, the genetics and prognosis may be clear, but in many cases neither prognosis nor genetic risk can be predicted.

## Treatment

In some patients, defects in gluconeogenesis can be treated with glucose administration, fructose avoidance, or administration of pharmacologic amounts of biotin. Modified ketogenic diet has been reported to be useful in some cases of proved or presumed pyruvate dehydrogenase deficiency. Other treatments are of theoretical value, with little data on efficacy. Thiamine and lipoic acid have been tried in patients who have pyruvate dehydrogenase complex deficiencies, and coenzyme Q and riboflavin have been reported to be helpful in some patients with respiratory chain defects. Dichloroacetic acid has been tried in pyruvate dehydrogenase complex deficiencies and in respiratory chain disorders, with variable clinical responses and adverse effects.

Borchert A et al Current concepts of mitochondrial disorders in childhood. Semin Pediatr Neurol 2002;9(2):151 [PMID: 12138999]

Chinnery PF, Turnbull DM: Epidemiology and treatment of mitochondrial disorders. Am J Med Genet 2001;106(1):94 [PMID: 11579428]

Darras BT Friedman NR: Metabolic myopathies: A clinical approach: Part I. Pediatr Neurol 2000;22:87 [PMID: 10738913].

Darras BT Friedman NR: Metabolic myopathies: A clinical approach: Part II. Pediatr Neurol 2000;22:171 [PMID: 10734246].

De Meirleir L: Defects of pyruvate metabolism and the Krebs cycle. J Child Neurol 2002;17 (Suppl 3):3S26; discussion 3S33 [PMID: 12597053].

DiMauro S et al: Diseases of oxidative phosphorylation due to mtDNA mutations. Semin Neurol 2001;21(3):251 [PMID: 11641815].

Gillis L, Kaye E: Diagnosis and management of mitochondrial diseases. Pediatr Clin North Am 2002;49(1):203 [PMID: 11826805].

Leonard JV, Schapira AH: Mitochondrial respiratory chain disorders I: Mitochondrial DNA defects. Lancet 2000;355:299 [PMID: 10675086].

Leonard JV, Schapira AH: Mitochondrial respiratory chain disorders II: Neurodegenerative disorders and nuclear gene defects. Lancet 2000;355:389 [PMID: 10665569].

Munnich A, Rustin P: Clinical spectrum and diagnosis of mitochondrial disorders. Am J Med Genet 2001;106(1):4 [PMID: 11579420].

Naviaux RK: Mitochondrial DNA disorders. Eur J Pediatr 2000;159 (Suppl 3):S219 [PMID: 11216904].

Schapira AH: Mitochondrial disorders. Curr Opin Neurol 2000; 13:527 [PMID: 11073358].

Schmiedel J et al: Mitochondrial cytopathies. J Neurol 2003; 250(3):267 [PMID: 12638015].

Singhal N et al: Mitochondrial diseases: An overview of genetics, pathogenesis, clinical features and an approach to diagnosis and treatment. J Postgrad Med 2000;46:224 [PMID: 11298479].

Smeitink J et al: The genetics and pathology of oxidative phosphorylation. Nat Rev Genet 2001; 2:342 [PMID: 11331900].

Vladutiu GD: The molecular diagnosis of metabolic myopathies. Neurol Clin 2000;18:53 [PMID: 10658169].

A patient/parent support group website with useful information for families: www.umdf.org

# ■ DISORDERS OF AMINO ACID METABOLISM

## DISORDERS OF THE UREA CYCLE

Ammonia is converted to an amino group in urea by enzymes of the urea cycle. Patients with defects in early urea cycle enzymes, such as carbamoyl phosphate synthetase or ornithine transcarbamoylase, usually present in infancy with severe and rapidly fatal hyperammonemia, vomiting, and encephalopathy, but the course may also be milder, with vomiting and encephalopathy following protein ingestion or infections. Although defects in argininosuccinic acid synthetase (citrullinemia) and argininosuccinic acid lyase (argininosuccinic acidemia) may also cause severe hyperammonemia in infancy, a chronic course with mental retardation is more usual in these conditions.

Except for ornithine transcarbamoylase deficiency, which is X-linked, urea cycle disorders are inherited as autosomal recessive traits. Citrullinemia and argininosuccinic acidemia can be diagnosed in utero by appropriate enzyme assays, but carbamoyl phosphate synthetase and ornithine transcarbamoylase deficiency can be diagnosed in utero only by using specific gene probes, and then only in certain families.

## Diagnosis

Blood ammonia levels should be measured in any newborn who is acutely ill without obvious cause. A urea cycle defect should be suspected when severe hyperammonemia is associated with respiratory alkalosis. Serum citrulline is low or undetectable in carbamoyl phosphate synthetase and ornithine transcarbamoylase deficiency, high in argininosuccinic acidemia, and very high in citrullinemia. Large amounts of argininosuccinic acid are found in the urine of patients with argininosuccinic acidemia. Urine orotic acid is increased in infants with ornithine transcarbamoylase deficiency, and there may also be a family history of male newborn deaths consistent with an X-linked genetic trait.

Age at onset of symptoms varies with residual enzyme activity, protein intake, growth, and stress such as infection. Even within a family, affected males may differ by decades in their age at onset of symptoms. Many female carriers of ornithine transcarbamoylase deficiency exhibit protein intolerance; some develop migraine-like symptoms after protein loads, and others develop potentially fatal episodes of vomiting and encephalopathy after protein ingestion, certain infections, or labor and delivery. Trichorrhexis nodosa is common in patients with the chronic form of argininosuccinic acidemia.

## Treatment

In the newborn, measures to reduce serum ammonia by hemodialysis, peritoneal dialysis, or double-volume exchange transfusion should be instituted as soon as hyperammonemia is documented. Protein intake should be stopped, and glucose should be given to reduce endogenous protein breakdown. Arginine should be given intravenously, both because it is an essential amino acid for patients with urea cycle defects and because it increases the excretion of waste nitrogen in patients with citrullinemia and argininosuccinic acidemia. Sodium benzoate, either alone or with sodium phenylacetate, can be given intravenously to treat hyperammonemic coma.

Long-term treatment includes oral administration of arginine (or citrulline), adherence to a low-protein diet, and administration of sodium benzoate and sodium phenylacetate or sodium phenylbutyrate to increase excretion of nitrogen as hippuric acid and phenylacetylglutamine. Females who are heterozygous for ornithine transcarbamoylase deficiency and who develop hyperammonemia should also receive such treatment. Liver transplantation may improve outcome.

The outcome of argininosuccinic acidemia and citrullinemia is better than that of ornithine transcarbamoylase and carbamoyl phosphate synthetase defi-

ciency. Most patients with urea cycle defects, no matter what the enzyme defect, develop permanent neurologic and intellectual impairments, with cortical atrophy and ventricular dilation seen on CT scan. The prognosis may be improved if the initial hyperammonemic episode is rapidly identified and treated.

Batshaw ML et al: Alternative pathway therapy for urea cycle disorders: Twenty years later. J Pediatr 2001;138 (Suppl 1):S46 [PMID: 11148549].

Berry GT, Steiner RD: Long-term management of patients with urea cycle disorders. J Pediatr 2001;138 (Suppl 1):S56 [PMID: 11148550].

Burton BK: Urea cycle disorders. Clin Liver Dis 2000;4:815 [PMID: 11232359].

Consensus statement from a conference for the management of patients with urea cycle disorders. J Pediatr 2001;138 (Suppl 1):S1 [PMID: 11148543].

Lee B, Goss J: Long-term correction of urea cycle disorders. J Pediatr 2001;138 (Suppl 1):S62 [PMID: 11148551].

Leonard JV: The nutritional management of urea cycle disorders. J Pediatr 2001;138 (Suppl 1):S40 [PMID: 11148548].

Leonard JV, Morris AA: Urea cycle disorders. Semin Neonatol 2002;7(1):27 [PMID: 12069536].

Nicolaides P et al: Neurological outcome in patients with ornithine carbamoyltransferase deficiency. Arch Dis Child 2002; 86(1):54 [PMID: 11806886].

Summar M: Current strategies for the management of neonatal urea cycle disorders. J Pediatr 2001;138 (Suppl 1):S30 [PMID: 11148547].

Summar M, Tuchman M: Proceedings of a consensus conference for the management of patients with urea cycle disorders. J Pediatr 2001;138 (Suppl 1):S6 [PMID: 11148544].

Steiner RD, Cedarbaum SD: Laboratory evaluation of urea cycle disorders. J Pediatr 2001;138 (Suppl 1):S21 [PMID: 11148546].

A patient/parent support group website with useful information for families: www.nucdf.org

## PHENYLKETONURIA & THE HYPERPHENYLALANINEMIAS

Probably the best-known disorder of amino acid metabolism is the classic form of phenylketonuria caused by decreased activity of phenylalanine hydroxylase, the enzyme that converts phenylalanine to tyrosine. Phenylketonuria is inherited as an autosomal recessive trait, with an incidence in whites of approximately 1:10,000 live births. On normal phenylalanine intake, affected patients develop hyperphenylalaninemia and produce and excrete phenylpyruvic, phenyllactic, phenylacetic, and 2-hydroxyphenylacetic acid. The patient with untreated phenylketonuria exhibits severe mental retardation, hyperactivity, seizures, a light complexion, and eczema. The patient's urine has a "mouse-like" odor.

Success in preventing severe mental retardation in phenylketonuric children by restricting phenylalanine from the diet starting in early infancy led to screening programs to detect the disease early. Because the outcome is best when treatment is begun in the first month of life, infants should be screened during the first few days. A second test is necessary when newborn screening is done before 24 hours of age, and in such cases the second test should be completed by the third week of life. Infants receiving hyperalimentation and premature infants should be screened at or near 7 days and rescreened if they were transfused or not fed at the time of the initial test.

Enzymes involved with the interconversion of phenylalanine and tyrosine and whose deficiencies can produce hyperphenylalaninemia are shown in Figure 32–1. In classic phenylketonuria, little or no phenylalanine hydroxylase activity is present, but in the less severe hyperphenylalaninemias significant residual activity does occur. Rare variants (also with autosomal recessive inheritance) can be due to deficiency of dihydrobiopterin reductase or to defects in biopterin synthesis.

Prenatal diagnosis of phenylketonuria is possible using DNA probes. Molecular approaches are replacing serum measurements of phenylalanine and tyrosine to determine carrier status. Prenatal diagnosis of defects in pterin metabolism can often be made.

## Diagnosis & Treatment

The diagnosis of phenylketonuria in a severely mentally retarded older child with typical biochemical and physi-

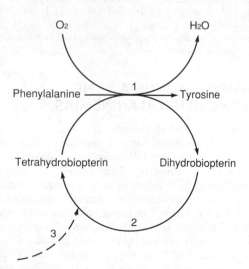

***Figure 32–1.*** Oxidation of phenylalanine to tyrosine. 1: Phenylalanine hydroxylase. 2: Dihydropteridine reductase. 3: Enzymes of biopterin biosynthesis.

cal characteristics is straightforward, but in the newborn period, especially when there is no family history, the condition must be differentiated from other forms of hyperphenylalaninemia. This is usually done by determining serum phenylalanine and tyrosine levels on a normal diet and by examining pterins in blood and urine.

### A. CLASSIC PHENYLKETONURIA

Findings include persistently elevated serum levels of phenylalanine (> 20 mg/dL on a regular diet), normal or low serum levels of tyrosine, urinary excretion of phenylpyruvic and 2-hydroxyphenylacetic acids, and normal pterins. Poor phenylalanine tolerance persists throughout life. Restriction of dietary phenylalanine intake (see Treatment section) is indicated, and a favorable outcome is the rule.

### B. PERSISTENT HYPERPHENYLALANINEMIA

In infants receiving a normal protein intake, serum phenylalanine levels are usually 4–20 mg/dL, and pterins are normal. Phenylalanine restriction may or may not be indicated, depending on the patient's phenylalanine tolerance.

### C. TRANSIENT HYPERPHENYLALANINEMIA

Serum phenylalanine levels are elevated early but progressively decline toward normal. Dietary restriction is only temporary, if required at all.

### D. DIHYDROPTERIDINE REDUCTASE DEFICIENCY

Serum phenylalanine levels vary. The pattern of pterin metabolites is abnormal. Seizures and psychomotor regression occur even with diet therapy, probably because the enzyme defect also causes neuronal deficiency of serotonin and dopamine. These deficiencies require treatment with levodopa, carbidopa, and 5-hydroxytryptophan, and possibly also with tetrahydrobiopterin.

### E. DEFECTS IN BIOPTERIN BIOSYNTHESIS

Serum phenylalanine levels vary. Total pterins are low, and their pattern may suggest the specific defect, which can be at one of several steps in the biosynthetic pathway. Clinical findings include myoclonus, tetraplegia, and other movement disorders. Treatment is the same as for dihydropteridine reductase deficiency but in general is not as effective.

### F. TYROSINEMIA OF THE NEWBORN

Serum phenylalanine levels are lower than those associated with phenylketonuria and are accompanied by marked hypertyrosinemia. Tyrosinemia of the newborn usually occurs in premature infants and is due to immaturity of 4-hydroxyphenylpyruvic acid oxidase. The condition resolves spontaneously within 3 months, almost always without sequelae. If necessary, oral administration of 50–200 mg ascorbic acid per day for 1–2 weeks will normalize serum tyrosine (and phenylalanine) levels.

### G. MATERNAL PHENYLKETONURIA

Offspring of phenylketonuric mothers may have transient hyperphenylalaninemia at birth. Elevated maternal phenylalanine causes mental retardation, microcephaly, growth retardation, and often congenital heart disease or other malformations. The risk to the fetus is lessened considerably if phenylalanine restriction is begun before conception and maintained throughout pregnancy.

## Treatment of Classic Phenylketonuria

Treatment of classic phenylketonuria is to limit dietary phenylalanine intake to amounts that permit normal growth and development. Metabolic formulas, deficient in phenylalanine, are available but must be supplemented with normal milk and other foods to supply enough phenylalanine to permit normal growth and development. Serum phenylalanine concentrations must be monitored frequently while ensuring that growth, development, and nutrition are adequate. This monitoring is best done in clinics experienced in dealing with such problems. Although dietary treatment is most effective when initiated during the first months of life, it may also be of benefit in reversing behaviors such as hyperactivity, irritability, and distractibility when started later in life.

Phenylalanine restriction should continue throughout life, both because of subtle changes in intellect and behavior in persons receiving treatment early who later stop the diet and because of the risk of late development of potentially irreversible neurologic damage after stopping the diet. Phenylketonuric females merit special attention during the childbearing years. Counseling should be given during adolescence, and the woman's diet should be monitored closely prior to conception and throughout pregnancy.

Children with classic phenylketonuria who receive treatment promptly after birth and achieve phenylalanine and tyrosine homeostasis will develop well physically and can be expected to have normal or nearly normal intellectual development.

American Academy of Pediatrics, Committee of Genetics: American Academy of Pediatrics: Maternal phenylketonuria. Pediatrics 2001;107:427 [PMID: 11158484].

Brenton DP, Pietz J: Adult care in phenylketonuria and hyperphenylalaninaemia: The relevance of neurological abnormalities. Eur J Pediatr 2000;159 (Suppl 2):S114 [PMID: 11043157].

Cederbaum S: Phenylketonuria: An update. Curr Opin Pediatr 2002;14(6):702 [PMID: 12436039].

Guttler F, Guldberg P: Mutation analysis anticipates dietary requirements in phenylketonuria. Eur J Pediatr 2000;159 (Suppl 2):S150 [PMID: 11043162].

Guttler F et al: Relationship among genotype, biochemical phenotype, and cognitive performance in females with phenylalanine hydroxylase deficiency: Report from the Maternal Phenylketonuria Collaborative Study. Pediatrics 1999;104: 258 [PMID: 10429004].

Huttenlocher PR: The neuropathology of phenylketonuria: Human and animal studies. Eur J Pediatr 2000;159 (Suppl 2):S102 [PMID: 11043154].

Koch R et al: Maternal phenylketonuria: An international study. Mol Genet Metab 2000;71:233 [PMID: 11001815].

Lucke T et al: BH4-sensitive hyperphenylalaninemia: New case and review of literature. Pediatr Neurol 2003;28(3):228 [PMID: 12770680]

MacDonald A: Diet and compliance in phenylketonuria. Eur J Pediatr 2000;159 (Suppl 2):S136 [PMID: 11043160].

National Institutes of Health Consensus Development Panel: National Institutes of Health Consensus Development Conference Statement: phenylketonuria: screening and management, October 16-18, 2000. Pediatrics 2001;108(4):972 [PMID: 11581453]

Smith I, Knowles J: Behaviour in early treated phenylketonuria: A systematic review. Eur J Pediatr 2000;159 (Suppl 2):S89 [PMID: 11043152].

Spaapen LJ, Rubio-Gozalbo ME: Tetrahydrobiopterin-responsive phenylalanine hydroxylase deficiency, state of the art. Mol Genet Metab 2003;78(2):93 [PMID: 12618080].

Surtees R, Blau N: The neurochemistry of phenylketonuria. Eur J Pediatr 2000;159 (Suppl 2):S109 [PMID: 11043156].

van Spronsen FJ et al: Phenylketonuria: Tyrosine beyond the phenylalanine-restricted diet. J Inherit Metab Dis 2001;24:1 [PMID: 11286377].

Patient/parent support group websites with useful information for families: www.pkunews.org and www.pkunetwork.org

## HEREDITARY TYROSINEMIA

Type 1 hereditary tyrosinemia is caused by deficiency of fumarylacetoacetase and is characterized by progressive hepatic parenchymal damage, renal tubular dystrophy with generalized aminoaciduria, hypophosphatemic rickets, hypermethioninemia, and the tyrosine metabolites, succinylacetone, and aminolevulinic acid in the urine. Liver failure may be rapidly fatal in infancy or somewhat more chronic, with liver cell carcinoma almost invariable in long-term survivors. The condition is inherited as an autosomal recessive trait and is especially common in Scandinavia and in the Chicoutimi–Lac St. Jean region of Quebec. Prenatal diagnosis can be established.

## Diagnosis

Similar clinical and biochemical findings may occur in galactosemia and hereditary fructose intolerance, but increased succinylacetone occurs only in fumarylace-toacetase deficiency, and diagnosis is based on demonstrating succinylacetone in urine.

## Treatment

A diet low in phenylalanine and tyrosine is indicated but not usually successful in preventing or reversing liver disease. Liver transplantation appears to be the only effective therapy for these children. Pharmacologic therapy to inhibit 4-hydroxyphenylpyruvate dehydrogenase using 2-(2-nitro-4-trifluoromethylbenzoyl)-1,3-cyclohexanedione (NTBC) decreases the production of toxic metabolites maleylacetoacetate and fumarylacetoacetate and improves the hepatic biochemical profile and clinical status. Studies are in progress to determine to what extent the risk of hepatocellular carcinoma is altered.

Grompe M: The pathophysiology and treatment of hereditary tyrosinemia type 1. Semin Liver Dis 2001;21(4):563 [PMID: 11745044].

Holme E, Lindstedt S: Nontransplant treatment of tyrosinemia. Clin Liver Dis 2000;4:805 [PMID: 11232358].

Pitkanen ST et al: Hereditary tyrosinaemia type I: From basics to progress in treatment. Ann Med 2000;32:530 [PMID: 11127930].

Russo PA et al: Tyrosinemia: A review. Pediatr Dev Pathol 2001;4(3):212-221. [PMID: 11370259].

## MAPLE SYRUP URINE DISEASE (Branched-Chain Ketoaciduria)

Maple syrup urine disease is due to deficiency of the enzyme that catalyzes oxidative decarboxylation of the branched-chain keto acid derivatives of leucine, isoleucine, and valine. The accumulated keto acids of leucine and isoleucine cause the characteristic odor, whereas only the keto acid of leucine has been implicated in causing CNS dysfunction. Many variants of this disorder have been described, including mild, intermittent, and thiamin-dependent forms, and all are inherited as autosomal recessive traits.

Patients with classic maple syrup urine disease are normal at birth but soon develop the characteristic odor, lethargy, feeding difficulties, coma, and seizures. Unless diagnosis is made and dietary restriction of branched-chain amino acids is begun, most will die in the first month of life, but nearly normal growth and development may be achieved if treatment is begun before about age 10 days.

## Diagnosis

Marked elevations of branched-chain amino acids (including alloisoleucine) in serum and urine are charac-teristic. Alloisoleucine, a transamination product of the keto acid of isoleucine, is almost pathognomonic. The magnitude and consistency of amino acid and organic acid changes are altered in mild and intermittent forms of the disease. Prenatal diagnosis is possible.

## Treatment

Metabolic formulas, deficient in branched-chain amino acids, are available but must be supplemented with normal milk and other foods to supply enough branched-chain amino acids to permit normal growth and development. Serum levels of branched-chain amino acids must be monitored frequently—even at intervals of 1 or 2 days—in the first months of life to deal with changing protein requirements. Acute episodes must be aggressively treated to prevent catabolism and negative nitrogen balance.

Morton DH et al: Diagnosis and treatment of maple syrup disease: A study of 36 patients. Pediatrics 2002;109(6):999 [PMID: 12042535].

Strauss KA, Morton DH: Branched-chain ketoacyl dehydrogenase deficiency: Maple syrup disease. Curr Treat Options Neurol 2003;5(4):329 [PMID: 12791200].

## HOMOCYSTINURIA

Homocystinuria is most often due to deficiency of cystathionine synthase, but it may also be due to deficiency of methylenetetrahydrofolate reductase (MTHR) or to defects in the biosynthesis of methyl-$B_{12}$, which is the coenzyme for $N^5$-methyltetrahydrofolate methyltransferase. All known inherited forms of homocystinuria are transmitted as autosomal recessive traits and can be diagnosed in the fetus.

About half of patients with untreated cystathionine synthase deficiency are mentally retarded, and most have arachnodactyly, osteoporosis, and a tendency to develop dislocated lenses and thromboembolic phenomena. Milder elevations of homocystine are increasingly recognized to be a factor in the etiology of vascular disease leading to myocardial infarction and stroke. These mild elevations are often caused by mutations leading to heat-sensitive defects in MTHR. Patients with remethylation defects usually exhibit failure to thrive and a variety of neurologic symptoms, including microcephaly and seizures in infancy and early childhood.

## Diagnosis

Diagnosis is made by demonstrating homocystinuria in a patient who is not severely deficient in vitamin $B_{12}$. Serum methionine levels are usually high in patients with cystathionine synthase deficiency and often low in patients with remethylation defects. When the remethylation defect is due to deficiency of methyl-$B_{12}$, megaloblastic anemia may be present, and an associated deficiency of adenosyl-$B_{12}$ may cause methylmalonic aciduria. Studies of cultured fibroblasts may be necessary to make a specific diagnosis.

## Treatment

About 50% of patients with cystathionine synthase deficiency respond to large oral doses of pyridoxine. Early treatment of pyridoxine nonresponders by dietary methionine restriction may prevent mental retardation and delay lens dislocations, perhaps justifying screening of newborn infants for the condition. Oral administration of betaine will increase methylation of homocystine to methionine in patients with remethylation defects and may also improve neurologic function. Large doses of vitamin $B_{12}$ (eg, 1 mg hydroxocobalamin administered intramuscularly) are indicated in some patients.

Smith DL, Bodamer OA: Practical management of combined methylmalonicaciduria and homocystinuria. J Child Neurol 2002;17(5):353 [PMID: 12150582].

Yap S et al: Vascular outcome in patients with homocystinuria due to cystathionine beta-synthase deficiency treated chronically: A multicenter observational study. Arterioscler Thromb Vasc Biol 2001;21(12):2080 [PMID: 11742888].

Yap S et al: Vascular complications of severe hyperhomocysteinemia in patients with homocystinuria due to cystathionine beta-synthase deficiency: Effects of homocysteine-lowering therapy. Semin Thromb Hemost 2000;26:335 [PMID: 11011851].

Yap S et al: The intellectual abilities of early-treated individuals with pyridoxine-nonresponsive homocystinuria due to cystathionine beta-synthase deficiency. J Inherit Metab Dis 2001;24(4):437 [PMID: 11596648].

## NONKETOTIC HYPERGLYCINEMIA

Inherited deficiency of various subunits of the glycine cleavage enzyme causes nonketotic hyperglycinemia. Glycine accumulation in the brain is thought to cause excessive stimulation of the N-methyl-D-aspartate (NMDA) receptor. In its most severe form, also termed glycine encephalopathy, the condition manifests in the newborn period as unremitting seizures, hypotonia, hiccups, a burst suppression pattern on electroencephalography, and (usually) death in infancy. Some patients with this disorder present with seizures later in infancy or with developmental delay in childhood. All forms of the condition are inherited as autosomal recessive traits.

### Diagnosis

Nonketotic hyperglycinemia should be suspected in any infant with intractable seizures, especially when hiccupping, and is confirmed by demonstrating a large increase in glycine in CSF, with the ratio of CSF glycine to serum glycine being abnormally high. Demonstration of the specific enzyme defect by liver biopsy is necessary only if the parents are contemplating having more children, because prenatal diagnosis is possible only by assaying the enzyme in chorionic villus samples.

### Treatment

Treatment is generally unsuccessful. Early efforts to use sodium benzoate therapy were thought to be without effect on long-term outcome, but recent studies suggest that this drug may be useful in seizure control. Dextromethorphan has also been advocated in the treatment of nonketotic hyperglycinemia with some evidence of improved seizure control and improved developmental progress.

Aliefendioglu D et al: Transient nonketotic hyperglycinemia: Two case reports and literature review. Pediatr Neurol 2003;28(2):151 [PMID: 12699870].

Applegarth DA, Toone JR: Nonketotic hyperglycinemia (glycine encephalopathy): Laboratory diagnosis. Mol Genet Metab 2001;74(1-2):139 [PMID: 11592811].

Toone JR et al: Biochemical and molecular investigations of patients with nonketotic hyperglycinemia. Mol Genet Metab 2000;70:116 [PMID: 10873393].

# ■ ORGANIC ACIDEMIAS

Organic acidemias are disorders of amino and fatty acid metabolism in which nonamino organic acids accumulate in serum and urine. These conditions are usually diagnosed by examining organic acids in urine, a complex procedure that requires considerable interpretive expertise and is usually performed only in specialized laboratories. Table 32–4 lists the clinical features of organic acidemias, together with the urine organic acid patterns typical of each. Additional details about some of the more important organic acidemias are provided in the sections that follow.

## KETOTIC HYPERGLYCINEMIAS (Propionic & Methylmalonic Acidemia)

Idiopathic hyperglycinemia was first reported in 1961 as a syndrome of mental retardation and episodic ketoacidosis, neutropenia, thrombocytopenia, osteoporosis, and hyperglycinemia induced by protein intake or infection. It was then renamed ketotic hyperglycinemia to distinguish it from nonketotic hyperglycinemia,

***Table 32–4.*** Clinical and laboratory features of organic acidemias.

| Disorder | Enzyme Defect | Clinical and Laboratory Features |
|---|---|---|
| Isovaleric acidemia | Isovaleryl-CoA dehydro-genase | Acidosis and odor of sweaty feet in infancy, or growth retardation and episodes of vomiting, lethargy, acidosis, and odor. Isovalerylglycine always present in urine, with 3-hydroxyisovaleric acid during acute episodes. |
| 3-Methylcrotonyl-CoA carboxylase deficiency | 3-Methylcrotonyl-CoA carboxylase | Acidosis and feeding problems in infancy, or Reye-like episodes in older child. 3-Methylcrotonylglycine in urine, usually with 3-hydroxyisovaleric acid. |
| Combined carboxylase deficiency | Holocarboxylase synthetase | Hypotonia and lactic acidosis in infancy. 3-Hydroxyisovaleric acid in urine, often with small amounts of 3-hydroxypropionic and methylcitric acids. Often biotin-responsive. |
| | Biotinidase | Alopecia, seborrheic rash, and ataxia in infancy or childhood. Urine organic acids as above. Usually biotin-responsive. |
| 3-Hydroxy-3-methylglutaric acidemia | Hydroxymethylglutaryl-CoA lyase | Hypoglycemia and acidosis in infancy; Reye-like episodes with non-ketotic hypoglycemia in older children. 3-Hydroxy-3-methylglutaric, 3-methylglutaconic, and 3-hydroxyisovaleric acids in urine. |
| 3-Ketothiolase deficiency | 3-Ketothiolase | Ketotic hyperglycinemia syndrome in infancy, or developmental and growth retardation with episodes of vomiting, acidosis, and encephalopathy. 2-Methyl-3-hydroxybutyric and 2-methylacetoacetic acids and tiglylglycine in urine, especially after isoleucine load. |
| Propionic acidemia | Propionyl-CoA car-boxylase | Hyperammonemia and metabolic acidosis in infancy; ketotic hyperglycinemia syndrome later. 3-Hydroxypropionic and methylcitric acids in urine, with 3-hydroxy- and 3-ketovaleric acids during ketotic episodes. |
| Methylmalonic acidemia | Methylmalonyl-CoA mutase | Clinical features same as in propionic acidemia. Methylmalonic acid in urine, often with 3-hydroxypropionic and methylcitric acids. |
| | Defects in $B_{12}$ biosynthesis | Clinical features same as above when only adenosyl-$B_{12}$ synthesis is decreased: early neurologic features prominent when accompanied by decreased synthesis of methyl-$B_{12}$. In latter instance, hypomethioninemia and homocystinuria accompany methylmalonic aciduria. |
| Pyroglutamic acidemia | Glutathione synthetase | Acidosis and hemolytic anemia in infancy; chronic acidosis later. Pyroglutamic acid in urine. |
| Glutaric acidemia type I | Glutaryl-CoA dehydro-genase | Progressive extrapyramidal movement disorder in childhood, with episodes of acidosis, vomiting, and encephalopathy. Glutaric acid in urine, usually with 3-hydroxyglutaric acid. |
| Glutaric acidemia type II | Electron transfer flavo-protein (ETF) ETF:ubiquinone oxido-reductase (ETF dehy-drogenase) | Hypoglycemia, acidosis, hyperammonemia, and odor of sweaty feet in infancy, often with polycystic and dysplastic kidneys. Later onset may be with episodes of hypoketotic hypoglycemia or slowly progressive skeletal myopathy. Glutaric, ethylmalonic, 3-hydroxyisovaleric, isovalerylglycine, and 2-hydroxyglutaric acids in urine, often with sarcosine in serum and urine. |
| 4-Hydroxybutyric acidemia | Succinic semialdehyde dehydrogenase | Seizures and developmental retardation. 4-Hydroxybutyric acid in urine. |

CoA = coenzyme A.

described in the preceding section. It is now known that the syndrome is almost always due to propionic or methylmalonic acidemia.

The oxidation of threonine, valine, methionine, and isoleucine through propionyl- and L-methylmalonyl-CoA is diagrammed in Figure 32–2. Propionic acidemia is due to a defect in the biotin-containing enzyme propionyl-CoA carboxylase, and methylmalonic acidemia is due to a defect in methylmalonyl-CoA mutase. In most cases the latter is due to a defect in the mutase apoenzyme, but in others it is due to a defect in the biosynthesis of its adenosyl-$B_{12}$ coenzyme. In some of these defects, only the synthesis of adenosyl-$B_{12}$ is blocked; in others, the synthesis of methyl-$B_{12}$ is also blocked.

Clinical symptoms in propionic and methylmalonic acidemia vary according to the location and severity of the enzyme block. Children with severe blocks present with acute, life-threatening metabolic acidemia and hyperammonemia early in infancy or with metabolic acidemia, vomiting, and failure to thrive during the first few months of life. Children with less severe blocks may present later with only mild or moderate mental retardation.

All known forms of propionic and methylmalonic acidemia are transmitted as autosomal recessive traits and can be diagnosed in utero.

## Diagnosis

Laboratory findings include hyperglycinemia and hyperglycinuria, increases in certain urinary organic acids (see Table 32–4), and, in some forms of abnormal $B_{12}$ metabolism, hypomethioninemic homocystinuria.

## Treatment

Patients with enzyme blocks in $B_{12}$ metabolism usually respond to massive doses of vitamin $B_{12}$ given intramuscularly, whereas nonresponders require amino acid restriction and correction of their rather constant metabolic acidemia. Secondary carnitine deficiency has been reported, and blood carnitine should be measured and supplemented if required. Liver transplantation may improve outcome.

Andersson HC et al: Long-term outcome in treated combined methylmalonic acidemia and homocystinemia. Genet Med 1999;1:146 [PMID: 11258350].

Ogier de Baulny H, Saudubray JM: Branched-chain organic acidurias. Semin Neonatol 2002;7(1):65 [PMID: 12069539].

Varvogli L et al: High cognitive outcome in an adolescent with mut-methylmalonic acidemia. Am J Med Genet 2000;96: 192 [PMID: 10893496].

patient/parent support group website with useful information for families:

www.oaanews.org

# ISOVALERIC ACIDEMIA

Isovaleric acidemia, due to deficiency of isovaleryl-CoA dehydrogenase in the leucine oxidative pathway, was the first organic acidemia to be described in humans. Patients with this disorder usually present with poor feeding, metabolic acidosis, seizures, and an odor of sweaty feet during the first few days of life, with coma and death occurring if the condition is not recognized and appropriate therapy started quickly. Other patients show a more chronic course, with episodes of vomiting, lethargy, and urine (and body) odor precipitated by intercurrent infections or increased protein intake. The condition is inherited as an autosomal recessive trait and can be diagnosed in utero.

## Diagnosis

Isovaleric acidemia and glutaric acidemia type II are the only conditions in which the characteristic odor of sweaty feet occurs. Isovalerylglycine is consistently detected in the urine by organic acid chromatography.

## Treatment

Providing a low-protein diet or diets low in leucine or all three branched-chain amino acids is effective. Oral administration of glycine appears to prevent complications during acute infections but poses a risk of neuro-

Threonine
Valine
Methionine
Isoleucine

Propionyl—CoA $\xrightarrow{1}$ D—Methylmalonyl—CoA → L—Methylmalonyl—CoA $\xrightarrow{2}$ Succinyl—CoA

Adenosyl—$B_{12}$

Vitamin $B_{12}$ —·—<

Methyl—$B_{12}$

*Figure 32–2.* Oxidation of propionyl-CoA to succinyl-CoA. **1:** Propionyl-CoA carboxylase. **2:** Methylmalonyl-CoA mutase.

toxicity due to severe hyperglycinemia. Oral administration of L-carnitine may also be indicated.

## COMBINED CARBOXYLASE DEFICIENCY

Holocarboxylase synthetase and biotinidase are two enzymes of biotin metabolism in mammals. Holocarboxylase synthetase covalently binds biotin to the apocarboxylases for pyruvate, 3-methylcrotonyl-CoA, and propionyl-CoA; and biotinidase releases biotin from these proteins and from proteins in the diet. Recessively inherited deficiency of either enzyme causes deficiency of all three carboxylases (ie, multiple carboxylase deficiency). Patients with holocarboxylase synthetase deficiency usually present in the neonatal period with hypotonia; those with biotinidase deficiency more often present somewhat later with a syndrome of ataxia, seborrhea, and alopecia. Because many patients with biotinidase deficiency do not have typical symptoms but do develop neurologic sequelae, newborn screening for the condition is justified.

### Diagnosis

This diagnosis should be considered in patients with typical symptoms or in those with primary lactic acidosis. Urine organic acids are usually but not always abnormal (see Table 32–4). Diagnosis is usually by enzyme assay. Biotinidase can be assayed in serum; holocarboxylase synthetase, in leukocytes or fibroblasts.

### Treatment

Oral administration of biotin in large doses often reverses the organic aciduria within days and the clinical symptoms within days to weeks. The incidence of hearing loss is high even in patients receiving treatment.

Gulati S et al: Biotinidase deficiency—A treatable entity. Indian J Pediatr 2000;67:464 [PMID: 10932969].

Morrone A et al: Clinical findings and biochemical and molecular analysis of four patients with holocarboxylase synthetase deficiency. Am J Med Genet 2002;111(1):10 [PMID: 12124727].

Muhl A et al: Molecular characterisation of 34 patients with biotinidase deficiency ascertained by newborn screening and family investigation. Eur J Hum Genet 2001;9:237 [PMID: 11313766].

Navarro PC et al: Cutaneous and neurologic manifestations of biotinidase deficiency. Int J Dermatol 2000;39:363 [PMID: 10849128].

Pacheco-Alvarez D et al: Biotin in metabolism and its relationship to human disease. Arch Med Res 2002;33(5):439 [PMID: 12459313].

## GLUTARIC ACIDEMIA TYPE I

Glutaric acidemia type I is due to deficiency of glutaryl-CoA dehydrogenase and causes a progressive extrapyramidal movement disorder in childhood, with dystonia and athetosis and neuronal degeneration in the caudate and putamen. Macrocephaly at birth is common. Death often occurs during the first decade, but the clinical course is highly variable, and several patients have had only mild neurologic abnormalities. Children with glutaric acidemia type I may present with retinal hemorrhages and intracranial bleeding, strongly resembling shaken baby syndrome. The condition is inherited as an autosomal recessive trait and prenatal diagnosis is possible.

### Diagnosis

Glutaric acidemia type I should be suspected in any patient with progressive dystonia or athetosis. The diagnosis is supported by demonstration of glutaric and 3-hydroxyglutaric acids in urine by organic acid analysis. Deficiency of glutaryl-CoA dehydrogenase can be demonstrated in fibroblasts, leukocytes, and, for prenatal diagnosis, amniotic cells.

### Treatment

Restriction of dietary lysine and tryptophan is indicated, but neurologic symptoms, once present, may not resolve. A variety of drugs that alter neurotransmitter levels, especially those of γ-aminobutyric acid, may be used to control dystonia. Studies suggest that early dietary treatment and aggressive management of intercurrent illness may prevent neurologic deterioration in some patients.

Bjugstad KB et al: Age at symptom onset predicts severity of motor impairment and clinical outcome of glutaric acidemia type 1. J Pediatr 2000;137:681 [PMID: 11060535].

Strauss KA et al: Type I glutaric aciduria, part 1: Natural history of 77 patients. Am J Med Genet 2003;121C(1):38 [PMID: 12888985].

Strauss KA, Morton DH: Type I glutaric aciduria, part 2: A model of acute striatal necrosis. Am J Med Genet 2003;121C(1): 53 [PMID: 12888986].

## ■ DISORDERS OF FATTY ACID OXIDATION & CARNITINE

### FATTY ACID OXIDATION DISORDERS

Deficiencies of very-long-chain and medium-chain acyl-CoA dehydrogenase (VLCAD, MCAD) and long-chain hydroxyacyl-CoA dehydrogenase (LCHAD), three enzymes of fatty acid β-oxidation, usually cause Reye-like episodes of hypoketotic hypoglycemia, mild hyperammonemia, hepatomegaly and encephalopathy, or, less often, sudden death in infancy. The long- and medium-chain defects can usually be distinguished clinically; the long-chain defects often cause early severe hypotonia and cardiomyopathy. MCAD deficiency is common, occurring in perhaps 1:9000 live births, and recent studies suggest that LCHAD deficiency may also be common. Although Reye-like episodes may be fatal, they tend to become less frequent and severe with time, and prolonged survival is typical of MCAD deficiency, with few deaths after diagnosis is made and treatment instituted. In VLCAD and LCHAD deficiencies, cardiomyopathy is the direct result of the defect in the oxidation of long-chain fatty acids, and progressive liver disease and renal tubular acidosis may also be present.

Short-chain acyl-CoA dehydrogenase (SCAD) deficiency is characterized by the presence of ethylmalonic acid in the urine, and although some patients have symptoms similar to those seen in MCAD deficiency, many remain asymptomatic. Glutaric acidemia type II results from defects in the transfer of electrons from fatty acid oxidation and some amino acid oxidation into the respiratory chain. Some patients with glutaric acidemia type II have a clinical presentation resembling MCAD deficiency. Other patients with glutaric acidemia type II, especially those with severe neonatal presentation, also have renal cystic disease and dysmorphic features.

These conditions are inherited as autosomal recessive traits. LCHAD deficiency is an example of a condition in which a heterozygous individual may manifest symptoms of disease. The pregnancies of mothers with LCHAD-deficient fetuses may be complicated by acute fatty liver of pregnancy (AFLP) or HELLP (hemolysis, elevated liver enzymes, and low platelets) syndrome.

## Diagnosis

Suspicion should be increased by the lack of an appropriate ketone response to fasting. Patients with MCAD deficiency may excrete phenylpropionylglycine and hexanoylglycine in the urine and have increased octanoylcarnitine in blood; urine and blood findings in glutaric acidemia type II and SCAD deficiency are often diagnostic, but are highly variable in VLCAD and LCHAD deficiencies. A common mutation has been found in MCAD deficiency, which may be useful in confirming the diagnosis; a common mutation in LCHAD deficiency may be similarly used. Assays of MCAD activity in fibroblasts are necessary only when typical biochemistry is not found. Fibroblast studies may be required for diagnosis of VLCAD, LCHAD, or

SCAD deficiencies. The finding of normal urine organic acids does not exclude these conditions, because excretion of dicarboxylic acids and other products of microsomal and peroxisomal oxidation of fatty acids can be intermittent.

## Treatment

Acute management is directed toward preventing or reversing catabolism and hypoglycemia. Long-term measures include providing carbohydrate snacks before bedtime and vigorous treatment of intercurrent infections. Because cardiomyopathy and muscle weakness in MCAD deficiency may be due to secondary carnitine deficiency, oral administration of carnitine is typically prescribed; carnitine use in VLCAD and LCHAD is controversial. Restriction of dietary long-chain fats is controversial in MCAD deficiency, but is required for VLCAD and LCHAD deficiencies. Medium-chain triglycerides are contraindicated in MCAD deficiency because they may cause serum octanoic acid to rise to neurotoxic concentrations, but are an essential energy source for patients with VLCAD and LCHAD deficiencies. Riboflavin may be very beneficial in some patients with glutaric acidemia type II.

Bennett MJ et al: Inborn errors of mitochondrial fatty acid oxidation. Crit Rev Clin Lab Sci 2000;37:1 [PMID: 10737439].

Gregersen N et al: Prevalent mutations in fatty acid oxidation disorders: Diagnostic considerations. Eur J Pediatr 2000;159 Suppl 3):S213 [PMID: 11216903].

Gregersen N et al: Mutation analysis in mitochondrial fatty acid oxidation defects: Exemplified by acyl-CoA dehydrogenase deficiencies, with special focus on genotype-phenotype relationship. Hum Mutat 2001;18(3):169 [PMID: 11524729].

Rakheja D et al: Long-chain L-3-hydroxyacyl-coenzyme a dehydrogenase deficiency: A molecular and biochemical review. Lab Invest 2002;82(7):815 [PMID: 12118083].

Rinaldo P, Matern D: Disorders of fatty acid transport and mitochondrial oxidation: Challenges and dilemmas of metabolic evaluation. Genet Med 2000;2:338.

Rinaldo P et al: Fatty acid oxidation disorders. Annu Rev Physiol 2002;64:477 [PMID: 11826276].

Sim KG et al: Strategies for the diagnosis of mitochondrial fatty acid beta-oxidation disorders. Clin Chim Acta 2002;323 (1-2):37 [PMID: 12135806].

Treem WR: Mitochondrial fatty acid oxidation and acute fatty liver of pregnancy. Semin Gastrointest Dis 2002;13(1):55 [PMID: 11944635].

Treem WR: New developments in the pathophysiology, clinical spectrum, and diagnosis of disorders of fatty acid oxidation. Curr Opin Pediatr 2000;12:463.

Vockley J, Whiteman DA: Defects of mitochondrial beta-oxidation: A growing group of disorders. Neuromuscul Disord 2002;12(3):235 [PMID: 11801395].

Patient/parent support group website with useful information for families: www.fodsupport.org

## CARNITINE

Carnitine is an essential nutrient found in highest concentrations in red meats. Its primary function is to transport long-chain fatty acids into mitochondria for oxidation. Primary defects of carnitine biosynthesis and transport (related to defects of carnitine palmitoyl transport protein I or II, or carnitine translocase) may manifest as Reye syndrome, myoglobinuria, hypotonia, or cardiomyopathy. These disorders are exceedingly rare compared with secondary carnitine deficiency or insufficiency, which may be due to diet (especially intravenous alimentation), renal losses, drug therapy (especially valproic acid), and other metabolic disorders (especially disorders of fatty acid oxidation and organic acidemias). The prognosis depends on the cause of the carnitine abnormality.

Carnitine can be measured in blood. Unless the purpose is solely to monitor dietary deficiency, amounts of free and esterified carnitine should be determined. In some situations, muscle carnitine may be low despite normal blood levels. Free and esterified carnitine also can be measured in urine, and specialized laboratories can identify the specific ester present. If carnitine insufficiency is suspected, the patient should be evaluated to rule out disorders that might cause secondary carnitine deficiency.

Oral levocarnitine is used in carnitine deficiency or insufficiency in doses of 25–100 mg/kg/d or higher. Levocarnitine may be added to intravenous alimentation solutions, and high-dose intravenous levocarnitine is available. Treatment is aimed at maintaining normal free carnitine levels. Carnitine supplementation in patients with some disorders of fatty acid oxidation and organic acidosis may also augment excretion of accumulated metabolites in addition to ameliorating carnitine insufficiency. Supplementation may not prevent metabolic crises in such patients, however, even when serum carnitine has been normalized.

Bartlett K, Pourfarzam M: Defects of beta-oxidation including carnitine deficiency. Int Rev Neurobiol 2002;53:469 [PMID: 12512350].

Evangeliou A, Vlassopoulos D: Carnitine metabolism and deficit— When supplementation is necessary? Curr Pharm Biotechnol 2003;4(3):211 [PMID: 12769764].

Kerner J, Hoppel C: Genetic disorders of carnitine metabolism and their nutritional management. Annu Rev Nutr 1998:18: 179 [PMID: 9706223].

Lopriore E et al: Carnitine-acylcarnitine translocase deficiency: Phenotype, residual enzyme activity and outcome. Eur J Pediatr 2001;160:101 [PMID: 11271379].

Roschinger W et al: Carnitine-acylcarnitine translocase deficiency: Metabolic consequences of an impaired mitochondrial carnitine cycle. Clin Chim Acta 2000;298:55 [PMID: 10876004].

Rubio-Gozalbo ME et al: Carnitine-acylcarnitine translocase deficiency: Case report and review of the literature. Acta Paediatr 2003;92(4):501 [PMID: 12801121].

Scaglia F, Longo N: Primary and secondary alterations of neonatal carnitine metabolism. Semin Perinatol 1999;23:152 [PMID: 10331466].

## HYPOXANTHINE–GUANINE PHOSPHORIBOSYLTRANSFERASE DEFICIENCY (Lesch–Nyhan Syndrome)

Hypoxanthine–guanine phosphoribosyltransferase (HPRT) is the enzyme that converts the purine bases hypoxanthine and guanine to inosine monophosphate (IMP) and guanosine monophosphate (GMP), respectively. The X-linked recessive disorder with complete deficiency is characterized by CNS dysfunction and purine overproduction with hyperuricemia and hyperuricuria. Depending on the residual activity of the mutant enzyme, male hemizygous individuals may be severely disabled and show choreoathetosis, spasticity, and compulsive, mutilating lip and finger biting, or they may present with only gouty arthritis and urate ureterolithiasis. The enzyme deficiency can be demonstrated in erythrocytes, fibroblasts, and cultured amniotic cells; this disorder can thus be diagnosed in utero.

Although the cause of the CNS dysfunction in Lesch–Nyhan syndrome remains obscure, the absent or less severe CNS manifestations of purine nucleoside phosphorylase deficiency suggest that the problem relates to accumulation of substrate behind the block.

### Diagnosis

Diagnosis is made by demonstrating an elevated uric acid:creatinine ratio in urine, followed by demonstration of enzyme deficiency in red blood cells or fibroblasts.

### Treatment

Allopurinol and probenecid may be given to reduce hyperuricemia but do not affect the neurologic status. Insertion of the HPRT gene into cultured cells from affected patients and into experimental animals has been effective, and such experiments offer promise as models for human gene therapy in the future.

Jinnah HA et al: The spectrum of inherited mutations causing HPRT deficiency: 75 new cases and a review of 196 previously reported cases. Mutat Res 2000;463:309 [PMID: 11018746].

Puig JG et al: The spectrum of hypoxanthine–guanine phosphoribosyltransferase (HPRT) deficiency: Clinical experience based on 22 patients from 18 Spanish families. Medicine 2001;80:102 [PMID: 11307586].

Saito Y, Takashima S: Neurotransmitter changes in the pathophysiology of Lesch-Nyhan syndrome. Brain Dev 2000;22 (Suppl 1):S122 [PMID: 10984673].

Schretlen DJ et al: Neurocognitive functioning in Lesch–Nyhan disease and partial hypoxanthine–guanine phosphoribosyltransferase deficiency. J Int Neuropsychol Soc 2001;7(7):805 [PMID: 11771623].

# LYSOSOMAL DISEASES

Lysosomes are cellular organelles in which complex macromolecules are degraded by specific acid hydrolases. Deficiency of a lysosomal enzyme causes its substrate to accumulate in lysosomes of tissues that degrade it, creating a characteristic clinical picture. These so-called storage disorders are classified as mucopolysaccharidoses, lipidoses, or mucolipidoses depending on the nature of the stored material. Two additional disorders, cystinosis and Salla disease, are caused by defects in lysosomal proteins that normally transport material from the lysosome to the cytoplasm. Table 32–5 lists clinical and laboratory features of these conditions. Most are inherited as autosomal recessive traits, and all can be diagnosed in utero.

The diagnosis of mucopolysaccharidosis is suggested by certain clinical and radiologic findings and urine screening tests. Further tests are needed to determine which mucopolysaccharides are present. Diagnosis should be confirmed by enzyme assays of cultured fibroblasts or leukocytes; this is especially important when the parents are contemplating having more children.

When a lipidosis or mucolipidosis is suspected, diagnosis is made by appropriate enzyme assays of biopsy specimens, cultured skin fibroblasts, and peripheral leukocytes.

Most of these conditions cannot be treated effectively, although increasing evidence indicates that hematopoietic stem cell transplantation may affect the course of some lysosomal diseases. Gaucher disease is treated effectively with infusions of natural enzyme modified to allow uptake of the enzyme by lysosomes. Enzyme replacement products have been developed to treat other lysosomal storage disorders, such as Pompe disease, Fabry disease, and several mucopolysaccharidoses, but data on long-term efficacy is not yet available.

Beck M: Variable clinical presentation in lysosomal storage disorders. J Inherit Metab Dis 2001;24 (Suppl 2):47; discussion 45 [PMID: 11758678].

Caillaud C, Poenaru L: Gene therapy in lysosomal diseases. Biomed Pharmacother 2000;54:505 [PMID: 11130848].

Charrow J et al: The Gaucher registry: Demographics and disease characteristics of 1698 patients with Gaucher disease. Arch Intern Med 2000;160:2835 [PMID: 11025794].

Charrow J et al: Gaucher disease: Recommendations on diagnosis, evaluation, and monitoring. Arch Intern Med 1998; 158:1754 [PMID: 9738604].

Desnick RJ et al: Fabry disease, an under-recognized multisystemic disorder: Expert recommendations for diagnosis, management, and enzyme replacement therapy. Ann Intern Med 2003;138(4):338 [PMID: 12585833].

Elstein D et al: Gaucher disease: Pediatric concerns. Paediatr Drugs 2002;4(7):417 [PMID: 12083970].

Krivit W: Stem cell bone marrow transplantation in patients with metabolic storage diseases. Adv Pediatr 2002;49:359 [PMID: 12214779].

Wenger DA et al: Insights into the diagnosis and treatment of lysosomal storage diseases. Arch Neurol 2003;60(3):322 [PMID: 12633142].

Wraith JE: Lysosomal disorders. Semin Neonatol 2002;7(1):75 [PMID: 12069540].

Patient/parent support group websites with useful information for families: www.mpssociety.org and www.ulf.org

# PEROXISOMAL DISEASES

Peroxisomes are intracellular organelles that contain a large number of enzymes, many of which are oxidases linked to catalase or peroxidase. Among the enzyme systems in peroxisomes is one for β-oxidation of very-long-chain fatty acids (which is analogous in many ways to the system for fatty acid oxidation in mitochondria) and another for plasmalogen biosynthesis. In addition, peroxisomes contain oxidases for D- and L-amino acids, pipecolic acid and phytanic acid, and an enzyme (alanine-glyoxylate aminotransferase) that effects transamination of glyoxylate to glycine.

In some peroxisomal diseases, many enzymes are deficient. Zellweger (cerebrohepatorenal) syndrome, the best known among these, can be caused by several defects in organelle assembly. Patients present in infancy with seizures, hypotonia, characteristic facies with a large forehead, and hepatomegaly; at autopsy renal cysts and absent peroxisomes are found. Neonatal adrenoleukodystrophy and hyperpipecolic acidemia have similar clinical and laboratory findings and multiple enzyme deficiencies in cultured fibroblasts, but peroxisomes are usually detected in tissues.

In other peroxisomal diseases, only a single enzyme is deficient. Primary hyperoxaluria (alanine-glyoxylate aminotransferase deficiency), X-linked adrenoleukodystrophy and adrenomyeloneuropathy (very-long-chain acyl-CoA ligase deficiency), and adult Refsum disease (phytanic acid oxidase deficiency) are disorders caused by deficiency of single peroxisomal enzymes.

Except for childhood adrenoleukodystrophy, which is X-linked, all peroxisomal diseases are transmitted as autosomal recessive traits and can be diagnosed in

***Table 32–5.*** Clinical and laboratory features of lysosomal storage diseases.

| Disorder | Enzyme Defect | Clinical and Laboratory Features |
|---|---|---|
| **I. Mucopolysaccharidoses** | | |
| Hurler syndrome | α-Iduronidase | Autosomal-recessive. Mental retardation, hepatosplenomegaly, umbilical hernia, coarse facies, corneal clouding, dorsolumbar gibbus, severe heart disease. Heparan sulfate and dermatan sulfate in urine. |
| Scheie syndrome | α-Iduronidase (incomplete) | Autosomal-recessive. Corneal clouding, stiff joints, normal intellect. Clinical types intermediate between Hurler and Scheie common. Heparan sulfate and dermatan sulfate in urine. |
| Hunter syndrome | Sulfoiduronate sulfatase | X-linked recessive. Coarse facies, hepatosplenomegaly, mental retardation variable. Corneal clouding and gibbus not present. Heparan sulfate and dermatan sulfate in urine. |
| Sanfilippo syndrome:<br>    Type A<br>    Type B<br><br>    Type C<br><br><br>    Type D | Sulfamidase<br>α-N-Acetylglucos-<br>    aminidase<br>Acetyl-CoA: α-<br>    glucosaminide-N-<br>    acetyltransferase<br>α-N-acetylglucosamine-<br>    6-sulfatase | Autosomal-recessive. Severe mental retardation with comparatively mild skeletal changes, visceromegaly, and facial coarseness. Types cannot be differentiated clinically. Heparan sulfate in urine. |
| Morquio syndrome | N-Acetylgalactosamine-<br>    6-sulfatase | Autosomal-recessive. Severe skeletal changes, platyspondylisis, corneal clouding. Keratan sulfate in urine. |
| Maroteaux–Lamy syndrome | N-Acetylgalactosamine-<br>    4-sulfatase | Autosomal-recessive. Coarse facies, growth retardation, dorsolumbar gibbus, corneal clouding, hepatosplenomegaly, normal intellect. Dermatan sulfate in urine. |
| β-Glucuronidase deficiency | β-Glucuronidase | Autosomal-recessive. Varies from mental retardation, dorsolumbar gibbus, corneal clouding, and hepatosplenomegaly to mild facial coarseness, retardation, and loose joints. Hearing loss common. Dermatan sulfate or heparan sulfate in urine. |
| **II. Mucolipidoses** | | |
| Mannosidosis | α-Mannosidase | Autosomal-recessive. Varies from severe mental retardation, coarse facies, short stature, skeletal changes, and hepatosplenomegaly to mild facial coarseness and loose joints. Hearing loss common. Abnormal oligosaccharides in urine. |
| Fucosidosis | α-Fucosidase | Autosomal-recessive. Variable: coarse facies, skeletal changes, hepatosplenomegaly, occasional angiokeratoma corporis diffusum. Abnormal oligosaccharides in urine. |
| I-cell disease (mucolipidosis II) | N-Acetylglucosaminyl-<br>    phosphotransferase | Autosomal-recessive; severe and mild forms known. Very short stature, mental retardation, early facial coarsening, clear cornea, stiffness of joints. Increased lysosomal enzymes in serum. Abnormal sialyl oligosaccharides in urine. |
| Sialidosis | N-Acetylineuraminidase<br>    (sialidase) | Autosomal-recessive. Mental retardation, coarse facies, skeletal dysplasia, myoclonic seizures, macular cherry-red spot. Abnormal sialyl oligosaccharides in urine. |

(continued)

***Table 32–5.*** Clinical and laboratory features of lysosomal storage diseases. (continued)

| Disorder | Enzyme Defect | Clinical and Laboratory Features |
|---|---|---|
| **III. Lipidoses** | | |
| Niemann–Pick disease | Sphingomyelinase | Autosomal recessive. Acute and chronic forms known. Acute neuronopathic form common in eastern European Jews. Accumulation of sphingomyelin in lysosomes of RE system and CNS. Hepatosplenomegaly, developmental retardation, macular cherry-red spot. Death by 1–4 y.. |
| Metachromatic leuko-dystrophy | Arylsulfatase A | Autosomal recessive. Late infantile form, with onset at 1–4 y, most common. Accumulation of sulfatide in white matter. Gait disturbances (ataxia), motor incoordination, and dementia. Death usually in first decade. |
| Krabbe disease (globoid cell leukodystrophy) | Galactocerebroside β-galactosidase | Autosomal recessive. Globoid cells in white matter. Onset at 3–6 mos with seizures, irritability, and retardation. Death by 1–2 y. Juvenile and adult forms are rare. |
| Fabry disease | α-Galactosidase A | X-linked recessive. Storage of trihexosylceramide in endothelial cells. Pain in extremities, angiokeratoma corporis diffusum and (later) poor vision, hypertension, and renal failure. |
| Farber disease | Ceramidase | Autosomal recessive. Storage of ceramide in tissues. Subcutaneous nodules, arthropathy with deformed and painful joints, and poor growth and development. Death within first year. |
| Gaucher disease | Glucocerebroside β-glucosidase | Autosomal recessive. Acute neuronopathic form: Accumulation of glucocerebroside in lysosomes of RE system and CNS. Retardation, hepatosplenomegaly, macular cherry-red spot, and Gaucher cells in bone marrow. Death by 1–2 y. Chronic form common in eastern European Jews. Accumulation of spingomyelin in lysosomes of RE system. Hepatosplenomegaly and flask-shaped osteolytic bone lesions. Consistent with normal life expectancy. |
| $G_{M1}$ gangliosidosis | $G_{M1}$ ganglioside β-galactosidase | Autosomal recessive. Accumulation of $G_{M1}$ ganglioside in lysosomes of RE system and CNS. Infantile form: Abnormalities at birth with dysostosis multiplex, hepatosplenomegaly, macular cherry-red spot, and death by 2 years. Juvenile form: Normal development to 1 year of age, then ataxia, weakness, dementia, and death by 4–5 y. Occasional inferior beaking of vertebral bodies of L1 and L2. |
| $G_{M2}$ gangliosidoses<br>Tay–Sachs disease<br><br>Sandhoff disease | β-N-Acetylhexos-aminidase A<br><br>β-N-Acetylhexos-aminidase A & B | Autosomal recessive. Tay-Sachs disease common in eastern European Jews; Sandhoff disease is panethnic. Clinical phenotypes are identical, with accumulation of $G_{M2}$ ganglioside in lysosomes of CNS. Onset at age 3–6 months, with hypotonia, hyperacusis, retardation, and macular cherry-red spot. Death by 2–3 years. Juvenile and adult onset forms of Tay-Sachs disease are rare. |
| Wolman disease | Acid lipase | Autosomal recessive. Accumulation of cholesterol esters and triglycerides in lysosomes of reticuloendothelial system. Onset in infancy with gastrointestinal symptoms and hepatosplenomegaly, and death by 3–6 mos. Adrenals commonly enlarged and calcified. |

CNS = central nervous system.

utero. Bone marrow transplantation may be effective treatment for some patients with adrenoleukodystrophy. Dietary treatment may have some promise for female carriers of X-linked adrenomyeloneuropathy, and diet therapy is being attempted in other peroxisomal disorders.

## Diagnosis

The best screening test for Zellweger syndrome, hyperpipecolic acidemia, X-linked adrenoleukodystrophy, neonatal adrenoleukodystrophy, and infantile Refsum disease is determination of very-long-chain fatty acids in serum or plasma; the levels of these acids are increased in all of these conditions. Urine bile acids are abnormal in other peroxisomal disorders; together, these studies identify most peroxisomal diseases. Tissue biopsy and appropriate enzyme assays are needed for confirmation, especially when the parents plan further pregnancies.

Baumgartner MR, Saudubray JM: Peroxisomal disorders. Semin Neonatol 2002;7(1):85 [PMID: 12069541].

Gartner J: Disorders related to peroxisomal membranes. J Inherit Metab Dis 2000;23:264[PMID: 10863942].

Gartner J: Organelle disease: Peroxisomal disorders. Eur J Pediatr 2000;159 (Suppl):S236[PMID: 11216907].

Gould SJ, Valle D: Peroxisome biogenesis disorders: Genetics and cell biology. Trends Genet 2000;16:340 [PMID: 10904262].

McGuinness MC et al: Therapeutic developments in peroxisome biogenesis disorders. Expert Opin Investig Drugs 2000;9: 1985 [PMID: 11060787].

Percy AK, Rutledge SL: Adrenoleukodystrophy and related disorders. Ment Retard Dev Disabil Res Rev 2001;7(3):179 [PMID: 11553934].

Suzuki Y et al: Clinical, biochemical and genetic aspects and neuronal migration in peroxisome biogenesis disorders. J Inherit Metab Dis 2001;24:151 [PMID: 11405337].

Suzuki Y et al: Genetic and molecular bases of peroxisome biogenesis disorders. Genet Med 2001;3(5):372 [PMID: 11545691].

# ■ CARBOHYDRATE-DEFICIENT GLYCOPROTEIN SYNDROMES

A variety of proteins, including many enzymes, require glycosylation with various carbohydrate moieties for normal function. The carbohydrate-deficient glycoprotein syndromes are a family of disorders that result from failures of glycosylation. Children with type I disease usually present with prenatal growth disturbance, often with abnormal fat distribution, cerebellar hypoplasia, typical facial dysmorphic features, and mental retardation. The typical course is remarkable for chronic liver disease, peripheral neuropathy, endocrinopathies, retinopathy, and, in some patients, acute life-threatening events. Biochemical differences and variations in clinical course (eg, the absence of peripheral neuropathy) characterize the other types. Pathophysiology probably relates to defects of those biochemical pathways that require glycosylated proteins. The syndromes appear so far to be inherited in an autosomal recessive manner, and frequency was initially estimated to be as high as 1:20,000 in northern Europe.

## Diagnosis

Diagnosis is supported by finding altered levels of glycosylated enzymes or other proteins such as transferrin, thyroxine-binding globulin, lysosomal enzymes, and clotting factors, but these levels may be normal in carbohydrate-deficient glycoprotein syndromes or altered in other conditions. Diagnosis is confirmed by demonstration of typical patterns of altered isoelectric focusing of selected proteins, with most diagnostic laboratories examining serum transferrin. Some patients with type I carbohydrate-deficient glycoprotein syndrome may exhibit deficient activity of phosphomannomutase in fibroblasts.

## Treatment

Treatment is supportive, with opportunity to monitor and provide early treatment for expected clinical features. Mannose supplementation has been beneficial in the treatment of patients with type 1b deficiency.

Grunewald S et al: Congenital disorders of glycosylation: A review. Pediatr Res 2002;52(5):618 [PMID: 12409504].

Jaeken J, Carchon H: Congenital disorders of glycosylation: The rapidly growing tip of the iceberg. Curr Opin Neurol 2001;14(6):811 [PMID: 11723393].

Marquardt T, Denecke J: Congenital disorders of glycosylation: Review of their molecular bases, clinical presentations, and specific therapies. Eur J Pediatr 2003;162(6):359 [PMID: 12756558].

Westphal V et al: Congenital disorders of glycosylation: Have you encountered them? Genet Med 2000; 2:329 [PMID: 11339653].

# ■ SMITH–LEMLI–OPITZ SYNDROME AND DISORDERS OF CHOLESTEROL SYNTHESIS

Several defects of cholesterol synthesis are associated with malformations and neurodevelopmental disability. For example, Smith–Lemli–Opitz (SLO) syndrome is an autosomal recessive disorder caused by a deficiency of the enzyme 7-dehydrocholesterol $\Delta^7$-reductase and is characterized by microcephaly, poor growth, mental retardation, typical dysmorphic features of face and extremities, and frequent malformations of the heart and genitourinary system. Severity ranges from survival with moderate to severe mental retardation to early death. Although deficient synthesis of cholesterol leads directly to deficiency of some hormones and bile acids, the pathophysiology of the malformations remains unclear. Frequency is estimated to be between 1:40,000 and 1:20,000.

## Diagnosis

Presence of abnormal cholesterol metabolites leads to diagnosis. In SLO, elevated 7- and 8-dehydrocholesterol in serum or other tissues, including amniotic fluid, is diagnostic. Serum cholesterol levels may be low, but may be in the normal range. Enzymes of cholesterol synthesis may be assayed in cultured fibroblasts or amniocytes.

## Treatment

Although postnatal treatment does not resolve prenatal injury, supplementation with cholesterol in SLO improves growth and behavior. The role of supplemental bile acids is controversial.

Battaile KP, Steiner RD: Smith–Lemli–Opitz syndrome: The first malformation syndrome associated with defective cholesterol synthesis. Mol Genet Metab 2000;71:154 [PMID: 11001806].

Haas D et al: Inherited disorders of cholesterol biosynthesis. Neuropediatrics 2001;32(3):113 [PMID: 11521206].

Kelley RI: Inborn errors of cholesterol biosynthesis. Adv Pediatr 2000;47:1 [PMID: 10959439].

Kelley RI, Hennekam RC: The Smith–Lemli–Opitz syndrome. J Med Genet 2000;37:321 [PMID: 10807690].

Nowaczyk M, Waye J: The Smith–Lemli–Opitz syndrome: A novel metabolic way of understanding developmental biology, embryogenesis, and dysmorphology. Clin Genet 2001;59:375 [PMID: 11453964].

Porter FD: Malformation syndromes due to inborn errors of cholesterol synthesis. J Clin Invest 2002;110(6):715 [PMID: 12235098].

Porter FD: RSH/Smith–Lemli–Opitz syndrome: A multiple congenital anomaly/mental retardation syndrome due to an inborn error of cholesterol biosynthesis. Mol Genet Metab 2000;71:163 [PMID: 11001807].

Starck L et al: Cholesterol treatment forever? The first Scandinavian trial of cholesterol supplementation in the cholesterol-synthesis defect Smith–Lemli–Opitz syndrome. J Intern Med 2002;252(4):314 [PMID: 12366604].

Tierney E et al: Behavioral phenotype of RSH/Smith–Lemli–Opitz syndrome. Ment Retard Dev Disabil Res Rev 2000;6:131 [PMID: 10899806].

Waterham HR, Wanders RJ: Biochemical and genetic aspects of 7-dehydrocholesterol reductase and Smith–Lemli–Opitz syndrome. Biochem Biophys Acta 2000;1529:340 [PMID: 11111101].

# ■ DISORDERS OF NEUROTRANSMITTER METABOLISM

Abnormalities of neurotransmitter metabolism are increasingly recognized as causes of significant neurodevelopmental disabilities, including in patients presenting with movement disorders (especially dystonia), seizures, abnormal tone, or mental retardation. Presentation ranges from mild (eg, adult onset dopa-responsive dystonia) to severe (eg, intractable seizures with profound mental retardation). In the most severe examples, the newborn has brain dysgenesis as a result of neurotransmitter deficiency in utero.

## Diagnosis

Although some disorders can be diagnosed by examining amino acids or neurotransmitter metabolites in blood or urine, in most cases, diagnosis requires analysis of CSF. Spinal fluid samples for neurotransmitter analysis require special collection and handling as the neurotransmitter levels are graduated along the axis of the CNS and are highly unstable once the sample is collected.

## Treatment

For some conditions, such as pyridoxine-responsive seizures or dopa-responsive dystonia, response to treatment can be dramatic. For others, response to therapy is less satisfactory, likely, in part, because of poor penetration of the blood–brain barrier.

Baxter P: Pyridoxine-dependent seizures: A clinical and biochemical conundrum. Biochim Biophys Acta 2003;1647(1–2):36 [PMID: 12686105].

Blau N et al: Tetrahydrobiopterin deficiencies without hyperphenylalaninemia: Diagnosis and genetics of dopa-responsive dystonia and sepiapterin reductase deficiency. Mol Genet Metab 2001;74(1–2):172 [PMID: 11592814].

Fiumara A et al: Aromatic L-amino acid decarboxylase deficiency with hyperdopaminuria: Clinical and laboratory findings in response to different therapies. Neuropediatrics 2002;33(4):203 [PMID: 12368991].

Hyland K, Arnold LA: Value of lumbar puncture in the diagnosis of infantile epilepsy and folinic acid-responsive seizures. J Child Neurol 2002;17(Suppl 3):3S48; discussion 3S56 [PMID 12597055].

Jaeken J: Genetic disorders of gamma-aminobutyric acid, glycine, and serine as causes of epilepsy. J Child Neurol 2002; 17 (Suppl 3):3S84; discussion 3S88 [PMID: 12597057].

Swoboda KJ, Hyland K: Diagnosis and treatment of neurotransmitter-related disorders. Neurol Clin 2002;20(4):1143 [PMID: 12616685].

# REFERENCES

Blau N et al (eds): *Physician's Guide to the Laboratory Diagnosis of Metabolic Diseases,* 2nd ed. Springer-Verlag, 2002.

Clark JTR: *A Clinical Guide to Inherited Metabolic Diseases.* Cambridge Univ Press, 1996.

Fernandez J et al (eds): *Inborn Metabolic Diseases: Diagnosis and Treatment,* 3rd ed. Springer-Verlag, 2000.

Lyon G et al: *Neurology of Hereditary Metabolic Diseases of Children,* 2nd ed. McGraw-Hill, 1996.

Nyhan WL, Ozand PT: *Atlas of Metabolic Diseases.* Chapman & Hall Medical, 1998.

Scriver CR et al (eds): *The Molecular and Metabolic Bases of Inherited Disease,* 8th ed. McGraw-Hill, 2001.

# Genetics & Dysmorphology    33

*Ellen Roy Elias, MD, Anne Chun-Hui Tsai, MD, MSc, & David K. Manchester, MD*

Genetics is a postmodern science, the applications of which are critical to all stages of life and to all manner of diseases. Many new technologies in molecular biology and biochemistry are allowing better understanding of the mechanisms inherent in genetic disorders and have led to new and better diagnostic tests and management options. However, some of these technologies and terms are unfamiliar to the clinician in practice. To best cover this complex and varied subject, this chapter contains two major parts. The first part serves as an introductory key, which reviews the basic principles of genetics. It starts from foundations of genetic diagnosis, and outlines basic knowledge of cytogenetics and molecular biology. It is then followed by a review of the principles of inherited human disorders, including different causes of genetic disorders, and finally a discussion of dysmorphology and teratology. The second part introduces common clinical disorders and includes descriptions of the diseases, with discussion of pathogenesis, diagnosis, and management.

## ■ PRINCIPLES OF GENETICS

## FOUNDATIONS OF GENETIC DIAGNOSIS

### CYTOGENETICS

Cytogenetics is the study of genetics at the chromosome level. Chromosomal anomalies occur in 0.4% of all live births and are a prevalent cause of mental retardation and congenital anomalies or birth defects. The prevalence of chromosomal anomalies is much higher among spontaneous abortions and stillbirths.

### Chromosomes

Human chromosomes consist of DNA (the blueprint of genetic material), specific proteins forming the backbone of the chromosome (called histones), and other chromatin structural and interactive proteins. Chromosomes contain most of the genetic information necessary for growth and differentiation. The nuclei of all normal human cells, with the exception of gametes, contain 46 chromosomes, consisting of 23 pairs (Figure 33–1). Of these, 22 pairs are called autosomes. They are numbered according to their size; chromosome 1 is the largest and chromosome 22 the smallest. In addition, there are two sex chromosomes: two X chromosomes in females and one X and one Y chromosome in males. The two members of a chromosome pair are called homologous chromosomes. One homolog of each chromosome pair is maternal in origin (from the egg); the second is paternal (from the sperm). The egg and sperm each contain 23 chromosomes (haploid cells). During formation of the zygote, they fuse into a cell with 46 chromosomes (diploid cell).

### Cell Division

Cells undergo cycles of growth and division that are controlled according to their needs and functions.

**Mitosis** is a kind of cell division, occurring in stages, during which DNA replication takes place and two daughter cells, genetically identical to the original parent cells, are formed. This cell division is typical for all somatic cells (cells other than the sperm or egg, which are called germline cells). There are four phases of mitosis: interphase, prophase, metaphase, and anaphase (Figure 33–2). In interphase, chromosomes are long, thin, and nonvisible. At this time, the genetic material is replicated. In prophase, the chromosomes are more condensed. During metaphase (the phase following DNA replication but preceding cell division), individual chromosomes can be visualized. Each arm consists of two identical parts, called chromatids. Chromatids of the same chromosome are called sister chromatids. In anaphase, the genetic material is separated into two cells.

**Meiosis** (Figure 33–3), during which eggs and sperm are formed, is cell division limited to gametes. During meiosis, three unique processes take place:

1. Crossing over of genetic material between two homologous chromosomes. This is proceeded by the pairing of both members of each chromosome pair, which facilitates the physical exchange of homologous genetic material.

2. Random assortment of maternally and paternally derived homologous chromosomes into the daughter cells. The distribution of maternal or paternal chromosomes to a particular daughter cell occurs independently in each cell.

**Normal Male**

**Normal Female**

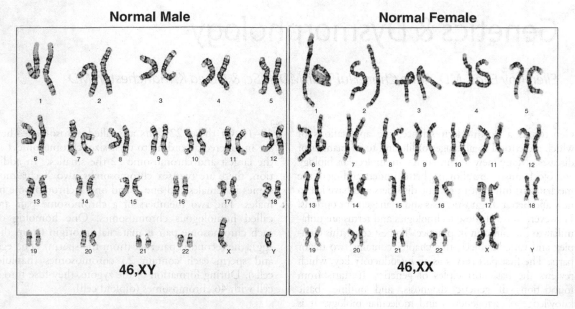

46,XY

46,XX

*Figure 33–1.* Normal male and female human karyotype. (Courtesy of Billie Carstens at CGL.)

3. Two cell divisions, the first of which is a reduction division—that is, separation between the homologous chromosomes. The second meiotic division is like mitosis, separating two sister chromatids into two genetically identical daughter cells.

## Chromosome Preparation & Analysis

Chromosome structure is visible only during mitosis, most often achieved in the laboratory by stimulating a blood lymphocyte culture with a mitogen for 3 days.

Other tissues used for this purpose include skin, products of conception, cartilage, and bone marrow. Chorionic villi or amniocytes are used for prenatal diagnosis. Spontaneously dividing cells without a mitogen are present in bone marrow, and historically, bone marrow biopsy was done when immediate identification of a pa-

Interphase

Interphase

Anaphase

Prophase

Metaphase

*Figure 33–2.* Stages of the mitotic cycle.

Homologous chromosomes one from each parent

Centromere

Sister chromatids

First meiotic division (reduction)

Second meiotic division similar to mitosis (separation of sister chromatids)

*Figure 33–3.* Meiosis—demonstrating conversion from the diploid somatic cell to the haploid gamete.

tient's chromosome constitution was necessary for appropriate management (eg, to rule out trisomy 13 in a newborn with a complex congenital heart disease). However, this invasive test has been replaced by the availability of the FISH technique (see following discussion).

Cells processed for routine chromosome analysis are stained on glass slides to yield a light-and-dark band pattern across the arms of the chromosomes (see Figure 33–1). This band pattern is characteristic and reproducible for each chromosome, allowing the chromosomes to be identified. Using different staining techniques, different banding patterns result: G, Q, and R banding. The most commonly used is G banding. The layout of chromosomes on a sheet of paper in a predetermined order is called a karyotype. High-resolution chromosome analysis is the study of more elongated chromosomes in prometaphase. In such an analysis, the bands can be visualized in greater detail, allowing detection of smaller, more subtle chromosomal rearrangements.

**Fluorescent in situ hybridization** (FISH) is a powerful technique that labels a known chromosome sequence with DNA probes attached to fluorescent dyes, thus enabling visualization of specific regions of chromosomes by fluorescent microscopy. There are many different kinds of probes, including paint probes (a mixture of sequences throughout one chromosome), sequence-specific probes, centromere probes, and telomere probes. A cocktail of differently colored probes, one color for each chromosome, called multicolor FISH, or M-FISH, can detect complex rearrangements between chromosomes. FISH can detect submicroscopic structural rearrangements undetectable by classic cytogenetic techniques and can identify marker chromosomes. For pictures of FISH studies see www.kumc.edu/gec/prof/cytogene.html

FISH also allows interphase cells (lymphocytes, amniocytes) to be screened for numerical abnormalities such as trisomy 13, 18, or 21, and sex chromosome anomalies. However, because of the possible background or contamination of the signal, the abnormality must be confirmed by conventional chromosome analysis.

Assessment of chromosome breaks and sister chromatid exchanges requires special techniques that lead to enhancement of the breaks, or special staining that allows visualization of the exchanged chromatids.

Luke S et al: FISH: Recent advances and diagnostic aspects. Cell Vis 1998;5:49 [PMID: 9660726].

## Chromosome Nomenclature

Visible under the microscope is a constriction site on the chromosome called the centromere, which separates the chromosome into two arms: p, for petite, refers to the short arm, and q, the letter following p, refers to the long arm. Each arm is further subdivided into numbered bands visible using different staining techniques. Centromeres are positioned at different sites on different chromosomes and are used to differentiate the chromosome structures seen during mitosis as **metacentric** (p arm and q arm of almost equal size), **submetacentric** (p arm shorter than q arm), and **acrocentric** (almost no p arm). The use of named chromosome arms and bands provides a universal method of chromosome description. Common symbols include *del* (deletion), *dup* (duplication), *inv* (inversion), *ish* (in situ hybridization), *i* (isochromosome), *pat* (paternal origin), *mat* (maternal origin), and *r* (ring chromosome). See the next section for definitions of these terms.

## Chromosomal Abnormalities

There are two types of chromosomal anomalies: numerical and structural.

### A. ABNORMALITIES OF CHROMOSOMAL NUMBER

When a human cell has 23 chromosomes, such as human ova or sperm, it is in the haploid state (n). After conception, in cells other than the reproductive cells, 46 chromosomes are present in the diploid state (2n). Any number that is an exact multiple of the haploid number [eg, 46(2n), 69(3n), or 92(4n)] is referred to as euploid. Polyploid cells are those that contain any number other than the usual diploid number of chromosomes. Polyploid conceptions are usually not viable except in a "mosaic state," with the presence of more than one cell line in the body. (See later text for details.)

Cells deviating from the multiple of the haploid number are called aneuploid, meaning not euploid, indicating an abnormal number of chromosomes. Trisomy, an example of aneuploidy, is the presence of three of a particular chromosome rather than two. It results from unequal division, called nondisjunction, of chromosomes into daughter cells. Trisomies are the most common numerical chromosomal anomalies found in humans [eg, trisomy 21 (Down syndrome), trisomy 18, and trisomy 13]. Monosomies, the presence of only one member of a chromosome pair, may be complete or partial. Complete monosomies may result from nondisjunction or anaphase lag. All complete autosomal monosomies appear to be lethal early in development and only survive in mosaic forms. Sex chromosome monosomy, however, can be viable.

### B. ABNORMALITIES OF CHROMOSOMAL STRUCTURE

Many different types of structural chromosomal anomalies exist. Figure 33–4 displays the formal

**Figure 33–4.** Examples of structural chromosomal abnormalities: deletion, duplication, inversion, ring chromosome, translocation, and insertion.

nomenclature as well as the ideogram demonstrating chromosomal anomalies. In clinical context, the sign (+) or (–) *preceding* the chromosome number indicates increased or decreased number, respectively, of that particular whole chromosome in a cell. For example, 47,XY+21 designates a male with three copies of chromosome 21. The sign (+) or (–) *after* the chromosome

number signifies extra material or missing material, respectively, on one of the arms of the chromosome. For example, 46,XX,8q– denotes a deletion on the long arm of chromosome 8. Detailed nomenclature, such as 8q11, is required to further demonstrate a specific missing region so that genetic counseling can be provided.

**1. Deletion (del) (see Figure 33–4A)**—This refers to an absence of normal chromosomal material. It may be terminal (at the end of a chromosome) or interstitial (within a chromosome). The missing part is described using the code "del," followed by the number of the chromosome involved in parentheses, and a description of the missing region of that chromosome, also in parentheses, for example, 46,XX,del(1)(p36.3). This chromosome nomenclature describes the loss of genetic material from band 36.3 of the short arm of chromosome 1, which results in 1p36.3 deletion syndrome. Some more common deletions result in clinically recognizable conditions associated with mental handicaps and characteristic facial features. For example, Wolf–Hirschhorn syndrome, del(4p), results in an unusual face with "Greek-helmet" appearance; Cri-du-chat syndrome, del(5p), is typified by an unusual high-pitched cry and dysmorphic features.

**2. Duplication (dup) (see Figure 33–4B)**—An extra copy of a chromosomal segment can be tandem (genetic material present in the original direction) or inverted (genetic material present in the opposite direction). A well-described duplication of chromosome 22q11 causes Cat eye syndrome, resulting in iris coloboma and anal or ear anomalies.

**3. Inversion (inv) (see Figure 33–4C)**—In this aberration, a rearranged section of a chromosome is inverted. It can be paracentric (not involving the centromere) or pericentric (involving the centromere).

**4. Ring chromosome (r) (see Figure 33–4D)**—Deletion of the normal telomeres (and possibly other subtelomeric sequences) leads to subsequent fusion of both ends to form a circular chromosome. Ring chromosomal anomalies often cause growth retardation and mental handicap.

**5. Translocation (trans) (see Figure 33–4E)**—This describes the interchromosomal rearrangement of genetic material. These may be balanced (the cell has a normal content of genetic material arranged in a structurally abnormal way) or unbalanced (the cell has gained or lost genetic material as a result of chromosomal interchange). Balanced translocations may further be described as reciprocal, the exchange of genetic material between two nonhomologous chromosomes, or robertsonian, the fusion of two acrocentric chromosomes.

**6. Insertion (ins) (see Figure 33–4F)**—Breakage within a chromosome at two points and incorporation of another piece of chromosomal material is called insertion. This requires three breakpoints and may occur between two chromosomes or within the same chromosome. The clinical presentation or phenotype depends on the origin of the inserted materials.

### C. Sex Chromosomal Anomalies

Abnormalities involving sex chromosomes, including aneuploidy and mosaicism, are relatively common in the general population. The most common sex chromosome anomalies include 45,X (Turner syndrome), 47,XXX, 47,XXY (Klinefelter syndrome), 47,XYY, and different mosaic states. (Please see later text for clinical discussion.)

### D. Mosaicism

**Mosaicism** is the presence of two or more different chromosome constitutions in different cells of the same individual. For example, a patient may have some cells with 47 chromosomes and others with 46 chromosomes (46,XX/47,XX,+21 indicates mosaicism for trisomy 21; similarly, 45,X/46,XX/47,XXX indicates mosaicism for a monosomy and a trisomy X). Mosaicism should be suspected if clinical symptoms are milder than expected in a nonmosaic patient with the same chromosomal abnormality, or if the patient's skin shows patchy or streaky hyper- or hypopigmentation. The prognosis is frequently better for a patient with mosaicism than for one with a corresponding chromosomal abnormality without mosaicism. In general, the smaller the proportion of the abnormal cell line, the better the prognosis. In the same patient, however, the proportion of normal and abnormal cells in various tissues, such as skin and peripheral blood, may be significantly different. The prognosis can seldom be assessed reliably based on the karyotype in one tissue alone, such as peripheral blood. Therefore, any prognosis should be made cautiously or even be deferred.

### E. Uniparental Disomy

Under normal circumstances, one member of each homologous pair of chromosomes is of maternal origin from the egg and the other is of paternal origin from the sperm (Figure 33–5A). In uniparental disomy (UPD), both copies of a particular chromosome pair originate from the same parent. If UPD is caused by chromosome error in the first meiotic division, both homologous chromosomes of that parent will be present in the gamete—a phenomenon called heterodisomy (see Figure 33–5B). If the disomy is caused by an error in the second meiotic division, two copies of the same chromosome will be present through the mechanism of rescue, duplication, and complementation (see Figure 33–5C–E)—a phenomenon called isodisomy. Isodisomy may also occur as a postfertilization error (see Figure 33–5F).

A chromosomal analysis would not reveal any abnormality, but DNA analysis would reveal that the child inherited two copies of DNA of a particular chromosome from one parent without the contribution

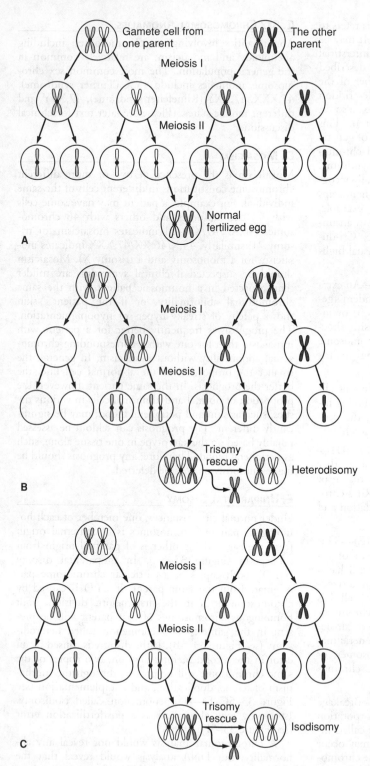

**Figure 33–5.** The assortment of homologous chromosomes during normal gametogenesis and uniparental disomy. **A:** Fertilization of normal gametes. **B:** Heterodisomy by trisomy rescue. **C:** Isodisomy by trisomy rescue.

**Figure 33–5.** (continued) **D:** Isodisomy by monosomy rescue (mitotic duplication). **E:** Gamete complementation. **F:** Postfertilization error.

from the other parent. UPD has been documented for human chromosomes, including chromosomes 7, 11, 15, and X. It has been found in patients with Prader–Willi, Angelman, and Beckwith–Wiedemann syndromes. In addition, cystic fibrosis with only one carrier parent (caused by maternal isodisomy) has been reported. UPD may cause severe prenatal and postnatal growth retardation. Furthermore, it is suspected that UPD of some chromosomes is lethal. The possible mechanisms for the adverse effects of UPD include possible homozygosity for deleterious recessive genes and the consequences of imprinting. (See principles of imprinting in the Imprinting section.)

## F. CONTIGUOUS GENE SYNDROMES

Contiguous gene syndromes result when a deletion causes the loss of genes adjacent to each other on a chromosome. Although many genes may be missing, the deletion may still be too small to be detected by routine karyotype. Therefore, contiguous gene syndromes are sometimes called "microdeletion syndromes." The genes involved in these syndromes are related only through their linear placement on the same chromosome segments and do not influence each other's functions directly. Table 33–1 lists examples of some currently known contiguous gene syndromes and their associated chromosomal abnormalities. In some of these syndromes, which usually occur sporadically but, in rare instances, are familial, high-resolution chromosome analysis can lead to identification of small interstitial deletions in affected individuals. In some patients with normal karyotypes, the deletion is submicroscopic and can be detected only with FISH or DNA analysis.

**Table 33–1.** Examples of contiguous gene syndromes.

| Syndrome | Abnormal Chromosome Segment |
| --- | --- |
| Prader–Willi/Angelman syndrome | del 15q11 |
| Shprintzen/DiGeorge spectrum | del 22q11 |
| Langer–Giedion syndrome | del 8q24 |
| Miller–Dieker syndrome | del 17p13 |
| Retinoblastoma/mental retardation | del 13q14 |
| Beckwith–Wiedemann syndrome | 11p15 |
| Wilms tumor with aniridia, genitourinary malformations, and mental retardation | del 11p13 |

## G. CHROMOSOME FRAGILITY

It is well known that environmental factors such as exposure to radiation, certain chemicals, and viruses contribute to chromosome breaks and rearrangements. However, some well-defined autosomal recessive syndromes with DNA repair defects are associated with a greatly increased risk of chromosome aberrations and are called chromosome instability or breakage syndromes. An example is Bloom syndrome, characterized clinically by small stature and development of telangiectasias on exposure to sunlight. It is caused by a defect in a DNA helicase that leads to increased somatic recombination and sister chromatid exchange. Other syndromes include the following:

- Fanconi anemia, often associated with radial ray defect, pigmentary changes, mild mental retardation, and development of pancytopenia
- Ataxia–telangiectasia (Louis–Bar syndrome), characterized by telangiectasia of the skin and eyes, immunodeficiency, and progressive ataxia, a DNA repair defect
- ICF syndrome, characterized by immunodeficiency, centromeric instability, and facial anomaly
- Roberts syndrome, characterized by growth retardation, developmental delay, and limb and craniofacial anomalies
- Xeroderma pigmentosum, resulting in formation of skin lesions secondary to sun exposure
- Werner syndrome, which is associated with premature senility.

The knowledge that specific chromosome aberrations are associated with these syndromes is often the basis for cytogenetic confirmation of their diagnosis. For example, in Fanconi anemia, after diepoxybutane (DEB) treatment, translocations between nonhomologous so-called quadriradii and chromosomal breakage increase, which confirms the diagnosis.

## H. CHROMOSOMAL ABNORMALITIES IN CANCER

Numerical and structural chromosomal abnormalities are often identified in hematopoietic and solid-tumor neoplasms in individuals with otherwise normal chromosomes. These cytogenetic abnormalities have been categorized as primary and secondary. In primary abnormalities, their presence is necessary for initiation of the cancer (eg, 13q– in retinoblastoma). Secondary abnormalities appear in somatic cells de novo only after the cancer has developed (eg, Philadelphia chromosome, t[9;22][q34;q11], in acute and chronic myeloid leukemia). "Cytogenetic noise" is the term used to denote a variety of random chromosomal abnormalities.

The primary and secondary chromosomal abnormalities are specific for particular neoplasms and can be used for diagnosis or prognosis. For example, the presence of the Philadelphia chromosome is a good prognostic sign in chronic myelogenous leukemia and indicates a poor prognosis in acute lymphoblastic leukemia. The sites of chromosome breaks coincide with the known loci of oncogenes and antioncogenes.

Jones KL: *Smith's Recognizable Patterns of Human Malformation*, 5th ed. WB Saunders, 1996.

## MOLECULAR GENETICS

The advances of molecular biology have been a major breakthrough for human genetics, because they allow for the localization, isolation, and characterization of the genes that encode protein sequences. As the Human Genome Project has moved into a postcloning era, the function of the gene products and their interaction with one another has become the main theme of molecular genetics. Also, molecular genetics can help explain the complex underlying biology involved in human diseases.

### Recombinant DNA Technology

Recombinant DNA technology was developed using restriction endonucleases, which cleave DNA at specific nucleotide sequences. A difference in DNA sequence caused by a normal variation of DNA or by a gene mutation either produces or eliminates an endonuclease recognition site, resulting in a DNA fragment of different size. Thus the number and arrangement of restriction sites (called a restriction map) are characteristic of a given DNA sequence.

Before a DNA fragment of interest can be analyzed, multiple copies of it must be produced. This can be achieved by incorporating the human DNA fragment into a vector (ie, a DNA segment containing the means of replication and selection in bacteria). The vector-containing human DNA insert is replicated, thus producing multiple copies of the segment of interest. The source of inserts can be genomic DNA, obtained directly from cleaving of the target organism, or complementary DNA (cDNA), obtained by copying messenger RNA (mRNA) into DNA by reverse transcription.

A genomic library can be assembled by fragmenting human genomic DNA with restriction enzymes and then inserting the fragments into a vector. Such a library contains large numbers of different DNA sequences. Some of these specific DNA fragments are used to manufacture human proteins (eg, insulin, growth hormone, interferon, and blood clotting factors) for pharmacologic applications; others are used as probes, which may be thought of as DNA segment-specific, radioactively labeled reagents for mapping and diagnosis.

Molecular genetic techniques are most commonly used to look for changes in genomic DNA detected by Southern blot analysis. But a similar technique with Northern blot analysis is being used increasingly to look for RNA abnormalities. Southern blot analysis relies on the use of restriction endonucleases to cleave human genomic DNA at specific nucleotide sequences and to produce DNA fragments of different lengths. These DNA fragments are then separated by agarose gel electrophoresis, transferred to a membrane, and overlaid with a radioactive probe. This fragment is identified by autoradiography, and its size is determined. Recently, non–radioisotope-based hybridization became available as an alternative to radioisotopes.

The **polymerase chain reaction (PCR)** replicates fragments of DNA between predetermined primers so that sufficient DNA is obtained for characterization or sequencing in the space of a few hours. For example, 20 cycles of synthesis will amplify DNA 1 millionfold. The disadvantage of PCR is that a small contamination with foreign DNA can result in an incorrect diagnosis.

### Application of Molecular Biology in Clinical Genetics and Genetic Diagnosis

Genetic diagnosis can be performed by direct detection of a mutant gene or by indirect methods. Direct detection is possible only when the gene causing the disease and the nature of the mutation are known. The advantage of a diagnostic study using the direct detection of the mutant gene is that it requires the affected individual only and need not involve the testing of other family members. Indirect detection of abnormal genes is used when the gene is known but there is extensive heterogeneity of the molecular defect between families, or when the gene responsible for a disease is unknown but its chromosome location is known.

The methods of direct DNA diagnosis include restriction analysis, single strand conformational polymorphism (SSCP) analysis, direct sequencing with assistance of PCR, heteroduplex assay, and protein truncation assay. The molecular mechanisms causing human diseases include point mutations, deletions, and insertions, and the unstable expansion of trinucleotide repeats, which leads to genetic anticipation (see previous sections and later discussion). Congenital adrenal hyperplasia secondary to 21-hydroxylase deficiency, Duchenne muscular dystrophy, hemophilias A and B, Lesch–Nyhan syndrome, fibroblast growth factor receptor (FGFR)-related craniosynostosis, cystic fibrosis, and fragile X syndrome are common examples of diseases caused by these mechanisms, for which direct DNA testing is available.

If the sequence or product of an abnormal gene cannot be studied, then the linkage analysis method may be applicable. Linkage traces the inheritance of the abnormal gene between members of a kindred. This method requires that the affected individual be studied, with parents and perhaps other relatives, both affected and unaffected.

Neurofibromatosis is an example of a disorder in which both the direct and indirect assay may be used. Because of the size and the heterogenous mutation pattern of the neurofibromin gene (*NFI*), the first step usually is the protein truncation assay, which is done via in vitro translation followed by analyzing the size of the protein. However, this method detects only two thirds of affected patients, in whom a nonsense mutation exists that truncates the gene message. All other cases must rely on linkage analysis, by using markers such as a restriction fragment length polymorphism (RFLP) or, increasingly, flanking microsatellite polymorphisms. The increase in density of polymorphisms discovered over the past few years means that the presence or absence of an abnormal copy of a gene in an individual can be predicted with a high degree of confidence, if the relatives have informative polymorphisms. Microsatellite polymorphisms are being used in sibling research studies to identify the multiple genes that contribute to polygenic traits such as diabetes and obesity. They are also used increasingly to identify gene changes in tumors.

## Application of Molecular Biology in Prevention of Human Diseases

Recombinant DNA technology has the potential for preventing genetic disease by facilitating the detection of carriers of defective genes and permitting prenatal diagnosis. Family studies can also clarify the mode of inheritance, thus allowing more accurate determination of recurrence risks and appropriate options. For example, differentiation of gonadal mosaicism from decreased penetrance of a dominant gene has important implications for genetic counseling. In the past, the diagnosis of a genetic disease characterized by late onset of symptoms (eg, Huntington disease) could not be made prior to the appearance of clinical symptoms. In some inborn errors of metabolism, diagnostic tests (eg, measurement of enzyme activities) could be conducted only on inaccessible tissues. Gene identification techniques can enormously enhance the ability to diagnose both symptomatic and presymptomatic individuals, as well as heterozygous carriers of the gene, and conduct prenatal diagnosis. However, presymptomatic DNA testing is associated with psychological, ethical, and legal implications and therefore should be used only with informed consent.

## Application of Molecular Biology in Treatment of Human Diseases

A normal gene introduced into an individual affected with a serious inherited disorder during embryonic life (germline therapy) in principle has the potential to be transmitted to future generations, whereas its introduction into somatic cells (somatic therapy) affects only the recipient. Experimental gene therapy by bone marrow transplantation is being tried for adenosine deaminase deficiency. Recombinant enzyme replacement has been successfully applied in treating the nonneurologic form of Gaucher disease and some types of lysosomal storage disease.

# PRINCIPLES OF INHERITED HUMAN DISORDERS
## MENDELIAN DISORDERS

Traditionally, autosomal single gene disorders follow the principles explained by Mendel's observations. To summarize, the inheritance of genetic traits through generations relies on segregation and independent assortment. **Segregation** is the process through which gene pairs are separated during gamete formation. Each gamete receives only one copy of each gene (allele). **Independent assortment** refers to the idea that the segregation of different alleles occurs independently.

Victor McKusick's catalog, *Mendelian Inheritance in Man,* lists more than 10,000 entries in which the mode of inheritance is presumed to be autosomal dominant, autosomal recessive, X-linked dominant, X-linked recessive, and Y-linked. Single genes at specific loci on one or a pair of chromosomes cause these disorders. An understanding of inheritance terminology is helpful in approaching mendelian disorders. Analysis of the pedigree and the pattern of transmission in the family, identification of a specific condition, and knowledge of that condition's mode of inheritance usually allows for explanation of the inheritance pattern.

## Terminology

The following terms are important in understanding heredity patterns.

**Dominant and Recessive**—As defined by Mendel, concepts for dominant and recessive refer to the **phenotypic expression** of alleles and are not intrinsic characteristics of gene loci. Therefore, it is inappropriate to discuss "a dominant locus.,"

**Genotype**—Genotype means the genetic status—that is, the alleles an individual carries.

**Phenotype**—Phenotype is the expression of an individual's genotype and may be modified by environment, that is, the structural or functional nature of an individual (appearance, physical features, organ structure, biochemical, physiologic nature).

**Pleiotropy**—Pleiotropy refers to the phenomenon whereby a single mutant allele can have widespread effects or expression in different tissues or organ systems. In other words, an allele may produce more than one effect on the phenotype. For example, Marfan syndrome has findings in different organ systems (skeletal, cardiac, ophthalmologic, etc) due to a single mutation within the *fibrillin* gene.

**Penetrance**—Penetrance refers to the proportion of individuals with a particular genotype that express the same phenotype. Penetrance is a proportion that ranges between 0 and 1.0 (or 0 and 100%). When 100% of mutant individuals express the phenotype, penetrance is **complete.** If some mutant individuals do not express the phenotype, penetrance is said to be **incomplete,** or **reduced.** Dominant conditions with incomplete penetrance, therefore, are characterized by "skipped" generations with unaffected, obligate gene carriers.

**Expressivity**—Expressivity refers to the variability in degree of phenotypic expression (severity) seen in different individuals with the same mutant genotype. Expressivity may be extremely variable or fairly consistent, both within and between families. Intrafamilial variability of expression may be due to factors such as epistasis, environment, true anticipation, presence of phenocopies, mosaicism, and chance (stochastic factors). Interfamilial variability of expression may be due to the previously mentioned factors as well, but may also be due to allelic or locus genetic heterogeneity.

**Genetic Heterogeneity**—A number of different genetic mutations may produce phenotypes that are identical or similar enough to have been traditionally considered as one diagnosis. The conditions of "anemia" and "mental retardation" are examples of this. There are two types of genetic heterogeneity, **allelic heterogeneity** and **locus heterogeneity.**

**Locus heterogeneity**—This describes a phenotype caused by mutations at more than one genetic locus; that is, mutations at different loci cause the same phenotype or a group of phenotypes that appear similar enough to have been previously classified as a single disease, clinical "entity," or diagnostic spectrum. An example would be Sanfilippo syndrome (mucopolysaccharidosis III A, B, C, and D), in which the same phenotype is produced by four different enzyme deficiencies.

**Allelic heterogeneity**—This term is applied to a phenotype caused by more than one genetic mutation at the same gene locus, that is, different mutations at a single gene locus. As an example, cystic fibrosis may be caused by many different genetic changes, such as homozygosity for the common $\Delta F 508$ mutation, or $\Delta F 508$ and a *R117H* mutation. The latter example represents compound heterozygosity.

**Phenotypic Heterogeneity or "Clinical Heterogeneity"**—This term describes the situation in which more than one phenotype is caused by different allelic mutations at a single locus. An example of phenotypic heterogeneity includes different mutations within the *Collagen II* gene, causing hypochondrogenesis, Kniest dysplasia, spondyloepiphyseal dysplasia congenita, and some cases of Stickler syndrome. Furthermore, different mutations in the *FGFR2* gene can cause different craniosynostosis disorders, including Crouzon syndrome, Jackson–Weiss syndrome, Pfeiffer syndrome, and Apert syndrome. These syndromes are clinically distinguishable and are due to the presence of a variety of genetic mutations within single genes.

**Homozygous**—A cell or organism that has identical alleles at a particular locus is said to be homozygous. For example, in an autosomal recessive disorder, the gene copies from both parents have to be inactivated to manifest the disease.

**Heterozygous**—A cell or organism that has nonidentical alleles at a genetic locus is said to be heterozygous. In autosomal dominant conditions, one copy of the gene pair is inactivated while the other is functional, resulting in a disease state. An individual who is heterozygous for a recessive disorder will not manifest symptoms.

Online Mendelian Inheritance in Man:
http://www.ncbi.nlm.nih.gov/entrez/query.fcgi?db=OMIM

## 1. Hereditary Patterns

### Autosomal Dominant Inheritance

Autosomal dominant inheritance has the following characteristics:

1.  Affected individuals in the same family may experience variable expressivity.

2.  Nonpenetrance is common, and the penetrance rate varies for each dominantly inherited condition.

3.  Both males and females can pass on the abnormal gene to children of either sex, although the manifestations may vary according to sex. For example, pattern baldness is a dominant trait but affects only males. In this case, the trait is said to be sex-limited.

4.  Dominant inheritance is typically said to be vertical, that is, the condition passes from one generation to the next in a vertical fashion (Figure 33–6).

5.  In some cases, the family history seems to be completely negative, and the patient appears to be the first affected individual. This spontaneous appearance may be caused by a new mutation. In some disorders, which tend to be more severe (eg,

LEGEND:

▢ Male    ◑ Scoliosis    ◨ Café au lait spots

◯ Female    ◔ Neurofibromata    ◰ Mental retardation

***Figure 33–6.*** Autosomal dominant inheritance. Variable expressivity in NF-1

achondroplasia) and therefore may decrease the reproductive fitness, there is a high rate of new mutations. The mutation rate varies with each dominant condition, and in some cases the mutation rate increases with advancing paternal age. Several other explanations for a negative family history are possible, however:

  a. Nonpaternity.

  b. Decreased penetrance or mild manifestations in one of the parents.

  c. Germline mosaicism (ie, mosaicism in the germ cell line of either parent), in which case the risk of recurrence increases. Germline mosaicism may mimic autosomal recessive inheritance, because it leads to situations in which two children of completely normal parents are affected with a genetic disorder. The best example of this is osteogenesis imperfecta type II. Laboratory studies have documented germline mosaicism by finding that only one allele of the paired collagen genes is abnormal in the severe form instead of both, as would be expected in a recessive disease. The recurrence risk in this form of osteogenesis imperfecta is 7%.

  d. The abnormality present in the patient may be a phenocopy, or it may be a similar but genetically different abnormality with a different mode of inheritance.

**6.** As a general rule, dominant traits are more often related to structural abnormalities of protein, as for example in Marfan syndrome.

**7.** For a parent who is affected, the risk of each offspring to inherit the abnormal dominant gene is 50%, or 1:2. This is true whether the gene is penetrant or not in the parent, and the severity of the condition in the offspring is not related to the severity in the affected parent. In some disorders, it may be related to the sex of the parent transmitting the gene. For example, if the gene for myotonic dystrophy is passed through the mother, there is a 10–20% chance that the child (regardless of sex) may have a severe congenital form of the disease. Conversely, if the gene for Huntington disease is passed through the father, the probability is 5–10% that the offspring may have the severe, rigid juvenile form. This has been attributed to imprinting, although we know in these two conditions that it is associated with expansion of the triplet repeats (see Genetic Anticipation section). If an abnormality represents a new mutation of a dominant trait, the parents of the affected individual run a low risk during subsequent pregnancies, but the risk for the offspring of the affected individual is 50%.

**8.** Prevention options available for future pregnancies include prenatal diagnosis, artificial insemination, and egg donation, depending on which parent has the abnormal gene.

## Autosomal Recessive Inheritance

Autosomal recessive inheritance also has some distinctive characteristics:

**1.** There is less variability among affected persons. Parents are carriers and are clinically normal. (There are exceptions to this rule, however. For example, sickle cell disease is considered recessive. Under normal circumstances, carriers—those with the sickle cell trait—are normal but may become symptomatic if they become hypoxic.)

**2.** Males and females are affected equally.

**3.** Inheritance is horizontal; siblings may be affected (Figure 33–7).

**4.** Recessive conditions are usually rare; the rarer the condition, the more likely it is that consanguinity is present. Conversely, if a child whose parents are related presents with an unrecognized abnormality, a recessive condition must be suspected.

**5.** The family history is usually negative, with the exception of siblings. However, in common conditions such as cystic fibrosis, a second- or third-degree relative may be affected.

**6.** Recessive conditions are frequently associated with enzyme defects.

**7.** The recurrence risk for parents of an affected child is 25%, or 1:4 for each pregnancy. The gene

LEGEND:

■ Affected (Cystic fibrosis)

◐ Carrier

□—○ Consanguineous marriage

***Figure 33–7.*** Autosomal recessive inheritance: cystic fibrosis.

carrier frequency in the general population can be used to assess the risk of having an affected child with a new partner, for unaffected siblings, and for the affected individuals themselves.

8. In rare instances, a child with a recessive disorder and a normal karyotype may have inherited both copies of the abnormal gene from one parent and none from the other. This uniparental disomy was first described in a girl with cystic fibrosis and growth retardation. This phenomenon is of unknown frequency, but it is more likely to be present in a child with several autosomal recessive conditions or in a patient with unexpected and seemingly unrelated abnormalities or severe growth retardation. Molecular testing can confirm the presence of uniparental disomy. The recurrence risk is obviously lower in such a situation, although the factors predisposing to uniparental disomy are unknown. Maternal age may play a role in these situations.

9. Options available for future pregnancies include prenatal diagnosis in many cases and artificial insemination.

## X-Linked Inheritance

When a gene for a specific disorder is on the X chromosome, the condition is said to be X-linked, or sex-linked. Females may be either homozygous or heterozygous, because they have two X chromosomes. Males, by contrast, have only one X, and a male is said to be hemizygous for any gene on his X chromosome. The severity of any disorder is greater in males than in females (within a specific family). According to the Lyon hypothesis, because one of the two X chromosomes in each cell is inactivated, and because this inactivation is random, the clinical picture in females depends on the percentage of mutant versus normal alleles inactivated. The X chromosome is not inactivated until about 14 days of gestation, and parts of the short arm remain active throughout life.

## X-Linked Recessive Inheritance

The following features are characteristic of X-linked recessive inheritance:

1. Males are affected, and heterozygous females are either normal or have mild manifestations.

2. Inheritance is diagonal through the maternal side of the family (Figure 33–8A).

3. A female carrier has a 50% chance that each daughter will be a carrier and a 50% chance that each son will be affected.

4. All of the daughters of an affected male are carriers, and none of his sons are affected. Because a father can give only his Y chromosome to his sons, male-to-male transmission excludes X-linked inheritance except in the rare case of uniparental disomy, in which a son receives both the X and the Y from his father.

5. The mutation rate is high in some X-linked disorders, particularly when the affected male dies or is so incapacitated by the disorder that reproduction is unlikely. In such instances, the mutation is thought to occur in the propositus in one third of cases, in the mother in one third of cases, and in earlier generations in one third of cases. For this reason, genetic counseling may be difficult in families with an isolated case.

6. On rare occasions, a female may be fully affected. Several possible mechanisms may account for a fully affected female: (a) unfavorable lyonization; (b) 45,X karyotype; (c) homozygosity for the abnormal gene; (d) an X-autosome translocation, or other structural abnormality of one X chromosome, in which the X chromosome of normal structure is preferentially inactivated; (e) uniparental disomy; and (f) nonrandom inactivation, which may be controlled by an autosomal gene.

A

LEGEND:

■ Duchenne-muscular dystrophy

◐ Carrier

† Deceased

B

LEGEND:

■ Affected male

● Affected female

**Figure 33–8. A:** X-linked recessive inheritance. **B:** X-linked dominant inheritance.

## X-Linked Dominant Inheritance

The X-linked dominant inheritance pattern is much less common than the X-linked recessive type. Examples include incontinentia pigmenti and hypophosphatemic or vitamin D-resistant rickets.

1. The heterozygous female is symptomatic, and the disease is twice as common in females because they have two X chromosomes that can have the mutation.

2. Clinical manifestations are more variable in females than in males.

3. The risk for the offspring of heterozygous females to be affected is 50% regardless of sex.

4. All of the daughters but none of the sons of affected males will have the disorder. (see Figure 33–8B)

5. Although a homozygous female is possible (particularly in an inbred population), she would be severely involved. All of her children would also be affected but more mildly.

6. Some disorders (eg, incontinentia pigmenti) are lethal in males (and in homozygous females). Affected women have twice as many daughters as sons and an increased incidence of miscarriages,

because affected males will be spontaneously aborted. A 47,XXY karyotype has allowed affected males to survive.

## Y-Linked Inheritance

Also known as "holandric" inheritance, these conditions are caused by genes located on the Y chromosome. These conditions are relatively rare with only about 40 entries listed in McKusick's catalog. Male-to-male transmission is seen in this category, with all sons of affected males being affected and no daughters or females being affected. Figure 33–9 shows a typical Y-linked inheritance pedigree.

## MULTIFACTORIAL INHERITANCE

Many common attributes, such as height, are familial, and are the result of the actions of multiple rather than single genes. Inheritance of these traits is described as **polygenic** or **multifactorial.** The latter term recognizes that environmental factors such as diet also contribute to these traits. As they begin to dissect the genetics of these traits in humans, geneticists are finding that multiple genes are often expressed in hierarchies in which the action of a small number of genes, two or three, explains much of the variation observed within affected populations.

Studies of twins have proven useful in determining the relative importance of genetic versus environmental factors in the expression of polygenic traits. If genetic factors are of little or no importance, then the concordance between monozygotic and dizygotic twins should be the same. (Dizygotic twins are no more genetically similar to each other than to other siblings.) If an abnormality is completely genetic, the concordance between identical twins should be 100%. In polygenic conditions, the concordance rate for identical twins is higher than that seen in dizygotic twins but still not 100%, indicating both genetic and environmental factors.

Many disorders and congenital abnormalities that are clearly familial but do not segregate as mendelian traits (eg, autosomal dominant, recessive, etc) show polygenic inheritance. For the most part, these conditions become manifest when thresholds of additive gene actions or contributing environmental factors are exceeded. Many common disorders ranging from hypertension, stroke, and thrombophlebitis to behavioral traits such as alcoholism demonstrate multifactorial (polygenic) inheritance. Some common birth defects, including isolated congenital heart disease, cleft lip and palate, and neural tube defects, also demonstrate polygenic inheritance. Neural tube defects provide a good model for how identification of both environmental and genetic contributions to multifactorial traits can lead to preventive measures.

Polygenic or multifactorial inheritance has several distinctive characteristics:

1. The risk for relatives of affected persons is increased, and the risk is higher for first-degree relatives (those who have 50% of their genes in common) and lower for more distant relations, although the risk for the latter is higher than for the general population (Table 33–2).

2. The recurrence risk varies with the number of affected family members. For example, after one child is born with a neural tube defect, the recurrence risk is 2–3%. If a second affected child is born, the risk for any future child increases to 10–12%. This is in contrast to single gene disorders, in which the risk is the same no matter how many family members are affected.

3. The risk is higher if the defect is more severe. In Hirschsprung disease, another polygenic condition, the longer the aganglionic segment, the higher the recurrence risk.

LEGEND:

 Affected male

*Figure 33–9.* Y-linked inheritance.

***Table 33–2.*** Empiric risks for some congenital disorders.

---

**Anencephaly and spina bifida:** Incidence (average) 1:1000
  One affected child: 2–3%
  Two affected children: 10–12%
  One affected parent: 4–5%
**Hydrocephalus:** Incidence 1:2000 newborns
  Occasional X-linked recessive
  Often associated with neural tube defect
  Some environmental etiologies (eg, toxoplasmosis)
  Recurrence risk, one affected child
    Hydrocephalus: 1%
    Some central nervous system abnormality: 3%
**Nonsyndromic cleft lip and/or palate:** Incidence (average) 1:1000
  One affected child: 2–4%
  One affected parent: 2–4%
  Two affected children: 10%
  One affected parent, one affected child: 10–20%
**Nonsyndromic cleft palate:** Incidence 1:2000
  One affected child: 2%
  Two affected children: 6–8%
  One affected parent: 4–6%
  One affected parent, one affected child: 15–20%
**Congenital heart disease:** Incidence 8:1000
  One affected child: 2–3%
  One affected parent, one affected child: 10%
**Clubfoot:** Incidence 1:1000 (male:female = 2:1)
  One affected child: 2–3%
**Congenital dislocated hip:** Incidence 1:1000
  (female > male) with marked regional variation
  One child affected: 2–14%
**Pyloric stenosis:** Incidence, males: 1:200; females: 1:1000
  Male index parent
    Brothers    3.2%
    Sons    6.8%
    Sisters    3.0%
    Daughters    1.2%
  Female index patient
    Brothers    13.2%
    Sons    20.5%
    Sisters    2.5%
    Daughters    11.1%

---

**4.** Sex ratios may not be equal. If a marked discrepancy exists, the recurrence risk is higher if a child of the less commonly affected sex has the disorder. This assumes that more genetic factors are required to raise the more resistant sex above the threshold. For example, pyloric stenosis is more common in males. If the first affected child is a female, the recurrence risk is higher than if the child is a male.

**5.** The risk for the offspring of an affected person is approximately the same as the risk for siblings, assuming that the spouse of the affected person has a negative family history. For many conditions, however, assortative mating, "like marrying like," adds to risks in offspring.

## NONMENDELIAN INHERITANCE

### Imprinting

Although the homologs of chromosome pairs may appear identical on routine karyotype analysis, it is now known that the parental origin of each homolog can effect which genes are actually transcribed and which are inactivated. The term "imprinting" refers to the process by which preferential transcription of certain genes takes place, depending on the parental origin, that is, which homolog (maternal or paternal) the gene is located on. Certain chromosomes, particularly chromosome X, and the autosomes 15, 11, and 7, have imprinted regions where certain genes are only read from one homolog (ie, either the maternal or paternal allele) under normal circumstances, and the gene on the other homolog is normally inactivated. Errors in imprinting may arise because of uniparental disomy (in which a copy from one parent is missing), by a chromosomal deletion causing loss of the gene normally transcribed, or by mutations in the imprinting genes that normally code for transcription or inactivation of other genes downstream. A good example of how imprinting may affect human disease is Beckwith–Wiedemann syndrome (BWS), the gene for which is located on chromosome 11p15.

Cohen MM et al: *Overgrowth Syndromes.* Oxford University Press, 2002.

### Genetic Anticipation

Geneticists coined the term "anticipation" to describe an unusual pattern of inheritance in which symptoms became manifest at earlier ages and with increasing severity as traits are passed to subsequent generations. Mapping of the genes responsible for these disorders led to the discovery that certain repeat sequences of DNA at disease loci were not stable when passed through meiosis. Repeated DNA sequences, in particular triplets (eg CGG, CAG), tended to increase their copy number. As these runs of triplets expanded they eventually affected the expression of genes and produced symptoms. Curiously, all the disorders undergoing triplet repeat expansion so far detected produce neurologic symptoms. Most are progressive. In general, the size of the triplet expansion is roughly correlated with the timing and severity of symptoms. The reasons for the meiotic instability of these sequences are not yet understood. The mechanisms appear to involve interactions between DNA structure (eg, formation of hairpin loops) and replication enzymes (DNA polymerase complexes) during meiosis.

Triplet repeat instability can modify the inheritance of autosomal dominant, autosomal recessive, and X-linked traits. Autosomal dominant disorders include several spinal cerebellar atrophies, Huntington disease, and myotonic dystrophy. Unstable triplet repeat expansion contributes to at least one autosomal recessive disorder, Friedreich ataxia. The most common X-linked disorder demonstrating triplet repeat instability and expansion is fragile X syndrome.

## Mitochondrial Inheritance

Mitochondrial DNA is double-stranded, circular, and smaller than nuclear DNA, and is found in the cytoplasm. It codes for enzymes involved in oxidative phosphorylation, which generates adenosine triphosphate (ATP). During the last decade of the twentieth century, enormous advances in technology and improved clinical documentation have led to a better understanding of the interesting disorders caused by mutations in mitochondrial DNA (mtDNA). It was initially appreciated that these unusual disorders seemed to be transmitted only by female members of a family and affected a high proportion of offspring, both male and female. Mitochondrial disorders have the following characteristics:

1. They show remarkable phenotypic variability.
2. They are maternally inherited, because only the egg has any cytoplasmic material.
3. In most mitochondrial disorders, cells are heteroplasmic. That is, all cells contain both normal and mutated or abnormal mtDNA. The proportion of normal to abnormal mtDNA in the mother's egg seems to determine the severity of the offspring's disease and the age at onset in most cases.
4. Those tissues with the highest ATP requirements—specifically, central nervous system (CNS) and skeletal muscle—seem to be most susceptible to mutations in mtDNA.
5. Somatic cells show an increase in mtDNA mutations and a decline in oxidative phosphorylation function with age. This explains the later onset of some of these disorders and may indeed be a clue to the whole aging process.

Mitochondrial disorders have been associated with deletions or duplications in mitochondrial DNA. Large deletions are usually sporadic, but smaller deletions may be secondary events due to defects in dominantly inherited nuclear genes. Mitochondrial dysfunction may also be caused by mutations in nuclear genes encoding mitochondrial proteins and can be inherited as dominant, recessive, or X-linked traits. Because of the difficulty in diagnosing mitochondrial disorders and the variability of the clinical course, it is often difficult to calculate specific recurrence risks.

## FAMILY HISTORY AND PEDIGREE

The first step in the collection of information regarding the genetics of a syndromic diagnosis is the construction of a family tree or pedigree. Underused by most medical personnel, the pedigree is a valuable record of genetic and medical information, which is much more useful in visual form than in list form. Tips for pedigree preparation include the following:

- Give simple instructions to the patient regarding the information desired.
- Use clearly defined symbols with a key for interpretation.
- Identify the informant, the historian, and the date of the interview.
- Start in the middle of the page to allow enough room for expansion.
- Start with the proband—the patient's siblings and parents.
- Always ask about consanguinity. Sometimes the question "Are you (the parents) related by blood?" will result in laughter but often yields potentially useful clues suggesting autosomal recessive inheritance. Ask for details such as place of birth, size of towns, and the presence of consanguinity. (These help to define recessive conditions and may increase suspicion of certain diseases that occur more frequently in particular ethnic backgrounds.)
- Obtain the maiden names of women in the family (particularly helpful for X-linked conditions).
- Obtain data from both sides of the family.
- Ask about spontaneous abortions, stillbirths, infertility, children relinquished for adoption, and deceased individuals. Such details are essential for understanding conditions that are lethal or are associated with reproductive losses.
- Even if the disease in question appears to be coming from one side of the family, always get the basic facts about the other side of the family as well. Sometimes unrelated data may be very important in interpreting the family's overall situation. In addition, obtaining data from both sides may avoid an inference of blame being placed on one family member.

In the course of taking the family history, one may find information that is not relevant in elucidating the cause of the patients' problem but may indicate a risk for other important health concerns. Such information should be appropriately followed and addressed. Such conditions that may arise are an overwhelming family history of early-onset breast and ovarian cancer, multiple pregnancy losses necessitating chromosome analyses, or symptoms of hemochromatosis, the common treatable disorder of iron metabolism.

# DYSMORPHOLOGY AND HUMAN EMBRYOLOGY

With advances in perinatal medicine and treatment of infectious diseases, birth defects have now become the leading cause of death in the neonatal period and first year of life. Birth defects are evident in 2–3% of newborns and will be detected in 7% of the adult population. The scientific investigation of the origins of birth defects is called teratology. Dysmorphology is its clinical arm.

## MECHANISMS

### Developmental Genetics

Most birth defects are multifactorial: They result from miscommunication between genetic processes and the environments in which they unfold. Specific causes of maldevelopment can be identified in about 30% of cases, but advances in developmental biology and human genetics promise better understanding. Single gene mutations and chromosomal abnormalities cause approximately 25% of birth defects. Specific genes or chromosome loci have now been identified for many recurring phenotypes, or syndromes.

Among the most fundamental genetic programs in cells are those that regulate cell division, proliferation, and those that program cell death, or apoptosis. Both proliferation and apoptosis are very active in embryogenesis. The balance between these processes is easily disrupted, and imbalances in regulation of cell cycles are an important determinant of birth defects.

Morphogenic processes and the genes that regulate them have been highly conserved through evolution. Thus experiments in lower organisms such as *Drosophila* (fruit flies) can be highly relevant to humans, because mutations producing abnormal development in less complex organisms identify candidate genes for human birth defects. Among the better examples of this connection are *pax* genes, involved in eye development in *Drosophila*. Mutations in one of these genes, *Pax 6*, produces "small eye" in mice, and aniridia and other abnormalities of the anterior chamber of the eye in humans.

Developmental biology is also taking advantage of two powerful technical advances: in situ hybridization for visualizing the expression of genes in embryos, and the production of transgenic animals in which genes of interest can be "knocked out" in order to determine their contributions to development. These techniques have uncovered, for example, very important regulatory pathways, such as the Hedgehog signaling pathway, which affects morphogenesis in organs as diverse as limbs, the heart, and the CNS. Human mutations in one of these evolutionarily conserved genes, sonic Hedgehog (*Shh*), can result in holoprosencephaly, a severe birth defect in which the CNS fails to complete hemispheric division.

## Cellular Interactions

The picture emerging from genetic studies of morphogenesis is one of a hierarchy of gene expression during development. Morphogenesis begins with expression of genes encoding transcription factors. These proteins bind to DNA in undifferentiated embryonic cells and recruit them into developmental fields, groups of cells primed to respond to specific signals later in development. This recruitment also establishes spatial relationships and orients cells with respect to their neighbors. As fields differentiate into identifiable tissues (eg, ectoderm, mesoderm, endoderm), cellular proliferation, migration, and further differentiation are mediated through genes encoding proteins that send signals through interactions with other proteins (receptors).

Products of these genes include growth factors and their receptors, cellular adhesion molecules, and extracellular matrix proteins that both provide structure and localize signals for further differentiation. Patterns in which fields of primed cells proliferate, migrate, and then interact through locally expressed growth factors and receptors occur repeatedly in mammalian development. Within these interactions are clues to understanding not only many human birth defects but also cancer. The genes that organize cell proliferation and differentiation during development are often precisely those that are knocked out or amplified by carcinogenic mutations.

## Epigenetic Regulation

Although development is regulated by genes, it is initiated and sustained by nongenetic processes. Epigenetic events are points of interaction between developmental programs and the physicochemical environments in differentiating cells. Genetic imprinting and DNA methylation are examples of epigenetic processes that affect development. Certain genes important in regulation of growth and differentiation are themselves regulated by chemical modification that occurs in specific patterns in gametes. For example, genes that are methylated are "turned off" and not transcribed. The pattern of which genes are methylated may be determined or affected by the sex of the parent of origin (see Imprinting section). Expression of imprinted genes may sometimes be limited to specific organs (eg, the brain), and imprinting may be relaxed and methyl groups lost as development progresses. Disruption of imprinting is now recognized as contributing to birth defect syndromes (described later in this chapter).

## Environmental Factors

The effects of exogenous agents during development are also mediated through genetically regulated pathways. At the cellular level, environmental effects occur because xenobiotics (compounds foreign to nature) either interact with signaling pathways or receptors and misdirect morphologically important cellular functions, or they are cytotoxic and lead to cell death in excess of the usual developmental program.

In general, drug receptors expressed in embryos and fetuses are the same molecules that mediate effects in adults. However, because differentiation pathways are active, and embryonic and fetal physiology differs from that of mature organisms, pharmacologic effector systems may be different.

To affect human embryonic and fetal tissues, xenobiotics must traverse the placenta. The human placenta is a relatively good barrier against microorganisms, but it is substantially less effective at excluding drugs and chemicals. The physicochemical properties (eg, molecular size, solubility, charge) that allow foreign chemicals to be absorbed into the maternal circulation also allow them to cross the placenta. Xenobiotic metabolism occurs in the human placenta, but the placenta is better able to metabolize steroid hormones and low-level environmental contaminants than drugs.

The timing of xenobiotic exposure is an important determinant of its effects. Individual organs express so-called critical periods of development, during which they are particularly susceptible to maldevelopment, if their programs for differentiation are disrupted or unbalanced. Figure 33–10 shows critical periods of development for several organs. These periods are not confined to early gestation. Note, for instance, that the developing brain is susceptible to toxicity throughout pregnancy.

Prescribed and over-the-counter drugs that reach pharmacologically active levels in maternal blood will, in general, equilibrate to the same levels across the placenta. Agents known to produce cytotoxicity in adults are therefore likely to be teratogenic. Abused substances achieve pharmacologically and toxicologically active levels on both sides of the placenta. Because they are frequently toxic to adults, they will be predictably toxic to embryos and fetuses. Drugs generally safe in adults will be generally safe for fetuses, but depending on specific drug-effector actions, some risk for abnormal development must always be considered. Risk assessment requires continuous monitoring of populations exposed to drugs during pregnancy.

Effects of environmental contaminants on the embryo and fetus are also dose-dependent. Thus the level of exposure frequently becomes the primary determinant of risk. In general, exposures producing symptoms in mothers can be assumed to be potentially toxic to the fetus.

Mutagens in the environment may be a special problem. Experiments at high levels of exposure indicate that mutagenic agents are also teratogenic. Specific phenotypes, however, are difficult to predict. Mutations induced in embryonic tissues result in mosaicism. These changes may not be visible but can contribute to diseases such as cancer later in life. DNA damage in developing cells can switch them into apoptotic pathways and may therefore have more immediate effects. The extent of this problem for humans is incompletely understood. Maternal exposure to mutagenic chemotherapy is predictably associated with abnormalities of fetal growth or birth defects. Evidence is also accumulating that transplacental exposures to environmental mutagens may affect brain growth. Not all transplacental pharmacologic effects are toxic. There is increasing potential for therapeutic transplacental uses of drugs in pregnancy. For example, folic acid supplementation can lower risks for birth defects such as spina bifida, and maternally administered corticosteroids induce fetal synthesis and secretion of surfactants prior to delivery.

## MECHANICAL FACTORS

Much of embryonic development and all of fetal growth occur normally with the conceptus surrounded by amniotic fluid. The low pressure and the space provided by this fluid are critical for the development of most organs. Disruption of the formation or integrity of placental membranes for whatever reason can lead to major, usually lethal, distortion of the embryo (early amnion disruption sequence) or to deformation or even amputation of fetal extremities (amniotic band sequence).

Fetal movement is also important for morphogenesis. Normal movement is necessary for normal development of joints and is the principal determinant of folds

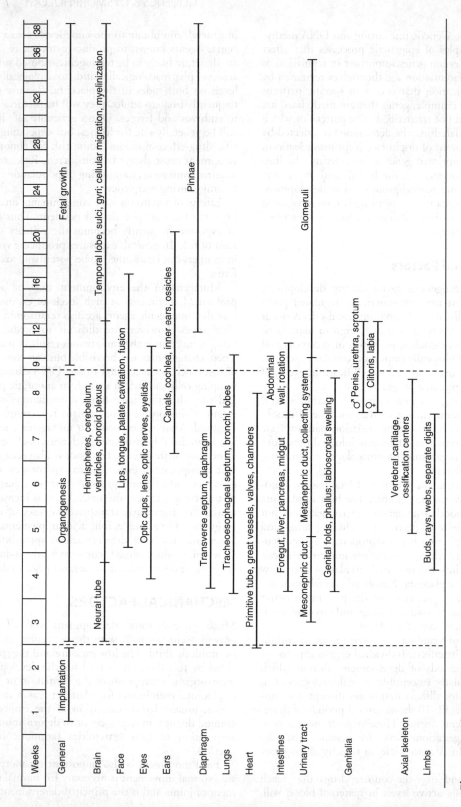

| Weeks | 1 | 2 | 3 | 4 | 5 | 6 | 7 | 8 | 9 | 12 | 16 | 20 | 24 | 28 | 32 | 36 | 38 |
|---|---|---|---|---|---|---|---|---|---|---|---|---|---|---|---|---|---|

General — Implantation — Organogenesis — Fetal growth

Brain — Neural tube — Hemispheres, cerebellum, ventricles, choroid plexus — Temporal lobe, sulci, gyri; cellular migration, myelinization

Face — Lips, tongue, palate: cavitation, fusion

Eyes — Optic cups, lens, optic nerves, eyelids

Ears — Canals, cochlea, inner ears, ossicles — Pinnae

Diaphragm — Transverse septum, diaphragm

Lungs — Tracheoesophageal septum, bronchi, lobes

Heart — Primitive tube, great vessels, valves, chambers

Intestines — Foregut, liver, pancreas, midgut — Abdominal wall; rotation

Urinary tract — Mesonephric duct — Metanephric duct, collecting system — Glomeruli

Genitalia — Genital folds, phallus; labioscrotal swelling — ♂ Penis, urethra, scrotum / ♀ Clitoris, labia

Axial skeleton — Vertebral cartilage, ossification centers

Limbs — Buds, rays, webs, separate digits

***Figure 33–10.*** Critical periods in human gestation.

and creases present at birth in the face, hands, feet, and other areas of the body. In the presence of fetal muscle weakness, for instance, developing joints conform to fetal position and shape of the uterus. Clubfoot, an etiologically heterogeneous condition in which the foot is malpositioned at birth, more often results from mechanical constraint secondary to intrauterine crowding, decreased muscle strength or tone, or abnormal neurologic function than from primary skeletal maldevelopment.

Lung and kidney development are particularly sensitive to mechanical forces. Constriction of the chest through maldevelopment of the ribs, lack of surrounding amniotic fluid, or lack of movement (fetal breathing) leads to varying degrees of pulmonary hypoplasia in which lungs are smaller than normal and develop fewer alveoli. Mechanically induced pulmonary hypoplasia is a common cause of respiratory distress at birth and may be lethal. Cystic renal dysplasia commonly accompanies birth defects that obstruct ureters or outflow from the bladder. In such cases, as the kidneys become functional, urinary pressure within obstructed collecting systems increases and is propagated back into developing tissues. This is a good example of how distortion of cell surface interactions and malalignment of extracellular matrix may lead to abnormal histogenesis. Developing kidneys exposed for long periods to increased internal pressures eventually become nonfunctional.

## PRENATAL DIAGNOSIS

To investigate fetal growth and development, prenatal visits should be noted and, with the aid of the obstetric wheel, a record should be made of the patterns of fetal growth, the onset of fetal movement (usually at 16 weeks), and the mother's perceptions of fetal movements. Normal fetal movement is usually strong enough to discomfort the mother and be visible to the father. Abnormal fetal movement may indicate neuromuscular dysfunction or fetal constraint. A history of decreased fetal movement will often distinguish neuromuscular abnormalities (which result in a low Apgar score) from intrapartum events (which depress the infant).

Abnormal patterns of uterine growth may also provide clues to fetal function. Increased uterine size may indicate accumulation of amniotic fluid (hydramnios). Fluid may accumulate if the fetus fails to swallow as a result of a neuromuscular disorder, obstruction of the fetal esophagus or proximal small bowel, or fetal heart failure. Hydramnios is also associated with diabetes and high-output renal failure in the fetus. Lack or delay of uterine growth may reflect fetal growth directly or may be a sign of too little amniotic fluid (oligohydramnios).

Amniotic fluid may be lost through premature rupture of membranes with or without formation of amniotic bands, or it may be the result of compromised function of fetal kidneys. The mother should be questioned about loss or leakage of amniotic fluid, which may have been mistaken for a vaginal discharge.

The history should also include details about the onset and progression of labor. Breech presentation at term may indicate a uterine anomaly or abnormality of the fetal CNS. Placental pathology should also be reviewed.

## CLINICAL DYSMORPHOLOGY

Classification of dysmorphic features is beginning to reflect better understanding of the mechanisms of maldevelopment. However, much of the nomenclature used to describe abnormal development remains historical, and reflects the fact that many patterns of birth defects were recognized prior to any understanding of their molecular biology.

Birth defects are referred to as **malformations** when they result from altered genetic or developmental processes. When physical forces interrupt or distort morphogenesis, their effects are termed **disruptions** and **deformations,** respectively. The term **dysplasia** is used to denote abnormal histogenesis. Malformations occurring together more frequently than would be expected by chance alone, whether within a currently recognized developmental field or not, may be classified as belonging to **associations.** Those in which the order of maldevelopment is understood may be referred to as **sequences.** For example, Robin sequence (Pierre Robin syndrome) is used to describe cleft palate that has occurred because poor growth of the jaw (retrognathia) has displaced the tongue and prevented posterior closure of the palate. **Syndromes** are simply recurrent patterns of maldevelopment.

### Evaluation of the Dysmorphic Infant

Physicians caring for infants with birth defects must frequently provide care and make accurate diagnoses under conditions of great stress. The extent of an infant's abnormalities may not be immediately apparent, and parents who feel grief and guilt are often desperate for information. As with any medical problem, however, the history and physical examination provide most of the clues to diagnosis. Special aspects of these procedures are outlined in the following sections.

#### A. HISTORY

Environmental, family, and pregnancy histories may contain important clues to the diagnosis. Parental recall after delivery of an infant with an anomaly is better than recall after a normal birth. An obstetric wheel can help document gestational age and events of the first trimester: the last menstrual period, the onset of symptoms of pregnancy, the date of diagnosis of the pregnancy, the date of the first prenatal visit, and the physician's impressions of fetal growth at that time.

Family histories should always be included and may provide important clues to genetic cause of the infant's issues. Finally, an environmental history that includes descriptions of parental habits, their work, and the home should be obtained.

### B. PHYSICAL EXAMINATION

Meticulous physical examination is crucial for accurate diagnosis in dysmorphic infants and children. In addition to the routine procedures described in Chapter 1, special attention should be paid to the neonate's physical measurements (Figure 33–11). Photographs are helpful and should include a scale of measurements for reference.

### C. IMAGING & LABORATORY STUDIES

Radiologic and ultrasonographic examinations can be extremely helpful in the evaluation of dysmorphic infants. In general, films of infants with apparent limb or skeletal anomalies should include views of the skull and all of the long bones in addition to frontal and lateral views of the axial skeleton. Chest and abdominal films should be obtained when indicated. The pediatrician should consult a radiologist for further work-up. Nuclear scans and imaging by computed tomography (CT), magnetic resonance imaging (MRI), and ultrasonography are all useful diagnostic tools, but their interpretation in the presence of birth defects may require considerable experience.

Cytogenetic analysis provides specific diagnoses in approximately 5% of dysmorphic infants who survive the newborn period. Chromosomal abnormalities are recognized in 10–15% of infants who die. Karyotypes can be determined rapidly through use of FISH. These allow limited interpretation and should always be accompanied by complete analysis of cultured cells. Any case requiring rapid diagnosis should be discussed with an experienced dysmorphologist. A normal karyotype does not rule out the presence of significant genetic disease.

### D. PERINATAL AUTOPSY

When a dysmorphic infant dies, postmortem examination can provide important diagnostic information and should include sampling of tissue for cytogenetic analysis. The pediatrician and the pathologist should consider whether samples of blood, urine, or tissue should be obtained for metabolic analyses.

| Measurement | Range (cm) | |
| --- | --- | --- |
| | **Term**<br>**(38–40 weeks)** | **Preterm**<br>**(32–33 weeks)** |
| 1 Head circumference | 32–37 | 27–32 |
| 2 Anterior fontanelle $\left(\frac{L-W}{2}\right)$ | 0.7–3.7 | . . . |
| 3 Interpupillary distance | 3.3–4.5 | 3.1–3.9 |
| 4 Palpebral fissure | 1.5–2.1 | 1.3–1.6 |
| 5 Inner canthal distance | 1.5–2.5 | 1.4–2.1 |
| 6 Outer canthal distance | 5.3–7.3 | 3.9–5.1 |
| 7 Philtrum | 0.6–1.2 | 0.5–0.9 |
| 8 Ear length | 3–4.3 | 2.4–3.5 |
| 9 Chest circumference | 28–38 | 23–29 |
| 10 Internipple distance* | 6.5–10 | 5–6.5 |
| 11 Height | 47–55 | 39–47 |
| 12<br>13 Ratio $\dfrac{\text{Upper body segment}}{\text{Lower body segment}}$ | 1.7 | . . . |
| 14 Hand (palm to middle finger) | 5.3–7.8 | 4.1–5.5 |
| 15 Ratio of middle finger to hand | 0.38–0.48 | 0.38–0.5 |
| 16 Penis (pubic bone to tip of glans) | 2.7–4.3 | 1.8–3.2 |

*Internipple distance should not exceed 25% of chest circumference.

***Figure 33–11.*** Neonatal measurements.

Radiologic studies should be done whenever limb anomalies or disproportionate growth is present. Placental as well as fetal tissue can be used for viral culture. The pediatrician should discuss the case thoroughly with the pathologist, and photographs should always be taken.

# ◼ CLINICAL FEATURES OF COMMON GENETIC DISORDERS

## CHROMOSOMAL DISORDERS: ABNORMAL NUMBER

### ANEUPLOIDY

#### Trisomy 21 (Down Syndrome)

Down syndrome occurs in about 1:600 newborns; however, the incidence is greater among children of mothers older than age 35 years. Mental retardation is characteristic of Down syndrome, with typical intelligence quotients (IQs) between 20 and 80 (mostly between 45 and 55). The principal physical findings include a small, brachycephalic head, characteristic facies (up-slanting palpebral fissures, epicanthal folds, midface hypoplasia, and small, dysplastic pinnae), and other dysmorphic features. About one third to one half of children with Down syndrome have congenital heart disease, most often an endocardial cushion defect or other septal defect. Anomalies of the gastrointestinal (GI) tract are seen in about 15% of cases, including esophageal and duodenal atresias. Generalized hypotonia is common. Sexual development is retarded, especially in males, who are usually sterile. The affected newborn may have prolonged physiologic jaundice, polycythemia, and a transient leukemoid reaction. Later, there is an increased tendency for thyroid dysfunction, hearing loss, celiac disease, and atlanto-occipital instability. Leukemia is 12–20 times more common in Down syndrome patients than in unaffected children.

#### Trisomy 18 Syndrome

The incidence of trisomy 18 syndrome is about 1:4000 live births, and the ratio of affected males to females is approximately 1:3. Trisomy 18 is characterized by prenatal and postnatal growth retardation that is often severe; hypertonicity; dysmorphic features, including a characteristic face (see the following website for clinical pictures:

medgen.genetics.utah.edu/photographs/pages/trisomy_18.htm

and extremities [overlapping fingers and rockerbottom feet]; and congenital heart disease [often ventricular septal defect or patent ductus arteriosus]). Complications are related to associated birth defects. Death is often caused by heart failure or pneumonia and usually occurs in infancy or early childhood, although a small percentage of patients reach adulthood. Surviving children show significant developmental delay and mental retardation.

#### Trisomy 13 Syndrome

The incidence of trisomy 13 is about 1:12,000 live births, and 60% of affected individuals are female. The mean maternal age is increased. The symptoms and signs include prenatal and postnatal growth deficiency (although, unlike trisomy 18, infants may have a normal birth weight), CNS malformations, arrhinencephaly, eye malformations (anophthalmia, colobomas), cleft lip and palate, polydactyly or syndactyly, and congenital heart disease (usually ventricular septal defect). The facies of an infant with trisomy 13 can be viewed on the following website:

medgen.genetics.utah. edu/photographs/pages/trisomy_13.htm

Surviving children demonstrate failure to thrive, developmental retardation, apneic spells, seizures, and deafness. Death usually occurs in early infancy or by the second year of life, commonly as a result of heart failure or infection.

### Treatment for Aneuploidies

There is no convincing documentation of the merit of any of the forms of specific therapy that have been attempted in Down syndrome, ranging from megadoses of vitamins to exercise programs proposed to overcome the physical and developmental abnormalities of the syndrome. Therapy is for specific problems: surgery or drugs for heart problems, antibiotics for infections and thyroid function tests, infant stimulation programs, special education, and occupational training as required. The goal of treatment is to help affected children develop to their full potential. Parents' participation in support groups such as the local chapter of the National Down Syndrome Congress should be encouraged. See the following website:

http://www. ndss.org/

There is no treatment, other than general supportive care, for trisomy 13 or 18. Because it is sometimes necessary to decide immediately after birth how extensive therapy should be for a severely malformed infant, trisomy 13 and 18 can be screened for in interphase nuclei of blood lymphocytes by FISH and confirmed by direct chromosome analysis of blood or bone marrow mitoses. A support group for families of children with trisomies 13 and 18 who survive beyond infancy is called SOFT. See the following website:

www.trisomy.org/

## Genetic Counseling

Most parents of trisomic babies have normal karyotypes. The risk of having a child affected with a trisomy varies with maternal age. For trisomy 21, age-specific risks are 1:2000 for mothers younger than age 25 years; 1:200 for mothers age 35 years; 1:100 for mothers age 40; and 1:10 for mothers older than age 45 years. The recurrence risk for trisomy in future pregnancies is equal to 1:100 plus the age-specific maternal risk (for example, a 40-year-old mother with a prior child with Down syndrome would have a risk of 1:100 for her age, plus 1:100 for her prior history, or 1:50). If the child has a trisomy resulting from a translocation, and the parent has an abnormal karyotype, the risks are increased.

When the mother is the carrier of a balanced 14/21 translocation, there is a 10–15% chance that the child will be affected and a 33% chance that the child will be a balanced translocation carrier. When the father is the carrier, there is a smaller than 0.5% chance of having another affected child. If the child has a 21/21 translocation and one parent has the translocation, the recurrence risk is 100%.

The recurrence risks in other trisomies are analogous to those for Down syndrome. The mother's age at the time of conception and the nature of the chromosomal abnormality are important in genetic counseling, which is indicated for prevention of all chromosomal abnormalities. Prenatal diagnosis is available.

## ■ SEX CHROMOSOMES

## Turner Syndrome (Monosomy X, Gonadal Dysgenesis)

The incidence of Turner syndrome is 1:10,000 females. However, it is estimated that 95% of conceptuses with monosomy X are miscarried and only 5% are liveborn. Newborns with Turner syndrome may have webbed neck, edema of the hands and feet, coarctation of the aorta, and a characteristic triangular facies. Later symptoms include short stature, a shield chest with wide-set nipples, streak ovaries, amenorrhea, absence of secondary sex characteristics, and infertility. Some affected girls, particularly those with mosaicism, have only short stature and amenorrhea, without dysmorphic features. Complications relate primarily to coarctation of the aorta, when present. Rarely, the dysgenetic gonads may become neoplastic (gonadoblastoma). The incidence of malformations of the urinary tract is increased. Learning disabilities are common, secondary to difficulties in perceptual motor integration. Patients with pseudohypoparathyroidism and Noonan syndrome have a similar phenotype to patients with Turner syndrome, but have normal chromosomes.

In Turner syndrome the identification and treatment of perceptual difficulties before they become problematic is very important. Teenage patients need counseling to cope with the stigma of their condition and to understand the need for hormone therapy. Estrogen replacement therapy will permit development of secondary sex characteristics and normal menstruation and prevent osteoporosis. Growth hormone therapy has been used to increase the height of affected girls. Females with 45,X or 45,X mosaicism have a low fertility rate, and those who become pregnant have a high risk of fetal wastage (spontaneous miscarriage, approximately 30%; stillbirth, 6–10%). Furthermore, their liveborn offspring have an increased frequency of chromosomal abnormalities involving either sex chromosomes or autosomes, and congenital malformations. Thus prenatal ultrasonography and chromosome analysis are indicated for the offspring of females with sex chromosome abnormalities.

## Klinefelter Syndrome (XXY)

The incidence of Klinefelter syndrome in the newborn population is roughly 1:1000, but it is about 1% among mentally retarded males and about 3% among males seen at infertility clinics. The maternal age at birth is often advanced. Unlike Turner syndrome, Klinefelter syndrome is rarely the cause of spontaneous abortions. The diagnosis is rarely made before puberty except as a result of prenatal diagnosis, because prepubertal boys have a normal phenotype. The characteristic findings after puberty include micro-orchidism associated with otherwise normal external genitalia, azoospermia, sterility, gynecomastia, normal to borderline IQ, diminished facial hair, lack of libido and potency, and a tall, eunuchoid build. In chromosome variants with three or four X chromosomes (XXXY and XXXXY), mental retardation may be severe, and radioulnar synostosis may be present as well as anomalies of the external genitalia and cryptorchidism. In the XXXXY cases, these findings are especially prominent, and microcephaly, short stature, and dysmorphic features also occur. In general, the physical and mental abnormalities associated with Klinefelter syndrome increase as the number of sex chromosomes increases. Males with Klinefelter syndrome require testosterone replacement therapy.

## XYY Syndrome

Newborns in general are normal. Affected individuals may on occasion exhibit an abnormal behavior pattern from early childhood and may have mild retardation. Fertility may be normal. Many males with an XYY karyotype are normal. There is no treatment. Long-term problems may relate to low IQ and environmental stress.

## XXX Syndrome

The incidence of females with an XXX karyotype is approximately 1:1000. Females with XXX are phenotypically normal. However, they tend to be taller than usual and to have lower IQs than their normal siblings. Learning and behavioral issues are relatively common. This is in contrast to individuals with XXXX, a much rarer condition causing more severe developmental issues, and a dysmorphic phenotype reminiscent of Down syndrome.

Gorlin RJ et al: *Syndromes of the Head and Neck,* 4th ed, Chapter 3. Oxford University Press, 2001.

Jones KL: *Smith's Recognizable Patterns of Human Malformation,* 5th ed. WB Saunders, 1996.

## MOSAICISM

Although most cases of severe chromosomal abnormality such as trisomy are lethal, some individuals may survive if the abnormality exists in mosaic form (ie, the patient has a mixture of trisomic and normal cells). Two disorders with this condition include trisomy 8 and Cat-eye syndromes.

## Trisomy 8 Syndrome

More than 100 cases of this condition have been reported. The phenotype is variable, but includes mildly dysmorphic features (deep-set eyes, hypertelorism, prominent pinnae, high arched or cleft palate), skeletal, cardiac, and renal malformations. Cognitively, the individuals have limitations ranging from mild to severe.

## Cat-Eye Syndrome

Cat-eye syndrome is caused by an extra chromosome, which is derived from a portion of chromosome 22 (the short arm, centromere, and a small piece of the long arm). The phenotype consists of iris coloboma (causing the appearance of the eye lending its name to the syndrome), dysmorphic features (down-slanting palpebral fissures, malformed pinnae), and anal atresia. Other common anomalies include those of the heart, kidneys, and GI tract. Intelligence is usually mildly impaired, but may be normal.

# ■ CHROMOSOMAL ABNORMALITIES: STRUCTURAL

Chromosomal abnormalities are most often present in newborns as multiple congenital anomalies in association with intrauterine growth retardation. Common aneuploid syndromes (trisomies 13, 18, and 21) were described earlier in this chapter. Several common chromosomal deletions produce contiguous gene syndromes recognizable in newborns. In the presence of apparently normal chromosomes, each of these conditions can be detected by FISH.

## Wolf–Hirschhorn Syndrome

Also known as 4p− (deletion of 4p16), this syndrome is characterized by microcephaly and unusual development of the nose and orbits that produces an appearance suggesting an ancient Greek warrior's helmet. Association with cleft lip and palate and other major organ anomalies, such as heart and renal structural anomalies and seizure disorders, are common. The majority of the patients have severe developmental delay and mental retardation. However, higher functioning individuals have been reported. A critical region defines the facial features of this syndrome and is detectable by FISH.

## Cri Du Chat Syndrome

Also known as 5p− (deletion of terminal chromosome 5p), this disorder is characterized by unique facial features, growth retardation, and microcephaly. Patients have an unusual cat-like cry. Most patients have major organ anomalies and significant developmental delay.

## Williams Syndrome

This, a contiguous gene disorder involving the elastin gene and other neighboring genes at 7q11.2, is characterized by short stature, congenital heart disease (supravalvular aortic stenosis), coarse, elfin-like facies with prominent lips, hypercalcemia or hypercalciuria in infancy, developmental delay, and neonatal irritability evolving into an overly friendly personality. Microdeletions of the elastin gene are diagnostic through FISH testing. However, individuals with smaller deletions require more specific probes to confirm the diagnosis. Calcium restriction may be necessary in early childhood to prevent nephrocalcinosis. Calcium determination is recommended in early infancy, and the hypercalcemia often resolves during the first year of life. The natural history includes progression of cardiac disease and predisposition to hypertension and spinal osteoarthritis in adults. Most patients have mild to moderate intellectual deficits.

## Langer–Giedion Syndrome

This syndrome, also known as trichorhinophalangeal syndrome type II, is caused by a deletion on the long arm of chromosome 8 (8q24.11–q24.13). Individuals with Langer–Giedion syndrome show unusual facial features (large, bulbous nose, large ears), and develop bony abnormalties including cone-shaped epiphyses and multiple bony exostoses. The skin may be loose and redundant, resembling the connective tissue disorder Ehlers–Danlos syndrome. Intelligence is impaired and hearing loss is common.

## Aniridia–Wilms Tumor Association (WAGR)

WAGR syndrome, which stands for **W**ilms tumor, **a**niridia, **g**enitourinary anomalies, and **r**etardation, is caused by a deletion of the short arm of chromosome 11 (11p13). In addition to the aniridia, other common eye defects include cataracts and ptosis. Many patients have visual impairment. About one half of patients develop Wilms tumor. Other anomalies include facial dysmorphism and genitourinary abnormalities.

## Miller–Dieker Syndrome

A contiguous gene syndrome involving 17p13, this abnormality is characterized by microcephaly and severe CNS dysgenesis. The most commonly seen CNS malformation is termed **lissencephaly** ("smooth brain" as the brain is lacking its normal convolutions and gyri). An unusually developed face and forehead reflect abnormal migration of neuronal germinal matrix cells. When the affected individuals cry, characteristic longitudinal groves appear in the forehead. Mutations in the gene *MDS1,* which is located in the critical region, can cause isolated lissencephaly, without the full picture of Miller–Dieker. Severe cognitive and developmental delay and seizure disorders are common. In the presence of apparently normal chromosomes, FISH can detect this condition.

## Smith–Magenis Syndrome

This syndrome is associated with microdeletion of 17p11 and is characterized by prominent forehead, deep-set eyes, cupid-shaped upper lip, self-mutilating behavior (pulling nails and hair, putting objects into body orifices), sleep disturbance, and developmental delay. Some patients also have seizure disorders. Melatonin has proven helpful in improving the abnormal sleep patterns and controlling the behavior. Some individuals with larger deletions involving *PMP22* can present with peripheral neuropathy.

## Del 22q11 Syndrome

Also known as DiGeorge syndrome, this abnormality was originally described in newborns presenting with cyanotic congenital heart disease, usually involving great vessel abnormalities; thymic hypoplasia leading to immunodeficiency; and hypocalcemia due to absent parathyroid glands. The disorder is now known to result most often from deletions of chromosome 22q11 and to be phenotypically highly variable. The less severe phenotypes include velocardiofacial syndrome (VCFS), Shprintzen syndrome, Cayler cardiofacial syndrome, and a subset of Opitz G and BBB syndromes. Characteristics include mild microcephaly; palatal clefting or incompetence; speech and language delays; congenital heart disease (ventricular or atrial septal defect); build-up of tissue lateral to the nose; long, tapering fingers; and emotional liability. Midline defects such as umbilical hernia and hypospadias can be associated anomalies. In some cases, individuals have an apparent predisposition to psychosis.

# MENDELIAN DISORDERS

## AUTOSOMAL DOMINANT INHERITANCE

### 1. Neurofibromatosis Type 1

**ESSENTIALS OF DIAGNOSIS & TYPICAL FEATURES**

*Minimal diagnostic criteria require two or more of the following:*

- *Six or more café au lait macules, at least 15 mm in diameter in postpubertal and 5 mm in prepubertal individuals.*
- *Two or more neurofibromas of any type or one plexiform neurofibroma.*
- *Axillary or inguinal freckling.*
- *Two or more Lisch nodules (iris hamartomas)*
- *Optic glioma*
- *Distinctive bony lesions such as sphenoid dysplasia or pseudarthrosis.*
- *An affected first-degree relative.*

## General Considerations

Neurofibromatosis 1 (NF-1) is one of the most common autosomal dominant disorders, occurring in 1:3000 births and seen in all races and ethnic groups. It has a wide range of clinical manifestations. In general, the disorder is progressive, and new manifestations appear over time. Neurofibromatosis 2, characterized by bilateral acoustic neuromas, with minimal or no skin manifestations, is a different disease caused by a different gene.

## Clinical Findings

Café au lait macules may be present at birth, and about 80% of individuals with neurofibromatosis 1 will have more than six by age 1 year. The typical skin lesion is 10–30 mm, ovoid, and smooth-bordered, but there is great variation. Neurofibromas are benign tumors consisting of Schwann cells, nerve fibers, and fibroblasts; they may be discrete or plexiform. Discrete tumors are more common and can occur at any age. They are well demarcated and can present in cutaneous, subcutaneous, or internal tissues. Plexiform neurofibromas are more diffuse and can invade normal tissue. They are congenital and are frequently detected during periods of rapid growth. If the face or a limb is involved, there may be associated hypertrophy or overgrowth. The incidence of Lisch nodules, which can be seen with a slit-lamp, also increases with age.

Common features of affected individuals include a large head (though only a small percentage have true hydrocephalus), bony abnormalities on radiographic studies, scoliosis, and a wide spectrum of developmental problems. The most common problems in childhood are secondary to plexiform neurofibromas and learning disabilities. Although the average IQ is within the normal range, it is lower than in unaffected family members. The common learning disabilities seen in patients with NF include dyslexia, dysgraphia, and disorders of visual perception.

## Differential Diagnosis

Areas of hyperpigmentation can occur in other conditions (eg, Albright, Noonan, and Leopard syndromes), but the lesions are either single or different in character. Isolated neurofibromas and familial café au lait spots as an autosomal dominant trait (fewer than six and with no other manifestations of NF) have been described. The relationship of such cases to classic NF-1 is uncertain.

## Complications

It is difficult to differentiate a complication from a rare manifestation of the underlying disorder. Seizures,

deafness, short stature, early puberty, and hypertension occur in less than 25% of persons with NF. Optic glioma seems to occur in about 15% of individuals with NF-1. Although the tumor may be apparent at an early age, it rarely causes functional problems and is usually nonprogressive. Patients have a slightly increased risk (5% life risk) for a variety of malignancies. Other tumors may be benign but may cause significant morbidity and mortality because of their size and location in a vital or enclosed space.

## Treatment

The therapy is symptomatic. Neurofibromas can be removed if they cause discomfort or are a cosmetic problem. The most important part of therapy is close, ongoing follow-up. Because this disorder is progressive, affected individuals should be seen at regular intervals and have regular monitoring of height, head circumference, blood pressure, and scoliosis. Additionally, eye examinations are necessary for early detection of changes associated with aggressive optic glioma. Developmental screening as well as other evaluations (eg, MRI scans) are done as indicated according to symptoms. Follow-up is best done in a multidisciplinary neurocutaneous clinic.

## Prognosis

Because NF varies so widely in its progress, assessing prognosis is difficult. However, most affected children have only skin lesions and few other problems. Severely affected individuals are rare in the pediatric age range, and close follow-up and early intervention may ameliorate some complications.

## Genetic Counseling

The gene for NF-1 is on the long arm of chromosome 17 and seems to code for a protein similar to a tumor suppresser factor. NF results from many different mutations of this gene. Approximately 50% of all cases of NF are caused by new mutations. Before attributing an individual case to a new mutation, however, both parents must be evaluated carefully, including a thorough examination of the skin and a slitlamp examination to look for Lisch nodules. Recent evidence suggests that penetrance is close to 100% in those who carry the gene if individuals are examined carefully.

## 2. Marfan Syndrome

Marfan syndrome is caused by mutations in genes coding for the connective tissue protein fibrillin, but laboratory detection of mutations in clinical practice remains, for the time being, difficult. Clinical diagnostic criteria have been developed that include disproportionate growth (arachnodactyly and tall stature), joint hyperextensibility, lens dislocation, and dilation of the aortic root. The latter two characteristics are considered major criteria and are diagnostic when accompanied by evidence of connective tissue involvement, usually joint hyperextensibility. The characteristic facies is long and thin, with down-slanting palpebral fissures. The palate is high arched, and dentition is often crowded. The most serious associated medical problems involve the heart. Many patients with Marfan syndrome have mitral valve prolapse. A potentially life-threatening cardiac problem is progressive aortic root dilatation, which may lead to aneurysmal rupture and death.

The diagnosis of Marfan syndrome is still made on a clinical basis, and many cases represent sporadic new mutations. Although the gene for fibrillin has been identified, many unique, family-specific mutations occur, making molecular confirmation difficult.

Medical treatment for patients with Marfan syndrome includes appropriate management of the ophthalmologic, orthopedic, and cardiac issues. Serial echocardiograms are indicated to diagnose and follow the degree of aortic root enlargement, which can be managed medically or surgically, in more severe cases. In individuals with marfanoid habitus and cognitive disabilities, homocystinuria should be excluded through careful metabolic testing. Another connective tissue disorder, Ehlers–Danlos syndrome (EDS), shares some features with Marfan syndrome, including joint hyperextensibility and skin fragility. The skin is the target organ for the most significant symptoms in EDS patients. At least nine forms of EDS occur, most inherited as dominant traits, but the biochemical causes have only been worked out for a few of the forms.

## 3. Achondroplasia

Achondroplasia is the most common form of skeletal dysplasia, like many forms of skeletal dysplasias is inherited as a dominant condition, and is caused by a mutation in *FGFR3*. The classic phenotype includes relative macrocephaly, midface hypoplasia, short-limbed dwarfism, and trident-shaped hands. The phenotype is apparent at birth and may be diagnosed prenatally on ultrasound. Individuals with achondroplasia are cognitively normal. Bony overgrowth at the level of the foramen magnum may lead to progressive hydrocephalus and may warrant neurosurgical intervention. Because of this, head circumference during infancy must be closely monitored and plotted on a diagnosis-specific head circumference chart. Serial head ultrasounds are helpful every few months. Orthopedic intervention is necessary for spinal problems including severe lumbar lordosis and gibbus deformity. Long bone lengthening surgery, such as the Ilizarov procedure, are used in some centers to increase height and upper extremity function, but their use is still controversial. Two hemizygous parents with achondroplasia have a 25% risk of having a child homozygous for *FGFR 3* mutations, which is a lethal disorder.

## 4. Osteogenesis Imperfecta

Osteogenesis imperfecta (OI), or brittle bone disease, is a relatively common autosomal dominant disorder, caused by mutations in type I collagen. Most patients with more severe disease represent new mutations for this disorder. There are four types of OI. Types I and IV are relatively mild and generally present with increased incidence of fracturing, but otherwise a fairly normal phenotype. Type II is generally lethal in the newborn period and is the most severe form. Formerly believed to be autosomal recessive, type II is now thought to be caused by a new dominant mutation, with multiple cases within a family attributed to parental germ cell mosaicism. Type III is the severe form causing significant bony deformity secondary to multiple fractures. A major advancement in the treatment of OI patients has been the use of pamidronate, a bisphosphonate compound, which has been reported to lead to a reduced incidence of fracture and improvement in bone density.

## 5. Craniosynostoses Syndromes

The craniosynostoses disorders are common dominant disorders associated with premature fusion of cranial sutures. This class of disorders is now known to be caused by mutations in *FGFR* genes. Crouzon syndrome is the most common of these disorders and is associated with multiple suture fusions, but with normal limbs. Common problems associated with craniosynostosis include shallow orbits leading to proptosis, midface narrowing that may result in upper airway obstruction, and hydrocephalus that may require shunting. Children with craniosynostosis undergo multiple staged craniofacial/neurosurgical procedures to address these issues. Other craniosynostosis disorders have limb as well as craniofacial anomalies, and include Pfeiffer, Apert, Jackson–Weiss, and Saethre–Chotzen syndromes.

## 6. Treacher Collins Syndrome

Treacher Collins syndrome is a dominant disorder, although more than half of the patients present as a result of new mutations. This is a craniofacial disorder associated with malar and mandibular hypoplasia, malformed ears with associated hearing loss, and abnormalities of the eye including lower lid coloboma and absent lashes. Airway anomalies may occur, causing life-threatening problems in the newborn period. Intelligence is generally normal. This disorder has been linked to chromosome 5q32–33.2 in some families.

## AUTOSOMAL RECESSIVE DISORDERS

### 1. Cystic Fibrosis

The gene for cystic fibrosis (CF), *CFTR*, is found on the long arm of chromosome 7. Approximately 1 in 22 persons are carriers. Over 600 different mutations have been identified: the most common in the Caucasian population, known as Δ F 508, is a three-base deletion coding for phenylalanine.

Cloning of the gene for CF and identification of the mutation in the majority of cases have completely changed genetic counseling and prenatal diagnosis for this disorder, although the sweat chloride assay is still important in confirming the diagnosis. The American College of Medical Genetics recommends the 25-mutation assay using PCR-based techniques, which can cover 85–90% of the mutations. If a mutation is found, carriers can be identified and specific prenatal diagnosis can be performed, identifying both carriers and affected fetuses. If a mutation cannot be identified, linkage analysis, DNA haplotyping, and amniotic fluid enzyme studies can be done.

The identification of the mutation in the CF gene has also raised the issue of mass newborn screening, because of the high frequency of this gene in the Caucasian population. Some states, such as Colorado, have offered newborn screening by trypsinogen assay, which can detect 70% of CF patients. Although the argument can be made for such screening (because early detection can ensure good nutritional status starting at birth, which is the key prognostic factor for the classic CF patient), newborn screening is controversial as there is no cure for CF. (For more details of medical management, please see Chapters 18 [Respiratory Tract & Mediastinum] and 20 [Gastrointestinal Tract] in this text).

### 2. Smith–Lemli–Opitz Syndrome

Smith–Lemli–Opitz (SLO) syndrome, a common autosomal recessive disorder, may have an incidence as high as 1:8000, and the carrier frequency may be as high as 1:31. In 1994, SLO was shown to be caused by a metabolic error in the final step of cholesterol production. This enzyme deficiency results in low cholesterol levels and accumulation of the precursor 7-dehydrocholesterol. Patients with SLO present with a characteristic phenotype, including dysmorphic facial features (Figure 33–12), multiple congenital anomalies (including

***Figure 33–12.*** Child with Smith–Lemli–Opitz syndrome, featuring bitemporal narrowing, upturned nares, ptosis, and small chin.

defects of the CNS, heart, cleft palate, cardiac, kidneys, genitalia and limbs), hypotonia, growth failure, and mental retardation. Treatment with cholesterol can ameliorate the growth failure and lead to improvement in behavior and developmental course, although treatment does not cure this complex disorder.

### 3. Sensorineural Hearing Loss

Nonsyndromic, recessively inherited deafness is the predominant form of severe inherited childhood deafness. There is marked genetic heterogeneity in causes of sensorineural hearing loss (SNHL), including autosomal dominant, recessive, and X-linked patterns. Of mutations known to cause SNHL, mutations of connexin 26 (*CX26*), a gap junction protein, are present in 49% of cases of prelingual deafness. Gap junctions are regionally specialized structures on plasma membranes of contacting adherent cells. These structures were shown to consist of cell-to-cell channels. Connexins are the proteins in the gap junctions. There are different kinds of connexins. Some mutations of connexin 26 can follow autosomal dominant inheritance, but the common mutations follow the recessive mode. Molecular testing is available.

Resendes BL et al: At the speed of sound: Gene discovery in the auditory system. Am J Hum Genet 2001;69:923 [PMID: 11577373].

## 4. Spinal Muscular Atrophy

Spinal muscular atrophy (SMA) is an autosomal recessive neuromuscular disorder in which anterior horn cells in the spinal cord degenerate. The molecular basis for loss of these cells is incompletely understood, but the mechanism appears to involve apoptosis of neurons in the absence of the product of the *SMN 1* (survival motor neuron) gene located on chromosome 5q. Loss of anterior horn cells leads to progressive atrophy of skeletal muscle. The disorder has an incidence of approximately 1 in 12,000, with the majority of the cases presenting in infancy. Carrier frequencies approach 1 in 50 in populations with European ancestry. Three clinical phenotypes are recognized based on age of onset and rate of progression. SMA I is the most devastating. Mild weakness may be present at birth, but is clearly evident by 3 months and is accompanied by loss of reflexes. Progression of the disorder leads to fasciculations and eventual respiratory failure, usually by age 1 year. Symptoms of SMA II begin later; with weakness and decreased reflexes generally apparent by 2 years of age. Children affected with SMA III begin to become weak as they approach adolescence.

The genetics of SMA are complex and relate to duplication, deletion, and gene conversion events in the region of the *SMN 1* gene. Homozygous deletion of exon 7 is detectable in more than 90% of all forms of SMA and constitutes a genetic test by which the clinical diagnosis can be confirmed. Variability in presentation appears to involve expression of neighboring genes including a more centromeric *SMN 2* pseudogene. The presence and expression of multiple copies of *SMN 2,* and a nearly complete copy of *SMN 1,* introduces complexity into molecular genetic analysis used to detect carriers. Prenatal diagnosis is available through analysis of *SMN 1* or genetic linkage, but carrier testing in individuals not related to affected patients known to have homozygous *SMN 1* deletions is not yet available.

## 5. Metabolic Disorders

Most inborn errors of metabolism are inherited in an autosomal recessive pattern. See Chapter 32 in this text for detailed explanations of these disorders.

## X-LINKED INHERITANCE

### 1. Duchenne-Type Muscular Dystrophy

Duchenne muscular dystrophy (DMD) results from failure of synthesis of the muscle cytoskeletal protein dystrophin, whose gene is located on the X chromosome, Xp12. Approximately 1 in 4000 male children are affected. Mutations in the same gene that result in partial expression of the dystrophin protein produce a less severe phenotype, Becker muscular dystrophy (BMD). In both disorders, progressive degeneration of skeletal muscle occurs. Cardiac muscle eventually also becomes involved. Boys with DMD exhibit proximal muscle weakness and pseudohypertrophy of calf muscles at age 5–6 years. Patients become nonambulatory at around age 13. Serum creatine kinase levels are markedly elevated. Affected boys frequently die in their early 20s of respiratory failure and cardiac dysfunction. The prognosis for BMD is more variable. Although corticosteroids are useful in maintaining strength, they do not slow progression of the disorder.

The gene for dystrophin is very large and a common target for mutation. Large deletions or duplications can be detected in the gene for dystrophin in 65% of cases. Demonstration of such a mutation provides a useful genetic marker for the disorder, but diagnosis and prognosis require muscle biopsy and immunohistochemistry for the dystrophin protein.

Theoretically, one third of DMD cases presenting with a negative family history are likely to be new mutations. When a mutation in the gene for dystrophin is detected, maternal carrier status is easily determined and work-up of the extended family is straightforward. Nonetheless, risk assessment and counseling must be approached with care since germline mosaicism for mutations in the gene for dystrophin occurs in approximately 15% of families. Thus, it is necessary to look for mutations in all sisters of affected boys. If a mutation has been detected, prenatal diagnosis is routinely offered to mothers regardless of their apparent carrier status based on analysis of blood samples. Since mutations are currently not detected in approximately 35% of cases, alternative approaches that estimate carrier risks based on creatine kinase levels and utilize genetic linkage for prenatal diagnosis remain useful. Counseling and prenatal diagnosis remain difficult in some families.

### 2. Hemophilia

Hemophilia A is an X-linked, recessive, bleeding disorder caused by a deficiency in the activity of coagulation factor VIII. Affected individuals develop a variable phenotype of hemorrhage into joints and muscles, easy bruising, and prolonged bleeding from wounds. The disorder is caused by heterogeneous mutations in the factor VIII gene, which maps to Xq28. Carrier detection and prenatal diagnosis can be done by direct detection of selected mutations, especially the inversions, the most common gene change, as well as indirectly by linkage analysis. Replacement of factor VIII is done using a variety of preparations derived from human plasma or recombinant techniques. Although replacement therapy is effective in most cases, 10–15% of treated individuals develop neutralizing antibodies that decrease its effectiveness.

### 3. Alport Syndrome

Alport syndrome is characterized by variable degrees of hearing loss and nephropathy. It is a clinically heterogeneous disease and at least six different variants have been reported. The most common type is X-linked due to mutations in the gene coding for the alpha chain of type IV collagen. Female carriers with collagen IVA5 mutations may manifest mild clinical findings such as hematuria and later-onset hearing loss. Affected males usually develop end-stage renal disease. Molecular testing for affected males is available, but no single test is available for female carriers.

### 4. Metabolic Disorders

Some important inborn errors are inherited as X-linked disorders, such as adrenoleukodystrophy. See Chapter 32 in this text for more detailed descriptions.

# NONMENDELIAN INHERITANCE
## DISORDERS OF IMPRINTING
### 1. Beckwith–Wiedemann Syndrome

The association of macrosomia (enlarged body size), macroglossia (enlarged tongue), and omphalocele constitutes the Beckwith–Wiedemann syndrome (BWS), now known to be related to abnormal expression of genes located at chromosome 11p15. Other associated findings include mild facial dysmorphism (hypertelorism, unusual ear creases), infantile hypoglycemia due to transient hyperinsulinemia, multiple congenital anomalies (cleft palate and genitourinary anomalies common), and increased risk for certain malignancies, especially Wilms tumor (7–10%). A growth factor gene, *IGF2* is normally imprinted such that the maternal allele is ordinarily not expressed during intrauterine development. Chromosomal abnormalities affecting expression of this gene, such as duplication of the paternal

11p15 region, are associated with BWS. Paternal UPD leading to duplication of transcription of *IGF2* on the paternal homolog, with loss of a tumor suppressor gene (*H19*) normally read from the maternal homolog, may lead to the macrosomia and an increased predisposition to cancer seen in this disorder. Supporting the role of imprinting in BWS is that paternal imprinting has been documented in about 10% of BWS patients, and that about 70% of Wilms tumors from BWS patients show loss of imprinting of the genes coding for IGF-2 and H19. Children affected with this condition should undergo ultrasound surveillance for abdominal tumors every 3 months until they reach age 7 years.

### 2. Prader–Willi Syndrome

Prader–Willi syndrome results from lack of expression of a number of imprinted genes, including *SNRPn*, located on chromosome 15q11. Clinical characteristics include severe hypotonia in infancy that often necessitates placement of a feeding gastrostomy tube. In older children, characteristic facies become obvious, with almond-shaped eyes, and frequent strabismus. Short stature, obesity, hypogenitalism, and small hands and feet with tapering fingers are now believed to be associated with growth hormone deficiency. Obsessive hyperphagia (usual onset 3–4 years) and type 2 (adult-onset) diabetes mellitus are common features.

Multiple chromosomal rearrangements and mutations have been reported to disrupt expression of the genes that contribute to this syndrome. Of these, deletion of paternal chromosome 15q11 is the most common, followed by maternal uniparental disomy. Molecular techniques that analyze patterns of methylation of involved DNA sequences provide a practical approach to diagnosis when clinical suspicion exists. But additional studies (eg, FISH) to determine the genetic mechanisms responsible are necessary in confirmed cases for reproductive risk counseling.

### 3. Angelman Syndrome

Angelman syndrome also involves imprinting and results from a variety of mutations that inactivate a ubiquitin–protein ligase gene, *UBE3A*, located in the same region of chromosome 15 as *SNRPn*, the maternally imprinted gene involved in Prader–Willi syndrome (see preceding section). *UBE3A* is paternally imprinted, and during normal development the maternal allele is expressed only in the brain. The classic phenotype includes severe mental retardation with prognathism, seizures, and marked delay in motor milestones, abnormal puppet-like gait and posturing, poor language development, and paroxysmal laughter and tongue thrusting.

Angelman syndrome is most commonly caused when sequences detectable by FISH on 15q11 are deleted from the maternal homolog. Uniparental paternal disomy 15 is the least common cause. Mutations in *UBE3A* cause the disorder in perhaps one fourth of cases.

With additional studies of mutations in the gene responsible for this syndrome, it is possible that its clinical description will be expanded to include less severely delayed individuals. Recurrence is possible when mothers carry mutations that are paternally imprinted and therefore silent until they are passed on as nonimprinted alleles.

## 4. UPD 7

Certain genes on chromosome 7 are now known to be imprinted. *UPD 7* has been reported to cause CF in a child who inherited two copies of the Δ F 508 deletion from one parent. That child also had Russell–Silver syndrome, a syndrome associated with intrauterine growth failure and dwarfism. Imprinting abnormalities and UPD may prove to be associated with growth abnormalities.

Elias ER et al: Beckwith–Wiedemann syndrome. In Jameson JL (ed): *Principles of Molecular Medicine.* Humana Press, 1998.

## DISORDERS ASSOCIATED WITH ANTICIPATION

### 1. (Autosomal Dominant) MYOTONIC DYSTROPHY

Internists are most likely to encounter families with myotonic dystrophy, a condition characterized by muscle weakness and tonic muscle spasms (myotonia) along with hypogonadism, frontal balding, cardiac conduction abnormalities, and cataracts. It is unclear how many genes are involved in this disorder. The critical region is on chromosome 19, where an amplified trinucleotide repeat (CTG) occurs in the 3′ untranslated region of a protein kinase gene. Normal individuals have from 5 to 30 CTG repeat copies. Repeat copies greater than 50 are meiotically unstable, but individuals carrying this number of repeats may be only mildly affected (eg, cataracts). Most individuals with repeat copies greater than 100 will have symptoms or electrical myotonia as adults. However, as copy numbers approach approximately 400, symptoms become evident in children. Expansion can progress to greater than 1000 copies and in doing so produce fetal and neonatal disease that is often lethal. As the copy numbers enlarge from generation to generation, they become more unstable through meiosis. Dramatic expansion from ap-

proximately 200 to 400 repeat copies, producing mild, often clinically undetected symptoms, to very large copy numbers (800–2000) associated with fetal manifestations (polyhydramnios and arthrogryposis) occur frequently when the expanded repeat copies are passed through female, but not male, meiosis. Therefore, an important component in the work-up of the floppy infant is a careful neurologic assessment of the mother for evidence of weakness or myotonia. Diagnostic molecular testing which measures the number of CTG repeats is now available.

### 2. (Autosomal Recessive) FRIEDREICH ATAXIA

Symptoms include progressive incoordination (cerebellar dysfunction) with both motor and sensory findings beginning in preadolescence and typically advancing through the teenage years. The gene involved, *FDRA,* is located on chromosome 9. Normal individuals carry 7–22 GAA repeats at this locus. Close to 75% of affected patients are homozygous for repeat expansions, having greater than 200 copies. Point mutations in the gene also occur. Meiotic instability of this repeat sequence is more variable than are others. Contractions occur more frequently than do expansions. Relationships between genotype and phenotype are also more complex. Molecular diagnostic testing requires careful interpretation with respect to prognosis and reproductive risks.

### 3. (X-Linked) FRAGILE X SYNDROME

Fragile X syndrome, present in approximately 1 in 1000 males, is the most common cause of mental retardation in males. The responsible gene is *FMR-1,* which has unstable CGG repeats at the 5′ end. Normal individuals have up to 55 CGG repeats. Individuals with 55–200 CGG repeats have a **premutation** and are generally phenotypically normal. Affected individuals with fragile X syndrome (full mutation) have greater than 200 CGG repeats and also have hypermethylation of both the CGG expansion and an adjacent CpG island. This methylation turns off the *FMR-1* gene. DNA analysis, rather than cytogenetic testing, is the method of choice for confirming the diagnosis of fragile X syndrome.

Most males with fragile X syndrome present with mental retardation, oblong face with large ears, and large testicles, especially after puberty. Other physical signs include symptoms suggestive of a connective tissue disorder (eg, hyperextensible joints, mitral valve prolapse). Many affected individuals are hyperactive and exhibit infantile autism or autistic-like behavior. Some males with the abnormal gene are of normal phenotype.

In contrast, about one half of females with the fragile X full mutation show normal intelligence, but often evidence learning disabilities and behavioral problems. About one half of females with the full mutation have lower IQs in the range of mental retardation and more severe behavioral problems. Females have more mild phenotypic changes than the males. Clinical expression of fragile X differs in male and female offspring depending on which parent is transmitting the gene. The premutation can change into the full mutation only when passed through a female. Identification of the abnormal DNA amplification by direct DNA analysis can confirm the diagnosis of fragile X in an affected individual and can detect asymptomatic gene carriers of both sexes. Therefore, DNA analysis is a reliable test for prenatal and postnatal diagnosis of fragile X syndrome and facilitates genetic counseling.

Cummings CJ, Zoghbi HY: Fourteen and counting: Unraveling trinucleotide repeat diseases. Hum Mol Genet 2000;9(6): 909 [PMID: 10767314].

## DISORDERS ASSOCIATED WITH MITOCHONDRIAL INHERITANCE

According to a special mitochondrial issue of the *Seminars in Medical Genetics,* published in the *American Journal of Medical Genetics,* Spring of 2001, more than 100 point mutations and rearrangements of mtDNA have been identified, which cause a large number of human diseases. Symptoms of the mitochondrial disorders are secondary to deficiency in the respiratory chain enzymes of oxidative phosphorylation, which supply energy to all cells. Mitochondrial diseases are progressive disorders with neurologic dysfunction including hypotonia, developmental delay, and seizures. Ophthalmologic issues, hearing loss, GI tract dysfunction with growth failure, renal, endocrine, cardiac, and autonomic dysfunction are some of the many issues which can affect patients with mitochondrial diseases. The following disorders are three of the more common ones.

### 1. MELAS

MELAS is an acronym for **m**itochondrial **e**ncephalopathy, **l**actic **a**cidosis, and **s**troke-like episodes. Symptoms occur in the pediatric age group and include recurrent episodes resembling stroke (blindness, paralysis), headache, vomiting, weakness of proximal muscles, and elevated blood lactate. (***Note:*** Lactate may be falsely elevated secondary to technical difficulties in obtaining a free-flowing blood specimen or delay in laboratory measurement.) The most common mutation causing MELAS is in the tRNA$^{Leu}$ gene (*A3243G*).

### 2. MERRF

MERRF is an acronym for **m**yoclonus **e**pilepsy with **r**agged **r**ed **f**ibers. Children with MERRF present with a variety of neurologic symptoms, including myoclonus, deafness, weakness of muscles, and seizures. Eighty percent of cases are due to a missense mutation in the mitochondrial tRNA$^{Lys}$ gene (*A8344G*).

### 3. LEIGH SUBACUTE NECROTIZING ENCEPHALOMYELOPATHY

Multiple different abnormalities in respiratory chain function lead to Leigh disease, a very severe disorder associated with progressive loss of developmental milestones associated with extrapyramidal symptoms, and brainstem dysfunction. Episodes of deterioration are frequently associated with an intercurrent febrile illness. Symptoms include hypotonia, unusual choreoathetoid hand movements, feeding dysfunction with failure to thrive, and seizures. Focal necrotic lesions of the brainstem and thalamus are hallmarks on MRI scan. Mitochondrial mutations affecting the respiratory chain, especially complexes I, II and IV, and nuclear DNA mutations affecting complex II have been identified as causing Leigh disease.

DiMauro S, Schon EA: Mitochondrial DNA mutations in human disease. Am J Med Genet 2001;106(1):18 [PMID: 11579421].

Munnich A, Rustin P: Clinical spectrum and diagnosis of mitochondrial disorders. Am J Med Genet 2001;106(1):4 [PMID: 11579420].

Smeitink J et al: The genetics and pathology of oxidative phosphorylation. Nat Rev Genet 2001;2:342 [PMID: 11331900].

## MULTIFACTORIAL INHERITANCE
### CLEFT LIP & CLEFT PALATE

From a genetic standpoint, cleft lip with or without cleft palate is distinct from isolated cleft palate. The former is more common in males, the latter in females. Although both can occur in a single family, particularly in association with certain syndromes, this pattern is unusual. Racial background is a factor in the incidence of facial clefting. Among Asians, Caucasians, and blacks, the incidence is 1.61, 0.9, and 0.31, respectively, per 1000 live births.

### Clinical Findings

A cleft lip may be unilateral or bilateral and complete or incomplete. It may occur with a cleft of the entire palate or just the primary (anterior and gingival ridge) or secondary (posterior) palate. An isolated cleft palate can involve only the soft palate or both the soft and hard palates. It can be a V-shaped or wide horseshoe cleft. When the cleft palate is associated with micrognathia and glossoptosis (a tongue that falls back and causes respiratory or feeding problems), it is called the Pierre Robin sequence. Among individuals with facial clefts—more commonly those with isolated cleft palate—the incidence of other congenital abnormalities is increased. The incidence of congenital heart disease, for example, is between 1–2% in liveborn infants, but among those with Pierre Robin sequence it can be as high as 15%. Associated abnormalities should be looked for in the period immediately after birth and before surgery.

## Differential Diagnosis

A facial cleft may occur in many different circumstances. It may be an isolated abnormality or part of a more generalized syndrome. Prognosis, management, and accurate determination of recurrence risks all depend on accurate diagnosis. In evaluating a child with a facial cleft, the physician must determine if the cleft is nonsyndromic or syndromic.

## Nonsyndromic

In the past, nonsyndromic cleft lip or cleft palate was considered a classic example of polygenic or multifactorial inheritance. More recently, however, this mode of inheritance has been questioned, and several studies have suggested one or more major autosomal loci, both recessive and dominant (or co-dominant). Empirically, however, the recurrence risk is still in the range of 2–3% because of nonpenetrance or the presence of other contributing genes.

## Syndromic

Cleft lip, with or without cleft palate, and isolated cleft palate may occur in a variety of syndromes that may be environmental, chromosomal, single gene, or of unknown origin (Table 33–3). Prognosis and accurate recurrence risks depend on the correct diagnosis.

## Complications & Treatment

Problems associated with facial clefts include early feeding difficulties, which may be severe; recurrent serous otitis media associated with fluctuating hearing and language delays; speech problems, including hypernasality and articulation errors; and dental and orthodontic complications. Long-term management ideally should be through a multidisciplinary cleft palate clinic.

**Table 33–3.** Syndromic isolated cleft palate (CP) and cleft lip with or without cleft palate (CL/CP).[a]

**Environmental**
  Maternal seizures, anticonvulsant usage (CL/CP or CP)
  Fetal alcohol syndrome (CP)
  Amniotic band syndrome (CL/CP)
**Chromosomal**
  Trisomies 13 and 18 (CL/CP)
  Wolf–Hirschorn or 4p– syndrome (CL/CP)
  Shprintzen or 22q11.2 deletion syndrome (CP)
**Single-gene disorders**
  Van der Woude syndrome, AD (CL/CP or CP)
  Treacher Collins syndrome, AD (CP)
  Stickler syndrome, AD (CP)
  Smith–Lemli-Opitz, AR (CP)[b]
**Unknown cause**
  Möbius syndrome (CP)
  Cornelia de Lange syndrome (CP)

[a]AD = autosomal-dominant.
[b]AR = autosomal-recessive.

## Genetic Counseling

Accurate counseling depends on accurate diagnosis and the differentiation of syndromic from nonsyndromic clefts. A complete family history must be taken, and the patient and both parents must be examined. The choice of laboratory studies is guided by the presence of other abnormalities and clinical suspicions. They may include chromosome analysis, including FISH, eye examination, and radiologic studies. When the risk for a facial cleft is known to be increased, clefts of both the lip and the palate have been sought and detected on ultrasound prenatally. Otherwise, intrauterine diagnosis of clefts is more likely to be established in syndromes in which the identification of other more serious abnormalities prompts the examiner to perform very detailed visualization of all organs.

## NEURAL TUBE DEFECTS

Neural tube defects comprise a variety of malformations, including anencephaly, encephalocele, spina bifida or myelomeningocele, sacral agenesis, sacral lipomas, and other spinal dysraphisms. Recent research suggests that the neural tube develops via closure at multiple rather than just two closure sites and that each closure site is probably mediated by different genes and affected by different teratogens. Hydrocephalus associated with the Arnold–Chiari type II malformation commonly occurs with myelomeningocele. Sacral agenesis, also called the caudal regression syndrome, occurs more frequently in infants of diabetic mothers.

## Clinical Findings

At birth, neural tube defects can present as an obvious rachischisis (open lesion) or as a more subtle skin-covered lesion associated with a fatty mass, a hemangioma, a tuft of hair, or asymmetrical buttock creases. In the latter case, computed tomography or MRI should be conducted to better define the anatomic defect. The extent of neurologic deficit depends on the level of the lesion and may include clubfeet, dislocated hips, or total flaccid paralysis below the level of the lesion. Hydrocephalus may be apparent at birth or may present with an increase in head circumference, irritability, and poor feeding, with vomiting shortly after the back has been repaired surgically. Neurogenic bladder and bowel are commonly seen. Other anomalies of the CNS may be present, as well as anomalies of the heart or kidneys.

## Differential Diagnosis

Neural tube defects (NTD) may occur in isolation or as part of a genetic syndrome. They may result from teratogenic exposure to alcohol or the anticonvulsant valproate. Any infant with dysmorphic features or other major anomalies in addition to the NTD should be evaluated by a geneticist, and a chromosome analysis should be performed.

## Complications & Management

### A. Neurosurgical

Infants with an open NTD should be placed in prone position, and the lesion kept moist with sterile dressing. Neurosurgical closure should occur within 24–48 hours after birth to reduce risk of infection. The infant should be monitored closely, and a ventriculoperitoneal shunt should be inserted as soon as signs of hydrocephalus become apparent. Shunts are required in about 85% of cases of myelomeningocele. Complications of the shunt include malfunction and infection. Symptoms of the Arnold–Chiari II malformation include feeding dysfunction, abducens nerve palsy, vocal cord paralysis with stridor, and apnea. Shunt malfunction may cause an acute worsening of Arnold–Chiari symptoms that may be life-threatening.

### B. Orthopedic

The child's ability to walk varies according to the level of the lesion. Children with low lumbar and sacral lesions walk with minimal support; those with high lumbar and thoracic lesions are rarely functional walkers; and in those with midlumbar lesions the effects are variable. Orthopedic surgery is necessary to get the child upright and ambulatory and to address foot deformities and scoliosis. Physical therapy services are indicated.

### C. Urologic

Neurogenic bladders have variable presentations. Urodynamic studies are recommended early on to define bladder function, and management is guided by the results of these studies. Continence can be achieved in a variety of ways, including use of anticholinergic or sympathomimetic agents, clean intermittent catheterization, and a variety of urologic procedures. Renal function should be monitored regularly, and an ultrasound examination should be periodically repeated. Symptomatic infections should be treated.

Symptoms of neurogenic bowel include incontinence and chronic constipation and are managed with a combination of dietary modifications, laxatives and stool softeners, and rectal stimulation. A recently developed surgical procedure called ACE (antegrade continence enema) uses the appendix to create a conduit from the upper colon to the surface at the umbilicus. An enema is then given through the conduit, cleaning out the colon from above rather than from below. Early results with respect to continence and patient satisfaction have been encouraging.

## Special Issues and Prognosis

All children requiring multiple surgical procedures (ie, patients with spina bifida or urinary tract anomalies) have a significant risk for developing hypersensitivity type I (IgE-mediated) allergic reactions to latex. For this reason, nonlatex medical products are now routinely used when caring for patients with NTDs. Most individuals with spina bifida are cognitively normal, but learning disabilities are common. Individuals with encephalocele or other CNS malformations generally have a much poorer intellectual outcome. Individuals with closed spinal cord abnormalities (eg, sacral lipomas) have more mild issues in general, and intelligence is usually normal. Problems in older patients include the development of spinal cord tethering, which usually presents with back pain, progressive scoliosis, and changes in bowel or bladder function. This often requires neurosurgical intervention. Individuals with NTDs have lifelong medical issues, which require the care of multiple medical and surgical specialists, as well as special educational and psychosocial issues requiring support for the patient and family. A good support for families is the national Spina Bifida Association, which has many local chapters. See the following website: sbaa.org

## Genetic Counseling

Recurrence risks vary according to the underlying cause, but most isolated NTDs are polygenic, with a recurrence risk of 2–3% for the parents in future pregnancies.

The recurrence risk for siblings of the parents and siblings of the patients is 1–2%. A patient with spina bifida has a 5% chance of having an affected child. Prenatal diagnosis is available, and pregnancies can be monitored in a variety of ways. In fetuses with open NTDs, maternal serum α-fetoprotein levels (AFP) measured at 16–18 weeks' gestation are elevated. AFP and acetylcholine esterase levels in amniotic fluid are also elevated. Ultrasound studies will detect approximately 90% of NTDs. Recent studies have shown that prophylactic folic acid can significantly lower the incidence and recurrence rate of NTDs, but the intake of the folic acid must start at least 3 months prior to conception and continue during the first month of pregnancy. It is now recommended that all women of childbearing age take 0.4 mg of folic acid daily. For the woman at increased risk because of a previous child with an NTD, the current recommendation is to increase folic acid intake to 4 mg daily when pregnancy is planned. Although the data are inconsistent, some evidence indicates that preconceptional folic acid supplementation may also lower the incidence of other congenital malformations such as conotruncal heart defects.

# ■ COMMON RECOGNIZABLE DISORDERS WITH VARIABLE OR UNKNOWN CAUSE

The text that follows describes several important and common human malformation syndromes. The emphasis is on clinical findings that should suggest their inclusion in differential diagnoses. Likely causes, if known, are also briefly explained. The best illustrations are in *Smith's Recognizable Patterns of Human Malformation*. An excellent Internet site at the University of Kansas Medical Center can be consulted for further information: http://www.kumc.edu/gec/support.

## Arthrogryposis Multiplex

Arthrogryposis multiplex is due to lack of fetal movement. Causes most often involve constraint, CNS maldevelopment or injury, and neuromuscular disorders. In the neuromuscular disorders, polyhydramnios is often present as a result of lack of fetal swallowing. Pulmonary hypoplasia may also be present, reflecting lack of fetal breathing. The work-up will usually include brain imaging, careful consideration of metabolic disease—especially peroxisomal disorders associated with elevated very-long-chain fatty acids—neurologic consultation, and, in some cases, electrophysiologic studies and muscle biopsy. The family history should be reviewed carefully for findings such as muscle weakness or cramping, cataracts, and early-onset heart disease, suggesting myotonic dystrophy. Parents should have careful neurologic examinations that include testing for myotonia.

## CHARGE Association

CHARGE association affects structures derived from rostral neural crest cells but also includes abnormal development of the eyes and midbrain. It is a sporadic condition whose cause is not understood. The acronym CHARGE serves as a mnemonic for associated abnormalities that include **c**olobomas, congenital **h**eart disease, choanal **a**tresia, growth **r**etardation, **g**enital abnormalities (hypogenitalism), and **e**ar abnormalities, with deafness.

Abnormal ear development always occurs in association with this condition. Whenever abnormal ears are encountered, careful physical assessment should follow, and ophthalmologic consultation should be considered. Facial asymmetry is a common finding. Studies of surviving patients indicate that neuronal damage due to airway and feeding complications contributes substantially to developmental delays. A number of other syndromes, some with much better prognoses, overlap with this condition. Chromosomal studies are normal but are usually necessary to distinguish this condition from other disorders. The following website of the Charge Syndrome Foundation, Inc, is a helpful source for additional information: http://www.chargesyndrome.org/.

## Cornelia De Lange Syndrome

Cornelia de Lange syndrome is a sporadically occurring malformation syndrome whose cause remains obscure. It is characterized by severe growth retardation; limb, especially hand, reduction defects (50%); congenital heart disease (25%); and stereotypical facies with hirsutism, medial fusion of eyebrows (synophrys), and thin, downturned lips.

The course and severity are variable, but the prognosis for survival and normal development is poor. Chromosomal analysis is usually normal.

## Goldenhar Syndrome

Goldenhar syndrome, also known as vertebroauriculofacial syndrome, is an association of multiple anomalies involving the head and neck. The classic phenotype includes hemifacial microsomia (one side of the face smaller than the other), with abnormalties of the pinna on the same side with associated deafness. Ear anomalies may be quite severe and include anotia. A characteristic benign fatty tumor in the outer eye, called an epibulbar dermoid, is frequently present, as are preauricular ear tags. Vertebral anomalies, particularly of the cervical vertebrae, are seen, and vertebral anomalies lower down are common. The Arnold–Chiari type I malformation (herniation of the cerebellum into the cervical spinal canal) is a common associated anomaly. Cardiac anomalies and hydrocephalus are seen in more severe cases. Most patients with Goldenhar syndrome have normal intelligence. The cause is unknown.

## Kabuki Syndrome

Kabuki syndrome is a disorder of unknown cause characterized by a distinctive facial appearance (hypertelorism with long palpebral fissures, large pinnae), developmental delay, and hearing loss. Most cases are sporadic although a few cases with dominant transmission have been reported. Anomalies of the heart and genitourinary system are occasionally seen.

## Noonan Syndrome

Noonan syndrome is an autosomal dominant disorder characterized by short stature, congenital heart disease, abnormalities of cardiac conduction and rhythm, webbed neck, down-slanting palpebral fissures, and low-set ears. Affected children may be large at birth and have mild subcutaneous edema. The phenotype evolves with age and may be difficult to recognize in older relatives. Mild developmental delays are often present. No genes have yet been identified, but a candidate locus has been mapped to chromosome 12q.

## Oligohydramnios Sequence (Potter Sequence)

This condition presents in newborns as severe respiratory distress due to pulmonary hypoplasia in association with positional deformities of the extremities, usually bilateral clubfeet, and typical facies consisting of suborbital creases, depressed nasal tip and low-set ears, and retrognathia. The sequence may be due to prolonged lack of amniotic fluid. Most often it is due to leakage, renal agenesis, or severe obstructive uropathy.

## Opitz G/BBB

Disrupted development of midline structures is a feature of several overlapping malformation syndromes, a number of them heritable. Hypertelorism (wide set eyes) is a unifying feature for these conditions, but it is the combined association of midbrain anomalies (agenesis of the corpus callosum), cardiac septal defects, and genitourinary tract anomalies, in particular, hypospadias, that has led to the recognition of a commonly disrupted midline developmental field. Current clinical genetic terminology refers to these conditions as Opitz G/BBB syndrome.

In addition to malformation of midline structures, hypotonia and problems with swallowing and gastroesophageal reflux are hallmark symptoms. Mentation is usually subnormal. Many cases are sporadic, but well-documented families with apparent autosomal dominant and X-linked inheritance identify the phenotype as genetically heterogeneous. Linkage studies have recently identified a candidate gene dubbed *M101* on the X chromosome. Mutations in this gene segregate with syndromic phenotypes in affected males. An additional X-chromosomal locus and an autosomal locus very close to the Shprintzen syndrome region, 22q11, are also under investigation. A number of Opitz G/BBB syndrome patients, in fact, have been shown by FISH to have deletions in this region. Additional resources include the Opitz Family Network and the OPITZ G/BBB Family Network and the following website: http://www.opitznet.org/joinus.html.

## Overgrowth Syndromes

Overgrowth syndromes are becoming increasingly recognized as important childhood conditions. They may present at birth and are characterized by macrocephaly, motor delays (cerebral hypotonia), and, in many cases, asymmetry of extremities. Bone age may be advanced. The most common overgrowth syndrome is Sotos syndrome. Patients with Sotos syndrome have a characteristic facies with a prominent forehead and down-slanting palpebral features. The cause of Sotos syndrome is unknown. There is a small but increased risk of cancer in patients with Sotos syndrome. Other overgrowth syndromes include Beckwith–Wiedemann syndrome (BWS), described in the section on imprinting, and two single gene disorders called Simpson–Golabi–Behmel syndrome and Bannayan–Riley–Ruvalcaba (BRR) syndrome. Simpson–Golabi–Behmel syndrome exhibits a BWS-like phenotype, but with additional anomalies including polydactyly and more severe facial dysmorphism. Unlike BWS patients who have normal intelligence, patients with Simpson–Golabi often have developmental delay. It is inherited as an X-linked disorder. Patients with BRR have macrosomia, macrocephaly, and unusual freckling of the penis. They have mild developmental issues. They may develop hemangiomatous/lymphangiomatous growths and have a predisposition to intestinal malignancies. The cause of BRR was recently found to be a mutation of the *PTEN* gene implicated in Cowden's syndrome, the association of intestinal polyposis with malignant potential.

## Rubenstein–Taybi Syndrome

Rubenstein–Taybi Syndrome is a genetic disorder of unknown cause, characterized by developmental delay;

growth failure; and a distinctive facial dysmorphology with microcephaly, prominent nose, and small chin. Feeding problems are common. About 25% of patients have been found with a microdeletion of chromosome 16 detectable by FISH, but most patients have a normal karyotype.

## Syndromic Short Stature

Short stature is an important component of numerous syndromes, or it may be an isolated finding. In the absence of nutritional deficiencies, endocrine abnormalities, evidence for skeletal dysplasia (disproportionate growth with abnormal skeletal films), or a positive family history, intrinsic short stature can be due to uniparental disomy (see previous discussion) such that only imprinted (silenced) copies of specific sequences are present. The phenotype of Russell–Silver syndrome—short stature with normal head growth (pseudohydrocephalus), normal development, and minor dysmorphic features (especially fifth finger clinodactyly)—has been associated in some cases with maternal uniparental disomy for chromosome 7.

## VACTERL Association

VACTERL association is described by an acronym denoting the association of **v**ertebral defects (segmentation anomalies), imperforate **a**nus, **c**ardiac malformation (most often ventricular septal defect), **t**racheoesophageal fistula, **r**enal anomalies, and **l**imb (most often radial ray) anomalies. The disorder is sporadic, and some of the defects may be life-threatening. The prognosis for normal development is good. The cause is unknown, but a high association with monozygotic twinning suggests a mechanism dating back to events perhaps as early as blastogenesis. Recently, disturbance of the sonic Hedgehog pathway was suggested to be part of the mechanism for VACTERL, based on a mouse model. Careful examination and follow-up are important, because numerous other syndromes with more complicated prognoses also include features present in VACTERL association. Chromosomal studies and genetic consultation are warranted.

Hall JG et al: *Handbook of Normal Physical Measurements.* Oxford Univ Press, 1989.

Spranger JW et al: *Bone Dysplasias: An Atlas of Genetic Disorders of Skeletal Development.* Oxford Univ Press, 2002.

# PERINATAL GENETICS

## TERATOGENS

### 1. Fetal Alcohol Syndrome

Fetal alcohol syndrome (FAS) results from excessive exposure to alcohol during gestation and affects 30–40% of offspring of mothers whose daily intake of alcohol exceeds 3 oz. Features of the syndrome include short stature; poor head growth (may be postnatal in onset), developmental delay, and midface hypoplasia characterized by a poorly developed long philtrum, narrow palpebral fissures, and short nose with anteverted nares. Facial findings may be subtle, but careful measurements and comparisons with standards (see Figure 33–11) can be useful. Structural abnormalities occur in half of affected children. Cardiac anomalies and NTDs are commonly seen. Genitourinary tract anomalies are frequent. Scientists and clinicians now agree that the term "fetal alcohol effect" may be misleading and should not be applied to apparently incomplete phenotypes. Careful evaluation for other syndromes and chromosomal disorders should be included in the work-up. Behavioral abnormalities in older children may or may not be directly attributable to alcohol, because psychiatric disorders, many with recognized inherited predisposition, affect a large number of women and their partners who abuse alcohol.

### 2. Maternal Anticonvulsant Effects

Anticonvulsant exposure during pregnancy is now recognized as being associated with adverse outcomes in approximately 10% of children born to women who are taking anticonvulsants. A syndrome characterized by small head circumference, anteverted nares, cleft lip and palate (occasionally), and distal digital hypoplasia was first described in association with maternal use of phenytoin but also occurs with other anticonvulsants. Risks for spina bifida are increased, especially in pregnancies exposed to valproic acid. Carbamazepine (Tegretol), felt to be less teratogenic than other anticonvulsants, has been associated with a characteristic dysmorphic facial appearance and developmental issues.

### 3. Retinoic Acid Embryopathy

Vitamin A and its analogs are potent morphogens that interact with specific receptors and therefore have considerable teratogenic potential. Developmental toxicity occurs in approximately one third of pregnancies exposed in the first trimester to the synthetic retinoid isotretinoin, commonly prescribed to treat acne. Exposure disrupts developmental fields to which rostral neural crest cells contribute and produces CNS maldevelopment, especially of the posterior fossa; ear anomalies (often absence of pinnae); congenital heart disease (great vessel anomalies); and tracheoesophageal fistula. These findings constitute a partial phenocopy of DiGeorge syndrome and demonstrate the continuum of contributing genetic and epigenetic factors in morphogenesis. It is now recognized that vitamin A itself, when taken during pregnancy in the active form of retinoic acid in doses exceeding 25,000 IU/d, can produce partially affected phenotypes. The limit is usually kept at 10,000 IU/d for safety, but evidence of problems is found at dosages above 25,000 IU/d. Maternal ingestion of even large amounts of vitamin A taken as retinol during pregnancy, however, does not increase risks, because conversion of this precursor to active retinoic acid is regulated by the body.

## 4. Maternal Substance Abuse

Maternal substance abuse is generally associated with increased risks for adverse perinatal outcomes, including miscarriage, preterm delivery, growth retardation, and increased risk for injury to the developing CNS. For most abused substances, the link between exposures and adverse outcomes is less well demonstrated than with alcohol. Multiple factors are probably involved, and it should be recognized that substance abuse often involves more than one drug. Maternal inhalant abuse appears to be associated with findings similar to those of FAS. Reports of abnormal outcomes following cocaine abuse (and the crack baby syndrome) have been contradicted by some studies that found no effects. In these cases the form of the drug used and its route of administration may be important determinants of risk.

Rimoin DL et al: *Emery and Rimoin's Principles and Practice of Medical Genetics,* 3rd ed. Churchill Livingstone, 2002.

Scriver CR (ed): *The Metabolic and Molecular Basis of Inherited Disease,* 8th ed, 4 vols. McGraw-Hill, 2001.

## PRENATAL DIAGNOSIS

Prenatal screening for birth defects in the form of analyte analyses in maternal blood, fetal and placental tissues, or ultrasound evaluation is now routinely offered to pregnant women. Prenatal diagnosis for specific genetic disorders is indicated in 7–8% of pregnancies. As technology improves, the indications for and the accuracy of prenatal diagnosis are expected to increase. Prenatal diagnosis introduces options for management including interruption of abnormal pregnancies, prenatal surgical and medical interventions, and preparation for specialized perinatal care.

## Methods

Prenatal diagnosis techniques analyze maternal blood, image the conceptus, and sample fetal and placental tissues (Table 33–4).

### A. MATERNAL BLOOD

The use of maternal serum AFP as a screening test was introduced because higher than normal values were found in association with open NTDs. It was later noted that 25% women who carried a fetus with Down syndrome had a 45% lower AFP value than those in whom the fetus was normal. Additional measurements of human chorionic gonadotropin and unconjugated estradiol (the "triple screen") can increase rates of detection for trisomy 21 to approximately 60% and predict many cases of trisomy 18 as well. Low estradiol levels can also predict cases of Smith–Lemli–Opitz, a devastating autosomal recessive disorder.

Fetal cells, including lymphocytes, trophoblasts, and nucleated red blood cells, are present in the maternal circulation. Research is being directed toward isolating these cells for prenatal diagnosis using culture, hybridization, and PCR-based techniques.

***Table 33–4.*** Prenatal diagnostic techniques.

| |
| --- |
| Maternal blood screening such as α-fetoprotein, estriol, hCG ("triple screen") |
|    Trisomies 21 and 18 |
|    Neural tube defects |
|    Smith–Lemli–Opitz syndrome |
| Fetal cells in maternal blood (research only) |
| Fetal ultrasound |
|    Structural defects |
|    Fetal hydrops |
|    Poly- or oligohydramnios |
| Fetal radiograph |
|    Skeletal defects |
| Fetal MRI |
| Amniocentesis |
|    Karyotyping |
|    Fetal cells for molecular or metabolic studies |
|    Amniotic fluid α-fetoprotein level for neural tube defects |
|    Biochemical studies on fluid |
| Chorionic villus sampling |
|    Karyotyping |
|    Fetal cells for molecular or metabolic studies |
| Fetal tissues |
|    Blood by percutaneous umbilical blood sampling |
|    Biopsy of other fetal tissues |
| Direct fetal visualization via fetoscopy (rarely used today because of the advances in fetal visualization by ultrasound and MRI) |

MRI = magnetic resonance imaging.

## B. TESTING OF FETAL TISSUE

**1. Amniocentesis**—This technique has been available for many years. Its accuracy and safety are well established. Fluid surrounding the fetus is sampled, and cells are cultured for cytogenetic, molecular, or metabolic analysis. AFP and other chemical markers can also be measured. This is a safe procedure with a complication rate (primarily for miscarriage) of less than 1% in experienced hands.

**2. Chorionic villus sampling (placental)**—This means of analysis is now available in most centers and is generally performed at 11–12 weeks' gestation. Tissue obtained by chorionic villus sampling (CVS) provides more DNA for molecular analysis and contains dividing cells (cytotrophoblasts) that can be rapidly karyotyped. However, direct cytogenetic preparations may be of poor quality. In addition, chromosomal abnormalities detected by this technique may be confined to the placenta (**confined placental mosaicism**). Cultured preparations may be more relevant. Certainly, if an unusual cytogenetic picture is found on CVS, further studies should be considered before management decisions are made. Numerous studies have been done comparing the safety of first-trimester CVS with amniocentesis. Of some concern is the possible association of CVS prior to 11 weeks with terminal transverse limb defects, perhaps secondary to vascular disruption.

Fetal blood can be sampled directly in late gestation through ultrasound-guided percutaneous umbilical blood sampling (PUBS).

It is occasionally necessary to biopsy fetal tissues such as liver or muscle for accurate prenatal diagnosis. These procedures are available in only a few perinatal centers.

Amniocentesis or CVS is indicated in the following circumstances:

1. Maternal age over 35 years.
2. Previous child with a chromosomal abnormality.
3. Either parent a translocation carrier. In this case, the risk for a fetus with an unbalanced chromosomal abnormality depends on the type of translocation.
4. A history of any genetic disorder diagnosable by biochemical techniques or by DNA analysis. The list of such conditions changes daily, and a genetic center should be contacted for the most recent information.
5. A request by the parents for fetal sex determination because of a history of an X-linked disorder that is not otherwise diagnosable.
6. Maternal blood testing (eg, triple screen) indicating increased risks for chromosomal abnormalities.

7. As part of the workup of fetal anomalies found by ultrasonography.

**3. Fetal ultrasonography**—Ultrasonography is indicated whenever an abnormality characterized by a structural defect is suspected. The defect may be suspected because of the family history, potential exposure to teratogens during pregnancy, or questionable abnormalities noted on a routine ultrasound examination done in the obstetrician's office. In any case, the patient should be referred for further evaluation to a medical center staffed by personnel experienced in fetal ultrasonography.

By 16–18 weeks' gestation, transabdominal real-time ultrasonography can visualize all major fetal organs, including the kidneys, heart, brain, spinal cord, bladder, and limbs. Beginning at 12 weeks' gestation, transvaginal ultrasonography can provide even earlier imaging. It is therefore possible to look for almost any genetic syndrome that includes a specific defect. Routine ultrasound screening has demonstrated many unexpected abnormalities. Most of these are major defects, however, and minor anomalies are easily missed, especially if unexpected.

Fetal motion has been a major deterrent to the use of MRI as a tool for prenatal diagnosis. However, new techniques are being developed to overcome this problem, making MRI a potentially valuable noninvasive means of fetal assessment.

Radiologic studies of the fetus are rarely necessary because ultrasonography has improved so greatly. If a skeletal abnormality or bone dysplasia is suspected, however, radiographic films may be helpful.

# EVALUATION OF THE DEVELOPMENTALLY DELAYED CHILD

Mental retardation or developmental delays affect 8% of the population. Disorders associated with symptoms of delayed development are heterogeneous but frequently include heritable components. Evaluation should be multidisciplinary; Table 33–5 lists its main features, emphasizing the major clinical and genetic considerations.

Discerning patterns and timing of growth and development are particularly important. For example, prenatal-onset growth retardation is less likely to have a metabolic origin than is postnatal growth delay. Loss of skills raises suspicion about possible metabolic or neurodegenerative disorders. Behavioral abnormalities are commonly associated with developmental delays, but behavioral diagnoses such as attention-deficit/hyperac-

**Table 33–5.** Evaluation of the child with developmental delay.

**History**
Pregnancy history
Growth parameters at birth
Neonatal complications
Feeding history
History of somatic growth
Motor, language, and psychosocial milestones
Seizures
Loss of skills
Abnormal movements
Results of previous tests and examinations

**Family history**
Developmental and educational histories
Psychiatric disorders
Pregnancy outcomes
Medical history
Consanguinity

**Physical examination**
General pediatric examination
Focused dysmorphologic evaluation including measurement of facial features and assessment of dermatoglyphics
Complete neurologic examination
Parental growth parameters (especially head circumferences) and dysmorphic features should also be assessed

**Imaging studies**
See text

**Laboratory assessment[a]**
Chromosomes (high-resolution analyses)
Fragile X testing (analysis of *FMR1* gene for triplet repeats)
FISH analyses guided by dysmorphic features
Other blood analyses: complete blood count, electrolytes, liver function tests, creatinine kinase (CK), lactate, pyruvate
Serum amino acid analysis
Urine amino and organic acid analyses
Urine analysis for mucopolysaccharides

[a]In many cases, negative results may be important.
FISH = fluorescent in situ hybridization.

tivity disorder, obsessive–compulsive disorder, autism, or autistic-like behaviors are better viewed as descriptive than as etiologically informative diagnoses.

Physical examination provides helpful clues. Close scrutiny for presence of dysmorphologic disorders is a clinical skill that requires practice. Referral to a clinical geneticist is indicated whenever unusual features are encountered. Neurologic, ophthalmologic, and audiologic consultation should be sought when indicated. Brain imaging should be requested in most cases involving otherwise unexplained deviations from normal head growth. Neuroimaging and skeletal studies may also be indicated when dysmorphic features are present. Neurologic consultation can often help sort through indications for imaging.

As molecular explanations for genetic disorders accumulate, opportunities for molecular genetic testing increase. Unlike the majority of the studies listed in Table 33–4, these are not screening tests—they may confirm but often do not entirely rule out specific diagnoses. In general, it will not be cost-effective to proceed with molecular genetic testing without clinical genetic consultation.

Metabolic and genetic testing procedures other than those listed in the table may also be indicated. Appropriate consultations should be sought to coordinate these investigations.

## Interpretation & Follow-Up

Clinical experience indicates that specific diagnoses can be made in approximately half of patients evaluated according to the protocol presented here. With specific diagnosis comes prognosis, ideas for management, and insight into recurrence risks. Prenatal diagnosis may also become possible.

Follow-up is important both for patients in whom diagnoses have been made and for those patients initially lacking a diagnosis. Genetic information is accumulating rapidly and can be translated into new diagnoses and better understanding with periodic review of clinical cases.

# Allergic Disorders

34

*Mark Boguniewicz, MD*

Allergic disorders are among the most common problems seen by pediatricians and primary care physicians, affecting over 25% of the population in developed countries. The economic impact of these illnesses can be measured in billions of dollars.

The prevalence of asthma, allergic rhinitis, and atopic dermatitis has increased in recent years. Among school-age children and adolescents, these illnesses result in significant morbidity and school absenteeism, with adverse consequences for school performance and quality of life, and may cause emotional stress. Understanding the language of allergy and the basic mechanisms involved may help physicians when treating these disorders. In this chapter, atopy refers to a genetically determined predisposition to develop IgE antibodies found in patients with asthma, allergic rhinitis, and atopic dermatitis. The Allergy Report is an easy-to-access compendium of allergic disorders that can be found on the Internet at www.TheAllergyReport.org.

## ■ THE ALLERGIC CASCADE

Allergic responses begin with sensitization to an allergen in a genetically susceptible host. The CD4 cells of allergic patients respond to allergens by producing interleukins, predominantly IL-3, IL-4, IL-5, and IL-13 (a so-called T helper cell-2, or TH2-type profile). These cytokines are involved in IgE synthesis and in the differentiation and activation of eosinophils (Figure 34–1).

Allergen-specific IgE binds to receptors on mast cells, basophils, and Langerhans cells distributed throughout the skin and respiratory tract and in the circulation. Cross-linking of receptor-bound IgE by allergen activates effector cells to release allergic mediators, including histamine and newly synthesized mediators such as prostaglandins and leukotrienes. Effector cells may also release other enzymes and cytokines. This immediate allergic reaction can cause sneezing, hives, wheezing, vomiting, or anaphylaxis. As part of the allergic cascade, mononuclear cells and eosinophils are recruited to the site of the acute reaction and can cause late phase responses. Activated eosinophils in particular release toxic mediators that cause many of the clinical

symptoms in allergic diseases. It is likely that a number of infiltrating cells such as monocytes, neutrophils, and basophils and resident cells such as epithelial cells and fibroblasts participate in perpetuating this inflammatory process even in the absence of allergens.

## ■ MAJOR ALLERGIC DISORDERS SEEN IN PEDIATRIC PRACTICE

### ASTHMA

### ESSENTIALS OF DIAGNOSIS & TYPICAL FEATURES

- *Episodic symptoms of airflow obstruction including wheezing, cough, and chest tightness.*
- *Airflow obstruction at least partially reversible.*
- *Exclusion of alternative diagnoses.*

### General Considerations

Asthma is the most common chronic disease of childhood, affecting over 5 million children in the United States. Despite advances in the understanding of asthma, associated morbidity has increased over the past decade and mortality rates have remained relatively stable. Asthma hospitalization rates are highest in the black population, with death rates consistently highest among African Americans age 15–24 years. The reasons for this are unclear but may be related to a combination of poor access to health care and environmental factors such as smoke and perennial allergen exposure. Alternatively, the "hygiene hypothesis" suggests that reduced exposure in early life to microbial organisms (or endotoxins) may account for the increase in atopic diseases, including asthma.

Up to 80% of children with asthma develop symptoms before their fifth birthday. Atopy is the strongest identifiable predisposing factor. Exposure to tobacco

*Figure 34–1.* Cellular interactions in allergic responses.

smoke, especially from the mother, is also a risk factor for asthma. About 40% of infants and young children who have wheezing with viral infections in the first few years of life will have continuing asthma through childhood. Sensitization to inhalant allergens increases over time and is found in the majority of children with asthma. The principal allergens associated with asthma are perennial aeroallergens such as dust mites, animal danders, cockroaches, and *Alternaria* (a soil mold). Of note, several recent studies suggest that exposure to high levels of cat allergen may have a protective effect against asthma. Rarely, foods may provoke isolated asthma symptoms. Other triggers include exercise, cold air, cigarette smoke, pollutants, strong chemical odors, and rapid changes in barometric pressure. Aspirin sensitivity is uncommon in children. Psychological factors may precipitate asthma exacerbations and place the patient at high risk from the disease.

Pathologic features of asthma include shedding of airway epithelium, edema, mucus plug formation, mast cell activation, and collagen deposition beneath the basement membrane. The inflammatory cell infiltrate includes eosinophils, lymphocytes, and neutrophils, especially in fatal asthma exacerbations. Airway inflammation contributes to airway hyperresponsiveness, airflow limitation, and disease chronicity. Persistent airway inflammation can lead to airway wall remodeling and irreversible changes.

## Clinical Findings

### A. SYMPTOMS AND SIGNS

Wheezing is the most characteristic sign of asthma, although it may be absent in some children, especially in those with cough-variant asthma. Patients may also have cough and shortness of breath. Complaints may include "chest congestion," prolonged cough, exercise intolerance, dyspnea, and recurrent bronchitis or pneumonia. If symptoms are absent or mild, chest auscultation during forced expiration may reveal prolongation of the expiratory phase and wheezing. As the obstruction becomes more severe, wheezes become more high-pitched and breath sounds diminished. With severe obstruction, wheezes may not be heard because of poor air movement. Flaring of nostrils, intercostal and suprasternal retractions, and use of accessory muscles of respiration are signs of severe obstruction. Flushed, moist skin may be noted, and mucous membranes may be dry. Cyanosis of the lips and nail beds may be seen with underlying hypoxia. Tachycardia and pulsus paradoxus also occur. Agitation and lethargy may be signs of impending respiratory failure.

## B. LABORATORY FINDINGS

Airway hyperresponsiveness to nonspecific stimuli is a hallmark of asthma. These include inhaled pharmacologic agents such as histamine and methacholine as well as physical stimuli such as exercise and cold air. Airways may exhibit hyperresponsiveness or twitchiness even when pulmonary function tests are normal. Giving increasing amounts of a bronchoconstrictive agent to induce a decrease in lung function (usually a 20% drop in forced expiratory volume in 1 second [$FEV_1$]) is the most common method of testing airway responsiveness. Hyperresponsiveness in normal children younger than age 5 years is greater than in older children. The level of airway hyperresponsiveness usually correlates with the severity of asthma.

During acute asthma exacerbations, $FEV_1$ is diminished and the flow-volume curve shows a "scooping out" of the distal portion of the expiratory portion of the loop (Figure 34–2). The residual volume, functional residual capacity, and total lung capacity are usually increased, while the vital capacity is decreased. Reversal or significant improvement of these abnormalities in response to inhaled bronchodilator therapy alone or with anti-inflammatory therapy is observed. Increased airway resistance also results in a decreased peak expiratory flow rate (PEFR). Diurnal variation in PEFR (ie, the difference between morning and evening measurements) of greater than 15–20% has been used as a defining feature of asthma. Significant changes in PEFR may occur before symptoms become evident. In more severe cases, PEFR monitoring enables earlier recognition of suboptimal asthma control. Exercise, cold air, and methacholine or histamine challenges may help to establish a diagnosis of asthma when the history, examination, and pulmonary function tests are not definitive. Alternatively, a diagnostic trial of inhaled bronchodilators and anti-inflammatory medica-

tions may be helpful, especially in infants and young children in whom underdiagnosis and undertreatment are common. Infant pulmonary function can be measured in sedated children with compression techniques. The forced oscillation technique can be used to measure airway resistance in younger children.

Hypoxemia is present early with a normal or low $PCO_2$ level and respiratory alkalosis. Hypoxemia may be aggravated during treatment with a $\beta_2$-agonist due to ventilation–perfusion mismatch. Oxygen saturation less than 91% is indicative of significant obstruction. Respiratory acidosis and increasing $CO_2$ tension may ensue with further airflow obstruction and signal impending respiratory failure. Hypercapnia is usually not seen until the $FEV_1$ falls below 20% of predicted value. Metabolic acidosis has also been noted in combination with respiratory acidosis in children with severe asthma and indicates imminent respiratory failure. A $PaO_2$ less than 60 mm Hg despite oxygen therapy and a $PaCO_2$ over 60 mm Hg and rising more than 5 mm Hg per hour are relative indications for mechanical ventilation in a child in status asthmaticus.

Pulsus paradoxus may be present with moderate or severe asthma. In moderate asthma in a child, this may be between 10 and 25 mm Hg, and in severe asthma between 20 and 40 mm Hg. Absence of pulsus paradoxus in a child with severe asthma exacerbation may signal respiratory muscle fatigue.

Clumps of eosinophils on sputum smear and blood eosinophilia are frequent findings. Their presence tends to reflect disease activity and does not necessarily mean that allergic factors are involved. Leukocytosis is common in acute severe asthma without evidence of bacterial infection and may be more pronounced after epinephrine administration. Hematocrit can be elevated with dehydration during prolonged exacerbations or in severe chronic disease. Potential noninvasive measures of airway inflammation include serum eosinophil

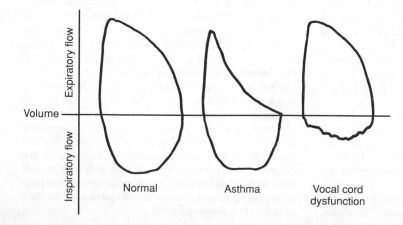

***Figure 34–2.*** Representative flow-volume loops in persons with normal lung function, asthma, and vocal cord dysfunction.

cationic protein levels, exhaled nitric oxide, and induced sputum. Each test has its strengths and weaknesses.

### C. IMAGING

On chest radiographs, bilateral hyperinflation with flattening of the diaphragms, peribronchial thickening, prominence of the pulmonary arteries and areas of patchy atelectasis may be present. Atelectasis is often misinterpreted as pneumonia.

Allergy testing is discussed in the General measures section under Treatment, Chronic Asthma.

## Differential Diagnosis

Diseases that may be mistaken for asthma are often related to the patient's age (Table 34–1). Congenital abnormalities must be excluded in infants and young children. Asthma can be confused with croup, acute bronchiolitis, pneumonia, and pertussis. Immunodeficiency may be associated with cough and wheezing. Foreign bodies in the airway may cause dyspnea or wheezing of sudden onset, and on auscultation wheezing may be unilateral. Asymmetry of the lungs secondary to air trapping may be seen on a chest radiograph, especially with forced expiration. Cystic fibrosis can be associated with or mistaken for asthma.

Vocal cord dysfunction is an important masquerader of asthma, although the two occasionally coexist. It is characterized by the paradoxic closure of the vocal cords that can result in dyspnea and wheezing. Diagnosis is made by direct visualization of the vocal cords. In normal individuals, the vocal cords abduct during inspiration and may adduct slightly during expiration. Asthmatic patients may have narrowing of the glottis during expiration as a physiologic adaptation to airway obstruction. In contrast, patients with isolated vocal

**Table 34–1.** Differential diagnosis of asthma in infants and children.

| |
| --- |
| Viral bronchiolitis |
| Aspiration |
| Laryngotracheomalacia |
| Vascular rings |
| Airway stenosis or web |
| Enlarged lymph nodes |
| Mediastinal mass |
| Foreign body |
| Bronchopulmonary dysplasia |
| Obliterative bronchiolitis |
| Cystic fibrosis |
| Vocal cord dysfunction |
| Cardiovascular disease |

cord dysfunction typically show adduction of the anterior two thirds of their vocal cords during inspiration, with a small diamond-shaped aperture posteriorly. Because this abnormal vocal cord pattern may be intermittently present, a normal examination does not exclude the diagnosis. Exercise or methacholine challenges can often precipitate symptoms of vocal cord dysfunction. The flow-volume loop may provide additional clues to the diagnosis of vocal cord dysfunction. Truncation of the inspiratory portion can be demonstrated in most patients during an acute episode, and some patients continue to show this pattern even when they are asymptomatic (see Figure 34–2). Children with vocal cord dysfunction, especially adolescents, tend to be overly competitive, primarily in athletics and scholastics. A psychiatric consultation may help define underlying psychological issues and provide appropriate therapy.

Treatment of isolated vocal cord dysfunction includes education regarding the syndrome and appropriate breathing exercises. Hypnosis, biofeedback, and psychotherapy have been effective for some patients. During an acute episode, a helium–oxygen mixture can be administered because the low density of the gas mixture facilitates movement of air through the adducted vocal cords.

## Conditions That May Increase Asthma Severity

Chronic hyperplastic sinusitis is frequently found in association with asthma. Upper airway inflammation has been shown to contribute to the pathogenesis of asthma, and asthma may improve after treatment of sinusitis. However, sinus surgery is usually not indicated for initial treatment of chronic mucosal disease associated with allergy.

A significant correlation has been observed between nocturnal asthma and gastroesophageal reflux. Patients may not complain of epigastric burning or have reflux symptoms—cough may be the only sign. For patients with poorly controlled asthma, particularly with a nocturnal component, investigation for gastroesophageal reflux may be warranted even in the absence of suggestive symptoms.

The risk factors for death from asthma include psychological and sociological factors. They are probably related to the consequences of illness denial as well as to nonadherence with prescribed therapy. Recent studies have shown that less than 50% of inhaled asthma medications are taken as prescribed and that compliance does not improve with increasing severity of illness. Moreover, children requiring hospitalization for asthma, or their caregivers, have often failed to institute appropriate home treatment.

## Complications

With acute asthma, complications are primarily related to hypoxemia and acidosis and can include generalized seizures. Pneumomediastinum or pneumothorax can be a complication in status asthmaticus. Recent studies point to airway wall remodeling and loss of pulmonary function with persistent airway inflammation. Childhood asthma independent of any corticosteroid therapy has been shown to be associated with delayed maturation and slowing of prepubertal growth velocity. However, attainment of final predicted adult height does not appear to be compromised.

## Treatment

### A. CHRONIC ASTHMA

**1. General measures**—Patients should avoid exposure to tobacco smoke and allergens to which they are sensitized, exertion outdoors when levels of air pollution are high, β-blockers, and sulfite-containing foods. Patients with persistent asthma should be given the inactivated influenza vaccine yearly unless they have a contraindication.

For patients with persistent asthma, the clinician should use the patient's history to assess sensitivity to seasonal allergens and *Alternaria* mold; use skin testing or in vitro testing to assess sensitivity to perennial indoor allergens; assess the significance of positive tests in the context of the patient's history; and identify relevant allergen exposures. For dust mite-allergic children, important environmental control measures include encasing the pillow and mattress in an allergen-impermeable cover and washing the sheets and blankets on the patient's bed weekly in hot water. Other measures include keeping indoor humidity below 50%, minimizing the number of stuffed toys, and washing such toys weekly in hot water. Children allergic to furred animals or feathers should avoid indoor exposure to pets, especially for prolonged periods of time. If removal of the pet is not possible, the animal should be kept out of the bedroom with the door closed. Carpeting and upholstered furniture should be removed. While a high-efficiency particle-arresting (HEPA) filter unit in the bedroom may reduce allergen levels, clinical symptoms may persist if the pet remains indoors. For cockroach-allergic children, control measures need to be instituted when infestation is present in the home. Poison baits, boric acid, and traps are preferred to chemical agents, which can be irritating if inhaled by asthmatic individuals. Indoor molds are especially prominent in humid environments or in homes with dampness. Measures to control dampness or fungal growth in the home may be of benefit. Patients can reduce exposure to outdoor allergens by staying in an air-conditioned environment.

Allergen immunotherapy may be useful for implicated aeroallergens that cannot be avoided. However, it should be administered only in facilities staffed and equipped to treat life-threatening reactions.

The patient and family must understand the role of asthma triggers, the importance of disease activity even without obvious symptoms, how to use objective measures to gauge disease activity, and the importance of airway inflammation—and they must learn to recognize the warning signs of worsening asthma, allowing for early intervention. A stepwise care plan should be developed for all patients with asthma. This educational process extends to school personnel and all those who care for children with asthma.

Because the degree of airflow limitation is poorly perceived by many patients, peak flow meters can aid in the assessment of airflow obstruction and day-to-day disease activity. Peak flow rates may provide early warning of worsening asthma. They are also helpful in monitoring the effects of medication changes. Spacer devices optimize delivery of medication from metered-dose inhalers to the lungs and, with inhaled steroids, minimize side effects. Large-volume spacers are preferred.

Patients should be treated for rhinitis, sinusitis, or gastroesophageal reflux, if present. Treatment of upper respiratory tract symptoms is an integral part of asthma management. Intranasal corticosteroids are recommended to treat chronic rhinitis in patients with persistent asthma because they reduce lower-airway hyperresponsiveness and asthma symptoms. Intranasal cromolyn reduces asthma symptoms during the ragweed season but less so than intranasal corticosteroids. Treatment of sinusitis includes medical measures to promote drainage and the use of antibiotics for acute bacterial infections. Medical management of gastroesophageal reflux includes avoiding eating or drinking 2 hours before bedtime, elevating the head of the bed with 6- to 8-inch blocks, and using appropriate pharmacologic therapy.

**2. Pharmacologic therapy**—A revised stepwise approach to pharmacologic therapy is recommended in the National Asthma Education and Prevention Program's *Expert Panel Report: Update on Selected Topics 2002* (www.nhlbi.nih.gov) (Tables 34–2 and 34–3). The choice of therapy is based on assessment of clinical features prior to treatment. The following key issues regarding pediatric asthma are discussed or updated compared with the 1997 guidelines:

1. Use of inhaled corticosteroids as the preferred treatment for mild or moderate persistent asthma.
2. Initiation of long-term controller therapy in infants or children who have risk factors for asthma (parental history of asthma or physician-diagnosed atopic dermatitis or two of the following:

***Table 34–2.*** Stepwise approach for treating infants and young children (5 years of age and younger) with acute or chronic asthma.

| Classify Severity: Clinical Features Before Treatment or Adequate Control | | Medications Required to Maintain Long-Term Control |
|---|---|---|
| | Symptoms/Day | |
| | Symptoms/Night | **Daily Medications** |
| Step 4: Severe persistent | Continual<br><br>Frequent | Preferred treatment:<br>  High-dose inhaled corticosteroids<br>  AND<br>  Long-acting inhaled $\beta_2$-agonists<br>  AND, if needed,<br>  Corticosteroid tablets or syrup long term (2 mg/kg/d generally do not exceed 60 mg/d). (Make repeat attempts to reduce systemic corticosteroids and maintain control with high-dose inhaled corticosteroids.) |
| Step 3: Moderate persistent | Daily<br><br>>1 night/wk | Preferred treatments:<br>  Low-dose inhaled corticosteroids and long-acting inhaled $\beta_2$-agonists<br>  OR<br>  Medium-dose inhaled corticosteroids.<br>Alternative treatment:<br>  Low-dose inhaled corticosteroids and either leukotriene receptor antagoinst or theophylline. |
| | | If needed (particularly in patients with recurring severe exacerbations):<br>Preferred treatment:<br>  Medium-dose inhaled corticosteroids and long-acting $\beta_2$-agonists.<br>Alternative treatment:<br>  Medium-dose inhaled corticosteroids and either leukotriene receptor antagonist or theophylline. |
| Step 2: Mild persistent | >2/wk but <1/d<br><br>>2 nights/mo | Preferred treatment:<br>  Low-dose inhaled corticosteroid (with nebulizer or MDI with holding chamber with or without face mask or DPI).<br>Alternative treatment (listed alphabetically):<br>  Cromolyn (nebulizer is preferred or MDI with holding chamber) OR leukotriene receptor antagonist. |
| Step 1: Mild intermittent | ≤2 d/wk<br><br>≤2 nights/mo | No daily medication needed. |
| All patients | | Bronchodilator as needed for symptoms ≤ 2 times a week. Intensity of treatment will depend upon severity of exacerbation.<br>  Preferred treatment: Inhaled short-acting $\beta_2$-agonist by nebulizer or face mask and space-holding chamber<br>  Alternative treatment: Oral $\beta_2$-agonist<br>With viral respiratory infection<br>  Bronchodilator q4–6h up to 24 h (longer with physician consult); in general no more than once every 6 wk<br>  Consider systemic corticosteroid if exacerbation is severe or patient has history of previous severe exacerbations<br>Use of short-acting $\beta_2$-agonist daily indicates the need to initiate or increase long-term control therapy |
| Step down | | Review treatment every 1–6 mos; a gradual stepwise reduction in treatment may be possible. |
| Step up | | If control is not maintained, consider step up. First, review patient medication technique, adherence, and environmental control. |

(*continued*)

***Table 34-2.*** Stepwise approach for treating infants and young children (5 years of age and younger) with acute or chronic asthma. (continued)

---

Minimal or no chronic symptoms day or night
Minimal or no exacerbations
No limitations on activities; no school/parent's work missed
Minimal use of inhaled short-acting $\beta_2$-agonist (< 1/d, < 1 canister/mo)
Minimal or no adverse effects from medications

---

**Notes**

The stepwise approach is intended to assist, not replace, the clinical decisionmaking required to meet individual patient needs.

Classify severity: assign patient to most severe step in which any feature occurs.

There are very few studies on asthma therapy for infants.

Gain control as quickly as possible (a course of short systemic corticosteroids may be required); then step down to the least medication necessary to maintain control.

Provide parent education on asthma management and controlling environmental factors that make asthma worse (e.g., allergies and irritants).

Consultation with an asthma specialist is recommended for patients with moderate or severe persistent asthma. Consider consultation for patients with mild persistent asthma.

Reprinted, with permission, from the National Asthma Education and Prevention Program: *Expert Panel Report: Update on Selected Topics 2002.*

physician-diagnosed allergic rhinitis, wheezing apart from colds, peripheral eosinophilia) with more than three episodes of wheezing over the past year that lasted longer than one day and affected sleep.

3. Benefits of inhaled corticosteroids at recommended doses (Table 34–4) versus potential risks.

4. Use of combination therapy including addition of long-acting inhaled $\beta_2$-agonists to low-to-medium doses of inhaled corticosteroids as the preferred treatment for children older than 5 years with moderate persistent asthma and either addition of long-acting inhaled $\beta_2$-agonists to a low dose of inhaled corticosteroids or medium-dose inhaled corticosteroids as monotherapy in children 5 years of age or younger. The preferred strategy is to initiate therapy at a higher level at the onset to gain prompt control and then step down, rather than gradually stepping up treatment if control is not achieved. A rescue course of systemic corticosteroids may be necessary at any step. A short course of systemic corticosteroids may be required for patients with intermittent asthma who experience infrequent but severe exacerbations—typically triggered by respiratory infections—with normal lung function between episodes.

Asthma medications are classified as long-term control medications and quick-relief medications. The for-

mer include anti-inflammatory agents, long-acting bronchodilators, and leukotriene modifiers. Inhaled corticosteroids delivered by aerosol, dry powder inhaler, or nebulizer are the most potent inhaled anti-inflammatory agents currently available. Recent data suggest that different inhaled corticosteroids are not equivalent on a per puff or microgram basis (see Table 34–4). Early intervention with inhaled corticosteroids can improve asthma control and may prevent airway remodeling. Inhaled corticosteroids may be associated with slowing of growth velocity in children, although a study of asthmatic children treated with budesonide (mean dose 412 µg/d) for a mean of 9.2 years showed no adverse effect on final adult height. Possible risks from inhaled corticosteroids need to be weighed against the risks from undertreated asthma. Only inhaled corticosteroids have been shown to be effective in long-term clinical studies with infants. Nebulized budesonide is approved for children as young as 12 months. The suspension (available in quantities of 0.25 mg/2 mL and 0.5 mg/2 mL) is usually administered at 0.5 mg/d, either once or twice a day in divided doses. Notably, this drug should not be given by ultrasonic nebulizer. Limited data suggest that inhaled corticosteroids may be effective even in very young children when delivered by metered-dose inhaler with a spacer with mask.

Fewer data are available with nedocromil, although comparative data from the Childhood Asthma Management Program study showed that an inhaled cortico-

***Table 34-3.*** Stepwise approach for managing asthma in adults and children older than 5 years of age: Treatment.

| Classify Severity: Clinical Features Before Treatment or Adequate Control | | | Medications Required to Maintain Long-Term Control |
|---|---|---|---|
| | Symptoms/Day<br>Symptoms/Night | PEF or FEV$_1$<br>PEF Variability | Daily Medications |
| Step 4: Severe persistent | Continual<br>Frequent | ≤ 60%<br>> 30% | Preferred treatment:<br>  High-dose inhaled corticosteroids<br>  AND<br>  Long-acting inhaled β$_2$-agonists<br>  AND, if needed,<br>  Corticosteroid tablets or syrup long term (2 mg/kg/d, generally do not exceed 60 mg/d). (Make repeat attempts to reduce systemic corticosteroids and maintain control with high-dose inhaled corticosteroids.) |
| Step 3: Moderate persistent | Daily<br>>1 night/wk | > 60%–< 80%<br>> 30% | Preferred treatment:<br>  Low-to-medium dose inhaled corticosteroids and long-acting inhaled β$_2$-agonists<br>Alternative treatment (listed alphabetically):<br>  Increase inhaled corticosteroids within medium-dose range<br>  OR<br>  Low-to-medium dose inhaled corticosteroids and either leukotriene modifier or theophylline. |
| | | | If needed (particularly in patients with recurring severe exacerbations):<br>**Preferred treatment:**<br>  Increase inhaled corticosteroids within medium-dose range, and add long-acting inhaled β$_2$-agonists.<br>Alternative treatment (listed alphabetically):<br>  Increase inhaled corticosteroids in medium-dose range, and add either leukotriene modifier or theophylline. |
| Step 2: Mild persistent | > 2/wk but < 1/d<br>> 2 nights/mo | ≥ 80%<br>20–30% | Preferred treatment:<br>  Low-dose inhaled corticosteroids<br>Alternative treatment (listed alphabetically): cromolyn, leukotriene modifier, nedocromil, OR sustained release theophylline to serum concentration of 5–15 μg/mL. |
| Step 1: Mild intermittent | ≤ 2 d/wk<br>≤ 2 nights/mo | ≥ 80%<br>< 20% | No daily medication needed.<br>Severe exacerbations may occur, separated by long periods of normal lung function and no symptoms. A course of systemic corticosteroids is recommended. |
| All patients | | | Short-acting bronchodilator: 2–4 puffs short-acting inhaled β$_2$-agonists as needed for symptoms.<br>Intensity of treatment will depend on severity of exacerbation: up to 3 treatments at 20-min intervals or a single nebulizer treatment as needed. Course of systemic corticosteroids may be needed.<br>Use of short-acting inhaled β$_2$-agonists on a daily basis, or increasing use, indicates the need to initiate or increase long-term control therapy. |
| Step down | | | Review treatment every 1–6 mos; a gradual stepwise reduction in treatment may be possible. |
| Step up | | | If control is not maintained, consider step up. First, review patient medication technique, adherence, and environmental control. |

*(continued)*

**Table 34–3.** Stepwise approach for managing asthma in adults and children older than 5 years of age: Treatment. (continued)

Minimal or no chronic symptoms day or night
Minimal or no exacerbations
No limitations on activities; no school/parent's work missed
Minimal use of inhaled short-acting $\beta_2$-agonist (< 1/d. < 1 canister/mo)
Minimal or no adverse effects from medications

**Notes**
The stepwise approach is intended to assist, not replace, the clinical decision making required to meet individual patient needs.
Classify severity: assign patient to most severe step in which any feature occurs (PEF is % of personal best; $FEV_1$ is % predicted).
Gain control as quickly as possible (consider a short course of systemic corticosteroids); then step down to the least medication necessary to maintain control.
Provide education on self-management and controlling environmental factors that make asthma worse (eg, allergens and irritants).
Refer to an asthma specialist if there are difficulties controlling asthma or if step 4 care is required. Referral may be considered if step 3 care is required.
Reprinted with permission. (See Table 34–2.)

steroid was superior to nedocromil with respect to a number of efficacy parameters, including rate of hospitalization, symptom-free days, need for albuterol rescue, and longer time to treatment with prednisone.

Sustained-release theophylline, an alternative long-term control medication for older children, may have particular risks of adverse side effects in infants, who frequently have febrile illnesses that increase theophylline concentrations.

Salmeterol, a long-acting $\beta_2$-agonist, is available as an inhalation powder (1 inhalation twice daily for patients age 4 years and older). Salmeterol in a metered-dose inhaler has recently been discontinued. Salmeterol can be used as adjunctive therapy with anti-inflammatory medications for long-term symptom control. Salmeterol should not be used for treatment of acute symptoms, and anti-inflammatory medication should not be discontinued when salmeterol is initiated, even if the patient feels better. Salmeterol, 50 µg, is available combined with fluticasone (100, 250, or 500 µg) in a dry powder inhaler. For children 12 years and older, one inhalation is taken twice daily. (*Note:* The 100/50 fluticasone/salmeterol combination is approved in children age 4 and older.) It can also be used 30 minutes before exercise (but not in addition to regularly used long-acting $\beta_2$-agonists). Formoterol is another long-acting $\beta_2$-agonist with a more rapid onset of action in a dry powder inhaler. It is approved for use in children 5 years and older, one inhala-

**Table 34–4.** Estimated comparative daily dosages for inhaled corticosteroids.

| Drug | Low Daily Dose Child | Medium Daily Dose Child | High Daily Dose Child |
|---|---|---|---|
| Beclomethasone CFC 42 or 84 µg/puff | 84–336 µg | 336–672 µg | > 672 µg |
| Beclomethasone HFA 40 or 80 µg/puff | 80–160 µg | 160–320 µg | > 320 µg |
| Budesonide DPI 200 µg/inhalation | 200–400 µg | 400–800 µg | > 800 µg |
| Budesonide suspension for nebulization (child dose) | 0.5 mg | 1.0 mg | 2.0 mg |
| Flunisolide 250 µg/puff | 500–750 µg | 1000–1250 µg | > 1,250 µg |
| Fluticasone<br>MDI: 44, 110, or 220 µg/puff<br>DPI: 50, 100, or 250 µg/inhalation | 88–176 µg | 176–440 µg | > 440 µg |
| Triamcinolone acetonide 100 µg/puff | 400–800 µg | 800–1200 µg | > 1200 µg |

tion (12 μg) twice daily. For long-term control, it should be used in combination with an anti-inflammatory agent. It can be used for exercise-induced bronchospasm in patents 12 years and older, 1 inhalation at least 15 minutes before exercise (but not in addition to regularly used long-acting $\beta_2$-agonists).

Montelukast and zafirlukast are leukotriene receptor antagonists available in oral formulations. Montelukast is given once daily and has been approved for children age 1 year and older. To date, no drug interactions have been noted. The dosage is 4 mg for children 1–5 years (oral granules are available for children 12–23 months), 5 mg for children age 6–14 years, and 10 mg for those age 15 years and older. The drug is given without regard to mealtimes, preferably in the evening. Zafirlukast is approved for patients age 5 years and older. The dose is 10 mg twice daily for 5–11 years and 20 mg twice daily for 12 years and older. It should be taken 1 hour before or 2 hours after meals. Rare cases of Churg–Strauss syndrome in adult patients with severe asthma whose steroids were being tapered have been reported with concomitant treatment with leukotriene receptor antagonists (but also with inhaled corticosteroids), and no causal link has been established.

Quick-relief medications include short-acting inhaled $\beta_2$-agonists such as albuterol, pirbuterol, or terbutaline, 1–2 puffs by inhaler. Albuterol HFA contains a nonchlorofluorocarbon propellant. Albuterol can be given by nebulizer, 0.05 mg/kg (with a minimal dose of 1.25 mg and a maximum of 2.5 mg) in 2–3 mL saline. It is better to use $\beta_2$-agonists as needed rather than on a regular basis. Increasing use, including more than one canister per month, may signify inadequate asthma control and the need to intensify anti-inflammatory therapy. Levalbuterol, the (*R*)-enantiomer of racemic albuterol, is available in solution for nebulization for patients age 6–11 years 0.31 mg tid and for patients 12 years and older 0.63–1.25 mg tid. Anticholinergic agents such as ipratropium, 1–3 puffs or 0.25–0.5 mg by nebulizer every 6 hours, may provide additive benefit when used together with inhaled $\beta_2$-agonists. Systemic corticosteroids such as prednisone, prednisolone, and methylprednisolone can be given in a dosage of 1–2 mg/kg, usually up to 60 mg/d in single or divided doses for 3–10 days. There is no evidence that tapering the dose following a "burst" prevents relapse.

Anti-IgE (omalizumab) is a recombinant DNA-derived humanized IgG$_1$ monoclonal antibody that selectively binds to human IgE. It inhibits the binding of IgE to the high-affinity IgE receptor (FcƐ-RI) on the surface of mast cells and basophils. Reduction in surface-bound IgE on FcƐRI-bearing cells limits the degree of release of mediators of the allergic response. Treatment with omalizumab also reduces the number of

FcƐRI receptors on basophils in atopic patients. Omalizumab is indicated for patients 12 years of age and older with moderate to severe persistent asthma who have a positive skin test or in vitro reactivity to a perennial aeroallergen with serum IgE ≤ 700 IU/mL and whose symptoms are inadequately controlled with inhaled corticosteroids. Omalizumab has been shown to decrease the incidence of asthma exacerbations in these patients. Dosing is based on the patient's weight and serum IgE level and is given subcutaneously every 2–4 weeks. Continual monitoring is necessary to ensure that control of asthma is achieved and sustained. Once control is established, gradual reduction in therapy is appropriate and may help determine the minimum amount of medication necessary to maintain control. Regular follow-up visits with the clinician are important to assess the degree of control and consider appropriate adjustments in therapy. At each step, patients should be instructed to avoid or control exposure to allergens, irritants, or other factors that contribute to asthma severity. Referral to an asthma specialist for consultation or comanagement is recommended if there are difficulties in achieving or maintaining control or if the patient has severe persistent asthma. Referral is also recommended if allergen immunotherapy is being considered.

Referral may be considered for patients with moderate persistent asthma. For children younger than age 3 years, referral is recommended if the patient requires step 3 or 4 care and should be considered if the patient requires step 2 care (see Table 34–3).

**3. Exercise induced bronchospasm**—Exercise-induced bronchospasm should be anticipated in all asthma patients. It typically occurs during or minutes after vigorous activity, reaches its peak 5–10 minutes after stopping the activity, and usually resolves over the next 20–30 minutes. Participation in physical activity should be encouraged in children with asthma, although the choice of activity may need to be modified based on the severity of illness, triggers such as cold air, and, rarely, confounding factors such as osteoporosis. Treatment immediately prior to vigorous activity or exercise is usually effective. Short-acting inhaled $\beta_2$-agonists, cromolyn or nedocromil can be used before exercise. The combination of a short-acting inhaled $\beta_2$-agonist with either cromolyn or nedocromil is more effective than either drug alone. Salmeterol and formoterol may block exercise-induced bronchospasm for up to 12 hours (as discussed earlier). Montelukast may be effective up to 24 hours. Occasionally an extended warm-up period may induce a refractory state, allowing patients to exercise without a need for repeat medications. If symptoms occur during usual play activities, a step-up in long-term therapy is warranted. Poor endurance or exercise-induced bronchospasm can be an indication of poorly controlled persistent asthma.

## B. ACUTE ASTHMA

**1. General measures**—The most effective strategy in managing asthma exacerbations involves early recognition of warning signs and early treatment. For patients with moderate or severe persistent asthma or a history of severe exacerbations, this should include a written action plan. The latter usually defines the patient's peak flow zones and what steps to take if peak flows are between 50% and 80% or below 50% of personal best. The child, parents, and other caregivers must be able to assess asthma severity accurately. Prompt communication with the clinician is indicated with severe symptoms or a drop in peak flow or with decreased response to short-acting inhaled $\beta_2$-agonists. At such times, intensification of therapy may include a short course of oral corticosteroids. The child should be removed from exposure to any irritants or allergens that could be contributing to the exacerbation.

**2. Management at home**—Early treatment of asthma exacerbations may prevent progression to severe disease. Initial treatment should be with a short-acting inhaled $\beta_2$-agonist such as albuterol; 2–4 puffs from a metered-dose inhaler can be given every 20 minutes up to three times, or a single treatment can be given by nebulizer (0.05 mg/kg; minimum 1.25 mg, maximum 2.5 mg of 0.5% solution of albuterol in 2–3 mL saline). If the response is good as assessed by sustained symptom relief or improvement in PEFR to over 80% of the patient's best, the short-acting $\beta_2$-agonist can be continued every 3–4 hours for 24–48 hours. For patients taking inhaled corticosteroids, the dose may be doubled for 7–10 days. If the patient does not completely improve from the initial therapy, with PEFR between 50% and 80%, the $\beta_2$-agonist should be continued, an oral corticosteroid should be added, and the patient should contact the physician. If the child experiences marked distress or if PEFR persists at under 50%, the patient should repeat the $\beta_2$-agonist immediately and go to the emergency department or call 911 or another emergency number for assistance.

**3. Management in the office or emergency department**—Functional assessment of the patient includes obtaining objective measures of airflow limitation with PEFR or $FEV_1$ and monitoring the patient's response to treatment. Other tests may include oxygen saturation and blood gases. If the initial $FEV_1$ or PEFR is over 50%, initial treatment can be with a $\beta_2$-agonist by inhaler (albuterol, 4–8 puffs) or nebulizer (0.15 mg/kg of albuterol 0.5% solution, minimum dose 2.5 mg), up to three doses in the first hour. Oxygen should be given to maintain oxygen saturation at greater than 90%. Oral corticosteroids (1 mg/kg q6h for 48 hours, then 1–2 mg/kg/d in divided doses, maximum 60 mg/d) should be instituted if the patient responds poorly to therapy or if the patient has been on oral corticosteroids recently. Sensitivity to adrenergic drugs may improve after initiation of corticosteroids. If the initial $FEV_1$ or PEFR is under 50%, initial treatment should be with a high-dose $\beta_2$-agonist by nebulizer every 20 minutes or continuously for the first hour (0.5 mg/kg/h). Ipratropium can be added to albuterol, 0.25 mg every 20 minutes for three doses, then every 2–4 hours. Oxygen should be given to maintain oxygen saturation at greater than 90%, and systemic corticosteroids should be instituted. For patients with severe asthma unresponsive to initial aerosolized therapy, or for those who cannot cooperate with or who resist inhalation therapy, epinephrine 1:1000 or terbutaline 1 mg/mL (both 0.01 mg/kg up to 0.3–0.5 mg) may be administered subcutaneously every 20 minutes for three doses. The role of theophylline or aminophylline remains questionable when added to optimal $\beta_2$-agonist therapy and may be associated with adverse events. For impending or ongoing respiratory arrest, patients should be intubated and ventilated with 100% oxygen and admitted to an intensive care unit (see Asthma (life-threatening) in Chapter 13). Further treatment is based on clinical response and objective laboratory findings. Hospitalization should be considered strongly for any patient with a history of respiratory failure.

**4. Hospital management**—For patients who do not respond to outpatient therapy, admission to the hospital becomes necessary for more aggressive care and support. Fluids should be given at maintenance requirements unless the patient has poor oral intake secondary to respiratory distress or vomiting, because overhydration may contribute to pulmonary edema associated with high intrapleural pressures generated in severe asthma. Potassium requirements should be kept in mind because both corticosteroids and $\beta_2$-agonists can cause potassium loss. Moisturized oxygen should be titrated by oximetry to maintain $SaO_2$ above 90%. Inhaled $\beta_2$-agonist should be continued by nebulization in single doses as needed or by continuous therapy, along with ipratropium and systemic corticosteroids (as discussed earlier). In addition, the role of methylxanthines in hospitalized children remains controversial. Antibiotics may be necessary to treat coexisting bacterial infection. Sedatives and anxiolytic agents are contraindicated in severely ill patients owing to their depressant effects on respiration. Chest physiotherapy is usually not recommended for acute exacerbations.

**5. Patient discharge**—Criteria for discharging patients home from the office or emergency department should include a sustained response of at least 1 hour to bronchodilator therapy with $FEV_1$ or PEFR greater than 70% and oxygen saturation greater than 90% in room air. Prior to discharge, the patient's or caregiver's ability to continue therapy and assess symptoms appropriately needs to be considered. Patients should be given an action plan for management of recurrent symptoms or exacerbations, and instructions about medications should be reviewed. The inhaled $\beta_2$-agonist and oral corticosteroids should be continued, the latter for 3–10 days. Finally, the patient or caregiver should be instructed about the follow-up visit, typically within 1 week. Hospitalized patients should receive more intensive education prior to discharge. Referral to an asthma specialist should be considered for all children with severe exacerbations or multiple emergency department visits or hospitalizations.

## Prognosis

Since the 1970s, morbidity and mortality rates for asthma have increased. Mortality statistics indicate that a high percentage of deaths have resulted from under-recognition of asthma severity and undertreatment, particularly in labile asthmatic patients and in asthmatic patients whose perception of pulmonary obstruction is poor. Long-term outcome studies suggest that children with mild symptoms generally outgrow their asthma, while patients with more severe symptoms, marked airway hyperresponsiveness, and a greater degree of atopy tend to have persistent disease. In a recently published unselected birth cohort from New Zealand, more than one in four children had wheezing that persisted from childhood to adulthood or that relapsed after remission. It is possible that early intervention with anti-inflammatory therapy and environmental control measures may alter the natural history of childhood asthma. In this respect, the pediatrician or primary care provider together with the asthma specialist has a critical opportunity to affect the course of this increasingly common disease.

Resources for health care providers, patients, and families:

Asthma and Allergy Foundation of America
1125 15th St NW, Suite 502
Washington, DC 20005; (800) 7-ASTHMA
Asthma and Allergy Network/Mothers of Asthmatics
3554 Chain Bridge Rd, Suite 200

Fairfax, VA 22030-2709; (800) 878-4403
Lung Line (800) 222-LUNG

Agertoft L, Pedersen S: Effect of long-term treatment with inhaled budesonide on adult height in children with asthma. N Engl J Med 2000;343:1064..

Berger W et al: Evaluation of long-term safety of the anti-IgE antibody, omalizumab, in children with allergic asthma. Ann Allergy Asthma Immunol 2003;91:182 [PMID: 12897737].

The Childhood Asthma Management Program Research Group: Long-term effects of budesonide or nedocromil in children with asthma. N Engl J Med 2000;343:1054.

Diette GB et al: Consistency of care with national guidelines for children with asthma in managed care. J Pediatr 2001; 138:59.

Liu AH et al: Advances in childhood asthma: Hygiene hypothesis, natural history, and management. J Allergy Clin Immunol 2003;111:S785 [PMID: 12612244].

National Asthma Education and Prevention Program: *Guidelines for the Diagnosis and Management of Asthma—Update on Selected Topics 2002.* NIH publication No. 02-5075. www.nhlbi.nih.gov.

Sears MR et al: A longitudinal, population-based, cohort study of childhood asthma followed to adulthood. N Engl J Med 2003;349:1414 [PMID: 14523172].

# ALLERGIC RHINOCONJUNCTIVITIS

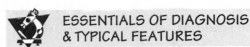

### ESSENTIALS OF DIAGNOSIS & TYPICAL FEATURES

*After exposure to allergen:*

• *Sneezing.*

• *Itching of nose and eyes.*

• *Clear rhinorrhea or nasal congestion.*

## General Considerations

Allergic rhinoconjunctivitis is the most common allergic disease and significantly affects quality of life as well as school performance and attendance. It frequently coexists with asthma and is a risk factor for subsequent development of asthma. Prevalence of this disease increases during childhood, peaking at 15% in the postadolescent years. Although allergic rhinoconjunctivitis is more common in boys during early childhood, there is little difference in incidence between the sexes after adolescence. Race and socioeconomic status are not considered to be important factors.

The pathologic changes in allergic rhinoconjunctivitis are chiefly hyperemia, edema, and increased serous and mucoid secretions caused by mediator release, all of which lead to variable degrees of nasal obstruction, pruritus, and rhinorrhea. This process may involve the eyes and other structures, including the sinuses and possibly the middle ear. Inhalant allergens are primarily responsible for symptoms, but food allergens can cause symptoms as well. Children with allergic rhinitis seem to be more susceptible to—or at least may experience more symptoms from—upper respiratory infections, which, in turn, may aggravate the allergic rhinitis.

Allergic rhinoconjunctivitis may be perennial, seasonal (hay fever), or episodic. Perennial allergic rhinitis occurs to some degree all year long but may be more severe in winter. Greater exposure to indoor allergens results from well-insulated homes, an increase in the amount of time spent indoors, and heating systems that disperse the allergens. Seasonal allergic rhinitis occurs as a result of exposure to specific aeroallergens, including pollens and molds. The major pollen groups in the temperate zones include trees (late winter to early spring), grasses (late spring to early summer), and weeds (late summer to early fall), but seasons can vary significantly in different parts of the country. Mold spores also cause seasonal allergic rhinitis, principally in the summer and fall. Seasonal allergy symptoms may be aggravated by coincident exposure to perennial allergens.

## Clinical Findings

### A. Symptoms and Signs

Patients may complain of itching of the nose, eyes, palate, or pharynx. Nasal itching can cause paroxysmal sneezing and epistaxis. Repeated rubbing of the nose (so-called allergic salute) may lead to a horizontal crease across the lower third of the nose. Nasal obstruction is associated with mouth breathing, nasal speech, allergic salute, and snoring. Nasal turbinates may appear pale blue and swollen, with dimpling, or injected, with minimal edema. Typically, clear and thin nasal secretions are increased, with anterior rhinorrhea, sniffling, postnasal drip, and congested cough. Nasal secretions often cause poor appetite, fatigue, and pharyngeal irritation. Conjunctival injection, tearing, periorbital edema, and infraorbital cyanosis (so-called allergic shiners) are frequently observed. Increased pharyngeal lymphoid tissue ("cobblestoning") from chronic drainage and enlarged tonsillar and adenoidal tissue may be present.

### B. Laboratory Findings

Eosinophilia often can be demonstrated on smears of nasal secretions or blood. This is a frequent but nonspecific finding and may occur in nonallergic conditions. Although serum IgE may be elevated, measurement of total IgE is a poor screening tool owing to the wide overlap between atopic and nonatopic subjects. Skin testing to identify allergen-specific IgE is the most sensitive and specific test for inhalant allergies; alternatively, radioallergosorbent assay test (RAST), ImmunoCAP, or other in vitro tests can be done for suspected allergens.

## Differential Diagnosis

Disorders that need to be differentiated from allergic rhinitis include infectious rhinitis and sinusitis. Foreign bodies and structural abnormalities such as choanal atresia, marked septal deviation, nasal polyps, and adenoidal hypertrophy may cause chronic symptoms. Overuse of topical nasal decongestants may result in rhinitis medicamentosa (rebound congestion). Use of medications such as propranolol, clonidine, and some psychoactive drugs may cause nasal congestion. Illicit drugs like cocaine can cause rhinorrhea. Spicy or hot foods may cause gustatory rhinitis. Nonallergic rhinitis with eosinophilia syndrome is usually not seen in young children. Vasomotor rhinitis is associated with persistent symptoms but without allergen exposure. Less common causes of symptoms that may be confused with allergic rhinitis include pregnancy, congenital syphilis, hypothyroidism, tumors, and cerebrospinal fluid rhinorrhea.

## Complications

Sinusitis may accompany allergic rhinitis. Allergic mucosal swelling of the sinus ostia can obstruct sinus drainage, interfering with normal sinus function and predisposing to chronic mucosal disease. Nasal polyps due to allergy are unusual in children, and cystic fibrosis should be considered if they are present.

## Treatment

### A. General Measures

The value of identification and avoidance of causative allergens cannot be overstated. Reducing indoor allergens through environmental control measures as discussed in the section on asthma can be very effective. Nasal saline irrigation may be useful.

### B. Pharmacologic Therapy

**1. Antihistamines**—Antihistamines help control itching, sneezing, and rhinorrhea. Sedating antihistamines include diphenhydramine, chlorpheniramine, hydroxyzine, and clemastine. Sedating antihistamines may cause daytime somnolence and negatively affect school performance and other activities, especially driving. Second-generation antihistamines include loratadine, desloratadine, cetirizine, and fexofenadine. Cetirizine is approved for use in children age 6–23 months (2.5 mg daily), 2–5 years (2.5–5 mg/d or 2.5 mg bid), and 6 years or older (5–10 mg/d). Loratadine is approved for use in children aged 2–5 years (5 mg/d) and 6 years or older (10 mg/d), and is available without prescription in tablet, rapidly disintegrating tablet, and liquid formulations. Desloratadine 5 mg/d is approved for patients 12 years and older. Fexofenadine is approved for children age 6–11 years (30 mg bid) and 12 years or older (60 mg bid or 180 mg once daily). Loratadine, fexofenadine, and cetirizine are available in combination with pseudoephedrine for patients age 12 years or older. Azelastine is available in a nasal spray and levocabastine as an ophthalmic preparation.

**2. Decongestants**—α-Adrenergic agents help to relieve nasal congestion. Topical decongestants such as phenylephrine and oxymetazoline should not be used for more than 4 days for severe episodes because prolonged use may be associated with rhinitis medicamentosa. Oral decongestants, including pseudoephedrine and phenylpropanolamine, are often combined with antihistamines or expectorants and cough suppressants in over-the-counter cold medications. They may cause insomnia, agitation, tachycardia, and, rarely, cardiac arrhythmias. Of note, the US Food and Drug Administration has recommended the removal of phenylpropanolamine from all drug products due to a public health advisory concerning the risk of hemorrhagic stroke associated with its use.

**3. Corticosteroids**—Intranasal corticosteroid sprays are effective in controlling allergic rhinitis if used chronically. They are minimally absorbed in usual doses and are available in pressurized nasal inhalers and aqueous sprays. Mometasone nasal spray has been approved for use in children as young as age 2 years (1 spray in each nostril once daily) and in children 12 years or older (2 sprays/nostril once daily). Fluticasone nasal spray is approved for children 4 years or older, and budesonide and triamcinolone nasal sprays are approved for 6 years or older, 1–2 sprays/nostril once daily. Flunisolide is approved for ages 6–14 years 1 spray/nostril tid or 2 sprays/nostril bid. Side effects include nasal irritation, soreness, and bleeding, although epistaxis occurs commonly in patients with allergic rhinitis if corticosteroids are used chronically. Rarely they can cause septal perforation. Excessive doses may produce systemic effects, especially if used together with orally inhaled steroids for asthma. Onset of action is within hours, although clinical benefit is usually not observed for a week or more. They may be effective alone or together with antihistamines.

**4. Other pharmacologic agents**—Montelukast is approved for seasonal allergic rhinitis in children 2 years and older in doses as discussed under the preceding section, Asthma Pharmacologic Therapy. Intranasal ipratropium can be used as adjunctive therapy for rhinorrhea. Intranasal cromolyn may be used alone or in conjunction with oral antihistamines and decongestants. It is most effective when used prophylactically, 1–2 sprays per nostril, qid. This dose may be tapered if symptom control is achieved. Rarely patients complain of nasal irritation or burning. Most patients find complying with four-times-daily dosing difficult. Cromolyn is also available in an ophthalmic solution (see also Chapter 15, Eye). Other ophthalmic mast cell stabilizers include lodoxamide 0.1% solution, 1–2 drops qid, and nedocromil, 1–2 drops bid. Olopatadine and ketotifen ophthalmic solutions have antihistamine and mast cell-stabilizing actions and can be given to children older than age 3 years as 1 drop bid (8 hours apart) and q8–12h, respectively.

### C. SURGICAL THERAPY

Surgical procedures, including turbinectomy, polypectomy, and functional endoscopic sinus surgery, are rarely indicated in allergic rhinitis or chronic hyperplastic sinusitis.

### D. IMMUNOTHERAPY

Allergen immunotherapy should be considered when symptoms are severe and due to unavoidable exposure to inhalant allergens, especially if symptomatic measures have failed. Immunotherapy is the only form of therapy that may alter the course of the disease. It should not be prescribed by sending the patient's serum to a laboratory where extracts based on in vitro tests are prepared for the patient (ie, the remote practice of allergy). Immunotherapy should be done in a facility where a physician prepared to treat anaphylaxis is present. Patients with concomitant asthma should not receive an injection if their asthma is not under good control (ie, peak flows preinjection are below 80% of personal best), and the patient should wait for 25–30 minutes after an injection before leaving the facility.

Outcomes with single allergen immunotherapy show success rates of approximately 80%. The optimal duration of therapy is unknown, but data suggest that immunotherapy for 3–5 years may have lasting benefit.

## Prognosis

Perennial allergic rhinoconjunctivitis tends to be protracted unless specific allergens can be identified and eliminated from the environment. In seasonal allergic rhinoconjunctivitis, symptoms are usually most severe from adolescence through mid adult life. After moving to a region devoid of problem allergens, patients may be symptom-free for several years, but they can develop new sensitivities to local aeroallergens.

Fireman P: Therapeutic approaches to allergic rhinitis: Treating the child. J Allergy Clin Immunol 2000;105:S616.

Simons FE: H1-antihistamines in children. Clin Allergy Immunol 2002;17:437 [PMID: 12063508].

# ATOPIC DERMATITIS

### ESSENTIALS OF DIAGNOSIS & TYPICAL FEATURES

- Pruritus.
- Facial and extensor involvement in infants and young children.
- Flexural lichenification in older children and adolescents.
- Chronic or relapsing dermatitis.
- Personal or family history of atopic disease.

## General Considerations

Atopic dermatitis is a chronically relapsing inflammatory skin disease typically associated with respiratory allergy. Over half of patients with atopic dermatitis will develop asthma and allergic rhinitis—often as they outgrow their atopic dermatitis. Atopic dermatitis may result in significant morbidity, leading to school absenteeism, occupational disability, and emotional stress. Atopic dermatitis presents in early childhood, with onset prior to age 5 years in approximately 90% of patients.

## Clinical Findings

### A. SYMPTOMS AND SIGNS

Atopic dermatitis has no pathognomonic skin lesions or laboratory parameters. Diagnosis is based on the clinical features, including severe pruritus, a chronically relapsing course, and typical morphology and distribution of the skin lesions. Acute atopic dermatitis is characterized by intensely pruritic, erythematous papules associated with excoriations, vesiculations, and serous exudate; subacute atopic dermatitis by erythematous, excoriated, scaling papules; chronic atopic dermatitis by thickened skin with accentuated markings (lichenification) and fibrotic papules. Patients with chronic atopic dermatitis may have all three types of lesions present concurrently. Patients usually have dry, "lackluster" skin. During infancy, atopic dermatitis involves primarily the face, scalp, and extensor surfaces of the extremities. The diaper area is usually spared. When involved, it may be secondarily infected with *Candida*. In older patients with long-standing disease, the flexural folds of the extremities are the predominant location of lesions.

### B. LABORATORY FINDINGS

Identification of allergens involves taking a careful history and performing selective immediate hypersensitivity skin tests or in vitro tests when appropriate. Negative skin tests with proper controls have a high predictive value for ruling out a suspected allergen. Positive skin tests have a lower correlation with clinical symptoms in suspected food allergen-induced atopic dermatitis and should be confirmed with double-blind, placebo-controlled food challenges unless there is a coincidental history of anaphylaxis to the suspected food. Alternatively, specific IgE levels to milk, egg, peanut, and fish proteins have been established with the Pharmacia ImmunoCAP assay correlating with a greater than 95% chance of a clinical reaction.

Elevated serum IgE levels can be demonstrated in 80–85% of patients with atopic dermatitis, and a similar number have positive immediate skin tests or in vitro tests with food and inhalant allergens. A number of well-controlled studies suggest that specific allergens can influence the course of this disease. However, triggers for clinical disease cannot be predicted simply by performing allergy testing. Double-blind, placebo-controlled food challenges show that food allergens can cause exacerbations in a subset of patients with atopic dermatitis. Although lesions induced by single positive challenges are usually transient, repeated challenges, more typical of real-life exposure, can result in eczematous lesions. Furthermore, elimination of food allergens results in amelioration of skin disease and a decrease in spontaneous basophil histamine release. Exacerbation of atopic dermatitis can occur with exposure to aeroallergens such as house dust mites, and environmental control measures have been shown to result in clinical improvement. Patients can make specific IgE directed at *Staphylococcus aureus* toxins secreted on the skin, and this correlates with clinical severity better than total serum IgE levels. Eosinophilia may occur. Routine skin biopsy does not differentiate atopic dermatitis from other eczematous processes and is not usually indicated.

## Differential Diagnosis

Scabies can present as a pruritic skin disease. However, distribution in the genital and axillary areas and the presence of linear lesions as well as skin scrapings may help to distinguish it from atopic dermatitis. Seborrheic dermatitis may be distinguished by a lack of significant pruritus; its predilection for the scalp (so-called cradle cap); and its coarse, yellowish scales. Allergic contact dermatitis may be suggested by the distribution of lesions with a greater demarcation of dermatitis than in atopic dermatitis. Occasionally, allergic contact dermatitis superimposed on atopic dermatitis may appear as an acute flare of the underlying disease. Nummular eczema is characterized by coin-shaped plaques. Although unusual in children, mycosis fungoides or cutaneous T-cell lymphoma has been described and is diagnosed by skin biopsy. Eczematous rash has been reported in patients with human immunodeficiency virus (HIV) infection. Other disorders that may resemble atopic dermatitis include Wiskott–Aldrich syndrome, severe combined immunodeficiency disease, hyper-IgE syndrome, zinc deficiency, phenylketonuria, and Letterer–Siwe disease.

## Complications

Ocular complications associated with atopic dermatitis can lead to significant morbidity. Atopic keratoconjunctivitis is always bilateral, and symptoms include itching, burning, tearing, and copious mucoid discharge. It is frequently associated with eyelid dermatitis and chronic blepharitis, and may result in visual impairment from corneal scarring. Vernal conjunctivitis is a severe bilateral recurrent chronic inflammatory process of the upper eyelid conjunctiva, occurring primarily in younger patients (see Chapter 15, Eye). It has a marked seasonal incidence, often in the spring. The associated intense pruritus is exacerbated by exposure to irritants, light, or perspiration. Examination of the eye reveals a papillary hypertrophy or cobblestoning of the upper inner eyelid surface. Keratoconus in atopic dermatitis is believed to result from persistent rubbing of the eyes in patients with atopic dermatitis and allergic rhinitis. Anterior subcapsular cataracts may develop during adolescence or early adult life.

Patients with atopic dermatitis have increased susceptibility to infection or colonization with a variety of organisms. These include viral infections with herpes simplex, molluscum contagiosum, and human papillomavirus. Of note, even a past history of atopic dermatitis is considered a contraindication for receiving the current smallpox (vaccinia) vaccine. Superimposed dermatophytosis may cause atopic dermatitis to flare.

*S aureus* can be cultured from the skin of more than 90% of patients with atopic dermatitis, compared with only 5% of normal subjects. Atopic dermatitis patients often have toxin-secreting *S aureus* cultured from their skin. These patients make specific IgE antibodies directed against the toxins found on their skin. *S aureus* toxins can act as superantigens, contributing to persis-

tent inflammation or exacerbations of atopic dermatitis. In addition, patients with atopic dermatitis may be predisposed to colonization and infections by *S aureus* and other microbial organism due to decreased synthesis of antimicrobial peptides in the skin, which may be mediated by increased levels of TH2-type cytokines. Patients without obvious superinfection may show a better response to combined antistaphylococcal and topical corticosteroid therapy than to corticosteroids alone. Although recurrent staphylococcal pustulosis can be a significant problem in atopic dermatitis, invasive *S aureus* infections occur rarely and should raise the possibility of an immunodeficiency such as hyper-IgE syndrome.

Patients with atopic dermatitis often have a nonspecific hand dermatitis. This is frequently irritating in nature and aggravated by repeated wetting, especially in the occupational setting.

Nutritional disturbances may result from unwarranted and unnecessarily vigorous dietary restrictions imposed by physicians and parents.

Poor academic performance and behavioral disturbances may be a result of uncontrolled intense or frequent itching, sleep loss, and poor self-image. Severe disease may lead to problems with social interactions and self-esteem.

## Treatment

### A. General Measures

Patients with atopic dermatitis have a lowered threshold of irritant responsiveness. Avoidance of irritants such as detergents, chemicals, and abrasive materials as well as extremes of temperature and humidity is important in managing this disease. New clothing should be washed to reduce the content of formaldehyde and other chemicals. Because residual laundry detergent in clothing may be irritating, using a liquid rather than a powder detergent and adding an extra rinse cycle is beneficial. Occlusive clothing should be avoided in favor of cotton or cotton blends. Temperature in the home and work environments should be controlled to minimize sweating. Swimming is usually well tolerated; however, because swimming pools are treated with chlorine or bromine, patients should shower and use a mild cleanser to remove these irritating chemicals, then apply a moisturizer or occlusive agent. Sunlight may be beneficial to some patients with atopic dermatitis, but nonsensitizing sunscreens should be used to avoid sunburn. Prolonged sun exposure can cause evaporative losses, overheating, and sweating, all of which can be irritating.

In children who have undergone controlled food challenges, eggs, milk, peanuts, soy, wheat, and fish account for approximately 90% of the food allergens that exacerbate atopic dermatitis. Avoidance of foods implicated in controlled challenges can lead to clinical improvement. Extensive elimination diets, which can be nutritionally unsound and burdensome, are almost never warranted because even patients with multiple positive skin tests rarely react to more than three foods on blinded challenges.

In patients who demonstrate specific IgE to dust mite allergen, environmental control measures aimed at reducing the dust mite load improve atopic dermatitis. These include use of dust mite-proof covers on pillows and mattresses, washing linens weekly in hot water, decreasing indoor humidity levels, and in some cases removing bedroom carpeting.

Counseling may be of benefit when dealing with the frustrations associated with atopic dermatitis. Relaxation, behavioral modification, or biofeedback training may help patients with habitual scratching. Patients with severe or disfiguring disease may require psychotherapy.

Clinicians should provide the patient and family with both general information and specific written skin care recommendations. The patient or parent should demonstrate an appropriate level of understanding to help ensure a good outcome. Educational pamphlets and a video about atopic dermatitis can be obtained from the Eczema Association for Science and Education, a national nonprofit, patient-oriented organization, at 1-800-818-7546 or at http://www.nationaleczema.org/.

## B. Hydration

Patients with atopic dermatitis have evaporative losses due to a defective skin barrier, so soaking the affected area or bathing for 15–20 minutes in warm water, then applying an occlusive agent to retain the absorbed water, is an essential component of therapy. Oatmeal or baking soda added to the bath may feel soothing to certain patients but does not improve water absorption. Atopic dermatitis of the face or neck can be treated by applying a wet facecloth or towel to the involved area for 15–20 minutes. The washcloth may be more readily accepted by a child if it is turned into a mask and also allows the older patient to remain functional. Lesions limited to the hands or feet can be treated by soaking in a basin. Daily baths may be needed and increased to several times daily during flares of atopic dermatitis, while showers may be adequate for patients with mild disease. It is important to use an occlusive preparation within a few minutes after soaking the skin to prevent evaporation, which is both drying and irritating.

## C. Moisturizers and Occlusives

An effective emollient combined with hydration therapy will help skin healing and can reduce the need for topical corticosteroids. Moisturizers are available as lotions, creams, and ointments. Because lotions contain more water than creams, they are more drying because of their evaporative effect. Preservatives and fragrances in lotions and creams may cause skin irritation. Moisturizers often need to be applied several times daily on a long-term basis and should be obtained in the largest size available. Crisco shortening can be substituted as an inexpensive alternative. Petroleum jelly (Vaseline) is an effective occlusive agent when used to seal in water after bathing.

## D. Corticosteroids

Corticosteroids reduce the inflammation and pruritus in atopic dermatitis. Topical corticosteroids can decrease *S aureus* colonization. Systemic corticosteroids, including oral prednisone, should be avoided in the management of this chronic relapsing disease. The dramatic improvement observed with systemic corticosteroids may be associated with an equally dramatic flaring of atopic dermatitis following their discontinuation. If a short course of oral corticosteroids is given, it is usually best to prescribe a tapering dose.

Topical corticosteroids are available in a wide variety of formulations, ranging from extremely high-potency to low-potency preparations (see Table 14–3). Choice of a particular product depends on the severity and distribution of skin lesions. Patients need to be counseled regarding the potency of their corticosteroid preparation and its potential side effects. In general, the least potent agent that is effective should be used. However, choosing a preparation that is too weak may result in persistence or worsening of the atopic dermatitis. Side effects include thinning of the skin, telangiectasias, bruising, hypopigmentation, acne, and striae, although these occur infrequently when low- to medium-potency topical corticosteroids are used appropriately. In contrast, use of potent topical corticosteroids for prolonged periods—especially under occlusion—may result in significant atrophic changes as well as systemic side effects. The face (especially the eyelids) and intertriginous areas are especially sensitive to corticosteroid side effects, and only low-potency preparations should be used routinely on these areas. Because topical corticosteroids are commercially available in a variety of bases, including ointments, creams, lotions, solutions, gels, and sprays, there is no need to compound them. Ointments are most occlusive and in general provide better delivery of the medication while preventing evaporative losses. However, in a humid environment, creams may be better tolerated than ointments because the increased occlusion may cause itching or even folliculitis. Creams and lotions, while easier to spread, can contribute to skin dryness and irritation. Solutions can be used on the scalp and hirsute areas, although they can be irritating, especially to open lesions. With clinical improvement, a less potent corticosteroid should be prescribed and the frequency of use decreased. Topical corticosteroids can be discontinued when inflammation resolves, but hydration and moisturizers need to be continued.

Of note, fluticasone 0.05% cream has been shown to be safe in infants as young as 3 months of age with extensive atopic dermatitis. In addition, several studies with fluticasone 0.05% cream have shown that once atopic dermatitis is stabilized, long-term control can be maintained with twice weekly therapy. Of note, during the maintenance phase, fluticasone 0.05% cream was also applied to areas that had healed, which resulted in delayed relapses.

### E. TOPICAL CALCINEURIN INHIBITORS

Tacrolimus and pimecrolimus are immunomodulatory agents that inhibit the transcription of proinflammatory cytokines as well as other allergic mediators and target key cells in allergic inflammation. They are available in topical formulations, and long-term studies up to 12 months have confirmed both efficacy and safety. Local burning at the site of application, which occurs more frequently with tacrolimus ointment, has been the most common side effect, although this is usually a transient problem. Tacrolimus ointment—0.03% for children 2–15 years of age and 0.1% for older patients—is approved for twice daily short term and intermittent long-term use in moderate-to-severe atopic dermatitis. Pimecrolimus 1% cream is approved for patients 2 years of age or older who have mild-to-moderate atopic dermatitis. As a precaution, patients should wear sunscreen with both drugs. More recently, several studies in children as young as 3 months of age with all disease severities have been performed for up to 12 months with pimecrolimus 1% cream used at the earliest sign of disease activity (eg, erythema, pruritus). With this early intervention approach, the need for topical steroid rescue was significantly decreased.

### F. TAR PREPARATIONS

Tar preparations are used primarily in shampoos and rarely as bath additives. Side effects associated with tar products include skin dryness or irritation, especially if applied to inflamed skin, and, less commonly, photosensitivity reactions and folliculitis.

### G. WET DRESSINGS

Wet dressings are used together with hydration and topical corticosteroids primarily for the treatment of severe atopic dermatitis. They can also serve as an effective barrier against the persistent scratching that often undermines therapy. Total body dressings can be applied by using wet pajamas or long underwear with dry pajamas or a sweat suit on top. Hands and feet can be covered by wet tube socks with dry tube socks on top. Alternatively, wet gauze with a layer of dry gauze over it can be used and secured in place with an elastic bandage. Dressings can be removed when they dry out, usually after several hours, and are often best tolerated at bedtime. Incorrect use of wet dressings can result in chilling, maceration of the skin, or secondary infection.

### H. ANTI-INFECTIVE THERAPY

Systemic antibiotic therapy may be important when treating atopic dermatitis secondarily infected with *S aureus*. For limited areas of involvement, a topical antibiotic such as mupirocin may be effective. First- or second-generation cephalosporins or a semisynthetic penicillin are usually the first choice for oral therapy, as erythromycin-resistant organisms are fairly common. Maintenance antibiotic therapy is rarely indicated and may result in colonization by methicillin-resistant bacteria.

Disseminated eczema herpeticum usually requires treatment with systemic acyclovir. Patients with recurrent cutaneous herpetic lesions can be given prophylactic oral acyclovir. Superficial dermatophytosis and *Pityrosporum ovale* infection can be treated with topical or (rarely) systemic antifungal agents.

### I. ANTIPRURITIC AGENTS

Pruritus is usually the least well tolerated symptom of atopic dermatitis. Oral antihistamines and anxiolytics may be effective owing to their tranquilizing and sedating effects and can be taken mostly in the evening to avoid daytime somnolence. Nonsedating antihistamines may be less effective in treating pruritus, although beneficial effects have been reported in blinded studies. Use of topical antihistamines and local anesthetics should be avoided because of potential sensitization.

### J. RECALCITRANT DISEASE

Patients who are erythrodermic or who appear toxic may need to be hospitalized. Hospitalization may also be appropriate for cases of severe disease that fail outpatient management. Marked clinical improvement often occurs when the patient is removed from environmental allergens or stressors. In the hospital, compliance with therapy can be monitored, the patient and family can receive intense education, and controlled provocative challenges can be conducted to help identify triggering factors.

Ultraviolet light therapy can be useful for chronic recalcitrant atopic dermatitis in a subset of patients under the supervision of a specialist. Photochemotherapy with oral methoxypsoralen therapy followed by UVA has been used in a limited number of children with severe atopic dermatitis unresponsive to other therapy, and significant improvement has been noted. However, the increased long-term risk of cutaneous malignancies from this therapy prevents its widespread use.

Limited published data are available on use of the systemic immunosuppressive agent cyclosporine. In an open study, children given oral cyclosporine, 5 mg/kg daily for 6 weeks, improved significantly and tolerated the treatment well. Unfortunately, discontinuation of treatment resulted in relapse, although the relapse rate was variable. Patients treated with this agent should have their dose titrated to the lowest effective dose after the disease is brought under control with appropriate monitoring, under the care of a specialist familiar with the drug.

### K. EXPERIMENTAL AND UNPROVED THERAPIES

A number of uncontrolled trials have suggested that desensitization to specific allergens may improve atopic dermatitis; however, controlled trials with standardized extracts of relevant allergens in atopic dermatitis are needed before this form of therapy can be recommended.

Traditional Chinese herbal therapy in the form of decoctions has also been proposed for atopic dermatitis. The herbs used may have antimicrobial, sedative, anti-inflammatory, and corticosteroid-like activities. Despite studies showing clinical efficacy, toxicity and idiosyncratic reactions remain a concern, and traditional Chinese herbal therapy should be considered investigational at best. Finally, although disturbances in the metabolism of essential fatty acids have been reported in patients with atopic dermatitis, well-controlled trials with fish oil and evening primrose have shown no clinical benefit.

### Prognosis

Although it has been held that most children outgrow atopic dermatitis by adolescence, recent studies present less optimistic outcomes. In one study, atopic dermatitis had disappeared in only 18% of children followed from infancy until age 13 years, although the symptoms had become less severe in 65%. In a prospective study from Finland, 77–91% of adolescent patients receiving treatment for moderate or severe atopic dermatitis had persistent or frequently relapsing dermatitis as adults, although only 6% had severe disease. More than half of adolescents receiving treatment for mild dermatitis experienced a relapse of disease as adults. Adults whose childhood atopic dermatitis has been in remission for a number of years may present with hand dermatitis, especially if daily activities require repeated hand wetting.

Boguniewicz M, Leung DYM: Pathophysiologic mechanisms in atopic dermatitis. Semin Cutan Med Surg 2001;20:217.

Eichenfield LF et al: Safety and efficacy of pimecrolimus (ASM 981) cream 1% in the treatment of mild and moderate atopic dermatitis in children and adolescents. J Am Acad Dermatol 2002;46:495 [PMID: 11892079].

Hanifin J et al: Intermittent dosing of fluticasone propionate cream for reducing the risk of relapse in atopic dermatitis patients. Br J Dermatol 2002;147:528 [PMID: 12169079].

Ho VC et al: Safety and efficacy of nonsteroid pimecrolimus cream 1% in the treatment of atopic dermatitis in infants. J Pediatr 2003;142:155 [PMID: 12507187].

Paller A et al: A 12-week study of tacrolimus ointment for the treatment of atopic dermatitis in pediatric patients. J Am Acad Dermatol 2001;44:S47.

## URTICARIA & ANGIOEDEMA

### ESSENTIALS OF DIAGNOSIS & TYPICAL FEATURES

- *Urticaria: Erythematous, blanchable, circumscribed, pruritic, edematous papules ranging from 1–2 mm to several centimeters in diameter and involving the superficial dermis. Individual lesions can coalesce.*
- *Angioedema: Edema extending into the deep dermis or subcutaneous tissues.*
- *Both resolve without sequelae—urticaria usually within hours (individual lesions rarely lasting up to 24 hours), angioedema within 72 hours.*

### General Considerations

Urticaria and angioedema are common dermatologic conditions, occurring at some time in up to 25% of the population. About half of patients will have concomitant urticaria and angioedema, whereas 40% will have only urticaria and 10% only angioedema. Urticarial lesions are arbitrarily designated as acute, lasting less than 6 weeks, or chronic, lasting more than 6 weeks. Acute versus chronic urticaria can also be distinguished by differences in histologic features. A history of atopy is common with acute urticaria or angioedema. In contrast, atopy does not appear to be a factor in chronic urticaria.

Mast cell degranulation, dilated venules, and dermal edema are present in most forms of urticaria or angioedema. The dermal inflammatory cells may be sparse or dense depending on the chronicity of the lesions. Mast cells are thought to play a critical role in the pathogenesis of urticaria or angioedema through release of a variety of vasoactive mediators. Mast cell activation and degranulation can be triggered by different stimuli, including cross-linking of Fc receptor-bound IgE by allergens or anti–FcεRI antibodies. Non–IgE-mediated mechanisms have also been identified, including complement anaphylatoxins (C3a, C5a), radiocontrast dyes, or physical stimuli. Chronic urticarial lesions have greater numbers of perivascular mononuclear cells, consisting primarily of T cells. There is also a marked increase in cutaneous mast cells. The cause of acute disease can be identified in about half of patients and include allergens such as foods, aeroallergens, latex, drugs, and insect venoms. Infectious agents, including streptococci, mycoplasmas, hepatitis B virus, and Epstein–Barr virus (EBV), can cause acute urticaria. Urticaria or angioedema can occur after the administration of blood products or immunoglobulin. This results from immune complex formation with complement activation, vascular alterations, and triggering of mast cells by anaphylatoxins. Opiate analgesics, polymyxin B, tubocurarine, and radiocontrast media can induce acute urticaria by direct mast cell activation. These disorders can also occur following ingestion of aspirin or nonsteroidal anti-inflammatory agents (see Adverse Reactions to Drugs & Biologicals section).

Physical urticarias represent a heterogeneous group of disorders in which urticaria or angioedema is triggered by physical stimuli, including pressure, cold, heat, water, or vibrations. Dermographism is the most common form of physical urticaria, affecting up to about 4% of the population and occurring at skin sites subjected to mechanical stimuli. Many physical urticarias are considered to be acute because the lesions are usually rapid in onset, with resolution within hours. However, symptoms can recur for months to years.

The cause of chronic urticaria is usually not due to allergies and typically cannot be determined. It can be associated with an underlying systemic disease such as thyroid disease. Some studies have demonstrated IgG autoantibodies directed at the high-affinity receptor for IgE or at IgE, suggesting that chronic urticaria may be an autoimmune disease.

## Clinical Findings

### A. SYMPTOMS AND SIGNS

Cold-induced urticaria or angioedema can occur within minutes of exposure to a decreased ambient temperature or as the skin is warmed following direct cold contact. Systemic features include headache, wheezing, and syncope. If the entire body is cooled, as may occur during swimming, hypotension and collapse can occur. Two forms of dominantly inherited cold urticaria have been described. The immediate form is known as familial cold urticaria, in which erythematous macules appear rather than wheals, along with fever, arthralgias,

and leukocytosis. The delayed form consists of erythematous, deep swellings that develop 9–18 hours after local cold challenge without immediate lesions.

In solar urticaria, which occurs within minutes after exposure to light of appropriate wavelength, pruritus is followed by morbilliform erythema and urticaria.

Cholinergic urticaria occurs after increases in core body and skin temperatures and typically develops after a warm bath or shower, exercise, or episodes of fever. Occasional episodes are triggered by stress or the ingestion of certain foods. The eruption appears as small punctate wheals surrounded by extensive areas of erythema. Rarely the urticarial lesions become confluent and angioedema develops. Associated features can include one or more of the following: headache, syncope, bronchospasm, abdominal pain, vomiting, and diarrhea. In severe cases, systemic anaphylaxis may develop. In pressure urticaria or angioedema, red, deep, painful swelling occurs immediately or 4–6 hours after the skin has been exposed to pressure. The immediate form is often associated with dermographism. The delayed form, which may be associated with fever, chills, and arthralgias, may be accompanied by elevated erythrocyte sedimentation rate and leukocytosis. Lesions are frequently diffuse, tender, and painful rather than pruritic. They typically resolve within 48 hours.

### B. LABORATORY FINDINGS

Laboratory tests are selected on the basis of the history and physical findings. Testing for specific IgE antibody to food or inhalant allergens may be helpful in implicating a potential cause. Specific tests for physical urticarias, such as an ice cube test or a pressure test, may be indicated. Intradermal injection of methacholine reproduces clinical symptoms locally in about one third of patients with cholinergic urticaria. A throat culture for streptococcal infection may be warranted with acute urticaria. In chronic urticaria, selected screening studies to look for an underlying disease may be indicated, including a complete blood count (CBC), erythrocyte sedimentation rate, biochemistry panel, and urinalysis. Antithyroid antibodies may be considered. Intradermal testing with the patient's serum has been suggested as a method of detecting histamine-releasing activity, including autoantibodies. Other tests should be done based on suspicion of a specific underlying disease. If the history or appearance of the urticarial lesions suggests vasculitis, a skin biopsy for immunofluorescence is indicated. Patient diaries occasionally may be helpful to determine the cause of recurrent hives. A trial of food or drug elimination may be considered.

## Differential Diagnosis

Urticarial lesions are usually easily recognized—the major dilemma is the etiologic diagnosis. Lesions of urticarial vasculitis typically last for more than 24 hours. "Papular urticaria" is a term used to characterize multiple papules from insect bites, found especially on the extremities, and is not true urticaria. Angioedema can be distinguished from other forms of edema because it is transient, asymmetrical, and nonpitting and does not occur predominantly in dependent areas. Hereditary angioedema is a rare autosomal dominant disorder caused by a quantitative or functional deficiency of C1-esterase inhibitor and characterized by episodic, frequently severe, nonpruritic angioedema of the skin, gastrointestinal tract, or upper respiratory tract. Life-threatening laryngeal angioedema may occur.

## Complications

In severe cases of cholinergic urticaria, systemic anaphylaxis may develop. In cold-induced disease, sudden cooling of the entire body as can occur with swimming can result in hypotension and collapse.

## Treatment

### A. GENERAL MEASURES

The most effective treatment is identification and avoidance of the triggering agent. Underlying infection should be treated appropriately. Patients with physical urticarias should avoid the relevant physical stimulus. Epinephrine can be used for treatment of acute episodes, especially when laryngeal edema complicates an attack (see Anaphylaxis section). Intubation may be indicated for life-threatening laryngeal edema.

### B. ANTIHISTAMINES

For the majority of patients, $H_1$ antihistamines given orally or systemically are the mainstay of therapy. Antihistamines are more effective when given on an ongoing basis rather than after lesions appear. For breakthrough symptoms, the dose may need to be increased. In the case of cold urticaria, the best treatment appears to be cyproheptadine. Cholinergic urticaria can be treated with hydroxyzine and dermographism with hydroxyzine or diphenhydramine. The addition of $H_2$ antihistamines may benefit some patients who fail to respond to $H_1$ receptor antagonists alone. Second-generation antihistamines (discussed previously under Allergic Rhinitis) are long acting, show good tissue levels, are non- or minimally sedating at usual dosing levels, and lack anticholinergic effects.

### C. CORTICOSTEROIDS

Although corticosteroids are usually not indicated in the treatment of acute or chronic urticaria, severe recalcitrant cases may require alternate-day therapy in an attempt to diminish disease activity and facilitate control

with antihistamines. Systemic corticosteroids may also be needed in the treatment of urticaria or angioedema secondary to necrotizing vasculitis, an uncommon occurrence in patients with serum sickness or collagen-vascular disease.

### D. OTHER PHARMACOLOGIC AGENTS

Limited studies suggest that some patients may benefit from treatment with a leukotriene receptor antagonist. The tricyclic antidepressant doxepin blocks both $H_1$ and $H_2$ histamine receptors and may be particularly useful in chronic urticaria, although its use may be limited by the sedating side effect. A limited number of patients—including euthyroid patients—with chronic urticaria and antithyroid antibodies have improved when given thyroid hormone. Treatment of chronic urticaria with hydroxychloroquine, nifedipine, colchicine, dapsone, sulfasalazine, cyclosporine, or intravenous immune globulin should be considered investigational.

## Prognosis

Spontaneous remission of urticaria and angioedema is frequent, but some patients have a prolonged course. Reassurance is important, because this disorder can cause significant frustration. Periodic follow-up is indicated, particularly for patients with laryngeal edema, to monitor for possible underlying cause.

Grattan C, et al: Management and diagnostic guidelines for urticaria and angio-oedema. Br J Dermatol 2001;144:708.

Leung DY, Boguniewicz M: Advances in allergic skin diseases. J Allergy Clin Immunol 2003;111:S805 [PMID: 12618744].

# ANAPHYLAXIS

## ESSENTIALS OF DIAGNOSIS & TYPICAL FEATURES

- *Rapid onset of allergic symptoms after exposure to allergen in a previously sensitized person.*
- *Generalized pruritus, anxiety, urticaria, angioedema, throat fullness, dyspnea, hypotension, and collapse.*

## General Considerations

Anaphylaxis is an acute life-threatening clinical syndrome that occurs when large quantities of inflammatory mediators are rapidly released from mast cells and basophils after exposure to an allergen in a previously sensitized patient. Anaphylactoid reactions mimic anaphylaxis but are not mediated by IgE. They may be mediated by anaphylatoxins such as C3a or C5a or through nonimmune mast cell degranulating agents. Some of the common causes of anaphylaxis or anaphylactoid reactions are listed in Table 34–5. Idiopathic anaphylaxis by definition has no recognized external cause.

## Clinical Findings

### A. SYMPTOMS AND SIGNS

The symptoms and signs of anaphylaxis or anaphylactoid reactions depend on the organs affected. Onset typically occurs within minutes after exposure to the offending agent and can be short-lived, protracted, or biphasic, with recurrence after several hours despite treatment. Patients may report generalized pruritus or a feeling of impending doom. Cutaneous signs include erythema, urticaria, and angioedema. Tearing, rhinorrhea, sneezing, and nasal congestion may occur. Respiratory symptoms include a sensation of having a lump in the throat or shortness of breath; signs include uvular edema, hoarseness, dysphonia, stridor, tachypnea, and wheezing. Cardiovascular findings include tachycardia, arrhythmias, hypotension, and collapse. The patient may complain of nausea and cramping pain with associated vomiting, and diarrhea. There may be anxiety or generalized seizures. Shock, upper airway edema, and bronchial obstruction are the principal life-threatening features.

**Table 34–5.** Common causes of systemic allergic and pseudoallergic reactions.

---

**Causes of anaphylaxis**
  Drugs
    Antibiotics
    Anesthetic agents
  Foods
    Peanuts, tree nuts, shellfish, and others
  Biologicals
    Latex
    Insulin
    Allergen extracts
    Antisera
    Blood products
    Enzymes
  Insect venoms
**Causes of anaphylactoid reactions**
  Radiocontrast media
  Aspirin and other nonsteroidal anti-inflammatory drugs
  Anesthetic agents

---

### B. LABORATORY FINDINGS

Tryptase released by mast cells can be measured in the serum and may remain elevated for up to 24 hours after an acute reaction. This may be helpful when the diagnosis of anaphylaxis is in question. The CBC may show an elevated hematocrit due to hemoconcentration. Elevation of serum creatine kinase, aspartate aminotransferase, and lactic dehydrogenase may be seen with myocardial involvement. Electrocardiographic abnormalities may include ST wave depression, bundle branch block, and various arrhythmias. Arterial blood gases may show hypoxemia, hypercapnia, and acidosis. The chest radiograph may show hyperinflation.

## Differential Diagnosis

Although shock may be the only sign of anaphylaxis, other diagnoses should be considered, especially in the setting of sudden collapse without typical allergic findings. Other causes of shock along with cardiac arrhythmias must be ruled out (see Chapters 11 and 13). Respiratory failure associated with asthma may be confused with anaphylaxis. Mastocytosis, hereditary angioedema, scombroid poisoning, vasovagal reactions, vocal cord dysfunction, and anxiety attacks may cause symptoms mistaken for anaphylaxis.

## Complications

Depending on the organs involved and the severity of the reaction, complications may vary from none to aspiration pneumonitis, acute tubular necrosis, bleeding diathesis, or sloughing of the intestinal mucosa. With irreversible shock, heart and brain damage can be terminal.

## Treatment

### A. GENERAL MEASURES

Anaphylaxis is a medical emergency that requires rapid assessment and treatment. Exposure to the triggering agent should be discontinued. Airway patency should be maintained and blood pressure and pulse monitored. The patient should be placed in a supine position with the legs elevated. Oxygen should be delivered by mask or nasal cannula with pulse oximetry monitoring. If the reaction is secondary to a sting or injection into an extremity, a tourniquet may be applied proximal to the site, briefly releasing it every 10–15 minutes.

### B. EPINEPHRINE

Epinephrine 1:1000, 0.01 mL/kg to a maximum of 0.3 mL, should be injected intramuscularly, without delay. This dose may be repeated at intervals of 15–20 minutes two or three times as necessary. If the precipitating allergen has been injected intradermally or subcutaneously, absorption may be delayed by giving 0.1 mL of epinephrine subcutaneously at the injection site unless the site is a digit.

### C. Antihistamines

Diphenhydramine, an $H_1$-blocker, 1–2 mg/kg up to 50 mg, can be given intramuscularly or intravenously. Intravenous antihistamines should be infused over a period of 5–10 minutes to avoid inducing hypotension. Addition of ranitidine, an $H_2$-blocker, 1 mg/kg up to 50 mg intravenously, may be more effective than an $H_1$-blocker alone, especially for hypotension.

### D. Fluids

Treatment of persistent hypotension requires restoration of intravascular volume by fluid replacement, initially with a crystalloid solution, 20–30 mL/kg in the first hour.

### E. Bronchodilators

Nebulized $\beta_2$-agonists such as albuterol 0.5% solution, 2.5 mg (0.5 mL) diluted in 2–3 mL saline, may be useful for reversing bronchospasm. Intravenous methylxanthines are generally not recommended because they provide little benefit over inhaled $\beta_2$-agonists and may contribute to toxicity.

### F. Corticosteroids

Although corticosteroids do not provide immediate benefit, when given early they may prevent protracted or biphasic anaphylaxis. Intravenous methylprednisolone, 1–2 mg/kg, or hydrocortisone, 5 mg/kg, can be given q4–6h.

### G. Vasopressors

Refractory hypotension should be treated with intravenous vasopressors such as dopamine or epinephrine (see Chapter 13).

### H. Observation

The patient should be monitored after the initial symptoms have subsided, because biphasic or protracted anaphylaxis can occur despite ongoing therapy.

## Prevention

Strict avoidance of the causative agent is extremely important. An effort to determine its cause should be made, beginning with a thorough history. Typically there is a strong temporal relationship between exposure and onset of symptoms. Testing for specific IgE to allergen with either in vitro or skin testing may be indicated. With exercise-induced anaphylaxis, patients should be instructed to exercise with another person and to stop exercising at the first sign of symptoms. If prior ingestion of food has been implicated, eating within 4 hours—perhaps up to 12 hours—before exercise should be avoided. Patients with a history of anaphylaxis should carry epinephrine for self-administration (eg, EpiPen, EpiPen Jr), and they and all caregivers should be instructed on its use. They should also carry an oral antihistamine such as diphenhydramine and wear a medical alert bracelet. Patients with idiopathic anaphylaxis may require prolonged treatment with oral corticosteroids. Specific measures for dealing with food, drug, latex, and insect venom allergies as well as radiocontrast media reactions are discussed in a later section.

## Prognosis

Anaphylaxis can be fatal. In one study of children and adolescents who died from food-induced anaphylaxis (eg, from peanuts, tree nuts, or egg), treatment with epinephrine was delayed for more than 1 hour after onset. The prognosis is good when signs and symptoms are recognized promptly and treated aggressively and the offending agent is avoided subsequently. Exercise-induced and idiopathic anaphylaxis may be recurrent. Because accidental exposure to the causative agent may occur, patients, parents, and caregivers must be prepared to recognize and treat anaphylaxis.

Sampson HA: Anaphylaxis and emergency treatment. Pediatrics 2003;111:1601 [PMID: 12667272].

## ADVERSE REACTIONS TO DRUGS & BIOLOGICALS

The majority of adverse drug reactions are not immunologically mediated and may be due to idiosyncratic reactions, overdosage, pharmacologic side effects, nonspecific release of pharmacologic effector molecules, or drug interactions.

Patients often describe themselves as being allergic to medications or biologicals, and clinicians may document a drug allergy in the patient's medical record based solely on this history. Adverse drug reactions are any undesirable and unintended response elicited by a drug. Allergic or hypersensitivity drug reactions are adverse reactions involving immune mechanisms. Although hypersensitivity reactions account for only 5–10% of all adverse drug reactions, they are the most serious, with 1:10,000 resulting in death.

### 1. Antibiotics

Antibiotics constitute the most frequent cause of allergic drug reactions. Amoxicillin, trimethoprim–sulfamethoxazole, and ampicillin are the most common causes of cutaneous drug reactions.

Most antibiotics and their metabolites are low-molecular-weight compounds that do not stimulate immunity until they have become covalently bound to a carrier protein. The penicillins and other β-lactam antibiotics, including cephalosporins, carbacephems, carbapenems, and monobactams, share a common β-lactam ring structure and a marked propensity to couple to carrier proteins. Penicilloyl is the predominant metabolite of penicillin and is called the major determinant. The other penicillin metabolites are present in low concentrations and are referred to as minor determinants. Sulfonamide reactions are mediated presumably by a reactive metabolite (hydroxylamine) produced by cytochrome P-450 oxidative metabolism. Slow acetylators appear to be at increased risk. Other risk factors for drug reactions include previous exposure, previous reaction, age (20–49 years), route (parenteral), and dose of administration (high, intermittent). Atopy does not predispose to development of a reaction, but atopic individuals have more severe reactions.

Immunopathologic reactions to antibiotics include type I (IgE-mediated) reactions resulting from a drug or metabolite interaction with preformed specific IgE bound to the surfaces of tissue mast cells or circulating basophils. Release of mediators such as histamine and leukotrienes contributes to the clinical development of angioedema, urticaria, bronchospasm, or anaphylaxis. Type II (cytotoxic) reactions involve IgG or IgM antibodies that recognize drug bound to cell membranes. In the presence of serum complement, the antibody-coated cell is either cleared or destroyed, causing drug-induced hemolytic anemia or thrombocytopenia. Type III (immune complex) reactions are caused by soluble complexes of drug or metabolite with IgG or IgM antibody. If the immune complex is deposited on blood vessel walls and activates the complement cascade, serum sickness may result. Type IV (T-cell-mediated) reactions require activated T lymphocytes that recognize a drug or its metabolite as seen in allergic contact dermatitis. Sensitization usually occurs via the topical route of administration. Immunopathologic reactions not fitting into the type I–IV classification include Stevens–Johnson syndrome, exfoliative dermatitis, and the maculopapular rash associated with penicillin or ampicillin. The prevalence of morbilliform rashes in patients given ampicillin is between 5.2% and 9.5% of treatment courses. However, patients given ampicillin during EBV and cytomegalovirus infections or with acute lymphoblastic anemia have a 69–100% incidence of non–IgE-mediated rash. Serum-sickness-like reactions resemble type III reactions, although immune complexes are not documented; β-lactams, especially cefaclor, and sulfonamides, have been implicated most often. They may result from an inherited propensity for hepatic biotransformation of drug into toxic or immunogenic metabolites. The incidence of "allergic" cutaneous reactions to trimethoprim–sulfamethoxazole in patients with acquired immunodeficiency syndrome (AIDS) has been reported to be as high as 70%. The mechanism is thought to relate to the severe immune dysregulation, although it may be due to glutathione deficiency resulting in toxic metabolites.

## Clinical Findings

### A. SYMPTOMS AND SIGNS

Allergic reactions can result in pruritus, urticaria, angioedema, or anaphylaxis. Serum sickness is characterized by fever, rash, lymphadenopathy, myalgias, and arthralgias. Cytotoxic drug reactions can result in symptoms and signs associated with the underlying anemia or thrombocytopenia. Delayed-type hypersensitivity may cause contact dermatitis.

### B. LABORATORY FINDINGS

Skin testing is the most rapid, useful, and sensitive method of demonstrating the presence of IgE antibody to a specific allergen. Skin testing to nonpenicillin antibiotics may be difficult, however, because many immunologic reactions are due to metabolites rather than to the parent drug and because the relevant metabolites for most drugs other than penicillin have not been identified. Because metabolites are usually low-molecular-weight haptens, they must combine with carrier proteins to be useful for diagnosis. In the case of contact sensitivity reactions to topical antibiotics, a 48-hour patch test can be useful.

Solid-phase in vitro immunoassays for IgE to penicillins are available for identification of IgE to penicilloyl but are considerably less sensitive and give less information than skin testing. Assays for specific IgG and IgM have been shown to correlate with a drug reaction in immune cytopenias, but in most other instances such assays are not clinically useful. Skin testing for immediate hypersensitivity is helpful only in predicting reactions caused by IgE antibodies. Most nonpruritic maculopapular rashes will not be predicted by skin testing.

Approximately 80% of patients with a history of penicillin allergy will have negative skin tests. Penicillin therapy in patients with a history of an immediate hypersensitivity reaction to penicillin, but with negative skin tests to both penicilloyl and the minor determinant mixture, is accompanied by a 1–3% chance of urticaria or other mild allergic reactions at some time during therapy, with anaphylaxis occurring in less than 0.1% of patients. In contrast, the predictive value of a positive skin test is approximately 60%. Testing with penicilloyl linked to polylysine (PPL) alone carries about a 76% sensitivity; use of both PPL and penicillin G (used as a minor determinant) increases sensitivity to about 95%. Not the using minor determinant mixture in skin testing can result in failure to predict potential anaphylactic reactions. Unfortunately the minor determinant mixture is still not commercially available, although most academic allergy centers make their own. Approximately 4% of subjects tested with no history of penicillin allergy have positive skin tests, and most fatalities occur in patients with no prior history of reaction. Rarely patients may have skin test reactivity only to a specific semisynthetic penicillin. Resensitization in skin-test-negative children occurs infrequently (< 1%) after a course of oral antibiotic.

The degree of cross-reactivity of determinants formed from cephalosporins with IgE to other β-lactam drugs remains unresolved, especially because haptens that may be unique to cephalosporin metabolism remain unknown. The degree of clinical cross-reactivity is much lower than the in vitro cross-reactivity. A clinical adverse reaction rate of 3–7% for cephalosporins may be expected in patients with positive histories of penicillin allergy. Antibodies to the second- and third-generation cephalosporins appear to be directed at the unique side chains rather than at the common ring structure. The present literature suggests that a positive skin test to a cephalosporin used at a concentration of 1 mg/mL would place the patient at increased risk for an allergic reaction to that antibiotic. However, a negative skin test would not exclude sensitivity to a potentially relevant metabolite. One review concluded that there is no increased incidence of allergy to second- and third-generation cephalosporins in patients with penicillin allergy and that penicillin skin testing does not identify patients who develop cephalosporin allergy. However, another study suggested that although only 2% of penicillin-allergic patients would react to a cephalosporin, they would be at risk for anaphylaxis.

Carbacephems (loracarbef) are similar to cephalosporins, although the degree of cross-reactivity is undetermined. Carbapenems (imipenem) represent another class of β-lactam antibiotics with a bicyclic nucleus and a high degree of cross-reactivity with penicillin. In contrast, monobactams (aztreonam) contain a monocyclic rather than bicyclic ring structure and limited data suggests that aztreonam can be safely administered to most penicillin-allergic subjects.

Skin testing for non–β-lactam antibiotics is less reliable, because the relevant degradation products are for the most part unknown or multivalent reagents are unavailable.

## Treatment

### A. GENERAL MEASURES

Withdrawal of the implicated drug is usually a central component of management. Acute IgE-mediated reactions such as anaphylaxis, urticaria, and angioedema are treated according to established therapeutic guidelines that include the use of epinephrine, $H_1$ and $H_2$ receptor blocking agents, volume replacement, and systemic corticosteroids (see previous sections). Antibiotic-induced immune cytopenias can be managed by withdrawal of the offending agent or reduction in dose. Drug-induced serum sickness can be suppressed by drug withdrawal, antihistamines, and corticosteroids. Contact allergy can be managed by avoidance and treatment with antihistamines and topical corticosteroids. Reactions such as toxic epidermal necrolysis and Stevens–Johnson syndrome require immediate drug withdrawal and supportive care.

### B. ALTERNATIVE THERAPY

If possible, subsequent therapy should be with an alternative drug that has therapeutic actions similar to the drug in question but with no immunologic cross-reactivity.

### C. DESENSITIZATION

Administering gradually increasing doses of an antibiotic either orally or parentally over a period of hours to days may be considered if alternative therapy is not acceptable. This should be done only by a physician familiar with desensitization, typically in an intensive care setting. Desensitization does not reduce or prevent non–IgE-mediated reactions. Patients with Stevens–Johnson syndrome should not be desensitized because of the high mortality rate.

## Prognosis

The prognosis is good when drug allergens are identified early and avoided. Stevens–Johnson syndrome and toxic epidermal necrolysis may be associated with a high mortality rate.

## 2. Latex Allergy

### ESSENTIALS OF DIAGNOSIS & TYPICAL FEATURES

- Immediate hypersensitivity reaction after exposure to latex, including airborne particles.
- Allergic contact dermatitis 24–48 hours after exposure to rubber accelerators or antioxidants.

## General Considerations

Allergic reactions to latex and rubber products have become increasingly common since the institution of universal precautions for exposure to bodily fluids. Children with spina bifida appear to have a unique sensitivity to latex, perhaps because of early and frequent latex exposure as well as altered neuroimmune interactions. Atopy—especially symptomatic latex allergy—appears to be significantly increased in patients with spina bifida experiencing anaphylaxis during general anesthesia. Other conditions requiring chronic or recurrent exposure to latex such as urogenital anomalies and ventriculoperitoneal shunt have also been associated with latex hypersensitivity. The combination of atopy and frequent exposure seems to synergistically increase the risk of latex hypersensitivity.

Latex is the milky fluid obtained by tapping the cultivated rubber tree, *Hevea brasiliensis.* During manufacture of latex products, various antioxidants and accelerators such as thiurams, carbamates, and mercaptobenzothiazoles are added. Latex products are typically produced by dipping a porcelain mold into a tank of latex and then vulcanizing it to enhance mechanical stability. The product is washed or "leached" of excess proteins, then dry-lubricated with a powder such as corn starch.

Latex is a complex biologic mixture composed of rubber particles in a phospholipoprotein envelope and a serum containing sugars, lipids, nucleic acids, minerals, and various proteins. The protein component is thought to contain the allergenic properties. Extra leaching steps may reduce the protein content and hence the allergenicity of the final product. IgE from latex-sensitized individuals reacts with different protein components, supporting the notion that more than one clinically important latex antigen exists. New allergenic epitopes are generated during the manufacturing process. Thus polypeptides from latex glove extracts vary both quantitatively and qualitatively with different brands and lots of gloves. Identification of the causative antigens is important because it may be possible to alter the manufacturing process to reduce the final allergen content.

Latex is ubiquitous in medical settings, and many sources may be inconspicuous. Synthetic alternatives to some latex products—including gloves, dressings, and tape—are available. Avoidance of contact with latex-containing items, however, may be insufficient to prevent allergic reactions, because lubricating powders may serve as vehicles for aerosolized latex antigens. The use of powder-free latex gloves is an important control measure for airborne latex allergen.

Nonmedical sources of latex are also common and include balloons, toys, rubber bands, erasers, condoms, and shoe soles. Pacifiers and bottle nipples have also been implicated as sources of latex allergen, although these products are molded rather than dipped, and allergic reactions to molded products are less common. Latex-allergic patients and their caregivers must be continuously vigilant for hidden sources of exposure.

## Clinical Findings

### A. SYMPTOMS AND SIGNS

The clinical manifestations of IgE-mediated reactions to latex can involve the full spectrum of symptoms associated with mast cell degranulation. Localized pruritus and urticaria occur after cutaneous contact; conjunctivitis and rhinitis can result from aerosol exposure or direct facial contact. Systemic reactions, including bronchospasm, laryngospasm, and hypotension, may occur with more substantial exposure or in extremely sensitive individuals. Finally, vascular collapse and shock leading to fatal cardiovascular events may occur. Intraoperative anaphylaxis represents a common and serious manifestation of latex allergy.

Allergic contact dermatitis to rubber products typically appears 24–48 hours after contact. The primary allergens include accelerators and antioxidants used in the manufacturing process. The diagnosis is established by patch testing. Shoe soles are an important source of exposure. The skin lesions appear primarily as a patchy eczema on exposed surfaces, although reactions can become generalized.

### B. LABORATORY FINDINGS

Epicutaneous prick testing is a rapid, inexpensive, and sensitive test that detects the presence of latex-specific IgE on skin mast cells. Obstacles to its use include lack of a standardized antigen. Reports of life-threatening anaphylactic events have been associated with skin testing to latex, and intradermal testing may be especially dangerous. A commercially available extract is pending FDA approval.

Immunoassay testing involves the in vitro measurement of specific IgE, which binds latex antigens. Antigen sources used for testing have included native plant extracts, raw latex, and finished products. When compared with a history of latex-induced symptoms or positive skin tests, the sensitivity of immunoassays testing for latex antigens ranges from 50% to 100% with specificity between 63% and 100%. These broad ranges may reflect the patient population studied and the source of latex antigen as well as the assay employed. A positive immunoassay test to latex in the presence of a highly suggestive latex allergy history is useful and may circumvent the potential concerns associated with prick skin testing in certain patients.

Cross-reactivity has been demonstrated between latex and a number of other antigens such as foods. Banana, avocado, and chestnut have been found to be antigenically similar to latex both immunologically and clinically.

## Complications

Complications may be similar to those caused by other allergens. Prolonged exposure to aerosolized latex may lead to persistent asthma. Chronic allergic contact dermatitis, especially on the hands, can lead to functional disability.

## Treatment

Avoidance remains the cornerstone of treatment for latex allergy. Prevention and supportive therapy are the most common methods for managing this problem. Patients identified as being allergic to latex may need to have a personal supply of vinyl or latex-free gloves for use when visiting a physician or dentist. "Hypoallergenic gloves" are poorly classified with respect to their ability to induce IgE-mediated reactions; the FDA currently uses this term to designate products that have a reduced capacity to induce contact dermatitis. Gloves made from synthetic materials include Neolon (Becton-Dickinson), Tactyl 1 (Smart Practice), and Elastyren (Hermal). Autoinjectable epinephrine and medical identification bracelets may be prescribed for latex-allergic patients along with avoidance counseling.

Prophylactic premedication of latex-allergic individuals has been used in some surgical patients at high risk for latex allergy. The rationale for this therapy is derived from the pretreatment protocols developed for iodinated radiocontrast media and anesthetic reactions. Although there has been some success using this regimen, anaphylaxis has occurred despite pretreatment. This approach should not substitute for careful avoidance measures.

## Prognosis

Owing to the ubiquitous nature of natural rubber, the prognosis is guarded for patients with severe latex allergy. Chronic exposure to airborne latex particles may lead to chronic asthma. Chronic dermatitis can lead to functional disability.

## 3. Vaccines

Mumps–measles–rubella (MMR) vaccine has been shown to be safe in egg-allergic patients (although rare reactions to gelatin or neomycin can occur). The ovalbumin content in influenza vaccine is variable, and skin testing with the specific vaccine lot is warranted in patients with egg allergy (*Note:* Some patients who tolerate cooked egg, that is, denatured protein, may still react to the vaccine). In addition, the newly introduced live intranasal influenza vaccine is contraindicated in egg-allergic children.

## 4. Radiocontrast Media

Non–IgE-mediated anaphylactoid reactions may occur with radiocontrast media with up to a 30% reaction rate on reexposure. Management involves using a low-molarity agent and premedication with prednisone, diphenhydramine, and possibly an $H_2$-blocker.

## 5. Insulin

Approximately 50% of patients receiving insulin have positive skin tests, but IgE-mediated reactions occur rarely. Insulin resistance is mediated by IgG. If less than 24 hours has elapsed after an allergic reaction to insulin, do not discontinue insulin but rather reduce the dose by one third, then increase by 2–5 units per injection. Skin testing and desensitization are necessary if the interval between the allergic reaction and subsequent dose is greater than 24 hours.

## 6. Local Anesthetics

Less than 1% of reactions to local anesthetics are IgE-mediated. Management involves selecting a local anesthetic from another class. Esters of benzoic acid include benzocaine and procaine; amides include lidocaine and mepivacaine. Alternatively, the patient can be skin tested with the suspected agent, followed by a provocative challenge. To rule out paraben sensitivity, skin testing can be done with 1% lidocaine from a multidose vial.

## 7. Aspirin & Other Nonsteroidal Anti-Inflammatory Drugs

Adverse reactions to aspirin and nonsteroidal anti-inflammatory drugs (NSAIDs) include urticaria and angioedema; rhinosinusitis, nasal polyps, and asthma; anaphylactoid reactions; and NSAID-related hypersensitivity pneumonitis. After a systemic reaction, a refractory period of 2–7 days occurs. Most aspirin-sensitive patients tolerate sodium salicylate. All NSAIDs inhibiting cyclooxygenase cross-react with aspirin. Cross-reactivity between aspirin and tartrazine (yellow dye No. 5) has not been substantiated in controlled trials. No skin test or in vitro test is available to diagnose aspirin sensitivity. Oral challenge can induce severe bronchospasm. Desensitization and cross-desensitization to NSAIDs can be achieved in most patients and maintained long-term. Leukotriene receptor antagonists or 5-lipoxyge-nase inhibitors attenuate the reaction to aspirin challenge and may be beneficial adjunct treatment in aspirin-sensitive asthmatic patients. Preliminary studies suggest that COX-2 inhibitors may be tolerated by patients with ASA-induced asthma.

Bohlke K et al: Risk of anaphylaxis after vaccination of children and adolescents. Pediatrics 2003;112:815 [PMID: 12952113].

Centers for Disease Control and Prevention, National Immunization Program: www.cdc.gov/nip.

Kelkar PS, Li JTC: Cephalosporin allergy. N Engl J Med 2001; 345:804.

Randolph C: Latex allergy in pediatrics. Curr Probl Pediatr 2001; 31:131.

Zeiger RS: Current issues with influenza vaccination in egg allergy. J Allergy Clin Immunol 2002;110:834 [PMID: 12373275].

# FOOD ALLERGY

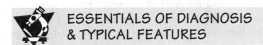

## ESSENTIALS OF DIAGNOSIS & TYPICAL FEATURES

- *Temporal relationship between ingestion of a suspected food and onset of allergic symptoms.*
- *Positive prick skin test or in vitro test to a suspected food allergen confirmed by a double-blind, placebo-controlled food challenge (except in cases of anaphylaxis).*

## General Considerations

Adverse reactions to foods are common in young children, especially in the first 3 years of life. The highest prevalence of food allergy is found in children with moderate-to-severe atopic dermatitis, with up to 33% affected. Up to 16% of children with asthma have been found to have food-induced wheezing in some studies. The most common food allergens in young children are eggs, milk, peanuts, soy, and wheat. In older children and adolescents, fish, shellfish, and nuts are most often involved in allergic reactions, and these may be lifelong.

Some reactions often diagnosed by patients or physicians as food allergy involve pharmacologic or metabolic mechanisms and reactions to food toxins. Foods containing significant amounts of vasoactive amines such as chocolate, cheese, and some wines and beers may precipitate migraine headaches in some patients. Claims that dyes, sugar, and food additives may contribute to hyperactivity in children with attention-deficit/hyperactivity disorder are controversial. In the occasional case in which a child appears to benefit from a restricted diet, there is no evidence for an IgE-mediated reaction.

## Clinical Findings

### A. SYMPTOMS AND SIGNS

Most reactions to foods occur minutes to 2 hours after ingestion. A history of a temporal relationship between the ingestion of a suspected food and onset of a reaction—as well as the nature and duration of symptoms observed—is important in establishing the diagnosis of food allergy. With chronic atopic dermatitis or persistent urticaria, the association with food may be less obvious (see Atopic Dermatitis and Urticaria sections). At times, acute symptoms may occur, but the cause may not be obvious because of hidden food allergens. A symptom diary kept for 7–14 days may be helpful in establishing an association between ingestion of foods and symptoms and also provides a baseline observation for the pattern of symptom expression. It is important to record both the form in which the food was ingested and the foods ingested concurrently.

Hives, flushing, facial angioedema, and mouth or throat itching are common. In severe cases, angioedema of the tongue, uvula, pharynx, or upper airway can occur. Contact urticaria can occur without systemic symptoms in some children. Gastrointestinal symptoms include abdominal discomfort or pain, nausea, vomiting, and diarrhea. Children with food allergy may occasionally have isolated rhinoconjunctivitis or wheezing. Rarely anaphylaxis to food may involve only cardiovascular collapse (see Anaphylaxis section). Anaphylactoid reactions can occur after ingestion of foods such as certain fish containing high amounts of histamine.

### B. LABORATORY FINDINGS

Typically, fewer than 50% of histories of food allergy will be confirmed by blinded challenge (although this percentage is much higher in food-induced anaphylaxis). Prick skin testing is useful to rule out a suspected food allergen, because the predictive value is high for a properly performed negative test with an extract of good quality. In contrast, the predictive value for a positive test is approximately 50%. RAST and other in vitro tests have lower specificity and positive predictive values. In contrast, specific IgE levels to milk, egg, peanut, and fish proteins have been established with the Pharmacia ImmunoCAP assay correlating with a greater than 95% chance of a clinical reaction. Measurement of IgG to foods is not clinically useful. Eosinophilia of stool mucus may be present in cases of gastrointestinal allergy; elevated circulating eosinophils may be present as well.

Double-blind, placebo-controlled food challenge is considered the standard method for diagnosing food allergy except in severe reactions. Even when multiple food allergies are suspected, most patients will be positive to three or fewer foods on blinded challenge. Therefore, extensive elimination diets are almost never indicated. Elimination without controlled challenge is a less desirable but at times more practical approach for suspected food allergy.

## Differential Diagnosis

Repeated vomiting in infancy may be due to pyloric stenosis or gastroesophageal reflux. With chronic gastrointestinal symptoms, enzyme deficiency (eg, lactase), cystic fibrosis, celiac disease, chronic intestinal infections, gastrointestinal malformations, and irritable bowel syndrome should be considered.

## Treatment

Treatment consists of eliminating and avoiding foods that have been documented to cause allergic reactions. This involves educating the patient, parent, and caregivers regarding hidden food allergens, the necessity for reading labels, and the signs and symptoms of food allergy and its appropriate management. Examples of ingredients that may indicate an implicated food protein include "emulsifier" (egg), "lecithin" (egg or soy), "natural flavoring" (milk), and "thickener" (soy). Consultation with a dietitian familiar with food allergy may be helpful, especially when common foods such as milk, egg, peanut, soy, or wheat are involved. Patients with a history of food-induced anaphylaxis or respiratory distress should carry epinephrine (see Anaphylaxis section). A study of peanut-allergic patients demonstrated that treatment with monoclonal anti-IgE significantly increased the threshold of sensitivity to peanut on oral food challenge, although this treatment is currently approved only for patients with asthma (see Asthma section).

## Prognosis

The prognosis is good if the offending food can be identified and avoided. Unfortunately, accidental exposure to food allergens in severely allergic patients can result in death. Most children outgrow their food allergies to egg, milk, or soy but not to peanut or tree nuts. The natural history of food allergy to milk, egg, peanut and fish proteins can be followed by measuring specific IgE levels by ImmunoCAP assay as discussed earlier. Approximately 2% will have food allergy as adults. Resources for food-allergic patients include the Food Al-

lergy and Anaphylaxis Network and the National Peanut and Tree Nut Registry (800-929-4040).

Leung DY et al: Effect of anti-IgE therapy in patients with peanut allergy. N Engl J Med 2003;348:986 [PMID: 12629027].

Sampson HA: Utility of food-specific IgE concentrations in predicting symptomatic food allergy. J Allergy Clin Immunol 2001;107:891.

Sicherer SH et al: Symposium: Pediatric food allergy. Pediatrics 2003;111(6pt3):1591 [PMID: 12777597].

# INSECT ALLERGY

Allergic reactions to insects include symptoms of respiratory allergy as a result of inhalation of particulate matter of insect origin, local cutaneous reactions to insect bites, and anaphylactic reactions to stings. The latter are almost exclusively caused by Hymenoptera and result in approximately 40 deaths each year in the United States. The order Hymenoptera includes honey bees, yellow jackets, yellow hornets, white-faced hornets, wasps, and fire ants. Africanized honey bees, also known as killer bees, are a concern because of their aggressive behavior and excessive swarming and not because their venom is more toxic. Rarely, patients sensitized to reduviid bugs (also known as kissing bugs) may have episodes of nocturnal anaphylaxis. Lepidopterism refers to adverse effects secondary to contact with larval or adult butterflies and moths. Salivary gland antigens are responsible for immediate and delayed skin reactions in mosquito-sensitive patients.

## Clinical Findings

### A. SYMPTOMS AND SIGNS

Insect bites or stings can cause local or systemic reactions ranging from mild to fatal responses in susceptible persons. The frequency increases in the summer months and with outdoor exposure. Local cutaneous reactions include urticaria as well as papulovesicular eruptions and lesions that resemble delayed hypersensitivity reactions. Papular urticaria is almost always the result of insect bites, especially of mosquitoes, fleas, and bedbugs. Toxic systemic reactions consisting of gastrointestinal symptoms, headache, vertigo, syncope, convulsions, or fever can occur following multiple stings. These reactions result from histamine-like substances in the venom. In children with hypersensitivity to fire ant venom, sterile pustules occur at sting sites on a nonimmunologic basis due to the inherent toxicity of piperidine alkaloids in the venom. Mild systemic reactions include itching, flushing, and urticaria. Severe systemic reactions may include dyspnea, wheezing, chest tightness, hoarseness, fullness in the throat, hypotension, loss of consciousness, incontinence, nausea, vomiting, and abdominal pain. Delayed systemic reactions occur from 2 hours to 3 weeks following the sting and include serum sickness, peripheral neuritis, allergic vasculitis, and coagulation defects.

## B. Laboratory Findings

Skin testing is indicated for children with systemic reactions. Venoms of honeybee, yellow jacket, yellow hornet, white-faced hornet, and wasp are available for skin testing and treatment. Fire ant venom is not yet commercially available, but an extract made from fire ant bodies appears adequate to establish the presence of IgE antibodies to fire ant venom. Of note, venom skin test results can be negative in patients with systemic allergic reactions, especially in the first few weeks after a sting, and the tests may need to be repeated. The presence of a positive skin test denotes prior sensitization but does not predict whether a reaction will occur with the patient's next sting, nor does it differentiate between local and systemic reactions. It is common for children who have had an allergic reaction to have positive skin tests to more than one venom. This might reflect sensitization from prior stings that did not result in an allergic reaction or cross-reactivity between closely related venoms. In vitro testing (compared with skin testing) has not substantially improved the ability to predict anaphylaxis. With venom RAST, there is a 15–20% incidence of both false-positive and false-negative results. Tests for mosquito saliva antigens or other insect allergy are not commercially available.

## Complications

Secondary infection can complicate allergic reactions to insect bites or stings. Serum sickness, nephrotic syndrome, vasculitis, neuritis, and encephalopathy may be seen as late sequelae of reactions to stinging insects.

## Treatment

For cutaneous reactions caused by biting insects, symptomatic therapy includes cold compresses, antipruritics (including antihistamines), and occasionally potent topical corticosteroids. Treatment of stings includes careful removal of the stinger, if present, by flicking it away from the wound and not by grasping in order to prevent further envenomation. Topical application of monosodium glutamate, baking soda, or vinegar compresses is of questionable efficacy. Local reactions can be treated with ice, elevation of the affected extremity, oral antihistamines, and NSAIDs as well as potent topical corticosteroids. Large local reactions in which swelling extends beyond two joints or an extremity, may require a short course of oral corticosteroids. Anaphylactic reactions following Hymenoptera stings should be managed essentially the same as anaphylaxis (see Anaphylaxis section). Children who have had severe or anaphylactic reactions to Hymenoptera stings—or their parents and caregivers—should be instructed in the use of epinephrine. Patients at risk for anaphylaxis from an insect sting should also wear a medical alert bracelet indicating their allergy. Children at risk from insect stings should avoid wearing bright-colored clothing and perfumes when outdoors and should wear long pants and shoes when walking in the grass. Patients who experience severe systemic reactions and have a positive skin test should receive venom immunotherapy. Immunotherapy is not indicated for children with only urticarial or local reactions.

## Prognosis

Children generally have milder reactions than adults after insect stings, and fatal reactions are extremely rare. Patients age 3–16 years with reactions limited to the skin, such as urticaria and angioedema, appear to be at low risk for more severe reactions with subsequent stings.

Golden DB: Stinging insect allergy. Am Fam Physician 2003;67:2541 [PMID: 12777600].

# Antimicrobial Therapy

*John W. Ogle, MD*

## PRINCIPLES OF ANTIMICROBIAL THERAPY

Antimicrobial therapy of bacterial infections is arguably the most important scientific development of twentieth-century medicine. It contributes significantly to the quality of life of many people and reduces the morbidity and mortality due to infectious disease. The remarkable success of antimicrobial therapy has been achieved with comparatively little toxicity and expense. The relative ease of administration and the widespread availability of these drugs have led many to adopt a philosophy of broad-spectrum empiric antimicrobial therapy for many common infections.

Unfortunately this era of cheap, safe, and reliable therapy may be coming to a close owing to the increasing frequency of antimicrobial resistance in previously susceptible microorganisms. The problem of antimicrobial resistance is certainly not new—resistance was recognized for sulfonamides and penicillins shortly after their introduction. What is new is the worldwide dissemination of resistant clones of microorganisms, such as *Streptococcus pneumoniae* and *Staphylococcus aureus,* which are inherently virulent and commonly cause serious infections, not only among hospitalized patients but also among outpatients.

Until recently the recognition of new resistant clones was balanced by the promise of newer and more potent antimicrobial agents. Today, because fewer new agents are under development, clinicians are beginning to encounter limitations in their ability to treat some serious bacterial infections. Many factors contribute to the selection of resistant clones. Our success in treating chronic diseases and immune-compromising conditions, which has resulted in additional years of life for patients, has increased opportunities for selection of resistant strains in inpatient units and chronic care facilities. Overuse of antimicrobial agents by well-intentioned clinicians also contributes to the selection of resistant strains. Examples include medications for mildly ill patients with self-limited conditions such as viral infections, and administration of broad-spectrum antimicrobials for patients whose condition can be treated with narrow-spectrum agents. Similarly, failure to document infection with cultures obtained prior to starting therapy limits our willingness to stop or narrow the spectrum of

antimicrobials. Little research has been conducted to determine the necessary duration of therapy, with the result that we probably often treat longer than is necessary. Prophylactic strategies, as used for prevention of recurrent otitis media or urinary tract infection, create a selection pressure for antibiotic resistance.

The decision-making process for choosing an appropriate antimicrobial agent is summarized in Table 35–1. Accurate clinical diagnosis is based on the history, physical examination, and initial laboratory tests. The clinical diagnosis then leads to a consideration of the organisms most commonly associated with the clinical condition, the usual pattern of antimicrobial susceptibility of these organisms, and past experience with successful treatment regimens.

Cultures should be obtained in potentially serious infections. Empiric antimicrobial therapy may be initiated, then modified according to the patient's response and the culture results. Often several equally safe and efficacious antimicrobials are available. In this circumstance, the relative cost and ease of administration of the different choices should be considered.

Other important considerations include the patient's age, immune status, and exposure history. Neonates and young infants may present with nonspecific signs of infection, making the differentiation of serious disease from mild illness difficult. In older children, clinical diagnosis is more precise, which may permit no therapy or use of a narrower-spectrum antibiotic. Immune deficiency may increase the number and types of potential infecting organisms that need to be considered, including organisms that are usually avirulent but that may cause infections that are serious and difficult to treat. An abnormal immune response may also diminish the severity of the clinical signs and symptoms of infection and thus lead to underestimation of the severity of illness. The exposure history may suggest the greater likelihood of certain types of infecting organisms. This history includes exposures from family members, classmates, and day care environments and exposure to unusual organisms by virtue of travel, diet, or contact with animals.

Final important considerations are the pace and seriousness of the illness. A rapidly progressive and severe illness should be treated initially with broad-spectrum antimicrobials until a specific etiologic diagnosis is

*Table 35–1.* Steps in decision making for use of antimicrobial agents.

| Step | Action | Example |
|---|---|---|
| 1 | Determine diagnosis. | Septic arthritis |
| 2 | Consider age and preexisting condition. | Previously healthy 2-year-old child |
| 3 | Consider common organisms. | *Staphylococus aureus, Kingella kingae* |
| 4 | Consider organism susceptibility. | Penicillin- or ampicillin-resistant, frequency MRSA[a] in community |
| 5 | Obtain proper cultures.[b] | Blood, joint fluid |
| 6 | Initiate empiric therapy based on above considerations and past experience (eg, personal, literature). | Nafcillin and cefotaxime, substitute vancomycin for nafcillin if obviously ill or MRSA prevalent. |
| 7 | Modify therapy based on culture results and patient response. | *S aureus* isolated. Discontinue cefotaxime. Substitute naficillin for vancomycin if susceptible. |
| 8 | Follow clinical response. | Interval physical examination |
| 9 | Stop therapy. | Clinically improved or well, minimum 3–4 weeks |

[a]Methicillin-resistant *S. aureus*.
[b]Indicated for serious or unusual infections or those with unpredictable clinical response to empiric therapy.

made. A mildly ill outpatient should receive treatment preferentially with narrow-spectrum antimicrobials.

Antimicrobial susceptibility, antimicrobial families, and dosing recommendations are listed in Tables 35–2 to 35–6.

## ANTIMICROBIAL SUSCEPTIBILITY TESTING

Cultures and other diagnostic material must be obtained prior to initiating antimicrobial therapy—especially when the patient has a serious infection, initial attempts at therapy have failed, or multiagent therapy is anticipated. Whenever cultures identify the causative organism, therapy can be narrowed or optimized according to susceptibility results. Antimicrobial susceptibility testing should be done in a laboratory using carefully defined procedures (National Committee for Clinical Laboratory Standards). The use of nonstandard media, inoculum size, or growth conditions may give markedly different and undependable results.

There are several ways to test antimicrobial susceptibility. Identification of an antibiotic-destroying enzyme (eg, β-lactamase) implies resistance to β–lactam-containing antimicrobial agents. Tube or microtiter broth dilution techniques can be used to determine the minimum inhibitory concentration (MIC) of antibiotic, which is the amount of antibiotic (in μg/mL) necessary to inhibit the organism under specific laboratory conditions. Disk susceptibility testing (also performed under carefully controlled conditions) yields similar results.

The E-test is a standardized test for some organisms that correlates well with MICs. Clinical laboratories usually define antimicrobial susceptibility (susceptible, intermediate, resistant) in relation to levels of the test antibiotic achievable in the blood (or serum).

Organisms are usually considered susceptible to an antibiotic if the MIC of the antibiotic for the organism is lower than levels of that agent achievable in the blood using appropriate parenteral dosages. This assumption of susceptibility should be reconsidered whenever the patient has a focus of infection (eg, meningitis, osteomyelitis, abscess) in which poor antibiotic penetration might occur, because the levels of antibiotic in such areas might be lower than the MIC. Conversely, although certain organisms may be reported resistant to an antibiotic because sufficiently high blood concentrations cannot be achieved, urine concentrations may be much higher. If so, a urinary tract infection might respond to an antibiotic that would not be adequate for treatment of septicemia.

Thus antimicrobial susceptibility testing, although a very important part of therapeutic decision making, reflects assumptions that the clinician must understand, especially for management of serious infections. Ultimately the true test of the efficacy of therapy is patient response. Patients who do not respond to seemingly appropriate therapy may require reassessment, including reconsidering the diagnosis, reculturing, and repeat susceptibility testing, to determine whether resistant strains have evolved or superinfection with a resistant organism is present. Antimicrobial therapy cannot be expected to cure some infections unless additional supportive treatment (usually surgical) is undertaken.

***Table 35–2.*** Susceptibility of some common pathogenic microorganisms to various antimicrobial drugs.

| Organism | Potentially Useful Antibiotics[a] |
|---|---|
| **BACTERIA** | |
| Anaerobic bacteria[b] | Cefoxitin,[c] cefotetan,[c] clindamycin, ertapenem,[c] imipenem,[c] meropenem, metronidazole, penicillins with or without β-lactamase inhibitor, trovofloxacin[c] |
| *Bacillus anthracis* | Amoxicillin, ciprofloxacin, clindamycin, doxycycline, rifampin |
| *Bartonella henselae* | Azithromycin, ciprofloxacin, clarithromycin, doxycycline, erythromycin |
| *Bordetella pertussis* | Amoxicillin, azithromycin, clarithromycin, erythromycin, trimethoprim–sulfamethoxazole |
| *Borrelia burgdorferi* | Amoxicillin, cefuroxime, cephalosporins (III),[h] clarithromycin, doxycycline |
| *Campylobacter* spp | Azithromycin, carbapenems, erythromycin, fluoroquinolones,[c,f] tetracyclines |
| *Clostridium* spp | Clindamycin, metronidazole, penicillins, tetracyclines |
| *Clostridium difficile* | Bacitracin (PO), metronidazole, vancomycin (PO) |
| *Corynebacterium diphtheriae* | Clindamycin, erythromycin, penicillins |
| Enterobacteriaceae[d] | Aminoglycosides,[e] ampicillin, aztreonam, cefepime, cephalosporins, ertapenem, imipenem, meropenem, fluoroquinolones,[c,f] trimethoprim–sulfamethoxazole |
| *Enterococcus* | Ampicillin (with aminoglycoside), carbapenems (not *E faecium*), vancomycin, linezolid,[c] quinupristin/dalfopristin[c] (*E faecium* only) |
| *Haemophilus influenzae* | Amoxicillin/clavulanate, ampicillin (if β-lactamase negative),[g] cephalosporins (II and III),[h] chloramphenicol, fluoroquinolones,[c,f] rifampin, trimethoprim–sulfamethoxazole |
| *Listeria monocytogenes* | Ampicillin with aminoglycoside, trimethoprim–sulfamethoxazole, vancomycin |
| *Moraxella catarrhalis* | Amoxicillin/clavulanate, ampicillins (if β-lactamase-negative),[g] cephalosporins (II, III),[h] erythromycin, fluorquinolones, trimethoprim-sulfamethoxazole |
| *Neisseria gonorrhoeae* | Ampicillin (if β-lactamase-negative),[g] cephalosporins (II and III),[h] penicillins, selected fluoroquinolones,[c,f] spectinomycin |
| *Neisseria meningitidis* | Ampicillin, cephalosporins (II and III),[h] chloramphenicol, fluoroquinolones[c,f] penicillins, rifampin |
| *Nocardia asteroides* | Tetracycline, trimethoprin–sulfamethoxazole (+ amikacin for severe infections); meropenem or cephalosporins (II)[h] for brain abscess |
| *Pasteurella multocida* | Amoxicillin/clavulanate, ampicillins, penicillins, tetracyclines |
| *Pseudomonas aeruginosa* | Aminoglycosides,[e] anti-*Pseudomonas* penicillins,[c] aztreonam, cefepime, ceftazidime, imipenem, meropenem, ciprofloxacin[c] |
| *Salmonella* spp | Ampicillin, azithromycin, cephalosporins (III),[h] fluoroquinolones,[c,f] trimethoprim–sulfamethoxazole |
| *Shigella* spp | Ampicillin, azithromycin cephalosporins (III),[h] fluoroquinolones,[c,f] tetracyclines, trimethoprim–sulfamethoxazole |
| *Staphylococcus aureus* | Antistaphylococcal penicillins,[j] cefepime, cephalosporins (I and II), ciprofloxacin, clindamycin, erythromycin, rifampin, trimethoprim–sulfamethoxazole, vancomycin |
| *S aureus* (methicillin-resistant) | Trimethoprim–sulfomethoxaole, vancomycin, linezolid,[c] quinupristin/dalfopristin[c] |
| Staphylococci (coagulase-negative) | Cephalosporins (I and II),[k] clindamycin, rifampin, vancomycin |
| Streptococci (most species) | Ampicillin, cephalosporins, clindamycin, enhanced fluoroquinolones,[c,n] erythromycin, meropenem, penicillins, vancomycin |
| *Streptococcus pneumoniae*[l] | Ampicillin, cephalosporins, enhanced fluoroquinolones,[c,n] erythromycin, meropenem, penicillin, vancomycin[12] |

*(continued)*

*Table 35–2.* Susceptibility of some common pathogenic microorganisms to various antimicrobial drugs (continued).

| Organism | Potentially Useful Antibiotics[a] |
|---|---|
| **INTERMEDIATE ORGANISMS** | |
| *Chlamydia* spp | Clarithromycin, erythromycin, levofloxacin,[c] ofloxacin[c,f] tetracyclines |
| *Mycoplasma* spp | Azithromycin, clarithromycin, erythromycin, fluoroquinolones,[c,f] tetracyclines |
| *Rickettsia* spp | Fluoroquinolones,[c,f] tetracyclines |
| **FUNGI** | |
| *Candida* spp | Amphotericin B, caspofungin; fluconazole, flucytosine, itraconazole, ketoconazole, voriconazole |
| Fungi, systemic[b] | Amphotericin B, caspofungin; fluconazole, itraconazole,[c] ketoconazole, miconazole, voriconazole |
| Dermatophytes | Butenafine, ciclopirox olamine, clotrimazole, econozole, fluconazole, griseofulvin, naftifine, itraconazole,[c] ketoconazole, miconazole, oxiconazole, sulconazole, terbinafine, torconazole |
| *Pneumocystis jiroveci* | Atovaquone, clindamycin+primaquin, dapsone, pentamidine, trimethoprim-sulfamethoxazole |
| **VIRUSES** | |
| Herpes simplex | Acyclovir, famciclovir,[c] foscarnet, trifluridine, valacyclovir[c] |
| Human immunodeficiency virus | Four classes: (1) nucleoside reverse transcriptase inhibitor (7 drugs); (2) non-nucleoside reverse transcriptase inhibitors (3 drugs); (3) protease inhibitors (7 drugs); (4) fusion inhibitors (1 drug). Generally in combinations of ≥ 3 drugs used (see Chapter 37). |
| Influenza virus | Amantadine,[o] oseltamivir, rimantidine,[o] zanamivir |
| Respiratory syncytial virus | Ribavirin[m] |
| Varicella-zoster virus | Acyclovir, famciclovir,[c] valacyclovir[c] |
| Cytomegalovirus | Cidofovir, foscarnet, ganciclovir, valgancyclovir |

[a]In alphabetical order. Selection depends on patient's age, diagnosis, site of infection, severity of illness, antimicrobial susceptibility of suspected organism, and drug risk.
[b]Species-dependent.
[c]Not FDA-approved for use in children.
[d]Includes *E coli, Klebsiella* spp, *Enterobacter* spp, and others; antimicrobial susceptibilities should always be measured.
[e]Amikacin, gentamicin, kanamycin, tobramycin.
[f]Includes ciprofloxacin, enoxacin, grepefloxacin, levofloxacin, lomefloxacin, norfloxacin, ofloxacin, sparfloxacin.
[g]Also applies to amoxicillin and related compounds.
[h]Refer to second- (II) or third- (III) generation cephalosporins.
[i]Carbenicillin, mezlocillin, piperacillin, ticarcillin.
[j]Cloxacillin, dicloxacillin, methicillin, nafcillin, oxacillin.
[k]Only if the coagulase-negative *Staphylococcus* is also methicillin- or oxacillin-sensitive.
[l]Because of increasing frequency of *S pneumoniae* strains resistant to penicillin and cephalosporins, therapy for presumed severe infections (eg, meningitis) should include vancomycin until susceptibility studies are available.
[m]FDA-approved for therapy of RSV by aerosol, but clinical studies show variable efficacy.
[n]Includes grepefloxacin, levofloxacin, lomefloxacin, sparfloxacin.
[o]Influenza A only.

# ALTERATION OF DOSE & MEASUREMENT OF BLOOD LEVELS

Certain antimicrobial agents have not been approved (and often not tested) for use in newborns. For those that have been approved, it is important to recognize that both dose and frequency of administration may need to be altered (see Tables 35–4 and 35–5), especially in young (7 days or younger) or low-birth-weight neonates (≤ 2000 g).

Antimicrobial agents are excreted or metabolized through various physiologic mechanisms (eg, renal, he-

**Table 35–3.** Groups of common antibacterial agents.

| Group | Examples | Some Common Susceptible Organisms[a] | Common Resistant Organisms | Common or Unique Adverse Reactions |
|---|---|---|---|---|
| **PENICILLIN GROUP** | | | | |
| Penicillins | Penicillin G, V | *Streptococcus, Neisseria* | *Staphylococcus, Haemophilus,* Enterobacteriaceae | Rash, anaphylaxis, drug fever, bone marrow suppression |
| Ampicillins | Ampicillin, amoxicillin | (Same as penicillins), plus *Haemophilus* (β-lactamase negative), *Escherichia coli, Enterococcus* | *Staphylococcus,* many Enterobacteriaceae | Diarrhea |
| Antistaphylococcal penicillins | Cloxacillin, dicloxacillin, methicillin, nafcillin, oxacillin | *Streptococcus, Staphylococcus aureus* | Gram-negative, *Staphylococcus* (coagulase-negative), *Enterococcus* | Renal (interstitial nephritis) |
| Anti-*Pseudomonas* penicillins | Azlocillin, piperacillin, ticarcillin | (Same as ampicillins), plus *Pseudomonas* | (Same as ampicillins) | Decreased platelet adhesiveness, hypokalemia, hypernatremia |
| Penicillin and β-lactamase inhibitor combination | Amoxicillin–clavulanate, ampicillin–sulbactam, ticarcillin–clavulanate | Broad-spectrum | Some enterobacteriaceae, *Pseudomonas* | Diarrhea |
| Carbapenems | Imipenem–cilastatin meropenem, ertapenem | Broad-spectrum, gram-negative rods, anaerobes, *Pseudomonas* | MRSA,[b] many enterococci | CNS, seizures |
| **CEPHALOSPORIN GROUP** | | | | |
| First generation (I) | Cefazolin, cephalexin, cephalothin, cephapirin, cephradine | Gram-positive | Gram-negative, *Enterococcus,* some *Staphylococcus* (coagulase-negative) | Rash; anaphylaxis, drug fever |
| Second generation (II) | Cefaclor, cefamandole, cefprozil, cefonicid, cefuroxime, loracarbef | Gram-positive, some *Haemophilus,* some Enterobacteriaceae | *Enterococcus, Pseudomonas,* some *Staphylococcus* (coagulase-negative) | Serum sickness (cefaclor) |
| | Cefoxitin, cefotetan | Same as second-generation plus anaerobes | | |
| Third generation (III) | Cefotaxime, ceftizoxime, ceftriaxone, cefpodoxime, ceftibuten, cefdinir | *Streptococcus, Haemophilus,* Enterobacteriaceae, *Neisseria* | *Pseudomonas, Staphylococcus* | Biliary sludging (ceftriaxone) rash |
| | Ceftazidime, cefepime | (Same as other third-generation cephalosporins), plus *Pseudomonas* | *Staphylococcus* | |
| **OTHER DRUGS** | | | | |
| Clindamycin | Clindamycin | Gram-positive, anaerobes | Gram-negative, *Enterococcus,* MRSA | Nausea, vomiting, hepatotoxicity |
| Vancomycin | Vancomycin | Gram-positive | Gram-negative | "Red man" syndrome, shock, ototoxicity, renal |

*(continued)*

***Table 35–3.*** Groups of common antibacterial agents. (continued)

| Group | Examples | Some Common Susceptible Organisms[a] | Common Resistant Organisms | Common or Unique Adverse Reactions |
|---|---|---|---|---|
| **OTHER DRUGS (*con't*)** | | | | |
| Macrolides and azilides | Erythromycin, clarithromycin, azithromycin | Gram-positive *Bordetella, Haemophilus, Mycoplasma, Chlamydia, Legionella* | Gram-negative | Nausea and vomiting |
| Monobactams | Aztreonam | Gram-negative aerobes, *Pseudomonas* | Gram-positive cocci | Rash, diarrhea |
| Oxazolidinones | Linezolid | Gram-positive aerobes | Gram-negative aerobes | Diarrhea Thrombocytopenia |
| Streptogamins | Quinupristin/ dalfopristin | Gram-positive aerobes | Gram-negative aerobes | Arthralgia myalgia |
| Fluoroquinolones[c] | Ciprofloxacin, ofloxacin | Gram-negative, *Chlamydia Pseudomonas* (ciprofloxacin) | *Enterococcus, Streptococcus, S pneumoniae,* anaerobes, *Staphylococcus* | GI, rash, CNS |
| | Norfloxacin (urinary tract infections only) | Gram-negative | *Enterococcus, Streptococcus, S pneumoniae,* anaerobes *Staphylococcus* | GI, rash, CNS |
| | Grepefloxacin, lomefloxacin, sparfloxacin | Gram-negative, streptococcus, some enterococci | Some *Enterococcus* | GI, rash, CNS |
| | Gatifloxacin, levofloxacin, moxifloxacin, trovofloxacin | Gram-negative, streptococci, *S pneumoniae,* staphylococci, anaerobes[e] | Some *Enterococcus* | GI, rash, CNS, severe hepatitis[e] |
| Tetracyclines | Chlortetracycline, tetracycline, doxycycline, minocycline | Anaerobes, *Mycoplasma, Chlamydia, Rickettsia, Ehrlichia* | Many Enterobacteriaceae, *Staphylococcus* | Teeth staining,[d] rash, flora overgrowth, hepatotoxicity, pseudotumor cerebri |
| Sulfonamides | Many | Gram-negative (urine) | Gram-positive | Rash, renal, bone marrow suppression, Stevens–Johnson syndrome |
| Trimethoprim–sulfamethoxazole | Trimethoprim-sulfamethoxazole | *S aureus,* gram-negative, *S pneumoniae H influenzae* | *Streptococcus, Pseudomonas,* anaerobes | Rash, renal, bone marrow suppression, Stevens–Johnson syndrome |
| Rifampin | Rifampin | *Neisseria, Haemophilus, Staphylococcus, Streptococcus* | Resistance develops rapidly if used as sole agent | Rash, GI, hepatotoxicity, CNS, bone marrow suppression, alters metabolism of other drugs |
| Aminoglycosides | Amikacin, gentamicin, kanamycin, streptomycin, tobramycin | Gram-negative, including *P aeruginosa* | Gram-positive, anaerobes, some pseudomonads | Nephrotoxicity, ototoxicity, potentiates neuromuscular blocking agents |

[a]Not all strains susceptible; always obtain antimicrobial susceptibility tests on significant isolates.
[b]MRSA = methicillin-resistant *S aureus.*
[c]Not approved for children.
[d]Dose-dependent in children < age 9 years.
[e]Trovofloxacin only.

**Table 35–4.** Guidelines for use of common parenteral antibacterial agents[a] in children age 1 month or older.

| | Route | Dose[b] (mg/kg/d) | Maximum Daily Dose | Interval (hours) | Adjustment[c] | Blood Levels[d] (µg/mL) Peak | Trough |
|---|---|---|---|---|---|---|---|
| Amikacin | IM, IV | 15–22.5 | 1.5 g | 8 | R | 15–25 | 5–10 |
| Ampicillin | IM, IV | 100–400 | 12 g | 4–6 | R | | |
| Aztreonam | IM, IV | 90–120 | 6 g | 6–8 | R | | |
| Cefazolin | IM, IV | 50–100 | 6 g | 8 | R | | |
| Cefepime[g] | IM, IV | 100–150 | 4–6 g | 8–12 | R | | |
| Cefotaxime | IM, IV | 100–200 | 12 g | 6–8 | R | | |
| Cefoxitin | IM, IV | 80–160 | 12 g | 4–6 | R | | |
| Ceftazidime | IM, IV | 100–150 | 6 g | 8 | R | | |
| Ceftizoxime | IM, IV | 150–200 | 12 g | 6–8 | R | | |
| Ceftriaxone | IM, IV | 50–100 | 4 g | 12–24 | R | | |
| Cefuroxime | IM, IV | 100–150 | 6 g | 6–8 | R | | |
| Cephalothin | IM, IV | 75–125 | 12 g | 4–6 | R | | |
| Cephradine | IM, IV | 50–100 | 8 g | 6 | R | | |
| Clindamycin | IM, IV | 25–40 | 4 g | 6–8 | R, H | | |
| Gentamicin | IM, IV | 3–7.5 | 300 mg | 8 | R | 5–10 | < 2 |
| Linezolid | IV, PO | 20 | 1.2 g | 12 | R | | |
| Meropenem | IV | 60–120 | 2 g | 8 | R | | |
| Metronidazole | IV | 30 | 4 g | 6 | H | | |
| Nafcillin | IM, IV | 150 | 12 g | 6 | H | | |
| Penicillin G | IM, IV | 100,000–250,000 units/kg | 20 million units | 4–6 | H, R | | |
| Penicillin G (benzathine) | IM | 50,000 units/kg | 2.4 million units | Single dose | None | | |
| Penicillin G (procaine) | IM | 25,000–50,000 units/kg | 4.8 million units | 12–24 | R | | |
| Tetracycline[e] | IV[e] | 20–30 | 2 g | 12 | R | | |
| Ticarcillin | IV | 200–300 | 24 g | 4–6 | R | | |
| Tobramycin | IM, IV | 3–6 | 300 mg | 8 | R | 5–10 | < 2 |
| Vancomycin | IV | 40–60 | 2 g | 6 | R | 20–40[f] | < 10[f] |

[a]Not including some newly released drugs, ones not recommended for use in children, or ones not widely used.
[b]Always consult package insert for complete prescribing information. Dosage may differ for alternative routes, newborns (see Table 34–6), or patients with liver or renal failure (see Adjustment column) and may not be recommended for use in pregnant women or newborns. Maximum dosage may be indicated only in severe infections or by parenteral routes.
[c]Mode of excretion (R = renal, H = hepatic) of antimicrobial agent should be assessed at the onset of therapy and dosage modified or levels determined as indicated in package insert.
[d]Suggested levels to reduce toxicity.
[e]Use with caution in children < age 9 years because of tooth staining with repeated doses.
[f]Target peak and trough vancomycin levels are not well correlated with either toxicity or outcome. Measure selectively in meningitis, impaired or changing renal function, or altered volume of distribution.
[g]Safety and efficacy are not established in chidlren < age 2 months.

**Table 35–5.** Guidelines for use of common oral antibacterial agents in children age 1 month or older.

| Agent[a] | Dose[b] (mg/kg/d) | Interval (hours) | Other Considerations |
|---|---|---|---|
| Amoxicillin | 40 | 8–12 | GI side effects |
| Amoxicillin[c] (high dose) | 80–90 | 12 | GI side effects |
| Amoxicillin-clavulanate | 45 | 12 | GI side effects |
| Ampicillin | 50 | 6 | GI side effects |
| Azithromycin | 10 (first dose) then 5; 12 for pharyngitis | 24 | GI side effects |
| Cefaclor | 40 | 8 | Serum sickness-like illness |
| Cefadroxil | 30 | 12 | |
| Cefpodoxime | 10 | 12 | Taste (suspension) |
| Cefprozil | 30 | 12 | GI side effects |
| Ceftibuten | 9 | 24 | GI side effects |
| Cefuroxime | 30–40 | 12 | GI side effects |
| Cephalexin | 25–50 | 6 | |
| Cephradine | 25–50 | 6 | |
| Clarithromycin | 15 | 12 | GI side effects |
| Clindamycin | 20–30 | 6 | GI side effects |
| Cloxacillin | 50–100 | 6 | GI side effects |
| Dicloxacillin | 12–25 | 6 | GI side effects |
| Doxycycline[d] | 2–4 | 12–24 | Tooth staining < 9 years |
| Erythromycin[e] | 20–50 | 6–12 | GI side effects |
| Erythromycin-sulfisoxazole | 40 (erythromycin) | 6–8 | |
| Furazolidone | 5–8 | 6 | |
| Linezolid | 20 | 12 | GI side effects |
| Loracarbef | 15; 30 for otitis | 12 | |
| Metronidazole | 15–35 | 8 | |
| Nitrofurantoin | 5–7 | 6 | |
| Oxacillin | 50–100 | 6 | |
| Penicillin V | 25–50 | 6 | Taste (suspension) |
| Rifampin | 10–20 | 12–24 | |
| Sulfisoxazole | 120–150 | 6 | |
| Tetracycline[d] | 25–50[c] | 6 | Teeth staining < 9 years |
| Trimethoprim-sulfamethoxazole | 8–12 (TMP) | 12 | Stevens–Johnson syndrome |

[a]Not including some newly released drugs, ones not recommended for use in children, or ones not widely used.
[b]Always consult package insert for complete prescribing information. Dosage may differ for alternative routes, newborns (see Table 34–6), or patients with liver or renal failure (see Table 34–4, Adjustment column) and may not be recommended for use in pregnant women or newborns. Maximum dosage may be indicated only in severe infections or by parenteral routes.
[c]Higher dose amoxicillin indicated for therapy of otitis media in regions where rates of penicillin-resistant S pneumoniae are common.
[d]Use with caution in children < age 9 years because of tooth staining with repeated doses.
[e]Preparation-dependent.

**Table 35–6.** Guidelines for use of selected antimicrobial agents in newborns.

| | Route | Body Wt (g) | Maximum Dosage (mg/kg/d) [Frequency] | | Blood Levels (µg/mL) | |
|---|---|---|---|---|---|---|
| | | | < 7 Days | 8–30 Days | Peak | Trough |
| Amikacin[a] | IV, IM | < 2000 | 15 [q12h] | 22.5 [q8h] | 15–25 | 5–10 |
| | | > 2000 | 20 [q12h] | 30 [q8h] | | |
| Ampicillin | IV, IM | < 2000 | 100 [q12h] | 150 [q8h] | | |
| | | > 2000 | 150 [q8h] | 200 [q6h] | | |
| Cefotaxime | IV, IM | | 100 [q12h] | 150 [q8h] | | |
| Ceftazidime | IV, IM | < 2000 | 100 [q12h] | 150 [q8h] | | |
| | | > 2000 | 100 [q8h] | 150 [q8h] | | |
| Clindamycin | IV, IM, PO | < 2000 | 10 [q12h] | 15 [q8h] | | |
| | | > 2000 | 15 [q8h] | 20 [q6h] | | |
| Erythromycin | PO | | 20 [q12h] | 30 [q8h] | | |
| Gentamicin[a] | IV, IM | | 5 [q12–18h] | 7.5 [q8h] | 5–10 | < 2 |
| Nafcillin | IV | < 2000 | 50 [q12h] | 75 [q8h] | | |
| | | > 2000 | 75 [q8h] | 150 [q6h] | | |
| Oxacillin | IV, IM | < 2000 | 100 [q12h] | 150 [q8h] | | |
| | | > 2000 | 50 [q8h] | 200 [q6h] | | |
| Penicillin G[b] | IV | < 2000 | 100,000 [q12h] | 150,000 [q8h] | | |
| | | > 2000 | 150,000 [q8h] | 200,000 [q6h] | | |
| Ticarcillin | IV, IM | < 2000 | 150 [q12h] | 225 [q8h] | | |
| | | > 2000 | 225 [q8h] | 300 [q6h] | | |
| Tobramycin[a] | IV, IM | | 5 [q12–18h] | 7.5 [q8h] | 5–10 | < 2 |
| Vancomycin[c] | IV | | 20 [q12h] | 30 [q8h] | 20–40 | |

[a]Neonates weighting < 1200 g may require even smaller doses. Antibiotic levels should be closely monitored.
[b]Penicillin dosages are in units/kg/d. Other preparations (eg, benzathine penicillin) may be given IM. See specific diseases for dosage.
[c]Target peak and trough vancomycin levels are not well correlated with either toxicity or outcome.

patic). It is important to consider these routes of excretion and alter the antimicrobial dosage appropriately in any patient with some degree of organ dysfunction (see Drug Therapy, Chapter 41). As indicated in Table 35–4, an assessment of renal or hepatic function may be routinely necessary for patients receiving certain drugs (eg, renal function for aminoglycosides, hepatic function for erythromycin or clindamycin); otherwise, harmful drug levels may accumulate. If significant organ dysfunction is present, drug clearance may be delayed and dosage modification may be necessary (see detailed descriptions in individual drug information packets), and measurement of drug levels may be indicated.

Serum levels of drugs posing a high risk of toxicity (eg, aminoglycosides) are ordinarily measured, and measurement of other drugs (eg, vancomycin) may be useful in selected circumstances (see following discussion). For certain other serious bacterial infections (eg, bacterial endocarditis), measurement of the serum concentration of an antimicrobial may be important to deliver optimal therapy.

Certain drug interactions may require modification of drug dosage or other therapeutic alterations. (See Chapter 41, Drug Therapy.) For example, rifampin stimulates the metabolism of warfarin, birth control pills, and anticonvulsants by stimulating the P-450 metabolic pathway. Dosage adjustments or alternative medications may be necessary to avoid significant adverse events. Another common example is erythromycin, which may inhibit the metabolism of theophylline, resulting in toxic theophylline levels. Although many drug interactions are known and well documented, it may be difficult to predict interactions that result from a combination of four, five, or more different medications. A high level of suspicion regarding adverse clinical events should be maintained.

## THE USE OF NEW ANTIMICROBIAL AGENTS

New antibiotics are introduced frequently, often with claims about unique features that distinguish these usually more expensive products from existing compounds. Often, these drugs share many properties with existing drugs. The role that any new antimicrobial will play can only be determined over time, during which new or previously unrecognized side effects might be described and the clinical efficacy established. Clinical trials may not be confirmed in the larger number of patients subsequently treated in practice. Because this may take many years, a conservative approach to using new antibiotics seems fitting, especially because their costs are often higher, and appropriate antimicrobial choices for most common infections already exist. It is appropriate to ask if a new antimicrobial has been proved to be as effective as (or more effective than) the current drug of choice, and whether its side effects are comparable or less common and its cost reasonable. The withdrawal of moxalactam and caution regarding use of trovafloxacin due to unexpected serious side effects, which were not anticipated despite extensive premarket testing, highlight the caution necessary before using new antimicrobials. The heavy marketing of new cephalosporins and fluoroquinolones, which are very similar to existing drugs, is typical of the difficulty faced by the primary physician in evaluating antimicrobials.

The development of new antibiotics is important as a response to the emergence of resistant organisms and for treatment of infections that are clinically difficult to treat (eg, viruses, fungi, and some resistant bacteria). Fortunately these infections are either rare or (usually) self-limited in immunocompetent hosts.

## PROPHYLACTIC ANTIMICROBIAL AGENTS

Antimicrobials can be used to decrease the incidence of postoperative infections (Table 35–7). A dose of an antimicrobial given 30 minutes to 2 hours prior to surgery can reduce postoperative wound infection. The goal is to achieve high levels in the serum at the time of incision and by this means—along with good surgical technique—to minimize bacterial contamination of the wound. During a lengthy procedure, a second dose may be given. No evidence exists that multiple subsequent doses of antimicrobials confer additional benefit. The

antimicrobial(s) used for prophylaxis are directed toward the flora that most commonly cause postoperative infection at a given anatomic site. Gram-positive cocci such as S aureus are usually targeted, and a first-generation cephalosporin (eg, cefazolin) is a cost-effective choice. Third-generation cephalosporins and other broad-spectrum agents are more expensive and offer less benefit because they are less active than cefazolin against S aureus. Cefoxitin or cefotetan is useful for procedures such as colorectal surgery, although cefazolin is appropriate for most gynecologic patients. In colorectal surgery, oral antimicrobials such as neomycin and erythromycin may be as effective as parenteral therapy.

In hospitals where the predominant S aureus strains are methicillin-resistant or in cases where the patient is allergic to penicillin and cephalosporins, vancomycin can be considered. However, prophylactic vancomycin has caused hypotension at the time of induction of general anesthesia. Frequent use of vancomycin as a prophylactic antimicrobial will contribute to the development of vancomycin-resistant strains such as Enterococcus faecalis. For these reasons, vancomycin should generally not be used for prophylaxis, although it might prove useful for individual patients at extremely high risk.

Prophylactic antimicrobials are given in several other circumstances. Endocarditis prophylaxis is indicated during dental and colorectal or genitourinary procedures in patients with high-risk heart lesions, such as prosthetic cardiac valves, surgically corrected systemic pulmonary shunts, and mitral valve prolapse with regurgitation. Patients with indwelling vascular catheters, such as Broviac catheters, should receive prophylaxis during similar procedures, which are likely to induce a transient bacteremia. Prophylaxis against infection with group A streptococci reduces the recurrence rate for acute rheumatic fever. Postexposure prophylaxis is given after exposure to pertussis, Haemophilus influenzae type b (HIB) infection (depending on age), meningococcus, gonococcus, tuberculosis (household exposure), plague, aerosolized tularemia, and other high-risk infections. Family or close contacts of patients with severe invasive streptococcal disease may benefit from prophylaxis. Silver nitrate, erythromycin, povidone–iodine, and tetracycline can be used in ophthalmic preparations for prevention of gonococcal ophthalmia neonatorum. Children with asplenia or sickle cell disease receive prophylactic penicillin to protect against overwhelming Streptococcus pneumoniae sepsis, usually started immediately with the onset of fever.

Prophylactic antimicrobials are sometimes used during the viral respiratory season in children at high risk for recurrent otitis media and for some children with recurrent urinary tract infection. However, because of the increasing frequency of resistant S pneumoniae, de-

***Table 35–7.*** Antimicrobial prophylaxis and preferred prophylactic agents: Selected conditions and pathogens.[a]

| Pathogen (Indication) | Prophylactic Agent |
| --- | --- |
| Bacillus anthracis[b] | Ciprofloxacin, doxycycline, amoxicillin (if proved susceptible) |
| Bacterial endocarditis[c] | Ampicillin, ampicillin and gentamicin, amoxicillin, or other approved regimens |
| *Bordetella pertussis* (exposure to respiratory secretions) | Azithromycin, clarithromycin, erythromycin |
| *Chlamydia trachomatis* (genital contact or neonate) | Erythromycin |
| *Haemophilus influenzae* type b[d] (household exposure) | Rifampin |
| *Mycobacterium tuberculosis* (household exposure) | Isoniazid |
| *Neisseria meningitidis* (household exposure) | Rifampin, sulfadiazine,[e] ciprofloxacin |
| *N gonorrhoeae* (ophthalmia neonatorum) | Erythromycin, silver nitrate ophthalmic |
| *N gonorrhoeae* (sexual contact) | Ceftriaxone, cefixime, cefpodoxime, fluoroquinolone |
| *Treponema pallidum* (sexual contact) | Penicillin |
| *Streptococcus pneumoniae* (sickle cell disease, asplenia) | Penicillin |
| Postoperative wound infection[f] | Cefazolin, other regimens[f] |
| Group A streptococci (rheumatic fever)[g] | Benzathine penicillin G, penicillin, sulfadiazine |
| Group B streptococcal sepsis | Ampicillin to mother prior to delivery |
| Pneumonic *Yersinia pestis*[h] (exposure) | Tetracycline,[i] |
| *Francisella tularensis*[h] (aerosolized exposure) | Tetracycline,[i] |
| *Vibrio cholera* | Tetracycline,[i] trimethoprim–sulfamethoxazole |
| Recurrent otitis media | Amoxicillin, sulfadiazine |
| Recurrent urinary tract infection | Nitrofurantoin, trimethoprim–sulfamethoxazole |
| *Pneumocystis jiroveci* (formerly *Pneumocystis carinii*)—(HIV, some immunocompromised patients) | Trimethoprim–sulfamethoxazole, pentamidine |

[a]Decisions for prophylaxis must take a number of factors into account, including the evidence for efficacy of therapy, the degree of the exposure to an infecting agent, the risk and consequences of infection, the susceptibility of the infecting agent to antimicrobials, and the patient's ability to tolerate and comply with the antimicrobial agent. See individual chapters of the text for discussion.
[b]Decisions for prophylaxis should be made in accordance with the responsible public health department recommendations.
[c]See discussion in Chapter 19.
[d]Prophylaxis provided to family if contacts include children < age 4 years. Some experts provide prophylaxis in day care settings after one case and some after two cases of HiB.
[e]Only for known sulfadiazine-susceptible strains.
[f]Alternative regimens may be used, depending on the site of surgery and the degree of contamination.
[g]Oral prophylaxis may be indicated in some patients. Alternative regimens indicated for penicillin-allergic patients. See discussion in chapter.
[h]Prophylaxis not well established. Carefully assess risk on a case-by-case basis.
[i]Usually not indicated for children < age 9 years because of tooth staining with repeated doses.

cisions for antimicrobial prophylaxis are generally discouraged and should be considered carefully for each child.

## INITIAL EMPIRIC ANTIMICROBIAL CHOICES FOR SELECTED CONDITIONS

General recommendations for specific conditions are as follows. A specific selection depends on the patient's age, diagnosis, site of infection, severity of illness, antimicrobial susceptibility of bacterial isolates, and history of drug allergy. Always consult the package insert for detailed prescribing information. Tables 35–2 to 35–6 include further information.

### Neonatal Sepsis & Meningitis

The newborn with sepsis may have signs of focal infection such as pneumonia or respiratory distress syndrome or may have subtle nonfocal signs. Group B streptococci, *Escherichia coli,* other gram-negative rods, and *Listeria monocytogenes* are commonly encountered. Ampicillin and gentamicin (or another aminoglycoside) are preferred. If meningitis is present, many clinicians substitute a third-generation cephalosporin for the aminoglycoside. *S pneumoniae* is an uncommon cause of meningitis in neonates. However, if the Gram stain shows gram-positive cocci suggesting *S pneumoniae,* substitution of vancomycin for ampicillin should be considered. In the newborn with cellulitis, *Staphylococcus aureus* and group A streptococci are additional considerations. Nafcillin, oxacillin, or a first-generation cephalosporin is usually added. Omphalitis is often polymicrobial, and *Enterococcus* species, gram-negative aerobes, and anaerobes may be causative. Clindamycin, ampicillin, and an aminoglycoside or cefotaxime cover the most likely organisms; early surgical intervention is indicated.

### Sepsis in an Infant

*S pneumoniae* and *Neisseria meningitidis* are most commonly encountered in infants. *H influenzae* type b infection may occur in unimmunized children. A third-generation cephalosporin is appropriate. Intermediate-level penicillin and cephalosporin resistance in *S pneumoniae* usually do not cause therapy to fail unless meningitis or another difficult-to-treat infection such as endocarditis or osteomyelitis is present.

Occult bacteremia may be encountered in young infants with high fever, and some experts recommend presumptive therapy to clear the bacteremia and to prevent complications. Prior to immunization with vaccines effective against HIB, persistent bacteremia and complications including meningitis were seen in approximately 50% of children infected with occult HIB

bacteremia. With widespread use of HIB vaccine, HIB is a very uncommon cause of occult bacteremia in young children with fever. *S pneumonia* bacteremia is demonstrated in 3–5% of infants age 3–36 months who have a fever of 39°C or greater, no identified source for fever on examination, and a white blood cell count (WBC) = 15,000/mm³. The risk of bacteremia increases to 6–10% in younger children with progressively high fever and high WBCs. The risk of developing meningitis due to persistent *S pneumoniae* is estimated at 3% of those who are known to be bacteremic. The risk of *S pneumoniae* bacteremia and its complications is currently decreasing due to widespread administration of a conjugate-7-valent pneumococcal vaccine. In clinical trials, this vaccine reduced the incidence of invasive pneumococcal diseases by approximately 90%. This decrease in the incidence of HIB and *S pneumoniae* occult bacteremia in young febrile children has led some experts to reconsider the recommendations for empiric presumptive therapy. Observation without antimicrobials, but with appropriate plans for follow-up examinations, is appropriate for most febrile young children who are fully immunized.

### Nosocomial Sepsis

Many bacterial pathogens can cause infection in hospitalized patients. Recent local experience is usually the best guide to etiologic diagnosis. For example, some neonatal units experience frequent infections due to *Enterobacter cloacae,* whereas in other units *Klebsiella pneumoniae* is the most common nosocomial isolate. Initial therapy should include antibiotics effective for methicillin-resistant *S aureus* (MRSA) and resistant *Pseudomonas aeruginosa* if these are frequent isolates. *Enterococcus faecalis* is a common cause of nosocomial bacteremia in patients with central catheters, particularly in units where cephalosporins are heavily used. Coagulase-negative staphylococci are commonly isolated from patients with indwelling central catheters. In seriously ill patients, when the local experience suggests that *Enterococcus* species or coagulase-negative staphylococci are common, the initial regimen should include vancomycin. Because *Enterococcus* species and coagulase-negative staphylococci commonly cause fever without significant morbidity or mortality, initial regimens without vancomycin are appropriate, with adjustment of treatment after susceptibility is known. If *P aeruginosa* or other resistant gram-negative rods are common, ceftazidime or cefepime should be included in initial therapy.

### Meningitis

Bacterial meningitis in neonates is usually caused by infection with group B streptococci, *E coli,* or *L monocy-*

*togenes*. A combination of ampicillin and gentamicin or another aminoglycoside—or ampicillin and a third-generation cephalosporin—is started initially. In an infant or older child, *S pneumoniae* or *N meningitidis* is the most common isolate. HIB is uncommon now because of widespread immunization. Increasingly, *S pneumoniae* with multiple resistances to penicillin, cephalosporins, and other drugs is isolated. In some communities, 30–40% of *S pneumoniae* isolates have intermediate susceptibility to penicillin (MIC between 0.1 and 2 μg/mL) and 5–10% of isolates may be highly resistant to penicillin (MIC > 2 μg/mL). Resistance to a third-generation cephalosporin (MIC > 2 μg/mL) may occur in 3–5% of isolates.

In bacterial meningitis, peak cerebrospinal fluid (CSF) antimicrobial concentrations 10 or more times greater than the MIC of the organism are desirable, but this may be difficult to achieve if organisms are resistant. The therapeutic problem is complicated if dexamethasone, which reduces the entry of some antimicrobials into the CSF, is also given.

Initial therapy of bacterial meningitis in an older child thus should include vancomycin and a third-generation cephalosporin. Alternatively, clinical experience with meropenem has also been successful. A lumbar puncture should be considered 24–48 hours after the start of therapy to assess the sterility of the CSF. Rifampin should be added if the Gram stain or cultures of CSF are positive on repeated lumbar puncture, if the child has failed to improve, or if an organism with a very high MIC to ceftriaxone is isolated. The optimal therapy of highly resistant *S pneumoniae* meningitis is not well established by clinical data.

Meningitis in a child with a ventriculoperitoneal shunt is most commonly caused by coagulase-negative staphylococci, many of which are methicillin-resistant, and *Corynebacterium* species, which are resistant to many antimicrobials. In many of these patients who are not seriously ill, therapy should be postponed while awaiting the appropriate shunt fluid for Gram stain and culture. Seriously ill patients should initially be given vancomycin and a third-generation cephalosporin, because *S aureus* and gram-negative rods are also possible and can cause serious infection.

## Urinary Tract Infection

*E coli* is the most common isolate from the urinary tract. Outpatients with symptoms of lower urinary tract disease or with mild illness can be given ampicillin, cephalexin, or a sulfonamide. Local experience and resistance rates should guide initial therapy. In selected patients with pyelonephritis, outpatient therapy is effective using parenteral aminoglycosides or ceftriaxone once per day. Oral cefixime has been used in place of ceftriaxone for outpatient therapy; unfortunately, cefixime is no longer available and there are little data on initial therapy with other third-generation cephalosporins. For hospitalized patients with genitourinary tract infection and suspected bacteremia, ampicillin and gentamicin or a third-generation cephalosporin is appropriate. Gram stain may be used to guide the initial choice. For patients with known or suspected resistant organisms, such as *P aeruginosa,* or for patients with urosepsis, an aminoglycoside and ceftazidime, cefepime, or ticarcillin may be started. Unit-specific data on typical bacterial species and their patterns of susceptibility should guide the antimicrobial choice for nosocomial urinary tract infections.

## Bacterial Pneumonia

Bacterial pneumonia in newborns generally should be treated the same as is sepsis. Infants and older children are frequently infected with *S pneumoniae*. Ampicillin and amoxicillin are effective in most patients eligible for outpatient therapy. Children who require hospitalization may benefit from a second- or third-generation cephalosporin. The broader initial coverage is indicated because of the greater severity of disease. A rapidly progressive pneumonia, with pneumatoceles or large pleural effusions, may be due to *S aureus* or group A streptococci, HIB, or another gram-negative rod. Oxacillin, nafcillin, or another effective antistaphylococcal agent should be used in addition to a third-generation cephalosporin.

Children age 6 years and older frequently have infection with *Mycoplasma pneumoniae, Chlamydia pneumoniae,* or *S pneumoniae*. Erythromycin, clarithromycin, or azithromycin is usually indicated for initial empiric therapy.

# ■ SPECIFIC ANTIMICROBIAL AGENTS

## PENICILLINS

### 1. Aminopenicillins

Penicillin remains the drug of choice for streptococcal infections, acute rheumatic fever prophylaxis, syphilis, oral anaerobic infections, dental infections, *N meningitidis* infection, leptospirosis, rat-bite fever, actinomycosis, and infections due to *Clostridium* and *Bacillus* species. For oral therapy of minor infections, amoxicillin or ampicillin is usually equivalent. For systemic therapy, aqueous penicillin G is preferable. Amoxicillin is preferred for oral therapy of Lyme disease in children.

For dog or cat bites, where *Pasteurella multocida* is commonly encountered, amoxicillin–clavulanate provides good coverage of *Pasteurella* as well as *Staphylococcus*. An alternative is separate prescriptions for penicillin and an antistaphylococcal drug such as cephalexin, or clindamycin and trimethoprim–sulfamethoxazole (TMP–SMX) in penicillin-allergic patients. As for human bites, amoxicillin–clavulanate provides adequate therapy for *Eikenella corrodens* and other mixed oral aerobes and anaerobes. The β-lactamase inhibitor sulbactam combined with ampicillin is given parenterally for human and animal bites, and some other infections due to organisms from the oral flora where mixed aerobic and anaerobic bacteria may be resistant to ampicillin due to β-lactamase production.

## 2. Penicillinase-Resistant Penicillins

*S aureus* is usually resistant to penicillin and amoxicillin owing to penicillinase production. Nafcillin, oxacillin, methicillin, and first- and second-generation cephalosporins are stable to penicillinase and are usually equivalent for intravenous therapy. Methicillin is associated with more frequent interstitial nephritis. Oxacillin and methicillin are renally excreted, whereas nafcillin is excreted through the biliary tract. These properties are occasionally considered in children with renal or liver failure. Cost should usually be the deciding factor for choosing an agent. Often both *S aureus* and *Streptococcus pyogenes* are suspected initially (eg, in cellulitis or postoperative wound infections). The penicillinase-resistant penicillins (PRPs) and first- and second-generation cephalosporins are efficacious for most streptococcal infections, although penicillin remains the drug of choice.

MRSA is an increasing community-acquired infection in children and may cause nosocomial infection. MRSA infections are also resistant to other PRPs and to first- and second-generation cephalosporins. Vancomycin is effective against MRSA and coagulase-negative staphylococci. *S aureus* infections range in severity from minor infections treated on an outpatient basis to life-threatening infections. However, progressively severe infections due to MRSA are a serious concern in some communities. It is important to culture and determine antimicrobial susceptibility of suspected *S aureus* infections in communities where MRSA is common. In communities with frequent MRSA infections in children, initial therapy of seriously ill children should include vancomycin. MRSA may also be resistant to macrolides and clindamycin by alteration in the bacterial 23S ribosomal RNA. Alternatively, strains with efflux mechanisms are frequently susceptible to clindamycin, but resistant to erythromycin. Inducible resistance to clindamycin may be detected in erythromycin-resistant MRSA that demonstrate a D-zone in disk susceptibility testing to clindamycin. Community-acquired MRSA are more likely to be susceptible to TMP–SMX, clindamycin and gentamicin than hospital-acquired infections.

For outpatient therapy, cloxacillin, dicloxacillin, and first- or second-generation cephalosporins are usually equally effective for infections due to susceptible *S aureus*. Cost may determine the choice between drugs.

## 3. Anti-Pseudomonas Penicillins

Ticarcillin, mezlocillin, and piperacillin are active intravenously against streptococci, ampicillin-susceptible enterococci, *H influenzae,* gram-negative rods (including more resistant gram-negative rods such as *Enterobacter, Proteus,* and *Pseudomonas aeruginosa*), and gram-negative anaerobes such as *Bacteroides fragilis. P aeruginosa* is inherently resistant to most antimicrobials, and high levels of these drugs are usually required. The combination of ticarcillin and an aminoglycoside is synergistic against *P aeruginosa* and many other enteric gram-negative rods. Ticarcillin in a fixed combination with clavulanic acid has activity against β-lactamase-producing strains of *Klebsiella, S aureus,* and *Bacteroides.* Piperacillin is more active in vitro against many gram-negative enteric infections and may be advantageous in some circumstances, but it is not approved in children. Piperacillin–tazobactam is another combination antimicrobial and β-lactamase inhibitor that has enhanced activity against many β-lactamase producers.

Antipseudomonal penicillins cause the same toxicities as penicillin and therefore are usually very safe. Carbenicillin, ticarcillin, and piperacillin contain large amounts of sodium, which may cause problems for some patients with cardiac or renal disease.

## GLYCOPEPTIDE AGENTS

Vancomycin and teicoplanin are glycopeptide antimicrobial agents active against the cell wall of gram-positive organisms. Only vancomycin is licensed in the United States. Vancomycin is useful for parenteral therapy of resistant gram-positive cocci such as penicillin- and cephalosporin-resistant *S pneumoniae*, MRSA, methicillin-resistant coagulase-negative staphylococci, and ampicillin-resistant enterococci. Vancomycin is also used orally for therapy of colitis due to *Clostridium difficile,* although it should not be used as the drug of first choice.

The empiric use of vancomycin has increased tremendously over the last several years. As a result, vancomycin-resistant enterococci (VRE) and coagulase-negative staphylococci have become problems, particularly in inpatient units, intensive care units, and oncology wards. *S aureus* with increased MICs to van-comycin has been reported in the United States and Japan. This resistance is of concern because of the in-herent virulence of many *S aureus* strains. Vancomycin use should be monitored carefully in hospitals and in their intensive care units. It should not be used empiri-cally when an infection is mild or when other antimi-crobial agents are likely to be effective. Vancomycin should be stopped promptly if infection is found to be due to organisms susceptible to other antimicrobials. Infection control guidelines for prevention of spread of VRE are published by the Centers for Disease Control and Prevention. Laboratory-based monitoring for VRE and vancomycin-resistant *S aureus* is warranted.

Rapid infusion of vancomycin is associated with the "red man syndrome," characterized by diffuse red flush-ing, at times pruritus, and occasionally tachycardia and hypotension. As a result, vancomycin is infused slowly over 1 hour or longer in some cases. Diphenhydramine or hydrocortisone (or both) may also be used as pre-medication.

Measurement of peak-and-trough serum van-comycin concentrations is not necessary in most clinical situations, because the levels achieved with standard dosing are usually predictable and nontoxic. Measure-ment of serum concentrations is helpful in patients with abnormal or unpredictable renal function; in those with altered volume of distribution, as occurs in nephrotic syndrome or shock; and in those receiving higher-dose therapy, for example, for meningitis or other difficult-to-treat infections. For patients receiving antimicrobials for weeks to months, weekly monitoring of clinical signs and symptoms and of urinalysis, creati-nine, and CBC will allow detection of toxicity.

## OXAZOLIDINONES

Linezolid is the first drug in this new class of antimicro-bials which have a distinct new mechanism of action; they bind to the 50s-ribosomal RNA subunit and pre-vent initiation of protein synthesis. Because of this unique mechanism, there is no cross-resistance with other classes of antimicrobials. The in vitro develop-ment of resistance has also been uncommon.

Linezolid is active against aerobic gram-positive or-ganisms, including streptococci, staphylococci, entero-cocci, and pneumococci. Because linezolid is active against gram-positive organisms resistant to other an-timicrobials (eg, MRSA, methicillin-resistant, coagu-lase-negative staphylococci, VRE, and penicillin-resis-tant *S pneumoniae*), it is a potentially useful rescue drug for these difficult-to-treat infections.

Linezolid is not approved for use in pediatrics, but in clinical studies has been safe and well tolerated. Gas-trointestinal symptoms are the most commonly en-countered side effect. Neutropenia and thrombocytope-nia have been reported, and linezolid should therefore be used with monitoring in patients at increased risk for these problems or in patients receiving therapy for 2 weeks or longer. Linezolid is an inhibitor of mono-anime oxidase (MAO) and should not be used with in-patients taking MAO inhibitors, or with patients taking phenylpropanolamine or pseudoephedrine.

Linezolid should be used only for infections due to a proven gram-positive pathogen that is known or strongly suspected to be resistant to other available agents.

## QUINUPRISTIN/DALFOPRISTIN

Quinupristin and dalfopristin are two antimicrobials of the streptogramin class, which individually are bacterio-static but in combination are synergistic and bacterioci-dal. These drugs are combined in a fixed ratio of 70:30, known as Synercid. Streptogramins inhibit protein syn-thesis by binding to the 50s ribosomal subunit. The streptogramins were discovered many years ago, but in-terest has increased only recently due to the activity of these agents against some very difficult-to-treat gram-positive infections.

The quinupristin/dalfopristin combination has ac-tivity against staphylococci, streptococci, pneumococci, and some enterococci. Quinupristin/dalfopristin is pri-marily indicated for serious infections due to van-comycin-resistant *Enterococcus faecium* and MRSA. Quinupristin/dalfopristin is not active against *E faecalis* and, therefore, differentiation of these strains from *E faecium* is important prior to initiating therapy.

Quinupristin/dalfopristin is not approved for ther-apy in children. Nonetheless, therapy has been initiated under a compassionate release program in some pedi-atric patients seriously ill with difficult-to-treat infec-tions due to resistant organisms.

Arthralgias and myalgias have at times been severe in adult patients. Other significant side effects include ele-vated bilirubin and inflammation at intravenous sites.

Quinupristin/dalfopristin is a significant inhibitor of P-450 3A4 and, therefore, must be used with caution in patients receiving drugs metabolized by this mecha-nism.

The use of quinupristin/dalfopristin should be lim-ited to serious infections due to proven *E faecium* or *S aureus* or infections due to proven gram-positive cocci that are resistant to other agents.

## CEPHALOSPORINS

Cephalosporin agents make up a large and often con-fusing group of antimicrobials. Many of these drugs are similar in antibacterial spectrum and side effects and may have similar names. Clinicians should learn well the properties of one or two drugs in each class. Cephalosporins are often grouped as "generations" to signify their similar antimicrobial activity. First-generation cephalosporins such as cefazolin intravenously and cephalexin orally are useful mainly for *S aureus* infection and urinary tract infection due to susceptible *E coli*. Second-generation cephalosporins, such as cefuroxime intravenously and cefprozil and cefuroxime orally, have somewhat reduced but acceptable activity against gram-positive cocci but greater activity against some gram-negative rods. They are active against *H influenzae* and *Moraxella catarrhalis*, including strains that produce β-lactamase capable of inactivating ampicillin. Third-generation cephalosporins have substantially less activity against gram-positive cocci such as *S aureus* but greatly augmented activity against aerobic gram-negative rods. Cefotaxime and ceftriaxone are examples of intravenous drugs, whereas cefpodoxime and ceftibuten are representative oral drugs. Cefepime is a new antimicrobial often described as fourth-generation because of its broad activity against gram-positive and gram-negative organisms, including *P aeruginosa*. Cefepime is stable to β-lactamase degradation and is a poor inducer of β-lactamase. Cefepime will be most useful for organisms resistant to other drugs. Cefepime is not approved for use in children younger than age 2 months.

No cephalosporin agent has substantial activity against *L monocytogenes,* enterococci, or MRSA. The only cephalosporins useful for treating anaerobic infections are cefoxitin and cefotetan, two second-generation cephalosporins with excellent activity against *B fragilis.* Ceftazidime is a third-generation cephalosporin with appreciable activity against *P aeruginosa.*

Allergy to β-lactam antimicrobials is reported commonly by parents, but the majority of children are not shown to be allergic when studied by skin test or oral challenge. Immediate hypersensitivity reactions, including anaphylaxis or hives, most commonly predict true allergy. In contrast, many delayed reactions and non-specific rashes are likely due to the underlying infection rather than allergy (see Chapter 34). Cephalosporins should be used with caution in children with immediate hypersensitivity reactions to penicillins or cephalosporins, because 10–15% will also be allergic to cephalosporins.

Cephalosporins are seldom the drug of choice for therapy of ambulatory infections, and despite their popularity they are often more expensive than other antimicrobials with similar side effects.

Resistance to cephalosporins is common among aerobic gram-negative rods. The presence of inducible cephalosporinases in the chromosome of some gram-negative rod organisms such as *P aeruginosa, Serratia marcescens, Citrobacter,* and *Enterobacter* has led to clinical failures because of the emergence of resistance during therapy. Extended spectrum β-lactamases mediate broad resistance to all β-lacatams. Many clinicians treat infections due to these organisms with a second effective drug to attempt to limit the emergence of resistant strains. Active laboratory-based surveillance is necessary to predict the usual susceptibility encountered in gram-negative infections.

## AZTREONAM

Aztreonam is the only monobactam antimicrobial agent approved in the United States. Although it is not approved for use in children, there is considerable pediatric experience with its use, including in neonates and premature infants. Aztreonam is active against aerobic gram-negative rods, including *P aeruginosa*. Aztreonam has activity against *H influenzae* and *M catarrhalis,* including those that are β-lactamase producers. Most patients with allergy to penicillin or cephalosporins are not sensitized to aztreonam, except that children with prior reactions to ceftazidime may have reactions to aztreonam because aztreonam and ceftazidime have a common side chain.

## CARBAPENEMS

Meropenem, ertapenem, and imipenem are broad-spectrum β-lactam antimicrobials. Imipenem–cilastatin is a combination of an active antibiotic and cilastatin, which inhibits the metabolism of imipenem in the kidney and thereby results in high serum and urine levels of imipenem. These carbapenems are also active against *S pneumoniae,* including many penicillin-resistant and cephalosporin-resistant strains. Carbapenems have been used successfully to treat meningitis and may be considered if vancomycin is not tolerated. An increased frequency of seizures is encountered when central nervous system infections are treated with carbapenems. These agents are broadly active against streptococci, methicillin-susceptible staphylococci, some enterococci, and gram-negative rods such as *P aeruginosa,* β-lactamase-producing *H influenzae,* and gram-negative anaerobes. Ertapenem has less activity against *P aeruginosa, Acinetobacter* sp., and *Enterococcus* sp. than meropenem and imipenem. Because carbapenems are active against so many species of bacteria, there is a strong temptation to use them as single-drug empiric therapy. Units that have used carbapenems heavily have encountered resistance in many different species of gram-negative rods. A more appropriate practice is to reserve carbapenems for patients who have infections that are unresponsive or resistant to other antimicrobial agents.

## MACROLIDES & AZILIDES

Erythromycin is the most commonly used macrolide antimicrobial agent. It is active against many bacteria that are resistant to cell wall-active antimicrobials and is the drug of choice for *Bordetella pertussis, Legionella pneumophila, Chlamydia pneumoniae, Mycoplasma pneumoniae,* and *C trachomatis* infections (in children in whom tetracycline is not an option). Erythromycin is used for outpatient therapy of streptococcal and staphylococcal infections and in patients with penicillin allergy. More serious infections due to streptococci and staphylococci are usually treated with penicillins, clindamycin, PRPs, or cephalosporins because of a significant incidence of erythromycin resistance in both species. *S pneumoniae* resistant to erythromycin and the related macrolides are now frequent in many communities. This limits the ability of macrolide antimicrobials for therapy of otitis media and sinusitis. Gastrointestinal side effects are common. Interactions with theophylline, carbamazepine, terfenadine, cycloserine, and other drugs may require dosage modifications of erythromycin and clarithromycin. Interactions with azithromycin are less common.

Erythromycin is available in many formulations, including the base, estolate, ethyl succinate, and stearate. Transient hepatic toxicity occurs in adults but is much less common in children. Erythromycin base and stearate should be taken with meals for best absorption.

Clarithromycin and azithromycin, macrolide and azilide antimicrobials, respectively, are much less likely than erythromycin to cause nausea, vomiting, and diarrhea. These agents are useful in children who cannot tolerate erythromycin. Clarithromycin is more active than erythromycin against *H influenzae, M catarrhalis,* and *N gonorrhoeae* and is the drug of choice, sometimes in combination, for some nontuberculous mycobacterial infections. Azithromycin has a prolonged tissue half-life that achieves a prolonged antimicrobial effect. Azithromycin is dosed once daily for 5 days but must be taken 1 hour before or 2 hours after meals because food interferes with absorption. Although azithromycin is active against *H influenzae,* some authors report delayed eradication of *H influenzae* from the middle ear. Azithromycin can be used for single-dose therapy of *C trachomatis* infections. It is beneficial in adolescents when compliance with erythromycin or tetracycline is a concern. Azithromycin is useful for therapy of *Shigella* and *Salmonella* infections including typhoid fever. Due to resistance of many strains to ampicillin and TMP–SMX, alternatives are needed in some cases. Cefixime is no longer available, and fluoroquinolones are not used generally in children. In these cases, azithromycin may be a useful alternative. Clarithromycin is effective against Lyme disease, but 7 days of azithromycin for that indication was inferior to amoxicillin. Clarithromycin and azithromycin are alternative drugs for toxoplasmosis in sulfonamide-allergic patients and as alternatives to erythromycin in legionellosis. In vitro and limited clinical experience in providing treatment to contacts of pertussis patients suggests efficacy equal to that of erythromycin. Clarithromycin and azithromycin are considerably more expensive than most erythromycin formulations, which for that reason are usually preferred, but they are advantageous by virtue of their twice-daily and once-daily dosing, respectively. Some failures of the newer macrolides have occurred in *S pneumoniae* sepsis and meningitis, perhaps because of low serum levels despite the high tissue levels achieved. High rates of resistance to macrolides and azilides have been encountered in some communities. The frequent use of azithromycin for respiratory infections and acute otitis media has contributed to selection of resistant strains.

## CLINDAMYCIN

Clindamycin is active against *Staphylococcus aureus, Streptococcus pyogenes,* other streptococcal species except enterococci, and both gram-positive and gram-negative anaerobes. Clindamycin or metronidazole is frequently combined with other antimicrobials for empiric therapy of suspected anaerobic or mixed anaerobic and aerobic infections. Examples are pelvic inflammatory disease, necrotizing enterocolitis, other infections in which the integrity of the gastrointestinal or genitourinary tracts is compromised, and sinusitis. Clindamycin does not achieve high levels in CSF, but brain abscesses, toxoplasmosis, and other central nervous system infections, where disruption of the blood–brain barrier occurs, may be successfully treated with clindamycin. Clindamycin may be superior for treatment of serious streptococcal infections that appear to be toxin-mediated. For the usual oral anaerobes, penicillin is more active than clindamycin. Empiric use of clindamycin is justified in suspected anaerobic infections because cultures frequently cannot be obtained and, if obtained, may be slow in confirming anaerobic infection. Clindamycin has been associated with the occurrence of pseudomembranous colitis. Although diarrhea is a frequent side effect, pseudomembranous colitis is uncommonly due to clindamycin in children.

## SULFONAMIDES

Sulfonamides—the oldest class of antimicrobials—remain useful for treatment of urinary tract infections. They are used also for other infections due to *E coli* and for *Nocardia.* Although useful for rheumatic fever prophylaxis in penicillin-allergic patients, sulfonamides fail to eradicate group A streptococci and cannot be used for treatment of acute infections.

Trimethoprim–sulfamethoxazole (TMP–SMZ) is a fixed combination that is more active than either drug alone. Gram-positive cocci, including *S pneumoniae,* many staphylococci, *Haemophilus,* and many gram-negative rods, are susceptible. Unfortunately, resistance to TMP–SMZ has developed in recent years. *S pneumoniae* resistant to penicillin and cephalosporins is often also resistant to TMP–SMZ and erythromycin. In some communities, *Shigella* and *Salmonella enteritidis* strains remain susceptible, as do most *E coli.* TMP–SMZ is therefore very useful for treatment of urinary tract infections and bacterial dysentery. TMP–SMZ is also the drug of choice for treatment or prophylaxis against *Pneumocystis jiroveci* (formerly *Pneumocystis carinii*) infection. Dermatologic and myelosuppressive side effects limit the use of TMP–SMZ in some children infected with HIV.

Sulfonamide is associated with several cutaneous reactions, including urticaria, photosensitivity, Stevens–Johnson syndrome, purpura, and maculopapular rashes. Hematologic side effects such as leukopenia, thrombocytopenia, and hemolytic anemia are uncommon. Common gastrointestinal side effects are nausea and vomiting. The dermatologic and hematologic side effects are thought to be more common and more severe with TMP–SMZ than with sulfonamide alone.

## TETRACYCLINES

Tetracyclines are effective against a broad range of bacteria but are not commonly used in children because alternative effective drugs are available. Many different tetracycline formulations are available. Tetracyclines are effective against *Bordetella pertussis* and *E coli* and many species of *Rickettsia, Chlamydia,* and *Mycoplasma.* Doxycycline or minocycline is the drug of choice for eradication of *Chlamydia trachomatis* in pelvic inflammatory disease and nongonococcal urethritis.

Staining of permanent teeth was noted in young children given repeated courses of tetracyclines. As a result, tetracyclines are generally not given to children younger than age 9 years unless alternative drugs are unavailable. A single course of tetracycline does not pose a significant risk of tooth staining. Mucous membrane candidiasis, photosensitivity, nausea, and vomiting are other common side effects. Tetracycline should be taken on an empty stomach, either 1 hour before or 2 hours after a meal. Doxycycline is well absorbed even in the presence of food; administration with food may minimize gastrointestinal side effects. Doxycycline is often preferred because it is better tolerated than tetracycline, and twice daily administration is convenient.

Tetracycline is used for therapy of rickettsial infections such as Rocky Mountain spotted fever, ehrlichiosis, rickettsialpox, murine typhus, and Q fever; as an alternative to erythromycin for *Mycoplasma pneumoniae* and *Chlamydia pneumoniae* infections; and for treatment of psittacosis, brucellosis, *Pasteurella multocida* infection, and relapsing fever.

## AMINOGLYCOSIDES

The aminoglycosides bind to ribosomal subunits and inhibit protein synthesis. They are active against aerobic gram-negative rods, including *P aeruginosa.* Streptomycin was the first drug in this class, but today it is used only to treat tuberculosis and the occasional cases of plague and tularemia.

Aminoglycosides are used to treat serious gram-negative infections and are given intravenously or intramuscularly. They are also used to treat pyelonephritis, suspected gram-negative sepsis, and in other settings where *P aeruginosa* infections are common, such as cystic fibrosis and burns. Aminoglycosides have activity against gram-positive organisms and, combined with penicillin or ampicillin, may achieve synergistic killing of *L monocytogenes* and group B streptococci. Penicillin, ampicillin, or vancomycin combined with gentamicin is indicated for therapy of serious enterococcal infections, such as sepsis or endocarditis because of more rapid clinical improvement with combined therapy. Aminoglycosides have activity against *S aureus* but are not used for therapy except in combination with other antistaphylococcal antibiotics.

Aminoglycosides are not active in an acidic environment and may not be effective against loculated abscesses. Aminoglycosides diffuse poorly into the CSF and achieve only about 10% of serum concentrations. As a result, a third-generation cephalosporin is preferred for treatment of bacillary meningitis.

Aminoglycosides kill bacteria in a concentration-dependent manner. They also have a prolonged suppressive effect on the regrowth of susceptible organisms (postantibiotic effect). These principles have led some investigators to establish guidelines for once-daily dosing of aminoglycosides, using larger initial doses given every 24 hours. Although aminoglycosides are associated with both renal and eighth nerve toxicity, the entry of the drug into renal and cochlear cells is saturable. It therefore was predicted that once-daily dosing would result in less toxicity than traditional twice-daily or three-times-daily dosing. Studies in adult patients confirm that once-daily dosing is as efficacious as traditional dosing and is associated with less toxicity. Although there is extensive experience with dosing intervals of 18–36 hours in premature babies, small total daily doses are customarily used (2–2.5 mg/kg/dose of gentamicin or tobramycin). A convenient and cost-effective approach in children is based on the experience with adult patients and uses larger daily doses (4–7 mg/kg/dose every 24 hours). Unfortunately, there is little published information on the efficacy and safety of this approach in children.

Accordingly, traditional twice-daily or three-times-daily dosing regimens of aminoglycosides, with monitoring of serum levels, are still widely used. Careful monitoring is necessary, particularly in children with abnormal or changing renal function, premature infants, and infants with rapidly changing volumes of distribution. Aminoglycosides are usually infused over 30–45 minutes, and the peak serum concentration is measured 30–45 minutes after the end of the infusion. A trough serum concentration is measured prior to the next dose. The efficacious and nontoxic serum concentrations for gentamicin and tobramycin are trough less than 2 μg/mL and peak 5–10 μg/mL; for amikacin, trough less than 10 μg/mL and peak 15–25 μg/mL (see Table 35–4). Aminoglycoside levels and creatinine levels should be measured in children expected to receive more than three days of therapy and weekly in children on long-term therapy even when renal function is normal and stable.

## FLUOROQUINOLONES

Nalidixic acid was the prototype quinolone antimicrobial, but it is not used today. Modification of the quinolone structure has led to the introduction of many new compounds called fluoroquinolones, which are well absorbed after oral administration and possess excellent antibacterial activity against resistant gram-negative pathogens. The nine currently available fluoroquinolones vary in their activity against specific organisms. Fluoroquinolones are active against most of the Enterobacteriaceae, including *Escherichia coli, Enterobacter, Klebsiella,* in some cases *P aeruginosa,* and many other gram-negative bacteria such as *H influenzae, M catarrhalis, N gonorrhoeae,* and *N meningitidis.* Some fluoroquinolones (ofloxacin, grepefloxacin) are active against *C trachomatis.* The fluoroquinolones are active against some enterococci, *S aureus,* and coagulase-negative staphylococci but not against MRSA. The newer quinolones have good activity against penicillin and cephalosporin-resistant *Streptococcus pneumoniae,* but clinical experience in children is limited.

Quinolones (except the otic and ophthalmic preparations) are currently not FDA-approved for use in children, although they often very attractive alternatives to approved agents. The objection to quinolones is based on the recognition that nalidixic acid and other quinolones cause arthropathy when used experimentally in newborn animals of many species. The fear that children would also be more susceptible than adults to cartilage injury has not been realized in clinical experience. Both retrospective long-term follow-up studies of children given nalidixic acid and prospective studies of children receiving treatment under protocols with fluoroquinolones have shown similar rates of toxicity compared with adult patients. Arthropathy occurs uncommonly, although tendon rupture is a reported rare, serious complication. For these reasons, quinolones should be considered for use in children when the benefit clearly outweighs the risk, when no alternative drug is available, and after discussion with the parents.

Ciprofloxacin is useful for oral therapy of resistant gram-negative urinary tract infections such as that caused by *P aeruginosa.* Ofloxacin, levofloxacin, ciprofloxacin, and gatifloxacin are useful for single-dose therapy of uncomplicated gonorrhea, and ofloxacin and levofloxacin are an alternative therapy for treating *Chlamydia* infections and pelvic inflammatory disease. Ciprofloxacin and ofloxacin are used as therapy of resistant cases of shigellosis. Levofloxacin and ciprofloxacin are usually the drugs of choice for treatment of traveler's diarrhea. Ciprofloxacin is useful for treatment of *P aeruginosa* infection in cystic fibrosis patients, and as therapy for chronic suppurative otitis media. Several quinolones are used as therapy for pneumonia due to *Legionella, Mycoplasma,* or *Chlamydia pneumoniae,* although a macrolide is often preferred, and as prophylactic therapy of meningococcal infection. Ofloxacin and levofloxacin are used for treatment of some cases of *Mycobacterium tuberculosis* and some atypical mycobacterial infections.

## METRONIDAZOLE

Metronidazole has excellent activity against most anaerobes, particularly gram-negative anaerobes such as *Bacteroides* and *Fusobacterium,* and against gram-positive anaerobes such as *Clostridium, Prevotella,* and *Porphyromonas.* Gram-positive anaerobic cocci such as *Peptococcus* and *Peptostreptococcus* are often more susceptible to penicillin or to clindamycin. Because metronidazole lacks activity against aerobic organisms, it is usually given with one or more other antibiotics. Metronidazole is well absorbed after oral administration and has excellent penetration into the central nervous system. Metronidazole is the drug of choice for bacterial vaginosis and for *C difficile* enterocolitis. It is active against many parasites, including *Giardia lamblia* and *Entamoeba histolytica.*

## DAPTOMYCIN

Daptomycin is a newly FDA-approved antimicrobial with bactericidal activity against gram-positive cocci.

Daptomycin is a lipopeptide that binds to bacterial cell membranes, resulting in membrane depolarization and cell death. Daptomycin is active against methicillin-sensitive and -resistant *Staphylococcus aureus, Streptococcus pyogenes,* and *Streptococcus agalactiae,* as well as *E faecium* (including vancomycin-resistant strains), and *E faecalis* (vancomycin-sensitive strains). Daptomycin is given as a once-daily intravenous infusion of 4 mg/kg, and is approved for therapy of complicated skin and soft tissue infections, but has not been sufficiently studied in children younger than 18 years to make recommendations for dosing and use. Daptomycin is excreted renally, so a modification of dosing is needed in patients with impaired renal function. It has significant interactions with aminoglycosides, so monitoring serum concentrations of aminoglycosides is necessary. Nausea, constipation, and headache are the most common side effects of therapy. In patients with muscle pain, monitoring creatinine phosphokinase (CPK) levels should be done.

## REFERENCES

Bradley JS, Nelson JB: *Nelson's Pocketbook of Pediatric Antimicrobial Therapy,* 15th ed. Lippincott, William & Williams, 2002.

Daum RS, Seal JB: Evolving antimicrobial chemotherapy for Staphylococcus aureus infections: Our backs to the wall. Crit Care Med 2001;29:S92 [PMID: 11292882].

Gilbert DN et al: *The Sanford Guide to Antimicrobial Therapy,* 33rd ed., 2003. Jeb C. Sanford Publiisher, Antimicrobial Therppy, Inc. Hyde Park, NY.

Kaplan SL et al: Linezolid versus vancomycin for treatment of resistant gram-positive infections in children. Pediatr Infect Dis J 2003;22(8):677 [PMID: 12913766].

Mainous AG 3rd et al: Trends in antimicrobial prescribing for bronchitis and upper respiratory infections among adults and children. Am J Public Health 2003;93(11):1910 [PMID 14600065].

Paterson DL et al: Outcome of cephalosporin treatment for serious infectious due to apparently susceptible organisms producing extended-spectrum beta-lactamases: Implications for the clinical microbiology laboratory. J Clin Microbiol 2001;39:2206 [PMID: 11376058].

Saiman L et al: Safety and tolerability of linezolid in children. Pediatr Infect Dis J 2003;22(9 Suppl):S193 [PMID: 14520146].

### Websites

http://www.cdc.gov/drugresistance
http://www.cdc.gov/ncidod/guidelines/guidelines_topic_ar.htm
http://www.tufts.edu/med/apua/index.html

# Infections: Viral & Rickettsial

**36**

*Myron J. Levin, MD, & Adriana Weinberg, MD*

## ▌ I. VIRAL INFECTIONS

Viruses cause most pediatric infections. Mixed viral or viral–bacterial infections of the respiratory and intestinal tracts are rather common, as is prolonged asymptomatic shedding of some viruses in childhood. Thus the detection of a virus is not always proof that it is the cause of a given illness. Viruses are often a predisposing factor for bacterial respiratory infections (eg, otitis, sinusitis, and pneumonia).

Many respiratory and herpes viruses can now be detected within 24–48 hours by combining culture and monoclonal antibody techniques ("rapid culture technique"). Diagnosis of many viral illnesses is also possible through antigen or nucleic acid detection techniques. These techniques are more rapid than isolation of viruses in tissue culture and in many cases are equally sensitive or more so. Polymerase chain reaction (PCR) amplification of viral genes has led to recognition of previously undetected infections. New diagnostic tests have changed some basic concepts about viral diseases and made diagnosis of viral infections both more certain and more complex. Only laboratories with excellent quality-control procedures should be used, and the results of new tests must be interpreted cautiously. The availability of specific antiviral agents increases the value of early diagnosis for some serious viral infections. Table 36–1 lists viral agents associated with common clinical signs, and Table 36–2 lists diagnostic tests. The viral diagnostic laboratory should be contacted for details regarding specimen collection, handling, and shipping. Table 36–3 lists common causes of red rashes in children that should be considered in the differential diagnosis of certain viral illnesses.

## RESPIRATORY INFECTIONS

Many virus infections cause upper or lower respiratory tract signs and symptoms. Those that produce a predominance of these signs and symptoms are described in the text that follows. Many so-called respiratory viruses can also produce distinct nonrespiratory disease (eg, enteritis or cystitis caused by adenoviruses; parotitis caused by parainfluenza viruses). Respiratory viruses can cause disease in any area of the respiratory tree. Thus they can cause coryza, pharyngitis, sinusitis, tracheitis, bronchitis, bronchiolitis, and pneumonia—although certain viruses tend to be closely associated with one anatomic area (eg, parainfluenza with croup, respiratory syncytial virus [RSV] with bronchiolitis) or discrete epidemics (eg, influenza, RSV, parainfluenza). Nevertheless it is impossible on clinical grounds to be certain of the viral cause of an infection in a given child. This information is provided by the virology laboratory and is often important for epidemiologic, therapeutic, and preventive reasons.

## VIRUSES CAUSING THE COMMON COLD

The common cold syndrome (also called upper respiratory infection) is characterized by combinations of runny nose, nasal congestion, sore throat, tearing, cough, and sneezing. Low-grade fever may be present. The causal agent is usually not sought or determined. Epidemiologic studies indicate that rhinoviruses, which are the most common cause (30–40%), are present throughout the year, but are more prevalent in the colder months in temperate climates. Adenoviruses also cause colds in all seasons, but epidemics are common. Respiratory syncytial, parainfluenza, and influenza viruses cause the cold syndrome during epidemics from late fall through winter. Coronaviruses ($\approx$10%) also cause colds in winter, and enteroviruses cause the "summer cold." One significance of these infections is morbidity continuing for 5–7 days. It is likely also that changes in respiratory epithelium, local obstruction, and altered local immunity are sometimes the precursors of more severe illnesses such as otitis media, pneumonia, and sinusitis. During and following a cold the bacterial flora changes, and bacteria are found in normally sterile areas of the upper airway. Asthma attacks are also provoked by viruses that cause the common cold. There is no evidence that antibiotics will prevent these complications, and the unjustified widespread use of antibiotics for cold symptoms has contributed to the emergence of antibiotic-resistant respiratory flora.

In 5–10% of children, symptoms from these virus infections persist for more than 10 days. This overlap

***Table 36–1.*** Some viral causes of clinical syndromes.

**Rash**
- Enterovirus
- Adenovirus
- Measles
- Rubella
- Human herpes virus type 6[a] or 7
- Varicella
- Parvovirus B19[b]
- Epstein–Barr virus
- Dengue
- Human immunodeficiency virus (acute syndrome)

**Fever**
- Enterovirus
- Epstein–Barr virus
- Human herpes virus type 6[a] or 7
- Cytomegalovirus
- Influenza
- Rhinovirus
- Most others

**Conjunctivitis**
- Adenovirus
- Enterovirus 70
- Measles
- Herpes simplex[c]

**Parotitis**
- Mumps
- Parainfluenza
- Enterovirus
- Cytomegalovirus
- Epstein–Barr virus
- Human immunodeficiency virus

**Pharyngitis**
- Adenovirus
- Enterovirus
- Epstein–Barr virus
- Herpes simplex virus[d]
- Influenza
- Other respiratory viruses

**Adenopathy**
- Epstein–Barr virus
- Cytomegalovirus
- Rubella[e]
- Human immunodeficiency virus

**Croup**
- Parainfluenza
- Influenza
- Adenovirus
- Measles

**Bronchiolitis**
- Respiratory syncytial virus[f]
- Adenovirus
- Parainfluenza
- Influenza

**Pneumonia**
- Respiratory syncytial virus
- Adenovirus
- Parainfluenza
- Hantavirus
- Measles
- Varicella[h]
- Cytomegalovirus[g,i]
- Influenza
- Severe acute respiratory syndrome (SARS)

**Enteritis**
- Rotavirus
- Enteric adenovirus
- Enterovirus
- Astrovirus
- Calicivirus
- Cytomegalovirus

**Hepatitis**
- Hepatitis A,[j] B, C, D, E
- Epstein–Barr virus
- Adenovirus
- Cytomegalovirus
- Varicella[k]
- Parvovirus B19

**Arthritis**
- Parvovirus B19
- Rubella
- Hepatitis B

**Congenital or perinatal infection**
- Adenovirus
- Cytomegalovirus
- Hepatitis B
- Hepatitis C[l]
- Rubella
- Human immunodeficiency virus
- Parvovirus B19
- Enterovirus
- Varicella
- Herpes simplex virus

**Meningoencephalitis**
- Enterovirus
- Mumps
- Arthropod-borne viruses
- Herpes simplex virus
- Cytomegalovirus
- Lymphocytic choriomeningitis virus
- Measles
- Varicella
- Adenovirus
- Human immunodeficiency virus
- Epstein–Barr virus
- Influenza
- West Nile virus

[a]Roseola agent.
[b]Erythema infectiosum agent.
[c]Conjunctivitis rare, only in primary infections; keratitis in older patients.
[d]May cause isolated pharyngeal vesicles at any age.
[e]May cause adenopathy without rash.
[f]Over 70% of cases.
[g]Usually only in young infants.
[h]Immunosuppressed, pregnant, rarely other adults.
[i]Severely immunosuppressed at risk.
[j]Anicteric cases more common in children; these may resemble viral gastroenteritis.
[k]Common, but only mild laboratory abnormalities.
[l]Especially when the mother is HIV-positive.

**Table 36–2.** Diagnostic tests for viral infections.

| Agent | Rapid Antigen Detection (Specimen) | Tissue Culture Mean Days to Positive (Range) | Acute | Paired | PCR[a] | Comments |
|---|---|---|---|---|---|---|
| Adenovirus | + (respiratory and enteric) | 10 (1–21) | – | + | + | "Enteric" strains detected by culture on special cell line, antigen detection, or PCR |
| Arboviruses | – | – | + | + | RL | Acute serum may diagnose many forms |
| Astrovirus | – | – | – | – | RL | Diagnosis by electron microscopy |
| Calicivirus | – | – | – | – | RL | Diagnosis by electron microscopy |
| Colorado tick virus | On RBC | – | – | RL, CDC | + | |
| Cytomegalovirus | + (tissue biopsy, blood, respiratory secretions) | 2 (2–28) | + | + | + | Diagnosis also by presence of IgM antibody |
| Enterovirus | – | 2 (2–14) | – | + | + | |
| Epstein–Barr virus | – | – | + | + | + | Single serologic panel defines infection status; heterophil antibodies less sensitive |
| Hantavirus | – | – | + | ND | RL | Diagnosis by presence of IgM antibody |
| Hepatitis A virus | – | – | + | ND | RL | Diagnosis by presence of IgM antibody |
| Hepatitis B virus | + (blood) | – | + | ND | + | Diagnosis by presence of surface antigen or anti-core IgM antibody |
| Hepatitis C virus | – | – | + | ND | + | Postitive serology suggests that hepatitis C may be the causative agent. PCR is confirmatory |
| Herpes simplex virus | + (mucosa, tissue biopsy, respiratory secretions skin) | 1 (1–7) | + | + | + | Serology rarely used for herpes simplex. IgM antibody used in selected cases |
| Human herpes-virus-6 | – | 2 | + | + | + | Roseola agent |
| Human immuno-deficiency virus | + (blood) (acid dissociation of immune complexes) | 15 (5–28) | + | ND | + | Antibody proves infection unless passively acquired (< age 15 mos); culture not widely available; PCR definitive for early diagnosis in infant |
| Human meta-pneumovirus | – | RL | – | + | + | |
| Influenza virus | + (respiratory secretions) | 2 (2–14) | – | + | + | Antigen detection 70–90% sensitive |
| Lymphocytic choriomeningitis virus | – | – | – | + | RL | Can be isolated in suckling mice |
| Measles virus | + (respiratory secretions) | – | + | + | RL | Difficult to grow; IgM serology diagnostic |
| Mumps virus | – | > 5 | + | + | RL | Complement fixation titers may allow single-specimen diagnosis |
| Parvovirus B19 | – | – | + | ND | + | Erythema infectiosum agent |

(continued)

***Table 36–2.*** Diagnostic tests for viral infections. (continued)

| Agent | Rapid Antigen Detection (Specimen) | Tissue Culture Mean Days to Positive (Range) | Acute | Paired | PCR[a] | Comments |
|---|---|---|---|---|---|---|
| Parainfluenza virus | + (respiratory secretions) | 2 (2–14) | – | + | + | |
| Rabies virus | + (skin, conjunctiva, tissue biopsy | – | + | + | CDC | Usually diagnosed by antigen detection |
| Respiratory syncytial virus | + (respiratory secretions) | 2 (2–21) | – | + | + | Rapid antigen detection; 90% sensitive |
| Rhinovirus | – | 4 (2–7) | – | – | RL | Too many strains to type serologically |
| Rotavirus | + (feces) | – | – | – | RL | Electron microscopy useful for many enteric viruses |
| Rubella virus | – | > 10 | + | + | RL | Recommended that paired sera be tested simultaneously |
| SARS coronavirus | — | RL | RL | RL | + | |
| Varicella-zoster virus | + (skin scraping) | 3 (3–21) | RL | + | + | |
| West Nile virus | — | RL | + | + | + | |

[a]Useful only when performed on selected specimens by qualified laboratories.

**Key:**

> **Plus signs** signify commercially or widely available; **minus signs** signify not commercially available. ***Note:*** Results from some commercial laboratories are unreliable.
>
> **RL, CDC:** Specific antibody titers or PCR available by arrangement with individual research laboratories or the Centers for Disease Control and Prevention.
>
> **ND:** Not done.

RBC = red blood cell; PCR = polymerase chain reaction.

with the symptoms of bacterial sinusitis presents a difficult problem for clinicians, especially because colds can produce an abnormal computed tomography (CT) scan of the sinuses. Viruses that cause a minor illness in immunocompetent children, such as rhinoviruses, can cause severe lower respiratory disease in immunologically or anatomically compromised children.

There is no evidence that symptomatic relief for children can be achieved with oral antihistamines, decongestants, or cough suppressants. Topical decongestants provide temporary improvement in nasal symptoms.

Cohen L, Castro M: The role of viral respiratory infections in the pathogenesis and exacerbation of asthma. Semin Resp Infect 2003;18:3 [PMID: 22539104].

Greenberg SB: Respiratory consequences of rhinovirus infection. Arch Intern Med 2003;278:278 [PMID: 22466407].

Gwaltney JM Jr: Nose blowing propels nasal fluid into the paranasal sinuses. Clin Infect Dis 2000;30:387 [PMID: 10671347].

Heikkinen T, Jarvinen A: The common cold. Lancet 2003; 361:51 [PMID: 22406053].

Sutter AI et al: Antihistamines for the common cold. Cochrane Database Syst Rev 2003;CD001267 [PMID: 22698575].

Taverner D et al: Nasal decongestants for the common cold. Cochrane Database Syst Rev 2000;(2): CD001953 [PMID: 10796673].

## INFECTIONS DUE TO ADENOVIRUSES

There are over 50 types of adenoviruses, which account for 5–10% of all respiratory illnesses in childhood, usually pharyngitis or tracheitis. Adenoviral infections are common early in life. Enteric adenoviruses are an important cause of childhood diarrhea. Epidemic respiratory disease occurs in winter and spring, especially in closed environments such as day care centers and institutions. Because of latent infection in lymphoid tissue, asymptomatic shedding from the respiratory or intestinal tract is common.

**Table 36–3.** Red rashes in children.

| Condition | Incubation Period (Days) | Prodrome | Rash | Laboratory Tests | Comments, Other Diagnostic Features |
|---|---|---|---|---|---|
| Adenovirus | 4–5 | URI; cough; fever | Morbilliform (may be petechial) | Normal; may see leukopenia or lymphocytosis | Respiratory symptoms are prominent. No Koplik spots. No desquamation |
| Measles | 9–14 | Cough, rhinitis, conjunctivitis | Maculopapular; face to trunk; lasts 7–10 d; Koplik spots in mouth | Leukopenia | Toxic. Bright red rash becomes confluent, may desquamate. Fever falls after rash appears. |
| Rubella | 14–21 | Usually none | Mild maculopapular; rapid spread face to extremities; gone by day 4 | Normal or leukopenia | Postauricular, occipital adenopathy common. Polyarthralgia in some older girls. Mild clinical illness. |
| Roseola (exanthem subitum) | 10–14 | Fever (3–4 d) | Pink, macular rash occurs at end of illness; transient | Normal | Fever often high; disappears when rash develops; child appears well. Usually occurs in children 6 mos to 2 y of age. Seizures may complicate. |
| Erythema infectiosum | 13–18 | None | Erythematous "slapped" cheeks; then reticular rash on extremities, trunk | Normal (reticulocytopenia) | Rash may reappear over weeks, especially with exposure to heat, sunlight. May cause arthralgia/arthritis, usually in older children or adults. Red cell maturation arrest in children with chronic hemolysis can cause aplastic crisis. |
| Enterovirus | 2–7 | Variable fever, chills, myalgia, sore throat | Usually macular, maculopapular on trunk or palms, soles; vesicles or petechiae also seen | Variable | Varied rashes may resemble those of many other infections. Pharyngeal or hand-foot-mouth vesicles may occur. |
| Streptococcal scarlet fever | 1–7 | Fever, abdominal pain, headache, sore throat | Diffuse erythema, "sandpaper" texture; neck, axillae, inguinal areas; spreads to rest of body; desquamates 7–14 d | Leukocytosis; positive group A streptococcus culture of throat or wound; positive streptococcal antigen test in pharynx | Strawberry tongue, red pharynx with or without exudate. Eyes, perioral and periorbital area, palms, and soles spared. Pastia's lines. Brief prodrome. Cervical adenopathy. Usually occurs in children 2–10 y of age. |
| Staphylococcal scarlet fever | 1–7 | Variable fever | Diffuse erythroderma; resembles streptococcal scarlet fever except eyes may be hyperemic, no "strawberry" tongue, pharynx spared | Variable leukocytosis if infected | Focal infection usually present. |

*(continued)*

| Disease | | Symptoms | Rash | Laboratory findings | Comments |
|---|---|---|---|---|---|
| Staphylococcal scalded skin | Variable | Irritability, absent to low fever | Painful erythroderma, followed in 1–2 d by cracking around eyes, mouth; bullae form with friction (Nikolsky sign) | Normal if only colonized by staphylococci; leukocytosis and sometimes bacteremia if infected | Normal pharynx. Look for focal staphylococcal infection. Usually occurs in infants. |
| Toxic shock syndrome | Variable | Fever, myalgia, headache, diarrhea, vomiting | Nontender erythroderma; red eyes, palms, soles, pharynx, lips | Leukocytosis; abnormal liver enzymes, coagulation tests; proteinuria | Staphylococcus aureus infection; toxin-mediated multiorgan involvement. Swollen hands, feet. Hypotension or shock. |
| Erythema multiforme | — | Usually none or related to underlying cause | Discrete, red maculopapular lesions; symmetrical, distal, palms and soles; target lesions classic | Normal or eosinophilia | Reaction to drugs (especially sulfonamides), or infectious agents (mycoplasma; herpes simplex virus). Urticaria, arthralgia also seen. |
| Stevens-Johnson syndrome | — | Pharyngitis, conjunctivitis, fever, malaise | Bullous erythema multiforme; may slough in large areas; hemorrhagic lips; purulent conjunctivitis | Leukocytosis | Classic precipitants are drugs (especially sulfonamides), *Mycoplasma pneumoniae* and herpes simplex infections. Pneumonitis and urethritis also seen. |
| Drug allergy | — | None, or fever alone, or with myalgia, pruritus | Macular, maculopapular, urticarial, or erythroderma | Leukopenia, eosinophilia | Rash variable. Severe reactions may resemble measles, scarlet fever; Kawasaki disease; marked toxicity possible. |
| Kawasaki disease | Unknown | Fever, cervical adenopathy, irritability | Polymorphous (may be erythroderma) on trunk and extremities; red palms and soles, conjunctiva, lips, tongue, pharynx. Desquamation is common | Leukocytosis, thrombocytosis, elevated ESR or C-reactive protein; pyuria; decreased albumin; negative cultures and streptococcal serology; resting tachycardia | Swollen hands, feet; prolonged illness; uveitis; aseptic meningitis; no response to antibiotics. Vasculitis and aneurysms of coronary and other arteries occur (cardiac ultrasound). |
| Leptospirosis | 4–19 | Fever (biphasic), myalgia, chills | Variable erythroderma | Leukocytosis; hematuria, proteinuria; hyperbilirubinemia | Conjunctivitis; hepatitis, aseptic meningitis may be seen. Rodent, dog contact. |

URI = upper respiratory infection; ESR = erythrocyte sedimentation rate.

## Specific Adenoviral Syndromes

### A. PHARYNGITIS

Pharyngitis is the most common adenoviral disease in children. Fever and adenopathy are common. Tonsillitis may be exudative. Rhinitis and an influenza-like systemic illness may be present. Laryngotracheitis or bronchitis may accompany pharyngitis.

### B. PHARYNGOCONJUNCTIVAL FEVER

Conjunctivitis may occur alone and be prolonged, but most often is associated with preauricular adenopathy, fever, pharyngitis, and cervical adenopathy. Foreign body sensation and other symptoms last less than a week. Lower respiratory symptoms are uncommon.

### C. EPIDEMIC KERATOCONJUNCTIVITIS

Symptoms are severe conjunctivitis with punctate keratitis and occasionally visual impairment. A foreign body sensation, photophobia, and swelling of conjunctiva and eyelids are characteristic. Preauricular adenopathy and subconjunctival hemorrhage are common.

### D. PNEUMONIA

Severe pneumonia may occur at all ages. It is especially common in young children (< age 3 years). Chest radiographs show bilateral peribronchial and patchy ground-glass interstitial infiltrates in the lower lobes. Symptoms persist for 2–4 weeks. Adenoviral pneumonia can be necrotizing and cause permanent lung damage, especially bronchiectasis. A pertussis-like syndrome with typical cough and lymphocytosis can occur with lower respiratory tract infection.

### E. RASH

A diffuse morbilliform (rarely petechial) rash resembling measles, rubella, or roseola may be present. Koplik spots are absent.

### F. DIARRHEA

Enteric adenoviruses (types 40 and 41) cause 3–5% of cases of short-lived diarrhea in afebrile children.

### G. MESENTERIC LYMPHADENITIS

Fever and abdominal pain may mimic appendicitis. Pharyngitis is often associated. Adenovirus-induced adenopathy may be a factor in appendicitis and intussusception.

### H. OTHER SYNDROMES

Immunosuppressed patients, including neonates, may develop severe or fatal pulmonary or gastrointestinal infections or multisystem disease. Other rare complications include encephalitis, hepatitis, and myocarditis. Adenoviruses have been implicated in the syndrome of idiopathic myocardiopathy. Hemorrhagic cystitis can be a serious problem in immunocompromised children.

## Diagnosis

Diagnosis is by culture of conjunctival, respiratory, or stool specimens. Several days to weeks are required for growth in conventional cultures. Viral culture using the rapid culture technique with immunodiagnostic reagents detects virus in 48 hours. Adenovirus infection can also be diagnosed using these reagents directly on respiratory secretions. This is quicker but less sensitive than the culture methods. PCR has now become an important, relatively rapid diagnostic method for adenovirus infections. Special cells are needed to isolate enteric adenoviruses. Enzyme-linked immunosorbent assay (ELISA) tests rapidly detect enteric adenoviruses in diarrheal specimens. Respiratory adenovirus infections can be detected retrospectively by comparing acute and convalescent sera, but this is not helpful during an acute illness.

## Treatment

There is no specific treatment for adenovirus infections. Intravenous immune globulin (IVIG) may be tried in immunocompromised patients with severe pneumonia. There are anecdotal reports of successful treatment of immunocompromised patients with ribavirin or cidofovir, but only cidofovir inhibits adenovirus in vitro.

Chuang YY et al: Severe adenovirus infection in children. J Microbiol Immunol Infect 2003;36:37 [PMID: 22626563].

Rieger-Fackeldey et al: Disseminated adenovirus infection in two premature infants. Infection 2000;28:237 [PMID: 10961532].

## INFLUENZA

Symptomatic infections are common in children because they lack immunologic experience with influenza viruses. Infection rates in children are greater than in adults and are instrumental in initiating community outbreaks. Three main types of influenza viruses (A/H1N1, A/H3N2, B) have caused most human epidemics, with the antigenic drift ensuring a supply of susceptible hosts of all ages. Recently, avian influenza A/H5N1 caused human outbreaks in Asia. Epidemics occur in fall and winter.

## Clinical Findings

Spread of influenza occurs by way of airborne respiratory secretions. The incubation period is 2–7 days.

## A. Symptoms and Signs

Influenza infection in older children and adults produces a characteristic syndrome of sudden onset of high fever, severe myalgia, headache, and chills. These symptoms overshadow the associated coryza, pharyngitis, and cough. Usually absent are rash, marked conjunctivitis, adenopathy, exudative pharyngitis, and dehydrating enteritis. Fever, diarrhea, vomiting, and abdominal pain are common in young children. Infants may develop a sepsis-like illness and apnea. Chest examination is usually unremarkable. Unusual clinical findings or variants include croup (most severe with type A influenza), exacerbation of asthma, myositis (especially calf muscles), myocarditis, parotitis, encephalopathy (distinct from Reye syndrome), nephritis, and a transient maculopapular rash. Acute illness lasts 2–5 days. Cough and fatigue may last several weeks. Viral shedding may persist for several weeks in young children.

## B. Laboratory Findings

The leukocyte count is normal to low, with variable shift. Influenza infections may be more difficult to recognize in children than in adults even during epidemics, and therefore a specific laboratory test is highly recommended. The virus may be found in respiratory secretions by direct fluorescent antibody staining of nasopharyngeal epithelial cells, ELISA, optic immunoassay (OIA), or PCR. It can also be cultured within 3–7 days from pharyngeal swabs or throat washings. Many laboratories use the rapid culture technique by centrifuging specimens onto cultured cell layers and detecting viral antigen after 48 hours. Other body fluids or tissues (except lung) rarely yield the virus in culture and are more appropriately tested by PCR, which, due to its high sensitivity, can increase influenza detection in respiratory specimens. A late diagnosis may be made with paired serology, using hemagglutination inhibition assays.

## C. Imaging

The chest radiograph is nonspecific; it may show hyperaeration, peribronchial thickening, diffuse interstitial infiltrates, or bronchopneumonia in severe cases. Hilar nodes are not enlarged. Pleural effusion is rare in uncomplicated influenza.

## Differential Diagnosis

The following may be considered: all other respiratory viruses, *Mycoplasma pneumoniae* or *Chlamydia pneumoniae* (longer incubation period, prolonged illness), streptococcal pharyngitis (pharyngeal exudate or petechiae, adenitis, no cough), bacterial sepsis (petechial or purpuric rash may occur), toxic shock syndrome (rash, hypotension), and rickettsial infections (rash, different season, insect exposure). High fever, the nature of preceding or concurrent illness in family members, and the presence of influenza in the community are distinguishing features from parainfluenza or respiratory syncytial virus infections.

## Complications & Sequelae

Lower respiratory tract symptoms are most common in children younger than age 5 years. Hospitalization rates are highest in children younger than 2 years. Influenza can cause croup in these children. Secondary bacterial infections (classically staphylococcal) of the middle ear, sinuses, or lungs are most common. Of the viral infections that precede Reye syndrome, varicella and influenza (usually type B) are most notable. During an influenza outbreak, ill children who develop protracted vomiting or irrational behavior should be evaluated for Reye syndrome (see Chapter 20). Influenza can also cause a viral or postviral encephalitis, with cerebral symptoms much more prominent than those of the accompanying respiratory infection. Although the myositis is usually mild and resolves promptly, severe rhabdomyolysis and renal failure have been reported.

Children with underlying cardiopulmonary, metabolic, neuromuscular, or immunosuppressive disease may develop severe viral pneumonia.

## Prevention

The inactivated influenza vaccine, which has been commercially available for many years, is moderately protective in older children (see Chapter 9). A new, live-attenuated influenza vaccine (Flumist), significantly more immunogenic in children, has been recently approved by the US Food and Drug Administration for use in immunocompetent children 5 years of age or older. All children between 6 and 23 months of age or those at high risk of developing severe complications should be immunized. Medical staff and family members should also be immunized to protect high-risk patients. Type A infections may be prevented by amantadine or rimantadine (5 mg/kg; maximum 150 mg/d < age 10 years; 200 mg/d if older). Amantadine is divided into two daily doses; rimantadine can be given in a single dose. Both influenza A and B can be prevented with the neuraminidase inhibitors zanamivir (2 inhalations bid if > 7 years of age) and oseltamivir (if child < 15 kg, 30 mg bid; 15–23 kg, 45 mg bid; 23–40 kg, 60 mg bid; > 40 kg, 75 mg bid). For outbreak prophylaxis, therapy should be maintained for 2 weeks or more and 1 week after the last case of influenza is diagnosed. Chemoprophylaxis should be considered during an epidemic for high-risk children who cannot be immunized or who have not yet developed immunity (about 6 weeks after primary vaccination or 2 weeks after a booster dose).

## Treatment & Prognosis

Treatment consists of general support and management of pulmonary complications, especially bacterial super-infections. Antivirals are of some benefit in immuno-competent hosts if begun within 48 hours after onset. Studies in lung transplant patients indicate that oseltamivir might be useful for treatment of influenza in this immunocompromised population. Resistance to amantadine and rimantadine develops within a couple of days of treatment. In contrast, neuraminidase inhibitors rarely select resistant isolates.

Recovery is usually complete unless severe cardiopulmonary or neurologic damage has occurred. Fatal cases occur in immunodeficient and anatomically compromised children.

Effective treatment or prophylaxis of influenza in children markedly reduces the incidence of acute otitis media and antibiotic usage during the flu season.

Advisory Committee on Immunization Practices (Centers for Disease Control and Prevention): Prevention and control of influenza. MMWR Morb Mortal Wkly Rep 2003;52:RR-8 (RR-4):1 [PMID: 12755288].

Peltola V et al: Influenza A and B virus infection in children. Clin Infect Dis 2003;36:299 [PMID: 12539071].

Steininger C et al: Acute encephalopathy associated with influenza A virus infections. Clin Infect Dis 2003;36: 567 [PMID: 12594636].

## PARAINFLUENZA

Parainfluenza viruses (types 1–4) are the most important cause of croup. Most infants are infected with type 3 within the first 3 years of life, often in the first year. Infection with types 1 and 2 is experienced gradually over the first 5 years of life. Types 1 and 2 occur in the fall; type 3 appears annually, with a peak in the spring or summer. Most primary infections are symptomatic and frequently involve the lower respiratory tract.

## Clinical Findings

### A. SYMPTOMS AND SIGNS

Clinical diseases include febrile upper respiratory infection (especially in older children with re-exposure), laryngitis, tracheobronchitis, croup, and bronchiolitis (second most common cause after respiratory syncytial virus). The relative incidence of these manifestations is type-specific. Parainfluenza viruses (especially type 1) cause 65% of cases of croup in young children, 25% of tracheobronchitis, and 50% of laryngitis. Types 1 and 2 are more likely to cause bronchiolitis. Pneumonia oc-

curs in infants and immunodeficient children, and it leads to particularly high mortality among stem cell recipients. Onset is acute. Most children are febrile. Symptoms of upper respiratory tract infection often accompany croup.

### B. LABORATORY FINDINGS

Diagnosis is often based on clinical findings. These viruses can be identified by conventional or rapid culture techniques (48 hours), by direct immunofluorescence on nasopharyngeal epithelial cells in respiratory secretions (< 3 hours), or by PCR (< 48 hours).

## Differential Diagnosis

Parainfluenza-induced respiratory syndromes are difficult to distinguish from those caused by other respiratory viruses. Croup must be distinguished from epiglottitis caused by *Haemophilus influenzae* (abrupt onset, toxicity, drooling, dyspnea, little cough, left shift of blood smear, and a history of inadequate immunization).

## Treatment

No specific therapy or vaccine is available. Croup management is discussed in Chapter 18. Ribavirin is active in vitro and has been used in immunocompromised children, but its efficacy is unproved.

Elizaga J et al: Parainfluenza virus 3 infection after stem cell transplant: Relevance to outcome of rapid diagnosis and ribavirin treatment. Clin Infect Dis 2001;32:413 [PMID: 11170949].

Mahdi SA et al. Severe lower respiratory tract infections associated with human parainfluenza viruses 1–3 in children infected and noninfected with HIV type 1. Eur J Clin Microbiol Infect Dis 2002;21:499 [PMID: 12172740].

Peltola V et al: Clinical courses of croup caused by influenza and parainfluenza viruses. Pediatr Infect Dis J 2002;21:76 [PMID: 11791108].

## RESPIRATORY SYNCYTIAL VIRUS DISEASE

### ESSENTIALS OF DIAGNOSIS & TYPICAL FEATURES

- *Diffuse wheezing and tachypnea following upper respiratory symptoms in an infant (bronchiolitis).*
- *Epidemics in late fall to early spring (January–February peak).*
- *Hyperinflation on chest radiograph.*
- *RSV antigen detected in nasal secretions.*

## General Considerations

RSV is the most important cause of lower respiratory tract illness in young children, accounting for more than 70% of cases of bronchiolitis and 40% of cases of pneumonia. Outbreaks occur annually, and attack rates are high; 60% of children are infected in the first year of life, and 90% by age 2 years. During peak season (cold weather in temperate climates), the clinical diagnosis of RSV infection in infants with bronchiolitis is as accurate as most laboratory tests. Despite the presence of serum antibody, reinfection is common. Distinct genotypes predominate in a community. Yearly shift in these is a partial explanation for reinfection. However, reinfection generally causes only upper respiratory symptoms in anatomically normal children. No vaccine is available. Immunosuppressed patients may develop progressive severe pneumonia. Children with congenital heart disease with increased pulmonary blood flow, children with chronic lung disease (eg, cystic fibrosis), and premature infants younger than age 6 months are also at higher risk for severe illness.

## Clinical Findings

### A. SYMPTOMS AND SIGNS

Initial symptoms are those of upper respiratory infection. Low-grade fever may be present. The classic disease is bronchiolitis, characterized by diffuse wheezing, variable fever, cough, tachypnea, difficulty feeding, and, in severe cases, cyanosis. Hyperinflation, crackles, prolonged expiration, wheezing, and retractions are present. The liver and spleen may be palpable because of lung hyperinflation but are not enlarged. The disease usually lasts 3–7 days in previously healthy children. Fever is present for 2–4 days; it does not correlate with pulmonary symptoms and may be absent during the height of lung involvement.

Apnea may be the presenting manifestation, especially in premature infants, in the first few months of life; it usually resolves after a few days, often being replaced by obvious signs of bronchiolitis. No explanation for apnea has been found.

RSV infection in subsequent years is more likely to cause tracheobronchitis or upper respiratory tract infection. Exceptions are immunocompromised hosts and children with severe chronic lung or heart disease, who may have especially severe or prolonged primary infections and are subject to additional attacks of severe pneumonitis.

### B. LABORATORY FINDINGS

Rapid detection of RSV antigen in nasal or pulmonary secretions by fluorescent antibody staining or ELISA requires only several hours and is more than 90% sensi-

tive and specific. Rapid tissue culture methods take 48 hours and have comparable sensitivity.

### C. IMAGING

Diffuse hyperinflation and peribronchiolar thickening are most common; atelectasis and patchy infiltrates also occur in uncomplicated infection, but pleural effusions are rare. Consolidation (usually subsegmental) occurs in 25% of children with lower respiratory tract disease.

## Differential Diagnosis

Although almost all cases of bronchiolitis are due to RSV during an epidemic, other viruses, particularly human metapneumovirus, cannot be excluded. Mixed infections with other viruses, chlamydiae, or bacteria can occur. Wheezing may be due to asthma, a foreign body, or other airway obstruction. RSV infection may closely resemble chlamydial pneumonitis when fine crackles are present and fever and wheezing are not prominent. The two may also coexist. Cystic fibrosis may resemble RSV infection; a positive family history or failure to thrive associated with hyponatremia or hypoalbuminemia should prompt a sweat chloride test. Pertussis should also be considered in this age group, especially if cough is prominent and if the infant is younger than age 6 months. A markedly elevated leukocyte count should suggest bacterial superinfection (neutrophilia) or pertussis (lymphocytosis).

## Complications

RSV commonly infects the middle ear. Symptomatic otitis media is more likely when secondary bacterial infection is present (usually due to pneumococci or *H influenzae*). This is the most common complication (10–20%). However, bacterial pneumonia occurs in only 0.5–1% of hospitalized patients. Sudden exacerbations of fever and leukocytosis should suggest bacterial infection. Respiratory failure or apnea may require mechanical ventilation, but occurs in less than 2% of hospitalized previously healthy full-term infants. Cardiac failure may occur as a complication of pulmonary disease or myocarditis. Respiratory syncytial virus—as well as parainfluenza and influenza viruses—commonly causes exacerbations of asthma. Nosocomial infection is so common during outbreaks that elective hospitalization or surgery, especially for those with underlying illness, should be postponed. Well-designed hospital programs to prevent nosocomial spread are imperative (see next section).

## Treatment & Prevention

Children who are very hypoxic or cannot feed because of respiratory distress must be hospitalized and given humidified oxygen and tube or intravenous feedings. Antibiotics, decongestants, and expectorants are of no value in routine infections. Such children should be kept in respiratory isolation. Cohorting ill infants in respiratory isolation during peak season (with or without rapid diagnostic attempts) and emphasizing good hand-washing may greatly decrease nosocomial transmission.

The utility of bronchodilator therapy has not been consistently demonstrated. Often a trial of bronchodilator therapy is given to determine response and is subsequently discontinued if there is no improvement. Racemic epinephrine occasionally works when albuterol fails. The use of corticosteroids is also controversial. A meta-analysis of numerous studies indicates a significant effect on hospital stay, especially in those most ill at the time of treatment. The use of steroids in the emergency room appears to speed improvement and prevent hospitalization.

Ribavirin is the only licensed antiviral therapy used for RSV infection. It is given by continuous aerosolization (6 g in a 300-mL vial of water) by a special nebulizer for 12–18 hours of every day for 3–5 days. This agent has minimal effect on virus shedding. There is great controversy about its efficacy, and its use is infrequent in infants without significant anatomic or immunologic defects. At best, there is a very modest effect on disease severity in immunocompetent infants with no underlying anatomic abnormality. Even in high-risk infants, clinical response to ribavirin therapy was not demonstrated in several studies. Nevertheless, ribavirin is sometimes used in severely ill children who are immunologically or anatomically compromised, in those with severe cardiac disease, and in those with evidence of severe RSV infection. Bronchospasm may be exacerbated by this drug, although randomized trials do not show a deterioration of pulmonary function in patients receiving ribavirin.

Monthly intramuscular administration of humanized RSV monoclonal antibody is now recommended to prevent severe disease in high-risk patients during epidemic periods. Monthly administration should be considered during the RSV season for high-risk children, as described in Chapter 9.

Use of passive immunization for immunocompromised children is logical but not established. RSV antibody is not effective for treatment of established infection.

## Prognosis

Although mild bronchiolitis does not produce long-term problems, 30–40% of patients hospitalized with this infection will wheeze later in childhood. Chronic restrictive lung disease and bronchiolitis obliterans are rare sequelae.

Black CO: Systematic review of the biology and medical management of respiratory syncytial virus infection. Respiratory Care 2003;48:209 [PMID: 12667273].

Hall CB: Respiratory syncytial virus and parainfluenza virus. N Engl J Med 2001;344:1917 [PMID: 11419430].

Ogra PL: From chimpanzee to palivizumab: Changing times for respiratory syncytial virus. Pediatr Infect Dis J 2000;19:774 [PMID: 10959757].

Panitch HB: Respiratory syncytial virus bronchiolitis: Supportive care and therapies designed to overcome airway obstruction. Pediatr Infect Dis J 2003;22:S83 [PMID: 12671457].

Welliver RC: Respiratory syncytial virus and other respiratory viruses. Pediatr Infect Dis J 2003;22:S6 [PMID: 12671447].

## Human Metapneumovirus

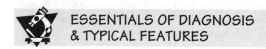

### ESSENTIALS OF DIAGNOSIS & TYPICAL FEATURES

- Cough, coryza, sore throat.
- Bronchiolitis.
- Positive hMPV PCR in respiratory secretion.

## General Considerations

After its discovery in 2001, human metapneumovirus (hMPV) was rapidly identified as a common agent of respiratory tract infections that is very similar to RSV in epidemiologic and clinical characteristics. Like RSV, parainfluenza, mumps, and measles, hMPV belongs to the paramyxovirus family. Humans are its only known reservoir. Seroepidemiologic surveys indicate that the virus has worldwide distribution. More than 90% of children contract hMPV infection by age 5 years, typically during late autumn through early spring outbreaks. hMPV accounts for 15–25% of the cases of bronchiolitis and pneumonia in children younger than 2 years of age. Older children and adults can also develop symptomatic infection.

## Clinical Characteristics

### A. SIGNS AND SYMPTOMS

The most common symptoms are fever, cough, rhinorrhea, and sore throat. Bronchiolitis and pneumonia occur in 40–70% of the children who acquire hMPV before the age of 2 years. Asymptomatic infection is uncommon. Other manifestations include otitis, conjunctivitis, diarrhea, and myalgia. Acute wheezing has been associated with hMPV in children of all ages, raising the possibility that this virus, like RSV, might trigger reactive airway disease. Dual infection with hMPV and RSV or other respiratory viruses seems to be a common occurrence and may increase morbidity and mortality.

### B. IMAGING STUDIES

Lower respiratory tract infection frequently shows hyperinflation and patchy pneumonitis on chest radiographs.

### C. LABORATORY DIAGNOSIS

The virus has very selective tissue culture tropism, which accounts for its late discovery in spite of its presence in archived specimens from the mid-1900s. The preferred method of diagnosis is PCR performed on respiratory specimens. Antibody tests are available, but are most appropriately used for epidemiologic studies.

## Prognosis & Treatment

No antiviral therapies are available to treat hMPV. Children with lower respiratory tract disease may require hospitalization and ventilatory support, but less frequently than with RSV-associated bronchiolitis. Duration of hospitalization with hMPV is typically shorter than with RSV.

Boivin G et al: Virological and clinical manifestations associated with human metapneumovirus: A new paramyxovirus responsible for acute respiratory tract infections in all age groups. J Infect Dis 2002;186:1330 [PMID: 12402203].

van den Hoogen BG et al: A newly discovered human pneumovirus. Nat Med 2001;7:719 [PMID: 11385510].

## SEVERE ACUTE RESPIRATORY SYNDROME (SARS)

### ESSENTIALS OF DIAGNOSIS & TYPICAL FEATURES

*Suspected case*
- *Febrile illness of unknown etiology with temperature above 38°C.*

*AND*
- *One or more clinical findings of respiratory illness (eg, cough, SOB, difficulty breathing, hypoxia).*

*AND*
- *Travel within 10 days of symptom onset to an area with documented/suspected community transmission of SARS.*

*OR*

- *Close contact within 10 days of onset of symptoms with a person with known or suspected SARS.*

*Probable Case*
- *Suspected case definition plus radiographic evidence of pneumonia.*

*OR*
- *Autopsy evidence of acute respiratory distress syndrome or pneumonia.*

## General Considerations

A new cause of atypical pneumonia arose in Asia in late 2002. Because of its severity it was named severe acute respiratory syndrome (SARS). During the following half year more than 8500 cases were documented. Many other countries reported cases from travelers, including 100 in the United States. A coronavirus (SARS-CoV) was isolated as the causative agent. This virus probably was acquired from indigenous wild animals sold in markets. Subsequent spread among close contacts, as well as within hospitals and by international travelers, extended the epidemic.

## Clinical Findings

### A. SYMPTOMS AND SIGNS

Initially, fever is accompanied by malaise, chills, headache, myalgia, dyspnea, and cough. Abnormal chest auscultation is noted in only 25% of cases and often is less prominent than would be expected from the chest radiograph. In two thirds of patients the pulmonary symptoms and signs progress, hypoxia occurs, and 20–30% require intensive care. Fatal respiratory failure ensues in a third to a half of these. A watery diarrhea is prominent in one quarter of the patients. The incubation period is 4–7 days (range is 2–10 days). The peak severity occurs at about 2 weeks after onset.

### B. LABORATORY

Leukopenia, lymphopenia, and thrombocytopenia occur in many patients. Lactate dehydrogenase (LDH), aspartate aminotransferase, and creatinine phosphokinase are often elevated. However, none of these changes are diagnostic. Virus can be isolated from respiratory secretions, saliva, urine, and feces. An RT-PCR is useful for diagnosis within 5 days of onset. Antibody can be detected by immunofluorescence assay at 10–14 days and by EIA about a week later.

### C. IMAGING

Most patients have an abnormal radiograph when first seen, typically with ground-glass opacities or focal consolidation. In severe cases this rapidly progresses to multiple bilateral consolidations.

## Differential Diagnosis

The initial onset is similar with that of other causes of atypical pneumonia (eg, *Mycoplasma, Chlamydia,* Q fever, *Legionella, C psittaci,* other viruses [especially influenza]). SARS differs from *Mycoplasma* and *Chlamydia* infections in the absence of significant coryza and sore throat. The seasonality of some viruses will suggest their exclusion from the diagnosis. The travel and contact history is a key factor in the diagnosis of SARS.

## Treatment

The management is largely supportive. Since no established therapy exists, potential approaches are still evolving. A SARS-specific immunoglobulin is under study.

## Prevention

Detailed surveillance and quarantine measures have evolved. These appear to have been important in limiting outbreaks. In addition, since spread within hospitals has been prominent, infection control and patient care rules for SARS are now in place.

## Prognosis

Ten to 20% of hospitalized cases are fatal. This rate is greatest in elderly people and those with other underlying illnesses. Children have milder disease and fewer radiographic abnormalities.

Abdullah AS et al: Lessons from the severe acute respiratory syndrome outbreak in Hong Kong. Emerg Infect Dis 2003; 9:1042 [PMID: 14519237].

Demmler GJ, Ligon BL: Severe acute respiratory syndrome (SARS): A review of the history, epidemiology, prevention and concerns for the future. Semin Pediatr Infect Dis 2003;14:240 [PMID: 12913837].

Peiris JSM et al: The severe acute respiratory syndrome. N Engl J Med 2003;349:2431 [PMID:14681510].

# INFECTIONS DUE TO ENTEROVIRUSES

Enteroviruses are a major cause of illness in young children. The multiple types are physically and biochemically similar and may produce identical syndromes. The multiplicity of types makes vaccine development impractical and has hindered development of antigen detection and serologic tests. However, common RNA sequences and group antigens have led to diagnostic tests for viral nucleic acid and proteins. A PCR assay is available in many medical centers, but tissue culture is the most commonly used diagnostic method for echoviruses, polioviruses, and coxsackie B viruses. Because cultures may turn positive in 2–4 days, they should be inoculated promptly and may be clinically useful, particularly in cases of meningoencephalitis. Many coxsackie A viruses fail to grow.

Transmission is fecal–oral or from upper respiratory secretions. Multiple enteroviruses circulate in the community at any one time; summer–fall outbreaks are common in temperate climates, but infections are seen year-round. After poliovirus, coxsackie B virus is most virulent, followed by echovirus. Neurologic, cardiac, and overwhelming neonatal infections are the most severe forms of illness.

## ACUTE FEBRILE ILLNESS

Accompanied by nonspecific upper respiratory or enteric symptoms, sudden onset of fever and irritability in infants or young children is often enteroviral in origin, especially in late summer and fall. More than 90% of enteroviral infections are not distinctive. Occasionally a petechial rash is seen; more often a diffuse maculopapular or morbilliform eruption (often prominent on palms and soles) occurs on the second to fourth day of fever. Rapid recovery is the rule. More than one febrile enteroviral illness can occur in the same patient in one season. The leukocyte count is usually normal. Infants, because of fever and irritability, may undergo an evaluation for bacteremia or meningitis and be hospitalized to rule out sepsis. Approximately one half of these infants have aseptic meningitis. In the summer months enterovirus infection is more likely than human herpesvirus 6 to cause an acute medical visit for fever. Duration of illness is 4–5 days.

Sawyer MH: Enterovirus infections: Diagnosis and treatment. Semin Pediatr Infect Dis 2002;13:40 [PMID: 12118843].

Stalkup JR, Chilukuri S: Enterovirus infections: A review of clinical presentation, diagnosis, and treatment. Dermatol Clin 2002;20:217 [PMID: 12120436].

## RESPIRATORY TRACT ILLNESSES

### 1. Febrile Illness with Pharyngitis

This syndrome is most common in older children, who complain of headache, sore throat, myalgia, and abdominal discomfort. The usual duration is 3–4 days. Vesicles or papules may be seen in the pharynx. There is no exudate. Occasionally, enteroviruses are the cause of croup, bronchitis, or pneumonia. They may also exacerbate asthma.

## 2. Herpangina

Herpangina is characterized by an acute onset of fever and posterior pharyngeal grayish white vesicles that quickly form ulcers (< 20 in number), often linearly arranged on the posterior palate, uvula, and tonsillar pillars. Bilateral faucial ulcers may also be seen. Dysphagia, vomiting, abdominal pain, and anorexia also occur and, rarely, parotitis or vaginal ulcers. Symptoms disappear in 4–5 days. The epidemic form is due to a variety of coxsackie A viruses; coxsackie B viruses and echoviruses cause sporadic cases.

The differential diagnosis includes primary herpes simplex gingivostomatitis (ulcers are more prominent anteriorly, and gingivitis is present), aphthous stomatitis (fever absent, recurrent episodes, anterior lesions), trauma, hand-foot-and-mouth disease (see later discussion), and Vincent angina (painful gingivitis spreading from the gum line, underlying dental disease). If the enanthema is missed, tonsillitis might be incorrectly diagnosed.

## 3. Acute Lymphonodular Pharyngitis

Coxsackievirus A10 has been associated with a febrile pharyngitis characterized by nonulcerative yellow-white posterior pharyngeal papules in the same distribution as herpangina. The duration is 1–2 weeks; therapy is supportive.

## 4. Pleurodynia (Bornholm Disease, Epidemic Myalgia)

Caused by coxsackie B virus (epidemic form) or many nonpolio enteroviruses (sporadic form), pleurodynia is associated with an abrupt onset of unilateral or bilateral spasmodic pain of variable intensity over the lower ribs or upper abdomen. Associated symptoms include headache, fever, vomiting, myalgias, and abdominal and neck pain. Physical findings include fever, chest muscle tenderness, decreased thoracic excursion, and occasionally a friction rub. The chest radiograph is normal. Hematologic tests are nondiagnostic. The illness generally lasts less than 1 week.

This is a disease of muscle, but the differential diagnosis includes bacterial pneumonia, empyema, tuberculosis, and endemic fungal infections (all excluded radiographically and by auscultation), costochondritis (no fever or other symptoms), and a variety of abdominal problems, especially those causing diaphragmatic irritation.

There is no specific therapy. Potent analgesic agents and chest splinting alleviate the pain.

## RASHES (Including Hand-Foot-and-Mouth Disease)

The rash may be macular, maculopapular, urticarial, scarlatiniform, petechial, or vesicular. One of the most characteristic is that of hand-foot-and-mouth disease (caused by coxsackieviruses, especially types A5, A10, and A16), in which vesicles or red papules are found on the tongue, oral mucosa, hands, and feet. Often they appear near the nails and on the heels. Associated fever, sore throat, and malaise are mild. The rash may appear when fever abates, simulating roseola.

## Cardiac Involvement

Myocarditis and pericarditis may be caused by a number of nonpolio enteroviruses, particularly type B coxsackieviruses. Most commonly, upper respiratory symptoms are followed by substernal pain, dyspnea, and exercise intolerance. A friction rub or gallop may be detected. Ultrasound will define ventricular dysfunction, and electrocardiography may show pericarditis or ventricular irritability. Creatine kinase may be elevated. The disease may be mild or fatal; most children recover completely. In infants, other organs may be involved at the same time; in older patients, cardiac disease is usually the sole manifestation (see Chapter 19 for therapy). Enteroviral RNA is present in cardiac tissue in some cases of dilated cardiomyopathy or myocarditis; the significance of this finding is unknown. Epidemics of enterovirus 71, which occur in Asia, as well as sporadic cases in the United States, are associated with severe left ventricular dysfunction and pulmonary edema following typical mucocutaneous manifestations of enterovirus infection.

## Severe Neonatal Infection

Sporadic and nosocomial nursery cases of severe systemic enteroviral disease occur. Clinical manifestations include combinations of fever, rash, pneumonitis, encephalitis, hepatitis, gastroenteritis, myocarditis, pancreatitis, and myositis. The infants, usually younger than 1 week old, may appear septic, with cyanosis, dyspnea, and seizures. The differential diagnosis includes bacterial and herpes simplex infections, necrotizing enterocolitis, other causes of heart or liver failure, and metabolic diseases. Diagnosis is suggested by the finding of cerebrospinal fluid (CSF) mononuclear pleocytosis and confirmed by the isolation of virus or detection of enteroviral RNA from urine, stool, CSF, or pharynx. Therapy is supportive. IVIG is often administered, but its value is uncertain. Passively acquired maternal antibody may protect newborns from severe disease. For this reason, labor should not be induced in pregnant women near term who have suspected enteroviral disease. Specific antiviral therapy (pleconaril) is being evaluated for severe enteroviral infection.

Huang F-L et al: Left ventricular dysfunction in children with fulminant enterovirus 71 infection: An evaluation of the clinical course. Clin Infect Dis 2002;34:1020 [PMID: 11880970].

# CENTRAL NERVOUS SYSTEM ILLNESSES

## 1. Poliomyelitis

### ESSENTIALS OF DIAGNOSIS & TYPICAL FEATURES

- *Inadequate immunization or underlying immune deficiency.*
- *Headache, fever, muscle weakness.*
- *Aseptic meningitis.*
- *Asymmetrical, flaccid paralysis; muscle tenderness and hyperesthesia; intact sensation; late atrophy.*

## General Considerations

Poliovirus infection is subclinical in 90–95% of cases; it causes nonspecific febrile illness in about 5% of cases and aseptic meningitis, with or without paralytic disease, in 1–3%. In endemic areas, most older children and adults are immune because of prior inapparent infections. Occasional cases in the United States occur in patients who have traveled to foreign countries. Most cases were in immunodeficient patients who received the oral poliovirus vaccine (OPV) or were exposed to recent vaccinees. Severe poliovirus infection was a rare complication of OPV vaccination as a result of reversion of the vaccine virus. The incidence of vaccine-associated paralytic poliomyelitis (VAPP) in the United States was 1:750,000 and 1:2.4 million doses for the first and second dose of OPV, respectively. Although rare, VAPP became more common than wild-type poliomyelitis in the United States in the 1980s. This led to change in the recommended immunization regimen, substituting inactivated poliovaccine (IPV) for OPV (see Chapter 9).

## Clinical Findings

### A. SYMPTOMS AND SIGNS

The initial symptoms are fever, myalgia, sore throat, and headache for 2–6 days. In less than 10% of infected children, several symptom-free days are followed by recurrent fever and signs of aseptic meningitis: headache, stiff neck, spinal rigidity, and nausea. Mild cases resolve completely. In only 1–2% of these children does high fever, severe myalgia, and anxiety portend progression to loss of reflexes and subsequent flaccid paralysis. Sensation remains intact, although hyperesthesia of skin overlying paralyzed muscles is common and pathognomonic.

Paralysis is usually asymmetrical. Proximal limb muscles are more often involved than distal, and lower limb involvement is more common. Bulbar involvement affects swallowing, speech, and cardiorespiratory function and accounts for most deaths. Bladder distention and marked constipation characteristically accompany lower limb paralysis. Paralysis is usually complete by the time the temperature normalizes. Weakness often resolves completely. Atrophy is usually apparent by 4–8 weeks. Most improvement of muscle paralysis will take place within 6 months.

### B. LABORATORY FINDINGS

In patients with meningeal symptoms, the CSF contains up to several hundred leukocytes (mostly lymphocytes) per microliter; the glucose level is normal, and protein concentration is mildly elevated. Poliovirus is easy to grow in cell culture and can be readily differentiated from other enteroviruses. It is rarely isolated from spinal fluid but is often present in the throat and stool for several weeks following infection. Paired serology is also diagnostic. Laboratory methods are available to differentiate wild from attenuated vaccine isolates.

## Differential Diagnosis

Aseptic meningitis due to poliovirus is indistinguishable from that due to other viruses. Paralytic disease in the United States is usually due to nonpolio enteroviruses. Polio may resemble Guillain–Barré syndrome (variable sensory loss, symmetrical loss of function; minimal pleocytosis, high protein concentration in spinal fluid), polyneuritis (sensory loss), pseudoparalysis due to bone or joint problems (eg, trauma, infection), botulism, or tick paralysis.

## Complications & Sequelae

Complications are the result of the acute and permanent effects of paralysis. Respiratory, pharyngeal, bladder, and bowel malfunction are most critical. Deaths are usually due to complications arising from respiratory dysfunction. Limbs injured near the time of infection, such as by intramuscular injections, excessive prior use, or trauma, tend to be most severely involved and have the worst prognosis for recovery (provocation paralysis). Postpolio muscular atrophy occurs in 30–40% of paralyzed limbs 20–30 years later, characterized by increasing weakness and fasciculations in previously affected, partially recovered limbs.

## Treatment & Prognosis

Therapy is supportive. Bed rest, fever and pain control (heat therapy is helpful), and careful attention to progression of weakness (particularly of respiratory muscles) are important. No intramuscular injections should be given during the acute phase. Intubation or tracheostomy for secretion control and catheter drainage of the bladder may be needed. Assisted ventilation and enteral feeding may also be needed. Pleconaril, which is an antiviral drug active against most enteroviruses, has no effect on polioviruses. Postpolio paralysis is mild in about 30%, permanent in 15%, and results in death in 5–10%. Disease is worse in adults and pregnant women than in children.

## 2. Nonpolio Viral Meningitis

Nonpolio enteroviruses cause over 80% of cases of aseptic meningitis at all ages. In the summer and fall, multiple cases may be seen associated with circulation of neurotropic strains. Nosocomial outbreaks also occur.

## Clinical Findings

The usual enteroviral incubation period is 4–6 days. Because many enteroviral infections are subclinical or not associated with central nervous system (CNS) symptoms, a history of contact with a patient with meningitis is unusual. Neonates may acquire infection from maternal blood, vaginal secretions, or feces at birth; occasionally the mother has had a febrile illness just prior to delivery.

### A. SYMPTOMS AND SIGNS

Onset is usually acute with variable fever, marked irritability, and lethargy in infants. Incidence is much greater in children younger than age 1 year. Older children also describe frontal headache, photophobia, and myalgia. Abdominal pain, diarrhea, and vomiting may occur. The incidence of rash varies with the infecting strain. If rash occurs, it is usually seen after several days of illness and is diffuse, macular or maculopapular, occasionally petechial, but not purpuric. Oropharyngeal vesicles and rash on the palms and soles suggest an enterovirus. The anterior fontanelle may be full. Meningismus may be present. The illness may be biphasic, with nonspecific symptoms and signs preceding those related to the CNS. In older children, it is easier to demonstrate meningeal signs. Seizures are unusual, and focal neurologic findings, which are rare, should lead to a search for an alternative cause. Frank encephalitis, which is also uncommon at any age, occurs most often in neonates. Because of the overall frequency of enteroviral disease in children, 10–20% of all cases of encephalitis of proved viral origin are caused by enteroviruses. In some areas of the world epidemics of enterovirus 71 that begin with typical mucocutaneous manifestations of enteroviruses are complicated by severe brainstem encephalitis and polio-like flaccid paralysis. Enterovirus 70 outbreaks have resulted in hemorrhagic conjunctivitis together with paralytic poliomyelitis. Such cases of enterovirus are now appearing in the United States. Other nonpolio enteroviruses cause sporadic cases of acute motor weakness similar to that seen with poliovirus infection. Children with congenital immune deficiency, especially agammaglobulinemia, are subject to chronic enteroviral meningoencephalitis that is often fatal or associated with severe sequellae.

### B. LABORATORY FINDINGS

Blood leukocyte counts are nonspecific and often normal. The spinal fluid leukocyte count is 100–1000/μL. Early in the illness, polymorphonuclear cells predominate; a shift to mononuclear cells occurs within 8–36 hours. In about 95% of cases, spinal fluid parameters include a total leukocyte count less than 3000/μL, protein less than 80 mg/dL, and glucose more than 60% of serum values. Marked deviation from any of these findings should prompt consideration of another diagnosis (see following section). The syndrome of inappropriate secretion of antidiuretic hormone may occur but is rarely clinically significant.

Culture of CSF may yield an enterovirus within a few days (<70%); virus may be found in acellular spinal fluids. PCR for enteroviruses is a useful diagnostic method in many centers (sensitivity > 90%). This test can give an answer within 24–48 hours. Isolation of an enterovirus from throat or stool suggests but does not prove enteroviral meningitis. Vaccine poliovirus present in feces in infants being evaluated for aseptic meningitis (outside of the United States) may confuse the diagnosis but can usually be distinguished by growth characteristics.

### C. IMAGING

Cerebral imaging is not often indicated; if done, it is usually normal. Subdural effusions, infarcts, edema, or focal abnormalities seen in bacterial meningitis are absent except for the rare case of focal encephalitis.

## Differential Diagnosis

In the prevaccine era, mumps and polio were leading causes of aseptic meningitis, but now this is usually caused by enteroviruses, especially in the summer and fall. Other causative viruses are mosquito-borne viruses (flavivirus, bunyavirus). These are usually considered during an investigation of encephalitis, but many of them are more likely to cause isolated meningitis and should be considered when seasonal clusters of viral meningitis occur. Primary herpes simplex infection can cause aseptic meningitis in adolescents who have a genital herpes infection. In neonates, early herpes simplex meningoencephalitis may mimic enteroviral disease (see section on Infections Due to Herpesviruses). This is an important alternative diagnosis to exclude because of the need for urgent specific therapy. Lymphocytic choriomeningitis virus causes meningitis in children in contact with rodents (pet or environmental exposure). Meningitis occurs in some patients at the time of infection with human immunodeficiency virus (HIV).

Other causes of aseptic meningitis that may resemble enteroviral infection include partially treated bacterial meningitis (recent antibiotic treatment; CSF parameters resembling those seen in bacterial disease and bacterial antigen sometimes present); parameningeal foci of bacterial infection such as brain abscess, subdural empyema, mastoiditis (predisposing factors, glucose level in CSF may be lower, focal neurologic signs, and characteristic imaging); tumors or cysts (malignant cells detected by cytologic examination, a history of neurologic symptoms, higher protein concentration or lower glucose level in CSF); trauma (presence, without exception, of red blood cells, which may be erroneously assumed to be due to traumatic lumbar puncture but are crenated and fail to clear); vasculitis (other systemic or neurologic signs, found in older children); tuberculous or fungal meningitis (see Chapters 38 and 39); cysticercosis; parainfectious encephalopathies (*Mycoplasma pneumoniae,* cat scratch disease, respiratory viruses [especially influenza]); Lyme disease; leptospirosis; and rickettsial diseases.

## Treatment & Prevention

No specific therapy exists. Infants are usually hospitalized, isolated, and treated with fluids and antipyretics. Moderately to severely ill infants are given appropriate antibiotics for bacterial pathogens until cultures are negative for 48–72 hours. This practice is changing somewhat, and hospital stay shortened, in areas where the PCR assay for enteroviruses is available. If patients—especially older children—are mildly ill, antibiotics may be withheld and the child observed. The illness usually lasts less than 1 week. Codeine compounds or other strong pain relievers may be needed. C-reactive protein and lactate levels are usually low in the CSF of children with viral meningitis; both may be elevated with bacterial infection. With clinical deterioration, repeat lumbar puncture, cerebral imaging, neurologic consultation, and more aggressive diagnostic tests should be considered. Herpesvirus encephalitis is an important consideration in such cases, particularly in infants younger than age 1 month. Newborns often receive empiric acyclovir therapy until an etiologic diagnosis is made. Specific antiviral therapy (pleconaril) is under study for the treatment of severe enteroviral infections.

Measures to prevent enteroviral infection include good hygiene, scrupulous hand washing, and proper isolation in the hospital.

## Prognosis

In general, enteroviral meningitis has no significant short-term neurologic or developmental sequelae. Developmental delay may follow severe neonatal infections. Unlike mumps, enterovirus infections rarely cause hearing loss.

Chang L-Y et al: Comparison of enterovirus 71 and coxsackie-virus A16 clinical illness during the Taiwan enterovirus epidemic, 1998. Pediatr Infect Dis J 1999;18:1092 [PMID: 10608631].

Romero JR, Newland JG: Viral meningitis and encephalitis: Traditional and emerging viral agents. Semin Pediatr Infect Dis 2003;14:72 [PMID: 12881794].

Stellrecht KA et al: The impact of an enteroviral RT-PCR on the diagnosis of aseptic meningitis and patient management. J Clin Virol 2002;25:S19.[PMID: 12091078].

# INFECTIONS DUE TO HERPESVIRUSES
## HERPES SIMPLEX

 **ESSENTIALS OF DIAGNOSIS & TYPICAL FEATURES**

- *Grouped vesicles on an erythematous base, typically in or around the mouth or genitals.*
- *Tender regional adenopathy, especially with primary infection.*
- *Fever and malaise with primary infection.*
- *Recurrent episodes in many patients.*

## General Considerations

There are two types of herpes simplex viruses. Type 1 (HSV-1) causes most cases of oral, skin, and cerebral disease. Type 2 (HSV-2) causes most (80–85%) genital and congenital infections. Latent infection in sensory ganglia routinely follows primary infection. Recurrences may be spontaneous or induced by external events (eg, fever, menstruation, or sunlight) or immunosuppression. Transmission is by direct contact with infected secretions. Herpes simplex viruses are very susceptible to antiviral drugs.

Primary infection with HSV-1 often occurs early in childhood, although many adults (20–50%) have never been infected. Primary infection with HSV-1 is subclinical in 80% of cases and causes gingivostomatitis in the remainder. HSV-2, which is transmitted sexually, is also usually (65%) subclinical or produces mild, nonspecific symptoms. Infection with one type of HSV may prevent or attenuate clinically apparent infection with the other type, but individuals can be infected at different times with both HSV-1 and HSV-2. Recurrent episodes are due to reactivation of latent HSV.

## Clinical Findings

The source of primary infection is often an asymptomatic excreter. Most previously infected individuals shed HSV at irregular intervals. At any one time (point prevalence), 2–4% of normal seropositive adults excrete HSV-1 in the saliva; the percentage is higher in recently infected children. HSV-2 shedding in genital secretions occurs with a point prevalence of 8–28%, depending on the method of detection (viral isolation vs PCR). A history of contact with an active HSV infection is unusual.

### A. SYMPTOMS AND SIGNS

**1. Gingivostomatitis**—High fever, irritability, and drooling occur in infants. Multiple oral ulcers are seen on the tongue and on the buccal and gingival mucosa, occasionally extending to the pharynx. Pharyngeal ulcers may predominate in older children and adolescents. Diffusely swollen red gums that are friable and bleed easily are typical. Cervical nodes are swollen and tender. Duration is 7–14 days. Herpangina, aphthous stomatitis, thrush, and Vincent angina should be excluded.

**2. Vulvovaginitis or urethritis**—Genital herpes (especially HSV-2) in a prepubertal child should suggest sexual abuse. Vesicles or painful ulcers on the vulva, vagina, or penis and tender adenopathy are seen. Systemic symptoms (fever, flu-like illness, myalgia) are common with the initial episode. Painful urination may cause retention. Primary infections last 10–21 days. Le-

sions may resemble trauma, syphilis (ulcers are painless), or chancroid (ulcers are painful and nodes are erythematous and fluctuant) in the adolescent, and bullous impetigo, trauma, and severe chemical irritation in younger children.

**3. Cutaneous infections**—Direct inoculation onto cuts or abrasions may produce localized vesicles or ulcers. A deep HSV infection on the fingers (called herpetic whitlow) may be mistaken for a bacterial felon or paronychia; surgical drainage is of no value and is contraindicated. HSV infection of eczematous skin may result in extensive areas of vesicles and shallow ulcers (eczema herpeticum), which may be mistaken for impetigo or varicella.

**4. Recurrent mucocutaneous infection**—Recurrent oral shedding is usually asymptomatic. Perioral recurrences often begin with a prodrome of tingling or burning limited to the vermilion border, followed by vesiculation, scabbing, and crusting around the lips over the next 3–5 days. Intraoral lesions rarely recur. Fever, adenopathy, and other symptoms are absent. Recurrent cutaneous herpes most closely resembles impetigo; the latter is often outside the perinasal and perioral region, responds to antibiotics, yields a positive Gram stain, and *Streptococcus pyogenes* or *Staphylococcus aureus* can be isolated. Recurrent genital disease is common after the initial infection with HSV-2. The disease is shorter (5–7 days) and milder (mean, four lesions) and is not associated with systemic symptoms.

**5. Keratoconjunctivitis**—Keratoconjunctivitis may be part of a primary infection due to spread from infected saliva. Most cases are caused by reactivation of virus latent in the ciliary ganglion. Keratoconjunctivitis produces photophobia, pain, and conjunctival irritation. With recurrences, dendritic corneal ulcers may be demonstrable with fluorescein staining. Stromal invasion may occur. Steroids should never be used for unilateral keratitis without ophthalmologic consultation. Other causes of these symptoms include trauma, bacterial infections, and other viral infections (especially adenovirus if pharyngitis is present; bilateral involvement makes HSV unlikely) (see Chapter 15).

**6. Encephalitis**—Although unusual in infants outside the neonatal period, encephalitis may occur at any age, usually without cutaneous herpes lesions. In older children, HSV encephalitis can follow a primary infection, but often represents reactivation of latent virus. HSV is the most common cause of sporadic severe encephalitis. It is the most important because it can be treated with specific antiviral therapy. Fever, headache, behavioral changes, and neurologic deficits or focal seizures occur. Mild mononuclear pleocytosis is typically present along with an elevated protein concentration, which continues to rise on repeat lumbar punctures. In older children hypodense areas with a medial and inferior temporal lobe predilection are seen on CT scan, especially after 3–5 days, but the findings in infants may be more diffuse. Magnetic resonance imaging (MRI) is more sensitive and is positive sooner. Periodic focal epileptiform discharges are seen on electroencephalograms but are not diagnostic of HSV infection. Viral cultures of CSF are rarely positive. The PCR assay to detect HSV DNA in CSF is a sensitive and specific rapid test. Without early antiviral therapy, the prognosis is poor. The differential diagnosis includes mumps, mosquito-borne and other viral encephalitides, parainfectious and postinfectious encephalopathy, brain abscess, acute demyelinating syndromes, and bacterial meningoencephalitis.

**7. Neonatal infections**—Infection is acquired by ascending spread prior to delivery (5–10% of cases) or at the time of vaginal delivery from a mother with genital infection. Occasionally the infection is acquired in the postpartum period from oral secretions of family members or hospital personnel. A history of genital herpes in the mother is usually absent. Within a few days and up to 4 weeks, skin vesicles (especially at sites of trauma, such as where scalp monitors were placed) appear. Some infants have infections limited to the skin, eye or mouth. Other infants are acutely ill, presenting with jaundice, shock, bleeding, or respiratory distress. Some infants appear well initially, but dissemination of the infection to the brain or other organs becomes evident during the ensuing week if it is untreated. HSV infection (and empiric therapy) should be considered in newborns with the sepsis syndrome who are unresponsive to antibiotic therapy and have negative bacterial cultures. Skin lesions may be absent at the time of presentation. Some infected infants exhibit only neurologic symptoms at 2–3 weeks after delivery: apnea, lethargy, fever, poor feeding, or persistent overt seizures. The brain infection in these children is often diffuse and is best diagnosed by MRI. The skin lesions may resemble impetigo, bacterial scalp abscesses, or miliaria; some children may fail to develop skin lesions. Skin lesions may recur over weeks or months after recovery from the acute illness. Progressive culture-negative pneumonitis is another manifestation of neonatal HSV.

### B. LABORATORY FINDINGS

With multisystem disease, abnormalities in platelets, clotting factors, and liver function tests are often present. A finding of lymphocytic pleocytosis and elevated CSF protein indicates aseptic meningitis or encephalitis. Virus may be cultured from infected epithelial sites (vesicles, ulcers, or conjunctival scrapings) and from in-fected tissue (skin, brain) obtained by biopsy. Cultures of CSF are positive in about 50% of neonatal cases, but uncommon in older children. HSV will be detected within 2 days by rapid tissue culture methods. Isolation from throat, eye, urine, or stool of a newborn is diagnostic. Vaginal culture of the mother may offer circumstantial evidence for the diagnosis, but may be negative.

Rapid diagnostic tests include immunofluorescent stains or ELISA to detect viral antigen. The PCR assay for HSV DNA is positive ($\approx$ 95%) in the CSF when there is brain involvement. Serum is often positive in the presence of multisystem disease.

## Complications, Sequelae, & Prognosis

Gingivostomatitis may result in dehydration due to dysphagia; severe chronic oral disease and esophageal involvement may occur in immunosuppressed patients. Primary vulvovaginitis may be associated with aseptic meningitis, paresthesias, autonomic dysfunction due to neuritis (urinary retention, constipation), and secondary candidal infection. Extensive cutaneous disease (as in eczema) may be associated with dissemination, and bacterial superinfection. Keratitis may result in corneal opacification or perforation. Untreated encephalitis is fatal in 70% of patients and causes severe damage in most of the remainder. When acyclovir treatment is instituted early, 20% die and 40% are neurologically impaired. Disseminated neonatal infection is often fatal in spite of therapy, and survivors are often impaired.

## Treatment

### A. SPECIFIC MEASURES

HSV is sensitive to antiviral therapy.

**1. Topical antivirals**—Antivirals are most effective for corneal disease and include 1% trifluridine, 5% acyclovir, and 3% vidarabine. Trifluridine appears superior; cure rates over 95% are reported. These agents should be used with the guidance of an ophthalmologist.

**2. Mucocutaneous HSV infections**—These respond to administration of oral nucleoside analogs (acyclovir, valacyclovir, or famciclovir). The main indications are severe genital HSV infection in adolescents (see Chapter 40) and severe gingivostomatitis in young children. Antiviral therapy is beneficial for primary disease when begun early. Recurrent disease rarely requires therapy. Frequent genital recurrences may be suppressed by oral administration of nucleoside analogs, but this approach should be used sparingly. Other forms of severe cutaneous disease, such as eczema herpeticum, respond to these antivirals. Intravenous acyclovir may be required when disease is extensive in immunocompromised children (500 mg/m² every 8 hours). Oral acyclovir, which is available in suspension, is also used within 72–96 hours for severe primary gingivostomatitis in immunocompetent young children (10 mg/kg per dose four times a day for 5–7 days). Antiviral therapy does not alter the incidence or severity of subsequent recurrences of oral or genital infection. Development of resistance to antivirals is very rare after treating immunocompetent patients, but is increasingly reported in immunocompromised patients who receive frequent and prolonged therapy.

**3. Encephalitis**—This is treated with intravenous acyclovir 500 mg/m² every 8 hours for 21 days.

**4. Neonatal infection**—Newborns receive 20 mg/kg intravenous acyclovir every 8 hours for 21 days (14 days if infection is limited to skin, eye, or mouth).

## B. GENERAL MEASURES

**1. Gingivostomatitis**—Gingivostomatitis is treated with pain relief and temperature control. Maintaining hydration is important because of the long duration of illness (7–14 days). Nonacidic, cool fluids are best. Topical anesthetic agents (eg, viscous lidocaine or an equal mixture of kaolin–attapulgite (Kaopectate), diphenhydramine, and viscous lidocaine may be used as a mouthwash for older children who will not swallow it; ingested lidocaine may be toxic to infants or may lead to aspiration. Antiviral therapy is indicated in normal hosts with severe disease. Antibiotics are not helpful.

**2. Genital infections**—Genital infections require pain relief, assistance with voiding (warm baths, topical anesthetics, rarely catheterization), and psychological support. Lesions should be kept clean; drying decreases the potential for spread and may shorten the duration of symptoms. Sexual contact should be avoided during the interval from prodrome to crusting stages.

**3. Cutaneous lesions**—Skin lesions should be kept clean, dry, and covered if possible to prevent spread. Systemic analgesics may be helpful. Secondary bacterial infection is uncommon in patients with lesions on the mucosa or involving small areas. Secondary infection should be considered and treated if necessary (usually with an antistaphylococcal agent) in patients with more extensive lesions. Candidal superinfection occurs in 10% of women with primary genital infections.

**4. Recurrent cutaneous disease**—Recurrent disease is usually milder than primary infection. Sun block lip balm helps prevent labial recurrences after intense sun exposure. There is no evidence that the many popular topical or vitamin therapies are efficacious.

**5. Keratoconjunctivitis**—An ophthalmologist should be consulted regarding the use of cycloplegics, anti-inflammatory agents, local debridement, and other therapies.

**6. Encephalitis**—Extensive support will be required for obtunded or comatose patients. Rehabilitation and psychological support are often needed for survivors.

**7. Neonatal infection**—The affected infant should be isolated and given acyclovir. Cesarean section is indicated if the mother has obvious cervical or vaginal lesions, especially if these represent primary infection (35–50% transmission rate). With infants born vaginally to mothers who have active lesions, appropriate cultures should be obtained at 24–48 hours after birth, and the infants should be observed closely. Treatment is given to babies whose culture results are positive or who have suggestive signs or symptoms. Babies born to mothers with obvious primary genital herpes should receive therapy before the culture results are known. For women with a history of genital herpes infection, but no genital lesions, vaginal delivery with peripartum cultures of maternal cervix is the standard. Clinical follow-up of the newborn is recommended when maternal culture results are positive. Repeated cervical cultures during pregnancy are not useful.

Amir J et al: The natural history of primary herpes simplex type 1 gingivostomatitis in children. Pediatr Dermatol 1999;16: 259 [PMID: 10469407].

Enright AM, Prober CG: Neonatal herpes infection: Diagnosis, treatment and prevention. Semin Neonatol 2002;7:283 [PMID: 12401298].

Kimberlin DW: Herpes simplex virus infections of the central nervous system. Semin Pediatr Infect Dis 2003;14:83 [PMID: 12881795].

Kohl S: The diagnosis and treatment of neonatal herpes simplex virus infection Pediatr Ann 2002;31:726 [PMID: 12455481].

Whitley RJ: Herpes simplex virus infection. Semin Pediatr Infect Dis 2002;13:6 [PMID: 12118847].

# VARICELLA & HERPES ZOSTER

 **ESSENTIALS OF DIAGNOSIS & TYPICAL FEATURES**

*Varicella (chickenpox):*

- *Exposure to varicella or herpes zoster 10–21 days previously; no prior history of varicella.*

- *Widely scattered red macules and papules concentrated on the face and trunk, rapidly progressing to clear vesicles, pustules, and then crusting,* over 5–6 days. Variable fever and nonspecific systemic symptoms.

*Herpes zoster (shingles):*

• *History of varicella.*

• *Local paresthesias and pain prior to eruption (more common in older children).*

• *Dermatomal distribution of grouped vesicles on an erythematous base.*

## General Considerations

Primary infection with varicella-zoster virus results in varicella, which almost always confers lifelong immunity; the virus remains latent in sensory ganglia. Herpes zoster, which represents reactivation of this latent virus, occurs in 15–20% of individuals some time in their life. The incidence of herpes zoster is highest in elderly individuals and in immunosuppressed patients. Spread of varicella from a contact is by respiratory secretions or fomites from vesicles or pustules, with a greater than 90% infection rate in susceptible persons. Herpes zoster is about one third as infectious. Over 95% of young adults with a history of varicella are immune, as are 90% of native-born Americans who are unaware of having had varicella. Many individuals from tropical or subtropical areas never have childhood exposure and are susceptible. Humans are the only reservoir.

## Clinical Findings

Exposure to varicella or herpes zoster has usually occurred 14–16 days previously (range, 10–21 days). Contact may not have been recognized, since the index case is infectious 1–2 days before rash appears. Although varicella is the most distinctive childhood exanthem, inexperienced observers may mistake other diseases for varicella. A 1- to 3-day prodrome of fever, respiratory symptoms, and headache may occur, especially in older children. The preeruptive pain of herpes zoster may last several days and be mistaken for other illnesses.

### A. Symptoms and Signs

**1. Varicella**—The usual case consists of mild systemic symptoms followed by crops of red macules that rapidly become small vesicles with surrounding erythema (described as a dew drop on a rose petal), form pustules, become crusted and then scab over, and leave no scar. The rash appears predominantly on the trunk and face. Lesions occur in the scalp, nose, mouth (where they are nonspecific ulcers), conjunctiva, and vagina. The magnitude of systemic symptoms usually parallels skin involvement. Up to five crops of lesions may be seen.

New crops usually stop forming after 5–7 days. Pruritus is often intense. If varicella occurs in the first few months of life, it is often mild as a result of persisting maternal antibody. Once crusting begins, the patient is no longer contagious.

**2. Herpes zoster**—The eruption of shingles involves a single dermatome, usually truncal or cranial. The rash does not cross the midline. Ophthalmic zoster may be associated with corneal involvement. The closely grouped vesicles, which resemble a localized version of varicella or herpes simplex, often coalesce. The duration is 7–10 days before crusting. Postherpetic neuralgia is rare in children. A few vesicles are occasionally seen outside the involved dermatome. Herpes zoster is a common problem in HIV-infected or other immunocompromised children. Herpes zoster is also common in children who had varicella in early infancy or whose mothers had varicella during pregnancy.

### B. Laboratory Findings

Leukocyte counts are normal or low. Leukocytosis suggests secondary bacterial infection. The virus can be identified by fluorescent antibody staining of a lesion smear. Rapid culture methods take 48 hours. Diagnosis can be made with paired serology. Serum aminotransferase levels may be modestly elevated during normal varicella.

### C. Imaging

Varicella pneumonia classically produces numerous bilateral nodular densities and hyperinflation. This is very rare in immunocompetent children. Abnormal chest radiographs are seen more frequently in adults.

## Differential Diagnosis

Varicella is usually distinctive. Similar rashes include those of coxsackievirus infection (fewer lesions, lack of crusting), impetigo (fewer lesions, smaller area, no classic vesicles, positive Gram stain, perioral or peripheral lesions), papular urticaria (insect bite history, nonvesicular rash), scabies (burrows, no typical vesicles), parapsoriasis (rare in children younger than age 10 years, chronic or recurrent, often a history of prior varicella), rickettsialpox (eschar where the mite bites, smaller lesions, no crusting), dermatitis herpetiformis (chronic, urticaria, residual pigmentation), and folliculitis. Herpes zoster is sometimes confused with a linear eruption of herpes simplex or a contact dermatitis (eg, *Rhus* dermatitis).

## Complications & Sequelae

### A. Varicella

Secondary bacterial infection with staphylococci or group A streptococci is most common, presenting as impetigo, cellulitis or fasciitis, abscesses, scarlet fever, or sepsis. Bacterial superinfection occurs in 2–3% of children. Hospitalization rates associated with varicella are 1:750–1:1000 cases in children and 10-fold higher in adults.

Protracted vomiting or a change in sensorium suggests Reye syndrome or encephalitis. Because Reye syndrome usually occurs in patients who are also using salicylates, these should be avoided in patients with varicella. Encephalitis occurs in less than 0.1% of cases, usually in the first week of illness. It is usually limited to cerebellitis with ataxia, which resolves completely. Diffuse encephalitis can be severe.

Varicella pneumonia usually afflicts immunocompromised children (especially those with leukemia or lymphoma or those receiving high doses of steroids or chemotherapy) and adults; pregnant women may be at special risk. Cough, dyspnea, tachypnea, rales, and cyanosis occur several days after onset of rash. Varicella may be life-threatening in immunosuppressed patients. Their disease is complicated by severe pneumonitis, hepatitis, and encephalitis. Varicella exposure in such patients must be evaluated immediately for postexposure prophylaxis (see Chapter 9).

Hemorrhagic varicella lesions may be seen without other complications. This is most often caused by autoimmune thrombocytopenia, but hemorrhagic lesions can occasionally represent idiopathic disseminated intravascular coagulation (purpura fulminans).

Neonates born to mothers who develop varicella from 5 days before to 2 days after delivery are at high risk for severe or fatal (5%) disease and must be given varicella-zoster immune globulin (VZIG) and followed closely (see Chapter 9).

Varicella occurring during the first 20 weeks of pregnancy may cause (2% incidence) congenital infection associated with cicatricial skin lesions, associated limb anomalies, and cortical atrophy.

Unusual complications of varicella include optic neuritis, myocarditis, transverse myelitis, orchitis, and arthritis.

### B. HERPES ZOSTER

Complications of herpes zoster include secondary bacterial infection, motor or cranial nerve paralysis (1 per 200 cases in adults), encephalitis, keratitis, and dissemination in immunosuppressed patients. These complications are rare in immunocompetent children, and they do not develop prolonged pain. Postherpetic neuralgia does occur in immunocompromised children.

## Treatment

### A. GENERAL MEASURES

Supportive measures include maintenance of hydration, administration of acetaminophen for discomfort, cool soaks or antipruritics for itching (diphenhydramine, 1.25 mg/kg every 6 hours, or hydroxyzine, 0.5 mg/kg every 6 hours), and observance of general hygiene measures (keep nails trimmed and skin clean). Care must be taken to avoid overdosage with antihistaminic agents. Topical or systemic antibiotics may be needed for bacterial superinfection.

### B. SPECIFIC MEASURES

Although acyclovir is more active against herpes simplex, it is the preferred drug for varicella and herpes zoster infections. Recommended parenteral acyclovir dosage for severe disease is 10 mg/kg (500 mg/m$^2$) intravenously every 8 hours, each dose infused over 1 hour. Parenteral therapy should be started early in immunosuppressed patients or high-risk infected neonates. VZIG is of no value for established disease. The effect of oral acyclovir (80 mg/kg/d, divided in four doses) on varicella in immunocompetent children was modestly beneficial and nontoxic, but only when administered within 24 hour after the onset of varicella. Oral acyclovir should be used selectively in immunocompetent children (eg, when intercurrent illness is present; possibly when second attacks occur in the household or when the patient is an adolescent—both of which are associated with more severe disease) and in children with underlying chronic illnesses. Valacyclovir and famciclovir are superior antiviral agents because of better absorption; acyclovir is available as a pediatric suspension. Herpes zoster in an immunocompromised child should be treated with intravenous acyclovir when it is severe. Oral valacyclovir or famciclovir can be used in immunocompromised children when the nature of the illness and the immune status support this decision.

## Prevention

VZIG is available for postexposure prevention of varicella in high-risk susceptible persons (see Chapter 9). Postexposure prophylaxis with acyclovir is effective when it is started at 8 or 9 days after exposure and is continued for 7 days. The live attenuated varicella vaccine should be given as part of routine childhood immunization, and "catch-up" immunization is recommended for all other susceptible children and adults. Varicella vaccine is also useful for postexposure prophylaxis when given within 3–5 days of the exposure.

## Prognosis

Except for secondary bacterial infections, serious complications are rare and recovery complete in immunocompetent hosts.

Varicella-related deaths—United States, 2002. MMWR- Morb Mortal Weekly Rep 2002;52:545 [PMID: 12803193].

# ROSEOLA INFANTUM (EXANTHEMA SUBITUM)

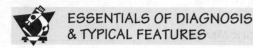

## ESSENTIALS OF DIAGNOSIS & TYPICAL FEATURES

- *High fever in a child age 6–36 months.*
- *Minimal toxicity.*
- *Rose-pink maculopapular rash appears when fever subsides.*

## General Considerations

Roseola infantum is a benign illness caused by human herpesviruses 6 (HHV-6) or 7 (HHV-7). HHV-6 is a major cause of acute febrile illness in young children. Its significance is its ability to mimic more serious causes of high fever and its role in inciting febrile seizures.

## Clinical Findings

The most prominent historical feature is the abrupt onset of fever, often reaching 40.6°C, which lasts up to 8 days (mean, 4 days) in an otherwise mildly ill child. The fever then ceases abruptly, and a characteristic rash may appear. Roseola occurs predominantly in children age 6 months to 3 years, with 90% of cases occurring before the second year. HHV-7 infection tends to occur somewhat later in childhood. These viruses are the most common recognized cause of exanthematous fever in this age group and are responsible for 20% of emergency room visits by children age 6–12 months.

### A. SYMPTOMS AND SIGNS

Mild lethargy and irritability may be present, but generally there is a dissociation between systemic symptoms and the febrile course. The pharynx, tonsils, and tympanic membranes may be injected. Conjunctivitis and pharyngeal exudate are notably absent. Diarrhea and vomiting occur in one third of patients. Adenopathy of the head and neck often occurs. The anterior fontanelle is bulging in one quarter of HHV-6-infected infants. If rash appears (20–30% incidence), it begins on the trunk and spreads to the face, neck, and extremities. Rose-pink macules or maculopapules, 2–3 mm in diameter, are nonpruritic, tend to coalesce, and disap-

pear in 1–2 days without pigmentation or desquamation. Rash may occur without fever.

### B. LABORATORY FINDINGS

Leukopenia and lymphocytopenia are present early. Laboratory evidence of hepatitis occurs in some patients, especially adults.

## Differential Diagnosis

The initial high fever may require exclusion of serious bacterial infection. The relative well-being of most children and the typical course and rash soon clarify the diagnosis. The erythrocyte sedimentation rate is normal. If the child has a febrile seizure, it is important to exclude bacterial meningitis. The CSF is normal in children with roseola. In children who receive antibiotics or other medication at the beginning of the fever, the rash may be attributed incorrectly to drug allergy.

## Complications & Sequelae

Febrile seizures occur in 10% of patients (even higher percentages in those with HHV-7 infections). There is evidence that HHV-6 can directly infect the CNS, causing meningoencephalitis or aseptic meningitis. Multiorgan disease (pneumonia, hepatitis, bone marrow suppression, encephalitis) may occur in immunocompromised patients.

## Treatment & Prognosis

Fever is managed readily with acetaminophen and sponge baths. Fever control should be a major consideration in children with a history of febrile seizures. Roseola infantum is otherwise entirely benign.

DeAraujo T et al: Human herpesviruses 6 and 7. Dermatol Clin 2002;20:301 [PMID: 12120443].

Jackson MA, Sommerauer JF: Human herpesviruses 6 and 7. Pediatr Infect Dis J 2002;21:566 [PMID: 12182383].

# CYTOMEGALOVIRUS INFECTIONS

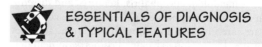

## ESSENTIALS OF DIAGNOSIS & TYPICAL FEATURES

*Primary Infection:*
- *Asymptomatic or minor illness in young children.*
- *Mononucleosis-like syndrome without pharyngitis in postpubertal individuals.*

*Congenital Infection:*
- *Intrauterine growth retardation.*

- Microcephaly with intracerebral calcifications and seizures.
- Retinitis and encephalitis.
- Hepatosplenomegaly with thrombocytopenia.
- "Blueberry muffin" rash.
- Sensorineural deafness.

Immunocompromised Hosts:

- Retinitis and encephalitis.
- Pneumonitis.
- Enteritis and hepatitis.
- Bone marrow suppression.

## General Considerations

Cytomegalovirus (CMV) is a ubiquitous herpesvirus transmitted by many routes. It can be acquired in utero following maternal viremia or postpartum from birth canal secretions or maternal milk. Young children are infected by the saliva of playmates; older individuals are infected by sexual partners (eg, from saliva, vaginal secretions, or semen). Transfused blood products and transplanted organs can be a source of CMV infection. Clinical illness is determined largely by the patient's immune competence. Immunocompetent individuals usually develop a mild self-limited illness, whereas immunocompromised children can develop severe, progressive, often multiorgan disease. In utero infection can be teratogenic.

## 1. In Utero Cytomegalovirus Infection

Approximately 0.5–1.5% of children are born with CMV infections acquired during maternal viremia. CMV infection is asymptomatic in over 90% of these children, who are usually born to mothers who had experienced reactivation of latent CMV infection during the pregnancy. Symptomatic infection occurs predominantly in infants born to mothers with primary CMV infection but can also result from recurrent, most likely, reinfection during pregnancy. Even when exposed to a primary maternal infection, less than 50% of fetuses are infected, and in only 10% of those infants is the infection symptomatic at birth. Primary infection in the first half of pregnancy poses the greatest risk for severe fetal damage.

## Clinical Findings

### A. SYMPTOMS AND SIGNS

Severely affected infants are born ill; they are often small for gestational age, floppy, and lethargic. They feed poorly and have poor temperature control. Hepatosplenomegaly, jaundice, petechiae, seizures, and microcephaly are common. Characteristic signs are a distinctive chorioretinitis and periventricular calcification. A purpuric (so-called blueberry muffin) rash similar to that seen with congenital rubella may be present. The mortality rate is 10–20%. Survivors usually have significant sequelae, especially mental retardation, neurologic deficits, retinopathy, and hearing loss. Isolated hepatosplenomegaly or thrombocytopenia may occur. Even mildly affected children may subsequently manifest mental retardation and psychomotor delay. However, most infected infants (90%) are born to mothers with preexisting immunity who had a reactivation of latent CMV during pregnancy. These children have no clinical manifestations at birth. Of these, 10–15% develop sensorineural hearing loss, which is often bilateral and may appear several years after birth.

### B. LABORATORY FINDINGS

In severely ill infants, anemia, thrombocytopenia, hyperbilirubinemia, and elevated aminotransferase levels are common. Lymphocytosis occurs occasionally. Pleocytosis and an elevated protein concentration are found in CSF. The diagnosis is readily confirmed by isolation of CMV from urine or saliva within 48 hours, using rapid culture methods combined with immunoassay. The presence in the infant of IgM-specific CMV antibodies suggests the diagnosis. Some commercial ELISA kits are 90% sensitive and specific for these antibodies.

### C. IMAGING

Head radiologic exams may show microcephaly, periventricular calcifications, and ventricular dilation. These findings strongly correlate with neurologic sequelae and retardation. Long bone radiographs may show the "celery stalk" pattern characteristic of congenital viral infections. Interstitial pneumonia may be present.

## Differential Diagnosis

CMV infection should be considered in any newborn who is seriously ill shortly after birth, especially once bacterial sepsis, metabolic disease, intracranial bleeding, and cardiac disease have been excluded. Other congenital infections to be considered in the differential diagnosis include toxoplasmosis (serology, more diffuse calcification of the CNS, specific type of retinitis, macrocephaly), rubella (serology, specific type of retinitis, cardiac lesions, eye abnormalities), enteroviral infections (time of year, maternal illness, severe hepatitis), herpes simplex (skin lesions, cultures, severe hepatitis), and syphilis (serology for both infant and mother, skin lesions, bone involvement).

## Treatment & Prevention

Support is rarely required for anemia and thrombocytopenia. Most children with symptoms at birth have significant neurologic, intellectual, visual, or auditory impairment. Ganciclovir, 5 mg/kg every 12 hours, is recommended for children with severe, life- or sight-threatening disease of if end-organ disease recurs or progresses. Duration is 2–3 weeks or until symptoms resolve. This approach decreases viral shedding and limits progression of symptoms, including hearing loss, during treatment. However, the therapeutic advantage is progressively lost over time after treatment is discontinued. Children who are asymptomatic at birth have a 10–15% incidence of hearing loss but few other sequelae. There is no evidence that early treatment prevents late-onset hearing loss. Delayed development and hearing loss should be looked for and treated as soon as possible.

## 2. Perinatal Cytomegalovirus Infection

CMV infection can be acquired from birth canal secretions or shortly after birth from maternal milk. In some socioeconomic groups, 10–20% of infants are infected at birth and excrete CMV for many months. Infection can also be acquired in the postnatal period from unscreened transfused blood products.

## Clinical Findings

### A. SYMPTOMS AND SIGNS

Ninety percent of immunocompetent infants infected by their mothers at birth develop subclinical illness (ie, virus excretion only) or a minor illness within 1–3 months. The remainder develop an illness lasting several weeks and characterized by hepatosplenomegaly, lymphadenopathy, and interstitial pneumonitis in various combinations. The severity of the pneumonitis may be increased by the simultaneous presence of *Chlamydia trachomatis*. Infants who receive blood products are often premature and immunologically impaired. If they are born to CMV-negative mothers and subsequently receive CMV-containing blood, they frequently develop severe infection and pneumonia after a 2- to 6-week incubation period.

### B. LABORATORY FINDINGS

Lymphocytosis, atypical lymphocytes, anemia, and thrombocytopenia may be present, especially in premature infants. Liver function is abnormal. CMV can be isolated from urine and saliva. Secretions obtained at bronchoscopy contain CMV and epithelial cells bearing CMV antigens. Serum levels of CMV antibody rise significantly.

### C. IMAGING

Chest radiographs show a diffuse interstitial pneumonitis in severely affected infants.

## Differential Diagnosis

CMV infection should be considered as a cause of any prolonged illness in early infancy, especially if hepatosplenomegaly, lymphadenopathy, or atypical lymphocytosis is present. This must be distinguished from granulomatous or malignant diseases and from congenital infections (syphilis, toxoplasmosis, hepatitis B) not previously diagnosed. Other viruses (Epstein–Barr virus [EBV], HIV, adenovirus) can cause this syndrome. CMV is a recognized cause of viral pneumonia in this age group. Because asymptomatic CMV excretion is common in early infancy, care must be taken to establish the diagnosis and to rule out concomitant pathogens such as *Chlamydia* and RSV. Severe CMV infection in early infancy may indicate that the child has a congenital or acquired immune deficiency.

## Treatment & Prevention

The self-limited disease of normal infants requires no therapy. Severe pneumonitis in premature infants requires oxygen administration and often intubation. Very ill infants should receive ganciclovir (6 mg/kg every 12 hours). CMV infection acquired by transfusion can be prevented by excluding CMV-seropositive blood donors. Milk donors should also be screened for prior CMV infection. It is likely that high-risk infants receiving large doses of IVIG for other reasons will be protected against severe CMV disease.

## 3. Cytomegalovirus Infection Acquired in Childhood & Adolescence

Young children are readily infected by playmates, especially because CMV continues to be excreted in saliva and urine for many months after infection. The cumulative annual incidence of CMV excretion by children in day care centers exceeds 75%. In fact, young children in a family are often the source of primary CMV infection of their mothers during subsequent pregnancies. An additional peak of CMV infection takes place when adolescents become sexually active. Sporadic acquisition of CMV occurs after blood transfusion and transplantation.

## Clinical Findings

### A. SYMPTOMS AND SIGNS

Most young children who acquire CMV are asymptomatic or have a minor febrile illness, occasionally with adenopathy. They provide an important reservoir of virus shedders that facilitates spread of CMV. Occasionally a child may have prolonged fever with hepatosplenomegaly and adenopathy. Older children and adults, many of whom are infected during sexual activity, are more likely to be symptomatic in this fashion and can present with a syndrome that mimics the infectious mononucleosis syndrome that follows EBV infection (1–2 weeks of fever, malaise, anorexia, splenomegaly, mild hepatitis, and some adenopathy; see next section). This syndrome can also occur 2–4 weeks after transfusion of CMV-infected blood.

### B. LABORATORY FINDINGS

In the CMV mononucleosis syndrome, lymphocytosis and atypical lymphocytes are common, as is a mild rise in aminotransferase levels. CMV is present in saliva and urine, and CMV DNA can be uniformly detected in plasma or blood.

## Differential Diagnosis

In older children, CMV infection should be included as a possible cause of fever of unknown origin, especially when lymphocytosis and atypical lymphocytes are present. CMV infection is distinguished from EBV infection by the absence of pharyngitis, the relatively minor adenopathy, and the absence of serologic evidence of acute EBV infection. Mononucleosis syndromes are also caused by *Toxoplasma gondii,* rubella virus, adenovirus, hepatitis A virus, and HIV.

## Prevention

Screening of transfused blood or filtering blood (thus removing CMV-containing white blood cells) prevents cases related to this source.

## 4. Cytomegalovirus Infection in Immunocompromised Children

In addition to symptoms experienced during primary infection, immunocompromised hosts develop symptoms with reinfection or reactivation of latent CMV. This is clearly seen in children with acquired immunodeficiency syndrome (AIDS), after transplantation, or with congenital immunodeficiencies. However, in most immunocompromised patients, primary infection is more likely to cause severe symptoms than is reactivation or reinfection. The severity of the resulting disease is generally proportionate to the degree of immunosuppression.

## Clinical Findings

### A. SYMPTOMS AND SIGNS

A mild febrile illness with myalgia, malaise, and arthralgia may occur, especially with reactivation disease. Severe disease often includes subacute onset of dyspnea and cyanosis as manifestations of interstitial pneumonitis. Auscultation reveals only coarse breath sounds and scattered rales. A rapid respiratory rate may precede clinical or radiographic evidence of pneumonia. Hepatitis without jaundice or hepatomegaly is common. Diarrhea, which can be severe, occurs with CMV colitis, and CMV can cause esophagitis with symptoms of odynophagia or dysphagia. These enteropathies are most common in AIDS, as is the presence of a retinitis that often progresses to blindness. Encephalitis and polyradiculitis also occur in AIDS.

### B. LABORATORY FINDINGS

Neutropenia and thrombocytopenia are common. Atypical lymphocytosis is infrequent. Serum aminotransferase levels are often elevated. The stools may contain occult blood if enteropathy is present. CMV is readily isolated from saliva, urine, buffy coat, and bronchial secretions. Results are available in 48 hours. Interpretation of positive cultures is made difficult by asymptomatic shedding of CMV in saliva and urine in many immunocompromised patients. CMV disease correlates more closely with the presence of CMV in the blood or lung lavage fluid. Monitoring for the appearance of CMV DNA in plasma or CMV antigen in blood mononuclear cells is used as a guide to early antiviral ("pre-emptive") therapy.

### C. IMAGING

Bilateral interstitial pneumonitis is present on chest radiographs.

## Differential Diagnosis

The initial febrile illness must be distinguished from treatable bacterial or fungal infection. Similarly the pulmonary disease must be distinguished from intrapulmonary hemorrhage; drug-induced or radiation pneumonitis; pulmonary edema; and bacterial, fungal, parasitic, and other viruses infection in this population. CMV infection is seen bilaterally and interstitially on chest radiographs, cough is nonproductive, chest pain is absent, and the patient is not usually toxic. *Pneumocystis jiroveci* (formerly *Pneumocystis carinii*) infection may have a similar presentation. These patients may have polymicrobial disease. It is suspected that bacterial and fungal infections are enhanced by the neutropenia that can accompany CMV infection. Infection of the gastrointestinal tract is diagnosed by endoscopy. This will exclude candidal, adenoviral, and herpes simplex infections and allows tissue confirmation of CMV-induced mucosal ulcerations.

## Treatment & Prevention

Blood donors should be screened to exclude those with prior CMV infection, or blood should be filtered. Ideally, seronegative transplant recipients should receive organs from seronegative donors. Severe symptoms, most commonly pneumonitis, often respond to early therapy with intravenous ganciclovir (5 mg/kg every 12 hours for 14–21 days). Neutropenia is a frequent side effect of this therapy. Foscarnet and cidofovir are alternative therapeutic agents recommended for patients with ganciclovir-resistant virus. Prophylactic use of oral or intravenous ganciclovir may prevent CMV infections in organ transplant recipients. Preemptive therapy can be used in some high-risk transplant recipients who are monitored for CMV antigen or DNA in their plasma or mononuclear cells and who receive antivirals when the test results reach a certain threshold or rapidly increase regardless of clinical signs or symptoms. CMV-seropositive children with AIDS and low CD4 counts (< 50/μL) should have funduscopic examinations and plasma CMV DNA measurements every 3 months.

Demmler G: Congenital cytomegalovirus infection and disease. Adv Pediatr Infect Dis 1996;11:135 [PMID: 8718462].

Kimberlin DW et al: Effect of ganciclovir therapy on hearing in symptomatic congenital CMV. J Pediatr 2003;143:17 [PMID: 12915819].

Michaels M et al: Treatment of children with congenital CMV with ganciclovir Pediatr Infect Dis J 2003;22:504 [PMID: 12799506].

# INFECTIOUS MONONUCLEOSIS (Epstein–Barr Virus)

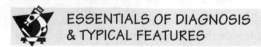

### ESSENTIALS OF DIAGNOSIS & TYPICAL FEATURES

- *Prolonged fever.*
- *Exudative pharyngitis.*
- *Generalized adenopathy.*
- *Hepatosplenomegaly.*
- *Atypical lymphocytes.*
- *Heterophil antibodies.*

## General Considerations

Mononucleosis is the most characteristic syndrome produced by EBV infection. Young children infected with EBV have either no symptoms or a mild nonspecific febrile illness. As the age of the host increases, EBV infection is more likely to produce the typical features of the mononucleosis syndrome in 20–25% of infected adolescents. EBV is acquired readily from asymptomatic carriers (15–20% of whom excrete the virus in saliva on any given day) and from recently ill patients, who excrete virus for many months. Young children are infected from the saliva of playmates and family members. Adolescents may be infected through sexual activity. EBV can also be transmitted by blood transfusion and organ transplantation.

## Clinical Findings

### A. SYMPTOMS AND SIGNS

After an incubation period of 1–2 months, a 2- to 3-day prodrome of malaise and anorexia yields, abruptly or insidiously, to a febrile illness with temperatures exceeding 39°C. The major complaint is pharyngitis, which is often (50%) exudative. Lymph nodes are enlarged, firm, and mildly tender. Any area may be affected, but posterior and anterior cervical nodes are almost always enlarged. Splenomegaly is present in 50–75% of patients. Hepatomegaly is common (30%), and the liver is frequently tender. Five percent of patients have a rash, which can be macular, scarlatiniform, or urticarial. Rash is almost universal in patients taking penicillin or ampicillin. Soft palate petechiae and eyelid edema are also observed.

### B. LABORATORY FINDINGS

**1. Peripheral blood**—Leukopenia may occur early, but an atypical lymphocytosis (comprising over 10% of the total leukocytes at some time in the illness) is most notable. Hematologic changes may not be seen until the third week of illness and may be entirely absent in some EBV syndromes (eg, neurologic ones).

**2. Heterophil antibodies**—These nonspecific antibodies appear in over 90% of older patients with mononucleosis but in fewer than 50% of children younger than age 5 years. They may not be detectable until the second week of illness and may persist for up to 12 months after recovery. Rapid screening tests (slide agglutination) are usually positive if the titer is significant; a positive result strongly suggests but does not prove EBV infection.

**3. Anti-EBV antibodies**—It may be necessary to measure specific antibody titers when heterophil antibodies fail to appear, as in young children. Acute EBV infection is established by detecting IgM antibody to the viral capsid antigen (VCA) or by detecting a fall over several weeks of IgG anti-VCA titers (IgG antibody peaks by the time symptoms appear).

**4. EBV PCR**—This assay detects EBV DNA. It is the method of choice for the diagnosis of CNS and ocular infections. Quantitative EBV PCR in peripheral blood mononuclear cells has been used to detect EBV-related lymphoproliferative disorders in transplant patients.

## Differential Diagnosis

Severe pharyngitis may suggest group A streptococcal infection. Enlargement of only the anterior cervical lymph nodes, a neutrophilic leukocytosis, and the absence of splenomegaly suggest bacterial infection. Although a child with a positive throat culture result for streptococcus usually requires therapy, up to 10% of children with mononucleosis are asymptomatic streptococcal carriers. In this group, penicillin therapy is unnecessary and often causes a rash. Severe primary herpes simplex pharyngitis, occurring in adolescence, may also mimic infectious mononucleosis. In this type of pharyngitis, some anterior mouth ulcerations should suggest the correct diagnosis. EBV infection should be considered in the differential diagnosis of any perplexing prolonged febrile illness. Similar illnesses that produce atypical lymphocytosis include rubella (pharyngitis not prominent, shorter illness, less adenopathy and splenomegaly), adenovirus (upper respiratory symptoms and cough, conjunctivitis, less adenopathy, fewer atypical lymphocytes), hepatitis A or B (more severe liver function abnormalities, no pharyngitis, no lymphadenopathy), and toxoplasmosis (negative heterophil test, less pharyngitis). Serum sickness-like drug reactions and leukemia (smear morphology is important) may be confused with infectious mononucleosis. CMV mononucleosis is a close mimic except for minimal pharyngitis and less adenopathy; it is much less common. Serologic tests for EBV and CMV should clarify the correct diagnosis. The acute initial manifestation of HIV infection is a mononucleosis-like syndrome in many patients.

## Complications

Splenic rupture is a rare complication, which usually follows significant trauma. Hematologic complications, including hemolytic anemia, thrombocytopenia, and neutropenia, are more common. Neurologic involvement can include aseptic meningitis, encephalitis, isolated neuropathy such as Bell palsy, and Guillain–Barré syndrome. Any of these may appear prior to or in the absence of the more typical signs and symptoms of infectious mononucleosis. Rare complications include myocarditis, pericarditis, and atypical pneumonia. Recurrence or persistence of EBV-associated symptoms for 6 months or longer characterizes chronic active EBV. This disease is due to continuous viral replication and warrants specific antiviral therapy. Rarely EBV infection becomes a progressive lymphoproliferative disorder characterized by persistent fever, multiple organ involvement, neutropenia or pancytopenia, and agammaglobulinemia. Hemocytophagia is often present in the bone marrow. An X-linked genetic defect in immune response has been inferred for some patients (Duncan syndrome, X-linked lymphoproliferative disorder). Children with other congenital immunodeficiencies or chemotherapy-induced immunosuppression can also develop progressive EBV infection, EBV-associated lymphoproliferative disorder or lymphoma, and other malignancies.

## Treatment & Prognosis

Bed rest may be necessary in severe cases. Acetaminophen controls high fever. Potential airway obstruction due to swollen pharyngeal lymphoid tissue responds rapidly to systemic corticosteroids. Corticosteroids may also be given for hematologic and neurologic complications, although no controlled trials have proved their efficacy in these conditions. Fever and pharyngitis disappear by 10–14 days. Adenopathy and splenomegaly can persist several weeks longer. Some patients complain of fatigue, malaise, or lack of well-being for several months. Although steroids may shorten the duration of fatigue and malaise, their long-term effects on this potentially oncogenic viral infection are unknown, and indiscriminate use is discouraged. Patients with splenic enlargement should avoid contact sports for 6–8 weeks. Acyclovir, valacyclovir, penciclovir, ganciclovir, and foscarnet are active against EBV and are indicated in the treatment of chronic active EBV.

Management of EBV-related lymphoproliferative disorders relies primarily on decreasing the immunosuppression whenever possible. Adjunctive therapy with acyclovir, ganciclovir, or another antiviral active against EBV as well as CMV hyperimmune globulin has been used without scientific evidence of efficacy.

Chetham MM, Roberts KB: Infectious mononucleosis in adolescents. Pediatr Ann 1991;20:206 [PMID: 1648197].

Kanegane H et al: Increased cell-free viral DNA in fatal cases of chronic active Epstein–Barr virus infection. Clin Infect Dis 1999;28:906 [PMID: 10825059].

Weinberg A et al: Quantitative CSF PCR in Epstein–Barr virus infections of the central nervous system. Ann Neurol 2002;52:543 [PMID: 12402250].

# VIRAL INFECTIONS SPREAD BY INSECT VECTORS

In the United States, mosquitoes are the most common insect vectors that spread viral infections (Table 36–4).

**Table 36–4.** Some virus diseases spread by insects in the United States.

| Disease | Natural Reservoir (Vector) | Geographic Distribution | Incubation Period | Clinical Presentations | Laboratory Findings | Complications, Sequelae | Diagnosis, Therapy, Comments |
|---|---|---|---|---|---|---|---|
| **FLAVIVIRUSES** | | | | | | | |
| St. Louis encephalitis (SLE) | Birds (Culex mosquitoes) | Southern Canada, central and southern United States Caribbean, South America | 2–5 d (up to 3 wk) | Abrupt onset of fever, chills, headache, nausea, vomiting; may develop generalized weakness, seizures, coma, ataxia, cranial nerve palsies. Aseptic meningitis is common in children | Modest leukocytosis, neutrophilia, elevated liver enzymes. CSF: 100–200 WBC/μL (PMNs predominate early). | Mortality rate 2–5% in children (especially < age 5). Neurologic sequelae in 1–20%. | 20–500 cases a year, < 2% symptomatic. (Worse in elderly.) Therapy: supportive. Diagnosis: serology. Specific antibody often present within 5 d. |
| Dengue | Humans (Aedes mosquitoes) | Asia, Africa, Central and South America, Caribbean; rarely in southern United States | 4–7 d (range 3–14 d) | Fever, headache, myalgia, joint and bone pain, retro-ocular pain, nausea and vomiting; maculopapular or petechial rash in 50%, sparing palms and soles; adenopathy. Meningoencephalitis in 5–10% of children. | Leukopenia, thrombocytopenia. CSF: 100–500 mononuclear cells/μL if neurologic signs are present. | Hemorrhagic fever, shock syndrome, prolonged weakness. | High infection rate. 50–150 cases occur in US travelers to endemic areas. Biphasic course may occur. Therapy: supportive. Diagnosis: serology; IgM-EIA antibody by day 6. |
| West Nile | Birds (Culex mosquitoes); small mammals | N. Africa, Middle East, parts of Asia, Europe, continental United States | 3–12 d | Abrupt onset of fever, headache, sore throat, myalgia, retro-ocular pain, conjunctivitis; 20–50% with rash; adenopathy. Encephalitis may be accompanied by muscle weakness, flaccid paralysis, or movement disorders. | Mild leukocytosis; 10–15% lymphopenic moderate CSF pleocytosis. | Mortality rate 10%, of those with CNS symptoms, especially in elderly; weakness and myalgia may persist for an extended period. | Most imortant mosquito-borne encephalitis in the United States. Diagnosis: IgM-EIA serology; cross-reacts with St. Louis encephalitis; positive by 6–8 d; definitive diagnosis by PCR. Therapy: supportive |
| **ALPHA TOGA VIRUSES** | | | | | | | |
| Western equine encephalitis | Birds (Culisata mosquitoes) | Canada, Mexico, and United States west of Mississippi River | 2–5 d | Similar to that of St. Louis encephalitis. Most infections are subclinical. | Variable white counts. CSF: 10–300 WBC/μL. | Permanent brain damage, 10% overall; most severe in older adults. | < 50 cases a year in the United States. Case/infection is 1:1000 for older adults and 1:1 for infants. Equine illness precedes human outbreaks. Diagnosis: IgM antibody in first week. Therapy: supportive |

| Disease | Reservoir (Vector) | Distribution | Incubation | Clinical features | Laboratory findings | Severity/Mortality | Comments |
|---|---|---|---|---|---|---|---|
| Eastern equine encephalitis | Birds (*Culisata* mosquitoes) | Eastern seaboard United States, Carribbean, South America | 2–5 d | Similar to that of St. Louis encephalitis but more severe. Progresses rapidly in one third to coma and death. | Leukocytosis with neutrophilia. CSF: 500–2000 WBC/μL; PMNs predominate early. | Mortality rate 20–50%; neurologic sequelae in over 50% of children. | Most severe mosquito-borne encephalitis in the United States. Fewer than 20 cases a year. Only 3–10% of cases are symptomatic. Therapy: supportive. Diagnosis: serology. Titers often positive in first week. Equine deaths may signal an outbreak. |
| Venezuelan equine encephalitis | Horses (ten species of mosquitoes) | South and Central America, Texas | 1–6 d | Similar to that of St. Louis encephalitis. | Lymphopenia, mild thrombocytopenia, abnormal liver function tests. CSF: 50–200 mononuclears/μL. | Severe disease more common in infants; 20% fatality rate for encephalitis. | Most infections do not cause encephalitis. Vaccination of horses will stop epidemic. Therapy: supportive. Diagnosis: IgM antibody (EIA). |
| **BUNYAVIRUS** | | | | | | | |
| California encephalitis (La Crosse, Jamestown Canyon, California) | Chipmunks and other small mammals (*Aedes* mosquitoes) | Northern and mid central United States, southern Canada | 3–7 d | Similar to that of St. Louis encephalitis; sore throat and respiratory symptoms are common; focal neurologic signs in up to 25%. Seizures prominent. Prepubertal children are most likely to have severe disease. Can mimic HSV encephalitis. | Variable white counts. CSF: 30–200 (up to 600) WBC/μL; variable PMNs; protein often normal. | Mortality rate < 1%. Seizure disorder may begin during acute illness. | About 100–150 cases a year in the United States, 5% symptomatic. > 10% with sequelae. Therapy: supportive. Diagnosis: serology. Up to 90% has specific IgM antibody in first week; 25% of population in certain regions has IgG antibody. |
| **COLTIVIRUS** | | | | | | | |
| Colorado tick fever | Small mammals (*Dermacentor andersoni*, or wood tick) | Rocky Mountain region of United States and Canada | 3–4 d (range, 2–14 d) | Fever, chills, myalgia, conjunctivitis, headache, retro-orbital pain; rash in < 10%. No respiratory symptoms. Biphasic fever in 50%. | Leukopenia (maximum at 4–6 d), mild thrombocytopenia. | Rare encephalitis, coagulopathy. | Patient may have no known tick bite. Acute illness lasts 7–10 d; prolonged fatigue in adults. Therapy: supportive. Diagnosis: serology, direct FA staining of red cells for viral antigen, PCR. |

CSF = cerebrospinal fluid; EIA = enzyme immunoassay; FA = fluorescent antibody; PCR = polymerase chain reaction; PMN = polymorphonuclear neutrophil; WBC = white blood cells; HSV = herpes simplex virus.

As a consequence, these infections—and others that are spread by ticks—tend to occur as summer–fall epidemics that coincide with the seasonal breeding and feeding habits of the vector, and the etiologic agent varies by region. Thus a careful travel and exposure history is critical for correct diagnostic work-up.

# ENCEPHALITIS

Encephalitis presents as fever, headache, and various combinations of sensorial or behavioral change, with or without focal neurological abnormalities (see Chapter 23). Evidence of meningitis is often present. CSF is abnormal, usually with mononuclear cell pleocytosis, elevated protein level, and normal sugar level. Neutrophils may be prominent in CSF early in the illness. Encephalitis is a common severe manifestation of many infections spread by insects (see Table 36–4). With many pathogens, the infection is most often subclinical, or mild CNS disease such as meningitis is present. These infections have some distinguishing features in terms of subclinical infection rate, unique neurologic syndromes, associated non-neurologic symptoms, and prognosis. The diagnosis is generally made clinically during recognized outbreaks and is confirmed by virus-specific serology. Prevention consists of control of mosquito vectors and precautions with proper clothing and insect repellents to minimize mosquito and tick bites.

## 1. West Nile Virus Encephalitis

This flavivirus is the most important arbovirus infection in the United States. Since it was described in 1999 in New York, it has spread to 47 states. In 2003, West Nile virus caused more than 8500 infections and 190 deaths, the largest epidemic of arboviral meningoencephalitis ever reported. Its reservoir includes more than 160 species of birds whose migration explain the rapid growth of the epidemic. During summer–fall epidemics most infected individuals are asymptomatic. Approximately 20% develop West Nile fever, which is characterized by fever, headache, retro-orbital pain, nausea and vomiting, lymphadenopathy, and a maculopapular rash (20–50%). Less than 1% of infected patients develop meningitis or encephalitis, but 10% of these cases are fatal (0.1% of all infections). The major risk factor for severe disease is age older than 50 years and immune compromise, although children develop West Nile fever and occasionally have neurologic disease. The neurologic manifestations are most often those found with other encephalitides. However, distinguishing atypical features include polio-like flaccid paralysis, movement disorders (parkinsonism, tremor, myoclonus), brainstem symptoms, polyneuropathy,

and optic neuritis. Muscle weakness, facial palsy, and hyporeflexia are common (20% of each finding). Diagnosis is best made by detecting IgM antibody (EIA) to the virus in CSF. This will be present by 2–3 days (95%) after onset. PCR is a specific diagnostic tool, but is less sensitive than antibody detection. Antibody rise in serum can also be used for diagnosis. Treatment is supportive, although various antivirals and specific immune globulin are being studied. The infection is not spread between contacts, but is spread by donated organs and blood and breast milk and transplacentally. The coming years will indicate if this virus will become a serious endemic problem in the United States.

Petersen LR et al: West Nile virus. JAMA 2003;290:524 [PMID: 2876096].

Solomon T et al: West Nile encephalitis. BMJ 2003;326:865 [PMID: 12702624].

# DENGUE

In endemic areas 50–100 million cases of dengue occur each year, often in severe forms. In the United States, 50–150 cases are diagnosed, most often in travelers from the Caribbean or Asia and less often in those visiting Central and South America. Texas has sporadic indigenous outbreaks of dengue. The spread of dengue requires the requisite species of mosquito, which transmits virus from a reservoir of viremic humans in endemic areas. Most patients have mild disease, especially young children, who may have a nonspecific fever and rash. Severity is a function of age and prior infection with other serotypes of dengue virus, a prerequisite for severe hemorrhagic complications.

## Clinical Findings

### A. SYMPTOMS AND SIGNS

Dengue fever begins abruptly 4–7 days after transmission (range, 3–14 days) with fever, chills, severe retro-orbital pain, severe muscle and joint pain, nausea, and vomiting. Erythema of the face and torso may occur early. After 3–4 days a centrifugal maculopapular rash appears in half of patients. The rash can become petechial, and mild hemorrhagic signs (epistaxis, gingival bleeding, microscopic blood in stool or urine) may be noted. The illness lasts 5–7 days, although rarely fever may reappear for several additional days.

### B. LABORATORY FINDINGS

Leukopenia and a mild drop in platelets are common. Liver function tests are usually normal. Diagnosis is made by viral culture of plasma (50% sensitive up to the fifth day), by detecting IgM-specific ELISA antibodies (90% sensitive at the sixth day), or by detecting a rise in type-specific antibody. PCR is available for diagnosis.

## Differential Diagnosis

This diagnosis should be considered for any traveler to an endemic area who has symptoms suggestive of a systemic viral illness, although less than 1 in 1000 travelers to these areas develop dengue. Often the areas visited have other unique viruses circulating and are potential sources of malaria, typhoid fever, leptospirosis, and measles. EBV, influenza, enteroviruses, and acute HIV infection may produce a similar illness. An illness that starts 2 weeks after the trip ends or that lasts longer than 2 weeks is not dengue.

## Complications

Rarely dengue fever is associated with meningoencephalitis (5–10%) or hepatic damage. More common in endemic areas is the appearance of dengue hemorrhagic fever, which is defined by significant thrombocytopenia, bleeding, and a plasma leak syndrome (hemoconcentration, hypoalbuminemia, and pleural or peritoneal effusions). This is the consequence of circulating antibody acquired from a prior heterotypic dengue virus infection; thus it is rarely seen in typical travelers. Failure to recognize and treat this complication may lead to dengue shock syndrome, which has a high fatality rate.

## Prevention

Prevention of dengue fever involves avoiding high-risk areas and using conventional mosquito avoidance measures. The main vector is a day-time feeder.

## Treatment

Dengue fever is treated by oral replacement of fluid lost from gastrointestinal symptoms. Analgesic therapy, which is often necessary, should not include drugs that affect platelet function. Recovery is complete without sequelae. The hemorrhagic syndrome requires prompt fluid therapy with plasma expanders and isotonic saline.

Gregson A, Edelman R: Dengue virus infection. Pediatr Infect Dis J 2003;22:179 [PMID:12586982].

## COLORADO TICK FEVER

Colorado tick fever, a tick-borne illness, is endemic in the high plains and mountains of the central and northern Rocky Mountains and northern Pacific coast of the United States. The reservoir of the virus consists of squirrels and chipmunks. Many hundreds of cases of Colorado tick fever occur each year in visitors or laborers entering this region, primarily from May through July.

## Clinical Findings

### A. SYMPTOMS AND SIGNS

After a 3- to 4-day incubation period (maximum, 14 days) fever begins suddenly together with chills, lethargy, headache, ocular pain, myalgia, abdominal pain, and nausea and vomiting. Conjunctivitis may be present. A nondistinctive maculopapular rash occurs in 5–10% of patients. The illness lasts 7–10 days, and half of patients have a biphasic fever curve with several afebrile days in the midst of the illness.

### B. LABORATORY FINDINGS

Leukopenia is characteristic early in the illness. Platelets are modestly decreased. Specific ELISA testing is available, but 3–4 weeks may elapse before seroconversion. Fluorescent antibody staining will detect virus-infected erythrocytes during the illness and for weeks after recovery.

## Differential Diagnosis

Early findings, especially if rash is present, may suggest enterovirus, measles, or rubella infection. Enteric fever may be an early consideration because of the presence of leukopenia and thrombocytopenia. A history of tick bite, which is often obtained, information about local risk, and the biphasic fever pattern will help with the diagnosis. Because of the wilderness exposure, diseases such as leptospirosis, borreliosis, tularemia, ehrlichiosis, and Rocky Mountain spotted fever will be considerations.

## Complications

Meningoencephalitis occurs in 3–7% of patients. Cardiac and pulmonary complications are rare.

## Prevention & Treatment

Prevention involves avoiding endemic areas and using conventional means to avoid tick bite. Therapy is supportive. Do not use analgesics that modify platelet function.

Klasco R: Colorado tick fever. Med Clin North Am 2002; 86:435 [PMID:11982311].

# OTHER MAJOR VIRAL CHILDHOOD EXANTHEMS

See Infections Due to Herpesvirus section for a discussion of varicella and roseola, two other major childhood exanthems.

## ERYTHEMA INFECTIOSUM

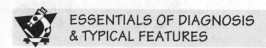

### ESSENTIALS OF DIAGNOSIS & TYPICAL FEATURES

- *Fever and rash with "slapped-cheek" appearance.*
- *Arthritis in older children.*
- *Profound anemia in patients with impaired erythrocyte production.*
- *Nonimmune hydrops fetalis.*

### General Considerations

This benign exanthematous illness of school-age children is caused by the human parvovirus designated B19. Spread is respiratory, occurring in winter–spring epidemics. A nonspecific mild flu-like illness may occur during the initial viremia at 7–10 days; the characteristic rash occurring at 10–17 days represents an immune response. The patient is viremic and contagious prior to—but not after—the onset of rash.

Approximately one half of infected individuals have a subclinical illness. Most cases (60%) occur in children between ages 5 and 15 years, with an additional 40% occurring later in life. Forty percent of adults are seronegative. The disease is mildly contagious; the secondary attack rate in a school or household setting is 50% among susceptible children and 20–30% among susceptible adults.

### Clinical Findings

Owing to the nonspecific nature of the exanthem and the many subclinical cases, a history of contact with an infected individual is often absent or unreliable. Recognition of the illness is easier during outbreaks.

#### A. SYMPTOMS AND SIGNS

Typically the first sign of illness is the rash, which begins as raised, fiery red maculopapular lesions on the cheeks that coalesce to give a "slapped-cheek" appearance. The lesions are warm, nontender, and sometimes pruritic. They may be scattered on the forehead, chin, and postauricular areas, but the circumoral region is spared. Within 1–2 days, similar lesions appear on the proximal extensor surfaces of the extremities and spread distally in a symmetrical fashion. Palms and soles are usually spared. The trunk, neck, and buttocks are also commonly involved. Central clearing of confluent lesions produces a characteristic lace-like pattern. The rash fades in several days to several weeks but frequently reappears in response to local irritation, heat (bathing), sunlight, and stress. Almost one half of infected children have some rash remaining (or recurring) for 10 days. Fine desquamation may be present. Mild systemic symptoms occur in up to 50% of children. These symptoms include low-grade fever (38–38.5°C), mild malaise, sore throat, and coryza. They appear for 2–3 days and are followed by a week-long asymptomatic phase before the rash appears.

Purpuric stocking-glove rashes, neurologic disease, and severe disorders resembling hemolytic–uremic syndrome have also been described in association with parvovirus B19.

#### B. LABORATORY FINDINGS

A mild leukopenia occurs early in some patients, followed by leukocytosis and lymphocytosis. Specific IgM and IgG serum antibody tests are available, but care must be used in choosing a reliable laboratory for this test. Nucleic acid detection tests are often definitive. The disease is not diagnosed by routine viral culture.

### Differential Diagnosis

In children immunized against measles and rubella, parvovirus B19 is the most frequent agent of morbilliform and rubelliform rashes. The characteristic rash and the mild nature of the illness distinguish erythema infectiosum from other childhood exanthems. It lacks the prodromal symptoms of measles and the lymphadenopathy of rubella. Systemic symptoms and pharyngitis are more prominent with enteroviral infections and scarlet fever.

### Complications & Sequelae

#### A. ARTHRITIS

Arthritis is more common in older patients, beginning with late adolescence. Approximately 10% of children have severe joint symptoms. Girls are affected more commonly than boys. Pain and stiffness occur symmetrically in the peripheral joints. Arthritis usually follows the rash and may persist for 2–6 weeks but resolves without permanent damage.

## B. Aplastic Crisis

Parvovirus B19 replicates primarily in erythroid progenitor cells. Consequently, reticulocytopenia occurs for approximately 1 week during the illness. This goes unnoticed in individuals with a normal erythrocyte half-life but results in severe anemia in patients with chronic hemolytic anemia. The rash of erythema infectiosum follows the hemolysis in these patients.

Pure red cell aplasia, leukopenia, pancytopenia, idiopathic thrombocytopenic purpura, and a hemophagocytic syndrome have also been described. Patients with AIDS and other immunosuppressive illnesses may develop prolonged anemia or pancytopenia. Patients with hemolytic anemia and aplastic crisis or immunosuppressed patients may still be contagious and should be isolated while in the hospital.

## C. Other End Organ Infections

Parvovirus is under study as a potential cause of a variety of collagen–vascular diseases, neurologic syndromes, hepatitis, and myocarditis.

## D. In Utero Infections

Infection of susceptible pregnant women may produce fetal infection with hydrops fetalis; fetal death occurs in about 6%, and most fatalities occur in the first 20 weeks—compared with a fetal loss of 3.5% in control subjects. The risk of fetal infection is unknown. Congenital anomalies have not been associated with parvovirus B19 infection during pregnancy.

## Treatment & Prognosis

Erythema infectiosum is a benign illness for immunocompetent individuals. Patients with aplastic crisis may require blood transfusions. It is unlikely that this complication can be prevented by quarantine measures, because acute parvovirus infection in contacts is often unrecognized and is most contagious prior to the rash. Pregnant women who are exposed to erythema infectiosum or who work in a setting in which an epidemic occurs should be tested for evidence of prior infection. Susceptible pregnant women should then be followed up for evidence of parvovirus infection. Approximately 1.5% of women of childbearing age are infected during pregnancy. If maternal infection occurs, the fetus should be followed up by ultrasonography for evidence of hydrops and distress. In utero transfusion or early delivery may salvage some fetuses. Pregnancies should not be terminated because of parvovirus infection. The risk of fetal death among exposed pregnant women of unknown serologic status is less than 2.5% for homemakers and less than 1.5% for schoolteachers.

Intramuscular immune globulin is not protective. High-dose IVIG has stopped viremia and led to mar-

row recovery in some cases of prolonged aplasia. Its role in immunocompetent patients and pregnant women is unknown.

Katta R: Parvovirus B19: A review. Dermatol Clin 2002;20: 333 [PMID:12120446].

Messina MF et al: Purpuric gloves and socks syndrome caused by parvovirus B19 infection. Pediatr Infect Dis J 2003;22: 755 [PMID: 12938681].

# MEASLES (RUBEOLA)

### ESSENTIALS OF DIAGNOSIS & TYPICAL FEATURES

- *Exposure to measles 9–14 days previously.*
- *Prodrome of fever, cough, conjunctivitis, and coryza.*
- *Koplik spots (few to many small white papules on a diffusely red base on the buccal mucosa) 1–2 days prior to and after onset of rash.*
- *Maculopapular rash spreading down from the face and hairline to the trunk over 3 days and later becoming confluent.*
- *Leukopenia.*

## General Considerations

This childhood exanthem is rarely seen in the United States because of universal vaccination (< 50 cases in 2003, all of which were imported or related to imported cases). Sporadic clusters of cases are the result of improper immunization more so than of vaccine failures, and are usually related to imported cases. It is recommended that all children be revaccinated on entrance into primary or secondary school (see Chapter 9). The attack rate in susceptible individuals is extremely high; spread is respiratory. Morbidity and mortality rates in the developing world are substantial because of underlying malnutrition and secondary infections. Because humans are the sole reservoir of measles, there is the potential to eliminate this disease worldwide.

## Clinical Findings

A history of contact with a suspected case may be absent because airborne spread is efficient and patients are contagious during the prodrome. Contact with an imported case may not be recognized. In temperate climates, epidemic measles is a winter–spring disease. Many suspected cases are misdiagnoses of other viral infections.

## A. SYMPTOMS AND SIGNS

High fever and lethargy are prominent. Sneezing, eyelid edema, tearing, copious coryza, photophobia, and harsh cough ensue and worsen. Koplik spots are white macular lesions on the buccal mucosa, typically opposite the lower molars. These are almost pathognomonic for rubeola, although they may be absent. A discrete maculopapular rash begins when the respiratory symptoms are maximal and spreads quickly over the face and trunk, coalescing to a bright red. As it involves the extremities, it fades from the face and is completely gone within 6 days; fine desquamation may occur. Fever peaks when the rash appears and usually falls 2–3 days thereafter.

## B. LABORATORY FINDINGS

Lymphopenia is characteristic. Total leukocyte counts may fall to 1500/μL. The diagnosis is usually made by detection of measles IgM antibody in serum drawn at least 3 days after the onset of rash or later by detection of a significant rise in antibody. Direct detection of measles antigen by fluorescent antibody staining of nasopharyngeal cells is a useful rapid method. PCR testing of oropharyngeal secretions or urine is extremely sensitive and specific and can detect infection up to 5 days before symptoms.

## C. IMAGING

Chest radiographs often show hyperinflation, perihilar infiltrates, or parenchymal patchy, fluffy densities. Secondary consolidation or effusion may be visible.

## Differential Diagnosis

Table 36–3 lists other illnesses that may resemble measles.

## Complications & Sequelae

### A. RESPIRATORY COMPLICATIONS

These complications occur in up to 15% of patients. Bacterial superinfections of lung, middle ear, sinus, and cervical nodes are most common. Fever that persists after the third or fourth day of rash suggests such a complication, as does leukocytosis. Bronchospasm, severe croup, and progressive viral pneumonia or bronchiolitis (in infants) also occur. Immunosuppressed patients are at much greater risk for fatal pneumonia than are immunocompetent patients.

### B. CEREBRAL COMPLICATIONS

Encephalitis occurs in 1 in 2000 cases. Onset is usually within a week after appearance of rash. Symptoms include combativeness, ataxia, vomiting, seizures, and coma. Lymphocytic pleocytosis and a mildly elevated protein concentration are usual CSF findings, but the fluid may be normal. Forty percent of patients so affected die or have severe neurologic sequelae.

Subacute sclerosing panencephalitis (SSPE) is a slow measles virus infection of the brain that becomes symptomatic years later in about 1 in 100,000 previously infected children. This progressive cerebral deterioration is associated with myoclonic jerks and a typical electroencephalographic pattern. It is fatal in 6–12 months. It rarely occurs following administration of vaccine; in fact, no case has been reported in recent years. High titers of measles antibody are present in serum and CSF.

### C. OTHER COMPLICATIONS

These include hemorrhagic measles (severe disease with multiorgan bleeding, fever, cerebral symptoms), thrombocytopenia, appendicitis, keratitis, myocarditis, and premature delivery or stillbirth. Mild liver function test elevation has been detected in up to 50% of cases in young adults; frank jaundice may also occur. Measles causes transient immunosuppression; thus, reactivation or progression of tuberculosis (including transient cutaneous anergy) occurs in untreated children.

## Treatment, Prognosis, & Prevention

Recovery generally occurs 7–10 days after onset of symptoms. Therapy is supportive: eye care, cough relief (avoid opioid suppressants in infants), and fever reduction (acetaminophen, lukewarm baths; avoid salicylates). Secondary bacterial infections should be treated promptly; antimicrobial prophylaxis is not indicated. Ribavirin is active in vitro and may be useful in infected immunocompromised children. High-dose intravenous ribavirin in combination with intrathecal interferon-α has been successfully used in the management of SSPE. In malnourished children, vitamin A supplementation should be given to attenuate the illness.

The current two-dose active vaccination strategy is successful. Vaccine should not be withheld for concurrent mild acute illness, tuberculosis or positive tuberculin skin test, breast-feeding, or exposure to an immunodeficient contact. The vaccine is recommended for HIV-infected children without severe HIV complications and adequate CD4 cells ($\geq$ 15%).

Vaccination prevents the disease in susceptible exposed individuals if given within 72 hours (see Chapter 9). Immune globulin (0.25 mL/kg intramuscularly; 0.5 mL/kg if immunocompromised) will prevent or modify measles if given within 6 days. Suspected cases should be diagnosed promptly and reported to the local health department.

Hosoya M et al: High-dose intravenous ribavirin therapy for subacute sclerosing panencephalitis. Antimicrob Agents Chemother 2001;45:943 [PMID: 11181386].

van Binnendijk RS et al: Evaluation of serological and virological tests in the diagnosis of clinical and subclinical measles virus infections during an outbreak of measles in the Netherlands. J Infect Dis 2003;188:898 [PMID: 12964122].

van den Hof et al: Measles epidemic in the Netherlands 1999–2000. J Infect Dis 2002;186:1483 [PMID: 12404165].

# RUBELLA

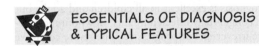

## ESSENTIALS OF DIAGNOSIS & TYPICAL FEATURES

- *History of rubella vaccination usually absent.*
- *Prodromal nonspecific respiratory symptoms and adenopathy (postauricular and occipital).*
- *Maculopapular rash beginning on face, rapidly spreading to the entire body, and disappearing by fourth day.*
- *Few systemic symptoms.*
- *Congenital infection.*
  *Retarded growth, development.*
  *Cataracts, retinopathy.*
  *Purpuric "blueberry muffin" rash at birth, jaundice, thrombocytopenia.*
  *Deafness.*
  *Congenital heart defect.*

## General Considerations

If it were not teratogenic, rubella would be of little clinical importance. Clinical diagnosis is difficult in some cases because of its variable expression. In one study, over 80% of infections were subclinical. Because of inadequate vaccination, outbreaks now occur in adolescents or adults. Rubella is transmitted by aerosolized respiratory secretions. Patients are infectious 5 days before until 5 days after the rash. Fewer than 10 cases were reported in the United States in 2003.

Congenital rubella, in infants both of unimmunized women and of women who have apparently been reinfected in pregnancy, is now rare (no cases in 2003).

## Clinical Findings

The incubation period is 14–21 days. The nondistinctive signs may make exposure history unreliable. A history of immunization makes rubella unlikely but still possible. Congenital rubella usually follows maternal infection in the first trimester.

### A. SYMPTOMS AND SIGNS

**1. Infection in children**—Young children may only have rash. Older patients often have a nonspecific prodrome of low-grade fever, ocular pain, sore throat, and myalgia. Postauricular and suboccipital adenopathy (sometimes generalized) is characteristic. This often precedes the rash or may occur without rash. The rash consists of erythematous discrete maculopapules beginning on the face. A "slapped-cheek" appearance or pruritus may occur. Scarlatiniform or morbilliform rash variants may occur. The rash spreads quickly to the trunk and extremities after it fades from the face; it is gone by the fourth day. Enanthema is usually absent.

**2. Congenital infection**—More than 80% of women infected in the first 4 months of gestation are delivered of affected infants; congenital disease occurs in less than 5% of women infected later in pregnancy. Later infections can result in isolated defects, such as deafness. The main manifestations are as follows:

**a. Growth retardation**—Between 50% and 85% of infants are small at birth and remain so.

**b. Cardiac anomalies**—Pulmonary artery stenosis, patent ductus arteriosus, ventricular septal defect.

**c. Ocular anomalies**—Cataracts, microphthalmia, glaucoma, retinitis.

**d. Deafness**

**e. Cerebral disorders**—Chronic encephalitis; retardation.

**f. Hematologic disorders**—Thrombocytopenia, dermal nests of extramedullary hematopoiesis or purpura ("blueberry muffin" rash), lymphopenia.

**g. Others**—Hepatitis, osteomyelitis, immune disorders, malabsorption, diabetes.

### B. LABORATORY FINDINGS

Leukopenia is common, and platelet counts may be low. Congenital infection is associated with low platelet counts, abnormal liver function tests, hemolytic anemia, pleocytosis, and very high rubella IgM antibody titers. Total serum IgM is elevated, and IgA and IgG levels may be depressed.

## C. IMAGING

Pneumonitis and bone metaphyseal longitudinal lucencies may be present in radiographs of children with congenital infection.

## Diagnosis & Differential Diagnosis

Virus may be isolated from throat or urine from 1 week before to 2 weeks after onset of rash. Children with congenital infection are infectious for months. The virus laboratory must be notified that rubella is suspected. Serologic diagnosis is best made by demonstrating a fourfold rise in antibody titer between specimens drawn 1–2 weeks apart. The first should be drawn promptly, because titers increase rapidly after onset of rash. Both specimens must be tested simultaneously by a single laboratory. Specific IgM antibody can be measured by immunoassay. Because the decision to terminate a pregnancy is usually based on serologic results, testing must be done carefully.

Rubella may resemble infections due to enterovirus, adenovirus, measles, EBV, roseola, parvovirus, *Toxoplasma gondii,* and *Mycoplasma.* Drug reactions may also mimic rubella. Because public health implications are great, sporadic suspected cases should be confirmed serologically or virologically.

Congenital rubella must be differentiated from congenital CMV infection, toxoplasmosis, and syphilis.

## Complications & Sequelae

### A. ARTHRALGIA AND ARTHRITIS

Both occur more often in adult women. Polyarticular involvement (fingers, knees, wrists), lasting a few days to weeks, is typical. Frank arthritis occurs in a small percentage of patients. It may resemble acute rheumatoid arthritis.

### B. ENCEPHALITIS

With an incidence of about 1:6000, this is a nonspecific parainfectious encephalitis associated with a low mortality rate. A syndrome resembling SSPE (see Measles section) has also been described in congenital rubella.

### C. RUBELLA IN PREGNANCY

Infection in the mother is self-limited and not severe.

## Prevention

Rubella is one of the infections that could be eradicated. See Chapter 9 for the indication and efficacy of rubella vaccine. Standard prenatal care should include rubella antibody testing. Seropositive mothers are at no risk; seronegative mothers are vaccinated after delivery.

A pregnant woman possibly exposed to rubella should be tested immediately; if seropositive, she is immune and need not worry. If she is seronegative, a second specimen should be drawn in 4 weeks, and both specimens should be tested simultaneously. Seroconversion in the first trimester suggests high fetal risk; such women require counseling regarding therapeutic abortion.

When pregnancy termination is not an option, some experts recommend intramuscular administration of 20 mL of immune globulin within 72 hours after exposure in an attempt to prevent infection. (This negates the value of subsequent antibody testing.) The efficacy of this practice is unknown.

## Treatment & Prognosis

Symptomatic therapy is sufficient. Arthritis may improve with administration of anti-inflammatory agents. The prognosis is excellent in all children and adults but poor in congenitally infected infants, in whom most defects are irreversible or progressive. The severe cognitive defects seem to correlate closely in these infants with the degree of growth failure.

Chantler JK et al: Persistent rubella virus infection associated with chronic arthritis in children. N Engl J Med 1985;313: 1117 [PMID: 4047116].

Freij BJ et al: Maternal rubella and the congenital rubella syndrome. Clin Perinatol 1988;15:247 [PMID: 3288422].

Kaplan KM et al: A profile of mothers giving birth to infants with congenital rubella syndrome: An assessment of risk factors. Am J Dis Child 1990;144:118 [PMID: 2294710].

Weber B et al: Congenital rubella syndrome after maternal reinfection. Infection 1993;21:118 [PMID: 8491520].

# INFECTIONS DUE TO OTHER VIRUSES

## HANTAVIRUS CARDIOPULMONARY SYNDROME

 **ESSENTIALS OF DIAGNOSIS & TYPICAL FEATURES**

- *Influenza-like prodrome (fever, myalgia, headache, cough).*
- *Rapid onset of unexplained pulmonary edema.*
- *Residence or travel in epidemic area; exposure to aerosols from deer mouse droppings or secretions.*

## General Considerations

Hantavirus cardiopulmonary syndrome is the first native bunyavirus infection endemic in this country. Hantavirus cardiopulmonary syndrome is distinctly different in mode of spread (no arthropod vector) and clinical picture from other bunyavirus diseases.

## Clinical Findings

The initial cases of hantavirus pulmonary syndrome involved travel to or residence in an area where New Mexico, Colorado, Utah, and Arizona are contiguous and involved potential exposure to the habitat of the reservoir, the deer mouse. This rodent and other selected rodents that harbor related hantaviruses live in many other locales. Thus, through 2003, more than 325 cases were confirmed in 29 other states, with additional cases in Canada. Epidemics occur when environmental conditions favor large increases in the rodent population and increased prevalence of virus in this reservoir.

### A. SYMPTOMS AND SIGNS

After an incubation period of 2–3 weeks, onset is sudden, with a nonspecific virus-like prodrome: fever; back, hip, and leg pain; chills; headache; and nausea and vomiting. Abdominal pain may be present. Sore throat, conjunctivitis, rash, and adenopathy are absent, and respiratory symptoms are absent or limited to a dry cough. After 1–10 days (usually 3–7), dyspnea, tachypnea, and evidence of a pulmonary capillary leak syndrome appear. This often progresses rapidly over a period of hours. Hypotension is common not only from hypoxemia but also from myocardial dysfunction. Copious, amber-colored, nonpurulent secretions are common. Decreased cardiac output and elevated systemic vascular resistance distinguish this disease from early bacterial sepsis.

### B. LABORATORY FINDINGS

The hemogram shows leukocytosis with a prominent left shift and immunoblasts, thrombocytopenia, and hemoconcentration. LDH is elevated, as are liver function tests; serum albumin is low. Creatinine is elevated in some patients, and proteinuria is common. Lactic acidosis and low venous bicarbonate are poor prognostic signs. A serum IgM ELISA test is positive early in the illness. Otherwise the diagnosis is made by specific staining of tissue or PCR, usually at autopsy.

### C. IMAGING

Initial chest radiographs are normal. This is followed by bilateral interstitial infiltrates with the typical butterfly pattern of acute pulmonary edema, bibasilar airspace disease, or both. Significant pleural effusions are often present. These findings contrast with those of other causes of acute respiratory distress syndrome.

## Differential Diagnosis

In some geographic areas, plague and tularemia may be possibilities. Infections with viral respiratory pathogens and *Mycoplasma* have a slower tempo, do not elevate the LDH, and do not cause the hematologic changes. Q fever, psittacosis, toxin exposure, legionellosis, and fungal infections are possibilities, but the history, tempo of the illness, and blood findings, as well as the exposure history, should be distinguishing features. Hantavirus cardiopulmonary syndrome is a consideration in previously healthy persons with a febrile illness associated with unexplained pulmonary edema.

## Treatment & Prognosis

When given early for other bunyavirus infections, intravenous ribavirin has been effective, and hantaviruses are sensitive in vitro to ribavirin. A trial of this therapy for hantavirus cardiopulmonary syndrome is under way. Management should concentrate on oxygen therapy and mechanical ventilation as required. Because of capillary leakage, Swan–Ganz catheterization to monitor cardiac output and inotropic support—rather than fluid therapy—should be used to maintain perfusion. Venoarterial extracorporeal membrane oxygenation can provide short-term support for selected patients. The virus is not spread by person-to-person contact. No isolation is required. Thus far, the case fatality rate is approximately 50%. Guidelines are available for reduction of exposure to the infectious agent.

Peters CJ, Khan AS: Hantavirus pulmonary syndrome: The new American hemorrhagic fever. Clin Infect Dis 2002:34: 1224 [PMID: 11941549].

## MUMPS

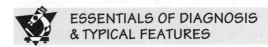

### ESSENTIALS OF DIAGNOSIS & TYPICAL FEATURES

- *No prior mumps immunization.*
- *Parotid gland swelling.*
- *Aseptic meningitis with or without parotitis.*

## General Considerations

Mumps was one of the classic childhood infections; virus spread by the respiratory route attacked almost all unimmunized children (asymptomatically in 30–40% of cases), and produced lifelong immunity. The vaccine is so efficacious that clinical disease is rare in immunized children. As a result of subclinical infections or childhood immunization, 95% of adults are immune. Infected patients can spread the infection from 1–2 days prior to the onset of symptoms and for 5 additional days. The incubation period is 14–21 days.

A history of exposure to a child with parotitis is not proof of mumps exposure. In an adequately immunized individual, parotitis is usually due to another cause. Currently in the United States less than 1 case is reported per 100,000 population.

## Clinical Findings

### A. SYMPTOMS AND SIGNS

**1. Salivary gland disease**—Tender swelling of one or more glands, variable fever, and facial lymphedema are typical. Parotid involvement is most common; signs are bilateral in 70% of patients. The ear is displaced upward and outward; the mandibular angle is obliterated. Systemic toxicity is usually absent. Parotid stimulation with sour foods may be quite painful. The orifice of the Stensen duct may be red and swollen; yellow secretions may be expressed, but pus is absent. Parotid swelling dissipates after 1 week.

**2. Meningoencephalitis**—Prior to widespread immunization, mumps was the most common cause of aseptic meningitis, which is usually manifested by mild headache or asymptomatic mononuclear pleocytosis. Fewer than 10% of patients have clinical meningitis or encephalitis. Cerebral symptoms do not correlate with parotid symptoms, which are absent in many patients with meningoencephalitis. Although neck stiffness, nausea, and vomiting can occur, encephalitic symptoms are rare (1:4000 cases of mumps); recovery in 3–10 days is the rule.

**3. Pancreatitis**—Abdominal pain may represent transient pancreatitis. Because salivary gland disease may elevate serum amylase, specific markers of pancreatic function (lipase, amylase isoenzymes) are required for assessing pancreatic involvement.

**4. Orchitis, oophoritis**—Involvement of the gonads is associated with fever, local tenderness, and swelling. Epididymitis is usually present. Orchitis is unusual in young children but occurs in up to one third of affected postpubertal males. Usually it is unilateral and resolves in 1–2 weeks. Although one third of infected testes atrophy, bilateral involvement and sterility are rare.

**5. Other**—Thyroiditis, mastitis (especially in adolescent females), arthritis, and presternal edema (occasionally with dysphagia or hoarseness) may be seen.

### B. LABORATORY FINDINGS

Peripheral blood leukocyte count is usually normal. Up to 1000 cells/$\mu$L (predominantly lymphocytes) may be present in the CSF, with mildly elevated protein and normal to slightly decreased glucose. Viral culture of saliva, throat, urine, or spinal fluid may be positive for at least 1 week after onset. Paired sera assayed by ELISA are currently used for diagnosis. Complement-fixing antibody to the soluble antigen disappears in several months; its presence in a single specimen thus indicates recent infection.

## Differential Diagnosis

Mumps parotitis may resemble the following: cervical adenitis (the jaw angle may be obliterated, but the ear does not usually protrude; the Stensen duct orifice is normal; leukocytosis and neutrophilia are observed); bacterial parotitis (pus in the Stensen duct, toxicity, exquisite tenderness); recurrent parotitis (idiopathic or associated with calculi); tumors or leukemia; and tooth infections. Many viruses, including parainfluenza, enteroviruses, EBV, CMV, and influenza virus, can cause parotitis. Parotid swelling in HIV infection is less painful and tends to be bilateral and chronic, but bacterial parotitis occurs in some children with HIV infection.

Unless parotitis is present, mumps meningitis resembles that caused by enteroviruses or early bacterial infection. An elevated amylase is a useful clue in this situation. Isolated pancreatitis is not distinguishable from many other causes of epigastric pain and vomiting. Mumps is a classic cause of orchitis, but torsion, bacterial or chlamydial epididymitis, *Mycoplasma* infection, other viral infections, hematomas, hernias, and tumors must also be considered.

## Complications

The major neurologic complication is nerve deafness (usually unilateral), which can result in inability to hear high tones. It may occur without meningitis. Permanent damage is rare, occurring in less than 0.1% of cases of mumps. Aqueductal stenosis and hydrocephalus (especially following congenital infection), myocarditis, transverse myelitis, and facial paralysis are other rare complications.

## Treatment & Prognosis

Treatment is supportive and includes provision of fluids, analgesics, and scrotal support for orchitis. Systemic steroids have been used for orchitis, but their value is anecdotal. Surgery is not recommended.

Caplan CE: Mumps in the era of vaccines. Can Med Assoc J 1999;160:865 [PMID: 10189437].

Hersh BS et al: Mumps outbreak in a highly vaccinated population. J Pediatr 1991;119:187 [PMID: 1861205].

Manson AL: Mumps orchitis. Urology 1990;36:355 [PMID: 2219620].

McDonald JC, Moore DL, Quennec P: Clinical and epidemiologic features of mumps meningoencephalitis and possible vaccine-related disease. Pediatr Infect Dis J 1989;8:751 [PMID: 2594449].

# RABIES

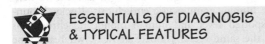

## ESSENTIALS OF DIAGNOSIS & TYPICAL FEATURES

- *History of animal bite 10 days to 1 year (usually less than 90 days) previously.*
- *Paresthesias or hyperesthesia in bite area.*
- *Progressive limb and facial weakness in some patients (dumb rabies; 30%).*
- *Irritability followed by fever, confusion, combativeness, muscle spasms (especially pharyngeal with swallowing) in all patients (furious rabies).*
- *Rabies antigen detected in corneal scrapings or tissue obtained by brain or skin biopsy; Negri bodies seen in brain tissue.*

## General Considerations

Rabies remains a potentially serious public health problem wherever animal immunization is not widely practiced or when humans play or work in areas with sylvan rabies. Although infection does not always follow a bite by a rabid animal (about 40% infection rate following rabid dog bites), infection is almost invariably fatal. Any warm-blooded animal may be infected, but susceptibility and transmissibility vary with different species. Bats often carry and excrete the virus in saliva or feces for prolonged periods; they are the major cause of rabies in the United States. Dogs and cats are usually clinically ill within 10 days after becoming contagious (the standard quarantine period for suspect animals). Valid quarantine periods or signs of illness are not fully known for many species. Rodents rarely transmit infection. Animal vaccines are very effective when properly administered, but a single inoculation may fail to produce immunity in up to 20% of dogs.

The risk is assessed according to the type of animal (bats always considered rabid; raccoons, skunks, foxes in many areas); wound extent and location (infection more common after head or hand bites, or if wounds have extensive salivary contamination or are not quickly and thoroughly cleaned); geographic area (urban rabies is rare to nonexistent in US cities; rural rabies is possible, especially outside the United States); and animal vaccination history (risk low if documented). Most rabies in the United States is with genotypes found in bats, yet a history of bat bite is rarely obtained. Aerosolized virus in caves inhabited by bats has caused infection.

## Clinical Findings

### A. Symptoms and Signs

Paresthesias at the bite site are usually the first symptoms. Nonspecific anxiety, excitability, or depression follows, then muscle spasms, drooling, hydrophobia, delirium, and lethargy. Swallowing or even the sensation of air blown on the face may cause pharyngeal spasms. Seizures, fever, cranial nerve palsies, coma, and death follow within 7–14 days after onset. In a minority of patients, the spastic components are initially absent and the symptoms are primarily flaccid paralysis and cranial nerve defects. The furious components appear subsequently.

### B. Laboratory Findings

Leukocytosis is common. CSF is usually normal or may show elevation of protein and mononuclear cell pleocytosis. Cerebral imaging and electroencephalography are not diagnostic.

Infection in an animal may be determined by use of the fluorescent antibody test to examine brain tissue for antigen. Rabies virus is excreted in the saliva of infected humans, but the diagnosis is usually made by antigen detection in scrapings or tissue samples of richly innervated epithelium, such as the cornea or the hairline of the neck. Classic Negri cytoplasmic inclusion bodies in brain tissue are not always present. Seroconversion occurs after 7–10 days.

## Differential Diagnosis

Failure to elicit the bite history in areas where rabies is rare may delay diagnosis. Other disorders to be considered include parainfectious encephalopathy; encephalitis due to herpes simplex, mosquito-borne viruses, other viruses; and Guillain–Barré syndrome.

## Prevention

See Chapter 9 for information regarding vaccination and postexposure prophylaxis. Rabies immune globulin and diploid cell vaccine have made prophylaxis more effective and minimally toxic; however, rare cases of prophylaxis failure are still being reported. Because rabies is almost always fatal, presumed exposures must be managed carefully.

## Treatment & Prognosis

Survival is rare but has been reported in four patients receiving meticulous intensive care. No antiviral preparations are of proved benefit. Early diagnosis is important for the protection and prophylaxis of individuals exposed to the patient.

Jackson AC et al: Management of rabies in humans. Clin Infect Dis 2003;36:60 [PMID: 12491203].

Messenger SL et al: Emerging epidemiology of bat-associated cryptic cases of rabies in humans in the United States. Clin Infect Dis 2002;35:738 [PMID: 12203172].

# ■ II. RICKETTSIAL INFECTIONS

Rickettsiae are pleomorphic, gram-negative coccobacilli which are obligate intracellular parasites. Rickettsial diseases are often included in the differential diagnosis of febrile rashes, although some (notably Q fever) are not characterized by rash. Severe headache is a prominent symptom. The endothelium is the primary target tissue, and the ensuing vasculitis is responsible for severe illness.

All rickettsioses except Q fever are transmitted by cutaneous arthropod contact, either by bite or contamination of skin breaks with tick feces. Evidence of such contact by history or physical examination may be completely lacking, especially in young children. The geographic distribution of the vector is often the primary determinant for suspicion of these infections. Therapy often must be empirical. Many new broadspectrum antimicrobials are inactive against these cell wall-deficient organisms; tetracycline is usually effective.

## HUMAN EHRLICHIOSIS

*Ehrlichia* species are responsible for febrile pancytopenia in animals. In humans, *Ehrlichia sennetsu* is responsible for a mononucleosis-like syndrome seen in Japan and Malaysia. One agent of North American human ehrlichiosis has been identified as *E chaffeensis*. The reservoir hosts are probably wild rodents, deer, and sheep; ticks are the vectors. Most cases caused by this agent are reported in the south central and middle to southern Atlantic states. Arkansas, Missouri, Oklahoma, and North Carolina are high-prevalence areas. Almost all cases occur between March and October, when ticks are active. A second ehrlichiosis syndrome, seen in the upper Midwest and Northeast (Connecticut, Wisconsin, Minnesota, and New York are high-prevalence areas), is caused by an organism closely related to *E phagocytophila* or *E equi*. These are known large animal pathogens. *E chaffeensis* has a predilection for mononuclear cells, whereas intracytoplasmic inclusions in granulocytes are common with the *E phagocytophila* and *E equi* infections. Hence diseases caused by these agents are referred to as human monocytic ehrlichiosis or human granulocytic ehrlichiosis, respectively. A newly discovered agent, *E ewingii*, also causes tickborne human granulocytic ehrlichiosis. Rocky Mountain spotted fever and human monocytic ehrlichiosis share the same vector (Lone Star tick), whereas Lyme disease and human granulocytic ehrlichiosis are both spread by the deer tick. Thus dual infections are common and should be considered in patients who fail to respond to therapy.

## Clinical Findings

In approximately 75% of patients, a history of tick bite can be elicited. The majority of the remaining patients report having been in a tick-infested area. The usual incubation period is 5–21 days.

### A. SYMPTOMS AND SIGNS

Fever and headache are universally present. Gastrointestinal symptoms (anorexia, nausea and vomiting) are reported in most pediatric patients. Distal limb edema may also occur in children. Chills, photophobia, conjunctivitis, myalgia, and arthralgia occur in more than half of patients. Rash occurs in one third of patients with monocytic ehrlichiosis but is less common (< 10%) in granulocytic ehrlichiosis. Rash may be erythematous, macular, papular, petechial, scarlatiniform, or vasculitic. Meningitis occurs. Interstitial pneumonitis, adult respiratory distress syndrome, and renal failure occur in severe cases. The physical examination reveals rash, mild cervical adenopathy, and hepatomegaly. Perinatal transmission has been documented. A child without a rash may present as a case of fever of unknown origin.

### B. LABORATORY FINDINGS

Laboratory abnormalities include leukopenia with left shift, lymphopenia, thrombocytopenia, and elevated aminotransferase levels. Disseminated intravascular coagulation can occur in severe cases. Anemia occurs in one third of patients. The definitive diagnosis is made serologically. The Centers for Disease Control and Prevention uses appropriate antigens in an immunofluorescent antibody test in order to distinguish between the etiologic agents. Intracytoplasmic inclusions (morulae) may occasionally be observed in mononuclear cells in monocytic ehrlichiosis and are usually observed in polymorphonuclear cells from the peripheral blood or bone marrow in granulocytic ehrlichiosis. Specific PCR is now available for diagnosis.

## Differential Diagnosis

The differential diagnosis includes septic or toxic shock, other rickettsial infections (especially Rocky Mountain spotted fever), Colorado tick fever, leptospirosis, Lyme borreliosis, relapsing fever, EBV, CMV, viral hepatitis and other viral infections, Kawasaki disease, systemic lupus erythematosus, and leukemia.

## Treatment & Prognosis

Although the disease may last several weeks, it is usually self-limited. Deaths do occur in children. Doxycycline, 2–4 mg/kg/d divided every 12 hours (maximum 100 mg/dose) for 7–10 days, is the treatment of choice. Fatal disease occurs in less than 3% of cases. Immune compromise is a risk factor for severe disease.

Jacobs RF: Human monocytic ehrlichiosis: Similar to Rocky Mountain spotted fever but different. Pediatr Ann 2002;31: 180 [PMID: 11905291].

Lantos P, Krause PJ: Ehrlichiosis in children. Semin Pediatr Infect Dis 2002;13:249-56 [PMID: 12491230].

Singh-Behl D et al: Tick-borne infections. Dermatol Clin 2003;21: 237 [PMID: 12757245].

## RICKETTSIALPOX

*Rickettsia akari* is transmitted by mites from infected house mice. Most cases in the United States have occurred in northeastern cities. The bite site becomes a papule, then a pustule; it ulcerates and then forms a characteristic black eschar at about the time fever develops at 9–14 days. Local adenopathy is the rule. Headache, myalgia, and photophobia are followed in 2–4 days by a generalized maculopapular rash. Palms and soles are usually spared. Vesicles develop on the papules. The fever lasts about a week. Diagnosis is established by serology.

The differential diagnosis includes varicella, enteroviral infections, other rickettsial spotted fevers, meningococcemia, and gonococcemia. Mild cases require no therapy. Tetracycline for 3 to 5 days is effective.

Paddock CD et al: Rickettsialpox in New York City: A persistent urban zoonosis. Ann NY Acad Sci 2003;990:36 [PMID:12860597].

## ROCKY MOUNTAIN SPOTTED FEVER

*Rickettsia rickettsii* causes one of many similar tickborne illnesses characterized by fever and rash that occur worldwide. Most are named for their geographic area. In all except Rocky Mountain spotted fever and murine typhus, there is a characteristic eschar at the bite site, called the *tache noire*. Dogs and rodents are reservoirs of *R rickettsii*.

Rocky Mountain spotted fever is the most severe of these infections and the most important (500–1000 cases per year) in the United States. It occurs predominantly in the eastern seaboard; in the southeastern states; and in Arkansas, Texas, Missouri, Kansas, and Oklahoma—much less common to the west. Most cases occur in children exposed in rural areas from April to September. Because tick attachment lasting 6 hours or longer is needed, frequent tick removal is a preventive measure.

## Clinical Findings

### A. SYMPTOMS AND SIGNS

After the incubation period of 3–12 days (mean, 7 days), there is high fever (over 40°C, often hectic), usually of abrupt onset, myalgia, severe and persistent headache (retro-orbital; less obvious in infants), toxicity, photophobia, vomiting, and diarrhea. The characteristic rash occurs in 85–90% of patients and appears 2–6 days after fever onset as macules and papules, especially prominent on the palms, soles, and extremities, becoming petechial and spreading centrally. Conjunctivitis, splenomegaly, edema, meningismus, irritability, and confusion may occur.

### B. LABORATORY FINDINGS

Laboratory findings are nonspecific and reflect diffuse vasculitis: thrombocytopenia, hyponatremia, early mild leukopenia, proteinuria, abnormal liver function tests, hypoalbuminemia, and hematuria. CSF pleocytosis is common. Serologic diagnosis is achieved with indirect fluorescent or latex agglutination antibody methods, but generally only 7–10 days after onset of the illness. Skin biopsy with specific fluorescent staining may give the diagnosis within the first week of the illness.

## Differential Diagnosis

The differential diagnosis includes meningococcemia, measles, meningitis, staphylococcal sepsis, enteroviral infection, leptospirosis, Colorado tick fever, scarlet fever, murine typhus, Kawasaki disease, and ehrlichiosis.

## Treatment & Prognosis

To be effective, therapy for Rocky Mountain spotted fever must be started early and is often based on a presumptive diagnosis in endemic areas prior to rash onset. It is important to remember that atypical presentations, such as the absence of pathognomonic rash, often lead to delay in appropriate therapy. Doxycycline is the agent of choice for children, regardless of age. Treatment should be continued for 2 or 3 days after the temperature has returned to normal for a full day. A minimum of 10 days of therapy is recommended.

Complications and death result from severe vasculitis, especially in the brain, heart, and lung. The mortality rate is 5–7%. Delay in therapy is an important determinant of mortality.

Masters EJ et al: Rocky Mountain spotted fever: A clinician's dilemma. Arch Intern Med 2003;163:769 [PMID: 12695267].

Sexton DJ, Kaye KS: Rocky mountain spotted fever. Med Clin North Am 2002;86:351 [PMID: 11982306].

## ENDEMIC TYPHUS (MURINE TYPHUS)

Endemic typhus is present in the southern United States, mainly in southern Texas, and in Southern California. The disease is transmitted by fleas from infected rodents, from their feces in scratches, or by inhalation. Domestic cats, dogs, and opossums may play a role in the transmission of suburban cases. No eschar appears at the inoculation site, which may go unnoticed. The incubation period is 6–14 days. Headache, myalgia, and chills slowly worsen. Fever may last 10–14 days. After 3–8 days, a rash appears. Truncal macules and papules spread to the extremities; the rash is rarely petechial. The location of the rash in typhus, with sparing of the palms and soles, is a distinction from Rocky Mountain spotted fever. Rash may be absent in 20–40% of patients. Hepatomegaly may be present. Intestinal and respiratory symptoms may occur. Mild thrombocytopenia and elevated liver enzymes may be present. The illness is usually self-limited and milder than epidemic typhus. More prolonged neurologic symptoms have been described. Therapy is usually not needed. Doxycycline is the drug of choice. Therapy for 3 days is usually sufficient. Fluorescent antibody and ELISA tests are available.

Fergie JE et al: Murine typhus in south Texas children. Pediatr Infect Dis J 2000;19:535 [PMID: 10877169].

## Q FEVER

*Coxiella burnetii* is transmitted by inhalation rather than by an arthropod bite. The birth tissues and excreta of domestic animals and of some rodents are the infectious source. Unpasteurized milk from infected animals may also transmit disease. Q fever is also distinguished from other rickettsial diseases by the infrequent occurrence of cutaneous manifestations and by the prominence of pulmonary disease.

## Clinical Findings

### A. SYMPTOMS AND SIGNS

Many patients have a self-limited flu-like syndrome of chills, fever, severe headache, and myalgia of abrupt onset occurring 10–30 days after exposure. Abdominal pain, vomiting, chest pain, and dry cough are prominent in children. Examination of the chest may produce few findings, as in other atypical pneumonias. Hepatosplenomegaly is common. The illness lasts 1–4 weeks, and frequently is associated with weight loss.

### B. LABORATORY FINDINGS

Leukopenia with left shift is characteristic. Thrombocytopenia is unusual and another distinction from other symptomatic rickettsial diseases. Aminotransferase and γ-glutamyl transferase levels are elevated. Diagnosis is made by finding a complement-fixing antibody response (fourfold rise or single high titer) to the phase II organism. Chronic infection is indicated by antibody against the phase I organism. IgM ELISA and specific PCR are also available.

### C. IMAGING

Pneumonitis occurs in 50% of patients. Multiple segmental infiltrates are common, but the radiographic appearance is not pathognomonic. Consolidation and pleural effusion are rare.

## Differential Diagnosis

In the appropriate epidemiologic setting, Q fever should be considered in evaluating causes of atypical pneumonias such as from *Mycoplasma pneumoniae*, viruses, *Legionella,* and *Chlamydia pneumoniae.* It should also be included among the causes of mild hepatitis without rash or adenopathy in children with exposure to farm animals.

## Treatment & Prognosis

Typically the illness lasts 1–2 weeks without therapy. One complication is chronic disease, which often implies myocarditis or granulomatous hepatitis. Meningoencephalitis is also a rare complication.

*C burnetii* is also one of the causes of so-called culture-negative endocarditis. Both types of complication are rare. Endocarditis is difficult to treat; mortality approaches 50%. The course of the uncomplicated illness is shortened with tetracycline; doxycycline is preferred.

Therapy is continued for several days after the patient becomes afebrile. Quinolones are also effective.

Marrie TJ, Raoult D: Update on Q fever, including Q fever endocarditis. Curr Clin Topics Infect Dis 2002;22:97 [PMID: 1250650].

Maltezou HC, Raoult D: Q fever in children. Lancet Infect Dis 2002;2:686 [PMID: 12409949].

# Human Immunodeficiency Virus Infection

**37**

*Elizabeth J. McFarland, MD*

## ESSENTIALS OF DIAGNOSIS & TYPICAL FEATURES

*Children younger than age 18 months:*

- *A child known to be HIV-seropositive or born to an HIV-infected mother.*

*And*

- *Has positive results on two separate determinations on blood or tissue (excluding cord blood) for one or more of the following HIV detection tests: HIV nucleic acid detection, HIV antigen (p24), HIV culture.*

*Or*

- *Meets criteria for AIDS diagnosis based on the 1987 Centers for Disease Control and Prevention (CDC) AIDS surveillance case (see Table 37–1 and CDC case definition, MMWR Morb Mortal Wkly Rep, 1994).*

*Or*

- *Has HIV antibody and evidence of cellular and humoral immunodeficiency (without another cause) and symptoms compatible with HIV infection.*

*Children older than age 18 months:*

- *HIV-seropositive by repeatedly reactive enzyme-linked immunosorbent assay and confirmatory test.*

*Or*

- *Meets any of the criteria listed for children younger than age 18 months.*

## General Considerations

Acquired immunodeficiency syndrome (AIDS) results from progression of human immunodeficiency virus (HIV) infection. HIV is a retrovirus that infects mainly helper T lymphocytes (CD4 lymphocytes), monocytes, and macrophages. In general, cells are infected after binding of the glycosylated envelope protein of HIV, gp120, to both the CD4 receptor protein and a chemokine receptor, which are found on the surface of the target cells. The function and number of CD4 lymphocytes and other affected cells are diminished by HIV infection, with profound effects on both humoral and cell-mediated immunity. Without treatment, HIV infection causes generalized immune incompetence and eventually AIDS. However, combination antiretroviral treatment is highly effective at delaying disease progression.

The clinical diagnosis of AIDS is made when an HIV-infected child develops any of the opportunistic infections, malignancies, or conditions listed in category C (Table 37–1). In adults and adolescents, the criteria for a diagnosis of AIDS also include absolute CD4 lymphocyte counts of 200/µL or less.

## Mode of Transmission

HIV is transmitted by sexual contact, percutaneous exposure to contaminated blood, and vertical transmission. Perinatal transmission may occur in utero, at the time of delivery, or via breast feeding. Indirect evidence suggests that about 30% of perinatal infections occur prior to birth. Risk factors associated with mother-to-infant transmission include high maternal plasma HIV RNA, advanced maternal disease stage, low CD4 lymphocyte count, and factors related to increased exposure to maternal blood or cervical secretions at the time of delivery (ie, duration of rupture of membranes, presence of blood in the infant's gastric secretions, first-born twin delivery).

In the United States, risk factors for HIV infection among adults include exposure to blood products from 1978 to early 1985, parenteral illicit drug use, multiple heterosexual or homosexual contacts, and a partner with any of the preceding risk factors. Casual, classroom, or household contact with an HIV-infected person poses no risk. Seroprevalence rates are highest among gay men and injecting drug users. However, the proportion of new AIDS cases in 2001 acquired by heterosexual contact was approximately equal to the proportion acquired by injecting drug use and only slightly

1174

**Table 37–1.** Clinical categories of children with HIV infection.

**Category N: Not symptomatic**
No signs or symptoms or only one of the conditions listed in category A

**Category A: Mildly symptomatic**
Having two or more of the following conditions:
Lymphadenopathy
Hepatomegaly
Splenomegaly
Dermatitis
Parotitis
Recurrent or persistent upper respiratory infection, sinusitis, or otitis media

**Category B: Moderately symptomatic**
Having symptoms attributed to HIV infections other than those in category A or C
*Examples:*
Anemia, neutropenia, thrombocytopenia
Bacterial meningitis, pneumonia, sepsis (single episode)
Candidiasis, oropharyngeal, persisting over 2 months
Cardiomyopathy
Cytomegalovirus infection with onset < 1 month of age
Diarrhea, recurrent or chronic
Hepatitis
Herpes simplex virus recurrent stomatitis, bronchitis, pneumonitis, esophagitis at < 1 month of age
Herpes zoster, two or more episodes or more than one dermatome
Leiomyosarcoma
Lymphoid interstitial pneumonia
Nephropathy
Nocardiosis
Persistent fever
Toxoplasmosis with onset < 1 month of age
Varicella, complicated

**Category C: Severely symptomatic**
Serious bacterial infections, multiple or recurrent
Candidiasis, esophageal or pulmonary
Coccidioidomycosis, disseminated
Cryptosporidiosis or isosporiasis with diarrhea > 1 month
Cytomegalovirus infection with onset > 1 month of age
Encephalopathy
Herpes simplex virus: persistent oral lesions, or bronchitis, pneumonitis, esophagitis at > 1 month of age
Histoplasmosis
Kaposi sarcoma
Lymphoma
*Mycobacterium tuberculosis,* extrapulmonary
*Mycobacterium* infection, other species, disseminated
*Pneumocystis jiroveci* pneumonia
Progressive multifocal leukoencephalopathy
*Salmonella* septicemia, recurrent
Toxoplasmosis of the brain with onset > 1 month of age
Wasting syndrome

Adapted from MMWR Morb Mortal Wkly Rep 1994;43(RR-12):6, 8.

less than the proportion acquired by men having sex with men. Youth (ages 13–24 years) and women of color are disproportionately represented among new cases. In developing nations, heterosexual contact is the most common mode of transmission among adults, and prevalence is similar in both genders.

Perinatal transmission accounts for over 90% of prepubertal AIDS cases in the United States and almost all new pediatric HIV infections. In the United States, the number of perinatally acquired AIDS cases declined 83% between 1992 (907 cases) and 2001 (150 cases). This decline reflects a decrease in perinatal transmission attributed primarily to zidovudine (ZDV) and other antiretroviral treatment during pregnancy. Without intervention, 15–30% of infants born to HIV-infected women will be infected. The rate of vertical transmission can be reduced to 5–8% by providing ZDV treatment to the mother during pregnancy and delivery and by providing additional prophylaxis to the infant during the first 6 weeks after birth. In the current era of combination therapy during pregnancy, transmission rates are as low as 1%. Most transmissions involve women not receiving therapy during pregnancy, either because the infection is undiagnosed or because of lack of prenatal care. Offering of HIV testing to all pregnant women is strongly recommended so that those who are HIV-infected can receive treatments to reduce perinatal transmission. Perinatal transmission rates in developing countries continue to be high. Worldwide, an estimated 3.2 million children are infected with HIV, most of them in Africa, India, Thailand, and parts of South America. In 2002, an estimated 800,000 new infections occurred in children younger than age 15 years. Studies of short-course medical treatment demonstrate reduced transmission rates, but have yet to be implemented on a wide-scale basis.

Currently, sexual activity (both heterosexual and homosexual) is the main mode of infection after puberty, with a smaller number of cases resulting from sharing of contaminated needles. The incidence among youth, especially minority youth, is increasing. As a result of careful donor screening and testing of the donated blood, HIV transmission resulting from blood products is now extremely rare (1:2,000,000 transfusions).

## Pathogenesis

At the time of initial HIV infection, high levels of HIV are detected in the bloodstream. In adults, the level of viremia declines without therapy concurrent with the appearance of an HIV-specific host immune response and plasma viremia usually reaches a steady-state level about 6–12 months after primary infection. The amount of virus present in the plasma at that point and thereafter is predictive of the rate of disease progression for the individual. Despite ongoing virus replication, a period of clinical latency occurs lasting from 1 year to more than 12 years during which the infected person is asymptomatic. The virus and anti-HIV immune responses are in a steady state, with high levels of virus production and destruction balanced against production and destruction of CD4 lymphocytes. Eventually, the balance favors the virus, and the viral burden increases as the CD4 lymphocyte count declines.

Approximately 30% of infants with vertically acquired HIV infection will have virus detectable in the blood at birth. This is thought to indicate infection acquired in utero. The remaining infected infants, probably acquiring HIV during labor and delivery, will test negative for HIV at birth but will soon have detectable virus, usually by 2–4 weeks. The level of viremia rises steeply, reaching a peak at age 1–2 months. In contrast with adults, infants will have a gradual decline in plasma viremia that extends beyond 2 years. Infants generally have plasma virus levels 10 times higher than those in adults.

Without treatment, about 20–30% of HIV-infected infants develop an AIDS-defining illness by age 1 year and die before age 2–3 years. High levels of viremia at age 1–2 months and over the first year of life characterize these infants. Other predictors of rapid progression are low absolute counts of CD4 and suppressor–killer T (CD8) lymphocytes in the first 6 months. In the remainder, the disease progresses more slowly, with a mortality rate of 3.5% per year between ages 1 and 7 years and median survival greater than 7 years. These so-called slow progressors will generally have lower virus levels and a more gradual decline in CD4 lymphocyte counts. There are rare instances of children and adults with untreated infection for 8–10 years or more with no evidence of immune suppression. Studies indicate that both viral and host genetic factors, not all fully defined, play a role in determining the rate of disease progression. The initiation of antiretroviral therapy

dramatically alters the natural history by slowing disease progression and permitting restoration of immune function.

## Clinical Findings

### A. SYMPTOMS AND SIGNS

The manifestations described in this section are likely to be observed in children with untreated infection or in those unresponsive to therapy. Children given effective antiretroviral therapy usually have few symptoms, most of which will be from the medications.

The CDC has developed disease staging criteria for HIV-infected children (see Tables 37–1 and 37–2). The criteria incorporate clinical symptoms ranging from no symptoms to mild, moderate, and severe symptoms (categories N, A, B, C, respectively) and age-adjusted CD4 lymphocyte counts (immunologic categories 1, 2, 3, corresponding to none, moderate, or severe immune suppression, respectively). Each child is classified both by CD4 lymphocyte count and by clinical category. Category C diagnoses are the diseases indicating an AIDS diagnosis, with the exception of lymphoid interstitial pneumonitis, which was included as an AIDS-defining illness but is not a sign of late-stage disease.

**1. Primary acute infection**—The incubation period is 2–4 weeks for primary infection acquired by adults and adolescents through high-risk behavior. Nonspecific symptoms occur in 30–90% of new infections (eg, flu or mild mononucleosis-like illness), and often are not brought to medical attention. Diagnosis requires a high index of suspicion. Infected persons may present with fever, fatigue, malaise, pharyngitis, enlarged lymph nodes, and hepatosplenomegaly. Signs seen less commonly but more specific to HIV are mild oral ulcerations; a diffuse macular, erythematous rash; and mild meningitis or encephalopathy. Occasionally, thrush,

**Table 37–2.** Immunologic categories based on age-specific CD4 lymphocyte counts and percentages of total lymphocytes.

| | Age of Child | | | | | |
|---|---|---|---|---|---|---|
| | **< 12 months** | | **1–5 years** | | **6–12 years** | |
| **Immunologic Category** | cells/µL | (%) | cells/µL | (%) | cells/µL | (%) |
| 1. No evidence of suppression | ≥ 1500 | (≥ 25) | ≥ 1000 | (≥ 25) | ≥ 500 | (≥ 25) |
| 2. Evidence of moderate suppression | 750–1499 | (15–24) | 500–999 | (15–24) | 200–499 | (15–24) |
| 3. Evidence of severe suppression | < 750 | (< 15) | < 500 | (< 15) | < 200 | (< 15) |

Adapted from MMWR Morb Mortal Wkly Rep 1994;43(RR-12):4.

*Candida* esophagitis, or genital ulcers are observed. These early symptoms of primary infection resolve spontaneously within 1–2 weeks, although some persons have fatigue and depression for weeks or months.

A primary infection syndrome is rarely recognized following perinatal acquisition. Newborns with perinatal HIV infection are rarely symptomatic (less than 7%) at birth. Size and physical features are not different from uninfected infants. However, 75–95% will demonstrate some sign (mostly nonspecific) by age 1 year.

**2. Nonspecific symptoms**—Nonspecific symptoms may be observed in early- or late-stage disease. Frequent illness (especially recurrent otitis media or sinusitis) is typical, in addition to poor weight gain, chronic cough, chronic diarrhea, developmental delay, unexplained fevers, night sweats, generalized lymphadenopathy, parotid swelling, or hepatosplenomegaly. Delayed growth may be observed as early as age 4 months in some infants. These common early findings may be present for years in an otherwise well child.

**3. Infections related to immunodeficiency**—Progressive immune dysfunction in both humoral and cell-mediated responses results in susceptibility to infections. Recurrent or serious bacterial infections are more common in children than in HIV-infected adults. Bouts of bacteremia, especially due to *Streptococcus pneumoniae,* can occur in children without suppressed CD4 T-cell counts. Infections with *Mycobacterium tuberculosis* (usually acquired from adults in the household) may be severe. Primary varicella-zoster (VZV) infections may be prolonged or severe. Recurrent herpes zoster (shingles) is common even in the era of combination therapy. Recurrent herpes simplex lesions may be large, painful, and persistent. Likewise, persistent aphthous ulcers may cause significant morbidity. Late-stage immunodeficiency is accompanied by susceptibility to a variety of opportunistic pathogens. Pneumonia caused by *Pneumocystis jiroveci* (formerly *Pneumocystis carinii*) is the most common AIDS-defining diagnosis in children with unrecognized HIV infection. The incidence is highest between ages 2 and 6 months and is often fatal during this period. Symptoms are difficult to distinguish from those of viral or atypical pneumonia. Patients typically have fever, tachypnea, intercostal retractions, progressive hypoxemia, and an elevated lactate dehydrogenase (LDH) concentration (see Chapter 39). Persistent candidal mucocutaneous infections (oral, skin, and vaginal) are common. Candidal esophagitis occurs with more advanced disease. In children with severe immunosuppression, cytomegalovirus (CMV) infections may result in disseminated disease, hepatitis, gastroenteritis, retinitis, and encephalitis.

Cryptococcal infections and histoplasmosis have been described, although much less frequently than among HIV-infected adults. Disseminated infection with *Mycobacterium avium* complex (MAC) occurs at the rate of 5 per 100 patient-years in infected children who have CD4 lymphocyte counts under 50–100/μL. Symptoms and signs associated with this opportunistic pathogen include fever, night sweats, weight loss, diarrhea, fatigue, lymphadenopathy, hepatomegaly, anemia, and granulocytopenia. A variety of diarrheal pathogens that cause mild, self-limited symptoms in healthy persons may result in severe, chronic diarrhea in HIV-infected persons. These include rotavirus, *Cryptosporidium parvum, Microsporidium, Cyclospora, Isospora belli, Giardia lamblia,* and bacterial pathogens. Chronic parvovirus infection manifested by anemia can occur. Reactivation of toxoplasmosis occurs rarely in children.

**4. Organ system disease**—HIV infection may cause a variety of organ system symptoms. In most cases, the pathogenesis is not fully understood; however, symptoms occurring in the absence of other pathogens are thought to result from HIV infection itself.

Prior to effective antiretroviral therapy, encephalopathy was a common problem, afflicting 20% or more of HIV-infected children. Following perinatal transmission, affected patients may present with acquired microcephaly, progressive motor deficit, ataxia, pseudobulbar palsy, and failure to attain (or loss of) developmental milestones. Children who are older may have symptoms similar to those observed in infected adults, such as gradual mental status changes initially affecting attention span and memory. However, other treatable causes of central nervous system disease should be sought, especially when an acute change in symptoms occurs.

Lymphoid interstitial pneumonitis is characterized by a diffuse peribronchial and interstitial infiltrate composed of lymphocytes and plasma cells. It may be asymptomatic or associated with dry cough, hypoxemia, dyspnea or wheezing on exertion, and clubbing of the digits. Auscultatory findings may be few. Children with this disorder frequently have enlargement of the parotid glands, generalized lymphadenopathy, and normal LDH (elevated in *Pneumocystis* pneumonia [PCP]). Although this diagnosis was originally classified as AIDS-defining because of specificity to HIV, the condition is associated with slow progression and is not an indicator of advanced disease.

Symptomatic cardiomyopathy is observed mainly in infants with rapid disease progression. Symptoms are those of congestive heart failure.

Mild to moderate elevation of liver enzymes is frequently observed, and, more rarely, overt clinical hepatitis occurs due to HIV infection itself. However, patients are often taking medications with potential hepatotoxicity, and superinfection with other pathogens (CMV, Epstein–Barr virus [EBV], MAC, hepatitis C, hepatitis B) that affect the liver is common. Thus the diagnosis of HIV hepatitis should be one of exclusion. Chronic diarrhea may occur with HIV infection; however, as with hepatitis, it is commonly associated with other gastrointestinal infections. Since these may respond to specific treatment, severe diarrhea warrants an aggressive evaluation, including cultures, microscopic examinations of stool, and often colonoscopy with biopsy. Nephropathy, myopathy, and neuropathy are all recognized in children but are relatively uncommon.

**5. Malignancy**—Children with HIV are at increased risk of malignancy, although even prior to effective therapy, malignancy was an uncommon AIDS-defining illness. The tumors most commonly associated with pediatric HIV infection are non-Hodgkin lymphomas. Unlike non-Hodgkin lymphomas in immunocompetent persons, these tumors commonly occur at extranodal sites (central nervous system, bone, gastrointestinal tract, liver, or lungs) and are usually high-grade and of B-cell origin. Cervical infection with human papillomavirus is more likely to progress to neoplasia in adolescent females with HIV infection. Kaposi sarcoma, a common malignancy among HIV-infected homosexual males, rarely occurs in children. There is an increased frequency of leiomyosarcomas.

**B. Laboratory Findings**

HIV antibody is measured by enzyme-linked immunosorbent assay (ELISA). A confirmatory test, usually a Western blot, must be performed because individuals occasionally have nonviral cross-reacting antibodies, which result in a false-positive ELISA. Rarely (in less than 1% of cases) an infected person may fail to make antibody. However, they are usually obviously ill, and tests for virus or viral antigen are positive. During the early weeks after nonvertical, primary infection, HIV antibody may be absent; tests for the presence of virus (nucleic acid detection or p24 antigen) are positive.

Infants born to HIV-infected mothers will have HIV antibody—regardless of infection status—owing to transplacental passage of maternal antibody. The median time to loss of maternal HIV antibody is 10 months; all children lose maternal antibody by 18 months. A diagnosis of HIV infection can be made in over 95% by age 2–4 months by detecting HIV in blood, with nucleic acid detection.

Approximately 70% of infected infants will have negative results with assays for HIV RNA and DNA at birth, presumably because of low viral burden, perhaps

indicating that the infection was acquired at the time of birth. Hence, negative tests during this early period do not rule out infection. Over the first 8 weeks, essentially all infected infants will become positive for HIV nucleic acid. An infant who is otherwise well and has had at least two negative HIV cultures or nucleic acid detection tests, both performed after age 1 month and at least one performed after age 3 months, is very unlikely to be infected. The infant should be followed-up for clinical symptoms and retested at ages 12, 15, and 18 months for reversion to seronegative status to confirm the absence of infection. The absolute number and percentage of CD4 lymphocytes decline with disease progression; CD8 lymphocytes may be increased. CD4 lymphocyte numbers and percentages in infants are normally much higher than in adults and decline to adult levels by age 6 years. Hence, age-adjusted values must be used in evaluating these tests (see Table 37–2).

Some children will have thrombocytopenia due to autoimmune antibodies at a relatively early stage of disease. As disease progresses, anemia and granulocytopenia become common. Patients are often also taking antiretroviral or prophylactic medication, which may result in bone marrow suppression; distinguishing between effects due to HIV or drug therapy may be difficult. Hypergammaglobulinemia is characteristic and may be observed as early as age 9 months. Some children fail to make specific antibody to antigens (eg, *Haemophilus influenzae* type b, *Streptococcus pneumoniae*), which contributes to subsequent infections. With brain involvement, the cerebrospinal fluid may be normal or the protein may be elevated and a mononuclear pleocytosis may be present.

**C. Imaging**

Cerebral images can demonstrate atrophy and calcification in the basal ganglia and frontal lobes in patients with encephalopathy. Chest radiographs of children with lymphoid interstitial pneumonitis show diffuse interstitial reticulonodular infiltrates, occasionally with hilar adenopathy. The chest radiograph in PCP typically demonstrates perihilar infiltrates progressing to bilateral diffuse alveolar disease.

**Differential Diagnosis**

Differential diagnosis of HIV infection will vary with the presenting sign or symptom. Infants with immunodeficiency may resemble infants with other types of congenital immunodeficiencies such as hypogammaglobulinemia or severe combined immunodeficiency syndrome (see Chapter 29). When poor growth is a prominent feature of the presentation, HIV infection may be confused with other causes of growth deficiency. Children or adolescents presenting with generalized lymphadenopathy or hepatosplenomegaly may resemble those infected with viruses such as EBV or CMV. The symptoms of acute primary infection in the adolescent may be similar to those of mononucleosis caused by EBV or CMV, toxoplasmosis, rubella, secondary syphilis, influenza, enterovirus, or viral hepatitis.

The diagnosis can be made or excluded with HIV antibody testing in a child older than age 18 months. In younger infants, a negative result usually excludes HIV infection, but a positive result must be followed by testing for the presence of virus. HIV-infected children with hypogammaglobulinemia occasionally have falsely negative antibody tests. Any child suspected of having HIV infection who has negative serologic tests should be tested by a nucleic acid-based test. Likewise, an adolescent with symptoms of primary infection should be tested for virus by nucleic acid detection.

## Prevention

The only 100% effective method of avoiding sexual transmission of HIV infection is abstinence or limiting sexual contact to a mutually monogamous partner who is not HIV-infected. However, condoms—used consistently and correctly—are highly effective in preventing transmission between stable, sexually active couples in which only one partner is HIV-infected. In two studies, seroconversions occurred in 0–2% of discordant couples using condoms consistently compared with 10–15% of couples with inconsistent condom use. A third study reported 1.1 seroconversions per 100 person-years of observation among consistent condom users compared with 9.7 seroconversions among inconsistent users. The CDC provides detailed instructions on correct condom use. Prompt treatment of other sexually transmitted diseases also reduces the risk of sexual transmission. Many experts have recently begun to offer antiretroviral medications as prophylaxis against HIV infection to people who are exposed to HIV in a circumstance that is not likely to recur (eg, sexual assault, condom rupture) although there are no official recommendations for or against this approach.

Vertical transmission can be substantially prevented by giving antiretroviral therapy to the mother during pregnancy and by providing prophylaxis of the newborn. Women with access to antiretroviral therapy should receive three-drug combination regimens during pregnancy. Zidovudine (ZDV) should be incorporated into the regimen if possible since this is the medication with the greatest amount of efficacy and safety data. Combination therapy that results in viral suppression to less than 1000 cp/mL reduces transmission rates to under 1%. Antiretroviral therapy begun later in pregnancy can also reduce transmission although less pro-

foundly. Studies have demonstrated the benefit of ZDV plus lamivudine, nevirapine plus ZDV, nevirapine alone, and even ZDV alone started as late as during labor. Short-course treatments can reduce transmission by 30–50%. Treatment of the infant for 1–2 weeks after birth is critical to preventing infection.

Elective cesarean section reduces the risk of transmission by 50% in women, with or without ZDV treatment. For women receiving combination therapy that suppresses viral load to less than 1000 cp/mL, cesarean section is unlikely to further decrease transmission appreciably.

The CDC and the American College of Obstetrics and Gynecology now recommend offering HIV testing with informed consent routinely to all pregnant women. Women found to be infected should be counseled regarding all HIV-related pregnancy care issues, including the benefits and risks of therapy with antiretroviral agents. Amniocentesis should be avoided if possible. Because breast milk can carry the virus, breastfeeding by HIV-infected mothers is contraindicated when access to safe formula can be ensured, as is the case in the United States.

Infected blood and secretions should be handled according to CDC recommendations.

The CDC recommends postexposure prophylaxis following occupational exposure. Recommended therapy is with ZDV and lamivudine (3TC), with or without a third agent, depending on the degree of risk associated with the exposure.

## Treatment

HIV infection calls for specific antiretroviral treatment to prevent progressive deterioration of the immune system as well as prophylactic measures at late stages of HIV infection to prevent opportunistic infections. Whenever possible, children should be enrolled in collaborative treatment studies. Current information on clinical trials may be obtained at:

http://aidsinfo.nih.gov/clinical_trials

Guidelines for the treatment of HIV developed by a national working group of pediatric HIV specialists are published by the United States Public Health System at:

http://aidsinfo.nih.gov/guidelines

The treatment paradigm changes frequently; therefore, prior to initiating treatment, expert consultation should be obtained.

## A. SPECIFIC MEASURES

**1. Principles of HIV treatment**—Treatment of HIV is aimed at suppressing viral replication. Numerous studies have demonstrated that the rate of disease progression is directly correlated with the number of HIV copies circulating in plasma. Antiretroviral treatment that reduces HIV replication is associated with increases in CD4 T-lymphocyte counts, reconstitution of immune function, and arrest of disease progression. Children have a remarkable ability to restore normal CD4 T-cell counts even when treatment is started at advanced disease stage. Highly active antiretroviral therapy (HAART) has been available for over 8 years, and, thus far, it appears that successful treatment may be able to prevent disease progression. However, it is clear that even the most potent regimens fail to eradicate virus. HIV persists in long-lived resting cells and cessation of antiretroviral treatment results in resumption of viremia and decline in CD4 lymphocytes. Therefore, treatment for HIV with currently available modalities must be continuous and lifelong.

Emergence of drug-resistant HIV during therapy is a major challenge. HIV has a high spontaneous mutation rate, and emergence of drug resistance during treatment is frequent. Many antiretroviral drugs select for resistant mutations in the virus within weeks to a few months when used as monotherapy. Prevention of resistance mutations requires complete suppression such that virus is not replicating and has no opportunity to generate new mutations. To date, achieving potent viral suppression requires a combination of at least three antiviral agents. Treatment with a combination of drugs with different mechanisms of action provides an additional barrier to resistance as the virus must be resistant to all the drugs in the combination. Finally, strict adherence to the prescribed treatment is critical. Studies demonstrate that more than 95% of the doses must be taken in order to maintain optimal viral suppression. Therefore programs and services that enhance adherence are essential adjuncts of any HAART regimen.

Determining the best time to initiate treatment is a subject of intense discussion and research. For children demonstrating HIV-related symptoms (clinical category C in Table 37–1) or evidence of immune suppression (CD4 lymphocyte counts in category 3; see Table 37–2) the consensus is that treatment should be started irrespective of age or HIV RNA level. In addition, children with a plasma HIV RNA over 100,000 copies/mL are at high risk of progression, so this is a well-accepted criterion for initiating treatment. In the United States, many experts recommend treatment for all HIV-infected infants younger than age 12 months because surrogate markers that reliably identify all infants at risk of rapid progression are lacking.

The best approach for the asymptomatic child with low or modest plasma viral load and without evidence of severe immune suppression is less clear. Such a child might live many years without HIV-related symptoms. It is possible that starting a complex medication regimen with associated toxicities and significant effect on quality of life could be delayed without detriment to the child's long-term prognosis. However, it can also be argued that early treatment will better preserve normal immune function and prevent effects on growth and development that may not be reversed when treatment is started. At present, for children older than age 12 months at diagnosis with mild to moderate clinical symptoms (clinical category A or B) or with moderate immunologic suppression (immune category 2), most experts would consider initiating therapy. For asymptomatic children, many experts favor close observation, with therapy initiated if declining CD4 lymphocyte counts or increasing HIV plasma RNA copy numbers are observed. Once therapy has been initiated, the patient should be monitored every 3 months for changes in plasma virus copy number, CD4 lymphocyte count, symptoms, and adverse drug effects.

**2. Considerations in selecting antiretroviral medications**—The process of selecting a combination of medications for a particular patient has become highly complex. The FDA has approved 20 drugs from four different classes for the treatment of HIV (Table 37–3). The clinician must consider the potency of the drugs, tolerability, simplicity of dosing, drug interactions, and viral resistance profiles.

Potency, the intrinsic ability of the regimen to fully suppress viral replication, is foremost because without complete suppression resistant virus will emerge. Tolerability is also critical because regimens that are poorly tolerated fail due to poor adherence. When selecting a tolerable regimen, the circumstances and priorities of each individual patient and family must be considered. Certain side effects may be acceptable to one person but for another person be intolerable. Likewise, for some patients the frequency of dosing may have the greatest effect on their compliance, whereas another may be satisfied with frequent dosing provided the number or size of pills taken is reduced. The most tolerable regimens are those with few adverse effects, simple dosing regimens, low number of different medications, few and small pills, and palatable taste. Unfortunately, many of the currently available medications lack these characteristics. However, the pharmaceutical industry is taking these characteristics into consideration in new drug development. Gradually, drugs that can be given once daily and require fewer total pills or liquids are becoming available.

***Table 37–3.*** Antiretroviral drugs approved by the US Food and Drug Administration.

| Drug Class or Drug Name | Potential Adverse Effects[1] | Mechanism of Action |
|---|---|---|
| Nucleoside/necleotide reverse transcriptase inhibitors | Lactic acidosis (rare but potentially fatal) | Chain termination of HIV DNA |
| Abacavir (ACC; Ziagen) | Hypersensitivity reaction | |
| Didanosin (ddl; Videx) | Pancreatitis, peripheral neuropathy, nausea, diarrhea | |
| Emtricitabine (FTC; Emtriva) | Minimal toxicity | |
| Lamivudine (3TC; Epivir) | Minimal toxicity | |
| Stavudine (d4T; Zerit) | Peripheral neuropathy, lipodystrophy, pancreatitis | |
| Tenofovir (TDF; Viread) | Headache, nausea, diarrhea, bone demineralization, renal insufficiency (rare) | |
| Zalcitabine (ddC; Hivid) | Peripheral neuropathy, stomatitis | |
| Zidovudine (ZDV, AZT; Retrovir) | Anemia, neutropenia, gastrointestinal intolerance, headache | |
| Zidovudine/lamivudine (CBV, Combivir) | See individual drugs | |
| Zidovudine/lamivudine/abacavir (TZV, Trizavir) | See individual drugs | |
| Non-nucleoside reverse transcriptase inhibitors | Rash, rarely Stevens–Johnson syndrome | Synthesis of HIV DNA inhibited |
| Delavirdine (Rescriptor) | Increased liver transaminases, headache | |
| Efavirenz (Sustiva) | Central nervous system symptoms, increased transaminases, teratogenic in monkeys | |
| Nevirapine (Viramune) | Hepatitis | |
| Protease inhibitors | Glucose intolerance, risk of bleeding in hemophilia, dyslipidemia, lipodystrophy, transaminase elevation | Production of noninfectious virions |
| Amprenavir (Agenerase) Fosamprenavir (Lexiva) | Rash, oral paresthesia | |
| Atazanavir (Reyataz) | Increased indirect bilirubin | |
| Indinavir (Crixivan) | Nephrolithiasis, increased indirect bilirubin | |
| Lopinavir/ritonavir (Kaletra) | Gastrointestinal intolerance | |
| Nelfinavir (Viracept) | Diarrhea | |
| Ritonavir (Norvir) | Nausea, circumoral paraesthesias, hepatitis, pancreatitis, taste perversion | |
| Saquinavir hard gel (Invirase) Saquinavir soft gel (Fortovase) | Gastrointestinal intolerance | |
| Fusion inhibitors | | Viral entry inhibited |
| Enfuvirtide (Fuzeon) | Injection site reactions, increased rate of bacterial pneumonias, hypersensitivity reactions (<1%) | |

[1]Relative incidence of adverse events depends on specific drug.

Drug interactions between different antiretroviral medications, and with other medications, are frequent and must be considered when selecting a combination of drugs. Most of the protease inhibitors and non-nucleoside reverse transcriptase inhibitors are metabolized by cytochrome P-450 isotypes and therefore can induce or inhibit the metabolism of other drugs that are me-

tabolized by that pathway. Some combinations lead to significant decreases or increases in drug levels, and combined use is contraindicated. On the other hand, drug interactions can also be advantageous. Certain combinations may inhibit metabolism, leading to increased plasma levels without requiring administration of higher doses. Drug absorption and metabolism can vary widely between individuals, especially for the protease inhibitor class. Therefore, therapeutic drug monitoring to determine the level of drug in serum and adjust doses to achieve therapeutic levels is recommended by some experts.

The potential for viral resistance should be evaluated when selecting a combination. Optimally, an initial regimen would select viral resistance mutations that do not confer cross-resistance to a large number of other drugs. This permits an opportunity to use alternative regimens if resistance to the initial regimen develops. The process is aided by laboratory methods (genotyping and phenotyping) to determine the presence of virus with specific drug resistance mutations in the patient.

**3. Specific antiretroviral medications—**

**a. Nucleoside and nucleotide reverse transcriptase inhibitors (NRTIs)**—The NRTIs act as nucleotide analogues, which are incorporated into HIV DNA during transcription by the HIV reverse transcriptase. The result is chain termination and failure to complete provirus, preventing incorporation of HIV genome into cellular DNA. The human mitochondrial DNA polymerase also has limited affinity for these analogues, the degree varying with the drug. Incorporation of the analogue into mitochondrial DNA is one mechanism thought to lead to adverse effects including pancreatitis, peripheral neuropathy, bone marrow suppression (anemia or neutropenia), and lipodystrophy (loss of peripheral fat and accumulation of visceral fat). Lactic acidosis with hepatic steatosis (fatty liver) is a rare but potentially fatal complication that may result from mitochondrial toxicity.

A hypersensitivity reaction to abacavir occurs in approximately 10% of patients. This adverse effect is not related to mitochondrial toxicity. The reaction, characterized by a flu-like syndrome with or without rash, may be fatal with continued treatment or rechallenge. The NRTIs vary widely with regard to antiviral activity, rates at which viral resistance occurs, and adverse effects. They are dosed either once or twice daily. Most NRTIs are available as liquids, and dosing recommendations for children have been determined for most.

**b. Nonnucleoside reverse transcriptase inhibitors (NNRTIs)**—NNRTIs also inhibit HIV DNA synthesis but act at a different site on the viral enzyme so no cross-resistance occurs with NRTI. The NNRTIs have potent antiretroviral activity, but single amino acid mutations in the viral reverse transcriptase protein often induce resistance to all three drugs in this class. The most common toxicity is rash. Stevens–Johnson syndrome has been reported, but rash is usually mild and often resolves without changing therapy. Efavirenz is associated with mild central nervous system symptoms

(ie, dizziness, confusion), which usually resolve after the initial weeks of use. Inflammation of the liver, rarely fatal, may occur with any of the drugs in the class but is more common with nevirapine. The NNRTI are dosed once or twice daily and the pill sizes are small. Pediatric dosing information is available for nevirapine and efavirenz.

**c. Protease inhibitors**—Protease inhibitors (PIs) are synthetic molecules designed to bind to the HIV protease. The protease is critical for the assembly of infectious virions. In the presence of PIs, progeny virus is released from the cell but cannot infect new cells. Acute adverse effects are mainly gastrointestinal intolerance as well as other effects specific to the particular drug (see Table 37–3). All PIs are associated with a risk of glucose intolerance and bleeding for hemophiliacs. Most are associated with dyslipidemia (elevated cholesterol and triglycerides) and may contribute to lipodystrophy. An exception is atazanavir, which is not associated with changes in serum lipids. As a rule, these drugs are highly potent and usually require multiple mutations for high-level resistance to develop. Cross-resistance is observed for some drugs in the class, but others have differing resistance mutations. Taste and pill burden limit tolerability of these medications. The PIs are metabolized by the hepatic P-450 cytochrome enzymes, resulting in many interactions with other drugs, including other antiretrovirals. Careful attention to drug interactions is necessary when treating a patient taking a PI. Regimens combining two PIs can take advantage of the drug interactions and improve the pharmacokinetic properties of the drugs.

**d. Fusion inhibitors**—Enfuvirtide is the first drug to be FDA-approved in this class. Enfuvirtide interferes with the fusion of the viral envelope and the cell plasma membrane, thereby preventing entry of the virus into the cell. Enfuvirtide must be administered parenterally, and local reactions at the injection site are common.

**B. GENERAL MEASURES**

**1. Immunizations**—Combined diphtheria–tetanus–acellular pertussis, inactivated poliovirus, conjugated *Haemophilus influenzae* type b, conjugated *Streptococcus pneumoniae,* and hepatitis B vaccines should be given as recommended for healthy children (see Chapter 9). A dose of 23-valent polysaccharide vaccine at 2 years and a booster after 3–5 years is recommended in addition to the conjugated pneumococcal vaccine series given in infancy. Infected children and their household contacts should receive inactivated influenza vaccine annually after age 6 months. In general, live virus vaccines should be avoided. However, the risk of measles is considered greater than the potential risk of the vaccine in asymptomatic children; thus measles–mumps–rubella vaccine should be given at age 12 months, with the second dose at 1 month later, provided the child does not have evidence of severe immunosuppression (category C or category 3). Varicella vaccine, also a live virus, is recommended for asymptomatic children without prior evidence of immunosuppression. Studies in progress preliminarily suggest that VZV vaccine will be safe in children with restored CD4 T-cells counts. Because antibody titers to vaccines decline with time and progressive immunodeficiency, prophylaxis with immune globulin for measles exposure and tetanus immune globulin for tetanus-prone wounds should be given regardless of immunization status. Varicella-zoster immune globulin should be considered after each varicella exposure for HIV-infected children with progressive HIV who have not had prior varicella or VZV vaccination.

**2. Prophylaxis for infections**—Children with suppressed CD4 lymphocyte numbers benefit from prophylactic treatment to prevent opportunistic infections. Children who have had their CD4 counts restored to category 1 or 2 for over 3–4 months can be taken off prophylactic treatments. Antibiotic prophylaxis for PCP has been extremely effective. Because this infection has its highest incidence during the first year of life, PCP prophylaxis is given to all infants born to HIV-infected mothers beginning at age 4–6 weeks. When tests for HIV DNA or RNA are demonstrated negative at age 3–4 months, the infant may discontinue prophylaxis. HIV-infected infants should continue on prophylactic drugs until age 12 months, when further treatment is based on assessment of symptoms and age-adjusted CD4 lymphocyte counts every 3 months. Published guidelines from the CDC for PCP prophylaxis are summarized in Table 37–4 and 37–5.

Children with hypogammaglobulinemia or a history of serious or multiple bacterial infections may benefit from monthly intravenous immune globulin (IVIG) if they are not receiving trimethoprim–sulfamethoxazole. Clarithromycin or azithromycin reduces the frequency of disseminated MAC with a survival benefit for children with very low CD4 counts.

Recurrent mucocutaneous and esophageal candidiasis can be prevented with nystatin, clotrimazole, or fluconazole treatment. Some patients suffer recurrent severe herpes simplex or VZV infections. These may be prevented with oral antiviral prophylaxis (acyclovir, valacyclovir, famciclovir).

HIV-infected children have a higher risk of progression of infections due to *M tuberculosis*. Because the child's infection is usually acquired from adult household contacts, other household members should be skin-tested for tuberculosis yearly. Adults and children found to have positive tuberculosis skin tests should be

**Table 37–4.** *Pneumocystis jiroveci*[a] (PCP) pneumonia prophylaxis for HIV-exposed and infected infants by age and HIV infection status.

| | |
|---|---|
| Birth to 4–6 wk | No prophylaxis |
| 4–6 wk to 4 mos | Prophylaxis |
| 4–12 mos | |
|   HIV-infected or indeterminate | Prophylaxis |
|   HIV infection reasonably excluded[b] | No prophylaxis |
| 1–5 y, HIV-infected | Prophylaxis if CD4 count < 500/μL or CD4 < 15%[c] |
| 6–12 y, HIV-infected | Prophylaxis if CD4 count < 200/μL or CD4 < 15%[c] |

[a]Formerly *Pneumocystis carinii*.
[b]Among children who have had two or more negative HIV cultures or PCR tests, both of which are performed at age 1 month and one of which is performed at age 3–4 months or older.
[c]Prophylaxis should be considered on a case-by-case basis for children who might otherwise be at risk for pneumocystis pneumonia, such as those with rapidly declining CD4 counts or percentages or children with category C conditions.
Adapted from 2001 USPHS/IDSA Guidelines for the Prevention of Opportunistic Infections in Persons Infected with Human Immunodeficiency Virus.
http://www.aidsinfo.nih.gov/guidelines

**Table 37–5.** Drug regimens for *Pneumocystis jirovaci* prophylaxis for children over age 4 weeks.

**Recommended regimen**
Trimethoprim–sulfamethoxazole, 150 mg TMP/m$^2$/d plus 750 mg SMX/m$^2$/d, administered orally, divided into two doses per day 3 days a week on consecutive days
Alternative (same total daily dosages):
  Single daily dose 3 days a week on consecutive days
  Divided twice-daily doses 7 days a week
  Divided twice-daily doses 3 days a week on alternate days

**Alternative if trimethoprim–sulfamethoxazole is not tolerated[a]**
Dapsone, 2 mg/kg/d (not to exceed 100 mg) orally once daily
Aerosolized pentamidine (children over age 5 years), 300 mg via Respirgard II inhaler monthly
Atovaquone, age 1–3 mos and > 24 mos, 30 mg/kg orally once daily; age 4–24 mos, 45 mg/kg orally once daily

[a]If dapsone, aerosolized pentamidine, or atovaquone is not tolerated, some clinicians use intravenous pentamidine 4 mg/kg every 2–4 wk.
Adapted from 2001 USPHS/IDSA Guidelines for the Prevention of Opportunistic Infections in Persons Infected with Human Immunodeficiency Virus.

evaluated further for disease and receive treatment according to their HIV status.

**3. Infections and other conditions**—Rates of bacteremia, especially pneumococcal bacteremia, and shingles are higher among HIV-infected children, even without severe suppression of CD4 counts. Therefore, blood cultures should be obtained liberally in ill-appearing or febrile HIV-infected children. VZV and herpes simplex virus infections are treated with acyclovir since symptoms may be prolonged in children with HIV. Short courses of valacyclovir or famciclovir—drugs with good bioavailability—are also effective, although not approved for children. Aphthous ulcers also occur in children, even when on suppressive antiretroviral drug therapy. Symptomatic CMV infection is treated with ganciclovir or foscarnet and requires ongoing secondary prophylaxis if CD4 lymphocytes counts remain low. MAC requires treatment with a multidrug regimen to delay the emergence of resistance. Lymphoid interstitial pneumonitis may respond to corticosteroid therapy. Chronic parvovirus as a cause of anemia should be investigated and can be treated with IVIG. Anemia and granulocytopenia, whether drug-induced or HIV-induced, may respond to epoetin alfa (erythropoietin) and filgrastim (granulocyte colony-stimulating factor, G-CSF), respectively. Rarely transfusions are needed; CMV-seronegative blood should be used.

**4. General support**—Growth failure (weight and height) is one of the earliest and most sensitive markers of disease progression. The cause is a combination of increased metabolic needs related to chronic infection and decreased caloric intake. Nutritional evaluation and counseling should be a part of early care before problems arise. When a child's routine diet fails to provide adequate nutrition, supplemental nutrition in the form of oral supplements and nutritious snacks is often required. Supplemental feeding by gastrointestinal tubes may be required for children who are unable to consume sufficient calories orally.

Evaluation and support for psychosocial needs of HIV-affected families is imperative. As with other chronic illnesses, HIV infection affects all family members, and it also carries an additional social stigma. Emotional concerns and financial needs are more prominent than medical needs at many stages of the disease process and influence the family's ability to comply with a medical treatment regimen. HIV-infected children often have comorbid mental health conditions. Ideally, care should be coordinated by a team of caregivers that is familiar with this disease and the newest therapies and that has access to community resources.

## Prognosis

Plasma viremia and age-adjusted CD4 lymphocyte count can be used to assess the risk of progression and complications of HIV. Poor prognosis in perinatal infection is associated with encephalopathy, infections with *P jiroveci*, early development of AIDS, and a rapidly declining CD4 lymphocyte count. Without treatment, approximately 30% of infected infants will progress to severe symptoms (class C) or death by 1 year of age. Among optimally treated children rates of progression and mortality are low.

## Public Health Issues

In general, the infant or child who is well enough to attend day care or school should be treated no differently from other children. The exception may be a toddler with uncontrollable biting behavior or bleeding lesions that cannot be covered adequately; in these situations, the child may be withheld from group day care. Routine good hygiene used for the prevention of transmission of other infectious diseases is appropriate for the prevention of common infections, which may be severe in the HIV-infected child. Optimally the school health care provider and teacher will be aware of the diagnosis, but there is no legal requirement that any individual at the school or day care center be informed. The parents and the child may prefer to keep the diagnosis confidential, because the stigma associated with HIV infection may be difficult to overcome. Adolescents with HIV should receive counseling on the risk of transmission through sexual activity and shared needles. Programs should be made available to encourage use of barrier protection and to develop strategies for disclosure to their partners and other friends.

Horizontal transmission (ie, in the absence of sexual contact or injecting drug use) of HIV is exceedingly rare and is associated with exposure of broken skin or mucous membranes to HIV-infected blood or bloody secretions. Because undiagnosed HIV-infected infants and children might be enrolled, all schools and day care centers should have policies with simple guidelines for using universal precautions to prevent transmission of HIV infection in these settings. Saliva, tears, urine, and stool are not contagious if there is no gross blood in these fluids. A barrier protection (eg, latex or rubber gloves, thick pads of fabric or paper) should be used when possible contact with blood or bloody body fluids may occur. Objects that might be contaminated with blood, such as razors or toothbrushes, should not be shared. No special care is required for dishes, towels, toys, or bedclothes. Blood-soiled clothing may be washed routinely with hot water and detergent. Contaminated surfaces may be disinfected easily with a variety of agents, including household bleach (1:10 dilution), some commercial disinfectants (eg, Lysol), or 70% isopropyl alcohol.

## Conclusion

Pediatric HIV infection is a complex and multifaceted disease. Many aspects of care are under intense investigation, and recommendations for clinical care change frequently. Updated information should be sought whenever a child is diagnosed with HIV infection. With recognition of the longer survival time in most infected children, this disease is now approached as a chronic illness. Many children, infected from birth, are entering adolescence and young adulthood. The complexity of antiretroviral drug therapy requires care from a provider with HIV expertise. Primary care physicians are encouraged to participate in the care of HIV-infected children in collaboration with centers staffed by personnel with expertise in pediatric HIV issues.

## REFERENCES

Abrams EJ et al. Maternal health factors and early pediatric antiretroviral therapy influence the rate of perinatal HIV-1 disease progression in children. AIDS 2003;17(6):867 [PMID: 12660534].

American Academy of Pediatrics, Committee of Pediatric AIDS and Committee on Infectious Diseases: Issues related to human immunodeficiency virus transmission in schools, child care, medical settings, the home, and community. Pediatrics 1999;104(2 Pt 1):318 [PMID: 10429018].

Centers for Disease Control and Prevention: 1994 Revised classification system for human immunodeficiency virus infection in children less than 13 years of age. MMWR Morb Mortal Wkly Rep 1994;43(RR-12):1 [PMID: 7908403].

Centers for Disease Control and Prevention: 1995 revised guidelines for prophylaxis against Pneumocystis carinii pneumonia for children infected with or perinatally exposed to human immunodeficiency virus. MMWR Morb Mortal Wkly Rep 1995;44(RR-4):1 [PMID: 7565543].

Centers for Disease Control and Prevention: Updated U.S. Public Health Service guidelines for the management of occupational exposures to HBV, HCV, and HIV and recommendations for postexposure prophylaxis. MMWR Morb Mortal Wkly Rep 2001;50(RR-11):1 [PMID: 11442229].

http://www.aidsinfo.nih.gov/guidelines/

Dankner WM et al: Pediatric AIDS Clinical Trials Group Protocol Teams 051, 128, 138, 144, 152, 179, 190, 220, 240, 245, 254, 300 and 327: Correlates of opportunistic infections in children infected with the human immunodeficiency virus managed before highly active antiretroviral therapy. Pediatr Infect Dis J 2001;20(1):40 [PMID: 11176565].

de Martino M et al: Reduction in mortality with availability of antiretroviral therapy for children with perinatal HIV-1 infection: Italian Register for HIV Infection in Children and the Italian National AIDS Registry. JAMA 2000;284(2): 190 [PMID: 10889592].

Fowler MG et al: Update on perinatal HIV transmission. Pediatr Clin North Am 2000;47:21 [PMID: 10697640].

Gray L et al: Fluctuations in symptoms in human immunodeficiency virus-infected children: The first 10 years of life. Pediatrics 2001;108(1):116 [PMID: 11433063].

Hirsch MS et al: Antiretroviral drug resistance testing in adults infected with human immunodeficiency virus type 1: 2003 recommendations of an International AIDS Society—USA Panel. Clin Infect Dis 2003;37(1):113 [PMID: 12830416].

Leonard EG, McComsey GA: Metabolic complications of antiretroviral therapy in children. Pediatr Infect Dis J 2003; 22(1):77 [PMID: 12544413].

Nesheim S et al: Quantitative RNA testing for diagnosis of HIV-infected infants. J Acquir Immune Defic Syndr 2003;32(2): 192 [PMID: 12571529].

Perinatal HIV Guidelines Working Group: Public Health Service Task Force recommendations for the use of antiretroviral drugs in pregnant women infected with HIV-1 for maternal health and interventions to reduce perinatal HIV-1 transmission in the United States.

http://www.aidsinfo.nih.gov/guidelines/

Pomerantz RJ: Residual HIV-1 infection during antiretroviral therapy: The challenge of viral persistence. AIDS 2001;15(10): 1201 [PMID: 11426065].

Weinberg GA: Postexposure prophylaxis against human immunodeficiency virus infection after sexual assault. Pediatr Infect Dis J 2002; 21(10):959 [PMID: 12394821].The Working Group on Antiretroviral Therapy and Medical Management of HIV-Infected Children: Guidelines for the use of antiretroviral agents in pediatric HIV infection.

http://www.aidsinfo.nih.gov/guidelines/

# Infections: Bacterial & Spirochetal

*John W. Ogle, MD, & Marsha S. Anderson, MD*

## ■ I. BACTERIAL INFECTIONS

### GROUP A STREPTOCOCCAL INFECTIONS

> **ESSENTIALS OF DIAGNOSIS & TYPICAL FEATURES**
>
> Streptococcal pharyngitis:
> - Clinical diagnosis based entirely on symptoms; signs and physical examination unreliable.
> - Throat culture or rapid antigen detection test positive for group A streptococci.
>
> Impetigo:
> - Rapidly spreading, highly infectious skin rash.
> - Erythematous denuded areas and honey-colored crusts.
> - On culture, group A streptococci are grown in most (not all) cases.

### General Considerations

Group A streptococci (GAS) are common gram-positive bacteria producing a wide variety of clinical illnesses, including acute pharyngitis, impetigo, cellulitis, and scarlet fever, the generalized illness caused by strains that elaborate erythrogenic toxin. Group A streptococci can also cause pneumonia, septic arthritis, osteomyelitis, meningitis, and other less common infections. GAS infections may also produce nonsuppurative sequelae (rheumatic fever, acute glomerulonephritis).

The cell walls of streptococci contain both carbohydrate and protein antigens. The C-carbohydrate antigen determines the group, and the M- or T-protein antigens determine the specific type. In most strains, the M protein appears to confer virulence, and antibod-

ies developed against the M protein are protective against reinfection with that type.

Group A streptococci are almost all β-hemolytic. These organisms may be carried without symptoms on the skin and in the pharynx, rectum, and vagina. Between 10% and 15% of school children in some studies are asymptomatic pharyngeal carriers of group A streptococci. Streptococcal carriers are individuals who do not mount an immune response to the organism and are therefore believed to be at low risk for nonsuppurative sequelae. All group A streptococci are sensitive to penicillin. Resistance to erythromycin is common in some countries and has increased in the United States.

### A. CLINICAL FINDINGS

#### 1. Respiratory infections—

**a. Infancy and early childhood (< age 3 years)—** The onset of infection is insidious, with mild symptoms (eg, low-grade fever, serous nasal discharge, and pallor). Otitis media is common. Pharyngitis with exudate and cervical adenitis are uncommon in this age group.

**b. Childhood type—** Onset is sudden, with fever and marked malaise and often with repeated vomiting. The pharynx is sore and edematous, and the tonsillar area generally shows exudate. Anterior cervical lymph nodes are tender and enlarged. Small petechiae are frequently seen on the soft palate. In scarlet fever, the skin is diffusely erythematous and appears sunburned and roughened (so-called sandpaper rash). The rash is most intense in the axillae and groin and on the abdomen and trunk. It blanches on pressure except in the skin folds, which do not blanch and are pigmented (Pastia sign). The rash usually appears 24 hours after the onset of fever and rapidly spreads over the next 1–2 days. Desquamation begins on the face at the end of the first week and becomes generalized by the third week. Early, the surface of the tongue is coated white, with the papillae enlarged and bright red (so-called white strawberry tongue). Subsequently desquamation occurs, and the tongue appears beefy red (strawberry tongue). The face generally shows circumoral pallor. Petechiae may be seen on all mucosal surfaces.

**c. Adult type**—The adult type is characterized by exudative or nonexudative tonsillitis with fewer systemic symptoms, lower fever, and no vomiting. Scarlet fever is uncommon in adults.

**2. Impetigo**—Streptococcal impetigo begins as a papule that vesiculates and then breaks, leaving a denuded area covered by a honey-colored crust. Both *Staphylococcus aureus* and group A streptococci are isolated in some cases. The lesions spread readily and diffusely. Local lymph nodes may become swollen and inflamed. Although the affected child often lacks systemic symptoms, occasionally a high fever and toxicity are present. If flaccid bullae are present, the disease is called bullous impetigo and is caused by an epidermolytic toxin-producing strain of *S aureus.*

**3. Cellulitis**—The portal of entry is often an insect bite or superficial abrasion on an extremity. A diffuse and rapidly spreading cellulitis occurs that involves the subcutaneous tissues and extends along the lymphatic pathways with only minimal local suppuration. Local acute lymphadenitis occurs. The child is usually acutely ill, with fever and malaise. In classic erysipelas, the involved area is bright red, swollen, warm, and very tender. The infection may extend rapidly from the lymphatics to the bloodstream.

Streptococcal perianal cellulitis is an entity peculiar to young children. Pain with defecation often leads to constipation, which may be the presenting complaint. The child is afebrile and otherwise well. Perianal erythema and tenderness and painful rectal examination are the only abnormal physical findings. Scant rectal bleeding with defecation may occur. Culture of a perianal swab specimen usually yields a heavy growth of group A streptococcus. A variant of this syndrome is streptococcal vaginitis in prepubertal girls. Symptoms are dysuria and pain; marked erythema and tenderness of the introitus and blood-tinged discharge are seen.

**4. Necrotizing fasciitis**—This dangerous disease is being reported more frequently, particularly as a complication of varicella infection. Only 20–40% of cases are due to GAS. About 30–40% are due to *S aureus* and the rest to mixed bacterial infections. The disease is characterized by extensive necrosis of superficial fasciae, with undermining of surrounding tissue and extreme systemic toxicity. Initially the skin overlying the infection is tender and pale red without distinct borders, resembling subcutaneous cellulitis. Blisters or bullae may appear. The color deepens to a distinct purple or in some cases becomes very pale. The involved area may develop mild to massive edema. Early recognition and aggressive debridement of necrotic tissue are essential.

**5. Group A streptococcal infections in newborn nurseries**—GAS epidemics occur occasionally in nurseries. The organism may be introduced into the nursery from the vaginal tract of a mother or from the throat or nose of a mother or a staff member. The organism then spreads from infant to infant. The umbilical stump is colonized while the infant is in the nursery. As is true also in staphylococcal infections, there may be no or few clinical manifestations while infants are still in the nursery. Most often, a colonized infant develops a chronic, oozing omphalitis days later at home. The organism may spread from the infant to other family members. More serious and even fatal infections may develop, including sepsis, meningitis, empyema, septic arthritis, and peritonitis.

**6. Streptococcal sepsis**—Serious illness from GAS sepsis is now more common both in children and in adults. Rash and scarlet fever may be present. Prostration and shock result in high mortality rates. Pharyngitis is uncommon as an antecedent illness. Underlying disease is a predisposing factor.

**7. Streptococcal toxic shock syndrome (STSS)**—A toxic shock syndrome caused by GAS has been defined. Like *S aureus*-associated toxic shock, multiorgan system involvement is a prominent part of the illness. The criteria for diagnosis include (1) isolation of GAS from a normally sterile site, hypotension or shock, and (2) at least two of the following: renal impairment (creatinine > 2 times the upper limit of normal for age), thrombocytopenia (< 100,000/mm$^3$) or coagulopathy, liver involvement (transaminases > 2 times normal), acute respiratory distress syndrome (ARDS), generalized erythematous macular rash, soft tissue necrosis (myositis, necrotizing fasciitis, gangrene). In cases that otherwise meet clinical criteria, isolation of GAS from a nonsterile site (throat, wound, vagina) is indicative of a probable cause.

**B. LABORATORY FINDINGS**

Leukocytosis with a marked shift to the left is seen early. Eosinophilia regularly appears during convalescence. β-Hemolytic streptococci are cultured from the throat. The organism may be cultured from the skin and by needle aspiration from subcutaneous tissues and other involved sites such as infected nodes. Occasionally blood cultures are positive. GAS may be identified most easily by their sensitivity to bacitracin. Rapid antigen detection tests are 60–95% sensitive and over 95% specific for detecting GAS in throat swabs. The predictive value of negative tests is about 80%, meaning that one in five patients with a positive throat culture will have a negative rapid antigen test. Rapid tests may be useful when early antibiotic therapy is considered, but because the currently available tests lack sensitivity, a standard culture should be done on specimens testing negative by the rapid test.

Antistreptolysin O (ASO) titers rise about 150 units within 2 weeks after an acute infection. Elevated ASO and anti-DNase B titers are useful in documenting prior throat infections in cases of acute rheumatic fever. The streptozyme test is a 2-minute slide test that detects antibodies to streptolysin O, hyaluronidase, streptokinase, DNase B, and NADase. It is somewhat more sensitive than the measurement of ASO titers.

Proteinuria, cylindruria, and minimal hematuria may be seen early in children with streptococcal infection. True poststreptococcal glomerulonephritis is seen 1–4 weeks after the respiratory or skin infection.

## Differential Diagnosis

Streptococcal infection in early childhood must be differentiated from adenovirus and other respiratory virus infections. The pharyngitis in herpangina (coxsackie A viruses) is vesicular or ulcerative. Herpes simplex also causes ulcerative lesions, which most commonly involve the anterior pharynx, tongue, and gums. In infectious mononucleosis, the pharyngitis is also exudative, but splenomegaly and generalized adenopathy are typical, and laboratory findings are often diagnostic (atypical lymphocytes, elevated liver enzymes, and a positive heterophil or other serologic test for mononucleosis). Uncomplicated streptococcal pharyngitis improves within 24–48 hours if penicillin is given and by 72–96 hours without antimicrobials.

Group G and group C streptococci are uncommon causes of pharyngitis but have been implicated in epidemics of sore throat in college students. Acute rheumatic fever does not occur following group G or group C infection, although acute glomerulonephritis is a complication. *Arcanobacterium hemolyticum* may cause pharyngitis with scarlatina-like or maculopapular truncal rash. In diphtheria, systemic symptoms, vomiting, and fever are less marked; pharyngeal pseudomembrane is confluent and adherent; the throat is less red; and cervical adenopathy is prominent. Pharyngeal tularemia causes white rather than yellow exudate. There is little erythema, and cultures for β-hemolytic streptococci are negative. A history of exposure to rabbits and a failure to respond to antimicrobials may suggest the diagnosis. Leukemia and agranulocytosis may present with pharyngitis and are diagnosed by bone marrow examination.

Scarlet fever must be differentiated from other exanthematous diseases (principally rubella), erythema due to sunburn, drug reactions, Kawasaki disease, toxic shock syndrome, and staphylococcal scalded skin syndrome (see also Table 36–3).

## Complications

Suppurative complications of GAS infections include sinusitis, otitis, mastoiditis, cervical lymphadenitis, pneumonia, empyema, septic arthritis, and meningitis. Spread of streptococcal infection from the throat to other sites—principally the skin (impetigo) and vagina—is common and should be considered in every instance of chronic vaginal discharge or chronic skin infection, such as that complicating childhood eczema. Both acute rheumatic fever and acute glomerulonephritis are nonsuppurative complications of GAS infections.

### A. ACUTE RHEUMATIC FEVER (SEE CHAPTER 19.)

### B. ACUTE GLOMERULONEPHRITIS

Acute glomerulonephritis can follow streptococcal infections of either the pharynx or the skin—in contrast to rheumatic fever, which follows pharyngeal infection only. Glomerulonephritis may occur at any age, even infancy. In most reports of acute glomerulonephritis, males predominate by a ratio of 2:1, whereas acute rheumatic fever occurs with equal frequency in both sexes. Certain M types are associated strongly with poststreptococcal glomerulonephritis (nephritogenic types). The serotypes resident on or producing disease on the skin often differ from those found in the pharynx.

The incidence of acute glomerulonephritis after streptococcal infection is variable and has ranged from nil to 28%. Several outbreaks of acute glomerulonephritis in families have involved 50–75% of siblings of affected patients in 1- to 7-week periods. Second attacks of glomerulonephritis are rare. The median latent period between infection and the development of glomerulonephritis is 10 days. In contrast, acute rheumatic fever occurs after a median latent period of 18 days.

## Treatment

### A. SPECIFIC MEASURES

Treatment is directed toward both eradication of acute infection and prevention of rheumatic fever. In patients with pharyngitis, antibiotics should be started early to relieve symptoms and should be continued for 10 days to prevent rheumatic fever. Although early therapy has not been shown to prevent glomerulonephritis, it seems advisable to treat impetigo promptly in sibling contacts of patients with poststreptococcal nephritis. Neither sulfonamides nor trimethoprim–sulfamethoxazole (TMP–SMX) is effective in the treatment of streptococcal infections. Although topical therapy for impetigo with antimicrobial ointments (especially mupirocin) is as effective as systemic therapy, it does not eradicate pharyngeal carriage and is less practical for extensive disease.

**1. Penicillin**—Except for penicillin-allergic patients, penicillin V (phenoxymethyl penicillin) is the drug of choice. Penicillin resistance has never been documented. For children weighing less than 27 kg, the regimen is 250 mg, given orally bid or tid for 10 days. For heavier children, adolescents, or adults, 500 mg bid–tid is recommended. Giving penicillin V (250 mg) bid is as effective as more frequent oral administration or intramuscular therapy, and it may lead to better compliance. Another alternative for treatment of pharyngitis and impetigo is a single dose of benzathine penicillin G, given intramuscularly (0.6 million units for children weighing < 60 lb [27.2 kg] and 1.2 million units for children weighing > 60 lb [27.2 kg]). Intramuscular delivery ensures compliance, but is painful. Parenteral therapy is indicated if vomiting or sepsis is present. Mild cellulitis due to GAS may be treated orally or intramuscularly as outlined earlier.

Cellulitis requiring hospitalization should be treated with aqueous penicillin G (150,000 units/kg/d, given intravenously in four to six divided doses) or procaine penicillin (50,000 units/kg, given intramuscularly once or twice a day) until there is marked improvement. Penicillin V, 125–250 mg q6h, may then be given orally to complete a 10-day course. Acute cervical lymphadenitis may require incision and drainage. Treatment of necrotizing fasciitis requires emergency surgical debridement followed by high-dose parenteral antibiotics appropriate to the organisms cultured.

**2. Other antibiotics**—For penicillin-allergic patients with pharyngitis or impetigo the following alternative regimens have been used: erythromycin estolate (20–40 mg/kg/d in two to four divided doses) for 10 days, clarithromycin (15 mg/kg/d in two divided doses) for 10 days, and azithromycin (12 mg/kg/d) once daily for 5 days. Erythromycin resistance, although not currently widespread in the United States, was reported in 48% of strains tested in Pittsburgh in 2001. Penicillin-allergic patients from areas with high rates of erythromycin resistance may require an alternative antibiotic. Clindamycin, cephalexin, ceftibuten, cefdinir, and cefadroxil are other effective oral antimicrobials. The dosage of clindamycin is 10–20 mg/kg/d orally in four divided doses. Each of these drugs should be given for 10 days. Patients with immediate, anaphylactic hypersensitivity to penicillin should not receive cephalosporins, because up to 15% will also be allergic to cephalosporins. In most studies, bacteriologic failures after cephalosporin therapy are less frequent than failures following penicillin. However, cephalosporins are far more expensive than penicillin. Additionally, there are few conclusive data on the ability of these agents to prevent rheumatic fever. Therefore, penicillin remains the agent of choice for nonallergic patients. Many strains are resistant to tetracycline.

For infections requiring intravenous therapy, aqueous penicillin G (250,000 units/kg in six divided doses given intravenously is usually the drug of choice. Cefazolin (100–150 mg/kg/d intravenously or intramuscularly in three divided doses), clindamycin (25–40 mg/kg/d intravenously in four divided doses), and vancomycin (40 mg/kg/d intravenously in four divided doses) are alternatives in penicillin-allergic patients. Clindamycin is preferred by many and may be superior to penicillin for necrotizing fasciitis. Clindamycin should not be used alone empirically for severe, suspected GAS infections because a small percentage of isolates in the United States are resistant to clindamycin. Some physicians use both penicillin and clindamycin in patients with STSS.

**3. Serious GAS disease**—Serious GAS infections, such as pneumonia, osteomyelitis, septic arthritis, sepsis, endocarditis, meningitis, and STSS, require parenteral antimicrobial therapy. Penicillin G is the drug of choice for these invasive infections. Clindamycin, in addition to penicillin G, is advocated by many experts for STSS or necrotizing fasciitis. Necrotizing fasciitis requires prompt surgical debridement. Patients with STSS need attention given to volume status and blood pressure and evaluation for a focus of infection, if not readily apparent. Intravenous immune globulin (in addition to antibiotics) has sometimes been used in severe cases.

**4. Treatment failure**—Even when compliance is perfect, organisms will be found cultures in 5–15% of children after cessation of therapy. Reculture is indicated only in the patient with pharyngitis or if the patient has a personal or family history of rheumatic fever. Repeat treatment at least once with an oral cephalosporin or clindamycin is indicated in patients with recurrent culture-positive pharyngitis.

**5. Prevention of recurrences in rheumatic individuals**—The preferred prophylaxis for rheumatic individuals is benzathine penicillin G, 1.2 million units intramuscularly every 4 weeks. If the risk of streptococcal exposure is high, every 3 week dosing is preferred. One of the following alternative oral prophylactic regimens may be used: sulfadiazine, 0.5 g (if < 27 kg) or 1 g (if > 27 kg)/d; penicillin V, 200,000 units bid; or erythromycin, 250 mg bid. Prophylaxis is continued for at least 5 years or until age 21 years (whichever is longer) if carditis is absent. Prophylaxis in these individuals should be continued if the risk of contact with persons with GAS is high (eg, parents of school-age children, pediatric nurses, teachers). In the presence of carditis without residual heart or valvular disease, a minimum of 10 years, (or well into adulthood, whichever is longer) is the minimum duration. If the patient has residual valvular heart disease, many recommend lifelong prophylaxis. These patients should be at least 10 years from their last episode of rheumatic disease and at least 40 years of age prior to considering discontinuation of prophylaxis. A similar approach to the prevention of recurrences of glomerulonephritis may be indicated during childhood when there is a suspicion that repeated streptococcal infections coincide with flare-ups of acute glomerulonephritis.

## B. GENERAL MEASURES

Acetaminophen is useful for pain or fever. Local treatment of impetigo may promote earlier healing. Crusts should first be soaked off. Areas beneath the crusts should then be washed with soap daily.

## C. TREATMENT OF COMPLICATIONS

Rheumatic fever is best prevented by early and adequate penicillin treatment of the streptococcal infection (see earlier discussion).

## D. TREATMENT OF CARRIERS

Identification and treatment of GAS carriers is difficult. There are no established clinical or serologic criteria for differentiating carriers from the truly infected. Some children receive multiple courses of antimicrobials, with persistence of GAS in the throat, leading to a so-called streptococcal neurosis on the part of families.

In certain circumstances, eradication of carriage may be desirable: (1) when a family member has a history of rheumatic fever, (2) when an episode of GAS toxic shock syndrome or necrotizing fasciitis has occurred in a household contact, (3) multiple, recurring, documented episodes of GAS in family members despite adequate therapy, and (4) during an outbreak of rheumatic fever or GAS-associated glomerulonephritis. Clindamycin (20 mg/kg/d, given orally in three divided doses, to a maximum of 1.8 g/d) or a combination of rifampin (20 mg/kg/d, given orally for 4 days) and penicillin in standard dosage given orally has been used to attempt eradication of carriage.

## Prognosis

Death is rare except in infants or young children with sepsis or pneumonia. The febrile course is shortened and complications eliminated by early and adequate treatment with penicillin.

Freeman AF, Shulman ST: Macrolide resistance in group A *Streptococcus*. Pediatr Infect Dis J 2002;21(12);1158 [PMID: 1248869].

Gerber MA, Tanz RR: New approaches to the treatment of group A streptococcal pharyngitis. Curr Opin Pediatr 2001;13; 51 [PMID:11176244].

Tanz RR: Convenient schedules and short course treatment of acute streptococcal pharyngitis: Pediatr Infect Dis J 2000;19: 560 [PMID:10877176]

The Working Group on Severe Streptococcal Infections: Defining the group A streptococcal toxic shock syndrome: Rationale and consensus definition. JAMA 1993;269:390 [PMID: 8418347].

# GROUP B STREPTOCOCCAL INFECTIONS

 **ESSENTIALS OF DIAGNOSIS & TYPICAL FEATURES**

*Early-onset neonatal infection:*

• *Newborn younger than age 7 days, with rapidly progressing overwhelming sepsis, with or without meningitis.*

• *Pneumonia with respiratory failure frequently present; chest radiograph resembles that seen in hyaline membrane disease.*

• *Leukopenia with a shift to the left.*

• *Blood or CSF cultures growing group B streptococci.*

*Late-onset infection:*

• *Meningitis, sepsis, or other focal infection in a child age 1–16 weeks with blood or CSF cultures growing group B streptococci.*

## General Considerations

Although most patients with group B streptococcal (GBS) disease are infants younger than age 3 months, cases are seen in infants age 4–5 months. Serious infection also occurs in women with puerperal sepsis, in immunocompromised patients, in patients with cirrhosis and spontaneous peritonitis, and in diabetic patients with cellulitis. GBS infections occur as frequently as gram-negative infections in the newborn period. Two distinct clinical syndromes distinguished by differing perinatal events, age at onset, and serotype of the infecting strain occur in these infants.

Risk factors for early-onset group GBS disease include maternal GBS colonization, gestational age less than 37 weeks, rupture of membranes more than 18 hours prior to presentation, young maternal age, black race, and low or absent maternal GBS anticapsular antibodies.

## Clinical Findings

Early-onset illness is observed in newborns younger than 7 days old. The onset of symptoms in the majority of these infants occurs in the first 48 hours of life, and most are ill within 6 hours. Apnea is often the first sign. Sepsis, meningitis, apnea, and pneumonia are the most common clinical presentations. There is a high incidence of associated maternal obstetric complications, especially premature labor and prolonged rupture of the membranes. Newborns with early-onset disease are severely ill at the time of diagnosis, and more than 50% die. Although most infants with early-onset infections are full-term, premature infants are at increased risk for the disease. Newborns with early-onset infection acquire GBS in utero as an ascending infection or during passage through the birth canal. When early-onset infection is complicated by meningitis, as occurs in approximately 30% of patients, more than 80% of the bacterial isolates belong to serotype III. Postmortem examination of infants with early-onset disease almost always reveals pulmonary inflammatory infiltrates and hyaline membranes containing large numbers of GBS.

Late-onset infection occurs in infants between ages 7 days and 4 months (median age at onset, about 4 weeks). Maternal obstetric complications are not usually associated with late-onset infection. These infants are usually not as ill at the time of diagnosis as those with early-onset disease, and the mortality rate is lower. In recent series, about 37% of patients have meningitis and 46% have sepsis. Septic arthritis and osteomyelitis, meningitis, occult bacteremia, otitis media, ethmoiditis, conjunctivitis, cellulitis (particularly of the face or submandibular area), lymphadenitis, breast abscess, empyema, and impetigo have been described. Strains of GBS possessing the capsular type III polysaccharide antigen are isolated from more than 95% of infants with late-onset disease, regardless of clinical manifestations. The exact mode of transmission of the organisms is not well defined.

## Diagnosis

Culture of GBS from a normally sterile site such as blood, pleural fluid, or cerebrospinal fluid (CSF) provides proof of diagnosis. Frequent false-positive results limit the usefulness of testing for GBS antigen in urine and CSF.

## Prevention

Many women of childbearing age possess type-specific circulating antibody to the polysaccharide antigens for GBS. These antibodies are transferred to the newborn via the placental circulation. Carriers delivering healthy infants have significant serum levels of IgG antibody to this antigen. In contrast, women delivering infants who develop GBS disease of either the early- or late-onset type rarely have detectable antibody in their sera.

Monovalent and bivalent vaccines with type II or III polysaccharide antigens have been studied in pregnant women, with 80–90% of bivalent conjugate vaccine recipients developing fourfold or greater increases in GBS capsular polysaccharide type II- or III-specific IgG. These reports are encouraging that a multivalent vaccine could be developed and given to pregnant women to prevent many cases of early-onset GBS disease.

The Centers for Disease Control (CDC) has issued culture-based maternal guidelines for the prevention of early-onset GBS disease.

## CDC Recommendations for Prevention of Perinatal GBS Disease

- All pregnant women should be screened at 35–37 weeks' gestation with a vaginal and rectal culture for GBS.

  Exceptions: women with known GBS bacteria during the current pregnancy or women who have delivered a previous infant with GBS disease do not need screening—all these women need intrapartum prophylaxis.

- If GBS status is unknown at onset of labor or rupture of membranes, intrapartum chemoprophylaxis should be administered to women with any of the following:

  Gestation less than 37 weeks.

  Rupture of membranes more than 18 hours

  Intrapartum temperature of greater than 38.0°C (> 100.4°F)

- Women with GBS colonization and a planned cesarean delivery done prior to labor and rupture of membranes do not routinely need intrapartum antibiotics

- Intrapartum antibiotic recommendations (Table 38–1).

- Empiric treatment of a neonate whose mother received intrapartum antibiotics (IAP) for prevention of GBS (Figure 38–1).

## Treatment of GBS Disease

Intravenous ampicillin and an aminoglycoside is the initial regimen of choice for newborns with presumptive invasive GBS disease. For neonates younger than 7 days of age with meningitis, the recommended ampicillin dosage is 200–300 mg/kg/d, given intravenously in 3 divided doses. For infants older than 7 days of age,

***Table 38–1.*** CDC recommended regimens for intrapartum prophylaxis for perinatal GBS disease.[a]

| Recommended | Penicillin G, 5 million units IV initial dose, then 2.5 million units IV q4h until delivery |
|---|---|
| Alternative | Ampicillin, 2 g IV initial dose, then 1 g IV q4h until delivery |
| If penicillin allergic[b] | |
|   Patients not at high risk for anaphylaxis | Cefazolin, 2 g IV initial dose, then 1 g IV q8h until delivery |
|   Patients at high risk for anaphylax[c] | |
|     GBS susceptible to clindamycin and erythromycin[d] | Clindamycin, 900 mg IV q8h until delivery |
| | OR |
| | Erythromycin, 500 mg IV q6h until delivery |
|     GBS resistant to clindamycin or erythromycin or susceptibility unknown | Vancomycin,[e] 1 g IV q12h until delivery |

[a]Broader-spectrum agents, including an agent active against GBS, may be necessary for treatment of chorioamnionitis.
[b]History of penicillin allergy should be assessed to determine whether a high risk for anaphylaxis is present. Penicillin-allergic patients at high risk for anapylaxis are those who have experienced immediate hypersensitivity to penicillin including a history of penicillin-related anaphylaxis; other high-risk patients are those with asthma or other diseases that would make anaphylaxis more dangerous or difficult to treat, such as persons being treated with beta-adrenergic-blocking agents.
[c]If laboratory facilities are adequate, clindamycin and erythromycin susceptibility testing should be performed on prenatal GBS isolates from penicillin allergic women at high risk for anaphylaxis.
[d]Resistance to erythromycin is often but not always associated with clindamycin resistance. If a strain is resistant to erythromycin but appears susceptible to clindamycin, it may have inducible resistance to clindamycin.
[e]Cefazolin is preferred over vancomycin for women with a history of penicillin allergy other than immediate hypersensitivity reactions, and pharmacologic data suggest it achieves effective intraamniotic concentrations. Vancomycin should be reserved for penicillin-allergic women at high risk for anaphylaxis.
Reprinted, with permission, from Schrag S et al: Prevention of perinatal Group B streptococcal disease, revised guidelines from CDC. MMWR 2002;51(RR11);1.

the recommended ampicillin dosage is 300 mg/kg/d, given intravenously in 4–6 divided doses. Penicillin G can be used once GBS is identified and clinical and microbiologic responses have occurred. GBS are less susceptible than other streptococci to penicillin, and high doses are recommended, especially for meningitis. In infants with meningitis, the recommended dosage of penicillin G varies with age: for infants age 7 days or younger, 250,000–450,000 units/kg/d, given intravenously in 3 divided doses; for infants older than age 7 days, 450,000–500,000 units/kg/d, given intravenously in 4–6 divided doses.

A second lumbar puncture after 24–48 hours of therapy is recommended by some experts to assess efficacy. Duration of therapy is 2–3 weeks for meningitis; at least 4 weeks for osteomyelitis, cerebritis, ventriculitis, or endocarditis; and 10–14 days for most other infections. Therapy does not eradicate carriage of the organism. Ceftriaxone is active in vitro against GBS, and because of its long serum half-life it may be given once or twice daily intramuscularly or intravenously.

Ceftriaxone is sometimes used to complete a course of therapy when intravenous access has become difficult. Ceftriaxone is usually not used in newborns because of associated cholestasis.

Baker CJ et al: Safety and immunogenicity of a bivalent group B streptococcal conjugate vaccine for serotypes II and III. J Infect Dis 2003;188(1);66 [PMID: 22708435].

Oddie S, Embleton ND: Risk factors for early onset neonatal group B streptococcal sepsis: Case-control study. BMJ 2000; 325(7359):308 [PMID 12169506].

Schrag S et al: Prevention of perinatal Group B streptococcal disease, revised guidelines from CDC. MMWR 2002;51(RR11);1.

Schrag SJ et al: Group B streptococcal disease in the era of intrapartum antibiotic prophylaxis. N Engl J Med 2000;342:15 [PMID: 10620644].

http://www.cdc.gov/mmwr/preview/mmwrhtml/rr5111a1.htm

# STREPTOCOCCAL INFECTIONS WITH ORGANISMS OTHER THAN GROUP A OR B

Streptococci of groups other than A and B are part of the normal flora of humans and can occasionally cause disease. Group C or group G organisms occasionally produce pharyngitis (with an ASO rise) but without risk of subsequent rheumatic fever. Acute glomerulonephritis may occasionally occur. Group D streptococci and *Enterococcus* species are normal inhabitants of the gastrointestinal tract and may produce urinary tract infections, meningitis, and sepsis in the newborn, as well as endocarditis. Nosocomial infections caused by *Enterococcus* are frequent in neonatal and oncology units and in patients with central venous catheters.

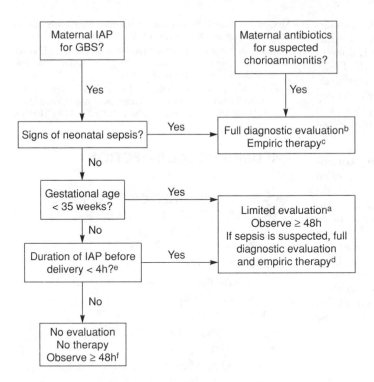

*Figure 38–1.* Algorithm for treatment of a newborn whose mother received intrapartum anitmicrobial prophylaxis for prevention of GBS or suspected chorioamonitis. This algorithm is not an exclusive course of management. Variations that incorporate individual circumstance or institutional preferences may be appropriate. (Reprinted, with permission, from Schrag S et al: Prevention of perinatal group B streptococcal disease, revised guidelines from CDC. MMWR 2002;51 (RR11):1.)

a If no maternal intrapartum prophylaxis for GBS was administered despite an indication being present. data are insufficient on which to recommend a single management strategy.

b Includes complete blood cell count and differential, blood culture, and chest radiograph if respiratory abnormalities are present. When signs of sepsis are present, a lumbar puncture, if feasible, should be performed.

c Duration of therapy varies depending on results of blood culture, cere-brospinal fluid findings, if obtained, and the clinical course of the infant. If laboratory results and clinical course do not indicate bacterial infection, duration may be as short as 48 h.

d CBC with differential and blood culture.

e Applies only to penicillin, ampicillin, or celazoin and assumes recommended dosing regimens.

f A healthy-appearing infant who was ≥ 38 weeks gestation at delivery and whose mother received ≥ 4 h of intrapartum prophylaxis before delivery may be discharged home after 24 h if other discharge criteria have been met and a person able to comply fully with instructions for home observation will be present. If any one of these conditions is not met, the infant should be observed in the hospital for at least 48 h and until criteria for discharge are achieved.

Nonhemolytic aerobic streptococci and β-hemolytic streptococci are normal flora of the mouth. They are involved in the production of dental plaque and probably dental caries and are the most common cause of subacute infective endocarditis. Finally, there are numerous anaerobic and microaerophilic streptococci, normal flora of the mouth, skin, and gastrointestinal tract, which alone or in combination with other bacteria may cause sinusitis, dental abscesses, brain abscesses, and intra-abdominal or lung abscesses.

## Treatment

### A. ENTEROCOCCAL INFECTIONS

**1. Infections with ampicillin-susceptible enterococci**—Lower tract urinary infections can be treated with oral amoxicillin alone. Pyelonephritis should be treated intravenously with ampicillin and gentamicin (gentamicin dosing may need to be adjusted for altered renal function). Sepsis or meningitis in the newborn should be treated intravenously with a combination of ampicillin (100–200 mg/kg/d in three divided doses) and gentamicin (6–7.5 mg/kg/d in three divided doses). Monitoring of aminoglycoside levels is done to avoid toxicity and to ensure therapeutic levels. Endocarditis requires 4–6 weeks of intravenous treatment. Penicillin G (250,000 units/kg/d in six to eight divided doses) plus streptomycin (30 mg/kg/d) or gentamicin (6–7.5 mg/kg/d in three divided doses) is most often used. Cephalosporins are not effective.

**2. Infections with ampicillin-resistant enterococci**—Ampicillin-resistant enterococci are often susceptible to vancomycin (40–60 mg/kg/d in four divided doses). Two agents are effective against vancomycin-resistant enterococci and approved for use in adults. Quinipristin/dalfopristin (Synercid) has been approved for infections with vancomycin-resistant *Enterococcus faecium* (not effective against *E faecalis*). Linezolid (Zyvox) is approved for vancomycin-resistant *E faecalis* and *E faecium* infections. Resistance to these newer agents has been rarely reported. Infectious disease consultation is recommended when use of these drugs is entertained.

### B. Viridans Streptococcal Infections (Subacute Infective Endocarditis)

It is important to determine the penicillin sensitivity of the infecting strain as early as possible in the treatment of viridans streptococcal endocarditis. Resistant organisms are most commonly seen in patients receiving penicillin prophylaxis for rheumatic heart disease. Strains sensitive to penicillin G (minimum inhibitory concentration [MIC] < 0.1 μg/mL) may be treated for 4 weeks with penicillin, 150,000–200,000 units/kg/d intravenously, with gentamicin added during the first 2 weeks. There is considerable experience with 2-week therapy in adult patients using penicillin and gentamicin. Similarly, excellent results have been obtained with ceftriaxone once daily for 4 weeks. If the MIC is 0.5 μg/mL or higher, longer therapy and higher doses of penicillin G must be used (200,000–300,000 units/kg/d intravenously in combination with streptomycin or gentamicin for 4–6 weeks). If the MIC is 0.1–0.5 μg/mL, penicillin G at the higher dose for a minimum of 4 weeks is recommended, with gentamicin added for the first 2 weeks. Vancomycin, 40 mg/kg/d, is usually preferred for resistant strains and patients allergic to penicillin.

Bratcher D: Vancomycin-resistant enterococci in the pediatric patient. Pediatr Infect Dis J 2001;20(6):621 [PMID: 11419507].

Das I, Gray J: Enterococcal bacteremia in children: A review of seventy five episodes in a pediatric hospital. Pediatr Infect Dis J 1998;17:1154 [PMID: 9877366].

McGeer AJ, Low DE: Vancomycin-resistant enterococci. Semin Respir Infect 2000;15:314 [PMID: 11220414].

Mutnick Ah, Jones RN: Linezolid resistance since 2001: SENTRY Anticmibrobial Surveillance Program. Ann Pharmac 2003;37(6):909 [PMID: 12773084].

Wilson WR et al: Antibiotic treatment of adults with infective endocarditis due to streptococci, enterococci, staphylococci, and HACEK microorganisms. JAMA 1995;274:1706 [PMID: 7474277].

# PNEUMOCOCCAL INFECTIONS

## ESSENTIALS OF DIAGNOSIS & TYPICAL FEATURES

*Bacteremia:*
- *High fever (> 39.4°C).*
- *Leukocytosis (> 15,000/μL).*
- *Age 6–24 months.*

*Pneumonia:*
- *Fever, leukocytosis, and tachypnea.*
- *Localized chest pain.*
- *Localized or diffuse rales. Chest radiograph may show lobar infiltrate (with effusion).*

*Meningitis:*
- *Fever, leukocytosis.*
- *Bulging fontanelle, neck stiffness.*
- *Irritability and lethargy.*

*All types:*
- *Diagnosis confirmed by cultures of blood, CSF, pleural fluid, or other body fluid.*

## General Considerations

Sepsis, sinusitis, otitis media, pneumonitis, meningitis, osteomyelitis, cellulitis, arthritis, vaginitis, and peritonitis are all part of a spectrum of pneumococcal infection. Clinical findings that correlate with occult bacteremia in ambulatory patients include age (6–24 months), degree of temperature elevation (> 39.4°C), and leukocytosis (>15,000/μL). Although each of these findings is in itself nonspecific, a combination of them should arouse suspicion. This constellation of findings in a child who has no focus of infection may be an indication for blood cultures and antibiotic therapy. The cause of most of such bacteremic episodes is pneumococci.

*Streptococcus pneumoniae* is the most common cause of acute purulent otitis media. Pneumococci are the organisms responsible for most cases of acute bacterial pneumonia in children. The disease is indistinguishable on clinical grounds from other bacterial pneumonias. Effusions are common, although frank empyema is less common. Abscesses also occasionally occur.

Pneumococcal meningitis is still more common than *H influenzae* type b meningitis. Pneumococcal meningitis, sometimes recurrent, may complicate serious head trauma, particularly if there is persistent leakage of CSF. This has led some physicians to recommend the prophylactic administration of penicillin or other antimicrobials in such cases.

Children with sickle cell disease, other hemoglobinopathies, congenital or acquired asplenia, and some immunoglobulin and complement deficiencies are unusually susceptible to pneumococcal sepsis and meningitis. These children often have a catastrophic illness with shock and disseminated intravascular coagulation (DIC). Even with excellent supportive care, the mortality rate is 20–50%. The spleen is important in the control of pneumococcal infection by clearing organisms from the blood and producing an opsonin that enhances phagocytosis. Autosplenectomy may explain why children with sickle cell disease are at increased risk for developing serious pneumococcal infections. Children with cochlear implants are at higher risk for pneumococcal meningitis. Children who have, or who are planning to receive, a cochlear implant should receive age-appropriate pneumococcal vaccination (> 2 weeks prior to surgery if possible).

*S pneumoniae* rarely causes serious disease in the neonate. Although *S pneumoniae* does not normally colonize the vagina, transient colonization does occur. Serious neonatal disease—including pneumonia, sepsis, and meningitis—may occur and clinically is similar to GBS infection.

Since being introduced in clinical medicine, penicillin has been the agent of choice for pneumococcal infections. Many strains are still highly susceptible to penicillin, and in those cases, penicillin is still the drug of choice. However, pneumococci with moderately increased resistance to penicillin are found in most communities, and reports of treatment failure, particularly in meningitis, are common. The prevalence of these relatively penicillin-resistant strains in North America varies geographically. Pneumococci with high-level resistance to penicillin and multiple other drugs are increasingly encountered throughout the United States. Pneumococci from normally sterile body fluids should be routinely tested for susceptibility to penicillin as well as other drugs.

Pneumococci have been classified into 90 serotypes based on capsular polysaccharide antigens. The frequency distribution of serotypes varies at different times, in different geographic areas, and with different sites of infection. Serotypes 4, 6B, 9V, 14, 18C, 19F, and 23F cause about 80–85% of invasive pneumococcal infections in young children. Similar serotypes, 6B, 9V, 14, 19A, 19F, and 23F, are responsible for most of the penicillin-resistant isolates. In February 2000, the first protein conjugate pneumococcal vaccine (Prevnar) received FDA approval for immunization of young children. It includes polysaccharide or oligosaccharide of seven different *S pneumoniae* serotypes conjugated to a protein carrier. The serotypes in the vaccine are those listed earlier, which cause the bulk of pediatric invasive pneumococcal disease. The development of this vaccine is important in the prevention of pneumococcal disease because young children (< age 2 years), who are most at risk for the disease, are unable to immunologically mount a predictable response to the 23-valent polysaccharide vaccine. This vaccine is discussed further in Chapter 9. For older children and adults, the 23-valent pneumococcal vaccine is generally recommended.

## Clinical Findings

### A. SYMPTOMS AND SIGNS

In pneumococcal sepsis, fever usually appears abruptly, often accompanied by chills. There may be no respiratory symptoms. In pneumococcal sinusitis, mucopurulent nasal discharge may occur. In infants and young children with pneumonia, fever and tachypnea without auscultatory changes are the usual presenting signs. Respiratory distress is manifested by nasal flaring, chest retractions, and tachypnea. Abdominal pain is common. In older children, the adult form of pneumococcal pneumonia with signs of lobar consolidation may occur, but sputum is rarely bloody. Thoracic pain resulting from pleural involvement is sometimes present, but less often in children than in adults. With involvement of the right hemidiaphragm, pain may be referred to the right lower quadrant, suggesting appendicitis. Vomiting is common at onset but seldom persists. Convulsions are relatively common at onset in infants.

Meningitis is characterized by fever, irritability, convulsions, and neck stiffness. The most important sign in very young infants is a tense, bulging anterior fontanelle. In older children, fever, chills, headache, and vomiting are common symptoms. Classic signs are nuchal rigidity associated with positive Brudzinski and Kernig signs. With progression of untreated disease, the child may develop opisthotonos, stupor, and coma.

### B. LABORATORY FINDINGS

Leukocytosis is often pronounced (20,000–45,000/µL), with 80–90% polymorphonuclear neutrophils. Neutropenia may be seen early in very serious infections. The presence of pneumococci in the nasopharynx is not a helpful finding, because up to 40%

of normal children carry pneumococci in the upper respiratory tract. Large numbers of organisms are seen on gram-stained smears of endotracheal aspirates from patients with pneumonia. In meningitis, CSF usually shows an elevated white blood cell (WBC) count of several thousand, chiefly polymorphonuclear neutrophils, with decreased glucose and elevated protein levels. Gram-positive diplococci are seen on stained smears of CSF sediment in 70–90% of cases in young children but are positive in only 50–65% of cases in adolescents and adults. Antigen detection tests are not useful.

## Differential Diagnosis

There are many causes of high fever and leukocytosis in young infants; 90% of children presenting with these features have a disease other than pneumococcal bacteremia such as herpesvirus 6, enterovirus, or other viral infection; urinary tract infection; unrecognized focal infection elsewhere in the body; or early acute shigellosis.

Infants with upper respiratory tract infection who subsequently develop signs and symptoms of lower respiratory disease are most likely to be infected with a respiratory virus. Hoarseness or wheezing is often present. A radiograph of the chest typically shows perihilar infiltrates and increased bronchovascular markings. Viral respiratory infection often precedes pneumococcal pneumonia; therefore, the clinical picture may be mixed.

Staphylococcal pneumonia may be indistinguishable early in its course from pneumococcal pneumonia. Later, pulmonary cavitation and empyema occur. Staphylococcal pneumonia is most common in infants.

In primary pulmonary tuberculosis, children do not have a toxic appearance, and radiographs show a primary focus associated with hilar adenopathy and often with pleural involvement. Miliary tuberculosis presents a classic radiographic appearance.

Pneumonia caused by *Mycoplasma pneumoniae* is most common in children age 5 years and older. Onset is insidious, with infrequent chills, low-grade fever, prominent headache and malaise, cough, and, often, striking radiographic changes. Marked leukocytosis (> 18,000/μL) is unusual.

Pneumococcal meningitis is diagnosed by lumbar puncture. Without a gram-stained smear and culture of CSF, it is not distinguishable from other types of acute bacterial meningitis.

## Complications

Complications of sepsis include meningitis and osteomyelitis; complications of pneumonia include empyema, parapneumonic effusion, and, rarely, lung abscess. Mastoiditis, subdural empyema, and brain abscess may follow untreated pneumococcal otitis media. Both pneumococcal meningitis and peritonitis are more likely to occur independently without coexisting pneumonia. Shock, DIC, and Waterhouse–Friderichsen syndrome resembling meningococcemia are occasionally seen in pneumococcal sepsis, particularly in asplenic patients. Hemolytic–uremic syndrome may occur as a complication of pneumococcal pneumonia or sepsis.

## Treatment

### A. SPECIFIC MEASURES

All *S pneumoniae* isolated from normally sterile sites should be tested for susceptibility to penicillin. Susceptible strains should be treated with penicillin, ampicillin, or amoxicillin. Penicillin-intermediate or penicillin-resistant strains should be tested for susceptibility to cephalosporins, vancomycin, and selected other drugs. Therapy with penicillin, amoxicillin, or cephalosporins will usually succeed in cases of bacteremia or pneumonia due to intermediate-resistant isolates because serum levels in excess of the MIC can be achieved. Therapy of meningitis, empyema, osteomyelitis, and endocarditis due to nonsusceptible *S pneumoniae* is more difficult, because penetration of antimicrobials to these sites is limited. Vancomycin and third-generation cephalosporins are indicated in these and other serious or life-threatening infections pending susceptibility test results.

**1. Bacteremia**—In studies done prior to immunization of young children with conjugated pneumococcal vaccine, 3–5% of blood cultures in patients younger than 2 years of age yielded *S pneumoniae*. These percentages are expected to decrease now that an effective vaccine is available. However, pneumococcal disease will not disappear, as the vaccine prevents only 85% of invasive disease. Many experts treat suspected bacteremia with ceftriaxone (50 mg/kg, given intramuscularly or intravenously). Compared with oral amoxicillin (80-90 mg/kg/d), ceftriaxone may reduce fever and the need for hospitalization. However, meningitis occurs with the same frequency despite presumptive therapy. The widespread use of ceftriaxone among young children has contributed significantly to antibiotic resistance in *S pneumoniae*. All children with blood cultures that grow pneumococci must be reexamined as soon as possible. The child who has a focal infection such as meningitis or who appears septic should be admitted to the hospital to receive parenteral antimicrobials. If the child is afebrile and appears well or mildly ill, management on an ambulatory basis is appropriate. If the physician is confident that close follow-up can be achieved, lumbar puncture is not mandatory.

**2. Pneumonia**—For infants, severely ill patients, and immunocompromised hosts, appropriate regimens include aqueous penicillin G (150,000–200,000 units/kg/d, given intravenously in four to six divided doses), cefotaxime (50 mg/kg, q8h), or cefuroxime (50 mg/kg, q8h). Mild pneumonia may be treated with amoxicillin (80–90 mg/kg/d) for 7–10 days. Alternative regimens include oral macrolides and cephalosporins.

**3. Otitis media**—Most experts recommend oral amoxicillin (80–90 mg/kg/d, divided in two doses) as first line therapy. The standard course of therapy is 10 days; however, many physicians have been treating uncomplicated cases for just 5 days, based on recent studies. Treatment failures may be treated with amoxicillin/clauvulanate (80–90 mg/kg/d of the amoxicillin component in the 7:1 formulation), intramuscular ceftriaxone, cefuroxime, axetil, or cefdinir. Clarithromycin or azithromycin can also be used.

**4. Meningitis**—Until bacteriologic confirmation and susceptibility testing are completed, patients should receive vancomycin (60 mg/kg/d, given intravenously in four divided doses) and cefotaxime (225–300 mg/kg/d intravenously in four divided doses), or vancomycin (see previous dosage) and ceftriaxone (100 mg/kg/d, given intravenously in two divided doses). Corticosteroids (dexamethasone, 0.6 mg/kg/d, in four divided doses for 4 days) are recommended by many experts as adjunctive therapy for pneumococcal meningitis. But they are controversial because they may reduce the entry of vancomycin into the CSF. Repeated lumbar puncture at 24–48 hours should be considered to ensure sterility of the CSF if dexamethasone is given or if resistant pneumococci are isolated.

If the isolate is determined to be penicillin-susceptible, aqueous penicillin G can be administered (300,000–400,000 units/kg/d, given intravenously in four to six divided doses for 10–14 days). Use of ceftriaxone or cefotaxime is acceptable alternative therapy in penicillin and cephalosporin-susceptible isolates. Consult an infectious disease specialist or the *Red Book* (American Academy of Pediatrics, 2003) for therapeutic options for isolates that are nonsusceptible to penicillin or cephalosporins.

## Prognosis

In children, case fatality rates of less than 1% should be achieved except in meningitis, in which rates of 5–20% still prevail. The presence of large numbers of organisms without a prominent CSF inflammatory response or meningitis due to a penicillin-resistant strain indicates a poor prognosis. Serious neurologic sequelae, particularly hearing loss, are frequent following pneumococcal meningitis.

Advisory Committee on Immunization Practices: Preventing pneumococcal disease among infants and young children. MMWR Morb Mortal Wkly Rep 2000;40:1 [PMID: 11055835].

Advisory Committee on Immunization Practices: Pneumococcal vaccination for cochlear implant candidates and recipients: Updated recommendations of the Advisory Committee on Immunization Practices. MMWR 2003;52(31):739 [PMID: 12908457].

Dowell S et al: Acute otitis media: Management and surveillance in an era of pneumococcal resistance: A report from the drug-resistant *Streptococcus pneumoniae* working group. Pediatr Infect Dis J 1999;18:1 [PMID: 9951971].

Shinefield HR et al: Safety and immunogenicity of heptavalent pneumococcal CRM 197 conjugate vaccine in infants and toddlers. Pediatr Infect Dis 1999;18:757 [PMID: 10493334].

Tan TQ: Antibiotic resistant infections due to *Streptococcus pneumoniae:* Impact on therapeutic options and clinical outcome. Curr Opin Infect Dis 2003;16(3):271 [PMID: 12821820].

# STAPHYLOCOCCAL INFECTIONS

Staphylococcal infections are common in childhood. Staphylococcal skin infections range from minor furuncles to the varied syndromes now collectively referred to as scalded skin syndrome. Staphylococci are the major cause of osteomyelitis and of septic arthritis as well as an uncommon but important cause of bacterial pneumonia. A toxin produced by certain strains causes staphylococcal food poisoning. Staphylococci are responsible for most infections of artificial heart valves. They cause toxic shock syndrome (see later discussion). Finally, they are found in infections at all ages and in multiple sites, particularly when infection is introduced from the skin or upper respiratory tract or when closed compartments become infected (pericarditis, sinusitis, cervical adenitis, surgical wounds, abscesses in the liver or brain, and abscesses elsewhere in the body).

Staphylococci that do not produce the enzyme coagulase are termed "coagulase-negative" and are seldom speciated in the clinical microbiology laboratory. Most *Staphylococcus aureus* strains produce coagulase. *S aureus* and coagulase-negative staphylococci are normal flora of the skin and respiratory tract. The latter rarely cause disease except in compromised hosts, the newborn, or patients with plastic indwelling lines.

Most strains of *S aureus* elaborate β-lactamase that confers penicillin resistance. This can be overcome in clinical practice by the use of a cephalosporin or a penicillinase-resistant penicillin such as methicillin, oxacillin, nafcillin, cloxacillin, or dicloxacillin. Methicillin-resistant strains of *S aureus* (MRSA) are found worldwide and are now common in certain hospitals and, increasingly, in community-acquired infections in some areas of the United States. Most MRSA retain β-lactamase production, and many are resistant to other antibiotics as well. MRSA are also resistant in vivo to all of the penicillinase-resistant penicillins and cephalosporins. Strains with intermediate susceptibility to vancomycin have been recovered in the United States and Japan. In addition there have been two reports of vancomycin-resistant strains. The existence of such strains is of concern because of the inherent virulence of most strains of *S aureus* and because of the limited choices for therapy. *S aureus* produces a variety of exotoxins, most of which are of uncertain importance. Two toxins are recognized as playing a central role in specific diseases: exfoliatin and staphylococcal enterotoxin. The former is largely responsible for the various clinical presentations of scalded skin syndrome. Most strains that elaborate exfoliatin are of phage group II. Enterotoxin causes staphylococcal food poisoning. The exoprotein toxin most commonly associated with toxic shock syndrome has been termed TSST-1.

## Clinical Findings

### A. SYMPTOMS AND SIGNS

**1. Staphylococcal skin diseases**—Dermal infection with *S aureus* causes furuncles or cellulitis. *S aureus* are often found along with streptococci in impetigo. If the strains produce exfoliatin, localized lesions become bullous (bullous impetigo).

Scalded skin syndrome is thought to be a systemic effect of exfoliatin. The initial infection may begin at any site but is in the respiratory tract in most cases. There is a prodromal phase of erythema, often beginning around the mouth, accompanied by fever and irritability. The involved skin becomes tender, and a sick infant will cry when picked up or touched. A day or so later, exfoliation begins, usually around the mouth. The inside of the mouth is red, and a peeling rash is present around the lips, often in a radial pattern. Generalized, painful peeling may follow, involving the limbs and trunk but often sparing the feet. More commonly, peeling is confined to areas around body orifices. If erythematous but unpeeled skin is rubbed sideways, superficial epidermal layers separate from deeper ones and slough (Nikolsky sign). In the newborn, the disease is termed Ritter disease and may be fulminant. If there is tender erythema but not exfoliation, the disease is termed nonstreptococcal scarlet fever. The scarlatiniform rash is sandpaper-like, but strawberry tongue is not seen, and cultures grow *S aureus* rather than streptococcus.

**2. Osteomyelitis and septic arthritis**—(See Chapter 24).

**3. Staphylococcal pneumonia**—Staphylococcal pneumonia in infancy is characterized by abdominal distention, high fever, respiratory distress, and toxemia. It often occurs without predisposing factors or after minor skin infections. The organism is necrotizing, producing bronchoalveolar destruction. Pneumatoceles, pyopneumothorax, and empyema are frequently encountered. Rapid progression of disease is characteristic. Frequent chest radiographs to monitor the progress of disease are indicated. Presenting symptoms may be typical of paralytic ileus, suggestive of an abdominal catastrophe.

Staphylococcal pneumonia usually is peribronchial, beginning with a focal infiltrative lesion progressing to patchy consolidation. Most often only one lung is involved (80%), more often the right. Purulent pericarditis occurs by direct extension in about 10% of cases, with or without empyema.

**4. Staphylococcal food poisoning**—Staphylococcal food poisoning is a result of ingestion of enterotoxin produced by staphylococci growing in uncooked and poorly refrigerated food. The disease is characterized by vomiting, prostration, and diarrhea occurring 2–6 hours after ingestion of contaminated foods.

**5. Staphylococcal endocarditis**—*S aureus* may produce infection of normal heart valves, of valves or endocardium in children with congenital or rheumatic heart disease, or of artificial valves. About 25% of all cases of endocarditis are due to *S aureus.* The great majority of artificial heart valve infections involve either *S aureus* or coagulase-negative staphylococci. Infection usually begins in an extracardiac focus, often the skin. Involvement of the endocardium must be suspected in every case of *S aureus* bacteremia, regardless of initial signs. Suspicion must be highest in the presence of congenital heart disease, particularly ventricular septal defects with aortic insufficiency but also simple ventricular septal defect, patent ductus arteriosus, and tetralogy of Fallot.

The presenting symptoms in staphylococcal endocarditis are fever, weight loss, weakness, muscle pain or diffuse skeletal pain, poor feeding, pallor, and cardiac decompensation. Signs include splenomegaly, cardiomegaly, petechiae, hematuria, and a new or changing murmur. The course of *S aureus* endocarditis is rapid, although subacute disease occurs occasionally. Peripheral septic embolization and uncontrollable cardiac failure are common, even when optimal antibiotic therapy is administered, and may be indications for surgical intervention (see later discussion).

**6. Toxic shock syndrome**—Toxic shock syndrome (TSS) is characterized by fever, blanching erythroderma, diarrhea, vomiting, myalgia, prostration, hypotension, and multiorgan dysfunction. It is due to *S aureus* focal infection, usually without bacteremia. Large numbers of cases have been described in menstruating adolescents and young women using vaginal tampons. TSS has also been reported in boys and girls with focal staphylococcal infections and in individuals with wound infections due to *S aureus*. Additional clinical features include sudden onset; conjunctival suffusion; mucosal hyperemia; desquamation of skin on the palms, soles, fingers, and toes during convalescence; DIC in severe cases; renal and hepatic functional abnormalities; and myolysis. The mortality rate with early treatment is now about 2%. Recurrences are seen during subsequent menstrual periods in as many as 60% of untreated women who continue to use tampons. Recurrences occur in up to 15% of women given antistaphylococcal antibiotics who stop using tampons. The disease is caused by strains of *S aureus* that produce TSST-1 or one of the related enterotoxins.

**7. Coagulase-negative staphylococcal infections—** Localized and systemic coagulase-negative staphylococcal infections occur primarily in immunocompromised patients, high-risk newborns, and patients with plastic prostheses or catheters. Coagulase-negative staphylococci are the most common nosocomial pathogen in hospitalized low-birth-weight neonates in the United States. Intravenous administration of lipid emulsions and indwelling central venous catheters are risk factors contributing to coagulase-negative staphylococcal bacteremia in newborn infants. In patients with an artificial heart valve, a Dacron patch, a ventriculoperitoneal shunt, or a central venous catheter, coagulase-negative staphylococci are a common cause of sepsis or catheter infection, often necessitating removal of the foreign material and protracted antibiotic therapy. Because blood cultures are frequently contaminated by this organism, diagnosis of genuine localized or systemic infection is often difficult.

### B. LABORATORY FINDINGS

Moderate leukocytosis (15,000–20,000/µL) with a shift to the left is occasionally found, although normal counts are common, particularly in infants. The sedimentation rate is elevated. Blood cultures are frequently positive in systemic staphylococcal disease and should always be obtained when it is suspected. Similarly, pus from sites of infection should always be aspirated or obtained surgically, examined with Gram stain, and cultured both aerobically and anaerobically. There are no useful serologic tests for staphylococcal disease.

## Differential Diagnosis

Staphylococcal skin disease takes many forms; therefore, the differential list is long. Bullous impetigo must be differentiated from chemical or thermal burns, from drug reactions, and, in the very young, from the various congenital epidermolytic syndromes or even herpes simplex infections. Staphylococcal scalded skin syndrome may resemble scarlet fever, Kawasaki disease,

Stevens–Johnson syndrome, erythema multiforme, and other drug reactions. A skin biopsy may be critical in establishing the correct diagnosis. The skin lesions of varicella may become superinfected with exfoliatin-producing staphylococci and produce a combination of the two diseases (bullous varicella).

Severe, rapidly progressing pneumonia with formation of abscesses, pneumatoceles, and empyemas is typical of *S aureus* infection and GAS but may occasionally be produced by pneumococci, *Haemophilus influenzae,* and GAS.

Staphylococcal food poisoning is often epidemic. It is differentiated from other common-source gastroenteritis syndromes (*Salmonella, Clostridium perfringens, Vibrio parahaemolyticus*) by the short incubation period (2–6 hours), the prominence of vomiting (as opposed to diarrhea), and the absence of fever.

Endocarditis must be suspected in any instance of *S aureus* bacteremia, particularly when a significant heart murmur or preexisting cardiac disease is present (see Chapter 19).

Newborn infections with *S aureus* can resemble infections with streptococci and a variety of gram-negative organisms. Umbilical and respiratory tract colonization occurs with many pathogenic organisms (GBS, *Escherichia coli, Klebsiella*), and both skin and systemic infections occur with virtually all of these organisms.

TSS must be differentiated from Rocky Mountain spotted fever, leptospirosis, Kawasaki disease, drug reactions, adenovirus, and measles (see also Table 36–3).

## Treatment

### A. SPECIFIC MEASURES

Community-acquired MRSA infections are on the rise. The incidence of community-acquired MRSA isolates varies greatly geographically. If the prevalence of MRSA isolates in the community is high or if the patient is seriously ill, vancomycin should be part of the empiric coverage in sick patients until culture results and susceptibility data are known. Currently, most community-acquired MRSA strains are susceptible to TMP–SMX and some are susceptible to clindamycin: Less serious infections in nontoxic patients may be initially treated using one of these agents while awaiting cultures and susceptibility data.

For methicillin-susceptible strains, a β-lactamase-resistant penicillin is the drug of choice (oxicllin, nafcillin, methicillin). In serious systemic disease, in osteomyelitis, and in the treatment of large abscesses, intravenous therapy is indicated initially (oxacillin or nafcillin, 100–150 mg/kg/d in four divided doses, or methicillin, 200–300 mg/kg/d in four divided doses). When high doses over a long period are required, it is preferable not to use methicillin, because of the frequency with which interstitial nephritis occurs. In life-threatening illness, an aminoglycoside antibiotic (gentamicin or tobramycin) or rifampin may be used in addition for its possible synergistic action.

Cephalosporins may be considered for patients with a history of penicillin sensitivity unless there is a history of type 1 hypersensitivity reaction (ie, anaphylaxis, wheezing, edema, hives: [cefazolin, 100–150 mg/kg/d, given intravenously in three divided doses] or cephalexin [50–100 mg/kg/d, given orally in four divided doses]) can be used once a child is able to take oral antibiotics. The third-generation cephalosporins should not generally be used for staphylococcal infections.

For nonmeningeal, suspected nosocomially acquired MRSA infections, vancomycin (40 mg/kg/d intravenously in three or four divided doses) should be used until susceptiblilities are available (these isolates are more frequently clindamycin- and TMP–SMX-resistant). Infections due to MRSA frequently do not respond to cephalosporins despite in vitro testing that suggests susceptibility. For treatment of meningitis, vancomycin must be given in higher doses (60 mg/kg/d divided into four doses). Combinations including rifampin may be either synergistic or antagonistic.

**1. Skin infections**—(See Chapter 14.)

**2. Osteomyelitis and septic arthritis**—Treatment should be begun intravenously, with antibiotics selected to cover the most likely organisms (staphylococci in hematogenous osteomyelitis; meningococci, pneumococci, staphylococci in children younger than age 3 years with septic arthritis; staphylococci and gonococci in older children with septic arthritis). Antibiotic levels should be kept high at all times.

In osteomyelitis, clinical studies support the use of intravenous treatment until fever and local symptoms and signs have subsided—usually after at least 3–5 days—followed by oral therapy (for susceptible strains, dicloxacillin, 100–150 mg/kg/d in four divided doses; or cephalexin, 100–150 mg/kg/d in four divided doses) for at least 3 additional weeks. Longer treatment may be required, particularly when radiographs show extensive involvement. Treatment of community acquired MRSA osteomyelitis should be based on susceptibility results; however, isolates are frequently susceptible to TMP–SMX or clindamycin. Vancomycin can be used as part of an empiric regimen while awaiting susceptiblilities in seriously ill patients or in areas where MRSA is likely as a pathogen. In arthritis, where drug diffusion into synovial fluid is good, intravenous therapy need be given only for a few days, followed by adequate oral therapy for at least 3 weeks. In all instances, oral therapy should be administered with careful attention to compliance, either in the hospital or at home with frequent support and reinforcement from physicians or visiting nurses. The erythrocyte sedimentation rate (ESR) is a good indicator of response to therapy. Surgical drainage of osteomyelitis or septic arthritis is often required (see Chapter 24).

**3. Staphylococcal pneumonia**—In areas of the country where MRSA is not prevalent, nafcillin and oxacillin are the usual drugs of choice. In sick patients, vancomycin should be used empirically until cultures and susceptibility results are obtained. Linezolid has recently been reported to be as efficacious as vancomycin in the treatment of resistant gram-positive pneumonia and soft tissue infections (cure rates: 95% linezolid vs 94% vancomycin).

Empyema and pyopneumothorax require drainage. The choice of chest tube drainage versus thoracoscopic drainage depends on the practitioner's experience and skill. If staphylococcal pneumonia is treated promptly and empyema drained promptly, resolution in children is almost always complete—despite evidence of widespread parenchymal destruction and the persistence of bullae, blebs, and even pockets of empyema or abscess fluid well into convalescence.

**4. Staphylococcal food poisoning**—Therapy is supportive and usually not required except in severe cases or for small infants with marked dehydration.

**5. Staphylococcal endocarditis**—As outlined earlier, high-dose, prolonged parenteral treatment is indicated. Methicillin-susceptible isolates are often treated with oxacillin or nafcillin. Some experts also recommend addition of gentamicin or rifampin for the first 5 days to 2 weeks. In penicillin-allergic patients (type 1 hypersensitivity, anaphylaxis) or patients with MRSA isolates, vancomycin should be used. With penicillin-sensitive organisms, penicillin G is the drug of choice. Therapy lasts in all instances for at least 6 weeks.

In some patients, medical treatment may fail. Signs of treatment failure are (1) recurrent fever without apparent treatable other cause (eg, thrombophlebitis, incidental respiratory or urinary tract infection, drug fever), (2) persistently positive blood cultures, (3) intractable and progressive congestive heart failure, and (4) recurrent (septic) embolization. In such circumstances—particularly (2), (3), and (4)—valve replacement becomes necessary. Antibiotics are continued for at least another 4 weeks. Persistent or recurrent infection may require a second surgical procedure.

**6. Toxic shock syndrome**—Treatment is aimed at expanding volume, maintaining perfusion pressure with inotropic agents as needed, prompt drainage of a focus of infection (or removal of tampons or foreign bodies), and giving intravenous antibiotics.

Vancomycin, in addition to a β-lactam antibiotic (oxacillin, nafcillin), can be used for empiric therapy. Some experts would use vancomycin and clindamycin, since clindamycin is a protein synthesis inhibitor and may turn off toxin production. Clindamycin should not be used empirically as a single agent until susceptibilities (if an isolate grows) are known; some strains of S aureus are clindamycin-resistant.

Intravenous immune globulin has been used as adjunctive therapy. Some experts believe that corticosteroid therapy may be effective if given to patients with severe illness early in the course of their disease. Antibiotic treatment reduces risk of recurrence.

**7. Coagulase-negative staphylococcal infections—** Bacteremia and other serious coagulase-negative staphylococcal infections are treated initially with vancomycin. Coagulase-negative staphylococci are uncommonly resistant to vancomycin (see Chapter 35 for dosing). Strains susceptible to methicillin are treated with methicillin, oxacillin, or cefazolin.

Eady EA, Cove JH: Staphylococcal resistance revisited: Community-acquired methicillin resistant *Staphylococcus aureus*—An emerging problem for the management of skin and soft tissue infections. Curr Opin Infect Dis 2003;16(2):103 [PMID: 12734443].

Kaplan SL: Use of linezolid in children. Pediatr Infect Dis J 2002;21(9):870 [PMID: 12352813].

Lowy FD: Staphylococcus aureus infections. N Engl J Med 1998; 339:520.

Marcinak JF, Frank AL: Treatment of community-acquired methicillin-resistant *Staphylococcus aureus* in children. Curr Opin Infect Dis 2003;16(3):265 [PMID: 12821819].

Naimi TS et al: Epidemiology and clonality of community-acquired methicillin-resistant *Staphylococcus aureus* in Minnesota, 1996–1998. Clin Infect Dis 2001;33(7):990 [PMID: 11528570].

Paradisi F et al: Antistaphylococcal (MSSA, MRSA, MSSE, MRSE) antibiotics. Med Clin North Am 2001;85:1 [PMID 11190346].

# MENINGOCOCCAL INFECTIONS

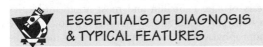

## ESSENTIALS OF DIAGNOSIS & TYPICAL FEATURES

- *Fever, headache, vomiting, convulsions, shock (meningitis).*
- *Fever, shock, petechial or purpuric skin rash (meningococcemia).*
- *Diagnosis confirmed by culture of normally sterile body fluids.*

## General Considerations

Meningococci (*Neisseria meningitidis*) may be carried asymptomatically for many months in the upper respiratory tract. Fewer than 1% of carriers develop disease. Meningitis and sepsis are the two most common forms of illness, but septic arthritis, pericarditis, pneumonia, chronic meningococcemia, otitis media, conjunctivitis, and vaginitis also occur. The highest attack rate for meningococcal meningitis is in the first year of life. The incidence in the United States is about 1.2 cases per 100,000 people. An estimated 2400–3000 cases occur in the United States annually.

Meningococci are gram-negative organisms containing endotoxin in their cell walls. Endotoxins may cause capillary vascular injury and leak and may also cause DIC. The development of irreversible shock with multiorgan failure is a significant factor in the fatal outcome of acute meningococcal infections. Meningococci are classified serologically into groups: A, B, C, Y, and W-135 are the groups most commonly implicated in systemic disease. The serologic groups serve as markers for studying outbreaks and transmission of disease. Currently in the United States, serogoups B, C, and Y each account for about one third of cases. Serogroup A, which causes periodic epidemics in developing countries, is responsible for only occasional cases of meningococcal disease in the United States. Sulfonamide resistance is common in non–serotype-A strains. *N meningitidis* with increased MICs to penicillin G are reported from South Africa and Spain. A small number of these isolates are reported in the United States. The resistance in these strains is low-level and not due to β-lactamase. Resistant isolates are susceptible to third-generation cephalosporins. Few isolates are resistant to rifampin.

Children develop immunity from asymptomatic carriage of meningococci (usually nontypable, nonpathogenic strains) or other cross-reacting bacteria. Patients deficient in one of the late components of complement (C6, C7, C8, or C9) are uniquely susceptible to meningococcal infection, particularly group A meningococci. Deficiencies of early and alternate pathway complement components are also associated with increased susceptibility.

## Clinical Findings

### A. SYMPTOMS AND SIGNS

Many children with clinical meningococcemia also have meningitis, and some have other foci of infection. All children with suspected meningococcemia should have a lumbar puncture.

**1. Meningococcemia—**A prodrome of upper respiratory infection is followed by high fever, headache, nausea, marked toxicity, and hypotension. Purpura, petechiae, and occasionally bright pink, tender macules or papules over the extremities and trunk are seen. The rash usually progresses rapidly. Occasional cases lack rash. Fulminant meningococcemia (Waterhouse–Friderichsen syndrome) progresses rapidly and is characterized by DIC, massive skin and mucosal hemorrhages, and shock. This syndrome also may be due to *H influenzae, S pneumoniae,* or other bacteria. Chronic meningococcemia is characterized by periodic bouts of fever, arthralgia or arthritis, and recurrent petechiae. Splenomegaly is often present. Patients may be free of symptoms between bouts. Chronic meningococcemia occurs primarily in adults and mimics Henoch–Schönlein purpura.

**2. Meningitis**—In many children, meningococcemia is followed within a few hours to several days by symptoms and signs of acute purulent meningitis, with severe headache, stiff neck, nausea, vomiting, and stupor. Children with meningitis generally fare better than children with meningococcemia alone, probably because they have survived long enough to develop clinical signs of meningitis.

### B. Laboratory Findings

The peripheral WBC count may be either low or elevated. Thrombocytopenia may be present with or without DIC (see Chapter 27). If petechial or hemorrhagic lesions are present, meningococci can sometimes be demonstrated on smear by puncturing the lesions and expressing a drop of tissue fluid. Organisms may be demonstrated by Gram stain of buffy coat preparations of blood. CSF is generally cloudy and contains more than 1000 WBCs per microliter, with many polymorphonuclear neutrophils and gram-negative intracellular diplococci. A total hemolytic complement assay may reveal absence of late components as an underlying cause.

## Differential Diagnosis

The skin lesions of *H influenzae* or pneumococci, enterovirus infection, endocarditis, leptospirosis, Rocky Mountain spotted fever, other rickettsial diseases, Henoch–Schönlein purpura, and blood dyscrasias may be similar to meningococcemia. Other causes of sepsis and meningitis are distinguished by appropriate Gram stain and cultures.

## Complications

Meningitis may lead to permanent central nervous system (CNS) damage, with deafness, convulsions, paralysis, or impairment of intellectual function. Hydrocephalus may develop and requires ventriculoperitoneal shunt. Subdural collections of fluid are common but

usually resolve spontaneously. Extensive skin necrosis, loss of digits or extremities, intestinal hemorrhage, and late adrenal insufficiency may complicate fulminant meningococcemia.

## Prevention

Household contacts, day care center contacts, and hospital personnel directly exposed to the respiratory secretions of patients are at increased risk for developing meningococcal infection and should be given chemoprophylaxis with rifampin. The secondary attack rate among household members is 1–5% during epidemics and less than 1% in nonepidemic situations. Children age 3 months to 2 years are at greatest risk, presumably because they lack protective antibodies. Secondary cases may occur in day care centers and in classrooms. Hospital personnel are not at increased risk unless they have had contact with a patient's oral secretions, for example, during mouth-to-mouth resuscitation, intubation, or suctioning procedures. Approximately 50% of secondary cases in households have their onset within 24 hours of identification of the index case. Exposed contacts should be examined promptly. If they are febrile, they should be fully evaluated and given high doses of penicillin or another effective antimicrobial pending the results of blood cultures.

All intimate contacts should receive chemoprophylaxis for meningococcal disease. The most commonly used agent is rifampin, given orally in the following dosages twice daily for 2 days: 600 mg for adults; 10 mg/kg for children younger than 1 month old (maximum dosage 600 mg); and 5 mg/kg for infants younger than 1 month. Rifampin may stain a patient's tears (and contact lenses), sweat, and urine orange; it may also affect the reliability of oral contraceptives, and alternative contraceptive measures should therefore be employed when rifampin is administered. Rifampin should not be given to pregnant women. Instead, intramuscular ceftriaxone is the preferred agent—125 mg given as a single dose if the patient is younger than 15 years; 250 mg given as a single dose if older than 15 years of age. Penicillin and most other antibiotics (even with parenteral administration) are not effective chemoprophylactic agents, because they do not eradicate upper respiratory tract carriage of meningococci. Ciprofloxacin effectively eradicates nasopharyngeal carriage in adults and children but is not approved for use in children or in pregnant women. Throat cultures to identify carriers are not useful. Meningococcal vaccine has been used increasingly for control of outbreaks. Patients with functional or anatomic asplenia, complement deficiencies, or properidin deficiency should be vaccinated.

## Treatment

Blood cultures should be obtained for all children with fever and purpura or other signs of meningococcemia, and antibiotics should be administered immediately as an emergency procedure. There is a good correlation between survival rates and prompt initiation of antibiotic therapy. Purpura and fever should be considered a medical emergency.

Children with meningococcemia or meningococcal meningitis should be treated as though shock were imminent even if their vital signs are stable when they are first seen. If hypotension already is present, supportive measures should be aggressive, because the prognosis is grave in such situations. It is optimal to initiate treatment in an intensive care setting. Treatment should not be delayed for the sake of transporting the patient. Shock may worsen following antimicrobial therapy due to endotoxin release. To minimize the risk of nosocomial transmission, patients should be placed in respiratory isolation for the first 24 hours of antibiotic treatment.

### A. SPECIFIC MEASURES

Antibiotics should be begun promptly. Because other bacteria, such as *S pneumoniae, S aureus,* or other gram-negative organisms, can cause identical syndromes, initial therapy should be broadly effective. Vancomycin and cefotaxime (or ceftriaxone) are preferred initial coverage. Once *N meningitidis* has been isolated, penicillin G, cefotaxime, and ceftriaxone intravenously for 7 days are the drugs of choice. Relative penicillin resistance is uncommon but has been reported in the United States.

### B. GENERAL MEASURES

Most cases of invasive meningococcal disease are treated with intravenous antibiotics for 7 days.

**1. Cardiovascular**—See Chapter 11 for management of septic shock. Corticosteroids are not beneficial. Sympathetic blockade and topically applied nitroglycerin have been used locally to improve perfusion.

**2. Hematologic**—Adjunctive therapy with heparin is controversial. Because hypercoagulability is frequently present in patients with meningococcemia, some experts believe heparin should be considered for those with DIC. A loading dose of 50 units/kg is followed by 15 units/kg/h as a continuous drip. The patient is monitored by following the partial thromboplastin time and heparin assay. Recombinant tissue plasminogen activator, concentrated antithrombin III, and recombinant protein C infusions have been tried experimentally to reverse coagulopathy. See Chapter 27 for the management of DIC.

## Prognosis

Unfavorable prognostic features include shock, DIC, and extensive skin lesions. The case fatality rate in fulminant meningococcemia is over 30%. In uncomplicated meningococcal meningitis, the fatality rate is much lower (10–20%).

## Vaccine

A quadrivalent vaccine prepared from purified meningococcal polysaccharides (A, C, Y, and W-135) is available in the United States for children younger than 2 years of age. This vaccine has been used for controlling outbreaks (ie, schools) and in special high-risk groups, such as patients with functional or anatomic asplenia and patients with complement or properidin deficiency. College students who will be residing in dormitories for the first time are at increased risk for meningococcal disease. Some states have mandated the meningococcal vaccine for new college students. College students and their parents should be educated about the availability of the meningococcal vaccine and immunized if they elect to receive it (see Chapter 9).

Harrison LH et al : Invasive meningococcal disease in adolescents and young adults. JAMA 2001;286(60):694 [PMID: 11495619].

Pathan N et al: Pathophysiology of meningococcal meningitis and septicaemia. Arch Dis Child 2003;88(7):601 [PMID: 12818907].

Recommendations of the Advisory Committee on Immunization Practices (ACIP): Meningococcal disease and college students. MMWR Morb Mortal Wkly Rep 2000; 49(RR-7):11 [PMID: 10902835].

Rosenstein NE et al: Meningococcal disease. N Engl J Med 2001;344(18):1378 [PMID:11333996].

Welch SB, Nadel S: Treatment of meningococcal infection. Arch Dis Child 2003;88(7):608 [PMID: 12818909].

## GONOCOCCAL INFECTIONS

 **ESSENTIALS OF DIAGNOSIS & TYPICAL FEATURES**

- *Purulent urethral discharge with intracellular gram-negative diplococci on smear in male patient (usually adolescent).*
- *Purulent, edematous, sometimes hemorrhagic conjunctivitis with intracellular gram-negative diplococci in infant age 2–4 days.*
- *Fever, arthritis (often polyarticular) or tenosynovitis, and maculopapular peripheral rash that may be vesiculopustular or hemorrhagic.*

• Positive culture of blood, pharyngeal, or genital secretions.

## General Considerations

*Neisseria gonorrhoeae* is a gram-negative diplococcus. Although morphologically similar to other neisseriae, it differs in its ability to grow on selective media and to ferment carbohydrates. The cell wall of *N gonorrhoeae* contains endotoxin, which is liberated when the organism dies and is responsible for the production of a cellular exudate. The incubation period is short, usually 2–5 days.

Antimicrobial-resistant gonococci are a serious problem. *N gonorrhoeae* resistant to tetracyclines, penicillins, or both are common. Fluoroquinolone-resistant strains are also increasing.

Gonococcal disease in children may be transmitted sexually or nonsexually. Prepubertal gonococcal infection outside the neonatal period should be considered presumptive evidence of sexual contact or child abuse. Prepubertal girls usually manifest gonococcal vulvovaginitis because of the neutral to alkaline pH of the vagina and thin vaginal mucosa.

In the adolescent or adult, the work-up of every case of gonorrhea should include a careful and accurate inquiry into the patient's sexual practices, because pharyngeal infection must be detected if present and may be difficult to eradicate. Efforts should be made to identify and provide treatment to all sexual contacts. When prepubertal children are infected, cultures should be obtained from family members, and epidemiologic investigation should be thorough.

Over 310,000 cases of gonorrhea were reported in 2003; increasing rates for the last several years are a source of concern because other sexually transmitted diseases often mirror changes in gonococcal incidence.

## Clinical Findings

### A. SYMPTOMS AND SIGNS

**1. Asymptomatic gonorrhea**—The ratio of asymptomatic to symptomatic gonorrheal infections in adolescents and adults is probably 3–4:1 in women and 0.5–1:1 in men. Asymptomatic infections are as infectious as symptomatic ones.

**2. Uncomplicated genital gonorrhea—**

**a. Male with urethritis**—Urethral discharge is sometimes painful and bloody and may be white, yellow, or green. There may be associated dysuria. The patient is usually afebrile.

**b. Prepubertal female with vaginitis**—The only clinical findings initially may be dysuria and polymorphonuclear neutrophils in the urine. Vulvitis characterized by erythema, edema, and excoriation accompanied by a purulent discharge may follow.

**c. Postpubertal female with cervicitis**—Symptomatic disease is characterized by a purulent, foul-smelling vaginal discharge, dysuria, and occasionally dyspareunia. Fever and abdominal pain are absent. The cervix is frequently hyperemic and tender when touched. This tenderness is not worsened by moving the cervix, nor are the adnexa tender to palpation.

**d. Rectal gonorrhea**—Rectal gonorrhea is often asymptomatic. There may be purulent discharge, edema, and pain during evacuation.

**3. Pharyngeal gonorrhea**—Pharyngeal infection is usually asymptomatic. There may be some sore throat and, rarely, acute exudative tonsillitis with bilateral cervical lymphadenopathy and fever.

**4. Conjunctivitis and iridocyclitis**—Copious exudate is characteristic of gonococcal conjunctivitis. Newborns are symptomatic on days 2–4 of life. In the adolescent or adult, infection probably is spread from infected genital secretions by the fingers.

**5. Pelvic inflammatory disease (salpingitis)**—The interval between initiation of genital infection and its ascent to the uterine tubes is variable and may range from days to months. Menses frequently are the initiating factor. With the onset of a menstrual period, gonococci invade the endometrium, causing transient endometritis. Subsequently salpingitis may occur, resulting in pyosalpinx or hydrosalpinx. Rarely infection progresses to peritonitis or perihepatitis. Gonococcal salpingitis occurs in an acute, subacute, or chronic form. All three forms have in common tenderness on gentle movement of the cervix and bilateral tubal tenderness during pelvic examination.

Gonococci or *Chlamydia trachomatis* are the cause of about 50% of cases of pelvic inflammatory disease. A mixed infection caused by enteric bacilli, *Bacteroides fragilis,* or other anaerobes occurs in the other 50%.

**6. Gonococcal perihepatitis (Fitz-Hugh and Curtis syndrome)**—In the typical clinical pattern, the patient presents with right upper quadrant tenderness in association with signs of acute or subacute salpingitis. Pain may be pleuritic and referred to the shoulder. Hepatic friction rub is a valuable but inconstant sign.

**7. Disseminated gonorrhea**—Dissemination follows asymptomatic more often than symptomatic genital infection and often results from gonococcal pharyngitis or anorectal gonorrhea. The most common form of disseminated gonorrhea is polyarthritis or polytenosynovitis, with or without dermatitis. Monarticular arthritis is less common, and gonococcal endocarditis and meningitis are fortunately rare.

**a. Polyarthritis**—Disease usually begins with the simultaneous onset of low-grade fever, polyarthralgia, and malaise. After a day or so, joint symptoms become acute. Swelling, redness, and tenderness occur, frequently over the wrists, ankles, and knees but also in the fingers, feet, and other peripheral joints. Skin lesions may be noted at the same time. Discrete, tender, maculopapular lesions 5–8 mm in diameter appear that may become vesicular, pustular, and then hemorrhagic. They are few in number and noted on the fingers, palms, feet, and other distal surfaces and may be single or multiple. In patients with this form of the disease, blood cultures are often positive, but joint fluid rarely yields organisms. Skin lesions often are positive by Gram stain but rarely by culture. Genital, rectal, and pharyngeal cultures must be performed.

**b. Monarticular arthritis**—In this somewhat less common form of disseminated gonorrhea, fever is often absent. Arthritis evolves in a single joint. Dermatitis usually does not occur. Systemic symptoms are minimal. Blood cultures are negative, but joint aspirates may yield gonococci on smear and culture. Genital, rectal, and pharyngeal cultures must be performed.

### B. LABORATORY FINDINGS

Demonstration of gram-negative, kidney-shaped diplococci in smears of urethral exudate in males is presumptive evidence of gonorrhea. Positive culture confirms the diagnosis. Negative smears do not rule out gonorrhea. Gram-stained smears of cervical or vaginal discharge in girls are more difficult to interpret because of normal gram-negative flora, but they may be useful when technical personnel are experienced. In girls with suspected gonorrhea, both the cervical os and the anus should be cultured. Gonococcal pharyngitis requires culture for diagnosis.

Cultures for *N gonorrhoeae* are plated on a selective chocolate agar containing antibiotics (eg, Thayer–Martin agar) to suppress normal flora. If bacteriologic diagnosis is critical, suspected material should be cultured on chocolate agar as well. Because gonococci are labile, agar plates should be inoculated immediately and placed without delay in an atmosphere containing $CO_2$ (candle jar). When transport of specimens is necessary, material should be inoculated directly into Transgrow medium prior to shipment to an appropriate laboratory. In cases of possible sexual molestation, notify the laboratory that definite speciation is needed, because nongonococcal *Neisseria* species can grow on the selective media.

Nucleic acid amplification tests on urine specimens now enable detection of *N gonorrhoeae* and *C trachomatis*. These tests have excellent sensitivity and are replacing culture in some settings. All children or adolescents with a suspected or established diagnosis of gonorrhea should have serologic tests for syphilis and HIV.

## Differential Diagnosis

Urethritis in the male may be gonococcal or nongonococcal (NGU). NGU is a syndrome characterized by discharge (rarely painful), mild dysuria, and a subacute course. The discharge is usually scant or moderate in amount but may be profuse. *C trachomatis* is the only proven cause of NGU. Doxycycline (100 mg orally bid for 7 days) is efficacious. Single-dose azithromycin, 1 g orally, may achieve better compliance. *C trachomatis* has been shown to cause epididymitis in males and salpingitis in females.

Vulvovaginitis in a prepubertal female may be due to infection caused by miscellaneous bacteria, including *Shigella* and GAS, *Candida,* and herpes simplex. Discharges may be caused by trichomonads, *Enterobius vermicularis* (pinworm), or foreign bodies. Symptom-free discharge (leukorrhea) normally accompanies rising estrogen levels.

Cervicitis in a postpubertal female, alone or in association with urethritis and involvement of Skene and Bartholin glands, may be due to infection caused by *Candida,* herpes simplex, *Trichomonas,* or discharge resulting from inflammation caused by foreign bodies (usually some form of contraceptive device). Leukorrhea may be associated with birth control pills.

Salpingitis may be due to infection with other organisms. The symptoms must be differentiated from those of appendicitis, urinary tract infection, ectopic pregnancy, endometriosis, or ovarian cysts or torsion.

Disseminated gonorrhea presents a differential diagnosis that includes meningococcemia, acute rheumatic fever, Henoch–Schönlein purpura, juvenile rheumatoid arthritis, lupus erythematosus, leptospirosis, secondary syphilis, certain viral infections (particularly rubella, but also enteroviruses and parvovirus), serum sickness, type B hepatitis (in the prodromal phase), infective endocarditis, and even acute leukemia and other types of cancer. The fully evolved skin lesions of disseminated gonorrhea are remarkably specific, and genital, rectal, or pharyngeal cultures, plus cultures of blood and joint fluid, usually yield gonococci from at least one source.

## Prevention

Prevention of gonorrhea is principally a matter of sex education, condom use, and identification and treatment of contacts.

## Treatment

### A. UNCOMPLICATED URETHRAL, ENDOCERVICAL, OR RECTAL GONOCOCCAL INFECTIONS IN ADOLESCENTS

Ceftriaxone (125 mg intramuscularly in a single dose), ciprofloxacin (500 mg orally in a single dose), ofloxacin (400 mg orally in a single dose), or levofloxacin (250 mg orally in a single dose) is preferred therapy. Doxycycline (100 mg orally bid for 7 days) or azithromycin (1 g orally in a single dose) is recommended unless *C trachomatis* is ruled out. Ceftizoxime, cefotaxime, and cefotetan parenterally are alternative single-dose therapies.

Quinolones and tetracyclines should be avoided in pregnancy. Quinolones are not approved for use in children, and repeated doses of tetracyclines may stain the teeth of young children. Erythromycin or amoxicillin is recommended for therapy of *C trachomatis* in pregnant women; azithromycin is an alternative regimen. Repeat testing 3 weeks after completion of therapy is recommended in pregnant women.

Spectinomycin (2 g intramuscularly in a single dose) is used for penicillin- and cephalosporin-allergic patients. Quinolone resistance is increasing and is common in Hawaii, Asia, and the Pacific. Quinolones are not recommended for therapy of patients or travelers from these areas. A repeat culture after completion of therapy is not necessary in asymptomatic adolescents after the ceftriaxone–doxycycline regimen. A repeat culture after completion of therapy should be obtained from infants and children.

### B. PHARYNGEAL GONOCOCCAL INFECTION

Ceftriaxone (125 mg intramuscularly in a single dose) should be used; ciprofloxacin (0.5 g orally in a single dose) is an alternative for adults and older adolescents. Neither spectinomycin nor amoxicillin is recommended. A repeat culture is recommended 4–7 days after therapy.

### C. DISSEMINATED GONORRHEA

Recommended regimens include ceftriaxone (1 g intramuscularly or intravenously once daily), cefotaxime (1 g intravenously q8h), ciprofloxacin (400 IV q12h), Ofloxacin (500 IV q12h), or levofloxacin (250 IV q24h). Oral therapy may follow parenteral therapy 24–48 hours after improvement. Recommended regimens include ciprofloxacin (0.5 g bid), ofloxacin (0.4 g bid), or levofloxacin (0.25 g orally once day) to complete 7 days of therapy. Fluoroquinolones are not used for pregnant patients. If concurrent infection with *Chlamydia* is present or has not been excluded, a course of doxycycline, azithromycin, or erythromycin should also be prescribed. Total duration of therapy is 7 days for disseminated infections.

### D. PELVIC INFLAMMATORY DISEASE

Doxycycline (100 mg bid orally) and either cefoxitin (2 g intramuscularly or intravenously q6h) or cefotetan (2 g intramuscularly or intravenously q12h) are given until the patient is clinically improved, then doxycycline is administered by mouth to complete 14 days of therapy. Clindamycin and gentamicin given intravenously until the patient is clinically improved may be used rather than cefoxitin. Many other regimens have been used for therapy of pelvic inflammatory disease, although comparative efficacy data is limited.

### E. PREPUBERTAL GONOCOCCAL INFECTIONS

**1. Uncomplicated genitourinary, rectal, or pharyngeal infections**—These infections may be treated with ceftriaxone (25–50 mg/kg/d to a maximum of 125 mg intramuscularly in a single dose). Children older than age 8 years should also receive doxycycline (100 mg orally bid for 7 days). The physician should evaluate all children for evidence of sexual abuse and coinfection with syphilis, *Chlamydia,* and HIV.

**2. Disseminated gonorrhea**—This should be treated with ceftriaxone (50 mg/kg once daily parenterally for 7 days).

Centers for Disease Control and Prevention: Sexually transmitted diseases treatment guidelines 2002. MMWR 2002;51(No. RR-6):1 [PMID: 12184549].

Palusci VJ: Testing for genital gonorrhea infections in prepubertal girls with suspected sexual abuse. Pediatr Infect Dis J 2003; 22(7):618 [PMID: 12867837].

www.cdc.gov/std/

# BOTULISM

## ESSENTIALS OF DIAGNOSIS & TYPICAL FEATURES

- *Dry mucous membranes.*
- *Nausea and vomiting.*
- *Diplopia; dilated, unreactive pupils.*
- *Descending paralysis.*
- *Difficulty in swallowing and speech occurring within 12–36 hours after ingestion of toxin-contaminated food.*
- *Multiple cases in a family or group.*
- *Hypotonia and constipation in infants.*
- *Diagnosis by clinical findings and identification of toxin in blood, stool, or implicated food.*

## General Considerations

Botulism is a paralytic disease caused by *Clostridium botulinum*, an anaerobic, gram-positive, spore-forming bacillus normally found in soil. The organism produces an extremely potent neurotoxin. Of the seven types of toxin (A–G), types A, B, and E cause most human diseases. The toxin, a polypeptide, is so potent that 0.1 mg is lethal for humans.

Food-borne botulism usually results from ingestion of toxin-containing food. Preformed toxin is absorbed from the gut and produces paralysis by preventing acetylcholine release from cholinergic fibers at myoneural junctions. In the United States, home-canned vegetables are usually the cause. Commercially canned foods rarely are responsible. Virtually any food will support the growth of *C botulinum* spores into vegetative toxin-producing bacilli if an anaerobic, nonacid environment is provided. The food may not appear or taste spoiled. The toxin is heat-labile, but the spores are heat-resistant. Inadequate heating during processing (temperature < 115°C) allows the spores to survive and later resume toxin production. Boiling of foods for 10 minutes or heating at 80°C for 30 minutes before eating will destroy the toxin.

Infant botulism is seen in infants younger than age 6 months (median, 10 weeks). The initial symptoms are usually constipation and severe hypotonia. Infants younger than age 2 weeks rarely develop botulism. The toxin appears to be produced by *C botulinum* organisms residing in the gastrointestinal tract. In some instances, honey has been the source of spores. Clinical findings include constipation, weak suck and cry, pooled oral secretions, cranial nerve deficits, generalized weakness, and, on occasion, apnea. The characteristic electromyographic pattern of brief, small, abundant motor-unit action potentials (BSAP) may help confirm the diagnosis.

Ten to 15 cases of wound botulism are reported yearly. Most cases occur in drug abusers with infection in intravenous or intramuscular injection sites.

Botulism, as a result of aerosolization of botulinum toxin, could also occur as the result of a bioterrorism event. Only three such cases of botulism have been reported; therefore, the incubation period is not well-defined, but was about 72 hours in the reported cases.

## Clinical Findings

### A. SYMPTOMS AND SIGNS

The incubation period for food-borne botulism is 8–36 hours. The initial symptoms are lethargy and headache. These are followed by double vision, dilated pupils, ptosis, and, within a few hours, difficulty with swallowing and speech. Pharyngeal paralysis occurs in some cases, and food may be regurgitated. The mucous membranes often are very dry. Descending skeletal muscle paralysis may be seen. Death usually results from respiratory failure.

Botulism patients present with a "classic triad": (1) afebrile; (2) symmetrical, flaccid, descending paralysis with prominent bulbar palsies; and (3) clear sensorium. Botulism is caused by a toxin, thus there is no fever unless secondary infection (eg, aspiration pneumonia) occurs. Common bulbar palsies seen include dysphonia, dysphagia, dysarthria, and diplopia (4 "D's"). Recognition of this triad is important in making the clinical diagnosis.

### B. LABORATORY FINDINGS

The diagnosis is made by demonstration of *C botulinum* toxin in stool, gastric aspirate/vomitus, or serum. Serum and stool samples can be sent for toxin confirmation (done by toxin neutralization mouse bioassay at CDC or state health departments). Foods that are suspected to be contaminated should be kept refrigerated and given to public health personnel for testing. Laboratory findings, including CSF examination, are usually normal. Electromyography suggests the diagnosis if the characteristic BSAP abnormalities are seen. A nondiagnostic electromyogram does not exclude the diagnosis.

## Differential Diagnosis

Guillain–Barré syndrome is characterized by ascending paralysis, sensory deficits, and elevated CSF protein without pleocytosis.

Other illnesses that should be considered include poliomyelitis, postdiphtheritic polyneuritis, certain chemical intoxications, tick paralysis, and myasthenia gravis. The history and elevated CSF protein characterize postdiphtheritic polyneuritis. Tick paralysis is characterized by a flaccid ascending motor paralysis. An attached tick should be sought. Myasthenia gravis usually occurs in adolescent girls. It is characterized by ocular and bulbar symptoms, with normal pupils, fluctuating weakness, absence of other neurologic signs, and clinical response to cholinesterase inhibitors.

## Complications

Difficulty in swallowing leads to aspiration pneumonia. Serious respiratory paralysis may be fatal despite assisted ventilation and intensive supportive measures.

## Treatment

### A. SPECIFIC MEASURES

Early treatment of botulism with antitoxin (food-borne or wound botulism) or passive human botulism immune globulin (infant botulism) is beneficial. Treatment should begin as soon as the clinical diagnosis is made (prior to microbiologic or toxin confirmation).

The current form of equine, trivalent antitoxin (types A, B, and E) is given by slow intravenous infusion. All patients need to be screened for hypersensitivity to the product prior to initiating the infusion; small challenge doses are given (see package insert). Patients who have reactions to the challenge doses are desensitized prior to receiving antitoxin infusion. The antitoxin, 24-hour diagnostic consultation, epidemic assistance, and laboratory testing services are available from the CDC through state and local health departments.

For treatment of infant botulism, intravenous human botulism immune globulin (BIG-IV) is available in California under a study protocol from the Infant Botulism Prevention Program (510-540-2646). Results of a placebo-controlled clinical trial of use in infant botulism showed reduction in the mean hospital stay in the BIG-IV–treated group (2.5 weeks) as compared with the placebo group (5.5 weeks). Equine botulinum antitoxin should not be used to treat infant botulism. BIG-IV is not available for use in any form of botulism (wound, food-borne) other than infant botulism.

### B. GENERAL MEASURES

General and supportive therapy consists of bed rest, ventilatory support (if necessary), fluid therapy, enteral or parenteral nutrition, and administration of purgatives and high enemas. Aminoglycoside antimicrobials and clindamycin may exacerbate neuromuscular blockage and should be avoided.

## Prognosis

The mortality rate has declined substantially in recent years and is currently at 6%. In nonfatal cases, symptoms subside over 2–3 months and recovery is usually complete.

Arnon SS et al: Botulinum toxin as a biological weapon. JAMA 2001;285(8):1059 [PMID: 11209178].

Centers for Disease Control and Prevention: Infant botulism–New York City, 2001–2002. JAMA 2003;289(7):834 [PMID: 12599363].

Robinson RF, Nahata MC: Management of botulism. Ann Pharmacother 2003;37(1):127 [PMID: 12503947].

# TETANUS

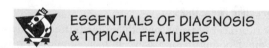

### ESSENTIALS OF DIAGNOSIS & TYPICAL FEATURES

- *Unimmunized or partially immunized patient.*
- *History of skin wound.*
- *Spasms of jaw muscles (trismus).*
- *Stiffness of neck, back, and abdominal muscles, with hyperirritability and hyperreflexia.*
- *Episodic, generalized muscle contractions.*
- *Diagnosis is based on clinical findings and the immunization history.*

## General Considerations

Tetanus is caused by *Clostridium tetani,* an anaerobic, gram-positive bacillus that produces a potent neurotoxin. In unimmunized or incompletely immunized individuals, infection follows contamination of a wound by soil containing clostridial spores from animal manure. The toxin reaches the CNS by retrograde axon transport, is bound to cerebral gangliosides, and is thought to increase reflex excitability in neurons of the spinal cord by blocking function of inhibitory synapses. Intense muscle spasms result. Two thirds of cases in the United States follow minor puncture wounds of the hands or feet. In many cases, no history of a wound can be obtained. In the newborn, usually in underdeveloped countries, infection generally results from contamination of the umbilical cord. The incubation period typically is 4–14 days but may be longer. Although 14 cases of tetanus were reported in the United States in 2003, an estimated 1 million cases per year occur globally. In the United States, cases in young children are due to failure to immunize. Eighty-five percent of cases occur in adults older than 25 years.

## Clinical Findings

### A. SYMPTOMS AND SIGNS

The first symptom is often mild pain at the site of inoculation, followed by hypertonicity and spasm of the regional muscles. Characteristically, difficulty in opening the mouth (trismus) is evident within 48 hours. In newborns, the first signs are irritability and inability to nurse. The infant may then develop stiffness of the jaw and neck, increasing dysphagia, and generalized hyperreflexia with rigidity and spasms of all muscles of the abdomen and back (opisthotonos). The facial distortion resembles a grimace (risus sardonicus). Difficulty in swallowing and convulsions triggered by minimal stimuli such as sound, light, or movement may occur. Individual spasms may last seconds or minutes. Recurrent spasms are seen several times each hour, or they may be almost continuous. In most cases, the temperature is normal or only mildly elevated. A high or subnormal temperature is a bad prognostic sign. Patients are fully conscious and lucid. A profound circulatory disturbance associated with sympathetic overactivity may occur on the second to fourth day, which may contribute to the mortality rate. This is characterized by elevated blood pressure, increased cardiac output, tachycardia (> 20 beats/min), and arrhythmia.

### B. LABORATORY FINDINGS

The diagnosis is made on clinical grounds. There may be a mild polymorphonuclear leukocytosis. The CSF is normal with the exception of mild elevation of opening pressure. Serum muscle enzymes may be elevated. Transient electrocardiographic and electroencephalographic abnormalities may occur. Anaerobic culture and microscopic examination of pus from the wound can be helpful, but *C tetani* is difficult to grow, and the drumstick-shaped gram-positive bacilli often cannot be found.

## Differential Diagnosis

Poliomyelitis is characterized by asymmetrical paralysis in an incompletely immunized child. The history of an animal bite and the absence of trismus may suggest rabies. Local infections of the throat and jaw should be easily recognized. Bacterial meningitis, phenothiazine reactions, decerebrate posturing, narcotic withdrawal, spondylitis, and hypocalcemic tetany may be confused with tetanus.

## Complications

Complications include sepsis, malnutrition, pneumonia, atelectasis, asphyxial spasms, decubitus ulcers, and fractures of the spine due to intense contractions. They can be prevented in part by skilled supportive care.

## Prevention

### A. TETANUS TOXOID

Active immunization with tetanus toxoid prevents tetanus (see Chapter 9). Immunity is almost always is achieved after the third dose of vaccine. A booster at the time of injury is needed if none has been given in the past 10 years—or within 5 years in case of a heavily contaminated wound. Nearly all cases of tetanus (99%) in the United States are in unimmunized or incompletely immunized individuals. Many adolescents and adults lack protective antibody.

### B. TETANUS ANTITOXIN

Human tetanus immune globulin (TIG) should be used in children with fewer than three previous tetanus toxoid immunizations (DPT, DPaT, DT, Td, etc) who have "tetanus-prone wounds." These include (1) wounds contaminated with soil, saliva, debris, or feces;

(2) crush wounds, puncture wounds, or wounds with avulsed or devitalized tissue; and (3) wounds due to thermal burns or frostbite. TIG should be administered to HIV-infected children with tetanus-prone wounds, regardless of their immunization history. When TIG is indicated, 250 units is given intramuscularly. If tetanus immunization is incomplete, a dose of age-appropriate vaccine should be given. When both are indicated, tetanus toxoid and TIG should be administered concurrently at different sites using different syringes.

### C. TREATMENT OF WOUNDS

Proper surgical cleansing and debridement of contaminated wounds will decrease the risk of tetanus.

### D. PROPHYLACTIC ANTIMICROBIALS

Prophylactic antimicrobials are useful if the child is unimmunized and TIG is not available.

## Treatment

### A. SPECIFIC MEASURES

Serotherapy lowers the mortality rate from tetanus, but not dramatically. Human TIG in a single dose of 3000–6000 units, intramuscularly, is given to children and adults. Doses of 500 units have been used in infants. Surgical debridement of wounds is indicated, but more extensive surgery or amputation to eliminate the site of infection is not necessary. Antibiotics are given to attempt to decrease the number of vegetative forms of the bacteria to decrease toxin production: oral metronidazole (30 mg/kg/d in four divided doses) for 10–14 days is the preferred agent.

### B. GENERAL MEASURES

The patient is kept in a quiet room with minimal stimulation. Control of spasms and prevention of hypoxic episodes are crucial. Diazepam or another anxiolytic is useful (0.6–1.2 mg/kg/d intravenously in six divided doses). In the newborn, two or three divided doses should be given. Large doses (up to 25 mg/kg/d) may be required for older children. Diazepam is given intravenously until muscular spasms become infrequent and the generalized muscular rigidity much less prominent. The drug may then be given orally and the dosage reduced as the child improves. Mechanical ventilation and muscle paralysis are necessary in severe cases. Nasogastric or intravenous feedings should be used to limit stimulation of feedings and prevent aspiration.

## Prognosis

The fatality rate in newborns and heroin-addicted individuals is high. The overall mortality rate in the United States is 11%. The fatality rate depends on the quality of supportive care, the patient's age, and the patient's vaccination history. Many deaths are due to pneumonia or respiratory failure. If the patient survives 1 week, recovery is likely.

Bunch TJ et al: Respiratory failure in tetanus: Case report and review of a 25-year experience. Chest 2002;122(4):1488 [PMID: 12377887].

Pascual FB et al: Tetanus surveillance–United States, 1998–2000. MMWR Surveill Summ 2003;52(3):1 [PMID: 12825541].

www.cdc.gov/nip/publications/pink/tetanus.pdf

# GAS GANGRENE

### ESSENTIALS OF DIAGNOSIS & TYPICAL FEATURES

- Contamination of a wound with soil or feces.
- Massive edema, skin discoloration, bleb formation, and pain in an area of trauma.
- Serosanguineous exudate from wound.
- Crepitation of subcutaneous tissue.
- Rapid progression of signs and symptoms.
- Clostridia cultured or seen on stained smears.

## General Considerations

Gas gangrene (clostridial myonecrosis) is a necrotizing infection that follows trauma or surgery and is caused by several anaerobic, gram-positive, spore-forming bacilli of the genus *Clostridium*. The spores are found in soil, feces, and vaginal secretions. In devitalized tissue, the spores germinate into vegetative bacilli that proliferate and produce toxins, causing thrombosis, hemolysis, and tissue necrosis. *Clostridium perfringens,* the species causing approximately 80% of cases of gas gangrene, produces at least eight such toxins. The areas involved most often are the extremities, abdomen, and uterus. *Clostridium septicum* may also cause myonecrosis and causes septicemia in patients with neutropenia. Nonclostridial infections with gas formation can mimic clostridial infections and are more common.

## Clinical Findings

### A. SYMPTOMS AND SIGNS

The onset of gas gangrene is sudden, usually 1–20 days (mean, 3–4 days) after trauma or surgery. The skin around the wound becomes discolored, with hemorrhagic bullae, serosanguineous exudate, and crepitation in the subcutaneous tissues. Pain and swelling are usually intense. Systemic illness appears early and progresses rapidly to intravascular hemolysis, jaundice, shock, toxic delirium, and renal failure.

### B. LABORATORY FINDINGS

Isolation of the organism requires anaerobic culture. Gram-stained smears may demonstrate many gram-positive rods and few inflammatory cells.

### C. IMAGING

Radiographs may demonstrate gas in tissues, but this is a late finding and is also seen in infections with other gas-forming organisms or may be due to air introduced into tissues during trauma or surgery.

### D. OPERATIVE FINDINGS

Direct visualization of the muscle at surgery may be necessary to diagnose gas gangrene. Early, the muscle is pale and edematous and does not contract normally; later, the muscle may be frankly gangrenous.

## Differential Diagnosis

Gangrene and cellulitis caused by other organisms and clostridial cellulitis (not myonecrosis) must be distinguished. Necrotizing fasciitis may resemble gas gangrene.

## Prevention

Gas gangrene can be prevented by the adequate cleansing and debridement of all wounds. It is essential that foreign bodies and dead tissue be removed. A clean wound does not provide a suitable anaerobic environment for the growth of clostridial species.

## Treatment

### A. SPECIFIC MEASURES

Penicillin G (300,000–400,000 units/kg/d intravenously in six divided doses) should be given, usually combined with clindamycin or metronidazole. Clindamycin, metronidazole, meropenem and imipenem–cilastatin are alternatives for penicillin-allergic patients.

### B. SURGICAL MEASURES

Surgery should be prompt and extensive, with removal of all necrotic tissue.

### C. HYPERBARIC OXYGEN

Hyperbaric oxygen therapy has been shown to be effective, but it is not a substitute for surgery. A patient may be exposed to 2–3 atm in pure oxygen for 1- to 2-hour periods for as many sessions as necessary until clinical remission occurs.

## Prognosis

Clostridial myonecrosis is fatal if untreated. With early diagnosis, antibiotics, and surgery, the mortality rate is 20–60%. Involvement of the abdominal wall, leukopenia, intravascular hemolysis, renal failure, and shock are ominous prognostic

Bryant P et al: Recurrent crepitant cellulitis caused by Clostridium perfringens. Pediatr Infect Dis J 2002;21(12):1173 [PMID 12506954].

Fielden MP et al: Hyperbaric oxygen therapy in the treatment of orbital gas gangrene. J AAPOS 2002;6(4):252 [PMID: 12185353].

Stevens DL, Bryant AE: The role of clostridial toxins in the pathogenesis of gas gangrene. Clin Infect Dis 2002;35 (Suppl 1):S93-S100 [PMID: 12173116].

# DIPHTHERIA

## ESSENTIALS OF DIAGNOSIS & TYPICAL FEATURES

- *A gray, adherent pseudomembrane, most often in the pharynx but also in the nasopharynx or trachea.*
- *Sore throat, serosanguineous nasal discharge, hoarseness, and fever in a nonimmunized child.*
- *Peripheral neuritis or myocarditis.*
- *Positive culture.*
- *Treatment should not be withheld pending culture results.*

## General Considerations

Diphtheria is an acute infection of the upper respiratory tract or skin caused by toxin-producing *Corynebacterium diphtheriae*. Diphtheria in the United States is rare; one case was reported in 2003, and only 48 cases were reported from 1980 to 1997. However, significant numbers of elderly adults and unimmunized children are susceptible to infection. Diphtheria still occurs in epidemics in countries where immunization is not universal. Travelers to these areas may acquire the disease. *Corynebacteria* are gram-positive club-shaped rods with a beaded appearance on Gram stain.

The capacity to produce exotoxin is conferred by a lysogenic bacteriophage and is not present in all strains of *C diphtheriae*. In immunized communities, infection probably occurs through spread of the phage among carriers of susceptible bacteria rather than through spread of phage-containing bacteria themselves. Diphtheria toxin kills susceptible cells by irreversible inhibition of protein synthesis.

The toxin is absorbed into the mucous membranes and causes destruction of epithelium and a superficial inflammatory response. The necrotic epithelium becomes embedded in exuding fibrin and red and white blood cells, forming a grayish pseudomembrane over the tonsils, pharynx, or larynx. Any attempt to remove the membrane exposes and tears the capillaries, resulting in bleeding. The diphtheria bacilli within the membrane continue to produce toxin, which is absorbed and may result in toxic injury to heart muscle, liver, kidneys, and adrenals, and is sometimes accompanied by hemorrhage. The toxin also produces neuritis, resulting in paralysis of the soft palate, eye muscles, or extremities. Death may occur as a result of respiratory obstruction or toxemia and circulatory collapse. The patient may succumb after a somewhat longer time as a result of cardiac damage. The incubation period is 2–7 days.

## Clinical Findings

### A. SYMPTOMS AND SIGNS

**1. Pharyngeal diphtheria**—Early manifestations of diphtheritic pharyngitis are mild sore throat, moderate fever, and malaise, followed fairly rapidly by prostration and circulatory collapse. The pulse is more rapid than the fever would seem to justify. A pharyngeal membrane forms and may spread into the nasopharynx or the trachea, producing respiratory obstruction. The membrane is tenacious and gray and is surrounded by a narrow zone of erythema and a broader zone of edema. The cervical lymph nodes become swollen, and swelling is associated with brawny edema of the neck (so-called bull neck). Laryngeal diphtheria presents with stridor, which can progress to obstruction of the airway.

**2. Other forms**—Cutaneous, vaginal, and wound diphtheria account for up to one third of cases and are characterized by ulcerative lesions with membrane formation.

### B. LABORATORY FINDINGS

Diagnosis is clinical. Direct smears are unreliable. Material is obtained from the nose, throat, or skin lesions, if present, for culture, but specialized culture media is required. Between 16 and 48 hours is required before identification of the organism. A toxigenicity test is then performed. Cultures may be negative in individuals who have received antibiotics. The WBC count is usually normal, but hemolytic anemia and thrombocytopenia are frequent.

## Differential Diagnosis

Pharyngeal diphtheria resembles pharyngitis secondary to β-hemolytic streptococcus, Epstein–Barr virus, or other viral respiratory pathogens. A nasal foreign body or purulent sinusitis may mimic nasal diphtheria. Other causes of laryngeal obstruction include epiglottitis and viral croup. Guillain–Barré syndrome, poliomyelitis, or acute poisoning may mimic the neuropathy of diphtheria.

## Complications

### A. MYOCARDITIS

Diphtheritic myocarditis is characterized by a rapid, thready pulse; indistinct heart sounds, ST-T wave changes, conduction abnormalities, dysrhythmias, or cardiac failure; hepatomegaly; and fluid retention. Myocardial dysfunction may occur from 2 to 40 days after the onset of pharyngitis.

### B. POLYNEURITIS

Neuritis of the palatal and pharyngeal nerves occurs during the first or second week. Nasal speech and regurgitation of food through the nose are seen. Diplopia and strabismus occur during the third week or later. Neuritis may also involve peripheral nerves supplying the intercostal muscles, diaphragm, and other muscle groups. Generalized paresis usually occurs after the fourth week.

### C. BRONCHOPNEUMONIA

Secondary pneumonia is common in fatal cases.

## Prevention

### A. IMMUNIZATION

Immunization with diphtheria toxoid combined with pertussis and tetanus toxoids (DTP) should be used routinely for infants and children (see Chapter 9).

### B. CARE OF EXPOSED SUSCEPTIBLES

Children exposed to diphtheria should be examined, and nose and throat cultures obtained. If signs and symptoms of early diphtheria are found, antibiotic treatment should be instituted. Immunized asymptomatic individuals should receive diphtheria toxoid if a booster has not been received within 5 years. Unimmunized close contacts should receive either erythromycin orally (40 mg/kg/d in four divided doses) for 7 days or benzathine penicillin G intramuscularly (25,000 units/kg), active immunization with diphtheria toxoid, and observation daily.

## Treatment

### A. SPECIFIC MEASURES

**1. Antitoxin**—To be effective, diphtheria antitoxin should be administered within 48 hours (see Chapter 9).

**2. Antibiotics**—Penicillin G (150,000 units/kg/d intravenously) should be given for 10 days. For penicillin-allergic patients, erythromycin (40 mg/kg/d) is given orally for 10 days.

### B. GENERAL MEASURES

Bed rest in the hospital for 10–14 days is usually required. All patients must be strictly isolated for 1–7 days until respiratory secretions are noncontagious. Isolation may be discontinued when three successive nose and throat cultures at 24-hour intervals are negative. These cultures should not be taken until at least 24 hours have elapsed since the cessation of antibiotic treatment.

### C. TREATMENT OF CARRIERS

All carriers should receive treatment. Erythromycin (40 mg/kg/d orally in three or four divided doses), penicillin V potassium (50 mg/kg/d for 10 days), or benzathine penicillin G (600,000–1,200,000 units intramuscularly) should be given. All carriers must be quarantined. Before they can be released, carriers must have three negative cultures of both the nose and the throat taken 24 hours apart and obtained at least 24 hours after the cessation of antibiotic therapy.

## Prognosis

Mortality varies from 3% to 25% and is particularly high in the presence of early myocarditis. Neuritis is reversible; it is fatal only if an intact airway and adequate respiration cannot be maintained. Permanent damage due to myocarditis occurs rarely.

Lumio J et al: Fatal case of diphtheria in an unvaccinated infant in Finland. Pediatr Infect Dis J 2003;22(9):844 [PMID: 14515838].

Munford L et al: Cardiac diphtheria in a previously immunized individual. J Natl Med Assoc 2003;95(9):875 [PMID: 14527057].

www.cdc.gov/nip/publications/pink/dip.pdf

# INFECTIONS DUE TO ENTEROBACTERIACEAE

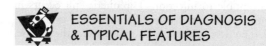

### ESSENTIALS OF DIAGNOSIS & TYPICAL FEATURES

- *Diarrhea by several different mechanisms due to Escherichia coli.*
- *Hemorrhagic colitis and hemolytic–uremic syndrome.*
- *Neonatal sepsis or meningitis.*

- *Urinary tract infection.*
- *Opportunistic infections.*
- *Diagnosis confirmed by culture.*

## General Considerations

Enterobacteriaceae are a family of gram-negative bacilli that are normal flora in the gastrointestinal tract and are also found in water and soil. They cause gastroenteritis, urinary tract infections, neonatal sepsis and meningitis, and opportunistic infections. *Escherichia coli* is the organism in this family that most commonly causes infection in children, but *Klebsiella, Morganella, Enterobacter, Serratia, Proteus,* and other genera are also important, particularly in the compromised host. *Shigella* and *Salmonella* are discussed in separate sections.

*E coli* strains capable of causing diarrhea were originally termed enteropathogenic (EPEC) and were recognized by serotype. It is now known that *E coli* may cause diarrhea by several distinct mechanisms. Classic EPEC strains cause a characteristic histologic injury in the small bowel termed "adherence and effacement." Enterotoxigenic *E coli* (ETEC) causes a secretory, watery diarrhea. ETEC adheres to enterocytes and secretes one or more plasmid-encoded enterotoxins. One of these, heat-labile toxin, resembles cholera toxin in structure, function, and mechanism of action. Enteroinvasive *E coli* (EIEC) is very similar to *Shigella* in pathogenetic mechanism. Enterohemorrhagic *E coli* (EHEC) is the cause of hemorrhagic colitis and the hemolytic–uremic syndrome. The most common EHEC serotype is O157:H7, although several other serotypes cause the same syndrome. These strains elaborate one of several cytotoxins, closely related to Shiga toxin produced by *S dysenteriae*. Outbreaks of hemolytic—uremic syndrome associated with EHEC have followed consumption of inadequately cooked ground beef. Thorough heating to 68–71°C is necessary. Unpasteurized fruit juice, various uncooked vegetables, and contaminated water have also caused infections and epidemics. The common source for EHEC in all of these foods and water is the feces of cattle. Person-to-person spread including spread in day care centers by the fecal–oral route has been reported.

*E coli* that aggregate on the surface of hep cells in tissue culture are termed enteroaggregative (EAggEC) *E coli*. EAggEC cause diarrhea by a distinct but unknown mechanism.

Eighty percent of *E coli* strains causing neonatal meningitis possess specific capsular polysaccharide (K1 antigen), which, alone or in association with spe-cific somatic antigens, confers virulence. K1 antigen is also present on approximately 40% of strains causing neonatal septicemia. The *E coli* K1 organisms do not appear to cause gastrointestinal disease.

Approximately 90% of urinary tract infections in children are caused by *E coli*. *E coli* binds to the uroepithelium by P-fimbriae, which are present in greater than 90% of *E coli* that cause pyelonephritis. Other bacterial cell surface structures, such as O and K antigens, and host factors are also important in the pathogenesis of urinary tract infections.

*Klebsiella, Enterobacter, Serratia,* and *Morganella* are normally found in the gastrointestinal tract and in soil and water. *Klebsiella* may cause a bronchopneumonia with cavity formation. *Klebsiella, Enterobacter,* and *Serratia* are often hospital-acquired opportunists associated with antibiotic usage, debilitated states, and chronic respiratory conditions. They frequently cause urinary tract infection or sepsis. In many newborn nurseries, nosocomial outbreaks caused by antimicrobial-resistant *Klebsiella* or *Enterobacter* sp. are a major problem.

Many of these infections are difficult to treat because of antibiotic resistance. Antibiotic susceptibility tests are necessary. Parenteral third-generation cephalosporins are usually more active than ampicillin, but resistance due to high-level production of chromosomal cephalosporinase may occur. *Enterobacter* and *Serratia* strains broadly resistant to cephalosporins also cause infections in hospitalized newborns and children. Aminoglycoside antibiotics are usually effective but require monitoring of serum levels to ensure therapeutic and nontoxic levels.

## Clinical Findings

### A. Symptoms and Signs:

**1. *E coli* gastroenteritis**—*E coli* may cause diarrhea of varying types and severity. ETEC usually produce mild, self-limiting illness without significant fever or systemic toxicity, often known as traveler's diarrhea. However, diarrhea may be severe in newborns and infants, and occasionally an older child or adult will have a cholera-like syndrome. EIEC strains cause a shigellosis-like illness, characterized by fever, systemic symptoms, blood and mucus in the stool, and leukocytosis, but currently are uncommon in the United States. EHEC strains cause hemorrhagic colitis. Diarrhea is initially watery, and fever is usually absent. Abdominal pain and cramping occur, and diarrhea progresses to blood streaking or grossly bloody stools. Hemolytic–uremic syndrome occurs within a few days of diarrhea in 2–5% of children and is characterized by microangiopathic hemolytic anemia, thrombocytopenia, and renal failure (see Chapter 22).

**2. Neonatal sepsis**—Findings include jaundice, hepatosplenomegaly, fever, temperature lability, apneic spells, irritability, and poor feeding. Meningitis is associated with sepsis in 25–40% of cases. Other metastatic foci of infection may be present, including pneumonia and pyelonephritis. Sepsis may lead to severe metabolic acidosis, shock, DIC, and death.

**3. Neonatal meningitis**—Findings include high fever, full fontanelles, vomiting, coma, convulsions, pareses or paralyses, poor or absent Moro reflex, opisthotonos, and occasionally hypertonia or hypotonia. Sepsis coexists or precedes meningitis in most cases. Thus signs of sepsis often accompany those of meningitis. CSF usually shows a cell count of over 1000/μL, mostly polymorphonuclear neutrophils, and bacteria on Gram stain. CSF glucose concentration is low (usually less than half that of blood), and the protein is elevated above the levels normally seen in newborns and premature infants (> 150 mg/dL).

**4. Acute urinary tract infection**—Symptoms include dysuria, increased urinary frequency, and fever in the older child. Nonspecific symptoms such as anorexia, vomiting, irritability, failure to thrive, and unexplained fever are seen in children younger than age 2 years. Young infants may present with jaundice. As many as 1% of girls of school age and 0.05% of boys have asymptomatic bacteriuria. Screening for and treatment of asymptomatic bacteriuria is not recommended.

## B. LABORATORY FINDINGS

Because *E coli* are normal flora in the stool, a positive stool culture alone does not prove that the *E coli* in the stool are causing disease. Serotyping, tests for enterotoxin production or invasiveness, and tests for P-fimbriae are performed in research laboratories. Mac-Conkey agar with sorbitol substituted for lactose (SMAC agar) is useful to screen stool for enterohemorrhagic *E coli*. Serotyping and testing for enterotoxin are available at many state health departments. Blood cultures are positive in neonatal sepsis. Cultures of CSF and urine should also be obtained. The diagnosis of urinary tract infections is discussed in Chapter 22.

## Differential Diagnosis

The clinical picture of EPEC infection may resemble that of salmonellosis, shigellosis, or viral gastroenteritis.

Neonatal sepsis and meningitis caused by *E coli* can be differentiated from other causes of neonatal infection only by blood and CSF culture.

## Treatment

### A. SPECIFIC MEASURES

**1. *E coli* gastroenteritis**—Gastroenteritis due to EPEC seldom requires antimicrobial treatment. Fluid and electrolyte therapy, preferably given orally, may be required to avoid dehydration. Bismuth subsalicylate reduces stool volume by about one-third in infants with watery diarrhea, probably including ETEC. In nursery outbreaks, *E coli* gastroenteritis has been treated with neomycin (100 mg/kg/d orally in three divided doses for 5 days). Clinical efficacy is not established. Traveler's diarrhea may be treated with TMP–SMX in children and with fluoroquinolones in adults. The risk of hemolytic–uremic syndrome increases following treatment of EHEC colitis, and antimicrobials should be withheld in suspected cases.

**2. *E coli* sepsis, pneumonia, or pyelonephritis**—The drugs of choice are ampicillin (150–200 mg/kg/d, given intravenously or intramuscularly in divided doses q4–6h), cefotaxime (150–200 mg/kg/d, given intravenously or intramuscularly in divided doses q6–8h), ceftriaxone (50–100 mg/kg/d, given intramuscularly as single dose or in two divided doses), and gentamicin (5–7.5 mg/kg/d, given intramuscularly or intravenously in divided doses q8h). Treatment is continued for 10–14 days. Amikacin or tobramycin may be used instead of gentamicin if the strain is susceptible. Third-generation cephalosporins are often an attractive alternative as single-drug therapy and do not require monitoring for toxicity.

**3. *E coli* meningitis**—Third-generation cephalosporins such as cefotaxime (200 mg/kg/d intravenously in four divided doses) are given for a minimum of 3 weeks. Ampicillin (200–300 mg/kg/d intravenously in four to six divided doses) and gentamicin (5–7.5 mg/kg/d intramuscularly or intravenously in three divided doses) are also effective. Treatment with intrathecal and intraventricular aminoglycosides does not improve outcome. Serum levels need to be monitored.

**4. Acute urinary tract infection**—See Chapter 22.

## Prognosis

Death due to gastroenteritis leading to dehydration can be prevented by early fluid and electrolyte therapy. Neonatal sepsis with meningitis is still associated with a mortality rate of over 50%. Most children with recurrent urinary tract infections do well if they have no underlying anatomic defects. The mortality rate in opportunistic infections usually depends on the severity of infection and the underlying condition.

Crump JA et al: An outbreak of Escherichia coli O157:H7 infections among visitors to the dairy farm. N Engl J Med 2002;347(8):555 [PMID: 12192014].

Klein EJ et al: Shiga toxin-producing *Escherichia coli* in children with diarrhea: A prospective point-of-care study. J Pediatr 2002;141(2):172 [PMID: 12183710].

Ladhani S, Gransden W: Increasing antibiotic resistance among urinary tract isolates. Arch Dis Child 2003;88(5):444 [PMID: 12716722].

Ochoa TJ, Cleary TG: Epidemiology and spectrum of disease of Escherichia coli O157. Curr Opin Infect Dis 2003;16(3):259 [PMID: 12821818].

Stoll BJ et al: Changes in pathogens causing early-onset sepsis in very-low-birth-weight infants. N Engl J Med 2002;347(4): 240 [PMID: 12140299].

Wong CS et al: The risk of the hemolytic uremic syndrome after antibiotic treatment of *Escherichia coli* 0157:H7 infections. N Engl J Med 2000;342:1930.

www.cdc.gov/ncidod/dbmd/diseaseinfo/diarrecoli_t.htm

# PSEUDOMONAS INFECTIONS

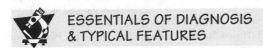

## ESSENTIALS OF DIAGNOSIS & TYPICAL FEATURES

- *Opportunistic infection.*
- *Confirmed by cultures.*

## General Considerations

*Pseudomonas aeruginosa* is an aerobic gram-negative rod with versatile metabolic requirements. *P aeruginosa* may grow in distilled water and in commonly used disinfectants, complicating infection control in medical facilities. *P aeruginosa* is both invasive and destructive to tissue, and toxigenic due to secreted exotoxins, all factors that contribute to virulence. Other genera previously classified as *Pseudomonas* occasionally cause nosocomial infections. *Stenotrophomonas maltophilia* (previously *P maltophilia*) and *Burkholderia cepacia* (previously *P cepacia*) are the most frequent.

*P aeruginosa* is an important cause of infection in children with cystic fibrosis, neoplastic disease, neutropenia, or extensive burns and in those receiving antibiotic therapy. Infections of the urinary and respiratory tracts, ears, mastoids, paranasal sinuses, eyes, skin, meninges, and bones are seen. *Pseudomonas* pneumonia is a common nosocomial infection in patients receiving assisted ventilation.

*P aeruginosa* sepsis may be accompanied by characteristic peripheral lesions called ecthyma gangrenosum. Ecthyma gangrenosum also may occur by direct invasion through intact skin in the groin, axilla, or other skinfolds. *P aeruginosa* is an infrequent cause of sepsis in previously healthy infants and may be the initial sign of underlying medical problems. *P aeruginosa* osteomyelitis often complicates puncture wounds of the feet. *P aeruginosa* is a frequent cause of malignant exter-nal otitis media and of chronic suppurative otitis media. Outbreaks of vesiculopustular skin rash have been associated with exposure to contaminated water in whirlpool baths and hot tubs.

*P aeruginosa* infects the tracheobronchial tree of nearly all patients with cystic fibrosis. Mucoid exopolysaccharide, an exuberant capsule, is characteristically overproduced by isolates from patients with cystic fibrosis. Although bacteremia seldom occurs, patients with cystic fibrosis ultimately succumb to chronic lung infection with *P aeruginosa*. Infection due to *B cepacia* has caused a rapidly progressive pulmonary disease in some colonized patients and may be spread by close contact.

## Clinical Findings

The clinical findings depend on the site of infection and the patient's underlying disease. Sepsis with these organisms resembles gram-negative sepsis with other organisms, although the presence of ecthyma gangrenosum suggests the diagnosis. The diagnosis is made by culture. *Pseudomonas* infection should be suspected in neonates and neutropenic patients with clinical sepsis. A severe necrotizing pneumonia occurs in patients on ventilators.

Patients with cystic fibrosis have a persistent bronchitis that progresses to bronchiectasis and ultimately to respiratory failure. During exacerbations of illness, cough and sputum production increase with low-grade fever, malaise, and diminished energy.

The purulent aural drainage without fever in patients with chronic suppurative otitis media is not distinguishable from that due to other cause.

## Prevention

### A. INFECTIONS IN DEBILITATED PATIENTS

Colonization of extensive second- and third-degree burns by *P aeruginosa* can lead to fatal septicemia. Aggressive debridement and topical treatment with 0.5% silver nitrate solution, 10% mafenide cream, or silver sulfadiazine will greatly inhibit *P aeruginosa* contamination of burns. (See Chapter 11 for a discussion of burn wound infections and prevention.)

### B. NOSOCOMIAL INFECTIONS

Faucet aerators, communal soap dispensers, disinfectants, improperly cleaned inhalation therapy equipment, infant incubators, and back rub lotions have all been associated with *Pseudomonas* epidemics. Infant-to-infant transmission by nursery personnel carrying *Pseudomonas* on the hands is frequent in neonatal units. Careful maintenance of equipment and enforcement of infection control procedures are essential to minimize nosocomial transmission.

## C. PATIENTS WITH CYSTIC FIBROSIS

Chronic infection of the lower respiratory tract occurs in nearly all patients with cystic fibrosis. The infecting organism is seldom cleared from the respiratory tract, even with intensive antimicrobial therapy, and the resultant injury to the lung eventually leads to pulmonary insufficiency. Treatment is aimed at controlling signs and symptoms of the infection.

## Treatment

*P aeruginosa* is inherently resistant to many antimicrobials and may develop resistance during therapy. Mortality rates in hospitalized patients exceed 50%, owing both to the severity of underlying illnesses in patients predisposed to *Pseudomonas* infection and to the limitations of therapy. Antibiotics effective against *Pseudomonas* include the aminoglycosides, ureidopenicillins (ticarcillin and piperacillin), β-lactamase inhibitor with a ureidopenicillin (ticarcillin–clavulanate and piperacillin–tazobactam), expanded-spectrum cephalosporins (ceftazidime and cefepime), imipenem, meropenem, and ciprofloxacin. Antimicrobial susceptibility patterns vary from area to area, and resistance tends to appear as new drugs become popular. Treatment of infections is best guided by clinical response and susceptibility tests.

Gentamicin or tobramycin (5–7.5 mg/kg/d, given intramuscularly or intravenously in three divided doses) or amikacin (15–22 mg/kg/d, given in two or three divided doses) in combination with ticarcillin (200–300 mg/kg/d, given intravenously in six divided doses) or with another antipseudomonal β-lactam antibiotic is recommended for treatment of serious *Pseudomonas* infections. Ceftazidime (150–200 mg/kg/d, given in four divided doses) or cefepime (150 mg/kg/d, given in three divided doses) has excellent activity against *P aeruginosa*. Treatment should be continued for 10–14 days. Treatment with two active drugs is recommended for all serious infections.

*Pseudomonas* osteomyelitis requires thorough surgical debridement and antimicrobial therapy for 2 weeks. *Pseudomonas* folliculitis does not require antibiotic therapy.

Oral or intravenous ciprofloxacin is also effective against susceptible *P aeruginosa*, but is not approved by the Food and Drug Administration for use in children because of concerns about skeletal toxicity. Nonetheless, in some circumstances of antimicrobial resistance, or when the benefits clearly outweigh the small risks, ciprofloxacin may be used.

Chronic suppurative otitis media responds to intravenous ceftazidime (150–200 mg/kg/d in three or four divided doses) given until the drainage has ceased for 3 days. Twice-daily ceftazidime with aural debridement and cleaning given on an outpatient basis has also been successful. Swimmer's ear may be caused by *P aeruginosa* and responds well to topical drying agents (alcohol–vinegar mix) and cleansing.

## Prognosis

Because debilitated patients are most frequently affected, the mortality rate is high. These infections may have a protracted course, and eradication of the organisms may be difficult.

Gendrel D et al: Fluoroquinolones in paediatrics: A risk for the patient or for the community? Lancet Infect Dis 2003(9): 537 [PMID: 12954559].

Maselli JH et al: Risk factors for initial acquisition of *Pseudomonas aeruginosa* in children with cystic fibrosis identified by newborn screening. Pediatr Pulmonol 2003;35(4):257 [PMID: 1269621].

Wisplinghoff H et al: Nosocomial bloodstream infections in pediatric patients in United States hospitals: Epidemiology, clinical features and susceptibilities. Pediatr Infect Dis J 2003; 22(8):686 [PMID: 1291376].

Zomorrodi A, Wald ER: Ecthyma gangrenosum: Considerations in a previously healthy child. Pediatr Infect Dis J 2002;21(12): 1161 [PMID: 12488670].

# *SALMONELLA* GASTROENTERITIS

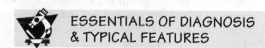

## ESSENTIALS OF DIAGNOSIS & TYPICAL FEATURES

- *Nausea, vomiting, headache, meningismus.*
- *Fever, diarrhea, abdominal pain.*
- *Culture or organism from stool, blood, or other specimens.*

## General Considerations

Salmonellae are gram-negative rods that frequently cause food-borne gastroenteritis and occasionally bacteremic infection of bone, meninges, and other foci. Three species—*Salmonella typhi*, *Salmonella cholerae-suis*, and *Salmonella enteritidis*—and approximately 2000 serotypes are recognized. *S typhimurium* is the most frequently isolated serotype in most parts of the world. An estimated 4 million cases of salmonellosis occur yearly in the United States, but only 45,000 are reported.

Salmonellae are able to penetrate the mucin layer of the small bowel and attach to epithelial cells. Organisms penetrate the epithelial cells and multiply in the submucosa. Infection results in fever, vomiting, watery diarrhea, and occasionally mucus and polymorphonuclear neutrophils in the stool. Although the small intestine is generally regarded as the principal site of infection, colitis also occurs. *S typhimurium* frequently involves the large bowel.

*Salmonella* infections in childhood occur in two major forms: (1) gastroenteritis (including food poisoning), which may be complicated by sepsis and focal suppurative complications; and (2) enteric fever (typhoid fever and paratyphoid fever) (see next section). Although the incidence of typhoid fever has decreased in the United States, the incidence of *Salmonella* gastroenteritis has greatly increased in the past 15–20 years. The highest attack rates occur in children younger than age 6 years, with a peak in the age group from 6 months to 2 years.

Salmonellae are widespread in nature, infecting domestic and wild animals. Fowl and reptiles have a particularly high carriage rate. Transmission results primarily from ingestion of contaminated food. Transmission from human to human occurs by the fecal–oral route via contaminated food, water, and fomites. Numerous foods, including meats, milk, cheese, ice cream, and chocolate, are associated with outbreaks. Contaminated egg powder and frozen whole egg preparations used to make ice cream, custards, and mayonnaise are responsible for outbreaks. Eggs with contaminated shells that are consumed raw or undercooked have been incriminated in outbreaks and sporadic cases.

Because salmonellae are susceptible to gastric acidity, the elderly, infants, and patients taking antacids or $H_2$-blocking drugs are at increased risk for infection. Most cases of *Salmonella* meningitis (80%) and bacteremia occur in infancy. Newborns may acquire the infection from their mothers during delivery and may precipitate outbreaks in nurseries. Newborns are at special risk for developing meningitis.

## Clinical Findings

### A. Symptoms and Signs

Infants usually develop fever, vomiting, and diarrhea. The older child may also complain of headache, nausea, and abdominal pain. Stools are often watery or may contain mucus and, in some instances, blood, suggesting shigellosis. Drowsiness and disorientation may be associated with meningismus. Convulsions occur less frequently than with shigellosis. Splenomegaly is occasionally noted. In the usual case, diarrhea is moderate and subsides after 4–5 days, but it may be protracted.

### B. Laboratory Findings

Diagnosis is made by isolation of the organism from stool, blood, or, in some cases, from urine, CSF, or pus from a suppurative lesion. The WBC count usually shows a polymorphonuclear leukocytosis but may show leukopenia. Typing of isolates is done with specific antisera. *Salmonella* isolates should be reported to public health authorities for epidemiologic purposes. Stool cultures are rarely positive when obtained from children who develop diarrhea after 3 days of hospitalization.

## Differential Diagnosis

In staphylococcal food poisoning, the incubation period is shorter (2–4 hours) than in *Salmonella* food poisoning (12–24 hours). Fever is absent, and vomiting rather than diarrhea is the main symptom. In shigellosis, many pus cells are likely to be seen on a stained smear of stool and there is more apt to be a marked shift to the left in the peripheral white count, although some cases of salmonellosis are indistinguishable from shigellosis. *Campylobacter* gastroenteritis commonly resembles salmonellosis clinically. Culture of the stools is necessary to distinguish the causes of bacterial gastroenteritis.

## Complications

Unlike most types of infectious diarrhea, salmonellosis is frequently accompanied by bacteremia, especially in newborns and infants. Septicemia with extraintestinal infection is seen, most commonly with *S choleraesuis* but also with *S enteritidis, S typhimurium,* and *S paratyphi* B and C. The organism may localize in any tissue and may cause arthritis, osteomyelitis, cholecystitis, endocarditis, meningitis, pericarditis, pneumonia, or pyelonephritis. Patients with sickle cell anemia or other hemoglobinopathies have a predilection for the development of osteomyelitis. Severe dehydration and shock are more likely to occur with shigellosis but may occur with *Salmonella* gastroenteritis.

## Prevention

Measures for the prevention of *Salmonella* infections include thorough cooking of foodstuffs derived from contaminated sources, adequate refrigeration, control of infection among domestic animals, and meticulous meat and poultry inspections. Raw and undercooked fresh eggs should be avoided. Food handlers and child care workers with salmonellosis should have three negative stool cultures before resuming work. Asymptomatic children, who have recovered from salmonella infection, do not need exclusion.

## Treatment

### A. SPECIFIC MEASURES

In uncomplicated *Salmonella* gastroenteritis, antibiotic treatment does not shorten the course of the clinical illness and may prolong convalescent carriage of the organism. Colitis or secretory diarrhea due to *Salmonella* may improve with antibiotic therapy.

Because of the higher risk of sepsis and focal disease, antibiotic treatment is recommended in infants younger than age 3 months; in severely ill children; and in children with sickle cell disease, liver disease, recent gastrointestinal surgery, cancer, depressed immunity, or chronic renal or cardiac disease. Infants younger than age 3 months with positive stool cultures or suspected salmonellosis sepsis should be admitted to hospital, evaluated for focal infection including cultures of blood and CSF, and given treatment intravenously. A third-generation cephalosporin is recommended due to frequent resistance to ampicillin and TMP–SMX. Older patients developing bacteremia during the course of gastroenteritis should receive parenteral treatment initially, and a careful search should be made for additional foci of infection. After signs and symptoms subside, these patients should receive oral medication. Parenteral and oral treatment should last a total of 7–10 days. Longer treatment is indicated for specific complications. If susceptibility tests indicate resistance to ampicillin, third-generation cephalosporins or TMP–SMX should be given. Fluoroquinolones also are efficacious but are not approved for administration to children. Fluoroquinolones are used for strains resistant to multiple other drugs.

*Salmonella* meningitis is best treated with ampicillin (200–300 mg/kg/d intravenously in four to six divided doses) and a third-generation cephalosporin (cefotaxime, ceftriaxone) for 3 weeks. If the child improves rapidly and the CSF is sterile, treatment may be completed with a single drug, the choice guided by results of susceptibility tests.

Outbreaks on pediatric wards are difficult to control. Strict hand washing, cohorting of patients and personnel, and ultimately closure of the unit may be necessary.

### B. TREATMENT OF THE CARRIER STATE

About half of patients may have positive stool cultures after 4 weeks. Infants tend to remain convalescent carriers for up to a year. Antibiotic treatment of carriers is not effective.

### C. GENERAL MEASURES

Careful attention must be given to maintaining fluid and electrolyte balance, especially in infants.

## Prognosis

In gastroenteritis, the prognosis is good. In sepsis with focal suppurative complications, the prognosis is more guarded. The case fatality rate of *Salmonella* meningitis is high in infants. There is a strong tendency to relapse if treatment is not continued for at least 14–21 days.

Fisker N et al: Clinical review of nontyphoid *Salmonella* infections from 1991 to 1999 in a Danish county. Clin Infect Dis 2003;37(4):e47 [PMID: 12905152].

Multistate outbreaks of *Salmonella* serotype Poona infections associated with eating cantaloupe from Mexico–United States and Canada, 2000–2002. MMWR 2002;51(46):1044 [PMID: 12487526].

Outbreak of multidrug-resistant *Salmonella* Newport–United States, January–April 2002. MMWR 2002;51(25):545 [PMID: 12118534].

Su FH et al: *Salmonella* retropharyngeal abscess in a child: Case report and literature review. Pediatr Infect Dis J 2003; 22(9):833 [PMID: 14506379].

Trevejo RT et al: Epidemiology of salmonellosis in California, 1990–1999: Morbidity, mortality, and hospitalization costs. Am J Epidemiol 2003;157(1):48 [PMID: 12505890].

White DG et al: The isolation of antibiotic-resistant salmonella from retail ground meats. N Eng J Med 2001;345:1147.

www.cdc.gov/ncidod/diseases/submenus/sub_salmonella.htm

# TYPHOID FEVER & PARATYPHOID FEVER

### ESSENTIALS OF DIAGNOSIS & TYPICAL FEATURES

- *Insidious or acute onset of headache, anorexia, vomiting, constipation or diarrhea, ileus, and high fever.*
- *Meningismus, splenomegaly, and rose spots.*
- *Leukopenia; positive blood, stool, bone marrow, and urine cultures.*

## General Considerations

Typhoid fever is caused by the gram-negative bacillus *Salmonella typhi*. Paratyphoid fevers, which are usually milder but may be clinically indistinguishable, are caused by *Salmonella paratyphi* A, *Salmonella schottmuelleri,* or *Salmonella hirschfeldii* (formerly *Salmonella paratyphi* A, B, and C). Children have a shorter incubation period than do adults (usually 5–8 days instead of 8–14 days). The organism enters the body through the walls of the intestinal tract and, following a transient bacteremia, multiplies in the reticuloendothelial cells of the liver and spleen. Persistent bacteremia and symptoms then follow. Reinfection of the intestine occurs as organisms are excreted in the bile. Bacterial emboli produce the characteristic skin lesions (rose spots). Symptoms in children may be mild or severe, but children younger than age 5 years rarely have severe typhoid fever.

Typhoid fever is transmitted by the fecal–oral route and by contamination of food or water. Unlike other Salmonella species, there are no animal reservoirs of *S typhi;* each case is the result of direct or indirect contact with the organism or with an individual who is actively infected or a chronic carrier.

About 350–450 cases per year are reported in the United States, 80% of which are acquired during foreign travel.

## Clinical Findings

### A. Symptoms and Signs

In children, the onset of typhoid fever is apt to be sudden rather than insidious, with malaise, headache, crampy abdominal pains and distention, and sometimes constipation followed within 48 hours by diarrhea, high fever, and toxemia. An encephalopathy may be seen with irritability, confusion, delirium, and stupor. Vomiting and meningismus may be prominent in infants and young children. The classic lengthy three-stage disease seen in adult patients is often shortened in children. The prodrome may last only 2–4 days, the toxic stage only 2–3 days, and the defervescence stage 1–2 weeks.

During the prodromal stage, physical findings may be absent, or there may merely be some abdominal distention and tenderness, meningismus, mild hepatomegaly, and minimal splenomegaly. The typical typhoidal rash (rose spots) is present in 10–15% of children. It appears during the second week of the disease and may erupt in crops for the succeeding 10–14 days. Rose spots are erythematous maculopapular lesions 2–3 mm in diameter that fade on pressure. They are found principally on the trunk and chest, and they generally disappear within 3–4 days. The lesions usually number fewer than 20.

### B. Laboratory Findings

Typhoid bacilli can be isolated from many sites, including blood, stool, urine, and bone marrow. Blood cultures are positive in 50–80% of cases during the first week and less often later in the illness. Stool cultures are positive in about 50% of cases after the first week. Urine and bone marrow cultures are also valuable. Most patients will have negative cultures (including stool) by the end of a 6-week period. Serologic tests (Widal reaction) are not as useful as cultures because both false-positive and false-negative results occur. A fourfold rise in titer of O (somatic) agglutinins is suggestive but not diagnostic of infection.

Leukopenia is common in the second week of the disease, but in the first week, leukocytosis may be seen. Proteinuria, mild elevation of liver enzymes, thrombocytopenia, and DIC are common.

## Differential Diagnosis

Typhoid and paratyphoid fevers must be distinguished from other serious prolonged fevers. These include typhus, brucellosis, malaria, tularemia, miliary tuberculosis, psittacosis, vasculitis, lymphoma, mononucleosis, and Kawasaki disease. The diagnosis of typhoid fever is often made clinically in developing countries, but the accuracy of clinical diagnosis is variable. In developed countries, where typhoid fever is uncommon and physicians are unfamiliar with the clinical picture, the diagnosis is often not suspected until late. Positive cultures confirm the diagnosis.

## Complications

The most serious complications of typhoid fever are gastrointestinal hemorrhage (2–10%) and perforation (1–3%). They occur toward the end of the second week or during the third week of the disease.

Intestinal perforation is one of the principal causes of death. The site of perforation generally is the terminal ileum or cecum. The clinical manifestations are indistinguishable from those of acute appendicitis, with pain, tenderness, and rigidity in the right lower quadrant. The radiographic finding of free air in the peritoneal cavity is diagnostic.

Bacterial pneumonia, meningitis, septic arthritis, abscesses, and osteomyelitis are uncommon complications, particularly if specific treatment is given promptly. Shock and electrolyte disturbances may lead to death.

About 1–3% of patients become chronic carriers of *S typhi*. Chronic carriage is defined as excretion of typhoid bacilli for more than a year, but carriage is often lifelong. Adults with underlying biliary or urinary tract disease are much more likely than children to become chronic carriers.

## Prevention

Routine typhoid vaccine is not recommended in the United States but should be considered for foreign travel to endemic areas. An attenuated oral typhoid vaccine produced from strain Ty21a has better efficacy and causes minimal side effects but is not approved for children younger than age 6 years. A capsular polysaccharide vaccine (ViCPS) requires one intramuscular injection and may be given to children age 2 years and older (see Chapter 9).

## Treatment

### A. SPECIFIC MEASURES

Antimicrobial susceptibility testing and local experience are used to guide therapy. Equally effective regimens for susceptible strains include the following: TMP–SMX (10 mg/kg trimethoprim and 50 mg/kg sulfamethoxazole per day orally in two or three divided doses), amoxicillin (100 mg/kg/d orally in four divided doses), and ampicillin (100–200 mg/kg/d intravenously in four divided doses). Aminoglycosides and first- and second-generation cephalosporins are clinically ineffective regardless of in vitro susceptibility results. Third-generation cephalosporins are used for resistant strains. Ceftriaxone and cefotaxime may be used parenterally. Ciprofloxacin or other fluoroquinolones are efficacious but not approved in children, but may be used for multiply resistant strains. Occasionally the presence of multiply resistant strains requires the use of chloramphenicol (50–100 mg/kg/d orally or intravenously in four doses). Treatment duration is 14–21 days. Patients remain febrile for 3–5 days even with appropriate therapy.

### B. GENERAL MEASURES

General support of the patient is exceedingly important and includes rest, good nutrition, and careful observation, with particular regard to evidence of intestinal bleeding or perforation. Blood transfusions may be needed even in the absence of frank hemorrhage.

## Prognosis

A prolonged convalescent carrier stage may occur in children. Three negative cultures after all antibiotics have been stopped are required before contact precautions are stopped. With early antibiotic therapy, the prognosis is excellent, and the mortality rate is less than 1%. Relapse occurs 1–3 weeks later in 10–20% of patients despite appropriate antibiotic treatment.

Crump JA et al: Estimating the incidence of typhoid fever and other febrile illnesses in developing countries. Emerg Infect Dis 2003;9(5):539. [PMID: 12737736].

Lin FYC et al: The efficacy of a Salmonella typhi Vi conjugate vaccine in two-to-five year old children. N Engl J Med 2001; 344:1263.

Mai NL et al: Persistent efficacy of Vi conjugate vaccine against typhoid fever in young children. N Engl J Med 2003;349(14): 1390 [PMID: 14523155].

Olsen SJ et al: Outbreaks of typhoid fever in the United States, 1960–99. Epidemiol Infect 2003;130(1):13 [PMID: 12613741].

Parry CM et al: Typhoid fever. N Engl J Med 2002;347(22):1770 [PMID:12456854].

Stormon M et al: Typhoid fever in children: Diagnostic and therapeutic difficulties. Pediatr Infect Dis J 1997;16:713.

# SHIGELLOSIS
# (BACILLARY DYSENTERY)

## ESSENTIALS OF DIAGNOSIS & TYPICAL FEATURES

- *Cramps and bloody diarrhea.*
- *High fever, malaise, convulsions.*
- *Pus and blood in diarrheal stools examined microscopically.*
- *Diagnosis confirmed by stool culture.*

## General Considerations

Shigellae are nonmotile gram-negative rods of the family Enterobacteriaceae and are closely related to *Escherichia coli*. The genus *Shigella* is divided into four major groups, A–D, representing *Shigella dysenteriae, Shigella flexneri, Shigella boydii,* and *Shigella sonnei*, respectively. Approximately 30,000 cases of shigellosis are reported each year in the United States. S sonnei followed by S flexneri are the most common isolates.

S dysenteriae, which causes the most severe diarrhea of all species and the greatest number of extraintestinal complications, accounts for fewer than 1% of all *Shigella* infections in the United States.

Shigellosis may be a serious disease, particularly in young children, and without supportive treatment an appreciable mortality rate results. In older children and adults, the disease tends to be self-limited and milder. Shigellosis is unusual in infants younger than age 3 months, although in rare cases shigellae may be transmitted from the mother to the newborn during delivery. Diarrhea and refusal to take feedings are the most common symptoms in neonatal shigellosis, and bloody diarrhea and fever occur less frequently. Vomiting, convulsions, or high fever is uncommon.

*Shigella* is usually transmitted by the fecal–oral route. Food- and water-borne outbreaks are increasing in occurrence, but are less important overall than person-to-person transmission. The disease is very communicable—as few as 200 bacteria can produce illness in an adult. The secondary attack rate in families is high, and shigellosis is a serious problem in day care centers and custodial institutions. *Shigella* organisms produce disease by invading the colonic mucosa, causing mucosal ulcerations and microabscesses. A plasmid-encoded gene is required for enterotoxin production, chromosomal genes are required for invasiveness, and smooth lipopolysaccharide are required for virulence. An experimental vaccine is under development and is safe and immunogenic in young children.

## Clinical Findings

### A. SYMPTOMS AND SIGNS

The incubation period of shigellosis is usually 2–4 days. Onset is abrupt, with abdominal cramps, urgency, tenesmus, chills, fever, malaise, and diarrhea. Hallucinations and seizures sometimes accompany high fever. In severe forms, blood and mucus are seen in small volume in the stool (dysentery), and meningismus and convulsions may occur. In older children, the disease may be mild and may be characterized by watery diarrhea without blood. In young children, a fever of 39.4–40°C is common. Rarely there is rectal prolapse. Symptoms generally last 3–7 days.

### B. LABORATORY FINDINGS

The total WBC count varies, but often there is a marked shift to the left. The stool may contain gross blood and mucus, and many neutrophils are seen if mucus from the stool is examined microscopically. Stool cultures are usually positive; however, they may be negative because the organism is somewhat fragile and present in small numbers late in the disease, and because laboratory techniques are suboptimal for the recovery of shigellae.

## Differential Diagnosis

Diarrhea due to rotavirus infection is a winter rather than a summer disease. Usually children with rotavirus infection are not as febrile or toxic as those with shigellosis, and in rotavirus infection, stool does not contain gross blood or neutrophils. Intestinal infections caused by *Salmonella* or *Campylobacter* are differentiated by culture. Grossly bloody stools in a patient without fever or stool leukocytes suggest *E coli* O:157 infection. Amebic dysentery is diagnosed by microscopic examination of fresh stools or sigmoidoscopy specimens. Intussusception is characterized by an abdominal mass, so-called currant jelly stools without leukocytes, and absence of fever. Mild shigellosis is not distinguishable clinically from other forms of infectious diarrhea.

## Complications

Dehydration, acidosis, shock, and renal failure are the major complications. In some cases, a chronic form of dysentery occurs, characterized by mucoid stools and poor nutrition. Bacteremia and metastatic infections are rare but serious complications. Febrile seizures are common. Fulminating fatal dysentery and hemolytic–uremic syndrome occur rarely.

## Treatment

### A. SPECIFIC MEASURES

Resistance to TMP–SMX (10 mg/kg/d trimethoprim and 50 mg/kg/d sulfamethoxazole, given in two divided doses orally for 5 days) is now commonly encountered in many communities and limits the use of this otherwise effective drug to cases where results of susceptibility testing are known. Amoxicillin is not effective. Ampicillin (100 mg/kg/d, given in four divided doses) is also efficacious if the strain is sensitive. Parenteral ceftriaxone and oral cefixime are both effective, although cefixime is now unavailable, and experience with other third-generation oral cephalosporins is limited. Azithromycin (12 mg/kg/d on day 1, then 6 mg/kg/d for four days) was superior to cefixime in one study. Ciprofloxacin (500 mg, given bid for 5 days) is efficacious in adults but is not approved for use in children. However, it may be used in children who remain symptomatic and in need of therapy, and when multiply resistant strains limit other preferred choices. Successful treatment reduces the duration of fever, cramping, and diarrhea and terminates fecal excretion of *Shigella*. Tetracycline and chloramphenicol are also effective, but resistance to them is common. Presumptive therapy should be limited to children with classic shigellosis or known outbreaks. Afebrile children with bloody diarrhea are more commonly infected with EHEC. Antimicrobial therapy of EHEC may increase the likelihood of hemolytic uremic syndrome.

### B. GENERAL MEASURES

In severe cases, immediate rehydration is critical. A mild form of chronic malabsorption syndrome may supervene and require prolonged dietary control.

## Prognosis

The prognosis is excellent if vascular collapse is treated promptly by adequate fluid therapy. The mortality rate is high in very young, malnourished infants who do not receive fluid and electrolyte therapy. Convalescent fecal excretion of *Shigella* lasts 1–4 weeks in patients not receiving antimicrobial therapy. Long-term carriers are rare.

Basualdo W, Arbo A: Randomized comparison of azithromycin versus cefixime for treatment of shigellosis in children. Pediatr Infect Dis J 2003;22(4):374 [PMID:12712971].

Bhattacharya SK, Sur D: An evaluation of current shigellosis treatment. Expert Opin Pharmacother 2003;4(8):1315 [PMID: 12877639].

Greenberg D et al: Shigella bacteremia: A retrospective study. Clin Pediatr (Phila) 2003;42(5):411 [PMID: 12862343].

Passwell JH et al: Safety and immunogenicity of *Shigella sonnei*-CRM9 and *Shigella flexneri* type 2a-rEPAsucc conjugate vaccines in one-to-four-year-old children. Pediatr Infect Dis J 2003;22(8):701 [PMID: 12913770].

# CHOLERA

### ESSENTIALS OF DIAGNOSIS & TYPICAL FEATURES

- *Sudden onset of severe watery diarrhea.*
- *Persistent vomiting without nausea or fever.*
- *Extreme and rapid dehydration and electrolyte loss, with rapid development of vascular collapse.*
- *Contact with a case of cholera or with shellfish, or the presence of cholera in the community.*
- *Diagnosis confirmed by stool culture.*

## General Considerations

Cholera is an acute diarrheal disease caused by the gram-negative organism *Vibrio cholerae*. It is transmitted by contaminated water or food, especially contaminated shellfish. Typical disease is generally so dramatic that in endemic areas the diagnosis is obvious. Individuals with mild illness and young children may play an important role in transmission of the infection.

Asymptomatic infection is far more common than clinical disease. In endemic areas, rising titers of vibriocidal antibody are seen with increasing age. Infection occurs in individuals with low titers. The age-specific attack rate is highest in children younger than age 5 years and declines with age. Cholera is unusual in infancy.

Cholera toxin is a protein enterotoxin that is primarily responsible for symptoms. Cholera toxin binds to a regulatory subunit of adenylyl cyclase in enterocytes, causing increased cAMP and an outpouring of NaCl and water into the lumen of the small bowel.

Nutritional status is an important factor determining the severity of the diarrhea. Duration of diarrhea is prolonged in adults and children with severe malnutrition.

Cholera is endemic in India and southern and Southeast Asia and in parts of Africa. The most recent pandemic, caused by the El Tor biotype of *V cholerae* 01, began in 1961 in Indonesia. Epidemic cholera spread in Central and South America, with a total of 1 million cases and 9500 deaths reported through 1994. Cases in the United States occurred in the course of foreign travel or as a result of consumption of contaminated imported food. Cholera is increasingly associated with consumption of shellfish. Interstate shipment of oysters has resulted in cholera in several inland states.

Several recent studies provide evidence that *V cholerae* is a natural inhabitant of shellfish and copepods in estuarine environments. Seasonal multiplication of *V cholerae* may provide a source of outbreaks in endemic areas. Chronic cholera carriers are rare. The incubation period is short, usually 1–3 days.

## Clinical Findings

### A. SYMPTOMS AND SIGNS

Many patients infected with *V cholerae* have mild disease, with 1–2% developing severe diarrhea. During severe cholera, there is a sudden onset of massive, frequent, watery stools, generally light gray in color (so-called rice-water stools) and containing some mucus but no pus. Vomiting may be projectile and is not accompanied by nausea. Within 2–3 hours, the tremendous loss of fluids results in life-threatening dehydration, hypochloremia, and hypokalemia, with marked weakness and collapse. Renal failure with uremia and irreversible peripheral vascular collapse will occur if fluid therapy is not administered. The illness lasts 1–7 days and is shortened by appropriate antibiotic therapy.

### B. LABORATORY FINDINGS

Markedly elevated hemoglobin (20 g/dL) and marked acidosis, hypochloremia, and hyponatremia are seen. Stool sodium concentration may range from 80 mEq/L to 120 mEq/L. Cultural confirmation using thiosulfate-citrate-bile salt-sucrose (TCBS) agar takes 16–18 hours for a presumptive diagnosis and 36–48 hours for a definitive bacteriologic diagnosis.

## Prevention

Cholera vaccine is available and provides 50% efficacy. Protection lasts 3–6 months. Cholera vaccine is not generally recommended for travelers. Tourists visiting endemic areas are at little risk if they exercise caution in what they eat and drink and maintain good personal hygiene. In endemic areas, all water and milk must be boiled, food protected from flies, and sanitary precautions observed. Simple filtration of water is highly effective in reducing cases. Thorough cooking of shellfish prevents transmission. All patients with cholera should be isolated.

Chemoprophylaxis is indicated for household and other close contacts of cholera patients. It should be initiated as soon as possible after the onset of the disease in the index patient. Tetracycline (500 mg/d for 5 days) is effective in preventing infection. TMP–SMX may be substituted in children.

## Treatment

Physiologic saline or lactated Ringer solution should be administered intravenously in large amounts to restore blood volume and urine output and prevent irreversible shock. Potassium supplements are required. Sodium bicarbonate, given intravenously, may also be needed initially to overcome profound acidosis. Moderate dehydration and acidosis can be corrected in 3–6 hours by oral therapy alone, because the active glucose transport system of the small bowel is normally functional. The optimal composition of the oral solution (in mEq/L) is as follows: $Na^+$, 90; $Cl^-$, 80; and $K^+$, 20 (with glucose, 110 mmol/L).

Treatment with tetracycline (50 mg/kg/d orally in four divided doses for 2–5 days) or azithromycin (10 mg/kg/d in one dose for 1–5 days) shortens the duration of the disease in children and prevents clinical relapse but is not as important as fluid and electrolyte therapy. Tetracycline resistance occurs in some regions, and ciprofloxacin may be used depending on local resistance patterns. TMP–SMX should be used in children younger than age 9 years.

## Prognosis

With early and rapid replacement of fluids and electrolytes, the case fatality rate is 1–2% in children. If significant symptoms appear and no treatment is given, the mortality rate is over 50%.

Bhattacharya MK et al: Azithromycin in the treatment of cholera in children. Acta Paediatr 2003;92(6):676 [PMID: 12856976].

Colwell RR et al: Reduction of cholera in Bangladeshi villages by simple filtration. Proc Natl Acad Sci U.S.A. 2003;100(3):1051 [PMID: 12529505].

Guerrant RL et al: Cholera, diarrhea and oral rehydration therapy: Triumph and indictment. Clin Infect Dis 2003;37(3):398 [PMID: 12884165].

Khan WA et al: Comparison of single-dose azithromycin and 12-dose, 3-day erythromycin for childhood cholera: A randomized, double-blind trial. Lancet 2002;360(9347):1722 [PMID: 12480424].

Kirkpatrick BG, Alston WK: Current immunizations for travel. Curr Opin Infect Dis 203;16(5):369 [PMID: 14501987].

Morris JG Jr: Cholera and other types of vibriosis: A story of human pandemic and oysters on the half shell. Clin Infect Dis 2003;37(2):272 [PMID: 12856219].

## *CAMPYLOBACTER* INFECTION

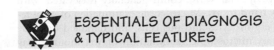

### ESSENTIALS OF DIAGNOSIS & TYPICAL FEATURES

- *Fever, vomiting, abdominal pain, diarrhea.*
- *Presumptive diagnosis by darkfield or phase contrast microscopy of stool wet mount or modified Gram stain.*
- *Definitive diagnosis by stool culture.*

## General Considerations

*Campylobacter* species are small gram-negative, curved or spiral bacilli that are commensals or pathogens in many animals. *Campylobacter jejuni* frequently causes acute enteritis in humans. In the 1990s, *C jejuni* was responsible for 3–11% of cases of acute gastroenteritis in North America and Europe. In many areas, enteritis due to *C jejuni* is more common than that due to *Salmonella* or *Shigella*. *Campylobacter fetus* causes bacteremia and meningitis in immunocompromised patients. *C fetus* may cause maternal fever, abortion, stillbirth, and severe neonatal infection. *Helicobacter pylori* (previously called *Campylobacter pylori*) causes most cases of gastritis and peptic ulcer disease in both adults and children (see Chapter 20).

*Campylobacter* colonizes domestic and wild animals, especially poultry. Numerous cases have been associated with sick puppies or other animal contacts. Contaminated food and water, improperly cooked poultry, and person-to-person spread by the fecal–oral route are common routes of transmission. Outbreaks associated with day care centers, contaminated water supplies, and raw milk have been reported. Newborns may acquire the organism from their mothers at delivery.

## Clinical Findings

### A. SYMPTOMS AND SIGNS

*C jejuni* enteritis can be mild or severe. In tropical countries, asymptomatic stool carriage is common. The incubation period is usually 1–7 days. The disease usually begins with sudden onset of high fever, malaise, headache, abdominal cramps, nausea, and vomiting. Diarrhea follows and may be watery or bile-stained, mucoid, and bloody. The illness is self-limiting, lasting 2–7 days, but relapses occur in 15–25% of cases. Without antimicrobial treatment, the organism remains in the stool for 1–6 weeks.

## B. LABORATORY FINDINGS

The peripheral WBC count generally is elevated, with many band forms. Microscopic examination of stool reveals erythrocytes and pus cells, and darkfield or phase contrast microscopic examination of wet mounts may reveal darting bacilli characteristic of *Campylobacter*. Other bacteria, particularly *Vibrio* species, may exhibit similar motility, but in areas where cholera and *Vibrio parahaemolyticus* diarrhea are rare, a positive darkfield examination has a predictive value of about 90%. Isolation of *C jejuni* from stool is not difficult but requires selective agar, incubation at 42°C rather than 35°C, and incubation in an atmosphere of about 5% oxygen and 5% $CO_2$ (candle jar is satisfactory).

## Differential Diagnosis

*Campylobacter* enteritis may resemble viral gastroenteritis, salmonellosis, shigellosis, amebiasis, or other infectious diarrheas. Because it also mimics ulcerative colitis, Crohn disease, intussusception, and appendicitis, mistaken diagnosis can lead to unnecessary surgery.

## Complications

The most common complication is dehydration. Other uncommon complications include erythema nodosum, convulsions, reactive arthritis, bacteremia, urinary tract infection, and cholecystitis. Guillain-Barré syndrome may follow *C jejuni* infection by 1–3 weeks.

## Prevention

No vaccine is available. Hand washing and adherence to basic food sanitation practices help prevent disease. Hand washing and cleaning of kitchen utensils after contact with raw poultry are important.

## Treatment

Treatment of fluid and electrolyte disturbances is important. Antimicrobial treatment with erythromycin in children (30–50 mg/kg/d orally in four divided doses for 5 days) or with ciprofloxacin in adults terminates fecal excretion and may prevent relapses. Fluoroquinolone-resistant *C jejuni* are now common worldwide. Therapy given early in the course of the illness will shorten the duration of symptoms but is unnecessary if given later. Antimicrobials used for shigellosis, such as TMP–SMX and ampicillin, are inactive against *Campylobacter*. Supportive therapy is sufficient in most cases.

## Prognosis

The outlook is excellent if dehydration is corrected and misdiagnosis does not lead to inappropriate diagnostic or surgical procedures.

Isenbarger DW et al: Comparative antibiotic resistance of diarrheal pathogens from Vietnam and Thailand, 1996–1999. Emerg Infect Dis 2002;8(2):175 [PMID: 11897070].

Sails AD et al: Utility of multilocus sequence typing as an epidemiological tool for investigation of outbreaks of gastroenteritis caused by *Campylobacter jejuni*. J Clin Microbiol 2003; 41(10):4733 [PMID: 14532212].

www.cdc.gov/ncidod/dbmd/diseaseinfo/campylobacter_g.htm

# TULAREMIA

### ESSENTIALS OF DIAGNOSIS & TYPICAL FEATURES

- A cutaneous or mucous membrane lesion at the site of inoculation and regional lymph node enlargement.
- Sudden onset of fever, chills, and prostration.
- History of contact with infected animals, principally wild rabbits, or history of tick exposure.
- Positive culture or immunofluorescence from mucocutaneous ulcer or regional lymph nodes.
- High serum antibody titer.

## General Considerations

Tularemia is caused by *Francisella tularensis,* a gram-negative organism usually acquired directly from infected animals, principally wild rabbits. Occasionally infection is acquired from infected domestic dogs or cats; by contamination of the skin or mucous membranes with infected blood or tissues; by inhalation of infected material; by bites of ticks, fleas, or deer flies that have been in contact with infected animals; or by ingestion of contaminated meat or water. The incubation period is short, usually 3–7 days, but may vary from 2 to 25 days.

Ticks are the most important vector. Rabbits are the classic vectors of tularemia. It is important to seek a history of rabbit hunting, skinning, or food preparation in any patient who has a febrile illness with tender lymphadenopathy, often in the region of a draining skin ulcer.

## Clinical Findings

### A. SYMPTOMS AND SIGNS

Several clinical types of tularemia occur in children. Sixty percent of infections are of the ulceroglandular form and start as a reddened papule that may be pruritic, quickly ulcerates, and is not very painful. Shortly thereafter, the regional lymph nodes become large and tender. Fluctuance quickly follows. At the same time, there may be marked systemic symptoms, including high fever, chills, weakness, and vomiting. Pneumonitis occasionally accompanies the ulceroglandular form or may be seen as the sole manifestation of infection (pneumonic form). A detectable skin lesion is occasionally absent, and localized lymphoid enlargement exists alone (glandular form). Oculoglandular and oropharyngeal forms also occur in children. The latter is characterized by tonsillitis, often with membrane formation, cervical adenopathy, and high fever. In the absence of any primary ulcer or localized lymphadenitis, a prolonged febrile disease reminiscent of typhoid fever can occur (typhoidal form). Splenomegaly is common in all forms.

### B. LABORATORY FINDINGS

*F tularensis* can be recovered from ulcers, regional lymph nodes, and sputum of patients with the pneumonic form. However, the organism grows only on an enriched medium (blood-cystine-glucose agar), and laboratory handling is dangerous owing to the risk of airborne transmission to laboratory personnel. Immunofluorescent staining of biopsy material or aspirates of involved lymph nodes is diagnostic, although it is not widely available.

The WBC count is not remarkable. Agglutinins are present after the second week of illness, and in the absence of a positive culture their development confirms the diagnosis. An agglutination titer of 1:160 or higher is considered positive.

## Differential Diagnosis

The typhoidal form of tularemia may mimic typhoid, brucellosis, miliary tuberculosis, Rocky Mountain spotted fever, and infectious mononucleosis. Pneumonic tularemia resembles atypical or mycotic pneumonitis. The ulceroglandular type of tularemia resembles pyoderma caused by staphylococci or streptococci, rat-bite fever, plague, anthrax, and cat-scratch fever. The oropharyngeal type must be distinguished from streptococcal or diphtheritic pharyngitis, infectious mononucleosis, herpangina, or other viral pharyngitides.

## Prevention

Children should be protected from insect bites, especially those of ticks, fleas, and deer flies, by the use of proper clothing and repellents. Because rabbits are the source of most human infections, the dressing and handling of such game should be performed with great care. If contact occurs, thorough washing with soap and water is indicated.

## Treatment

### A. SPECIFIC MEASURES

Historically, streptomycin was the drug of choice (30 mg/kg/d, given intramuscularly in two divided doses, to a maximum dose of 1 g). Gentamicin and amikacin are also efficacious, more available, and familiar to clinicians. Doxycycline is effective, but relapse rates are higher. Chloramphenicol therapy is also associated with a higher relapse rate. Failures occur with ceftriaxone.

### B. GENERAL MEASURES

Antipyretics and analgesics may be given as necessary. Skin lesions are best left open. Glandular lesions occasionally require incision and drainage.

## Prognosis

The prognosis is excellent in cases of tularemia that are recognized early and treated appropriately.

Ellis J et al: Tularemia. Clin Microbiol Rev 2002;15(4):631 [PMID: 12364373].

Parola P, Raoult D: Ticks and tickborne bacterial diseases in humans: An emerging infectious threat. Clin Infect Dis 2001; 32(6):897 [PMID: 11247714].

# PLAGUE

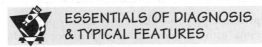

## ESSENTIALS OF DIAGNOSIS & TYPICAL FEATURES

- *Sudden onset of fever, chills, and prostration.*
- *Regional lymphadenitis with suppuration of nodes (bubonic form).*
- *Hemorrhage into skin and mucous membranes and shock (septicemia).*
- *Cough, dyspnea, cyanosis, and hemoptysis (pneumonia).*
- *History of exposure to infected animals.*

## General Considerations

Plague is an extremely serious acute infection caused by a gram-negative bacillus, *Yersinia pestis.* It is a disease of rodents that is transmitted to humans by flea bites. Plague bacilli have been isolated from rodents in 15 of the western states in the United States. Direct contact with rodents, rabbits, or domestic cats may transmit fleas infected with plague bacilli. Most cases occur from June through September. Human plague in the United States appears to occur in cycles that reflect cycles in wild animal reservoirs.

## Clinical Findings

### A. SYMPTOMS AND SIGNS

Plague assumes several clinical forms, the two most common being bubonic and septicemic. Pneumonic plague, the form that occurs when organisms enter the body through the respiratory tract, is uncommon.

**1. Bubonic plague**—Bubonic plague begins after an incubation period of 6 days with a sudden onset of high fever, chills, headache, vomiting, and marked delirium or clouding of consciousness. A less severe form also exists, with a less precipitous onset, but with progression over several days to severe symptoms. Although the flea bite is rarely seen, the regional lymph node, usually inguinal and unilateral, is painful and tender, 1–5 cm in diameter. The node usually suppurates and drains spontaneously after 1 week. The plague bacillus produces endotoxin that causes vascular necrosis. Bacilli may overwhelm regional lymph nodes and enter the circulation to produce septicemia. Severe vascular necrosis results in widely disseminated hemorrhage in skin, mucous membranes, liver, and spleen. Myocarditis and circulatory collapse may result from damage by the endotoxin. Plague meningitis or pneumonia may occur following bacteremic spread from an infected lymph node.

**2. Septicemic plague**—Plague may initially present as septicemia without evidence of lymphadenopathy. In some series, 25% of cases are initially septicemic. Septicemia plague carries a worse prognosis than bubonic plague, largely because it is not recognized and treated early. Patients may present initially with a nonspecific febrile illness characterized by fever, myalgia, chills, and anorexia. Plague is frequently complicated by secondary seeding of the lung causing plague pneumonia.

**3. Primary pneumonic plague**—Inhalation of *Y pestis* bacilli causes primary plague pneumonia. This form of plague has been transmitted to humans from cats with pneumonic plague and would be the form of plague most likely seen after aerosolized release of *Y pestis* in a bioterrorist incident. After an incubation of 1–6 days, the patient develops fever, cough, shortness of breath, and the production of bloody, watery, or purulent sputum. Gastrointestinal symptoms are sometimes prominent. Because the initial focus of infection is the lung, buboes are usually absent; occasionally cervical buboes may be seen.

### B. LABORATORY FINDINGS

Aspirate from a bubo contains bipolar staining gram-negative bacilli. Pus, sputum, and blood all yield the organism. Laboratory infections are common enough to make isolation dangerous. A buffy coat Gram stain may reveal the organism, and blood-agar cultures yield positive results in 48 hours. The WBC count is markedly elevated, with a shift to the left. Paired acute and convalescent sera may be tested for an antibody rise in those cases with negative cultures.

## Differential Diagnosis

The septic phase of the disease may be confused with illnesses such as meningococcemia, sepsis, and rickettsioses. The bubonic form resembles tularemia, anthrax, cat-scratch fever, streptococcal adenitis, and cellulitis. Primary gastroenteritis and appendicitis may have to be distinguished.

## Prevention

Proper disposal of household and commercial wastes and chemical control of rats are basic elements of plague prevention. Flea control is instituted and maintained with liberal use of insecticides. Children vacationing in remote camping areas should be warned not to handle dead or dying animals. Domestic cats that roam freely in suburban areas may contact infected wild animals and acquire infected fleas. There is no commercially available vaccine for plague.

## Treatment

### A. SPECIFIC MEASURES

Streptomycin (20–40 mg/kg/d intramuscularly) or gentamicin (7.5 mg/kg/d) in three divided doses for 7–10 days after defervescence is effective. For patients not requiring parenteral therapy, doxycycline may be given. Doxycycline is not usually recommended for children younger than 8 years of age unless benefits of use outway the risk of dental staining. Plague bacilli that are multiply resistant to antimicrobials are uncommon but of serious concern.

Mortality is extremely high in septicemic and pneumonic plague if specific antibiotic treatment is not started in the first 24 hours of the disease.

Every effort should be made to effect resolution of buboes without surgery. Pus from draining lymph nodes should be handled with gloves.

## B. GENERAL MEASURES

Pneumonic plague is highly infectious, and droplet isolation is required until the patient has been on effective antimicrobial therapy for 48 hours. All contacts should receive prophylaxis with oral doxycycline 2.2 mg/kg/dose (maximum dose 100 mg) given bid for 7 days. State health officials should be notified immediately about suspected plague cases.

## Prognosis

The mortality rate in untreated bubonic plague is about 50%. The mortality rate for treated pneumonic plague is 50–60%. Recent mortality rates in New Mexico were 3% for bubonic plague and 71% for the septicemic form.

Gage KL et al: Cases of cat-associated human plague in the Western US, 1977–1998. Clin Infect Dis 2000;30(6):893.

Inglesby T et al: Plague as a biological weapon: Medical and public health management. JAMA 2000;283(17):2281 [PMID: 10807389].

http://www.cdc.gov/ncidod/dvbid/plague

# HAEMOPHILUS INFLUENZAE TYPE B INFECTIONS

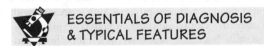

### ESSENTIALS OF DIAGNOSIS & TYPICAL FEATURES

- Purulent meningitis in children younger than age 4 years with direct smears of CSF showing gram-negative pleomorphic rods.
- Acute epiglottitis: High fever, drooling, dysphagia, aphonia, and stridor.
- Septic arthritis: Fever, local redness, swelling, heat, and pain with active or passive motion of the involved joint in a child age 4 months to 4 years.
- Cellulitis: Sudden onset of fever and distinctive cellulitis in an infant, often involving the cheek or periorbital area.
- In all cases, a positive culture from the blood, CSF, or aspirated pus confirms the diagnosis.

## General Considerations

*H influenzae* type b (Hib) has become uncommon because of widespread immunization in early infancy.

The 99% reduction in incidence seen in many parts of the United States is due to high rates of vaccine coverage and reduced nasopharyngeal carriage after vaccination. Forty percent of cases occur in children younger than 6 months who are too young to have completed a primary immunization series. Hib may cause meningitis, bacteremia, epiglottitis (supraglottic croup), septic arthritis, periorbital and facial cellulitis, pneumonia, and pericarditis.

Disease due to *H influenzae* types A, C, D, E, F, or unencapsulated strains is rare, but it now accounts for a larger proportion of positive culture results. Third-generation cephalosporins are preferred for initial therapy of Hib infections. Ampicillin is adequate for culture-proved Hib susceptible strains.

Unencapsulated, nontypable *H influenzae* frequently colonizes the mucous membranes and causes otitis media, sinusitis, bronchitis, and pneumonia in children and adults. Bacteremia is uncommon. Neonatal sepsis similar to early-onset GBS is recognized. Obstetric complications of chorioamnionitis and bacteremia are usually the source of neonatal cases.

Ampicillin resistance occurs in 25–40% of nontypable *H influenzae*.

## Clinical Findings

### A. SYMPTOMS AND SIGNS

**1. Meningitis**—Infants usually present with fever, irritability, lethargy, poor feeding with or without vomiting, and a high-pitched cry.

**2. Acute epiglottitis**—The most useful clinical finding in the early diagnosis of Hib epiglottitis is evidence of dysphagia, characterized by a refusal to eat or swallow saliva and by drooling. This finding, plus the presence of a high fever in a "toxic" child—even in the absence of a cherry-red epiglottis on direct examination—should strongly suggest the diagnosis and lead to prompt intubation. Stridor is a late sign. (See Chapter 17 for details.)

**3. Septic arthritis**—Hib is a common cause of septic arthritis in unimmunized children younger than age 4 years in the United States. The child is febrile and refuses to move the involved joint and limb because of pain. Examination reveals swelling, warmth, redness, tenderness on palpation, and severe pain on attempted movement of the joint.

**4. Cellulitis**—Cellulitis due to Hib occurs almost exclusively in the age group from 3 months to 4 years but is now uncommon as a result of immunization. Fever is usually noted at the same time as the cellulitis, and many infants appear toxic. The cheek or periorbital (preseptal) area is usually involved.

### B. Laboratory Findings

The WBC count in Hib infections may be high or normal with a shift to the left. Blood culture is frequently positive. Positive culture of aspirated pus or fluid from the involved site proves the diagnosis. In untreated meningitis, CSF smear may show the characteristic pleomorphic gram-negative rods.

### C. Imaging

A lateral view of the neck may suggest the diagnosis in suspected acute epiglottitis, but misinterpretation is common. Intubation should not be delayed to obtain radiographs. Haziness of maxillary and ethmoid sinuses occurs with orbital cellulitis.

## Differential Diagnosis

### A. Meningitis

Meningitis must be differentiated from head injury, brain abscess, tumor, lead encephalopathy, and other forms of meningoencephalitis, including mycobacterial, viral, fungal, and bacterial agents.

### B. Acute Epiglottitis

In croup caused by viral agents (parainfluenza 1, 2, and 3, respiratory syncytial virus, influenza A, adenovirus), the child has more definite upper respiratory symptoms, cough, hoarseness, slower progression of obstructive signs, and lower fever. Spasmodic croup occurs typically at night in a child with a history of previous attacks. A history of sudden onset of choking and paroxysmal coughing suggests aspiration of a foreign body. Retropharyngeal abscess may have to be differentiated from epiglottitis.

### C. Septic Arthritis

Differential diagnosis includes acute osteomyelitis, prepatellar bursitis, cellulitis, rheumatic fever, and fractures and sprains.

### D. Cellulitis

Erysipelas, streptococcal cellulitis, insect bites, and trauma (including Popsicle panniculitis or other types of freezing injury) may mimic Hib cellulitis. Periorbital cellulitis must be differentiated from paranasal sinus disease without cellulitis, allergic inflammatory disease of the lids, conjunctivitis, and herpes zoster infection.

## Complications

### A. Meningitis (See Chapter 23.)

### B. Acute Epiglottitis

The disease may rapidly progress to complete airway obstruction with complications owing to hypoxia. Mediastinal emphysema and pneumothorax may occur.

### C. Septic Arthritis

Septic arthritis may result in rapid destruction of cartilage and ankylosis if diagnosis and treatment are delayed. Even with early treatment, the incidence of residual damage and disability after septic arthritis in weight-bearing joints may be as high as 25%.

### D. Cellulitis

Bacteremia may lead to meningitis or pyarthrosis.

## Prevention

The risk of invasive Hib disease is highest in unimmunized, or partially immunized, household contacts who are younger than 4 years of age. The following situations require rifampin chemoprophylaxis of all household contacts to eradicate potential naspopharyngeal colonization with Hib and limit risk of invasive disease: (1) families where at least one household contact is younger than 4 years of age and either unimmunized or incompletely immunized against Hib, (2) an immunocompromised child (of any age or immunization status) resides in the household, or (3) a child younger than 12 months of age resides in the home and has not received three doses of the Hib vaccine. Preschool and day care center contacts may need prophylaxis if more than one case has occurred in the center in the previous 60 days (discuss with state health officials). The index case also needs chemoprophylaxis unless treated with ceftriaxone or cefotaxime (both are effective in eradication of Hib from the nasopharynx). Household contacts and index cases who are younger than 1 month of age needing chemoprophylaxis should be given rifampin, 20 mg/kg/dose (maximum adult dose 600 mg), orally, once daily for 4 successive days. Persons younger than 1 month of age should be given oral rifampin 10 mg/kg/dose once daily for 4 days. Rifampin should not be used in pregnant females.

## Treatment

All patients with bacteremic or potentially bacteremic Hib diseases require hospitalization for treatment. The drugs of choice in hospitalized patients are a third-generation cephalosporin (cefotaxime or ceftriaxone) until the sensitivity of the organism is known.

### A. Meningitis

Therapy is begun as soon as bacterial meningitis has been identified and CSF, blood, and other appropriate cultures have been obtained. Therapy is begun with cefotaxime (50 mg/kg intravenously q6h) or ceftriaxone (50 mg/kg intravenously q12h). If the organism is sensitive to ampicillin, it is the drug of choice. Therapy should preferably be given intravenously for the entire course. Ceftriaxone may be given intramuscularly if venous access becomes difficult.

Duration of therapy is 10 days. Longer treatment is reserved for children who respond slowly or in whom septic complications have occurred.

Repeated lumbar punctures are usually not necessary in Hib meningitis. They should be obtained in the following circumstances: unsatisfactory or questionable clinical response, seizure occurring after several days of therapy, and prolonged (7 days) or recurrent fever if the neurologic examination is abnormal or difficult to evaluate. Dexamethasone given immediately after diagnosis and continued for 2–4 days may reduce the incidence of hearing loss in children with Hib meningitis. The use of dexamethasone is controversial, but when it is used the dosage is 0.6 mg/kg/d in four divided doses for 4 days.

### B. Acute Epiglottitis (See Chapter 17.)

### C. Septic Arthritis

Initial therapy should include nafcillin (or another effective antistaphylococcal antibiotic), 150 mg/kg/d in four divided doses, and cefotaxime or ceftriaxone (dosage as for meningitis). If the isolate is sensitive to ampicillin, it is given in a dosage of 200–300 mg/kg/d intravenously in four divided doses. If a child is improved following initial intravenous therapy, oral amoxicillin (75–100 mg/kg/d in four divided doses q6h) may be administered under careful supervision to complete a 2-week course. Alternative oral agents for ampicillin-resistant organisms include amoxicillin–clavulanic acid or second- or third-generation cephalosporins. Ideally, susceptibility to these agents should be proved prior to use. Drainage of infected joint fluid is an essential part of treatment. In joints other than the hip, this can often be accomplished by one or more needle aspirations. In hip infections—and in arthritis of other joints where treatment is delayed or clinical response is slow—surgical drainage is advised. The joint should be immobilized.

### D. Cellulitis, Including Orbital Cellulitis

Initial therapy should include an agent effective against staphylococci in combination with cefotaxime or ceftriaxone. Ampicillin may be used if the isolate is shown to be susceptible. Therapy is given parenterally for 3–7 days, followed by oral treatment as for septic arthritis, and supportive and symptomatic treatment as required. There is usually marked improvement after 72 hours of treatment. Antibiotics should be given for 10–14 days.

### Prognosis

The case fatality rate for Hib meningitis is less than 5%. Young infants have the highest mortality rate. One of the most common neurologic sequelae, developing in 5–10% of patients with Hib meningitis, is sensorineural hearing loss. All patients with Hib meningitis should have their hearing checked during the course of the illness or shortly after recovery. Children in whom invasive Hib infection develops despite appropriate immunization should have tests to investigate immune function and to rule out HIV. The case fatality rate in acute epiglottitis is 2–5%. Deaths are associated with bacteremia and the rapid development of airway obstruction. The prognosis for the other diseases requiring hospitalization is good with the institution of early and adequate antibiotic therapy.

### Vaccines

There are currently four separate carbohydrate protein conjugate Hib vaccines available (see Chapter 9).

Heath PT et al: Non-type b *Haemophilus influenzae* disease: Clinical and epidemiologic characteristics in the *Haemophilus influenzae* type b vaccine era. Pediatr Infect Dis J 2001;20:300.

Lucas AH, Granoff DM: Imperfect memory and the development of *Haemophilus influenzae* type b disease. Pediatr Infect Dis J 2001,20.235.

Rosenstein N, Perkins B: Update of *Haemophilus influenzae* serotype B and meningococcal vaccines. Pediatr Clin North Am 2000;47(2):337 [PMID: 10761507].

## PERTUSSIS (WHOOPING COUGH)

### ESSENTIALS OF DIAGNOSIS & TYPICAL FEATURES

- *Prodromal catarrhal stage (1–3 weeks) characterized by mild cough, coryza, without fever.*
- *Persistent staccato, paroxysmal cough ending with a high-pitched inspiratory "whoop."*
- *Leukocytosis with absolute lymphocytosis.*
- *Diagnosis confirmed by PCR or culture of nasopharyngeal secretions.*

### General Considerations

Pertussis is an acute, highly communicable infection of the respiratory tract caused by *Bordetella pertussis* and characterized by severe bronchitis. Children usually acquire the disease from symptomatic family contacts.

Adults who have mild respiratory illness, not recognized as pertussis, frequently are the source of infection. Asymptomatic carriage of *B pertussis* is not recognized. Infectivity is greatest during the catarrhal and early paroxysmal cough stage (for about 4 weeks after onset).

Pertussis cases have increased in the United States since 1980. In 2003, about 8000 cases were reported with 30% in older children and adolescents age 10–19 years. The morbidity and mortality of pertussis is greatest in young children. Fifty percent of children younger than age 1 year with a diagnosis of pertussis are hospitalized. Of 17 deaths reported in 1996 and 1997, 11 were in children younger than age 6 months.

Active immunity follows natural pertussis. Reinfections occur years to decades later but are usually milder. Immunity following vaccination wanes in 5–10 years. The majority of young adults in the United States are susceptible to pertussis infection, and disease is probably common but unrecognized.

*Bordetella parapertussis* causes a similar but milder syndrome and is reported frequently in Central Europe.

*B pertussis* organisms attach to the ciliated respiratory epithelium and multiply there; deeper invasion does not occur. Disease is due to several bacterial toxins, the most potent of which is pertussis toxin, which is responsible for lymphocytosis and many of the symptoms of pertussis.

## Clinical Findings

### A. SYMPTOMS AND SIGNS

The onset of pertussis is insidious, with catarrhal upper respiratory tract symptoms (rhinitis, sneezing, and an irritating cough). Slight fever may be present; temperature greater than 38.3°C suggests bacterial superinfection or another cause of respiratory tract infection. After about 2 weeks, cough becomes paroxysmal, characterized by 10–30 forceful coughs ending with a loud inspiration (the whoop). Infants and adults with otherwise typical severe pertussis often lack characteristic whooping. Vomiting commonly follows a paroxysm. Coughing is accompanied by cyanosis, sweating, prostration, and exhaustion. This stage lasts for 2–4 weeks, with gradual improvement. Cough suggestive of chronic bronchitis lasts for another 2–3 weeks. Paroxysmal coughing may continue for some months and may worsen with intercurrent viral respiratory infection. In adults, older children, and partially immunized individuals, symptoms may consist only of irritating cough lasting 1–2 weeks. In the younger unimmunized child, symptoms of pertussis last about 8 weeks or longer. Clinical pertussis is milder in immunized children.

### B. LABORATORY FINDINGS

WBC counts of 20,000–30,000/μL with 70–80% lymphocytes typically appear near the end of the catarrhal stage. Many older children and adults with mild infections never demonstrate lymphocytosis. The blood picture may resemble lymphocytic leukemia or leukemoid reactions. Identification of *B pertussis* by culture or polymerase chain reaction (PCR) from nasopharyngeal swabs or nasal wash specimens proves the diagnosis. The organism may be found in the respiratory tract in diminishing numbers beginning in the catarrhal stage and ending about 2 weeks after the beginning of the paroxysmal stage. After 4–5 weeks of symptoms, cultures and fluorescent antibody tests are almost always negative. Charcoal agar containing an antimicrobial should be inoculated as soon as possible; *B pertussis* does not tolerate drying or prolonged transport PCR detection is replacing culture in most pediatric centers because of improved sensitivity, decreased time to diagnosis, and cost. Enzyme-linked immunosorbent assays (ELISA) for detection of antibody to pertussis toxin or filamentous hemagglutinin may be useful for diagnosis but are currently not widely available, and interpretation of antibody titers may be difficult in previously immunized patients. The chest radiograph reveals thickened bronchi and sometimes shows a "shaggy" heart border.

## Differential Diagnosis

The differential diagnosis of pertussis includes bacterial, tuberculous, chlamydial, and viral pneumonia. Cystic fibrosis and foreign body aspiration may be considerations. Adenoviruses and respiratory syncytial virus may cause paroxysmal coughing with an associated elevation of lymphocytes in the peripheral blood, mimicking pertussis.

## Complications

Bronchopneumonia due to superinfection is the most common serious complication. It is characterized by abrupt clinical deterioration during the paroxysmal stage, accompanied by high fever and sometimes a striking leukemoid reaction with a shift to predominantly polymorphonuclear neutrophils. Atelectasis is a second common pulmonary complication. Atelectasis may be patchy or extensive and may shift rapidly to involve different areas of lung. Intercurrent viral respiratory infection is also a common complication and may provoke worsening or recurrence of paroxysmal coughing. Otitis media is common. Residual chronic bronchiectasis is infrequent despite the severity of the illness. Apnea and sudden death may occur during a particularly severe paroxysm. Seizures complicate 1.5% of cases, and encephalopathy occurs in 0.1%. The encephalopathy frequently is fatal. Anoxic brain damage, cerebral hemorrhage, or pertussis neurotoxins are hypothesized, but anoxia is most likely the cause. Epistaxis and subconjunctival hemorrhages are common.

## Prevention

Active immunization (see Chapter 9) with DTP vaccine should be given in early infancy. Acellular pertussis (DTaP) vaccines cause less fever and fewer local and febrile systemic reactions and have replaced the former whole cell vaccines. The recent increase in incidence of pertussis is primarily due to increased recognition of disease in adolescents and adults.

Chemoprophylaxis with erythromycin should be given to exposed family and hospital contacts, particularly those younger than age 2 years. Hospitalized children with pertussis should be isolated because of the great risk of transmission to patients and staff. Several large hospital outbreaks have been reported.

## Treatment

### A. SPECIFIC MEASURES

Antibiotics may ameliorate early infections but have no effect on clinical symptoms in the paroxysmal stage. Erythromycin is the drug of choice because it promptly terminates respiratory tract carriage of *B pertussis*. Resistance to macrolides has been rarely reported. Patients should be given erythromycin estolate (40–50 mg/kg/24 h in four divided doses for 14 days). Erythromycin ethylsuccinate is efficacious, but the higher dose recommended causes considerable gastrointestinal intolerance. A recent study suggests that 7 days and 14 days of treatment are equally effective. Treatment with clarithromycin for 7 days and azithromycin for 5 days was equal to erythromycin for 14 days, with fewer gastrointestinal side effects. Ampicillin (100 mg/kg/d in four divided doses) may also be used for erythromycin-intolerant patients. Household or other close contacts (eg, in day care centers) should be given erythromycin to reduce secondary transmission. This prophylaxis should be used regardless of age or immunization status.

Corticosteroids reduce the severity of disease but may mask signs of bacterial superinfection. Albuterol (0.3–0.5 mg/kg/d in four doses) has reduced the severity of illness, but tachycardia is common when the drug is given orally, and aerosol administration may precipitate paroxysms.

### B. GENERAL MEASURES

Nutritional support during the paroxysmal phase is important. Frequent small feedings, tube feeding, or parenteral fluid supplementation may be needed. Minimizing stimuli that trigger paroxysms is probably the

best way of controlling cough. In general, cough suppressants are of little benefit.

### C. TREATMENT OF COMPLICATIONS

Respiratory insufficiency due to pneumonia or other pulmonary complications should be treated with oxygen and assisted ventilation if necessary. Convulsions are treated with oxygen and anticonvulsants. Bacterial pneumonia or otitis media requires additional antibiotics.

## Prognosis

The prognosis for patients with pertussis has improved in recent years because of excellent nursing care, treatment of complications, attention to nutrition, and modern intensive care. However, the disease is still very serious in infants younger than age 1 year; most deaths occur in this age group. Children with encephalopathy have a poor prognosis.

Cherry JD: The science and fiction of the "resurgence" of pertussis. Pediatrics 2003;112(2):405 [PMID: 12897292].

Crowcroft NS et al: Severe and unrecognized: pertussis in UK patients. Arch Dis Child 2003;88(9):802 [PMID: 12937105].

Ntezayabo B et al: Pertussis resurgence in Canada largely caused by a cohort effect. Pediatr Infect Dis J 2003;22(1):22 [PMID: 12544404].

Vitek CR et al: Increase in deaths from pertussis among young infants in the United States in the 1990s. Pediatr Infect Dis J 2003;22(7):628 [PMID: 12867839].

Senzilet LD et al: Pertussis is a frequent cause of prolonged cough illness in adults and adolescents. Clin Infect Dis 2001;32:1691.

## LISTERIOSIS

## ESSENTIALS OF DIAGNOSIS & TYPICAL FEATURES

*Early-onset neonatal disease:*
- *Signs of sepsis a few hours after birth in an infant born with fetal distress and hepatosplenomegaly; maternal fever.*

*Late-onset neonatal disease:*
- *Meningitis, sometimes with monocytosis in the CSF and peripheral blood. Onset at age 9–30 days.*

## General Considerations

*Listeria monocytogenes* is a gram-positive, non–spore-forming aerobic rod distributed widely in the animal kingdom and in food, dust, and soil. It causes systemic infections in newborn infants and immunosuppressed older children. In pregnant women, infection is relatively mild, with fever, aches, and chills, but is accompanied by bacteremia and sometimes results in intrauterine or perinatal infection with grave consequences for the fetus or newborn. One fourth of cases occur in pregnant women, and 20% of their pregnancies end in stillbirth or neonatal death. Listeria is present in the stool of approximately 10% of the healthy population. Persons in contact with animals are at greater risk. Outbreaks of listeriosis have been traced to contaminated cabbage in coleslaw, soft cheese, hot dogs, luncheon meats, and milk. *Listeria* infections have decreased since the adoption of strict regulations for ready-to-eat foods.

Like GBS infections, listeria infections in the newborn can be divided into early and late forms. Early infections are more common, leading to a severe congenital form of infection. Later infections are often characterized by meningitis.

## Clinical Findings

### A. SYMPTOMS AND SIGNS

In the early neonatal form, symptoms of listeriosis usually appear on the first day of life and always by the third day. Fetal distress is common, and infants frequently have signs of severe disease at birth. Respiratory distress, diarrhea, and fever occur. On examination, hepatosplenomegaly and a papular rash are found. A history of maternal fever is common. Meningitis may accompany the septic course. The late neonatal form usually occurs after age 9 days and can occur as late as 5 weeks. Meningitis is common, characterized by irritability, fever, and poor feeding.

*Listeria* infections are rare in older children and are usually associated with immunodeficiency. Several recent cases are associated with tumor necrosis factor-α neutralizing agents. Signs and symptoms are those of meningitis, usually with insidious onset.

### B. LABORATORY FINDINGS

In all patients except those receiving white cell depressant drugs, the WBC count is elevated, with 10–20% monocytes. When meningitis is found, the characteristic CSF cell count is high (> 500/μL) with a predominance of polymorphonuclear neutrophils in 70% of cases. Monocytes may predominate in up to 30% of cases. Gram-stained smears of CSF are usually negative, but short gram-positive rods may be seen. The chief pathologic feature in severe neonatal sepsis is miliary granulomatosis with microabscesses in liver, spleen, CNS, lung, and bowel.

Cultures are frequently positive from multiple sites, including blood from the infant and the mother. The organisms form small, weakly hemolytic colonies on blood agar and may be mistaken for streptococci.

## Differential Diagnosis

Early-onset neonatal disease resembles hemolytic disease of the newborn, GBS sepsis or severe cytomegalovirus infection, rubella, or toxoplasmosis. Late-onset disease must be differentiated from meningitis due to echovirus and coxsackievirus, GBS, and gram-negative enteric bacteria.

## Prevention

Immunosuppressed, pregnant, and elderly patients can decrease the risk of *Listeria* infection by avoiding soft cheeses, by thoroughly reheating or avoiding delicatessen and ready-to-eat foods, by avoiding raw meat and milk, and by thoroughly washing fresh vegetables.

## Treatment

Ampicillin (150–300 mg/kg/d q6h intravenously) is the drug of choice in most cases of listeriosis. Gentamicin (2.5 mg/kg q8h intravenously) has a synergistic effect with ampicillin and should be given in serious infections and to patients with immune deficits. If ampicillin cannot be used, TMP–SMX is also effective. Cephalosporins are not effective. Treatment of severe disease should continue for at least 2 weeks.

## Prognosis

In a recent outbreak of early-onset neonatal disease, the mortality rate was 27% despite aggressive and appropriate management. Meningitis in older infants has a good prognosis. In immunosuppressed children, prognosis depends to a great extent on that of the underlying illness.

Braden CR: Listeriosis. Pediatr Infect Dis J 2003;22(8):745 [PMID: 12913780].

Colodner R et al: Listeria monocytogenes cross-contamination in a nursery. Am J Infect Control 2003;31(5):322 [PMID: 12888770].

Das A et al: Meningoencephalitis in a previously healthy nine-year-old girl. Pediatr Infect Dis J 2003;22(8):757,761 [PMID: 12938682].

Safdar A, Armstrong D: Listeriosis in patients at a comprehensive cancer center, 1955–1997. Clin Infect Dis 2003;37(3):359 [PMID: 12884160].

Rocourt J, Jacquet C, Reilly A: Epidemiology of human listeriosis and seafoods. Int J Food Microbiol 2000;62(3):197.

# TUBERCULOSIS

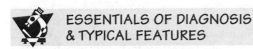

## ESSENTIALS OF DIAGNOSIS & TYPICAL FEATURES

- *All types: Positive tuberculin test in patient or members of household, suggestive chest radiograph, history of contact, and demonstration of organism by stain and culture.*
- *Pulmonary: Fatigue, irritability, and undernutrition, with or without fever and cough.*
- *Glandular: Chronic cervical adenitis.*
- *Miliary: Classic snowstorm appearance of chest radiograph; choroidal tubercles.*
- *Meningitis: Fever and manifestations of meningeal irritation and increased intracranial pressure. Characteristic CSF.*

## General Considerations

Tuberculosis is a granulomatous disease caused by *Mycobacterium tuberculosis*. It is a leading cause of death throughout the world. Children younger than age 3 years are most susceptible. Lymphohematogenous dissemination through the lungs to extrapulmonary sites, including the brain and meninges, eyes, bones and joints, lymph nodes, kidneys, intestines, larynx, and skin, is more likely to occur in infants. Increased susceptibility occurs again in adolescence, particularly in girls within 2 years of menarche. Following substantial increases in disease during the 1980s, tuberculosis incidence has decreased since 1992 due to increased control measures. Eleven thousand three hundred new cases were reported in 2003 High-risk groups include ethnic minorities, foreign-born persons, prisoners, residents of nursing homes, indigents, migrant workers, and health care providers. However, 50% of cases in 2001 occurred in United States-born persons. HIV infection is an important risk factor for both development and spread of disease. Pediatric tuberculosis incidence mirrors the trends seen in adults.

Exposure to an infected adult is the most common risk factor in children. The primary complex in infancy and childhood consists of a small parenchymal lesion in any area of the lung with caseation of regional nodes and calcification. Postprimary tuberculosis in adolescents and adults occurs in the apices of the lungs and is likely to cause chronic progressive cavitary pulmonary disease with less tendency for hematogenous dissemination. *Mycobacterium bovis* infection is clinically identi-cal to *M tuberculosis*. *M bovis* may be acquired from unpasteurized dairy products obtained outside the United States.

## Clinical Findings

### A. SYMPTOMS AND SIGNS

**1. Pulmonary**—See Chapter 18.

**2. Miliary**—Diagnosis is usually based on the classic "snowstorm" or "millet seed" appearance of lung fields on radiograph, although early in the course of disseminated tuberculosis, the chest radiograph may show no or only subtle abnormalities. The majority of patients have a fresh primary complex and pleural effusion. Choroidal tubercles are sometimes seen on funduscopic examination. Other lesions may be present and produce osteomyelitis, arthritis, meningitis, tuberculomas of the brain, enteritis, or infection of the kidneys and liver.

**3. Meningitis**—Symptoms include fever, vomiting, headache, lethargy, and irritability, with signs of meningeal irritation and increased intracranial pressure, cranial nerve palsies, convulsions, and coma.

**4. Lymphatic**—The primary complex may be associated with a skin lesion drained by regional nodes or chronic cervical node enlargement or infection of the tonsils. Involved nodes may become fixed to the overlying skin, suppurate, and drain.

### B. LABORATORY FINDINGS

The Mantoux test (0.1 mL of intermediate-strength purified protein derivative [PPD] [5 TU] inoculated intradermally) is positive at 48–72 hours if there is significant induration (Table 38–2). Parental reporting of skin test results is often inaccurate. All tests should be read by professionals trained to interpret Mantoux tests. False-negative results occur in malnourished patients, in those with overwhelming disease, and in 10% of children with isolated pulmonary disease. Temporary suppression of tuberculin reactivity may be seen with viral infections (eg, measles, influenza, varicella, mumps), after live virus immunization, and during corticosteroid or other immunosuppressive drug therapy. For these reasons, a negative Mantoux test does not exclude the diagnosis of tuberculosis. When tuberculosis is suspected in a child, household members and adult contacts (eg, teachers, caregivers) should also be tested immediately. Multiple puncture tests (tine tests) should not be used because they are associated with false-negative and false-positive reactions, and because standards for interpretation of positive results do not exist. The ESR is usually elevated. Cultures of pooled early morning gastric aspirates from three successive days will yield *M tuberculosis* in about 40% of cases. Biopsy may be necessary to establish the diagnosis. Therapy should not

***Table 38–2.*** Interpretation of tuberculin skin test reactions.[a]

| Degree of Risk | Risk Factors | Positive Reaction |
|---|---|---|
| High | Recent close contact with a case of active tuberculosis; chest x-ray compatible with tuberculosis; immunocompromise; HIV infection | ≥ 5 mm induration |
| Medium | Current or previous residence in high-prevalence area (Asia, Africa, Latin America); skin test converters within past 2 years; intravenous drug use; homelessness or residence in a correctional institution; recent weight loss or malnutrition; leukemia, Hodgkin disease, diabetes mellitus; age < 4 years | ≥ 10 mm induration |
| Low | Children ≥ 4 years without any risk factor | ≥ 15 mm induration |

[a]Standard intradermal Mantoux test, 5 test units.

be delayed in suspected cases. The CSF in tuberculous meningitis shows slight to moderate pleocytosis (50–300 WBCs/μL, predominantly lymphocytes), decreased glucose, and increased protein.

The direct detection of mycobacteria in body fluids or discharges is best done by staining specimens with auramine-rhodamine and examining them with fluorescence microscopy; this method is superior to the Ziehl–Neelsen method.

### C. IMAGING

Chest radiograph should be obtained in all children with suspicion of tuberculosis at any site or with a positive skin test. Segmental consolidation with some volume loss and hilar adenopathy are common findings in children. Pleural effusion also occurs with primary infection. Cavities and apical disease are unusual in children but are common in adolescents and adults.

## Differential Diagnosis

Pulmonary tuberculosis must be differentiated from fungal, parasitic, mycoplasmal, and bacterial pneumonias; lung abscess; foreign body aspiration; lipoid pneumonia; sarcoidosis; and mediastinal cancer. Cervical lymphadenitis is most likely due to streptococcal or staphylococcal infections. Cat-scratch fever and infection with atypical mycobacteria may need to be distinguished from tuberculous lymphadenitis. Viral meningoencephalitis, head trauma (child abuse), lead poisoning, brain abscess, acute bacterial meningitis, brain tumor, and disseminated fungal infections must be excluded in tuberculous meningitis. The skin test in the patient or family contacts is frequently valuable in differentiating these conditions from tuberculosis.

## Prevention

### A. BCG VACCINE

Bacille Calmette–Guérin (BCG) vaccines are live attenuated strains of *M bovis*. Although neonatal and childhood administration of BCG is carried out in countries with a high prevalence of tuberculosis, protective efficacy varies greatly with vaccine potency and method of delivery. Because the great majority of children who have received BCG still have negative Mantoux tests, the past history of BCG vaccination should be ignored in interpreting the skin test. In the United States, BCG vaccination is given only to tuberculin-negative children and neonates in high-risk situations who are HIV-negative, who are unlikely to receive isoniazid prophylaxis or close follow-up, or who are at high risk for exposure to persons infected with *M tuberculosis* resistant to isoniazid and rifampin (see Chapter 9).

### B. ISONIAZID CHEMOPROPHYLAXIS

Daily administration of isoniazid (10 mg/kg/d orally; maximum 300 mg) is advised for children who cannot avoid intimate household contact with adolescents or adults with active disease. Isoniazid is given until 3 months after last contact. At the end of this time, a Mantoux test should be done, and therapy should be continued for an additional 6 months if the test is positive.

### C. OTHER MEASURES

Tuberculosis in infants and young children is evidence of recent exposure to active infection in an adult, usually a family member or household contact. The source contact (index case) should be identified, isolated, and given treatment to prevent other secondary cases. Reporting cases to local health departments is essential for contact tracing. Exposed tuberculin-negative children should usually receive isoniazid chemoprophylaxis. If a repeated skin test is negative 2–3 months following the last exposure, isoniazid may be stopped. Routine tuberculin skin testing is no longer recommended for children without risk factors who reside in communities with a low incidence of tuberculosis. Children with no personal risk for tuberculosis but who reside in communities with a high incidence of tuberculosis should be given a skin test at school entry and then again at age 11–16 years. Children with a risk factor for acquiring tuberculosis should be tested every 2–3 years. Incarcerated adolescents and children living in a household with HIV-infected persons should have annual skin tests.

Children who immigrate from a country with a high incidence of infection should receive a skin test on entry to the United States or upon presentation to health care providers. A past history of BCG vaccine should not delay skin testing.

## Treatment

### A. SPECIFIC MEASURES

Most children with tuberculosis in the United States are hospitalized initially. If the infecting organism has not been isolated from the presumed contact for susceptibility testing, reasonable attempts should be made to obtain it from the child using morning gastric aspirates, sputum, bronchoscopy, thoracentesis, or biopsy when appropriate. Unfortunately, cultures are frequently negative in children, and the risk of these procedures must be weighed against the yield. Therapy is given daily for 2–4 weeks and then reduced to 2–3 times per week for the duration of the course. Directly observed administration of all doses of antituberculosis therapy by a trained health care professional is essential to ensure compliance with therapy.

All children with positive skin tests (see Table 38–2) without evidence of active disease have latent tuberculosis and should receive 9 months of isoniazid (10 mg/kg/d orally; maximum 300 mg) therapy. In children with active pulmonary disease, therapy for 6 months using isoniazid (10 mg/kg/d), rifampin (15 mg/kg/d), and pyrazinamide (25–30 mg/kg/d) in a single daily oral dose for 2 months, followed by isoniazid plus rifampin (either in a daily or twice-weekly regimen) for 4 months appears effective for eliminating isoniazid-susceptible organisms. For more severe disease, such as miliary or CNS infection, duration is increased to 12 months or more, and a fourth drug (streptomycin or ethambutol) is added for the first 2 months. In communities with resistance rates greater than 4%, initial therapy should usually include four drugs.

**1. Isoniazid**—The hepatotoxicity from isoniazid seen in adults and some adolescents is rare in children. Transient elevation of aminotransferases (up to three times normal) may be seen at 6–12 weeks, but therapy is continued unless clinical illness occurs. Routine monitoring of liver function tests is unnecessary unless prior hepatic disease is known or the child is severely ill. Peripheral neuropathy associated with pyridoxine deficiency is rare in children, and it is not necessary to add pyridoxine unless significant malnutrition coexists.

**2. Rifampin**—Although it is an excellent bactericidal agent, rifampin is never used alone owing to rapid development of resistance. Hepatotoxicity may occur but rarely with recommended doses. The orange discoloration of secretions is benign but may stain contact lenses or clothes.

**3. Pyrazinamide**—This excellent sterilizing agent is most effective during the first 2 months of therapy. With the recommended duration and dosing, it is well tolerated. Although pyrazinamide elevates the uric acid level, it rarely causes symptoms of hyperuricemia in children. Use of this drug is now common for tuberculous disease in children, and resistance is almost unknown. Oral acceptance and CNS penetration are good.

**4. Ethambutol**—Because optic neuritis is the major side effect in adults, ethambutol has usually been given only to children whose vision can be reliably tested for loss of color differentiation. Optic neuritis is rare and usually occurs in those receiving more than the recommended dosage of 25 mg/kg/d. Documentation of optic toxicity in children is lacking despite considerable worldwide experience. Therefore, many four-drug regimens for children now include ethambutol.

**5. Streptomycin**—Streptomycin (20–30 mg/kg/d, given intramuscularly in one or two doses) should be given for 1 or 2 months in severe disease. The child's hearing should be tested periodically during use.

### B. CHEMOTHERAPY FOR DRUG-RESISTANT TUBERCULOSIS

The incidence of drug resistance is increasing and reaches 10–20% in some areas of the United States. Transmission of multiply drug-resistant strains to contacts has occurred in some epidemics. All patients with resistant strains should be given at least two effective drugs. In areas with rates of resistance greater than 4%, initial therapy should include four drugs pending susceptibility testing. Consultation with local experts in treating tuberculosis is important in these difficult cases. Therapy should continue for 12 months or longer.

### C. GENERAL MEASURES

**1. Corticosteroids**—These drugs may be used for suppressing inflammatory reactions in meningeal, pleural, and pericardial tuberculosis and for the relief of bronchial obstruction due to hilar adenopathy. Prednisone is given orally, 1 mg/kg/d for 6–8 weeks, with gradual withdrawal at the end of that time. The use of corticosteroids may mask progression of disease. Accordingly, the clinician needs to be sure that an effective regimen is being used.

**2. Bed rest**—Rest in bed is indicated only while the child feels ill. Isolation is necessary only for children with draining lesions or renal disease and for those with chronic pulmonary tuberculosis. Most children with tuberculosis are noninfectious and can attend school while receiving treatment.

## Prognosis

If bacteria are sensitive and treatment is completed, most children are cured with minimal sequelae. Repeat treatment is more difficult and less successful. With antituberculosis chemotherapy (especially isoniazid), there should now be nearly 100% recovery in miliary tuberculosis. Without treatment, the mortality rate in both miliary tuberculosis and tuberculous meningitis is almost 100%. In the latter form, about two thirds of patients receiving treatment survive. There may be a high incidence of neurologic abnormalities among survivors if treatment is started late.

American Thoracic Society, CDC, Infectious Diseases Society of America: Treatment of tuberculosis. MMWR Recomm Rep 2003;52(RR-11):1 [PMID: 12836625].

Gounder CR et al: Tuberculin testing and risk of tuberculosis infection among New York City schoolchildren. Pediatrics 2003;111(4):e309 [PMID: 12671144].

Jasmer RM et al: Latent tuberculosis infection. N Engl J Med 2002;347(23):1860 [PMID: 12466511].

Khan K et al: Global drug-resistance patterns and the management of latent tuberculosis infection in immigrants to the United States. N Engl J Med 2002;347(23):1850 [PMID: 12466510].

Lienhardt C et al: Risk factors for tuberculosis infection in children in contact with infectious tuberculosis cases in The Gambia, West Africa. Pediatrics 203;111(5):e608 [PMID: 12728119].

Mongkolrattanothai K et al: Tuberculous otitis media with mastoiditis and central nervous system involvement. Pediatr Infect Dis J 2003;22(5):453 [PMID: 12792390].

# INFECTIONS WITH NONTUBERCULOUS MYCOBACTERIA

 **ESSENTIALS OF DIAGNOSIS & TYPICAL FEATURES**

- *Chronic unilateral cervical lymphadenitis.*
- *Granulomas of the skin.*
- *Chronic bone lesion with draining sinus (chronic osteomyelitis).*
- *Reaction to PPD-S (standard) of 5–8 mm, negative chest radiograph, and negative history of contact with tuberculosis.*
- *Diagnosis by positive acid-fast stain or culture.*
- *Disseminated infection in patients with AIDS.*

## General Considerations

Various species of acid-fast mycobacteria other than *Mycobacterium tuberculosis* may cause subclinical infections and occasionally clinical disease resembling tuberculosis. Strains of nontuberculous mycobacteria are common in soil, food, and water. Organisms enter the host by small abrasions in skin, oral mucosa, or gastrointestinal mucosa. Strain cross-reactivity with *M tuberculosis* can be demonstrated by simultaneous skin testing (Mantoux) with PPD-S (standard) and PPD prepared from one of the atypical antigens. Unfortunately, reagents prepared for routine non-tuberculosis skin testing are not available to clinicians.

The Runyon classification of mycobacteria includes the following:

**Group I. Photochromogens (PPD-Y):** (*M kansasii* and *M marinum*) Yellow color develops on exposure to light in previously white colony grown 2–4 weeks in the dark.

**Group II. Scotochromogens (PPD-G):** (*M scrofulaceum*) Colonies are definitely yellow-orange after incubation in the dark. Organisms may be found in small numbers in the normal flora of some human saliva and gastric contents. Subclinical infection is widespread in the United States, but clinical disease appears rarely.

**Group III. Nonphotochromogens (PPD-B):** "Battey avian-swine group" grows as small white colonies after incubation in the dark, with no significant development of pigment on exposure to light. Infection with *Mycobacterium avium* complex (MAC) is prevalent on the East Coast of the United States, particularly the Southeast, and in patients with AIDS.

**Group IV. "Rapid growers":** (*M fortuitum, M chelonei*) Within 1 week after inoculation they form colonies closely resembling *M tuberculosis* morphologically.

## Clinical Findings

### A. SYMPTOMS AND SIGNS

**1. Lymphadenitis**—In children, the most common form of infection due to mycobacteria other than *M tuberculosis* is cervical lymphadenitis. MAC is the most common organism. A submandibular or cervical node swells slowly and is firm and initially somewhat tender. Low-grade fever may occur. Over time, the node suppurates and may drain chronically. Nodes in other areas of the head and neck and elsewhere are sometimes involved.

**2. Pulmonary disease**—In the western United States, pulmonary disease is usually due to *M kansasii*. In the eastern United States, it may be due to MAC. In other countries, disease is usually caused by MAC. In adults, there is usually underlying chronic pulmonary disease. Immunologic deficiency may be present. Presentation is clinically indistinguishable from that of tuberculosis.

Adolescents with cystic fibrosis may be infected with nontuberculous mycobacteria.

**3. Swimming pool granuloma**—This is due to *M marinum.* A solitary chronic granulomatous lesion with satellite lesions develops after minor trauma in infected swimming pools. Minor trauma in home aquariums or other aquatic environments also may lead to infection.

**4. Chronic osteomyelitis**—Osteomyelitis is caused by *M kansasii, M fortuitum,* or other rapid growers. Findings include swelling and pain over a distal extremity, radiolucent defects in bone, fever, and clinical and radiographic evidence of bronchopneumonia. Such cases are rare.

**5. Meningitis**—Disease is due to *M kansasii* and may be indistinguishable from tuberculous meningitis.

**6. Disseminated infection**—Rarely, apparently immunologically normal children develop disseminated infection due to nontuberculous mycobacteria. Children are ill, with fever and hepatosplenomegaly, and organisms are demonstrated in bone lesions, lymph nodes, or liver. Chest radiographs are usually normal. Between 60% and 80% of patients with AIDS will acquire MAC infection, characterized by fever, night sweats, weight loss, and diarrhea. Infection usually indicates severe immune dysfunction and is associated with CD4 lymphocyte counts less than 50/µL.

**B. LABORATORY FINDINGS**

In most cases, there is a small reaction (<10 mm) when Mantoux testing is done. Larger reactions may be seen. The chest radiograph is negative, and there is no history of contact with tuberculosis. Needle aspiration of the node excludes bacterial infection and may yield acid-fast bacilli on stain or culture. Fistulization should not be a problem because total excision is usually recommended for infection due to atypical mycobacteria. Cultures of any normally sterile body site will yield MAC in immunocompromised patients with disseminated disease. Blood cultures are positive, with a large density of bacteria.

## Differential Diagnosis

See section on differential diagnosis in the previous discussion of tuberculosis and in Chapter 18.

## Treatment

**A. SPECIFIC MEASURES**

The usual treatment of lymphadenitis is complete surgical excision. Occasionally excision is impossible because of proximity to branches of the facial nerve. Chemotherapy may then be necessary. Response of extensive adenopathy or other forms of infection varies according to the infecting species and susceptibility. Usually, combinations of two to four medications administered for months are required. Isoniazid, rifampin, ethambutol (depending on sensitivity to isoniazid) will result in a favorable response in almost all patients with *M kansasii* infection. Chemotherapeutic treatment of MAC is much less satisfactory because resistance to isoniazid, rifampin, and pyrazinamide is common. Susceptibility testing is necessary to optimize therapy. Most clinicians favor surgical excision of involved tissue if possible and treatment with at least three drugs to which the organism has been shown to be sensitive. Disseminated disease in patients with AIDS calls for a combination of three or more active drugs. Clarithromycin or azithromycin and ethambutol, in addition to one or more of the following drugs, is started: ethionamide, capreomycin, amikacin, rifabutin, or ciprofloxacin. *M fortuitum* and *M chelonei* are usually susceptible to amikacin plus cefoxitin followed by erythromycin, clarithromycin, azithromycin, or doxycycline and may be successfully treated with such combinations. Swimming pool granuloma due to *M marinum* is usually treated with doxycycline (in children > age 9 years) or rifampin, plus ethambutol, clarithromycin, or TMP–SMX for a minimum of 3 months. Surgery may also be beneficial.

**B. GENERAL MEASURES**

Isolation of the patient is usually not necessary. General supportive care is indicated for the child with disseminated disease.

## Prognosis

The prognosis is good for localized disease, although fatalities occur in immunocompromised children who have disseminated disease.

Albright JT, Pransky SM: Nontuberculous mycobacterial infections of the head and neck. Pediatr Clin North Am 2003;59(2): 503 [PMID: 12809337].

Chesny PJ: Nontuberculous mycobacteria. Pediatr Rev 2002;23(9): 300 [PMID: 12205297].

Panesar J et al: Nontuberculous mycobacterial cervical adenitis: A ten-year retrospective study. Laryngoscope 2003;13(1):149 [PMID: 12514400].

Oliver A et al: Non-tuberculous mycobacteria in patients with cystic fibrosis. Clin Infect Dis 2001;32:1298.

## *LEGIONELLA* INFECTION

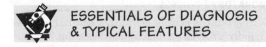

### ESSENTIALS OF DIAGNOSIS & TYPICAL FEATURES

- *Severe progressive pneumonia in a child with compromised immunity.*

- Diarrhea and neurologic signs are common.
- Positive culture requires buffered charcoal yeast extract media and proves infection.
- Direct fluorescent antibody staining of respiratory secretions proves infection.

## General Considerations

*Legionella pneumophila* is a ubiquitous gram-negative bacillus that causes two distinct clinical syndromes: Legionnaire disease and Pontiac fever. Usually Legionnaire disease is an acute, severe pneumonia that is frequently fatal in immunocompromised patients. Pontiac fever is a mild, flu-like illness that spares the lungs and is characterized by fever, headache, myalgia, and arthralgia. The disease is self-limited and is described in outbreaks in otherwise healthy adults.

Over forty species of *Legionella* have been discovered, but not all cause disease in humans. *L pneumophila* causes most infections. *Legionella* is present in many natural water sources as well as domestic water supplies (faucets, showers). Contaminated cooling towers and heat exchangers have been implicated in several large institutional outbreaks. Person-to-person transmission has not been documented.

Few cases of Legionnaire disease have been reported in children. Most were in children with compromised cellular immunity. In adults, risk factors include smoking, underlying cardiopulmonary or renal disease, alcoholism, and diabetes.

*L pneumophila* is thought to be acquired by inhalation of a contaminated aerosol. The bacteria are phagocytosed but proliferate within macrophages. Cell-mediated immunity is necessary to activate macrophages to kill intracellular bacteria.

## Clinical Findings

### A. SYMPTOMS AND SIGNS

Onset of fever, chills, anorexia, and headache is abrupt. Pulmonary symptoms appear within 2–3 days and progress rapidly. The cough is nonproductive early. Purulent sputum occurs late. Hemoptysis, diarrhea, and neurologic signs (including lethargy, irritability, tremors, and delirium) are seen.

### B. LABORATORY FINDINGS

The WBC count is usually elevated. Chest radiographs show rapidly progressive patchy consolidation. Cavitation and large pleural effusions are uncommon. Cultures from sputum, tracheal aspirates, or bronchoscopic specimens, when grown on buffered yeast charcoal extract media, are positive in 70–80% of patients at 3–7 days. Direct fluorescent antibody staining of sputum or other respiratory specimens is only 50–70% sensitive but 95% specific. Thus a negative culture or direct fluorescent antibody staining of sputum or tracheal secretions does not rule out Legionnaire disease. A urine test for Legionella antigen detects 80% of infecting species. Serologic tests are available and aid in diagnosis, but a maximum rise in titer may require 6–8 weeks.

## Differential Diagnosis

Legionnaire disease is usually a rapidly progressive pneumonia in a patient who appears very ill with unremitting fevers. Other bacterial pneumonias, viral pneumonias, *Mycoplasma* pneumonia, and fungal disease are all possibilities and may be difficult to differentiate on clinical grounds in an immunocompromised patient.

## Complications

In sporadic untreated cases, mortality rates are 5–25%. In immunocompromised patients with untreated disease, mortality approaches 80%. Hematogenous dissemination may result in extrapulmonary foci of infection, including pericardium, myocardium, and kidneys. *Legionella* may be the cause of culture-negative endocarditis.

## Prevention

No vaccine is available. Hyperchlorination and periodic superheating of water supplies in hospitals have been shown to reduce the number of organisms and the risk of infection.

## Treatment

Intravenous azithromycin 10 mg/kg/d given as a once daily intravenous dose (maximum dose 500 mg) is the drug of choice. Rifampin (20 mg/kg/d divided in two doses) may be added to the regimen in gravely ill patients. Ciprofloxacin and levofloxacin are also effective in adults, but are not approved for use in children. Duration of therapy is 5–10 days if azithromycin is used; for other antibiotics a 14–21-day course is recommended. Oral therapy may be substituted for intravenous therapy as the patient's condition improves.

## Prognosis

Mortality rate is high if treatment is delayed. Malaise, problems with memory, and fatigue are common problems after recovery.

Campins M et al: Nosocomial Legionnaire's disease in a children's hospital. Pediatric Infect Dis J 2000;19:228.

Roig J et al: *Legionella* spp.: Community acquired and nosocomial infections. Curr Opin Infect Dis 2003;16(2):145 [PMID: 12734447].

# PSITTACOSIS (ORNITHOSIS) & *CHLAMYDIA PNEUMONIAE* INFECTION

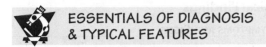

## ESSENTIALS OF DIAGNOSIS & TYPICAL FEATURES

- *Fever, cough, malaise, chills, headache.*
- *Diffuse rales; no consolidation.*
- *Long-lasting radiographic findings of bronchopneumonia.*
- *Isolation of the organism or rising titer of complement-fixing antibodies.*
- *Exposure to infected birds (ornithosis).*

## General Considerations

Psittacosis is caused by *Chlamydia psittaci*. When the agent is transmitted to humans from psittacine birds (parrots, parakeets, cockatoos, and budgerigars), the disease is often called psittacosis or parrot fever. However, other avian genera (pigeons, turkeys) are common sources of infection in the United States, and the general term "ornithosis" is often used. The agent is an obligate intracellular parasite. Human-to-human spread occurs rarely. The incubation period is 5–14 days. The bird from which the disease was transmitted may not be clinically ill.

*C pneumoniae* may cause atypical pneumonia similar to that due to *Mycoplasma pneumoniae*. Transmission is by respiratory spread. Infection appears to be most prevalent during the second decade; half of surveyed adults are seropositive. Only a small percentage of infections result in clinical pneumonia. The disease may be more common than atypical pneumonia due to *M pneumoniae*. Lower respiratory tract infection due to *C pneumoniae* is uncommon in infants and young children.

## Clinical Findings

### A. SYMPTOMS AND SIGNS

**1. *C psittaci*—**The disease is extremely variable but tends to be mild in children. The onset is rapid or insidious, with fever, chills, headache, backache, malaise, myalgia, and dry cough. Signs include pneumonitis, alteration of percussion note and breath sounds, and rales. Pulmonary findings may be absent early. Dyspnea

and cyanosis may occur later. Splenomegaly, epistaxis, prostration, and meningismus are occasionally seen. Delirium, constipation or diarrhea, and abdominal distress may occur.

**2. *C pneumoniae*—**Clinically, *C pneumoniae* infection is similar to *M pneumoniae* infection. Most are mild upper respiratory infections. Lower respiratory tract infection is characterized by fever, sore throat (perhaps more severe with *C pneumoniae*), cough, and bilateral pulmonary findings and infiltrates.

### B. LABORATORY FINDINGS

**1. *C psittaci*—**In psittacosis, the WBC count is normal or decreased, often with a shift to the left. Proteinuria is frequently present. *C psittaci* is present in the blood and sputum during the first 2 weeks of illness and can be isolated by inoculation of specimens into mice or embryonated eggs, but culture is available only in research laboratories. A fourfold rise in complement fixation titers in specimens obtained at least 2 weeks apart or a single titer above 1:32 is considered evidence of infection. The rise in titer may be minimized or delayed by therapy. Infection with *C pneumoniae* may lead to diagnostic confusion because cross-reactive antibody may cause falsely positive *C psittaci* titers. Microimmunofluorescence and PCR assays are specific but usually not commercially available for *C psittaci*.

**2. *C pneumoniae*—**A fourfold rise in IgG titer (microimmunoflouresence antibody test) or an IgM above 16 is evidence of infection. IgG antibody peaks 6–8 weeks after infection. *C pneumoniae* can be isolated from nasal wash or throat swab specimens after inoculation into cell culture. A PCR assay is also available.

### C. IMAGING

The radiographic findings in psittacosis are those of central pneumonia, which later becomes widespread or migratory. Psittacosis is indistinguishable from viral pneumonias by radiograph. Signs of pneumonitis may appear on radiograph in the absence of clinical suspicion of pulmonary involvement.

## Differential Diagnosis

Psittacosis can be differentiated from acute viral or mycoplasmal pneumonias only by the history of contact with potentially infected birds. In severe or prolonged cases with extrapulmonary involvement, the differential diagnosis includes a wide spectrum of diseases including typhoid fever, brucellosis, and rheumatic fever.

## Complications

Complications of psittacosis include myocarditis, endocarditis, hepatitis, pancreatitis, and secondary bacterial pneumonia. *C pneumoniae* infection may be prolonged or may recur.

## Treatment

Doxycycline should be given for 14 days after defervescence to patients older than age 8 years with psittacosis. Alternatively, erythromycin, azithromycin, or clarithromycin may be used in children younger than age 8 years. Supportive oxygen may be needed. The patient should be kept in isolation. *C pneumoniae* responds to macrolides or doxycycline: a 14-day course is recommended.

Centers for Disease Control and Prevention: Compendium of measures to control *Chlamydia psittaci* infection among humans (psittacosis) and pet birds (avian chlamydiosis), 2000. MMWR 2000;49(RR-8):3.

File TM Jr et al: The role of atypical pathogens: *Mycoplasma pneumoniae, Chlamydia pneumoniae,* and *Legionella pneumophila* in respiratory infection. Infect Dis Clin North Am 1998; 12:569.

# CAT-SCRATCH DISEASE

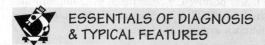

### ESSENTIALS OF DIAGNOSIS & TYPICAL FEATURES

- *History of a cat scratch or cat contact.*
- *Primary lesion (papule, pustule, conjunctivitis) at site of inoculation.*
- *Acute or subacute regional lymphadenopathy.*
- *Aspiration of sterile pus from a node.*
- *Laboratory studies excluding other causes.*
- *Biopsy of node or papule showing histopathologic findings consistent with cat-scratch disease and occasionally characteristic bacilli on Warthin–Starry stain.*
- *Positive cat-scratch serology (antibody to Bartonella henselae).*

## General Considerations

The causative agent of cat-scratch disease is *Bartonella henselae,* a gram-negative bacillus that also causes bacillary angiomatosis. Cat-scratch disease is a benign, self-limited form of lymphadenitis. Patients often report a cat scratch (67%) or contact with a cat or kitten (90%). The cat almost invariably is healthy. The clinical picture is that of a regional lymphadenitis associated with an erythematous papular skin lesion without intervening lymphangitis. The disease occurs worldwide and is more common in the fall and winter. It is estimated that more than 20,000 cases per year occur in the United States. The most common systemic complication is encephalitis.

## Clinical Findings

### A. SYMPTOMS AND SIGNS

About 50% of patients with cat-scratch disease develop a primary lesion at the site of inoculation. The lesion usually is a papule or pustule that appears 3–10 days after injury and is located most often on the arm or hand (50%), head or leg (30%), or trunk or neck (10%). The lesion may be conjunctival (10%). Regional lymphadenopathy appears 10–50 days later and may be accompanied by mild malaise, lassitude, headache, and fever. Multiple sites are seen in about 10% of cases. Involved nodes may be hard or soft and 1–6 cm in diameter. They are usually tender, and 10–20% of them suppurate. The overlying skin may be inflamed. Lymphadenopathy usually resolves in about 2 months but may persist for up to 8 months.

Unusual manifestations include erythema nodosum, thrombocytopenic purpura, conjunctivitis (Parinaud oculoglandular fever), parotid swelling, pneumonia, osteolytic lesions, mesenteric and mediastinal adenitis, neuroretinitis, peripheral neuritis, hepatitis, granulomata of the liver and spleen, and encephalitis.

Immunocompetent patients may develop an atypical systemic form of cat-scratch disease. These patients have prolonged fever, fatigue, and malaise. Lymphadenopathy may be present. Hepatosplenomegaly or low-density hepatic or splenic lesions visualized by ultrasound or computed tomography scan are seen in some patients.

Infection in immunocompromised individuals may take the form of bacillary angiomatosis, presenting as vascular tumors of the skin and subcutaneous tissues. Immunocompromised patients may also have bacteremia or infection of the liver (peliosis hepatis).

### B. LABORATORY FINDINGS

Serologic evidence of *Bartonella* infection by indirect fluorescent antibody or enzyme-linked immunosorbent assay with a titer above 1:64 is supportive of the diagnosis. PCR assays are available commercially. Cat-scratch skin test antigens are not recommended.

Histopathologic examination of involved tissue may show pyogenic granulomas or bacillary forms demonstrated by Warthin–Starry silver stain. There is usually some elevation in the ESR. In patients with CNS involvement, the CSF is usually normal but may show a slight pleocytosis and modest elevation of protein.

## Differential Diagnosis

Cat-scratch disease must be distinguished from pyogenic adenitis, tuberculosis (typical and atypical), tularemia, plague, brucellosis, lymphoma, primary toxoplasmosis, infectious mononucleosis, lymphogranuloma venereum, and fungal infections.

## Treatment

Treatment of cat-scratch disease adenopathy is controversial because the disease usually resolves without therapy and the patient is typically not exceedingly ill. Treatment of typical cat-scratch disease with a 5-day course of azithromycin has been shown to speed resolution of lymphadenopathy in some patients. The best therapy is reassurance that the adenopathy is benign and will subside spontaneously with time (mean duration of illness is 14 weeks). In cases of suppuration, node aspiration under local anesthesia with an 18- to 19-gauge needle relieves the pain. Excision of the involved node is indicated in cases of chronic adenitis. In some reports, gentamicin, ciprofloxacin, and TMP–SMX have been useful. Immunocompromised patients with evidence of infection should be treated with antibiotics: long-term therapy (months) in these patients with azithromycin, erythromycin, or doxycycline is often needed to prevent relapses.

## Prognosis

The prognosis is good if complications do not occur.

Bass JW et al: Prospective randomized double blind placebo-controlled evaluation of azithromycin for treatment of cat scratch disease. Pediatr Infect Dis J 1998;17:447 [PMID:9655532].

Conrad DA: Treatment of cat-scratch disease. Curr Opin Pediatr 2001;13:56 [PMID: 1117624].

Schutze GE: Diagnosis and treatment of *Bartonella henselae* infections. Pediatr Infect Dis J 2000;19:1185 [PMID: 11144381].

Windsor JJ: Cat-scratch disease: Epidemiology, aetiology and treatment. Br J Biomed Sci 2001;58:101 [PMID: 11440202].

# ■ II. SPIROCHETAL INFECTIONS

## SYPHILIS

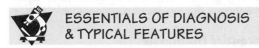

### ESSENTIALS OF DIAGNOSIS & TYPICAL FEATURES

*Congenital:*

- *All types: History of untreated maternal syphilis, a positive serologic test, and a positive darkfield examination.*

- *Newborn: Hepatosplenomegaly, characteristic radiographic bone changes, anemia, increased nucleated red cells, thrombocytopenia, abnormal spinal fluid, jaundice, edema.*
- *Young infant (3–12 weeks): Snuffles, maculopapular skin rash, mucocutaneous lesions, pseudoparalysis (in addition to radiographic bone changes).*
- *Children: Stigmata of early congenital syphilis, interstitial keratitis, saber shins, gummas of nose and palate.*

*Acquired:*

- *Chancre of genitals, lip, or anus in child or adolescent. History of sexual contact.*

## General Considerations

Syphilis is a chronic, generalized infectious disease caused by a spirochete, *Treponema pallidum.* In the acquired form, the disease is transmitted by sexual contact. Primary syphilis is characterized by the presence of an indurated painless chancre, which heals in 7–10 days. A secondary eruption involving the skin and mucous membranes appears in 4–6 weeks. After a long latency period, late lesions of tertiary syphilis involve the eyes, skin, bones, viscera, CNS, and cardiovascular system.

Congenital syphilis results from transplacental infection. Infection may result in stillbirth or produce illness in the newborn, in early infancy, or later in childhood. First-trimester fetal infection has been found in the products of conception in therapeutic abortions. Syphilis occurring in the newborn and young infant is comparable to secondary disease in the adult but is more severe and life-threatening. Late congenital syphilis (developing in childhood) is comparable to tertiary disease.

Congenital syphilis is increasing in the United States due to increasing primary and secondary syphilis in women of childbearing age, and perhaps due to inadequate diagnosis and treatment of syphilis in prenatal care programs.

## Clinical Findings

### A. SYMPTOMS AND SIGNS

#### 1. Congenital syphilis—

a. **Newborns**—Most newborns with congenital syphilis are asymptomatic. If not detected and treated, symptoms develop within weeks to months. When clinical signs are present, they usually consist of jaundice, anemia with or without thrombocytopenia, increase in nucleated red blood cells, hepatosplenomegaly, and edema. Overt signs of meningitis (bulging fontanelle, opisthotonos) may be present, but subclinical infection with CSF abnormalities is more likely.

**b. Young infants (3–12 weeks)**—The infant may appear normal for the first few weeks of life only to develop mucocutaneous lesions and pseudoparalysis of the arms or legs. Shotty lymphadenopathy may be felt. Hepatomegaly is universal, with splenomegaly in 50% of patients. Other signs of disease similar to those seen in the newborn may be present. Anemia has been reported as the only presenting manifestation of congenital syphilis in this age group. "Snuffles" (rhinitis), characterized by a profuse mucopurulent discharge that excoriates the upper lip, is present in 25% of patients. A syphilitic rash is common on the palms and soles but may occur anywhere on the body. The rash consists of bright red, raised maculopapular lesions that gradually fade. Moist lesions occur at the mucocutaneous junctions (nose, mouth, anus, genitals) and lead to fissuring and bleeding.

Syphilis in the young infant may lead to stigmata recognizable in later childhood, such as rhagades (scars) around the mouth or nose, a depressed bridge of the nose (saddle nose), and a high forehead (secondary to mild hydrocephalus associated with low-grade meningitis and frontal periostitis). The permanent upper central incisors may be peg-shaped with a central notch (Hutchinson teeth), and the cusps of the sixth-year molars may have a lobulated mulberry appearance.

**c. Children**—Bilateral interstitial keratitis (at age 6–12 years) is characterized by photophobia, increased lacrimation, and vascularization of the cornea associated with exudation. Chorioretinitis and optic atrophy may also be seen. Meningovascular syphilis (at age 2–10 years) is usually slowly progressive, with mental retardation, spasticity, abnormal pupillary response, speech defects, and abnormal CSF. Deafness sometimes occurs. Thickening of the periosteum of the anterior tibias produces saber shins. A bilateral effusion into the knee joints (Clutton joints) may occur but is not associated with sequelae. Gummas may develop in the nasal septum, palate, long bones, and subcutaneous tissues.

**2. Acquired syphilis**—The primary chancre of the genitals, mouth, or anus may occur as a result of intimate sexual contact. If the chancre is missed, signs of secondary syphilis, such as rash, fever, headache, and malaise, may be the first manifestation of the disease.

**B. LABORATORY FINDINGS**

**1. Darkfield microscopy**—Treponemes can be seen in scrapings from a chancre and from moist lesions.

**2. Serologic tests for syphilis**—There are two general types of serologic tests for syphilis: treponemal and nontreponemal. The latter (Venereal Disease Research Laboratory, or VDRL) is useful for screening and follow-up of known cases. A rapid test (the rapid plasma reagin, or RPR) is useful for screening, but positive sera should be examined further by quantitative nontreponemal and treponemal tests. Positive nontreponemal tests are confirmed with more specific fluorescent treponemal antibody absorbed, or FTA-ABS test. False-positive FTA-ABS tests are uncommon except with other spirochetal disease.

One or two weeks after the onset of primary syphilis (chancre), the FTA-ABS test becomes positive. The VDRL or a similar nontreponemal test usually turns positive a few days later. By the time the secondary stage has been reached, virtually all patients show both positive FTA-ABS and positive nontreponemal tests. During latent and tertiary syphilis, the VDRL may become negative, but the FTA-ABS test usually remains positive. The quantitative VDRL or a similar nontreponemal test should be used to follow-up treated cases (see following discussion).

Positive serologic tests in cord sera may represent passively transferred antibody rather than congenital infection and therefore must be supplemented by a combination of clinical and laboratory data. Elevated total cord IgM is a helpful but nonspecific finding. A specific IgM–FTA-ABS is available, but negative results are not conclusive and should not be relied on. Demonstration of characteristic treponemes by darkfield examination of material from a moist lesion (skin; nasal or other mucous membranes) is definitive. Serial measurement of quantitative VDRL is also very useful, because passively transferred antibody in the absence of active infection should decay with a normal half-life of about 18 days.

In one study, 15% of infants with congenital syphilis had negative cord blood serology, presumably due to maternal infection late in pregnancy.

**C. IMAGING**

Radiographic abnormalities are present in 90% of infants with symptoms of congenital syphilis and in 20% of asymptomatic infants. Metaphyseal lucent bands, periostitis, and a widened zone of provisional calcification may be present. Bilateral symmetrical osteomyelitis with pathologic fractures of the medial tibial metaphyses (Wimberger sign) is almost pathognomonic.

**Differential Diagnosis**

**A. CONGENITAL SYPHILIS**

**1. Newborns**—Sepsis, congestive heart failure, congenital rubella, toxoplasmosis, disseminated herpes simplex, cytomegalovirus infection, and hemolytic disease of the newborn have to be differentiated. A positive Coombs test and blood group incompatibility distinguish hemolytic disease.

**2. Young infants**—Injury to the brachial plexus, poliomyelitis, acute osteomyelitis, and septic arthritis must be differentiated from pseudoparalysis. Coryza due to viral infection often responds to symptomatic treatment. Rash (ammoniacal diaper rash) and scabies may be confused with a syphilitic eruption.

**3. Children**—Interstitial keratitis and bone lesions of tuberculosis are distinguished by positive tuberculin reaction and chest radiograph. Arthritis associated with syphilis is unaccompanied by systemic signs, and joints are nontender. Mental retardation, spasticity, and hyperactivity are shown to be of syphilitic origin by strongly positive serologic tests.

### B. ACQUIRED SYPHILIS

Herpes genitalis, traumatic lesions, and other venereal diseases must be differentiated.

## Prevention

A serologic test for syphilis should be performed at the initiation of prenatal care and repeated at delivery. In mothers at high risk for syphilis, repeated tests may be necessary. Serologic tests for syphilis may be negative on both the mother and the baby at the time of birth if the mother acquires syphilis near term. Adequate treatment of mothers with secondary syphilis before the last month of pregnancy reduces the incidence of congenital syphilis from 90% to less than 2%. Examination and serologic testing of sexual partners and siblings should also be done.

## Treatment

### A. SPECIFIC MEASURES

Penicillin is the drug of choice for *T pallidum* infection. If the patient is allergic to penicillin, erythromycin or one of the tetracyclines may be used.

**1. Congenital syphilis**—Infants born to seropositive mothers require careful examination and quantitative antitreponemal (VDRL, RPR) syphilis testing. The same quantitative antitreponemal test should be done on the infant as the one done on the mother so the titers can be compared. Maternal records regarding the diagnosis of syphilis, treatment, and follow-up titers should be reviewed. Infants should be further evaluated for congenital syphilis for any of the following circumstances:

- The maternal titer has increased fourfold.
- The infant's titer is at least fourfold greater than the maternal titer.

- Signs of syphilis are found on examination.
- Maternal syphilis was not treated or inadequately treated during pregnancy.
- Maternal treatment of syphilis with a nonpenicillin regimen, or the regimen or dose of medication is undocumented.
- Maternal syphilis treated during pregnancy, but therapy completed less than 4 weeks prior to delivery.
- Maternal syphilis treated appropriately during pregnancy, but without the appropriate decrease in maternal nontreponemal titers after treatment.

The complete evaluation of an infant for possible congenital syphilis includes complete blood count, liver function tests, long bone radiographs, CSF examination (cell counts, glucose, protein), CSF VDRL, and quantitative serologic tests. In addition, the placenta and umbilical cord should be examined pathologically using fluorescent antitreponemal antibody.

Treatment for congenital syphilis is indicated for infants with physical signs, umbilical cord or placenta positive for DFA-TP staining or darkfield examination, abnormal radiographs, elevated CSF protein or cell counts, reactive CSF VDRL, or serum quantitative nontreponemal titer that is more than fourfold higher than the maternal titer (using same test). Infants with proved or suspected congenital syphilis should receive either (1) aqueous crystalline penicillin G, 50,000 units/kg/dose intravenously q12h (if <1 week old) or q8h (if 1–4 weeks old) for 10 days; or (2) aqueous procaine penicillin G, 50,000 units/kg/dose intramuscularly once daily for 10 days. All infants diagnosed after age 4 weeks receive 50,000–60,000 units/kg/dose aqueous crystalline penicillin intravenously q6h for 10 days.

Additionally, treatment should be given to infants whose mothers have inadequately treated syphilis, to those whose mothers received treatment less than 1 month before delivery, to those whose mothers have undocumented or inadequate serologic response to therapy, and to those whose mothers were given nonpenicillin drugs to treat syphilis. In these instances, if the infant is asymptomatic, has a normal physical exam, normal CSF parameters, nonreactive CSF VDRL, normal bone films, quantitative nontreponemal titer less than fourfold of the mother's titer, and good follow-up is certain, some experts would give a single dose of penicillin G benzathine 50,000 units/kg intramuscularly. If there is any abnormality in the preceding evaluation or if the CSF testing is not interpretable, the full 10 days of intravenous penicillin should be given. Close clinical and serologic follow-up monthly is necessary.

Asymptomatic, seropositive, infants with normal physical examinations born to mothers who received adequate syphilis treatment (completed > 4 weeks prior to delivery) and whose mothers have an appropriate serologic response (fourfold or greater decrease in titer) to treatment may be at lower risk for congenital syphilis. Some experts believe complete laboratory and radiographic evaluation in these infants (CSF, long bone films) is not necessary. Those infants who meet the preceding criteria, have nontreponemal titers less than fourfold higher than maternal titers, and for whom follow-up is certain can be given benzathine penicillin G, 50,000 units/kg, administered intramuscularly in a single dose. Subsequently, the infants should be followed with quantitative serologic tests and physical examinations until the nontreponemal serologic test is negative (see follow-up). Rising titers or clinical signs usually occur within 4 months in infected infants, requiring a full evaluation (including CSF studies and long bone radiographs) and institution of intravenous penicillin therapy.

**a. Follow-up for congenital syphilis**—Children treated for congenital syphilis need physical examinations at 1 and 2 months after completion of therapy, and both physical examinations and quantitative VDRL or RPR tests should be performed at 3, 6, and 12 months after the end of therapy or until the tests become nonreactive. Repeat CSF examination, including a CSF VDRL test, every 6 months until normal is indicated for infants with a positive CSF VDRL reaction. A reactive CSF VDRL test at the 6-month interval is an indication for retreatment. Titers decline with treatment and are usually negative by 6 months. Repeat treatment is indicated for children with rising titers or stable titers that do not decline.

**2. Acquired syphilis of less than one year's duration**—Benzathine penicillin G (50,000 units/kg, given intramuscularly, to a maximum of 2.4 million units) is given to adolescents with primary, secondary, or latent disease of less than 1 year's duration. All children should have a CSF examination (with CSF VDRL) prior to commencing therapy, to exclude neurosyphilis. Adolescents and adults need a CSF examination if clinical signs or symptoms suggest neurologic involvement.

**3. Syphilis of more than one year's duration (late latent disease)**—Syphilis of more than 1 year's duration (without evidence of neurosyphilis) requires weekly intramuscular benzathine penicillin G therapy for 3 weeks. CSF examination and VDRL test should be done on all children and patients with coexisting HIV infection or neurologic symptoms. In addition, patients who have failed treatment or who were previously treated with an agent other than penicillin need a CSF examination and CSF VDRL.

**4. Neurosyphilis**—Aqueous crystalline penicillin G is recommended, 200,000–300,000 U/kg/d in four to six divided doses, given intravenously for 10–14 days. The maximum adult dose is 4 million units/dose. This regimen should possibly be followed by an intramuscular course of benzathine G penicillin, 50,000 U/kg given once a week for 3 consecutive weeks, to a maximum dose of 2.4 million units.

**B. GENERAL MEASURES**

Penicillin treatment of early congenital or secondary syphilis may result in a febrile Jarisch–Herxheimer reaction. Treatment is symptomatic, with careful follow-up and aspirin or acetaminophen, although transfusion may be necessary in infants with severe hemolytic anemia.

## Prognosis

Severe disease, if undiagnosed, may be fatal in the newborn. Complete cure can be expected if the young infant is given penicillin. Serologic reversal usually occurs within 1 year. Treatment of primary syphilis with penicillin is curative. Permanent neurologic sequelae may occur in meningovascular syphilis.

Centers for Disease Control and Prevention: Congenital syphilis–United States, 2000. JAMA 2001;286(5):529 [PMID: 11508285].

Guidelines for treatment of sexually transmitted diseases. MMWR 1998;47(RR-1):28.

# RELAPSING FEVER

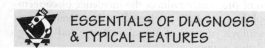

### ESSENTIALS OF DIAGNOSIS & TYPICAL FEATURES

- *Episodes of fever, chills, malaise.*
- *Occasional rash, arthritis, cough, hepatosplenomegaly, conjunctivitis.*
- *Diagnosis confirmed by direct microscopic identification of spirochetes in smears of peripheral blood.*

## General Considerations

Relapsing fever is a vector-borne disease caused by spirochetes of the genus *Borrelia*. Epidemic relapsing fever is transmitted to humans by body lice (*Pediculus humanus*) and endemic relapsing fever by soft-bodied ticks (genus *Ornithodoros*). Tick-borne relapsing fever is endemic in the western United States. Transmission usually takes place during the warm months, when ticks are active and recreation or work brings people into contact with *Ornithodoros* ticks. Infection is often acquired in mountain camping areas and cabins. The ticks are nocturnal feeders and remain attached for only 5–20 minutes. Consequently the patient seldom remembers a tick bite. Rarely, neonatal relapsing fever results from transplacental transmission of *Borrelia.* Both louse-borne and tick-borne relapsing fever may be acquired during foreign travel.

## Clinical Findings

### A. SYMPTOMS AND SIGNS

The incubation period is 4–18 days. The attack is sudden, with high fever, chills, tachycardia, nausea and vomiting, headache, myalgia, arthralgia, bronchitis, and a dry, nonproductive cough. Hepatomegaly and splenomegaly appear later. Meningeal irritation may be present. An erythematous rash may be seen over the trunk and extremities, and petechiae may be present. After 3–10 days, the fever falls by crisis. Jaundice, iritis, conjunctivitis, cranial nerve palsies, and hemorrhage occur more commonly during relapses.

The disease is characterized by relapses at intervals of 1–2 weeks and lasting 3–5 days. The relapses duplicate the initial attack but become progressively less severe. In louse-borne relapsing fever, there is usually a single relapse. In tick-borne infection, two to six relapses occur.

### B. LABORATORY FINDINGS

During febrile episodes, the patient's urine contains protein, casts, and occasionally erythrocytes; a marked polymorphonuclear leukocytosis is present; and, in about 25% of cases, the patient has a false-positive serologic test for syphilis. Examination of the peripheral blood smear is the diagnostic test of choice. Spirochetes can be found in the peripheral blood by direct microscopy in approximately 70% of cases by darkfield examination or by Wright, Giemsa, or acridine orange staining of thick and thin smears. Spirochetes are not found during afebrile periods. Immunofluorescent antibody (or ELISA confirmed by Western blot) can sometimes help establish the diagnosis serologically. However, high titers of *Borrelia hermsii* can cross-react with *Borrelia burgdorferi* (the agent in Lyme disease) in immunofluorescent antibody assay, ELISA, and Western blots. Serologic specimens can be sent to the Division of Vector-Borne Infectious Diseases, Centers for Disease Control and Prevention, Fort Collins, CO 80522.

## Differential Diagnosis

Relapsing fever may be confused with malaria, leptospirosis, dengue, typhus, rat-bite fever, Colorado tick fever, Rocky Mountain spotted fever, collagen vascular disease, or any fever of unknown origin.

## Complications

Complications include facial paralysis, iridocyclitis, optic atrophy, hypochromic anemia, pneumonia, nephritis, myocarditis, endocarditis, and seizures. CNS involvement occurs in 10–30% of patients.

## Treatment

For children younger than age 8 years who have tick-borne relapsing fever, standard dosages of penicillin or erythromycin should be given for 10 days. Older children may be given doxycycline. Chloramphenicol is also efficacious. Patients who are unable to take oral medications may be given intravenous penicillin G. In louse-borne relapsing fever, a single dose of tetracycline or erythromycin has been effective.

Severely ill patients should be hospitalized. Antibiotic treatment should be started after the fever has dropped, to reduce the risk of severe Jarisch–Herxheimer reaction. Isolation precautions are not necessary for relapsing fever. Contact precautions are recommended for patients with louse infestations.

## Prognosis

The mortality rate in treated cases of relapsing fever is very low, except in debilitated or very young children. With treatment, the initial attack is shortened and relapses prevented. The response to antimicrobial therapy is dramatic.

Cadavid D, Barbour AG: Neuroborreliosis during relapsing fever: Review of the clinical manifestations, pathology, and treatment of infections in humans and experimental animals. Clin Infect Dis 1998; 26:151.

Tickborne relapsing fever outbreak after a family gathering—New Mexico, August 2002. MMWR 2003;52(34):809.

## LEPTOSPIROSIS

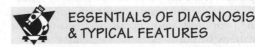

### ESSENTIALS OF DIAGNOSIS & TYPICAL FEATURES

- *Biphasic course lasting 2 or 3 weeks.*
- *Initial phase: high fever, headache, myalgia, and conjunctivitis.*
- *Apparent recovery for 2–3 days.*
- *Return of fever associated with meningitis.*

- *Jaundice, hemorrhages, and renal insufficiency (severe cases).*
- *Culture of organism from blood and CSF (early) and from urine (later), or direct microscopy of urine or CSF.*
- *Positive leptospiral agglutination test.*

## General Considerations

Leptospirosis is a zoonosis caused by many antigenically distinct but morphologically similar spirochetes. The organism enters through the skin or respiratory tract. Classically the severe form (Weil disease), with jaundice and a high mortality rate, was associated with infection with *Leptospira icterohaemorrhagiae* after immersion in water contaminated with rat urine. It is now known that a variety of animals (eg, dogs, rats, cattle) may serve as reservoirs for pathogenic *Leptospira,* that a given serogroup may have multiple animal species as hosts, and that severe disease may be caused by many different serogroups.

In the United States, leptospirosis usually occurs after contact with dogs. Cattle, swine, or rodents may transmit the organism. Sewer workers, farmers, abattoir workers, animal handlers, and soldiers are at risk for occupational exposure. Outbreaks have resulted from swimming in contaminated streams and harvesting field crops. In the United States, about 100 cases are reported yearly, and about one third are in children.

## Clinical Findings

### A. Symptoms and Signs

**1. Initial phase**—The incubation period is 4–19 days (mean, 10 days). Chills, fever, headache, myalgia, conjunctivitis (episcleral injection), photophobia, cervical lymphadenopathy, and pharyngitis occur commonly. The initial leptospiremic phase lasts for 3–7 days.

**2. Phase of apparent recovery**—Symptoms typically (but not always) subside for 2–3 days.

**3. Systemic phase**—Fever reappears and is associated with headache, muscular pain and tenderness in the abdomen and back, and nausea and vomiting. Lung, heart, and joint involvement occasionally occurs. These manifestations are due to extensive vasculitis.

   **a. Central nervous system involvement**—The CNS is involved in 50–90% of cases. Severe headache and mild nuchal rigidity are usual, but delirium, coma, and focal neurologic signs may be seen.

   **b. Renal and hepatic involvement**—In about 50% of cases, the kidney or liver is affected. Gross hematuria and oliguria or anuria is sometimes seen. Jaundice may be associated with an enlarged and tender liver.

   **c. Gallbladder involvement**—Leptospirosis may cause acalculous cholecystitis in children, demonstrable by abdominal ultrasound as a dilated, nonfunctioning gallbladder. Pancreatitis is unusual.

   **d. Hemorrhage**—Petechiae, ecchymoses, and gastrointestinal bleeding may be severe.

   **e. Rash**—A rash is seen in 10–30% of cases. It may be maculopapular and generalized or may be petechial or purpuric. Occasionally erythema nodosum is seen. Peripheral desquamation of the rash may occur. Gangrenous areas are sometimes noted over the distal extremities. In such cases, skin biopsy demonstrates the presence of severe vasculitis involving both the arterial and the venous circulations.

### B. Laboratory Findings

Leptospires are present in the blood and CSF only during the first 10 days of illness. They appear in the urine during the second week, where they may persist for 30 days or longer. The organism can be isolated from blood inoculated into Fletcher's semisolid medium or Ellinghausen–McCullough–Johnson–Harris (EMJH) semisolid medium, but culture techniques are slow (7–10 days), difficult, and not generally available.

The WBC count is often elevated, especially when there is liver involvement. Serum bilirubin levels usually remain below 20 mg/dL. Other liver function tests may be abnormal, although the aspartate transaminase (AST) usually is elevated only slightly. An elevated serum creatine kinase is frequently found. CSF shows moderate pleocytosis (<500/μL)—predominantly mononuclear cells—increased protein (50–100 mg/dL), and normal glucose. Urine often shows microscopic pyuria, hematuria, and, less often, moderate proteinuria (++ or greater). The ESR is elevated markedly. Chest radiograph may show pneumonitis.

Serologic antibodies measured by enzyme immunoassay may be demonstrated during or after the second week of illness. The serologic test of choice is a microscopic agglutination test using live organisms (performed at the CDC, Atlanta, GA 30333). Leptospiral agglutinins generally reach peak levels by the third to fourth week. A 1:100 titer is considered suspicious; a fourfold or greater rise is diagnostic. A PCR assay may be available at specialized research centers or through the CDC.

## Differential Diagnosis

Fever and myalgia associated with the characteristic episcleral injection should suggest leptospirosis. During the prodrome, malaria, typhoid fever, typhus, rheumatoid arthritis, brucellosis, and influenza may be suspected. Later, depending on the organ systems involved, a variety of other diseases need to be distinguished, including encephalitis, viral or tuberculous meningitis, viral hepatitis, glomerulonephritis, viral or bacterial pneumonia, rheumatic fever, subacute infective endocarditis, acute surgical abdomen, and Kawasaki disease (see Table 36–3).

## Prevention

Preventive measures include avoidance of contaminated water and soil, rodent control, immunization of dogs and other domestic animals, and good sanitation. Immunization or antimicrobial prophylaxis with doxycycline may be of value to certain high-risk occupational groups.

## Treatment

### A. SPECIFIC MEASURES

Aqueous penicillin G (150,000 units/kg/d, given in four to six divided doses intravenously for 7–10 days) should be given when the diagnosis is suspected. Studies in severely ill patients indicate a benefit even if treatment is started 4 days after onset. A Jarisch–Herxheimer reaction may occur. Oral doxycycline may be used for mildly ill patients.

### B. GENERAL MEASURES

Symptomatic and supportive care is indicated, particularly for renal and hepatic failure and hemorrhage.

## Prognosis

Leptospirosis is usually self-limiting and not characterized by jaundice. The disease usually lasts 1–3 weeks but may be more prolonged. Relapse may occur. There are usually no permanent sequelae associated with CNS infection, although headache may persist. The mortality rate in reported cases in the United States is 5%, usually from renal failure. The mortality rate may reach 20% or more in elderly patients who have severe kidney and hepatic involvement.

Levett PN: Leptospirosis. Clin Microbiol Rev 2001;14:296 [PMID: 11292640].

Plank R, Dean D: Overview of the epidemiology, microbiology, and pathogenesis of *Leptospira* spp. in humans. Microbes Infect 2000;2:1265 [PMID: 11008116].

Sertour N et al: Cluster of leptospirosis cases among children in France. Eur J Clin Microbiol Infect Dis 2002;21(7):560 [PMID: 12172752].

# LYME DISEASE

## ESSENTIALS OF DIAGNOSIS & TYPICAL FEATURES

- *Characteristic skin lesion (erythema migrans) 3–30 days after tick bite.*
- *Arthritis, usually pauciarticular, occurring about 4 weeks after appearance of skin lesion. Headache, chills, and fever.*
- *Residence or travel in an endemic area during the late spring to early fall.*

## General Considerations

Lyme disease is a subacute or chronic spirochetal infection caused by *Borrelia burgdorferi* and transmitted by the bite of an infected deer tick (*Ixodes* species). The disease was known in Europe for many years as tickborne encephalomyelitis, often associated with a characteristic rash (erythema migrans). Discovery of the agent and vector followed investigation of an outbreak of pauciarticular arthritis in Lyme, Connecticut, in 1977.

Although cases are reported from many countries, the most prominent endemic areas in the United States include the Northeast, upper Midwest, and West Coast. The northern European countries also have high rates of infection. More than 17,000 cases were reported in the United States in 2003. The disease is spreading as a result of increased infection in and distribution of the tick vector. Most cases with rash are recognized in spring and summer, when most tick bites occur; however, because the incubation period for joint and neurologic disease may be months, cases may present at any time. *Ixodes* ticks are very small, and their bite is often unrecognized.

## Clinical Findings

### A. SYMPTOMS AND SIGNS

Erythema migrans, the most characteristic feature of Lyme disease, develops in 60–80% of patients. Between 3 and 30 days after the bite, a ring of erythema develops at the site and spreads over days. It may attain a diameter of 20 cm. The center of the lesion may clear (resembling tinea corporis), remain red, or become raised (suggesting a chemical or infectious cellulitis). Many patients are otherwise asymptomatic. Some have fever (usually low-grade), headache, and myalgias. Multiple satellite skin lesions, urticaria, or diffuse erythema may occur. Untreated, the rash lasts days to 3 weeks.

In up to 50% of patients, arthritis develops several weeks to months after the bite. Recurrent attacks of migratory, monarticular, or pauciarticular arthritis involving the knees and other large joints occur. Each attack lasts for days to a few weeks. Fever is common and may be high. Complete resolution between attacks is typical. Chronic arthritis develops in less than 10% of patients, more often in those with the DR4 haplotype.

Neurologic manifestations develop in up to 20% of patients and usually consist of Bell palsy, aseptic meningitis (which may be indistinguishable from viral meningitis), or polyradiculitis. Peripheral neuritis, Guillain–Barré syndrome, encephalitis, ataxia, chorea, and other cranial neuropathies are less common. Seizures suggest another diagnosis. Untreated, the neurologic symptoms are usually self-limited but may be chronic or permanent. Although the fatigue and nonspecific neurologic symptoms may be prolonged in a few patients, Lyme disease is not proved to be a cause of chronic fatigue syndrome.

Self-limited heart block or myocardial dysfunction occurs in about 5% of patients.

## B. LABORATORY FINDINGS

Most patients with only rash have normal laboratory tests. Children with arthritis may have moderately elevated ESRs and WBC counts; the antinuclear antibodies and rheumatoid factor tests are negative or nonspecific; streptococcal antibodies are not elevated. Circulating IgM cryoglobulins may be present. Joint fluid may show up to 100,000 cells with a polymorphonuclear predominance, normal glucose, and elevated protein and immune complexes; Gram stain and culture are negative. In patients with CNS involvement, the CSF may show lymphocytic pleocytosis and elevated protein; the glucose and all cultures and stains are normal or negative. Abnormal nerve conduction may be present with peripheral neuropathy.

## Diagnosis

Lyme disease is a clinical diagnosis. History, physical examination, and laboratory features are important to consider. The causative organism is difficult to culture. Serologic testing may support the clinical diagnosis. Antibody testing should be performed in experienced laboratories. Serologic diagnosis of Lyme disease is based on a two-test approach: an ELISA and an immunoblot to confirm a positive or indeterminate ELISA. Antibodies may not be detectable until several weeks after infection has occurred; therefore, serologic testing in children with a typical rash is not recommended. Therapy early in disease may blunt antibody

titers. Recent studies have shown considerable intralaboratory and interlaboratory variability in titers reported. Overdiagnosis of Lyme disease based on atypical symptoms and positive serology appears to be common. Sera from patients with syphilis, HIV, and leptospirosis may give false-positive results for Lyme disease. Patients who receive appropriate treatment for Lyme disease may remain seropositive for several years. Diagnosis of CNS disease requires objective abnormalities of the neurologic examination, laboratory or radiographic studies, and consistent positive serology.

## Differential Diagnosis

Aside from the disorders already mentioned, the rash may resemble pityriasis, erythema multiforme, a drug eruption, or erythema nodosum. Erythema migrans is nonscaly, minimally tender or nontender, and persists longer in the same place than many of the more common childhood erythematous rashes. The arthritis may resemble juvenile rheumatoid arthritis, reactive arthritis, septic arthritis, reactive effusion from a contiguous osteomyelitis, rheumatic fever, leukemic arthritis, systemic lupus erythematosus, and Henoch–Schönlein purpura. Spontaneous resolution in a few days to weeks helps differentiate Lyme disease from juvenile rheumatoid arthritis, in which arthritis lasting a minimum of 6 weeks is required for diagnosis. The neurologic signs may suggest idiopathic Bell palsy, viral or parainfectious meningitis or meningoencephalitis, lead poisoning, psychosomatic illness, and many other conditions.

## Prevention

Prevention consists of avoidance of endemic areas, wearing long sleeves and pants, frequent checks for ticks, and application of tick repellents. Ticks usually are attached for 24–48 hours before transmission of Lyme disease occurs. Ticks should be removed with a tweezer by pulling gently without twisting or excessive squeezing of the tick. Permethrin sprayed on clothing decreases tick attachment. Repellents containing high concentrations of DEET may be neurotoxic and should be used cautiously and washed off when tick exposure ends. The CDC does not recommend prophylactic antibiotics for tick bites in asymptomatic individuals.

A Lyme vaccine was licensed for use in persons age 15–70 years, but was withdrawn and is not available.

## Treatment

Antimicrobial therapy is beneficial in most cases of Lyme disease. It is most effective if started early. Prolonged treatment is important for all forms. Relapses occur in some patients on all regimens.

## A. RASH, OTHER EARLY INFECTIONS

Amoxicillin, 25–50 mg/kg/d, given orally in two divided doses (to a maximum of 2 g/d) for 14–21 days can be used for children of all ages. Doxycycline (100 mg, given orally bid) for 14–21 days may be used for children older than age 8 years. Erythromycin (30 mg/kg/d) or cefuroxime is used in penicillin-allergic children, although erythromycin may be less effective than amoxicillin.

## B. ARTHRITIS

The amoxicillin or doxycycline regimen (same dosage as for the rash) should be used, but treatment should continue for 4 weeks. Parenteral ceftriaxone (75–100 mg/kg/d) or penicillin G (300,000 units/kg/d, given intravenously in four divided doses for 2–4 weeks) is used for persistent arthritis.

## C. BELL PALSY

The same oral drug regimens may be used for 3–4 weeks.

## D. OTHER NEUROLOGIC DISEASE OR CARDIAC DISEASE

Parenteral therapy for 2–3 weeks is recommended with either ceftriaxone (75–100 kg/d in one daily dose) or penicillin G (300,000 units/kg/d intravenously in four divided doses).

Eppes SC: Diagnosis, treatment and prevention of Lyme disease in children. Paediatr Drugs 2003;5(6):363 [PMID: 12765486].

Eppes SC, Childs JA: Comparative study of cefuroxime axetil versus amoxicillin in children with early Lyme disease. Pediatrics 2002;109(6):1173 [PMID: 12042561].

Moss WJ, Dumler JS: Simultaneous infection with *Borrelia burgdorferi* and human granulocytic ehrlichiosis. Pediatr Infect Dis J 2003;22(1):91 [PMID: 12553302].

Thorstrand C et al: Successful treatment of neuroborreliosis with ten day regimens. Pediatr Infect Dis J 2002;21(12):1142 [PMID: 12488665].

Vazquez M et al: Long-term neuropsychologic and health outcomes of children with facial nerve palsy attributable to Lyme disease. Pediatrics 2003;112(2):e93 [PMID: 12897313].

http://www.cdc.gov/ncidod/dvbid/lyme

## REFERENCES

Pickering LK et al (eds): *2003 Red Book: Report of the Committee on Infectious Diseases,* 26th ed. American Academy of Pediatrics, 2003.

# Infections: Parasitic & Mycotic   39

*Adriana Weinberg, MD, & Myron J. Levin, MD*

---

## ■ I. INFECTIONS: PARASITIC

Parasitic diseases are common and may present clinically in a variety of ways (Table 39–1). Although travel to endemic areas suggests particular infections, many are transmitted through fomites or acquired from contact with human carriers and can occur anywhere. Some of the less common parasitic infections and those seen primarily in the developing world are presented in abbreviated form in Table 39–2.

### Selection of Patients for Evaluation

The incidence of parasitic infections varies greatly with geographic area. Children who have traveled or lived in areas where parasitic infections are endemic are at risk for infection with a variety of intestinal and tissue parasites. Children who have resided only in developed countries are usually free of tissue parasites (except *Toxoplasma*). Searching for intestinal parasites is expensive for the patient and time-consuming for the laboratory. More than 90% of ova and parasite examinations performed in most hospital laboratories in the United States are negative; many have been ordered inappropriately. An approach to determining which children with diarrhea need such examinations is presented in Figure 39–1. It can be more cost-effective to treat symptomatic US immigrants with albendazole or nitazoxanide, broad-spectrum antiparasitic drugs, and to investigate only those whose symptoms persist.

Immunodeficient children are very susceptible to protozoal intestinal infections. Multiple opportunists are frequently identified, and the threshold for ordering tests should be low for these children.

### Specimen Processing

For tissue parasites, contact the laboratory for proper collection procedures. Diarrheal stools may contain trophozoites that die rapidly during transport. The specimen should be either examined immediately or placed in a stool fixative such as polyvinyl alcohol. Fixative vials for home collection of stool are available. They may contain toxic compounds, so they should be stored safely. Fixed specimens are stable at room temperature. Formed stools usually contain cysts that are more stable. It is best to fix these also after collection, but they may be reliably examined after transport at room temperature.

### Eosinophilia & Parasitic Infections

Although parasites commonly cause eosinophilia, in developed countries other causes are much more common and include allergies, drugs, and other infections. Heavy intestinal nematode infections cause eosinophilia; they are easily detected on a single ova and parasite examination. Light nematode infections and common protozoal infections—giardiasis, cryptosporidiosis, and amebiasis—rarely cause eosinophilia. Eosinophilia is also unusual or minimal in more serious infections such as amebic liver abscess, toxoplasmosis, and malaria.

The most common parasitic infection in the United States that causes significant eosinophilia with negative stool examination is toxocariasis. In a young child with unexplained eosinophilia and a negative stool examination, a serologic test for *Toxocara* may be the next appropriate test. Trichinosis is a rare cause of marked eosinophilia; strongyloidiasis is a cause of eosinophilia that may be difficult to diagnose with stool examinations. The differential diagnosis of eosinophilia is broad for patients who have been in developing countries.

Muening P et al: The cost effectiveness of strategies for the treatment of intestinal parasites in immigrants. N Engl J Med 1999;340:773 [PMID: 10072413].

***Table 39–1.*** Symptoms of parasitic infection.

| Sign | Agent | Comments[a] |
|------|-------|-------------|
| Abdominal pain | *Anisakis* | Shortly after raw fish ingestion. |
| | *Ascaris* | Heavy infection may obstruct bowel, biliary tract. |
| | *Clonorchis* | Heavy, early infection. Hepatomegaly later. |
| | *Entamoeba histolytica* | Hematochezia, variable fever, diarrhea. |
| | *Fasciola hepatica* | Diarrhea, vomiting. |
| | Hookworm | Iron deficiency anemia with heavy infection. |
| | *Strongyloides* | Eosinophilia, pruritus. May resemble peptic disease. |
| | *Trichinella* | Myalgia, periorbital edema, eosinophilia. |
| | *Trichuris* | Diarrhea, dysentery with heavy infection. |
| Cough | *Ascaris* | Wheezing, eosinophilia during migration phase. |
| | *Paragonimus westermani* | Hemoptysis; chronic. May mimic tuberculosis. |
| | *Strongyloides* | Wheezing, pruritus, eosinophilia during migration or dissemination. |
| | *Toxocara* | Affects ages 1–5 y; hepatosplenomegaly; eosinophilia. |
| | Tropical eosinophilia | Pulmonary infiltrates, eosinophilia. |
| Diarrhea | *Blastocystis* | Possibly with heavy infection in immunosuppressed or immunocompetent individuals. |
| | *Cryptosporidium* | Watery; prolonged in normals, chronic in immunosuppressed individuals. |
| | *Dientamoeba fragilis* | Only with heavy infection. |
| | *Entamoeba histolytica* | Hematochezia, variable fever; no eosinophilia. |
| | *Giardia* | Afebrile, chronic; anorexia; no hematochezia or eosinophilia. |
| | *Schistosoma* | Chronic; hepatosplenomegaly (some types). |
| | *Strongyloides* | Abdominal pain; eosinophilia. |
| | *Trichinella* | Myalgia, periorbital edema, eosinophilia. |
| | *Trichuris* | With heavy infection. |
| Dysentery | *Balantidium coli* | Swine contact. |
| | *Entamoeba histolytica* | Few to no leukocytes in stool; fever; hematochezia. |
| | *Schistosoma* | During acute infection. |
| | *Trichuris* | With heavy infection. |
| Dysuria | *Enterobius* | Usually girls with worms in urethra, bladder; nocturnal, perianal pruritus. |
| | *Schistosoma* | Hematuria. Exclude bacteriuria, stones (some types). |
| Headache | *Angiostrongylus* | Eosinophilic meningitis. |
| (and other cerebral | *Naegleria* | Fresh-water swimming; rapidly progressive meningoencephalitis. |
| symptoms) | *Plasmodium* | Fever, chills, jaundice, splenomegaly. Cerebral ischemia (with *P falciparum*). |
| | *Taenia solium* | Cysticercosis. Focal seizures, deficits; hydrocephalus, aseptic meningitis. |
| | *Toxoplasma* | Meningoencephalitis (especially in the immunosuppressed); hydrocephalus in infants. |
| | *Trypanosoma* | African forms. Chronic lethargy (sleeping sickness). |

*(continued)*

*Table 39–1.* Symptoms of parasitic infection. (continued)

| Sign | Agent | Comments[a] |
|------|-------|-------------|
| Pruritus | *Ancylostoma braziliense* | Creeping eruption; dermal serpiginous burrow. |
| | *Enterobius* | Perianal, nocturnal. |
| | Filaria | Variable; seen in many filarial diseases. |
| | Hookworm | Local at penetration site in heavy exposure. |
| | *Strongyloides* | Diffuse with migration; may be recurrent. |
| | *Trypanosoma* | African forms; one of many nonspecific symptoms. |
| Fever | *Entamoeba histolytica* | With acute dysentery or liver abscess. |
| | *Leishmania donovani* | Hepatosplenomegaly, anemia, leukopenia. |
| | *Plasmodium* | Chills, headache, jaundice; periodic. |
| | *Toxocara* | Cough, hepatosplenomegaly, eosinophilia. |
| | *Toxoplasma* | Generalized adenopathy; splenomegaly. |
| | *Trichinella* | Myalgia, periorbital edema, eosinophilia. |
| | *Trypanosoma* | Early stage, African forms; lymphadenopathy. |
| Anemia | *Diphyllobothrium* | Megaloblastic due to $B_{12}$ deficiency; rare. |
| | Hookworm | Iron deficiency. |
| | *Leishmania donovani* | Fever, hepatosplenomegaly, leukopenia (kala-azar). |
| | *Plasmodium* | Hemolysis. |
| | *Trichuris* | Heavy infection due to iron loss. |
| Eosinophilia | *Angiostrongylus* | Eosinophilic meningitis. |
| | *Fasciola* | Abdominal pain. |
| | Filaria | Microfilariae in blood. Lymphadenopathy. |
| | *Onchocerca* | Skin nodules, keratitis. |
| | *Schistosoma* | Chronic; intestinal or genitourinary symptoms. |
| | *Strongyloides* | Abdominal pain, diarrhea. |
| | *Toxocara* | Hepatosplenomegaly, cough; affects ages 1–5 y. |
| | *Trichinella* | Myalgia, periorbital edema. |
| | Tropical pulmonary eosinophilia | Cough. |
| Hematuria | *Schistosoma* | *S haematobium.* Bladder, urethral granulomas. Exclude stones, bacteriuria. |
| Hemoptysis | *Paragonimus westermani* | Lung fluke. Variable chest pain; chronic. |
| Hepatomegaly | *Clonorchis* | Heavy infection. Tenderness early; cirrhosis late. |
| | *Echinococcus* | Chronic; cysts. |
| | *Entamoeba histolytica* | Toxic hepatitis or abscess. No eosinophilia. |
| | *Leishmania donovani* | Splenomegaly, fever, pancytopenia. |
| | *Schistosoma* | Chronic; hepatic fibrosis, splenomegaly (some types). |
| | *Toxocara* | Splenomegaly, eosinophilia, cough; no adenopathy. |

(continued)

***Table 39–1.*** Symptoms of parasitic infection. (continued)

| Sign | Agent | Comments[a] |
|---|---|---|
| Splenomegaly | *Leishmania donovani* | Hepatomegaly, fever, anemia. |
| | *Plasmodium* | Fever, chills, jaundice, headache. |
| | *Schistosoma* | Hepatomegaly. |
| | *Toxocara* | Eosinophilia, hepatomegaly. |
| | *Toxoplasma* | Lymphadenopathy, other symptoms. |
| Lymphadenopathy | Filaria | Inguinal typical; chronic. |
| | *Leishmania donovani* | Hepatosplenomegaly, pancytopenia, fever. |
| | *Schistosoma* | Acute infection; fever, rash, arthralgia, hepatosplenomegaly. |
| | *Toxoplasma* | Cervical common; may involve single site; splenomegaly. |
| | *Trypanosoma* | Localized near bite or generalized hepatosplenomegaly (Chagas disease); generalized (especially posterior cervical) in African forms. |

[a]Symptoms usually related to degree of infestation. Infestation with small numbers of organisms is often asymptomatic.

# PROTOZOAL INFECTIONS

## SYSTEMIC INFECTIONS

### 1. Malaria

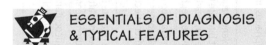

### ESSENTIALS OF DIAGNOSIS & TYPICAL FEATURES

- *Residence in or travel to an endemic area.*
- *Cyclic paroxysms of chills, fever, and intense sweating.*
- *Headache, backache, cough, abdominal pain, nausea, vomiting, diarrhea.*
- *Coma, seizures.*
- *Splenomegaly, anemia.*
- *Malaria parasites in peripheral blood smear.*

## General Considerations

Malaria kills a million children worldwide each year and is undergoing a resurgence in areas where it was previously controlled. Approximately 1000 imported cases are diagnosed in the United States each year, but local transmission may also occasionally take place. The female anopheline mosquito transmits the parasites—*Plasmodium vivax* (most common), *P falciparum* (most virulent), *P ovale* (similar to *P vivax*), and *P malariae*.

The gametocytes ingested from an infected human form sporozoites in the mosquito; when inoculated into a susceptible host, these sporozoites infect hepatocytes. The preerythrocytic phase (hepatic) is about 1–2 weeks for all but *P malariae* infection (3–5 weeks), but the initial symptoms may be delayed for up to a year in *P falciparum*, 4 years in *P vivax*, and decades in *P malariae* infections. Merozoites released into the circulation from hepatocytes infect red cells (young cells by *P vivax* and *P ovale*, old cells by *P malariae*, and all cells by *P falciparum*) and begin the synchronous erythrocytic cycles—rupturing the infected cells at regular 48- or 72-h intervals. Asynchronous cycles causing daily fevers are most common in early stages of infection. Survival is associated with a progressive decrease in intensity of cycles; relapses years later may occur from persistent hepatic infection, which occurs in *P vivax* and *P ovale* infections. Infection acquired congenitally or from transfusions or needle sticks does not result in a hepatic phase.

Susceptibility varies genetically; certain red cell phenotypes are partially resistant to *P falciparum* infection (hemoglobin S, hemoglobin F, thalassemia, and possibly glucose-6-phosphate dehydrogenase deficiency). The worldwide distribution of the four species is determined, to some extent, by host genetic factors. The absence of *P vivax* from Africa reflects the lack of specific Duffy blood group substances among most native Africans. Recurrent infections result in some natural species-specific immunity; this does not prevent infection but does decrease parasitemia and symptoms. Normal splenic function is an important factor because of

**Table 39–2.** Some parasitic infections seen less commonly in developed regions.

| Agent (Disease) | Geographic Region | Vector | Symptoms and Signs | Laboratory Findings | Diagnosis | Therapy and Comments |
|---|---|---|---|---|---|---|
| *Trypanosoma cruzi* (Chagas disease) | South and Central America, Mexico | Reduviid bug | Acute: painful red nodule at bite site, conjunctivitis, periorbital edema (Romaña sign), fever, local ± generalized adenitis. Late: myocarditis, megaesophagus, megacolon. | Mononuclear leukocytosis | Organisms in peripheral blood. Positive serology. | Nifurtimox or benznidazole may help early. No therapy for late disease. May be transmitted by blood transfusion or congenitally. |
| *Trypanosoma brucei* (sleeping sickness) | Africa | Tsetse fly | Hepatosplenomegaly, adenopathy. Nodule at bite site (resolves). Recurrent fever, headache, myalgia, progressive encephalitis. | Elevated ESR, anemia, CSF pleocytosis | Organisms in blood, CSF, marrow, nodes. Positive serology. | Suramin, eflornithine, fentamidine, Melortopol. |
| *Leishmania donovani* (kala-azar) | Mideast, India, Mediterranean, South and Central America | Sandfly | Fever, generalized adenopathy, hepatosplenomegaly weeks to months after infection. | Pancytopenia, hypergammaglobulinemia | Organisms in marrow, nodes, spleen. Positive serology. | Sodium stibogluconate, meglumine antimonate, pentamidine, amphotericin B. |
| *Leishmania tropica* (Oriental sore) | Asia, India, North Africa | Sandfly | Papule at bite site (usually on face, limbs) develops after weeks to months, then ulcerates and scars. | — | Organisms in skin biopsy. Positive skin test, serology. | Same as for *L donovani*. |
| *Leishmania braziliensis*, *L mexicana* (chiclero ulcer) | South America | Sandfly | Painful mucocutaneous ulcers or granulomas. Nasolabial lesions common. | — | Skin biopsy. Positive skin test, serology. | Same as for *L donovani*; ketoconazole. |

| | | | | | | |
|---|---|---|---|---|---|---|
| Wuchereria, Brugia (filariasis) | Tropics, subtropics | Mosquito | Chronic adenopathy, often inguinal. Obstructive lymphedema. | Eosinophilia | Concentrated blood smears for larvae. Positive serology. | Ivermectin, diethylcarbamazine kill larvae. Surgery for lymphatic obstruction. |
| Angiostrongylus cantonensis (eosinophilic meningitis) | Hawaii, Asia, Pacific Islands | Snails, slugs | Ingestion (usually inadvertent) followed in 1–4 wk by meningitis of variable severity. Paresthesias. | Eosinophils in CSF and blood | Positive serology. Larvae may be present in CSF. | Fever absent or low. No focal lesions on CNS imaging. No specific therapy. Steroids may be beneficial. Mebendazole may help. |
| Paragonimus westermani (lung fluke infection) | Asia, South America, Africa | Raw crabs, crustaceans | Cough, hemoptysis. Rarely seizures, other CNS signs if migration to brain occurs. | — | Large ova in concentrated specimens, feces. Cystic nodular lesions on chest radiograph or CNS imaging. | Resembles pulmonary tuberculosis. Praziquantel very effective. |
| Clonorchis sinensis (liver fluke infection) | Asia | Raw fish | Adult flukes obstruct biliary tree. Acute: hepatomegaly, fever, jaundice, urticaria. Late: cirrhosis, carcinoma. | Variable liver function abnormalities | Ova in feces. | Praziquantel. Advanced disease not treatable. Liver transplant. |

CNS = central nervous system; ESR = erythrocyte sedimentation rate.

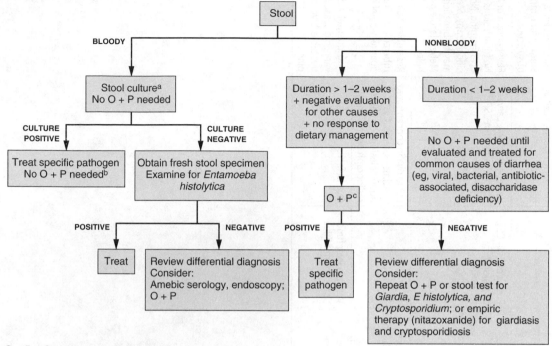

**Figure 39–1.** Parasitologic evaluation of acute diarrhea.

O + P = Ova and parasite examination.

[a] *Shigella, Salmonella, Campylobacter, E. coli (Escherichia coli)* 0157, *Yersinia*; assay for *Clostridium difficile* toxin if recent antimicrobial use.

[b] Unless critically ill, from endemic area for amebiasis, or unresponsive to standard therapy.

[c] Include examination for *Cryptosporidium and cyclospora*; immediate stool fixation needed if stool is diarrheal.

the immunologic and filter function of the spleen. Asplenic persons develop rapidly progressive malaria with many circulating infected erythrocytes (including mature forms of *P falciparum*). Maternal immunity protects the neonate.

## Clinical Findings

### A. Symptoms and Signs

Clinical manifestations vary according to species, strain, and host immunity. The infant presents with recurrent bouts of fever, irritability, poor feeding, vomiting, jaundice, and splenomegaly. Rash is usually absent, which helps distinguish malaria from viral infections in patients presenting with similar symptoms. In older children, the pathognomonic constellation of headache, backache, chills, myalgia, and fatigue is more easily elicited. Fever may be cyclic (every 48 hours for all but *P malariae* infection, in which it occurs every 72 hours) or irregular (most commonly observed with *P falciparum*). Between attacks, patients may look quite well. If the disease is untreated, relapses cease within a year in

*P falciparum* and within several years in *P vivax* infections but may recur decades later with *P malariae* infection. Infection during pregnancy often causes intrauterine growth retardation or premature delivery but rarely true fetal infection.

Physical examination in patients with uncomplicated cases may show only mild splenomegaly and anemia.

### B. Laboratory Findings

The diagnosis of malaria relies on detection of one or more of the four human plasmodia in blood smears. Most acute infections are caused by *P vivax, P ovale,* or *P falciparum,* although 5–7% are due to multiple species. Giemsa-stained thick smears offer the highest diagnostic accuracy for malaria parasites. Identification of the *Plasmodium* species relies on morphologic criteria (Table 39–3) and requires an experienced observer.

Alternative techniques of similar or higher diagnostic accuracy for *P falciparum* include enzyme-linked immunosorbent assay (ELISA), DNA hybridization, and polymerase chain reactors (PCR). A unique feature of

**Table 39–3.** Differentiation of malaria parasites on blood smears.

|  | *Plasmodium falciparum* | *P vivax, P ovale* |
|---|---|---|
| Multiple infected erythrocytes | Common | Rare |
| Mature trophozoites or schizonts | Absent[a] | Common |
| Schüffner dots | Absent | Common |
| Enlarged erythrocytes | Absent | Common |
| Banana-shaped gametocytes | Common | Absent |

[a]Usually sequestered in the microcirculation. Rare cases with circulating forms have extremely high parasitemia and a poor prognosis.

the microscopic examination is the semiquantitative estimate of the parasitemia, which is best done on thin smears. This information is particularly useful in the management of infections caused by *P falciparum,* in which high parasitemia (more than 10% infected erythrocytes or more than 500,000 infected erythrocytes/μL) is associated with high morbidity and mortality and requires hospitalization. Treatment response of *P falciparum* and chloroquine-resistant *P vivax* infections is best monitored by daily parasitemia assays: Constant or increased number of infected erythrocytes after 48 hours of treatment or after the second hemolytic crisis suggests an inadequate therapeutic response. Other laboratory findings that reflect the severity of hemolysis include decreased hematocrit, hemoglobin, and haptoglobin levels; increased reticulocyte count; and hyperbilirubinemia and increased lactate dehydrogenase (LDH). Thrombocytopenia is common, but the incidence of leukocytosis is variable.

## Differential Diagnosis

Relapsing fever may be associated with borreliosis, brucellosis, sequential common infections, Hodgkin disease, juvenile rheumatoid arthritis, rat-bite fever, or one of the idiopathic periodic fevers. Other common causes of high fever and headache include influenza, *Mycoplasma pneumoniae* or enteroviral infection, sinusitis, meningitis, enteric fever, tuberculosis, occult pneumonia, or bacteremia. Fever, headache, and jaundice in a patient returning from tropical areas indicate that leptospirosis and yellow fever should be included in the differential diagnosis. Malaria may also coexist with other diseases.

## Complications & Sequelae

Severe complications are limited to *P falciparum* infection and result from microvascular obstruction and tissue ischemia. Impaired consciousness and seizures are the most common complications of malaria in children. In addition, respiratory failure, renal impairment, severe bleeding, and shock are associated with a poor prognosis. Among the laboratory abnormalities, hypoglycemia, acidosis, elevated aminotransferases, and parasitemia greater than 10% characterize severe malaria.

## Prevention

Malaria chemoprophylaxis should be instituted 2 weeks (weekly regimens) to 2 days (daily regimens) before traveling to an area of endemic infection to permit changes if the drug is not tolerated. Because the antimalarial drugs recommended for prophylaxis do not kill sporozoites, therapy should be continued for 1 week (atovaquone/proguanil) or 4 weeks (all other regimens) after returning from an endemic area to cover infection acquired at departure.

Chloroquine is the drug of choice for prophylaxis of *P vivax, P ovale, P malariae,* and chloroquine-sensitive *P falciparum* (Table 39–4). Chloroquine is safe for all ages and during pregnancy. Side effects (dizziness, blurred vision, headache) can be reduced by administering half of the weekly dose twice per week. Effects of chloroquine on heart rhythm are infrequent and are typically associated with rapid intravenous infusion or overdosage. Chloroquine has immunosuppressive properties and has been reported to impair immunization against rabies but not against yellow fever.

For chloroquine-resistant *P falciparum,* the regimens of choice are weekly mefloquine, daily doxycycline, or daily atovaquone/proguanil. The side effects of mefloquine are headache, dizziness, and blurred vision. This drug is now considered safe during pregnancy but is not used in children weighing less than 15 kg. Daily doxycycline is recommended for patients older than age 8 years who are unable to tolerate mefloquine. Women on prolonged doxycycline therapy tend to develop yeast vaginitis, and it is advisable to supply them with nystatin suppositories. Atovaquone/proguanil is better tolerated than mefloquine. For optimal absorption, this drug should be administered with food or no later than 45 minutes after a meal. Daily primaquine is also effective. Primaquine is also used to prevent relapse of *P vivax* or *P ovale* infections. Primaquine is contraindicated for patients with glucose-6-phosphate dehydrogenase (G6PD) deficiency, in whom it induces hemolysis. Less effective alternatives include chloroquine plus proguanil or chloroquine alone, with one therapeutic dose of pyrimethamine/sulfadoxine made available for

***Table 39–4.*** Chemoprophylaxis of malaria.[a]

| Drug | Dosage |
|---|---|
| **Chloroquine-sensitive areas**[b] | |
| Chloroquine | 5 mg base/kg/wk up to 300 mg (adult dose) |
| **Chloroquine-resistant areas** | |
| Mefloquine | 0.25 tablet (62.5 mg) once a week (15–19 kg)<br>0.5 tablet (125 mg) (20–30 kg)<br>0.75 tablet (187.5 mg) (31–45 kg)<br>1 tablet (250 mg) (> 45 kg) |
| Doxycycline | 2 mg/kg/d (age > 8 years) up to 100 mg (adult dose) |
| Atovaquone/proguanil | 11–20 kg: 62.5 mg/25 mg daily<br>21–30 kg: 125 mg/50 mg<br>31–40 kg: 187.5 mg/75 mg<br>> 40 kg: 250 mg/100 mg |
| Primaquine | 0.5 mg/kg base daily up to 30 mg (adult dose) |
| Chloroquine | As above |
| **plus** | |
| Proguanil | 50 mg daily (age < 2 y)<br>100 mg (age 2–6 y)<br>150 mg (age 7–10 y)<br>200 mg (age > 10 y) |
| **or** | |
| Pyrimethamine-sulfadoxine for presumptive treatment (carry a single dose for self-treatment of febrile illness when medical care is not immediately available) | < 1 y: 1/4 tablet<br>1–3 y: 1/2 tablet<br>4–8 y: 1 tablet<br>9–14 y: 2 tablets<br>> 14 y: 3 tablets |
| **Relapse of *P vivax* or *P ovale*[c]** | |
| Primaquine | 0.3 mg base/kg/d up to 15 mg (adult dose) during the last 2 wk of prophylaxis |

[a]Updated malaria chemoprophylaxis information may be obtained by calling the Centers for Disease Control and Prevention Hot Line at 404-332-4555 or on the web at www.cdc.gov.
[b]Chloroquine-resistant *Plasmodium falciparum* has not yet been identified in Central America west of the Panama Canal zone, Haiti, Dominican Republic, Mexico, and most of the Middle East.
[c]Optional. Observation and prompt initiation of treatment when relapse occurs is sufficient.

self-treatment in the advent of potential breakthrough, signaled by fever, in areas where medical attention is not readily available.

No drug regimen guarantees protection against malaria. If fever develops within 1 year (particularly within 2 months) after travel to an endemic area, patients should be advised to seek medical attention. Insect repellents, insecticide-impregnated bed nets, and proper clothing are important adjuncts for malaria prophylaxis.

## Treatment

Treatment for malaria includes a variety of supportive strategies in addition to the antimalarial drugs. It is advisable to hospitalize nonimmune patients infected with *P falciparum* until a decrease in parasitemia is demonstrated, indicating that treatment is effective and severe complications are unlikely to occur.

Partially immune patients with uncomplicated *P falciparum* infection and nonimmune persons infected with *P vivax, P ovale,* or *P malariae* can receive treatment as outpatients if follow-up is reliable. For children, hydration and treatment of hypoglycemia are of utmost importance. Anemia, seizures, pulmonary edema, and renal failure require conventional management. Corticosteroids are contraindicated for cerebral malaria because of increased mortality. In severe malaria, exchange transfusion can be life-saving, particularly in nonimmune persons with parasitemia greater than 15%.

Chloroquine is the drug of choice for treatment of infection with chloroquine-sensitive plasmodia (Table 39–5). For patients unable to take oral medication, intravenous chloroquine or quinidine can be administered with careful monitoring for potential arrhythmogenic effects. Therapy can later be converted to oral chloroquine. For chloroquine-resistant *P falciparum* infection, oral therapy includes quinine with pyrimethamine/sulfadoxine, tetracycline, doxycycline, or clindamycin. Two-drug treatment shortens the quinine course from 7 to 3 days unless the malaria is severe or was acquired in areas of multidrug-resistant *P falciparum* (South America and Southeast Asia). Other options are mefloquine, halofantrine, and atovaquone/proguanil. Artemether* and artesunate* are very effective against *P falciparum,* including quinine-resistant strains. However, cardiovascular toxicity might be a limiting factor. If chemoprophylaxis failed to protect the patient, the same drug should not be used for treatment. Halofantrine should not be used as treatment for persons who failed mefloquine chemoprophylaxis, because the two drugs exhibit cross-resistance. Patients in-

---

*Not licensed in USA

**Table 39–5.** Treatment of malaria.

| Drug | Dosage |
|---|---|
| **Chloroquine-sensitive plasmodia** | |
| Chloroquine | 10 mg base/kg up to 600 mg, followed either by 5 mg base/kg after 6, 24, and 48 h, or 5 mg base/kg after 12, 24, and 36 h |
| **Chloroquine-resistant *P falciparum*** | |
| **A. Oral regimens** | |
| 1. Quinine sulfate | 25 mg/kg/d up to 2g/d in three doses for 3–7 d |
| **plus** | |
| Pyrimethamine-sulfadoxine | ¼ tablet on the last day of quinine (age < 1 y) ½ tablet (age 1–3 y) 1 tablet (age 4–8 y) 2 tablets (age 9–14 y) 3 tablets (age > 15 y) |
| **or** | |
| Tetracycline | 20 mg/kg/d up to 1 g/d in four doses for 7 d |
| **or** | |
| Doxycycline | 3 mg/kg/d up to 100 mg as single daily dose for 7 d |
| **or** | |
| Clindamycin | 20–40 mg/kg/d up to 2700 mg in three doses for 3 d |
| 2. Mefloquine | 25 mg/kg up to 1250 mg as a single dose |
| 3. Halofantrine | 8 mg/kg up to 500 mg every 6 h for three doses; repeat in 1 wk |
| 4. Atovaquone/proguanil | 11–20 kg: 1 tablet (250 mg/100 mg daily for 3 d) 21–30 kg: 2 tablets 31–40 kg: 3 tablets > 40 kg: 4 tablets |
| **B. Parenteral regimen** | |
| Quinidine gluconate | 10 mg/kg up to 600 mg as loading dose IV in normal saline slowly over 1–2 h followed by continuous infusion of 0.02 mg/kg/min until oral therapy can be started |
| **Chloroquine-resistant *P vivax*** | |
| Mefloquine | 25 mg/kg up to 1250 mg in a single dose |
| Halofantrine | 8 mg/kg up to 500 mg/kg every 6 h for three doses; repeat in 1 week |
| **Prevention of relapse with *P vivax* or *P ovale*** | |
| Primaquine phosphate[a] | 0.3 mg base/kg/d up to 15 mg base/d for 14 d |

[a]Screen for glucose-6-phosphate dehydrogenase deficiency.

fected with chloroquine-resistant *P falciparum* who cannot take oral medication should receive intravenous quinidine, which is two or three times more active than quinine. Serum levels of quinidine can be measured in most North American hospitals. Chloroquine-resistant *P vivax* infection, which has been identified in Papua New Guinea, Irian Jaya (in Indonesia), India, Brazil, and Colombia, can be treated with mefloquine or halofantrine. *P vivax* or *P ovale* infections in persons living in nonendemic areas are usually treated with primaquine to prevent late relapse.

Centers for Disease Control and Prevention Web site: www.cdc.gov

Fischer PR et al: Prevention of malaria in children. Clin Infect Dis 2002;34:493 [PMID: 11797176].

Malecki JM et al: Local transmission of Plasmodium vivax malaria—Palm Beach County, Florida, 2003. MMWR 2003; 52:908 [PMID: 14508439].

Stauffer W et al: Diagnosis and treatment of malaria in children. Clin Infect Dis 2003;37:1340 [PMID: 14583868].

## 2. Babesiosis

*Babesia microti* is a malaria-like protozoan that infects and lyses erythrocytes of wild and domestic animals in North America and Europe. In the United States, human babesiosis occurs in the coastal areas of Massachusetts, Rhode Island, and New York. Humans accidentally enter the cycle when bitten by *Ixodes scapularis,* one of the intermediate hosts and vectors of *B microti.* After inoculation, the protozoan penetrates the erythrocytes and starts an asynchronous cycle that causes hemolysis.

## Clinical Findings

The incubation period is 1–3 weeks but may extend up to 6 weeks. Many times the tick bite is unnoticed. Symptoms are nonspecific and include sustained or cyclic fever up to 40°C, shaking chills, malaise, myalgias, headache, and dark urine. Hepatosplenomegaly is an uncommon finding. The disease is usually self-limited, but severe cases have been described in asplenic patients and immunocompromised hosts. Because *Babesia* and *Borrelia burgdorferi* share another vector, *Ixodes dammini,* dual infection may occur.

## Diagnosis

Microscopic evaluation of thin or thick blood smears reveals the intraerythrocytic organisms that resemble *P falciparum* ring forms. Specific serology is also available through the Centers for Disease Control and Prevention. IgG titers greater than or equal to 1:1024 are diagnostic of acute infection.

## Treatment

Clindamycin (20 mg/kg/d, up to 600 mg every 6 hours) or azithromycin (500 mg on the first day, followed by 250 mg/d) in combination with quinine (25 mg/kg/d, up to 650 mg every 6–8 hours) or azithromycin and atovaquone (750 mg bid) for 7–10 days is the treatment of choice. Other antimalarial drugs, including chloroquine, have been unsuccessful.

Krause PJ et al: Atovaquone and azithromycin for the treatment of babesiosis. N Engl J Med 2000;343:1454 [PMID: 11078770].

Lantos PM et al: Babesiosis: Similar to malaria but different. Pediatr Ann 2002;31:192 [PMID: 11905293].

## 3. Toxoplasmosis

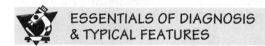

### ESSENTIALS OF DIAGNOSIS & TYPICAL FEATURES

- *Congenital toxoplasmosis: chorioretinitis, microphthalmia, strabismus, microcephaly, hydrocephaly, convulsions, psychomotor retardation, intracranial calcifications, jaundice, hepatosplenomegaly, abnormal blood cell counts.*
- *Acquired toxoplasmosis in an immunocompetent host: lymphadenopathy, hepatosplenomegaly, rash.*
- *Acquired or reactivated toxoplasmosis in an immunocompromised host: encephalitis, chorioretinitis, myocarditis, and pneumonitis.*
- *Ocular toxoplasmosis: chorioretinitis.*
- *Serologic evidence of infection with Toxoplasma gondii or demonstration of the agent in tissue or body fluids.*

## General Considerations

*Toxoplasma gondii* is a worldwide parasite of animals and birds. Felines, the definitive hosts, excrete oocysts in their feces. Ingested mature oocysts or tissue cysts lead to tachyzoite invasion of the intestinal cells. Intracellular replication of the tachyzoites cause cell lysis and spread of the infection to adjacent cells or to other tissues via the bloodstream. In chronic infection, *T gondii* appears as bradyzoite-containing tissue cysts that do not trigger an inflammatory reaction. In immunocompromised hosts, tachyzoites are released from the cysts and begin a new cycle of infection. The two major routes of *Toxoplasma* transmission to humans are oral (including pica)

and congenital. Oocysts survive for up to 18 months in moist soil. Oral infection occurs after ingestion of cyst-containing undercooked meat or other food products. Oocyst survival is limited in dry, very cold, or very hot conditions, and at high altitude, which probably accounts for the lower incidence of toxoplasmosis in these climatic regions. In the United States, less than 1% of cattle and 25% of sheep and pigs are infected with toxoplasmosis. In humans, depending on geographic area, seropositivity increases with age from nil–10% in children younger than age 10 years to 3–70% in adults. Congenital transmission occurs during acute infection of pregnant women; this occurs in 0.2–1% of all pregnancies in the United States. Rarely, fetal infection has been documented in immunocompromised mothers who have chronic toxoplasmosis. The rate of vertical transmission in patients with untreated toxoplasmosis increases from 10% in the first trimester to 60% in the third. Symptomatic disease, however, is more likely to follow infection in early gestation (20–25%) compared with late gestation (less than 11%). Treatment during pregnancy decreases transmission by 60%.

## Clinical Findings

### A. CONGENITAL TOXOPLASMOSIS

Congenital toxoplasmosis has a variety of manifestations, including miscarriage, prematurity, and stillbirth. Most frequently, symptomatic infants present with a combination of fever, microcephaly or hydrocephaly, hepatosplenomegaly, jaundice, chorioretinitis, convulsions, abnormal cerebrospinal fluid (CSF) (xanthochromia and mononuclear pleocytosis), and cerebral calcifications. Other findings include strabismus, eye palsy, maculopapular rash, pneumonitis, myocarditis, thrombocytopenia, lymphocytosis and monocytosis, and an erythroblastosis-like syndrome. The overall mortality rate for congenital toxoplasmosis, which is approximately 10%, is higher in neonates who are symptomatic at birth. Congenital toxoplasmosis must be differentiated from cytomegalovirus infection, rubella, herpes simplex infection, syphilis, Lyme disease, listeriosis, erythroblastosis, and the encephalopathies that accompany degenerative diseases.

### B. ACQUIRED TOXOPLASMA INFECTION IN THE IMMUNOCOMPETENT HOST

Only 10–20% of acute *Toxoplasma* infections produce symptoms. Patients usually present with lymphadenopathy without fever. The nodes are discrete, variably tender, and do not suppurate. Cervical lymph nodes are most frequently involved, but any nodes may be enlarged. Less common findings include fever, malaise, myalgias, fatigue, hepatosplenomegaly, low lymphocyte counts (usually less than 10%), and liver enzyme elevations. Unilateral chorioretinitis may occur. The disease is self-limited, although lymph node enlargement may persist or may wax and wane for a few months to 1 or even more years. Rarely, an apparently healthy child may develop severe disseminated disease associated with myocarditis, pneumonitis, or encephalitis.

Toxoplasmic lymphadenitis must be distinguished from other causes of infectious mononucleosis-like syndromes (< 1% are caused by *Toxoplasma*).

## C. ACUTE TOXOPLASMOSIS
### IN THE IMMUNODEFICIENT HOST

Patients with human immunodeficiency virus (HIV), lymphoma, leukemia, or transplantation are at high risk for developing severe disease (encephalitis, chorioretinitis, myocarditis, or pneumonitis) following acute infection or reactivation. Children born to HIV- and *Toxoplasma*-infected mothers may acquire both pathogens in utero.

### D. OCULAR TOXOPLASMOSIS

In active congenital toxoplasmosis, chorioretinitis is usually bilateral and shows acute inflammatory foci on funduscopic examination. This generally resolves, leaving depigmented scars of the retina surrounded by areas of hyperpigmentation. Chorioretinitis may reactivate in a single eye later in life. The appearance of the ocular lesion is not specific and mimics other granulomatous ocular diseases.

## Diagnosis

Active infection is diagnosed by demonstration of *T gondii* or its DNA in blood or body fluids; seeing tachyzoites in histologic sections or cytology preparations; cysts in placenta or fetal tissues; characteristic lymph node histology; or typical serology (most commonly used). IgG antibodies, measured by the Sabin–Feldman dye test, immunofluorescence, ELISA, or particle agglutination, become detectable 1–2 weeks after infection, peak at 1–2 months, and, after decreasing at variable speed, persist for life. IgM antibodies, measured by ELISA or particle agglutination, appear earlier and decline faster than IgG antibodies. Absence of both serum IgG and IgM virtually rules out the diagnosis of toxoplasmosis. Acute toxoplasmosis in an immunocompetent host is best documented by analyzing IgG and IgM in paired blood samples drawn 3 weeks apart. Because high antibody titers (IgM or IgG) can persist for several months after acute infection, a single high-titer determination is nonspecific. However, seroconversion or a fourfold increase in titer confirms the diagnosis.

In the immunocompromised host, serology is not sensitive, and active infection is documented by PCR or finding tachyzoites by histologic examination.

Patients with *Toxoplasma* chorioretinitis typically have low levels of specific IgG and absent IgM. The diagnosis can be confirmed by demonstrating high antibody titers in aqueous fluid.

Congenital infection is documented by anti-*Toxoplasma* IgM or IgA antibodies in the blood of the neonate. Prenatal diagnosis of congenital infection requires a combination of ultrasonography (to detect ventricle enlargement) and amniotic fluid PCR or cord blood serology. Amniotic fluid PCR is highly sensitive and carries fewer risks than cord puncture.

## Differential Diagnosis

Congenital infection may resemble that due to cytomegalovirus, syphilis, rubella, or herpes simplex. Acquired infection mimics viral, bacterial, or lymphoproliferative disorders.

## Prevention

Pregnant women and immunocompromised patients should wash hands thoroughly after handling raw meat, cook meat to 66°C or greater, wash fruits and vegetables before consumption, and avoid contact with cat feces. Serologic screening of pregnant women is warranted in areas of high prevalence. A first test should be performed by 10–12 weeks of pregnancy. Seronegative patients should be retested at 20–22 weeks' gestation and near term. Seroconverters require specific therapy.

## Treatment

Treatment does not reverse central nervous system (CNS) damage in neonates but does markedly decrease late sequelae. A year of treatment is recommended for all congenitally infected infants; symptomatic patients receive 6 months of pyrimethamine and sulfadiazine, followed by alternating spiramycin and pyrimethamine–sulfadiazine monthly for the next 6 months. Subclinical infection is treated with pyrimethamine and sulfadiazine for 6 weeks, followed by alternating spiramycin for 6 weeks with pyrimethamine–sulfadiazine for 4 weeks.

Oral pyrimethamine at 1 mg/kg/d (maximum 25 mg) causes gastrointestinal upset, leukopenia, thrombocytopenia, and, rarely, agranulocytosis. Frequent blood counts should be performed to guide therapy. Leucovorin calcium (folinic acid), 5 mg given intramuscularly every 3 days, decreases myelotoxicity. The dosage of sulfadiazine or trisulfapyrimidines is 40–45 mg/kg twice a day orally (maximum 8 g/d). Clindamycin can be substituted for sulfadiazine in patients who cannot tolerate sulfonamides. Spiramycin and trimethoprim–sulfamethoxazole are less active.

In acquired infection, usually self-limited, the potentially toxic therapy should be prescribed with discretion, only if the illness is complicated.

In chorioretinitis, antimicrobial therapy is used for 4 weeks. A course of corticosteroids (prednisone, 1.5 mg/kg up to 75 mg) is recommended when lesions involve the macula or the optic nerve. Lesions tend to improve after 10 days of therapy.

In primary infection during pregnancy, spiramycin is started immediately. Pyrimethamine plus sulfadiazine, alternating every 3 weeks with spiramycin, are used when fetal infection has been documented.

Montoya JG: Laboratory diagnosis of *Toxoplasma gondii* infection and toxoplasmosis. J Infect Dis 2002;185 (Suppl): S73 [PMID: 11865443].

# GASTROINTESTINAL INFECTIONS

## 1. Amebiasis

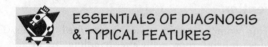
### ESSENTIALS OF DIAGNOSIS & TYPICAL FEATURES

*Acute dysentery: diarrhea with blood and mucus, abdominal pain, tenesmus.*

*or*

- *Chronic nondysenteric diarrhea.*

*or*

- *Hepatic abscess.*
- *Amebas or cysts in stool or abscesses; amebic antigen in stool.*
- *Serologic evidence of amebic infection.*

## General Considerations

Amebiasis, caused by *Entamoeba histolytica,* is a common problem in areas with poor hygiene. An estimated 10% of the world's population is infected with *E histolytica* or *Entamoeba dispar,* and an estimated 100,000 people die of amebic infection each year. Amebiasis should be suspected in patients with a history of travel to, or contact with individuals who may be asymptomatic carriers from, endemic areas. In the United States, amebiasis may occur in homes for the handicapped, where poor hygiene fosters the spread of enteric pathogens. *E histolytica* has been found in the stools of as many as 30% of homosexual men. Individuals of any age may be infected. Transmission is usually fecal–oral, often from asymptomatic carriers who pass cysts. Trophozoites are killed by stomach acid and are not infectious. Infection with *E dispar,* which is morphologically identical to *E histolytica* but results only in asymptomatic carriage, is ten times more

common than infection with *E histolytica.* Furthermore, only 10% of *E histolytica* infections result in gastrointestinal or other symptoms.

## Clinical Findings

Patients with intestinal amebiasis can present with asymptomatic cyst passage, acute amebic proctocolitis, chronic nondysenteric colitis, or ameboma. Because all *E dispar* infections and up to 90% of *E histolytica* infections are asymptomatic, carriage is the most common manifestation of amebiasis. Patients with acute amebic colitis typically have a 1- to 2-week history of watery stools containing blood and mucus, abdominal pain, and tenesmus. A minority of patients are febrile or dehydrated. Abdominal examination may reveal pain over the lower abdominal quadrants. Fulminant colitis is an unusual complication of amebic dysentery and is associated with a grave prognosis (more than 50% mortality). Patients with fulminant colitis present with severe bloody diarrhea, fever, and diffuse abdominal pain. Children younger than age 2 years appear to be at increased risk for this condition. Chronic amebic colitis is clinically indistinguishable from idiopathic inflammatory bowel disease; patients present with recurrent episodes of bloody diarrhea over a period of years. Ameboma is a localized amebic infection, usually in the cecum or ascending colon, which presents as a painful abdominal mass.

The most common complication of intestinal amebiasis is intestinal perforation and peritonitis. Perianal ulcers, a less common complication, are painful, punched-out lesions that usually respond to medical therapy. Infrequently, colonic strictures may develop following colitis.

Extraintestinal amebiasis can result in liver, lung, and cerebral abscesses and, rarely, genitourinary disease. Patients with amebic liver abscess, the most common form of extraintestinal amebiasis, present with recent-onset fever and right upper quadrant tenderness. The pain may be dull or pleuritic or referred to the right shoulder. Physical examination reveals liver enlargement in less than 50% of affected patients. Some patients have a subacute presentation lasting 2 weeks to 6 months. In these patients, hepatomegaly, anemia and weight loss are common findings, and fever is less common. Jaundice and diarrhea are rarely associated with an amebic liver abscess.

The most common complication of amebic liver abscess is pleuropulmonary amebiasis due to rupture of a right liver lobe. Lung abscesses may occur from hematogenous spread. Cough, dyspnea, and pleuritic pain can also be caused by the serous pleural effusions and atelectasis that frequently accompany amebic liver abscesses. Rupture of hepatic abscesses can lead to peritonitis and more rarely to pericarditis. Cerebral amebiasis is an infrequent manifestation. Genitourinary amebiasis, which is also uncommon, results from rupture of a liver abscess, hematogenous dissemination, or lymphatic spread.

## Diagnosis

Intestinal amebiasis is diagnosed by detecting the parasite on stool examination or mucosal biopsy. The differential diagnosis of acute amebic colitis includes bacillary diarrhea and perhaps infection with *Balantidium coli* and *Dientamoeba fragilis,* which have occasionally been associated with acute diarrhea but whose pathogenic role remains controversial. Chronic amebic colitis has to be distinguished from inflammatory bowel disease, *Cyclospora,* and perhaps *B coli.* Occult blood is present in virtually all cases of amebic colitis and can be used as an inexpensive screening test. Fecal leukocytes are uncommon. The presence of hematophagous trophozoites in feces indicates pathogenic *E histolytica* infection.

Ideally, a wet mount of the stool should be examined no longer than 20 minutes after collection to detect motile trophozoites. Otherwise, specimens should be fixed with polyvinyl alcohol or refrigerated to avoid disintegration of the trophozoites. The use of three separate stool examinations has 90% sensitivity for the diagnosis of amebic dysentery. However, infection of the ascending colon, amebomas, and extraintestinal infections frequently yield negative stool examinations. The antigen detection test for stool is very sensitive and more specific, because it detects *E histolytica*-specific antigens that do not cross-react with *E dispar.* Colonoscopy and biopsy are most helpful in diagnosing amebic colitis when stool samples lack ova or parasites. Barium studies are contraindicated for patients with suspected acute amebic colitis because of the risk of perforation.

The presence of antibodies against *E histolytica* can differentiate *E histolytica* from *E dispar* infections. The antibody response follows both intestinal and extraintestinal invasive amebiasis and can be used for diagnostic purposes. ELISA and indirect hemagglutination assays are positive in 85–95% of invasive *E histolytica* colitis or amebic abscess. However, these antibodies persist for years, and a positive result does not distinguish between acute and past infection. Noninvasive imaging studies have greatly improved the diagnosis of hepatic abscesses. Ultrasonographic examination and computed tomography (CT) are sensitive techniques that can guide fine-needle aspiration to obtain specimens for definitive diagnosis. Because an amebic abscess may take up to 2 years to completely resolve on CT scans, imaging techniques are not recommended for therapeutic evaluation.

***Table 39–6.*** Treatment of amebiasis.

| Type of Infection | Drug of Choice | Dosage |
|---|---|---|
| Asymptomatic | Iodoquinol | 30–40 mg/kg/d up to 2 g/d in three doses for 20 d |
| | **or** | |
| | Paromomycin | 25–35 mg/kg/d in three doses for 7 d |
| | **or** | |
| | Diloxanide furoate[a] | 20 mg/kg/d up to 1.5 g/d in three doses for 10 d |
| Intestinal disease and hepatic abscess[b] | Metronidazole **or** Tinidazole[c] | 35–50 mg/kg/d up to 2.25 g/d in three doses for 10 d |
| | | 50 or 60 mg/kg up to 2 g/d for 3 d |

[a]Diloxanide furoate is available from the CDC Drug Service, 404-639-3670.
[b]Treatment should be followed by iodoquinol or another intraluminal cysticidal agent.
[c]Not marketed in the United States; higher dosage is for hepatic abscess.

## Treatment & Prevention

Treatment of amebic infection is complex because different agents are required for eradicating the parasite from the bowel or tissue (Table 39–6). Whether treatment of asymptomatic cyst passers is indicated is a controversial issue. The prevalent opinion is that asymptomatic infection with *E histolytica,* as evidenced by amebic cysts in the stool and a positive serologic test, should be treated in nonendemic areas. If serology is negative, the cysts are more likely to represent infection with the nonpathogenic *E dispar,* which does not require treatment. Among the drugs active against intraluminal cysts, iodoquinol is the most readily available but also the most toxic (causing prominent gastrointestinal side effects, interfering with thyroid function, and causing dose-dependent optic neuritis). Paromomycin, a nonabsorbable aminoglycoside, can be used safely during pregnancy and has only mild intestinal side effects, including flatulence and increased number of stools. Diloxanide furoate is relatively nontoxic and used widely outside the United States. The treatment of invasive amebiasis requires metronidazole. Metronidazole has a disulfiram-like effect and should be avoided in patients receiving ethanol-containing medications. Tinidazole, a more potent nitroimidazole against amebic infection can be used for shorter treatment courses and is well tolerated in children.

In patients who cannot tolerate metronidazole or tinidazole, erythromycin and tetracycline are active against intestinal trophozoites but are inactive against trophozoites in liver abscesses. Conversely, chloroquine is active only against hepatic amebiasis. Treatment of invasive amebiasis should always be followed with an intraluminal cysticidal agent, even if the stool examination is negative. Patients with large, thin-walled hepatic abscesses may need therapeutic aspiration to avoid abscess rupture. Patients with amebiasis should be placed under enteric precautions. Travelers to endemic areas need to follow the precautions designed to prevent enteric infections—drink bottled or boiled water and eat cooked or peeled vegetables and fruits.

Thielman NM et al: Acute infectious diarrhea. N Engl J Med 2004;350:38 [PMID: 14702426].

## 2. Giardiasis

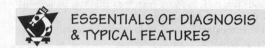

### ESSENTIALS OF DIAGNOSIS & TYPICAL FEATURES

- Chronic relapsing diarrhea, flatulence, bloating, anorexia, poor weight gain.
- Absence of fever and hematochezia.
- Detection of trophozoites, cysts, or Giardia antigens in stool.

## General Considerations

Giardiasis is the most common intestinal protozoal infection in children in the United States and in most of the world. It is caused by *Giardia lamblia.* Endemic worldwide, the infection is classically associated with drinking contaminated water, either in rural areas or in areas with faulty purification systems. But even ostensibly clean urban water supplies can be contaminated intermittently. Persons have acquired the infection in swimming pools. Fecal–oral contamination allows person-to-person spread. Day care centers have become a major source of infection, with an incidence of up to 50% reported in some centers. No symptoms occur in 25% of infected persons, facilitating spread to household contacts. Food-borne outbreaks also occur. Although infection is rare in neonates, giardiasis may occur at any age.

## Clinical Findings

### A. SYMPTOMS AND SIGNS

*Giardia* infection is followed by asymptomatic cyst passage, acute self-limited diarrhea, or a chronic syndrome of diarrhea, malabsorption, and weight loss. Acute diarrhea occurs 1–2 weeks after infection and is characterized by abrupt onset of diarrhea with greasy, malodorous stools; malaise; flatulence; bloating; and nausea. Fever and vomiting occur in a minority of patients. Urticaria, reactive arthritis, biliary tract disease, gastric infection, and constipation have occasionally been reported. The disease has a protracted course (> 1 week) and frequently leads to weight loss. Patients who develop chronic diarrhea complain of profound malaise, lassitude, headache, and diffuse abdominal pain in association with bouts of diarrhea—most typically foul-smelling, greasy stools—intercalated with periods of constipation or normal bowel habits. This syndrome can persist for months until specific therapy is administered or until it subsides spontaneously. Chronic diarrhea frequently leads to malabsorption, steatorrhea, vitamin A and vitamin $B_{12}$ deficiencies, and disaccharidase depletion. Lactose intolerance, which develops in 20–40% of patients, can persist for several weeks after treatment and needs to be differentiated from relapsing giardiasis or reinfection.

### B. LABORATORY FINDINGS

The diagnosis of giardiasis relies on finding the parasite in stool or duodenal aspirates or detecting *Giardia* antigen in feces. For ova and parasite examination, a fresh stool provides the best examination results. Liquid stools have the highest yield of trophozoites, which are more readily found on wet mounts. With semiformed stools, the examiner should look for cysts in fresh or fixed specimens, preferably using a concentration technique. When these techniques are applied carefully, one examination has a 50–70% sensitivity; three examinations increase the sensitivity to 90%. Antigen assays detect *Giardia* by means of immunofluorescence or ELISA. They are comparable in cost to a stool ova and parasite examination and are 85–90% sensitive and 95–100% specific. With a careful stool ova and parasite examination or with the use of a new antigen test, direct sampling of the duodenal contents should be restricted to particularly difficult cases. Three methods are currently available: the string test (Entero-Test), duodenal aspiration, and duodenal biopsy.

## Treatment & Prevention

Metronidazole is the drug of choice for treatment of giardiasis. When given at 5 mg/kg (up to 250 mg) three times daily for 5 days, metronidazole has 80–95% efficacy. The drug is well tolerated in children. It has a disulfiram-like effect and should be avoided in patients receiving ethanol-containing medication. Metronidazole can be administered safely during pregnancy. Furazolidone is frequently used in children as an alternative drug because it is available in suspension. Administered at 1.5 mg/kg (up to 100 mg) four times daily for 7–10 days, it has only 80% efficacy. Furazolidone may cause gastrointestinal side effects, turn urine red, and cause mild hemolysis in patients with G6PD deficiency. For patients who do not respond to metronidazole or furazolidone or who suffer relapse, a second course with the same drug or switching to the other drug is equally effective. In cases of repeated treatment failure, albendazole (400 mg/day for 5–10 days), although not specifically released in the United States for the treatment of giardiasis, is an effective option. Tinidazole, which is not available in the United States, and the recently FDA-approved broad-spectrum antiparasitic nitazoxanide have higher efficacy than any of the drugs already mentioned. Furthermore, nitazoxanide is available in liquid formulation and reduces the duration of treatment to 3 days. Recommended doses are 100 mg (5 mL) every 12 hours for children 12–4 months of age and 200 mg (10 mL) for 4- to 11-year-olds.

The prevention of giardiasis requires proper treatment of water supplies and interruption of person-to-person transmission. Travelers to developing countries or wilderness areas should halogenate or boil (for over 10 minutes) drinking water and avoid uncooked foods that might have been washed with contaminated water. Sexual transmission is prevented by avoiding oral–anal and oral–genital sex. Interrupting fecal–oral transmission requires strict hand washing. However, outbreaks of diarrhea in day care centers might be particularly difficult to eradicate, and reinforcing hand-washing and treating the disease in both symptomatic and asymptomatic carriers may be necessary.

Abboud P et al: Successful treatment of metronidazole- and albendazole-resistant giardiasis with nitazoxanide in a patient with acquired immunodeficiency syndrome. Clin Infect Dis 2001;32:1792 [PMID: 11360222].

Thielman NM et al: Acute infectious diarrhea. N Engl J Med 2004;350:38 [PMID: 14702426].

## 3. Cryptosporidiosis

*Cryptosporidium parvum* is an intracellular protozoan that has gained importance because it causes severe diarrhea in patients with acquired immunodeficiency syndrome (AIDS) and in other immunodeficient persons. The parasite is ubiquitous and infects and reproduces itself in the epithelial cell lining of the digestive and respiratory tracts of humans and most other vertebrate animals. Humans acquire the infection from contaminated water supplies or from close contact with infected humans or animals.

## Clinical Findings

### A. SYMPTOMS AND SIGNS

Immunocompetent persons infected with *Cryptosporidium* usually develop self-limited diarrhea (2–26 days) with or without abdominal cramps. Diarrhea is intermittent and scant or continuous, watery, and voluminous. Low-grade fever, nausea, vomiting, loss of appetite, and malaise may accompany the diarrhea. Young children (< age 2 years) appear more susceptible to infection than are older children. Immunocompromised patients (either cellular or humoral deficiency) tend to develop prolonged disease, which usually subsides only after the immunodeficiency is corrected. Other clinical manifestations associated with cryptosporidiosis in immunocompromised hosts include cholecystitis, pancreatitis, hepatitis, and respiratory symptoms.

### B. LABORATORY FINDINGS

Cryptosporidiosis has no characteristic laboratory features other than identification of the microorganism in feces or on biopsy. ELISA and PCR tests are more sensitive than staining of stool specimens or concentrates.

## Treatment & Prevention

Immunocompetent patients and those with temporary immunodeficiencies may benefit from treatment with nitazoxanide, antidiarrheal agents, and hydration. Immunocompromised patients usually require more intense supportive care with parenteral nutrition in addition to hydration and nonspecific antidiarrheal agents. Octreotide acetate, a synthetic analogue of somatostatin that inhibits secretory diarrhea, has been associated with symptomatic improvement but not with parasitologic cure. Among the antiparasitic agents, nitazoxanide, paromomycin/azithromycin, rifabutin, and hyperimmune bovine colostrum, in that order, have met with success. For patients with AIDS, institution of effective antiretroviral therapy eliminates symptomatic cryptosporidiosis. Prevention of *Cryptosporidium* infection is limited by oocyst resistance to some of the standard water purification procedures and to common disinfectants. Enteric precautions are recommended for infected persons. Boiled or bottled drinking water may be considered for those at high risk for developing chronic infection (eg, patients with AIDS).

Amadi B et al: Effect of nitazoxanide on morbidity and mortality in Zambian children with cryptosporidiosis: A randomized controlled trial. Lancet 2002;360:1375 [PMID: 12423984].

Chen X et al: Cryptosporidiosis. N Engl J Med 2002;346:1723 [PMID: 12037153].

## 4. Cyclosporiasis

*Cyclospora* is a coccidian with worldwide distribution that infects both humans and animals. It causes food-associated outbreaks, characterized by an incubation period of 2–11 days followed by watery diarrhea in relapsing patterns, sometimes alternating with constipation. Other symptoms include profound fatigue, vomiting, and myalgias. Although the illness is self-limited, it may last for several weeks. Diagnosis is based on finding oocysts 8–10 mm in diameter on examination of stool specimens stained with acid-fast stain. The treatment of choice is trimethoprim–sulfamethoxazole for 7 days.

Herwaldt BL: Cyclospora cayetanensis: A review, focusing on the outbreaks of cyclosporiasis in the 1990s. Clin Infect Dis 2000;31:1040 [PMID: 11049789].

## 5. Free-Living Amebas

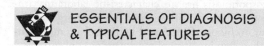

> **ESSENTIALS OF DIAGNOSIS & TYPICAL FEATURES**
>
> • *Acute meningoencephalitis: fever, headache, meningismus, acute mental deterioration.*
> • *Swimming in warm, fresh water in endemic areas.*
> • *Chronic granulomatous encephalitis: insidious onset of focal neurologic deficits.*
> • *Keratitis: pain, photophobia, conjunctivitis, blurred vision.*

### General Considerations

Infections with free-living amebas are uncommon. *Naegleria* species, *Acanthamoeba* species, and *Balamuthia* (previously called leptomyxid) amebas have been associated with human disease.

Acute meningoencephalitis, caused by *N fowleri,* occurs mostly in children and young adults. Patients present with abrupt fever, headache, nausea and vomiting, meningismus, and decreased mental status a few days to 2 weeks after swimming in warm fresh-water lakes. Swimming history may be absent. CNS invasion occurs after nasal inoculation of *N fowleri.* The disease is rapidly progressive, and death ensues within 1 week of onset.

Chronic granulomatous encephalitis, caused by *Acanthamoeba* or *Balamuthia,* occurs most commonly in patients who are immunocompromised from corticosteroid use, chemotherapy, or AIDS. There is no association with fresh-water swimming. This disease has

an insidious onset of focal neurologic deficits, and approximately 50% of patients present with headache. Skin, sinus, or lung infections with *Acanthamoeba* precede many of the CNS infections and may still be present at the onset of neurologic disease. The granulomatous encephalitis progresses to fatal outcome over a period of weeks to months (average 6 weeks).

*Acanthamoeba* keratitis is a corneal infection associated with minor trauma or use of soft contact lenses in otherwise healthy persons. Frequently misdiagnosed as herpes simplex or bacterial keratitis, *Acanthamoeba* keratitis has a characteristic dendriform epithelial pattern that suggests the diagnosis.

### Diagnosis

Amebic encephalitis should be included in the differential diagnosis of acute meningoencephalitis in children with a history of recent fresh-water swimming. The CSF is usually hemorrhagic, with leukocyte counts that may be normal early in the disease but later range from 400 to 2600/μL with neutrophil predominance, low to normal glucose, and elevated protein. The etiologic diagnosis relies on finding trophozoites on a wet mount of the CSF.

Granulomatous encephalitis is diagnosed by brain biopsy of CT-identified nonenhancing lucent areas. The CSF of these patients is usually nondiagnostic with intermediate white blood cell counts, elevated protein, and decreased glucose. *Acanthamoeba* or leptomyxid amebas have not been found in the CSF; however, they can be visualized in biopsies or grown from brain or other infected tissues.

*Acanthamoeba* keratitis is diagnosed by finding the trophozoites in corneal scrapings or by isolating the parasite from corneal specimens or contact lens cultures.

### Treatment & Prevention

The few patients who have survived acute amebic meningoencephalitis received high-dose intravenous and intrathecal amphotericin B, accompanied by miconazole, rifampin, and sulfisoxazole in some cases. The first two cases of successful treatment of *Balamuthia* encephalitis were reported after combination therapy with flucytosine, pentamidine, fluconazole, sulfadiazine, and a macrolide.

*Acanthamoeba* keratitis responds well to surgical debridement followed by 3–4 weeks of topical 1% miconazole; 0.1% propamidine isethionate; and polymyxin B sufate, neomycin, bacitracin (Neosporin).

Because primary amebic meningitis occurs infrequently, active surveillance of lakes for *N fowleri* is not warranted. However, in the presence of a documented case, it is advisable to close the implicated lake to swimming. *Acanthamoeba* keratitis can be prevented by heat disinfection of contact lenses, by storage of lenses in sterile solutions, and by not wearing lenses when swimming in fresh water.

Deetz TR et al: Successful treatment of *Balamuthia* amoebic encephalitis: Presentation of two cases. Clin Infect Dis 2003; 37:1304 [PMID: 14583863].

Kumar R et al: Recent advances in the treatment of *Acanthamoeba* keratitis. Clin Infect Dis 2002;35:434 [PMID: 12145728].

McKee T et al: Primary amebic meningoencephalitis—Georgia, 2002. MMWR 2003;52:962 [PMID: 14534512].

## TRICHOMONIASIS

*Trichomonas vaginalis* is discussed in Chapter 40.

# METAZOAL INFECTIONS

## NEMATODE INFECTIONS

### 1. Enterobiasis (Pinworms)

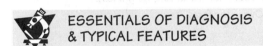

ESSENTIALS OF DIAGNOSIS
& TYPICAL FEATURES

- *Anal pruritus.*
- *Worms in the stool or eggs on perianal skin.*

## General Considerations

This worldwide infection is caused by *Enterobius vermicularis*. The adult worms are about 5–10 mm long and live in the colon; females deposit eggs on the perianal area, primarily at night, causing intense pruritus. Scratching contaminates the fingers and allows transmission back to the host (autoinfection) or to contacts.

## Clinical Findings

### A. SYMPTOMS AND SIGNS

Although blamed for myriad symptoms, pinworms are definitely associated only with localized pruritus. Adult worms may migrate within the colon or up the urethra or vagina in girls. They can be found within the bowel wall, in the lumen of the appendix (usually an incidental finding by the pathologist), in the bladder, and even in the peritoneal cavity of girls. The granulomatous reaction that may be present around these ectopic worms is usually asymptomatic. Worm eradication may correspond with the cure of recurrent urinary tract infections in some young girls.

### B. LABORATORY FINDINGS

The usual diagnostic test consists of pressing a piece of transparent tape on the child's anus in the morning prior to bathing, then placing it on a drop of xylene on a slide. Microscopic examination under low power usually demonstrates the ova. Occasionally eggs or adult worms are seen in fecal specimens. Parents may also notice adult worms.

## Differential Diagnosis

Nonspecific irritation or vaginitis, streptococcal perianal cellulitis (usually painful; marked erythema), and vaginal or urinary bacterial infections may at times resemble pinworm infection, although the symptoms of pinworms are often so suggestive that a therapeutic trial is justified without a confirmed diagnosis.

## Treatment

### A. SPECIFIC MEASURES

Treat all household members at the same time to prevent reinfections. Because the drugs are not active against the eggs, therapy should be repeated after 2 weeks to kill the recently hatched adults.

Pyrantel pamoate is given as a single dose (11 mg/kg, maximum 1 g); it is safe and very effective. Mebendazole and albendazole are highly effective for this and other helminthic infections. A single oral dose of 100 mg mebendazole or 400 mg albendazole is used for all ages.

### B. GENERAL MEASURES

Personal hygiene must be emphasized. Nails should be kept short and clean. Children should wear undergarments to bed to diminish contamination of fingers; bedclothes should be laundered frequently. Although eggs may be widely dispersed in the house and multiple family members infected, the disease is mild and treatable. Avoid creating in the parents an excessive concern with contamination.

St Georgiev V: Chemotherapy of enterobiasis (oxyuriasis). Expert Opin Pharmacother 2001;2:267 [PMID: 11336585].

### 2. Ascariasis

ESSENTIALS OF DIAGNOSIS
& TYPICAL FEATURES

- *Abdominal cramps and discomfort.*
- *Large, white or reddish, round worms, or ova in the feces.*

## General Considerations

*Ascaris lumbricoides* is a worldwide human parasite. Ova passed by carriers may remain viable for months under the proper soil conditions. The ova contaminate food or fingers and are subsequently ingested by a new host. The larvae hatch, penetrate the intestinal wall, enter the venous system, reach the alveoli, are coughed up, and return to the small intestine, where they mature. The female lays thousands of eggs daily.

## Clinical Findings

### A. SYMPTOMS AND SIGNS

Infections usually remain asymptomatic; severe cases, however, can be associated with pain, weight loss, anorexia, diarrhea, or vomiting. Adult worms may be seen in feces or vomitus. Rarely, they perforate or obstruct the small bowel, biliary system, or appendix. Large numbers of larvae migrating through the lungs may cause an acute, transient eosinophilic pneumonia (Löffler syndrome).

### B. LABORATORY FINDINGS

The diagnosis is made by observing the large round worms in the stool or by microscopic detection of the ova.

## Treatment

Because the adult worms live less than a year, asymptomatic infection need not be treated. Mebendazole (100 mg twice daily for 3 days), pyrantel pamoate (a single dose of 11 mg/kg, maximum 1 g), and albendazole (400 mg in a single dose) are highly and equally effective. In cases of intestinal or biliary obstruction, piperazine (150 mg/kg initially, followed by six doses of 65 mg/kg every 12 hours by nasogastric tube) is recommended because it narcotizes the worms and helps relieve obstruction. However, surgical removal is occasionally required.

## 3. Trichuriasis (Whipworm)

*Trichuris trichiura* is a widespread human and animal parasite common in children living in warm, humid areas conducive to survival of the ova. The adult worms live in the cecum and colon; the ova are passed and become infectious after several weeks in the soil. Ingested infective eggs hatch in the upper small intestine. Unlike *Ascaris*, *Trichuris* does not have a migratory tissue phase. Symptoms are not present unless the infection is severe, in which case pain, diarrhea, and mild abdominal distention are present. Massive infections may also cause rectal prolapse and dysentery. Detection of the

characteristic barrel-shaped ova in the feces confirms the diagnosis. Adult worms may be seen in the prolapsed rectum or at proctoscopy; their thin heads are buried in the mucosa, and the thicker posterior portions extrude. Mild to moderate eosinophilia may be present.

Mebendazole (100 mg orally twice daily for 3 days) or albendazole (400 mg in a single dose) improves gastrointestinal symptoms and terminates constitutional symptoms.

Crompton DW et al: Nutritional impact of intestinal helminthiasis. Ann Rev Nutr 2002;22:35 [PMID: 12055337].

## 4. Hookworm

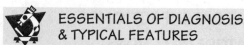

### ESSENTIALS OF DIAGNOSIS & TYPICAL FEATURES

- Iron deficiency anemia.
- Abdominal discomfort, weight loss.
- Ova in the feces.

## General Considerations

The common human hookworms are *Ancylostoma duodenale* and *Necator americanus*. Both are widespread in the tropics and subtropics. The larger *A duodenale* is more pathogenic because it consumes more blood, up to 0.5 mL per worm per day.

The adults live in the jejunum. Eggs are passed in the feces and develop and hatch into infective larvae in warm, damp soil within 2 weeks. The larvae penetrate human skin on contact, enter the blood, reach the alveoli, are coughed up and swallowed, and develop into adults in the intestine. The adult worms attach with their mouth parts to the mucosa, from which they suck blood. Blood loss is the major sequela of infection. Infection rates reach 90% in areas without sanitation.

A separate species, *A braziliense* (dog or cat hookworm), causes creeping eruption (cutaneous larva migrans). This disease occurs mainly on the warm-water American coasts.

## Clinical Findings

### A. SYMPTOMS AND SIGNS

The larvae usually penetrate the skin of the feet and cause intense local itching (ground itch). This subsides as the larvae continue their migration. Löffler syndrome may supervene during lung migration. In creeping eruption, the nonhuman *Ancylostoma* larvae migrate blindly in the skin before dying, creating serpiginous burrows.

Mild intestinal infections produce no symptoms. Severe infections cause iron deficiency anemia and malnutrition. Occasionally abdominal pain and diarrhea may be observed.

### B. LABORATORY FINDINGS

The large ova of both species of hookworm are found in feces and are indistinguishable. Microcytic anemia, hypoalbuminemia, eosinophilia, and hematochezia occur in severe cases.

## Prevention

Fecal contamination of soil and skin contact with potentially contaminated soil should be avoided.

## Treatment

### A. SPECIFIC MEASURES

Mebendazole (100 mg orally twice daily for 3 days) and pyrantel pamoate (11 mg/kg, maximum 1 g, daily for 3 days) are the drugs of choice. Topical thiabendazole or albendazole or oral thiabendazole are useful for creeping eruption.

### B. GENERAL MEASURES

Iron therapy may be as important as worm eradication.

## Prognosis

The outcome is usually excellent.

Caumes E: Treatment of cutaneous larva migrans. Clin Infect Dis 2000;30:811 [PMID: 10816151].

## 5. *Strongyloidiasis*

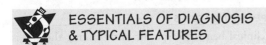

ESSENTIALS OF DIAGNOSIS
& TYPICAL FEATURES

- *Abdominal pain, diarrhea.*
- *Eosinophilia.*
- *Larvae in stools and duodenal aspirates.*
- *Serum antibodies.*

## General Considerations

*Strongyloides stercoralis* is unique in having both parasitic and free-living forms; the latter can survive in the soil for several generations. The parasite is found in most tropical and subtropical regions of the world. The adults live in the submucosal tissue of the duodenum and occasionally elsewhere in the intestines. Eggs deposited in the mucosa hatch rapidly; the first-stage (rhabditiform) larvae, therefore, are the predominant form found in duodenal aspirates and feces. The larvae mature rapidly to the tissue-penetrating filariform stage and initiate internal autoinfection. The filariform larvae also inhabit the soil and can penetrate the skin of another host, subsequently migrating into veins and pulmonary alveoli, reaching the intestine when coughed up and swallowed.

Older children and adults are infected more often than are young children. Even low worm burden can result in significant clinical symptoms. Infestations due to poor sanitation and hygiene in homes for the retarded are noteworthy. Immunosuppressed patients may develop fatal disseminated strongyloidiasis, known as the hyperinfection syndrome.

## Clinical Findings

### A. SYMPTOMS AND SIGNS

At the site of the skin penetration, a pruritic rash may occur. Large numbers of migrating larvae can cause wheezing, cough, and hemoptysis. Although one third of intestinal infections are asymptomatic, the most prominent features of strongyloidiasis include abdominal pain, distention, diarrhea, vomiting, and occasionally malabsorption.

Patients with cellular immunodeficiencies and those on steroid therapy may develop disseminated infection involving the intestine, the lungs, and the meninges. Gram-negative sepsis may complicate disseminated strongyloidiasis.

### B. LABORATORY FINDINGS

Finding larvae in the feces, in duodenal aspirates, on a string test (Entero-Test), or in sputum is diagnostic. IgG antibodies measured by ELISA or immunoblot are sensitive and specific for *Strongyloides*. These persist after successful therapy. Marked eosinophilia is common.

## Differential Diagnosis

Strongyloidiasis should be differentiated from peptic disease, celiac disease, regional or tuberculous enteritis, hookworm infection, and other causes of intestinal symptoms or malabsorption. The pulmonary phase may mimic asthma or bronchopneumonia. Patients with severe infection can present with as an acute abdomen.

## Treatment & Prevention

Thiabendazole (25 mg/kg orally twice daily for 2 days; maximum 3 g/d) and ivermectin (200 mg/kg/d for 1 or 2 days) are the drugs of choice. Relapses are common. In the hyperinfection syndrome, 2–3 weeks of therapy may be necessary. Patients from endemic areas should be tested for specific antibodies and receive treatment before undergoing immunosuppression.

Keiser PB et al: Strongyloides stercoralis in the immunocompromised population. Clin Microbiol Rev 2004;17:208 [PMID: 14726461].

## 6. Visceral Larva Migrans (Toxocariasis)

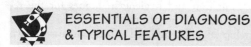

### ESSENTIALS OF DIAGNOSIS & TYPICAL FEATURES

- Visceral involvement including hepatomegaly, marked eosinophilia, and anemia.
- Posterior or peripheral ocular inflammatory mass.
- Elevated antibody titers in serum or aqueous fluid; demonstration of Toxocara larvae on biopsy.

## General Considerations

Visceral larva migrans is a worldwide disease. The agent is the cosmopolitan intestinal ascarid of dogs and cats, *Toxocara canis* or *Toxocara cati*. The eggs passed by infected animals contaminate parks and other areas that young children frequent. Children with pica are at increased risk. In the United States, seropositivity ranges from 2.8% in unselected populations to 23% in southern states to 54% in rural areas. Ingested eggs hatch and penetrate the intestinal wall, then migrate to the liver, lungs, eyes, and other organs, where they die and incite a granulomatous inflammatory reaction.

## Clinical Findings & Diagnosis

### A. VISCERAL LARVA MIGRANS

Toxocariasis is usually asymptomatic, but young children (age 1–5 years) sometimes present with anorexia, fever, fatigue, pallor, abdominal distention, abdominal pain, nausea, vomiting, and cough. Hepatomegaly is common, splenomegaly is unusual, and adenopathy is absent. Lung involvement, usually asymptomatic, can be demonstrated readily by radiologic examination. Seizures are common, but more severe neurologic abnormalities are infrequent. Eosinophilia with leukocytosis, anemia, and elevated liver function tests are typical laboratory findings. ELISA is sensitive, specific, and useful in confirming the clinical diagnosis. Most patients recover spontaneously, but disease may last up to 6 months.

### B. OCULAR LARVA MIGRANS

This condition occurs in older children and adults who present with a unilateral posterior or peripheral inflammatory mass. History of visceral larva migrans and eosinophilia are typically absent. Anti-*Toxocara* antibody titers are low in the serum and high in vitreous and aqueous fluids.

## Diagnosis

Hypergammaglobulinemia and elevated isohemagglutinins sometimes result from cross-reactivity between *Toxocara* antigens and human group A and B blood antigens. The diagnosis is confirmed by finding larvae in granulomatous lesions. Positive serology in high titers (optical density ≥ 0.5) and the exclusion of other causes of hypereosinophilia allow a presumptive diagnosis to be made in typical cases.

## Differential Diagnosis

Diseases associated with hypereosinophilia must be considered. These include trichinosis (enlarged liver not common; muscle tenderness common), eosinophilic leukemia (rare in children; eosinophils are abnormal in appearance), collagen–vascular disease (those associated with eosinophilia are rare in young children), strongyloidiasis (no organomegaly; enteric symptoms are common), early ascariasis, tropical eosinophilia (occurring mainly in India), allergies, and hypersensitivity syndromes.

## Treatment & Prevention

### A. SPECIFIC MEASURES

The clinical benefit of specific anthelmintic therapy is not defined. Treatment with thiabendazole (25 mg/kg—maximum 3 g/d orally twice a day for 5–7 days), diethylcarbamazine (2 mg/kg three times a day orally for 7–10 days), albendazole (400 mg twice a day for 3–5 days), or mebendazole (100–200 mg twice a day for 5 days) is indicated for severe complications of brain, lung, or heart.

### B. GENERAL MEASURES

Treating any cause of pica, such as iron deficiency, is important. Corticosteroids are used to treat marked inflammation of lung, eye, or other organs. Pets should be dewormed routinely. Other children in the household may be infected. Mild eosinophilia and positive serologic tests may be the only clue to their infection. Therapy is not necessary for these individuals.

## 7. Trichinosis

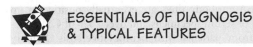

> **ESSENTIALS OF DIAGNOSIS & TYPICAL FEATURES**
>
> - *Vomiting, diarrhea, and pain within 1 week of eating infected meat.*
> - *Fever, periorbital edema, myalgia, and marked eosinophilia.*

### General Considerations

*Trichinella spiralis* is a small roundworm that inhabits hogs and several other meat-eating animals. The human cycle begins with ingestion of viable larvae in undercooked meat. In the intestine, the larvae develop into adult worms which mate and produce hundreds of larvae. The larvae enter the bloodstream and migrate to the striated muscle where they continue to grow and eventually encyst. Symptoms are caused by the inflammatory response in the intestines or muscle.

### Clinical Findings

#### A. SYMPTOMS AND SIGNS

Most infections are asymptomatic. The initial bowel penetration may cause nausea, vomiting, diarrhea, and cramps within 1 week after ingestion of contaminated meat. This may progress to the classic myopathic form, which consists of fever, periorbital edema, myalgia, and weakness. Many organs may be infected by the migrating larvae: diaphragm, heart, lungs, kidneys, spleen, skin, and brain. Severe cerebral involvement may be fatal. Myocarditis may also be severe or fatal. Symptoms usually peak after 2–3 weeks but may last months.

#### B. LABORATORY FINDINGS

Marked eosinophilia is the rule. Serology confirms the diagnosis. Muscle biopsy is rarely necessary.

### Differential Diagnosis

The classic symptoms are pathognomonic if one is aware of this disease. It has to be distinguished from dermatomyositis, typhoid fever, sinusitis, influenza with myopathy, and angioneurotic edema.

### Prevention

Because a microscopic examination must be performed, meat in the United States is not inspected for trichinosis. Although all states require the cooking of hog swill, hog-to-hog or hog-to-rat cycles may continue. All pork and sylvatic meat (eg, bear or walrus) should be heated to at least 65°C. Freezing meat to at least –15°C for 3 weeks may also prevent transmission. Animals used for food should not be fed or allowed access to raw meat.

### Treatment

Mebendazole has activity against the intestinal, circulating, and tissue stages of infection. The adult dose is 200–400 mg three times daily for 3 days followed by 400–500 mg three times daily for 10 days. Pediatric dosing has not been standardized. Concurrent corticosteroids are used in an attempt to prevent the Herxheimer reaction associated with treatment.

### Prognosis

Death may occur within the first weeks, but most infections are self-limited.

Bruschi F et al: New aspects of human trichinellosis: The impact of new *Trichinella* species. Postgrad Med J 2002;78:15 [PMID: 11796866].

## CESTODE INFECTIONS (FLUKES)

## 1. Taeniasis & Cysticercosis

> **ESSENTIALS OF DIAGNOSIS & TYPICAL FEATURES**
>
> - *Mild abdominal pain; passage of worm segments (taeniasis).*
> - *Focal seizures, headaches (neurocysticercosis).*
> - *Cysticerci present in biopsy specimens, on plain films (as calcified masses), or on CT scan or magnetic resonance imaging.*
> - *Proglottids and eggs in feces; specific antibodies in serum or CSF.*

## General Considerations

Both the beef tapeworm (*Taenia saginata*) and the pork tapeworm (*Taenia solium*) cause taeniasis. The adults live in the intestines of humans; the egg-laden distal segments, or proglottids, break off and are passed in feces, disintegrating and releasing the ova in the soil. After ingestion in food or water by cattle or pigs, the eggs hatch and the larvae migrate to and encyst in skeletal muscle. Encysted larvae in meat ingested by humans mature into adults.

Humans can be an intermediate host for *T solium* (but not *T saginata*), and the larvae released from ingested eggs encyst in a variety of tissues, especially muscle and brain. Full larval maturation occurs in 2 months, but the cysts cause little inflammation until they die months to years later. Inflammatory edema ensues with calcification or disappearance of the cyst. A slowly expanding mass of sterile cysts at the base of the brain may cause obstructive hydrocephalus (racemose cysticercosis).

Both parasites are distributed worldwide. Contamination of foods by eggs in human feces allows infection without exposure to meat or travel to endemic areas. Asymptomatic cases are common, but neurocysticercosis is a leading cause of seizures in endemic areas.

Person-to-person spread may occur, resulting in infection of individuals with no exposure to infected meat.

## Clinical Findings

### A. SYMPTOMS AND SIGNS

**1. Taeniasis**—In most tapeworm infections, the only clinical manifestation is the passage of fecal proglottids, white, motile bodies 1–2 cm in size. They occasionally crawl out onto the skin and down the leg, especially the larger *T saginata*. Children may harbor the adult worm for years and complain of abdominal pain, anorexia, and diarrhea.

**2. Cysticercosis**—Most cases are asymptomatic. Subcutaneous nodules of 1–2 cm may be the only sign. After several years, the cysticerci calcify and appear as radiographic opacities. Brain cysts may remain silent or cause seizures, headache, hydrocephalus, and basilar meningitis. Rarely, the spinal cord is involved. Neurocysticercosis manifests an average of 5 years after exposure but may cause symptoms in the first year of life. In the eye, cysts cause bleeding, retinal detachment, and uveitis. Definitive diagnosis requires histologic demonstration of larvae or cyst membrane. Presumptive diagnosis is often made by the characteristics of the cysts seen on CT scan or magnetic resonance imaging; the differential diagnosis may include tuberculoma, brain abscess, arachnoid cyst, and tumor. The presence of *T*

*solium* eggs in feces is uncommon but supports the diagnosis.

### B. LABORATORY FINDINGS

Eggs or proglottids may be found in feces or on the perianal skin (using the tape method employed for pinworms). Eggs of both *Taenia* species are identical. The species are identified by examination of proglottids.

Peripheral eosinophilia is minimal or absent. CSF eosinophilia is seen in 10–75% of cases of neurocysticercosis; its presence supports an otherwise presumptive diagnosis.

ELISA antibody titers are eventually positive in up to 98% of serum specimens and over 75% of CSF specimens from patients with neurocysticercosis. Solitary cysts are associated with seropositivity less often than are multiple cysts. High titers tend to correlate with more severe disease. CSF titers are higher if cysts are near the meninges.

## Treatment

### A. TAENIASIS

Praziquantel (5–10 mg/kg once) and albendazole are equally effective. Feces free of segments or ova for 3 months suggest cure.

### B. CYSTICERCOSIS

Specific treatment is reserved for patients with meningitis or parenchymal cysts. In contrast, those with inactive disease require only symptomatic treatment (anticonvulsants). Praziquantel and albendazole cause disappearance of noninflamed cysts and possibly more rapid resolution of inflamed ring-enhancing cysts. Albendazole, 15 mg/kg divided into three doses daily for 8 days, is the treatment of choice. Larval death may result in clinical worsening because of inflammatory edema. A short course of dexamethasone may decrease these symptoms. Giant subarachnoidal cysts may require more than one cycle of therapy or surgery (or both). Follow-up scans every several months help assess the response to therapy. Treatment of patients with calcified lesions and seizure disorder results in a decrease of generalized seizures.

## Prevention

The incidence in the United States is low, because beef and pork are inspected for taeniasis. Prevention requires proper cooking of meat, careful washing of raw vegetables and fruits, treatment of intestinal carriers, avoiding the use of human excrement for fertilizer, and providing proper sanitary facilities.

## Prognosis

The prognosis is good in intestinal taeniasis. Symptoms associated with a few cerebral cysts may disappear in a few months; heavy brain infections may cause death or chronic neurologic impairment.

Garcia HH et al: A trial of antiparasitic treatment to reduce the rate of seizures due to cerebral cysticercosis. N Engl J Med 2004;350:249 [PMID: 14724304].

Proano JV et al: Medical treatment for neurocysticercosis characterized by giant subarachnoid cysts. N Engl J Med 2001;345: 879 [PMID: 11565520].

## 2. Hymenolepiasis

*Hymenolepis nana,* the cosmopolitan human tapeworm, is a common parasite of children; *Hymenolepis diminuta,* the rat tapeworm, is rare. The former is capable of causing autoinfection. Larvae hatched from ingested eggs penetrate the intestinal wall and then reenter the lumen to mature into adults. Their eggs are immediately infectious for the same or a new host. The adult is only a few centimeters long. Finding the characteristic eggs in feces is diagnostic.

*H diminuta* has an intermediate stage in rat fleas and other insects; children are infected when they ingest these insects.

Light infections with either tapeworm are usually asymptomatic; heavy infection can cause diarrhea and abdominal pain. Therapy is with praziquantel (25 mg/kg once).

## 3. Echinococcosis

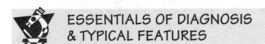

### ESSENTIALS OF DIAGNOSIS & TYPICAL FEATURES

- Cystic tumors of liver, lung, kidney, bone, brain, and other organs.
- Eosinophilia.
- Urticaria and pruritus if cysts rupture.
- Protoscoleces or daughter cysts in the primary cyst.
- Positive serology.
- Epidemiologic evidence of exposure

## General Considerations

Dogs, cats, and other carnivores are the hosts for *Echinococcus granulosus.* Endemic areas include Aus-

tralia, New Zealand, and the southwestern United States, including Native American reservations where shepherding is practiced. The adult tapeworm lives in sheep intestines, and eggs are passed in the feces. When ingested by humans, the eggs hatch, and the larvae penetrate the intestinal mucosa and disseminate in the bloodstream. The larvae produce cysts; the primary sites of involvement are the liver (60–70%) and the lungs (20–25%). A unilocular cyst is most common. Over years, the cyst may reach 25 cm in diameter, although most are much smaller. The cysts of *Echinococcus multilocularis* are multilocular and demonstrate more rapid growth.

## Clinical Findings

### A. SYMPTOMS AND SIGNS

Clinical disease is due to pressure from the enlarging cysts, vessel erosion, and sensitization to cyst or worm antigens. Liver cysts present as slowly expanding tumors that may cause biliary obstruction. Most are in the right lobe and extend inferiorly; 25% are on the upper surface and may be asymptomatic for years. Omental torsion or hemorrhage from vessel erosion may occur.

Rupture of a pulmonary cyst causes coughing, dyspnea, wheezing, urticaria, chest pain, and hemoptysis; cyst and worm remnants are found in sputum. Brain cysts may cause focal neurologic signs and convulsions; renal cysts cause pain and hematuria; bone cysts cause pain.

### B. LABORATORY FINDINGS

Presumptive diagnosis is made by a combination of radiographic or ultrasonographic and serologic findings. ELISA, which is the method most widely used for antibody testing, is highly sensitive but has only limited specificity. Confirmation may be obtained by ultrasonography-guided fine-needle aspiration coupled with parasitologic exam for protoscoleces, rostellar hooks, antigens, or DNA. Eosinophilia is variable and may be absent. Serologic tests are useful for diagnosis and follow-up of therapy.

### C. IMAGING

Pulmonary or bone cysts may be visible on plain films. Other imaging techniques are preferred for cysts in other organs. Visualization of daughter cysts is highly suggestive of echinococcosis.

## Differential Diagnosis

Tumors, bacterial or amebic abscess, and tuberculosis (pulmonary) must be considered.

## Complications

Sudden cyst rupture with anaphylaxis, and death is the worst complication. If the patient survives, secondary infections from seeding of daughter cysts may occur. Segmental lung collapse, secondary bacterial infections, effects of increased intracranial pressure, and severe renal damage due to renal cysts are other potential complications.

## Treatment

Definitive therapy of *E multilocularis* requires meticulous surgical removal of the cysts, preceded by careful injection of the cyst with formalin, iodine, or 95% alcohol solution to sterilize infectious protoscoleces, freezing the cyst wall and injecting silver nitrate prior to its removal, or puncture-aspiration/injection-reaspiration technique, which is best suited for treatment of multiple cysts. A surgeon familiar with this disease should be consulted. Medical therapy may be of additional benefit, particularly in disseminated disease. Albendazole (15 mg/kg/d for 28 days with repeat courses as necessary following a 14-day rest period) is effective in many cases of *E granulosus* infection (hydatid disease). If the cyst leaks or ruptures, the allergic symptoms must be managed immediately.

## Prognosis

Patients with large liver cysts may be asymptomatic for years. Surgery is often curative for lung and liver cysts but not always for cysts in other locations. Secondary disease has a much worse prognosis; about 15% of patients with this disease die.

Eckert J et al: Biological, epidemiological, and clinical aspects of echinococcosis, a zoonosis of increasing concern. Clin Microbiol Rev 2004;17:107 [PMID: 14726458].

Smego RA et al: Percutaneous aspiration–injection–reaspiration drainage plus albendazole or mebendazole for hepatic cystic echinococcosis: A meta-analysis. Clin Infect Dis 2003;37:83 [PMID: 14523772].

# TREMATODE INFECTIONS

## *Schistosomiasis*

### ESSENTIALS OF DIAGNOSIS & TYPICAL FEATURES

- Transient pruritic rash after exposure to fresh water.
- Fever, urticaria, arthralgias, cough, lymphadenitis, and eosinophilia.
- Weight loss, anorexia, hepatosplenomegaly.
- Hematuria, dysuria.
- Eggs in stool, urine, or rectal biopsy specimens.

## General Considerations

One of the most common serious parasitic diseases, schistosomiasis, is caused by several species of *Schistosoma* flukes. *Schistosoma japonicum, S mekongi,* and *S mansoni* involve the intestines and *S haematobium* the urinary tract. The first two are found in eastern and southeastern Asia; *S mansoni* in tropical Africa, the Caribbean, and parts of South America; and *S haematobium* in northern Africa.

Infection is caused by free-swimming larvae (cercariae), which emerge from the intermediate hosts, certain species of fresh-water snails. The cercariae penetrate human skin, migrate to the liver, and mature into adults, which then migrate through the portal vein to lodge in the bladder veins (*S haematobium*), superior mesenteric veins (*S mekongi, S japonicum*), or inferior mesenteric veins (*S mansoni*). Clinical disease results primarily from inflammation caused by the many eggs that are laid in the perivascular tissues or that embolize to the liver. Escape of ova into bowel or bladder lumen allows microscopic visualization and diagnosis from stool or urine specimens, as well as contamination of fresh water and infection of the snail hosts that ingest them.

## Clinical Findings

Much of the population in endemic areas is infected but asymptomatic. Only heavy infections produce symptoms.

### A. SYMPTOMS AND SIGNS

The cercarial penetration may cause a pruritic rash; larval migration may cause fever, urticaria, and cough; the maturation phase may cause tender hepatosplenomegaly followed by days to weeks of fever and malaise as the worms migrate to their final destination. Bladder infection results in dysuria, hematuria, reflux, stones, and incontinence. Secondary pyelonephritis and ureteral obstruction may occur. Intestinal infection is usually asymptomatic. The final stages of disease are characterized by hepatic fibrosis, portal hypertension, splenomegaly, ascites, and bleeding from esophageal varices. The chronic inflammation in the urinary tract associated with *S haematobium* infections may result in obstructive uropathy, stones, infection, bladder cancer, fistulas, and anemia due to chronic hematuria. Spinal cord granulomas and paraplegia due to egg embolization into the Batson plexus have been reported.

### B. LABORATORY FINDINGS

The diagnosis is made by finding the species-specific eggs in feces (*S japonicum, S mekongi, S mansoni,* and occasionally *S haematobium*) or urine (*S haematobium* and occasionally *S mansoni*). A rectal biopsy may reveal *S mansoni* and should be done if other specimens are negative. Peripheral eosinophilia is common, and eosinophils may be seen in urine.

## Prevention

The best prevention is to avoid contact with contaminated fresh water in endemic areas. Efforts to destroy the snail hosts have been successful in areas of accelerated economic development.

## Treatment

### A. SPECIFIC MEASURES

Praziquantel is the treatment of choice for schistosomiasis. A dosage of 40 mg/kg/d in two divided doses (*S mansoni* or *S haematobium*) or 20 mg/kg three times in 1 day (*S japonicum* or *S mekongi*) is very effective and nontoxic. Oxamniquine (20 mg/kg/d in two doses once per day) is an alternative regimen for treatment of *S mansoni* infection. Arthameter, 6 mg/kg every 3 weeks, may prevent new infections or reinfection after curative treatment.

### B. GENERAL MEASURES

Medical therapy of nutritional deficiency or secondary bacterial infections may be needed. The patient's urinary tract should be evaluated carefully in *S haematobium* infection; reconstructive surgery may be needed. Hepatic fibrosis requires careful evaluation of the portal venous system and surgical management of portal hypertension when appropriate.

## Prognosis

Medical therapy decreases the worm infection and liver size, despite continued exposure in endemic areas. Early disease responds well to therapy, but once significant scarring or severe inflammation has occurred, eradication of the parasites is of little benefit.

Corachan M: Schistosomiasis and international travel. Clin Infect Dis 2002;35:446 [PMID: 12145730].

Utzinger J et al: Oral artemeter for prevention of Schistosoma mansoni infection: Randomised controlled trial. Lancet 2000; 355:1320 [PMID: 10776745].

# ■ II. INFECTIONS: MYCOTIC

Fungi can be classified as yeasts, which are unicellular and reproduce by budding; as molds, which are multicellular and consist of tubular structures (hyphae) and grow by elongation and branching; or as dimorphic fungi, which can exist either as yeasts or molds depending on environmental conditions. Fungal infections can be categorized as shown in Table 39–7.

In the United States, systemic disease in normal hosts is commonly caused by three organisms—*Coccidioides, Histoplasma,* and *Blastomyces*—which are restricted to certain geographic areas. Prior residence in or travel to these areas, even for a brief time, is a prerequisite for inclusion in a differential diagnosis. Of these three, *Histoplasma* most often relapses years later in patients who are immunosuppressed.

Immunosuppression, foreign bodies (eg, central catheters), ulceration of gastrointestinal and respiratory mucosae, broad-spectrum antimicrobial therapy, malnutrition, HIV infection, and neutrophil defects or depletion are major risk factors for opportunistic fungal disease.

Laboratory diagnosis may be difficult because of the small number of fungi present in some lesions, slow growth of some organisms, and difficulty in distinguishing normal colonization of mucosal surfaces from infection. A tissue biopsy with fungal stains and culture is the best method for diagnosing systemic disease. Repeat blood cultures may be negative even in the presence of intravascular infections. Serology is useful for diagnosing coccidioidomycosis and histoplasmosis, and antigen detection is useful for diagnosing histoplasmosis and cryptococcosis.

The risk of empiric treatment is greater for fungal than for bacterial infections because of the toxicity of some antifungals (especially amphotericin B), the frequent need for prolonged parenteral administration, and the limited data available for choosing the best dose

*Table 39–7.* Pediatric fungal infections.

| Type | Agents | Incidence | Diagnosis | Diagnostic Tests | Therapy | Prognosis |
|------|--------|-----------|-----------|------------------|---------|-----------|
| Superficial | *Candida* *Dermatophytes* *Malassezia* | Very common | Simple | KOH prep | Topical | Good |
| Subcutaneous | *Sporothrix*[b] | Uncommon | Simple[a] | Culture | Oral | Good |
| Systemic: normal host | *Coccidioides* *Histoplasma* *Blastomyces* | Common: regional | Often presumptive | Chest radiograph Serology, antigen detection (histoplasmosis) Histology Culture of body fluids or tissue | None[c] or systemic | Good |
| Systemic: opportunistic infection | *Candida*[b] *Pneumocystis*[d] *Aspergillus* *Malassezia* *Pseudallescheria* *Cryptococcus* | Uncommon | Difficult[e] | Tissue biopsy, culture, antigen detection (cryptococcosis) | Systemic, prolonged | Poor if therapy delayed and in severely immunocompromised patients |

[a]Sporotrichosis may require biopsy for diagnosis.
[b]*Candida* and *Sporothrix* in immunocompromised patients may cause severe, rapidly progressive disease and require systemic therapy.
[c]Often self-limited in normal host.
[d]Now reclassified as a fungus. May infect many normal hosts.
[e]Except *Cryptococcus,* which is often diagnosed by antigen detection.

or regimen. Delay in treating systemic disease, however, may prove fatal.

Susceptibility testing of *Candida* species with some drugs is now available, but testing of other organisms, especially molds, and testing with additional antifungal agents, is not well standardized.

The common superficial fungal infections of the hair and skin are discussed in Chapter 14.

# BLASTOMYCOSIS

## General Considerations

The causative fungus, *Blastomyces dermatitidis,* is found in soil primarily in the Mississippi and Ohio River valleys, additional southeastern and south central states, and the states bordering the Great Lakes. Transmission is by inhalation of spores. Subclinical disease is common. Severe disease is much more common in adults and males. In children, infection rates are similar in both sexes.

## Clinical Findings

### A. SYMPTOMS AND SIGNS

Primary infection is unrecognized or produces pneumonia. Acute symptoms include cough, chest pain,

headache, weight loss, and fever occurring several weeks to months after inoculation. Infection is usually self-limited in immunocompetent patients (50%). In some patients an indolent progressive pulmonary disease occurs after an incubation period of 30–45 days. Cutaneous lesions usually represent disseminated disease; local primary inoculation is rare. Slowly progressive ulcerating lesions with a sharp, heaped-up border or verrucous lesions occur. Bone disease resembles other forms of chronic osteomyelitis. Lytic skull lesions in children are typical, but long bones, vertebrae, and the pelvis may be involved. Extrapulmonary disease occurs in 25–40% of patients. A total body radiographic examination is advisable when blastomycosis is diagnosed in the skin or another nonpulmonary site. The genitourinary tract involvement characteristic of dissemination in adults is rare in prepubertal children. Lymph nodes, brain, and kidneys may be involved.

### B. LABORATORY FINDINGS

Diagnosis requires isolation or visualization of the fungus. Pulmonary specimens (sputum, tracheal aspirates, lung biopsy) may be positive with conventional stains or fungal cell wall stains. An initial suppurative response is followed by an increase in the number of mononuclear cells, and then formation of noncaseating granulomas. On microscopic examination, the budding yeasts are thick-walled, have refractile walls, and are very large and distinctive. Sputum specimens are positive in 50–80% of cases; skin lesions are positive in 80–100%. The fungus can be grown readily in most laboratories, but 2–4 weeks are required. Serologic tests are generally not helpful for diagnosis.

### C. IMAGING

Radiographic consolidation and fibronodular interstitial and alveolar infiltrates are typical; effusions, hilar nodes, and cavities are less common. The paucity of cavitation distinguishes acute blastomycosis from histoplasmosis and tuberculosis. Miliary patterns also occur with acute infection. Chronic disease can develop in the upper lobes, with cavities and fibronodular infiltrations similar to that seen in tuberculosis, but, unlike in tuberculosis or histoplasmosis, these lesions rarely caseate or calcify.

## Differential Diagnosis

Primary pulmonary infection resembles acute viral, bacterial, or mycoplasmal infections. Blastomycosis should be considered when a significant pulmonary infection in an endemic area fails to respond to antibiotic therapy. Subacute infection mimics tuberculosis, histoplasmosis, and coccidioidomycosis. Chronic pulmonary or disseminated disease must be differentiated from cancer, tuberculosis, or other fungal infections.

## Treatment

Mild pulmonary blastomycosis does not require treatment; indeed, it is rarely recognized. Recommended therapy for life-threatening (especially in the immuncompromised patient) or CNS infections is amphotericin B (0.7–1.0 mg/kg intravenously for a total of 1.5–2.0 g). Itraconazole (6–8 mg/kg/d for 6 months) is preferred for other forms of blastomycosis. Bone disease may require a full year of itraconazole therapy. Surgical debridement is required for devitalized bone, drainage of large abscesses, and pulmonary lesions not responding to medical therapy.

Bradsher RW et al: Blastomycosis. Infect Dis Clin North Am 2003;17:21 [PMID: 12751259].

# CANDIDIASIS

## ESSENTIALS OF DIAGNOSIS & TYPICAL FEATURES

- *In normal or immunosuppressed individuals: superficial infections (oral thrush or ulcerations; vulvovaginitis; erythematous intertriginous rash with satellite lesions); fungemia related to intravascular devices.*
- *In immunosuppressed individuals: systemic infections (renal, hepatic, splenic, pulmonary, or cerebral abscesses); cotton-wool retinal lesions; cutaneous nodules.*
- *In either patient population: budding yeast and pseudohyphae seen in biopsy specimens, body fluids, or scrapings of lesions; positive culture.*

## General Considerations

Disease due to *Candida* is caused by *Candida albicans* in 60–80% of cases; similar systemic infection may be due to *C tropicalis, C parapsilosis, C glabrata,* and a few other *Candida* species. Speciation is important because of differences in pathogenicity and response to azole therapy. In tissue, pseudohyphae or budding yeast (or both) are seen. *Candida* grows on routine media more slowly than bacteria; growth is usually evident on agar after 2–3 days and in blood culture media in 2–7 days.

*C albicans* is ubiquitous and often present in small numbers on skin, mucous membranes, or in the intestinal tract. Normal bacterial flora, intact epithelial barriers, neutrophils and macrophages in conjunction with antibody and complement, and normal lymphocyte function (manifested by skin test reactivity) are factors in preventing invasion. Disseminated infection is almost always preceded by prolonged broad-spectrum antibiotic therapy, instrumentation (including intravascular catheters), or immunosuppression. Patients with diabetes mellitus are especially prone to superficial *Candida* infection, for whom thrush and vaginitis are most common. *Candida* is the third most common blood isolate in hospitals in the United States and is a common cause of catheter-related urinary tract infection.

## Clinical Findings

### A. SYMPTOMS AND SIGNS

**1. Oral candidiasis (thrush)**—Adherent creamy white plaques on the buccal, gingival, or lingual mucosa are seen. These may be painful. Lesions may be few and asymptomatic, or they may be extensive, extending into the esophagus. Thrush is very common in otherwise normal infants in the first weeks of life; it may last weeks despite topical therapy. Spontaneous thrush in older children is unusual unless they have recently received antimicrobials. Steroid inhalation for asthma predisposes patients to thrush. HIV infection should be considered if there is no other reason for oral thrush, or if it is persistent or recurrent. *Angular cheilitis* is the name given to painful erythematous fissures caused by *Candida* at the corners of the mouth, often in association with a vitamin or iron deficiency.

**2. Vaginal infection**—Vulvovaginitis occurs in sexually active girls, in diabetic patients, and in girls receiving antibiotics. Thick, odorless, cheesy discharge with intense pruritus is typical. The vagina and labia are usually erythematous and swollen. Outbreaks are more frequent before menses.

**3. Skin infection—**

**a. Diaper dermatitis**—Diaper dermatitis is often due entirely or partly to *Candida*. Pronounced erythema with a sharply defined margin and satellite lesions is typical. Pustules, vesicles, papules, or scales may be seen. Weeping, eroded lesions with a scalloped border are common. Any moist area, such as axillae or neck folds, may be involved.

**b. Congenital skin lesions**—These lesions may be seen in infants born to women with *Candida* amnionitis. A red maculopapular or pustular rash is seen. Dissemination may occur in premature babies or infants after prolonged rupture of membranes.

**c. Scattered red papules or nodules**—Such findings may represent cutaneous dissemination.

**d. Paronychia and onychomycosis**—These conditions occur in immunocompetent children but are often associated with immunosuppression, hypoparathyroidism, or adrenal insufficiency (*Candida* endocrinopathy syndrome). The selective abscence of specific T-cell responses to *Candida* can lead to marked, chronic skin and nail infections called *chronic mucocutaneous candidiasis*.

**e. Chronic draining otitis media**—This problem may occur in patients who have received multiple courses of antibiotics and are superinfected with *Candida*.

**4. Enteric infection**—Esophageal involvement in immunosuppressed patients is the most common enteric manifestation. It is manifested by substernal pain, dysphagia, painful swallowing, and anorexia. Nausea and vomiting are common in young children. Most patients do not have thrush. Stomach or intestinal ulcers also occur. A syndrome of mild diarrhea in normal individuals who have predominant *Candida* on stool culture has also been described, although *Candida* is not considered a true enteric pathogen. Its presence more often reflects recent antimicrobial therapy.

**5. Pulmonary infection**—Because the organism frequently colonizes the respiratory tract, it is commonly isolated from respiratory secretions. Thus demonstration of tissue invasion is needed to diagnose *Candida* pneumonia or tracheitis. It is rare, being seen in immunosuppressed patients and patients intubated for long periods, usually while taking antibiotics. The infection may cause fever, cough, abscesses, nodular infiltrates, and effusion.

**6. Renal infection**—Candiduria may be the only manifestation of disseminated disease. More often, candiduria is associated with instrumentation, an indwelling catheter, or anatomic abnormality of the urinary tract. Symptoms of cystitis may be present. Masses of *Candida* may obstruct ureters and cause obstructive nephropathy. *Candida* casts in the urine suggest renal tissue infection.

**7. Other infections**—Endocarditis, myocarditis, meningitis, and osteomyelitis usually occur only in immunocompromised patients or neonates.

**8. Disseminated candidiasis**—Skin and mucosal colonization precedes but does not predict dissemination. Too often, dissemination is confused with bacterial sepsis. This occurs in neonates—especially premature infants—in an intensive care unit setting, and is recognized when the infant fails to respond to antibiotics or when candidemia is documented. A careful search should be carried out for lesions suggestive of disseminated *Candida* (retinal cotton-wool spots or nodular dermal abscesses). If these findings are absent, diagnosis is often based presumptively on the presence of a compatible illness in an immunocompromised patient, a burn patient, or a patient with prolonged postsurgical or intensive care unit course who has no other cause for the symptoms; who fails to respond to antimicrobials; and who usually has *Candida* colonization of mucosal surfaces. Treatment for presumptive infection is often undertaken because candidemia is not identified antemortem in many such patients.

Hepatosplenic candidiasis occurs in immunosuppressed patients. The typical case consists of a severely neutropenic patient who develops chronic fever, variable abdominal pain, and abnormal liver function tests. No bacteria are isolated, and there is no response to antimicrobials. Symptoms persist even when neutrophils return. Ultrasound or CT scan of the liver and spleen demonstrates multiple round lesions. Biopsy is needed to confirm the diagnosis.

## B. LABORATORY FINDINGS

Budding yeast cells are easily seen in scrapings or other samples. A wet mount of vaginal secretions is 40–50% sensitive; this is increased to 50–70% with the addition of 10% KOH. The use of a Gram-stain smear is 70–100% sensitive. The presence of pseudohyphae suggests tissue invasion. Culture is definitive. Ninety-five percent of positive blood cultures will be detected within 3 days, but cultures may remain negative (10–40%), even with disseminated disease or endocarditis. *Candida* should never be considered a contaminant in cultures from normally sterile sites. *Candida* in any number in appropriately collected urine suggests true infection. Antigen tests are not sensitive or specific enough for clinical use. Antibody tests are not useful. The ability of yeast to form germ tubes when incubated in human serum gives a presumptive speciation for *C albicans*.

## Differential Diagnosis

Thrush may resemble formula (which can be easily wiped away with a tongue blade or swab, revealing normal mucosa without underlying erythema or erosion), other types of ulcers (including herpes), or burns. Skin lesions may resemble contact, allergic, chemical, or bacterial dermatitis; miliaria; folliculitis; or eczema. Candidemia and systemic infection should be considered in any seriously ill patient with the risk factors previously mentioned.

## Complications

Failure to recognize disseminated disease early is the greatest complication. Osteoarthritis and meningitis occur more often in neonates than in older children. Blindness from retinitis, massive emboli from large vegetations of endocarditis, and abscesses in any organ are other complications; the greater the length or degree of immunosuppression and the longer the delay before therapy, the more complications are seen.

## Treatment

### A. ORAL CANDIDIASIS

In infants, oral nystatin suspension (100,000 units four to six times a day in the buccal fold after feeding until resolution) usually suffices. Nystatin must come in contact with the lesions because it is not absorbed systemically. Older children may use it as a mouthwash (200,000–500,000 units four times a day), although it is poorly tolerated because of its taste. Clotrimazole troches (10 mg) four times a day are an alternative in older children. Prolonged therapy with either agent or more frequent dosing may be needed. Painting the lesions with a cotton swab dipped in gentian violet

(0.5–1%) is visually dramatic and messy but may help refractory cases. Eradication of *Candida* from pacifiers, bottle nipples, toys, or the mother's breasts (if the infant is breast-feeding and there is candidal infection of the nipples) may be helpful.

Oral azoles—ketoconazole (200 mg/m$^2$ in divided doses every 12 hours for 5–7 days) and fluconazole (6 mg/kg/d)—are effective in older children with candidal infection refractory to nystatin. Discontinuation of antibiotics or corticosteroids is advised when possible.

### B. SKIN INFECTION

Cutaneous infection usually responds to a cream or lotion containing nystatin, amphotericin B, or an imidazole. Associated inflammation, such as severe diaper dermatitis, is also helped by concurrent use of a topical mild corticosteroid cream, such as 1% hydrocortisone. One approach is to keep the involved area dry; a heat lamp and nystatin powder may be used. Cornstarch is a yeast nutrient and should not be used as a drying agent.

Suppression of intestinal *Candida* with nystatin and eradicating thrush may speed recovery and prevent recurrence of the diaper dermatitis.

### C. VAGINAL INFECTIONS

Vaginal infection (see Chapter 40) is treated with clotrimazole, miconazole, triazoles, or nystatin (cheapest if generic is used) suppositories or creams, usually applied once nightly for 3–7 days. In general, nystatin is less effective and longer therapy is required. A high-dose clotrimazole formulation need be given for only a single night. *Candida balanitis* in sexual partners should be treated. Oral azole therapy is equally effective. A single 150-mg oral dose of fluconazole is effective for vaginitis. It is more expensive but very convenient. No controlled study has shown that treating colonization of male sexual partners prevents recurrence in females. Frequent recurrent infections may require elimination of risk factors, the use of oral therapy, or some prophylactic antifungal therapy, such as a single dose of fluconazole weekly.

### D. RENAL INFECTION

Candiduria limited to the bladder may be treated with amphotericin B bladder irrigation (if a catheter is already in place). A more effective approach is a 7- to 14-day course of fluconazole, which is concentrated in the urine. Renal abscesses or ureteral fungus balls require systemic antifungal therapy. Surgical debridement may be required. Removal of an indwelling catheter is imperative. Amphotericin B may improve poor renal function caused by renal candidiasis, even though the drug is nephrotoxic.

### E. SYSTEMIC INFECTION

Systemic infection is dangerous and resistant to therapy. Surgical drainage of abscesses and removal of all infected tissue (eg, a heart valve) are required for cure. Hepatosplenic candidiasis should be treated until all lesions have disappeared or are calcified on imaging studies. Systemic infection is optimally treated with amphotericin B or a lipid formulation. Lipid forms of amphotericin B retain the antifungal potency of the free drug but are much better tolerated. Although they are much more expensive than amphotericin B, they are indicated for patients who are intolerant of conventional therapy, for those whose infection is refractory to treatment, or for those who have a high likelihood of developing renal toxicity from such therapy.

Correction of predisposing factors is important (eg, discontinuing antibiotics and immunosuppressives and improving control of diabetes). Addition of flucytosine (50–75 mg/kg/d orally in four doses; keep serum levels below 75 µg/mL) may help. This is frequently added to treat neonatal infections, but clinical outcome seems to be similar when amphotericin B is used alone. Unlike amphotericin B, flucytosine penetrates tissues well; it is also synergistic with amphotericin B against many organisms. It should not be used as a single agent in serious infections because resistance develops rapidly.

Fluconazole is an acceptable alternative for serious *C albicans* infections in nonneutropenic patients and is often effective as first-line therapy in immunocompromised patients. However, the decision to use fluconazole must include consideration of the local experience with fluconazole-resistant *Candida*. Susceptibility testing for *Candida* species is now available to guide this decision. *C glabrata* and *C krusei* are common isolates that may be resistant to azoles. Infected central venous lines must be removed immediately; this alone often is curative. Persistent fever and candidemia suggest infected thrombus, endocarditis, or tissue infection. If the infection is considered limited to the line and environs, a 14-day course (after the last positive culture) of an antifungal agent such as amphotericin B or fluconazole following line removal is recommended for immunocompromised patients. Fluconazole should also be considered for immunocompetent patients with candidemia, because of the late occurrence of focal *Candida* infection in some cases.

Fluconazole is well absorbed (oral and intravenous therapy are equivalent), reasonably nontoxic, and effective for a variety of *Candida* infections. It is the treatment of choice if amphotericin B is not tolerated. The dosage is 8–12 mg/kg/d in a single daily dose for initial therapy of severely ill children. Selected patients with prolonged immunosuppression (eg, after bone marrow transplantation) should receive fluconazole, itraconazole, or intermittent amphotericin B prophylaxis. Treatment of azole-resistant *Candida* is now facilitated by the availability of voriconazole and by the first licensed echinocandin, caspofungin, which is active against these organisms. These drugs are less expensive than the lipid formulations of amphotericin and are becoming first-line alternatives.

## Prognosis

Superficial disease in normal hosts has a good prognosis; in abnormal hosts, it may be refractory to therapy. Early therapy of systemic disease is often curative if the underlying immune response is adequate. The outcome is poor when therapy is delayed or when host response is inadequate.

Chapman RL: *Candida* infections in the neonate. Curr Opin Pediatr 2003;15:97 [PMID: 12544279].

Kalfa VC et al: The syndrome of chronic mucocutaneous candidiasis with selective antibody deficiency. Ann Allergy Asthma Immunol 2003;90:259 [PMID: 12602677].

Moylett EH: Neonatal *Candida* meningitis. Semin Pediatr Infect Dis 2003;14:115 [PMID: 1281799].

Williams K: Lipid amphotericin preparations. Pediatr Infect Dis J 2000;19:567 [PMID: 10877175].

# COCCIDIOIDOMYCOSIS

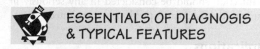

### ESSENTIALS OF DIAGNOSIS & TYPICAL FEATURES

- *Residence in or travel to an endemic area.*
- *Primary pulmonary form: fever, chest pain, cough, anorexia, weight loss, and often a macular rash or erythema nodosum or multiforme.*
- *Primary cutaneous form: trauma followed in 1–3 weeks by an ulcer and regional adenopathy.*
- *Spherules seen in pus, sputum, CSF, joint fluid; positive culture.*
- *Appearance of precipitating (early) and complement-fixing antibodies (late).*

## General Considerations

Coccidioidomycosis is caused by the dimorphic fungus *Coccidioides immitis,* which is endemic in the Sonoran Desert areas of western and southern parts of Texas, New Mexico, and Arizona, southern California, northern Mexico, and South America. Infection results from inhalation or inoculation of arthrospores (highly contagious and readily airborne in the dry climate). Even brief travel in or through an endemic area, especially during windy seasons, may allow infection. Human-to-human transmission does not occur. More than half of all infections are asymptomatic, and fewer than 5–10% are associated with significant pulmonary disease. Chronic pulmonary disease or dissemination occurs in less than 1% of cases.

## Clinical Findings

### A. SYMPTOMS AND SIGNS

**1. Primary disease**—The incubation period is 10–16 days (range, 7–28 days). Symptoms vary from those of a mild fever and arthralgia to severe influenza-like illness with high fever, nonproductive cough, pleurisy, myalgias, arthralgias, headache, night sweats, and anorexia. Upper respiratory tract signs are not common. Severe pleuritic chest pain suggests this diagnosis. Signs vary from none to rash, rales, pleural rubs, and signs of pulmonary consolidation. Weight loss may occur.

**2. Skin disease**—Up to 10% of children develop erythema nodosum or multiforme. These manifestations imply a favorable host response to the organism. Less specific maculopapular eruptions occur in a larger number of children. Skin lesions can occur following fungemia. Primary skin inoculation sites develop indurated ulcers with local adenopathy. Contiguous involvement of skin from deep infection in nodes or bone also occurs. The presence of chronic skin lesions with this fungus should lead to a search for other areas of infection (eg, lung).

**3. Chronic pulmonary disease**—This is uncommon in children. Chronic disease is manifested by chronic cough (occasionally with hemoptysis), weight loss, pulmonary consolidation, effusion, cavitation, or pneumothorax.

**4. Disseminated disease**—This is less common in children than adults. It is more common in infants, neonates, pregnant women (especially during the third trimester), blacks, Filipinos, American Indians, and patients with HIV or any other type of immunosuppression. One or more organs may be involved. The most common sites involved are bone or joint (usually a single bone or joint; subacute or chronic swelling, pain, redness); nodes, meninges (slowly progressive meningeal signs, ataxia, vomiting, headache, cranial neuropathies); and kidney (dysuria, urinary frequency). As with most fungal diseases, the evolution of the illness is usually slow.

### B. LABORATORY FINDINGS

Direct examination of respiratory secretions, pus, CSF, or tissue may reveal large spherules (30–60 mm) containing endospores. These are the product of coccidioidal spores germinating in tissue. Phase-contrast microscopy is useful for demonstrating these refractile bodies; Gram or methylene blue stains are not helpful, but periodic acid–Schiff reagent, methenamine silver, and calcofluor stains are. Fluffy, gray-white colonies grow within 2–5 days on routine fungal and many other media. They are highly infectious. CSF cultures are often negative.

Routine laboratory tests are nonspecific. The sedimentation rate is usually elevated. Eosinophilia may occur, particularly prior to dissemination and is more common in coccidioidomycosis than in many other conditions with similar symptoms. Meningitis causes a mononuclear pleocytosis (70% with eosinophils) with elevated protein and mild hypoglycorrhachia.

Within 2–21 days, most patients develop a delayed hypersensitivity reaction to coccidioidin skin test antigen (Spherulin 0.1 mL, intradermally, should produce 5-mm induration at 48 hours). Erythema nodosum predicts strong reactivity; when this reaction is present the antigen should be diluted 10–100 times before use. The skin test may be negative in immunocompromised patients or in those with disseminated disease. Positive reactions may remain for years and do not prove active infection.

Antibodies consist of precipitins (usually measurable by 2–3 weeks in 90% of cases and gone by 12 weeks) and complement-fixing antibodies (delayed for several weeks; appear as the precipitins are falling and disappear by 8 months, unless dissemination or chronic infection occurs). The extent of the complement-fixing antibody response reflects the severity of infection. Persistent high levels suggest dissemination. Serum precipitins usually indicate acute infection. Excellent ELISA assays are now available to detect IgM and IgG antibodies against the precipitin and complement-fixing antigens. The presence of antibody in CSF indicates CNS infection.

### C. IMAGING

Approximately half of symptomatic infections are associated with abnormal chest radiographs—usually infiltrates with hilar adenopathy. Pulmonary consolidation, effusion, and thin-walled cavities may be seen. About 5% of infected patients have asymptomatic nodules or cysts after recovery. Unlike reactivation tuberculosis, apical disease is not prominent. Bone infection causes osteolysis that enhances with technetium. Cerebral imaging may show hydrocephalus and meningitis; intracranial abscesses and calcifications are unusual. Radiographic evolution of all lesions is slow.

## Differential Diagnosis

Primary pulmonary infection resembles acute viral, bacterial, or mycoplasmal infections; subacute presentation mimics tuberculosis, histoplasmosis, and blastomycosis. Chronic pulmonary or disseminated disease must be differentiated from cancer, tuberculosis, or other fungal infections.

## Complications

Dissemination of primary pulmonary disease is associated with ethnic background, prolonged fever (> 1 month), a negative skin test, high complement-fixation antibody titer, and marked hilar adenopathy. Local pulmonary complications include effusion, empyema, and pneumothorax. Cerebral infection can cause noncommunicating hydrocephalus due to basilar meningitis.

## Treatment

### A. SPECIFIC MEASURES

Mild pulmonary infections in most normal hosts require no therapy. These patients should be assessed for 1–2 years to document resolution and to identify any complications early. Antifungal therapy is used for prolonged fever, weight loss, prolonged duration of night sweats, severe pneumonitis (especially if persisting for 4–6 weeks), or any form of disseminated disease. Neonates, those with genetic risk factors, pregnant women, and those with high antibody titer also receive treatment.

Amphotericin B is used to treat severe disease (1 mg/kg/d until better; then reduce dose; total duration, 2–3 months). For less severe disease and for meningeal disease, fluconazole is preferred (duration of therapy is more than 6 months). Chronic fibrocavitary pneumonia is treated for at least 12 months. Lifelong suppressive therapy is recommended after treating coccidioidal meningitis. Itraconazole may be superior to fluconazole. Refractory meningitis may require prolonged intrathecal or intraventricular amphotericin B therapy. Pregnant patients should not receive azoles.

### B. GENERAL MEASURES

Most pulmonary infections require only symptomatic therapy, self-limited activity, and good nutrition. They are not contagious.

### C. SURGICAL MEASURES

Excision of chronic pulmonary cavities or abscesses may be needed. Infected nodes, sinus tracts, and bone are other operable lesions. Azole therapy should be given prior to surgery to prevent dissemination; it is contin-

ued for 4 weeks arbitrarily or until other criteria for cure are met.

## Prognosis

Most patients recover. Even with amphotericin B, however, disseminated disease may be fatal, especially in those racially predisposed to severe disease. Reversion of the skin test to negative or a rising complement-fixing antibody titer is an ominous sign. Individuals who later in life undergo immunosuppressive therapy may experience reactivation of dormant disease.

Chiller TM et al: Coccidioidomycosis. Infect Dis Clin North Am 2003;17:41 [PMID: 12751260].

Cortez KJ et al: Successful treatment of coccidioidal meningitis with voriconazole. Clin Infect Dis 2003;36;1619 [PMID:12802765].

# CRYPTOCOCCOSIS

## ESSENTIALS OF DIAGNOSIS & TYPICAL FEATURES

- *Acute pneumonitis in immunocompetent individuals.*
- *Immunosuppressed patients especially vulnerable to CNS infection (headache, vomiting, cranial nerve palsies, meningeal signs; mononuclear cell pleocytosis).*
- *Cryptococcal antigen detected in CSF; also in serum and urine in some patients.*
- *Readily isolated on routine media.*

## General Considerations

*Cryptococcus neoformans* is a ubiquitous soil yeast. It appears to survive better in soil contaminated with bird excrement, especially that of pigeons. However, most infections in humans are not associated with a history of significant contact with birds. Inhalation is the presumed route of inoculation. Infections in children are rare, even in heavily immunocompromised patients such as those with HIV infection. Immunocompetent individuals can also be infected. Asymptomatic carriage does not occur.

## Clinical Findings

### A. SYMPTOMS AND SIGNS

**1. Pulmonary disease**—Pulmonary infection precedes dissemination to other organs. It is frequently asymptomatic (most older children and adults have serologic evidence of prior infection) and less often clinically apparent than cryptococcal meningitis. Pneumonia is the primary manifestation in one third of patients and CNS disease in 50%; cryptococcal pneumonia may coexist with cerebral involvement. Symptoms are nonspecific and subacute—cough, weight loss, and fatigue. The fungus can persist in a latent form in subpleural granulomas.

**2. Meningitis**—The most common clinical disease is meningitis, which follows hematogenous spread from a pulmonary focus. Symptoms of headache, vomiting, and fever occur over days to months. Meningeal signs and papilledema are common. Cranial nerve dysfunction and seizures may occur.

**3. Other forms**—Cutaneous forms are usually secondary to dissemination. Papules, pustules, and ulcerating nodules are typical. Bones (rarely joints) may be infected; osteolytic areas are seen, and the process may resemble osteosarcoma. Many other organs, especially the eye, can be involved with dissemination.

### B. LABORATORY FINDINGS

The CSF usually has a lymphocytic pleocytosis; it may be completely normal in immunosuppressed patients who have cryptococcal meningitis. Direct microscopy may reveal organisms in sputum, CSF, or other specimens. The capsular antigen can be detected by latex agglutination or ELISA, which are both sensitive (> 90%) and specific. Serum, CSF, and urine may be tested. The serum may be negative if the only organ infected is the lung. False-negative CSF tests have been reported. The organism grows well after several days on many routine media; for optimal culture, collecting and concentrating a large amount of CSF ($\leq$ 10 mL) is recommended, because the number of organisms may be low.

### C. IMAGING

Radiographic findings are usually lower lobe infiltrates or nodular densities; less often effusions; and rarely cavitation, hilar adenopathy, or calcification. Single or multiple focal mass lesions (cryptococcoma) may be detected in the CNS on CT or magnetic resonance imaging scan.

## Differential Diagnosis

Cryptococcal meningitis may mimic tuberculosis, viral meningoencephalitis, meningitis due to other fungi, or a space-occupying CNS lesion. Lung infection is difficult to differentiate from many causes of pneumonia.

## Complications

Hydrocephalus may be caused by chronic basilar meningitis. Symptomatic intracranial hypertension is common. Significant pulmonary or osseous disease may accompany the primary infection or dissemination.

## Treatment

Patients with symptomatic pulmonary disease should receive fluconazole for 3–6 months. All such immunocompromised patients should have a lumbar puncture to rule out CNS infection; this should also be done for immunocompetent patients with cryptococcal antigen in the serum. Severely ill patients should instead receive amphotericin B (0.7 mg/kg/d). Meningitis is treated with amphotericin B and flucytosine (100 mg/kg/d). The combination is synergistic and allows lower doses of amphotericin B to be used. Therapy is usually 6 weeks for cerebral infections (or for 1 month after sterilization) and 8 weeks for osteomyelitis. An alternative is to substitute fluconazole after 2 weeks of the combination therapy and continue fluconazole alone for 8–10 weeks. Fluconazole is the preferred maintenance therapy to prevent relapses in high-risk (HIV) patients. CSF antigen levels should be checked after 2 weeks of therapy. Intracranial hypertension is treated by frequent spinal taps or a lumbar drain.

## Prognosis

Treatment failure, including death, is common in immunosuppressed patients, especially those with AIDS. Lifelong maintenance therapy is required in these patients. Poor prognostic signs are the presence of extrameningeal disease; fewer than 20 cells/μL of initial CSF; and initial CSF antigen titer greater than 1:32.

Perfect TF, Casadevall A: Cryptococcosis. Infect Dis Clin North Am 2002;16:837 [PMID:12512184].

# HISTOPLASMOSIS

**ESSENTIALS OF DIAGNOSIS & TYPICAL FEATURES**

- *Residence in or travel to endemic areas.*
- *Pneumonia with flu-like illness.*
- *Hepatosplenomegaly, anemia, leukopenia if disseminated.*
- *Histoplasmal antigen in urine, blood, or CSF.*
- *Detection of the organism in smears or tissue or by culture.*

## General Considerations

The dimorphic fungus *Histoplasma capsulatum* is found in the central and eastern United States (Ohio and Mississippi River valleys), Mexico, and most of South America. Soil contamination is enhanced by the presence of bat or bird feces. The small yeast form (2–4 mm) is seen in tissue, especially within macrophages. Infection is acquired by inhaling spores that transform into the pathogenic yeast phase. Infections in endemic areas are very common at all ages and are usually asymptomatic. Over two thirds of children are infected in these areas. Reactivation is very rare in children; it may occur years later, usually owing to significant immunosuppression. Reinfection also occurs. The extent of symptoms with primary or reinfection is influenced by the size of the infecting inoculum.

## Clinical Findings

Because human-to-human transmission does not occur, infection requires exposure in the endemic area—usually within prior weeks or months. Congenital infection does not occur.

### A. SYMPTOMS AND SIGNS

**1. Asymptomatic infection (50% of infections)—** Asymptomatic histoplasmosis is usually diagnosed by the presence of scattered calcifications in lungs or spleen and a positive skin test. The calcification may resemble that caused by tuberculosis but may be more extensive than the usual Ghon complex.

**2. Pneumonia—**Approximately 45% of patients have mild to moderate disease. Most of these patients are not recognized as having a histoplasmal infection. Acute pulmonary disease may resemble influenza, with fever, myalgia, arthralgia, and cough occurring 1–3 weeks after exposure; the subacute form resembles infections such as tuberculosis, with cough, weight loss, night sweats, and pleurisy. Chronic disease is unusual in children. Physical examination may be normal, or rales may be heard. A small number of patients may have immune-mediated signs such as arthritis, pericarditis, and erythema nodosum. The usual duration of the disease is less than 2 weeks, followed by complete resolution. Symptoms may last several months and still resolve without antifungal therapy.

**3. Disseminated infection (5% of infections)—** Fungemia during primary infection probably occurs in the first 2 weeks of all infections, including those with minimal symptoms. Transient hepatosplenomegaly may occur, but resolution is the rule in immunocompetent individuals. Heavy exposure, severe underlying pulmonary disease, and immunosuppression are risk factors for progressive reticuloendothelial cell infection, with anemia, fever, weight loss, organomegaly, bone marrow involvement, and death. Dissemination may occur in otherwise immunocompetent children; usually they are younger than age 2 years.

**4. Other forms—**Ocular involvement consists of multifocal choroiditis. This usually occurs in immunocompetent adults who exhibit other evidence of disseminated disease. Brain, heart valve, pericardium, intestine, and skin (oral ulcers, nodules) are other involved sites. Adrenal gland involvement is common with systemic disease.

### B. LABORATORY FINDINGS

Routine tests are normal or nonspecific in the benign forms. Pancytopenia is present in many patients with disseminated disease. The diagnosis can be made by demonstrating the organism by histology or culture. Tissue yeast forms are small and may be mistaken for artifact. They are usually found in macrophages, occasionally in peripheral blood leukocytes in severe disease, but rarely in sputum, urine, or CSF. Cultures of infected fluids or tissues may yield the organism after 1–6 weeks of incubation on fungal media, but even cultures of bronchoalveolar lavage or transbronchial biopsy specimens in immunocompromised patients are often negative (15%). Thus bone marrow and tissue specimens are needed. Detection of histoplasmal antigen in blood, urine, CSF, and bronchoalveolar lavage is probably the most sensitive diagnostic test (90% positive in the urine with disseminated disease; 75% positive with acute pneumonia). The level of antigen correlates with the extent of the infection, and antigen levels can be used to follow the response to therapy and to indicate low-grade infection persisting after completion of therapy (eg, in a child with HIV infection).

Antibodies may be detected by immunodiffusion, complement fixation, and precipitation; the latter two measures rise in the first 2–6 weeks of illness and fall unless dissemination occurs. Cross-reactions occur with some other endemic fungi. A single high titer or rising titer indicates a high likelihood of disease. Antigen detection has replaced serology as a rapid diagnostic test.

### C. IMAGING

Scattered pulmonary calcifications in a well child are typical of past infection. Bronchopneumonia (focal midlung infiltrates) occurs with acute disease, often with hilar and mediastinal adenopathy, occasionally with nodules, but seldom with effusion. Apical cavitation occurs with chronic infection, often on the background of preexisting pulmonary infection.

## Differential Diagnosis

Pulmonary disease resembles viral infection, tuberculosis, coccidioidomycosis, and blastomycosis. Systemic disease resembles disseminated fungal or mycobacterial infection, leukemia, histiocytosis, or cancer.

## Treatment

Mild infections do not require therapy. Treatment is indicated for severe pulmonary disease (diffuse radiographic involvement), disseminated disease, when endovascular, CNS, or chronic pulmonary disease is present, and for children younger than age 1 year. Treatment should also be considered for patients who show no clinical improvement after 1 month. Disseminated disease in infants may respond to as little as 10 days of amphotericin B, although 4–6 weeks (or 30 mg/kg total dosage) is usually recommended. Amphotericin B is the preferred therapy for moderately severe forms of the disease. Patients with severe disease may benefit from a short course of steroid therapy (see also section on *Pneumocystis jiroveci,* formerly *Pneumocystis carinii*). Surgical excision of chronic pulmonary lesions is rarely required. Itraconazole (3–5 mg/kg/d for 6–12 weeks; achieve peak serum level of > 1.0 μg/mL) appears to be equivalent to amphotericin B therapy for mild disease and can be substituted for amphotericin B in severe disease after a favorable initial response has occurred. With chronic pulmonary, CNS, or disseminated disease, therapy may be required for prolonged periods.

Quantification of fungal antigen is useful for directing therapy. Histoplasmosis can reactivate in previously infected individuals who subsequently become immunosuppressed. Chronically immunosuppressed patients (eg, those with HIV) may require lifelong maintenance therapy with an azole.

## Prognosis

Mild and moderately severe infections have a good prognosis. With early diagnosis and treatment, infants with disseminated disease usually recover; the prognosis worsens if the immune response is poor.

Johnson PC et al: Safety and efficacy of liposomal amphotericin B compared with conventional amphotericin B for induction therapy of histoplasmosis in patients with AIDS. Ann Intern Med 2002;137:105 [PMID: 12118965].

Wheat LJ, Kauffman CA: Infect Dis Clin North Am 2003;17:1 [PMID: 1271258].

# SPOROTRICHOSIS

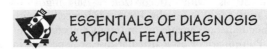

### ESSENTIALS OF DIAGNOSIS & TYPICAL FEATURES

- *Subacute cutaneous ulcers.*
- *New lesions appearing proximal to existing lesions along a draining lymphatic.*
- *Absence of systemic symptoms.*
- *Isolation of* Sporothrix schenckii *from wound drainage or biopsy.*

## General Considerations

Sporotrichosis is caused by *Sporothrix schenckii,* a dimorphic fungus present as a mold in soil, plants, and plant products from most areas of North and South America. Spores of the fungus can cause infection when they breach the skin at areas of minor trauma. Sporotrichosis has been transmitted from cutaneous lesions of pets.

## Clinical Findings

Cutaneous disease is by far the most common manifestation. Typically at the site of inapparent skin injury an initial papular lesion will slowly become nodular and ulcerate. Subsequent new lesions develop in a similar fashion proximally along lymphatics draining the primary lesion. This sequence of developing painless, chronic ulcers in a linear pattern is strongly suggestive of the diagnosis. Solitary lesions may exist and some lesions may develop a verrucous character. Systemic symptoms are absent and laboratory evaluations are normal, except for acute phase reactants. The fungus rarely disseminates in immunocompetent hosts, but bone and joint infections have been described. Cavitary pneumonia is an uncommon manifestation when patients inhale the spores. Immunocompromised patients, especially those with HIV infection, may develop multiorgan disease and extensive pneumonia.

## Diagnosis

The differential diagnosis of nodular lymphangitis (sporotrichoid infection) includes other endemic fungi and some bacteria, especially atypical mycobacteria. Diagnosis is made by culture. Biopsy of skin lesions will demonstrate a suppurative response with granulomas and provides the best source for laboratory isolation. Occasionally the characteristic yeast will be seen in the biopsy.

## Treatment & Prognosis

Treatment is with itraconazole (100 mg/d or 5 mg/kg/d) for 3–6 months. Prognosis is excellent with lymphocutaneous disease in immunocompetent children. Pulmonary or osteoarticular disease, especially in immunocompromised individuals, requires longer therapy, and surgical debridement may be required.

Burch JM et al: Unsuspected sporotrichosis in childhood. Pediatr Infect Dis J 2001;20:442 [PMID: 11332673].

Queiroz-Telles F et al: Subcutaneous mycoses. Infect Dis Clin North Am 2003;17;59 [PMID: 12751261].

## OPPORTUNISTIC FUNGAL INFECTIONS

These infections occur most commonly when therapy with steroids, antineoplastic drugs, or radiation is used for treatment, thereby reducing the number or function of neutrophils and competent T lymphocytes. Inborn errors in immune function (combined immune deficiency; chronic granulomatous disease) may also be complicated by these fungal infections. Infection is also facilitated by altering the normal flora with antibiotics and by disruption of mucus membranes or skin with antineoplastic therapy and with indwelling lines and tubes.

Table 39–8 indicates that filamentous fungi are prominent causes of severe systemic fungal disease in immunocompromised patients. *Aspergillus* species (usually *fumigatus*) and *Zygomycetes* (usually *mucorales*) cause subacute pneumonia and sinusitis and should be considered when these conditions do not respond to antibiotics in immunocompromised patients. Mucormycosis is especially likely to produce severe sinusitis in patients with chronic acidosis, usually because of poorly controlled diabetes. This fungus may invade the orbit and cause brain infection. Mucormycosis also occurs in patients receiving iron chelation therapy. These fungal infections may disseminate widely. They are best diagnosed by aspiration or biopsy of infected tissues. *Cryptococcus,* which can cause disease in the immunocompetent host, is more likely to be clinically apparent and severe in immunocompromised patients. This yeast causes pneumonia and is a prominent cause of fungal meningitis. *Candida* species in these patients cause fungemia and multiorgan disease, with lung, esophagus, liver and spleen frequently affected.

*Malassezia furfur* is a yeast that normally causes the superficial skin infection known as tinea versicolor (see Chapter 14). This organism is considered an opportunist when it is associated with prolonged intravenous therapy, especially central lines used for hyperalimentation. The yeast, which requires skin lipids for its growth, can infect lines when lipids are present in the infusate. Some species will grow in the absence of lipids. Unexplained fever and thrombocytopenia are common. Pulmonary infiltrates may be present. The diagnosis is facilitated by alerting the bacteriology laboratory to add olive oil to culture media. The infection will respond to removal of the line or the lipid supplement. Amphotericin B may hasten resolution.

Opportunistic fungal infections are always in the differential diagnosis for immunocompromised patients with unexplained fever or pulmonary infiltrates. These pathogens should be aggressively pursued with imaging studies and with tissue sampling when clues are available. These infections are difficult to treat. Amphotericin B and appropriate triazole drugs are usually indicated. Caspofungin is a member of a new class of drugs now available to treat *Candida* and *Aspergillus* infections. Voriconazole is a new triazole available for first-line treatment of resistant *Candida* infections and infections caused by *Aspergillus* species. Combinations of these antifungal drugs are being tested in order to improve the outcome. Many children who will have depressed phagocytic and T-cell-mediated immune function for long periods should receive antifungal prophylaxis, most often itraconazole.

Gonzalez CE et al: Zygomycosis. Infect Dis Clin North Am 2002;16:895 [PMID: 12512186].

Marr KA et al: *Aspergillus* pathogenesis, clinical manifestations, and therapy. Infect Dis Clin North Am 2002;16:875 [PMID: 12512185].

## *PNEUMOCYSTIS JIROVECI* INFECTION

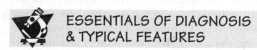

### ESSENTIALS OF DIAGNOSIS & TYPICAL FEATURES

- *Significant immunosuppression.*
- *Fever, tachypnea, cough, dyspnea.*
- *Hypoxemia; diffuse interstitial infiltrates.*

### General Considerations

Although classified as a fungus on the basis of structural and nucleic acid characteristics, *Pneumocystis* responds readily to antiprotozoal drugs and antifols. It is a ubiquitous pathogen. Infection is presumed to occur via inhalation, usually in early childhood. With normal immune function, clinical disease rarely occurs. A syndrome of afebrile pneumonia similar to that caused by *Chlamydia trachomatis* in normal infants has been described but is rarely diagnosed. Organisms dormant in the lung may be reactivated in heavily immunosup-

*Table 39–8.* Unusual fungal infections in children.

| Organism | Predisposing Factors | Route of Infection | Clinical Disease | Diagnostic Tests | Therapy and Comments |
|---|---|---|---|---|---|
| *Aspergillus* species | None | Inhalation of spores | Allergic bronchopulmonary aspergillosis; wheezing, cough, migratory infiltrates, eosinophilia. | Organisms in sputum; positive skin test; specific IgE antibody; elevated IgE levels. | Hypersensitivity to fungal antigens. Use steroids. Antifungals may not be needed. |
| | Immuno-suppression | Inhalation of spores | Progressive pulmonary disease: consolidation, nodules, abscesses. Sinusitis. Disseminated disease: usually lung, brain; occasionally intestine, kidney, heart, bone. Invades blood vessels. | Demonstrate fungus in tissues by stain or culture; septate hyphae branching at 45-degree angle. | Amphotericin B and voriconazole are effective therapies. Caspfungin may be equally effective and can be used in combination with either of the other drugs. |
| *Malassezia furfur, M pachyder-matis* | Central venous catheter, usually lipid infusion (can occur in the absence of lipid) | Line infection from skin colonization | Sepsis; pneumonitis, thrombocytopenia. | Culture of catheter or blood on lipid-enriched media (for *M furfur; M pachydermatis* does not need lipid). Fungus may be seen in buffy coat. | Discontinuation of lipid may be sufficient. Remove catheter. Short-term amphotericin B may be added. Organism ubiquitous on normal skin; requires long-chain fatty acids for growth. |
| *Mucorales (Mucor, Rhizopus, Absidia)* | Immunosuppression, diabetic acidosis, iron chelation therapy | Inhalation, mucosal colonization | Rhinocerebral: sinus, nose, necrotizing vasculitis; central nervous system spread. Pulmonary. Disseminated: any organ. | Broad aseptate hyphae branching at 90-degree angles seen on tissue stains. Culture: rapidly growing, fluffy fungus. | Amphotericin B, surgical debridement; itraconazole may be a second agent for combined therapy. Poor prognosis. |
| *Pseudalles-cheria boydii* | Immuno-suppression | Inhalation | Disseminated abscesses (lung, brain, liver, spleen, other). | Culture of pus or tissue. | Surgical drainage; Voriconazole or caspofungin |
| | Minor trauma | Cutaneous | Mycetoma (most common). | Yellow-white granules in pus. Culture. | Aggressive surgery. Amputation may be needed. |
| *Sporothrix schenckii* | Minor trauma (thorns, splinters) | Cutaneous | Chronic skin ulcers, subcutaneous nodules along lymphatics. Rarely pneumonia, osteomyelitis, arthritis. Disseminated disease in immunocompromised host. | Gram or fungal stain of pus or tissue may show "hockey stick" organisms. Culture of pus, tissue. | Itraconazole, drainage, debridement. |

pressed children, chiefly those with abnormal T-cell function such as occurs with HIV infection, hematologic malignancies, and organ transplantation. Environmental exposure is also presumed to cause infection in immunocompromised children. Prolonged, high-dose corticosteroid therapy is a risk factor; onset of illness as steroids are tapered is a typical presentation. Severely malnourished infants with no underlying illness may also develop this infection, as can those with congenital humoral or cellular immune deficiency. The incubation period is usually at least 1 month after onset of immunosuppression.

*Pneumocystis* pneumonia is a common complication of advanced HIV infection and is one of the diseases that defines AIDS. Prophylaxis usually prevents this infection (see Chapter 37).

Infection is generally limited to the lower respiratory tract. In advanced disease, spread to other organs occurs.

## Clinical Findings

### A. SYMPTOMS AND SIGNS

In most patients, a gradual onset of fever, tachypnea, dyspnea, and mild cough occurs over 1–4 weeks. Initially the chest is clear, although retractions and nasal flaring are present. At this stage, the illness is nonspecific. Hypoxemia out of proportion to the clinical and radiographic signs is an early finding, however, and even minimally decreased arterial $PaO_2$ values should suggest this diagnosis in immunosuppressed children. Tachypnea, nonproductive cough, and dyspnea progress. Respiratory failure and death occur without treatment. In some children with AIDS or severe immunosuppression from chemotherapy or organ transplantation, the onset may be abrupt and progression more rapid.

The general examination is unremarkable. There are no upper respiratory signs, conjunctivitis, organomegaly, enanthem, or rash.

### B. LABORATORY FINDINGS

Laboratory findings reflect the individual child's underlying illness and are not specific. Serum lactate dehydrogenase levels may be elevated markedly as a result of pulmonary damage. In moderately severe cases, the $PaO_2$ is less than 70 mm Hg or the A-a gradient is less than 35 mm Hg.

### C. IMAGING

Early chest radiographs are normal. The classic pattern in later films is that of bilateral, interstitial, lower lobe alveolar disease starting in the perihilar regions, without effusion, consolidation, or hilar adenopathy. Older HIV-infected patients present with other patterns, including nodular infiltrates, lobar pneumonia, cavities, and upper lobe infiltrates.

## Diagnosis

Diagnosis requires finding characteristic round (6–8 mm) cysts in a lung biopsy specimen, bronchial brushings or alveolar washings, induced sputum, or tracheal aspirates. The latter specimens are less sensitive but are more rapidly and easily obtained. They are more often negative in children with leukemia compared with those with HIV infection; presumably, greater immunosuppression results in larger numbers of organisms. Because pneumonia in immunosuppressed patients may have many causes, negative results from tracheal secretions should prompt more aggressive diagnostic attempts. Bronchial washing using fiberoptic bronchoscopy is usually well tolerated and rapidly performed.

Several rapid stains—as well as the standard methenamine silver stain—are useful. The indirect fluorescent antibody method is most sensitive. These methods require competent laboratory evaluation, because few organisms may be present and many artifacts may be found.

## Differential Diagnosis

In immunocompetent infants, *C trachomatis* pneumonia is the most common cause of the afebrile pneumonia syndrome described for *Pneumocystis*. In older immunocompromised children, the differential diagnosis includes influenza, respiratory syncytial virus, cytomegalovirus, adenovirus, and other viral infections; bacterial and fungal pneumonia; pulmonary emboli or hemorrhage; congestive heart failure; and *Chlamydia pneumoniae* and *Mycoplasma pneumoniae* infections. Lymphoid interstitial pneumonitis, which occurs in older infants with HIV infection, is more indolent and the patient's lactate dehydrogenase level is normal (see Chapter 37). *Pneumocystis* pneumonia is uncommon in children who are complying with prophylactic regimens.

## Prevention

Children at high risk for developing *Pneumocystis* infection should receive prophylactic therapy. Children at risk include those with hematologic malignancies or other reasons for receiving intensive chemotherapy or high-dose corticosteroids and children with organ transplants or advanced HIV infection. All children born to HIV-infected mothers should receive prophylaxis against *Pneumocystis* starting at age 6 weeks. Prophylaxis should be maintained until HIV infection has been ruled out or, if the infant is infected, until the patient's immunologic status has been clarified (see Chapter 37). The prophylaxis of choice is trimethoprim–sulfamethoxazole (150 mg/m$^2$/d of trimethoprim and 750 mg/m$^2$/d of sulfamethoxazole) for 3 consecutive days of each week. Alternatives to this prophylaxis regimen are described in Chapter 37.

## Treatment

### A. GENERAL MEASURES

Supplemental oxygen and nutritional support may be needed. Bronchodilators may be tried but are usually not helpful. The patient should be in respiratory isolation.

## B. Specific Measures

Trimethoprim–sulfamethoxazole (20 mg/kg/d of trimethoprim and 100 mg/kg/d of sulfamethoxazole in four divided doses intravenously or orally if well tolerated) is the treatment of choice. Improvement may not be seen for 3–5 days. Duration of treatment is 3 weeks in HIV-infected children. Methylprednisolone (2–4 mg/kg/d in four divided doses intravenously) should also be given to HIV-infected patients with moderate to severe infection for the first 5 days of treatment. The dosage is reduced 50% for the next 5 days, and further reduced by 50% until antibiotic treatment is completed. If trimethoprim–sulfamethoxazole is not tolerated or there is no clinical response in 5 days, pentamidine isethionate (4 mg/kg once daily by slow intravenous infusion) should be given. Clinical efficacy is similar with pentamidine, but adverse reactions are more common. These reactions include dysglycemia, pancreatitis, nephrotoxicity, and leukopenia. Other effective alternatives in adults include atovaquone, trimethoprim–dapsone, and primaquine plus clindamycin.

## Prognosis

The mortality rate is high in immunosuppressed patients who receive treatment late in the illness.

Hidalgo A et al. Accuracy of high-resolution CT in distinguishing between *Pneumocystis carinii* pneumonia and non-*Pneumocystis carinii* pneumonia in AIDS patients. Eur Radiol 2003;13:1179 [PMID: 12695843].

LaRocque RC et al: The utility of sputum induction for diagnosis of *Pneumocystis* pneumonia in immunocompromised patients without human immunodeficiency virus. Clin Infect Dis 2003;37:1380. [PMID: 1453873].

Mahindra AD, Grossman SA: *Pneumocystis carinii* pneumonia in HIV negative patients with primary brain tumors. J Neurooncol 2003;63:263 [PMID: 12892232].

## REFERENCES

### Parasitic Infections

Drugs for parasitic infections: Med Lett Drugs Ther 1998;40:1 [PMID: 9442765].

Liu LY, Weller PF: Antiparasitic drugs. N Engl J Med 1996; 334:1178 [PMID: 8602186].

### Mycotic Infections

Deresinski SC, Stevens DA: Caspofungin. Clin Infect Dis 2003;36:1445 [PMID: 12766841]

Groll AH et al: Clinical pharmacology of antifungal compounds. Infect Dis Clinics North Am 2003;17:159 [PMID: 12751265].

Johnson LB, Kauffman CA: Voriconazole: A new triazole antifungal agent. Clin Infect Dis 2003;36:630 [PMID: 12594645].

Voriconazole. Med Lett Drugs Ther 2002;44:63 [PMID: 12138377].

# Sexually Transmitted Infections

**40**

*Ann-Christine Nyquist, MD, MSPH, Myron J. Levin, MD, & Eric J. Sigel, MD*

The rate of sexually transmitted infections (STIs) acquired during adolescence remains high despite widespread educational programs and increased access to health care. The highest age-specific rates for gonorrhea, chlamydia, and human papillomavirus infection occur in adolescents. By age 18 years, half of youth will have had sexual intercourse. One quarter of those having intercourse will develop an STI—an estimated 3 million teenagers per year. Adolescents contract STIs at a higher rate than adults because of sexual risk-taking, age-related biologic factors, and barriers to health care access. Providers need to comply with state-sanctioned confidentiality laws covering STI-related services, while recognizing the importance of confidentiality to adolescents. Except in a few states, adolescents can provide consent for the diagnosis and confidential treatment of STIs without parental consent or knowledge. In many states, adolescents can also provide consent for HIV counseling and testing.

Providers should screen sexually experienced adolescents for STIs and use this opportunity to discuss risk reduction. Health education counseling should be nonjudgmental and appropriate for the developmental level, yet sufficiently thorough to identify risk behaviors because many adolescents may not readily acknowledge engaging in these behaviors.

## ADOLESCENT SEXUALITY

The spectrum of sexual behavior includes romance—holding hands and kissing; touching, including mutual masturbation; oral–genital contact; and vaginal and anal intercourse. Each has its associated risks. A small but statistically significant trend has occurred in the epidemiology of sexual risk taking toward less sexual involvement and later onset of vaginal intercourse. The most recent Youth Risk Behavior Survey reports that 46% of high school students have had vaginal intercourse during their lifetime; down from 50% in 1999. Seven percent of teenagers have initiated sex by age 13. Significant racial differences exist, with 16% of black students, 7% of Hispanics, and 5% of whites having initiated sex by age 13. Thirty-three percent of students have had sex in the last 3 months—48% of twelfth-graders and 23% of ninth-graders. Condom use has increased, with 58% of youth reporting that either they

or their partner had used a condom during their last sexual intercourse, compared with 42% in 1999. Paradoxically, condom use decreases with age—67% of ninth-graders report condom use at last intercourse compared with 49% of twelfth-graders.

Oral sex has not been as well studied. A recent study reports that 38% of boys, and 42% of girls in the tenth grade engaged in oral sex, with only 17% using any protection.

A significant number of teenagers exhibit higher risk sexual behavior: 22% of high school seniors have had four or more sexual partners. One million teenagers become pregnant annually. Eight percent of students have had sex forced on them—10% of females and 5% of males. Anal intercourse occurs in both heterosexual and homosexual populations.

Adolescents may not yet identify themselves as gay, lesbian, or bisexual but continue to be questioning and engage in high-risk behaviors with multiple partners. Anywhere from 10% to 30% of males experiment with same-sex partners in some fashion, with 4–10% practicing anal sex. Frequently teenage males have their first same-sex experience with partners who are significantly older, which puts them at higher risk for STIs. Lesbians often experiment with male partners during their teen years as they sort out their sexual orientation, placing them at increased risk for pregnancy and STIs.

Impaired judgment related to alcohol or drug use creates an environment for unsafe sexual experimentation. Eighty-two percent of high school students have experimented with alcohol; 50% of high school senior boys have been drunk in the last 30 days. Nationwide, among students who were currently having sexual intercourse, one fourth (25%) used alcohol or drugs the last time they had sex. This additional barrier to decision-making ability results in decreased condom use and an increased incidence of forced sex.

## RISK FACTORS

Certain behaviors and experiences put the adolescent at higher risk for developing STIs. These include early age at sexual debut, lack of condom use, multiple partners, prior STI, history of STI in a partner, and sex with a partner who is 3 or more years older. The type of sex affects risk as well, with intercourse being riskier than oral sex. Other risk-taking behaviors associated with STIs in adolescents are smoking, alcohol use, drug use, dropping out of school, pregnancy, and watching X-rated movies.

Biologically the adolescent female is predisposed to chlamydia, gonorrhea, and human papillomavirus (HPV) infection because the cervix during adolescence has an exposed squamocolumnar junction. The rapidly dividing cells in this area are especially susceptible to microorganism attachment and infection. During early to midpuberty this junction slowly invaginates as the uterus and cervix matures, and by the late teens to early 20s the squamocolumnar junction is inside the cervix.

Grunbaum JA et al: Youth risk behavior surveillance, United States, 2001. MMWR Surveill Summ 2002;51(SS04):1 [PMID: 12102329].

Prinstein MJ et al: Adolescent oral sex, peer popularity, and perceptions of best friend's sexual behavior. J Pediatr Psychol 2003;28:243 [PMID: 22616299].

Sieving R et al: Cognitive and behavioral predictors of sexually transmitted disease: Risk behavior among sexually active adolescents. Arch Pediatr Adolesc Med 1997;151:243 [PMID: 97236012].

## PREVENTION OF SEXUALLY TRANSMITTED INFECTIONS

Efforts to reduce STI risk behavior should begin before the onset of sexual experimentation, first by helping youth personalize their risk for STIs and encouraging positive behaviors that minimize these risks, and then by helping them develop communication skills with sexual partners about STI prevention, abstinence, and condom use.

*Primary prevention* focuses largely on education and risk-reduction techniques. Health care providers should routinely discuss these as part of well adolescent checkups. Nationwide, greater than 90% of students have been taught about acquired immunodeficiency syndrome (AIDS) or human immunodeficiency virus (HIV) infection in school. Although adolescents may be aware of HIV/AIDS or other STIs, they still have a difficult time personalizing risk. Discussing prevalence, symptoms, and sequelae of STIs can raise awareness and help teenagers make informed decisions about whether to initiate sexual activity and what safer sex techniques they should use. Making condoms available reiterates the message that safer sex is vital to health. Discussing condoms, dental dams, and the proper use of lubrication also facilitates safer sex practices. Condoms prevent infections with HIV, gonorrhea, *Chlamydia,* and herpes simplex. They are probably effective in preventing other STIs, as well.

*Secondary prevention* requires identifying and treating STIs (see Screening section) before infected individuals transmit infection to others. Access to medical care is critical to this objective. Identifying and treating STIs in partners are essential in limiting the spread of these infections. Cooperation with the state or county health department is valuable, because these agencies assume the responsibility for locating the contacts of infected persons and ensuring appropriate treatment.

*Tertiary prevention* is directed toward complications of a specific illness. Examples of tertiary prevention would be treating pelvic inflammatory disease (PID) before infertility develops; following the serologic response to syphilis to prevent late-stage syphilis; treating cervicitis to prevent PID; or treating a chlamydial infection before epididymitis ensues.

Finally, preexposure vaccination against hepatitis B or hepatitis A reduces the risk for these preventable STIs. All adolescents should have prior or current immunization against hepatitis B. However, because hepatitis B infection is frequently sexually transmitted, this vaccine is especially critical for all unvaccinated patients being evaluated for an STI. Hepatitis A vaccination is recommended for men who have sex with men and for injection drug users.

## SCREENING FOR SEXUALLY TRANSMITTED INFECTIONS

An essential part of screening is by history. Teenagers should be asked open-ended questions about their sexual experiences to assess their risk for STIs. The ability of the health care provider to obtain an accurate sexual history is crucial in prevention and control efforts. Questions must be explicit and understandable to the teen. If the adolescent has ever engaged in sexual activity, the provider needs to determine what kind of sexual activity (mutual masturbation, oral, anal, or vaginal sex); whether it has been heterosexual, homosexual, or both; whether birth control and condoms were used; and whether it has been consensual or forced. During the interview, to assess degree of risk, the clinician should take the opportunity to discuss risk-reduction techniques. Importantly, female health care providers are twice as likely as male providers to screen female teenagers for STIs, so male health care providers need to better use screening opportunities.

A routine laboratory screening process is warranted if the patient has engaged in intercourse, presents with STI symptoms, or reports a partner with an STI. The availability of nucleic acid amplification tests (NAAT), primarily for *Chlamydia* and *Neisseria gonorrhoeae,* has changed the nature of STI screening and intervention. These amplification tests are more than 95% sensitive and more than 99% specific, using either urine or cervical/urethral swabs.

Initial screening for urethritis in males begins with a physical exam. If there are no signs (urethral discharge/lesions) or symptoms, then a first-catch urine sample (the first 10–40 mL of voided urine collected after not voiding for 2 hours) should be sent for *Chlamydia* testing. If signs or symptoms are present, then either the urine or a urethral swab should be sent to test for both *Neisseria gonorrhoeae* and *Chlamydia*. A wet prep should then be done on a spun urine sample or from urethral discharge, evaluating for the presence of *Trichomonas vaginalis.*

For females, screening asymptomatic patients has become more complicated because a variety of approaches are available. Generally, either a first-void urine specimen or a cervical swab is used to screen for *Chlamydia* and *N gonorrhoeae* by NAAT. When screening for *N gonorrhoeae,* it is important to recognize that certain NAATs are less sensitive when using urine compared with a cervical swab, and the specific test available should guide the screening procedure. A wet mount of the vaginal secretions should be performed annually to check for bacterial vaginosis and trichomoniasis, and a potassium hydroxide (KOH) preparation to screen for yeast infections. The Papanicolaou (Pap) smear serves to evaluate the cervix for the presence of HPV or other cervical cytopathology. Recent availability of Thin Prep, which accomplishes HPV typing, along with an increased understanding of the progression of abnormal cervical changes, has led to a change in the recommendations for performing Pap smears. Though there is not an absolute consensus it appears that the initial Pap smear does not need to be done until 3 years after initiation of sexual intercourse, or by age 21.

For both sexes if high-risk behavior is present (three or more partners in the last 6 months or more than two partners per year for several years), then screening for hepatitis B surface antigen is warranted. In communities with a high prevalence of hepatitis B, practitioners should test for hepatitis B infection once in patients who have previously received the hepatitis B vaccine to detect anyone who was infected before receiving the vaccine. The presence of hepatitis B surface antigen indicates either the carrier state or active infection. Presence of only hepatitis B surface antibody identifies vaccinated individuals, whereas hepatitis B core antibody identifies individuals with past infection (see Chapter 21).

In urban areas with a relatively high rate of syphilis, an RPR/VDRL (rapid plasma reagin/Venereal Disease Research Laboratory) test should be drawn yearly. RPR should be done in all cases in which a concomitant STI is present. HIV antibody determination should be considered for any sexually active adolescent and is strongly recommended for patients engaging in high-risk behaviors.

Nelson HD, Helfand M: Screening for chlamydial infection. Am J Prev Med 2001;20(3 Suppl):95 [PMID: 21203146].

Serlin M et al. What sexually transmitted disease screening method does the adolescent prefer? Adolescents' attitudes toward first-void urine, self-collected vaginal swab, and pelvic examination. Arch Pediatr Adolesc Med 2002:156;588 [PMID: 22035040].

## SIGNS & SYMPTOMS

For males, the most common symptoms are dysuria and penile discharge resulting from urethral inflammation. Less common symptoms are scrotal pain, hematuria, proctitis, and pruritus in the pubic region. Signs include epididymitis, orchitis, and urethral discharge. Rarely do males develop systemic symptoms. For females, the most common symptoms are vaginal discharge and dysuria. Vaginal itching and irregular menses or spotting are also common. Abdominal pain, fever, and vomiting, though less common, are signs of PID. Pain in the genital region and dyspareunia may be present.

Signs that can be found in both males and females with an STI include genital ulcerations, adenopathy, and genital warts.

# ■ THE MOST COMMON ANTIBIOTIC-RESPONSIVE SEXUALLY TRANSMITTED INFECTIONS

*Chlamydia trachomatis* and *Neisseria gonorrhoeae* are sexually transmitted infections that are epidemic in the United States and are readily treated when appropriate antibiotics are administered in a timely fashion.

## *CHLAMYDIA TRACHOMATIS* INFECTION

### General Considerations

*Chlamydia* is the most common bacterial cause of STIs in the United States. Three million cases are estimated to occur annually in adolescents and young adults. *Chlamydia trachomatis* is an obligate intracellular bacterium that replicates within the cytoplasm of host cells. Destruction of *Chlamydia*-infected cells is mediated by host immune responses.

## Clinical Findings

### A. SYMPTOMS AND SIGNS

Clinical infection in females manifests as dysuria, urethritis, vaginal discharge, cervicitis, or PID. The presence of mucopus at the cervical os (mucopurulent cervicitis) is a sign of *Chlamydia* infection or gonorrhea. *Chlamydia* infection is asymptomatic in 75% of females.

Clamydial infection may be asymptomatic in 70% of males or manifest as dysuria, urethritis, or epididymitis. Some patients complain of urethral discharge. On clinical exam a clear white discharge may be found after milking the penis. Proctitis or proctocolitis from *Chlamydia* may occur in adolescents practicing receptive anal intercourse.

### B. LABORATORY FINDINGS

NAAT (polymerase or ligase chain reaction) is the most sensitive (93–97%) way to detect *Chlamydia*. ELISA or direct fluorescent antibody tests are less sensitive but may be the only testing option in some centers. Culture is mandated for sexual abuse cases.

A cervical swab, using the manufacturer's swab provided with the specific test, or first-void urine specimen should be obtained. Often a single swab can be used to collect both the *Chlamydia* and *N gonorrhoeae* specimen. To optimize detection of *Chlamydia* from the cervix, columnar cells need to be collected by inserting the swab in the os and rotating it 360 degrees. If rectal symptoms are present, a rectal specimen should be obtained.

The first-void urine test for leukocyte esterase was previously used for screening asymptomatic, sexually active males. Due to the high false-positive rate, this screening technique is now less commonly used. In symptomatic males, examination of the urine sediment for white blood cells (WBCs) can provide evidence of urethritis, though it is often impractical to perform in a clinical setting. In general, a first-void urine sample, or urethral swab for NAAT should be done at least annually. Some studies suggest that more frequent screenings—every 6 months—in higher prevalence populations can decrease the rate of chlamydial infection. Evaluation of the symptomatic male patient or an asymptomatic contact for *Chlamydia* is the same.

For both males and females, testing urine allows for more frequent screening and simplifies screening in schools, the military, or other groups.

## Complications

Epididymitis is a complication in males. Reiter syndrome occurs in association with chlamydial urethritis (see Chapter 26). This should be suspected in male patients who are sexually active and present with low back pain (sacroiliitis), arthritis (polyarticular), characteristic mucocutaneous lesions, and conjunctivitis. PID is an important complication in females.

## Treatment

Infected patients and their contacts, regardless of the extent of signs or symptoms, need to receive treatment (Table 40–1). Because adolescents have a high risk of acquiring a repeat *Chlamydia* infection within several months of the first infection, all infected females should be rescreened 3–4 months after treatment.

Guaschino S, DeSeta F: Update on *Chlamydia trachomatis.* Ann N Y Acad Sci 2000;900:293 [PMID: 20278358].

Watson EJ et al: The accuracy and efficacy of screening tests for *Chlamydia trachomatis:* A systematic review. J Med Microbiol 2002:51;1021 [PMID: 22354463].

## *NEISSERIA GONORRHOEAE* INFECTION

### General Considerations

Gonorrhea is the second most prevalent bacterial STI. Sites of infection include the cervix, urethra, rectum, and pharynx. In addition, gonorrhea is a cause of PID. Humans are the natural reservoir. Gonococci are present in the exudate and secretions of infected mucus membranes.

### Clinical Findings

#### A. SYMPTOMS AND SIGNS

In uncomplicated gonococcal cervicitis, females are symptomatic 57% of the time, presenting with vaginal discharge and dysuria. Urethritis and pyuria may be present. Mucopurulent cervicitis with a yellowish discharge may be found, and the cervix may be edematous and friable. Other symptoms include abnormal menstrual periods and dyspareunia. Approximately 15% of women with endocervical gonorrhea will have signs of involvement of the upper genital tract. Compared with *Chlamydia* infection, pelvic inflammation with gonorrhea often has a shorter duration but an increased intensity of symptoms and is more often associated with fever. Ninety-five percent of males with gonorrhea are symptomatic, with a yellowish green urethral discharge and burning on urination. Both males and females can develop gonococcal proctitis and pharyngitis after exposure.

#### B. LABORATORY FINDINGS

A cervical swab from females should be sent for NAAT or cultured on Thayer–Martin agar. Obtaining specimens from the rectum or pharynx when clinically indi-

***Table 40–1.*** Treatment regimens

| Disease | Recommended Regimens | Pregnancy[a] |
|---|---|---|
| **Pelvic inflammatory disease (PID)**<br>Inpatient therapy regimen A<br>***Note:*** Therapy should be continued for 24–48 h after the patient has improved; therapy can then be switched to either oral regimen to complete a 14-d course.<br>Inpatient therapy regimen B<br>***Note:*** Once clinically improved for 48 h, patients can be discharged and continue doxycycline 100 mg PO bid for 14 days total.[b] | Cefotetan, 2 g IV q6 h | Safe [B] |
| | or | |
| | Cefoxitin, 2 g IV q12 h | Safe [B] |
| | plus | |
| | Doxycycline, 100 mg IV or PO bid | Contraindicated [D] |
| | Clindamycin, 900 mg IV q8 h | Safe [B] |
| | plus | |
| | Gentamicin, 2 mg/kg IV loading dose, then 1.5 mg/kg IV q8 h | Safe [B] |
| Alternative parenteral regimens | Ofloxacin, 400 mg IV q12 h[c] | Contraindicated [C] |
| | or | |
| | Levofloxacin, 500 mg IV once daily[c] | Contraindicated [C] |
| | with or without Metronidazole, 500 mg IV q8h | Safe[d] [B] |
| | or | |
| | Ampicillin/sulbactam, 3 g IV q6 h | Safe [A] |
| | plus | |
| | Doxycycline, 100 mg IV or PO q12 h | Contraindicated [D] |
| Outpatient therapy regimen A | Ofloxacin, 400 mg PO bid for 14 d[c] | Contraindicated [C] |
| | or | |
| | Levofloxacin, 500 mg PO, once a day for 14 d[c] with or without | Contraindicated [C] |
| Out patient therapy regimen B<br>***Note:*** Pregnant patients with PID should be hospitalized and given parenteral antibiotics.[b] | Ceftriaxone, 250 mg IM once | Safe [B] |
| | or | |
| | Cefoxitin, 2 g IM once plus probenicid, 1 g PO | Safe [B] |
| | or | |
| | Third generation cephalosporin | Safe [B] |
| | plus | |
| | Doxycycline, 100 mg, PO bid for 14 d | Contraindicated [D] |
| | with or without | |
| | Metronidazole, 500 mg PO bid for 14 d | Safe[d] [B] |
| **Gonorrhea, uncomplicated**<br>Cervicitis, urethritis<br>***Note:*** Empiric treatment for *Chlamydia trachomatis* with azithromycin or doxycycline is recommended due to coexisting infection in 20–40% of patients with gonorrhea infection. | Cefixime, 400 mg PO as single dose | Safe [B] |
| | or | |
| | Ceftriaxone, 125 mg IM as single dose | Safe [B] |
| | or | |
| | Ciprofloxacin, 500 mg PO in a single dose | Contraindicated [C] |
| | or | |
| | Ofloxacin, 400 mg PO as single dose[c] | Contraindicated [C] |
| | or | |
| | Levofloxacin, 250 mg PO as single dose[c] | Contraindicated [C] |
| Pharyngitis | Ceftriaxone, 125 mg IM once | Safe [B] |
| | or | |
| | Ciprofloxacin, 500 mg PO once[c] | Contraindicated [C] |
| Gonorrea disseminated<br>***Note:*** Treat IV until clinically improved (usually 48h; then switch to PO) | Ceftriaxone, 1 g IV or IM every 24 h | Safe [B] |
| | or | |
| | Ceftizoxime, 1 g IV every 8 h | Safe [B] |
| | or | |
| | Ciprofloxacin, 400 mg IV every 12 h | Contraindicated [C] |
| | or | |

*(continued)*

*Table 40–1.* Treatment regimens (continued)

| Disease | Recommended Regimens | Pregnancy[1] |
|---|---|---|
| | Complete at least a 7 d course with cefixime, 400 mg PO bid<br>or<br>Ciprofloxacin, 500 mg PO bid<br>or<br>Ofloxacin, 400 mg PO bid<br>or<br>Levofloxacin, 500 mg PO once daily | |
| **Nongonococcal, nonchlamydial urethritis** | Azithromycin, 1 g PO as single dose<br>or<br>Doxycycline, 100 mg PO bid for 7 d | |
| Alternative regimens | Erythromycin base, 500 mg PO qid for 7 d<br>or<br>Erythromycin ethylsuccinate, 800 mg PO qid for 7 d<br>or<br>Ofloxacin, 300 mg PO bid for 7 d[c]<br>or<br>Levofloxacin, 500 mg PO once daily for 7 d[c] | |
| Recurrent or persistent urethritis | Metronidazole, 2 g PO as single dose<br>plus<br>Erythromycin base, 500 mg PO quid for 7 d<br>or<br>Erythromycin ethylsuccinate, 800 mg PO qid for 7 d | |
| **Proctitis, proctocolitis, and enteritis** | Ceftriaxone 125 mg IM<br>plus<br>Doxycycline, 100 mg PO bid for 7 d | Safe [B]<br><br>Contraindicated [D] |
| *Trichomonas vaginalis* **vaginitis or urethritis** | Metronidazole, 2 g PO as single dose<br>or<br>Metronidazole, 500 mg PO bid for 7d | Safe[d] [B]<br><br>Safe[d] [B] |
| **Bacterial vaginosis** | Metronidazole, 500 mg PO bid for 7 d<br>or<br>Metronidazole, 0.75% gel, 5 g intravaginally bid for 5 d<br>or<br>Clindamycin cream, 2%, one applicator intravaginally at bedtime for 5 d<br>or<br>Clindamycin ovules 100 mg intravaginal for 3 d | Safe[d] [B]<br><br>Safe[d] [B]<br><br>Safe [B] |
| Alternative regimen | Metronidazole, 2 g PO as single dose<br>or<br>Clindamycin, 300 mg PO bid for 7 d<br>or<br>Clindamycin 100 mg intravaginally once at bedtime for 3d | Safe[d] [B]<br><br>Safe [B] |
| **Vulvovaginal candidiasis** | Butoconazole, clotrimazole, miconazole, terconazole or tioconazole, intravaginal for 1, 3, or 7 d<br>Butoconazole sustained release, 5 g once intravaginally<br>or<br>Fluconazole, 150 mg oral tablet, in single dose | Safe [B]<br><br>Safe [B]<br><br>Contraindicated [C] |

(*continued*)

***Table 40–1.*** Treatment regimens (continued)

| Disease | Recommended Regimens | Pregnancy[a] |
|---|---|---|
| **Syphilis**<br>Early (primary, secondary, or latent < 1 y) | Benzathine penicillin G, 2.4 million units IM (for patients > 40 kg) | Safe [B] |
| | Benzathine penicillin G, 50,000 units/kg IM (for patients < 40 kg); up to 2.4 million units in one dose<br>or | Safe [B] |
| | Doxycycline, 100 mg PO bid for 14 d | Contraindicated [D] |
| **Epididymitis**<br>  Most likely caused by gonococcal or chlamydial infection | Ceftriaxone, 250 mg IM as single dose<br>plus<br>Doxycycline, 100 mg PO bid for 14 d | |
| Most likely caused by enteric organisms, Patient older than 35 y old or allergies to cephalosporins and/or tetracyclines | Ofloxacin, 300 mg PO bid for 14 d<br>or<br>Levofloxacin, 500 mg PO once daily for 14 d | |
| ***Chlamydia trachomatis***<br>Cervicitis or urethritis | Azithromycin, 1 g PO as single dose<br>or | Safe [B] |
| | Erythromycin, 500 mg PO qid for 7 d | Safe [B] |
| Alternative regimen[b] | Doxycycline, 100 mg PO bid for 7d<br>or | Contraindicated [D] |
| | Ofloxacin, 300 mg PO bid for 7 d<br>or levofloxacin 500 mg<br>PO once daily for 7 d | Contraindicated [C]<br>Contraindicated [C] |
| Late (more than 1 y duration) | Benzathine penicillin G, 2.4 million units IM (for patients > 40 kg) once a week for 3 consecutive weeks<br>or | Safe [B] |
| | Benzathine penicillin G, 50,000 units/kg IM (for patients < 40 kg) once a week for 3 consecutive weeks; up to 2.4 million units in one dose<br>or | |
| | Doxycycline, 100 mg PO bid for 4 wk | Contraindicated [D] |
| **Granuloma inguinale** | Doxycycline, 100 mg PO bid for 3 wk or longer<br>or | Contraindicated [D] |
| | Trimethoprim–sulfamethoxazole, one double-strength tablet PO bid for 3 weeks or longer | Safe [B] |
| Alternative regimen | Ciprofloxacin, 750 mg PO bid for at least 3 wk<br>or | Contraindicated [C] |
| | Erythromycin base, 500 mg PO four times daily for at least 3 wk<br>or | Safe [B] |
| | Azithromycin, 1 g PO once per week for at least 3 wk | Safe [B] |
| **Lymphogranuloma venereum** | Doxycycline, 100 mg PO bid for 3 wk<br>or | Contraindicated [D] |
| | Erythromycin, 500 mg PO qid for 3 wk | Safe [B] |
| **Herpes simplex**<br>First episode, genital | Acyclovir, 400 mg PO tid for 7–10 d<br>or | Safe [B] |
| | Famciclovir, 250 mg PO tid for 7–10 d<br>or | |
| | Valacyclovir, 1 g PO bid for 7–10 d | |

(continued)

*Table 40–1.* Treatment regimens (continued)

| Disease | Recommended Regimens | Pregnancy[1] |
|---|---|---|
| Recurrent | Acyclovir, 400 mg PO tid for 5 d<br>or<br>Acyclovir, 800 mg PO bid for 5 d<br>or<br>Famciclovir, 125 mg PO bid for 5 d<br>or<br>Valacyclovir, 500 mg PO bid for 5 d<br>or<br>Valacyclovir, 1 g PO once a day for 5 d | |
| Suppression | Acyclovir, 400 mg PO bid<br>or<br>Famciclovir, 250 mg PO bid<br>or<br>Valacyclovir, 500 mg PO daily (if < 10 recurrences per year; if ≥ 10 recurrences use 1 g daily) | Safe [B] |
| **Chancroid** | Azithromycin, 1 g PO as single dose | Safe [B] |
| | or | |
| | Ceftriaxone 250 mg IM once | Safe [B] |
| | or | |
| | Ciprofloxacin, 500 mg PO bid for 3 d | Contraindicated [D] |
| | or | |
| | Erythromycin, 500 mg PO tid for 7 d | Safe [B] |
| **Human papillomavirus**<br>External lesions<br>*Note:* Topical therapies usually require weekly treatments for 4 consecutive weeks | Podophyllin, 25% in benzoin tincture applied directly to warts; wash off in 1–4 h [contraindicated for urethral or intravaginal lesions] | Contraindicated [X] |
| | or | |
| | Trichloroacetic acid (85%); apply directly to warts; wash off in 6–8 h | Safe |
| | or | |
| | Podofilox, 0.5% solution; apply bid for 3 d; used by the patient at home; practitioner needs to demonstrate how compound is applied (to be used only on external lesions) | Contraindicated [C] |
| | or | |
| | Imiquimod 5% cream, applied three times per week overnight (maximum of 16 weeks) | Contraindicated [B] |
| | Cryotherapy: liquid nitrogen, cryoprobe<br>Electrocautery | Safe |
| **Ectoparasitic infections**<br>**Pediculosis pubis**[e] | Permethrin 1% cream rinse: wash off after 10 min | Safe [B] |
| | or | |
| | Lindane 1% shampoo: apply for 4 min, then wash off | Contraindicated [B] |
| | or | |
| | Pyrethins with piperonyl butoxide: apply, wash off after 10 min | Safe [B] |

***Table 40–1.*** Treatment regimens (continued)

| Disease | Recommended Regimens | Pregnancy[a] |
|---------|---------------------|-------------|
| Scabies | Permethrin cream 5%: apply to entire body from the neck down | Safe [B] |
| | or | |
| | Ivermectin 200 mg/kg orally, repeat in 2 weeks | Contraindicated [C] |

[a]FDA use in pregnancy ratings: [A] *Controlled studies show no risk.* Adequate, well-controlled studies in pregnant women have failed to demonstrate a risk to the fetus in any trimester of pregnancy. [B] *No evidence of risk in humans.* Adequate, well-controlled studies in pregnant women have not shown increased risk of fetal abnormalities despite adverse findings in animals, or, in the absence of adequate human studies, animal studies show no fetal risk. The chance of fetal harm is remote but remains a possibility. [C] *Risk cannot be ruled out.* Adequate, well-controlled human studies are lacking, and animal studies have shown a risk to the fetus or are lacking as well. There is a chance of fetal harm if the drug is administered during pregnancy; but the potential benefits outweigh the potential risk. [D] *Positive evidence of risk.* Studies in humans, or investigational or post-marketing data, have demonstrated fetal risk. Nevertheless, potential benefits from the use of the drug may outweigh the potential risk. For example, the drug may be acceptable if needed in a life-threatening situation or serious disease for which safer drugs cannot be used or are ineffective. [X] *Contraindicated in pregnancy.* Studies in animals or humans, or despite adverse findings in animals, or investigational or post-marketing reports have demonstrated positive evidence of fetal abnormalities or risk that clearly outweighs any possible benefit to the patient.

[b]Doxycycline is contraindicated in pregnancy. Alternative therapies during pregnancy which include erythromycin, azithromycin, and amoxicillin are not as effective, but are clinically useful if the recommended regimens cannot be used due to allergy or pregnancy.

[c]Quinolones should not be used in areas with increased prevalence of quinolone resistance (ie, Asia, the Pacific, Hawaii, California).

[d]Previously metronidazole was contraindicated in the first trimester.

[e]Bedding and clothing need to be decontaminated by washing in hot water or by dry cleaning. Regimen may be repeated in 1 week if complete response is not achieved.

[f]These are oil-based and should not be used with latex benion imfrocep.

cated will increase the likelihood of positive results. Pharyngeal infection requires more intensive therapy. Nongonococcal *Neisseria* species reside in the vagina, thereby negating the value of the Gram stain in a female.

Culture or NAAT for *N gonorrhoeae* in males can be achieved with a swab of the urethra or first-void urine. Gram stain of urethral discharge showing gram-negative intracellular diplococci indicates gonorrhoeae in a male.

If proctitis is present appropriate cultures should be obtained and treatment for both gonorrhoeae and *Chlamydia* infection given. If oral exposure to gonorrhoeae is suspected cultures should be taken and the patient given empiric treatment.

## Differential Diagnosis

Gonococcal pharyngitis needs to be differentiated from streptococcal infection, herpes simplex pharyngitis, and infectious mononucleosis. *Chlamydia* infection needs to be differentiated from gonococcal infection.

## Complications

Disseminated gonococcal infection occurs in a minority (0.5–3%) of patients with untreated gonorrhoeae. Hematogenous spread most commonly causes arthritis and dermatitis. The joints most frequently involved are the wrist, metacarpophalangeal joints, knee, and ankle. Skin lesions are typically tender, hemorrhagic or necrotic pustules or bullae on an erythematous base occurring on the distal extremities. Disseminated disease occurs more frequently in women than in men. Risk factors include pregnancy and gonococcal pharyngitis. Gonorrhoeae is complicated occasionally by perihepatitis and very rarely by endocarditis or meningitis.

## Treatment

Because chlamydial and gonorrhoeael infections coexist 20–40% of the time, both infections should be treated when one infection is diagnosed.

Centers for Disease Control and Prevention (CDC) guidelines state that *N gonorrhoeae* and *C trachomatis* do not require tests of cure when they are treated with first-line medications, unless the patient remains symptomatic. If rescreening is indicated it should be delayed for 1 month after completion of therapy if NAATs are used to document a test of cure. Rescreening might also be considered for sexually active adolescents likely to be reinfected. Patients should be advised to abstain from sexual intercourse until both they and their partners have completed a course of treatment. Treatment for disseminated disease may require hospitalization (see Table 40–1).

# ■ THE SPECTRUM OF SEXUALLY TRANSMITTED INFECTIONS

The patient presenting with an STI usually has one or more of the signs or symptoms presented in this section. Management considerations for STIs include assessing the patient's adherence to therapy and ensuring follow-up, treating STIs in partners, and determining pregnancy risk. Treatment of each STI is detailed in Table 40–1.

## MUCOPURULENT CERVICITIS

### General Considerations

Mucopurulent cervicitis (MPC) is caused by *C trachomatis* or *N gonorrhoeae* approximately 30% of the time. Herpes simplex virus and *Mycoplasma genitalium* are less common causes. MPC can also be present without an STI.

### Clinical Findings

#### A. SYMPTOMS AND SIGNS

MPC is often asymptomatic, but many women have an abnormal vaginal discharge or postcoital bleeding. MPC is characterized by a purulent or mucopurulent endocervical exudate visible in the endocervical canal or on an endocervical swab specimen. The cervix is often friable with easily induced bleeding.

#### B. LABORATORY FINDINGS

Although endocervical Gram stain may show an increased number of polymorphonuclear leukocytes, it has a low positive predictive value and is not recommended for diagnosis. Patients who have MPC should be tested for *C trachomatis* and *N gonorrhoeae* by using the most sensitive and specific tests available at the site.

### Complications

Persistent MPC is difficult to manage and requires reassessment of the initial diagnosis. MPC can persist despite repeated courses of antimicrobial therapy. Presence of a large ectropion can contribute to persistent MPC.

### Treatment

Empiric treatment for both gonorrhea and *Chlamydia* infection is recommended when the prospect of follow-up is questionable or the patient is part of a high-risk population. If the patient is asymptomatic aside from MPC, then treatment may wait until diagnostic tests are back (see Table 40–1). Follow-up is recommended if symptoms persist. Patients should be instructed to abstain from sexual intercourse until they and their sex partners are cured and treatment is completed.

## PELVIC INFLAMMATORY DISEASE

### General Considerations

PID is defined as inflammation of the upper female genital tract and may include endometritis, salpingitis, tubo-ovarian abscess, and pelvic peritonitis. It is the most common gynecologic disorder necessitating hospitalization for women of reproductive age in the United States. Over 1 million women develop PID annually, and 275,000 are hospitalized. The incidence is highest in the teen population. Teenage girls who are sexually active have a high risk (1 in 8) of developing PID, whereas women in their 20s have one tenth the risk. Predisposing risk factors include number of partners, younger age of initiating sexual intercourse, and lack of condom use. Lack of protective antibody from previous exposure to sexually transmitted organisms and cervical ectopy contribute to the development of PID. Many adolescents with subacute or asymptomatic disease are never identified.

PID is often polymicrobial. Causative agents include *N gonorrhoeae*, *Chlamydia*, anaerobic bacteria that reside in the vagina, and genital mycoplasmas. Vaginal douching and other mechanical factors such as an intrauterine device or prior gynecologic surgery increase the risk of PID by providing access of lower genital tract organisms to pelvic organs. Recent menses and bacterial vaginosis have been associated with the development of PID.

### Clinical Findings

#### A. SYMPTOMS AND SIGNS

Acute PID is difficult to diagnose because of the wide variation in the symptoms and signs. No single historical, clinical, or laboratory finding has both high sensitivity and specificity for the diagnosis of PID. Diagnosis of PID is usually made clinically (Table 40–2). Typical patients have lower abdominal pain, nausea, vomiting, and fever. However, the patient may be afebrile. Vaginal discharge is variable. Cervical motion tenderness, uterine or adnexal tenderness, or signs of peritonitis are present. Mucopurulent cervicitis is present in 50% of patients. Tubo-ovarian abscesses can be detected by careful physical examination (feeling a mass or fullness in the adnexa).

***Table 40–2.*** Diagnostic criteria for pelvic inflammatory disease (PID).

---

**Minimum criteria**
Empiric treatment of PID should be initiated in sexually active young women and others at risk for sexually transmitted infections if all the following minimum criteria are present and no other cause(s) for the illness can be identified:
    Lower abdominal tenderness
    Uterine adnexal tenderness
    Cervical motion tenderness
**Additional supportive criteria**
Oral temperature >38.3°C (101°F)
Abnormal cervical or vaginal mucopurulent discharge
Presence of WBCs on saline microscopy of vaginal secretions
Elevated erythrocyte sedimentation rate or elevated C-reactive protein
Laboratory documentation of infection with *N gonorrhoeae* or *C trachomatis*
**Definitive criteria [selected cases]**
Histopathologic evidence of endometritis on endometrial biopsy
Tubo-ovarian abscess on sonography or other radiologic tests
Laparoscopic abnormalities consistent with PID

---

Adapted, with permission, from Centers for Disease Control and Prevention. Sexually transmitted diseases treatment guidelines 2002. MMWR 2002;51(No. RR-6):48–51.

Laparoscopy is the gold standard for detecting salpingitis; it can be used if the diagnosis is in question or to help differentiate PID from an ectopic pregnancy, ovarian cysts, or adnexal torsion. The clinical diagnosis of PID has a positive predictive value for salpingitis of 65–90% in comparison with laparoscopy. Pelvic ultrasonography also is helpful in detecting tubo-ovarian abscesses, which are found in almost 20% of teens with PID. Transvaginal ultrasound is more sensitive than abdominal ultrasound.

### B. LABORATORY FINDINGS

Laboratory findings include elevated WBCs with a left shift and elevated acute-phase reactants (erythrocyte sedimentation rate or C-reactive protein). A positive test for *N gonorrhoeae* or *C trachomatis* is supportive, although 25% of the time neither of these bacteria is detected. Pregnancy needs to be ruled out, because patients with an ectopic pregnancy can present with abdominal pain.

## Differential Diagnosis

Differential diagnosis includes other gynecologic illnesses (ectopic pregnancy, threatened or septic abortion, adnexal torsion, ruptured and hemorrhagic ovarian cysts, dysmenorrhea, endometriosis, mittelschmerz); gastrointestinal illnesses (appendicitis, cholecystitis, hepatitis, gastroenteritis, inflammatory bowel disease); and genitourinary illnesses (cystitis, pyelonephritis, urinary calculi).

## Complications

Scarring of the fallopian tubes is one of the major sequelae of PID. With one episode of PID, 17% of patients become infertile, 17% develop chronic pelvic pain, and 10% will have an ectopic pregnancy. Infertility rates increase with each episode of PID; three episodes of PID result in a 73% infertility rate. Fitz-Hugh–Curtis syndrome is inflammation of the liver capsule (perihepatitis) from either hematogenous or lymphatic spread of organisms from the fallopian tubes. This results in right upper quadrant pain and elevation of liver function tests.

## Treatment

The objective of treatment is to achieve a clinical cure and prevent long-term sequelae. The ability of various therapeutic regimens in preventing sequelae has not been compared. PID is frequently managed at the outpatient level, although some clinicians argue that all adolescents with PID should be hospitalized because of the rate of complications. Severe systemic symptoms and toxicity, signs of peritonitis, inability to take fluids, pregnancy, and elevated WBCs and erythrocyte sedimentation rate support hospitalization. In addition, if the practitioner believes that the patient will not comply with medication, hospitalization is warranted. Surgical drainage may be required to ensure adequate treatment of tubo-ovarian abscesses.

The treatment regimens described in Table 40–1 are broad spectrum to cover the numerous microorganisms associated with PID. Outpatient treatment should be reserved for compliant patients who have classic signs of PID without systemic symptoms. Patients with PID who receive treatment as an outpatient should be reexamined within 24–48 hours, with phone contact in the interim, to detect persistent disease or treatment failure. Patients should have substantial improvement within 48–72 hours. An adolescent should be reexamined 7–10 days after the completion of therapy to ensure the resolution of symptoms.

Eissa MA, Cromwell PF: Diagnosis and management of pelvic inflammatory disease in adolescents. J Pediatr Health Care 2003;17:145 [PMID: 22620085].

Ness RB et al: Effectiveness of inpatient and outpatient treatment strategies for women with pelvic inflammatory disease: Results from the Pelvic Inflammatory Disease Evaluation and

Clinical Health (PEACH) Randomized Trial. Am J Obstet Gynecol 2002;186;929 [PMID: 22009815].

# URETHRITIS

## General Considerations

Common bacterial causes of urethritis in men are *N gonorrhoeae* and *C trachomatis.* Additionally, *Trichomonas vaginalis,* herpes simplex virus (HSV), *Ureaplasma urealyticum,* and *Mycoplasma genitalium* cause urethritis. Coliforms may cause urethritis in men practicing insertive anal intercourse. Mechanical manipulation or contact with irritants can also cause transient urethritis.

Women often present with symptoms of a urinary tract infection from which no enteric bacterial pathogens are isolated. These women often have urethritis caused by the organisms just mentioned.

## Clinical Findings

### A. SYMPTOMS AND SIGNS

Most commonly in men, a clear or purulent discharge from the urethra is present with dysuria. Hematuria and associated inguinal adenopathy can occur. Fifty percent of infections caused by *C trachomatis* and *T vaginalis* are asymptomatic, whereas 95% of gonococcal urethritis is symptomatic.

### B. LABORATORY FINDINGS

In a symptomatic male a positive leukocyte esterase test on first-void urine, or microscopic examination of first-void urine demonstrating more than 10 WBCs per high-power field, is suggestive of urethritis. Gram stain of urethral secretions demonstrating more than 5 WBCs per high-power field is also suggestive. Gonococcal urethritis is established by documenting the presence of WBCs containing intracellular gram-negative diplococci. Urethral swab or first-void urine for culture or NAAT should be sent to the laboratory to detect *N gonorrhoeae* and *Chlamydia.* Evaluation for *T vaginalis* by a wet preparation of either urethral discharge or spun urine should be considered when the other test results are negative.

## Complications

Complications include recurrent or persistent urethritis or epididymitis.

## Treatment

Patients with evidence of urethritis should receive empiric treatment for gonorrhea and *Chlamydia* infection. If the infection is unresponsive and culture negative, the syndrome of nongonococcal, nonchlamydial urethritis is often associated with *Mycoplasma genitalium* or *Ureaplasma urealyticum.* Approximately half of males with this syndrome have no identified pathogen. Trichomoniasis should be excluded. Patients should be instructed to return for evaluation if symptoms persist or recur after completion of initial empiric therapy. Symptoms alone, without documentation of signs or laboratory evidence of urethral inflammation, are not a sufficient basis for retreatment (see Table 40–1). Azithromycin is the initial recommended therapy for persistence of symptoms and urethritis.

McKee KT et al: Features of urethritis in a cohort of male soldiers. Clin Infect Dis 2000;30;736 [PMID: 20233758].

Totten PA et al: Association of *Mycoplasma genitalium* with non-gonococcal urethritis in heterosexual men. J Infect Dis 2001:183(2);269 [PMID: 21063472].

# EPIDIDYMUS

## General Considerations

Epididymitis is most often caused by *C trachomatis* or *N gonorrhoeae.* Epididymitis caused by *Escherichia coli* occurs among homosexual men who are the insertive partners during anal intercourse and in men who have urinary tract abnormalities.

## Clinical Findings

### A. SYMPTOMS AND SIGNS

Epididymitis is associated with unilateral testicular pain and tenderness. Palpable, tender swelling of the epididymitis is usually present. Often these symptoms are accompanied by asymptomatic urethritis.

### B. LABORATORY FINDINGS

Diagnosis is made clinically. Additional evaluation is similar to that described for suspected urethritis (see Urethritis section).

## Differential Diagnosis

Acute epididymitis associated with sexual activity must be distinguished from orchitis due to infarct, testicular torsion, or viral infection.

## Complications

Infertility is rare, and chronic local pain is uncommon.

## Treatment

Empiric therapy is indicated before culture results are available. As an adjunct to therapy, bed rest, scrotal elevation, and analgesics are recommended until fever and local inflammation subside. Lack of improvement of swelling and tenderness within 3 days requires reevaluation of both the diagnosis and therapy (see Table 40–1).

# PROCTITIS, PROCTOCOLITIS, AND ENTERITIS

## General Considerations

Proctitis occurs predominantly among persons who participate in anal intercourse. Enteritis occurs among those whose sexual practices include oral–fecal contact. Proctocolitis can be acquired by either route depending on the pathogen. Common sexually transmitted pathogens causing proctitis or proctocolitis include *C trachomatis, Treponema pallidum,* HSV, *N gonorrhoeae, Giardia lamblia,* and enteric organisms.

## Clinical Findings

### A. SYMPTOMS AND SIGNS

Proctitis, defined as inflammation limited to the distal 10–12 cm of the rectum, is associated with anorectal pain, tenesmus, and rectal discharge. Acute proctitis among persons who have recently practiced receptive anal intercourse is most often sexually transmitted. The symptoms of proctocolitis combine those of proctitis, plus diarrhea or abdominal cramps (or both), because of inflamed colonic mucosa more than 12 cm from the anus. Enteritis usually results in diarrhea and abdominal cramping without signs of proctitis or proctocolitis.

### B. LABORATORY FINDINGS

Evaluation may include anoscopy or sigmoidoscopy, stool exam, and culture for appropriate organisms and serology for syphilis.

## Treatment

Management will be determined by the etiologic agent (See Table 40–1 and Chapters 20 and 38). Reinfection may be difficult to distinguish from treatment failure.

Rompalo AM: Diagnosis and treatment of sexually acquired proctitis and proctocolitis: An update. Clin Infect Dis 1999; 28(Suppl 1):S84 [PMID: 99152439].

# VAGINAL DISCHARGE

Adolescent girls may have a normal physiologic leukorrhea, secondary to turnover of vaginal epithelium. Infectious causes of discharge include *T vaginalis, C trachomatis, N gonorrhoeae,* and bacterial pathogens for vaginosis. Candidiasis is a yeast infection that produces vaginal discharge but is not usually sexually transmitted.

Vaginitis is characterized by vaginal discharge, vulvar itching and irritation; the discharge may be foul-smelling. Discharge may be white, gray, or yellow. Physiologic leukorrhea is usually white, homogeneous, and not associated with itching, irritation, or foul odor.

Mechanical, chemical, allergic, or other noninfectious irritants of the vagina may cause vaginal discharge.

## 1. Bacterial Vaginosis

### General Considerations

Bacterial vaginosis (BV) is a polymicrobial infection of the vagina caused by an imbalance of the normal bacterial vaginal flora. The altered flora has a paucity of hydrogen peroxide-producing lactobacilli and increased concentrations of *Mycoplasma hominis* and anaerobes, such as *Gardnerella vaginalis* and *Mobiluncus.* It is unclear whether BV is sexually transmitted, but it is associated with having multiple sex partners.

### Clinical Findings

#### A. SYMPTOMS AND SIGNS

The most common symptom is a heavy, malodorous, homogeneous gray-white vaginal discharge. Patients may report vaginal itching or dysuria. The fishy odor may be more noticeable after intercourse or during menses, when the high pH of blood or semen volatilizes the amines.

#### B. LABORATORY FINDINGS

BV is most often diagnosed by the use of clinical criteria, which include (1) presence of gray-white discharge; (2) fishy odor before or after the addition of 10% KOH (whiff test); (3) pH of vaginal fluid greater than 4.5 determined with narrow range pH paper; and (4) presence of greater than 20% "clue cells." Clue cells are squamous epithelial cells that have multiple bacteria adhering to them, making their borders irregular and giving them a speckled appearance. Diagnosis requires three out of four criteria, although many women who fulfill these criteria have no discharge or other symptoms.

### Complications

BV during pregnancy is associated with adverse outcomes such as premature labor, preterm delivery, and postpartum endometritis. In the nonpregnant individual, it may be associated with PID and urinary tract infections.

## Treatment

All women who have symptomatic disease should receive treatment to relieve vaginal symptoms and signs of infection (see Table 40–1). Additional goals for pregnant women include prevention of adverse outcomes of pregnancy. Treatment for patients who do not complain of vaginal discharge or itching, but who demonstrate BV on routine pelvic examination, is unclear. Because some studies associate BV and PID, the recommendation is to have a low threshold for treating asymptomatic BV. Follow-up visits are unnecessary if symptoms resolve. Recurrence of BV is not unusual. Follow-up examination 1-month after treatment for high-risk pregnant women is recommended.

Males do not develop infection equivalent to BV. Treatment of male partners has no effect on the course of infection in females.

Koumans EH et al: Indications for therapy and treatment recommendations for bacterial vaginosis in nonpregnant and pregnant women: A synthesis of data. Clin Infect Dis 2002;35;S152 [PMID: 12353202].

Schwebke JR: Bacterial vaginosis. Curr Infect Dis Rep 2000;2:14 [PMID: 11095832].

## 2. Trichomonas Vaginalis Infection

### General Considerations

Trichomoniasis is caused by *T vaginalis,* a flagellated protozoan that infects 2.5–3 million people annually.

### Clinical Findings

#### A. SYMPTOMS AND SIGNS

Fifty percent of females with trichomoniasis develop a symptomatic vaginitis with vaginal itching; a green-gray, malodorous frothy discharge; and dysuria. Occasionally postcoital bleeding and dyspareunia may be present. The vulva may be erythematous and the cervix friable. Half of men with trichomoniasis will have urethritis.

#### B. LABORATORY FINDINGS

Mixing the discharge with normal saline facilitates detection of the flagellated protozoan on microscopic examination (wet preparation). The infection may be detected by the pathologist when reviewing the Pap smear. The InPouch TV system is available for culture when the diagnosis is unclear. Culture and antigen detection are sensitive, but expensive and not readily available. Trichomonal urethritis frequently causes a positive urine leukocyte esterase test or WBCs on urethral smear.

## Complications

Male partners of females diagnosed with trichomoniasis have a 22% chance of having trichomoniasis. *Trichomonas* infection in women has been associated with adverse pregnancy outcomes.

## Treatment (See Table 40–1.)

Schwebke JR, Hook EW 3rd: High rates of *Trichomonas vaginalis* among men attending a sexually transmitted diseases clinic: Implications for screening and urethritis management. J Infect Dis 2003;188:465 [PMID: 22751764].

## 3. Vulvovaginal Candidiasis

### General Considerations

Vulvovaginal candidiasis is caused by *Candida albicans* in 85–90% of cases. Most women will have at least one episode of vulvovaginal candidiasis, and almost half will have two or more episodes. The highest incidence is between ages 16 and 30 years. Predisposing factors include recent use of antibiotics, diabetes, pregnancy, and HIV. Risk factors include vaginal intercourse, use of oral contraceptives, and use of spermicide. This is rarely a sexually transmitted infection. Recurrences generally reflect reactivation of colonization.

### Clinical Findings

#### A. SYMPTOMS AND SIGNS

Typical symptoms include pruritus and a white, "cottage cheese"-like vaginal discharge without odor. The itching is more common midcycle and shortly after menses. Other symptoms include vaginal soreness, vulvar burning, vulvar edema and redness, dyspareunia, and dysuria (especially after intercourse).

#### B. LABORATORY FINDINGS

The diagnosis is usually made by visualizing yeast or pseudohyphae with 10% KOH (90% sensitive) or Gram stain (77% sensitive) in the vaginal discharge. Fungal culture can be used if symptoms and microscopy are not definitive, although colonization is common in asymptomatic women. Vaginal pH is normal with yeast infections.

## Complications

The only complication of vulvovaginal candidiasis is recurrent infections (ie, four or more episodes annually).

## Treatment

Topical formulations effectively treat vaginal yeast infections. The topically applied azole drugs are more effective than nystatin. Treatment with azoles results in relief of symptoms and negative cultures in 80–90% of patients who complete therapy. Oral fluconazole as a one-time dose is an effective oral medication. Patients should be instructed to return for follow-up visits only if symptoms persist or recur. Six-month prophylaxis regimens have been effective in many women with persistent or recurrent yeast infection. Recurrent disease is usually due to *C albicans* that remains susceptible to azoles, and should be treated for 14 days with oral azoles. Some non-albicans *Candida* will respond to itraconazole. Boric acid capsules (600 mg daily for 14 days) intravaginally are effective. Treatment of sex partners is not recommended but may be considered for women who have recurrent infection (see Table 40–1).

Drugs for vulvovaginal candidiasis. Med Lett Drugs Ther 2001; 43:3 [PMID: 20583850].

Sobel JD: Management of patients with recurrent vulvovaginal candidiasis. Drugs 2003;63:1059 [PMID: 22635335].

## GENITAL ULCERATIONS

In the United States, young, sexually active patients who have genital ulcers have genital herpes, syphilis, or chancroid. The relative frequency of each disease differs by geographic area and patient population; however, in most areas of the United States, genital herpes is the most prevalent of these diseases. More than one of these diseases could be present in a patient with genital ulcers. All ulcerative diseases are associated with an increased risk for HIV infection. The acute retroviral syndrome of HIV infection may be accompanied with oral and genital ulcers.

Ulcers are vaginal, vulvar, or cervical in females, and on any part of the penis in males. Oral lesions may occur concomitant with genital ulcerations in HSV and syphilis. Each etiologic agent has specific characteristics that are described in the following sections. Lesion pain, inguinal lymphadenopathy, and urethritis may be found in association with the ulcers.

### 1. Herpes Simplex Virus

#### General Considerations

HSV is the most common cause of visible genital ulcers. At least 50 million people are infected with HSV-2 in the United States. Approximately 0.5–1.5 million new cases occur each year. As with oral HSV infections, many primary genital infections are asymptomatic (60–80%) or not recognizable as herpetic in origin.

## Clinical Findings

### A. Symptoms and Signs

Symptomatic initial HSV infection causes vesicles of the external genitalia, quickly followed by shallow, painful ulcerations. These may occur in the vulva, vagina, cervix, penis, rectum, or urethra. Atypical presentation of HSV infection includes vulvar erythema and fissures. Urethritis may occur. Initial infection can be severe, lasting up to 3 weeks, and be associated with fever and malaise, as well as localized tender adenopathy. The pain and dysuria can be extremely uncomfortable, requiring sitz baths, topical anesthetics, and occasionally catheterization for urinary retention.

HSV-2 is the most common cause of genital herpes (80%). Symptoms tend to be more severe in females. Recurrence in the genital area with HSV-2 is likely (65–80%). Recurrent genital herpes is of shorter duration (7–10 days), with fewer lesions and usually no systemic symptoms. Prodromal pain in the genital, buttock, or pelvic region is common prior to recurrences. HSV-1, which accounts for 20% of first-episode genital herpes infections, is usually the consequence of oral–genital sex. Primary HSV-1 infection is as severe as HSV-2 infection, and treatment is the same. HSV-1 is associated with recurrent genital disease much less often (< 10%) than is HSV-2.

### B. Laboratory Findings

Diagnosis of genital HSV is often made presumptively, but in one large series this diagnosis was incorrect for 20% of cases. Culture or antigen testing of the vesicles confirms the diagnosis; recurrent genital ulceration is suggestive of HSV infection.

## Differential Diagnosis

Any genital ulcer should be cultured for HSV and differentiated from syphilis and chancroid ulcers. The character of the ulcers and inguinal nodes differ in these diseases. (See Chancroid and Syphilis sections).

## Complications

Complications, usually with the first episode of genital HSV, include viral meningitis, urinary retention, transmission to newborns at birth, and pharyngitis.

## Prevention

All patients with active lesions should be counseled to abstain from sexual contact. Most patients have periodic asymptomatic shedding of HSV, and many cases of genital HSV are transmitted by persons who are unaware that they have the infection or are asymptomatic when transmission occurs. Reactivation can occur in individuals who never had symptomatic disease. Individuals with prior HSV infection should be encouraged to always use condoms to protect susceptible partners. Antiviral prophylaxis of infected individuals reduces shedding and significantly reduces the chance of transmission to their sexual partners.

## Treatment

Antivirals administered within the first 5 days of primary infection decrease the duration and severity of HSV infection (see Table 40–1). The effect of antivirals on the severity or duration of recurrent disease is limited. For best results, therapy should be started with the prodrome or during the first day of the attack. Although the current recommendations are for 5 days of therapy for recurrences, new information suggests that 3 days of therapy may be sufficient. If recurrences are frequent and cause significant physical or emotional discomfort, patients may elect to take antiviral prophylaxis on a daily basis to reduce the frequency (75% decrease) and duration of recurrences. Treatment of first or subsequent attacks will not prevent future attacks, but recurrence frequency decreases in many individuals over time.

Corey L: Challenges in genital herpes simplex virus management. J Infect Dis 2002;186 (Suppl):S29-33 [PMID: 22239185].

Whitley RJ: Herpes simplex virus infection. Semin Pediatric Infect Dis 2002;13: 6-11 [PMID: 22409051].

## 2. Syphilis

### General Considerations

Syphilis is an acute and chronic STI caused by infection with *T pallidum*. The overall rate of syphilis has increased since 1999 to 2.4/100,000 with rates of 3.8/100,000 in men, predominantly those who have sex with men. The South and certain urban areas continue to have high rates of syphilis.

### Clinical Findings

#### A. SYMPTOMS AND SIGNS

Skin and mucous membrane lesions characterize the acute phase of primary and secondary syphilis. Lesions of the bone, viscera, aorta, and central nervous system predominate in the chronic phase (tertiary syphilis) (see Chapter 38). Prevention of syphilis is also important because syphilitic mucosal lesions facilitate transmission of HIV.

Primary syphilis usually presents as a solitary chancre—a painless ulcer with an indurated base and associated nontender, firm adenopathy. The chancre appears 10–90 days after exposure and resolves spontaneously

4–8 weeks later. Because it is painless, it may go undetected, especially if the lesion is within the vagina. Chancres may occur on the genitalia, lips, or anus. Secondary syphilis occurs 4–10 weeks after the chancre appears, with generalized malaise, adenopathy, and a nonpruritic maculopapular rash that often includes the palms and soles. Secondary syphilis resolves in 1–3 months but can recur. Verrucous lesions known as condyloma lata may develop on the genitalia. These must be distinguished from genital warts.

#### B. LABORATORY FINDINGS

If the patient has a suspect primary lesion, is at high risk, is a contact, or may have secondary syphilis, a nontreponemal serum screen—either RPR or VDRL—should be performed. If the nontreponemal test is positive, then a specific treponemal test, a fluorescent treponemal antibody-absorbed (FTA-ABS) or microhemagglutination–*Treponema pallidum* (MHA-TP) test, is done to confirm the diagnosis. An additional diagnostic tool is darkfield microscopy, which can be used to detect spirochetes in scrapings of the chancre base. Darkfield examinations and direct fluorescent antibody tests of lesion exudate or tissue are the definitive methods for diagnosing early syphilis.

If a patient is engaging in high-risk sexual behavior or is living in an urban area in which syphilis is endemic, RPRs should be drawn yearly to screen for asymptomatic infection. Syphilis is reportable to state health departments, and all contacts need to be evaluated. Patients also need to be evaluated for other STIs, including HIV.

### Complications

Untreated syphilis can lead to tertiary complications with serious multiorgan involvement, including aortitis and neurosyphilis. Transmission to the fetus can occur from an untreated pregnant woman (see Chapters 1 and 38).

### Treatment

See Table 40–1. Patients should be reexamined clinically and serologically with nontreponemal tests at 6 months and 12 months after treatment. If signs or symptoms persist or recur, or patients do not have a fourfold decrease in their nontreponemal test titer, they should be considered to have failed treatment, or be reinfected, and need retreatment.

Golden MR et al: Update on syphilis: Resurgence of an old problem. JAMA 2003;290;1510 [PMID: 13129993].

Primary and secondary syphilis–United States, 2002. MMWR Morb Mortal Wkly Rep 2003;52:1117 [PMID: 14627949].

## 3. Chancroid

### General Considerations

Chancroid is caused by *Haemophilus ducreyi*. It is relatively rare but endemic in some urban areas and has been associated with HIV infection, drug use, and prostitution. Ten percent of patients with chancroid are coinfected with HSV or syphilis.

### Clinical Findings

#### A. SYMPTOMS AND SIGNS

The typical lesion begins as a papule that erodes after 24–48 hours into an ulcer. The ulcer has ragged, sharply demarcated edges and a purulent base, is painful (unlike syphilis), solitary, and somewhat deeper than HSV infection. Tender, fluctuant (unlike syphilis and HSV) inguinal adenopathy is present in one third of patients. A painful ulcer in combination with suppurative inguinal adenopathy is very often chancroid.

#### B. LABORATORY FINDINGS

Gram stain shows gram-positive cocci arranged in a boxcar formation. Culture can be performed on special culture media that is available in academic centers. Other causes of genital ulceration should be excluded.

### Differential Diagnosis

Chancroid is distinguished from syphilis by the painful nature of the ulcer and the associated tender suppurative adenopathy. HSV vesicles often produce painful ulcers, but these are multiple, smaller, and shallower than chancroid ulcers. Adenopathy associated with initial HSV infection does not suppurate. A presumptive diagnosis of chancroid should be considered in a patient with typical painful genital ulcers and regional adenopathy, if the test results for syphilis and HSV are negative.

### Treatment

Symptoms improve within 3 days after therapy (see Table 40–1). Most ulcers resolve in 7 days, although large ulcers may take 2 weeks to heal. All sexual contacts need to be examined and given treatment, even if asymptomatic.

Lewis DA: Chancroid: Clinical manifestations, diagnosis, and management. Sex Trans Infect 2003;79:68 [PMID: 22465222].

## 4. Other Ulcerations

Lymphogranuloma venereum (LGV), caused by *C trachomatis* serovars L1, L2, or L3, is rare in the United States. Patients with LGV present with a painless vesicle or ulcer that heals spontaneously, followed by development of tender adenopathy, either unilateral or bilateral. A classic finding is the groove sign—an inguinal crease created by concomitant involvement of inguinal and femoral nodes. These become matted and fluctuant and may rupture. LGV can cause proctocolitis, fistulas, and strictures in patients with anal involvement. Diagnosis can be made by culturing a node aspirate for *Chlamydia* or by serology. Differential diagnosis during the adenopathy phase includes bacterial adenitis, lymphoma, and cat-scratch disease. Differential diagnosis during the ulcerative phase encompasses all causes of genital ulcers. Treatment is with doxycycline, 100 mg twice daily for 21 days.

Granuloma inguinale, or donovanosis, is caused by *Calymmatobacterium granulomatis,* a gram-negative bacillus that is rare in the United States. An indurated subcutaneous nodule erodes to form a painless, friable ulcer with granulation tissue. Diagnosis is based on clinical suspicion and supported by a Wright or Giemsa stain of the granulation tissue that reveals intracytoplasmic rods (Donovan bodies) in mononuclear cells. See Table 40–1 for treatment recommendations.

Mabey D, Peeling RW: Lymphogranuloma venereum. Sex Transm Dis 2002;78:90 [PMID: 22075989].

Resnick SD: Skin signs of sexually transmitted diseases in adolescents. Adolesc Med 2001;12:285 [PMID: 21296765].

## GENITAL WARTS (HUMAN PAPILLOMAVIRUS)

### General Considerations

Condylomata acuminata, or genital warts, are caused by HPV, which can also cause cervical dysplasia. Estimates suggest that up to one third of adolescent females having sexual intercourse in the United States have HPV infections. HPV is transmitted sexually: 30–60% of males whose partners have HPV have evidence of condylomata on examination.

HPV has multiple serotypes. Types 6 and 11 are detected most frequently in genital warts, whereas 16 and 18 cause more than 70% of cervical dysplasia. The infection is more common in persons with multiple partners and in women who have previously had an abnormal Pap smear or genital warts. Cervical HPV is relatively more common in the adolescent population because of increased susceptibility of the cervical transition zone.

The American Cancer Society indicates that there is little risk of missing an important cervical lesion until 3–5 years after initiation of intercourse. Pap smears should be obtained after this time or by age 21. Thereafter, annual cervical screening should be performed using conventional Pap smears or every 2 years if using liquid-based cytology (Thin Prep), which can type HPV.

## Clinical Findings

### A. SYMPTOMS AND SIGNS

For males, verrucous lesions are found on the shaft or corona of the penis. Lesions also may develop in the urethra or rectum. Lesions do not produce discomfort. They may be single or found in clusters. Females develop verrucous lesions on any genital mucosal surface, either internally or externally. In women, cervical HPV infection may only be detected by cytology.

### B. LABORATORY FINDINGS

External, visible lesions have unique characteristics that make the diagnosis straightforward. Condylomata acuminata can be distinguished from condylomata lata (syphilis), skin tags, and molluscum contagiosum by application of 5% acetic acid solution. Aceto-whitening is used to indicate the extent of cervical infection.

Pap smears detect cervical abnormalities. HPV infection is the most frequent cause of an abnormal smear. Pap smear findings are graded by the atypical nature of the cervical cells. These changes range from atypical squamous cells of undetermined significance (ASCUS) to low-grade squamous interepithelial lesions (LSIL) and high-grade squamous interepithelial lesions (HSIL). LSIL encompasses cellular changes associated with HPV and mild dysplasia. HSIL includes moderate dysplasia, severe dysplasia, and carcinoma in situ.

Follow-up for ASCUS is controversial, as only 25% progress to dysplasia, and the remainder either demonstrate no progression or regress. If ASCUS is present, the laboratory should be instructed to do HPV typing on Thin Prep Pap smears. If HSIL are found, colposcopy should be performed. If LSIL are detected, colposcopy is not needed and a repeat Pap smear should be done in 1 year. If LSIL or HSIL are subsequently detected, the patient is also referred for colposcopy for direct visualization or biopsy of the cervix (or both). If a Pap smear shows signs of inflammation only, and concomitant infection such as vaginitis or cervicitis is present, the smear should be repeated after the infection has cleared.

## Differential Diagnosis

The differential diagnosis includes normal anatomic structures (pearly penile papules, vestibular papillae, sebaceous glands), molluscum contagiosum, seborrheic keratosis, and syphilis.

## Complications

Because genital warts can proliferate and become friable during pregnancy, many experts advocate their removal during pregnancy. HPV types 6 and 11 can cause laryngeal papillomatosis in infants and children. Complications of appropriate treatment include scarring with changes in skin pigmentation or chronic pain at the treatment site. Cervical cancer is the most common and important sequel of HPV.

## Prevention

The use of condoms may reduce, but does not eliminate, the risk for transmission to uninfected partners.

## Treatment

All penile and external vaginal or vulvar lesions can be treated topically. Treatment should be for 4–6 weeks to clear the infection. An experienced practitioner should treat internal and cervical lesions (See Table 40–1).

Warts may resolve or remain unchanged if left untreated or they may increase in size or number. Treatment can induce wart-free periods in most patients. Most recurrences occur within the 3 months following completion of a treatment regimen. Appropriate follow-up of abnormal Pap smears is essential to detect any progression to malignancy.

Kahn JA: An update on human papillomavirus infection and Papanicolaou smears in adolescents. Curr Opin Pediatr 2001; 13:303 [PMID: 21573855].

Moscicki AB: Human papillomavirus infection in adolescents. Pediatr Clin North Am 1999;46:4:783 [PMID: 99424044].

Moscicki AB et al: Risks for incident human papillomavirus infection and low-grade squamous intraepithelial lesion development in young females. JAMA 2001:285;2995 [PMID: 11410098].

Saslow D et al: American Cancer Society Guideline for the early detection of cervical neoplasia and cancer CA. Cancer J Clin 2002;52:342 [PMID: 12469763].

Wiley DJ et al: External genital warts: Diagnosis, treatment, and prevention. Clin Infect Dis 2002:35;S210 [PMID: 12353208].

# OTHER VIRAL INFECTIONS

## 1. Hepatitis (See Chapters 21 and 36)

### General Considerations

Hepatitis B and hepatitis C are often STIs. Hepatitis B is at least 10 times more common than HIV in the adolescent population. Since 1998, sexual transmission has accounted for approximately 50% of the estimated 181,000 new hepatitis B infections that occur annually in the United States. Heterosexuals who have unprotected sex with multiple partners and men who have sex with men are the groups at highest risk for sexual transmission.

Hepatitis C generally is transmitted through blood products and shared intravenous needles, although about 10% of hepatitis C infections have been linked to sexual transmission. Hepatitis C needs to be considered in teenagers who are symptomatic and engage in high-risk sexual behavior or intravenous drug use. Outbreaks of sexually transmitted hepatitis A infection have occurred among men who have sex with men, although the efficiency of sexual transmission is low.

## Clinical Findings

### A. Symptoms and Signs

Symptoms, diagnosis, and treatment are described in Chapter 36.

### B. Laboratory Findings

Adolescents with high-risk behaviors need to be screened for hepatitis B virus (see Screening section). If hepatitis B surface antigen test is present, the patient should be followed to distinguish acute from chronic infection and to provide appropriate management of chronic infection.

## Complications

Hepatocellular carcinoma and chronic liver disease are complications of hepatitis B and C infections.

## Prevention

Hepatitis B vaccination is the most effective means of preventing infection. All unvaccinated youth should be immunized. A simpler two-dose regimen is available for this age group. Vaccination against hepatitis A virus is recommended for travelers to high-prevalence areas, intravenous drug users, men who have sex with men, and individuals with chronic liver disease of other etiologies.

## Treatment

See Chapters 21 and 36.

## 2. Human Immunodeficiency Virus (See Chapter 37.)

### General Considerations

One in four new HIV infections in the United States is acquired by a person age 22 years or younger. Each hour two new young people in the United States become infected with HIV. Because of the long latency period between infection with HIV and progression to AIDS, it is felt that many HIV-positive young adults contracted HIV during adolescence. The number of females who become HIV-positive has increased dramatically, representing almost half of teenagers with HIV infection.

Risk factors for contracting HIV include a prior STI, infrequent condom use, practicing insertive or receptive anal sex (both males and females), practicing survival sex (ie, trading sex for money or drugs), intravenous drug or crack cocaine use, homelessness, and being the victim of sexual abuse (males). HIV infection should be considered in any sexual risk-taking youths, whether they are practicing heterosexual or homosexual sex.

## Clinical Findings

### A. Symptoms and Signs

Adolescents may be asymptomatic with recent HIV infection or may present with the acute retroviral syndrome, which is evident 2–6 weeks after exposure. Fever, malaise, lymphadenopathy, rash, upper respiratory symptoms, oral and genital ulcerations, aseptic meningitis, and thrush may occur. If HIV infection is suspected, diagnosis is made in the acute period by p24 antigen detection or HIV polymerase chain reaction.

### B. Laboratory Findings

Screening for HIV by serology should include risk-taking youths and those with any STI. Adolescents may also present to the office requesting an HIV test. In either case, a careful history of sexual behavior should be obtained to assess risk and intervene with risk-reduction counseling. It is also necessary to determine how teens may respond to being told they are HIV-positive and what support systems they have in place. If an adolescent is homeless; does not have emotional support from family, friends, or a counselor; or threatens suicide or homicide in response to the idea of being HIV-positive, then testing should be deferred until the practitioner is confident that the youth will be safe if the test is positive.

## Treatment

Many experts recommend aggressive antiretroviral treatment of patients diagnosed with acute retroviral syndrome.

Guidelines for the Use of Antiretroviral Agents in HIV-Infected Adults and Adolescents:
http://www.aidsinfo.nih.gov
Futterman D et al: HIV and AIDS in adolescents. Pediatr Clin North Am 2000;47:171 [PMID: 20162755].

### 3. HIV Postsexual Exposure Prophylaxis

The risk of acquiring HIV infection through sexual assault or abuse is low but present. The risk for HIV transmission per episode of receptive penile–anal sexual exposure is estimated at 0.1–0.3%; the risk per episode of receptive vaginal exposure is estimated at less than 0.1–0.15%. For males practicing vaginal intercourse, the risk is somewhat less (0.03–0.1%). HIV transmission also occurs from receptive oral exposure, but the risk is unknown.

Health care providers who consider offering postexposure therapy should take into account the likelihood that exposure to HIV occurred, the potential benefits and risks of such therapy, and the interval between the exposure and initiation of therapy. It will be helpful to know the HIV status of the sexual contact. In general, postexposure therapy is not recommended for exposures to noninfectious fluids or exposures to intact skin and when more than 72 hours has passed since exposure. If the patient decides to take postexposure therapy, clinical management should be implemented according to CDC guidelines for occupational mucous membrane exposure.

CDC: Updated US Public Health Service guidelines for the management of occupational exposures to HBV, HCV, and HIV and recommendations for postexposure prophylaxis. MMWR Recomm Rep 2001;50 (RR-11):1 [PMID: 11442229].

Havens PL et al: Postexposure prophylaxis in children and adolescents for nonoccupational exposure to human immunodeficiency virus. Pediatrics 2003;111:1475 [PMID: 22662832].

## ECTOPARASITIC INFECTIONS

### 1. Pubic Lice

*Phthirus pubis,* or pubic lice, live in the pubic hair. The louse or the nits can be transmitted by close contact from person to person. Patients complain of itching, and they may report having seen the insect. Examination of the pubic hair may reveal the louse crawling around or attached to the hair. Closer inspection may reveal the nit or sack of eggs, which is a gelatinous material (1–2 mm) stuck to the hair shaft.

### 2. Scabies

*Sarcoptes scabiei,* or scabies, is an organism smaller than the louse. It can be identified by the classic burrow, created by the organism laying eggs and traveling just below the skin surface. Scabies can be sexually transmitted by close contact and can be found in the pubic region, groin, lower abdomen, or upper thighs. The rash is intensely pruritic, erythematous, and scaly.

See Table 40–1 for treatment options. The entire area needs to be covered with the lotion or shampoo for the time specified by the manufacturer. One treatment usually clears the infestation, although a second treatment may be necessary. Bed sheets and clothes must be washed in hot water. Both sexual and close personal or household contacts within the preceding month should be examined and treated.

Wendel K, Rompalo A: Scabies and pediculosis pubis: An update of treatment regimens and general review. Clin Infect Dis 2002:35:S146 [PMID: 12353201].

## ■ EVALUATION OF SEXUALLY TRANSMITTED INFECTIONS IN SEXUAL ABUSE AND ASSAULT

Sexual abuse is common: 25% of females and 12% of males will have suffered some form of sexual violence by age 18 years. Half of rape victims are younger than age 18 years. Rape is both a medical and a psychological emergency. Evaluation and treatment after sexual abuse or assault depends on the patient's age, his or her ability to communicate what occurred, and the timing of the abuse.

Teenagers usually can describe the kind of abuse (eg, oral, anal, vaginal; receptive or insertive), and evaluation needs to be directed accordingly. If the abuse has occurred in the preceding 72 hours, most states require, for legal purposes, that a rape kit be used. All practitioners should have access to a rape kit, which guides the practitioner through a stepwise collection of evidence and cultures. A thorough physical examination is indicated to evaluate for other signs of trauma.

Beyond 72 hours, evaluation is tailored to the history provided. The involved orifices should be cultured for *N gonorrhoeae* and *Chlamydia* (NAAT is not admissible in court), and vaginal secretions evaluated for *Trichomonas*. RPR, hepatitis B, and HIV serology should be drawn at baseline and repeated in 2–3 months. Pregnancy testing should be done as indicated.

Trichomoniasis, BV, chlamydia, and gonorrhea are the most frequently diagnosed infections among women who have been sexually assaulted. Because the prevalence of these STIs is substantial among sexually experienced women, their presence after an assault does not necessarily signify acquisition during the assault.

Prophylactic therapy should be offered when patients present within the incubation time of any of the disease processes: oral ceftriaxone for gonorrhea and azithromycin or doxycycline for *Chlamydia* infection. If a person is exposed and does not have anti-HBs antibody, give hepatitis B immune globulin (HBIG) and vaccine. The efficacy of HBIG for sexual exposure is diminished if delay is greater than 7 days after exposure, and the value after 14 days is uncertain. No effective prophylaxis is available for hepatitis C. Evaluating the perpetrator for STI, if possible, can help determine risk exposure and guide prophylaxis. HIV prophylaxis should be considered in certain circumstances (discussed earlier). Emergency contraception should be given if the abuse occurred within 72 hours. Psychological assessment at the time of presentation, as well as over the next several months, is a top priority. Any suspected abuse must reported to the local authorities.

All younger children should be referred to child abuse multidisciplinary teams that help with the psychological aspect of the abuse and are well versed in helping children communicate what may have occurred. Colposcopic examination is critical in determining the extent of damage and provide documentation for the legal system.

Although it is often difficult for persons to comply with follow-up examinations weeks after an assault, such examinations are essential in detecting new infections, complete immunization with hepatitis B vaccination if needed, and continued psychological support.

American Academy of Pediatrics: Committee on Adolescence: Care of the adolescent sexual assault victim. Pediatrics 2001;107: 1476 [PMID: 21293379].

# REFERENCES

Braverman PK: Sexually transmitted disease in adolescents. Med Clin North Am 2000;84:869 [PMID: 20383328].

Burstein GR, Workowski KA: Sexually transmitted disease treatment guidelines. Curr Opin Pediatr 2003;15:391 [PMID: 12891051].

CDC Sexually Transmitted Infections: http://www.cdc.gov/std/.

Centers for Disease Control and Prevention: Sexually transmitted diseases treatment guidelines 2002. MMWR 2002;51(No. RR-6):1 [PMID: 12184549].

# Drug Therapy

**41**

*Patricia Orma, PharmD, Jerrod Milton, PharmD, & Douglas N. Fish, PharmD*

Choosing a safe and effective treatment regimen for pediatric patients can be challenging. New medications and new approaches to drug dosing often originate from adult patient care and are then adapted to the care of pediatric patients. However, it is apparent that simply scaling down drug dosages to allow for differences in weight is not an optimal method of providing effective drug therapy to children. The process of physiologic growth and development is dynamic and extremely complex, resulting in equally dynamic changes in the disposition of drugs and subsequent response to therapies. Multiple patient-specific variables, such as developmental physiology, past medical history, pharmacokinetic and pharmacodynamic properties, desired therapeutic outcomes, and psychosocial issues, need to be considered when designing appropriate drug therapy regimens for children. Unfortunately, there is still a relative deficiency of information regarding exactly how these factors should best be considered when developing regimens that provide adequate therapeutic responses while minimizing potential adverse effects. This chapter provides a brief overview of those issues and how they apply in developing pediatric drug regimens and offers suggestions on how to avoid common medication-related errors.

## DEVELOPING A PEDIATRIC DRUG REGIMEN

The various components of a drug therapy regimen—dose, route, frequency, and treatment duration—are dictated by the pharmacokinetic and pharmacodynamic properties of the drug.

### Pharmacokinetic Considerations

Pharmacokinetic properties include absorption, distribution, metabolism, and elimination. These properties have not always been well described in terms of changes occurring during specific periods in the life of the child and the physiologic reasons for those changes.

### A. ABSORPTION

Oral drug absorption in neonates, infants, and children can be unpredictable owing to variations in gastric pH, gastric emptying time, and intestinal transit time. At birth, gastric pH approaches neutral, but becomes more acidic as acid secretory mechanisms become more functional, usually within hours of birth. An infant's gastric pH is closer to an adult's by 3 months of age. Gastric emptying in neonates and infants is often considerably prolonged (up to 8 hours or more) but approaches adult values by 6 to 8 months of age. Intestinal transit time is similarly prolonged, and peristaltic mechanisms may be quite erratic.

Elevated gastric pH, together with decreased gastric emptying time and intestinal transit time, may significantly affect a drug's absorption, depending on its physiochemical properties. Weak acids such as phenytoin, phenobarbital, and acetaminophen may be more slowly and incompletely absorbed due to decreased gastric acidity, whereas weak bases such as penicillin G and ampicillin may demonstrate increased bioavailability and more rapid absorption. Sustained release products (eg, theophylline) should be used with care due to the unpredictable and inconsistent absorption that may occur.

### B. DISTRIBUTION

Drugs given intravenously (IV), intramuscularly (IM), subcutaneously (SC), topically (TP), or transdermally (TD) may have erratic and unpredictable distribution, especially in neonates. This may be due to poor perfusion (IV, IM, SC, TP, TD), decreased muscle mass (IM, SC), or differences in percentage of total body water (IM, SC, TP, TD). Premature and full-term infants may have body water percentages of 75–85% compared with the more normal adults values of 55–60%. These changes in body water result in significantly increased volumes of distribution and may cause concentrations of water-soluble drugs such as aminoglycoside antibiotics and theophylline to be unusually low with customary doses, whereas the lower volumes of distribution associated with fat-soluble agents such as antiepileptic agents may cause drug concentrations to reach toxic ranges. The reduction in total body water is rapid during the first year of life and reaches adult values by approximately 10–12 years of age.

Another physiologic factor that may affect a drug's distributive properties is the plasma protein (ie, albumin) concentration. Because this concentration in the neonate is lower, drugs such as phenytoin, which is highly protein bound, will have more unbound or active drug circulating. This can result in more adverse effects even with an apparent therapeutic blood level. Unbound drugs also have greater membrane permeability, and changes in protein binding may also be at least partially responsible for increased toxicities observed with some centrally acting agents such as analgesics or antiepileptic drugs. Plasma proteins approach normal adult values by 10–12 months of life.

### C. METABOLISM

Although a normal, healthy neonate is born with the same hepatic enzymes important for drug metabolism that an adult has, a reduced ability to metabolize drugs is present in the postnatal period. Hepatic enzyme activity is generally reduced in the neonate. As the infant ages, his or her ability to metabolize medications increases. It is interesting to note that, although total metabolic capacity is reduced in neonates and infants, certain metabolic pathways may actually be much more active than in adults and some medications may be metabolized through alternative pathways. Nevertheless, care should be taken during the postnatal period when using medications, such as phenytoin, phenobarbital, and diazepam, that are primarily hepatically metabolized.

### D. ELIMINATION

The kidney is responsible for elimination of the majority of drugs and their metabolites from the body. At birth, glomerular filtration rate (GFR) is less than 50% of what it will be eventually. Renal tubular secretory pathways are also relatively immature and decreased in function. Consequently, elimination is prolonged and the dose or dosing intervals (or both) for renally eliminated drugs, such as vancomycin, ranitidine, gentamicin, and ampicillin, need to be adjusted accordingly (see Chapter 35). By age 6 months, the infant's GFR has matured to about 90% of the adult level.

## Pharmacodynamic Considerations

Pharmacodynamics describes the relationship between concentrations of drug at the site of drug action and the magnitude of the resulting pharmacologic effect. In contrast to pharmacokinetics, which only considers the disposition of drug within the body, pharmacodynamics relates to how the pharmacokinetics of the drug interact with the target organ or microorganism to cause a drug effect. The purpose of characterizing the pharmacodynamics of drugs is to maximize drug effect and minimize drug toxicities by being able to anticipate the intensity as well as the time course of pharmacologic effects.

For example, the bactericidal effects of aminoglycoside antibiotics are maximized when high plasma concentrations of the drug are achieved rapidly; this pharmacodynamic property is referred to as **concentration-dependent** killing. Rapid bacterial killing and extended drug effects occur when peak plasma concentrations of 10–12 times the minimum inhibitory concentration (MIC) of the microbe are achieved. Thus, providing relatively large doses of a drug to achieve high concentrations optimizes the effectiveness of aminoglycosides. In contrast, the pharmacodynamic properties of β-lactam antibiotics (ie, penicillins, cephalosporins) are characterized as **time-dependent.** These drugs kill most effectively when blood levels above the MIC are achieved throughout the interval between drug doses. Thus, relatively smaller doses administered more frequently (every 8 hours or every 6 hours) provide an optimal pharmacodynamic setting.

Antimicrobial treatment is one of the best characterized and most commonly applied examples of pharmacodynamics in the clinical setting. An understanding of the relationship between drug concentration and drug effect is useful for many other drug classes. Theophylline requires approximately 1 hour after a dose for initial effects on pulmonary function to be seen and 12–24 hours after a dose to achieve maximum effects; these effects are not directly correlated with the pharmacokinetic properties of the drug. Maximum anti-inflammatory effects of prednisone or prednisolone occur 6–8 hours after the dose and return to baseline by 24–36 hours, long after blood concentrations of the drug become undetectable. Knowledge of the pharmacodynamics of commonly used agents may assist clinicians in anticipating when desired therapeutic responses will occur or in explaining unusual responses to drug therapy that may be inconsistent with the drug's systemic concentrations.

The pharmacodynamics of most drugs have not been well studied in children. Characterization of the pharmacodynamic properties of drugs in adults is usually based on the assumption that drug-binding receptors present at the site of drug action are stable in number and function. However, it has been demonstrated that certain receptors such as β-adrenergic receptors are quite variable in number and binding affinity, and that this variability is age-related. Further research pertaining to the pharmacodynamics of drugs in children will yield important information that will allow medications to be used more effectively and safely.

## 1. Therapeutic Drug Monitoring

Many factors can affect a patient's response to a medication, and individualized dosage adjustments may be necessary to achieve the desired response or outcome. Drugs that require routine blood concentration monitoring may require a patient-specific dose adjustment in

**Figure 41–1.** Differences between linear and nonlinear concentration–dose profiles. Drugs with nonlinear pharmacokinetics can produce unexpected toxic concentrations with only small incremental changes in dose.

order to achieve therapeutic and nontoxic concentrations (Figure 41–1). Three important pharmacokinetic principles govern appropriate individualization of drug doses based on blood concentration determinations.

**Steady state** is the time it takes for the drug concentration to reach physiologic equilibrium in the body and is directly related to the drug's elimination half-life. In general, a drug is considered to be at steady state after it has been administered continuously at the same dosage and interval (eg, gentamicin, 25 mg every 8 hours) for at least three to five half-lives. For some drugs, the half-life may be short (eg, gentamicin's half-life is 2–4 hours), and steady state is achieved in 1 day. Some drugs have a long half-life (eg, the half-life of phenobarbital is 24–36 hours) and require days or weeks to achieve steady state. Interpreting drug levels and making dosage adjustments on the basis of blood concentrations that are not at steady state can lead to overdosing and subsequent toxicity. Likewise, after a dosage adjustment has been made, sufficient time must be allowed (an additional three to five half-lives) and a new steady state must be achieved before rechecking the blood concentration and making additional clinical decisions based on the result.

A second principle is the **linear relationship** between the blood concentration of most drugs at steady state and the dose administered (eg, vancomycin, theophylline, phenobarbital). Therefore, if a steady-state blood concentration is 50% of that eventually desired, doubling the dosage will achieve the desired concentration after the drug achieves its new pharmacokinetic steady state.

A third concept is the **nonlinear relationship** among clearance, dosing rate, and blood concentration that exists for a select group of drugs (salicylates, ethanol, phenytoin). These drugs do not have a predictable correlation between dosing rate and steady-state blood concentration. Doubling the daily dosage of one of these drugs may result in a three- to fourfold increase in concentrations, overshooting the desired concentrations and resulting in exaggerated response or undesirable toxicities. Drugs with nonlinear pharmacokinetics thus require close drug monitoring by clinicians experienced with these drugs (Table 41–1).

It should be noted that the therapeutic blood levels shown in Table 41–1 are not absolute numbers that will produce desired responses in all patients. Recommended blood concentrations are based on the *probability* of a drug producing the desired response at those levels. Most patients will have good drug responses and therapeutic outcomes when blood concentrations are in the desired ranges. However, some patients may achieve adequate responses at less-than-recommended blood concentrations, while other patients may require concentrations far in excess of those normally required. Likewise, unacceptable drug toxicities may occur in some patients at concentrations less than those normally recommended, whereas others will tolerate high concentrations of drugs relatively well. The tremendous variability among patients requires that blood concentrations be interpreted in the overall context of a patient's clinical response rather than solely on the basis of recommended blood concentrations.

## 2. Drug Selection

### Patient-Specific Factors

The patient's age is one of the most important parameters to consider when developing a drug therapy regimen. Additionally, physiologic and psychological age should influence the choice of drug, the route of administration, the dosing regimen, and the monitoring parameters. Physiologic factors such as the inability of newborns and infants to reliably absorb oral medications limit this route of administration. Psychological issues are more important when considering treatment for older children and adolescents or when the parents of a young child have limited cognitive functioning. The ability of the patient or parent to accurately administer a drug therapy can affect its efficacy and safety. Factors to keep in mind when selecting drug therapy are given in Table 41–2.

Because nearly all drugs are primarily eliminated from the body by the liver and kidneys, the function of these organs should be assessed before selecting drug therapy and throughout the treatment course. Renal

**Table 41–1.** Therapeutic blood levels.[a]

| Drug | Therapeutic Range |
|------|-------------------|
| Acetaminophen | 10–20 μg/mL |
| Amikacin | 15–30 μg/mL (peak)<br>< 5 μg/mL (trough) |
| Aspirin | 150–300 μg/mL |
| Carbamazepine | 4–12 μg/mL |
| Cyclosporine | 50–250 mg/mL[b] |
| Digoxin | 0.9–2.4 ng/mL |
| Ethanol | 1000 μg/mL |
| Ethosuximide | 40–100 μg/mL |
| Flucytosine | < 100 μg/mL<br>< 80 μg/mL in newborns and infants |
| Gentamicin | 6–10 μg/mL (peak)<br>< 2 μg/mL (trough) |
| Lidocaine | < 100 ng/mL (newborn)<br>1.5–2.5 μg/mL (adult) |
| Methsuximide as the metabolite of N-desmethsuximide | 10–40 μg/mL |
| Phenobarbital | 15–40 μg/mL |
| Phenytoin | 10–20 μg/mL |
| Primidone | 4–12 μg/mL |
| Procainamide | 4–6 μg/mL |
| Quinidine | 3–5 μg/mL |
| Theophylline | 5–20 μg/mL |
| Tobramycin | 6–10 μg/mL (peak)<br>< 2 μg/mL (trough) |
| Valproic acid | 50–120 μg/mL |
| Vancomycin | 20–40 μg/mL (peak)<br>4–12 μg/mL (trough) |

[a]Therapeutic level or range for drugs that can be routinely analyzed.
[b]Therapeutic ranges will differ depending on type of cyclosporine assay used (eg, monoclonal versus polyclonal whole blood TDx assays) and the type of transplant (ie, heart, kidney, bone marrow).

function can be assessed easily by using serum creatinine concentrations to estimate GFR.

Since most of the renal dosing adjustment guidelines are derived from adult experience, it is necessary to calculate an infant's adjusted GFR by using his or her body surface area (BSA). This subsequently will better simulate adult values and allow for more accurate adjustments of pediatric doses to account for renal dysfunction. Close monitoring for drug toxicity is necessary when decreased hepatic metabolism is suspected in patients receiving hepatically metabolized drugs. Table 41–3 lists some commonly used drugs and their primary route of elimination.

The acuteness of the patient's condition should always be considered. Drug therapy may not be appropriate when the child has mild symptoms because drug side effects may be worse than the disease (eg, decongestant use in infants with a cold).

## Drug-Specific Factors

Individualization of drug therapy requires specific knowledge about the patient and the potential drug treatment alternatives. The therapeutic index (Figure 41–2) is the ratio of the maximum tolerated dose to the minimum curative dose. It is a measure of the relative benefits and risks of a selected drug regimen. A drug with a wide therapeutic index has a greater margin of safety than one with a narrow index (Table 41–4). As with the relationship between drug blood concentrations and patient response, the therapeutic index for any specific drug is characterized by significant variation among individuals. However, this variability is usually more problematic in the clinical use of a drug with a narrow therapeutic index. Drugs with wide therapeutic indices are therefore usually selected for initial treatment if possible. Close patient monitoring is required to ensure an acceptable clinical response to drug therapy.

## 3. Routes Of Administration
### Oral Route

Oral administration is the easiest, least expensive, and most convenient route of drug administration in children. Oral therapy is sometimes not the most appropriate in very young infants (younger than age 1–2 months) or in children with short bowel syndrome because of unpredictable absorption. Oral therapy is also not initially indicated for a severely ill child. When oral therapy is chosen, the desired dosage form for the child's age should be selected. Oral suspensions and liquids are available for many medications and are preferred for infants and young children. A number of drugs are not available in liquid formulations but can be compounded by pharmacies (Table 41–5). Several "sprinkle" formulations are available that can be added to foods. Chewable tablets can be used beginning at about age 12–18 months.

Absorption of orally administered medications can be affected by dietary factors. Recommendations for administration with or without food are specific for each drug and should be followed.

*Table 41–2.* Factors that can affect drug therapy selection and decision making.

| Factors | Concerns |
|---|---|
| **PHYSIOLOGIC**<br>Hyperbilirubinemia | Drugs such as ceftriaxone and sulfisoxazole can displace bilirubin and induce kernicterus in newborns. |
| Newborn immaturity<br>　GI malabsorption<br>　Renal insufficiency<br><br>　Hepatic insufficiency | Oral antibiotics are unreliably absorbed during the first month of life<br>Renal-eliminated drugs such as the penicillins and aminoglycosides in newborns require extended dosing intervals<br>Hepatic-eliminated drugs such as phenobarbital, morphine, and diazepam in newborns require lower doses and extended intervals. |
| Malnutrition (decreased albumin) | Drugs such as phenytoin, warfarin, and ibuprofen can have enhanced pharmacologic action due to decreased protein binding and increased free drug concentrations. |
| Short bowel syndrome | Oral medications of all types can have erratic absorption when the amount of bowel (especially duodenum) available to absorb drug is reduced. |
| Coordination of swallow | Solid oral medications (capsules, tablets) can be swallowed by children as young as 3 years |
| **PSYCHOLOGICAL**<br>Cognitive ability | Decreased understanding of directions, indications, or monitoring of drug therapy can lead to noncompliance or delayed recognition of side effects. |
| **PSYCHOSOCIAL** | Patients with a chaotic home situation, those with multiple caregivers, and those in daycare or school can have difficulty with dosing regimens. Low-income families may have problems paying for expensive drug therapies. |
| **COMPLIANCE**<br>Palatability<br>Schedule<br><br>Timing with respect<br>　to eating<br>Volume<br>Side effects | Liquid oral medications with an unpleasant taste, texture, or aftertaste.<br>Dosing regimens with complicated schedules (tapering doses) or high-frequency intervals (four times daily).<br>Requirement to dose on empty stomach or with food.<br><br>Liquid oral medications with large volume doses (> 10 ml).<br>Medications with undesirable side effects (eg, diarrhea). |
| **MISCELLANEOUS**<br>Availability | The dosage form needs to be available either commercially or by extemporaneous preparation or by splitting a commercially available tablet. |

## Rectal Route

Rectal administration of medications should be reserved for children who cannot take oral medications. Incomplete dose administration can occur if the suppository does not remain in the rectum for sufficient time. Drug distribution within a suppository may not be uniform; therefore, administering half of a suppository may not provide half the dose, leading to either a subtherapeutic or a toxic response in the child.

## Parenteral Route

Intravenous administration of drugs is the most reliable method of delivery and is preferred in severely ill children. Many physical incompatibilities have been identified with the coadministration of intravenous medications and maintenance fluids. If an incompatibility is suspected, a pharmacist should be contacted for documentation and management of the incompatibility. Although IV administration is the most direct way to deliver a medication, it is not without risks. Complications such as thrombophlebitis and extravasation, in addition to IV access itself, can be painful and detrimental to the child.

## 4. Drug Dosing

### Methods Based on Weight

Nearly every drug that has been safely used in pediatric patients has an established milligram-per-kilogram dos-

**Table 41–3.** Primary route of elimination for drugs commonly used in pediatrics.

| Renal Elimination | Hepatic Elimination |
|---|---|
| Acyclovir | Acetaminophen |
| Aminoglycosides | Anticonvulsants (phenytoin, carbamazepine) |
| Cephalosporins | |
| Digoxin | Antidepressants (imipramine, fluoxetine) |
| Fluconazole | |
| Furosemide | Benzodiazepines (diazepam, lorazepam) |
| Penicillins | |
| Ranitidine and cimetidine | Clindamycin |
| | Erythromycin |
| | Opiates (morphine, codeine) |
| | Steroids (anti-inflammatory and hormonal) |
| | Theophylline |

**Table 41–4.** Therapeutic indices of selected drugs.

| Wide[a] | Narrow[b] |
|---|---|
| Acetaminophen | Aminoglycosides |
| Benzodiazepines | Amphotericin B |
| Cephalosporins | Anticonvulsants |
| Decongestants and antihistamines | Cancer chemotherapy agents |
| | Catecholamines (dopamine, epinephrine) |
| Ibuprofen | |
| Penicillins | Digoxin |
| Ranitidine and cimetidine | Heparin and warfarin |
| | Lidocaine |
| Sucralfate | Opiate narcotics (morphine, codeine) |
| | Theophylline |
| | Vancomycin and immunosuppressants (cyclosporine) |

[a]Relatively safe; can round doses.
[b]Increased toxicity; requires specific dosing.

ing range. Drug dosing based on a child's weight in kilograms is simple, convenient, and widely accepted. In general, drugs with a wide therapeutic index have wider dosing ranges, and rounding of doses to a standard dose (eg, amoxicillin 250 mg rather than 236 mg) is recommended.

Drugs with a narrow therapeutic index should be dosed based on the specific mg/kg dosing guidelines and adjusted during therapy with serum drug level monitoring, if available. Frequent recalculation of dosages should be incorporated into the care of children receiving long-term drug therapy because their growth will eventually necessitate increased dosages.

## Methods Based on Body Surface Area

Drug dosing based on BSA may be more accurate. Many drugs with a narrow therapeutic index have dosing guidelines based on patient BSA. Antineoplastic (chemotherapy) drugs used to treat cancer in pediatric patients, antiretroviral drugs used to treat HIV infection, and some other antiviral agents are a few of the commonly prescribed pediatric drugs that are dosed according to BSA measurements. With some drugs (eg, acyclovir), dosing recommendations are based both on mg/kg and BSA, and the calculated dosages by the two methods can be discrepant. Limited data are available

A    Narrow therapeutic index

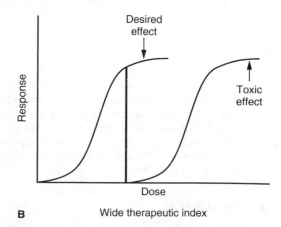

B    Wide therapeutic index

**Figure 41–2.** Graphs of therapeutic index defined as the difference between desired (therapeutic) effect and toxic effect of a drug at a given dose. **A:** Narrow therapeutic index. **B:** Wide therapeutic index.

**Table 41–5.** Common drugs that can be compounded into suspensions or liquids for oral administration.

| | |
|---|---|
| Amlodipine | Metolazone |
| Azathioprine | Metronidazole |
| Baclofen | Omeprazole |
| Caffeine | Phenazopyridine |
| Captopril | Rifampin |
| Clonidine | Sotolol |
| Dipyridamole | Spironolactone |
| Enalapril | Ursodiol |
| Ganciclovir | Verapamil |

evaluating the differences in efficacy and safety of drugs dosed by each method; however, many clinicians believe that dosing based on BSA is a more accurate method.

### Methods Based on Age

Drug dosing based on age is the least accurate method for determining the appropriate dose for a pediatric patient. This method can result in a child receiving a dose that is too high if the child is small for his or her age. This type of dosing method is appropriate only for children who are of average weight and height (ie, 50th percentile) or for medications with a wide therapeutic range. Over-the-counter medications are a class of drugs most commonly dosed based on the age method.

## DRUG INTERACTIONS

Drug interactions can occur between several drugs or between drugs and food. Table 41–6 lists pediatric drugs that have known drug–drug interactions (see Table 41–7 for other sources for this information).

**Table 41–6.** Pediatric drugs commonly associated with drug interactions.

| Inducers[a] | Inhibitors[b] |
|---|---|
| Carbamazepine | Cimetidine |
| Phenobarbital | Cisapride |
| Phenytoin | Erythromycin/clarithromycin |
| Rifampin | Fluconazole/itraconazole |
| | Valproate |
| | Ritonavir |

[a]Inducers increase the metabolism of other medications, thus decreasing plasma levels.
[b]Inhibitors decrease the metabolism of other medications, thus increasing plasma levels.

Drug interactions are usually a direct result of the "overlapping" of the metabolism of two drugs. Most drugs undergo biotransformation to active metabolites in the liver. The liver can transform drugs in many ways. The cytochrome P-450 monooxygenase system contributes to the mechanism of many drug interactions. When evaluating drug combinations for safety, the physician must determine conflicting routes of metabolism. This is paramount when more than one hepatically metabolized drug is prescribed.

Drug interactions are not necessarily a contraindication to use of the drugs. With appropriate identification, proper dosage adjustment, and close therapeutic monitoring, some potentially interacting drug regimens can safely be used concurrently.

## PREVENTING MEDICATION ERRORS

*Primum non nocere*—the first rule of medicine most certainly applies to the application of pharmacotherapy. Avoiding medication error is critical, especially in pediatric patients, in whom the margin of error is typically less. Prescribing errors can be reduced by a number of simple steps.

### Decimal Point Placement

For doses less than one, always put a leading zero before the decimal point (ie, write 0.1 mg not .1 mg). Likewise, if the dose is a fractional whole number, never place a decimal point and a zero after the number (ie, write 1 mg not 1.0 mg). Decimal points can easily be overlooked or misinterpreted. This can result in a tenfold dosing error, either underdose or overdose.

### Abbreviations

Abbreviations should be avoided. This includes the common use of Latin abbreviations and the use of abbreviations in reference to drug names (eg, qid, qd, $MSO_4$, $MgSO_4$). Abbreviations can have multiple meanings or be mistaken for numbers. For example, using the letter "u" to indicate units can be misinterpreted as a zero when closely following a number (ie, write 10 units not 10 u). The handwritten symbol "μg" commonly used as an abbreviation for microgram can be confused with another commonly used symbol "mg" for milligram (note 1000-fold difference). Prescribers are encouraged to use the abbreviation "mcg" for micrograms to avoid confusion and resulting dosing errors.

### Legibility

Writing neat, legible orders will minimize the need for interpretation or clarification of orders. Additionally,

*Table 41–7.* Important drug and herbal product information resources for pediatric practitioners.

| Resource | Information Content | Cost[a] | Availability |
|---|---|---|---|
| Pediatric Dosage Handbook (Lexicomp, Inc.) www.lexi.com ISBN: 1930598750 | Alphabetized drug monographs; reasonably comprehensive; referenced; current, inexpensive, includes OTCs. | Textbook: $45 PDA: $75 CD: $70 Online subscription: $150 | Pocket-size textbook, Palm OS/Pocket PC, CDRom, Online |
| American Hospital Formulary Service (American Society of Health-System Pharmacists) www.ashp.org ISBN: 1585280399 | Most pediatric dosing, very comprehensive specific evaluative data, authored/published by over 500 experts, includes off-label use and dosing, current, includes OTCs, parenteral nutritionals. | Full Text: $199 Condensed Text: $45 Multimedia card: $100 | Large soft-cover book, (condensed handbook size also available), Multimedia card for PDA, Online |
| Drugs in Pregnancy and Lactation: A Reference Guide to Fetal and Neonatal Risk (Lippincott Williams and Wilkins) www.barnesandnoble.com ISBN: 0781732034 | *The book* on drugs used during pregnancy and lactation. No dosing, but well referenced with primary literature, current. | $99 | Hardcover text |
| Drug Facts and Comparisons (publisher Facts & Comparisons) www.factsand comparisons.com ISBN: 157439178x | Comprehensive, organized by disorder, differentiates between OTC and Rx; monthly updates available in print, extensive charts and tables, contact information to all major pharmaceutical manufacturers. | Hardcover: $205 Looseleaf: $398 Online subscription: $380 | Hardcover Text, Looseleaf Text (monthly updates), Online subscription |
| Teddy Bear Book, Pediatric Injectable Drugs (American Society of Health-System Pharmacists) www.ashp.org ISBN: 1585280542 | Exclusively dedicated to pediatric intravenous drug therapy guidelines, neonate through adolescent, 170 drug monographs including common pediatric dosing, dosage adjustment in organ dysfunction, administration routes and rates (IV push vs continuous infusion vs IM), maximum concentration, additives, and precautions. | $69 | Spiral-bound, soft-cover text. |
| Natural Medicines Comprehensive Database (Pharmacist's Letter/Prescriber's Letter) www.naturaldatabase.com ISBN: 0967613647 | Alphabetical index, comprehensive, scientific information, authored/researched by numerous clinical contributors, includes common and scientific nomenclature, also known as, extensive common indications, safety data, effectiveness, possible mechanism of action, active ingredient(s), adverse reactions, known allergies, possible interactions, drugs' influence on nutrient levels and depletion, dosing information, among more. | Online Web Access: $92 Textbook with Web Access: $40 Textbood without Web Access: $92 PDA with Web Access: $60 PDA without Web Access: $92 | Large soft-cover text, PDA, Online |

[a]Approximate, as of January, 2004.

the use of institutionally approved preprinted order forms can increase legibility and decrease the chance of medication errors occurring. Unfortunately, many look-alike, sound-alike drug names exist (eg, Celexa, Cerebyx, Celebrex), and poor legibility can lead to mixups with these products.

## Maximum Dosing

In older children weighing more than 40–50 kg, in whom pediatric doses based on body weight might exceed the normal adult dose, the normal adult dosage should be used as the upper limit to prevent toxicity and achieve desired efficacy.

## SOURCES OF PEDIATRIC DRUG INFORMATION

### The Pharmacist

Pharmacists—particularly those who practice in a pediatric care environment—are extremely useful sources of pediatric drug information. They often know drug doses, side effects, and practical issues regarding the appropriate therapeutic uses of pharmaceuticals in children. Their services are usually available at any hour, 7 days a week, at no cost to the patient.

### References at Work

Table 41–7 summarizes useful pediatric-based drug references. Clinicians who care for pediatric patients should be familiar with these resources.

### The Federal Drug Administration (FDA)

In 1997, the Food and Drug Modernization Act of 1997 was signed into law. The purpose behind this law was to remedy the lack of pediatric information avail-able for many medications being prescribed for children. A list of drugs was created and, after consultation with pediatric experts, was posted on the FDA website, www.fda.gov. These medications have been targeted so that research surrounding their use in pediatric patients will be performed, thus providing clinicians with timely pediatric drug information. The hope is that enforcement of this act will lead to new and helpful prescribing guidelines that are more accessible to pediatric clinicians.

## REFERENCES

Carr RR, Ensom MHH: Drug disposition and therapy in adolescence: The effects of puberty. J Pediatr Pharmacol Ther 2003:8;86-96.

Gelman CR, Rumack BH (eds): *DRUGDEX Information Systems.* Micromedex, 1999.

Gilman AG et al: *Goodman & Gilman's The Pharmacological Basis of Therapeutics,* 9th ed. McGraw-Hill, 1996.

Radde IC, MacLeod SM: *Pediatric Pharmacology & Therapeutics,* 2nd ed. Mosby, 1993.

Reiter PD: Neonatal pharmacology and pharmacokinetics. *NeoReviews* 2002:3(11);229.

# Fluid, Electrolyte, & Acid–Base Disorders & Therapy

**42**

*Douglas M. Ford, MD*

## REGULATION OF BODY FLUIDS, ELECTROLYTES, & TONICITY

Total body water (TBW) constitutes 50–75% of the total body mass depending on age, sex, and fat content. After an initial postnatal diuresis, the TBW slowly decreases to the adult range near puberty (Figure 42–1). TBW is divided into the intracellular and extracellular spaces. Intracellular fluid (ICF) accounts for two thirds of the TBW, or roughly 50% of total body mass. Extracellular fluid (ECF) constitutes one third of the TBW and 25% of total body mass. The ECF is further compartmentalized into plasma (intravascular) volume and interstitial fluid (ISF).

The principal constituents of plasma are sodium, chloride, bicarbonate, and protein (primarily albumin). The ISF is similar to plasma but lacks significant amounts of protein (Figure 42–2). Conversely, the ICF is rich in potassium, magnesium, phosphates, sulfates, and protein.

An understanding of osmotic shifts between the ECF and ICF is fundamental to understanding disorders of fluid balance. Iso-osmolality is generally maintained between fluid compartments. Because the cell membrane is water-permeable, abnormal fluid shifts occur if the concentration of solutes that cannot permeate the cell membrane in the ECF does not equal the concentration of such solutes in the ICF. Thus, NaCl, mannitol, and glucose (in the setting of hyperglycemia) remain restricted to the ECF space and contribute effective osmoles by obligating water to remain in the ECF compartment. In contrast, a freely permeable solute, such as urea, does not contribute effective osmoles because it is not restricted to the ECF and readily crosses cell membranes. Tonicity, or effective osmolality, differs from measured osmolality in that it accounts only for osmotically active impermeable solutes rather than all osmotically active solutes, including those that are permeable to cell membranes. Osmolality may be estimated by the following formula:

$$\text{mOsm/kg} = 2(\text{Na}^+, \text{mEq/L}) + \frac{\text{Glucose, mg/dL}}{18} + \frac{\text{BUN, mg/dL}}{2.8}$$

Although osmolality and osmolarity differ, the former being an expression of osmotic activity per weight (kg) and the latter per volume (L) of solution, for clinical purposes they are similar and occasionally used interchangeably. Oncotic pressure represents the osmotic activity of macromolecular constituents such as albumin in the plasma and body fluids.

The principal mechanisms that regulate ECF volume and tonicity are antidiuretic hormone (ADH), thirst, aldosterone, and atrial natriuretic factor (ANF).

### Antidiuretic Hormone

In the kidney, ADH increases water reabsorption in the cortical and medullary collecting ducts, leading to formation of a concentrated urine. In the absence of ADH, a dilute urine is produced. Under normal conditions, ADH secretion is regulated by the tonicity of body fluids rather than the fluid volume and becomes detectable at a plasma osmolality of 280 mOsm/kg or greater. However, tonicity may be sacrificed to preserve ECF volume, as in the case of hyponatremic dehydration, wherein ADH secretion and renal water retention are maximal.

### Thirst

Water intake is commonly determined by cultural factors rather than by thirst. Thirst is not physiologically stimulated until plasma osmolality reaches 290 mOsm/kg, a level at which ADH levels are sufficient to induce maximal antidiuresis. Thirst provides control over a wide range of fluid volumes and can even be a response to absence of ADH with attendant production of copious and dilute urine. One who cannot perceive thirst develops profound problems with fluid balance.

### Aldosterone

Aldosterone—released from the adrenal cortex in response to decreased effective circulating volume and stimulation of the renin–angiotensin–aldosterone axis or in response to increasing plasma $K^+$—enhances renal tubular reabsorption of $Na^+$ in exchange for $K^+$ and, to

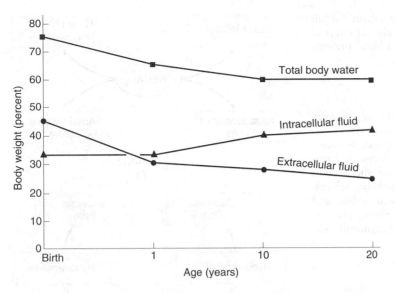

**Figure 42–1.** Body water compartments related to age. (Modified, with permission, from Friis-Hansen B: Body water compartments in children: Changes during growth and related changes in body composition. Pediatrics 1961;28:169.)

a lesser degree, $H^+$. At a constant osmolality, retention of $Na^+$ leads to expansion of ECF volume and suppression of aldosterone release.

## Atrial Natriuretic Factor

ANF, a polypeptide hormone secreted principally by the cardiac atria in response to atrial dilatation, plays an important role in regulation of blood volume and blood pressure. ANF inhibits renin secretion and aldosterone synthesis and causes an increase in glomerular filtration rate and renal sodium excretion. ANF also guards against excessive plasma volume expansion in the face of increased ECF volume by shifting fluid from the vascular to the interstitial compartment. ANF inhibits angiotensin II- and norepinephrine-induced vasoconstric-

**Figure 42–2.** Composition of body fluids. ICF = intracellular fluid; ISF = interstitial fluid.

tion and acts in the brain to decrease the desire for salt and inhibit the release of ADH. Thus the net effect of ANF is a decrease in blood volume and blood pressure associated with natriuresis and diuresis.

## ACID–BASE BALANCE

The pH of arterial blood is maintained between 7.38 and 7.42 to ensure that pH-sensitive enzyme systems function normally. Acid–base balance is maintained by interaction of the lungs, kidneys, and systemic buffering systems. Over 50% of the blood's buffering capacity is provided by the carbonic acid/bicarbonate system, roughly 30% by hemoglobin, and the remainder by phosphates and ammonium. The carbonic acid/bicarbonate system, depicted chemically as:

$$CO_2 + H_2O \rightleftharpoons H_2CO_3 \leftrightarrow H^+ + HCO_3$$

interacts with the lungs, kidneys, and nonbicarbonate systems to stabilize systemic pH. The concentration of dissolved $CO_2$ in blood is established by the respiratory system and that of $HCO_3^-$ by the kidneys. Disturbances in acid–base balance are initially stabilized by chemical buffering, compensated for by pulmonary or renal regulation of $CO_2$ or $HCO_3^-$, and ultimately corrected when the primary cause of the acid–base disturbance is eliminated.

Renal regulation of acid–base balance is accomplished by the reabsorption of filtered $HCO_3^-$ and the excretion of $H^+$ or $HCO_3^-$ to match the net input of acid or base. When urine is alkalinized, $HCO_3^-$ enters the kidney and is ultimately lost in the urine. Alkalinization of the urine may occur when an absolute or relative excess of bicarbonate exists. However, urinary alkalinization will not occur if there is a deficiency of $Na^+$ or $K^+$, because $HCO_3^-$ must also be retained to maintain electroneutrality. In contrast, the urine may be acidified if an absolute or relative decrease occurs in systemic $HCO_3^-$. In this setting, proximal tubular $HCO_3^-$ reabsorption and distal tubular $H^+$ excretion are maximal. Some of the processes involved in acid–base regulation are shown in Figure 42–3.

## ▪ FLUID & ELECTROLYTE MANAGEMENT

Therapy of fluid and electrolyte disorders is directed toward providing maintenance fluid and electrolyte requirements, replenishing prior losses, and replacing persistent abnormal losses. Therapy should be phased

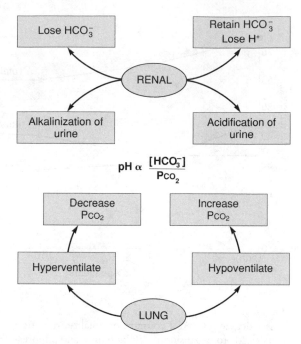

**Figure 42–3.** Maintaining metabolic stability via compensatory mechanisms.

to (1) rapidly expand the ECF volume and restore tissue perfusion, (2) replenish fluid and electrolyte deficits while correcting attendant acid–base abnormalities, (3) meet the patient's nutritional needs, and (4) replace ongoing losses.

The cornerstone of therapy involves an understanding of maintenance fluid and electrolyte requirements. Maintenance requirements call for provision of enough water, glucose, and electrolytes to prevent deterioration of body stores. During short-term parenteral therapy, sufficient glucose is provided to prevent ketosis and limit protein catabolism, although this is usually little more than 20% of the patient's true caloric needs. Prior to the administration of maintenance fluids, it is important to consider the patient's volume status and to determine whether intravenous fluids are needed at all.

Various models have been devised to facilitate calculation of maintenance requirements based on body surface area, weight, and caloric expenditure. A system based on caloric expenditure is most helpful, because 1 mL of water is needed for each kilocalorie expended. The system presented in Table 42–1 is based on caloric needs and is applicable to children weighing more than 3 kg.

As depicted in Table 42–1, a child weighing 30 kg would need 1700 kcal and 1700 mL of water daily. If

**Table 42–1.** Caloric and water needs per unit of body weight.

| Body Weight (kg) | kcal/kg | mL of Water/kg |
|---|---|---|
| 3–10 kg | 100 | 100 |
| 11–20 kg | 1000 kcal + 50 kcal/kg for each kg > 10 kg | 1000 mL + 50 mL/kg for each kg > 10 kg |
| >20 kg | 1500 kcal + 20 kcal/kg for each kg > 20 kg | 1500 mL + 20 mL/kg for each kg > 20 kg |

Adapted, with permission, from Holliday MA, Segar WE: The maintenance need for water in parenteral fluid therapy. Pediatrics 1957;19:823.

the child received parenteral fluids for 2 days, the fluid would usually contain 5% glucose, which would provide 340 kcal/d, or 20% of the maintenance caloric needs. Maintenance fluid requirements take into account normal insensible water losses and water lost in sweat, urine, and stool and assume the patient to be afebrile and relatively inactive. Maintenance requirements are greater for low-birth-weight and preterm infants. Table 42–2 lists other factors that commonly alter fluid and caloric needs.

Electrolyte losses occur primarily through the urinary tract and to a lesser degree via the skin and stool. Although maintenance electrolyte estimates vary, reasonable approximations for maintenance needs are 3 mEq $Na^+$/100 kcal and 2 mEq $K^+$/100 kcal or 30 mEq $Na^+$/L and 20 mEq $K^+$/L, respectively, of intravenous fluid.

It is helpful to monitor the patient's daily weight, urinary output, fluid input, and urine specific gravity. If fluid or electrolyte balance is abnormal, serial determination of electrolyte concentrations, blood urea nitrogen (BUN), and creatinine may be necessary. In patients with significant burns, anuria, oliguria, or persistent abnormal losses (eg, from a stoma, or polyuria secondary to a renal concentrating defect), it is important to measure output and, if needed, its components so that appropriate replacement can be provided.

# DEHYDRATION

Depletion of body fluids is one of the most commonly encountered problems in clinical pediatrics. Children have a high incidence of gastrointestinal diseases, including gastroenteritis, and may demonstrate gastrointestinal symptoms in nongastrointestinal conditions. Infants and young children often decrease their oral intake when ill, and their high ratio of surface area to weight promotes significant evaporative losses. Renal concentrating mechanisms do not maximally conserve water in early life, and fever may significantly increase fluid needs. Dehydration decreases ECF volume, leading to decreased tissue perfusion, impaired renal function, compensatory tachycardia, and lactic acidosis. The clinical effects of dehydration relate to the degree of dehydration and to the relative amounts of salt and water lost. Caregivers must be particularly aware of dehydration occurring in breast-fed newborn infants who go home soon after birth and whose mothers fail to produce enough milk. This problem is more common in the hot summer months and has been associated with severe dehydration, brain damage, and death.

The clinical evaluation of a child with dehydration should focus on the composition and volume of fluid intake; the frequency and amount of vomiting, diarrhea, and urine output; the degree and duration of fever; the nature of any administered medications; and the existence of underlying medical conditions. A recently recorded weight, if known, can be very helpful in calculating the magnitude of dehydration. Important clinical features in estimating the degree of dehydration include the capillary refill time, postural blood pressure, and heart rate changes; dryness of the lips and mucous membranes; lack of tears; lack of external jugular venous filling when supine; a sunken fontanelle in an infant; oliguria; and altered mental status (Table 42–3). Children generally respond to a decrease in circulating volume with a compensatory increase in pulse rate and may maintain their blood pressure in the face of severe dehydration. A low or falling blood pressure is, therefore, a late sign of shock in children, and when present should prompt emergent treatment. Salient laboratory parameters include a high urine specific gravity (in the absence of an underlying renal concentrating defect), a relatively greater elevation in BUN than in creatinine, a low urinary $[Na^+]$ excretion (< 15 mEq/L), and an ele-

**Table 42–2.** Alterations of maintenance fluid requirements.

| Factor | Altered Requirement |
|---|---|
| Fever | 12% per °C[a] |
| Hyperventilation | 10–60 mL/100 kcal |
| Sweating | 10–25 mL/100 kcal |
| Hyperthyroidism | Variable: 25–50% |
| Gastrointestinal loss and renal disease | Monitor and analyze output. Adjust therapy accordingly. |

[a]Do not correct for 38°C; correct 24% for 39°C.

***Table 42-3.*** Clinical manifestations of dehydration.

| Clinical Signs | Degree of Dehydration | | |
| --- | --- | --- | --- |
| | Mild | Moderate | Severe |
| Decrease in body weight | 3–5% | 6–10% | 11–15% |
| Skin | | | |
|   Turgor | Normal (+/−) | Decreased | Markedly decreased |
|   Color | Normal | Pale | Markedly decreased |
|   Mucous membranes | Dry ⟶ | | Mottled or gray; parched |
| Hemodynamic signs | | | |
|   Pulse | Normal | Slight increase | Tachycardia |
|   Capillary refill | 2–3 sec | 3–4 sec | > 4 sec |
|   Blood pressure | Normal ⟶ | | Low |
|   Perfusion | Normal ⟶ | | Circulatory collapse |
| Fluid loss | | | |
|   Urinary output | Mild oliguria | Oliguria | Anuria |
|   Tears | Decreased ⟶ | | Absent |
| Urinary indices | | | |
|   Specific gravity | > 1.020 ⟶ | | Anuria |
|   Urine [$Na^+$] | < 20 mEq/L ⟶ | | Anuria |

vated hematocrit or serum albumin level secondary to hemoconcentration.

Emergent intravenous therapy is indicated when there is evidence of compromised perfusion (inadequate capillary refill, tachycardia, poor color, oliguria, or hypotension). The initial goal is to rapidly expand the plasma volume and to prevent circulatory collapse. A 20 mL/kg bolus of isotonic fluid should be given intravenously as rapidly as possible. Either colloid (5% albumin) or crystalloid (normal saline or Ringer lactate) may be used. Colloid is particularly useful in hypernatremic patients in shock, in malnourished infants, and in neonates. If no intravenous site is available, fluid may be administered intraosseously through the marrow space of the tibia. If there is no response to the first fluid bolus, a second bolus may be given. When adequate tissue perfusion is demonstrated by improved capillary refill, decreased pulse rate and urine output, and improved mental status, deficit replacement may be instituted. If adequate perfusion is not restored after 40 mL/kg of isotonic fluids, other pathologic processes must be considered such as sepsis, occult hemorrhage, or cardiogenic shock. Isotonic dehydration may be treated by providing half of the remaining fluid deficit over 8 hours and the second half over the ensuing 16 hours in the form of 5% dextrose with 0.2–0.45%

saline containing 20 mEq/L KCl. In the presence of metabolic acidosis, $K^+$ acetate may be considered. Maintenance fluids and replacement of ongoing losses should also be provided. Typical electrolyte compositions of various body fluids are depicted in Table 42–4, although it may be necessary to measure the specific constituents of a patient's fluid losses to guide therapy. If the patient is unable to eat for a prolonged period, nutritional needs must be met through hyperalimentation or enteral tube feedings.

Oral rehydration may be provided to children with mild to moderate dehydration. Clear liquid beverages found in the home, such as broth, soda, juice, and tea, are inappropriate for the treatment of dehydration. Commercially available solutions provide 45–75 mEq/L of $Na^+$, 20–25 mEq/L of $K^+$, 30–34 mEq/L of citrate or bicarbonate, and 2–2.5% glucose. Frequent small aliquots (5–15 mL) should be given to provide approximately 50 mL/kg over 4 hours for mild dehydration and up to 100 mL/kg over 6 hours for moderate dehydration. Oral rehydration is contraindicated in children with altered levels of consciousness or respiratory distress who cannot drink freely; in children suspected of having an acute surgical abdomen; in infants with greater than 10% volume depletion; in children with hemodynamic instability; and in the setting of se-

**Table 42–4.** Typical electrolyte compositions of various body fluids.

| | $Na^+$ (mEq/L) | $K^+$ (mEq/L) | $HCO_3^-$ (mEq/L) |
|---|---|---|---|
| Diarrhea | 10–90 | 10–80 | 40 |
| Gastric | 20–80 | 5–20 | 0 |
| Small intestine | 100–140 | 5–15 | 40 |
| Ileostomy | 45–135 | 3–15 | 40 |

Adapted, with permission, from Winters RW: *Principles of Pediatric Fluid Therapy*. Little, Brown, 1973.

vere hyponatremia ($[Na^+] < 120$ mEq/L) or hypernatremia ($[Na^+] > 160$ mEq/L). Failure of oral rehydration due to persistent vomiting or inability to keep up with losses mandates intravenous therapy. Successful oral rehydration requires explicit instructions to caregivers.

The type of dehydration is characterized by the serum $[Na^+]$. If relatively more solute is lost than water, the $[Na^+]$ falls, and hyponatremic dehydration ($[Na^+] < 130$ mEq/L) ensues. This is important clinically because hypotonicity of the plasma contributes to further volume loss from the ECF into the intracellular space. Thus tissue perfusion is more significantly impaired for a given degree of hyponatremic dehydration than for a comparable degree of isotonic or hypertonic dehydration. It is important to note, however, that significant solute losses also occur in hypernatremic dehydration. Furthermore, because plasma volume is somewhat protected in hypernatremic dehydration, it poses the risk of underestimating the severity of dehydration. Typical fluid and electrolyte losses associated with each form of dehydration are shown in Table 42–5.

**Table 42–5.** Estimated water and electrolyte deficits in dehydration (moderate to severe).

| Type of Dehydration | $H_2O$ (mL/kg) | $Na^+$ (mEq/kg) | $K^+$ (mEq/kg) | $Cl^-$ and $HCO_3^-$ (mEq/kg) |
|---|---|---|---|---|
| Isotonic | 100–150 | 8–10 | 8–10 | 16–20 |
| Hypotonic | 50–100 | 10–14 | 10–14 | 20–28 |
| Hypertonic | 120–180 | 2–5 | 2–5 | 4–10 |

Adapted, with permission, from Winters RW: *Principles of Pediatric Fluid Therapy*. Little, Brown, 1982.

## HYPONATREMIA

Hyponatremia may be factitious in the presence of high plasma lipids or proteins, which decrease the percentage of plasma volume that is water. Hyponatremia in the absence of hypotonicity also occurs when an osmotically active solute, such as glucose or mannitol, is added to the ECF. Water drawn from the ICF dilutes the serum $[Na^+]$ despite isotonicity or hypertonicity.

Patients with hyponatremic dehydration generally demonstrate typical signs and symptoms of dehydration (see Table 41–3), because the vascular space is compromised as water leaves the ECF to maintain osmotic neutrality. The treatment of hyponatremic dehydration is fairly straightforward. The magnitude of the sodium deficit may be calculated by the following formula:

$$Na^+ \text{ deficit} = (Na^+ \text{ desired} - Na^+ \text{ observed}) \times \text{Body weight (kg)} \times 0.6$$

One half of the deficit is replenished in the first 8 hours of therapy, and the remainder is given over the following 16 hours. Maintenance and replacement fluids should also be provided. The deficit plus maintenance calculations generally approximate 5% dextrose with 0.45% saline. The rise in serum $[Na^+]$ should not exceed 2 mEq/L/h. The dangers of too rapid correction of hyponatremia include cerebral dehydration and injury due to fluid shifts from the ICF compartment.

Hypovolemic hyponatremia also occurs in cerebral salt wasting associated with central nervous system (CNS) insults, a condition characterized by high urine output and elevated urinary $[Na^+]$ ($> 80$ mEq/L) due to an increase in ANF. This must be distinguished from the syndrome of inappropriate ADH (SIADH), which may also become manifest in CNS conditions and certain pulmonary disorders. In contrast to cerebral salt wasting, SIADH is characterized by euvolemia or mild volume expansion and relatively low urine output due to ADH-induced water retention. Urinary $[Na^+]$ is high in both conditions, though generally not as high in SIADH. It is important to distinguish between these two conditions, because the treatment of the former involves replacement of urinary salt and water losses, whereas the treatment of SIADH involves water restriction.

In cases of severe hyponatremia (serum $[Na^+] < 120$ mEq/L) with CNS symptoms, intravenous 3% NaCl may be given over 1 hour to raise the $[Na^+]$ to 120 mEq/L, to alleviate CNS manifestations and sequelae. In general, 6 mL/kg of 3% NaCl will raise the serum $[Na^+]$ by 5 mEq/L. If 3% NaCl is administered, estimated $Na^+$ and fluid deficits should be adjusted accordingly. Further correction should proceed slowly, as outlined earlier.

Hypervolemic hyponatremia may occur in edematous disorders such as nephrotic syndrome, congestive heart failure, and cirrhosis, wherein water is retained in excess of salt. Treatment involves restriction of $Na^+$ and water and correction of the underlying disorder. Hypervolemic hyponatremia due to water intoxication is characterized by a maximally dilute urine (specific gravity < 1.003) and is also treated with water restriction.

## HYPERNATREMIA

Although diarrhea is commonly associated with hyponatremic or isonatremic dehydration, hypernatremia may develop in the presence of persistent fever or decreased fluid intake or in response to improperly mixed rehydration solutions. Extreme care is required to treat hypernatremic dehydration appropriately. If the serum $[Na^+]$ falls precipitously, the osmolality of the ECF drops more rapidly than that of the CNS. Water shifts from the ECF compartment into the CNS to maintain osmotic neutrality. If hypertonicity is corrected too rapidly (a drop in $[Na^+]$ of greater than 0.5–1 mEq/L/h), cerebral edema, seizures, and CNS injury may occur. Thus, following the initial restoration of adequate tissue perfusion using isotonic fluids, a gradual decrease in serum $[Na^+]$ is desired (10–15 mEq/L/d). This is commonly achieved using 5% dextrose with 0.2% saline to replace the calculated fluid deficit over 48 hours. Maintenance and replacement fluids should also be provided. If the serum $[Na^+]$ is not correcting appropriately, the free water deficit may be estimated as 4 mL/kg of free water for each milliequivalent of serum $[Na^+]$ above 145 and provided as 5% dextrose over 48 hours. If metabolic acidosis is also present, it must be corrected slowly to avoid CNS irritability. Potassium is provided as indicated—as the acetate salt if necessary. Electrolyte concentrations should be assessed every 2 hours in order to control the decline in serum $[Na^+]$. Elevations of blood glucose and BUN may worsen the hyperosmolar state in hypernatremic dehydration and should also be monitored closely. Hyperglycemia is often associated with hypernatremic dehydration and may necessitate lower intravenous glucose concentrations (eg, 2.5%).

Patients with diabetes insipidus, whether nephrogenic or central in origin, are prone to develop profound hypernatremic dehydration as a result of unremitting urinary free water losses (urine specific gravity < 1.010), particularly during superimposed gastrointestinal illnesses associated with vomiting or diarrhea. Treatment involves restoration of fluid and electrolyte deficits as described earlier as well as replacement of excessive water losses, with subsequent water deprivation

testing during daylight hours to distinguish responsiveness to ADH. The evaluation and treatment of nephrogenic and central diabetes insipidus are discussed in detail in Chapters 22 and 30, respectively.

Hypervolemic hypernatremia (salt poisoning), associated with excess total body salt and water, may occur as a consequence of providing improperly mixed formula, excessive NaCl or $NaHCO_3$ administration, or as a feature of primary hyperaldosteronism. Treatment includes the use of diuretics and, potentially, concomitant water replacement or even dialysis.

## POTASSIUM DISORDERS

The predominantly intracellular distribution of potassium is maintained by the actions of $Na^+/K^+$ ATPase in the cell membranes. Potassium is shifted into the ECF and plasma by acidemia and into the ICF in the setting of alkalosis, hypochloremia, or in conjunction with insulin-induced tissue glucose uptake. The ratio of intracellular to extracellular $K^+$ is the major determinant of the cellular resting membrane potential and contributes to the action potential in neural and muscular tissue. Abnormalities of $K^+$ balance are potentially life-threatening. In the kidney, $K^+$ is filtered at the glomerulus, reabsorbed in the proximal tubule, and excreted in the distal tubule. Distal tubular $K^+$ excretion is regulated primarily by aldosterone. Renal $K^+$ excretion continues for significant periods even after the intake of $K^+$ is decreased. Thus, by the time urinary $[K^+]$ decreases, the systemic $K^+$ pool has been depleted significantly.

The causes of net $K^+$ loss are primarily renal in origin. Gastrointestinal losses through nasogastric suction or vomiting reduce total body $K^+$ to some degree. However, the attendant volume depletion results in an increase in plasma aldosterone, promoting renal excretion of $K^+$ in exchange for $Na^+$. Diuretics (especially thiazides), mineralocorticoids, and intrinsic renal tubular diseases (eg, Bartter syndrome) enhance the renal excretion of $K^+$. Clinically, hypokalemia is associated with neuromuscular excitability, decreased peristalsis or ileus, hyporeflexia, paralysis, rhabdomyolysis, and arrhythmias. Electrocardiographic changes include flattened T waves, a shortened PR interval, and the appearance of U waves. Arrhythmias associated with hypokalemia include premature ventricular contractions; atrial, nodal, or ventricular tachycardia; and ventricular fibrillation. Hypokalemia increases responsiveness to digitalis and may precipitate overt digitalis toxicity. In the presence of arrhythmias, extreme muscle weakness, or respiratory compromise, intravenous $K^+$ should be given. If the patient is hypophosphatemic ($[PO_4^{-3}]$ < 2 mg/dL), a phosphate salt may be used. The first priority in the treatment of hypokalemia is the restoration of an adequate serum $[K^+]$. Providing maintenance amounts of $K^+$ is usually sufficient; however, when the serum $[K^+]$ is dangerously low and $K^+$ must be administered intravenously, it is imperative that the patient have a cardiac monitor. Intravenous $K^+$ should generally not be given faster than at a rate of 0.5 mEq/kg/h. Oral $K^+$ supplements may be needed for weeks to replenish depleted body stores.

Hyperkalemia—due to decreased renal $K^+$ excretion, mineralocorticoid deficiency or unresponsiveness, or $K^+$ release from the ICF compartment—is characterized by muscle weakness, paresthesias, and tetany; ascending paralysis; and arrhythmias. Electrocardiographic changes associated with hyperkalemia include peaked T waves, widening of the QRS complex, and arrhythmias such as sinus bradycardia or sinus arrest, atrioventricular block, nodal or idioventricular rhythms, and ventricular tachycardia or fibrillation. The severity of hyperkalemia depends on the electrocardiographic changes, the status of the other electrolytes, and the stability of the underlying disorder. A rhythm strip should be obtained when significant hyperkalemia is suspected. If the serum $[K^+]$ is less than 6.5 mEq/L, discontinuing $K^+$ supplementation is usually sufficient. If the serum $[K^+]$ is greater than 7 mEq/L or if potentiating factors such as hyponatremia, digitalis toxicity, and renal failure are present, more aggressive therapy is needed. If electrocardiographic changes or arrhythmias are present, treatment must be initiated promptly. Intravenous 10% calcium gluconate (0.2–0.5 mL/kg over 2–10 minutes) will rapidly ameliorate depolarization and may be repeated after 5 minutes if electrocardiographic changes persist. Calcium should be given only with a cardiac monitor in place and should be discontinued if bradycardia develops. The intravenous administration of a diuretic that acts in the loop of Henle, such as furosemide (1–2 mg/kg), will augment renal $K^+$ excretion and can be very helpful in lowering serum and total body $[K^+]$. Administering $Na^+$ and increasing systemic pH with bicarbonate therapy (1–2 mEq/kg) will shift $K^+$ from the ECF to the ICF compartment, as will therapy with a β-agonist such as albuterol. In nondiabetic patients, 0.5 g/kg of glucose over 1–2 hours will enhance endogenous insulin secretion, lowering serum $[K^+]$ 1–2 mEq/L. Administration of intravenous glucose and insulin may be needed as a simultaneous drip (0.5–1 g/kg glucose and 0.3 units of regular insulin per gram of glucose) given over 2 hours with monitoring of the serum glucose level every 15 minutes.

The therapies outlined provide transient benefits. Ultimately, $K^+$ must be reduced to normal levels by reestablishing adequate renal excretion using diuretics or optimizing urinary flow, using ion exchange resins such as sodium polystyrene sulfonate orally or as a retention enema (0.2–0.5 g/kg orally or 1 g/kg as an enema), or by dialysis.

# ACID–BASE DISTURBANCES

When evaluating a disturbance in acid–base balance, the systemic pH, $P_{CO_2}$, serum $[HCO_3^-]$, and anion gap must be considered. The anion gap, $Na^+ - (Cl^- + HCO_3^-)$, is an expression of the unmeasured anions in the plasma and is normally $12 \pm 4$ mEq/L. An increase above normal suggests the presence of an unmeasured anion, such as occurs in diabetic ketoacidosis, lactic acidosis, salicylate intoxication, and so on. Although the base excess (or deficit) is also used clinically, it is important to recall that this expression of acid–base balance is influenced by the renal response to respiratory disorders and cannot be interpreted independently (as in a compensated respiratory acidosis, wherein the base excess may be quite large).

## METABOLIC ACIDOSIS

Metabolic acidosis is characterized by a primary decrease in serum $[HCO_3^-]$ and systemic pH due to the loss of $HCO_3^-$ from the kidneys or gastrointestinal tract, the addition of an acid (from external sources or via altered metabolic processes), or the rapid dilution of the ECF with nonbicarbonate containing solution (usually normal saline). When $HCO_3^-$ is lost through the kidneys or gastrointestinal tract, $Cl^-$ must be reabsorbed with $Na^+$ disproportionately, resulting in a hyperchloremic acidosis with a normal anion gap. Thus a normal anion gap acidosis in the absence of diarrhea or other bicarbonate-rich gastrointestinal losses suggests the possibility of renal tubular acidosis and should be evaluated appropriately (see Chapter 21). In contrast, acidosis that results from addition of an unmeasured acid is associated with a widened anion gap. Examples are diabetic ketoacidosis, lactic acidosis, starvation, uremia, toxin ingestion (salicylates, ethylene glycol, methanol), and certain inborn errors of organic or amino acid metabolism. Dehydration may also result in a widened anion gap acidosis as a result of inadequate tissue perfusion, decreased $O_2$ delivery, and subsequent lactic and keto acid production. Respiratory compensation is accomplished through an increase in minute ventilation and a decrease in $P_{CO_2}$. The patient's history, physical findings, and laboratory features should lead to the appropriate diagnosis.

The ingestion of unknown toxins or the possibility of an inborn error of metabolism (see Chapter 32) must be considered in children without an obvious cause for a widened anion gap acidosis. Unfortunately, some hospital laboratories fail to include ethylene glycol or methanol in their standard toxicology screens, so that these toxins must be requested specifically. This is of grave importance when therapy with ethanol must be considered for either ingestion—and instituted quickly to head off profound toxicity. Ethylene glycol (eg, antifreeze) is particularly worrisome because of its sweet taste and accounts for a significant number of toxin ingestions. Screening by fluorescence of urine under a Wood lamp is relatively simple but does not replace specific laboratory assessment. Salicylate intoxication has a stimulatory effect on the respiratory center of the CNS; thus, patients may initially present with respiratory alkalosis or mixed respiratory alkalosis and widened anion gap acidosis.

Most types of metabolic acidosis will resolve with correction of the underlying disorder, improved renal perfusion, and acid excretion. Intravenous $NaHCO_3$ administration may be considered in the setting of metabolic acidosis when the pH is less than 7.0 or the $[HCO_3^-]$ is less than 5 mEq/L, but only if adequate ventilation is ensured. The dose (in mEq) of $NaHCO_3$ may be calculated as:

$$\text{Weight (kg)} \times \text{Base deficit} \times 0.3$$

and given as a continuous infusion over 1 hour. The effect of $NaHCO_3$ in lowering serum potassium and ionized calcium concentrations must also be considered and monitored.

## METABOLIC ALKALOSIS

Metabolic alkalosis is characterized by a primary increase in $[HCO_3^-]$ and pH resulting from a loss of strong acid or gain of buffer base. The most common cause for a metabolic alkalosis is the loss of gastric juice via nasogastric suction or vomiting. This results in a $Cl^-$-responsive alkalosis, characterized by a low urinary $[Cl^-]$ (< 20 mEq/L) indicative of a volume-contracted state that will be responsive to the provision of adequate $Cl^-$ salt (usually in the form of normal saline). Cystic fibrosis is also commonly associated with a $Cl^-$-responsive alkalosis due to the high losses of NaCl through the sweat, whereas congenital $Cl^-$-losing diarrhea is a rare cause of $Cl^-$-responsive alkalosis. Chloride-resistant alkaloses are characterized by a urinary $[Cl^-]$ greater than 20 mEq/L and include Bartter syndrome, Cushing syndrome, and primary hyperaldosteronism, conditions associated with primary increases in urinary $[Cl^-]$, or volume-expanded states lacking stimuli for $Cl^-$ reabsorption. Thus the urinary $[Cl^-]$ is helpful in distinguishing the nature of a metabolic alkalosis but must be specifically requested in many laboratories because it is not routinely included in urine electrolyte screens. The serum $[K^+]$ is also low in these settings (hypokalemic metabolic alkalosis) owing to a combination of increased mineralocorticoid activity associated with volume contraction, the shift of $K^+$ to the ICF compartment, preferential reabsorption of $Na^+$ rather than $K^+$ to preserve intravascular volume, or primary mineralocorticoid excess.

## RESPIRATORY ACIDOSIS

Respiratory acidosis develops when alveolar ventilation is decreased, increasing $P_{CO_2}$ and lowering systemic pH. The kidneys compensate for a respiratory acidosis by increasing $HCO_3^-$ reabsorption, a process that takes several days to manifest. Patients with acute respiratory acidoses frequently demonstrate air-hunger with retractions and the use of accessory respiratory muscles. Respiratory acidoses occur in upper or lower airway obstruction, ventilation–perfusion disturbances, CNS depression, and neuromuscular defects. Hypercapnia is not as detrimental as the hypoxia that usually accompanies these disorders. The goal of therapy is to correct or compensate for the underlying pathologic process, to improve alveolar ventilation. Bicarbonate therapy is not indicated in a pure respiratory acidosis, because it will worsen the acidosis by shifting the equilibrium of the carbonic acid–bicarbonate buffer system to increase $P_{CO_2}$.

## RESPIRATORY ALKALOSIS

Respiratory alkalosis occurs when hyperventilation results in a decrease in $P_{CO_2}$ and an increase in pH. Patients may experience tingling, paresthesias, dizziness, palpitations, syncope, or even tetany and seizures due to the associated decrease in ionized calcium. Causes of respiratory alkalosis include psychobehavioral disturbances, CNS irritation from meningitis or encephalitis, and salicylate intoxication. Therapy is directed toward the causal process. Rebreathing into a paper bag will decrease the severity of symptoms in acute hyperventilation.

## REFERENCES

Adrogue JA, Madias NE: Management of life-threatening acid–base disorders: Parts 1 and 2. N Engl J Med 1998:338: 26,107 [PMID: 9414329].

Avner ED: Clinical disorders of water metabolism: Hyponatremia and hypernatremia. Pediatr Ann 1995;24:23 [PMID: 7715960].

Finberg L et al: *Water and Electrolytes in Pediatrics: Physiology, Pathophysiology and Treatment,* 2nd ed. WB Saunders, 1993.

Hellerstein S: Fluids and electrolytes: Physiology. Pediatr Rev 1993;14:70 [PMID: 8493184].

Jospe N, Forbes G: Fluids and electrolytes: Clinical aspects. Pediatr Rev 1996;17:395 [PMID: 8937172].

Kappy MS, Ganong CA: Cerebral salt wasting in children: The role of atrial natriuretic hormone. Adv Pediatr 1996;43:271 [PMID: 8794180].

Liebelt EL: Clinical and laboratory evaluation and management of children with vomiting, diarrhea, and dehydration. Curr Opin Pediatr 1998:10:461 [PMID: 9818241].

McDonald RA: Disorders of potassium balance. Pediatr Ann 1995;24:31 [PMID: 7715961].

Watkins SL: The basics of fluid and electrolyte therapy. Pediatr Ann 1995;24:16 [PMID: 7715959].

# Information Technology in Pediatrics

# 43

*Carol S. Kamin, MS, EdD, & David W. Kaplan, MD, MPH*

Increasing numbers of physicians and patients are taking advantage of technologic resources, especially those available on the Internet. Nearly 100% of physicians report access to the Internet through office, hospital, or home connections. In a survey of British physicians conducted in June 2000, 88% of pediatricians reported using the Internet, with 50% using it both at work and at home (www.rsm.ac.uk/new/websurvey.htm). A global study done in 1998 found in phase-one telephone interviews that 80% of physicians in 11 North American, European, and Asian countries own a computer and 44% of them access the Internet. In phase two, 2,500 Internet-connected physicians from 105 countries were surveyed. Ninety-five percent of these physicians said they use the Internet to access disease information, 88% read medical journals online, and 86% said they use the Internet to obtain drug information. Sixty-three percent have visited a pharmaceutical company's Website, 62% have referred their patients to medical information on the web, and 33% report that patients have brought medical or health related information from the Internet to their office (www.xpresspress.com/news/physiciansurvey.html). Because the Internet has such an abundance of information, navigating its terrain is problematic. Increasingly, sites are being created as indexes of multiple Websites of interest to a particular population (eg, www. generalpediatrics.com). Keeping these indexes current is a relentless task since new sites are added daily and old sites may be removed or changed. However, this changing Internet landscape can provide opportunities to improve health by supporting and educating both providers and patients.

*Note:* When typing the address of a Website into your browser, always use the site's exact designation, which may or may not start with www. Websites listed in this chapter that omit www should be typed exactly that way, as in pediatrics.about.com. Your browser will automatically add the familiar tag, http://.

## CONTINUING MEDICAL EDUCATION

The numbers of continuing medical education (CME) Websites and continuing education online providers are increasing (Table 43–1). In 2000, 96 CME sites were available; in 2001, this number increased to 200 (www.netcantina.com). By 2004, one Website linked to 270 online CME sites with more than 12,000 courses (www.cmelist.com/list.htm). An example of an award-winning free Website is the one on breastfeeding at www.breastfeedingbasics.org. Accreditation Council for Continuing Medical Education (ACCME) requirements are still grounded in conferences and have been slow to adopt regulations regarding CME credit for computer-based educational materials. In addition, limited educational strategies have been applied to those that are available. For the most part, existing programs and lectures have been transferred to the Internet without much thought about how the medium could best be used to improve the instruction, evidenced by the fact that most CME Websites are text-based with only 20% containing interactive components. Cases and tutorials on CD-ROMs can provide more interactivity and video images than the Internet bandwidth can currently manage, but this could change quickly.

In a 2002 survey of 2200 US office-based physicians, the most common reason physicians look for Internet-based CME is to solve a specific patient problem. They expect these programs to be easy to use, relevant, and credible. An example of the potential for case-based CME is an award-winning CME program on genetic counseling produced by the Dartmouth Interactive Media Laboratory. This highly interactive program incorporates multiple learning strategies with rich video cases (Available at no cost from iml.dartmouth.edu/education/cme/index.html).

Casebeer L et al: Physician Internet medical information seeking and online continuing education use patterns. J Contin Educ Health Prof 2002;22:33 [PMID: 12004639].

## Conferences

Today's busy clinical practice makes it difficult to attend local and national conferences. The Internet offers opportunities to make conference materials available to those unable to attend. These may include PowerPoint

**Table 43–1.** CME resources.

| | |
|---|---|
| AAP CME Course Calendar | www.pedialink.org/pedialink/cme/coursefinder/index.htm |
| Pediatric emergency medicine site with cases of the week | www.pediatric-emergency.com |
| CME Web—The Global CME Resource with 1300 credit hours in 21 specialties | www.cmeweb.com |
| Pediatric Development and Behavior CME Course (case discussions) | www.dbpeds.org/CME |
| CME web | www.cmeweb.com |
| American Academy of Pediatrics home site | pedialink.org/index.cfm |
| Pediatrics in Review CME | pedsinreview. aapjournals.org/cme |
| CME at the Virtual Lecture Hall | www.vih.com |
| Online CME for the Pediatric Professional | www.pedseducation.org/main/index.htm |
| Links to 200 CME sites, up to 4000 courses and 8000 ACCME accredited hours | www.cmelist.com |
| Electronic CME: Online and Software Resources—Very comprehensive site | www.medicalcomputingtoday.com/0listcme.html |

slides with audio tracks, streaming video, or papers. You can see an example of streaming video at the University of Nebraska site that has a Grand Round lecture series (www.unmc.edu/Pediatrics/GrandRounds/home.htm).

Many Websites include directories of medical meetings. One example is the Physician's Guide to the Internet, at www.physiciansguide.com. In addition to announcements of CME events and national conferences, this site contains sections on professional opportunities, clinical practice guidelines, and practical advice (eg, repaying medical loans).

## Consultation

With electronic access to experts and colleagues readily available, it is not surprising that clinicians and patients seek advice over the Internet. This may be done directly by e-mail or as part of an asynchronous discussion group or listserv. To have e-mail service, you must have an account with an Internet service provider who has an address (a server) or mailbox where you receive incoming mail. Listservs use e-mail technology to allow users to subscribe to discussion groups (Table 43–2). If you subscribe to a listserv, you receive a copy of every message sent to the group. Some of these services offer the option of receiving messages in a digest form that compiles several messages into one. Some of them also keep an archive of old messages that can be searched by key words. A listserv may be moderated to ensure that messages are appropriate for its audience. Discussion groups are slightly different from listservs. The messages are posted on restricted (password-protected) Websites. Users log into the site to read or add messages. Younger age, urban setting, private practice, and infrequent consultation with colleagues were found to be the most common characteristics of the users of the discussion groups on Physicians' Online, an Internet-based information and communication network with more than 200,000 members.

Angelo SJ, Citkowitz E: An electronic survey of physicians using online clinical discussion groups. Conn Med 2001;65(3): 135 [PMID: 11291565].

## Self-Study

Scientific information is growing exponentially, and most physicians have difficulty managing and evaluating this abundance of information. The Internet provides access to tools to help the practitioner manage the information overload. In addition to exclusively online journals, many print journals now have subscription online versions that can be searched by keywords (Table 43–3). Electronic newsletters inform subscribers of the latest research findings. Abstracts can be sent to an e-mail account on topics the subscriber selects. You can find the latest pediatric practice guidelines online (Table 43–4). Do you have questions about a new drug? Information on specific drugs is available online. In fact, some Websites have e-detailing, which provides multimedia presentations of new drugs. If you still have questions about the drug, you can create an online request for a call from a drug representative.

**Table 43–2.** Listservs and discussion groups.

| | |
|---|---|
| Listing of parent discussion groups | www.med.stanford.edu/touchstone/listserv.html |
| PedTalk—for general pediatric discussions | www.pcc.com/lists/pedtalk |
| This is a site with many different types of discussion groups including those for pediatricians | Pediatrics.about.com |
| Disability/Medical related discussion lists | www.makoa.org/listserv.htm |
| Spina Bifida/Hydrocephalus | www.waisman.wisc.edu/~rowley/sb_sourc.htm |
| SJU celiac—wheat and gluten intolerance list | www.lsoft.com/scripts/wl.exe?SLI=CELIAC&H=MAELSTROM.STJOHNS.EDU |
| Cystic fibrosis list | www.esiason.org/newsResourcesMail.html |
| Diabetes list | Listserv@lehigh.edu/lists/diabetic |

A new service being subscribed to by individual practitioners and institutions is UpToDate (www.uptodate.com). Over 3000 authors contribute to this growing database of expert clinical information. Some studies report that this resource is used more frequently than any other electronic clinical reference. It can also be accessed on wireless PDAs. CME credit is available.

The pressure to practice evidence-based medicine (EBM) is growing, by integrating individual clinical expertise with the best available external clinical evidence from systematic research. Clinical databases, like PubMed (www.ncbi.nlm.nih.gov/PubMed), a Web-based resource of Medline, is a service of the National Library of Medicine and can offer access to over 11 million citations. Before conducting your search, identify key concepts you are interested in and consider alternative phrasing of those concepts. Next, limit your search by refining the dates, gender and age if possible, and the type of publication (clinical trials, editorials, letters, meta-analysis, practice guidelines, randomized control trials, or reviews). Boolean logic represents the relationship between more than one keyword. Use AND (in all caps) to retrieve citations which contain all of the search terms. Use OR to retrieve citations that contain at least one of the search terms. Use NOT to exclude the retrieval of terms from your search (eg, lead poison-

**Table 43–3.** Journal Websites.

| | |
|---|---|
| *AAP News* | www.aapnews.org |
| *Archives of Pediatrics and Adolescent Medicine* | archpedi.ama-assn.org |
| *JAMA* | jama.ama-assn.org |
| *Journal of Pediatrics* | www.harcourthealth.com/scripts/om.dll/serve?action=searchDB&searchDBfor=home&id=pd |
| *Journal of the American Academy of Child and Adolescent Health* | www.jaacap.com |
| *Pediatrics* | www.pediatrics.org |
| *Pediatrics—Subspecialty Collections* | www.pediatrics.org/collections |
| *The New England Journal of Medicine* | www.nejm.org |
| *Pediatric Research* | www.pedresearch.org |
| *British Medical Journal* | www.bmj.com/index.dtl |
| *Morbidity and Mortality Weekly Report* | www.cdc.gov/mmwr |
| *Annals of Internal Medicine* | http://www.annals.org/ |

***Table 43–4.*** Online clinical practice guidelines.

| | |
|---|---|
| AAP Guidelines | aap.org/policy/paramtoc.html |
| Agency for Health Care Policy and Research | www.ahrq.gov |
| Bright Futures Searchable database | www.brightfutures.org |
| Centers for Disease Control and Prevention Guidelines | http://www.phppo.cdc.gov/cdc/Recommends/AdvSearchV.asp |
| National Guideline Clearinghouse | www.guideline.gov |
| ACEP Policy Statements | www.acep.org/1,193,0.html |
| American Heart Association scientific statements | www.americanheart.org/presenter.jhtml?identifier=120003 |
| Society for Adolescent Medicine Position Statements | www.adolescenthealth.org/html/summary_statements.html |
| National Cancer Institute | cancernet.nci.nih.gov |
| AHRQ clinical practice guidelines | www.ahrq.gov/clinic/cpgsix.htm |
| AMA Policy finder | www.ama-assn.org/apps/pf_online/pf_online |
| U.S. Preventive Services Task Force guidelines | www.ahrq.gov/clinic/uspstfix.htm |

ing NOT adults). Under clinical queries, you can use filters to limit your search to therapy, etiology, diagnosis, or prognosis. An example of results using these strategies for a search on Otitis Media is found in Table 43–5. What you hope to find is a manageable number of articles that match your clinical question as closely as possible. You still must evaluate the studies and determine whether they offer any new information for your patients.

Systematic reviews and meta-analyses of the literature are available in evidence-based medicine databases

***Table 43–5.*** Sample Pub-Med search on otitis media.

| Search Terms and Limits | Number of Citations |
|---|---|
| Otitis media (no limits) | 14,477 |
| Limit to <23 months, human, English | 165 |
| Add AND antibiotics to above | 50 |
| Limit to meta analysis | 6 |
| Otitis media plus clinical filter for therapy with above limits | 3 |
| Otitis media plus clinical filter for prognosis, with above limits plus limited to review articles | 6 |
| Otitis media plus clinical filter for diagnosis with above limits | 6 |

that have been contributed by EBM experts. Most of these services require a fee. However, as medical schools struggle to enhance clinical sites to provide experience to students and residents, one of the fringe benefits increasingly provided to preceptors is access to library resources that may include EBM databases. Critically appraised topics (CATS) Websites offer opportunities to read others' appraisals of the literature or tools to contribute your own. Additional EBM resources are listed in Table 43–6.

Sackett D et al: Evidence-based medicine: What it is and what it isn't (editorial). Br Med J 1996;312:71 [PMID: 8555924].

## CLINICAL SUPPORT

### E-Mail

Corresponding through e-mail is becoming commonplace in clinical practice communication. The utility of e-mail is its asynchronous nature. It provides a permanent form of documentation and helps prevent "telephone tag." The use of e-mail has dramatically increased, with over 100 million users in year 2000 in the United States. E-mail communication is being used for consultation, patient communication, and practice management. With the growing use of e-mail in clinical practice, the American Medical Informatics Association has published guidelines for the use of electronic mail with patients for clinical purposes:

• Establish turnaround time for messages. Do not use e-mail for urgent matters.

• Inform patients about privacy issues.

***Table 43–6.*** EBM Resources.

| Tools to improve search strategies—Note the second link, an excellent tutorial from the National Library of Medicine | www.urmc.rochester.edu/miner/Educ/Expertsearch.html<br>www.nlm.nih.gov/bsd/pubmed_tutorial/m1001.html |
|---|---|
| Critically Appraised Topics (CATS) in Pediatrics | PedsCCM.wustl.edu/EBJ/EB_Resources.html<br>www.med.umich.edu/pediatrics/ebm/CAT.htm |
| CAT Tools | www.cebm.net/cats.asp<br>www.hsc.usf.edu/~bdjulbeg/Programs/evidencetable.htm |

- Determine who besides the addressee on the receiving end processes messages.
- Include messages as part of the medical record.
- Establish acceptable types of transactions (prescription refill, appointment scheduling, etc), and discourage e-mail communications on sensitive matters (eg, HIV, mental health).
- Instruct patients to put the type of transaction in the subject line for triaging: "prescription," "appointment," "medical advice," "billing question."
- Request that patients put their name and medical record or patient identification number in the body of the message.
- Configure an automatic reply to acknowledge receipt of message.
- Print all messages with replies and confirmation of receipt and place the e-mail in the patient's paper chart.
- Send a message to inform the patient of completion of the request.
- Request that the patients reply to the provider's message, to acknowledge receipt.
- Configure e-mail messages so that, when broadcasting to a group of patients, individual recipients are not visible to others on the mailing list.
- Pay attention to the tone of your message. Avoid anger, sarcasm, harsh criticism.

In addition, the American Medical Informatics Association recommended the following medicolegal and administrative guidelines:

- Consider obtaining the patient's informed consent for the use of e-mail. The consent form should include the communication guidelines, provide instructions for when and how to escalate to phone calls and office visits, describe security mechanisms in place, indemnify the health care institution for information lost due to technical failures, and waive encryption requirement, if any, at the patient's insistence.

- Use password-protected workstations in the clinical setting.
- Never forward patient identifiable information to a third party without the patient's express permission.
- Never use the patient's e-mail address for marketing.
- Use encrypted secure e-mail that is user friendly and practical.
- Regularly back up e-mail onto long-term storage.

E-mail is used for patient education, including distribution of disease specific "handouts," and for conveying medication information, gathering references for current medical research, and sharing Internet resources. It is used for monitoring such markers of chronic illness as peak flow measurements, weight, blood pressure, and glucose levels. Finally, e-mail is used for administrative information including requests for referrals, address changes, and other demographic updates along with requests for prescription refills, laboratory test results, and reminders about appointments and vaccinations.

As the volume of e-mail begins to increase, providers may resist the burden of this new form of communication. It is not known if physicians will begin to provide e-mail care when it is reimbursed.

Kane B, Sands DZ: Guidelines for the clinical use of electronic mail with patients: The AMIA Internet Working Group, Task Force on Guidelines for the Use of Clinic-Patient Electronic Mail. J Am Med Inform Assoc 1998;5:104 [PMID: 9452989].

Kohn L et al (eds): *To Err Is Human: Building a Safer Health System.* Committee on Quality of Health Care in America. Institute of Medicine. National Academy Press, 1999.

## Electronic Medical Records

Electronic medical record (EMR) systems, also known as digital health records (DHR), are systems that provide quicker retrieval of patient data with the potential for greater accuracy. The Institute of Medicine (IOM) has produced two companion reports. The first, entitled "To Err is Human: Building a Safer Health System," concluded that "reorganization and reform are urgently needed to fix what is now a disjointed and inefficient health care system." Studies estimate that between 44,000 and 98,000 patients die each year as a result of medical errors, and preventable medication errors occur in 7.3% of hospital admissions. Even using the lower estimate for deaths, more people die in a given year as a result of medical errors than from motor vehicle accidents, breast cancer, or AIDS. The decentralized and fragmented nature of the health care delivery system contributes to unsafe conditions for patients, and serves as an impediment to efforts to improve safety.

The second IOM report, "Crossing the Quality Chasm: A New Health System for the Twenty-First Century," calls for action to improve health care over the next decade and emphasizes the use of information technology as key to a comprehensive strategy. The IOM committee believes that "information technology must play a central role in the redesign of the health care system if substantial improvement in quality is to be achieved in the coming decade." Health care delivery has been relatively untouched by the revolution in information technology that has been transforming nearly every other aspect of society. Health care organizations are only beginning to apply technologic advances. Patient information typically is dispersed in a collection of paper records, which often are poorly organized, illegible, and not easy to retrieve, making it nearly impossible to manage various chronic illnesses that require frequent monitoring and ongoing patient support.

Growth in clinical knowledge and technology has been profound, yet many health care settings lack basic computer systems to provide clinical information or support clinical decision making. The implementation of an electronic clinical information system offers the potential for improved patient safety, efficiency, and effectiveness. Standardized data collection can assist in implementing consistent care pathways and eliminating the need for data interpretation after the fact. The general attributes of a computer-based patient record should include the following:

• Problem list
• Measurement and recording of health status and functional level
• Statements about the logical basis for all diagnoses and conclusions
• Linkage with all of the patient's clinical records across settings and time periods
• Assurance of confidentiality
• Widespread accessibility
• Selective retrieval and formatting
• Linkage to local and remote knowledge sources

• Structured data collection using a defined vocabulary
• Expandability to meet evolving needs

Features specific for pediatrics include the following:

• Ability to calculate, display, and compare a child's growth percentiles and body mass index with normal ranges
• Special terminology and information to document developmental milestones and physical findings in infants and children
• Age-based normal ranges for vital signs and other physiologic parameters
• Prescribing medications based on age, weight, and body surface area of the child

Tools such as clinical alerts, ordering guidelines, care paths, and structured clinical documentation can provide clinicians with assistance in ordering and delivering health care. Clinical data repositories designed to capture, store, and analyze extensive patient information can form the foundation for effective care decisions. When automated documentation becomes part of the workflow, effective data collection becomes a byproduct rather than an additional task.

Although all-inclusive, computer-based patient records are still rare, especially outside the area of primary care, the benefits of an electronic patient record system are significant:

• Convenient access to patient data from a variety of locations, whenever it is needed. With the advent of the Internet, remote access to clinical data has been further simplified.
• Electronic access to clinical data allows for rapid filtering, sorting, and searching for specific information. Numeric data such as height, weight, and blood pressure can be graphed.
• Automated alerts, reminders, and suggestions can be built into clinical orders and decision points.
• Population-based data are available for clinical research, epidemiologic studies, and the development of quality measures.
• Clinical patient records offer the potential of coordinated information collected at all points of care, incorporating primary care, consultation, hospitalization, laboratory and radiology data, transcription, rehabilitation, and home care.

Bates DW et al: Relationship between medication errors and adverse drug events. J Gen Intern Med 1995;10:199 [PMID: 7790981].

Committee on Quality of Health Care in America: *Crossing the Quality Chasm: A New Health System for the 21st Century.* National Academy Press, 1999.

Dick RS et al (eds): *The Computer Based Patient Record: An Essential Technology for Health Care,* in The Institute of Medicine. National Academy Press, 1997.

Kaushal R et al: Medication errors and adverse drug events in pediatric inpatients. JAMA 2001;285:2114 [PMID: 11311101].

Special Requirements for the Electronic Medical Records Systems in Pediatrics—American Academy of Pediatrics: Task Force on Medical Informatics. Pediatrics 2001;108:513 [PMID: 11483828].

# Telemedicine

Telemedicine uses telecommunications technology for medical diagnostic, monitoring, and therapeutic purposes when distance separates the users. There are three general categories of telemedicine: (1) store-and-forward, (2) self-monitoring and testing, and (3) clinical interactive services. Store-and-forward telemedicine services collect data, store them, and then forward them for interpretation later. The store-and-forward system eliminates the need for the patient and clinician to be available at the same time and place. It is generally used in clinical consultation. Self-monitoring and testing enable providers to monitor physiologic measurements, test results, images, and sounds, usually collected in another care facility or the patient's residence. This modality is used to monitor patients with chronic illnesses and those whose conditions limit their mobility. In the United States more than 450 telemedicine programs exist. The most common activities are consultation or second opinions, diagnostic test interpretation, chronic disease management, and posthospitalization or postoperative follow-up.

Telemedicine is being used in a wide variety of clinical settings, some examples of which are disasters and emergencies; home care and home nursing; new neurologic out-patient referrals; psychiatric and neuropsychological evaluation; hypertension and diabetes management; and surgical consultation. In addition to a growing number of programs in western countries, it is being used to assist in delivering health services in other parts of the globe, such as northwest Russia, Bangladesh, Thailand, Taiwan, and Africa.

In pediatrics, telemedicine is being used in a range of subspecialties for consultation. Among these is remote echocardiographic diagnosis of congenital heart defects. In one 2-year study in Halifax, the telemedicine network saved a necessary patient transfer in 31 cases and avoided over $100,000 in additional costs. Use of the Internet and telemedicine has been studied as an adjunct in improving care for high-risk infants. The technology was used to enhance interactions among families, staff, and community providers. A video conferencing module allowed for virtual visits and distance learning from a family's home during an infant's hospitalization, as well as for virtual house calls and remote monitoring after discharge. In a randomized study of very low birth weight infants, the study group (Baby CareLink) reported a higher overall quality of care and greater satisfaction. Although the length of hospitalization was similar between the study and control groups, all of the study infants were discharged directly to home, whereas 20% of the control infants were transferred to a community hospital before discharge.

A number of questions remain for clinical telemedicine consultation and monitoring. What are the geographic limits for reimbursement? Which practitioners are eligible to present patients? Which practitioners are eligible to act as consultants? What teleconsultative services will be covered? What technologies will be covered? One reason for the lack of coverage of telemedicine has been an uncertainty about its efficacy and cost. In a systematic review of clinical outcomes resulting from telemedicine interventions commissioned by the US Health Care Financing Agency and the Agency for Healthcare Research and Quality, evidence concerning the benefits of its use exists in only a small number of health care areas despite widespread use of telemedicine.

Reimbursement for telemedicine services varies among states and insurers. Presently in the United States, at least 18 states are allowing reimbursement through Medicaid for services provided via telemedicine, for reasons that include improved access to specialists for rural communities and reduced transportation costs.

With faster and less expensive computers and greater access to high bandwidth, telemedicine should continue to improve in quality and ease of use. As the use of telemedicine matures, essential elements to improve performance will include the following:

1. Licensing and credentialing. Telemedicine overcomes geographic boundaries but may be constrained by state laws.
2. Data security and privacy. Telemedicine consultation records need to be stored to document clinical decisions, especially for risk management.
3. Informed consent.
4. Peer-reviewed quality assessment.

Hersh WR et al: Clinical outcomes resulting from telemedicine interventions: A systematic review. BMC Med Inform Decis Mak 2001;1(1):5. Epub 2001 Nov 26 [PMID: 11737882].

## Personal Digital Assistants

PDAs, also know as Palm-tops or handheld computers, have grown in popularity, and as they have so have their software applications. Harris Interactive Polls conducted interviews with 834 practicing US physicians and found that the use of PDAs increased from 15% in 1999 to 26% in 2001. The number using PDAs as an integral part of their practice almost doubled from 10%

to 18%. This use is higher among doctors younger than 45 (33%) than among older doctors (21%). It is also higher among wholly or partly hospital-based physicians (33% and 29%) than among those who are mostly office-based (23%).

Sittig and colleagues conducted a study to determine what physicians wanted from a PDA. Important tasks cited included checking drug information and treatment regimens, viewing patient data, and looking up diagnostic codes and laboratory values. New PDA software is being created specifically for pediatricians, with database-driven tools for basic vital signs, lab values for all ages, growth and development tools, vaccine recommendations, electrocardiographic findings, resuscitation dosage codes, and more (see www .kidometer.com). PediSuite, a suite of seven modules providing calculations and other information, recently won the RNpalm NFP award (see www.rnpalm.com/ pedisuite_review.htm). Downloadable database programs using JFile or HanDBase can be found at www.keepkidshealthy.com/pediatricpilotpage/jfile.html. To find out more about pediatric-specific PDA software, see the comprehensive Website at www .pediatricsonhand.com where software is organized by subspecialty and other specific areas of interest.

As wireless PDAs increase in popularity, we could see applications proliferate. Currently users can subscribe to channels of information. For information about software for physicians in any specialty, check out PdaMD.com. Many software developers creating PDA applications for physicians are developing companion products for patients. One example includes award-winning PediSuite by Medical Wizards, who have also created PediParents. Instead of keeping paper diaries, physicians can monitor electronic diaries kept by their patients with asthma on PDAs and specialized software (eg, asthma application at www.HealthEngage .com/healthengageasthma.html).

Johns Hopkins Department of Pediatrics describes their progress in the use of PDAs as well as some of the clinical applications they have developed at www.welch.jhu.edu/about/mac2002_pdas.pdf.

Sittig DF et al: Techniques for identifying the applicability of new information management technologies in the clinical setting: An example focusing on handheld computers (Proceedings). AMIA Symposium 2000;20 (Suppl):804 [PMID: 11079995].

## Security

Although the principles of protecting the confidentiality and privacy of medical records apply to all forms of personally identifiable information, whether communicated on paper, orally, or electronically, the electronic dissemination of patient data is of special concern. Computerization makes it much easier to acquire, manipulate, and disseminate vast amounts of personal health information rapidly. Highly sensitive health data flow through employer-sponsored health plans, managed care organizations, hospitals, pharmacies, laboratories, and physicians' offices. These data are used for numerous health-related purposes, including clinical care, quality assurance, utilization review, reimbursement, research, and public health. In 1996, the Health Insurance Portability and Accountability Act (HIPAA) authorized the federal government to establish a national standard for medical record privacy either by legislative or regulatory action. In 1999, the Department of Health and Human Services published regulations to guarantee patients new rights and protections against the misuse or disclosure of their health records. The regulations apply to what are called "covered entities": healthcare providers, health plans, and healthcare clearinghouses that transmit health information in electronic form. The regulations are made up of three distinct parts: transaction standards, privacy, and security. The transactions standards call for use of common electronic claims standards, common code sets, and unique identifiers for all healthcare payers and providers. The privacy rules govern the release of individually identifiable health information, specifying how health providers must provide notice of privacy policies and procedures to patients, obtain consent and authorization for use of information; tell how information is generally shared; and how patients can access, inspect, copy and amend their own medical record. The security regulations dictate the kind of administrative procedures and physical safeguards covered entities must have in place to ensure the confidentiality and integrity of protected health information. All medical records and other individually identifiable health information used or disclosed by a covered entity in any form, whether electronically, on paper, or orally, are covered by the new rule. Providers and health plans will be required to give patients a clear written explanation of how their health data may be used and their health information disclosed. In general, the disclosure of health information will be limited to the minimum amount necessary for purposes of the disclosure. In very limited circumstances, health information may be disclosed in emergencies, for public health concerns, and for research when a waiver of authorization is independently approved by a privacy board or institutional review board.

## PATIENT EDUCATION

Patients are accessing many kinds of Websites that offer information about their conditions. Home usage of the

Internet is more common among highly educated and wealthier individuals, with no difference based on gender or community size. Sixty-three percent of women and 46% of male Internet users use the Internet to get medical information on a regular basis (www .pewinternet. org/reports/toc.asp?Report=26). How might this change the patient–physician relationship? A study of patients with breast cancer who participated in online education and support groups reported that patients increased their confidence in their physicians and their competence to participate in their own care. A Harris online poll found that patients who used the Internet to look for health information were more likely to ask informed questions of their physicians and were more likely to comply with prescribed treatment plans. Similar results have been reported in studies of patients with cystic fibrosis and amyotrophic lateral sclerosis (ALS).

In addition to changing the relationship between physician and patient, patient outcomes can improve as a result of online patient education. In a study of patients participating in an online diabetes education and support group, patients lowered their blood glucose level more than the control group.

Physicians can help their patients evaluate the accuracy of information found on the Web and provide links to reliable patient education resources. General sites, like Medline Plus (www.nlm.nih.gov/medlineplus), provide a great deal of reliable information indexed at one site by the National Library of Medicine. Specialty listservs or discussion groups for parents are also available.

A recent review of online pediatric patient education materials suggests that the majority of materials are not written at an appropriate reading level for the average adult (eighth to ninth grade). If your practice is interested in hosting a patient education Website, consider the following guidelines:

- Write patient guidelines clearly, make them highly visible, and ensure that all parties read and understand them before they use the resource.

- Present a statement about the intent and limitations of the resource, and provide contact information should the user have questions.

- Address concerns about privacy; identify possible security breaches and the steps users must take to protect their information.

- Define and clarify which areas of the resource are for posting private messages to providers containing health information, and which areas are public.

- Define the patient's rights and responsibilities, and provide examples of queries that should be posted and those situations that require more immediate medical attention.

- Define the provider's responsibilities.

Because a mixture of high-quality and low-quality resources are available for patients on the Web, it is important that physicians are aware of Web-based resources and have reliable sites to recommend to an increasingly sophisticated population.

Technology and the Internet are changing our culture as well as medical education and healthcare delivery. Properly implemented and adopted, these new applications offer physicians the opportunity to harness the technology for better and more efficient patient care.

Alessandro DM et al: The readability of pediatric patient education materials on the world wide web. Arch Pediatr Adolesc Med 2001;155:807 [PMID: 11434848].

Characteristics and Choices of Internet Users: Report to the Ranking Minority Member Subcommittee on Telecommunications Committee on Energy and Commerce, House of Representatives. United States General Accounting Office, February 2001.

Feenberg AL et al: The online patient meeting. J Neurol Sci 1996;139 (Suppl):129 [PMID: 8899672].

Gustafson DH et al: Effect of computer support on younger women with breast cancer. J Gen Intern Med 2001;16(7):435 [PMID: 11520380].

Harris Interactive: The increasing impact of eHealth on consumer behavior. Health Care News 2001;1(21):1.

Johnson KB et al: Hopkins Teen central: Assessment of an Internet-based support system for children with cystic fibrosis. Pediatrics 2001;107(2):E24 [PMID: 11158498].

McKay HG et al: The diabetes network Internet-based physical activity intervention: A randomized pilot study. Diabetes Care 2001;24(8):1328 [PMID: 11473065].

Prady SL et al: Expanding the guidelines for electronic communication with patients. JAMA 2001;8:344 [PMID: 11418540].

# Chemistry & Hematology Reference Ranges

**44**

*Iris M. Osberg, MT*

Pediatricians and other health professionals caring for children have the responsibility to insist on accurate, rapid, and comprehensive laboratory testing. Collecting large blood samples for biochemical assay is not suitable for the proper care of children, especially for premature infants or older children in intensive care units, where repetitive sampling may be essential.

In infants and young children, blood samples taken by heel-prick are better collected by laboratory personnel than by physicians or nurses.

## INTERPRETATION OF LABORATORY VALUES

Accreditation by the College of American Pathologists and by state or federal agencies has done much to ensure standardized laboratory performance. Methods used in various laboratories differ, as do reference (normal) values for the methods. Reference (normal) range is, of course, a combination of biologic variation and intrinsic laboratory variation; thus, an acceptable range of reference (normal) values should ideally be composed of data developed within the laboratory for the population it serves. Any laboratory should be able to provide information on the coefficient of variation and standard deviation applicable to each test performed in that laboratory. Each laboratory should maintain a rigorous procedure of checks with daily standards and quality control specimens. Errors may still occur but can usually be detected by retesting before a questionable result is reported. Fortunately, errors occur much less commonly today than in the past.

The clinical value of a test is related to its sensitivity and specificity. Sensitivity is an expression of the incidence of positive test results in those who have the disease. Specificity is an expression of the incidence of negative test results in those free of the disease. Sensitivity and specificity are calculated as follows:

$$\text{Sensitivity (\%)} = \frac{TP}{TP + FN} \times 100$$

(ie, the percentage of TP detected by the test in those with the disease)

$$\text{Specificity (\%)} = \frac{TN}{TN + FP} \times 100$$

(ie, the percentage of TN detected by the test in those without the disease)

where TP = a true-positive result, FP = a false-positive result, TN = a true-negative result, and FN = a false-negative result.

Screening tests must be interpreted with appreciation of sensitivity and specificity. These expressions are illustrated in Figure 44–1 in terms of a screening test for phenylketonuria in newborns. The values are not strictly correct but serve the purpose of illustration. According to Figure 44–1, a blood phenylalanine level of 4 mg/dL is the discriminating point above which all infants are presumed to have the disease and below which they are presumed to be normal. However, no test is ever quite that exact. Some normal infants will have levels above 4 mg/dL; the test results in these will be false-positive. Some abnormal infants will have levels below 4 mg/dL; the test results in these infants will be false-negative. The discriminating point is a compromise between sensitivity and specificity. Moving the point to 2 mg/dL would effect 100% sensitivity, but there would be a large increase in the number of false-positive results. Moving it to 6 mg/dL would make it very specific, but this would increase the number of false-negative responses, which would result in failure to detect phenylketonuria in a much larger proportion of affected children.

These concepts can be viewed in yet another way. Suppose that this test were set at a specificity of

**1339**

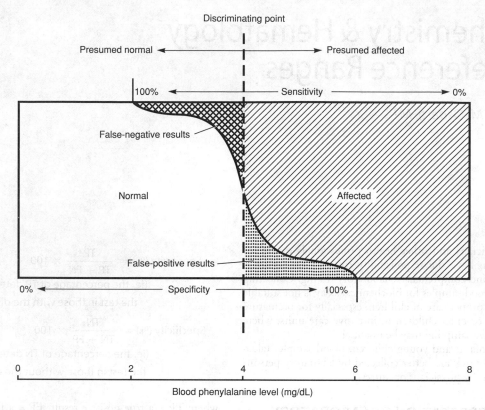

*Figure 44–1.* Screening test for phenylketonuria in newborns. Data have been simplified to illustrate the concepts of sensitivity and specificity (see text).

99.9%. This would mean that in a sample of 10,000 tests, there would be 10 false-positive results. In a rare condition such as phenylketonuria, however, the true incidence of the disease may be only 1:12,000. The ratio of true-positive to false-positive results is thus 1:12; this is a reflection of the low incidence of the disease and the relatively high incidence of false-positive results because of the nature of the assay. These consid-

erations, of course, apply to the interpretation of all laboratory tests.

## LABORATORY VALUES

Blood chemistry and miscellaneous other laboratory reference ranges are shown in Tables 44–1 to 44–3.

***Table 44–1.*** Normal blood chemistry values and miscellaneous other hematologic values. (Values may vary with the procedure used.)

| Determinations for | |
|---|---|
| (S) = Serum | (P) = Plasma |
| (B) = Whole blood | (RBC) = Red blood cells |

**Acid Phosphatase (S, P)**
Values using *p*-nitrophenyl phosphate buffered with citrate (end-point determination)
Newborns: 7.4–19.4 IU/L at 37 °C
2–13 y: 6.4–15.2 IU/L at 37 °C
Adult males: 0.5–11 IU/L at 37 °C
Adult females: 0.2–9.5 IU/L at 37 °C

**Alanine Aminotransferase (ALT, SGPT) (S)**
Newborns (1–3 d): 1–25 IU/L at 37 °C
Adult males: 7–46 IU/L at 37 °C
Adult females: 4–35 IU/L at 37 °C

**Alkaline Phosphatase (S)**
Values in IU/L at 37 °C using *p*-nitrophenyl phosphate buffered with AMP (kinetic)

| Group | Males | Females |
|---|---|---|
| Newborns (1–3 d) | 95–368 | 95–368 |
| 2–24 mo | 115–460 | 115–460 |
| 2–5 y | 115–391 | 115–391 |
| 6–7 y | 115–460 | 115–460 |
| 8–9 y | 115–345 | 115–345 |
| 10–11 y | 115–336 | 115–437 |
| 12–13 y | 127–403 | 92–336 |
| 14–15 y | 79–446 | 78–212 |
| 16–18 y | 58–331 | 35–124 |
| Adults | 41–137 | 39–118 |

**Ammonia (P)**
Newborns: 90–150 µg/dL (53–88 µmol/L); higher in premature and jaundiced infants
Thereafter: 0–60 µg/dL (0–35 µmol/L) when blood is drawn with proper precautions

**Amylase (S)**
Values using maltotetrose substrate (kinetic)
Neonates: Undetectable
2–12 mo: Levels increase slowly to adult levels
Adults: 28–108 IU/L 37 °C

**Anticoagulation Factors (P)**
Values in U/mL. Shown are mean values and 2 SD or lower range (in parentheses)

**Anticoagulation Factors (P)**

| Factor | Preterm (25–32 wk) | Term Infant | Infant (6 mos) | Adult |
|---|---|---|---|---|
| AT III | 0.35 (0.20) | 0.56 (0.32) | 1.04 (0.84) | 1.0 (0.8) |
| PC | 0.29 (0.20) | 0.50 (0.30) | 0.59 (0.37) | 1.0 (0.6) |
| PS, total | . . . | 0.24 (0.10) | 0.87 (0.55) | 1.0 (0.6) |
| PS, free | 0.48 | 0.42 | . . . | 1.0 (0.5) |
| HCF II | 0.25 (0.10) | 0.49 (0.36) | 0.97 (0.59) | 1.0 (0.7) |

AT III = antithrombin III, PC = protein C, PS = protein S, HCf II = heparin cofactor II.

**$\alpha_1$-Antitrypsin (antiprotease) (S)**
1–3 mo: 127–404 mg/dL
3–12 mo: 145–362 mg/dL
1–2 y: 160–382 mg/dL
2–15 y: 148–394 mg/dL

**Ascorbic Acid:** See Vitamin C.

**Aspartate Aminotransferase (AST, SGOT) (S)**
Newborns (1–3 d): 16–74 IU/L at 37 °C
Adult males: 8–46 IU/L at 37 °C
Adult females: 7–34 IU/L at 37 °C

**Bicarbonate, Actual (P)**
Calculated from pH and $Pa_{CO_2}$
Newborns: 17.2–23.6 mmol/L
2 mos–2 y: 19–24 mmol/L
Children: 18–25 mmol/L
Adult males: 20.1–28.9 mmol/L
Adult females: 18.4–28.8 mmol/L

**Bile Acids, Total[a] (S)**
Values in µmol/L
1 mo     11–69
3 mos    1–41
6–12 mos 1–37

**Bilirubin (S)**
Values in mg/dL (µmol/L)
Levels after 1 mo are as follows:
Conjugated: 0–0.3 mg/dL (0–5 µmol/L)
Unconjugated: 0.1–0.7 mg/dL (2–12 µmol/L)

**Blood Volume**
Premature infants: 98 mL/kg
At 1 y: 86 mL/kg (range, 69–112 mL/kg)
Older children: 70 mL/kg (range, 51–86 mL/kg)

(continued)

***Table 44–1.*** Normal blood chemistry values and miscellaneous other hematologic values. (Values may vary with the procedure used.) (continued)

---

**BUN:** See Urea Nitrogen.

**C Peptide (S)**
5–15 y (8:00 am fasting): 1–4 ng/mL
Adults (8:00 am fasting): < 4 ng/mL
Adults (nonfasting): < 8 ng/mL

**C-Reactive Protein (S)**
3–16 y: 0.1–1.5 mg/dL

**Calcium, Ionized (P)**
0–2 d: 1.1–1.4 mmol/L
3–4 d: 1.1–1.5 mmol/L
5–8 d: 1.2–1.5 mmol/L
9–14 d: 1.3–1.6 mmol/L
2 mo–18 y: 1.2–1.4 mmol/L

**Calcium, Total (S)**
Premature infants (first week): 3.5–4.5 mEq/L (1.7–2.3 mmol/L)
Full-term infants (first week): 4–5 mEq/L (2–2.5 mmol/L)
Thereafter: 4.4–5.3 mEq/L (2.2–2.7 mmol/L)

**Carbon Dioxide, Total (S, P)**
Cord blood: 15–20.2 mmol/L
Children: 18–27 mmol/L
Adults: 24–35 mmol/L

**Carnitine (P)**
Values in mmol/L, measured by an enzymatic radioisotopic method:

| Age | Total Carnitine | Free Carnitine | Acyl-carnitine | AC/FC Ratio |
|-----|-----|-----|-----|-----|
| 1 day | 23.3–67.9 | 11.5–36.0 | 7.0–36.6 | 0.37–1.68 |
| 2–7 d | 17.4–40.6 | 10.1–21.0 | 2.9–23.8 | 0.15–1.44 |
| 8–28 d | 18.5–58.7 | 12.3–46.2 | 4.1–14.5 | 0.11–0.65 |
| 1 mo–1 y | 38.1–68.0 | 26.9–49.0 | 7.4–19.0 | 0.23–0.50 |
| 1–6 y | 34.6–83.6 | 24.3–62.5 | 4.0–28.3 | 0.11–0.83 |
| 6–10 y | 27.8–82.9 | 21.7–66.4 | 3.1–32.1 | 0.08–0.87 |
| 10–17 y | 33.7–77.0 | 21.6–64.5 | 3.7–29.2 | 0.09–0.88 |
| 22–60 y | 33.8–77.5 | 25.4–54.1 | 5.4–30.1 | 0.11–0.78 |

**Cation–Anion Gap (S, P)**
5–15 mmol/L

**Ceruloplasmin (Copper Oxidase) (S, P)**
21–43 mg/dL (1.3–2.7 μmol/L)

**Chloride (S, P)**
Premature infants: 95–110 mmol/L
Full-term infants: 96–116 mmol/L
Children: 98–105 mmol/L
Adults: 98–108 mmol/L

**Cholesterol, Total (S, P)**
Values in mg/dL (mmol/L)

| Group | Males | Females |
|-----|-----|-----|
| 6–7 y | 115–197 (2.97–5.09) | 126–199 (3.25–5.14) |
| 8–9 y | 112–199 (2.89–5.14) | 124–208 (3.20–5.37) |
| 10–11 y | 108–220 (2.79–5.68) | 115–208 (2.97–5.37) |
| 12–13 y | 117–202 (3.02–5.21) | 114–207 (2.94–5.34) |
| 14–15 y | 103–207 (2.66–5.34) | 102–208 (2.63–5.37) |
| 16–17 y | 107–198 (2.76–5.11) | 106–213 (2.73–5.50) |

**Coagulation Factors (P)**
Values in U/mL. Shown are mean values and –2 SD or lower range (in parentheses).

| Factor | Preterm (25–32 wk) | Term Infant | Infant (6 mos) | Adult |
|-----|-----|-----|-----|-----|
| II | 0.32 (0.18) | 0.52 (0.25) | 0.88 (0.60) | 1.0 (0.7) |
| V | 0.80 (0.43) | 1.00 (0.54) | 0.91 (0.55) | 1.0 (0.6) |
| VII | 0.37 (0.24) | 0.57 (0.35) | 0.87 (0.50) | 1.0 (0.6) |
| VIII | 0.75 (0.40) | 1.50 (0.55) | 0.90 (0.50) | 1.0 (0.6) |
| vWF | 1.50 (0.90) | 1.60 (0.84) | 1.07 (0.60) | 1.0 (0.6) |
| IX | 0.22 (0.17) | 0.35 (0.15) | 0.86 (0.36) | 1.0 (0.5) |
| X | 0.38 (0.20) | 0.45 (0.30) | 0.78 (0.38) | 1.0 (0.6) |
| XI | 0.20 (0.12) | 0.42 (0.20) | 0.86 (0.38) | 1.0 (0.6) |
| XII | 0.22 (0.09) | 0.44 (0.16) | 0.77 (0.39) | 1.0 (0.6) |
| XIII | ... | 0.61 (0.36) | 1.04 (0.50) | 1.0 (0.6) |
| PreK | 0.26 (0.14) | 0.35 (0.16) | 0.86 (0.56) | 1.1 (0.6) |

vWF = von Willebrand factor, PreK = prekallikrein.

**Complement (S)**
C3: 96–195 mg/dL
C4: 15–20 mg/dL

**Copper (S)**
Cord blood: 26–32 μg/dL (4.1–5.2 μmol/L)
Newborns: 26–32 μg/dL (4.1–5.2 μmol/L)
1 mo: 73–93 μg/dL (11.5–14.6 μmol/L)
2 mo: 59–69 μg/dL (9.3–10.9 μmol/L)
6 mo–5 y: 27–153 μg/dL (4.2–24.1 μmol/L)
5–17 y: 94–234 μg/dL (14.8–36.8 μmol/L)
Adults: 70–118 μg/dL (11–18.6 μmol/L)

**Copper Oxidase:** See Ceruloplasmin.

**Cortisol (S, P)**
Morning (8:00 am): 5–25 μg/dL (0.14–0.68 μmol/L)
Evening: 5–15 μg/dL (0.14–0.41 μmol/L)

**Creatine (S, P)**
0.2–0.8 mg/dL (15.2–61 mmol/L)

(continued)

**Table 44–1.** Normal blood chemistry values and miscellaneous other hematologic values. (Values may vary with the procedure used.) (continued)

---

**Creatine Kinase (S, P)**
Newborns (1–3 d): 40–474 IU/L at 37 °C
Adult males: 30–210 IU/L at 37 °C
Adult females: 20–128 IU/L at 37 °C

**Creatinine (S,P)**
Values in mg/dL (μmol/L)

| Group | Males | Females |
|---|---|---|
| Newborns (1–3 d)* | 0.2–1.0 (17.7–88.4) | 0.2–1.0 (17.7–88.4) |
| 1 y | 0.2–0.6 (17.7–53.0) | 0.2–0.5 (17.7–44.2) |
| 2–3 y | 0.2–0.7 (17.7–61.9) | 0.3–0.6 (26.5–53.0) |
| 4–7 y | 0.2–0.8 (17.7–70.7) | 0.2–0.7 (17.7–61.9) |
| 8–10 y | 0.3–0.9 (26.5–79.6) | 0.3–0.8 (26.5–70.7) |
| 11–12 y | 0.3–1.0 (26.5–88.4) | 0.3–0.9 (26.5–79.6) |
| 13–17 y | 0.3–1.2 (26.5–106.1) | 0.3–1.1 (26.5–97.2) |
| 18–20 y | 0.5–1.3 (44.2–115.0) | 0.3–1.1 (26.5–97.2) |

*Values may be higher in premature newborns.

**Creatinine Clearance**
Values show great variability and depend on the specificity of the analytical methods used.
Newborns (1 d): 5–50 mL/min/1.73 m (mean, 18 mL/min/1.73 m)
Newborns (6 d): 15–90 mL/min/1.73 $m^2$ (mean, 36 mL/min/1.73 $m^2$)
Adult males: 85–125 mL/min/1.73 $m^2$
Adult females: 75–115 mL/min/1.73 $m^2$

**2,3-Diphosphoglycerate (B)**
Values vary with the method used and with altitude.
4.5–6 mmol/L

**Factor:** See Anticoagulation Factors and Coagulation Factors.

**Fatty Acids, "Free" (P)**
Newborns: 435–1375 μEq/L
4 mo–10 y (14-h fast): 500–900 μEq/L
4 mo–10 y (19-h fast): 730–1200 μEq/L
Adults (14-h fast): 310–590 μEq/L
Adults (19-h fast): 405–720 μEq/L

**Ferritin (S)**
Newborns: 20–200 ng/mL (mean, 117 ng/mL)
1 mo: 60–550 ng/mL (mean, 350 ng/mL)
1–15 y: 7–140 ng/mL (mean, 31 ng/mL)
Adult males: 50–225 ng/mL (mean, 140 ng/mL)
Adult females: 10–150 ng/mL (mean, 40 ng/mL)

**Fibrinogen (P)**
200–500 mg/dL (5.9–14.7 μmol/L)

**Galactose (S, P)**
1.1–2.1 mg/dL (0.06–0.12 mmol/L)

**Galactose 1-Phosphate (RBC)**
Normal: 1 mg/dL of packed erythrocyte lysate; slightly higher in cord blood
Infants with congenital galactosemia on a milk-free diet: < 2 mg/dL
Infants with congenital galactosemia taking milk: 9–20 mg/dL

**Galactose-1-Phosphate Uridyl Transferase (RBC)**
Normal: 308–475 mIU/g of hemoglobin
Heterozygous for Duarte variant: 225–308 mIU/g of hemoglobin
Homozygous for Duarte variant: 142–225 mIU/g of hemoglobin
Heterozygous for congenital galactosemia: 142–225 mIU/g of hemoglobin
Homozygous for congenital galactosemia: < 8 mIU/g of hemoglobin

**Glomerular Filtration Rate**
Newborns: About 50% of values for older children and adults
Older children and adults: 75–165 mL/min/1.73 $m^2$ (levels reached by about 6 mo)

**Glucose (S, P)**
Premature infants: 20–80 mg/dL (1.11–4.44 mmol/L)
Full-term infants: 30–100 mg/dL (1.67–5.56 mmol/L)
Children and adults (fasting): 60–105 mg/dL (3.33–5.88 mmol/L)

**Glucose-6-Phosphate Dehydrogenase (RBC)**
150–215 U/dL

(continued)

***Table 44–1.*** Normal blood chemistry values and miscellaneous other hematologic values. (Values may vary with the procedure used.) (continued)

**Glucose Tolerance Test (S):**

**Glucose tolerance test results in serum.**

Normal levels based on results in 13 normal children given glucose. 1.75 g/kg orally in one dose, after 2 wk on a high-carbohydrate diet.

| Time | Glucose mg/dL | Glucose mmol/L | Insulin μU/mL | Insulin pmol/L | Phosphorus mg/dL | Phosphorus mmol/L |
|---|---|---|---|---|---|---|
| Fasting | 59–96 | 3.11–5.33 | 5–40 | 36–287 | 3.2–4.9 | 1.03–1.58 |
| 30 min | 91–185 | 5.05–10.27 | 36–110 | 258–789 | 2.0–4.4 | 0.64–1.42 |
| 60 min | 66–164 | 3.66–9.10 | 22–124 | 158–890 | 1.8–3.6 | 0.58–1.16 |
| 90 min | 68–148 | 3.77–8.22 | 17–105 | 122–753 | 1.8–3.6 | 0.58–1.16 |
| 2 h | 66–122 | 3.66–6.77 | 6–84 | 43–603 | 1.8–4.2 | 0.58–1.36 |
| 3 h | 47–99 | 2.61–5.49 | 2–46 | 14–330 | 2.0–4.6 | 0.64–1.48 |
| 4 h | 61–93 | 3.39–5.16 | 3–32 | 21–230 | 2.7–4.3 | 0.87–1.39 |
| 5 h | 63–86 | 3.50–4.77 | 5–37 | 36–265 | 2.9–4.4 | 0.94–1.42 |

**γ-Glutamyl Transpeptidase (S)**
0–1 mo: 12–271 IU/L at 37 °C (kinetic)
1–2 mo: 9–159 IU/L at 37 °C (kinetic)
2–4 mo: 7–98 IU/L at 37 °C (kinetic)
4–7 mo: 5–45 IU/L at 37 °C (kinetic)
7–12 mo: 4–27 IU/L at 37 °C (kinetic)
1–15 y: 3–30 IU/L at 37 °C (kinetic)
Adult males: 9–69 IU/L at 37 °C (kinetic)
Adult females: 3–33 IU/L at 37 °C (kinetic)

**Glycohemoglobin (Hemoglobin A$_{1c}$) (B)**
Normal: 6.3–8.2% of total hemoglobin
Diabetic patients in good control of their condition ordinarily have levels < 10%
Values tend to be lower during pregnancy; they also vary with technique

**Growth Hormone (GH) (S)**
After infancy (fasting specimen): 0–5 ng/mL
In response to natural and artificial provocation (eg, sleep, arginine, insulin, hypoglycemia): > 8 ng/mL
During the newborn period (fasting specimen), GH levels are high (15–40 ng/mL) and responses to provocation are variable

**Haptoglobin (S)**
50–150 mg/dL has hemoglobin-binding capacity.

**Hematocrit (B)**
At birth: 44–64%
14–90 d: 35–49%
6 mo–1 y: 30–40%
4–10 y: 31–43%

**Hemoglobin A$_{1c}$:** See Glycohemoglobin

**Hemoglobin Electrophoresis (B)**
A$_1$ hemoglobin: 96–98.5% of total hemoglobin
A$_2$ hemoglobin: 1.5–4% of total hemoglobin

**Hemoglobin, Fetal (B)**
At birth: 50–85% of total hemoglobin
At 1 y: < 15% of total hemoglobin
Up to 2 y: Up to 5% of total hemoglobin
Thereafter: < 2% of total hemoglobin

**Immunoglobulins (S)**
Values in mg/dL

| Group | IgG | IgA | IgM |
|---|---|---|---|
| Cord blood | 766–1693 | 0.04–9 | 4–26 |
| 2 wk–3 mo | 299–852 | 3–66 | 15–149 |
| 3–6 mo | 142–988 | 4–90 | 18–118 |
| 6–12 mo | 418–1142 | 14–95 | 43–223 |
| 1–2 y | 356–1204 | 13–118 | 37–239 |
| 2–3 y | 492–1269 | 23–137 | 49–204 |
| 3–6 y | 564–1381 | 35–209 | 51–214 |
| 6–9 y | 658–1535 | 29–384 | 50–228 |
| 9–12 y | 625–1598 | 60–294 | 64–278 |
| 12–16 y | 660–1548 | 81–252 | 45–256 |

**Immunoreactive Trypsinogen[d,e] (IRT) (P)(S)**
Normal controls             10–57 ng/ml
Chronic pancreatitis     < 1.5–47 ng/ml
Acute pancreatitis         92–850 ng/ml
Total pancreatectomy   < 1.5 ng/ml

(continued)

**Table 44–1.** Normal blood chemistry values and miscellaneous other hematologic values. (Values may vary with the procedure used.) (continued)

---

**Insulin**

**Insulin Clearance**
< 1 mo: 29–88 mL/min/1.73 m$^2$
1–6 mos: 40–112 mL/min/1.73 m$^2$
6–12 mos: 62–121 mL/min/1.73 m$^2$
< 1 y: 78–164 mL/min/1.73 m$^2$

**Iron (S, P)**
Newborns: 20–157 μg/dL (3.6–28.1 μmol/L)
6 wk –3 y: 20–115 μg/dL (3.6–20.6 μmol/L)
3–9 y: 20–141 μg/dL (3.6–25.2 μmol/L)
9–14 y: 21–151 μg/dL (3.8–27 μmol/L)
14–16 y: 20–181 μg/dL (3.6–32.4 μmol/L)
Adults: 44–196 μg/dL (7.2–31.3 μmol/L)

**Iron-Binding Capacity (S, P)**
Newborns: 59–175 μg/dL (10.6–31.3 μmol/L)
Children and adults: 275–458 μg/dL (45–72 μmol/L)

**Lactate (B)**
Venous blood: 5–18 mg/dL (0.5–2 mmol/L)
Arterial blood: 3–7 mg/dL (0.3–0.8 mmol/L)

**Lactate Dehydrogenase (LDH) (S, P)**
Values using lactate substrate (kinetic)
Newborns (1–3 d): 40–348 IU/L at 37 °C
1 mo–5 y: 150–360 IU/L at 37 °C
5–8 y: 150–300 IU/L at 37 °C
8–12 y: 130–300 IU/L at 37 °C
12–14 y: 130–280 IU/L at 37 °C
14–16 y: 130–230 IU/L at 37 °C
Adult males: 70–178 IU/L at 37 °C
Adult females: 42–166 IU/L at 37 °C

**LDH:** See Lactate Dehydrogenase.

**Lead (B)**
< 10 μg/dL (< 0.48 mmol/L)
When a large proportion of a population of children have blood lead levels in the range of 10–19 μg/dL (0.48–0.92 μmol/L), communitywide childhood lead poisoning activities are warranted.

Levels > 20 μg/dL (> 0.97 μmol/L) indicate the need for medical and environmental evaluation and possible pharmalogic intervention.
Levels > 70 μg/dL (> 3.38 μmol/L) indicate the immediate need for medical and environmental management.

**Lipase (S, P)**
20–136 IU/L based on 4-h incubation

**Lipoprotein Cholesterol, High-Density (HDL) (S)**
Values in mg/dL (mmol/L)

| Group | Males | Females |
|---|---|---|
| 6–7 y | 35–77 (0.90–1.98) | 24–76 (0.62–1.96) |
| 8–9 y | 31–80 (0.80–2.06) | 34–77 (0.87–1.98) |
| 10–11 y | 34–81 (0.87–1.09) | 30–74 (0.77–1.91) |
| 12–13 y | 30–82 (0.77–2.11) | 33–73 (0.85–1.88) |
| 14–15 y | 26–72 (0.67–1.86) | 29–73 (0.74–1.88) |
| 16–17 y | 25–66 (0.72–1.70) | 27–78 (0.69–2.01) |

**Lipoprotein Cholesterol, Low-Density (LDL) (S)**
Values in mg/dL (mmol/L)

| Group | Males | Females |
|---|---|---|
| 6–7 y | 56–134 (1.44–3.46) | 52–149 (1.34–3.85) |
| 8–9 y | 52–129 (1.34–3.33) | 57–143 (1.47–3.69) |
| 10–11 y | 45–149 (1.16–3.85) | 56–140 (1.44–3.61) |
| 12–13 y | 55–135 (1.42–3.48) | 58–138 (1.49–3.56) |
| 14–15 y | 48–143 (1.24–3.69) | 47–140 (1.21–3.61) |
| 16–17 y | 53–134 (1.36–3.36) | 44–147 (1.13–3.79) |

**Magnesium (S, P)**
Newborns: 1.5–2.3 mEq/L (0.75–1.15 mmol/L)
Adults: 1.4–2 mEq/L (0.7–1 mmol/L)

**Methemoglobin (B)**
0–0.3 g/dL (0–186 μmol/L)

**Osmolality (S, P)**
270–290 mOsm/kg

(continued)

---

**Proteins in serum.**

Values are for cellulose acetate electrophoresis and are in g/dL. SI conversion factor: g/dL × 10 = g/L.

| Group | Total Protein | Albumin | $\alpha_1$-Globulin | $\alpha_2$-Globulin | β-Globulin | γ-Globulin |
|---|---|---|---|---|---|---|
| At birth | 4.6–7.0 | 3.2–4.8 | 0.1–0.3 | 0.2–0.3 | 0.3–0.6 | 0.6–1.2 |
| 3 mos | 4.5–6.5 | 3.2–4.8 | 0.1–0.3 | 0.3–0.7 | 0.3–0.7 | 0.2–0.7 |
| 1 y | 5.4–7.5 | 3.7–5.7 | 0.1–0.3 | 0.5–1.1 | 0.4–1.0 | 0.2–0.9 |
| >4 y | 5.9–8.0 | 3.8–5.4 | 0.1–0.3 | 0.4–0.8 | 0.5–1.0 | 0.4–1.3 |

*Table 44–1.* Normal blood chemistry values and miscellaneous other hematologic values. (Values may vary with the procedure used.) (continued)

**Oxygen Capacity (B)**
1.34 mL/g of hemoglobin

**Oxygen Saturation (B)**
Newborns: 30–80% (0.3–0.8 mol/mol of venous blood)
Thereafter: 65–85% (0.65–0.85 mol/mol of venous blood)

**Partial Thromboplastin Time (P)**
Children: 42–54 s

**Phenylalanine (S, P)**
0.7–3.5 mg/dL (0.04–0.21 mmol/L)

**Phosphatase:** See Acid Phosphatase and Alkaline Phosphatase.

**Phosphorus, Inorganic (S, P)**
Premature infants:
At birth: 5.6–8 mg/dL (1.81–2.58 mmol/L)
6–10 d: 6.1–11.7 mg/dL (1.97–3.78 mmol/L)
20–25 d: 6.6–9.4 mg/dL (2.13–3.04 mmol/L)
Full-term infants:
At birth: 5–7.8 mg/dL (1.61–2.52 mmol/L)
3 d: 5.8–9 mg/dL (1.87–2.91 mmol/L)
6–12 d: 4.9–8.9 mg/dL (1.58–2.87 mmol/L)
Children:
1 y: 3.8–6.2 mg/dL (1.23–2 mmol/L)
10 y: 3.6–5.6 mg/dL (1.16–1.81 mmol/L)
Adults: 3.1–5.1 mg/dL (1–1.65 mmol/L)
(See also Glucose Tolerance Test.)

**Potassium (S, P)**
Premature infants: 4.5–7.2 mmol/L
Full-term infants: 3.7–5.2 mmol/L
Children: 3.5–5.8 mmol/L
Adults: 3.5–5.5 mmol/L

**Prealbumin:** See Transthyretin.

**Proteins (S):** See table (top of page).

**Prothrombin Time (P)**
Children: 11–15 s

**Protoporphyrin, "Free" (FEP, ZPP) (B)**
Values for free erythrocyte protoporphyrin (FEP) and zinc protoporphyrin (ZPP) are 1.2–2.7 µg/g of hemoglobin.

**Pyruvate (B)**
Resting adult males (arterial blood): 50.5–60.1 µmol/L
Adults (venous blood): 34–102 µmol/L

**Retinol-Binding Protein (S)**

| | |
|---|---|
| 3–5 y | 1.0–5.0 mg/dL |
| 6–8 y | 1.5–5.9 mg/dL |
| 9–11 y | 1.5–6.5 mg/dL |
| 12–16 y | 1.5–7.0 mg/dL |

**Sedimentation Rate (Micro) (B)**
< 2 y: 1–5 mm/h
> 2 y: 1–8 mm/h

**SGOT:** See Aspartate Aminotransferase.

**SGPT:** See Alanine Aminotransferase.

**Sodium (S, P)**
Children and adults: 135–148 mmol/L

**Sugar:** See Glucose.

**T$_3$:** See Triiodothyronine.

**T$_4$:** See Thyroxine.

**TBG:** See Thyroxine-Binding Globulin.

**Thrombin Time (P)**
Children: 12–16 s

**Thyroid-Stimulating Hormone (TSH) (S)**
Values in µIU/mL

| | **Males** | **Females** |
|---|---|---|
| 1–30 d | 0.52–16.0 | 0.72–13.1 |
| 1 mo–5 y | 0.55–7.1 | 0.46–8.1 |
| 6–18 y | 0.37–6.0 | 0.36–5.8 |

**Thyroxine (T$_4$) (S)**
1–2 d: 11.4–25.5 µg/dL (147–328 nmol/L)
3–4 d: 9.8–25.2 µg/dL (126–324 nmol/L)
1–6 y: 5–15.2 µg/dL (64–196 nmol/L)
11–13 y: 4–13 µg/dL (51–167 nmol/L)
> 18 y: 4.7–11 µg/dL (60–142 nmol/L)

**Thyroxine, "Free" (Free T$_4$) (S)**
1–2.3 ng/dL

**Thyroxine-Binding Globulin (TBG) (S)**
1–7 mos: 2.9–6 mg/dL
7–12 mos: 2.1–5.9 mg/dL
Prepubertal children: 2–5.3 mg/dL
Pubertal children and adults: 1.8–4.2 mg/dL

*(continued)*

**Table 44–1.** Normal blood chemistry values and miscellaneous other hematologic values. (Values may vary with the procedure used.) (continued)

α-**Tocopherol:** See Vitamin E.

**Transaminase:** See Alanine Aminotransferase and Aspartate Aminotransferase.

**Transthyretin (prealbumin) (S, P)**
2–5 mos: 14–33 mg/dL
6–11 mos: 12–27 mg/dL
12–17 mos: 11–26 mg/dL
18–23 mos: 14–24 mg/dL
24–36 mos: 11–26 mg/dL
3–5 y: 9.1–33.0 mg/dL
6–8 y: 15.3–45.5 mg/dL
9–11 y: 16.0–47.6 mg/dL
12–16 y: 19.0–50.0 mg/dL

**Triglyceride (S, P)**
Fasting (> 12 h) values in mg/mL (mmol/L)

| Group | Males | Females |
| --- | --- | --- |
| 6–7 y | 32–79 (0.36–0.89) | 24–128 (0.27–1.44) |
| 8–9 y | 28–105 (0.31–1.18) | 34–115 (0.38–1.29) |
| 10–11 y | 30–115 (0.33–1.29) | 39–131 (0.44–1.48) |
| 12–13 y | 33–112 (0.37–1.26) | 36–125 (0.40–1.41) |
| 14–15 y | 35–136 (0.39–1.53) | 36–122 (0.40–1.37) |
| 16–17 y | 38–167 (0.42–1.88) | 34–136 (0.38–1.53) |

**Note:** Lower values represent the 5th percentile, whereas upper values are calculated from the mean + 2 SD.

**Triiodothyronine (T$_3$) (S)**
1–3 d: 89–405 ng/dL
1 wk: 91–300 ng/dL
1–12 mos: 85–250 ng/dL
Prepubertal children: 119–218 ng/dL
Pubertal children and adults: 55–170 ng/dL

**Tyrosine (S, P)**
Premature infants: 3–30.2 mg/dL (0.17–1.67 mmol/L)
Full-term infants: 1.7–4.7 mg/dL (0.09–0.26 mmol/L)
1–12 y: 1.4–3.4 mg/dL (0.08–0.19 mmol/L)
Adults: 0.6–1.6 mg/dL (0.03–0.09 mmol/L)

**Ubiquinone, Total[b] (Coenzyme Q10) (S)**
Values in μg/mL
1 mo–< 8 years 0.40–1.19 (0.46–1.38 μmol/L)
8–18 y 0.29–0.89 (0.34–1.03 μmol/L)

**Urea Clearance**
Premature infants: 3.5–17.3 mL/min/1.73 m$^2$
Newborns: 8.7–33 mL/min/1.73 m$^2$
2–12 mos: 40–95 mL/min/1.73 m$^2$
≥ 2 y: > 52 mL/min/1.73 m$^2$

**Urea Nitrogen (S, P)**
1–2 y: 5–15 mg/dL (1.8–5.4 mmol/L)
Thereafter: 10–20 mg/dL (3.5–7.1 mmol/L)

**Uric Acid (S, P)**
Males:
0–14 y: 2–7 mg/dL (119–416 μmol/L)
> 14 y: 3–8 mg/dL (178–476 μmol/L)
Females:
0–14 y: 2–7 mg/dL (119–416 μmol/L)
> 14 y: 2–7 mg/dL (119–416 μmol/L)

**Vitamin A (Retinol) (S, P)**
Total vitamin A: 19–81 μg/dL (0.66–2.82 μmol/L)
Retinol: 19–77 μg/dL (0.66–2.68 μmol/L)
Retinyl esters: 0.1–4.7 μg/dL (0.01–0.16 μmol/L)

**Vitamin C (Ascorbic Acid) (S, P)**
0.2–2 mg/dL (11–114 μmol/L)

**Vitamin D (S)**
1,25-Dihydroxycholecalciferol:
Normal: 37 ± 12 pg/mL
X-linked vitamin D–resistant disease: 16 ± 8 pg/mL
Vitamin D dependency: 9.5 ± 3 pg/mL in type I. Normal in type II.
Hypophosphatemic bone disease: 30 ± 6 pg/mL
Lead poisoning: 20 ± 1 pg/mL
25-Hydroxycholecalciferol:
Normal: 26–31 ng/mL

**Vitamin E (Tocopherol) (S, P)**
α-Tocopherol:
<12 y: 3.8–15.5 μg/mL (9.1–37.2 μmol/L)
>12 y: 4.7–203 μg/mL (11.3–48.7 μmol/L)
γ-Tocopherol:
The γ isomer contributes 10–20% of the total tocopherols in plasma but is only 10% as active as the α form in vivo.
Vitamin E status is best assessed by performing chromatographic separation of the isomers and determining both α- and γ-tocopherol levels. Levels should be expressed in terms of vitamin E/total lipid ratio:
< 12 y: > 0.6 mg/g (> 1.4 μmol/g)
> 12 y: > 0.8 mg/g (> 1.9 μmol/g)

**Volume (B)**
Premature infants: 98 mL/kg (mean)
Full-term infants: 75–100 mL/kg
1 y: 69–112 mL/kg (mean, 86 mL/kg)
Older children: 51–86 mL/kg (mean, 70 mL/kg)

(continued)

***Table 44–1.*** Normal blood chemistry values and miscellaneous other hematologic values.[1] (Values may vary with the procedure used.) (continued)

**Volume (P)**

Full-term neonates: 39–77 mL/kg

Infants: 40–50 mL/kg

Older children: 30–54 mL/kg

**Water (B, S, RBC)**

Whole blood: 79–81 g/dL

Serum: 91–92 g/dL

Red blood cells: 64–65 g/dL

**Xylose Absorption Test (B)**

Following a 5-g loading dose, the laboratory will report the D-xylose concentration of the baseline and 60-min samples in mg/dL. The difference between these two values should be corrected to a constant surface area of 1.73 m$^2$ according to the formula shown below.

The actual surface area can be derived from a number of available nomograms using the patient's weight and height.

Normal corrected blood values[c]: 9.8–20 mg/dL

Effect of age and sex: No significant differences between males and females. No significant differences in ages 14–92 y.

**Zinc (S)**

Males: 83–88 µg/dL (12.7–13.5 µmol/L)

Females: 85–91 µg/dL (13–13.9 µmol/L)

Females taking oral contraceptives: 86–93 µg/dL (13.2–14.2 µmol/L)

At 16 wk of gestation: 66–70 µg/dL (10.1–10.7 µmol/L)

At 38 wk of gestation: 54–58 µg/dL (8.3–8.9 µmol/L)

---

[a]McGraw C et al: Reference ranges for total serum bile acids in infants. Clin Chem 1996;42:S30.

[b]Artuch R et al: Serum Ubiquinone-10 in a pediatric population. Clin Chem 1998;44:2378.

[c]
$$\text{Corrected blood value} = \frac{(\text{value}_{60\ \text{min}} - \text{value}_{\text{baseline}}) \times \text{actual surface area}}{1.73}$$

[d]Adrian, TE et al: Plasma trypsin in chronic pancreatitis and pancreatic adenocarcinoma. Clin Chim Acta 97:205 (1979).

[e]Andriulli, A et al: Clinical evaluation of serum cathodic trypsin-like immunoreactivity in patients with differnet pancreatic diseases. Ital J Gastroenterol 12:260 (1980).

Adapted, with permission, from Meites S (ed): *Pediatric Clinical Chemistry,* 2nd ed. American Association for Clinical Chemistry, 1982, and many other sources.

***Table 44–2.*** Normal values: urine, duodenal fluid, feces, sweat, and miscellaneous.

---

### URINE

**Addis Count**
Red blood cells (12-h specimen): < 1 million
White blood cells (12-h specimen): < 2 million
Casts (12-h specimen): < 10,000
Protein (12-h specimen): < 55 mg

**Albumin**
First mo: 1–100 mg/L
Second month: 0.2–34 mg/L
2–12 mos: 0.5–19 mg/L

**δ-Aminolevulinic Acid:** See Porphyrins.

**Ammonia**
2–12 mos: 4–20 μEq/min/m$^2$
1–16 y: 6–16 μEq/min/m$^2$

**Calcium**
4–12 y: 4–8 meq/L (2–4 mmol/L)

**Catecholamines (Norepinephrine, Epinephrine)**
Values in μg/24 h (nmol/24 h)
(See table, bottom of page.)

**Chloride**
Infants: 1.7–8.5 mmol/24 h
Children: 17–34 mmol/24 h
Adults: 140–240 mmol/24 h

**Copper**
0–30 μg/24 h

**Coproporphyrin:** See Porphyrins.

**Creatine**
18–58 mg/L (1.37–4.42 mmol/L)

**Creatinine**
Newborns: 7–10 mg/kg/24 h
Children: 20–30 mg/kg/24 h
Adult males: 21–26 mg/kg/24 h
Adult females: 16–22 mg/kg/24 h

**Epinephrine:** See Catecholamines.

**Homovanillic Acid (HVA)**
Children: 3–16 μg/mg of creatinine
Adults: 2–4 μg/mg of creatinine

**5-Hydroxyindoleacetic Acid**
0.11–0.61 μmol/kg/7 h, based on results in 15 well-nourished,
apparently healthy, mentally defective
children on a tryptophan load

**Hydroxyproline, Total**
5–14 y: 38–126 mg/24 h (290–961 μmol/24 h)

**Mercury**
< 50 μg/24 h (249 nmol/24 h)

**Metanephrine and Normetanephrine**
< 2 y: < 4.6 μg/mg of creatinine (23.3 nmol)
2–10 y: < 3 μg/mg of creatinine (15.2 nmol)
10–15 y: < 2 μg/mg of creatinine (10.3 nmol)
> 15 y: < 1 μg/mg of creatinine (5.1 nmol)

**Mucopolysaccharides**
Acid mucopolysaccharide screen should yield negative
results. Positive results after dialysis of the urine
should be followed up with a thin-layer chromatogram
for evaluation of the acid mucopolysaccharide excretion
pattern.

**Norepinephrine:** See Catecholamines.

**Normetanephrine:** See Metanephrine and Normetanephrine.

**Osmolality**
Infants: 50–600 mosm/L
Older children: 50–1400 mosm/L
**Phosphorus, Tubular Reabsorption**
78–97%

**Porphobilinogen:** See Porphyrins.

---

#### Catecholamines in urine.

| Group | Total Catecholamines | Norepinephrine | Epinephrine |
|---|---|---|---|
| < 1 y | 20 | 5.4–15.9 (32–94) | 0.1–4.3 (0.5–23.5) |
| 1–5 y | 40 | 8.1–30.8 (48–182) | 0.8–9.1 (4.4–49.7) |
| 6–15 y | 80 | 19.0–71.1 (112–421) | 1.3–10.5 (7.1–57.3) |
| > 15 y | 100 | 34.4–87.0 (203–514) | 3.5–13.2 (19.1–72.1) |

(*continued*)

***Table 44–2.*** Normal values: urine, duodenal fluid, feces, sweat, and miscellaneous. (continued)

**Porphyrins**
δ-Aminolevulinic acid: 0–7 mg/24 h (0–53.4 µmol/24 h)
Porphobilinogen: 0–2 mg/24 h (0–8.8 µmol/24 h)
Coproporphyrin: 0–160 µg/24 h (0–244 nmol/24 h)
Uroporphyrin: 0–26 µg/24 h (0–31 nmol/24 h)

**Potassium**
26–123 mmol/L

**Sodium**
Infants: 0.3–3.5 mmol/24 h (6–10 mmol/m$^2$)
Children and adults: 5.6–17 mmol/24 h

**Urobilinogen**
< 3 mg/24 h (< 5.1 µmol/24 h)

**Uroporphyrin:** See Porphyrins.

**Vanillylmandelic Acid (VMA)**
· Because of the difficulty in obtaining an accurately timed
    24-h collection, values based on micrograms per
    milligram of creatinine are the most reliable indications
    of VMA excretion in young children.
1–12 mos: 1–35 µg/mg of creatinine
    (31–135 µg/kg/24 h)
1–2 y: 1–30 µg/mg of creatinine
2–5 y: 1–15 µg/mg of creatinine
5–10 y: 1–14 µg/mg of creatinine
10–15 y: 1–10 µg/mg of creatinine (1–7 mg/24 h;
    5–35 µmol/24 h)
Adults: 1–7 µg/mg of creatinine (1–7 mg/24 h;
    5–35 µmol/24 h)

**VMA:** See Vanillylmandelic Acid.

**Xylose Absorption Test**
Mean 5-h excretion expressed as a percentage
    of the ingested load
< 6 mos: 11–30%
6–12 mos: 20–32%
1–3 y: 20–42%
3–10 y: 25–45%
> 10 y: 25–50%
Or: % excretion > (0.2 × age [mo]) + 12

**DUODENAL FLUID**

**Enzymes**
Amylase: (Anderson)
    0–2 mos: 0–10 U/mL
    2–6 mos: 10–20 U/mL
    6–12 mos: 40–150 U/mL
    1–2 y: 100–225 U/mL
    2–5 y: 125–275 U/mL

Carboxypeptidase:
    0.4–1 U (Ravin)
Chymotrypsin:
    11–65 U (Ravin)
Protease:
    18–70 U (Free-Meyers)
Trypsin: (Anderson or as noted)
    0–2 mos: 110–160 U/mL
    2–6 mos: 115–160 U/mL
    6–12 mos: 120–290 U/mL; 3–10 U
        (Nothman et al)
    1–2 y: 200–300 U/mL
    2–5 y: 200–275 U/mL

**pH**
6–8.4

**FECES**

**Fat, Total**
2–6 mos: 0.3–1.3 g/d
6 mos–1 y: < 4 g/d
Children: < 3 g/d
Adolescents: < 5 g/d
Adults: < 7 g/d

**Lipids, Split Fat**
Adults: > 40% of total lipids

**Lipids, Total**
Adults: Up to 7 g/d on normal diet, 10–27% of dry weight

**Nitrogen**
Infants: < 1 g/d
Children: < 1.2 g/d
Adults: < 3 g/d

**Pancreatic Elastase-1[a,b] (E1)**
Normal                              200 to >500 µg E1/g stool
Moderate to mild exocrine 100–200 µg E1/g stool
    pancreatic insufficiency
Severe exocrine pancreatic <100 µgE1/g stool
    insufficiency

**SWEAT**

**Electrolytes**
Values for chloride. Elevated values in the presence of a
    family history or clinical findings of cystic fibrosis are
    diagnostic of cystic fibrosis.
Normal: < 40 mmol/L
Borderline: 40–60 mmol/L
Elevated: > 60 mmol/L

*(continued)*

**Table 44–2.** Normal values: urine, duodenal fluid, feces, sweat, and miscellaneous.[1] (continued)

| MISCELLANEOUS | |
|---|---|
| **Amylo-1,6-Glucosidase Debrancher (Liver)** | **Potassium** |
| >1 µmol/min/g of wet tissue | Breast milk: 12–17 mmol/L |
| | Cow's milk: 20–45 mmol/L |
| **Chloride** | Muscle: 160–180 mmol/kg of wet fat-free tissue |
| Breast milk: 2.5–30 mmol/L | |
| Cow's milk: 20–80 mmol/L | **Proteins (Cerebrospinal Fluid)** |
| Muscle: 20–26 mmol/kg of wet fat-free tissue | Total proteins: |
| Spinal fluid: 120–128 mmol/L | Newborn: 40–120 mg/dL (0.4–1.2 g/L) |
| | 1 mo: 20–70 mg/dL (0.2–0.7 g/L) |
| **Copper (Liver)** | Thereafter: 15–40 mg/dL (0.15–0.4 g/L) |
| < 20 µg/g of wet tissue | γ-globulin: |
| | Children: Up to 9% of total |
| **Glucose-6-Phosphatase (Liver)** | Adults: Up to 14% of total |
| > 5 µmol/min/g of wet tissue | |
| | **Sodium** |
| **Lactate Dehydrogenase (LDH) (Cerebrospinal Fluid)** | Breast milk: 4.7–8.3 mmol/L |
| 17–59 IU/L at 37 °C | Cow's milk: 22–26 mmol/L |
| | Muscle: 33–43 mmol/kg of wet fat-free tissue |

[a]Cade, A et al: Evaluation of fecal pancreatic elastase 1 as a measure of pancreatic exocrine function in children with cystic fibrosis. Pedr Pulmonol 2000;29(3):172–176.

[b]Dominguez-Monoz, JE et al: Fecal elastase test: Evaluation of a new noninvasive pancreatic function test. Am J Gastroenterol 1995;90:1834–1837.

Adapted from Meites S (ed): *Pediatric Clinical Chemistry*, 2nd ed. American Association for Clinical Chemistry, 1982, and many other sources.

**Table 44–3.** Normal values: common hematologic measurements and indices.

### RED BLOOD CELL VALUES AT VARIOUS AGES: MEAN AND LOWER LIMIT OF NORMAL (−2 SD)[a]

| Age | Hemoglobin (g/dL) Mean | −2 SD | Hematocrit (%) Mean | −2 SD | Red Cell Count ($10^{12}$/L) Mean | −2 SD | MCV (fl) Mean | −2 SD | MCH (pg) Mean | −2 SD | MCHC (g/dL) Mean | −2 SD |
|---|---|---|---|---|---|---|---|---|---|---|---|---|
| Birth (cord blood) | 16.5 | 13.5 | 51 | 42 | 4.7 | 3.9 | 108 | 98 | 34 | 31 | 33 | 30 |
| 1–3 d (capillary) | 18.5 | 14.5 | 56 | 45 | 5.3 | 4.0 | 108 | 95 | 34 | 31 | 33 | 29 |
| 1 wk | 17.5 | 13.5 | 54 | 42 | 5.1 | 3.9 | 107 | 88 | 34 | 28 | 33 | 28 |
| 2 wk | 16.5 | 12.5 | 51 | 39 | 4.9 | 3.6 | 105 | 86 | 34 | 28 | 33 | 28 |
| 1 mo | 14.0 | 10.0 | 43 | 31 | 4.2 | 3.0 | 104 | 85 | 34 | 28 | 33 | 29 |
| 2 mo | 11.5 | 9.0 | 35 | 28 | 3.8 | 2.7 | 96 | 77 | 30 | 26 | 33 | 29 |
| 3–6 mo | 11.5 | 9.5 | 35 | 29 | 3.8 | 3.1 | 91 | 74 | 30 | 25 | 33 | 30 |
| 0.5–2 y | 12.0 | 10.5 | 36 | 33 | 4.5 | 3.7 | 78 | 70 | 27 | 23 | 33 | 30 |
| 2–6 y | 12.5 | 11.5 | 37 | 34 | 4.6 | 3.9 | 81 | 75 | 27 | 24 | 34 | 31 |
| 6–12 y | 13.5 | 11.5 | 40 | 35 | 4.6 | 4.0 | 86 | 77 | 29 | 25 | 34 | 31 |
| 12–18 y | | | | | | | | | | | | |
| Female | 14.0 | 12.0 | 41 | 36 | 4.6 | 4.1 | 90 | 78 | 30 | 25 | 34 | 31 |
| Male | 14.5 | 13.0 | 43 | 37 | 4.9 | 4.5 | 88 | 78 | 30 | 25 | 34 | 31 |
| 18–49 y | | | | | | | | | | | | |
| Female | 14.0 | 12.0 | 41 | 36 | 4.6 | 4.0 | 90 | 80 | 30 | 26 | 34 | 31 |
| Male | 15.5 | 13.5 | 47 | 41 | 5.2 | 4.5 | 90 | 80 | 30 | 26 | 34 | 31 |

### NORMAL LEUKOCYTE COUNTS[b]

| Age | Total Leukocytes Mean | (Range) | Neutrophils Mean | (Range) | % | Lymphocytes Mean | (Range) | % | Monocytes Mean | % | Eosinophils Mean | % |
|---|---|---|---|---|---|---|---|---|---|---|---|---|
| Birth | 18.1 | (9.0–30.0) | 11.0 | (6.0–26.0) | 61 | 5.5 | (2.0–11.0) | 31 | 1.1 | 6 | 0.4 | 2 |
| 12 h | 22.8 | (13.0–38.0) | 15.5 | (6.0–28.0) | 68 | 5.5 | (2.0–11.0) | 24 | 1.2 | 5 | 0.5 | 2 |
| 24 h | 18.9 | (9.4–34.0) | 11.5 | (5.0–21.0) | 61 | 5.8 | (2.0–11.5) | 31 | 1.1 | 6 | 0.5 | 2 |
| 1 wk | 12.2 | (5.0–21.0) | 5.5 | (1.5–10.0) | 45 | 5.0 | (2.0–17.0) | 41 | 1.1 | 9 | 0.5 | 4 |
| 2 wk | 11.4 | (5.0–20.0) | 4.5 | (1.0–9.5) | 40 | 5.5 | (2.0–17.0) | 48 | 1.0 | 9 | 0.4 | 3 |
| 1 mo | 10.8 | (5.0–19.5) | 3.8 | (1.0–9.0) | 35 | 6.0 | (2.5–16.5) | 56 | 0.7 | 7 | 0.3 | 3 |
| 6 mos | 11.9 | (6.0–17.5) | 3.8 | (1.0–8.5) | 32 | 7.3 | (4.0–13.5) | 61 | 0.6 | 5 | 0.3 | 3 |
| 1 y | 11.4 | (6.0–17.5) | 3.5 | (1.5–8.5) | 31 | 7.0 | (4.0–10.5) | 61 | 0.6 | 5 | 0.3 | 3 |
| 2 y | 10.6 | (6.0–17.0) | 3.5 | (1.5–8.5) | 33 | 6.3 | (3.0–9.5) | 59 | 0.5 | 5 | 0.3 | 3 |
| 4 y | 9.1 | (5.5–15.5) | 3.8 | (1.5–8.5) | 42 | 4.5 | (2.0–8.0) | 50 | 0.5 | 5 | 0.3 | 3 |
| 6 y | 8.5 | (5.0–14.5) | 4.3 | (1.5–8.0) | 51 | 3.5 | (1.5–7.0) | 42 | 0.4 | 5 | 0.2 | 3 |
| 8 y | 8.3 | (4.5–13.5) | 4.4 | (1.5–8.0) | 53 | 3.3 | (1.5–6.8) | 39 | 0.4 | 4 | 0.2 | 2 |
| 10 y | 8.1 | (4.5–13.5) | 4.4 | (1.8–8.0) | 54 | 3.1 | (1.5–6.5) | 38 | 0.4 | 4 | 0.2 | 2 |
| 16 y | 7.8 | (4.5–13.0) | 4.4 | (1.8–8.0) | 57 | 2.8 | (1.2–5.2) | 35 | 0.4 | 5 | 0.2 | 3 |
| 21 y | 7.4 | (4.5–11.0) | 4.4 | (1.8–7.7) | 59 | 2.5 | (1.0–4.8) | 34 | 0.3 | 4 | 0.2 | 3 |

[a]These data have been compiled from several sources. Emphasis is given to recent studies using electronic counters and to the selection of populations that are likely to exclude individuals with iron deficiency. The mean ± 2 SD can be expected to include 95% of the observations in a normal population.
(Based on Cairo MS: In: Rudolph AM [ed]: *Pediatrics,* 20th ed. Appleton & Lange, 1996:1222. As modified in Lubin BH: Reference values in infancy and childhood. In: Nathan DG, Oski FA [eds]: *Hematology of Infancy and Childhood,* 4th ed. WB Saunders, 1993:Appendix iii.)

[b]Numbers of leukocytes are in thousands per cubic millimeter, ranges are estimates of 95% confidence limits, and percentages refer to differential counts. Neutrophils include band cells at all ages and a small number of metamyelocytes and myelocytes in the first few days of life.
From Cairo MS: In: Rudolph AM [ed]: *Pediatrics,* 20th ed. Appleton & Lange, 1996. As modified in Lubin BH: Reference values in infancy and childhood. In: Nathan DG, Oski FA [eds]: *Hematology of Infancy and Childhood,* 4th ed. WB Saunders, 1993: Appendix xi.)

MCV = mean corpuscular volume; MCH = mean corpuscular hemoglobin; MCHC = mean corpuscular hemoglobin concentration.

# Index

NOTE: Page numbers in **boldface** type indicate a major discussion. A *t* following a page number indicates tabular material, and an *f* following a page number indicates a figure. Drugs are listed under their generic names. When a drug trade name is listed, the reader is referred to the generic name.

Kearns-Sayre, 798t–799t
Keloids, 428
Keratitis
  corneal, *Acanthamoeba,* 450
  ocular, 450
  ultraviolet, 439
Keratoconjunctivitis. *See also*
      Conjunctivitis
  epidemic, from adenovirus, 1136
  herpesvirus, 1147
    treatment of, 1149
Keratolytic agents. *See also* specific agents
  for keratosis pilaris, 427
  topical, for acne, 419
Keratosis pilaris, 427
Kerion, 421
Kerosene poisoning, 359–360
Keshan disease, 292
Ketamine
  for burn patients, 333
  for controlled intubation, 376t
  in critical care, 407–408
Ketoacidosis, in diabetes mellitus, 1012
Ketoaciduria, branched-chain, 1026
Ketoconazole
  for candidiasis, oral (thrush), 1279
  for precocious puberty in
      McCune–Albright
      syndrome, 991, 992–993
Ketogenic diet, for seizure disorders, 759
Ketonemia, in diabetes mellitus,
    1011–1012
Ketonuria, in diabetes mellitus,
    1011–1012
Ketorolac tromethamine, for
      conjunctivitis, allergic, 446,
      446t
Ketotic hyperglycinemias, 1027–1029,
    1028t, 1029f
Ketotifen, for allergic rhinoconjunctivitis,
    1093
Kidney, solitary, sports and, 835t
Kidney & urinary tract disorders,
    **707–731.** *See also* Renal
  evaluation of, **707–711**
    glomerular filtration rate in,
      707–708
    history in, 707
    immunologic function in, 710–711
    isolated proteinuria in, 708–709,
      710f
    microhematuria in, 708, 709t
    physical examination in, 707
    radiographic, 711
    renal biopsy in, 711
    serum analysis in, 707
    urinalysis in, 707
    urine concentrating ability in, 708

hematuria & glomerular disease,
    **712–716** (*See also*
      Glomerulonephritis;
      Hematuria)
  acute interstitial nephritis,
      **714–715**
  congenital nephrosis, **715**
  focal glomerular sclerosis, **716**
  glomerulonephritis, **713–714,**
      714t (*See also*
      Glomerulonephritis)
  idiopathic nephrotic syndrome of
      childhood, **715–716**
  membranous nephropathy, **716**
  mesangial nephropathy, **716**
  proteinuria & renal disease, 710f,
      **715**
renal failure, **718–725**
  acute, **718–720,** 718t, 719t
  chronic, **720–722**
  classification of, 718t
renal hypertension, **722–724,** 723f
renal parenchymal anomalies,
    **711–712**
renal vessel diseases, **716–718**
  hemolytic-uremic syndrome,
      **717–718**
  renal arterial disease, **717**
  renal vein thrombosis, **716–717**
urinary tract anomalies
  congenital, **711–712** (*See also*
      Urinary tract anomalies,
      congenital)
  inherited or developmental,
      **725–729,** 725t (*See also*
      Urinary tract anomalies)
Kinky hair disease, 778t
Kinky hair syndrome, 292
Klinefelter syndrome (XXY syndrome),
    **1062**
  ambiguous genitalia in, 988
  gynecomastia in, 995
  sex chromosomal anomalies in, 1043
Klippel–Feil syndrome, 813
Klippel-Trénaunay syndrome, port-wine
      stain birthmark with, 415
Knee, internal derangements of, 818
Knee injuries, sports-related, 841–843
  anterior cruciate ligament, 842
  anterior knee pain, 841–842
  lateral knee pain, 842
  medial & lateral collateral ligaments,
      842–843
  meniscal, 842
  posterior cruciate ligament, 842
Knee sprains, 818
Knock-knee, 816
Koplik spots, 1163, 1164

Krabbe disease (leukodystrophy), 775t,
    1033, 1035t
Kugelburg–Welander disease, 796t–797t
Kwashiorkor, 304

L
Labetalol, for renal hypertension, 724t
Labial sucking tubercle, **503**
Laboratory screening. *See* Screening,
      laboratory
Laboratory values. *See also* specific
      disorders; specific values
  interpretation of, 1339–1340, 1341f
  normal, 1341t–1352t
    blood chemistry & other
      hematologic, 1341t–1348t
    common hematologic measurements
      and indices, 1352t
    duodenal, 1350t
    feces, 1350t
    sweat, 1350t–1351t
    urine, 1349t–1350t
Lacerations, of eye, 439, 439f
Lack-of-breast-milk jaundice, **14–15,** 15t
LaCross encephalitis, 1159t
β-Lactam antibiotics, allergic reactions
      to, 1102–1104
β-Lactamase inhibitor, and penicillin,
      1114t
β-Lactamase-resistant penicillins, for
      impetigo, 420
Lactase, 288
  deficiency of, 647–648
Lactate, normal blood values for, 1345t
Lactate dehydrogenase (LDH)
  CSF, values for, 1351t
  normal blood values for, 1345t
Lactic acid, topical, for keratosis pilaris,
      427
Lactic acidemia, primary, 1015t–1016t,
      1021–1022, 1021t
Lactobacilli, vaginosis from, 146
Lactose intolerance, 288
Lamellar ichthyosis, 417, 417t
Lamivudine
  for AIDS, 1181t, 1182
  for hepatitis B, 676
Lamotrigine, for seizure disorders, 757t
Landouzy–Déjérine muscular dystrophy,
      796t–797t
Landry–Guillain-Barré syndrome,
      790–794, 792t–793t
Langer–Giedion syndrome, 1046t, **1064**
Langerhans cell histiocytosis, **938**
Language
  at ages 1-4, 79t, 81f, 82–83, 84f
  disorders of, in adolescents, 124t
  in first year of life, 75, 76t–79t, 81f